CURRENT
Diagnosis & Treatment
Surgery

13TH EDITION

Edited by

Gerard M. Doherty, MD
N.W. Thompson, Professor of Surgery
Chief, Division of Endocrine Surgery
Section Head, General Surgery
University of Michigan
Ann Arbor, Michigan

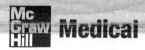
McGraw Hill **Medical**

New York   Chicago   San Francisco   Lisbon   London   Madrid   Mexico City
Milan   New Delhi   San Juan   Seoul   Singapore   Sydney   Toronto

Current Diagnosis & Treatment: Surgery, Thirteenth Edition

Copyright © 2010 by The McGraw-Hill Companies, Inc. All rights reserved. Printed in the United States of America. Except as permitted under the United States Copyright Act of 1976, no part of this publication may be reproduced or distributed in any form or by any means, or stored in a data base or retrieval system, without the prior written permission of the publisher.

Previous editions copyright ©2006; ©2003; ©1994, 1991 by Appleton & Lange; ©1973–1985 by Lange Medical Publications.

1 2 3 4 5 6 7 8 9 10   DOC DOC   12 11 10 9

Set ISBN 978-0-07-163515-8; MHID 0-07-163515-7
Book ISBN 978-0-07-159087-7; MHID 0-07-159087-0
CD ISBN 978-0-07-162953-9; MHID 0-07-162953-X
ISSN: 0894-227

Notice

Medicine is an ever-changing science. As new research and clinical experience broaden our knowledge, changes in treatment and drug therapy are required. The authors and the publisher of this work have checked with sources believed to be reliable in their efforts to provide information that is complete and generally in accord with the standards accepted at the time of publication. However, in view of the possibility of human error or changes in medical sciences, neither the authors nor the publisher nor any other party who has been involved in the preparation or publication of this work warrants that the information contained herein is in every respect accurate or complete, and they disclaim all responsibility for any errors or omissions or for the results obtained from use of the information contained in this work. Readers are encouraged to confirm the information contained herein with other sources. For example and in particular, readers are advised to check the product information sheet included in the package of each drug they plan to administer to be certain that the information contained in this work is accurate and that changes have not been made in the recommended dose or in the contraindications for administration. This recommendation is of particular importance in connection with new or infrequently used drugs.

This book was set in Minion by Silverchair Science & Communications, Inc.
The editors were Marsha S. Loeb and Karen Davis.
The production supervisor was Catherine H. Saggese.
Project management was provided by Marsha Hall, Progressive Publishing Alternatives.
The cover art director was Margaret Webster-Shapiro. The cover designer was Mary McKeon.
The index was prepared by Progressive Publishing Alternatives.
RR Donnelley was the printer and binder.

This book is printed on acid-free paper.

International Edition ISBN 978-0-07-163849-4; MHID 0-07-163849-0
Copyright © 2010. Exclusive rights by The McGraw-Hill Companies, Inc., for manufacture and export. This book cannot be re-exported from the country to which it is consigned by McGraw-Hill. The International Edition is not available in North America.

Contents

Authors

Craig T. Albanese, MD
Professor of Surgery and Pediatrics
Department of Surgery
Lucile Packard Children's Hospital at Stanford
Stanford, California
Chapter 43: Pediatric Surgery

John T. Anderson, MD
Associate Professor
Department of Surgery
Division of Trauma & Emergency Surgery
University of California, Davis
Davis, California
*Chapter 12: Shock & Acute Pulmonary Failure
in Surgical Patients*

English F. Barbour, RD, LD, CNSD
Nutrition Support Dietitian
Digestive Disease Center / Nutrition Services
Medical University of South Carolina
Charleston, South Carolina
Chapter 10: Surgical Metabolism & Nutrition

John R. Barbour, MD
Chief Resident
Department of Surgery
Medical University of South Carolina
Charleston, South Carolina
Chapter 10: Surgical Metabolism & Nutrition

Edward L. Bove, MD
Professor
Pediatric Cardiac Surgery, Section of
   Cardiac Surgery
University of Michigan
Ann Arbor, Michigan
*Chapter 19: The Heart: Part II. Congenital
   Heart Disease*

George J. Chang, MD, MS
Assistant Professor
Surgical Oncology
University of Texas, M.D. Anderson Cancer Center
   Houston, Texas
Chapter 29: Small Intestine
Chapter 30: Large Intestine
Chapter 31: Anorectum

Orlo H. Clark, MD
Professor and Vice Chair
Department of Surgery
University of California, San Francisco
San Francisco, California
Chapter 16: Thyroid & Parathyroid

Christopher S. Cooper, MD
Associate Professor of Pediatric Urology
Department of Urology
University of Iowa College of Medicine and
   Children's Hospital of Iowa
Iowa City, Iowa
Chapter 38: Urology

John A. Cowan Jr., MD
Department of Neurosurgery
Harbin Clinic
Rome, Georgia
Chapter 36: Neurosurgery

K. Barrett Deatrick, MD
House Officer
Resident in Surgery
University of Michigan
Ann Arbor, Michigan
Chapter 7: Power Sources in Surgery

Robert H. Demling, MD
Professor
Department of Surgery
Harvard Medical
Boston, Massachusetts
Chapter 14: Burns & Other Thermal Injuries

Eric J. Devaney, MD
Associate Professor of Surgery
Department of Surgery, Division of Cardiac Surgery
University of Michigan
Ann Arbor, Michigan
Chapter 19: The Heart: Part II. Congenital Heart Disease

Karen E. Deveney, MD
Professor
Department of Surgery
Oregon Health & Science University
Portland, Oregon
*Chapter 32: Hernias & Other Lesions of the
   Abdominal Wall*

Gerard M. Doherty, MD
N.W. Thompson, Professor of Surgery
Chief, Division of Endocrine Surgery
Section Head, General Surgery
University of Michigan
Ann Arbor, Michigan
Chapter 2: Training, Communication, Professionalism, and
  Systems-based Practice
Chapter 3: Preoperative Care
Chapter 4: Postoperative Care
Chapter 5: Postoperative Complications
Chapter 7: Power Sources in Surgery
Chapter 8: Inflammation, Infection, & Antimicrobial Therapy
Chapter 9: Fluid & Electrolyte Management
Chapter 21: The Acute Abdomen
Chapter 22: Peritoneal Cavity
Chapter 23: Stomach & Duodenum
Chapter 25: Biliary Tract
Chapter 26: Pancreas
Chapter 28: Appendix

Quan-Yang Duh, MD
Professor
Department of Surgery
University of California, San Francisco
San Francisco, California
Chapter 33: Adrenals

J. Englebert Dunphy, MD*
Formerly Professor of Surgery Emeritus
University of California, San Francisco
Chapter 1: Approach to the Surgical Patient

Piero M. Fisichella, MD
Assistant Professor of Surgery
Director, Swallowing Center
Department of Surgery, Stritch School of Medicine
Loyola University Medical Center
Maywood, Illinois
Chapter 20: Esophagus & Diaphragm

Douglas L. Fraker, MD
Jonathan E. Rhoads Associate Professor of Surgery
Vice-Chair, Clinical Affairs & Director,
  General Surgery
Chief, Division of Surgical Oncology
The University of Pennsylvania
Philadelphia, Pennsylvania
Chapter 27: Spleen

Michael G. Franz, MD
Associate Professor
Department of Surgery
University of Michigan
Ann Arbor, Michigan
Chapter 6: Wound Healing

Armando E. Giuliano, MD
Chief of Science and Medicine
Director, John Wayne Cancer Institute
  Breast Center
John Wayne Cancer Institute
Santa Monica, California
Chapter 17: Breast Disorders

Ameen Habash, MD
Chief Resident
Department of General Surgery, Division of
  Plastic Surgery
University of Kentucky
Lexington, Kentucky
Chapter 41: Plastic & Reconstructive Surgery

Jonathan W. Haft, MD
Assistant Professor
Department of Surgery
University of Michigan
Ann Arbor, Michigan
Chapter 19: The Heart: Part I. Surgical Treatment
  of Acquired Cardiac Disease

Scott L. Hansen, MD
Assistant Professor of Surgery
Department of Surgery
University of California, San Francisco
San Francisco, California
Chapter 42: Hand Surgery

Mark R. Hemmila, MD
Associate Professor
Department of Surgery
University of Michigan
Ann Arbor, Michigan
Chapter 13: Management of the Injured Patient

Virginia M. Hermann, MD
Professor
Department of Surgery
Medical University of South Carolina
Charleston, South Carolina
Chapter 10: Surgical Metabolism & Nutrition

*Deceased.

Jennifer C. Hirsch, MD, MS
Lecturer
Department of Surgery
University of Michigan
Ann Arbor, Michigan
Chapter 19: The Heart: Part II. Congenital Heart Disease

James W. Holcroft, MD
Professor
Department of Surgery
University of California, Davis
Davis, California
*Chapter 12: Shock & Acute Pulmonary Failure
    in Surgical Patients*

David Jablons, MD
Professor of Surgery
University of California, San Francisco
San Francisco, California
*Chapter 18: Thoracic Wall, Pleura, Mediastinum,
    & Lung*

William R. Jarnagin, MD
Professor of Surgery, Chief HPB Service
Department of Surgery
Memorial Sloan-Kettering Cancer Center, Weill Medical
    College of Cornell University
New York, New York
Chapter 24: Liver & Portal Venous System

Fadi N. Joudi, MD
Assistant Professor
Department of Urology
University of Iowa
Iowa City, Iowa
Chapter 38: Urology

Stephen A. Kamenetzky, MD
Clinical Professor
Department of Ophthalmology and Visual Science
Washington University School of Medicine
St. Louis, Missouri
Chapter 37: The Eye & Ocular Adnexa

Chienying Liu, MD
Assistant Clinical Professor of Medicine
University of California, San Francisco
San Francisco, California
Chapter 33: Adrenals

Paul V. Loar III, MD
Texas Oncology
Austin, Texas
Chapter 39: Gynecology

Jason MacTaggart, MD
Clinical Instructor
Division of Vascular Surgery
University of California, San Francisco
School of Medicine
San Francisco, California
Chapter 34: Arteries

Louis M. Messina, MD
Professor and Chief
Division of Vascular Surgery
University of Massachusetts Medical School
Worcester, Massachusetts
Chapter 35: Veins & Lymphatics

Linda M. Mundy, MD
Doctoral Student
Epidemiology
St. Louis University School of Public Health
St. Louis, Missouri
Chapter 8: Inflammation, Infection, & Antimicrobial Therapy

Richard G. Ohye, MD
Associate Professor
Department of Surgery
University of Michigan
Ann Arbor, Michigan
Chapter 19: The Heart: Part II. Congenital Heart Disease

Marco G. Patti, MD
Professor
Department of Surgery
University of Chicago Pritzker School of Medicine
Chicago, Illinois
Chapter 20: Esophagus & Diaphragm

Carlos E. Pineda, MD
Resident
Department of Surgery
Stanford University School of Medicine
Stanford, California
Chapter 31: Anorectum

Jeffrey D. Punch, MD
Associate Professor of Surgery
Chief, Division of Transplantation
University of Michigan
Ann Arbor, Michigan
Chapter 45: Organ Transplantation

Joseph H. Rapp, MD
Professor of Surgery in Residence
University of California, San Francisco
Chief, Vascular Surgery Service
San Francisco Veterans Administration Medical Center
San Francisco, California
Chapter 34: Arteries

John R. Rectenwald, MD
Assistant Professor
Department of Surgery
University of Michigan
Ann Arbor, Michigan
Chapter 35: Veins & Lymphatics

R. Kevin Reynolds, MD
The George W. Morley Professor and Chief,
    Division of Gyn Oncology
Director, Gynecologic Oncology Fellowship
Department of Obstetrics and Gynecology
The University of Michigan
Ann Arbor, Michigan
Chapter 39: Gynecology

Michael S. Sabel, MD
Associate Professor
Department of Surgery
University of Michigan
Ann Arbor, Michigan
Chapter 44: Oncology

Theodore J. Sanford Jr., MD
The Georgine M. Stuede Professor of
    Anethesiology Education
Professor of Clinical Anesthesiology
University of Michigan
Ann Arbor, Michigan
Chapter 11: Anesthesia

Matthew J. Sena, MD
Assistant Professor
Division of Trauma and Emergency Surgery
University of California, Davis Medical Center
Sacramento, California
*Chapter 12: Shock & Acute Pulmonary Failure
    in Surgical Patients*

Andrew A. Shelton, MD
Assistant Professor of Surgery (General Surgery)
Stanford University School of Medicine
Stanford, California
Chapter 29: Small Intestine
Chapter 30: Large Intestine
Chapter 31: Anorectum

Ramesh C. Srinivasan, MD
House Officer
Orthopaedic Surgery
University of Michigan
Ann Arbor, Michigan
Chapter 40: Orthopedic Surgery

Karl G. Sylvester, MD
Assistant Professor
Department of Surgery
Stanford University School of Medicine
Stanford, California
Chapter 43: Pediatric Surgery

David J. Terris, MD
Porubsky Distinguished Professor and Chairman
Department of Otolaryngology—Head and
    Neck Surgery
Medical College of Georgia
Augusta, Georgia
Chapter 15: Otolaryngology—Head & Neck Surgery

Pierre R. Theodore, MD
Assistant Professor of Surgery
Division of Cardiothoracic Surgery
Department of Surgery
University of California, San Francisco
San Francisco, California
*Chapter 18: Thoracic Wall, Pleura, Mediastinum,
    & Lung*

B. Gregory Thompson, MD
Professor of Neurosurgery, Otolaryngology
    and Radiology
Department of Neurosurgery
University of Michigan
Ann Arbor, Michigan
Chapter 36: Neurosurgery

Stephen Tolhurst, MD
House Officer
Department of Orthopaedic Surgery
University of Michigan
Ann Arbor, Michigan
Chapter 40: Orthopedic Surgery

Linda M. Tsai, MD
Associate Professor
Department of Ophthalmology and
    Visual Sciences
Washington University
St. Louis, Missouri
Chapter 37: The Eye & Ocular Adnexa

J. Blake Tyrrell, MD
Clinical Professor
Division of Endocrinology and Metabolism
University of California
San Francisco, California
Chapter 33: Adrenals

Kelly L. Vanderhave, MD
Assistant Professor
Orthopaedic Surgery
University of Michigan
Ann Arbor, Michigan
Chapter 40: Orthopedic Surgery

Henry C. Vasconez, MD
Professor of Surgery and Pediatrics, William S. Farish
    Endowed Chair of Plastic Surgery
Department of Surgery—Division of Plastic Surgery
University of Kentucky
Lexington, Kentucky
Chapter 41: Plastic & Reconstructive Surgery

Wendy L. Wahl, MD
Associate Professor of Surgery
Director, Trauma Burn Intensive Care Unit
University of Michigan
Ann Arbor, Michigan
Chapter 13: Management of the Injured Patient

Thomas W. Wakefield, MD
S. Martin Lindenauer Professor of Surgery
Section Head, Vascular Surgery
Department of Surgery
University of Michigan
Ann Arbor, Michigan
Chapter 35: Veins & Lymphatics

Lawrence W. Way, MD
Professor
Department of Surgery
University of California, San Francisco
San Francisco, California
Chapter 1: Approach to the Surgical Patient
Chapter 23: Stomach & Duodenum
Chapter 26: Pancreas

Paul M. Weinberger, MD
Resident
Otolaryngology/Head and Neck Surgery
Medical College of Georgia
Augusta, Georgia
Chapter 15: Otolaryngology—Head & Neck Surgery

Mark L. Welton, MD
Associate Professor & Chief
Section of Colon & Rectal Surgery
Department of Surgery
Stanford University School of Medicine
Stanford, California
Chapter 29: Small Intestine
Chapter 30: Large Intestine
Chapter 31: Anorectum

Richard D. Williams, MD
Rubin H. Flocks Chair & Professor
Department of Urology
University of Iowa College of Medicine
Iowa City, Iowa
Chapter 38: Urology

David M. Young, MD
Professor, Plastic Surgery
University of California, San Francisco
San Francisco, California
Chapter 42: Hand Surgery

Preface

Current Diagnosis & Treatment: Surgery is a ready source of information about diseases managed by surgeons. Like other books in this Lange series, it emphasizes quick recall of major diagnostic features and brief descriptions of disease processes, followed by approaches for definitive diagnosis and treatment. Epidemiology, pathophysiology, and pathology are discussed to the extent that they contribute to the ultimate purpose of the book, which is guidance for patient care. About one-third of the book is focused on general medical and surgical topics important in the management of all patients.

The book also includes limited current references to journal literature for the reader who wishes to pursue specific additional detail. Because of the concise nature of this text, more focused exploration may be useful to gain detail in specific areas.

OUTSTANDING FEATURES

- To maintain currency of the information, this text is revised and updated frequently. The most recent edition was published in 2006. With each revision, particular subjects are completely, substantially, partially, or minimally rewritten as indicated by the progress in each field. New authors and chapters are introduced for the text as needed.
- This edition includes major revisions of many chapters, and entirely new chapters on
  - Training, Communication, Professionalism and Systems-based Practice
  - Wound Healing
  - Anesthesia
  - Otolaryngology/Head & Neck Tumors
  - The Heart, for both Acquired and Congenital Diseases
  - Neurosurgery & Surgery of the Pituitary
  - Gynecology
    and
  - Orthopedics
- Illustrations have been judiciously chosen to demonstrate anatomic and surgical concepts, and color has been added in this edition for additional clarity.
- Over 1,000 diseases and disorders are covered.
- Thorough coverage of minimally invasive surgical procedures.

INTENDED AUDIENCE

- Students: this is an authoritative introduction to surgery as the discipline is taught and practiced at major teaching institutions.
- Residents: this is a ready reference for concise discussions of the diseases faced each day as well as the less common ones calling for quick study.
- Medical practitioners: those who have occasion to counsel patients needing surgical referrals appreciate the concise readability of this book.
- Practicing surgeons: a most useful guide to current management strategies.

ORGANIZATION

This book is organized chiefly by organ system. Lists of subjects taken up in the longer chapters are presented in the Table of Contents, but for some users the more convenient portal of entry to the text is the Index.

Early chapters provide general information about the relationship between surgeons and their patients (Chapter 1), training and professionalism (Chapter 2), preoperative care (Chapter 3), postoperative care (Chapter 4), and surgical complications (Chapter 5). Subsequent chapters deal with wound healing, inflammation, infection, antibiotics, fluid and electrolyte management, and surgical metabolism and nutrition. The main series of body systems topics begins with the chapter on head and neck tumors and ends with the chapter on hand surgery. Further chapters on pediatric surgery, oncology, and organ transplantation complete the coverage.

NEW TO THIS EDITION

Along with the customary revision of all sections as called for by changing concepts in each field covered, the following major changes have been made.

- This has been a particularly complete revision with extensive changes to every chapter to update the material, and the addition of several new chapters as detailed above.
- The work is now presented in a two-color format to clarify the organizational levels, and with color added to the artwork.
- A CD of "Quick Answers: Surgery" is included for a quick look-up of surgical diagnosis & treatment.

ACKNOWLEDGMENTS

The editor and contributors continue to acknowledge their gratitude to J. Englebert Dunphy, MD for the inspiration to begin the first edition of this text, and his lifetime of service to the practice and teaching of surgery, and to Lawrence W. Way, the long-time editor of editions Two through Twelve, and conscience of the UCSF surgical training program. As a mentor to generations of surgical residents at UCSF, Dr. Way has had an immeasurable impact on American Surgery. I am particularly grateful for the important contributions that the staff at McGraw-Hill has made to ensuring an accurate, high-quality text. In particular, Marsha Loeb and Karen Davis have been extremely supportive and helpful. I am also grateful to colleagues and readers who have offered comments and criticisms to guide preparation for future editions. I hope that anyone with an idea, suggestion, or criticism regarding this book will contact me.

Gerard M. Doherty, MD
Ann Arbor, Michigan
July 2009

Approach to the Surgical Patient

J. Englebert Dunphy, MD[*]
Lawrence W. Way, MD

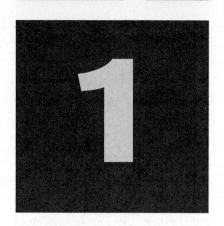

The management of surgical disorders requires not only the application of technical skills and training in the basic sciences to the problems of diagnosis and treatment but also a genuine sympathy and indeed love for the patient. The surgeon must be a doctor in the old-fashioned sense, an applied scientist, an engineer, an artist, and a minister to his or her fellow human beings. Because life or death often depends upon the validity of surgical decisions, the surgeon's judgment must be matched by courage in action and by a high degree of technical proficiency.

THE HISTORY

At their first contact, the surgeon must gain the patient's confidence and convey the assurance that help is available and will be provided. The surgeon must demonstrate concern for the patient as a person who needs help and not just as a "case" to be processed. This is not always easy to do, and there are no rules of conduct except to be gentle and considerate. Most patients are eager to like and trust their doctors and respond gratefully to a sympathetic and understanding person. Some surgeons are able to establish a confident relationship with the first few words of greeting; others can do so only by means of a stylized and carefully acquired bedside manner. It does not matter how it is done, so long as an atmosphere of sympathy, personal interest, and understanding is created. Even under emergency circumstances, this subtle message of sympathetic concern must be conveyed.

Eventually, all histories must be formally structured, but much can be learned by letting the patient ramble a little. Discrepancies and omissions in the history are often due as much to overstructuring and leading questions as to the unreliability of the patient. The enthusiastic novice asks leading questions; the cooperative patient gives the answer

that seems to be wanted; and the interview concludes on a note of mutual satisfaction with the wrong answer thus developed.

BUILDING THE HISTORY

History taking is detective work. Preconceived ideas, snap judgments, and hasty conclusions have no place in this process. The diagnosis must be established by inductive reasoning. The interviewer must first determine the facts and then search for essential clues, realizing that the patient may conceal the most important symptom—eg, the passage of blood by rectum—in the hope (born of fear) that if it is not specifically inquired about or if nothing is found to account for it in the physical examination, it cannot be very serious.

Common symptoms of surgical conditions that require special emphasis in the history taking are discussed in the following paragraphs.

▶ Pain

A careful analysis of the nature of pain is one of the most important features of a surgical history. The examiner must first ascertain how the pain began. Was it explosive in onset, rapid, or gradual? What is the precise character of the pain? Is it so severe that it cannot be relieved by medication? Is it constant or intermittent? Are there classic associations, such as the rhythmic pattern of small bowel obstruction or the onset of pain preceding the limp of intermittent claudication?

One of the most important aspects of pain is the patient's reaction to it. The overreactor's description of pain is often obviously inappropriate, and so is a description of "excruciating" pain offered in a casual or jovial manner. A patient who shrieks and thrashes about is either grossly overreacting or suffering from renal or biliary colic. Very severe pain—due to infection, inflammation, or vascular disease—usually forces the patient to restrict all movement as much as possible.

Moderate pain is made agonizing by fear and anxiety. Reassurance of a sort calculated to restore the patient's

[*]Deceased

confidence in the care being given is often a more effective analgesic than an injection of morphine.

Vomiting

What did the patient vomit? How much? How often? What did the vomitus look like? Was vomiting projectile? It is especially helpful for the examiner to see the vomitus.

Change in Bowel Habits

A change in bowel habits is a common complaint that is often of no significance. However, when a person who has always had regular evacuations notices a distinct change, particularly toward intermittent alternations of constipation and diarrhea, colon cancer must be suspected. Too much emphasis is placed on the size and shape of the stool—eg, many patients who normally have well-formed stools may complain of irregular small stools when their routine is disturbed by travel or a change in diet.

Hematemesis or Hematochezia

Bleeding from any orifice demands the most critical analysis and can never be dismissed as due to some immediately obvious cause. The most common error is to assume that bleeding from the rectum is attributable to hemorrhoids. The character of the blood can be of great significance. Does it clot? Is it bright or dark red? Is it changed in any way, as in the coffee-ground vomitus of slow gastric bleeding or the dark, tarry stool of upper gastrointestinal bleeding? The full details and variations cannot be included here but are emphasized under separate headings elsewhere.

Trauma

Trauma occurs so commonly that it is often difficult to establish a relationship between the chief complaint and an episode of trauma. Children in particular are subject to all kinds of minor trauma, and the family may attribute the onset of an illness to a specific recent injury. On the other hand, children may be subjected to severe trauma though their parents are unaware of it. The possibility of trauma having been inflicted by a parent must not be overlooked.

When there is a history of trauma, the details must be established as precisely as possible. What was the patient's position when the accident occurred? Was consciousness lost? Retrograde amnesia (inability to remember events just preceding the accident) always indicates some degree of cerebral damage. If a patient can remember every detail of an accident, has not lost consciousness, and has no evidence of external injury to the head, brain damage can be excluded.

In the case of gunshot wounds and stab wounds, knowing the nature of the weapon, its size and shape, the probable trajectory, and the position of the patient when hit may be very helpful in evaluating the nature of the resultant injury.

The possibility that an accident might have been caused by preexisting disease such as epilepsy, diabetes, coronary artery disease, or hypoglycemia must be explored.

When all of the facts and essential clues have been gathered, the examiner is in a position to complete the study of the present illness. By this time, it may be possible to rule out (by inductive reasoning) all but a few diagnoses. A novice diagnostician asked to evaluate the causes of shoulder pain in a given patient might include ruptured ectopic pregnancy in the list of possibilities. The experienced physician will automatically exclude that possibility on the basis of gender or age.

Family History

The family history is of great significance in a number of surgical conditions. Polyposis of the colon is a classic example, but diabetes, Peutz-Jeghers syndrome, chronic pancreatitis, multiglandular syndromes, other endocrine abnormalities, and cancer are often better understood and better evaluated in the light of a careful family history.

Past History

The details of the past history may illuminate obscure areas of the present illness. It has been said that people who are well are almost never sick, and people who are sick are almost never well. It is true that a patient with a long and complicated history of diseases and injuries is likely to be a much poorer risk than even a very old patient experiencing a major surgical illness for the first time.

In order to make certain that important details of the past history will not be overlooked, the system review must be formalized and thorough. By always reviewing the past history in the same way, the experienced examiner never omits significant details. Many skilled examiners find it easy to review the past history by inquiring about each system as they perform the physical examination on that part of the body.

In reviewing the past history, it is important to consider the nutritional background of the patient. There is a clear awareness throughout the world that the underprivileged, malnourished patient responds poorly to disease, injury, and operation. Malnourishment may not be obvious on physical examination and must be elicited by questioning.

Acute nutritional deficiencies, particularly fluid and electrolyte losses, can be understood only in the light of the total (including nutritional) history. For example, low serum sodium may be due to the use of diuretics or a sodium-restricted diet rather than to acute loss. In this connection, the use of any medications must be carefully recorded and interpreted.

A detailed history of acute losses by vomiting and diarrhea—and the nature of the losses—is helpful in estimating the probable trends in serum electrolytes. Thus, the patient who has been vomiting persistently with no evidence of bile in the vomitus is likely to have acute pyloric stenosis associated with benign ulcer, and hypochloremic alkalosis must be anticipated. Chronic vomiting without bile—and particularly with evidence of changed and previously digested food—is suggestive of chronic obstruction, and the possibility of carcinoma should be considered.

It is essential for the surgeon to think in terms of nutritional balance. It is often possible to begin therapy before the results of laboratory tests have been obtained, because the specific nature and probable extent of fluid and electrolyte losses can often be estimated on the basis of the history and the physician's clinical experience. Laboratory data should be obtained as soon as possible, but knowledge of the probable level of the obstruction and of the concentration of the electrolytes in the gastrointestinal fluids will provide sufficient grounds for the institution of appropriate immediate therapy.

▶ The Patient's Emotional Background

Psychiatric consultation is seldom required in the management of surgical patients, but there are times when it is of great help. Emotionally and mentally disturbed patients require surgical operations as often as do others, and full cooperation between psychiatrist and surgeon is essential. Furthermore, either before or after an operation, a patient may develop a major psychotic disturbance that is beyond the ability of the surgeon to appraise or manage. Prognosis, drug therapy, and overall management require the participation of a psychiatrist.

On the other hand, there are many situations in which the surgeon can and should deal with the emotional aspects of the patient's illness rather than resorting to psychiatric assistance. Most psychiatrists prefer not to be brought in to deal with minor anxiety states. As long as the surgeon accepts the responsibility for the care of the whole patient, such services are superfluous.

This is particularly true in the care of patients with malignant disease or those who must undergo mutilating operations such as amputation of an extremity, ileostomy, or colostomy. In these situations, the patient can be supported far more effectively by the surgeon and the surgical team than by a consulting psychiatrist.

Surgeons are increasingly aware of the importance of psychosocial factors in surgical convalescence. Recovery from a major operation is greatly enhanced if the patient is not worn down with worry about emotional, social, and economic problems that have nothing to do with the illness itself. Incorporation of these factors into the record contributes to better total care of the surgical patient.

THE PHYSICAL EXAMINATION

The complete examination of the surgical patient includes the physical examination, certain special procedures such as gastroscopy and esophagoscopy, laboratory tests, x-ray examination, and follow-up examination. In some cases, all of these may be necessary; in others, special examinations and laboratory tests can be kept to a minimum. It is just as poor practice to insist on unnecessary thoroughness as it is to overlook procedures that may contribute to the diagnosis. Painful, inconvenient, and costly procedures should not be ordered unless there is a reasonable chance that the information gained will be useful in making clinical decisions.

THE ELECTIVE PHYSICAL EXAMINATION

The elective physical examination should be done in an orderly and detailed fashion. One should acquire the habit of performing a complete examination in exactly the same sequence, so that no step is omitted. When the routine must be modified, as in an emergency, the examiner recalls without conscious effort what must be done to complete the examination later. The regular performance of complete examinations has the added advantage of familiarizing the beginner with what is normal so that what is abnormal can be more readily recognized.

All patients are sensitive and somewhat embarrassed at being examined. It is both courteous and clinically useful to put the patient at ease. The examining room and table should be comfortable, and drapes should be used if the patient is required to strip for the examination. Most patients will relax if they are allowed to talk a bit during the examination, which is another reason for taking the past history while the examination is being done.

A useful rule is to first observe the patient's general physique and habitus and then to carefully inspect the hands. Many systemic diseases show themselves in the hands (cirrhosis of the liver, hyperthyroidism, Raynaud disease, pulmonary insufficiency, heart disease, and nutritional disorders).

Details of the examination cannot be included here. The beginner is urged to consult special texts.

Inspection, palpation, and auscultation are the time-honored essential steps in appraising both the normal and the abnormal. Comparison of the two sides of the body often suggests a specific abnormality. The slight droop of one eyelid characteristic of Horner syndrome can only be recognized by comparison with the opposite side. Inspection of the female breasts, particularly as the patient raises and lowers her arms, will often reveal slight dimpling indicative of an infiltrating carcinoma barely detectable on palpation.

Successful palpation requires skill and gentleness. Spasm, tension, and anxiety caused by painful examination procedures may make an adequate examination almost impossible, particularly in children.

Another important feature of palpation is the laying on of hands that has been called part of the ministry of medicine. A disappointed and critical patient often will say of a doctor, "He hardly touched me." Careful, precise, and gentle palpation not only gives the physician the information being sought but also inspires confidence and trust.

When examining for areas of tenderness, it may be necessary to use only one finger in order to precisely localize the extent of the tenderness. This is of particular importance in examination of the acute abdomen.

Auscultation, once thought to be the exclusive province of the physician, is now more important in surgery than it is in medicine. Radiologic examinations, including cardiac catheterization, have relegated auscultation of the heart and lungs to the status of preliminary scanning procedures in medicine. In surgery, however, auscultation of the abdomen and peripheral vessels has become absolutely essential. The nature of ileus and the presence of a variety of vascular lesions are revealed by auscultation. Bizarre abdominal pain in a young woman can easily be ascribed to hysteria or anxiety on the basis of a negative physical examination and x-rays of the gastrointestinal tract. Auscultation of the epigastrium, however, may reveal a murmur due to obstruction of the celiac artery.

▶ Examination of the Body Orifices

Thorough examination of the ears, mouth, rectum, and pelvis is accepted as part of a complete examination. Palpation of the mouth and tongue is as essential as inspection. Every surgeon should acquire familiarity with the use of the ophthalmoscope and sigmoidoscope and should use them regularly in doing complete physical examinations.

THE EMERGENCY PHYSICAL EXAMINATION

In an emergency, the routine of the physical examination must be altered to fit the circumstances. The history may be limited to a single sentence, or there may be no history if the patient is unconscious and there are no other informants. Although the details of an accident or injury may be very useful in the total appraisal of the patient, they must be left for later consideration. The primary considerations are the following: Is the patient breathing? Is the airway open? Is there a palpable pulse? Is the heart beating? Is massive bleeding occurring?

If the patient is not breathing, airway obstruction must be ruled out by thrusting the fingers into the mouth and pulling the tongue forward. If the patient is unconscious, the respiratory tract should be intubated and mouth-to-mouth respiration started. If there is no pulse or heartbeat, start cardiac resuscitation.

Serious external loss of blood from an extremity can be controlled by elevation and pressure. Tourniquets are rarely required.

Every victim of major blunt trauma should be suspected of having a vertebral injury capable of causing damage to the spinal cord unless rough handling is avoided.

Some injuries are so life threatening that action must be taken before even a limited physical examination is done. Penetrating wounds of the heart; large, open, sucking wounds of the chest; massive crush injuries with flail chest; and massive external bleeding all require emergency treatment before any further examination can be done.

In most emergencies, however, after it has been established that the airway is open, the heart is beating, and there is no massive external hemorrhage—and after antishock measures have been instituted, if necessary—a rapid survey examination must be done. Failure to perform such an examination can lead to serious mistakes in the care of the patient. It takes no more than 2 or 3 minutes to carefully examine the head, thorax, abdomen, extremities, genitalia (particularly in females), and back. If cervical cord damage has been ruled out, it is essential to turn the injured patient and carefully inspect the back, buttocks, and perineum.

Tension pneumothorax and cardiac tamponade may easily be overlooked if there are multiple injuries.

Upon completion of the survey examination, control of pain, splinting of fractured limbs, suturing of lacerations, and other types of emergency treatment can be started.

▼ LABORATORY & OTHER EXAMINATIONS

▶ Laboratory Examination

Laboratory examinations in surgical patients have the following objectives: (1) screening for asymptomatic disease that may affect the surgical result (eg, unsuspected anemia or diabetes); (2) appraisal of diseases that may contraindicate elective surgery or require treatment before surgery (eg, diabetes, heart failure); (3) diagnosis of disorders that require surgery (eg, hyperparathyroidism, pheochromocytoma); and (4) evaluation of the nature and extent of metabolic or septic complications.

Patients undergoing major surgery, even though they seem to be in excellent health except for their surgical disease, should have age-appropriate laboratory examination. A history of renal, hepatic, or heart disease requires detailed studies. Medical consultation may be helpful in the total preoperative appraisal of the surgical patient. It is essential, however, that the surgeon not become totally dependent upon a medical consultant for the preoperative evaluation and management of the patient. The total management must be the surgeon's responsibility and is not to be delegated. Moreover, the surgeon is the only one with the experience and background to interpret the meaning of laboratory tests in the light of other features of the case—particularly the history and physical findings.

▶ Imaging Studies

Modern patient care calls for a variety of critical radiologic examinations. The closest cooperation between the radiologist and the surgeon is essential if serious mistakes are to be avoided. This means that the surgeon must not refer the patient to the radiologist, requesting a particular examination, without providing an adequate account of the history and physical findings. Particularly in emergencies, review of the films and consultation are needed.

When the radiologic diagnosis is not definitive, the examinations must be repeated in the light of the history and physical examination. Despite the great accuracy of x-ray diagnosis, a negative gastrointestinal study still does not exclude either ulcer or a neoplasm; particularly in the right colon, small lesions are easily overlooked. At times, the history and physical findings are so clearly diagnostic that operation is justifiable despite negative imaging studies.

Special Examinations

Special examinations such as cystoscopy, gastroscopy, esophagoscopy, colonoscopy, angiography, and bronchoscopy are often required in the diagnostic appraisal of surgical disorders. The surgeon must be familiar with the indications and limitations of these procedures and be prepared to consult with colleagues in medicine and the surgical specialties as required.

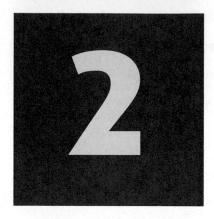

Training, Communication, Professionalism, and Systems-based Practice

Gerard M. Doherty, MD

TRAINING

The process of medical education and surgical training in the United States is overseen by an interconnected group of organizations. Each of these organizations has a specific focus; however, their common theme is continuous process improvement encouraged by intermittent external review (Table 2–1). Their ultimate goal is to provide a consistent, qualified, and professional workforce for medical care in the United States.

▶ Medical Student Education

The Liaison Committee on Medical Education (LCME) provides accreditation for medical schools in the United States and Canada. Accreditation is the process of quality assurance in postsecondary education that assesses whether an institution meets established standards. Accreditation by the LCME is effectively necessary for schools to function in the United States. Without accreditation, the schools cannot receive federal grants for medical education or participate in federal loan programs. Graduation from an LCME-accredited school enables students to sit for medical licensing examinations (the USMLE) and to achieve licensure in most US states. Graduation from an LCME-accredited medical school is also necessary for acceptance into an Accreditation Council for Graduate Medical Education (ACGME)–accredited residency program for graduates of US medical schools. The authority for the LCME to provide this accreditation is delegated by the US Department of Education in the United States and the Committee on Accreditation of Canadian Medical Schools (CACMS) in Canada.

Each accredited medical school is reviewed annually for appropriateness of its function, structure, and performance. Formal site visits are conducted periodically with more in-depth review and reaccreditation at that time. The usual period of full accreditation is 8 years. At the time of this in-depth accreditation visit, and in the intervals between, the LCME works to disseminate best practices and approve the overall quality of education leading to the MD degree.

▶ Graduate Medical Education

The ACGME is responsible for the accreditation of post-MD medical training programs within the United States. Accreditation is accomplished through a peer review process based on established standards and guidelines. The member organizations of the ACGME as an accrediting group are the American Board of Medical Specialties (ABMS), the American Hospital Association (AHA), the American Medical Association (AMA), the Association of American Medical Colleges (AAMC), and the Council of Medical Specialty Societies. The ACGME oversees a variety of graduate medical education programs in specific specialties. These ACGME-accredited residency programs must adhere to the ACGME common program requirements that apply to all residencies as well as specific program requirements that apply to each training program. The hospitals that house the training programs must also meet institutional requirements set by the ACGME.

The ACGME has identified 6 general competency areas that must be addressed during every graduate residency training program (Table 2–2). The specific application of these competency areas varies widely among training programs. However, each rotation of each residency must include attention to and assessment of progress in fulfilling the general competency requirements.

The review and accreditation of specialty residency programs is undertaken by a committee specific for that field. In surgery, the group is the Residency Review Committee for Surgery (RRC-S). The RRC-S assesses program compliance with accreditation standards at both the common program requirements and the program-specific levels. Programs are typically fully accredited on a 5-year cycle, with annual updates and questionnaires in the interim. Early site visits can be triggered by a variety of events, including significant changes in the program or its leadership. The Residency Review Committees also control the number of positions that each program is accredited to have. This effectively sets the maximum number of graduates that can finish from a given training program in any given year.

Table 2–1. US Organization with Medical Education Oversight.

Organization	Acronym and Web Site	Purpose
Liaison Committee on Medical Education	LCME www.lcme.org	Accreditation of medical schools in United States and Canada
Accreditation Council for Graduate Medical Education	ACGME www.acgme.org	Accreditation of post-MD training programs in some specialties
American Board of Surgery	ABS www.absurgery.org	Certification and recertification of individual surgeons who meet standards of education, training, and knowledge
American College of Surgeons	ACS www.facs.org	Scientific and educational association of surgeons to improve the quality of care for the surgical patient

American Board of Surgery

The American Board of Surgery (ABS) is an independent, nonprofit organization with the purpose of certifying individual surgeons who have met defined standards of education, training, and knowledge. The distinction between the ACGME and the ABS is that the ACGME accredits training programs, while the ABS certifies individuals. This distinction is similar for specialty boards in other disciplines as well. The ABS also recertifies practicing surgeons and is making a fundamental philosophical change from periodic retesting for recertification to a more continuous maintenance of certification (MOC) plan.

The ACGME and the specialty boards interact. The success of individuals in achieving board certification is an important measure of graduate medical education program success, and the measures required for board certification must also reflect the education that is offered to individuals through their graduate medical education. Thus, although these entities have different purposes, they must mesh their efforts constructively.

Board certification within a defined period after completing residency is necessary for privileging to perform surgery in many US hospitals. Thus, the most straightforward route into surgical practice in the United States includes graduation from an LCME-accredited medical school, completion of an ACGME-accredited residency training program, and satisfactory completion of the Qualifying Examination (written boards) and Certifying Examination (oral boards) of the ABS.

There are other entry points into surgical practice in the United States, most prominently by physicians who have graduated from medical schools in countries outside the United States and Canada. These graduates can be certified by the Educational Commission for Foreign Medical Graduates (ECFMG). Once a graduate is certified by the ECFMG, he or she is eligible to train in an ACGME-approved residency training program and can thus be eligible for board certification.

American College of Surgeons

The American College of Surgeons (ACS) is a scientific and educational association of surgeons whose mission is to improve the quality of care for the surgical patient by setting high standards for surgical education and practice. ACS members, known as fellows, are entitled to use the letters FACS after their name. Membership as a fellow implies that the surgeon has met standards of education, training, professional qualifications, surgical competence, and ethical conduct. However, despite these requirements, the ACS is a voluntary professional membership group and does not certify individuals for practice. The ACS sponsors a wide variety of educational and professional support programs for both practicing surgeons and trainees. In addition, it offers membership for surgeons in training (Resident Membership) and students (Medical Student Membership) and for those surgeons who have completed training but have not yet met all the requirements for fellowship (Associate Fellow). The ACS also engages in important advocacy roles on behalf of patients and the surgeon members.

COMMUNICATION

Efficient and effective communication skills are a critical resource for all clinicians, including surgeons. A surgeon must be able to establish rapport with the patient and family quickly and reliably. Mutual respect is critical to a therapeutic relationship. The patient and family must be confident of the competence of the surgeon in order to participate in the recommended management and recovery. Judgments about a surgeon's competence frequently are made within the first few moments of interaction based on the surgeon's ability to communicate. In addition to communicating with patients,

Table 2–2. ACGME General Competencies for Graduate Medical Education.

General Competency
Medical knowledge
Interpersonal and communication skills
Professionalism
Practice-based learning
Systems-based practice

clinicians must communicate with referring and collaborating physicians and also within their own health care teams.

Communication with Patients

Communication with patients requires attention to several aspects. First, the clinician must demonstrate respect for the patient as a person. Second, the clinician must display effective listening to the patient's message and empathy for the patient's situation or concerns. Finally, the clinician must be clear in his or her response. If any of these items are neglected, the interaction will be less effective than it otherwise could be. Many surgeons try to jump straight to a very clear, concise statement of the plan, but unless the first three steps have occurred, the patient may not listen to the plan at all.

Respect

It is crucial to show respect for the patient and family as persons. The health care environment is often inconvenient and encountered during a time of stress. Patients are out of their normal venue and comfort zone. They are often frightened by the prospect of what they may learn. Showing respect for their identity helps put patients at ease and encourages their trusting communication with the clinician. Failing to show respect has the opposite effect. For instance, meeting adults for the first time and addressing them by their first name may put some patients on guard with respect to their personal independence and control. Similarly, referring to the mother of a pediatric patient as "Mom" rather than using her name implies lack of attention to her as an individual. On initial meetings, the clinician should use the patient's last name preceded by an honorific title (Mr Smith or Ms Jones). If uncertain whether a woman prefers Mrs or Ms, the clinician should ask her. In contemporary US society, a woman over 18 years old is never referred to as Miss.

Engaging in brief small talk regarding some aspect of a patient's life other than the medical matter at hand can help put the person at ease ("It must be interesting to be a dog trainer. What is your favorite breed?"). These efforts will be rewarded by a more trusting patient, a more efficient interview, and a better therapeutic relationship over the long term.

Listening

Listening to the patient is critical to establishing a correct diagnosis and appropriate therapeutic plan for the individual. All patients have a story to tell, and it is important to let them do so. They are likely to reveal critical issues regarding the clinical matter as they tell their story. Patients often need to tell their story in their own words, without interruption, so they feel confident they have provided details that might be missed if the interview is limited to simply answering the clinician's questions. Encouraging them to do so at the beginning of the interview relieves them of this burden of information and allows the clinician to move on to interpretation.

Listening should be an active, engaged activity. The clinician should appear comfortable, settled, and as close as possible to eye level with the patient. It is important not to appear rushed, inattentive, or bored by the patient's account. Interjecting questions for clarity or intermittent, brief verbal encouragements reassures the patient that the clinician is engaged with the problem.

It may be helpful at the outset of the listening phase to let the patient know what materials have been reviewed. For example, telling the patient that the clinician has reviewed the referral letter from the primary physician, the results of the last two operations, and his or her recent laboratory work may help the patient to be more concise in the discussion.

Empathy

Once the patient has recounted his or her history, and the other aspects of examination and data review have been completed, it is important to review this material with the patient in a way that demonstrates empathy with his or her situation. A surgeon's understanding of the problem is important for the patient, but the problem is not confined to the medical issue: It must be understood in the context of the patient. Therefore, demonstration of empathy is important to the patient's trust of the physician. Establishing this connection is crucial to engaging the patient in the process of care.

Clarity

Having established respect for the patient, heard and understood the patient's story, and empathized with his or her situation, the physician must speak clearly, in a vocabulary understood by the individual, about the recommendations for further evaluation or care. This part of the conversation should include a clear distinction between what is known about the patient's diagnosis or condition and what is not known but might be anticipated. When appropriate, likelihoods of various outcomes should be estimated in a way that the patient can grasp. The recommended approach to next steps should be listed clearly, along with alternative approaches. Patients always have at least one alternative to the recommended choice, even if only to decide not to have further medical care. The conversation can be augmented with illustrations or models that may improve the patient's understanding. Reviewing radiological studies directly with the patient or family also can help their understanding.

Failing to establish a comfortable, mutually respectful relationship with the patient can lead to errors in judgment about diagnosis or management. It also precludes the opportunity to engage the patient as an ally in his or her care. And if treatment goes badly, it can make communication about problems or complications difficult or impossible. Finally, the surgeon who communicates poorly excludes himself or herself from enjoying a personally and professionally satisfying physician-patient relationship.

Communication with Collaborating Physicians

Surgeons often work with other physicians in collaboration of care for patients. Communication in these settings is important to the overall patient outcome, particularly when the surgeon is involved in the patient's care for some defined interval that was preceded and will be followed by the ongoing care provided by the primary care physician. In this situation, there are two basic types of communication: routine and urgent. Routine communication of reasonably expected information that does not need to be acted on urgently can take place in a variety of ways depending on the health care setting. It is typically asynchronous and written, and it may take the form of a note in the patient's electronic medical record or a letter sent to the physician's office. For example, regarding a patient who is referred to a surgeon for cholecystectomy and who has a plan made for the operation, communication between the surgeon and referring physician can be routine.

Urgent communication should occur between or among the collaborating physicians when unexpected or adverse outcomes occur. Again, a variety of communication modes may be utilized, but the communication is more often synchronous via a direct conversation either in person or by telephone. The communication is more than courtesy to the collaborating physicians, as knowledge of these events allows them to participate constructively on behalf of the patient. Examples of situations that warrant more urgent communication include new diagnosis of significant cancers, life-altering complications from interventions, and certainly death of the patient.

Clarity in transfer-of-care responsibility is critical to the continuous optimal care of the patient. Therefore, any communication with the collaborating physicians should indicate either the ongoing role of the surgeon in the patient's care or the deliberate transfer of responsibility for ongoing care issues back to other collaborating physicians.

Communication within Teams

Surgical care is often provided in a team setting. Current surgical teams typically include physicians, nonphysician midlevel providers (often physician assistants or nurse practitioners), and a variety of students. The student trainees may include students in medical school, physician assistant programs, or nursing school. These teams have become increasingly complex, and the information they manipulate as a team to provide patient care is voluminous. In addition, the transfer of information from one provider to another as shifts or rotations change is recognized as a weak point in the patient care continuum.

With these complex teams and extensive information, the keys to efficient and effective team processes appear to be clarity of roles and processes that involve writing things down only once. The advent of electronic medical records has allowed the generation of electronic tools to transfer information among team members. Such tools may be useful to facilitate team processes. Careful attention to transfers of care from one provider to another and explicit recognition that this is a potential time for errors is important.

PROFESSIONALISM

Professionalism denotes behavior that characterizes a person as a professional. A professional is implied to possess the specialized knowledge of and to have gone through intensive academic preparation for his or her vocation. Because conduct affects all interactions, for optimal effectiveness, the surgeon should behave professionally with patients with other health care professionals and in the broader context of their institutions. The AMA has promulgated a set of medical ethical principles that apply equally well to surgical practice and that can help to guide professional behavior (Table 2–3).

The ethics of surgical practice are complex and can be approached from a variety of theoretical frameworks. The most commonly applied framework for the evaluation of ethical dilemmas for individual patient decisions in medi-

Table 2–3. AMA Principles of Medical Ethics.

1. A physician shall be dedicated to providing competent medical care, with compassion and respect for human dignity and rights.
2. A physician shall uphold the standards of professionalism, be honest in all professional interactions, and strive to report physicians deficient in character or competence, or engaging in fraud or deception, to appropriate entities.
3. A physician shall respect the law and also recognize a responsibility to seek changes in those requirements which are contrary to the best interests of the patient.
4. A physician shall respect the rights of patients, colleagues, and other health professionals, and shall safeguard patient confidences and privacy within the constraints of the law.
5. A physician shall continue to study, apply, and advance scientific knowledge, maintain a commitment to medical education, make relevant information available to patients, colleagues, and the public, obtain consultation, and use the talents of other health professionals when indicated.
6. A physician shall, in the provision of appropriate patient care, except in emergencies, be free to choose whom to serve, with whom to associate, and the environment in which to provide medical care.
7. A physician shall recognize a responsibility to participate in activities contributing to the improvement of the community and the betterment of public health.
8. A physician shall, while caring for a patient, regard responsibility to the patient as paramount.
9. A physician shall support access to medical care for all people.

From "Principles of Medical Ethics," adopted by the AMA's House of Delegates, June 17, 2001. Available at www.ama-assn.org/ama/pub/category/2512.html.

cine, known as "the principles approach," involves four principles: autonomy, beneficence, nonmaleficence, and justice, as promulgated by Beauchamp and Childress (2001); see Table 2–4. A detailed analysis of these principles is beyond the scope here; however, the need for a code of medical ethics that is distinct from general societal ethics is the basis for medical professionalism. Five features of medical relationships provide the moral imperatives that underlie the requirement for a professional ethical code separate from other forms of business: (1) the inequality in medical knowledge, and attendant vulnerability, of the patient; (2) the requirement for the patient to trust the physician, known as the fiduciary nature of the relationship; (3) the moral nature of medical decisions that encompass both the technical aspects of health management and the ultimate effect on the patient's life; (4) the nature of medical knowledge as a public property that physicians receive in order to apply to the practical improvement of patients' lives; and (5) the moral complicity of the physician in the outcome of the prescribed care in that no formal medical care can take place without the physician's collusion. Because of these characteristics of the relationship between physicians and their patients, physicians must adhere to a set of ethical constraints specific to their profession.

While these imperatives are not generally understood explicitly by patients, patients can clearly grasp when these principles are in danger. They may even be suspicious that their physician or surgeon has competing motives to the patient's best interest. One of the goals of the physician-patient interaction is to allay these fears and construct a trusting relationship based on the patient's needs, within the principles noted above.

Interaction with Patients

Interactions with patients should be characterized by polite and possibly somewhat formal manners. Such manners aid professionals in their communication efforts and help them to meet patient expectations. Socially acceptable manners put patients at ease that the physician is an empathetic person with the self-awareness to recognize the way he or she appears to other people. The physician's manners affect his or her credibility in subsequent interactions. These conventions extend to the type of dress that is worn in a professional setting. Whether a physician wears a white coat or formal business clothing (suits, ties, pantsuits, blouses, skirts, etc.) is best left to local custom and practice. However, the mode of dress in general should be neat, clean, formal rather than casual, and not distracting to the interaction.

Another aspect of professionalism is the physician's ability to do the right thing for the patient and the family even when that course is difficult or unpleasant. This includes such situations as frankly and openly disclosing errors made during care or delivering bad news about new or unexpected diagnoses. While human nature can make these interactions difficult, the professional must rise to the task and perform it

Table 2–4. Principles of Medical Ethics.

Principle	Definition
Autonomy	Deliberated self-rule; the patient has the right to choose or refuse treatments; requires physicians to consult the patient and obtain patient's agreement before administering care
Beneficence	A practitioner should act in the best interest of the patient without regard to physician self-interest
Nonmaleficence	Do no harm; the practitioner should avoid treatments that harm the patient
Justice	Rendering what is due to others; affects the distribution of medical care among patients and populations

well. Avoiding the opportunity to do so not only obviates the professional's role as advisor on the issue at hand but affects the physician's credibility in the remainder of that therapeutic relationship.

Interactions with Health Care Personnel

Surgeons frequently work in complex, multilayered organizations. The behavior of the surgeon within this group should always remain productive and patient centered. In any complex organization with multiple people and personalities, conflicts arise. When they do, the surgeon should not shrink from the conflict but rather should take up the role of constructive evaluator and team builder to resolve the issue. At all times, the surgeon must avoid personal attacks based on individuals' personal characteristics, but he or she may legitimately criticize behavior and ideas. Professional comportment in these matters will be rewarded with progress in resolving the issue.

Reputation is a fragile and valuable commodity, as valuable to the clinician as his or her education or certification. All health care professionals have a reputation, and it works either for or against them in achieving their patient care and professional goals. Careful adherence to professional behavior in dress, speech, manners, and conflict resolution will create the most advantageous professional reputation for the surgeon. With a positive reputation, the surgeon's behavior in ambiguous situations will be interpreted in a benevolent way.

SYSTEMS-BASED PRACTICE

Systems-based practice is one of the core competencies defined by the ACGME as a necessary skill to be developed by graduate medical trainees. Residents must demonstrate an awareness of and responsiveness to the larger context and system of health care and the ability to effectively call on system resources to provide optimal care. The process of teaching and learning systems-based practice has been in place for many years. It is what might be considered the practical part of graduate medical training. However, only fairly recently has it become a focus and metric for performance by training programs.

As a part of training, then, residents must learn how different types of medical practice and health care delivery systems differ from one another, including methods for controlling health care costs and allocating resources. They must use this knowledge to practice cost-effective health care and resource allocation that limits the compromise of quality of care. They must advocate for quality patient care and assist patients in dealing with complexities of the health care delivery system. They must also understand how to work with health care managers and other collaborating health care providers to assess, coordinate, and improve health care for patients.

The role of the resident in identifying both the health care needs of the patient and the capability of the system to meet those needs is well established. Surgery residents in their senior years are often important resources for hospital systems because they understand how to manipulate the system to meet the needs of the patient. Medical students and surgical trainees must also recognize their role as a part of these complex systems.

[Accreditation Council for Graduate Medical Education] www.acgme.org

[American Board of Surgery] www.absurgery.org

[American College of Surgeons, "Why Is Professionalism Important Now, and How Does It Affect You?" by Paul Friedman] www.facs.org/spring_meeting/2003/gs07friedmann.pdf

Beauchamp TL, Childress JF: *Principles of Biomedical Ethics*, 6th ed. Oxford University Press, 2001.

Council on Ethical and Judicial Affairs: *Code of Medical Ethics of the American Medical Association: Current Opinions with Annotations.* AMA Press, 2008.

Fox S. *Business Etiquette for Dummies.* Wiley, 2008.

Greenberg JA et al. The ACGME competencies in the operating room. Surgery 2007;142:180.

Pellegrino ED, Thomasma DC. *The Virtues in Medical Practice.* Oxford University Press, 1993.

Rowland PA, Lang NP. *Communication & Professionalism Competencies: A Guide for Surgeons.* Cine-Med, 2007.

www.lcmc.org

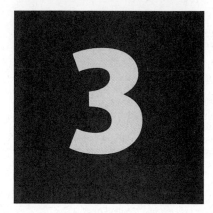

Preoperative Care

Gerard M. Doherty, MD

The care of the patient with a major surgical problem commonly involves distinct phases of management that occur in the following sequence:

1. Preoperative care
   Diagnostic workup
   Preoperative evaluation
   Preoperative preparation
2. Anesthesia and operation
3. Postoperative care
   Postanesthetic observation
   Intensive care
   Intermediate care
   Convalescent care

DEFINITIONS & OBJECTIVES

Preoperative Care

The **diagnostic workup** is concerned primarily with determining the cause and extent of the present illness. **Preoperative evaluation** consists of an overall assessment of the patient's general health in order to identify significant abnormalities that might increase operative risk or adversely influence recovery. **Preoperative preparation** includes interventions dictated by the findings on diagnostic workup and preoperative evaluation and by the nature of the expected operation. This includes interventions specifically imposed to modify the risk of perioperative complications.

Postoperative Care

The **postanesthetic observation** phase of management is the few hours immediately after operation during which the acute reaction to operation and the residual effects of anesthesia subside. A postanesthetic recovery unit with special staff and equipment is usually provided for this purpose. Patients who need continued cardiopulmonary support or

continued invasive monitoring to avoid major morbidity and death should be transferred to an intensive care unit.

Intermediate care is usually provided on an inpatient nursing unit until the patient's recovery can continue at home during the convalescent phase.

The Continuum of Surgical Care

The continuum of surgical care is represented above as progressing through a series of preoperative and postoperative phases. In practice, these phases merge, overlap, and vary in relative importance from patient to patient. Complications, death, and the therapeutic end result in the surgical patient depend upon the competence with which each succeeding phase is managed. The rapid progression and severe episodic stress of major surgical illness leave small margin for errors in management. The care immediately preceding and following operation, which includes preoperative evaluation and preparation and postanesthetic observation and intensive care, is especially critical. The increased complexity of surgical critical care has resulted in a team approach to the ICU patient, with management directed by the primary surgeon and the critical care specialists in the ICU, whose role it is to maintain optimum care.

PREOPERATIVE EVALUATION

General Health Assessment

The initial diagnostic workup of the surgical patient is focused on the cause of the presenting complaints. Except in strictly minor surgical illness, this initial workup should be supplemented by a complete assessment of the patient's general health. This evaluation, which should be completed prior to all major operations, seeks to identify abnormalities that may influence operative risk or may have a bearing on the patient's future well-being. Preoperative evaluation includes at least a complete history and physical examination. The evaluation should initially focus on the clinical assessment of risk based on the patient's history and current symptoms. This assessment should guide the remainder of the evaluation. Bleeding tendencies, medications currently being taken, and allergies and reactions to antibiotics and other agents should be noted and prominently displayed on the chart. Previous personal or familial complications such as venous thromboembolism affect the risk of similar complications going forward and require active management to decrease the risk.

The physical examination should be thorough and must include neurologic examination and assessment of peripheral arterial pulses (carotid, radial, femoral, popliteal, posterior tibial, and dorsalis pedis). The adequacy of circulating blood volume can be determined by the adequacy of peripheral perfusion, the fullness of neck veins in the supine and partially erect positions, and tests for orthostatic changes in blood pressure and pulse. Severe cardiovascular disease will make these parameters much more difficult to interpret. Patients who are prone to a hypovolemic state include those with significant weight loss as a result of cancer, gastrointestinal disease, or drugs such as diuretics. Peripheral vascular disease should be suspected if there is a history of transient ischemic attacks, claudication, or diabetes. If a carotid bruit is found, other studies may be indicated to specifically evaluate for stenosis. Rectal examination and pelvic examination should be performed as dictated by the patient's specific disease and health-maintenance examination schedule.

All significant complaints, physical findings, and test abnormalities should be adequately evaluated by appropriate further tests, examinations, and consultations. Practice in the United States has generally included a complete blood count and serum electrolyte measurements for patients over 40 and a chest x-ray and electrocardiogram for those over 50. Although these recommendations are simple to apply, they are not entirely supported by the medical literature and may result in more testing than is absolutely necessary. All test results must be interpreted in the context of the individual patient. For example, a hemoglobin of 8 g/dL is generally physiologically safe for tissue oxygen delivery but may be inadequate in the patient with reduced cardiac output. The adequacy of liver and kidney function should be tested if impairment is suspected, because each organ plays a major role in the response to and clearance of various anesthetic agents both preoperatively and intraoperatively. Selection of the ideal agent depends on recognition of liver or renal impairment in the preoperative period. Psychiatric consultation should be considered in patients with a history of significant mental disorder that may be exacerbated by operation and in patients whose complaints may have a psychoneurotic basis.

If the scheduled procedure will or may require blood replacement, the preoperative preparation should include planning for that possibility. Appropriate strategies may include storing autologous blood in the weeks prior to operation to allow reinfusion, directed-donor blood storage for transfusion, or phlebotomy and hemodilution immediately preoperatively with subsequent reinfusion.

In summary, the preoperative evaluation should be comprehensive to assess the patient's overall state of health, to determine the risk of the impending surgical treatment, and to guide the preoperative preparation.

Garcia-Miguel FJ, Serrano-Aguilar PG, Lopez-Bastida J: Preoperative assessment. Lancet 2003;362:1749.
Halaszynski TM, Juda R, Silverman DG: Optimizing postoperative outcomes with efficient preoperative assessment and management. Crit Care Med 2004;32:S76.

▶ Specific Factors Affecting Operative Risk

A. The Compromised or Altered Host

Patients may be considered compromised or altered hosts if significant impairment of systems and tissues does not permit a normal response to operative trauma or infection. Preoperative recognition of an abnormal nutritional or immune state is of obvious importance.

1. Nutritional assessment—Malnutrition leads to a significant increase in the operative death rate. Weight loss of more than 20% caused by illness such as cancer or intestinal disease not only results in a higher death rate but also a greater than threefold increase in the postoperative infection rate. There is no one best way to determine nutritional status, but it is clear that dietary history is of major importance in the assessment, as is a working knowledge of the basic nutritional deficiencies associated with certain disease states, particularly vitamin deficiencies. Standard biochemical parameters that indicate impairment in the visceral protein mass include a serum albumin of less than 3 g/dL or a serum transferrin of less than 150 mg/dL.

Even when malnutrition is diagnosed, the utility of short-term (7–10 days) preoperative hyperalimentation is not clear. It is known that nutrition can improve wound healing and immune function. Current indications for supportive measures before elective surgery include a history of weight loss in excess of 10% of body weight or an anticipated prolonged postoperative recovery period during which the patient will not be fed orally.

2. Assessment of immune competence—Increased knowledge and appreciation of immune defenses has led to a greater awareness of the increased postoperative rates of complications and death due to infection in patients with immune deficiency disorders. Many immune deficiency states are linked to malnutrition. Total lymphocyte count and cell-mediated immunity measurement are the two most commonly performed tests. Anergy or impaired immunity is diagnosed if no response is noted to any of the skin tests, whereas a positive response (5 mm or more of induration at the test site) to one or more skin tests indicates normal lymphocyte activity. Anergy is associated with an increased susceptibility to infectious complications. Other more specific tests include neutrophil chemotaxis and measurements of specific lymphocyte populations. Patients at high risk for immune deficiency in whom this information is helpful include elderly patients and those with malnutrition, severe trauma or burns, or cancer.

3. Other factors leading to increased infection—Certain drugs may reduce the patient's resistance to infection by interfering with host defense mechanisms. Corticosteroids, immunosuppressive agents, cytotoxic drugs, and prolonged antibiotic therapy are associated with an increased incidence of invasion by fungi and other organisms not commonly encountered in infections. A high rate of wound, pulmonary, and other infections is observed in renal failure, presumably as a result of decreased host resistance. Granulocytopenia and diseases that may produce immunologic deficiency—eg, lymphomas, leukemias, and hypogammaglobulinemia—are frequently associated with septic complications. The uncontrolled diabetic patient is also more susceptible to infection.

B. Pulmonary Dysfunction

The patient with compromised preoperative pulmonary function is susceptible to postoperative pulmonary complications, including hypoxia, atelectasis, and pneumonia. Preoperative evaluation of the degree of respiratory impairment is necessary in patients at high risk for postoperative complications. This evaluation includes a history of heavy smoking and cough, obesity, advanced age, and known pulmonary disease, particularly before major intrathoracic or upper abdominal surgery. Pertinent factors in the history include the presence and character of cough and excessive sputum production, history of wheezing, and exercise tolerance. Pertinent physical findings include the presence of wheezing or prolonged expiration. A chest x-ray, ECG, blood gases, and some basic pulmonary function tests are useful preoperative studies in these patients. Although evaluation of arterial oxygen tension is helpful, the main reason for obtaining preoperative blood gases is to evaluate for CO_2 retention, which indicates severe pulmonary dysfunction. If surgery is necessary, supplemental oxygen must be used carefully in the postoperative period, because overuse may accentuate CO_2 retention and aggravate concomitant respiratory acidosis. The most helpful screening pulmonary function tests are forced vital capacity (FVC) and forced expiratory volume in 1 second (FEV_1). Values less than 50% of predicted, based on age and body size, indicate significant airway disease with a high risk for complications.

Preoperative pulmonary preparation for a period as short as 48 hours has been shown to significantly decrease postoperative complications. Even a few days of abstinence from smoking will decrease sputum production. Oral or inhaled bronchodilators along with twice-daily chest physical therapy and postural drainage will help clear inspissated secretions from the airway. Before operation, patients should be instructed in techniques of coughing, deep breathing, and

use of one of the incentive spirometry devices that increase inspiratory effort.

Lawrence VA, Cornell JE, Smetana GW: Strategies to reduce postoperative pulmonary complications after noncardiothoracic surgery: systematic review for the American College of Physicians. Ann Intern Med 2006;144:596.

C. Delayed Wound Healing

This problem can be anticipated in certain categories of patients whose tissue repair process may be compromised. Important factors include protein depletion, ascorbic acid deficiency, marked dehydration or edema, severe anemia, diabetes mellitus, and smoking. The most important component is maintenance of adequate blood volume and perfusion. Decreased perfusion results in a marked decrease in tissue oxygen tension, which in turn correlates with delayed wound healing or infection. Often the decrease is not clinically evident, but it can be expected to occur in patients receiving chronic diuretic therapy or those with underlying myocardial dysfunction. Large doses of corticosteroids depress wound healing in humans. Wounds in patients who have received appreciable doses of corticosteroids preoperatively should be closed with special care to prevent disruption and managed postoperatively as though healing will be delayed.

Operation can be required on a patient receiving cytotoxic chemotherapy for malignancy. These drugs usually interfere with cell proliferation and tend to decrease the tensile strength of the surgical wound. Although experimental evidence to support this assumption is equivocal, it is wise to manage wounds in patients receiving cytotoxic drugs as though healing will be slower than normal.

Decreased vascularity and other local changes occur after a few weeks or months in tissues that have been heavily irradiated. These are potential deterrents to wound healing; surgical incisions in patients who have been irradiated must be planned to avoid complications due to delayed healing in these areas if possible. Radiation therapy at levels of 3000 cGy or more are injurious to skin and to connective and vascular tissues. Chronic changes include scarring, damage to fibroblasts and collagen, and degenerative changes with subsequent hyalinization in the walls of blood vessels. Angiogenesis, observable as the capillary budding in granulation tissue and collagen formation, is inhibited when these changes are well established, so that surgical wounds in heavily irradiated tissues will heal slowly or may break down in the presence of infection. When radiation is given prior to operation, there is an optimal delay period (2–12 weeks) after completion of the radiation therapy before operation is performed in order to minimize wound complications. Technical problems in correctly timed operations for cancer are not usually increased by low-dosage (2000–4000 cGy) adjunctive radiotherapy. With radiation dosage in the therapeutic range (5000–6000 cGy), there is an increased incidence of wound complications, though this can be minimized by careful surgical technique and proper timing.

D. Drug Effects

Drug allergies, sensitivities, and incompatibilities and adverse drug effects that may be precipitated by operation must be foreseen and, if possible, prevented. A history of skin or other untoward reactions or sickness after injection, oral administration, or other use of any of the following substances should be noted so they can be avoided:

Penicillin or other antibiotic

Morphine, codeine, meperidine, or other opioid

Procaine or other anesthetic

Aspirin or other analgesic

Barbiturates

Sulfonamides

Tetanus antitoxin or other serum

Iodine, thimerosal (Merthiolate), or other germicide

Any other medication

Any foods such as eggs, milk, or chocolate

Adhesive tape

A personal or strong family history of asthma, hay fever, or other allergic disorder should alert the surgeon to possible hypersensitivity to drugs.

Drugs currently or recently taken by the patient may require continuation, dosage adjustment, or discontinuation.

E. Perioperative Management of Chronic Medications

Cardiovascular

Beta blockers (metoprolol, atenolol, others)
- Should be continued until and including the day of operation

Ace inhibitors (ACEI) & angiotensin receptor blockers (ARB) (captopril, lisinopril, losartan, candesartan, others)
- Patients booked for general anesthesia should continue these medications until the day before the operation but discontinue them on the day of the operation; patients booked for monitored anesthesia patient support (MAPS) should continue these medications until and including the day of the operation

Calcium channel blockers (nifedipine, diltiazem, others)
- Should be continued until and including the day of the operation

Nitrates (nitroglycerin, isosorbide, others)
- Should be continued until and including the day of the operation

Alpha-2 agonists (clonidine, others)
- Should be continued until and including the day of the operation

Aspirin or clopidogrel (Plavix)
- Should be discontinued at least 1 week prior to the planned operation if bleeding is a significant risk or concern; may be continued usually at the discretion of the surgeon

Oral anticoagulants (warfarin, coumadin)
- Should be discontinued at least 5 days prior to the planned operation unless specifically stated otherwise by the surgical service

Diuretics (furosemide, hydrochlorothiazide, others)
- Should be taken until the day before the operation but discontinued the day of the operation

Cardiac rhythm management medications (digoxin, beta-blockers, quinidine, amiodarone, others)
- Should be continued until and including the day of the operation

Statins (atorvastatin, simvastatin, others)
- Should be continued until and including the day of the operation

Cholesterol-lowering medications
- Should be taken until the day before the operation but discontinued the day of the operation

Central Nervous System Medications

Anticonvulsants (phenytoin, Tegretol, others)
- Should be continued until and including the day of the operation

Antidepressants (imipramine, sertraline, others)
- Should be continued until and including the day of the operation

Monoamine oxidase inhibitors (very rarely used)
- Should be discontinued at least 2 full weeks prior to the planned operation

Antianxiety medications (diazepam, lorazepam, others)
- Should be continued until and including the day of the operation

Antipsychotics (haloperidol, Risperdal, others)
- Should be continued until and including the day of the operation

Lithium
- Should be continued until and including the day of the operation

Antiparkinson drugs (Sinemet, others)
- Should be continued until and including the day of the operation

Recreational drugs (marijuana, cocaine, others)
- Should be discontinued as soon as possible prior to any planned elective operation

Vitamins/Nutritional Supplements

Over-the-counter vitamins
- May be continued until the day before the planned operation except preparations containing vitamin E, which should be discontinued 1 week prior to the planned operation

Herbal/alternative preparations
- Should be discontinued at least 1 full week prior to the planned surgical procedure

Pulmonary Medications

Asthma medications (theophylline, inhaled steroids, others)
- Should be continued until and including the day of the operation

Chronic obstructive pulmonary disease (COPD) medications (theophylline, ipratropium, inhaled steroids, others)
- Should be continued until and including the day of the operation

Pulmonary hypertension medications (sildenafil, prostacyclin, others)
- Should be continued until and including the day of the operation

Endocrine

Insulin

Night before procedure

Patient taking evening or bedtime insulin
- Neutral protamine Hagedorn (NPH)/Levemir (detemir): give usual dose
- Mixed insulins (70/30, 75/25, etc): give usual dose
- Lantus (glargine): give 80% of usual dose

Patients using insulin pump
- Continue basal rate

Morning of procedure (for patients who are NPO)

Morning insulin injections

Morning intermediate or long-acting insulin
- NPH/Levemir (detemir): give one half usual morning dose
- Lantus (glargine): give 80% of usual morning dose
- Mixed insulin: give one third usual morning dose

Morning short-acting insulin (Novolog, Humalog, Apidra, regular)
- Hold all short-acting insulin

Patients using insulin pump
- Continue basal insulin rate
- Intraoperative and postoperative use of the pump must be addressed on an individual basis

Oral hypoglycemics
- Should be taken until the day before the operation but discontinued the day of the operation

Thyroid medications (Synthroid, desiccated thyroid, propylthiouracil, others)
- Should be continued until and including the day of the operation

Steroids (prednisone, Cortef, others)
- Should be continued until and including the day of the operation

Oral contraceptives
- Should be continued until and including the day of the operation

Renal

Phosphate binders, renal vitamins, iron, erythropoietin, others
- Should be taken until the day before the operation but discontinued the day of the operation

Gynecology/Urology

Prostate medications (terazosin, tamsulozsin, others)
- Should be continued until and including the day of the operation

Hormonal medications
- Should be continued until and including the day of the operation

Oral contraceptives
- Should be continued until and including the day of the operation

Analgesics

Opiate-containing analgesics (Vicodin, Tylox, methadone, others)
- Should be continued until and including the day of the operation without exception

Nonsteroidal anti-inflammatory compounds (ibuprofen, naproxen, others)
- Should be discontinued at least 5 days prior to the planned surgical procedure

Sublingual buprenorphine (Suboxone and Subutex)
- Should be discontinued as soon as possible prior to any planned elective operation; if used within 5 days of surgery, opioids will be ineffective pain relief

Gastrointestinal

Gastroesophageal reflux disease (GERD) medications (ranitidine, omeprazole, others)
- Should be continued until and including the day of the operation

Antiemetics (ondansetron, metaclopramide, others)
- Should be continued until and including the day of the operation

F. Risks of Thromboembolism

Increased risk factors for deep vein thrombophlebitis and pulmonary embolus include cancer, obesity, myocardial dysfunction, age over 45 years, and a prior history of thrombosis. Prophylaxis and treatment of venous thrombotic disease are discussed in Chapter 35.

G. The Elderly Patient

Operative risk should be judged on the basis of physiologic rather than chronologic age, and an elderly patient should not be denied a needed operation because of age alone. The hazard of the average major operation for the patient over age 60 years is increased only slightly provided there is no cardiovascular, renal, or other serious systemic disease. Assume that every patient over 60—even in the absence of symptoms and physical signs—has some generalized arteriosclerosis and potential limitation of myocardial and renal reserve. Accordingly, the preoperative evaluation should be comprehensive.

Administer intravenous fluids with care so as not to overload the circulation. Monitoring of intake, output, body weight, serum electrolytes, and central venous pressure is important in evaluating cardiorenal response and tolerance in this age group.

Aged patients generally require smaller doses of strong narcotics and are frequently depressed by routine doses. Codeine is usually well tolerated. Sedative and hypnotic drugs often cause restlessness, mental confusion, and uncooperative behavior in the elderly and should be used cautiously. Preanesthetic medications should be limited to atropine or scopolamine in the debilitated elderly patient, and anesthetic agents should be administered in minimal amounts.

H. The Obese Patient

Obese patients have an increased frequency of concomitant disease and a high incidence of postoperative wound complications. A controlled preoperative weight loss program is often beneficial before elective procedures.

Halaszynski TM, Juda R, Silverman DG: Optimizing postoperative outcomes with efficient preoperative assessment and management. Crit Care Med 2004;32:S76.

I. Preoperative Hemostatic Evaluation

Surgery challenges hemostasis. A patient's risk of bleeding from surgery depends not only on any preexisting hemostatic defect but also on the extent, site, and type of surgical procedure being performed. All patients should be evaluated for their risk of bleeding based on the specific surgery being planned.

Preoperative hemostatic assessment begins with a comprehensive personal history for bleeding tendencies. This provides the basis for further diagnostic studies and helps assess the probability of future bleeding. Patients should be asked about epistaxis, gingival bleeding, bruising, ecchymoses, and menorrhagia. A history of mucocutaneous bleeding at these sites suggests von Willebrand disease (vWD), thrombocytopenia, or functional platelet disorders. A history of excessive bleeding during or following circumcision, tonsillectomy, tooth extraction, other surgeries, or during childbirth can be very helpful in uncovering a hemostatic disorder. It is important to obtain an accurate history of drug intake, as medications like aspirin, nonsteroidal anti-inflammatory drugs (NSAIDs), clopidogrel, and warfarin impair hemostasis.

Routine preoperative prothrombin time (PT) and activated partial thromboplastin time (aPTT) testing is unnecessary in patients scheduled for low-risk surgery and can be reserved for the preoperative workup in patients scheduled for high-risk surgery. Initial laboratory testing includes PT, aPTT, complete blood count (CBC), examination of the blood smear, and biochemical tests of hepatic and renal function. Bleeding time does not predict abnormal surgical bleeding and is not routinely recommended. If a screening test is positive, specific tests to rule out deficiencies of individual coagulation factors, von Willebrand factor (vWF), and platelet function defects are performed. Laboratory workup and diagnosis during the initial assessment allows for appropriate perioperative management.

Dagi TF: The management of postoperative bleeding. Surg Clin North Am 2005;85:1191.

▶ Consultations

The opinion of a qualified consultant should be obtained when it may be of benefit to the patient, when requested by the patient or family members, or when it may be of medicolegal importance. The physician should take the initiative in arranging consultation when the treatment proposed is controversial or exceptionally risky, when dangerous complications occur, or when the physician senses that the patient or family members are unduly apprehensive regarding the plan of management or the course of events. Consultation with cardiac or other medical or surgical specialists preoperatively is important if the patient has abnormal findings in their fields of competence. It is also beneficial for the specialist consultant to become acquainted with the patient and the condition preoperatively when the possibility exists that the consultant will be called upon for advice later in connection with a postoperative complication or development.

PREOPERATIVE PREPARATION

Major operations create surgical wounds and cause severe stress, subjecting the patient to the hazard of infection and metabolic and other derangements. Appropriate preoperative preparation facilitates wound healing and systemic recovery by making certain that the patient's condition is optimal. Operation also results in psychic trauma to the patient and to family members and has significant medicolegal implications, all of which deserve special consideration preoperatively to avoid postoperative repercussions. In emergency conditions, time for preparation is limited but is usually sufficient to permit the principles of good surgical preparation to be followed. In elective operation, meticulous preoperative preparation is both possible and mandatory and includes the following steps.

Informing the Patient

Surgery is a frightening prospect for both patient and family. Their psychologic preparation and reassurance should begin at the initial contact with the surgeon. Appropriate explanation of the nature and purpose of preoperative studies and treatments establishes confidence. When all pertinent information has been gathered, it is the surgeon's responsibility to describe the planned surgical procedure, any alternatives, and its risks and possible consequences in understandable terms to the patient and usually also to the next of kin. The potential need for blood transfusion must be addressed. This discussion must be documented in the chart. It is also very helpful to explain to the patient what will happen in the operating room before induction of anesthesia and in the recovery room. Similarly, prompt postoperative interpretation of pertinent findings and prospects to patient and family contributes to rapport and to cooperation during the recovery period.

Operative Permit

The patient or the patient's legal guardian must sign (in advance) a permit authorizing a major or minor operation. The nature, risk, and probable result of the operation or procedure must be made clear to the patient or a legally responsible relative or guardian so that the signed permit will document the informed consent to the procedure. A signed consent is not valid except for the specific operation or procedure for which it was obtained.

Emergency lifesaving operations or procedures may have to be done without a permit. In such cases, every effort should be made to obtain adequate consultation. The situation should be carefully documented in the chart.

Legal and institutional requirements regarding permits vary. It is essential that the physician understand and follow local regulations.

Asepsis & Antisepsis in the Prevention of Wound Infection

Protection of the surgical patient from infection is a primary consideration throughout the preoperative, operative, and postoperative phases of care. The factor of host resistance that influences the individual patient's susceptibility to infection was discussed above. The incidence and severity of infection, particularly wound sepsis, are related also to the bacteriologic status of the hospital environment and to the care with which basic principles of asepsis, antisepsis, and surgical technique are implemented. The entire hospital environment must be protected from undue bacterial contamination in order to avoid colonization and cross-infection of surgical patients with virulent strains of bacteria that will invade surgical wounds in the operating room in spite of

aseptic precautions taken during operation. Prevention of wound infection therefore involves both application of general concepts and techniques of antisepsis and asepsis in the hospital at large and the use of specific procedures in preparation for operation.

A. Sterilization

The only completely reliable methods of sterilization in wide current use for surgical instruments and supplies are (1) steam under pressure (autoclaving), (2) dry heat, and (3) ethylene oxide gas.

1. Autoclaving—Saturated steam at a pressure of 750 mm Hg (14.5 psi above atmospheric pressure) at a temperature of 120 °C destroys all vegetative bacteria and most resistant dry spores in 13 minutes. Sterilization time is markedly shortened by the high-vacuum or high-pressure autoclaves now widely used.

2. Dry heat—Exposure to continuous dry heat at 170 °C for 1 hour will sterilize articles that would be spoiled by moist heat or are more conveniently kept dry. If grease or oil is present on instruments, safe sterilization calls for a 4-hour exposure at 160 °C.

3. Gas sterilization—Liquid and gaseous ethylene oxide as a sterilizing agent will destroy bacteria, viruses, molds, pathogenic fungi, and spores. It is also flammable and toxic, and it will cause severe burns if it comes in contact with the skin. Gas sterilization with ethylene oxide is an excellent method for sterilization of most heat-sensitive materials, including telescopic instruments, plastic and rubber goods, sharp and delicate instruments, and miscellaneous items such as electric cords and sealed ampules. It has largely replaced soaking in antiseptics as a means of sterilizing materials that cannot withstand autoclaving. Gas sterilization is normally carried out in a pressure vessel (gas autoclave) at slightly elevated pressure and temperature. Following sterilization, a variable period of time is required for dissipation of the gas from the materials sterilized. Solid metal or glass items such as knives, drills, and thermometers may be used immediately following sterilization. Lensed instruments and packs including cloth, paper, rubber, and other porous items must usually be kept on the shelf exposed to air for 24–48 hours before use. Certain types of materials or complex instruments, such as a cardiac pacemaker, may require 7 days of exposure to air before use.

B. Skin Antiseptics

The most important applications of skin antiseptics are the hand scrub of the operating team and the preparation of the operative field on the patient.

1. Hand scrub routine—Although the duration of the hand scrub is not universally defined, a 5-minute scrub before the first case—provided a brush is used—appears to be sufficient. Greatest attention should be paid to the fingertips and nails, since these areas harbor the greatest numbers of bacteria. A 2-minute scrub is adequate between cases. Solutions containing chlorhexidine or one of the iodophors appear to be most effective. Other skin antisepsis techniques, such as the use of alcohol-based skin lotions applied to clean hands for 1 minute and allowed to dry on the skin, also are effective at decreasing skin colonization.

2. Preparation of the operative field—Initial preparation of the skin is usually done the afternoon or evening before operation. The area should be washed with soap and water, making sure that it is grossly quite clean. A shower is satisfactory. The type of soap used makes little difference. Soap is a weak antiseptic and is useful because of its nonirritating detergent action, especially when washing is combined with mechanical friction.

For elective operations involving areas with high levels of resident bacteria (eg, hands, feet) or likely to be irritated by strong antiseptics (eg, face, genitalia), preoperative degerming of the skin can be improved by repeated use of chlorhexidine gluconate (Hibiclens). Instruct the patient to wash the area several times daily with one of these preparations (and with nothing else) for 3–5 days before the scheduled day of operation. It has been established that shaving the surgical area the night before or within several hours before surgery increases the skin bacterial flora. Therefore, it is recommended that if necessary at all, shaving be performed immediately before the operation, preferably in an adjacent preparation area. Shaving may be eliminated if only fine hairs are present, as their presence has not been found to increase the incidence of infection.

3. In the operating room—A 1-minute skin preparation using either 70% alcohol or 2% iodine in 90% alcohol—followed by a polyester adherent wound drape—has been shown to be as effective in controlling wound infections as the more traditional 5- to 10-minute wound scrub with povidone-iodine. However, the alcohol-based solutions also carry some risk of ignition and operating room fire.

Iodine is one of the most efficient skin antiseptics available. It rarely causes skin reactions in this concentration. Avoid streaming of iodine outside of the operative field. Do not use iodine on the perineum, genitalia, or face; on irritated or delicate skin (eg, small children); or when the patient has a history of iodine sensitivity. For iodine-sensitive patients, one can use 80% isopropyl or 70% ethyl alcohol. Apply to the skin with a gauze swab for 3 minutes and allow to dry before draping. Alternatively, tinted tincture of benzalkonium (1:750) may be used.

For sensitive areas (perineum, around the eyes, etc), apply iodophor, chlorhexidine, or 1:1000 aqueous benzalkonium solution.

Disease transmission to patients and health care workers—especially with the hepatitis virus and the AIDS virus—is a major problem in the operating room environment.

Both can be transmitted to the patient and care providers by blood. Transmission to the surgeon or nurse via a needle or cut is of major concern because of the frequent occurrence of accidental punctures. Since the infected patient cannot readily be detected in the absence of a mandatory preoperative testing program, universal precautions are required, including the following:

a. All health care workers should routinely use appropriate barrier precautions—gloves, masks, goggles, etc—to prevent skin and mucous membrane exposure when contact with blood or body fluids is anticipated.

b. Immediate hand and other skin surface washing is necessary if contamination occurs.

c. Special precautions must be taken to avoid accidental injuries, eg, needle punctures and cuts.

d. Workers who have any open wounds should avoid direct patient contact.

e. If a glove is torn, it should be removed and changed as promptly as patient safety permits and the needle or instrument removed from the sterile field.

C. Control of Hospital Environment

Hospital cross-infection with hemolytic, coagulase-positive *Staphylococcus aureus* and other organisms is always a potential problem. Strains endemic in hospitals are often resistant to many antimicrobial drugs as a consequence of the widespread use of these agents. Relaxation of aseptic precautions in the operating room and an unwarranted reliance on "prophylactic" antibiotics contribute to the development of resistant strains. The result may be a significant increase in the incidence of hospital-acquired wound infection, pneumonitis, and septicemia, the latter two complications especially affecting infants, the aged, and the debilitated.

Although pyogenic cocci are major offenders, enteric gram-negative bacteria (particularly the coliform and proteus groups and *Pseudomonas aeruginosa*) are increasingly prominent in hospital-acquired infections. Gastrointestinal infection with *Clostridium difficile* has become endemic in some hospitals including the development of drug-resistant strains.

1. Hospital administration

a. The surgical infection control program should be coordinated closely with that of other services through a hospital infection committee set up to promulgate and enforce regulations.

b. All significant infections must be reported immediately. A clean wound infection rate of more than 1% indicates a need for more effective control measures. The wound infection rate should be continuously monitored on the surgical services.

2. Cultures—Obtain culture and antibiotic sensitivity studies on all significant infections.

3. Isolation—Isolate every patient with a significant source of communicable bacteria; every case of suspected communicable infection until the diagnosis has been ruled out; and every patient in whom cross-infection will be serious.

4. Aseptic technique

A. OPERATING ROOM—The operating room should be considered an isolation zone that may be entered only by persons wearing clean operating attire (which may not be worn elsewhere).

B. PATIENT UNIT PROCEDURES—All open wounds should be aseptically dressed to protect them from cross-infection and to prevent heavy contamination of the environment. Eliminate dressing carts containing supplies and equipment for multiple bedside dressings.

C. HAND WASHING—Hand washing before and after each contact with a patient is a simple but important routine measure in control of infection. Alcohol-based hand antiseptics are useful but do not eliminate *C difficile* contamination.

5. Antibiotics—Prophylactic antibiotics are indicated for clean contaminated or contaminated cases. Even for clean cases, prophylactic antibiotics may decrease the rate of infection for procedures at significant risk. When possible, antibiotic therapy should be based on sensitivity studies. Antibiotics should be given in adequate doses, redosed at appropriate intraoperative intervals, and discontinued as soon as it is appropriate to do so (usually within 24 hours of operation).

6. Epidemiology

a. Personnel with active staphylococcal infections should be excluded from patient contact until they have recovered. Personnel carrying staphylococci in their nasal passages or gastrointestinal tracts must observe personal hygiene but need not be removed from duty unless they prove to be a focus of infection. The advisability of treatment of the carrier is uncertain, since the carrier state is frequently transient or recurrent in spite of treatment.

b. Every significant infection acquired in the hospital should be investigated to determine its origin and spread, possible contacts and carriers, and whether improper techniques may have been responsible.

Association of periOperative Registered Nurses: Recommended practices for cleaning and caring for surgical instruments and powered equipment. AORN J 2002;75:627.

Association of periOperative Registered Nurses: Recommended practices for surgical hand antisepsis/hand scrubs. AORN J 2004;79:416.

Bolding B: Flash sterilization (steam). Can Oper Room Nurs J 2003;21:31.

Mangram AJ et al: Guideline for prevention of surgical site infection, 1999. Am J Infect Control 1999;27:97.

National Nosocomial Infections Surveillance (NNIS) System Report: Data summary from January 1992 through June 2003, issued August 2003. Am J Infect Control 2003;31:481.

DIABETES MELLITUS

Diabetic patients undergo more surgical procedures than do nondiabetics, and management of the diabetic patient before, during, and after surgery is an important responsibility of the surgeon. Fortunately, because close control of fluids, electrolytes, glucose, and insulin is now possible in the operating room, control of blood glucose levels during the perioperative period is usually relatively simple. Marked hyperglycemia should be avoided during surgery; the greater danger, however, is from severe unrecognized hypoglycemia.

▶ Preoperative Workup

Blood glucose concentrations may be elevated in diabetic patients during the preoperative period. Physical trauma, if present, combined with the emotional and physiologic stress of the illness may cause epinephrine and cortisol levels to rise, in each case resulting in increased blood glucose levels. If exogenous cortisol is being administered (eg, to a renal or pancreatic transplant recipient), marked insulin resistance and elevations of blood glucose levels regularly result. Infections may also increase blood glucose concentrations, occasionally to dangerous levels. Inactivity in bedridden patients can increase blood glucose levels by causing insulin resistance. Hypokalemia—frequently the result of diuretic therapy but also of epinephrine release induced by trauma—may prevent B cells from secreting adequate amounts of insulin and may thereby raise blood glucose levels in patients with type 2 diabetes.

The preoperative workup of patients with diabetes mellitus includes a thorough physical examination with special care to discover occult infections, an ECG to rule out myocardial infarction, and a chest x-ray to identify hidden pneumonia or pulmonary edema. A complete urinalysis can rule out urinary tract infection and proteinuria, the earliest signs of diabetic renal disease. Serum potassium levels are measured to check for hypokalemia or hyperkalemia, the latter usually resulting from hyporeninemic hypoaldosteronism, a relatively common syndrome in diabetics. Serum creatinine levels are used to assess renal function. The serum glucose concentration should ideally be between 100 and 200 mg/dL, but operation can be safely performed in patients whose serum glucose is as high as 350–400 mg/dL preoperatively.

▶ Preoperative & Intraoperative Management of Diabetic Patients

A. Type 2 (Non-Insulin-Dependent) Diabetes Mellitus

Approximately 85% of diabetics over age 50 years have only a moderately decreased ability to produce and secrete insulin, and when at home they can usually be controlled by diet or by sulfonylureas. If the serum glucose level is below 250 mg/dL on the morning of surgery, sulfonylureas should be withheld, long-acting sulfonylurea drugs—glipizide, glyburide, and chlorpropamide—should be discontinued on the day before surgery, and 5% glucose solution should be administered intravenously at a rate of about 100 mL/h. This means that over a 10-hour period, only 50 g of glucose would be given; by contrast, during an average day, a diabetic on a normal diet would consume four to five times as much carbohydrate (ie, 200–250 g). During any but the most extensive surgery, the pancreas should be able to produce enough insulin to handle this modest glucose load and at the same time prevent undue gluconeogenesis.

If the fasting glucose level is above 250–300 mg/dL or if the patient is taking small doses of insulin but does not actually require insulin to prevent ketoacidosis, an alternative approach is to add 5 units of insulin directly to each liter of 5% glucose solution being given at 100 mL/h. If the operation is lengthy, blood glucose levels should be measured every 3–4 hours during surgery to ensure adequate glucose control. The goal is to maintain glucose levels between 100 and 200 mg/dL, but there is little immediate metabolic harm in allowing levels to go as high as 250 mg/dL.

B. Type 1 (Insulin-Dependent) Diabetes Mellitus

Type 1 patients require insulin during surgery. It can be administered by any of the following methods: (1) subcutaneous administration of long-acting insulin, (2) constant infusion of a mixture of glucose and insulin, or (3) separate infusions of glucose and insulin. Intravenous boluses of regular insulin are rarely, if ever, indicated. The effect of single boluses of insulin given intravenously typically lasts only minutes, leading to the danger of acute hypoglycemia followed shortly thereafter by recurrent hyperglycemia. With either technique, blood glucose levels should be monitored at least every 2 hours during the procedure to avoid hypoglycemia below 60 mg/dL and hyperglycemia above 250 mg/dL. Blood glucose levels can be measured rapidly during surgery with a portable electronic glucose analyzer.

1. Conventional procedure for insulin administration—
The first and still most widely used method of controlling blood glucose levels during surgery is to administer subcutaneously, on the morning of the operation, one-third to one-half the patient's usual dose of long-acting insulin plus one-third to one-half the usual dose of short-acting insulin. This is followed by intravenous infusion of 5% or even 10% glucose at a rate of 100 mL/h preoperatively and intraoperatively. If the operation is prolonged, potassium chloride should be added at a rate of 20 meq/h.

There are a number of disadvantages to this procedure, which results in giving the full day's insulin requirement preoperatively. First, after subcutaneous administration, the absorption of NPH and regular insulin varies greatly in individual patients, especially when they are inactive. Second, although surgeons may prefer that operations on diabetics be scheduled early in the day, often the procedure must be delayed until afternoon. The relatively small

amounts of glucose being administered are then inadequate to compensate for the 18–20 hours the patient has been without food, with the result that the insulin causes severe afternoon hypoglycemia. In the average diabetic, the peak action of regular insulin occurs about 6 hours after its administration. Therefore, if regular insulin is given subcutaneously at 7 AM, its peak action in an average patient will occur at about 1 PM. As a result, following subcutaneous administration of regular insulin in the early morning, the patient's glucose concentration may be inadequately controlled early in the morning; and if surgery is delayed, the peak action of regular insulin in the early afternoon and of NPH insulin in the later afternoon may result in severe hypoglycemia. If surgery must be delayed, it is imperative that blood glucose levels be carefully monitored for hypoglycemia and additional glucose given as necessary.

2. Intravenous infusion of insulin in glucose solution—
Another option is to treat type 1 diabetics undergoing surgery by giving an infusion of 5% or 10% glucose solution containing 5, 10, or even 15 units of insulin per liter, depending on the patient's initial blood glucose concentration. At an infusion rate of 100 mL/h, the insulin is administered at a rate of 0.5, 1, or 1.5 units/h respectively. In patients receiving corticosteroids, as much as 20 units per liter of insulin may be required.

There are a number of advantages to this regimen. First, the problem of absorption of insulin is avoided, since it is given intravenously. As a result, instead of an average 6-hour lag for maximal response to regular insulin, the effect starts within 10–15 minutes and is relatively constant. Second, unlike the fixed insulin dose with subcutaneous administration, the insulin infusion can be changed at any time in response to changes in blood glucose levels. Third, the dangers of hypoglycemia and hyperglycemia are minimized, because if the intravenous solution is stopped (if the needle is inadvertently removed or the tubing clamped), both the glucose and the insulin are discontinued simultaneously. Since only about 10% of insulin adsorbs to glass or plastic, the resulting reduction in dosage is of little therapeutic importance. A similar continuous intravenous infusion of insulin has also become a common way to treat diabetic ketoacidosis.

3. Use of insulin piggy-backed into the glucose infusion—
Instead of mixing insulin in the same bottle as the glucose, an insulin solution is infused ("piggy-backed") into the tubing delivering the 5% or 10% glucose. Generally, 50 units of regular insulin are mixed with 500 mL of normal saline—a solution containing 1 unit of insulin per 10 mL of solution. The glucose solution is given at a rate of 100 mL/h, and the insulin infusion is adjusted (usually by IVAC pump) to deliver a total of 5 mL (0.5 units), 10 mL (1 unit), 30 mL (30 units) per hour, etc, depending on the results of blood glucose determinations obtained approximately hourly during the surgical procedure. Of the three techniques, this is

the most flexible and allows the closest control of blood glucose levels. It requires careful monitoring of the pump delivery rate, because too rapid infusion of insulin will cause hypoglycemia. A number of simple algorithms have been recommended for adjusting the rate of insulin infusion according to the previous plasma glucose levels. This approach is especially useful during prolonged operations. The simplest and most practical procedure is to give no insulin if plasma glucose is less than 90 mg/dL. Above values of 90 mg/dL, the dosage of regular insulin in units per hour should equal 1% of the previous hour's plasma glucose (mg/dL)—eg, at a glucose level of 200 mg/dL, give 2 units/h; at 300 mg/dL, give 3 units/h, etc.

▶ Postoperative Care

With either of the intravenous infusion techniques, it is best to continue the glucose-insulin infusion until the patient is eating. Hypoglycemia, the most common postoperative complication, most often follows the use of long-acting insulin given subcutaneously before surgery. Although hypoglycemia may also occur if the intravenous insulin infusion is excessive in relation to that of the glucose, an infusion of 1.5 units or less of insulin per hour, when given with 5% glucose, rarely results in hypoglycemia. Blood glucose levels should be measured every 2–4 hours and the patient monitored for signs and symptoms of hypoglycemia (eg, anxiety, tremulousness, profuse sweating without fever). When hypoglycemia is detected, the amount of glucose infused should be promptly increased and the insulin decreased. It is rarely advisable to stop the insulin infusion completely for mild hypoglycemia, since a smoother transition to euglycemia results if the insulin is continued but at a lower dose.

A marked increase in glucose and insulin requirements postoperatively suggests the presence of occult infection (eg, wound infection, cellulitis at the intravenous site, urinary tract infection, or unrecognized aspiration pneumonia).

Adjustments in the rate of glucose or insulin administration must be based on *blood* glucose levels.

▶ Hyperosmolar Coma

Hyperosmolar coma, the result of severe dehydration, may occur in undiagnosed diabetics who have been given large amounts of glucose during surgery. The resulting osmotic diuresis leads to disproportionate water loss, dehydration, and hyperosmolarity. Hyperosmolar coma rarely occurs until the serum glucose level exceeds 800 mg/dL and the osmolarity exceeds 340 meq/L. Hyperosmolar coma is best avoided by monitoring fluid input and output, measuring blood glucose levels, and instituting treatment promptly if the value exceeds 400 mg/dL.

Golden SH et al: Perioperative glycemic control and the risk of infectious complications in a cohort of adults with diabetes. Diabetes Care 1999;22:1408.

Hirsch IB et al: Diabetes management in special situations. Endocrinol Metab Clin North Am 1997;26:631.
Kaufman FR et al: Perioperative management with prolonged intravenous insulin infusion versus subcutaneous insulin in children with type I diabetes mellitus. J Diabetes Complications 1996;10:6.
Vanhaeverbeek M: Peri-operative care: management of the diabetic patient. A novel controversy about tight glycemic control. Acta Clin Belg 1997;52:313.

THYROID DISEASE

Both hyper- and hypothyroidism represent serious problems for patients undergoing surgery. It may be difficult to establish an adequate airway in patients with large goiters. The hyperthyroid patient undergoing surgery is apt to develop hypertension, severe cardiac dysrhythmias, congestive heart failure, and hyperthermia.

Life-threatening thyrotoxicosis (thyroid storm) may be precipitated by any operation but especially by thyroidectomy, which accentuates thyroxine release. It is therefore preferable to bring hyperthyroid patients into a euthyroid state before surgery. This takes 1–6 weeks and is best accomplished by treatment with propylthiouracil, 800–1000 mg/d for about 1 week, followed by a maintenance dose of 200–400 mg/d. If emergency surgery is required, adequate sedation and potassium iodide plus a β-adrenergic blocking agent such as propranolol should be given in addition to propylthiouracil.

Hypothyroid patients are subject to acute hypotension, shock, and hypothermia during surgery; if the patient is allowed to breathe spontaneously, severe CO_2 retention may result from hypoventilation. **Myxedema coma** should be suspected in patients who fail to awaken promptly from anesthesia and who manifest CO_2 retention, even to the point of CO_2 narcosis, accompanied by hypothermia. Increased tissue friability, poor wound healing, and even wound dehiscence may also occur. It is highly advisable to treat myxedematous patients with levothyroxine before elective surgery. In an emergency (eg, severe myxedema requiring immediate surgery), treatment should consist of levothyroxine sodium, 500 μg (0.5 mg) intravenously, by nasogastric tube, or orally. If there is no emergency, the euthyroid state may be gradually restored with levothyroxine, 25 μg/d, with the dose increased over several weeks to a maintenance dose of 150–200 μg/d. It is also always advisable to obtain a baseline cortisol level before treatment of myxedema to rule out coexistent Addison disease (Schmidt syndrome), since levothyroxine therapy can precipitate addisonian crisis in this setting.

Attia J et al: Diagnosis of thyroid disease in hospitalized patients: a systematic review. Arch Intern Med 1999;159:658.
Cooper DS: Antithyroid drugs for the treatment of hyperthyroidism caused by Graves disease. Emerg Med Clin North Am 1998;27:225.

Kahaly GJ et al: Cardiac risks of hyperthyroidism in the elderly. Thyroid 1998;8:1165.

Koutras DA: Subclinical hyperthyroidism. Thyroid 1999;9:311.

Ladenson PW et al: Complications of surgery in hypothyroid patients. Am J Med 1984;77:261.

ADRENAL INSUFFICIENCY

Patients with adrenal insufficiency undergoing the stress of operation are at risk of addisonian crisis, manifested by salt wastage, decreased blood volume, hypotension, shock, and death. For at least 2–3 days preoperatively, they should receive fluid and sodium chloride replacement intravenously (usually 1–3 L of normal saline per day) and cortisol therapy (20 mg each morning and 10 mg each afternoon). On the day of surgery, 100 mg of cortisol is administered intramuscularly or intravenously just before the operation, followed by 50–100 mg every 6 hours during surgery—a regimen that mimics the normal endogenous cortisol response to stress (up to 300 mg/d). Saline is continued postoperatively at a rate of at least 2–3 L/d, with careful monitoring of blood pressure, serum electrolyte concentrations, and urine output. In the absence of complications, the cortisol dosage can be decreased by half each day until the usual maintenance dose of about 30 mg/d is reached.

Patients receiving chronic corticosteroid therapy may present with severe hypokalemia and at times serious hypertension, both of which should be corrected before surgery. Stress doses of cortisol (approximately 300 mg/d) must be administered during surgery according to the protocol described for addisonian patients. If the patient is diabetic, large doses of insulin (eg, 3 units/h) may be required to control blood glucose levels during surgery. Postoperatively, slow wound healing and a predisposition to infection should be anticipated. Infections in these patients may occur without fever.

Postoperative Care

Gerard M. Doherty, MD

The recovery from major surgery can be divided into three phases: (1) an immediate, or postanesthetic, phase; (2) an intermediate phase, encompassing the hospitalization period; and (3) a convalescent phase. During the first two phases, care is principally directed at maintenance of homeostasis, treatment of pain, and prevention and early detection of complications. The convalescent phase is a transition period from the time of hospital discharge to full recovery. The trend toward earlier postoperative discharge after major surgery has shifted the venue of this period.

THE IMMEDIATE POSTOPERATIVE PERIOD

The primary causes of early complications and death following major surgery are acute pulmonary, cardiovascular, and fluid derangements. The postanesthesia care unit (PACU) is staffed by specially trained personnel and provided with equipment for early detection and treatment of these problems. All patients should be monitored in this specialized unit initially following major procedures unless they are transported directly to an intensive care unit. While en route from the operating room to the PACU, the patient should be accompanied by a physician and other qualified attendants. In the PACU, the anesthesiology service generally exercises primary responsibility for cardiopulmonary function. The surgeon is responsible for the operative site and all other aspects of the care not directly related to the effects of anesthesia. The patient can be discharged from the recovery room when cardiovascular, pulmonary, and neurologic function have returned to baseline, which usually occurs 1–3 hours following operation. Patients who require continuing ventilatory or circulatory support or who have other conditions that require frequent monitoring are transferred to an intensive care unit. In this setting, nursing personnel specially trained in the management of respiratory and cardiovascular emergencies are available, and the staff-to-patient ratio is higher than it is on the wards. Monitoring equipment is available to enable early detection of cardiorespiratory derangements.

▶ Postoperative Orders

Detailed treatment orders are necessary to direct postoperative care. The transfer of the patient from OR to PACU requires reiteration of any patient care orders. Unusual or particularly important orders should also be communicated to the nursing team orally. The nursing team must also be advised of the nature of the operation and the patient's condition. Errors in postoperative orders, including medication errors and omission of important orders, are diminished by electronic order entry systems that can contain postoperative order sets. Postoperative orders should cover the following:

A. Monitoring

1. Vital signs—Blood pressure, pulse, and respiration should be recorded frequently until stable and then regularly until the patient is discharged from the recovery room. The frequency of vital sign measurements thereafter depends upon the nature of the operation and the course in the PACU. When an arterial catheter is in place, blood pressure and pulse should be monitored continuously. Continuous electrocardiographic monitoring is indicated for most patients in the PACU. Any major changes in vital signs should be communicated to the anesthesiologist and surgeon immediately.

2. Central venous pressure—Central venous pressure should be recorded periodically in the early postoperative period if the operation has entailed large blood losses or fluid shifts, and invasive monitoring is available. A Swan-Ganz catheter for measurement of pulmonary artery wedge pressure is indicated under these conditions if the patient has compromised cardiac or respiratory function.

3. Fluid balance—The anesthetic record includes all fluid administered as well as blood loss and urine output during the operation. This record should be continued in the postoperative period and should also include fluid losses from drains and stomas. This aids in assessing hydration and helps to guide intravenous fluid replacement. A bladder catheter can be placed for frequent measurement of urine output. In the absence of a bladder catheter, the surgeon should be notified if the patient is unable to void within 6–8 hours after operation.

4. Other types of monitoring—Depending on the nature of the operation and the patient's preexisting conditions, other types of monitoring may be necessary. Examples include measurement of intracranial pressure and level of consciousness following cranial surgery and monitoring of distal pulses following vascular surgery or in patients with casts.

B. Respiratory Care

In the early postoperative period, the patient may remain mechanically ventilated or be treated with supplemental oxygen by mask or nasal prongs. These orders should be specified. For intubated patients, tracheal suctioning or other forms of respiratory therapy must be specified as required. Patients who are not intubated should do deep breathing exercises frequently to prevent atelectasis.

C. Position in Bed and Mobilization

The postoperative orders should describe any required special positioning of the patient. Unless doing so is contraindicated, the patient should be turned from side to side every 30 minutes until conscious and then hourly for the first 8–12 hours to minimize atelectasis. Early ambulation is encouraged to reduce venous stasis; the upright position helps to increase diaphragmatic excursion. Venous stasis may also be minimized by intermittent compression of the calf by pneumatic stockings.

D. Diet

Patients at risk for emesis and pulmonary aspiration should have nothing by mouth until some gastrointestinal function has returned (usually within 4 days). Most patients can tolerate liquids by mouth shortly after return to full consciousness.

E. Administration of Fluid and Electrolytes

Orders for postoperative intravenous fluids should be based on maintenance needs and the replacement of gastrointestinal losses from drains, fistulas, or stomas.

F. Drainage Tubes

Drain care should be included in the postoperative orders. Details such as type and pressure of suction, irrigation fluid and frequency, and skin exit site care should be specified. The surgeon should examine drains frequently, since the character or quantity of drain output may herald the development of postoperative complications such as bleeding or fistulas.

G. Medications

Orders should be written for antibiotics, analgesics, gastric acid suppression, deep vein thrombosis prophylaxis, and sedatives. If appropriate, preoperative medications should be reinstituted. Careful attention should be paid to replacement of corticosteroids in patients at risk, since postoperative adrenal insufficiency may be life threatening. Other medications such as antipyretics, laxatives, and stool softeners should be used selectively as indicated.

H. Laboratory Examinations and Imaging

Postoperative laboratory and radiographic examinations should be used to detect specific abnormalities in high-risk groups. The routine use of daily chest radiographs, blood counts, electrolytes, and renal or liver function panels is not useful.

THE INTERMEDIATE POSTOPERATIVE PERIOD

The intermediate phase starts with complete recovery from anesthesia and lasts for the rest of the hospital stay. During this time, the patient recovers most basic functions and becomes self-sufficient and able to continue convalescence at home.

▶ Care of the Wound

Within hours after a wound is closed, the wound space fills with an inflammatory exudate. Epidermal cells at the edges of the wound begin to divide and migrate across the wound surface. By 48 hours after closure, deeper structures are completely sealed off from the external environment. Sterile dressings applied in the operating room provide protection during this period. Dressings over closed wounds should be removed on the third or fourth postoperative day. If the wound is dry, dressings need not be reapplied; this simplifies periodic inspection. Dressings should be removed earlier if they are wet, because soaked dressings increase bacterial contamination of the wound. Dressings should also be removed if the patient has manifestations of infection (such as fever or increasing wound pain). The wound should then be inspected and the adjacent area gently compressed. Any drainage from the wound should be examined by culture and Gram-stained smear. Removal of the dressing and handling of the wound during the first 24 hours should be done with aseptic technique. Medical personnel should wash their hands before and after caring for any surgical wound. Gloves should always be used when there is contact with open wounds or fresh wounds.

Generally, skin sutures or skin staples may be removed by the fifth postoperative day and replaced by tapes. Sutures should be left in longer (eg, for 2 weeks) for incisions that cross creases (eg, groin, popliteal area), for incisions closed under tension, for some incisions in the extremities (eg, the hand), and for incisions of any kind in debilitated patients.

Sutures should be removed if suture tracts show signs of infection. If the incision is healing normally, the patient may be allowed to shower or bathe by the seventh postoperative day.

Management of Drains

Drains are used either to prevent or to treat an unwanted accumulation of fluid such as pus, blood, or serum. Drains are also used to evacuate air from the pleural cavity so that the lungs can reexpand. When used prophylactically, drains are usually placed in a sterile location. Strict precautions must be taken to prevent bacteria from entering the body through the drainage tract in these situations. The external portion of the drain must be handled with aseptic technique, and the drain must be removed as soon as it is no longer useful. When drains have been placed in an infected area, there is a smaller risk of retrograde infection of the peritoneal cavity, since the infected area is usually walled off. Drains should usually be brought out through a separate incision, because drains through the operative wound increase the risk of wound infection. Closed drains connected to suction devices (Jackson-Pratt or Blake drains are two examples) are preferable to open drains (such as Penrose) that predispose to wound contamination. The quantity and quality of drainage should be recorded and contamination minimized. When drains are no longer needed, they may be withdrawn entirely at one time if there has been little or no drainage or may be progressively withdrawn over a period of a few days.

Sump drains (such as Davol drains) have an airflow system that keeps the lumen of the drain open when fluid is not passing through it, and they must be attached to a suction device. Sump drains are especially useful when the amount of drainage is large or when drainage is likely to plug other kinds of drains. Some sump drains have an extra lumen through which saline solution can be infused to aid in keeping the tube clear. After infection has been controlled and the discharge is no longer purulent, the large-bore catheter is progressively replaced with smaller catheters, and the cavity eventually closes.

Postoperative Pulmonary Care

The changes in pulmonary function observed following anesthesia and surgery are principally the result of decreased vital capacity, functional residual capacity (FRC), and pulmonary edema. Vital capacity decreases to about 40% of the preoperative level within 1–4 hours after major intra-abdominal surgery. It remains at this level for 12–14 hours, slowly increases to 60–70% of the preoperative value by 7 days, and returns to the baseline level during the ensuing week. FRC is affected to a lesser extent. Immediately after surgery, FRC is near the preoperative level, but by 24 hours postoperatively, it has decreased to about 70% of the preoperative level. It remains depressed for several days and then gradually returns to its preoperative value by the tenth day.

These changes are accentuated in patients who are obese, who smoke heavily, or who have preexisting lung disease. Elderly patients are particularly vulnerable because they have decreased compliance, increased closing volume, increased residual volume, and increased dead space, all of which enhance the risk of postoperative atelectasis. In addition, reduced forced expiratory volume in 1 second (FEV_1) impairs the aged patient's ability to clear secretions and increases the chance of infection postoperatively.

The postoperative decrease in FRC is caused by a breathing pattern consisting of shallow tidal breaths without periodic maximal inflation. Normal human respiration includes inspiration to total lung capacity several times each hour. If these maximal inflations are eliminated, alveolar collapse begins to occur within a few hours, and atelectasis with transpulmonary shunting is evident shortly thereafter. Pain is thought to be one of the main causes of shallow breathing postoperatively. Complete abolition of pain, however, does not completely restore pulmonary function. Neural reflexes, abdominal distention, obesity, and other factors that limit diaphragmatic excursion appear to be as important.

The principal means of minimizing atelectasis is deep inspiration. Periodic hyperinflation can be facilitated by using an incentive spirometer. This is particularly useful in patients with a higher risk of pulmonary complications (eg, elderly, debilitated, or markedly obese patients). Early mobilization, encouragement to take deep breaths (especially when standing), and good coaching by the nursing staff suffice for most patients.

Postoperative pulmonary edema is caused by high hydrostatic pressures (due to left ventricular failure, fluid overload, decreased oncotic pressure, etc), increased capillary permeability, or both. Edema of the lung parenchyma narrows small bronchi and increases resistance in the pulmonary vasculature. In addition, pulmonary edema may increase the risk of pulmonary infection. Adequate management of fluids postoperatively and early treatment of cardiac failure are important preventive measures.

Systemic sepsis increases capillary permeability and can lead to pulmonary edema. In the absence of deranged cardiac function or fluid overload, the development of pulmonary edema postoperatively should be regarded as evidence of sepsis.

RESPIRATORY FAILURE

Most patients tolerate the postoperative changes in pulmonary function described above and recover from them without difficulty. Patients who have marginal preoperative pulmonary function may be unable to maintain adequate ventilation in the immediate postoperative period and may develop respiratory failure. In these patients, the operative trauma and the effects of anesthesia reduce respiratory reserve below levels that can provide adequate gas exchange. In contrast to acute respiratory distress syndrome (see Chapter 12), early postoperative respiratory failure (which develops within 48 hours after the operation) is usually only a mechanical problem, ie, there are minimal alterations of the lung parenchyma. However, this problem is life threatening and requires immediate attention.

Early respiratory failure develops most commonly in association with major operations (especially on the chest or upper abdomen), severe trauma, and preexisting lung disease. In most of these patients, respiratory failure develops over a short period (minutes to 1–2 hours) without evidence of a precipitating cause. By contrast, late postoperative respiratory failure (which develops beyond 48 hours after the operation) is usually triggered by an intercurrent event such as pulmonary embolism, abdominal distention, or opioid overdose.

Respiratory failure is manifested by tachypnea of 25–30 breaths per minute with a low tidal volume of less than 4 mL/kg. Laboratory indications are acute elevation of PCO_2 above 45 mm Hg, depression of PO_2 below 60 mm Hg, or evidence of low cardiac output. Treatment consists of immediate endotracheal intubation and ventilatory support to ensure adequate alveolar ventilation. As soon as the patient is intubated, it is important to determine whether there are any associated pulmonary problems such as atelectasis, pneumonia, or pneumothorax that require immediate treatment.

Prevention of respiratory failure requires careful postoperative pulmonary care. Atelectasis must be minimized using the techniques described above. Patients with preexisting pulmonary disease must be carefully hydrated to avoid hypovolemia. These patients must hyperventilate in order to compensate for the inefficiency of the lungs. This extra work causes greater evaporation of water and dehydration. Hypovolemia leads to dry secretions and thick sputum, which are difficult to clear from the airway. High fraction of inspired oxygen (FIO_2) in these patients removes the stabilizing gas nitrogen from the alveoli, predisposing to alveolar collapse. In addition, it may impair the function of the respiratory center, which is driven by the relative hypoxemia, and thus further decrease ventilation. The use of epidural blocks or other methods of local analgesia in patients with chronic obstructive pulmonary disease (COPD) may prevent respiratory failure by relieving pain and permitting effective respiratory muscle function.

▶ Postoperative Fluid & Electrolyte Management

Postoperative fluid replacement should be based on the following considerations: (1) maintenance requirements, (2) extra needs resulting from systemic factors (eg, fever, burns), (3) losses from drains, and (4) requirements resulting from tissue edema and ileus (third space losses). Daily maintenance requirements for sensible and insensible loss in the adult are about 1500–2500 mL depending on the patient's age, gender, weight, and body surface area. A rough estimate can be obtained by multiplying the patient's weight in kilograms times 30 (eg, 1800 mL/24 h in a 60-kg patient). Maintenance requirements are increased by fever, hyperventilation, and conditions that increase the catabolic rate.

For patients requiring intravenous fluid replacement for a short period (most postoperative patients), it is not necessary to measure serum electrolytes at any time during the postoperative period, but measurement is indicated in more complicated patients (those with extra fluid losses, sepsis, preexisting electrolyte abnormalities, or other factors). Assessment of the status of fluid balance requires accurate records of fluid intake and output and is aided by weighing the patient daily.

As a rule, 2000–2500 mL of 5% dextrose in normal saline or in lactated Ringer solution is given daily (Table 4–1). Potassium should usually not be added during the first 24 hours after surgery, because increased amounts of potassium enter the circulation during this time as a result of operative trauma and increased aldosterone activity.

In most patients, fluid loss through a nasogastric tube is less than 500 mL/d and can be replaced by increasing the infusion used for maintenance by a similar amount. About 20 meq of potassium should be added to every liter of fluid used to replace these losses. However, with the exception of urine, body fluids are isosmolar, and if large volumes of gastric or intestinal juice are replaced with normal saline solution, electrolyte imbalance will eventually result. When-

Table 4–1. Composition of Frequently Used Intravenous Solutions.

Solution	Glucose (g/dL)	Na⁺ (meq/L)	Cl⁻ (meq/L)	HCO₃⁻ (meq/L)	K⁺ (meq/L)
Dextrose 5% in water	50	...	...	...	...
Dextrose 5% and sodium chloride 0.45%	50	77	77	...	...
Sodium chloride 0.9%	...	154	154	...	...
Sodium chloride 0.45%	...	77	77	...	...
Lactated Ringer's solution	...	130	109	28	4
Sodium chloride 3%	...	513	513	...	...

ever external losses from any site amount to 1500 mL/d or more, electrolyte concentrations in the fluid should be measured periodically, and the amount of replacement fluids should be adjusted to equal the amount lost. Table 4–1 lists the compositions of the most frequently used solutions.

Losses that result from fluid sequestration at the operative site are usually adequately replaced during operation, but in a patient with a large retroperitoneal dissection, severe pancreatitis, etc, third space losses may be substantial and should be considered when postoperative fluids are given.

Fluid requirements must be evaluated frequently. Intravenous orders should be rewritten every 24 hours or more often if indicated by special circumstances. Following an extensive operation, fluid needs on the first day should be reevaluated every 4–6 hours.

▶ Postoperative Care of the Gastrointestinal Tract

Following laparotomy, gastrointestinal peristalsis temporarily decreases. Peristalsis returns in the small intestine within 24 hours, but gastric peristalsis may return more slowly. Function returns in the right colon by 48 hours and in the left colon by 72 hours. After operations on the stomach and upper intestine, propulsive activity of the upper gut can remain disorganized for 3–4 days. In the immediate postoperative period, the stomach may be decompressed with a nasogastric tube. Nasogastric intubation was once used in almost all patients undergoing laparotomy to avoid gastric distention and vomiting, but it is now recognized that routine nasogastric intubation is unnecessary and may cause postoperative atelectasis and pneumonia. For example, following cholecystectomy, pelvic operations, and colonic resections, nasogastric intubation is not needed in the average patient, and it is probably of marginal benefit following operations on the small bowel. On the other hand, nasogastric intubation is probably useful after esophageal and gastric resections and should always be used in patients with marked ileus or a very low level of consciousness (to avoid aspiration) and in patients who manifest acute gastric distention or vomiting postoperatively.

The nasogastric tube should be connected to low intermittent suction and irrigated frequently to ensure patency. The tube should be left in place for 2–3 days or until there is evidence that normal peristalsis has returned (eg, return of appetite, audible peristalsis, or passage of flatus). The nasogastric tube enhances gastroesophageal reflux, and if it is clamped overnight for assessment of residual volume, there is a slight risk of aspiration.

Once the nasogastric tube has been withdrawn, fasting is usually continued for another 24 hours, and the patient is then started on a liquid diet. Opioids may interfere with gastric motility and should be stopped in patients who have evidence of gastroparesis beyond the first postoperative week.

Gastrostomy and jejunostomy tubes should be connected to low intermittent suction or dependent drainage for the first 24 hours after surgery. Absorption of nutrients and fluids by the small intestine is not affected by laparotomy, and enteral nutrition through a jejunostomy feeding tube may therefore be started on the second postoperative day even if motility is not entirely normal. Gastrostomy or jejunostomy tubes should not be removed before the third postoperative week, because firm adhesions should be allowed to develop between the viscera and the parietal peritoneum.

After most operations in areas other than the peritoneal cavity, the patient may be allowed to resume a regular diet as soon as the effects of anesthesia have completely resolved.

TRANSFUSION THERAPY

▶ Whole Blood

Whole blood is composed of 450–500 mL of donor blood, containing RBCs (hematocrit, 35–45%), plasma, clotting factors (reduced levels of labile factors V and VIII), and anticoagulant. Platelets and granulocytes are not functional. It is indicated for red cell replacement in massive blood loss with pronounced hypovolemia. However, it is not routinely available.

▶ Red Blood Cells (RBCs)

RBCs are obtained by apheresis collection or prepared from whole blood by centrifugation and removal of plasma, followed by supplementation with 100 mL of adenine-containing red cell nutrient solution. The hematocrit is 55–60%, and the volume is 300–350 mL. RBCs collected in CPDA-1 anticoagulant have a hematocrit of 65–80% and a storage volume of 250–300 mL. RBC transfusions are indicated to increase oxygen-carrying capacity in anemic patients. Hemoglobin levels of 7–9 g/dL are well tolerated by most asymptomatic patients. A transfusion trigger of 7g/dL is commonly used in most stable patients. Symptomatic patients with cardiac, pulmonary, or cerebrovascular disease may require RBC transfusions at higher hemoglobin levels. In a nonbleeding 70-kg recipient, transfusion of one unit of RBCs should increase hemoglobin level by 1 g/dL and the hematocrit by 3%.

▶ Washed Red Blood Cells

RBCs are washed with saline to remove more than 98% of plasma proteins and resuspended in approximately 180 mL of saline, at an approximate hematocrit of 75%. Anemic patients with recurrent or severe allergic reactions benefit from washed RBCs. Patients with severe IgA deficiency who test positive for anti-IgA antibodies should receive RBCs washed with 2–3 L of saline or receive blood collected from IgA-deficient donors.

Leukocyte-Reduced Red Blood Cells

Third-generation leukocyte reduction filters remove more than 99.9% of the contaminating leukocytes, leaving less than 5×10^6 white blood cells per unit. Filtration done soon after collection (prestorage leukoreduction) is more effective than bedside filtration. Patients experiencing recurrent febrile nonhemolytic transfusion reactions (FNHTRs) to RBCs or platelets should receive leukocyte-reduced products. The prophylactic use of leukoreduced RBCs and platelets in patients with long-term transfusion needs decreases the likelihood of human leukocyte antigens (HLA) alloimmunization and protects from immune platelet refractoriness and recurrent FNHTRs. Leukoreduction also decreases the risk of transmission of cytomegalovirus (CMV) infection in immunosuppressed CMV-seronegative patients.

Irradiated Red Blood Cells

RBCs are irradiated with 25 Gy of gamma irradiation. All cellular products should be irradiated for patients who are at risk for transfusion-associated graft versus host disease (TA-GVHD). Adult patients at risk for TA-GVHD include, but are not limited to, the following: those with congenital severe immunodeficiency, hematological malignancy receiving intensive chemoradiotherapy, Hodgkin and non-Hodgkin lymphoma, certain solid tumors (neuroblastoma and sarcoma), peripheral blood stem cell and marrow transplants, or recipients of fludarabine-based chemotherapy and those receiving directed donations from blood relatives or HLA-matched platelets. Acellular products like fresh frozen plasma and cryoprecipitate are not irradiated. Leukoreduction is not an acceptable substitute for irradiation.

Frozen-Deglycerolized Red Blood Cells

RBCs frozen in glycerol are washed extensively in normal saline to remove the cryoprotectant and then resuspended in saline at a hematocrit of approximately 75%. More than 99.9% of the plasma is removed, and few leukocytes remain in the product. Patients who are alloimmunized to multiple antigens or those with antibodies against high-frequency antigens are supported with blood collected from donors with rare phenotypes. Most patients with severe IgA deficiency can safely receive RBCs washed with 2 L or more of saline. Frozen-deglycerolized RBCs are an equally safe and effective, albeit more cumbersome, alternative for these patients. Rarely, patients may require RBCs collected from IgA-deficient donors. A national rare donor program facilitates the collection and storage of rare blood types.

Platelets

Apheresis platelets are collected from single donors by apheresis and contain at least 3×10^{11} platelets in 250–300 mL plasma. Random-donor platelets (RDP) are platelet concentrates prepared from whole blood and contain 5.5×10^{10} platelets suspended in approximately 50 mL of plasma. Five to six units of RDP are pooled into a single pack to provide an adult dose. Platelet transfusions are indicated for the management of active bleeding in thrombocytopenic patients. Nonthrombocytopenic patients with congenital or acquired disorders of platelet function may also require platelets to stop bleeding manifestations. Platelet transfusions are also indicated prophylactically in patients requiring line placement or minor surgery when the platelet counts are less than 50,000/μL and in patients undergoing major surgical procedures when the count falls below 75,000/μL. Patients scheduled for ophthalmic, upper airway, or neurosurgical procedures should have platelet counts above 100,000/μL. Platelets are not usually recommended for the correction of thrombocytopenia in patients with heparin-induced thrombocytopenia (HIT), type IIB von Willebrand disease (vWD), idiopathic thrombocytopenic purpura (ITP), or thrombotic thrombocytopenic purpura (TTP). The clinical indications for the use of washed, irradiated, and leukoreduced platelets are analogous to those described in the section on RBCs. Patients with platelet refractoriness secondary to HLA alloimmunization should be supported with HLA-matched platelets.

Fresh Frozen Plasma

Fresh frozen plasma (FFP) is obtained by apheresis or prepared by centrifugation of whole blood and frozen within 8 hours of collection. It contains normal levels of all clotting factors, albumin, and fibrinogen. FFP is indicated for the replacement of coagulation factors in patients with deficiencies of multiple clotting factors as seen in the coagulopathy of liver disease, disseminated intravascular coagulation (DIC), warfarin overdose, and massive transfusions. One mL of FFP contains one unit of coagulation factor activity; soon after the infusion of a 10–15 mL/kg dose, the activity of all coagulation factors increases by 20–30%. Coagulation tests should be monitored to determine efficacy and appropriate dosing intervals. FFP should be used only if the INR is greater than 1.5 or the PT/aPTT are elevated more than 1.5 times the normal. Patients with liver disease who have minimally altered PT/aPTT and nominal bleeding should initially be managed with vitamin K replacement. Similarly, most patients with warfarin overdose can be managed by stopping warfarin for 48 hours and monitoring coagulation tests until they return to baseline levels. FFP is indicated only for active bleeding or if there is a risk for bleeding from an emergent procedure. FFP is the only replacement product currently available for patients with rare disorders like isolated factor deficiencies (V, X, XI) or C-1 esterase inhibitor deficiency. Patients with severe IgA deficiency should be supported with IgA-deficient plasma. FFP is the first choice for fluid replacement in patients with TTP undergoing therapeutic plasma exchange. FFP is not indicated for volume replacement, nutritional support, or replacement of immunoglobulins.

Cryoprecipitate

Cryoprecipitate is the cold-insoluble precipitate formed when FFP is thawed at 1–6 °C. This is then resuspended in 10–15 mL plasma. It contains 150 mg or more of fibrinogen, 80 IU or more of factor VIII, 40–70% of vWF and 20–30% of factor XIII present in the initial unit of FFP, and 30–60 mg of fibronectin. Each unit (bag) of cryoprecipitate increases fibrinogen level by 5–10 mg/dL. Eight to 10 bags are pooled and infused as a single dose in a 70-kg adult. Cryoprecipitate is indicated for the correction of hypofibrinogenemia in dilutional coagulopathy and the hypofibrinogenemia/dysfibrinogenemias of liver disease and DIC. Cryoprecipitate improves platelet aggregation and adhesion and decreases bleeding in uremic patients. It has been used for the correction of factor XIII deficiency, and it is the source of fibrinogen in the 2-component fibrin sealant (Tisseel). Cryoprecipitate is no longer used to treat patients with hemophilia A or vWD.

Granulocyte Transfusions

Granulocytes are collected by leukapheresis from donors stimulated with granulocyte colony-stimulating factor (G-CSF) and steroids to mobilize neutrophils from the marrow storage pool into peripheral blood. On average they contain 1×10^{10} or more granulocytes suspended in 200–300 mL plasma. About $1-3 \times 10^{11}$ platelets and 10–30 mL RBCs are also present in the product. Granulocyte transfusions are indicated in severely neutropenic (absolute neutrophil count $< 0.5 \times 10^3/\mu L$) patients with bacterial sepsis who have not responded to optimum antibiotic therapy after 48–72 hours, provided there is a reasonable expectation of recovery of bone marrow function. Transfusions are given daily until clinical improvement or neutrophil recovery occurs.

Postoperative Pain

Severe pain is a common sequela of intrathoracic, intra-abdominal, and major bone or joint procedures. About 60% of such patients perceive their pain to be severe, 25% moderate, and 15% mild. In contrast, following superficial operations on the head and neck, limbs, or abdominal wall, less than 15% of patients characterize their pain as severe. The factors responsible for these differences include duration of surgery, degree of operative trauma, type of incision, and magnitude of intraoperative retraction. Gentle handling of tissues, expedient operations, and good muscle relaxation help lessen the severity of postoperative pain.

While factors related to the nature of the operation influence postoperative pain, it is also true that the same operation produces different amounts of pain in different patients. This varies according to individual physical, emotional, and cultural characteristics. Much of the emotional aspect of pain can be traced to anxiety. Feelings such as helplessness, fear, and uncertainty contribute to anxiety and may heighten the patient's perception of pain.

It was once thought that anesthesia and analgesia in neonates and infants was too risky and that these young patients did not perceive pain. It is now known that reduction of pain with appropriate techniques actually decreases morbidity from major surgery in this age group.

The physiology of postoperative pain involves transmission of pain impulses via splanchnic (not vagal) afferent fibers to the central nervous system, where they initiate spinal, brain stem, and cortical reflexes. Spinal responses result from stimulation of neurons in the anterior horn, resulting in skeletal muscle spasm, vasospasm, and gastrointestinal ileus. Brain stem responses to pain include alterations in ventilation, blood pressure, and endocrine function. Cortical responses include voluntary movements and psychologic changes, such as fear and apprehension. These emotional responses facilitate nociceptive spinal transmission, lower the threshold for pain perception, and perpetuate the pain experience.

Postoperative pain serves no useful purpose and may cause alterations in pulmonary, circulatory, gastrointestinal, and skeletal muscle function that set the stage for postoperative complications. Pain following thoracic and upper abdominal operations, for example, causes voluntary and involuntary splinting of thoracic and abdominal muscles and the diaphragm. The patient may be reluctant to breathe deeply, promoting atelectasis. The limitation in motion due to pain sets the stage for venous stasis, thrombosis, and embolism. Release of catecholamines and other stress hormones by postoperative pain causes vasospasm and hypertension, which may in turn lead to complications such as stroke, myocardial infarction, and bleeding. Prevention of postoperative pain is thus important for reasons other than the pain itself. Effective pain control may improve the outcome of major operations.

A. Physician-Patient Communication

Close attention to the patient's needs, frequent reassurance, and genuine concern help minimize postoperative pain. Spending a few minutes with the patient every day in frank discussions of progress and any complications does more to relieve pain than many physicians realize.

B. Parenteral Opioids

Opioids are the mainstay of therapy for postoperative pain. Their analgesic effect is via two mechanisms: (1) a direct effect on opioid receptors and (2) stimulation of a descending brain stem system that contributes to pain inhibition. Although substantial relief of pain may be achieved with opioids, they do not modify reflex phenomena associated with pain, such as muscle spasm. Opioids administered intramuscularly, while convenient, result in wide variations in plasma concentrations. This, as well as the wide variations in dosage required for analgesia among patients, reduces analgesic efficacy. Physician and nurse attitudes reflect a persistent misunderstanding of the pharmacology and psychology of pain control. Frequently, the dose of opioid prescribed or administered is too small and too infrequent. When opioid usage is limited to temporary treatment of postoperative pain, drug addiction is extremely rare.

Morphine is the most widely used opioid for treatment of postoperative pain. Morphine may be administered intravenously, either intermittently or continuously. Except as discussed below in the section on patient-controlled analgesia, these last methods require close supervision and are impractical except in the PACU or intensive care unit. Side effects of morphine include respiratory depression, nausea and vomiting, and clouded sensorium. In the setting of severe postoperative pain, however, respiratory depression is rare, because pain itself is a powerful respiratory stimulant.

Meperidine is an opioid with about one-eighth the potency of morphine. It provides a similar quality of pain control with similar side effects. The duration of pain relief is somewhat shorter than with morphine. Like morphine, meperidine may be given intravenously, but the same requirements for monitoring apply.

Other opioids useful for postoperative analgesia include hydromorphone and methadone. Hydromorphone is usually administered in a dose of 1–2 mg intramuscularly every 2–3 hours. Methadone is given intramuscularly or orally in an average dose of 10 mg every 4–6 hours. The main advantage of methadone is its long half-life (6–10 hours) and its ability to prevent withdrawal symptoms in patients with morphine dependence.

C. Nonopioid Parenteral Analgesics

Ketorolac tromethamine is a nonsteroidal anti-inflammatory drug (NSAID) with potent analgesic and moderate anti-inflammatory activities. It is available in injectable form suitable for postoperative use. In controlled trials, ketorolac (30 mg) has demonstrated analgesic efficacy roughly equivalent to that of morphine (10 mg). A potential advantage over morphine is its lack of respiratory depression. Gastrointestinal ulceration, impaired coagulation, and reduced renal function—all potential complications of NSAID use—have not yet been reported with short-term perioperative use of ketorolac.

D. Oral Analgesics

Within several days following most abdominal surgical procedures, the severity of pain decreases to a point where oral analgesics suffice. Aspirin should be avoided as an analgesic postoperatively, since it interferes with platelet function, prolongs bleeding time, and interferes with the effects of anticoagulants. For most patients, a combination of acetaminophen with codeine (eg, Tylenol No. 3) or propoxyphene (Darvocet-N 50 or -N 100) suffices. Hydrocodone with acetaminophen (Vicodin) is a synthetic opioid with properties similar to those of codeine. For more severe pain, oxycodone is available in combination with aspirin (Percodan) or acetaminophen (Percocet, Tylox). Oxycodone is an opioid with slightly less potency than morphine. As with all opioids, tolerance develops with long-term use.

E. Patient-Controlled Analgesia

Patient-controlled analgesia (PCA) puts the frequency of analgesic administration under the patient's control but within safe limits. A device containing a timing unit, a pump, and the analgesic medication is connected to an intravenous line. By pressing a button, the patient delivers a predetermined dose of analgesic (usually morphine, 1–3 mg). The timing unit prevents overdosage by interposing an inactivation period (usually 6–8 minutes) between patient-initiated doses. The possibility of overdosage is also limited by the fact that the patient must be awake in order to search for and push the button that delivers the morphine. The dose and timing can be changed by medical personnel to accommodate the needs of the patient. This method appears to improve pain control and even reduces the total dose of opioid given in a 24-hour period. The addition of a background continuous infusion to the patient-directed administration of analgesic appears to offer no advantage over PCA alone.

F. Continuous Epidural Analgesia

Opioids are also effective when administered directly into the epidural space. Topical morphine does not depress proprioceptive pathways in the dorsal horn, but it does affect nociceptive pathways by interacting with opioid receptors. Therefore, epidural opioids produce intense, prolonged segmental analgesia with relatively less respiratory depression or sympathetic, motor, or other sensory disturbances. In comparison with parenteral administration, epidural administration requires similar dosage for control of pain, has a slightly delayed onset of action, provides substantially longer pain relief, and is associated with better preservation of pulmonary function. Epidural morphine is usually administered as a continuous infusion at a rate of 0.2–0.8 mg/h with or without the addition of 0.25% bupivacaine. Analgesia produced by this technique is superior to that of intravenous or intramuscular opioids. Patients managed in this way are more alert and have better gastrointestinal function. Side effects of continuous epidural administration of morphine include pruritus, nausea, and urinary retention. Respiratory depression may occur. Because the patient is unable to urinate, bladder catheterization is almost always required.

G. Intercostal Block

Intercostal block may be used to decrease pain following thoracic and abdominal operations. Since the block does not include the visceral afferents, it does not relieve pain completely, but it does eliminate muscle spasm induced by cutaneous pain and helps to restore respiratory function. It does not carry the risk of hypotension—as does continuous epidural analgesia—and it produces analgesia for periods of 3–12 hours. The main disadvantage of intercostal blocks is the risk of pneumothorax and the need for repeated injections. These problems can be minimized by placing a catheter in the intercostal space or in the pleura through which a continuous infusion of bupivacaine 0.5% is delivered at a rate of 3–8 mL/h.

▶ References

Wound Healing

Clark MA, Plank LD, Hill GL: Wound healing associated with severe surgical illness. World J Surg 2000;24:648.
Hunt TK, Hopf HW: Wound healing and wound infection. What surgeons and anesthesiologists can do. Surg Clin North Am 1997;77:587.
Singer AJ, Clark RA: Cutaneous wound healing. N Engl J Med 1999;341:738.
Wilmore DW: Metabolic response to severe surgical illness: overview. World J Surg 2000;24:705.
Witte MB, Barbul A: General principles of wound healing. Surg Clin North Am 1997;77:509.

Fluid Therapy

Kim PK, Deutschman CS: Inflammatory responses and mediators. Surg Clin North Am 2000;80:885.
Plank LD, Hill GL: Sequential metabolic changes following induction of systemic inflammatory response in patients with severe sepsis or major blunt trauma. World J Surg 2000;24:630.
Rooke GA: Autonomic and cardiovascular function in the geriatric patient. Anesthesiol Clin North Am 2000;18:31.

Transfusion Therapy

Corwin HL et al: The CRIT study: anemia and blood transfusion in the critically ill—current clinical practice in the United States. Crit Care Med 2004;32:39.
Napolitano LM, Corwin HL: Efficacy of red blood cell transfusion in the critically ill. Crit Care Clin 2004;20:255.
Stroncek DF, Rebulla P: Platelet transfusions. Lancet 2007;370:427.
Klein HG, Spahn DR, Carson JL: Red blood cell transfusion in clinical practice. Lancet 2007;370:415.

Pain

Austrup ML, Korean G: Analgesic agents for the postoperative period. Opioids. Surg Clin North Am 1999;79:253.
Buggy DJ, Smith G: Epidural anaesthesia and analgesia: better outcome after major surgery? Growing evidence suggests so. BMJ 1999;319:530.
Etches RC: Patient-controlled analgesia. Surg Clin North Am 1999;79:297.
Grass JA: The role of epidural anesthesia and analgesia in postoperative outcome. Anesthesiol Clin North Am 2000;18:407.
Krauss B, Green SM: Sedation and analgesia for procedures in children. N Engl J Med 2000;342:938.
Power I, Barratt S: Analgesic agents for the postoperative period. Nonopioids. Surg Clin North Am 1999;79:275.
Rawal N: Epidural and spinal agents for postoperative analgesia. Surg Clin North Am 1999;79:313.
Sorkin LS, Wallace MS: Acute pain mechanisms. Surg Clin North Am 1999;79:213.
Wiklund RA, Rosenbaum SH: Anesthesiology. First of two parts. N Engl J Med 1997;337:1132.
Wiklund RA, Rosenbaum SH: Anesthesiology. Second of two parts. N Engl J Med 1997;337:1215.

Postoperative Complications

Gerard M. Doherty, MD

Postoperative complications may result from the primary disease, the operation, or unrelated factors. Occasionally, one complication results from another previous one (eg, myocardial infarction following massive postoperative bleeding). The clinical signs of disease are often blurred in the postoperative period. Early detection of postoperative complications requires repeated evaluation of the patient by the operating surgeon and other team members.

Prevention of complications starts in the preoperative period with evaluation of the patient's disease and risk factors. Improving the health of the patient before surgery is one goal of the preoperative evaluation. For example, cessation of smoking for 6 weeks before surgery decreases the incidence of postoperative pulmonary complications from 50% to 10%. Correction of gross obesity decreases intra-abdominal pressure and the risk of wound and respiratory complications and improves ventilation postoperatively.

The surgeon should explain the operation and the expected postoperative course to the patient and family. The preoperative hospital stay, if one is necessary, should be as short as possible both to reduce costs and to minimize exposure to antibiotic-resistant microorganisms. Adequate training in respiratory exercises planned for the postoperative period substantially decreases the incidence of postoperative pulmonary complications.

Early mobilization, proper respiratory care, and careful attention to fluid and electrolyte needs are important. On the evening after surgery the patient should be encouraged to sit up, cough, breathe deeply, and walk, if possible. The upright position permits expansion of basilar lung segments, and walking increases the circulation of the lower extremities and lessens the danger of venous thromboembolism. In severely ill patients, continuous monitoring of systemic blood pressure and cardiac performance enables identification and correction of mild derangements before they become severe.

WOUND COMPLICATIONS

▶ Hematoma

Wound hematoma, a collection of blood and clot in the wound, is one of the most common wound complications and is almost always caused by imperfect hemostasis. Patients receiving aspirin or low-dose heparin have a slightly higher risk of developing this complication. The risk is much higher in patients who have been given systemically effective doses of anticoagulants and those with preexisting coagulopathies. Vigorous coughing or marked arterial hypertension immediately after surgery may contribute to the formation of a wound hematoma.

Hematomas produce elevation and discoloration of the wound edges, discomfort, and swelling. Blood sometimes leaks through skin sutures. Neck hematomas following operations on the thyroid, parathyroid, or carotid artery are particularly dangerous, because they may expand rapidly and compromise the airway. Small hematomas may resorb, but they increase the incidence of wound infection. Treatment in most cases consists of evacuation of the clot under sterile conditions, ligation of bleeding vessels, and reclosure of the wound.

▶ Seroma

A seroma is a fluid collection in the wound other than pus or blood. Seromas often follow operations that involve elevation of skin flaps and transection of numerous lymphatic channels (eg, mastectomy, operations in the groin). Seromas delay healing and increase the risk of wound infection. Those located under skin flaps can usually be evacuated by needle aspiration. Compression dressings should then be applied to seal lymphatic leaks and prevent reaccumulation. Small seromas that recur may be treated by repeated evacuation. Seromas of the groin, which are common after vascular operations, are best left to resorb without aspiration, since the risks of introducing a needle (infection, disruption of vascular structures, etc) are greater than the risk associated with the seroma itself. If seromas persist—or if they start leaking through the wound—the wound should be explored in the operating room and the lymphatics ligated. Open wounds with persistent lymph leaks can be treated with wound vacuum devices.

▶ Wound Dehiscence

Wound dehiscence is partial or total disruption of any or all layers of the operative wound. Rupture of all layers of the abdominal wall and extrusion of abdominal viscera is evisceration. Wound dehiscence occurs in 1–3% of abdominal surgical procedures. Systemic and local factors contribute to the development of this complication.

A. Systemic Risk Factors

Dehiscence is rare in patients under age 30 but affects about 5% of patients over age 60 having laparotomy. It is more common in patients with diabetes mellitus, uremia, immunosuppression, jaundice, sepsis, hypoalbuminemia, and cancer; in obese patients; and in those receiving corticosteroids.

B. Local Risk Factors

The three most important local factors predisposing to wound dehiscence are inadequate closure, increased intra-abdominal pressure, and deficient wound healing. Dehiscence often results from a combination of these factors rather than from a single one. The type of incision (transverse, midline, etc) does not influence the incidence of dehiscence.

1. Adequacy of closure—This is the single most important factor. The fascial layers give strength to a closure, and when fascia disrupts, the wound separates. Accurate approximation of anatomic layers is essential for adequate wound closure. Most wounds that dehisce do so because the sutures tear through the fascia. Prevention of this problem includes performing a neat incision, avoiding devitalization of the fascial edges by careful handling of tissues during the operation, placing and tying sutures correctly, and selecting the proper suture material. Sutures must be placed 2–3 cm from the wound edge and about 1 cm apart. *Dehiscence is often the result of using too few stitches and placing them too close to the edge of the fascia.* It is unusual for dehiscence to recur following reclosure, implying that adequate closure was technically possible at the initial procedure. In patients with risk factors for dehiscence, the surgeon should "do the second closure at the first operation," ie, take extra care to prevent dehiscence. Modern synthetic suture materials (polyglycolic acid, polypropylene, and others) are clearly superior to catgut for fascial closure. In infected wounds, polypropylene sutures are more resistant to degradation than polyglycolic acid sutures and have lower rates of wound disruption. Wound complications are decreased by obliteration of dead space. Ostomies and drains should be brought out through separate incisions to reduce the rate of wound infection and disruption.

2. Intra-abdominal pressure—After most intra-abdominal operations, some degree of ileus exists, which may increase pressure by causing distention of the bowel. High abdominal pressures can also occur in patients with chronic obstructive pulmonary disease who use their abdominal muscles as accessory muscles of respiration. In addition, coughing produces sudden increases in intra-abdominal pressure. Other factors contributing to increased abdominal pressure are postoperative bowel obstruction, obesity, and cirrhosis with ascites formation. Extra precautions are necessary to avoid dehiscence in such patients.

3. Deficient wound healing—Infection is an associated factor in more than half of wounds that rupture. The presence of drains, seromas, and wound hematomas also delays healing. Normally, a "healing ridge" (a palpable thickening extending about 0.5 cm on each side of the incision) appears near the end of the first week after operation. The presence of this ridge is clinical evidence that healing is adequate, and it is invariably absent from wounds that rupture.

C. Diagnosis and Management

Although wound dehiscence may occur at any time following wound closure, it is most commonly observed between the fifth and eighth postoperative days, when the strength of the wound is at a minimum. Wound dehiscence may occasionally be the first manifestation of an intra-abdominal abscess. The first sign of dehiscence is discharge of serosanguineous fluid from the wound or, in some cases, sudden evisceration. The patient often describes a popping sensation associated with severe coughing or retching. Thoracic wounds, with the exception of sternal wounds, are much less prone to dehiscence than are abdominal wounds. When a thoracotomy closure ruptures, it is heralded by leakage of pleural fluid or air and paradoxic motion of the chest wall. Sternal dehiscences, which are almost always associated with infection, produce an unstable chest and require early treatment. If infection is not overwhelming and there is minimal osteomyelitis of the adjacent sternum, the patient may be returned to the operating room for reclosure. Continuous mediastinal irrigation through small tubes left at the time of closure appears to reduce the failure rate. In cases of overwhelming infection, the wound is best treated by debridement and closure with a pectoralis major muscle flap, which resists further infection by increasing vascular supply to the area.

Patients with dehiscence of a laparotomy wound and evisceration should be returned to bed and the wound covered with moist towels. With the patient under general anesthesia, any exposed bowel or omentum should be rinsed with lactated Ringer solution containing antibiotics and then returned to the abdomen. After mechanical cleansing and copious irrigation of the wound, the previous sutures should be removed and the wound reclosed using additional measures to prevent recurrent dehiscence, such as full-thickness retention sutures of No. 22 wire or heavy nylon. Evisceration carries a 10% mortality rate due both to contributing factors (eg, sepsis and cancer) and to resulting local infection.

Wound dehiscence without evisceration is best managed by prompt elective reclosure of the incision. If a partial disruption (ie, the skin is intact) is stable and the patient is a poor operative risk, treatment may be delayed and the resulting incisional hernia accepted. It is important in these patients that skin stitches not be removed before the end of the second postoperative week and that the abdomen be wrapped with a binder or corset to prevent further enlargement of the fascial defect or sudden disruption of the covering skin. When partial dehiscence is discovered during treatment of a wound infection, repair should be delayed if possible until the infection has been controlled, the wound has healed, and 6–7 months have elapsed. In these cases, antibiotics specific for the organisms isolated from the previous wound infection must be given at the time of hernia repair.

Recurrence of evisceration after reclosure of disrupted wounds is rare, though incisional hernias are later found in about 20% of such patients—usually those with wound infection in addition to dehiscence.

▶ Miscellaneous Problems of the Operative Wound

Every new operative wound is painful, but those subject to continuous motion (eg, incisions that cross the costal margin) may be more painful than others. In general, the pain of an operative wound decreases substantially during the first 4–6 postoperative days. Chronic pain localized to one portion of an apparently healed wound may indicate the presence of a stitch abscess, a granuloma, or an occult incisional hernia. Abnormalities on examination of the wound usually allow for easy diagnosis; when this is difficult, ultrasound scanning may help detect a fascial defect or a collection of fluid associated with granulomas or abscesses. Rarely, a neuroma in the wound is responsible for focal pain and tenderness late in the postoperative course. Persistent localized pain is best treated by exploring the area, usually under local anesthesia, and removing a stitch, draining an abscess, or closing a hernia defect. Small sinus tracts usually result from stitch abscesses. The infected stitch can usually be removed with a clamp or crochet hook passed down the tract. If drainage continues, it is occasionally necessary to reopen the skin for better exposure and to remove a series of infected stitches.

Patients with ascites are at risk of fluid leak through the wound. Left untreated, **ascitic leaks** increase the incidence of wound infection and, through retrograde contamination, may result in peritonitis. Prevention in susceptible patients involves closing at least one layer of the wound with a continuous suture and taking measures to avoid the accumulation of ascites postoperatively. If an ascitic leak develops, the wound should be explored and the fascial defect closed. The rest of the wound, including the skin, should also be closed.

RESPIRATORY COMPLICATIONS

Respiratory complications are the most common single cause of morbidity after major surgical procedures and the second most common cause of postoperative deaths in patients older than 60 years. Patients undergoing chest and upper abdominal operations are particularly prone to pulmonary complications. The incidence is lower after pelvic surgery and even lower after extremity or head and neck procedures. Pulmonary complications are more common after emergency operations. Special hazards are posed by preexisting chronic obstructive pulmonary disease (chronic bronchitis, emphysema, asthma, pulmonary fibrosis). Elderly patients are at much higher risk because they have decreased compliance, increased closing and residual volumes, and increased dead space, all of which predispose to atelectasis.

▶ Atelectasis

Atelectasis, the most common pulmonary complication, affects 25% of patients who have abdominal surgery. It is more common in patients who are elderly or overweight and in those who smoke or have symptoms of respiratory disease. It appears most frequently in the first 48 hours after operation and is responsible for over 90% of febrile episodes during that period. In most cases, the course is self-limited and recovery uneventful.

The pathogenesis of atelectasis involves obstructive and nonobstructive factors. Obstruction may be caused by secretions resulting from chronic obstructive pulmonary disease, intubation, or anesthetic agents. Occasional cases may be due to blood clots or malposition of the endotracheal tube. In most instances, however, the cause is not obstruction but closure of the bronchioles. Small bronchioles ($\leq$ 1 mm) are prone to close when lung volume reaches a critical point ("closing volume"). Portions of the lung that are dependent or compressed are the first to experience bronchiole closure, since their regional volume is less than that of nondependent portions. Shallow breathing and failure to periodically hyperinflate the lung result in small alveolar size and decreased volume. The closing volume is higher in older patients and in smokers owing to the loss of elastic recoil of the lung. Other nonobstructive factors contributing to atelectasis include decreased functional residual capacity and loss of pulmonary surfactant.

The air in the atelectatic portion of the lung is absorbed, and since there is minimal change in perfusion, a ventilation/perfusion mismatch results. The immediate effect of atelectasis is decreased oxygenation of blood; its clinical significance depends on the respiratory and cardiac reserve of the patient. A later effect is the propensity of the atelectatic segment to become infected. In general, if a pulmonary segment remains atelectatic for over 72 hours, pneumonia is almost certain to occur.

Atelectasis is usually manifested by fever (pathogenesis unknown), tachypnea, and tachycardia. Physical examination may show elevation of the diaphragm, scattered rales, and decreased breath sounds, but it is often normal. Postoperative atelectasis can be largely prevented by early mobilization, frequent changes in position, encouragement to cough, and use of an incentive spirometer. Preoperative teaching of respiratory exercises and postoperative execution of these exercises prevents atelectasis in patients without preexisting lung disease. Intermittent positive pressure breathing is expensive and less effective than these simpler exercises.

Treatment consists of clearing the airway by chest percussion, coughing, or nasotracheal suction. Bronchodilators and mucolytic agents given by nebulizer may help in patients with severe chronic obstructive pulmonary disease. Atelectasis from obstruction of a major airway may require intrabronchial suction through an endoscope, a procedure that can usually be performed at the bedside with mild sedation.

▶ Pulmonary Aspiration

Aspiration of oropharyngeal and gastric contents is normally prevented by the gastroesophageal and pharyngoesophageal sphincters. Insertion of nasogastric and endotracheal tubes and depression of the central nervous system by drugs interfere with these defenses and predispose to aspiration. Other factors, such as gastroesophageal reflux, food in the stomach, or position of the patient, may play a role. Trauma victims are particularly likely to aspirate regurgitated gastric contents when consciousness is depressed. Patients with intestinal obstruction and pregnant women—who have increased intra-abdominal pressure and decreased gastric motility—are also at high risk of aspiration. Two-thirds of cases of aspiration follow thoracic or abdominal surgery, and of these, one-half result in pneumonia. The death rate for grossly evident aspiration and subsequent pneumonia is about 50%.

Minor amounts of aspiration are frequent during surgery and are apparently well tolerated. Methylene blue placed in the stomach of patients undergoing abdominal operations can be found in the trachea at completion of the procedure in 15% of cases. Radionuclide techniques have shown aspiration of gastric contents in 45% of normal volunteers during sleep.

The magnitude of pulmonary injury produced by aspiration of fluid, usually from gastric contents, is determined by the volume aspirated, its pH, and the frequency of the event. If the aspirate has a pH of 2.5 or less, it causes immediate chemical pneumonitis, which results in local edema and inflammation, changes that increase the risk of secondary infection. Aspiration of solid matter can produce airway obstruction. Obstruction of distal bronchi, though well tolerated initially, can lead to atelectasis and pulmonary abscess formation. The basal segments are affected most often. Tachypnea, rales, and hypoxia are usually present within hours; less frequently, cyanosis, wheezing, and apnea may appear. In patients with massive aspiration, hypovolemia caused by excessive fluid and colloid loss into the injured lung may lead to hypotension and shock.

Aspiration has been found in 80% of patients with tracheostomies and may account for the predisposition to pulmonary infection in this group. Patients who must remain intubated for long periods should have a low-pressure, high-volume type of cuff on their tube, which helps to prevent aspiration and limits the risk of pressure necrosis of the trachea.

Aspiration can be prevented by preoperative fasting, proper positioning of the patient, and careful intubation. A single dose of H_2-blocker or proton pump inhibitor before induction of anesthesia may be of value in situations where the risk of aspiration is high. Treatment of aspiration involves reestablishing patency of the airway and preventing further damage to the lung. Endotracheal suction should be performed immediately, as this procedure confirms the diagnosis and stimulates coughing, which helps to clear the airway. Bronchoscopy may be required to remove solid matter. Fluid resuscitation should be undertaken concomitantly. Antibiotics are used initially when the aspirate is heavily contaminated; they are used later to treat pneumonia.

▶ Postoperative Pneumonia

Pneumonia is the most common pulmonary complication among patients who die after surgery. It is directly responsible for death—or is a contributory factor—in more than half of these patients. Patients with peritoneal infection and those requiring prolonged ventilatory support are at highest risk for developing postoperative pneumonia. Atelectasis, aspiration, and copious secretions are important predisposing factors.

Host defenses against pneumonitis include the cough reflex, the mucociliary system, and the activity of alveolar macrophages. After surgery, cough is usually weak and may not effectively clear the bronchial tree. The mucociliary transport mechanism is damaged by endotracheal intubation, and the functional ability of the alveolar macrophage is compromised by a number of factors that may be present during and after surgery (oxygen, pulmonary edema, aspiration, corticosteroid therapy, etc). In addition, squamous metaplasia and loss of ciliary coordination further hamper antibacterial defenses. More than half of the pulmonary infections that follow surgery are caused by gram-negative bacilli. They are frequently polymicrobial and usually acquired by aspiration of oropharyngeal secretions. Although colonization of the oropharynx with gram-negative bacteria occurs in only 20% of normal individuals, it is frequent after major surgery as a result of impaired oropharyngeal clearing mechanisms. Aggravating factors are azotemia, prolonged endotracheal intubation, and severe associated infection.

Occasionally, infecting bacteria reach the lung by inhalation—eg, from respirators. *Pseudomonas aeruginosa* and klebsiella can survive in the moist reservoirs of these machines, and these pathogens have been the source of epidemic infections in intensive care units. Rarely, contamination of the lung may result from direct hematogenous spread from distant septic foci.

The clinical manifestations of postoperative pneumonia are fever, tachypnea, increased secretions, and physical changes suggestive of pulmonary consolidation. A chest x-ray usually shows localized parenchymal consolidation. Overall mortality rates for postoperative pneumonia vary from 20% to 40%. Rates are higher when pneumonia develops in patients who had emergency operations, are on respirators, or develop remote organ failure, positive blood cultures, or infection of the second lung.

Maintaining the airway clear of secretions is of paramount concern in the prevention of postoperative pneumonia. Respiratory exercises, deep breathing, and coughing help prevent atelectasis, which is a precursor of pneumonia. Although postoperative pain is thought to contribute to shallow breathing, neither intercostal blocks nor epidural narcotics prevent atelectasis and pneumonia when compared with traditional methods of postoperative pain control. The prophylactic use of antibiotics does not decrease the incidence of gram-negative colonization of the oropharynx or that of pneumonia. Treatment consists of measures to aid the clearing of secretions and administration of antibiotics. Sputum obtained directly from the trachea, usually by endotracheal suctioning, is required for specific identification of the infecting organism.

▶ Postoperative Pleural Effusion & Pneumothorax

Formation of a very small pleural effusion is fairly common immediately after upper abdominal operations and is of no clinical significance. Patients with free peritoneal fluid at the time of surgery and those with postoperative atelectasis are more prone to develop effusions. In the absence of cardiac failure or a pulmonary lesion, appearance of a pleural effusion late in the postoperative course suggests the presence of subdiaphragmatic inflammation (subphrenic abscess, acute pancreatitis, etc). Effusions that do not compromise respiratory function should be left undisturbed. If there is a suspicion of infection, the effusion should be sampled by needle aspiration. When an effusion produces respiratory compromise, it should be drained with a thoracostomy tube.

Postoperative pneumothorax may follow insertion of a subclavian catheter or positive-pressure ventilation, but it sometimes appears after an operation during which the pleura has been injured (eg, nephrectomy or adrenalectomy). Pneumothorax should be treated with a thoracostomy tube.

FAT EMBOLISM

Fat embolism is relatively common but only rarely causes symptoms. Fat particles can be found in the pulmonary vascular bed in 90% of patients who have had fractures of long bones or joint replacements. Fat embolism can also be caused by exogenous sources of fat, such as blood transfusions, intravenous fat emulsion, or bone marrow transplantation. **Fat embolism syndrome** consists of neurologic dysfunction, respiratory insufficiency, and petechiae of the axillae, chest, and proximal arms. It was originally described in trauma victims—especially those with long bone fractures—and was thought to be a result of bone marrow embolization. However, the principal clinical manifestations of fat embolism are seen in other conditions. The existence of fat embolism as an entity distinct from posttraumatic pulmonary insufficiency has been questioned.

Fat embolism syndrome characteristically begins 12–72 hours after injury but may be delayed for several days. The diagnosis is clinical. The finding of fat droplets in sputum and urine is common after trauma and is not specific. Decreased hematocrit, thrombocytopenia, and other changes in coagulation parameters are usually seen.

Once symptoms develop, supportive treatment should be provided until respiratory insufficiency and central nervous system manifestations subside. Respiratory insufficiency is treated with positive end-expiratory pressure ventilation and diuretics. The prognosis is related to the severity of the pulmonary insufficiency.

CARDIAC COMPLICATIONS

Cardiac complications following surgery may be life threatening. Their incidence is reduced by appropriate preoperative preparation.

Dysrhythmias, unstable angina, heart failure, or severe hypertension should be corrected before surgery whenever possible. Valvular disease—especially aortic stenosis—limits the ability of the heart to respond to increased demand during operation or in the immediate postoperative period. When aortic stenosis is recognized preoperatively—and assuming that the patient is monitored adequately (Swan-Ganz catheterization, central venous pressure, etc)—the incidence of major perioperative complications is small. Thus, patients with preexisting heart disease should be evaluated by a cardiologist preoperatively. Determination of cardiac function, including indirect evaluation of the left ventricular ejection fraction, identifies patients at higher risk for cardiac complications. Continuous electrocardiographic monitoring during the first 3–4 postoperative days detects episodes of ischemia or dysrhythmia in about a third of these patients. Oral anticoagulant drugs should be stopped 3–5 days before surgery, and the prothrombin time should be allowed to return to normal. Patients at high risk of thromboembolic disease should receive heparin until approximately 6 hours before the operation, when heparin should be stopped. If needed, heparin can be restarted 36–48 hours after surgery along with oral anticoagulation.

General anesthesia depresses the myocardium, and some anesthetic agents predispose to dysrhythmias by sensitizing the myocardium to catecholamines. Monitoring of cardiac activity and blood pressure during the operation detects dysrhythmias and hypotension early. In patients with a high cardiac risk, regional anesthesia may be safer than general anesthesia for procedures below the umbilicus.

The duration and urgency of the operation and uncontrolled bleeding with hypotension have been individually shown to correlate positively with the development of serious postoperative cardiac problems. In patients with pacemakers, the electrocautery current may be sensed by the intracardiac electrode, causing inappropriate pacemaker function.

Noncardiac complications may affect the development of cardiac complications by increasing cardiac demands in patients with a limited reserve. Postoperative sepsis and hypoxemia are foremost. Fluid overload can produce acute left ventricular failure. Patients with coronary artery disease, dysrhythmias, or low cardiac output should be monitored postoperatively in an intensive care unit.

Dysrhythmias

Most dysrhythmias appear during the operation or within the first 3 postoperative days. They are especially likely to occur after thoracic procedures.

A. Intraoperative Dysrhythmias

The overall incidence of intraoperative cardiac dysrhythmias is 20%; most are self-limited. The incidence is higher in patients with preexisting dysrhythmias and in those with known heart disease (35%). About one-third of dysrhythmias occur during induction of anesthesia. These dysrhythmias are usually related to anesthetic agents (eg, halothane, cyclopropane), sympathomimetic drugs, digitalis toxicity, and hypercapnia.

B. Postoperative Dysrhythmias

These dysrhythmias are generally related to reversible factors such as hypokalemia, hypoxemia, alkalosis, digitalis toxicity, and stress during emergence from anesthesia. Occasionally, postoperative dysrhythmias may be the first sign of myocardial infarction. Most postoperative dysrhythmias are asymptomatic, but occasionally the patient complains of chest pain, palpitations, or dyspnea.

Supraventricular dysrhythmias usually have few serious consequences but may decrease cardiac output and coronary blood flow. Patients with atrial flutter or fibrillation with a rapid ventricular response and who are in shock require cardioversion. If they are hemodynamically stable, they should have the heart rate controlled with digitalis, beta-blockers, or calcium channel blockers. Associated hypokalemia should be treated promptly.

Ventricular premature beats are often precipitated by hypercapnia, hypoxemia, pain, or fluid overload. They should be treated with oxygen, sedation, analgesia, and correction of fluid losses or electrolyte abnormalities. Ventricular dysrhythmias have a more profound effect on cardiac function than supraventricular dysrhythmias and may lead to fatal ventricular fibrillation. Immediate treatment is with lidocaine, 1 mg/kg intravenously as a bolus, repeated as necessary to a total dose of 250 mg, followed by a slow intravenous infusion at a rate of 1–2 mg/min. Higher doses of lidocaine may cause seizures.

Postoperative complete heart block is usually due to serious cardiac disease and calls for the immediate insertion of a pacemaker. First- or second-degree heart block is usually well tolerated.

Postoperative Myocardial Infarction

Approximately 0.4% of all patients undergoing an operation in the United States develop postoperative myocardial infarction. The incidence increases to 5–12% in patients undergoing operations for other manifestations of atherosclerosis (eg, carotid endarterectomy, aortoiliac graft). Other important risk factors include preoperative congestive heart failure, ischemia identified on dipyridamole-thallium scan or treadmill exercise test, and age over 70 years. In selected patients with angina, consideration should be given to coronary revascularization before proceeding with a major elective operation on another organ.

Postoperative myocardial infarction may be precipitated by factors such as hypotension or hypoxemia. Clinical manifestations include chest pain, hypotension, and cardiac dysrhythmias. Over half of postoperative myocardial infarctions, however, are asymptomatic. The absence of symptoms is thought to be due to the residual effects of anesthesia and to analgesics administered postoperatively.

Diagnosis is substantiated by electrocardiographic changes, elevated serum creatine kinase levels—especially the MB isoenzyme—and serum troponin I levels. The mortality rate of postoperative myocardial infarction is as high as 67% in high-risk groups. The prognosis is better if it is the first infarction and worse if there have been previous infarctions. Prevention of this complication includes postponing elective operations for 3 months or preferably 6 months after myocardial infarction, treating congestive heart failure preoperatively, and controlling hypertension perioperatively.

Patients with postoperative myocardial infarction should be monitored in the intensive care unit and provided with adequate oxygenation and precise fluid and electrolyte replacement. Anticoagulation, though not always feasible after major surgery, prevents the development of mural thrombosis and arterial embolism after myocardial infarction. Congestive heart failure should be treated with digitalis, diuretics, and vasodilators as needed.

Postoperative Cardiac Failure

Left ventricular failure and pulmonary edema appear in 4% of patients over age 40 undergoing general surgical procedures with general anesthesia. Fluid overload in patients with limited myocardial reserve is the most common cause. Postoperative myocardial infarction and dysrhythmias producing a high ventricular rate are other causes. Clinical manifestations are progressive dyspnea, hypoxemia with normal CO_2 tension, and diffuse congestion on chest x-ray.

Clinically inapparent ventricular failure is frequent, especially when other factors predisposing to pulmonary edema are present (massive trauma, multiple transfusions, sepsis, etc). The diagnosis may be suspected from a decreased PaO_2, abnormal chest x-ray, or elevated pulmonary artery wedge pressure. The treatment of left ventricular failure depends on the hemodynamic state of the patient. Those who are in shock require transfer to the intensive care unit, placement of a pulmonary artery line, monitoring of filling pressures, and immediate preload and afterload reduction. Preload reduction is achieved by diuretics (and nitroglycerin if needed); afterload reduction, by administration of sodium nitroprusside. Patients who are not in shock may instead be digitalized. Rapid digitalization (eg, divided intravenous doses of digoxin to a total of 1–1.5 mg over 24 hours, with careful monitoring of the serum potassium level), fluid restriction, and diuretics may be enough in these cases. Fluids should be restricted, and diuretics may be given. Respiratory insufficiency calls for ventilatory support with endotracheal intubation and a mechanical respirator. Although pulmonary function may improve with the use of positive end-expiratory pressure, hemodynamic derangements and decreased myocardial reserve preclude it in most cases.

PERITONEAL COMPLICATIONS

Hemoperitoneum

Bleeding is the most common cause of shock in the first 24 hours after abdominal surgery. Postoperative hemoperitoneum—a rapidly evolving, life-threatening complication—is usually the result of a technical problem with hemostasis, but coagulation disorders may play a role. For example, many of these patients have experienced substantial intraoperative blood loss, and several transfusions have been already given. As a consequence, changes usually observed after transfusion, such as thrombocytopenia, may be present. Other causes of coagulopathy, such as mismatched transfusion, administration of heparin, etc, should also be considered. In these cases, bleeding tends to be more generalized, occurring in the wound, venipuncture sites, etc.

Hemoperitoneum usually becomes apparent within 24 hours after the operation. Its manifestations are those of intravascular hypovolemia: tachycardia, decreased blood pressure, decreased urine output, and peripheral vasoconstriction. If bleeding continues, abdominal girth may increase. Changes in the hematocrit are usually not obvious for 4–6 hours and are of limited diagnostic help in patients who sustain rapid blood loss.

The manifestations may be so subtle that the diagnosis is overlooked. Only a high index of suspicion, frequent examination of patients at risk, and a systematic investigation of patients with postoperative hypotension will result in early recognition of the problem. Preexisting disease and drugs taken before surgery as well as those administered during the operation may cause hypotension. The differential diagnosis

of immediate postoperative circulatory collapse also includes pulmonary embolism, cardiac dysrhythmias, pneumothorax, myocardial infarction, and severe allergic reactions. Infusions to expand the intravascular volume should be started as soon as other diseases have been ruled out. If hypotension or other signs of hypovolemia persist, one must reoperate promptly. At operation, bleeding should be stopped, clots evacuated, and the peritoneal cavity rinsed with saline solution.

Complications of Drains

Postoperative drainage of the peritoneal cavity is indicated to prevent fluid accumulation such as bile or pancreatic fluid or to treat established abscesses. Drains may be left to evacuate small amounts of blood, but drain output cannot be used to provide a reliable estimate of the rate of bleeding. The use of drains in operations not expected to have fluid leaks (such as cholecystectomy, splenectomy, and colectomy) increases the rate of postoperative intra-abdominal and wound infection. Latex Penrose drains, which were once used frequently, should generally be avoided because of the risk of introducing infection. Large rigid drains may erode into adjacent viscera or vessels and cause fistula formation or bleeding. This risk is lessened with the use of softer Silastic drains, and removing them as early as possible. Drains should not be left in contact with intestinal anastomoses, as they promote anastomotic leakage and fistula formation.

POSTOPERATIVE PAROTITIS

Postoperative parotitis—a rare but serious staphylococcal infection of the parotid gland—is limited almost entirely to elderly, debilitated, malnourished patients with poor oral hygiene. It appears in the second postoperative week and is associated with prolonged nasogastric intubation. The triggering factors are dehydration and poor oral hygiene, and the pathogenesis consists of a decrease in the secretory activity of the gland with inspissation of parotid secretions that become infected by staphylococci or gram-negative bacteria from the oral cavity. This results in inflammation, accumulation of cells that obstruct large and medium-sized ducts, and eventually formation of multiple small abscesses. These lobular abscesses, separated by fibrous bands, may dissect through the capsule and spread to the periglandular tissues to involve the auditory canal, the superficial skin, and the neck. If the disease is not treated at this stage, it may produce acute respiratory failure from tracheal obstruction.

Clinically, parotitis first appears as pain or tenderness at the angle of the jaw. With progression, high fever and leukocytosis develop, and there is swelling and redness in the parotid area. The parotid usually feels firm, and even after abscesses have formed, fluctuance is uncommon.

Prophylaxis includes adequate fluid intake, avoiding the use of anticholinergics, minimizing trauma during intubation, and, most importantly, good oral hygiene (frequent gargles, mouth irrigation, and other mouth cleansing and moistening measures). Stimulation of salivary flow with chewing gum, hard candy, etc, may also be useful. Routine observance of these simple preventive measures has virtually eliminated parotitis, which was once a common postoperative complication.

When signs of acute parotitis appear, fluid obtained from the Stensen duct by gentle compression of the gland should be cultured. Vancomycin should be started while the results of cultures are awaited. Warm moist packs and mouth irrigations may be helpful. In most instances, the disease responds promptly to these measures. If the disease progresses, the parotid must be surgically drained. The procedure consists of elevating a skin flap over the gland and making multiple small incisions parallel to the branches of the facial nerve. The wound is then packed open.

COMPLICATIONS CAUSED BY POSTOPERATIVE ALTERATIONS OF GASTROINTESTINAL MOTILITY

The presence, strength, and direction of normal peristalsis are governed by the enteric nervous system. Anesthesia and surgical manipulation result in a decrease of the normal propulsive activity of the gut, or postoperative ileus. Several factors worsen ileus or prolong its course. These include medications—especially opioids—electrolyte abnormalities, inflammatory conditions such as pancreatitis or peritonitis, and pain. The degree of ileus is related to the extent of operative manipulation.

Gastrointestinal peristalsis returns within 24 hours after most operations that do not involve the abdominal cavity. In general, laparoscopic approaches cause less ileus than open procedures. After laparotomy, gastric peristalsis returns in about 48 hours. Colonic activity returns after 48 hours, starting at the cecum and progressing caudally. The motility of the small intestine is affected to a lesser degree, except in patients who have had small bowel resection or who were operated on to relieve bowel obstruction. Normal postoperative ileus leads to slight abdominal distention and absent bowel sounds. Return of peristalsis is often noted by the patient as mild cramps, passage of flatus, and return of appetite. Feedings should be withheld until there is evidence of return of normal gastrointestinal motility. There is no specific therapy for postoperative ileus.

► Gastric Dilation

Gastric dilation, a rare life-threatening complication, consists of massive distention of the stomach by gas and fluid. Predisposing factors include asthma, recent surgery, gastric outlet obstruction, and absence of the spleen. Infants and children in whom oxygen masks are used in the immediate postoperative period and adults subjected to forceful assisted respiration during resuscitation are also at risk. Occasionally, gastric dilation develops in patients with anorexia nervosa or during serious illnesses without a specific intercurrent event.

As the air-filled stomach grows larger, it hangs down across the duodenum, producing a mechanical gastric outlet obstruction that contributes further to the problem. The increased intragastric pressure produces venous obstruction of the mucosa, causing mucosal engorgement and bleeding and, if allowed to continue, ischemic necrosis and perforation. The distended stomach pushes the diaphragm upward, which causes collapse of the lower lobe of the left lung, rotation of the heart, and obstruction of the inferior vena cava. The acutely dilated stomach is also prone to undergo volvulus.

The patient appears ill, with abdominal distention and hiccup. Hypochloremia, hypokalemia, and alkalosis may result from fluid and electrolyte losses. When the problem is recognized early, treatment consists of gastric decompression with a nasogastric tube. In the late stage, gastric necrosis may require gastrectomy.

► Bowel Obstruction

Failure of postoperative return of bowel function may be the result of paralytic ileus or mechanical obstruction. Mechanical obstruction is most often caused by postoperative adhesions or an internal (mesenteric) hernia. Most of these patients experience a short period of apparently normal intestinal function before manifestations of obstruction supervene. About half of cases of early postoperative small bowel obstruction follow colorectal surgery.

Diagnosis may be difficult because the symptoms are difficult to differentiate from those of paralytic ileus. If plain films of the abdomen show air-fluid levels in loops of small bowel, mechanical obstruction is a more likely diagnosis than ileus. Enteroclysis or an ordinary small bowel series with barium sulfate may aid diagnosis.

Strangulation is uncommon because the adhesive bands are broader and less rigid than is typical of late small bowel obstruction. The death rate is high (about 15%), however, probably because of delay in diagnosis and the postoperative state. Treatment consists of nasogastric suction for several days and, if the obstruction does not resolve spontaneously, laparotomy.

Small bowel intussusception is an uncommon cause of early postoperative obstruction in adults but accounts for 10% of cases in the pediatric age group. Ninety percent of postoperative intussusceptions occur during the first 2 postoperative weeks, and more than half in the first week. Unlike idiopathic ileocolic intussusception, most postoperative intussusceptions are ileoileal or jejunojejunal. They most often follow retroperitoneal and pelvic operations. The cause is unknown. The symptom complex is not typical, and x-ray studies are of limited help. The physician should be aware that intussusception is a possible explanation for vomiting, distention, and abdominal pain after laparotomy in children and that early reoperation will avoid the complications of perforation and peritonitis. Operation is the only treatment, and if the bowel is viable, reduction of the intussusception is all that is needed.

Postoperative Fecal Impaction

Fecal impaction after operative procedures is the result of colonic ileus and impaired perception of rectal fullness. It is principally a disease of the elderly but may occur in younger patients who have predisposing conditions such as megacolon or paraplegia. Postoperative ileus and the use of opioid analgesics and anticholinergic drugs are aggravating factors. Early manifestations are anorexia and obstipation or diarrhea. In advanced cases, marked distention may cause colonic perforation. The diagnosis of postoperative fecal impaction is made by rectal examination. The impaction should be manually removed, enemas given, and digital examination then repeated.

Barium remaining in the colon from an examination done before surgery may harden and produce barium impaction. This usually occurs in the right colon, where most of the water is absorbed, and is a more difficult management problem than fecal impaction. The clinical manifestations are those of bowel obstruction. Treatment includes enemas and purgation with polyethylene glycol-electrolyte solution (eg, CoLyte, GoLYTELY). Diatrizoate sodium (Hypaque), a hyperosmolar solution that stimulates peristalsis and increases intraluminal fluid, may be effective by enema if other solutions fail. Operation is rarely needed.

POSTOPERATIVE PANCREATITIS

Postoperative pancreatitis accounts for 10% of all cases of acute pancreatitis. It occurs in 1–3% of patients who have operations in the vicinity of the pancreas and with higher frequency after operations on the biliary tract. For example, pancreatitis occurs in about 1% of patients undergoing cholecystectomy and in 8% of patients undergoing common bile duct exploration. In the latter cases, it does not appear to be related to the performance of intraoperative cholangiograms or choledochoscopy. Postoperative pancreatitis after biliary surgery is worse in patients who have had biliary pancreatitis preoperatively. Pancreatitis occasionally occurs following cardiopulmonary bypass, parathyroid surgery, and renal transplantation. Postoperative pancreatitis is frequently of the necrotizing type. Infected pancreatic necrosis and other complications of pancreatitis develop with a frequency three to four times greater than in biliary and alcoholic pancreatitis. The reason postoperative pancreatitis is so severe is unknown, but the mortality rate is 30–40%.

The pathogenesis in most cases appears to be mechanical trauma to the pancreas or its blood supply. Nevertheless, manipulation, biopsy, and partial resection of the pancreas are usually well tolerated, so the reasons that some patients develop pancreatitis are unclear. Prevention of this complication includes careful handling of the pancreas and avoidance of forceful dilation of the choledochal sphincter or obstruction of the pancreatic duct. The 2% incidence of pancreatitis following renal transplantation is probably related to special risk factors such as use of corticosteroids or azathioprine, secondary hyperparathyroidism, or viral infection. Acute changes in serum calcium are thought to be responsible for pancreatitis following parathyroid surgery. Hyperamylasemia develops in about half of patients undergoing heart surgery with extracorporeal bypass, but clinical evidence of pancreatitis is present in only 5% of these patients.

The diagnosis of postoperative pancreatitis may be difficult in patients who have recently had an abdominal operation. Hyperamylasemia may or may not be present. One must be alert to renal and respiratory complications and the consequences of necrotizing or hemorrhagic pancreatitis. Because of the high frequency with which complications develop, frequent monitoring of the pancreas and retroperitoneum with CT scans is useful.

POSTOPERATIVE HEPATIC DYSFUNCTION

Hepatic dysfunction, ranging from mild jaundice to life-threatening hepatic failure, follows 1% of surgical procedures performed under general anesthesia. The incidence is greater following pancreatectomy, biliary bypass operations, and portacaval shunt. Postoperative hyperbilirubinemia may be categorized as prehepatic jaundice, hepatocellular insufficiency, and posthepatic obstruction (Table 5–1).

Prehepatic Jaundice

Prehepatic jaundice is caused by bilirubin overload, most often from hemolysis or reabsorption of hematomas. Fasting, malnutrition, hepatotoxic drugs, and anesthesia are among the factors that impair the ability of the liver to excrete increased loads of bilirubin in the postoperative period.

Increased hemolysis may result from transfusion of incompatible blood but more often reflects destruction of fragile transfused red blood cells. Other causes include extra-

Table 5–1. Causes of Postoperative Jaundice.

Prehepatic jaundice (bilirubin overload)
Hemolysis (drugs, transfusions, sickle cell crisis)
Reabsorption of hematomas
Hepatocellular insufficiency
Viral hepatitis
Drug-induced (anesthesia, others)
Ischemia (shock, hypoxia, low-output states)
Sepsis
Liver resection (loss of parenchyma)
Others (total parenteral nutrition, malnutrition)
Posthepatic obstruction (to bile flow)
Retained stones
Injury to ducts
Tumor (unrecognized or untreated)
Cholecystitis
Pancreatitis
Occlusion of biliary stents

corporeal circulation, congenital hemolytic disease (eg, sickle cell disease), and effects of drugs.

Hepatocellular Insufficiency

Hepatocellular insufficiency, the most common cause of postoperative jaundice, occurs as a consequence of hepatic cell necrosis, inflammation, or massive hepatic resection. Drugs, hypotension, hypoxia, and sepsis are among the injurious factors. Although posttransfusion hepatitis is usually observed much later, this complication may occur as early as the third postoperative week.

Benign postoperative intrahepatic cholestasis is a vague term used to denote jaundice following operations that often involve hypotension and multiple transfusions. Serum bilirubin ranges from 2 to 20 mg/dL and serum alkaline phosphatase is usually high, but the patient is afebrile and postoperative convalescence is otherwise smooth. The diagnosis is one of exclusion. Jaundice clears by the third postoperative week.

Hepatocellular damage occasionally occurs after intestinal bypass procedures for morbid obesity. Cholestatic jaundice may develop in patients receiving total parenteral nutrition.

Posthepatic Obstruction

Posthepatic obstruction can be caused by direct surgical injury to the bile ducts, retained common duct stones, tumor obstruction of the bile duct, or pancreatitis. Acute postoperative cholecystitis is associated with jaundice in one-third of cases, though mechanical obstruction of the common duct is usually not apparent.

One must determine if a patient with postoperative jaundice has a correctable cause that requires treatment. This is particularly true for sepsis (when decreased liver function may sometimes be an early sign), lesions that obstruct the bile duct, and postoperative cholecystitis. Liver function tests are not helpful in determining the cause and do not usually reflect the severity of disease. Liver biopsy, ultrasound and CT scans, and transhepatic or endoscopic retrograde cholangiograms are the tests most likely to sort out the diagnostic possibilities. Renal function must be monitored closely, since renal failure may develop in these patients. Treatment is otherwise expectant.

POSTOPERATIVE CHOLECYSTITIS

Acute postoperative cholecystitis may follow any kind of operation but is more common after gastrointestinal procedures. Acute cholecystitis develops shortly after endoscopic sphincterotomy in 3–5% of patients. Chemical cholecystitis occurs in patients undergoing hepatic arterial chemotherapy with mitomycin and floxuridine with such frequency that cholecystectomy should always be performed before infusion of these agents is begun. Fulminant cholecystitis with gallbladder infarction may follow percutaneous embolization of the hepatic artery for malignant tumors of the liver or for arteriovenous malformation involving this artery.

Postoperative cholecystitis differs in several respects from the common form of acute cholecystitis: It is frequently acalculous (70–80%), more common in males (75%), progresses rapidly to gallbladder necrosis, and is not likely to respond to conservative therapy. The cause is clear in cases of chemical or ischemic cholecystitis but not in other forms. Factors thought to play a role include biliary stasis (with formation of sludge), biliary infection, and ischemia.

CLOSTRIDIUM DIFFICILE COLITIS

Postoperative diarrhea due to *Clostridium difficile* is a common nosocomial infection in surgical patients. The spectrum of illness ranges from asymptomatic colonization to—rarely—severe toxic colitis. Transmission from hospital personnel probably occurs. The main risk factor is perioperative antibiotic use. The diagnosis is established by identification of a specific cytopathic toxin in the stool or culture of the organism from stool samples or rectal swabs. In severely affected patients, colonoscopy reveals pseudomembranes. Prevention is accomplished by strict handwashing, enteric precautions, and minimizing antibiotic use. Treatment of established infection is with intravenous metronidazole or, for infections with resistant pathogens, oral vancomycin.

URINARY COMPLICATIONS

Postoperative Urinary Retention

Inability to void postoperatively is common, especially after pelvic and perineal operations or operations conducted under spinal anesthesia. Factors responsible for postoperative urinary retention are interference with the neural mechanisms responsible for normal emptying of the bladder and overdistention of the urinary bladder. When its normal capacity of approximately 500 mL is exceeded, bladder contraction is inhibited. Prophylactic bladder catheterization should be performed whenever an operation is likely to last 3 hours or longer or when large volumes of intravenous fluids are anticipated. The catheter can be removed at the end of the operation if the patient is expected to be able to ambulate within a few hours. When bladder catheterization is not performed, the patient should be encouraged to void immediately before coming to the operating room and as soon as possible after the operation. During abdominoperineal resection, operative trauma to the sacral plexus alters bladder function enough so that an indwelling catheter should be left in place for 4–5 days. Patients with inguinal hernia who strain to void as a manifestation of prostatic hypertrophy should have the prostate treated before the hernia.

The treatment of acute urinary retention is catheterization of the bladder. In the absence of factors that suggest the need for prolonged decompression, such as the presence of 1000 mL of urine or more, the catheter may be removed.

Urinary Tract Infection

Infection of the lower urinary tract is the most frequently acquired nosocomial infection. Preexisting contamination of the urinary tract, urinary retention, and instrumentation are the principal contributing factors. Bacteriuria is present in about 5% of patients who undergo short-term (< 48 hours) bladder catheterization, though clinical signs of urinary tract infection occur in only 1%. Cystitis is manifested by dysuria and mild fever and pyelonephritis by high fever, flank tenderness, and occasionally ileus. Diagnosis is made by examination of the urine and confirmed by cultures. Prevention involves treating urinary tract contamination before surgery, prevention or prompt treatment of urinary retention, and careful instrumentation when needed. Treatment includes adequate hydration, proper drainage of the bladder, and specific antibiotics.

CENTRAL NERVOUS SYSTEM COMPLICATIONS

Postoperative Cerebrovascular Accidents

Postoperative cerebrovascular accidents are almost always the result of ischemic neural damage due to poor perfusion. They often occur in elderly patients with severe atherosclerosis who become hypotensive during or after surgery (from sepsis, bleeding, cardiac arrest, etc). Normal regulatory mechanisms of the cerebral vasculature can maintain blood flow over a wide range of blood pressures down to a mean pressure of about 55 mm Hg. Abrupt hypotension, however, is less well tolerated than a more gradual pressure change. Irreversible brain damage occurs after about 4 minutes of total ischemia.

Strokes occur in 1–3% of patients after carotid endarterectomy and other reconstructive operations of the extracranial portion of the carotid system. Embolization from atherosclerotic plaques, ischemia during carotid clamping, and postoperative thrombosis at the site of the arteriotomy or of an intimal flap are usually responsible. Aspirin, which inhibits platelet aggregation, may prevent immediate postoperative thrombosis.

Open heart surgery using extracorporeal circulation or deep cooling is also occasionally followed by stroke. The pathogenesis of stroke is thought to be related to hypoxemia, emboli, or poor perfusion. The presence of a carotid bruit preoperatively increases the risk of postoperative stroke after coronary bypass by a factor of 4. Previous stroke or transient ischemic attacks and postoperative atrial fibrillation also increase the risk. For patients undergoing noncardiac, noncarotid surgery, the risk of stroke is about 0.2%. Predictors of risk in these patients are the presence of cerebrovascular, cardiac, or peripheral vascular disease and arterial hypertension.

Seizures

Epilepsy, metabolic derangements, and medications may lead to seizures in the postoperative period. For unknown reasons, patients with ulcerative colitis and Crohn disease are peculiarly susceptible to seizures with loss of consciousness after surgery. Seizures should be treated as soon as possible to minimize their harmful effects.

PSYCHIATRIC COMPLICATIONS

Anxiety and fear are normal in patients undergoing surgery. The degree to which these emotions are experienced depends upon diverse cultural and psychologic variables. Underlying depression or a history of chronic pain may serve to exaggerate the patient's response to surgery. The boundary between the normal manifestations of stress and **postoperative psychosis** is difficult to establish, since the latter is not really a distinct clinical entity.

Postoperative psychosis (so-called) develops in about 0.5% of patients having abdominal operations. It is more common after thoracic surgery, in the elderly, and in those with chronic disease. About half of these patients suffer from mood disturbances (usually severe depression). Twenty percent have delirium. Drugs given in the postoperative period may play a role in the development of psychosis; meperidine, cimetidine, and corticosteroids are most commonly implicated. Patients who develop postoperative psychosis have higher plasma levels of β-endorphin and cortisol than those who do not. These patients also lose, temporarily, the normal circadian rhythms of β-endorphin and cortisol. Specific psychiatric syndromes may follow specific procedures, such as visual hallucinations and the "black patch syndrome" after ophthalmic surgery. Preexisting psychiatric disorders not apparent before the operation sometimes contribute to the motivation for surgery (eg, circumcision or cosmetic operations in schizophrenics).

Clinical manifestations are rare on the first postoperative day. During this period, patients appear emotionless and unconcerned about changes in the environment or in themselves. Most overt psychiatric derangements are observed after the third postoperative day. The symptoms are variable but often include confusion, fear, and disorientation as to time and place. Delirium presents as altered consciousness with cognitive impairment. These symptoms may not be readily apparent to the surgeon, as this problem usually occurs in sick patients whose other problems may mask the manifestations of psychosis. Early psychiatric consultation should be obtained when psychosis is suspected so that adequate and prompt assessment of consciousness and cognitive function can be done and treatment instituted. The earlier the psychosis is recognized, the easier it is to correct. Metabolic derangements or early sepsis (especially in burn patients) must be ruled out as the cause. Severe postoperative emotional disturbances may be avoided by appropriate preoperative counseling of the patient by the surgeon. This includes a thorough discussion of the operation and the expected outcome, acquainting the patient with the intensive care unit, etc. Postoperatively, the surgeon must attend to the patient's emotional needs, offering frequent reassurance, explaining the postoperative course, and discussing the prognosis and the outcome of the operation.

Special Psychiatric Problems

A. The ICU Syndrome

The continuous internal vigilance that results from pain and fear and the sleep deprivation from bright lights, monitoring equipment, and continuous noise cause a psychologic disorganization known as ICU psychosis. The patient whose level of consciousness is already decreased by illness and drugs is more susceptible than a normal individual, and the result is decreased ability to think, perceive, and remember. When the cognitive processes are thoroughly disorganized, delirium occurs. The manifestations include distorted visual, auditory, and tactile perception; confusion and restlessness; and inability to differentiate reality from fantasy. Prevention includes isolation from the environment, decreased noise levels, adequate sleep, and removal from the intensive care unit as soon as possible.

B. Postcardiotomy Delirium

Mental changes that occasionally follow open heart surgery include impairment of memory, attention, cognition, and perception and occasionally hysteria, depressive reaction, and anxiety crisis. The symptoms most often appear after the third postoperative day. The type of operation, the presence of organic brain disease, prolonged medical illness, and the length of time on extracorporeal circulation are related to the development of postcardiotomy psychosis. Mild sedation and measures to prevent the ICU syndrome may prevent this complication. In more severe cases, haloperidol (Haldol) in doses of 1–5 mg given orally, intramuscularly, or intravenously may be required. Haloperidol is preferred over phenothiazines in these patients because it is associated with a lower incidence of cardiovascular side effects.

C. Delirium Tremens

Delirium tremens occurs in alcoholics who stop drinking suddenly. Hyperventilation and metabolic alkalosis contribute to the development of the full-blown syndrome. Hypomagnesemia and hypokalemia secondary to alkalosis or nutritional deficits may precipitate seizures. Readaptation to ethanol-free metabolism requires about 2 weeks, and it is during this period that alcoholics are at greatest risk of developing delirium tremens.

The prodrome includes personality changes, anxiety, and tremor. The complete syndrome is characterized by agitation, hallucinations, restlessness, confusion, overactivity, and occasionally seizures and hyperthermia. The syndrome also causes a hyperdynamic cardiorespiratory and metabolic state. For example, cardiac index, oxygen delivery, and oxygen consumption double during delirium tremens and

return to normal 24–48 hours after resolution. The wild behavior may precipitate dehiscence of a fresh laparotomy incision. Diaphoresis and dehydration are common, and exhaustion may herald death.

Withdrawal symptoms may be prevented by giving small amounts of alcohol, but benzodiazepines are the treatment of choice. Vitamin B_1 (thiamine) and magnesium sulfate should also be given.

The aims of treatment are to reduce agitation and anxiety as soon as possible and to prevent the development of other complications (eg, seizures, aspiration pneumonia). General measures should include frequent assessment of vital signs, restoration of nutrition, administration of vitamin B, correction of electrolyte imbalance or other metabolic derangements, and adequate hydration. Physical restraint, though necessary for seriously violent behavior, should be as limited as possible. With proper care, most patients improve within 72 hours.

D. Sexual Dysfunction

Sexual problems commonly occur after certain kinds of operations, such as prostatectomy, heart surgery, and aortic reconstruction. The pathogenesis can be due to injury to nerves necessary for sexual function, though in other cases the etiology is unclear. In abdominoperineal resection, severance of the peripheral branches of the sacral plexus may cause impotence. It is important to discuss this possibility with the patient before any operation with a risk of impotence is performed. When sexual dysfunction is psychogenic, reassurance is usually all that is needed. If impotence persists beyond 4–6 weeks, appropriate consultation is indicated.

COMPLICATIONS OF INTRAVENOUS THERAPY & HEMODYNAMIC MONITORING

Air Embolism

Air embolism may occur during or after insertion of a venous catheter or as a result of accidental introduction of air into the line. Intravenous air lodges in the right atrium, preventing adequate filling of the right heart. This is manifested by hypotension, jugular venous distention, and tachycardia. This complication can be avoided by placing the patient in the Trendelenburg position when a central venous line is inserted. Emergency treatment consists of aspiration of the air with a syringe. If this is unsuccessful, the patient should be positioned right side up and head down, which will help dislodge the air from the right atrium and return circulatory dynamics to normal.

Phlebitis

A needle or a catheter inserted into a vein and left in place will in time cause inflammation at the entry site. When this process involves the vein, it is called phlebitis. Factors determining the degree of inflammation are the nature of the cannula, the solution infused, bacterial infection, and venous thrombosis. Phlebitis is one of the most common causes of fever after the third postoperative day. The symptomatic triad of induration, edema, and tenderness is characteristic. Visible signs may be minimal. Prevention of phlebitis is best accomplished by observance of aseptic techniques during insertion of venous catheters, frequent change of tubing (ie, every 48–72 hours), and rotation of insertion sites (ie, every 4 days). Silastic catheters, which are the least reactive, should be used when the line must be left in for a long time. Hypertonic solutions should be infused only into veins with substantial flow, such as the subclavian, jugular, or vena cava. Venous catheters should be removed at the first sign of redness, induration, or edema. Because phlebitis is most frequent with cannulation of veins in the lower extremities, this route should be used only when upper extremity veins are unavailable. Removal of the catheter is adequate treatment.

Suppurative phlebitis may result from the presence of an infected thrombus around the indwelling catheter. Staphylococci are the most common causative organisms. Local signs of inflammation are present, and pus may be expressed from the venipuncture site. High fever and positive blood cultures are common. Treatment consists of excising the affected vein, extending the incision proximally to the first open collateral, and leaving the wound open.

▶ Cardiopulmonary Complications

Perforation of the right atrium with cardiac tamponade has been associated with the use of central venous lines. This complication can be avoided by checking the position of the tip of the line, which should be in the superior vena cava, not the right atrium. Complications associated with the use of the flow-directed balloon-tipped (Swan-Ganz) catheter include cardiac perforation (usually of the right atrium), intracardiac knotting of the catheter, and cardiac dysrhythmias. Pulmonary hemorrhage may result from disruption of a branch of the pulmonary artery during balloon inflation and may be fatal in patients with pulmonary hypertension. Steps in prevention include careful placement, advancement under continuous pressure monitoring, and checking the position of the tip before inflating the balloon.

▶ Ischemic Necrosis of the Finger

Continuous monitoring of arterial blood pressure during the operation and in the intensive care unit requires insertion of a radial or femoral arterial line. The hand receives its blood supply from the radial and ulnar arteries, and because of the anatomy of the palmar arches, patency of one of these vessels is usually enough to provide adequate blood flow through the hand. Occasionally, ischemic necrosis of the finger has followed use of an indwelling catheter in the radial artery. This serious complication may be avoided by evaluating the patency of the ulnar artery (Allen test) before establishing

the radial line and by changing arterial line sites every 3–4 days. After an arterial catheter is withdrawn, a pressure dressing should be applied to avoid formation of an arterial pseudoaneurysm.

POSTOPERATIVE FEVER

Fever occurs in about 40% of patients after major surgery. In most patients the temperature elevation resolves without specific treatment. However, postoperative fever may herald a serious infection, and it is therefore important to evaluate the patient clinically. Features often associated with an infectious origin of the fever include preoperative trauma, ASA class above 2, fever onset after the second postoperative day, an initial temperature elevation above 38.6 °C, a postoperative white blood cell count greater than 10,000/μL, and a postoperative serum urea nitrogen of 15 mg/dL or greater. If three or more of the above are present, the likelihood of associated bacterial infection is nearly 100%.

Fever within 48 hours after surgery is usually caused by atelectasis. Reexpansion of the lung causes body temperature to return to normal. Because laboratory and radiologic investigations are usually unrevealing, an extensive evaluation of early postoperative fever is rarely appropriate if the patient's convalescence is otherwise smooth.

When fever appears after the second postoperative day, atelectasis is a less likely explanation. The differential diagnosis of fever at this time includes catheter-related phlebitis, pneumonia, and urinary tract infection. A directed history and physical examination complemented by focused laboratory and radiologic studies usually determine the cause.

Patients without infection are rarely febrile after the fifth postoperative day. Fever this late suggests wound infection or, less often, anastomotic breakdown and intra-abdominal abscesses. A diagnostic workup directed to the detection of intra-abdominal sepsis is indicated in patients who have high temperatures (> 39 °C) and wounds without evidence of infection 5 or more days postoperatively. CT scan of the abdomen and pelvis is the test of choice and should be performed early, before overt organ failure occurs.

Fever is rare after the first week in patients who had a normal convalescence. Allergy to drugs, transfusion-related fever, septic pelvic vein thrombosis, and intra-abdominal abscesses should be considered.

Biscione FM et al: Factors influencing the risk of surgical site infection following diagnostic exploration of the abdominal cavity. J Infect 2007;55:317.

Fleisher LA et al: ACC/AHA 2007 guidelines on perioperative cardiovascular evaluation and care for noncardiac surgery: a report of the American College of Cardiology/American Heart Association Task Force on Practice Guidelines. J Am Coll Cardiol 2007;50:e159.

Moller AM et al: Effect of preoperative smoking intervention on postoperative complications: a randomised clinical trial. Lancet 2002;359:114.

National Nosocomial Infection Surveillance (NNIS) System Report, data summary from January 1992 through June 2004, issued October 2004. Available at: http://www.cdc.gov/ncidod/dhqp/pdf/nnis/2004NNISreport.pdf. Accessed November 15, 2008.

Rabinowitz RP, Caplan ES: Management of infections in the trauma patient. Surg Clin North Am 1999;79:1373.

Sitges-Serra A, Girvent M: Catheter-related bloodstream infections. World J Surg 1999;23:589.

van 't Riet M et al: Meta-analysis of techniques for closure of midline abdominal incisions. Br J Surg 2002;89:1350.

Wound Healing

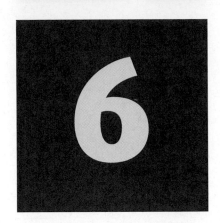

Michael G. Franz, MD

ESSENTIALS OF DIAGNOSIS

▶ Types of Wounds
  • Acute wound
  • Chronic wound

Acute Wound

An acute wound results from the sudden loss of anatomic structure in tissue following the transfer of kinetic, chemical, or thermal energy. Functionally, an acute wound should pass predictably through the phases of wound healing to result in complete and sustained repair. Acute wounds typically occur in recently uninjured and otherwise normal tissue. Acute wound healing is timely and reliable, completing the entire process within 6–12 weeks. Most surgical wounds are acute wounds.

▶ Chronic Wound

Wound healing fails in a chronic wound. The process of tissue repair is prolonged and pathologic. The usual mechanism is dysregulation of one of the phases of normal acute wound healing. Most often, healing arrest occurs in an inflammatory phase. This prolonged inflammatory phase may be due to wound infection or another form of chronic irritation. Tissue and wound hypoxia is the other important mechanism for the development of a chronic wound. Failed epithelialization due to repeat trauma or desiccation may also result in a chronic partial thickness wound. Surgeons may sharply convert a chronic wound into an acute wound.

GENERAL CONSIDERATIONS

▶ Clinical Wound Healing

Surgeons often describe wound healing as primary or secondary. **Primary healing** occurs when tissue is cleanly incised and anatomically reapproximated. It is also referred to as healing by primary intention, and tissue repair usually proceeds without complication. **Secondary healing** occurs in wounds left open through the formation of granulation tissue and eventual coverage of the defect by migration of epithelial cells. Granulation tissue is composed of new capillaries, fibroblasts, and a provisional extracellular matrix that forms at the base of the early wound. This process is also referred to as healing by secondary intention. Most infected wounds and burns heal in this manner. Primary healing is simpler and requires less time and tissue synthesis than secondary healing. A wound healing primarily repairs a smaller volume than an open wound healing secondarily. The principles of primary and secondary healing are combined in **delayed primary closure,** when a wound is left open to heal under a carefully maintained, moist wound healing environment for approximately 5 days and is then closed as if primarily. Wounds treated with delayed primary closure are less likely to become infected than if closed immediately because bacterial balance is achieved and oxygen requirements are optimized through capillary formation in the granulation tissue.

▶ The Mechanism of Wound Healing

The complex process of wound healing normally proceeds from coagulation and inflammation through fibroplasia, matrix deposition, angiogenesis, epithelialization, collagen maturation, and finally wound contraction (Figure 6–1). Wound healing signals include peptide growth factors, complement, cytokine inflammatory mediators, and metabolic signals such as hypoxia and accumulated lactate. Many of these cellular signaling pathways are redundant and pleiotropic.

Hemostasis and Inflammation

Following injury, a wound must stop bleeding in order to heal and for the injured host to survive. It is therefore not surprising that cellular and molecular elements involved in hemostasis also signal tissue repair. Immediately after injury,

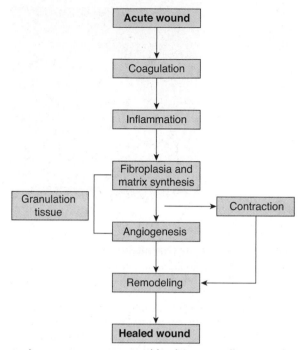

```
          Acute wound
               │
               ▼
          Coagulation
               │
               ▼
          Inflammation
               │
               ▼
      Fibroplasia and
      matrix synthesis
               │
  Granulation  │          Contraction
    tissue     │              ▲
               ▼              │
          Angiogenesis ───────┘
               │
               ▼
          Remodeling ◄──────
               │
               ▼
          Healed wound
```

▲ **Figure 6–1.** Acute wound healing normally proceeds from coagulation and inflammation, through angiogenesis, fibroplasia, matrix deposition (granulation tissue formation), collagen maturation, epithelialization, and finally wound contraction. A chronic wound fails to heal anywhere along this wound healing pathway.

the coagulation products fibrin, fibrinopeptides, thrombin split products, and complement components attract inflammatory cells into the wound. Platelets activated by thrombin release insulinlike growth factor 1 (IGF-1), transforming growth factor α (TGF-α), transforming growth factor β (TGF-β), and platelet-derived growth factor (PDGF), which attract leukocytes, particularly macrophages, and fibroblasts into the wound. Damaged endothelial cells respond to a signal cascade involving the complement products C5a, tumor necrosis factor α (TNF-α), interleukin-1 (IL-1), and interleukin-8 (IL-8) and express receptors for integrin molecules on the cell membranes of leukocytes. Circulating leukocytes then adhere to the endothelium and migrate into the wounded tissue. Interleukins and other inflammatory components, such as histamine, serotonin, and bradykinin, cause vessels first to constrict for hemostasis and later to dilate, becoming porous so that blood plasma and leukocytes can migrate into the injured area.

The very early wound inflammatory cells increase metabolic demand. Since the local microvasculature is damaged, a local energy sink results, and PaO_2 falls while CO_2 accumulates. Lactate in particular plays a critical role, since its source is mainly aerobic, and its level is tightly regulated by tissue

oxygen levels. Oxidative stress is an important signal for tissue repair. These conditions trigger reparative processes and stimulate their propagation.

Macrophages assume a dominant role in the synthesis of wound healing molecules as coagulation-mediated tissue repair signals fall. Importantly, macrophages, stimulated by fibrin, continue to release large quantities of lactate. This process continues even as oxygen levels begin to rise, thereby maintaining the "environment of injury." Lactate alone stimulates angiogenesis and collagen deposition through the sustained production of growth factors. Unless the wound becomes infected, the granulocyte population that dominated the first days diminishes. Macrophages now cover the injured surface. Fibroblasts begin to organize, mixed with buds of new blood vessels. It has been shown that circulating stem cells, such as bone marrow–derived mesenchymal stem cells, contribute fibroblasts to the healing wound, but the extent of this process is as yet unknown.

Fibroplasia and Matrix Synthesis

Fibroplasia—Throughout wound healing, fibroplasia (the replication of fibroblasts) is stimulated by multiple mechanisms, starting with PDGF, IGF-1, and TGF-β released by platelets and later by the continual release of numerous peptide growth factors from macrophages and even fibroblasts within the wound. Growth factors and cytokines shown to stimulate fibroplasia and wound healing include fibroblast growth factor (FGF), IGF-1, vascular endothelial growth factor (VEGF), IL-1, IL-2, IL-8, PDGF, TGF-α, TGF-β, and TNF-α. Dividing fibroblasts localize near the wound edge, an active tissue repair environment with tissue oxygen tensions of approximately 40 mm Hg in normally healing wounds. In cell culture, this PaO_2 is optimum for fibroblast replication. Smooth muscle cells are also likely progenitors because fibroblasts seem to migrate from the adventitia and media of wound vessels. Lipocytes, pericytes, and other cell sources may exist for terminal differentiation into repair fibroblasts.

Matrix synthesis—Fibroblasts secrete the collagen and proteoglycans of the connective tissue matrix that hold wound edges together and embed cells of the healing wound matrix. These extracellular molecules assume polymeric forms and become the physical basis of wound strength (Figure 6–2). Collagen synthesis is not a constitutive property of fibroblasts but must be signaled. The mechanisms that regulate the stimulation and synthesis of collagen are multifactorial and include both growth factors and metabolic inputs such as lactate. The collagen gene promoter has regulatory binding sites to stress corticoids, the TGF-β signaling pathway, and retinoids, which control collagen gene expression. Other growth factors regulate glycosaminoglycans, tissue inhibitors of metalloproteinase (TIMP), and fibronectin synthesis. The accumulation of lactate in the extracellular environment is shown to directly stimulate transcription of collagen genes as well as posttranslational processing of collagen peptides. It is

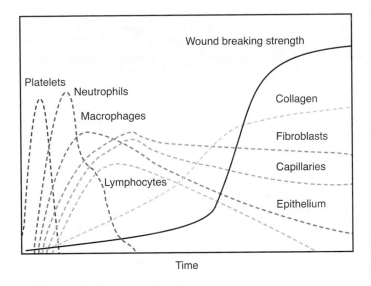

▲ Figure 6–2. The fundamental cellular and molecular elements activated during normal wound healing.

clear that the redox state and energy stores of repair cells occupying the wound regulate collagen synthesis.

The increase in collagen messenger RNA (mRNA) leads to an increased procollagen peptide. This, however, is not sufficient to increase collagen deposition because procollagen peptide cannot be transported from the cell to the extracellular space until, in a posttranslational step, a proportion of its proline amino acids are hydroxylated. In this reaction, catalyzed by prolyl hydroxylase, an oxygen atom derived from dissolved O_2 is inserted (as a hydroxyl group) into selected collagen prolines in the presence of the cofactors ascorbic acid, iron, and α-ketoglutarate. Thus, accumulation of lactate, or any other process that decreases the nicotinamide adenine dinucleotide (NAD^+) pool, leads to production of collagen mRNAs, increased collagen peptide synthesis, and (provided enough ascorbate and oxygen is present) increased posttranslational modification and secretion of collagen monomers into the extracellular space.

Another enzyme, lysyl hydroxylase, hydroxylates many of the procollagen lysines. A lysyl-to-lysyl covalent link then occurs between collagen molecules, maximizing mature collagen fiber strength. This process, too, requires adequate amounts of ascorbate and oxygen. These oxygenase reactions (and therefore collagen deposition) are rate limited by tissue oxygen level, PaO_2. The rates are half-maximal at about 20 mm Hg and maximal at about 200 mm Hg. Hydroxylation can be "forced" to supernormal rates by tissue hyperoxia. Collagen deposition, wound strength, and angiogenesis rates may be increased and accelerated as tissue PaO_2 is elevated.

Angiogenesis

Angiogenesis is required for wound healing. It is clinically evident about 4 days following injury but begins earlier when new capillaries sprout from preexisting venules and grow toward the injury in response to chemoattractants released by platelets and macrophages. In primarily closed wounds, budding vessels soon meet and fuse with counterparts migrating from the other side of the wound, establishing blood flow across the wound. In wounds left open, newly forming capillaries connect with adjacent capillaries migrating in the same direction, and granulation tissue forms. Numerous growth factors and cytokines are observed to stimulate angiogenesis, but animal experiments indicate that the dominant angiogenic stimulants in wounds are derived first from platelets in response to coagulation and then from macrophages in response to hypoxia or high lactate, fibrin and its products.

Epithelialization

Epithelial cells respond to several of the same stimuli as fibroblasts and endothelial cells within the mesenchymal area of a wound. A variety of growth factors also regulate epithelial cell replication. TGF-α and keratinocyte growth factor (KGF), for instance, are potent epithelial cell mitogens. TGF-β tends to inhibit epithelial cells from differentiating and thus may potentiate and perpetuate mitogenesis, though it is itself not a mitogen for these cells. During wound healing, mitoses appear in the epithelium a few cells away from the wound edge. The new cells migrate over the cells at the edge and into the unhealed area and anchor to the first unepithelialized matrix position encountered. The PaO_2 on the underside of the cell at the anchor point is usually low. Low PaO_2 stimulates squamous epithelial cells to produce TGF-β, likely suppressing terminal differentiation and again supporting further mitosis. This process of epidermal-mesenchymal communication repeats itself until the wound is closed.

Squamous epithelialization and differentiation proceed maximally when surface wounds are kept moist. It is clear that even short periods of drying impairs the process, and therefore wounds should not be allowed to desiccate. The exudates from acute, uninfected superficial wounds also contain growth factors and lactate and therefore recapitulate the growth environment found at the base of the wound.

Collagen Fiber Remodeling and Wound Contraction

Remodeling of the wound extracellular matrix is also a well-regulated process. First, fibroblasts replace the provisional fibrin matrix with collagen monomers. Extracellular enzymes, some of which are PaO_2-dependent, quickly polymerize these monomers, initially in a pattern that is more random than in uninjured tissue, predisposing early wound to mechanical failure. Progressively, the very early provisional matrix is replaced with a more mature one by forming larger, better organized, stronger, and more durable collagen fibers. The very early wound provisional matrix usually mechanically fails within the matrix itself (days 0–5). Next, mechanical failure occurs at the matrix-tissue interface or fusion point (Figure 6–3). The mechanism for connecting the wound matrix to the uninjured tissue border is poorly understood.

Reorganization of the new matrix is an important feature of healing, and fibroblasts and leukocytes secrete collagenases that ensure the lytic component. Turnover occurs rapidly at first and then more slowly. Even in simple wounds, wound matrix turnover can be detected chemically for as long as 18 months. Healing is successful when a net excess of matrix is deposited despite concomitant lysis. Lysis, in contrast to anabolic synthesis, is less dependent upon energy and nutrition. If synthesis is impaired, however, lysis weakens wounds.

During rapid turnover, wounds normally gain strength and durability but are vulnerable to contraction or stretching. Fibroblasts exert the force for contraction. Fibroblasts attach to collagen and each other and pull the collagen network together when the cell membranes shorten as the fibroblasts migrate. The wound myofibroblast, a specialized phenotype, expresses intracellular actin filaments that also contribute force to fibroblast-mediated wound contraction. The collagen fibers are then fixed in the packed positions by a variety of cross-linking mechanisms. Both open and closed wounds tend to contract if not subjected to a superior counterforce. The phenomenon is best seen in surface wounds, which may close 90% or more by contraction alone in loose skin. For example, the residual of a large open wound on the back of the neck may be only a small area of epithelialization. On the back, the buttock, or the neck, this is often a beneficial process, whereas in the face and around joints, the results may be disabling or disfiguring. Pathological wound contraction is usually termed a contracture or a stricture. Skin grafts, especially thick ones, may minimize or prevent disabling wound contractures. Dynamic splints, passive or active stretching, or insertion of flaps containing dermis and subdermis also counteract contraction. Prevention of a stricture often depends on ensuring that opposing tissue edges are well perfused so that healing can proceed

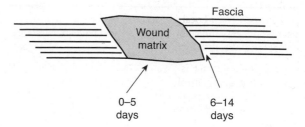

▲ **Figure 6–3.** The very early wound matrix is weak and susceptible to mechanical failure, especially in load-bearing tissues like the abdominal wall. After 5 days, mechanical failure occurs at the interface of the wound matrix and the uninjured surrounding tissue.

quickly to completion and contraction stops. Healing wounds may also stretch during active turnover when tension overcomes contraction. This may account for the laxity of scars in ligaments of injured but unsplinted joints and the tendency for incisional hernia formation in abdominal wounds of obese patients.

Healing of Specialized Tissues

Tissue other than skin heals generally by the same fundamental pathways. Although tissue structure may be specialized, the initial repair processes are shared. It does appear that the rate and efficiency of wound healing in different tissue types depends in large part on total collagen content, collagen organization, and blood supply.

Gastrointestinal tract—The rate of repair varies from one part of the intestine to the other in proportion to blood supply. Anastomoses of the colon and esophagus heal least reliably and are most likely to leak, whereas failure of stomach or small intestine anastomoses is rare. Intestinal anastomoses regain strength rapidly when compared to skin wounds. After 1 week, bursting strength may exceed the uninjured surrounding intestine. However, the surrounding intestine also participates in the reaction to injury, initially losing collagen by lysis, and as a result may lose strength. For this reason, leakage can occur a few millimeters from the anastomosis. A tight suture line causing ischemia will exacerbate this surgical problem.

The mesothelial cell lining of the peritoneum also is important for healing in the abdomen and GI tract. The esophagus and retroperitoneal colon lack a serosal mesothelial lining, which may contribute to failed wound healing. There is evidence that mesothelial cells signal the repair of peritoneal linings and are a source of repair cells.

Comorbidities that delay collagen synthesis or stimulate collagen lysis are likely to increase the risk of perforation and leakage. The danger of leakage is greatest from the fourth to seventh days, when tensile strength normally would rise rapidly but may be impeded by impaired collagen deposition or increased lysis. Local infection, which most often occurs near esophageal and colonic anastomoses, promotes lysis and delays synthesis, thus increasing the likelihood of perforation.

Bone—Bone healing is controlled by many of the same mechanisms that control soft tissue healing. It too occurs in predictable, morphologic stages: inflammation, fibroplasia, and remodeling. The duration of each stage varies depending on the location and extent of the fracture.

Injury (fracture) causes hematoma formation from the damaged blood vessels of the periosteum, endosteum, and surrounding tissues. Within hours, an inflammatory infiltrate of neutrophils and macrophages is recruited into the hematoma as in soft tissue injuries. Monocytes and granulocytes debride and digest necrotic tissue and debris, including bone, on the fracture surface. This process continues for days to weeks depending on the amount of necrotic tissue. As inflammation progresses to fibroplasia, the hematoma is progressively replaced by granulation tissue that can form bone. This bone wound tissue, known as callus, develops from both sides of the fracture and is composed of fibroblasts, endothelial cells, and bone-forming cells (chondroblasts, osteoblasts). As macrophages (osteoclasts) phagocytose the hematoma and injured tissue, fibroblasts (osteocytes) deposit a collagenous matrix, and chondroblasts deposit proteoglycans in a process called enchondral bone formation. This step, prominent in some bones, is then converted to bone as osteoblasts condense hydroxyapatite crystals at specific points on the collagen fibers. Endothelial cells form a vasculature structure characteristic of uninjured bone. Eventually the fibrovascular callus is completely replaced by new bone. Unlike healing of soft tissue, bone healing has features of regeneration, and bone often heals without leaving a scar.

Bone healing also depends on blood supply. Following injury, the ends of fractured bone are avascular. Osteocyte and blood vessel lacunae become vacant for several millimeters from the fracture. New blood vessels must sprout from preexisting ones and migrate into the area of injury. As new blood vessels cross the bone ends, they are preceded by osteoclasts just as macrophages precede them in soft tissue repair. In bone, this unit is called the cutting cone because it bores its way through bone in the process of connecting with other vessels. Excessive movement of the bone ends during this revascularization stage will break the delicate new vessels and delay healing. Osteomyelitis originates most often in ischemic bone fragments. Hyperoxygenation optimizes fracture healing and aids in the cure (and potentially the prevention) of osteomyelitis. Acute or chronic hypoxia slows bone repair.

Bone repair may occur through primary or secondary intention. Primary repair can occur only when the fracture is stable and aligned and its surfaces closely apposed. This is the goal of rigid plate fixation or rod fixation of fractures. When these conditions are met, capillaries can grow across the fracture and rapidly reestablish a vascular supply. Little or no callus forms. Secondary repair with callus formation is more common. Once the fracture has been bridged, the new bone remodels in response to the mechanical stresses upon it, with restoration to normal or near-normal strength. During this process, as in soft tissue, preexisting bone and its vascular network are simultaneously removed and replaced. Increased bone turnover may be detected as long as 10 years after injury. Although remodeling is efficient, it cannot correct deformities of angulation or rotation in misaligned fractures. Careful fracture reduction is still important.

Bone repair can be manipulated. Electrical stimulation, growth factors, and distraction osteogenesis are three tools for this purpose. Electrical currents applied directly (through implanted electrodes) or induced by external alternating electromagnetic fields accelerate repair by inducing new bone formation in much the same way as small piezoelectric currents produced by mechanical deformation of intact bone controls remodeling along lines of stress. Electrical stimulation has been used successfully to treat nonunion of bone (where new bone formation between bone ends fails, often requiring long periods of bed rest). Bone morphogenetic protein (BMP)-impregnated implants have accelerated bone healing in animals and have been used with encouraging results to treat large bony defects and nonunions, including during spinal fusion.

The **Ilizarov technique,** linear distraction osteogenesis, can lengthen bones, stimulate bone growth across a defect, or correct defects of angulation. The Ilizarov device is an external fixator attached to the bones through metal pins or wires. A surgical break is created and then slowly pulled apart (1 mm/d) or slowly reangulated. The vascular supply and subsequent new bone formation migrate along with the moving segment of bone.

Franz MG et al: The use of the wound healing trajectory as an outcome determinant for acute wound healing. Wound Repair Regen 2001;8:511.

Robson MC et al: Wound healing: biology and approaches to maximize healing trajectories. Curr Probl Surg 2001;38:61.

PATHOGENESIS

▶ Effect of Tissue Hypoxia

Impaired perfusion and inadequate oxygenation are the most frequent causes of healing failure. Oxygen is required for successful inflammation, bactericidal activity, angiogenesis, epithelialization, and matrix (collagen) deposition. The critical collagen oxygenases involved have Km values for oxygen of about 20 mm Hg and maximums of about 200 mm Hg, meaning that reaction rates are regulated by PaO_2 and blood perfusion throughout the entire physiologic range. The PaO_2 of wound fluid in human incisions is about 30–40 mm Hg, suggesting that these enzymes normally function just beyond half capacity. Wound PaO_2 is depressed by hypovolemia, catecholamine infusion, stress, fear, or cold. Under ideal conditions, wound fluid PaO_2 can be raised above 100 mm Hg by improved perfusion and breathing of oxygen. Human healing is profoundly influenced by local blood supply, vasoconstriction, and all other factors that govern perfusion and blood oxygenation. Wounds in well vascularized tissues (e.g., head, anus) heal rapidly and are remarkably resistant to infection (Figure 6–4).

Dysregulated Inflammation during Impaired Wound Healing

Molecular growth signals and lytic enzymes released by inflammatory cells are necessary for repair. Inhibited or excessive inflammatory responses lead to wound complications. Failure to heal is common in patients taking anti-inflammatory corticosteroids, immune suppressants, or cancer chemotherapeutic agents that inhibit inflammatory cells. Open wounds are more effected than primarily repaired wounds. Anti-inflammatory drugs impair the wound less after the third day of healing, as the normal level of inflammation in wound healing is reduced. Inflammation may also be excessive. Increased wound inflammation (eg, in response to infection and endotoxin or foreign bodies like mesh implants during hernia repair) can stimulate inflammatory cells to produce cytolytic cytokines and excessive proteases with the consequence of pathologic lysis of newly formed tissue. A pathological cycle of wound healing may ensue and result in an impaired quantity and quality of wound scar.

Impaired Healing Due to Malnutrition

Malnutrition impairs healing, since healing depends on nucleic acid and protein synthesis, cell replication, specific organ function (liver, heart, lungs), and extracellular matrix production. Weight loss and protein depletion have been shown experimentally and clinically to be risk factors for poor healing. Deficient healing is seen mainly in patients with acute malnutrition (ie, in the weeks just before or after an injury or operation). Even a few days of starvation measurably impairs healing, and an equally short period of repletion can reverse the deficit. Wound complications increase in severe malnutrition. A period of preoperative corrective nutrition is generally helpful for patients who have recently lost 10% or more of their body weight.

Scar Formation versus Regeneration

In excessive healing or proliferative scarring, it is as if the equilibrium point between collagen deposition and collagen lysis is never reached. It is unclear why some wounds seem to continue in the dysregulated repair process. Upregulation of fibroplastic growth factors like TGF-β is implicated during hypertrophic or keloid scar formation. Because the mechanism of excessive scar formation is unknown, there is no universally accepted treatment regimen. In a recent meta-analysis of pathologic scar treatments, the mean amount of improvement to be expected was only 60%. Hypertrophic scars are generally self-limited, are related to residual inflam-

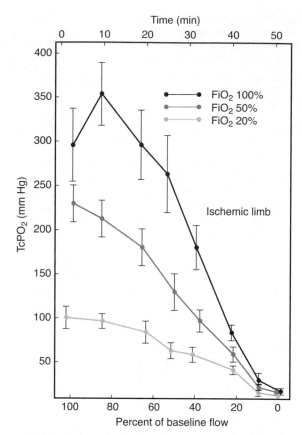

▲ **Figure 6–4.** Tissue oxygen concentration (TcPO$_2$) is a critical determinant of wound healing. Human healing is profoundly influenced by local blood supply, vasoconstriction, and all other factors that govern perfusion and blood oxygenation. Despite raising FiO$_2$ to 50% or 100%, the TcPO$_2$ remains in the ischemic range when flow is reduced to less than 25% of baseline. Supplementing the FiO$_2$ of oxygen will not benefit healing of ischemic ulcers. Flow must be increased to improve the TcPO$_2$.

mation, and may regress after a year or so. Keloids by definition extend beyond the borders of the wound and are most common in pigmented skin. The last areas of a burn to heal are the most often hypertrophic, possibly due to traction, reinjury, and tension. Immune mechanisms may also contribute to pathological scar. Prolonged inflammatory reactions potentiate scar. Therapy includes intralesional injection of anti-inflammatory steroids and dressing with Silastic sheets, which are shown to increase protease-based lytic activity in the scar. Excessive or hypertrophic scarring is rare in burn injuries that heal within 21 days. Pressure garments or compression dressings are effective in decreasing scarring in burn injuries that require more than 21 days to heal. The exact mechanism by which pressure is effective is unknown.

Braga M et al: Nutritional approach in malnourished surgical patients: a prospective randomized study. Arch Surg 2002;137:174.

Carlson MA: Acute wound failure. Wound healing. Surg Clin N Am 2001;77:607.

Collins CE et al: Effect of nutritional supplements on wound healing in home-nursed elderly: a randomized trial. Nutrition 2005;21:147.

Farreras N et al: Effect of early postoperative enteral immunonutrition on wound healing in patients undergoing surgery for gastric cancer. Clin Nutrition 2005;24:55.

Ngo BT et al: Manifestations of cutaneous diabetic microangiopathy. Am J Clin Dermatol 2005;6:225.

Robson MC: Proliferative scarring. Surg Clin N Amer 2003;83:557.

Sahota PS et al: Approaches to improve angiogenesis in tissue engineered skin. Wound Repair Regen 2004;12:635.

Sorensen LT et al: Abstinence from smoking reduces incisional wound infection: a randomized controlled trial. Ann Surg 2003;238:1.

Williams JG et al: Nutrition and wound healing. Surg Clin N Amer 2003;83:571.

CLINICAL FINDINGS

Impediments to wound healing may be broadly categorized as those local to the wound and those that are systemic comorbidities and diseases. Often, a clinical intervention is possible to minimize or eliminate these obstacles to tissue repair (see Table 6–1).

▶ Acute Wounds

Acute wounds express normal wound healing pathways and are expected to heal. Over days and weeks, the undisturbed acute wound can be observed to progress reliably through the phases of hemostasis, normal inflammation, normal fibroplasia, and ultimately scar maturation with epithelialization. The most common acute wound complications are pain, infection, mechanical dehiscence, and hypertrophic scar.

▶ Chronic Wounds & Decubiti
Chronic Wounds

Chronically unhealed wounds, especially on the lower extremity, are common in the setting of vascular, immunologic, and neurologic disease. Venous ulcers, largely of the lower leg, reflect poor perfusion and perivascular leakage of plasma into tissue. The extravasation of plasma proteins into the soft tissue stimulates chronic inflammation. This is the result of venous hypertension produced by incompetent venous valves. Most venous ulcers will heal if the venous congestion and edema are relieved by leg elevation, compression stockings, or surgical procedures that eliminate or repair incompetent veins or their valves.

Arterial or ischemic ulcers, which tend to occur on the lateral ankle or foot, are best treated by revascularization. Hyperbaric oxygen, which provides a temporary source of enhanced oxygenation that stimulates angiogenesis, is an effective though expensive alternative when revascularization is not possible. Useful information can be obtained by transcutaneous oximetry. Tissues with a low PaO_2 will not heal

Table 6–1. Local and Systemic Impediments to Wound Healing.

Systemic	Local
Malnutrition	Wound infection
Diabetes mellitus	Wound necrosis
Drugs (steroids, cytotoxins)	Foreign bodies
Obesity	Wound hypoperfusion and hypoxia
Shock	Repeat trauma
Immunodeficiency	Irradiated tissue
Renal failure	Neoplasm

spontaneously. However, if oxygen tension can be raised into a relatively normal range by oxygen administration even intermittently, the wound may respond to oxygen therapy.

Sensory loss, especially of the feet, can lead to ulceration. Bony deformities due to chronic fractures, like the Charcot deformity, cause pathologic pressure on wounded tissue. Ulcers in patients with diabetes mellitus may have two causes. Patients with neuropathic ulcers usually have good circulation, and their lesions will heal if protected from trauma by offloading, special shoes, or splints. Recurrences are common, however. Diabetics with ischemic disease, whether they have neuropathy or not, are at risk for gangrene, and they frequently require amputation when revascularization is not possible.

In pyoderma gangrenosum, granulomatous inflammation, with or without arteritis, causes skin necrosis, possibly by a mechanism involving excess cytokine release. These ulcers are associated with inflammatory bowel disease and certain types of arthritis and chondritis. Corticosteroids or other anti-inflammatory drugs are helpful. However, anti-inflammatory corticosteroids can also contribute to poor healing by inhibiting cytokine release and collagen synthesis.

Decubiti

Decubitus ulcers can be major complications of immobilization. The morbidity of decubitus ulcers lengthens hospital stays and increases health care costs. They result from prolonged pressure that reduces tissue blood supply, irritative or contaminated injections, and prolonged contact with moisture, urine, or feces. Most patients who develop decubitus ulcers are also poorly nourished. Pressure ulcers are common in paraplegics, immobile elderly patients following fractures, and intensive care unit patients. The ulcers vary in depth and often extend from skin to a bony pressure point such as the greater trochanter, the sacrum, the heels, or the head. Most decubitus ulcers are preventable. Hospital-acquired ulcers are nearly always the result of immobilization, unprotected positioning on operating tables, and ill-fitting casts or other orthopedic appliances.

COMPLICATIONS

▶ Wound Infection

A wound infection results when bacterial proliferation and invasion overcomes wound immune defense mechanisms. When an imbalance in this quantitative equilibrium results in infection, a delay in wound healing occurs. Therefore, prevention and treatment of wound infection involves maintenance or reestablishment of the balanced equilibrium.

Wounds containing more than 10^5 bacteria/gram of tissue or any tissue level of β-hemolytic streptococci are at high risk for wound infection if closed by direct wound edge approximation, skin graft, pedicled, or free flap. Clean-contaminated and contaminated wounds result in high rates of postoperative infection (6–15%), while clean cases have lower infection rates (1–3%). When wounds are considered at risk for having a significant bacterial bioburden (clean-contaminated or contaminated cases), prophylactic operative antibiotics reduce wound infection rates. Wounds following clean cases with negligible bacterial bioburden do not clearly benefit from prophylactic antibiotics except when implanted prosthetic materials are used.

▶ Mechanical Wound Failure

Mechanical factors play an important and often underappreciated role in acute wound healing. Primary closure of an incision stabilizes distractive forces to allow wound healing and an optimized anatomic result (Figure 6–5). Cellular studies confirm that mechanical load forces are an important signal for acute wound repair. When anatomic stability of a wound is achieved, a particular suture material or suturing technique is of secondary importance. The increased use of foreign material implants, like meshes for hernia repair, are suggested to manipulate the mechanical environment of the acute wound, even to the point of promoting "tension-free" wound healing. Negative pressure wound therapy is increasingly applied to stabilize acute wounds and to support acute wound healing. Mechanical microdeformation of repair cells in the wound bed is thought to stimulate acute wound healing.

Mechanical signaling pathways are important for the regulation of tissue repair, especially in load-bearing structures like the abdominal wall and Achilles tendon. From this perspective, the midline fascia behaves more like a ligament or tendon than skin, for example. It is observed that scars placed under mechanical loads ultimately will assume the morphology and function of tendons and, conversely, that incisions placed under "low" loads organize scars with reduced tensile strengths. The empiric observation that a suture length (SL)–wound length (WL) ratio of 4:1 results in the most reliable midline abdominal wall closure may reflect the technique resulting in establishing the optimal acute wound healing–load set point for the abdominal wall. When a laparotomy wound mechanically fails, a fundamental repair signal may be lost, contributing to the biology of hernia formation. Clinically, laparotomy dehiscence of only 12 mm on postoperative day 30 predicts a 94% incisional hernia rate after 3 years.

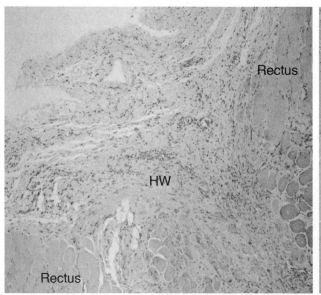
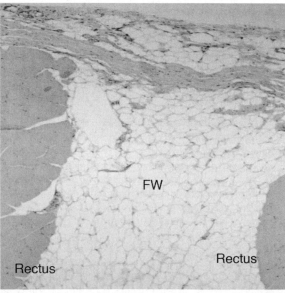

A

B

▲ **Figure 6–5.** **A:** In a healing laparotomy wound (HW), fibroplasia, matrix synthesis, and angiogenesis stabilize the rectus muscles at the wound edges until repair is complete. **B:** When laparotomy wounds fail to heal (FW), there is an absence of fibroplasia and herniated preperitoneal fat occupies the wound space.

Bratzler DW et al: Antimicrobial prophylaxis for surgery: an advisory statement from the National Surgical Infection Prevention Project. Clin Infect Dis 2004;38:1706.

DuBay D et al: Acute wound healing: the biology of acute wound failure. Surg Clin N Am 2003;83:463.

Franz MG: The biology of hernia formation. Surg Clin N Am 2008;88:1.

Franz MG: The biology of hernias and the abdominal wall. Hernia 2006;10:462.

Franz MG et al: Optimizing healing of the acute wound by minimizing complications. Curr Prob Surg 2007;44:1.

Pollock AV et al: Early prediction of late incisional hernias. Br J Surg 1989;76:953.

Sanchez-Manuel FJ et al: Antibiotic prophylaxis for hernia repair. Cochrane Database Syst Rev 2007;3:CD003769.

TREATMENT

▶ Acute Wounds

Sutures

The ideal suture material is flexible, strong, easily tied, and securely knotted. It stimulates little tissue reaction and does not serve as a nidus for infection.

Silk is an animal protein but is relatively inert in human tissue. It is commonly used because of its track record and favorable handling characteristics. It loses strength over long periods and is unsuitable for suturing arteries to plastic grafts or for insertion of prosthetic cardiac valves. Silk sutures are multifilament, providing mechanical immune barriers for bacteria. Occasionally, silk sutures form a focus for small abscesses that migrate and "spit" through the skin, forming small sinuses that will not heal until the suture is removed.

Synthetic nonabsorbable sutures are generally inert polymers that retain strength. However, their handling characteristics are not as good as those of silk, and they must usually be knotted at least four times, resulting in increased amounts of retained foreign material. Multifilament plastic sutures may also become infected and migrate to the surface like silk sutures. Monofilament plastics will not harbor bacteria. Nylon monofilament is extremely nonreactive, but it is difficult to tie. Monofilament polypropylene is intermediate in these properties. Vascular anastomoses to prosthetic vascular grafts rely indefinitely on the strength of sutures; therefore, use of absorbable sutures may lead to aneurysm formation.

Synthetic absorbable sutures are strong, have predictable rates of loss of tensile strength, incite a minimal inflammatory reaction, and have special usefulness in gastrointestinal, urologic, and gynecologic operations that are contaminated. Polyglycolic acid and polyglactin retain tensile strength longer in gastrointestinal anastomoses. Polydioxanone sulfate and polyglycolate are monofilament and lose about half their strength in 50 days, thus solving the problem of premature breakage in fascial closures. Poliglecaprone monofilament synthetic sutures have faster reabsorption, retaining 50% tensile strength at 7 days and 0% at 21 days. This suture is suitable for low-load soft tissue approximation but is not intended for fascial closure.

Stainless steel wire is inert and maintains strength for a long time. It is difficult to tie and may have to be removed late postoperatively because of pain. It does not harbor bacteria, and it can be left in granulating wounds, when necessary, and will be covered by granulation tissue without causing abscesses. However, sinuses due to motion are fairly common.

Catgut (now made from the submucosa of bovine intestine) will eventually resorb, but the resorption time is highly variable. It stimulates a considerable inflammatory reaction and tends to potentiate infections. Catgut also loses strength rapidly and unpredictably in the intestine and in infected wounds as a consequence of acid and enzyme hydrolysis.

Staples, whether for internal use or skin closure, are mainly steel-tantalum alloys that incite a minimal tissue reaction. The technique of staple placement is different from that of sutures, but the same basic rules pertain. There are no real differences in the healing that follows sutured or stapled closures. Stapling devices tend to minimize errors in technique, but at the same time, they do not offer a feel for tissue and have limited ability to accommodate to exceptional circumstances. Staples are preferable to sutures for skin closure, since they do not provide a conduit for contaminating organisms. There is no reliable evidence that absorbable sutures lead to more incisional hernias or gastrointestinal anastamotic leaks.

Surgical glues or **tissue adhesives** are now established as safe and effective for the repair of small skin incisions. The most common forms are cyanoacrylate-based glues. Tissue adhesives are often less painful than sutures or staples, and the seal can serve as the wound dressing as well.

▶ Surgical Technique

Primarily closed wounds are of a smaller volume and heal mainly by the synthesis of a new matrix. Wound contraction and epithelialization, as in an open wound healing by secondary intent, contribute a small part to primary wound healing. An open wound, healing by secondary intent, must synthesize granulation tissue to fill in the wound bed, contract at the wound periphery, and cover the surface area with epithelial cells. Wounds heal faster following delayed primary closure than by secondary intent, as well. The mechanical load forces transmitted through a primarily reconstructed wound will stimulate repair. Successful delayed primary closure requires that the acute wound be in bacterial balance. Primary repair should approximate, but not strangulate, the incision. The type of suture material used does not matter, as long as the primary repair is anatomic and perfused.

The most important means of achieving optimal healing after operation is good surgical technique. Many cases of surgical wound failure are due to technical errors. Tissue should be protected from drying and contamination. The surgeon should use fine instruments; should perform clean, sharp dissection; and should make minimal, skillful use of electrocautery, ligatures, and sutures. All these precautions contribute to the most important goal of surgical technique, gentle handling of tissue. Anatomic tissue approximation should be achieved when possible but optimum tissue perfusion preserved.

Wound Closure

As with many surgical techniques, the exact method of wound closure may be less important than how well it is performed. The tearing strength of sutures in fascia is no greater than 4 kg. There is little reason to use sutures of greater strength than this. Excessively tight closure strangulates tissue, likely leading to hernia formation or infection.

The most reliable laparotomy closure uses a continuous technique at SL-WL ratio of 4:1, which allows for the normal 10% strain that occurs along the length of the incision, while maintaining mechanical integrity. A 4:1 SL-WL ratio is achieved with suture placed 1 cm deep on normal fascia (the bite) followed by 1 cm of progress. The depth of the suture-line bite must extend beyond the wound lytic zone. Normal collagen lysis occurs for approximately 5 mm perpendicular to the incision, weakening the adjacent fascia. The most common technical causes of dehiscence are an SL-WL ratio less than 4:1, infection, and excessively tight sutures. Tight suture lines impair wound perfusion and oxygen delivery that is required for wound healing. If wound healing is impaired, wider, interrupted internal retention sutures may be added, although improved outcomes are not proven (Figure 6–6).

Delayed primary closure is a technique by which the subcutaneous portion of the wound is left open for 4–5 days prior to primary repair. During the delay period, angiogenesis and fibroplasia start, and bacteria are cleared from the wound. The success of this method depends on the ability of the surgeon to detect the signs of wound infection. Merely leaving the wound open for 4 days does not guarantee that it will not become infected. Some wounds (eg, fibrin-covered or inflamed wounds) should not be closed but should be left open for secondary closure. Quantitative bacterial counts less than 10^5 non-β-hemolytic streptococcus organisms per gram of wound tissue predict successful healing after delayed primary closure. Any level of β-hemolytic streptococcal wound infection predicts delayed wound healing.

▶ Implantable Materials

Soft tissue prostheses reduce the incidence of wound failure and recurrence following hernia repair. The recurrence rate following inguinal hernia repairs using autologous tissues ranges from 5% to 25% in most series. The recurrence rate following primary incisional hernia repair using autologous tissues is even worse, ranging from 20% to 60%. The introduction of synthetic soft tissue prostheses to inguinal and incisional hernia repair has significantly reduced recurrence rates across general surgery. The prevailing view is that the mechanism for the reduced hernia recurrence rates is the

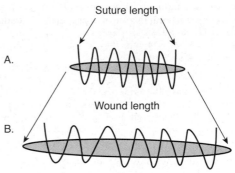

▲ **Figure 6–6.** The most reliable laparotomy closure uses a continuous technique at a suture length–wound length ratio of 4:1. **A:** This allows for the normal 10% strain that occurs along the length of the incision, while maintaining mechanical integrity (**B**).

reduction of tension along suture lines when using mesh and the replacement abnormal tissue.

No implantable prosthesis is ideal in regard to tissue compatibility, permanent fixation, and resistance to infection. Two principles are paramount: biocompatibility and a material that is incorporated into tissue. Both specific and nonspecific immune mechanisms are involved in the inflammatory reaction to foreign materials. Highly incompatible materials, such as wood splinters, elicit an acute inflammatory process that includes massive local release of proteolytic enzymes (inflammation). Consequently, the foreign body is never incorporated and instead is isolated loosely in a fibrous pocket. In less severe incompatibility, rejection is not so vigorous and proteolysis not so prominent. Mononuclear cells and lymphocytes, the major components of wound inflammatory tissue, direct a response that creates a fibrous capsule that may be acceptable in a joint replacement but may distort a breast reconstruction (encapsulation). Newer biological prostheses are composed of acellularized tissue to abrogate the immune response. The expectation is that these materials recellularize with host cells and blood vessels during incorporation and assume a more physiological function (regeneration).

Most implants must become anchored to adjacent normal tissues through fibrous tissue ingrowth. This process requires biocompatibility and interstices large enough to permit repair fibroblast migration, just as in a wound, and to allow pedicles of vascularized tissue to enter and join similar units. In bone, this tissue incorporation imparts stability. In vascular grafts, the invading tissue supports neointima formation, which retards mural thrombosis and distal embolization. Soft tissue will grow into pores larger than about 50 μm in diameter. Of the vascular prostheses, woven Dacron is best for tissue incorporation. In bone, sintered, porous metallic surfaces are best. Large-screen polypropylene mesh can be used to support the abdominal wall or chest and is usually well incorporated into the granulation tissue that penetrates the mesh. Mesh porosity is increasingly recognized as an important design element for reliable implantation and wound healing. Microporous polytetrafluoroethylene (PTFE) sheets are often not well incorporated and are not suitable for use in infected tissues.

The implantation space remains vulnerable to infection for years and is a particular problem in implants that cross the body surface. Mesh cuffs around vascular access devices that incite incorporation have successfully forestalled infection for months, but infections that arise from bacteria entering the body along "permanently" implanted foreign bodies traversing the skin surface, such as ventricular assist devices, remain an unsolved problem.

▶ Negative Pressure Wound Therapy

Negative pressure therapy (NPWT) mechanically stabilizes the distractive forces of an open acute wound and supports healing. Distractive tissue forces keep a wound open with force vectors that oppose wound contraction, thereby delaying healing. NPWT also reduces periwound edema and improves wound perfusion. NPWT may directly stimulate repair fibroblast activity through mechanical microdeformation of the cell surface.

NPWT can also stabilize a therapeutically open abdomen (laparostomy), minimizing wound size and supporting closure of the abdominal wall. Distractive force from the rectus muscle components and lateral oblique muscles act to keep the laparostomy open, leading to incisional hernia formation and potentially loss of abdominal, peritoneal volume (domain) (Figure 6–7).

Chronic Wounds

The first principle in managing chronic wounds is to diagnose and treat tissue hypoxia, such as underlying circulatory disease. The second principle is never to allow open wounds to dry—ie, use moist dressings, which may also relieve pain. A third principle is to control any infection with topical or systemic antibiotics. A fourth principle is to recognize that chronically scarred or necrotic tissue is usually poorly perfused. Debridement of unhealthy tissue, often followed by skin grafting, may be required for healing. A fifth principle is to reduce autonomic vasoconstriction by means of warmth, moisture, and pain relief.

A number of growth factors have been shown to accelerate healing of acute wounds in animals. They include FGFs, TGF-β, IGF-1, PDGF, and epidermal growth factor (EGF). However, in the setting of chronic human wounds, with the perfusion problems noted above and the hostile wound environ-

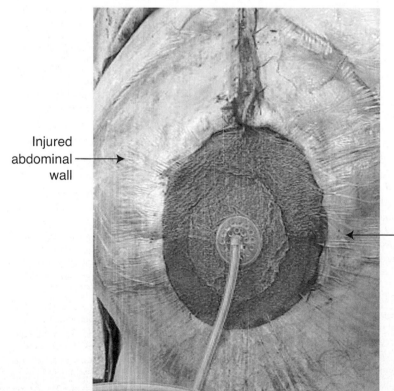

Injured abdominal wall

Negative pressure wound therapy

▲ **Figure 6–7.** Negative pressure dressings oppose distractive soft tissue vectors and mechanically stabilize a wound.

ment with elevated protease levels, proof of efficacy has been difficult to develop, and no clear-cut advantage to any formulation has yet been convincingly demonstrated. The one exception is the randomized, prospective, double-blind, placebo-controlled multicenter trial by the Diabetic Ulcer Study Group, which demonstrated that daily topical application of recombinant human PDGF-BB homodimer moderately accelerated healing and resulted in more wounds that healed completely.

Ducubiti

The first principle is to incise and drain any infected spaces or debride necrotic tissue. Dead tissue is debrided until the exposed surfaces are viable. Sources of pressure must again be unloaded. Many will then heal spontaneously. However, deep ulcers may require surgical closure, sometimes with removal of underlying bone. The defect may require closure by judicious movement of thick, well-vascularized tissue into the affected area. Musculocutaneous flaps are the treatment of choice when chronic infection and significant tissue loss are combined. However, recurrence is common because the flaps are usually insensate.

▶ Postoperative Care

Optimum postoperative care of the wound requires cleanliness, maintenance of a moist wound environment, protection from trauma, and support of the patient. Even closed wounds can be infected by surface contamination, particularly within the first 2–3 days. Bacteria gain entrance most easily through suture tracts. If a wound is likely to be traumatized or contaminated, it should be protected during this time. Such protection may require special dressings such as occlusive dressings or sprays and repeated cleansing.

Some mechanical stress enhances healing. Even fracture callus formation is greater if slight motion is allowed. Patients should move and stress their wounds a little. Early ambulation and return to normal activity are, in general, good for repair.

The appearance of delayed wound infections, weeks to years after operation, reinforces that all wounds are contaminated and may harbor bacteria. Most frequently, poor tissue perfusion and oxygenation of the wound during the postoperative period weakens host resistance. Regulation of perfusion is largely due to sympathetic nervous activity. The major stimuli of vasoconstriction are cold, pain, hypovolemia, cigarette smoking, and hypoxemia. Recent studies show that efforts to limit these impediments to wound healing reduce the wound infection rate by more than half. Maintenance of intraoperative normothermia and blood volume is particularly important. Appropriate assurance that peripheral perfusion is adequate is best obtained from peripheral tissues rather than urine output, central venous pressure, or wedge pressure, none of which correlate with peripheral wound tissue oxygenation. What does correlate with tissue oxygenation is the capillary refill time on the forehead or patella, which should be

less than 2 s and 5 s respectively. Collagen deposition is increased also by the addition of oxygen breathing (nasal prongs or light mask) but only in well-perfused patients.

The ideal care of the wound begins in the preoperative period and ends only months later. The patient must be prepared so that optimal conditions exist when the wound is made. Surgical technique must be clean, gentle, and skillful. Nutrition should be optimized preoperatively when possible. Cessation of cigarette smoking will improve wound outcomes. Postoperatively, wound care includes maintenance of nutrition, blood volume, oxygenation, and careful restriction of immunosuppressant drugs when possible. Although wound healing is in many ways a local phenomenon, ideal care of the wound is essentially ideal care of the patient.

Armstrong DG et al, for the Diabetic Foot Study Consortium: Negative pressure wound therapy after partial diabetic foot amputation: a multicentre randomised controlled trial. Lancet 2005;366:1704.

Bennett MH et al: Hyperbaric oxygen therapy for late radiation tissue injury. Cochrane Database Syst Rev 2005;3: CD005005.

Brown SR et al: Transverse verses midline incisions for abdominal surgery. Cochrane Database Syst Rev 2005;4:CD005199.

Burger WA et al: Long-term follow-up of a randomized controlled trial of suture versus mesh repair of incisional hernia. Ann Surg 2004;24:578.

Coulthard P et al. Tissue adhesives for closure of surgical incisions. Cochrane Database Syst Rev 2004;2:CD004287.

Friedman HI et al: An evidence-based appraisal of the use of hyperbaric oxygen on flaps and grafts. Plast Reconstr Surg 2006;117(7 suppl):175S.

Garcia-Covarrubias L et al: Adjuvant hyperbaric oxygen therapy in the management of crush injury and traumatic ischemia: an evidence-based approach. Am J Surg 2005;71:144.

Luijendijk RW et al: A comparison of suture repair with mesh repair for incisional hernia. NEJM 2000;343:392.

O'Brien L et al: Silicon gel sheeting for preventing and treating hypertrophic and keloid scars. Cochrane Database Syst Rev 2006;1:CD003826.

Perez D et al: Prospective evaluation of vacuum-assisted closure in abdominal compartment syndrome and severe abdominal sepsis. J Am Coll Surg 2007;205:586.

Robson MC et al: Guidelines for the best care of chronic wounds. Wound Rep Regen 2006;14:647.

Steed DL: Debridement. Am J Surg 2004;187(5A suppl):71S.

Steed DL et al: Guidelines for the treatment of diabetic ulcers. Wound Rep Reg 2006;14:680.

Teodorescu V et al: Detailed protocol of ischemia and the use of noninvasive vascular laboratory testing in diabetic foot ulcers. Am J Surg 2004;187(5A suppl):75S.

Van den Kerckhove E et al: The assessment of erythema and thickness on burn related scars during pressure garment therapy as a preventive measure for hypertrophic scarring. Burns 2005;31:696.

van't Riet M et al: Meta-analysis of techniques for closure of midline abdominal incisions. Br J Surg 2002;89:1350.

Wackenfors A et al: Effects of vacuum-assisted closure therapy on inguinal wound edge microvascular blood flow. Wound Repair Regen 2004;12:600.

Ziegler UE. International clinical recommendations on scar management. Zentralbl Chir 2004;129:296.

Power Sources in Surgery

K. Barrett Deatrick, MD

Gerard M. Doherty, MD

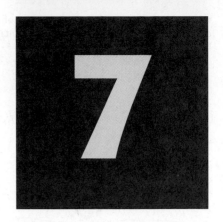

INTRODUCTION

Modern surgery has been redefined by powered instruments, technological tools that in many ways have revolutionized the delicacy, precision, and accuracy of the various operations performed. Yet many people who use these implements every day have very little understanding of the technology behind these tools. Although a complete treatise on electromagnetic generation of heat and the physics of current generation are beyond the scope of this chapter (and are available elsewhere), understanding some fundamental rules governing the behavior of electrical currents and some relatively straightforward principles helps guide the use of these technologies.

ELECTROSURGERY

▶ Principles of Electricity

An electrical **circuit** is any pathway that allows the uninterrupted flow of electrons. Electrical **current** is the flow of electricity (the number of electrons) in a given circuit over a constant period of time and is measured in **amperes** (A). Current can be supplied either as direct current (DC) with constant positive and negative terminals or as alternating current (AC) with constantly reversing poles. The electromotive force, or **voltage,** is a measurement of the force that propels the current of electrons and is related to the difference in potential energy between two terminals. The **resistance** is the tendency of any component of a circuit to resist the flow of electrons and applies to DC circuits. The equivalent of this tendency in an AC circuit is known as impedance. Any electromagnetic wave, from household electricity to radio broadcasts to visible light, can be described by three components: speed, frequency, and wavelength. Because all electromagnetic waves travel at the speed of light, which is a constant, these waves depend on the relationship between their frequency and wavelength. Since these three characteristics are defined by the equation:

$$c = f\lambda$$

(where c is the speed of light, 2.998×10^8 m/s)

frequency (f) and wavelength (λ) are inversely related; ie, as frequency increases, wavelength decreases, and vice versa. The ability to pass high-frequency current through the human body without causing excess damage makes electrosurgery possible.

▶ Electrocautery

Electrosurgery is often incorrectly termed electrocautery, which is a separate technique. Electrocautery is a closed-circuit DC device in which current is passed through an exposed wire offering resistance to the current (Figure 7–1). The resistance causes some of the electrical energy to be dissipated as heat, increasing the temperature of the wire, which then heats tissue. In true electrocautery, *no current passes through the patient.* Electrocautery is primarily applied for microsurgery, such as ophthalmologic procedures, where a very small amount of heat will produce the desired effect or where more heat or current may be dangerous.

▶ Principles of Electrosurgery

True electrosurgery, colloquially referred to as the "Bovie" (following its inventor, William T. Bovie, engineer and collaborator of Harvey Cushing), is perhaps the most ubiquitous power source in surgery. While the principle of using heat to cauterize bleeding wounds dates back to the third millennium BC, the directed use of electrical current to produce these effects is a far more recent development. While other scientists and engineers made significant contributions to the development of this new technology, it was Bovie who refined the electrical generator and made it practical and applicable to everyday surgery. At the most fundamental level, electrosurgery uses high-frequency (radiofrequency) electromagnetic waves to produce a local-

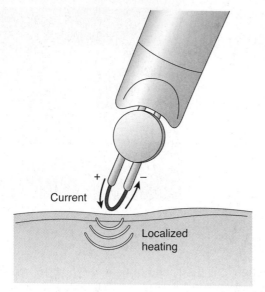

+ −
Current
Localized heating

▲ **Figure 7-1.** In electrocautery, current passes through a wire loop and heats it. This heat cauterizes tissue. No current passes through the patient.

ized heating of tissues, leading to localized tissue destruction. The effect produced (cutting vs. coagulation) depends on how this energy is supplied.

A useful exercise to understand the way electrosurgery works is to follow the flow of current from the power outlet as it travels through the patient and returns to the wall outlet. By convention, charge is depicted as moving from positive (cathode) to negative (anode) despite that the particles that are actually moving are electrons, which have a negative charge. These descriptions are based on that convention, following the flow of positive charge.

Monopolar Circuits

The electrosurgical circuit consists of four primary parts: the electrosurgical generator, the active electrode, the patient, and the return electrode. Current flows from the electrosurgical generator after it is modulated to a high-frequency, short wavelength current and where multiple waveforms can be produced. (The importance of the waveform is discussed in later sections.) The current flows from the machine, through the handpiece, out the tip of the device, to the patient. If the patient were not connected in some way either to a negative terminal or to ground, no current would flow, as there would be no way to complete the circuit, hence nowhere for the charge to go. However, the patient is always connected to the electrosurgical generator by a return electrode, which allows the charge delivered by the electrosurgical probe to pass through the patient, exerting its effect, and back to the generator, completing the circuit. In reality, the

term *monopolar circuit* is incorrect, as there are in fact two poles (the active and return electrodes); it is distinguished from bipolar electrosurgery in which both electrodes are under the surgeon's direct control (Figure 7–2A).

Bipolar Circuits

The essential components of the bipolar electrosurgical circuit are the same as those in the monopolar circuit; however, in this system, the active and return electrodes are in the same surgical instrument. In this technique, high-frequency current is passed through the active electrode and through the patient to heat and disrupt tissue. In this arrangement, however, the return electrode is in the handpiece, as the opposite pole of the active electrode. This method enables the surgeon to heat only a discrete amount of tissue (Figure 7–2B).

▶ The Electromagnetic Spectrum and Tissue Effects

The current that powers the electrosurgical generator is supplied at a frequency of 60 Hz. This type of electromagnetic energy can indeed cause very strong (potentially lethal) neuromuscular stimulation, making it unsuitable for use in its pure form. Muscle and nerve stimulation, however, ceases at around 100 kHz. Current with a frequency above this threshold can be delivered safely, without the risk of electrocution. The outputs of electrosurgical generators deliver current with a frequency greater than 200 kHz. Current at this frequency is known as **radiofrequency** (RF); it is in the same portion of the spectrum as some radio transmitters. This level of RF, released from a radio antenna, can produce serious RF burns if the proper precautions are not taken.

Applying electrosurgical current to a patient produces localized tissue destruction via intense heat production, yet barring a mishap, no other lesions are produced during application of this technique. The reason the effect is exerted only at the site where the surgeon is operating, and not at the site of the return electrode, is that the surface area by which the charge is delivered is much smaller than that to which it returns. Thus, there is a far greater **density of charge** at the site of the handpiece ("active" electrode) contact than there is at the site of return. If there is another connection between the patient and ground that offers less resistance to the flow of current, and if it also comprises a relatively small surface area, then the patient could be in danger of suffering an electrosurgical burn. Similarly, it is possible that if the return electrode were to be damaged, or if contact was not maintained, a burn could occur in this area. The possibility of a burn at the site of the return electrode is eliminated in most modern machines by the presence of a monitoring system that assesses the completeness of contact (by maintaining a smaller, secondary circuit) and automatically disables power if full contact of the pad is lost (as could be caused by tripping over a wire and tearing the return pad).

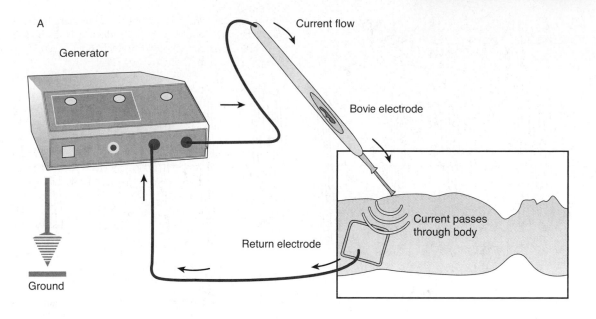

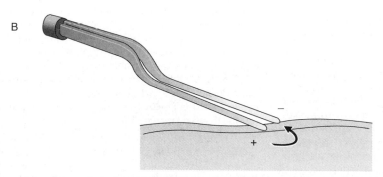

▲ **Figure 7–2.** **A:** In monopolar electrosurgery, current from an electrosurgical generator passes from an active electrode (the "Bovie" tip) through the patient to a return electrode of greater area. **B:** In bipolar electrosurgery, the active and return electrodes are in the handpiece, and current only flows through the surgical site.

▶ Types of Electrosurgery

All types of electrosurgery exert their effects via the localized production of heat and the subsequent changes in the heated tissue. Therefore, the different effects produced by electrosurgical instruments are created by altering the manner in which this heat is produced and delivered. Adjustment is made possible by altering the wave pattern of the current.

Cutting

Cutting depends on the production of a continuous sine wave of current (Figure 7–3A). Compared with coagulation current (discussed later), cutting current has a relatively low

voltage and a relatively high crest factor, which is the ratio of the peak voltage to the mean (root mean square) voltage of the current. Additionally, it has a relatively high "duty cycle"—ie, once the current is applied, the current is actively flowing during the entire application. In this technique, the tip of the electrode is held just slightly off the surface of the tissue. The flow of the high-frequency current through the resistance of the patient's tissue at a very small site produces intense heat, vaporizing water and exploding the cells in the immediate vicinity of the current. Thus, cutting occurs with minimal coagulum production and consequently minimal hemostasis. A combination of coagulation and cutting can be produced by setting the electrosurgical generator to **blend,**

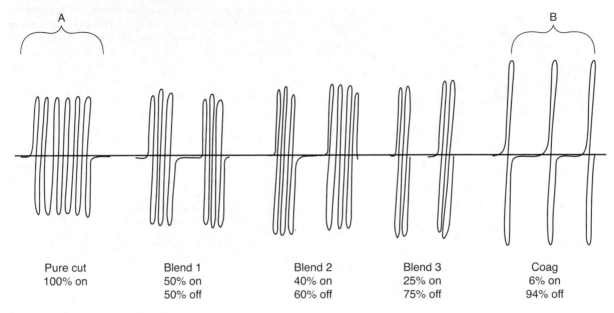

Pure cut	Blend 1	Blend 2	Blend 3	Coag
100% on	50% on	40% on	25% on	6% on
	50% off	60% off	75% off	94% off

▲ **Figure 7–3.** Electrosurgical waveforms. **A:** Cutting current. **B:** Coagulation current.

which damps down a portion of the waveform, allowing greater formation of a coagulum and consequently more control of local bleeding.

Coagulation: Desiccation and Fulguration

In contrast with cutting currents, **coagulation** currents do not produce a constant waveform. Rather, they rely on spikes of electric wave activity (Figure 7–3B). Although these currents produce less heat overall than the direct sine wave, enough heat is produced to disrupt the normal cellular architecture. Because the cells are not instantly vaporized, however, the cellular debris remains associated with the edge of the wound, and the heat produced is enough to denature the cellular protein. This accounts for the formation of a coagulum, a protein-rich mixture that allows sealing of smaller blood vessels and control of local bleeding. Compared to cutting, coagulation currents have a higher crest factor and a shorter duty cycle (94% off, 6% on). In part, the increased voltage is necessary to overcome the impedance of air during the process of arcing current to the tissues. Coagulation can be accomplished in one of two ways. With **desiccation,** the conductive tip is placed in direct contact with the tissue. Direct contact of the electrode with tissue reduces the concentration of the current; less heat is generated, and no cutting action occurs. A relatively low power setting is used, resulting in a limited area of tissue ablation with coagulation. Desiccation is achieved most efficiently with the cutting current. The cells dry out and form a coagulum rather than vaporize and explode.

In **fulguration,** the tip of the active electrode is not actually brought into contact with the tissues but rather is held just off the surface, and following activation, the current arcs through the air to the target. Again, this process disrupts normal cellular protein to form a coagulum; the tissue is charred, and a black eschar forms at the site of operation. It is possible to cut with the coagulation current and, conversely, to coagulate with the cutting current by holding the electrode in direct contact with tissue. It may be necessary to adjust power settings and electrode size to achieve the desired surgical effect. The benefit of using the cutting current is that far less voltage is needed, an important consideration during minimally invasive procedures.

Variables

Just as the power setting and the waveform affect the results of the current application, any change in the circuit that influences the impedance of the system will influence the tissue effect. These include the size of the electrode, the position of the electrode, the type of tissue, and the formation of eschar.

Size of the electrode—The smaller the electrode, the higher the current concentration. Consequently, the same tissue effect can be achieved with a smaller electrode, even though the power setting is reduced. At any given setting, the longer the generator is activated, the more heat is produced. The greater the heat, the farther it will travel to adjacent tissue (thermal spread). (See various electrodes, Figure 7–4.)

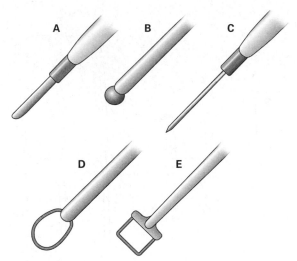

▲ **Figure 7–4. A:** Knife electrode. **B:** Ball electrode.
C: Needle electrode. **D:** Loop electrode. **E:** Wire electrode.

Placement of the electrode—Placement can determine whether vaporization or coagulation occurs. Which one occurs is a function of current density and the heat produced while sparking to tissue versus holding the electrode in direct contact.

Type of Tissue—Tissues vary widely in resistance.

Eschar—Eschar is relatively high in resistance to current. Electrodes should be kept clean and free of eschar, maintaining lower resistance within the surgical circuit.

Disadvantages and Potential Hazards

Alternate site burns—Early electrosurgical generators used a **ground referenced** circuit design. In this type of construction, grounded current from the wall outlet was directly modulated, and it was assumed that it would return to the generator via the return electrode. With this type of system, however, any path of low resistance to ground, including metal instruments, EKG leads, and other wire and conductive surfaces, can complete the circuit. The ground referenced circuit design presented a relatively high hazard for alternate site burns when current was not distributed over a great enough area to dissipate the current.

Modern electrosurgical units use isolated generator technology. The isolated generator separates the therapeutic current from ground by referencing it within the generator circuitry. In an isolated electrosurgical system, the circuit is completed by the generator, and electrosurgical current from isolated generators will not recognize grounded objects as pathways to complete the circuit. Isolated electrosurgical energy recognizes the patient return electrode as the preferred pathway back to the generator. Since the ground is not

the reference for completion of the circuit, the potential for alternate site burns is greatly reduced. However, if the return electrode were to become partially disconnected, a burn could occur at the site of the return electrode if the area was too small to distribute the current widely enough to prevent heating of the tissue or if the impedance was too high. It is important to place the return electrode over a well-vascularized tissue mass, not over areas of vascular insufficiency or over bony prominences where contact might be compromised. Therefore, some electrosurgical generators use a monitoring system that assesses the quality of the contact between the return electrode and the patient by monitoring impedance, which is related to surface area. Any loss of contact between the electrode and the generator results in interruption of the circuit and deactivation of the system.

Surgical fires—In any setting with high heat sources and an ample supply of oxygen, vigilance against combustion is essential. Drapes, gowns, gas (particularly in bowel surgery and cases involving the upper airway), and hair, for example, are flammable and must be kept away from heat sources. Careful application of electrosurgery and use of a protective holster to store the electrode while not in use are important to minimize the risk of fire.

Minimally invasive surgery—Several safety concerns are unique to minimally invasive surgery, given the limited and relatively tight environment in which operations occur. One potential danger is that of direct coupling between the electrode and other conductive instruments, leading to inadvertent tissue damage. Another is the risk, with the use of high-voltage currents (especially those used for coagulation), of breakdown in the insulation, resulting in arcing from an exposed conductor to adjacent tissue, again, causing unwanted tissue damage. The risk can be reduced by using cutting current instead of coagulation current to lower the voltage used.

Yet another unique hazard is the potential for creating a capacitor with the cannula. A capacitor is any conductor separated from another conductor by a dielectric. The conductive electrode separated from either a metal cannula or the abdominal wall (both good conductors) can induce capacitance in either of these structures. For maximum safety, an all-metal cannula (by which current can escape to the rest of the body) rather than a combination of metal and plastic should be used, and vigilance must be maintained at all times.

Principal Applications for Electrosurgery

Electrosurgery is ubiquitous in its presence within the modern operating room. In its earliest use by Dr. Cushing, it allowed surgery on previously inoperable vascular tumors in neurosurgery. Today, electrosurgery is an essential component of all types of surgery. Applications include dissection in general and vascular surgery, allowing tissue to be resected with minimal blood loss. Additionally, use in urology facilitates transurethral prostatectomy (TURP) and other procedures. In gynecologic practice, electrosurgical instruments are essential in cervical resections and biopsies.

Argon Beam Coagulation
Principles

Argon beam coagulation is closely related to basic electrosurgery. Argon beam coagulation uses a coaxial flow of argon gas to conduct monopolar RF current to the target tissue. Argon is an inert gas that is easily ionized by the application of an electrical current. When ionized, argon gas becomes far more conductive (has less impedance) than normal air and provides a more efficient pathway for transmitting current from the electrode to tissues (Figure 7–5). The current arcs along the pathway of the ionized gas, which is heavier than both oxygen and nitrogen, and thereby displaces air. Whereas current can sometimes follow unpredictable pathways while arcing through the air, the argon gas allows more accurate placement of current flow. Once the current arrives at the tissue, it produces its coagulating effect in the same manner as conventional electrosurgery. Argon beam coagulation devices can operate only in two modes: pinpoint coagulation and spray coagulation. The method does not cut even the most delicate tissue.

Advantages

There are multiple advantages to this type of electrosurgical current delivery. First, it allows use of the coagulation mode without contact of the electrode. This prevents buildup of eschar, which diminishes electrode efficiency, on the electrode tip. Second, there is generally less smoke and less odor from coagulating with this type of current. Third, tissue loss and tissue damage are reduced when the current is more accurately targeted. Fourth, because the argon gas is delivered at room temperature, there is less danger of the instrument igniting gowns or drapes. Finally, the beam of coagulation generally improves coagulation and reduces blood loss and the risk of rebleeding.

Disadvantages

Argon beam coagulation cannot be used to produce a cutting effect in the same manner as other types of electrosurgical equipment. Also, the nozzle for gas delivery can become clogged, reducing its efficiency, and just as with other electrosurgical instruments, if it is used for a prolonged period of time, it may overheat and cause inadvertent damage when set aside.

Applications

Argon beam coagulation is especially useful for procedures in which the surgeon must rapidly and efficiently coagulate a wide area of tissue. It is especially suited to dissecting very vascular tissues and organs, such as the liver. Its efficient

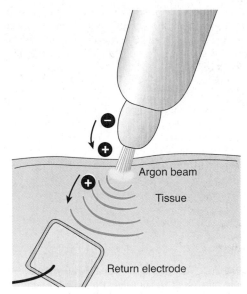

▲ **Figure 7–5.** Ionized argon gas facilitates the flow of current from the handpiece to the tissue.

delivery of a consistent current load and its inability to become occluded with eschar are advantageous for operation with a significant risk of hemorrhage.

MECHANICAL (ULTRASONIC) TISSUE DISRUPTION

Apart from passing current through the patient to produce localized heating and tissue destruction (either cutting or coagulation), there are other means of transforming electrical potential energy into energy for surgery. Two of the most prominent technologies depend on the production of ultrasonic vibrations, although each produces its effect in a unique manner.

Ultrasonic Scalpels and Clamps
Principles

Several types of ultrasonic "scalpels" and clamps allow cutting and coagulation of tissue in a technique completely different from that employed in electrosurgery. In this type of an instrument, electrical energy from a power source is transformed into ultrasonic vibrations by a transducer, a unit that expands and contracts in response to electrical current at a frequency of up to 55.5 kHz/sec. The vibration is amplified in the shaft of the instrument to magnify the vibrating distance of the blade, which moves longitudinally. The blade tip vibrates through an amplitude of around 200 μm. As the blade tip vibrates, it produces cellular friction and denatures proteins. The denatured proteins form a coagulum, which allows sealing of coapted blood vessels. With longer instrument applications, significant secondary heat is produced, and larger blood vessels may be sealed by coagulation of tissue at a small distance from the instrument. By producing cellular disruption in this fashion, the temperatures achieved are between 50 °C and 100 °C. In contrast, in conventional electrosurgery, tissues are subjected to temperatures between 150 °C and 400 °C. Thus, with an ultrasonic device, tissues can be dissected without burning or oxidizing tissues and without producing an eschar; there is also less potential to disrupt the coagulum when removing the instrument. When cutting using the clamp portion of the instrument, energy is transferred to the tissue through the active blade under applied force, minimizing lateral spread. Additionally, the motion of the blade induces cavitation along the cell surfaces, whereby low pressure causes cell fluid to vaporize and rupture (Figure 7–6).

Advantages

The advantages of an ultrasonic scalpel system are clearest when operating in tight spaces with the attendant risks of damage to adjacent structures. Ultrasonic instruments are especially suited for laparoscopic and other types of minimally invasive procedures. While the potential still exists for damaging adjacent tissue by inadvertently touching it with an active tip, there is no risk of current inadvertently arcing to adjacent structures, since the current is converted into mechanical energy in the handpiece. Further, there is no neuromuscular stimulation produced, since no current passes through the patient. Because the tissue effects are exerted through mechanical disruption of the cells, and coagulation occurs at much lower temperatures than used in conventional electrosurgery, lateral thermal tissue damage is minimized. And because tissue is not heated to the point of combustion or carbonization of proteins, there is no eschar formation on the blade, and less smoke is produced.

Disadvantages

A primary disadvantage of ultrasonic scalpels and clamps is that the components are more expensive than those used for conventional electrosurgery, and with more mechanical parts, there are more potential points of equipment failure. Further, whereas electrosurgery can be applied throughout an operation, ultrasonic scalpels are typically used for more controlled dissection around the site of interest.

Applications

The primary applications of ultrasonic instruments are found when traditional electrosurgery is unsuitable or undesirable. As mentioned, they are particularly useful during minimally invasive procedures because they mitigate the risk of running an active electrode through a cannula and into a body cavity. Additionally, the reduced smoke production by instruments of this type is advantageous in this setting. When electrophysiology is involved (such as in patients with

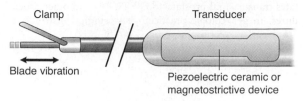

▲ **Figure 7–6.** Ultrasonic scalpel.

implantable cardiac defibrillators or pacemakers), ultrasonic instruments eliminate a source of concern by avoiding the hazard of passing current through the patient's body.

▶ Cavitational Ultrasonic Surgical Aspiration

Principles

Cavitational ultrasonic surgical aspirators work on many of the same principles as ultrasonic scalpels. In the handpiece, current passes through a coil and induces a magnetic field. The magnetic field excites a transducer of a nickel alloy (either a piezoelectric or magnetostrictive device), expanding and contracting to produce an oscillating motion (vibration) in the longitudinal axis with a frequency of 23 or 36 kHz. These ultrasonic mechanical vibrations are magnified over the length of the handpiece. The amount of oscillation varies: with low frequency, there is greater amplitude; with high frequency, there is lower amplitude. The oscillating tip, when brought into contact with tissue, causes fragmentation of tissue by producing cavitation at the cell surface, with low pressure outside the cell leading to cellular disruption. This high-frequency vibration produces heat, which is reduced via a closed, recirculating cooling-water system. This system maintains the temperature of the tip at approximately 40 °C. As tissue is fragmented, the debris must be carried away, which is another function of the cavitational ultrasonic surgical aspirator, as its name implies. For irrigation, IV fluid (water or saline) is fed through tubing to the handpiece, where it irrigates the surgical site and suspends the fragmented tissue debris. Removal of this debris is possible because the instrument contains a vacuum pump that provides suction. Suction pulls irrigation fluid, fragmented tissue, and other material through the distal tip of the handpiece. The material is contained in a separate canister.

Some ultrasonic surgical aspirator instruments enable the surgeon to influence the selectivity of the disruption induced by the instrument itself. Some surgeons attempt to gain extra control by lowering the amplitude of the tip oscillations. Lowering amplitude to gain greater selectivity when fragmenting tissue near critical structures, however, only results in reduced speed of tissue removal. By using a mode in which on/off power intervals are supplied, the reserve power (which governs the tip response when encountering tissue) is reduced. The total amount of power in the oscillating hollow

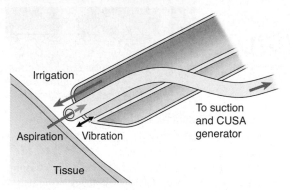

▲ Figure 7–7. Cavitational ultrasonic surgical aspirator.

tip is determined by the amount of reserve power available. Reserve power maintains tip oscillation when a resistive load is placed on the tip, as occurs when it contacts tissue. As the resistance increases, more power is supplied to the tip (Figure 7–7).

Applications

Ultrasonic surgical aspirator systems are primarily applicable in situations where fragmentation, emulsification, and aspiration of a significant amount of tissue is desirable. Since minimal additional hemostasis is provided, this instrument is not as versatile in its application to general surgery as electrosurgery or the more high-power ultrasonic scalpel. In general surgery, its primary application is in liver resection, where it can disrupt parenchyma while leaving major vasculature and the biliary ducts intact.

ConMed: *Electrosurgical Generator + ABC Mode Operator's Manual.* Conmed Corporation, 1999.

Duffy S, Cobb GV: *Practical Electrosurgery.* Chapman & Hall Medical, 1995.

Johnson & Johnson Gateway: Technology Overview. 2008. Available at: http://www.jnjgateway.com : accessed 12/8/2008.

Pearce JA: *Electrosurgery.* Chapman & Hall, 1986.

Valleylab. Principles of Electrosurgery Online. 2008. Available at: http://www.valleylab.com/education/poes/index.html accessed 12/8/2008.

Valleylab. *CUSA Excel System User's Guide.* Tyco Healthcare Group, 2000.

Inflammation, Infection, & Antimicrobial Therapy

Linda M. Mundy, MD
Gerard M. Doherty, MD

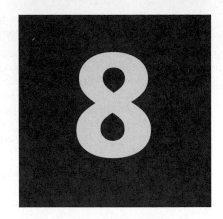

SURGICAL INFECTIONS

A surgical infection is an infection that (1) is unlikely to respond to nonsurgical treatment (it usually must be excised or drained) and occupies an unvascularized space in tissue or (2) occurs in an operated site. Common examples of the first group are appendicitis, empyema, gas gangrene, and most abscesses.

Surgeons are regrettably familiar with the vicious circle of operation or injury, infection, malnutrition, immunosuppression, organ failure, reoperation, further malnutrition, and further infection. One of the fine arts of surgery is to know when to intervene with excision, drainage, physiologic support, antibiotic therapy, and nutritional therapy. For infections arising in a space or in dead tissue, by far the most important aspect of treatment is to establish surgical drainage.

▶ Pathogenesis

Three elements are common to surgical infections: (1) an infectious agent, (2) a susceptible host, and (3) a closed, unperfused space.

A. The Infectious Agent

Although a few pathogens cause most surgical infections, many organisms are capable of doing so. Among the aerobic organisms, streptococci may invade even minor breaks in the skin and spread through connective tissue planes and lymphatics. *Staphylococcus aureus* is the most common pathogen in wound infections and around foreign bodies. Klebsiella often invades the inner ear and enteric tissues as well as the lung. Enteric organisms, especially the Enterobacteriaceae and enterococci, are often found together with anaerobes. Among the anaerobes, bacteroides species and *Peptostreptococci* are often present in surgical infections, and clostridium species are major pathogens in ischemic tissue.

Pseudomonas and serratia are usually nonpathogenic surface contaminants but may be opportunistic and even lethal invaders in critically ill or immunosuppressed patients. Some fungi (histoplasma, coccidioides) and yeasts (candida), along with nocardia and actinomyces, cause abscesses and sinus tracts, and even animal parasites (amebas and echinococcus) may cause abscesses, especially in the liver. Destructive granulomas, such as tuberculosis, once required excision, but antibiotic therapy has now superseded operation for this purpose in most cases. Other rare diseases such as cat-scratch fever, psittacosis, and tularemia may cause suppurative lymphadenitis and require drainage or excision.

Identification of the pathogen by smear and culture remains a cardinal step in therapeutic decision making. The surgeon must inform the microbiologist of peculiar circumstances associated with any given specimen, so that appropriate smears and cultures can be done; serious errors may otherwise result.

B. The Susceptible Host

Surgical infections such as appendicitis and furuncles occur in patients whose only defect in immunity is a closed space in tissue. However, patients with suppressed immune systems are being seen with increasing frequency, and their problems have become a major surgical challenge. **Immunosuppression** seems a simple concept but in fact usually represents a combination of defects of the multifaceted immune mechanism.

1. Specific immunity—The immune process that depends upon prior exposure to an antigen involves detection and processing of antigen by macrophages, mobilization of T and B lymphocytes, synthesis of specific antibody, and other functions. Its importance is illustrated in AIDS, transplant immunosuppression, and agammaglobulinemia, each of which is associated with only a slight increase in the frequency and severity of some surgical infections. In general, isolated defects contribute little to the severity of ordinary surgical infections. Major defects contribute substantially to morbidity, mortality, and resource consumption.

2. Nonspecific immunity—Innate or nonspecific immunity serves to limit damage during the first few hours after infection. Despite the emphasis in the literature on specific immune mechanisms, nonspecific immunity, which depends on phagocytic leukocyte migration, ingestion, and cidal activity for microorganisms, is the principal means by which the host defends against abscess-forming and necrotizing infections.

A. Chemoattraction and phagocytosis—Invading microbes display molecular patterns that are shared among groups of pathogens. Examples include lipopolysaccharides (LPS) of gram-negative bacteria, lipoteichoic acid of gram-positive bacteria, mannans of yeast, and double-stranded RNA of certain viruses. To control infection, the host uses an array of pattern recognition receptors (complement, adhesins, collectins, bactericidal permeability-increasing protein [BPI], LPS-binding protein [LBP]) that bind to these molecular moieties, acting together with effector cells to eliminate them. Typically, granulocytes internalize these pattern-receptor complexes by engulfment into a phagocytic vacuole. The subsequent release of chemoattractants causes the movement (diapedesis) of leukocytes from the bloodstream to the tissue, increasing leukocyte numbers locally and the likelihood that the invading microbe will be destroyed. These steps require little or no oxygen, but chemotaxis is vulnerable to a number of disorders, particularly anti-inflammatory steroid hormones and malnutrition, which reduce the number of granulocytes that arrive at a contaminated site in a given time.

B. Killing mechanisms—Once the phagosome is formed, other cytoplasmic granules (lysosomes) fuse with it and release into it preformed and increasingly acidic proteolytic solutions that kill most bacteria and fungi.

A second process, "oxidative killing," is particularly important to the killing of organisms such as staphylococci, which are commonly responsible for surgical infections. This mechanism consumes and requires molecular oxygen, which it converts to superoxide anion. In this process, a membrane-bound NADPH oxidase is activated, and a burst of respiration (oxygen consumption) follows. Part of the consumed oxygen is converted to a series of oxygen radicals (including superoxide, hydroxyl radical, and hypochlorite), which are released into phagosomes and assist in bacterial killing. This process is progressively inhibited when extracellular oxygen tension falls below about 30 mm Hg. When oxygen tension is 0 mm Hg, the antibacterial capacity of normal granulocytes for *S aureus* and *E coli,* for instance, falls by half—to the same capacity observed in granulocytes taken from victims of chronic granulomatous disease, which results from the genetic absence of membrane-bound oxidase and which without aggressive antibiotic therapy is lethal in early childhood.

Whether a given inoculum will establish an infection and become invasive depends to a great extent on how well tissue perfusion—and therefore oxygenation—can meet the increased metabolic demands of the granulocytes. Inflammatory signals from complement factors and histamine, for instance, dilate vessels and help direct blood flow to infected areas, but if blood volume or regional vascular supply is so poor that tissue perfusion cannot increase, invasive infection ensues. Tissue oxygen supplies can often be raised by increasing blood volume and arterial P_{O_2} and are lowered by hypovolemia and pulmonary insufficiency.

Patients with pulmonary disease, severe trauma, congestive heart failure, hypovolemia, or excessive levels of vasopressin, angiotensin, or catecholamines have hypoxic peripheral tissues and are unusually susceptible to infection. They are truly immunosuppressed. Support of the circulation is just as important to immune defense as is nutrition or antibiotic therapy.

3. Anergy—Anergy is defined as the lack of inflammatory response to skin test antigens. It characterizes a population of immunosuppressed patients who tend to develop infections and die from them. The skin tests used to diagnose anergy are those often used to test recall antigens and delayed hypersensitivity—but in fact they test much of the spectrum of antibacterial immunologic events, including antigen detection and processing by macrophages, release of lymphokines, antibody synthesis, and the inflammatory response, including leukocyte chemotaxis. One event they do not detect is, conspicuously, the final crucial step of actually killing bacteria. Anergy has many causes, including defective T and B lymphocytes, the presence of excess anti-inflammatory corticosteroids, defective antigen processing, and increased numbers of suppressor T cells. Among surgical patients, severe malnutrition, trauma, shock, and sepsis suppress skin test responses, which become active again after resolution of the acute process.

4. Immunity in diabetes mellitus—Diabetes mellitus impairs immunity. Well-controlled diabetics resist infection normally except in tissues made ischemic by arterial disease, while uncontrolled diabetics do not. The mechanism is unknown, except that leukocytes from poorly controlled diabetics adhere, migrate, and kill bacteria poorly. They improve their performance when glucose control is regained. Leukocytes also function poorly without insulin, and insulin is consumed in wounds and other poorly perfused spaces, resulting in low ambient insulin levels.

C. The Closed Space

Most surgical infections start in a susceptible, usually poorly vascularized place in tissue such as a wound or a natural space. The common denominators are poor perfusion, local hypoxia, hypercapnia, and acidosis. Some natural spaces with narrow outlets, such as those of the appendix, gallbladder, ureters, and intestines, are especially prone to becoming obstructed and then infected.

The peritoneal and pleural cavities are potential spaces, and their surfaces slide over one another, thereby dispersing contaminating bacteria. Foreign bodies, dead tissue, and injuries interfere with this mechanism and predispose to infection. Fibrin inhibits the clearing of bacteria. It polymerizes around bacteria, trapping them; this encourages abscess formation but at the same time prevents dangerous spread of infection.

Foreign bodies may have spaces in which bacteria can reside. Infarcted tissue is markedly susceptible to infection. Thrombosed veins, for example, rarely become infected unless intravenous catheters enter them and act as entry points for bacteria.

▶ Spread of Surgical Infections

Surgical infections usually originate as a single focus and become life threatening by spreading and releasing toxins. Spreading occurs by several mechanisms.

A. Necrotizing Infections

Necrotizing infections tend to spread along anatomically defined paths. Necrotizing fasciitis spreads along poorly perfused fascial and subcutaneous planes, its toxins causing thrombosis even of large vessels ahead of the necrotic area, thus creating more ischemic and vulnerable tissue.

B. Abscesses

If not promptly drained, abscesses enlarge, killing more tissue in the process. Leukocytes contribute to necrosis by releasing lysosomal enzymes during phagocytosis. Natural boundaries can be breached; eg, intestinal cutaneous fistulas may form, or blood vessel walls may be penetrated.

C. Phlegmons and Superficial Infections

Phlegmons contain little pus but much edema. They spread along fat planes and by contiguous necrosis, combining features of both of the above kinds of spread. Retroperitoneal peripancreatic inflammation or infection is typical. Superficial infections may spread along skin not only by contiguous necrosis but also by metastasis.

D. Spread of Infection Via the Lymphatic System

Lymphangiitis produces red streaks in the skin and travels proximally along major lymph vessels. However, it may also occur in hidden places such as the retroperitoneum in puerperal sepsis.

E. Spread of Infection Via the Bloodstream

Empyema and endocarditis caused by intravenously injected contaminated recreational drugs are now common. Brain abscesses resulting from infections elsewhere in the body (especially the face) occur in infants and diabetics. Liver abscesses may complicate appendicitis and inflammatory bowel disease, sometimes as a result of suppurative phlebitis of the portal vein (pylephlebitis).

▶ Complications

A. Fistulas and Sinus Tracts

Fistulas and sinus tracts often result when abdominal abscesses contiguous to bowel open to the skin. When tissue necrosis compounds the development of sinus tracts and erodes major blood vessels, severe bleeding may occur. This is most troublesome in irradiated tissue of nonhealing neck wounds and in infected groin wounds after vascular surgery.

Some intestinal fistulas originate in poorly fashioned or necrotic suture lines, and some result from contiguous abscesses that eventually penetrate both bowel and skin, often helped along by the surgeon who must drain the abscess.

B. Suppressed Wound Healing

Suppressed wound healing is a consequence of infection. The mechanism is probably stimulation by bacteria of cytokines, which in turn stimulates proteolysis, especially collagenase production.

C. Immunosuppression and Superinfection

Immunosuppression is a common consequence of injury, which includes surgery, trauma, shock, or infection or sepsis. Superinfection occurs when immunosuppression provides an opportunity for invasion by opportunistic, often antibiotic-resistant organisms.

D. Bacteremia

Bacteremia is the presence of bacteria in blood. The significance of bacteremia is variable. Bacteremia that follows dental work is usually rapidly cleared and harmless, except in patients with damaged heart valves; cardiac, vascular, or orthopedic prostheses; or impaired immunity. It occurs predictably during instrumentation of the gastrointestinal tract or infected urinary tract. Patients in these groups are at increased risk and should receive an appropriate prophylactic antibiotic regimen.

E. Organ Dysfunction, Sepsis, and the Systemic Inflammatory Response Syndrome

Infection and tissue damage initiate the inflammatory response, a very tightly controlled, adaptive response to eliminate dead or infected tissue. At the site of injury, endothelial cells and leukocytes coordinate the local release of mediators of the inflammatory response, including cytokines (tumor necrosis factor-α), interleukins, interferons, leukotrienes, prostaglandins, nitric oxide, reactive oxygen species, and products of the classic inflammatory pathway (complement, histamine, and bradykinin) (Table 8–1). When local-

Table 8–1. Cytokines and Growth Factors.

Peptide	Site of Synthesis	Regulation	Target Cells	Effects
G-CSF	Fibroblasts, monocytes	Induced by IL-1, LPS, IFN-α	Committed neutrophil progenitors (CFU-G, Gran)	Supports the proliferation of neutrophil-forming colonies. Stimulates respiratory burst.
GM-CSF (IL-3 has almost identical effects)	Endothelial cells, fibroblasts, macrophages, T lymphocytes, bone marrow	Induced by IL-1, TNF	Granulocyte-erythrocyte-monocyte-megakaryocyte progenitor cells (CFU-GEMM, CFU-MEG, CFU-Eo, CFU-GM)	Supports the proliferation of macrophage-, eosinophil-, neutrophil-, and monocyte-containing colonies.
IFN-α, IFN-β, IFN-γ	Epithelial cells, fibroblasts, lymphocytes, macrophages, neutrophils	Induced by viruses (foreign nucleic acids), microbes, microbial foreign antigens, cancer cells	Lymphocytes, macrophages, infected cells, cancer cells	Inhibits viral multiplication. Activates defective phagocytes, direct inhibition of cancer cell multiplication, activation of killer leukocytes, inhibition of collagen synthesis.
IL-1	Endothelial cells, keratinocytes, lymphocytes, macrophages	Induced by TNF-α, IL-1, IL-2, C5a; suppressed by IL-4, TGF-β	Monocytes, macrophages, T cells, B cells, NK cells, LAK cells	Stimulates T cells, B cells, NK cells, LAK cells. Induces tumoricidal activity and production to other cytokines, endogenous pyrogen (via PGE_2 release). Induces steroidogenesis, acute phase proteins, hypotension; chemotactic neutrophils. Stimulates respiratory burst.
IL-1ra	Monocytes	Induced by GM-CSF, LPS, IgG	Blocks type 1 IL-1 receptors on T cells, fibroblasts, chondrocytes, endothelial cells	Blocks type 1 IL-1 receptors on T cells, chondrocytes, endothelial cells. Ameliorates animal models of arthritis, septic shock, and inflammatory bowel disease.
IL-2	Lymphocytes	Induced by IL-1, IL-6	T cells, NK cells, B cells, activated monocytes	Stimulates growth of T cells, NK cells, and B cells
IL-4	T cells, NK cells, mast cells	Induced by cell activation, IL-1	All hematopoietic cells and many others express receptors	Stimulates B cell and T cell growth. Induces HLA class II molecules.
IL-6	Endothelial cells, fibroblasts, lymphocytes, some tumors	Induced by IL-1, TNF-α	T cells, B cells, plasma cells, keratinocytes, hepatocytes, stem cells	B cell differentiation. Induction of acute phase proteins, growth of keratinocytes. Stimulates growth of T cells and hematopoietic stem cells.
IL-8	Endothelial cells, fibroblasts, lymphocytes, monocytes	Induced by TNF, IL-1, LPS, cell adherence (monocytes)	Basophils, neutrophils, T cells	Induces expression of endothelial cell LECAM-1 receptors, β_2 integrins, and neutrophil transmigration. Stimulates respiratory burst.
M-CSF	Endothelial cells, fibroblasts, monocytes	Induced by IL-1, LPS, IFN-α	Committed monocyte progenitors (CFU-M, mono)	Supports the proliferation of monocyte-forming colonies. Activates macrophages.
MCP-1, MCAF	Monocytes; some tumors secrete a similar peptide	Induced by IL-1, LPS, PHA	Unstimulated monocytes	Chemoattractant specific for monocytes
TNF-α (LT has almost identical effects)	Macrophages, NK cells, T cells, transformed cell lines, B cells (LT)	Suppressed by PGE_2, TGF-β, IL-4; induced by LPS	Endothelial cells, monocytes, neutrophils	Stimulates T cell growth. Direct cytotoxin to some tumor cells. Profound proinflammatory effect via induction of IL-1 and PGE_2. systemic administration produces many symptoms of sepsis. Stimulates respiratory burst and phagocytosis.

CFU = colony-forming unit; G-CSF = granulocyte colony-stimulating factor; GM-CSF = granulocyte-macrophage colony-stimulating factor; IFN = interferon; IL = interleukin; IL1ra = interleukin-1 receptor antagonist; LPS = lipopolysaccharide; LT = lymphotoxin; MCAF = Monocyte chemotactic and activating factor; M-CSF = macrophage colony-stimulating factor; MCPO-1 = monocyte chemotactic peptide-1; NK = natural killer (cell); PHA = phytohemagglutinin; TGF-β = transforming growth factor beta; TNF-α = tumor necrosis factor alpha.

ized to diseased tissue, these mediators are highly effective at recruiting and arming cells of the innate and adaptive immune systems to destroy invading organisms and elicit reparative mechanisms in wounded tissue. However, if the degree of the infectious or traumatic insult exceeds the ability of the host to contain it, the inflammatory response becomes systemic. The result is whole-body activation of the inflammatory response, with resultant disruption of normal cellular metabolism and microcirculatory perfusion. This leads to clinical deterioration, manifested as dysfunction of the brain (delirium), lungs (hypoxia), heart and blood vessels (shock and edema), kidneys (oliguria), intestines (ileus), liver (hyperbilirubinemia), and the hematologic (coagulopathy, anemia) and immunologic systems (immunosuppression). This syndrome is referred to as **multiple organ dysfunction syndrome** (**MODS**). The risks of organ failure in general are directly proportionate to the duration and severity of shock and inversely proportionate to the age and underlying health of the patient. It is frequently difficult or impossible to determine whether the cause of organ dysfunction in critically ill patients is severe infection or inflammation. The term **sepsis** is used when the systemic response results from infection. In contrast, when the systemic response occurs in the absence of infection, as it does in severe burns, trauma, and pancreatitis, it is called **systemic inflammatory response syndrome** (**SIRS**). The interrelationships among infection, bacteremia, sepsis, and SIRS are depicted in Figure 8–1.

▶ Diagnosis

The aim of management is to detect and treat sepsis before it evolves into more advanced stages.

A. Physical Examination

Physical examination is the easiest way to localize a surgical infection. When infection is suspected but cannot be identified initially, repeated examination will often reveal subtle warmth, erythema, induration, tenderness, or splinting due to a developing abscess. Failure to repeat the physical examination is the most common reason for delayed diagnosis and therapy.

B. Laboratory Findings

1. General findings—Laboratory data are of limited value. Leukocytosis may give way to leukopenia when the infection is severe. Acidosis is helpful in diagnosis, and signs of disseminated intravascular coagulation are useful as well. Otherwise unexplained respiratory, hepatic, renal, and gastric (ie, stress ulcers) failure is strong evidence for sepsis.

2. Cultures—Positive cultures help to differentiate SIRS from sepsis even though 50% of cases of sepsis are culture-negative. If infection is suspected, cultures of blood, sputum, and urine are collected routinely initially, especially in hospitalized patients given the high frequency of nosoco-

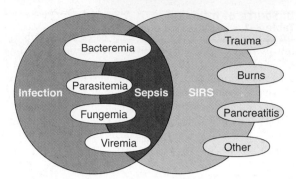

▲ **Figure 8–1.** Interrelationships among systemic inflammatory response syndrome (SIRS), sepsis, and infection. (Modified, with permission, from Crit Care Med 1992;20:864.)

mial pneumonia and urinary tract infections (see below). This is particularly important because data from the Centers for Disease Control and Prevention (CDC) suggest that 70% of the bacteria causing hospital-associated infections are resistant to at least one of the drugs most commonly used to treat them. Other fluids, such as cerebrospinal fluid, pleural and joint effusions, and ascites, can be aspirated and cultured on the basis of signs or symptoms that specifically indicate these sites as potential sources of infection. In general, pus from abscesses should be cultured unless the causative organism is known. In rapidly advancing cases, two separate blood cultures should be taken within 15 minutes. In less urgent situations, cultures should be taken over a 24-hour period, and up to six cultures should be taken if the patient has enigmatic fevers and either a cardiac or joint prosthesis or vascular shunt. False-negative blood culture results occur in about 20% of cases. False-positive results are difficult to define, since skin commensals (even some diphtheroids and *Staphylococcus epidermidis*), regarded as contaminants in the past, have proved occasionally to be true pathogens. Arterial blood cultures may be necessary to detect fungal endocarditis.

C. Imaging Studies

Radiologic examination is frequently helpful, particularly for the diagnosis of pulmonary infections. Whenever infection is close to bone, radiologic examination is indicated to detect early signs of osteomyelitis, which might require more aggressive surgical or antibiotic therapy. MRI imaging is most useful in detecting bone edema, an early sign of osteomyelitis. For detecting abscesses in solid organs, CT scanning is useful. CT scanning and ultrasonography are particularly useful in localizing occult infection.

Numerous radionuclide scans have been tested, all with fair results. The best radionuclides for labeling leukocytes are gallium (^{67}Ga) and indium (^{111}In). Nuclear imaging modalities are rarely used today for localization of infection.

D. Source of Infection

An early diagnosis of sepsis is usually based on a combination of suspicion and inconclusive evidence, since the results of blood cultures are often unavailable during this stage. An important initial step is to identify the source. Surgical or traumatic wounds, surgical infections in the abdomen or thorax, and clostridial infections are all common, but so are urinary tract infections, pneumonia, and even sinus infections. Once identified, any septic focus amenable to surgical therapy should be excised or drained.

▶ Treatment

A. Incision and Drainage

Abscesses must be opened and bacteria, necrotic tissue, and toxins drained to the outside. The pressure and the number of bacteria in the infected space are lowered; this decreases the spread of toxins and bacteria. An abscess with systemic manifestations is a surgical emergency.

Fluctuation is a reliable but late sign of a subcutaneous abscess. Abscesses in the parotid or perianal area may never become fluctuant, and if the surgeon waits for this sign, serious sepsis may result. Drainage creates an open wound, but the tissue will heal by second intention with remarkably little scarring. Deep abscesses difficult to drain surgically may be drained by a catheter placed percutaneously under guidance by CT scanning or ultrasonography.

It may appear that a patient with sepsis cannot withstand operation. In fact, operation to drain an abscess may be the most important of all therapeutic measures. One can hardly imagine delaying removal of infarcted bowel because the patient is in shock. There is no substitute for obliteration of the focus of infection when it is surgically accessible.

B. Excision

Some surgical infections may be excised (eg, an infected appendix or gallbladder). In these cases, drainage may not be necessary, and the patient is cured on the operating table. Clostridial myositis may require amputation of the infected limb. The success of such operations is greatly facilitated by intensive specific adjuvant antimicrobial therapy.

C. Circulatory Enhancement

Just as infections due to vascular ischemia are cured by restoring arterial patency, chronic infections in poorly vascularized areas, as in osteoradionecrosis, may be cured by transplanting a functioning vascular bed (eg, a musculocutaneous flap or omental transposition) into the affected area.

D. Antimicrobial Therapy

Antimicrobial agents are not necessary for simple surgical infections that respond to incision and drainage alone—furuncles and uncomplicated wound infections. Infections likely to spread or persist require antimicrobial therapy, best chosen on the basis of therapy targeted to the evidence of pathogen(s) via cultures and sensitivity tests. In "toxic" infections, including septic shock, antimicrobial therapy must be started promptly; empiric regimens can be modified later based on procured specimen results. The preemptive or empiric choice of drugs must take into account the organisms most often cultured from similar infections in previous patients, the results of body fluid Gram stains, and specific characteristics of the patient.

E. Nutritional Support

In malnourished, septic, or severely traumatized patients, the ability to ward off or recover from infection is often enhanced by aggressive nutritional therapy. Specific measurable effects include improved immunocompetency and blunting or reversal of catabolism. Protection or restoration of visceral and skeletal muscle allows the patient to cough better and be more mobile.

▶ Prognosis

The mortality rate ranges from 10% in septic patients with manifestations limited to fever, chills, and toxicity, to almost 100% in those who manifest shock and multiple organ failure. Factors that have independent influences on outcome include the causative microorganism, blood pressure, body temperature (inverse relationship), primary site of infection, age, predisposing factors, and place of acquisition of infection (hospital or home). Of patients with low-grade fever and an elevated leukocyte count after antibiotics have been discontinued, 60% will have a relapse. Nevertheless, continuation of antibiotics in questionable cases is often contraindicated because it only delays recognition of infection and may enhance morbidity as well as increase antibiotic resistance.

Bone RC: Sir Isaac Newton, sepsis, SIRS, and CARS. Crit Care Med 1996;24:1125.

Bone RC et al: Definitions for sepsis and organ failure and guidelines for the use of innovative therapies in sepsis. The ACCP/SCCM Consensus Conference Committee: American College of Chest Physicians/Society of Critical Care Medicine. Chest 1992;101:1644.

Lederer JA et al: The effects of injury on the adaptive immune response. Shock 1999;11:153.

O'Grady NP et al: Practice parameters for evaluating new fever in critically ill adult patients. Task Force of the American College of Critical Care Medicine of the Society of Critical Care Medicine in collaboration with the Infectious Disease Society of America. Crit Care Med 1998;26:392.

NOSOCOMIAL INFECTIONS & INFECTION CONTROL

Nosocomial infections affect approximately 2 million patients annually in the United States and add approximately $3.5 billion to the cost of health care. Patients may acquire infection in hospital through contact with personnel or from a nonsterile environment, or infection may develop from bacteria harbored by the patient before operation.

Hospital Personnel as a Source of Infection

Most nosocomially acquired bacteria are transmitted through human contact. In order to minimize transmission in hospital, rules made for behavior, dress, and hygiene should be obeyed.

Unwashed hands are by far the most frequent sources of nosocomial infections such as pneumonia, intravenous catheter-related sepsis, burn wound infections, and even pseudomembranous colitis. Therefore, hand washing is the single most important procedure for preventing nosocomial infections. Routine hand washing should be a matter of reflex conditioning. In today's atmosphere, failure to wash one's hands between patient contacts in a hospital is essentially an unethical act.

The Operating Room as a Source of Infection

Any break in operative technique noted by any member of the operating team should be corrected immediately. Members of the team should not operate if they have cutaneous infections or upper respiratory or viral infections that may cause sneezing or coughing.

Scrub suits should be worn only in the operating room and not in other areas of the hospital. If they must be worn outside the operating room, they should be changed before reentering. Physicians and nurses should always wash their hands between patients. Careful hand washing should follow all contact with infected patients. For preoperative preparation, hands and forearms up to the elbows should be scrubbed for 2–5 minutes with any approved agent if the surgeon has not scrubbed within the past week. Shorter scrubs are allowable between operations. Traffic and talking in the operating room should be minimized.

Though many parts of the operating environment are sterile, the operative field is not—it is merely as sterile as it can be made. Attempts to achieve a level of sterility beyond normal standards have not led to further reductions in wound infection rates. This reflects the fact that bacteria are also present in the patient, and host defense mechanisms are also important determinants of infection not affected by more aggressive attempts to achieve sterility.

Many special and expensive techniques have been devised to minimize bacterial contamination in the operating room. Ultraviolet light, laminar flow ventilation, and elaborate architectural and ventilation schemes have been advocated, but none have been definitively proved more effective than observation of current infection control guidelines and surgical discipline.

The only completely reliable methods for sterilization of surgical instruments and supplies are steam under pressure (autoclaving), dry heat, and ethylene oxide gas. Saturated steam at 2 atm pressure and a temperature of 120 °C destroys all vegetative bacteria and most resistant dry spores in 13 minutes, but exposure of surgical instrument packs should usually be extended to 30 minutes to allow heat and moisture to penetrate to the center of the package. Shorter times are allowable for unwrapped instruments with the vacuum-cycle or high-pressure autoclaves now widely used. Continuous dry heat at 170 °C for 1 hour sterilizes articles that cannot tolerate moist heat. If grease or oil is present on instruments, safe dry-heat sterilization requires 4 hours at 160 °C.

Gaseous ethylene oxide destroys bacteria, viruses, fungi, and various spores. It is used for heat-sensitive materials, including telescopic instruments, plastic and rubber goods, sharp and delicate instruments, electrical cords, and sealed ampules. It damages certain plastics and pharmaceuticals. The technique requires a special pressurized-gas autoclave, with 12% ethylene oxide and 88% Freon-12 at 55 °C, 8 psi pressure above atmospheric pressure. Most items must be aerated in sterile packages on the shelf for 24–48 hours before use in order to rid them of the dissolved gas. Implanted plastics should be stored for 7 days before use. Ethylene oxide is toxic and represents a safety hazard unless it is used according to strict regulations.

Miscellaneous sterilization procedures include soaking in antiseptics such as 2% glutaraldehyde to remove viruses from instruments with lenses. Total sterilization by this method requires 10 hours. Chemical antiseptics are often used to clean operating room surfaces and instruments that need not be totally sterile. Other disinfectant solutions include synthetic phenolics, polybrominated salicylanilides, iodophors, alcohols, other glutaraldehyde preparations, and 6% stabilized hydrogen peroxide. These agents maintain high potency in the presence of organic matter and usually leave effective residual antibacterial activity on surfaces. They are also used to clean anesthetic equipment that cannot be sterilized. Prepackaged instruments and supplies can be sterilized with gamma radiation by manufacturers. Synthetic fabrics have now proved to be superior barriers to bacteria and less costly than the traditional cotton. They can be used in gowns and drapes.

The Patient as a Source of Infection

When possible, preexisting infections should be treated before operation. Secretions from patients with a history of respiratory tract infections should be cultured and appropriate treatment given. The urinary tract should be cultured and specific antibiotics administered before instruments are introduced; this precaution has eliminated septic shock as a complication of urologic surgery. The colon should be prepared as discussed in Chapter 31. Dental extractions for caries are imperative prior to cardiac valve replacement.

Bacteria on the patient's skin are a common cause of infection. Preoperative showers or baths with antiseptic soap reduce the infection rate in clean wounds by 50%. Shaving of the operative field hours prior to incision is associated with a 50% increase in wound infection rates and should not be done. If the patient has a heavy growth of hair, an area just large enough to accommodate the wound and its closure should be clipped rather than shaved immediately before operation. Razor shaving more than a few minutes before operation raises the wound infection rate.

The skin to be included in the operative field should be cleansed with antiseptic. Nonirritating agents such as benzalkonium salts should be used in or around the nose or eyes. For other skin areas, the iodophors (eg, povidone-iodine) and chlorhexidine are used most commonly.

▶ Isolation Procedures: Universal Precautions

Traditionally, patients with infection were individually isolated. Since 1985—partly in response to the HIV epidemic—a more general kind of isolation called "universal precautions" has been substituted. In this system, *any* procedure involving close contact with *any* patient—and especially those involving contact with blood—is performed by hospital personnel wearing gloves and other protective devices. The concept of universal precautions emphasizes (1) prevention of needlestick injuries, (2) the use of traditional barriers such as gloves and gowns, (3) the use of masks and eye coverings to prevent mucous membrane exposure during procedures, and (4) the use of individual ventilation devices when the need for resuscitation is predictable. The CDC recommends that universal precautions apply to blood, semen, and vaginal secretions; to amniotic, cerebrospinal, pericardial, peritoneal, pleural, and synovial fluids; and to other body fluids contaminated with blood. Universal precautions are not recommended for feces, nasal secretions, sputum, sweat, tears, urine, or vomitus unless they contain visible blood. The need for hand washing is not diminished by this system.

http://www.cdc.gov/ncidod/hip/isolat/isolat.htm

▶ Antibiotic Prophylaxis Against Surgical Infections

Prophylactic use of antibiotics can decrease the incidence of infections, especially surgical site infections, but at the risk of toxic and allergic reactions to the drug, drug interactions, bacterial resistance, and superinfection. The principles of antibiotic prophylaxis are simple: (1) Choose antibiotics effective against the expected type of contamination. (2) Use antibiotics only if the risk of infection justifies doing so. (3) Give antibiotics in appropriate doses and at appropriate times. (4) Stop dosing before the risk of side effects outweighs benefits.

Antibiotics for preventive use must not be highly toxic and should not be "first-line" antibiotics for treatment of established infection. Because resistance to antibiotics may develop quickly, agents that have been used frequently for prophylaxis are likely to lose their effectiveness for later treatment. Prophylactic agents should be chosen for cost-effectiveness and safety as well as for efficacy.

Prophylactic antibiotics should be selected to target the organisms most likely to be encountered in the anticipated operative procedure. A first-generation cephalosporin (eg, cefazolin) is preferred for most procedures, since it is effective against common gram-positive and gram-negative bacteria and has a moderately long serum half-life. The routine use of vancomycin for prophylaxis is discouraged in light of the emergence of vancomycin-resistant organisms—especially enterococcus and staphylococcus. Agents with better gram-negative and anaerobic bacterial activity (eg, cefoxitin, cefotetan) are preferred for colorectal and gynecologic procedures. A single dose of antibiotic given 30 minutes prior to making the skin incision should provide adequate tissue concentrations for most procedures. Additional doses are advisable for longer procedures (over 4 hours) or those that require large volumes of resuscitative fluids (larger volume of distribution). Postoperative doses of prophylactic antibiotics are usually not necessary; in general, no prophylactic antibiotics should be given after wound closure. The American Heart Association recommends that patients with valvular heart disease or prosthetic heart valves receive antibiotics prior to procedures that result in bacteremia in order to prevent endocarditis. A similar argument has been made for patients with indwelling prosthetic joints.

Antibiotic prophylaxis cannot and is not intended to eliminate bacteria. Use of multiple antibiotics increases the risk of drug reactions, diminishes effectiveness in the long run by promoting the emergence of resistant strains, and increases costs. Antibiotics should be given only when a significant rate of infection is encountered without them or when the consequences of infection would be disastrous, as with placement of vascular, cardiac, or joint prostheses.

The surgeon may be tempted to give every patient antibiotics in order to have an infection-free record, but this strategy is inappropriate for several reasons: (1) Clean wounds may become infected with organisms for which prophylactic antibiotics are ineffective. (2) Resistant organisms will eventually develop, creating a higher risk of infection within the hospital. (3) The expense and risks associated with antibiotics (eg, kidney failure, hearing loss, anaphylaxis, skin rashes, fungal infections, enterocolitis) overshadow the minimal beneficial effects of using antibiotics in clean cases. The number of antibiotic-resistant strains has been correlated with the number of kilograms of antibiotics used in any given hospital.

▶ Control of Infection within the Hospital

Considering the cost of hospital-associated infections, infection control is a very sound investment. Data indicate that infection control programs can prevent approximately one-third of nosocomial infections. Consequently, the Joint Commission on Accreditation of Healthcare Organizations in the United States requires each hospital to have an infection control committee with established infection control procedures. This multidisciplinary committee establishes rules for isolation of infected patients and for protection of hospital personnel exposed to infection, procedures for disposal of materials contaminated by bacteria, and guidelines for limiting the spread of infection. Infection control specialists usually record and analyze patterns of infection. Isolates of bacteria cultured from patients are routinely analyzed for potential significance to the hospital environment. Attempts are made to determine the source of "epidemics." These efforts are coordinated at the national level by the CDC to monitor and report nosocomial infection trends. These data are then used to generate recommendations and guidelines to improve outcomes.

Antimicrobial prophylaxis in surgery. Med Lett Drugs Ther 1999;41:75.

CDC Guidelines on Prevention of Nosocomial Infections, Hospital Infections Program, Centers for Disease Control and Prevention: http://www.cdc.gov/ncidod/hip/

▼ SPECIFIC TYPES OF INFECTIONS

SURGICAL SITE INFECTIONS

Surgical site infections, previously called postoperative wound infections, result from bacterial contamination during or after a surgical procedure. The most recent data from the National Nosocomial Infection Surveillance (NNIS) of the CDC indicate that surgical site infections are the third most frequently reported hospital-associated infection, accounting for 14–16% of all infections in hospitalized patients. Among surgical patients, surgical site infections are the most frequent cause of hospital-associated infections, accounting for 38% of the total.

Infection usually is confined to the subcutaneous tissues. Despite every effort to maintain asepsis, most surgical wounds are contaminated to some extent. However, infection rarely develops if contamination is minimal, if the wound has been made without undue injury, if the subcutaneous tissue is well perfused and well oxygenated, and if there is no dead space. The criteria used to define surgical site infections have been standardized and describe three different anatomic levels of infection (see Table 8–2).

Table 8–2. Types of Surgical Site Infections (SSIs).

Incisional SSIs
  Superficial: Incisional (skin and subcutaneous tissues)
  Deep: Incisional (deeper soft deep fascia, muscles, and tissues beneath subcutaneous tissue of the incision)
Organ/space SSIs
  Any part of the anatomy other than body wall layers that was manipulated during the procedure

The degree of intraoperative contamination can be divided into four categories: (1) clean (no gross contamination from exogenous or endogenous sources), (2) lightly contaminated (clean-contaminated), (3) heavily contaminated, and (4) infected (in which obvious infection has been encountered during operation). The infection rate is about 1.5% in clean cases. Clean-contaminated wounds (eg, with gastric or biliary surgery) are infected about 2–5% of the time. Heavily contaminated wounds, as in operations on the unprepared colon or emergency operations for intestinal bleeding or perforation, may have an infection risk of 5–30%. Wise use of isolation techniques, preoperative antibiotics, and delayed primary closure will keep rates of surgical site infections within acceptable limits. Since even a minor surgical site infection significantly prolongs hospitalization and increases economic loss, all reasonable efforts must be made to keep the infection rate as low as possible.

The risk of wound infection is influenced but not entirely determined by the degree of contamination. Multiple patient risk factors and perioperative characteristics can increase the likelihood of surgical site infections (Table 8–3).

The susceptibility of the host is usually but not always local. Susceptibility is also proportionate to the oxygen tension in the operative wound. Wound tissue P_{O_2} in turn is proportionate to arterial P_{O_2} and the perfusion rate. The perfusion rate is generally determined by the cardiac output and by the tone of the sympathetic nervous system. Sympathetic tone, ie, the degree of peripheral vasoconstriction, is determined by the patient's surface temperature, the degree of pain, the blood volume, and the degree of fear. Therefore, susceptibility to infection can be reduced by such simple methods as rapid infusion of additional fluids, warming, better pain control, and oxygen administration (but only after perfusion has been ensured). Contrary to popular

Table 8–3. Surgical Site Infection Risk Factors.

Host factors
  Diabetes mellitus
  Hypoxemia
  Hypothermia
  Leukopenia
  Nicotine (tobacco smoking)
  Long-term use of steroid or immunosuppressive agents
  Malnutrition
  Nares colonization with *S aureus*
  Poor skin hygiene
Perioperative factors
  Operative site shaving
  Breaks in operative sterile technique
  Early or delayed initiation of antimicrobial prophylaxis
  Inadequate intraoperative dosing of antimicrobial prophylaxis
  Infected or colonized surgical personnel (skin or surgical attire)
  Prolonged hypotension
  Poor operating room air quality (contaminated ventilation)
  Contaminated operating room instruments or environment
  Poor wound care postoperatively

opinion, urinary output correlates poorly with the incidence of wound infection. When the infection risk is high, wound tissue P_{O_2} can be measured, monitored, and supported. Appropriate technology is available.

Clinical Findings

Wound infections usually appear between the fifth and tenth days after surgery, but they may appear as early as the first postoperative day or even years later. The first sign is usually fever, and postoperative fever requires inspection of the wound. The patient may complain of pain at the surgical site. The wound rarely appears severely inflamed, but edema may be obvious because the skin sutures appear tight.

Palpation of the wound may disclose an abscess. A good method is to pour surgical soap on the wound and, using it as a lubricant, palpate gently with the gloved hand. Firm or fluctuant areas, crepitus, or tenderness can be detected with minimal pain and contamination. The rare infection deep to the fascia may be difficult to recognize. In doubtful cases, one can carefully open the wound in the suspicious area using meticulous sterile technique. If no pus is present, the wound can be closed immediately with skin tapes. Cultures even of clean wounds that are successfully reclosed are often positive.

Differential Diagnosis

Differential diagnosis includes all other causes of postoperative fever, wound dehiscence, and wound herniation (see Chapter 5).

Prevention

Detailed recommendations for the prevention of surgical site infections (and the relevant supporting data) have been published by the CDC. In general, there are three main aspects to prevention of infection: (1) careful, gentle, clean surgery; (2) reduction of contamination; and (3) support of the patient's defenses, including use of prophylactic antibiotics. The surgeon who traumatizes tissue, leaves foreign bodies or hematomas in wounds, uses too many ligatures, and exposes the wound to drying or pressure from retractors is exposing patients to needless risks of infection.

The purpose of sutures is to approximate tissues and hold them securely, and the right number to use is as few as will accomplish this aim. Since sutures strangulate tissue, they should be tied as loosely as the requirements of approximation permit. Subcutaneous sutures should be used rarely. Using skin tapes instead of skin sutures or staples lowers infection rates, especially in contaminated wounds.

Severely contaminated wounds in which subcutaneous infection is likely to develop are best left open initially and managed by delayed primary closure. This means that the deep layers are closed while skin and subcutaneous tissues are left open, dressed with sterile gauze, inspected on the fourth or fifth day, and then closed (preferably with skin tapes) if no sign of infection is seen. A clean granulating open wound is preferable to a wound infection. Scarring from secondary healing is usually minimal.

Prophylactic antibiotics are indicated whenever wound contamination during the operation can be predicted to be high (eg, operations on the colon). Excessively liberal use of antibiotics is not reasonable. The incidence of postoperative infections in clean operations is not diminished by administration of antimicrobials, and the prophylactic use of these drugs must be reserved for selected cases at high risk for infection.

Treatment

The basic treatment of established wound infection is to open the wound and allow it to drain. Antibiotics are not necessary unless the infection is invasive, manifested by a surrounding zone of soft tissue inflammation (erythema and edema). Culture should be performed to help locate the source and prevent further infection in other patients, to gain a preview of bacterial flora in case other infections develop deep to the wound or in case the existing infection becomes invasive, and to select preoperative antibiotics in case the wound must be entered again.

Prognosis

Most wound infections make illness more severe. Wound infection correlates positively with death rates but is not often the cause of death. It may tip the scales against successful operation.

Bergamini TM et al: The importance of tissue antibiotic activity in the prevention of operative wound infection. J Antimicrob Chemother 1989;23:303.
Culver DH et al: Surgical wound infection rates by wound class, operative procedure, and patient risk index. National Nosocomial Infections Surveillance System. Am J Med 1991;91:152S.

CELLULITIS

Cellulitis is a common, invasive, nonsuppurative infection of connective tissue. The term is loosely used and often misapplied. The microscopic picture is one of severe inflammation of the dermal and subcutaneous tissues. Although PMNs predominate on Gram stain, there is no gross suppuration except perhaps at the portal of entry.

Clinical Findings

Cellulitis usually appears on an extremity as a brawny red or reddish-brown area of edematous skin. It advances rapidly from its starting point, and the advancing edge may be vague or sharply defined (eg, in erysipelas). A surgical wound, puncture, skin ulcer, or patch of dermatitis is usually identifiable as a portal of entry. The disease often occurs in susceptible patients, eg, alcoholics with postphlebitic leg ulcers. Most cases are caused by streptococci or staphylococci, but other bacteria have been involved. A moderate or high fever is almost always present.

Lymphangitis arising from cellulitis produces red, warm, tender streaks 3–4 mm wide leading from the infection along lymphatic vessels to the regional lymph nodes. There is no suppuration. Bacteria are difficult to obtain for culture, but blood culture is sometimes positive.

Differential Diagnosis

Since the visible features of cellulitis are all due to inflammation, the words inflammation and cellulitis have sometimes been used imprecisely as synonyms. Some forms of inflammation are associated with suppuration requiring incision and drainage, whereas cellulitis as such is not.

Thrombophlebitis is often difficult to differentiate from cellulitis, but phlebitic swelling is usually greater, and tenderness may localize over a vein. Homans sign does not always make the differentiation—nor does lymphadenopathy. Fever is usually greater with cellulitis, and pulmonary embolization does not occur in cellulitis.

Contact allergy, such as poison oak, may mimic cellulitis in its early phase, but dense nonhemorrhagic vesiculation soon discloses the allergic cause.

Chemical inflammation due to drug injection may also mimic streptococcal cellulitis.

The appearance of hemorrhagic bullae and skin necrosis suggests necrotizing fasciitis.

Treatment

Therapy should consist of rest, elevation, warm packs, and an oral or intravenous antibiotic. Warm packs elevate subcutaneous tissue temperature, and if regional blood supply is normal, they can raise local oxygen tension, which should support clearing of infection. Semisynthetic penicillins or first-generation cephalosporins are usually effective. If a clear response has not occurred in 12–24 hours, one should suspect an abscess or consider the possibility that the causative agent is a gram-negative rod or resistant organism. The patient must be examined once daily or more often to detect a hidden abscess masquerading within or under an area of cellulitis.

DIFFUSE NECROTIZING INFECTIONS

These infections are particularly dangerous because they frequently are difficult to diagnose, are extremely toxic, and spread rapidly, often leading to limb amputation. Hence, the popular press has characterized the causative bacteria as "flesh-eating" or "meat-eating." Although several classification systems for diffuse necrotizing infections have been published, most are not practical because they are based on historical descriptions and eponyms. The American College of Surgeons recently published a classification system based on clinical presentation, anatomic site of primary tissue involvement, and the microbiology of the causative organisms (Table 8–4). The four known pathogenic factors are the presence of an anaerobic wound, bacterial exotoxins, bacterial synergy, and thrombosis of nutrient bridging vessels.

Table 8–4. Classification of Diffuse Necrotizing Infections.

Clostridial
Necrotizing cellulitis
Myositis
Nonclostridial
Necrotizing fasciitis
Streptococcal gangrene

Classification & Clinical Findings
A. Clostridial Infections

Clostridia are saprophytes. Vegetative and spore forms are widespread in soil, sand, clothing, and feces. They are generally fastidious anaerobes requiring a low redox potential to grow and to initiate conversion of the spores into vegetative, toxin-producing pathogens. Tissue redox potentials in vivo are diminished by impaired blood supply, muscle injury, pressure from casts, severe local edema, foreign bodies, or oxygen-consuming organisms. On Gram stain they appear as relatively large, gram-positive, rod-shaped bacteria. Clostridial infections frequently occur in the presence of other bacteria, especially gram-negative bacilli. A broad spectrum of disease is caused by clostridia, ranging from negligible surface contamination to invasive cellulitis of connective tissue to invasive anaerobic infection of muscle with massive tissue necrosis and profound shock. Six species cause infection in humans; *Clostridium perfringens* (80% of cases), *C novyi*, and *C septicum* are the species most frequently isolated.

Clostridia proliferate and produce toxins that diffuse into the surrounding tissue. *C tetani* and *C botulinum* produce extremely potent biologic toxins. As the pathogens responsible for tetanus and food-borne botulism, respectively, they owe their virulence to toxin production (see below). Other clostridia, however, are highly invasive. For example, *C perfringens* produces a large number of exotoxins that destroy the local microcirculation. This allows further invasion, which can advance at an astonishing rate. The alpha toxin, a necrotizing lecithinase, is thought to be particularly important in this sequence, but other toxins, including collagenase, hyaluronidase, leukocidin, protease, lipase, and hemolysin, also contribute. When the disease has advanced sufficiently, toxins enter the systemic circulation, causing the features of SIRS and, if untreated, ultimately septic shock, MODS, and death. The severity and progress of the local lesion can be judged by the general state of the patient as well as by the local signs of infection. Immunosuppressed patients are particularly susceptible.

Many open wounds are superficially infected or contaminated with clostridia without developing significant infections. The condition is not invasive because the surrounding tissue is basically healthy and the clostridia are confined to necrotic surface tissue. Debridement of dead surface tissue is usually the only treatment necessary. A crepitant abscess or cellulitis has a characteristic brown seropurulent exudate and mousy odor. Invasion is usually superficial to the deep fascia and may spread very quickly, producing discoloration of the skin. Delayed or inadequate debridement of injured tissue after devascularizing injury is the most common setting. Severe pain suggests extension into muscle compartments (myositis). The disease characteristically progresses rapidly, with loss of blood supply to the infected muscle. Profound shock can appear early, rapidly leading to organ dysfunction (MODS). Air bubbles—often visible on plain radiographs (gas gangrene)—and crepitus may be present. However, gas in the tissues is not a good differentiating point because some clostridial species do not produce gas (eg, *C novyi*), nonclostridial organisms often produce gas (eg, *E coli*), and air can enter tissues through a penetrating wound.

B. Nonclostridial Infections

Necrotizing fasciitis is caused by multiple nonclostridial bacterial pathogens. Infection usually involves a mixed microbial flora, often including microaerophilic streptococci, staphylococci, aerobic gram-negative bacteria, and anaerobes, especially *Peptostreptococci* and bacteroides. Fasciitis usually begins in a localized area such as a puncture wound, leg ulcer, or surgical wound. The infection spreads along the relatively ischemic fascial planes, leading to thrombosis of penetrating vessels. Overlying subcutaneous tissue and skin are thus devascularized. Externally, hemorrhagic bullae are usually the first sign of skin death. The skin is usually anesthetic, and crepitus is occasionally present. The fascial necrosis is usually wider than the skin appearance indicates. The patient often seems alert and unconcerned but appears toxic. At operation, the finding of edematous, dull-gray, and necrotic fascia and subcutaneous tissue confirms the diagnosis. Thrombi in penetrating vessels are often visible.

Group A streptococcus (*S pyogenes*) is a bacterium frequently found on the skin and in the throat. Severe invasive infections with group A streptococci associated with shock and organ failure (streptococcal gangrene) are uncommon but have been reported with increasing frequency since the 1980s. This type of infection is also referred to as streptococcal toxic shock syndrome. The incidence of these infections was 1 to 10 cases per 100,000 population in the United States in 1998. Those with chronic immunosuppressive illnesses such as cancer, diabetes, and end-stage renal disease and those taking corticosteroids are at increased risk.

Streptococcal organisms release at least five different types of exotoxins. The sudden onset of severe pain is the most common presenting symptom, usually in an extremity associated with a wound. Fever and other signs of systemic infection are frequently present at the time of presentation. Shock and renal dysfunction are usually present within the first 24 hours after admission. Invasion of deeper layers, especially muscle, is uncommon.

▶ Treatment

The major emphasis in treatment is inevitably surgical. Suspicion should be directed toward any wound incurred out of doors and contaminated with a foreign body, soil, or feces and any wound in which tissue (particularly muscle) has been extensively injured. This type of wound should be carefully examined, with the patient under sufficient anesthesia to permit full inspection and debridement of devitalized tissue, including muscle.

It is often difficult to distinguish necrotic from edematous tissue. Careful daily inspections of the wound will determine whether repeated debridement will be necessary. Daily debridement under anesthesia may be required, since these lesions are extensive and the degree of tissue viability is often difficult to assess in the operating room. Tight fascial compartments must be decompressed. Wide-open drainage is essential and may require extensive denudation. A functional extremity can usually be salvaged in fasciitis; if not, amputation can be safely performed later.

It is important to avoid confusing fasciitis with deep gangrene. It is a tragic error to amputate an extremity when removal of dead skin and fascia will suffice. Immediate amputation is necessary when there is diffuse myositis with complete loss of blood supply or when adequate debridement would clearly leave a useless limb. When viability of the remaining tissue is assured and the infection has been controlled, soft tissue deficits can be covered with skin grafts.

Antibiotics are often essential but are ineffective without primary surgical intervention. Given the polymicrobial nature of many necrotizing infections and the difficulty of distinguishing them clinically, broad-spectrum antibiotic therapy is indicated. Broad empiric regimens include intravenous (1) penicillin and an aminoglycoside plus clindamycin, (2) imipenem-cilastatin, or (3) ampicillin plus sulbactam (Unasyn) plus an aminoglycoside. Some authorities recommend also giving immune globulin (400 mg/kg/d intravenously for 5 days) for documented streptococcal toxic shock syndrome. Gram stain and intraoperative culture of the infected tissue will help to narrow the antibiotic spectrum once bacterial sensitivities are available.

In severe cases of infection, the importance of resuscitative therapy cannot be overemphasized. Debridement often leaves a large raw surface that may bleed extensively and contribute to massive insensible water losses. Intravascular volume must be maintained by infusions of crystalloid; plasma and blood are transfused as needed to correct coagulopathy or anemia. Diabetes mellitus, if present, must be treated aggressively.

Hyperbaric oxygenation has been reported anecdotally to be beneficial adjuvant therapy for clostridial infections, but it cannot replace the primary role of surgical intervention, as no amount of increased arterial PO_2 can force oxygen into dead tissue. Hyperbaric oxygen inhibits bacterial invasion but does not eliminate the focus of infection.

Prognosis

Diffuse necrotizing infections are potentially lethal diseases. With adequate treatment, deaths should occur only when treatment is delayed or when patients are already severely ill with other comorbidities (eg, diabetes mellitus) or have advanced bacterial invasion of vital structures. About 20% of patients with necrotizing fasciitis and more than half of patients with streptococcal toxic shock syndrome die. The prognosis for salvage of functioning limbs is not favorable. Limbs affected with myonecrosis often become useless and must be amputated to save life.

Stevens DL: Streptococcal toxic-shock syndrome: spectrum of disease, pathogenesis, and new concepts in treatment. Emerg Infect Dis 1995;1:69.

FURUNCLE, CARBUNCLE, & HIDRADENITIS

Furuncles and carbuncles are cutaneous abscesses (primary pyodermas) that begin in skin glands and hair follicles. Hair follicles normally contain bacteria. Furuncles (boils) usually start in infected hair follicles, though some are caused by retained foreign bodies and other injuries. If the pilosebaceous apparatus becomes obstructed at the skin level, the development of a furuncle can be anticipated. Because the base of the hair follicle may lie in subcutaneous tissue, the infection can spread as cellulitis or it can form a subcutaneous abscess. If a furuncle results from confluent infection of hair follicles, a central core of skin may become necrotic and will slough when the abscess is drained. Furuncles may take a phlegmonous form, ie, extend into the subcutaneous tissue, forming a long, flat abscess. A carbuncle is a deep-seated mass of fistulous tracts between infected hair follicles. Furuncles are the most common surgical infections, but carbuncles are rare.

Furuncles can be multiple and recurrent (furunculosis). Furunculosis usually occurs in young adults and is associated with hormonal changes resulting in impaired skin function. The commonest organisms are staphylococci and anaerobic diphtheroids.

Hidradenitis suppurativa is a serious skin infection of the axillae or groin consisting of multiple abscesses of the apocrine sweat glands. The condition often becomes chronic and disabling. The cause is unknown but may involve a defect of terminal follicular epithelium.

Clinical Findings

Furuncles itch and cause pain. The skin first becomes red and then turns white and necrotic over the top of the abscess. There is usually some surrounding erythema and induration. Regional nodes may become enlarged. Systemic symptoms are rare.

Carbuncles usually start as furuncles, but the infection dissects through the dermis and subcutaneous tissue in a myriad of connecting tunnels. Many of these small extensions open to the surface, giving the appearance of large furuncles with many pustular openings. As carbuncles enlarge, the blood supply to the skin is destroyed and the central tissue becomes necrotic. Carbuncles on the back of the neck are seen almost exclusively in diabetic patients or other relatively immunocompromised patients. The patient is usually febrile and mildly toxic. This is a serious problem that demands immediate surgical attention. Diabetes or some other immunosuppressive condition (eg, HIV disease) must be suspected and treated when a carbuncle is found.

Differential Diagnosis

On occasion, the surgeon may be confronted with a localized area of erythema and induration without obvious suppuration. Many such lesions will go on to central suppuration and become obvious furuncles. On the other hand, when these lesions are located near joints or over the tibia or when they are widely distributed, one must consider such differential diagnoses as rheumatoid nodules, gout, bursitis, synovitis, erythema nodosum, fungal infections, some benign or malignant skin tumors, and inflamed (but not usually infected) sebaceous or epithelial inclusion cysts.

Hidradenitis is differentiated from furunculosis by skin biopsy, which shows typical involvement of the apocrine sweat glands. One suspects hidradenitis when abscesses are concentrated in the apocrine gland areas, ie, the axillae, groin, and perineum. Carbuncles are rarely confused with any other condition.

Complications

Any of these infections may cause suppurative phlebitis when located near major veins. This is particularly important when the infection is located near the nose or eyes. Central venous thrombosis in the brain is a serious complication, and abscesses on the face usually must be treated with antibiotics as well as by prompt incision and drainage.

Hidradenitis may disable the patient but rarely has systemic manifestations. Carbuncles on the back of the neck may in rare cases lead to epidural abscess and meningitis.

Treatment

The classic therapy for furuncle is drainage, not antibiotics. Invasive carbuncles, however, must be treated by excision and adjuvant antibiotic therapy. Between these two extremes, the use of antibiotics depends on the location of the abscess and the extent of infection.

Patients with recurrent furunculosis may be diabetic or immunodeficient. Approximately 50% of patients in a recent study had impaired neutrophil function; treatment with vitamin C appeared to improve neutrophil function and the clinical response. Frequent washing with soaps containing hexachlorophene or other disinfectants is advisable. It may also be necessary to advise extensive laundering of all personal clothing and disinfection of the patient's living quarters in order to reduce the reservoirs of bacteria.

When an abscess fails to resolve after a superficial incision, the surgeon must look for a small opening to a deeper and larger subcutaneous abscess, ie, a **collar-button abscess.**

Carbuncles are often more extensive than the external appearance indicates. Incision alone is almost always inadequate, and excision with electrocautery is required. Excision is continued until the many sinus tracts are removed—usually far beyond the cutaneous evidence of suppuration. It is sometimes necessary to produce a large open wound. This may appear to be drastic treatment, but it achieves rapid cure and prevents further spread. The large wound usually contracts to a small scar and does not usually require skin grafting, because carbuncles tend to occur in loose skin on the back of the neck and on the buttocks, where contraction is the predominant form of repair.

Hidradenitis is usually treated by drainage of the individual abscess followed by careful hygiene. The patient must avoid astringent antiperspirants and deodorants. Painting with mild disinfectants is sometimes helpful. Fungal infections should be searched for if healing after drainage does not occur promptly. If none of these measures is successful, the apocrine sweat-bearing skin must be excised; if the deficit is large, closure with a skin graft may be indicated. The choice of antibiotic must reflect the frequent polymicrobial origin of these infections, including mixed aerobic and anaerobic bacteria. Topical clindamycin was beneficial in a randomized controlled trial. In a separate trial, systemic therapy with tetracycline yielded similar results when compared with topical clindamycin. Isotretinoin may be useful in some cases.

Brook I et al: Aerobic and anaerobic microbiology of axillary hidradenitis suppurativa. J Med Microbiol 1999;48:103.
Brown TJ et al: Hidradenitis suppurativa. South Med J 1998;91:1107.
Jemec GB et al: Topical clindamycin versus systemic tetracycline in the treatment of hidradenitis suppurativa. J Am Acad Dermatol 1998;39:971.
Levy R et al: Vitamin C for the treatment of recurrent furunculosis in patients with impaired neutrophil functions. J Infect Dis 1996;173:1502.

ANTIBIOTIC-ASSOCIATED COLITIS

The incidence of colonic dysfunction secondary to antibiotic use has increased over the past decade. Although all antimicrobial agents are implicated, aminopenicillins, cephalosporins, and clindamycin are commonly used in clinical care and thus are most often implicated. Illness results from antibiotic-induced relative changes in normal colonic flora, with resultant overgrowth of some commensals, usually *Clostridium difficile.* These bacteria, normally present in the feces of 5% of healthy persons, can be induced to release two types of toxins (cytotoxin A and cytotoxin B) that induce inflammation and mucosal damage. The spectrum of disease ranges from diarrhea to severe, potentially life-threatening colitis associated with mucosal ulceration, bacteremia, and septic shock. The pathognomonic finding on colonoscopy is an elevated, yellow pseudomembrane of necrotic mucosa ("pseudomembranous colitis"). The clinical presentation is characterized by fever, abdominal distention, and usually copious diarrhea in postoperative patients who have recently been exposed to antimicrobial therapy. Although not commonly assessed, stool smear shows numerous fecal leukocytes. *C difficile* toxin A and B can be readily detected by commercially available cytotoxic assays or enzyme immunoassays (EIA). Other organisms that rarely cause colitis include salmonella species, *Clostridium perfringens, Candida albicans,* and *Staphylococcus aureus.*

Treatment includes intravenous fluid resuscitation, correction of electrolyte disorders, and withdrawal of antibiotics if possible. Moderate to severe cases are treated with metronidazole, 250 mg orally three to four times per day for 14 days. Oral vancomycin is also effective, but current guidelines suggest that use be reserved for those who are critically ill or who have not responded to metronidazole—or in whom this agent is contraindicated because of allergy. Recurrence of symptoms, which occurs in up to 20% of cases, requires repeated antibiotic treatment; many experts also recommend adjunctive attempts to normalize colonic flora with either probiotic therapy or fecal instillations.

Environmental spread of *C difficile* has been reported, poor hand washing has been implicated, and use of hypochlorite solution as an environmental control strategy has been an effective intervention to control high rates of endemicity.

Cleary RK: *Clostridium difficile*-associated diarrhea and colitis: clinical manifestations, diagnosis, and treatment. Dis Colon Rectum 1998;41:1435.
Cunha BA: Nosocomial diarrhea. Crit Care Clin 1998;14:329.
Frost F et al: Increasing hospitalization and death possibly due to *Clostridium difficile* diarrheal disease. Emerg Infect Dis 1998;4:619.
Mayfield JL et al: Environmental control to reduce transmission of *Clostridium difficile.* Clin Infect Dis 2000;31:995.
Surawicz CM et al: Pseudomembranous colitis: causes and cures. Digestion 1999;60:91.

TETANUS

Tetanus is a specific anaerobic infection mediated by a neurotoxin that causes nervous irritability and tetanic muscular contractions. The causative organism, *Clostridium tetani,* enters and flourishes in hypoxic wounds contaminated with soil or feces (eg, deep puncture from stepping on a nail). The tetanus-prone wound is usually a puncture wound or one containing devitalized tissue or a foreign body. The occurrence of tetanus in the United States has dropped over the last 5 decades. This improvement is attributed to the increasingly widespread use of tetanus toxoid and improved wound management including the use of prophylaxis against tetanus in emergency rooms. Tetanus continues to be a severe disease primarily of older adults who are unvaccinated or inadequately vaccinated; during 1995–1997, a disproportionately high number of cases (35%) were reported in persons aged 60 or older.

Tetanus is a clinical diagnosis, as confirmatory laboratory tests are not routinely available. Wound isolation of the organism is neither sensitive nor specific. Symptoms of tetanus may occur as soon as 1 day following exposure or as long as several months later; the median incubation period is 7 days. The first symptoms are usually pain or tingling in the area of injury, limitation of movements of the jaw ("lockjaw"), and spasms of the facial muscles (risus sardonicus). These are followed typically by stiffness of the neck, dysphagia, and laryngospasm. In more severe cases, spasms of the muscles of the back produce opisthotonos. As chest and diaphragm spasms occur, increasingly longer periods of apnea follow. The temperature is normal or slightly elevated. The severity of cases varies widely; some are very mild and barely recognizable.

The CDC regularly revises its recommendations for the prevention and treatment of tetanus (www.cdc.gov/nip). Importantly, serosurveys indicate that at least 40% of adults over the age of 60 may lack protective levels of circulating tetanus antitoxin. Because people of all ages are exposed to tetanus, each person should be actively immunized with tetanus toxoid, beginning with routine childhood immunization and continuing with booster injections every 10 years (Table 8–5). It is thus imperative that all patients with traumatic wounds be queried regarding previous tetanus prophylaxis. Tetanus prophylaxis in injured patients depends on the history of immunization and the type of wound. A tetanus-diphtheria (Td) booster (active immunization for clean wounds), tetanus immune globulin (TIG; passive immunization for contaminated wounds), or both may be indicated.

If established tetanus is suspected, intensive treatment should be started immediately. Mainstays of therapy include neutralization of the toxin with TIG, excision and debridement of the suspected wound, intravenous high-dose penicillin, ventilatory support if indicated, and protection from sudden stimuli. The death rate is approximately 18% in established tetanus. An attack of tetanus does not confer lasting immunity, and patients who have recovered from the disease require active immunization according to the usual recommended schedules.

[CDC National Immunization Program—Epidemiology and Prevention of Vaccine-Preventable Diseases] http://www.cdc.gov/nip/publications/pink/tetanus.pdf
Diphtheria, tetanus, and pertussis: recommendations for vaccine use and other preventive measures: recommendations of the Immunization Practices Advisory Committee (ACIP), Centers for Disease Control and Prevention. MMWR Morb Mortal Wkly Rep 1991;40(RR-10):1.
Tetanus surveillance: United States, 1995–1997. MMWR Morb Mortal Wkly Rep 1998;47(SS-2):1.
Tetanus surveillance: United States, 1991–1994. MMWR Morb Mortal Wkly Rep 1997;46(SS-2):15.

Table 8–5. Tetanus Immunization and Prophylaxis.

Indication	Immunization or Prophylaxis[1]
Routine adult immunization	Td 0.5 mL every 10 years (or a single booster at age 50)[2]
Clean minor wounds	
Prior immunization unknown or < 3 doses	Td 0.5 mL
Prior immunization > 3 doses	Td 0.5 mL if last dose > 10 years ago
Other wounds	
Prior immunization unknown or < 3 doses	Td 0.5 mL and TIG
Prior immunization > 3 doses	Td 0.5 mL (unless last dose < 5 years ago)

[1]Td – adult tetanus-diphtheria booster; TIG = tetanus immune globulin 250 units IM. If given concurrently with Td, give at separate site.
[2]Patients who have never received an initial vaccination series should receive the complete series.

RABIES

Rabies is a preventable viral encephalitis of mammals transmitted through the saliva of an infected animal. Humans are usually inoculated by the bite of a rabid bat, raccoon, skunk, fox, or other wild animal; however, about 30% of victims have no memory or evidence of a bite. Other reported modes of transmission include mucous membranes (eyes, nose, mouth), aerosolization, and corneal transplantation. In 1997, there were 8513 reported cases of rabies (93% in wild animals), but only four were in humans. The number of human deaths due to rabies in the United States decreased dramatically during the 20th century, down to one to four deaths per year in the late 1990s.

Since the established disease is almost invariably fatal, early preventive measures are essential. The wound should be washed thoroughly with soap and water. Information useful in determining the risk of potential rabies infection includes the geographic location of the incident, the type of animal involved, how the exposure occurred, the vaccination status of the animal, and whether it can be safely captured and tested for rabies. Rabies prophylaxis has proved nearly 100% successful, as most human deaths now occur in people who fail to seek medical assistance. Each year, approximately 18,000 people receive rabies vaccine prophylaxis before exposure, and an additional 40,000 receive prophylaxis (vaccine plus immune globin) after exposure. The latest information regarding both pre- and postexposure prophylaxis is available at the CDC's Rabies Section web site (http://www.cdc.gov/ncidod/dvrd/rabies).

The rabies virus has a distinctive bullet shape and a nonsegmented, negative-stranded RNA genome. After local (primary) infection, the virus enters peripheral nerves and is transported to the central nervous system, making it difficult to detect (eclipse phase). The subsequent incubation period varies in humans from several days to typically 1–3 months. Clinical symptoms begin with pain and numbness around the site of the wound, followed by nonspecific flulike symptoms of fever, irritability, malaise, and progressive cerebral dysfunction. Delirium, hallucinations, insomnia, paralysis, and convulsions occur terminally.

The direct fluorescent antibody (DFA) test on brain tissue is used most frequently to diagnose rabies in animals. A complement of tests are used routinely in humans, because no single test can rule out rabies absolutely: Serum and cerebrospinal fluid are tested for antibodies, skin biopsy is examined by DFA, and saliva can be tested by nested reverse transcriptase polymerase chain reaction (RT-PCR).

Rabies Section, Viral and Rickettsial Zoonoses Branch, Division of Viral and Rickettsial Diseases, National Center for Infectious Diseases, Centers for Disease Control and Prevention, Atlanta, Georgia. http://www.cdc.gov/ncidod/dvrd/rabies

ECHINOCOCCOSIS

Echinococcosis (hydatid disease) is caused by the microscopic cestode parasites *Echinococcus granulosus* and *E multilocularis* (1–4 mm tapeworms), which form larval cysts in mammalian tissue. Foxes, coyotes, dogs, and cats are the definitive hosts that harbor the adult tapeworms in their intestines; these animals are not harmed by the worms and have no symptoms. Ova are passed in the feces and are ingested by intermediate hosts such as cattle, humans, rodents, and particularly sheep. The ova penetrate the intestine and pass via the portal vein to the liver (75%) and then to the lung (15%) or other tissues. In the liver, the ovum typically develops into a cyst filled with clear fluid. Brood capsules containing scoleces bud into the cyst lumen. Such "endocysts" may cause secondary intraperitoneal cyst formation if spilled into the peritoneal cavity. Because the cysts grow slowly, patients may be asymptomatic for several years. Pain or discomfort in the upper abdominal region and weight loss may occur as a result of the cyst enlarging. Eosinophilia is present in about 40% of patients. Serologic diagnosis may be substantiated by immunoassays. Ultrasonography and CT scanning readily demonstrate cysts. In some patients, the parasite dies, the cyst wall calcifies, and therapy is not required. However, surgery is most often required, though removal of the cyst is not usually 100% effective for eradication of infection. Excision of the cyst intact, if practical, is preferred. Because of the dangers of anaphylaxis or implantation, care must be taken to avoid rupturing the cyst and spilling its contents into the peritoneal cavity. In some cases, the cyst fluid can be aspirated and replaced by a scolicidal agent (hypertonic

sodium chloride solution or sodium hypochlorite solution). After surgery, albendazole or mebendazole may be necessary to keep the cyst from growing back. The overall death rate is about 15%, but it is only 4% in surgically treated cases.

Ammann RW et al: Cestodes. Echinococcus. Gastroenterol Clin North Am 1996;25:655.
Clarkson MJ: Hydatid disease. J Med Microbiol 1997;46:24.
http://www.dpd.cdc.gov/dpdx/HTML/Echinococcosis.htm
Taylor BR et al: Current surgical management of hepatic cyst disease. Adv Surg 1997;31:127.

ACTINOMYCOSIS & NOCARDIOSIS

Actinomycosis and nocardiosis are chronic, slowly progressive infections that may involve many tissues, resulting in the formation of granulomas and abscesses that drain through sinuses and fistulas. Although the causative organisms are true bacteria, the lesions resemble those produced by mycobacteria, fungi, and cancer, making accurate diagnosis difficult.

Actinomyces israelii is a gram-positive, non-acid-fast, filamentous organism that usually shows branching and may break up into short bacterial forms. It is a strict anaerobe and part of the normal flora of the human oropharynx and upper intestinal tract. Inflammatory nodular masses, abscesses, and draining sinuses occur most commonly in the head and neck. One-fifth of patients with actinomycosis have primary lesions in the chest and an equal proportion in the abdomen, most commonly involving the appendix and cecum. Multiple sinuses are commonly formed, and the pus may contain yellow "sulfur granules" of tangled filaments. The inflammatory lesions are often hard and relatively painless and nontender. Systemic symptoms, including fever, are variably present. The discharging sinus tracts or fistulas usually become secondarily infected with other bacteria. Abdominal actinomycosis may produce an abdominal mass mimicking a malignant process or may give rise to appendicitis. If the appendix perforates, multiple lesions and sinuses of the abdominal wall form. Thoracic actinomycosis may give rise to cough, pleural pain, fever, and weight loss, simulating mycobacterial or mycotic infection. Later in the course of the disease, the sinuses perforate the pleural cavity and the chest wall, often involving ribs or vertebrae. CT scanning and needle aspiration may be helpful diagnostically. All forms of actinomycosis are treated with penicillin G for many weeks. Although long-term antibiotic therapy appears to be very successful and can preclude the need for operation, preoperative exclusion of other diagnoses is difficult. Surgical extirpation or drainage of lesions therefore is frequently performed.

Nocardiae are gram-positive, branching, filamentous organisms that may be acid-fast; *Nocardia asteroides* is the most common isolate. The filaments often fragment into bacillary forms. They are aerobes rarely found in the normal flora of the respiratory tract. Nocardiosis may present in two forms. One is localized, chronic granuloma with suppuration, abscess, and sinus tract formation resembling actinomycosis. A specialized disorder occurs in the extremities as Madura foot (mycetoma), with extensive bone destruction but little systemic illness. The second form is a systemic infection, usually beginning as pneumonitis with suppuration and progressing via the bloodstream to involvement of other organs, eg, meninges or brain. Systemic nocardiosis produces fever, cough, and weight loss and resembles mycobacterial or mycotic infections. The mortality rate of nocardial bacteremia is as high as 50%. It is particularly apt to occur as a complication of immunodeficiency in patients with chronic obstructive pulmonary disease, cancer, chronic granulomatous disease, HIV-associated disease, or immunoremittive drug regimens. Nocardiosis is best treated with sulfonamides (eg, sulfadiazine or trimethoprim-sulfamethoxazole) or, when severe, with imipenem and amikacin, for many weeks. Surgical drainage of abscesses, excision of fistulas, and repair of defects are essential features of management.

Cintron JR et al: Abdominal actinomycosis. Dis Colon Rectum 1996;39:105.
Conant EF et al: Actinomycosis and nocardiosis of the lung. J Thorac Imaging 1992;7:75.
Kontoyiannis DP et al: *Nocardia* bacteremia. Report of 4 cases and review of the literature. Medicine 1998;77:255.
Lerner PI: Nocardiosis. Clin Infect Dis 1996;22:891.
Menendez R et al: Pulmonary infection with *Nocardia* species: a report of 10 cases and review. Eur Respir J 1997;10:1542.
Smego R Jr et al: Actinomycosis. Clin Infect Dis 1998;26:1255.
Tarabichi M, Schloss M: Actinomycosis otomastoiditis. Arch Otolaryngol 1993;119:561.
Threlkeld SC et al: Update on management of patients with *Nocardia* infection. Curr Clin Top Infect Dis 1997;17:1.
Warren NG: Actinomycosis, nocardiosis, and actinomycetoma. Dermatol Clin 1996;14:85.

VENOMOUS BITE INJURIES

SNAKEBITE

About 8000 people a year in the United States are bitten by venomous snakes. About one-third of these snakebites do not result in envenomation, as the snake may bite but not inject venom or may eject it onto the skin in a superficial fashion. Death from serious envenomation occurs in only 9–15 victims per year in the United States. In comparison, there are about 120 US deaths a year from wasp and bee stings and about 150 deaths per year from lightning.

Identification of Snake

The vast majority of snakebites in the United States are from nonvenomous snakes. Distinguishing whether the patient has been bitten and envenomed by a venomous snake, bitten but not envenomed, or bitten by a nonvenomous snake is critical prior to starting treatments that may not only cause discomfort but may also produce serious side effects. These distinctions require identification of the attacking snake through knowledge of snake taxonomy, anatomy, and geographic distribution. Coloration patterns and fang or tooth marks are deceptive and unreliable identification criteria.

There are about 120 species of snakes in the United States, of which 26 are venomous. The indigenous venomous snakes of North America can be placed in four groups. Three groups are pit vipers of the subfamily Crotalidae: rattlesnakes, with multiple species within the two genera (*Crotalus* and *Sistrurus*); the cottonmouth or water moccasin (*Agkistrodon piscivorus*); and the copperhead (*Agkistrodon contortrix*). Pit vipers can be distinguished from nonvenomous snakes by a round mouth and a pit between the eyes and the nares on each side. They have retractable canaliculated fangs that can rapidly spring into biting position and deliver venom. The large venom glands also give the head a triangular or diamond appearance. North American pit vipers have vertically oriented elliptiform irises. Most North American pit vipers have a primarily hemotoxic venom, but some, particularly the Mojave rattlesnake, have primarily neurotoxic venom.

The coral snake is in the fourth group of indigenous North American venomous snakes. It is a member of the family Elapidae, which also includes the much more dangerous cobras and kraits. Two different genera of coral snakes (the Western coral snake, *Micruroides euryxanthus,* and the Eastern coral snake, *Micrurus fulvius*) are found chiefly in the western and southern states, respectively, with distinct nonoverlapping geographic distributions. Coral snakes have small mouths, short teeth, and deliver secreted venom into prey through created lacerations. A coral snake bite lacks the characteristic fang marks of bites by pit vipers, sometimes making the bite hard to detect. The degree of envenomation depends upon the size of the snake and the duration of contact; rapid removal of the snake from the victim reduces the risk of significant poisoning. Coral snake venom is primarily neurotoxic and unrelated to that of the pit vipers. Victims may experience respiratory paralysis, one of the hazards of neurotoxic venom.

Some nonpoisonous snakes such as the red milk snake and the scarlet king snake mimic the bright red, yellow, and black coloration of the coral snake. True coral snakes will have red bands immediately adjacent to yellow bands; the nonvenomous mimics will have black bands immediately adjacent to the red bands, thus giving rise to the colloquial mnemonic: "Red on black, venom lack; red on yellow, kill a fellow." This rhyming maxim applies only to North American coral snakes.

The family Elapidae includes the cobras, kraits, and mambas, common in Asia and Africa. Their fangs are at the front of the mouth and are small to moderate in size. Cobra venoms are quite toxic and internationally are a major cause of human snakebite morbidity and mortality.

Sea snakes of the family Hydrophiidae are closely related to the cobras. They are native to the Indian and Pacific oceans, live primarily in an aquatic—usually marine—environment, and have short fixed fangs and flattened tails. Their venom is quite toxic, and envenomation is a significant risk for fishermen in areas where these snakes are indigenous.

The family Atractaspididae consists of the side-fanged vipers, including mole vipers and stiletto snakes. They are confined to Africa and the Middle East. Their venom contains sarafotoxins, which are endothelinlike compounds causing potent smooth muscle contraction and vasoconstriction.

▶ Snake Venom

The poison glands of snakes are modified salivary glands that secrete a complex mixture of specialized proteins and enzymes. Snake venom has several functions, including rapid immobilization of prey, predigestion of prey, and defense against predators. Snake venom effects are often broadly and superficially classified as primarily hemotoxic or neurotoxic. Caution should be used, as a combination of multiple effects may present either concurrently or consecutively.

Hemotoxic effects are mediated by proteolytic enzymes, peptides, and metalloproteins that can cause local tissue destruction directly and by intimal injury to blood vessels, followed by thrombosis and necrosis. Activation of the coagulation cascade can occur at multiple points, resulting in net anticoagulation. Direct lysis of red blood cells can cause acute hemolytic anemia and produce acute tubular necrosis. Bites on extremities may cause subcutaneous tissue destruction and loss of digits. Myotoxins can cause compromise of muscle compartments from direct myonecrosis as well as from local pressure effects. Secondary edema can develop rapidly in tissues from both cytokine release and from hemorrhage into local tissues. Systemic effects can include pulmonary edema. Intravascular injection can cause a more severe systemic reaction, with diffuse bleeding from thrombocytopenia and hypofibrinogenemia.

Snake venom neurotoxins often act upon the acetylcholine receptor system, with different components causing postsynaptic antagonism and acetylcholinesterase activity. Other components may cause direct presynaptic nerve cell destruction.

▶ Clinical Findings

Bites by nonvenomous snakes are much more common than bites by venomous snakes. These should be treated as simple puncture wounds, employing an appropriate antitetanus agent.

The excitement and hysteria associated with any snakebite may give rise to symptoms of disorientation, faintness, dizziness, hyperventilation, a rapid pulse, and primary shock even with nonvenomous snakebites.

A bite by a venomous snake results in envenomation in only 50–70% of cases. Envenomation may be classified as mild (scratch followed by minimal swelling and not much pain), moderate (fang marks, local swelling, and definite pain), or severe (fang marks, severe and progressive swelling and pain).

Most rattlesnakes, copperheads, water moccasins, and coral snakes tend to bite superficially, but a few bites penetrate muscle. The severity of the poisoning will depend upon the species and size of the snake; the age and size of the victim; the location, depth, nature, and number of bites; the amount of venom injected; the victim's sensitivity to the venom; the microbes present in the snake's mouth; and the availability of appropriate first-aid treatment and subsequent medical care.

Local signs of envenomation include puncture marks, local ecchymosis and discoloration, vesicles and bullae, and rapid appearance of swelling and edema at the injured area, with further progression to adjacent areas. The pain of the bite can be quite severe. Additional signs of hypotension, diaphoresis, nausea, weakness, and faintness are common. Perioral or peripheral paresthesias, taste changes, and fasciculations can be seen. Signs suggestive of neurotoxic envenomation include dysphagia, dysphonia, diplopia, headache, weakness, and respiratory distress. Laboratory findings may include hemoconcentration initially due to fluid shifts, with later decreases in red blood cells and platelets. Urinalysis may show hematuria, glycosuria, and proteinuria. Prothrombin and partial thromboplastin times are often abnormal.

▶ Treatment

The presence and degree of envenomation dictate treatment measures; other factors, such as time elapsed since being bitten, prehospital care, and the age and size of the victim, are also critical.

Wash the bite with soap and water or an antiseptic if available. Apply a broad, firm compressing bandage over the bite which does not restrict arterial and venous blood flow, and immobilize the bitten area at a level below the heart. Remove rings and constrictive devices, and keep the victim at rest and warm. Popular conceptions of first-aid measures including tourniquets, wound incision and suction, application of ice, cryotherapy, electrical shock, and ingestion of alcohol are of no proved value and may be hazardous to both the patient and the caregiver, particularly in the field setting. Transporting the patient to a medical facility is an important field management objective. Identification of the snake is helpful but of lower priority.

Standard evaluation and support of respiratory and cardiovascular function are initial priorities. Laboratory evaluation should include blood typing and crossmatching, coagulation studies, a complete blood count, and urinalysis. Local wound management includes cleansing and disinfection. Systemic measures include administration of antitetanus agent for tetanus prophylaxis and broad-spectrum antibiotic therapy. Fasciotomy should be reserved only for the uncommon compartment syndrome with compartment pressures documented above 30–40 mm Hg. Local bite area excision is not useful and should not be done.

The decision to use antivenin is based upon identification of the offending snake as venomous, discernment of the degree and manifestations of envenomation, time elapsed since the bite, and laboratory abnormalities. Several grading systems have been proposed but are inadequate at present, and the decision to use antivenin must be individualized to each patient and his or her specific reaction to the snakebite.

Effective specific antivenins are available for the bites of both pit vipers and Eastern coral snakes. Crotalidae polyvalent antivenin is effective against all North American pit vipers; North American coral snake antivenin is effective only for the Eastern coral snake. Because these equine antivenins have serious potential side effects, including both allergic reactions and serum sickness, their administration should be reserved for patients with significant bites or after early signs of envenomation have appeared.

Antivenin should ideally be administered early and as a diluted continuous intravenous infusion; local injection in or around the bite is contraindicated. Crotalidae polyvalent antivenin is most effective if given within 4 hours after a bite, of less value after 8 hours, and of questionable value after 30 hours. Severe envenomations may require over 30 vials; antivenin may be appropriate for moderate envenomation, but the risks outweigh the benefits if envenomation is minimal. Coral snake antivenin may be started prior to any neurologic symptoms if the offending snake is suspected or confirmed to be a coral snake.

Chippaux JP et al: Venoms, antivenoms and immunotherapy. Toxicon 1998;36:823.

Holstege CP et al: Crotalid snake envenomation. Crit Care Clin 1997;13:889.

Thwin MM et al: Snake envenomation and protective natural endogenous proteins: a mini review of the recent developments (1991–1997). Toxicon 1998;36:1471.

ARTHROPOD BITES

Stings and bites of arthropods are most often merely a nuisance. Some arthropods, however, can produce death by direct toxicity or by hypersensitivity reactions. Because of their prevalence and numbers, bees and wasps kill more people than do any other venomous animal, including snakes.

▶ Bees & Wasps

When a bee stings, it becomes anchored by the two barbed lancets, so that withdrawal is impossible. In the struggle, a bee will usually avulse its stinging apparatus and die. After being stung by a bee, one should scrape the exuded poison sac with a sharp knife. Any attempt to pull the poison apparatus out will simply cause more venom to be squeezed into the tissue. The stinger, once embedded, remains present. If this has occurred in an eyelid, it may irritate the globe of the eye months after the sting.

The stinging lancets of the wasp are not barbed and can easily be withdrawn by the insect to allow it to reinsert or to escape. It is unusual, therefore, to find a stinger left in place after a wasp sting. The females of the variety called yellow jackets are very aggressive. These insects sometimes bite before stinging.

The venom of bees and wasps contains histamine, basic protein components of high molecular weight, free amino acids, hyaluronidase, and acetylcholine. Antigenic proteins are species-specific and may lead to cross-reactivity between insects. Symptoms of arthropod stings may vary from minimal erythema to a marked local reaction of severe systemic toxicity (especially from multiple stings). Infection may occur. A generalized allergic reaction has been described that resembles serum sickness.

Early application of ice packs to reduce swelling is indicated. Elevation of the extremity is also useful. Oral antihistamines may be of some use in reducing urticaria. Parenteral corticosteroids may reduce delayed inflammation. If infection occurs, treatment consists of local debridement and antibiotics. Moderately severe reactions will present as generalized syncope or urticarial reactions. If an anaphylactic reaction or severe reaction is present, aqueous epinephrine, 0.5–1 mL of 1:1000 solution, should be given intramuscularly. A repeat dose may be given in 5–10 minutes, followed by 5–20 mg of diphenhydramine slowly intravenously. Administration of corticosteroids and general supportive measures such as oxygen administration, plasma expanders, and pressor agents may be required in case of shock. Previously sensitized patients should carry identifying tags and a kit for emergency intramuscular injection of epinephrine.

It is possible to immunize persons against bee and wasp stings, but cost-benefit analyses indicate that this is rarely if ever indicated.

▶ Spiders

While all spiders have poison glands and use venom for killing prey, only a few spider venoms are harmful to humans. As with all toxic exposures, the very young, the elderly, and patients with comorbid medical conditions are at greatest risk for adverse outcomes.

A. Lactrodectism

The bite of the *Lactrodectus* species of spiders (widow and red-back spiders), including the black widow (*Latrodectus mactans*) and the red-backed spider (*L hasseltii*), has primarily systemic neurotoxic effects. The female black widow spider can be identified by its characteristic black body with a red hourglass-like pattern on the abdomen; the male of the species does not bite and is smaller. The potent venom of this genus acts by destabilization of cell membranes and degranulation at nerve terminals with release of neurotransmitters. Neuromuscular toxic effects of black widow venom occur by presynaptic motor end plate neurotransmitter release, with release of norepinephrine and acetylcholine causing excessive stimulation and eventual fatigue of the motor end plate and muscle.

Symptoms of envenomation begin with pain at the bite location, followed by later development of abdominal wall muscle rigidity, abdominal pain and cramping, respiratory difficulty with potential paralysis, and lower extremity weakness. Massive hemolysis, severe hypotension, and cardiovascular collapse can be seen. Local skin changes are often minimal and can make identification of the bite difficult.

Intravenous administration of calcium gluconate may relieve muscle pain and spasm, but similar relief can be obtained from intravenous opioids and benzodiazepines. Ice packs may improve localized pain from the bite. Most symptoms are self-limited and, with appropriate supportive therapy, resolve within 48 hours, though full recovery may take over a week. A horse antivenin is available but may cause allergic reactions. Antivenin may be indicated in severely symptomatic patients to speed recovery and perhaps to prevent development of long-term symptoms related to neurologic dysfunction.

B. Loxoscelism

The brown recluse spider (*Loxosceles reclusa*) is dark tan and has a violin-shaped mark on the back of the main body. Envenomation can have significant and prolonged local dermonecrotic effects, with development of deep necrotic wounds at the bite site that are very slow to heal. Systemic loxoscelism with intravascular coagulation and renal failure has been seen but is uncommon. The venom appears to cause local tissue necrosis by dissociating normal neutrophil responses of adhesion and degranulation from transmigration and shape changes. Phospholipase D and sphingomyelinase D also contribute to the local necrosis, as well as venom-induced platelet aggregation. Alterations in complement activation and binding of venom to erythrocyte membranes contribute to hemolysis.

The bite may have local signs of erythema and edema but usually minimal associated pain. With serious envenomation, hemorrhagic bullae surrounded by localized ischemia develop over 24–48 hours. The local lesion usually progresses to a very slowly healing ulcer. Systemic effects of fever, urticaria, lymphangitis, nausea, and emesis can develop. Hemolysis and disseminated intravascular coagulation are rare.

Loxoscelism is managed by supportive measures. Cleansing of the bite, rest, and elevation of the affected area are appropriate. While tissue loss is common, early excision of lesions is also associated with poor wound healing. Conflicting data exist regarding systemic treatment with corticosteroids; evidence for efficacy of dapsone treatment (50–100 mg/d) remains anecdotal.

Anderson PC: Spider bites in the United States. Dermatol Clin 1997;15:307.
Bond GR: Snake, spider, and scorpion envenomation in North America. Pediatr Rev 1999;20:147.
Clark RF et al: Clinical presentation and treatment of black widow spider envenomation: a review of 163 cases. Ann Emerg Med 1992;21:782.
Gendron B: *Loxosceles reclusa* envenomation. Am J Emerg Med 1990;8:51.
Gomez HF et al: Loxosceles spider venom induces the production of alpha and beta chemokines: implications for the pathogenesis of dermonecrotic arachnidism. Inflammation 1999;23:207.
Hobbs GD et al: Comparison of hyperbaric oxygen and dapsone therapy for Loxsceles envenomation. Acad Emerg Med 1996;3:758.
Phillips S et al: Therapy of brown spider envenomation: a controlled trial of hyperbaric oxygen, dapsone, and cyproheptadine. Ann Emerg Med 1995;25:363.
Wilson DC et al: Spiders and spider bites. Dermatol Clin 1990;8:277.
Wright SW et al: Clinical presentation and outcome of brown recluse spider bite. Ann Emerg Med 1997;30:28.

▼ ANTIMICROBIAL CHEMOTHERAPY

PRINCIPLES OF SELECTION OF ANTIMICROBIAL DRUGS

▶ Initial & Subsequent Selection of Antimicrobial Agents

The decisions to initiate, continue, and stop antimicrobial chemotherapy should be prudently determined. These decisions entail (1) clinical judgment that a microbial infection probably exists, (2) formulation of a differential diagnosis with associated microbial pathogens, (3) procurement of specimens likely to provide evidence for a microbiologic diagnosis, (4) prompt initiation of empiric therapy presumed effective against the suspected organisms, (5) observation of the clinical response to the prescribed antimicrobial and laboratory identification of a putative microbial pathogen, and (6) continuation of the empiric regimen or a switch to pathogen-directed therapy. The clinical status of the patient contributes to the time to initiation of empiric therapy, the route of administration, and the type of therapy. Although laboratory data need not overrule a decision based on clinical and empiric grounds, judicious targeted use of antimicrobial therapy minimizes drug exposure, adverse events, the emergence of multidrug-resistant organisms (MDROs), and excess costs.

▶ Selection of an Antimicrobial Drug by Laboratory Tests

When an organism has been identified from a clinical specimen, it is often possible to select the drug of choice on the basis of current clinical experience (see Table 8–6). Given the rising rates of MDROs and geographic differences in antibiogram data (tables of pathogen-specific antibiotic sensitivities), laboratory tests for antimicrobial drug susceptibility are necessary, particularly if the isolated organism is of a type that often exhibits drug resistance, eg, enteric gram-negative rods. The US Clinical and Laboratory Standards Institute (CLSI) has published several consensus recommendations, with updates, for quality control of com-

Table 8–6. Antimicrobial Drugs of Choice for Suspected and Empiric Regimens. Pathogen-Directed Therapy Should Utilize Antibiogram Data from Regional Clinical Microbiology Laboratory.[*]

Suspected or Confirmed Etiologic Agent		Alternative Drugs
Gram-negative cocci		
Moraxella catarrhalis	Amoxicillin-clavulanic acid or TMP-SMZ[1]	Cephalosporins,[2] erythromycin,[3] tetracycline[4]
Gonococcus	Ceftriaxone	Cefixime, ciprofloxacin, spectinomycin
Meningococcus	Penicillin[5]	Cephalosporins,[2] ampicillin, chloramphenicol
Gram-positive cocci		
Streptococcus pneumoniae (penicillin-susceptible)	Penicillin,[5] ceftriaxone ± vancomycin (especially for CNS) macrolide,	Erythromycin,[3] cephalosporin,[6] vancomycin (combination therapy may be indicated)
S pneumoniae (penicillin-resistant)	Ceftriaxone ± vancomycin (especially for CNS)	Vancomycin (combination therapy may be indicated)
Streptococcus, hemolytic, groups A, B, C, G	Penicillin[5]	Erythromycin,[3] cephalosporin,[6] vancomycin
Viridans streptococci	Penicillin[5] ± aminoglycosides[7]	Cephalosporin,[6] vancomycin
Staphylococcus, methicillin-resistant	Vancomycin + gentamicin or rifampin (or both)	TMP-SMZ, ciprofloxacin
Staphylococcus, non-penicillinase-producing	Penicillin	Cephalosporin, vancomycin
Staphylococcus, penicillinase-producing	Penicillinase-resistant penicillin[8]	Vancomycin, cephalosporin[6]
Enterococci	Ampicillin ± gentamicin	Vancomycin + gentamicin
Gram-negative rods		
Acinetobacter	Aminoglycoside[7] + imipenem	Minocycline, TMP-SMZ[1]
Bacteroides, oropharyngeal strains	Penicillin,[5] clindamycin	Metronidazole, cephalosporin[2,6]
Bacteroides, gastrointestinal strains	Metronidazole	Cefoxitin, chloramphenicol, clindamycin, TMP-SMZ[1]
Brucella	Tetracycline[4] + streptomycin	Tetracycline,[4] ciprofloxacin
Campylobacter	Third-generation fluoroquinolone	Imipenem, newer cephalosporins[2]
Enterobacter	TMP-SMZ,[1] aminoglycoside[7]	Ampicillin, TMP-SMZ[1]
Escherichia coli (sepsis)	Aminoglycoside,[7] newer cephalosporins[2]	Ampicillin, cephalosporin[6]
E coli (first urinary infection)	Sulfonamide,[9] TMP-SMZ[1]	Ampicillin and chloramphenicol,[1] second- or third-generation fluoroquinolone
Haemophilus (meningitis, respiratory infections)	Cephalosporins[2]	TMP-SMZ,[1] aminoglycoside[7]
Klebsiella	Cephalosporins[2]	TMP-SMZ
Legionella pneumonia	Macrolide + rifampin	Chloramphenicol
Pasteurella (Yersinia)	Streptomycin, tetracycline[4]	Cephalosporins,[2] aminoglycoside[7]
Proteus mirabilis	Ampicillin	Aminoglycoside[7]
Proteus vulgaris and other species	Newer cephalosporins[2]	Ceftazidime or cefoperazone + aminoglycoside; imipenem + aminoglycoside; aztreonam
Pseudomonas aeruginosa	Aminoglycoside[7] + antipseudomonal penicillin[10]	Carbapenemase, tetracycline,[4] TMP-SMZ
Burkholderia pseudomallei (melioidosis)	Ceftazidime	Chloramphenicol + streptomycin
Burkholderia mallei (glanders)	Streptomycin + tetracycline[4]	TMP-SMZ,[1] ciprofloxacin, ampicillin, chloramphenicol
Salmonella	Ceftriaxone	TMP-SMZ[1]
Serratia, Providencia	Cephalosporins,[2] aminoglycoside[7]	Ampicillin, tetracycline,[4] ciprofloxacin, chloramphenicol
Shigella	TMP-SMZ[1]	

(continued)

Table 8–6. Antimicrobial Drugs of Choice for Suspected and Empiric Regimens. Pathogen-Directed Therapy Should Utilize Antibiogram Data from Regional Clinical Microbiology Laboratory.* *(Continued)*

Suspected or Confirmed Etiologic Agent		Alternative Drugs
Stenotrophomonas maltophilia	TMP-SMZ[1]	
Vibrio (cholera, sepsis)	Tetracycline[4]	TMP-SMZ[1]
Gram-positive rods		
Actinomyces	Penicillin[5]	Tetracycline[4]
Bacillus (eg, Anthrax)	Penicillin[5]	Erythromycin[3]
Clostridium (eg, gas gangrene, tetanus)	Penicillin[5]	Metronidazole, chloramphenicol, clindamycin
Corynebacterium diphtheriae	Erythromycin[3]	Penicillin[5]
Corynebacterium jeikeium	Vancomycin	Ciprofloxacin
Listeria	Ampicillin + aminoglycoside[7]	TMP-SMZ[1]
Acid-fast rods		
Mycobacterium tuberculosis	INH + rifampin + pyrazinamide + ethambutol	Other antituberculosis drugs
Mycobacterium leprae	Dapsone + rifampin, clofazimine	Ethionamide
Mycobacterium kansasii	INH + rifampin + ethambutol	Other antituberculosis drugs
Mycobacterium aviumintracellulare	Ethambutol + rifampin + clarithromycin	Other antituberculosis drugs
Mycobacterium fortuitumchelonei	Amikacin + doxycycline	Cefoxitin, erythromycin, sulfonamide
Nocardia	Sulfonamide,[9] TMP-SMZ[1]	Minocycline
Spirochetes		
Borrelia (Lyme disease, relapsing fever)	Tetracycline,[4] ceftriaxone	Penicillin,[5] erythromycin[3]
Leptospira	Penicillin[5]	Tetracycline[4]
Treponema (syphilis, yaws, etc)	Penicillin[5]	Erythromycin,[3] tetracycline[4]
Mycoplasmas	Macrolide or tetracycline[4]	
Chlamydiae		
C psittaci	Tetracycline[4]	Chloramphenicol
C trachomatis (urethritis or pelvic inflammatory disease)	Doxycycline or erythromycin[3]	Ofloxacin or azithromycin
C pneumoniae	Tetracycline[4]	Erythromycin[3]
Rickettsiae	Tetracycline[4]	Chloramphenicol

*N Engl J Med 1997;336:708. (From the New England Journal of Medicine. Copyright © 1997 Massachusetts Medical Society. All rights reserved.)
[1]TMP-SMZ is a mixture of 1 part trimethoprim and 5 parts sulfamethoxazole.
[2]Cephalosporins include cefotaxime, cefuroxime, ceftriaxone, ceftazidime, ceftizoxime, and others.
[3]Erythromycin estolate is best absorbed orally but carries the highest risk of hepatitis; erythromycin stearate and erythromycin ethyl succinate are also available.
[4]All tetracyclines have similar activity against microorganisms. Dosage is determined by rates of absorption and excretion of various preparations.
[5]Penicillin G is preferred for parenteral injection; penicillin V for oral administration—to be used only in treating infections due to highly sensitive organisms.
[6]Older cephalosporins are cephalothin, cefazolin, cephapirin, and cefoxitin for parenteral injection; cephalexin and cephradine can be given orally.
[7]Aminoglycosides—gentamicin, tobramycin, amikacin, netilmicin—should be chosen on the basis of local patterns of susceptibility.
[8]Parenteral nafcillin or oxacillin; oral dicloxacillin, cloxacillin, or oxacillin.
[9]Oral sulfisoxazole and trisulfapyrimidines are highly soluble in urine; parenteral sodium sulfadiazine can be injected intravenously in treating severely ill patients.
[10]Antipseudomonal penicillins: ticarcillin, carbenicillin, mezlocillin, azlocillin, piperacillin.
[11]First choice for previously untreated urinary tract infection is a highly soluble sulfonamide or TMP-SMZ.

mercial microbial identification systems and antimicrobial susceptibility testing (www.clsi.org). Susceptibility testing methods include disk diffusion and dilution (broth microdilution, plates, and E-tests) procedures. Disk diffusion tests indicate whether a microbial culture is susceptible or resistant to serum-achievable, in vivo drug concentrations with conventional dosage regimens. In contrast, dilution procedures allow report of the minimal inhibitory concentration

(MIC) and minimal bactericidal concentration (MBC). The MIC is the lowest concentration of a specific antimicrobial agent that inhibits the test organism, while the MBC is the lowest concentration of a specific antimicrobial agent that kills the test organism. Reporting of susceptibility via disk diffusion or MIC, over MBC, is recommended. The duration of appropriate therapy depends on the nature of the infection and the severity of the clinical presentation. When clinical improvement does not occur after initiation of putatively appropriate antimicrobial therapy, possible explanations include the following:

1. The organism isolated from the specimen may not be the one responsible for the infectious process.

2. There may have been failure to drain a collection of pus, debride necrotic tissue, or remove a foreign body. Antimicrobials can never take the place of surgical drainage and removal.

3. Superinfection in the course of prolonged antimicrobial chemotherapy. New or drug-resistant microorganisms may have replaced the original infectious agent. This is particularly common with open wounds or sinus tracts.

4. The drug may not reach the site of active infection in adequate concentration. The pharmacologic properties of antimicrobials determine their absorption and distribution. Certain drugs penetrate phagocytic cells poorly and thus may not reach intracellular organisms. Some drugs may diffuse poorly into the eye, central nervous system, or pleural space unless injected directly into the area.

5. At times, two or more microorganisms participate in an infectious process but only one may have been isolated from the specimen. The antimicrobial being used may be effective only against the less virulent organism.

6. In the course of drug administration, resistant microorganisms may have been selected from a mixed population, and these drug-resistant organisms continue to grow in the presence of the drug.

Assessment of Drug & Dosage

An adequate therapeutic response is an important but not always sufficient indication that the right drug is being given in the right dosage. Proof of drug activity in serum against the original infecting organisms may provide important support for a selected drug regimen even if fever or other signs of infection are continuing. In sepsis, extended-interval administration of aminoglycosides has efficacy and toxicity similar to that associated with traditional dosing regimens, but costs are less and convenience is increased. This dosing regimen is not recommended for patients with endocarditis, pregnancy, cystic fibrosis, burns covering more than 20% of body surface area, mycobacterial infections, or anasarca. The initial dose is gentamicin or tobramycin, 5 mg/kg intravenously, or amikacin, 15 mg/kg intravenously. A follow-up

random serum drug level 6–14 hours later is compared with a nomogram to determine follow-up dosing intervals.

Determining Duration of Therapy

The duration of drug therapy depends on the nature of the infection and the severity of the clinical presentation. Treatment of acute uncomplicated infections should be continued until the patient has been afebrile and clinically well for at least 72 hours. Infections at certain sites (eg, endocarditis, septic arthritis, osteomyelitis) require more prolonged therapy. In evaluating the patient's clinical response, the possibility of adverse reactions to drugs must be considered. Such reactions may mimic continuing activity of the infectious process by causing fever, skin rashes, central nervous system disturbances, and changes in blood and urine. In the case of many drugs, it is desirable to assess hepatic and renal function at intervals. Adverse events may require dose reduction or drug discontinuation.

Oliguria & Renal Failure

Oliguria and renal failure have an important influence on antimicrobial drug dosage, since most of these drugs are excreted—to a greater or lesser extent—by the kidneys. Some drugs require minor adjustments in dosage or frequency of administration. Others, such as vancomycin, penicillins, aminoglycosides, and tetracyclines, must be reduced in dosage or frequency of administration to avert toxicity in the presence of nitrogen retention. General guidelines for the administration of such drugs to patients with renal failure are set forth in Table 8–7. The administration of potentially nephrotoxic antimicrobial agents, such as aminoglycosides, to patients in renal failure require guidance by direct assays of serum drug concentrations. In the newborn or premature infant, excretory mechanisms for some antimicrobials are poorly developed and special dosage schedules must therefore be used in order to avoid accumulation of drugs.

Prevention & Control of Spread of Drug-Resistant Genes

In an attempt to prevent the emergence of and control the spread of drug-resistant transmissible agents and genes, judicious selection and continued use of antimicrobial therapy is warranted.

Vancomycin should not be used routinely (1) for surgical prophylaxis in a patient without a severe β-lactam allergy, (2) for empiric therapy of a febrile neutropenic patient unless initial evidence suggests an infection with gram-positive bacteria, (3) for treatment of a single positive blood culture with a coagulase-negative staphylococcus, (4) for continued empiric administration against presumed infection when cultures do not confirm a β-lactam-resistant gram-positive organism, (5) as prophylaxis against infection of a central or peripheral intravascular catheter, and (6) for topical application or irrigation.

Table 8–7. Use of Antibiotics in Patients with Renal Failure and Hepatic Failure.

	Principal Mode of Excretion or Detoxification	Approximate Half-Life in Serum		Proposed Dosage Regimen in Renal Failure		Removal of Drugs by Hemodialysis	Dose After Hemodialysis	Dosage in Hepatic Failure[3]
		Normal	Renal Failure[1]	Initial Dose[2]	Maintenance Dose			
Acyclovir	Renal	2.5–3.5 h	20 h	2.5 mg/kg	2.5 mg/kg q24h	Yes	2.5 mg/kg	NC
Ampicillin	Tubular secretion	0.5–1 h	8–12 h	1 g	1 g q8–12h	Yes	1 g	NC
Azlo-, mezlo-, piperacillin	Renal 50–70%; biliary 20–30%	1 h	3–6 h	3 g	2 g q6–8h	Yes	1 g	1–2 g q8h
Azithromycin	Mainly liver/biliary	> 24 h	> 24 h	500 mg	250 mg/d	No	No	NC
Carbenicillin	Tubular secretion	1 h	16 h	4 g	2 g q12h	Yes	2 g	NC
Chloramphenicol	Mainly hepatic	3 h	4 h	0.5 g	0.5 g q6h	Yes	0.5 g	0.25–0.5 g q12h
Ciprofloxacin	Renal and hepatic	4 h	8.5 h	0.5 g	0.25–0.75 g q24h	No	None	NC
Clindamycin	Hepatic	2–4 h	2.4 h	0.6 g IV	0.6 g q8h	No	None	0.3–0.6 q8h
Erythromycin	Mainly hepatic	1.5 h	1.5 h	0.5–1 g	0.5–1 g q6h	No	None	0.25–0.5 g q6h
Fluconazole	Renal	30 h	98 h	0.2 g	0.1 g q24h	Yes	Give q24h dose	NC
Ganciclovir	Renal	3 h	11–28 h	1.25 mg/kg	1.25 mg/kg q24h	Yes	Give q24h dose	NC
Imipenem	Glomerular filtration	1 h	3 h	0.5 g	0.25–0.5 g q12h	Yes	0.25–0.5 g	NC
Levofloxacin		360–480 min	360–480 min	250–500 mg	250–500 mg/d	No	No	Avoid use
Meropenem		60 min	180 min	1000 mg	1000 mg q8h	Yes	500 mg q4h	NC
Metronidazole	Hepatic	6–10 h	6–10 h	0.5 g IV	0.5 g qh	Yes	0.25 g	0.25 g q12h
Moxifloxacin	Renal	720 min	720 min	400 mg	400 mg	No	No	Avoid use
Nafcillin	Hepatic 80%, kidney 20%	0.75 h	1.5 h	1.5 g	1.5 g q5h	No	None	2–3 g q12h
Penicillin G	Tubular secretion	0.5 h	7–10 h	1–2 million units	1 million units q8h	Yes	500,000 units	NC
Ticarcillin	Tubular secretion	1.1 h	15–20 h	3 g	2 g q6–8h	Yes	1 g	NC
Trimethoprim-sulfamethoxazole	Some hepatic	TMP 10–12 h; SMZ 8–10 h	TMP 24–48 h; SMZ 18–24 h	320 mg TMP + 1600 mg SMZ	80 mg TMP + 400 mg SMZ q12h	Yes	80 mg TMP + 400 mg SMZ	NC
Vancomycin	Glomerular filtration	6 h	6–10 days	1 g	1 g q6–10 days based on serum levels	None	None	NC
Voriconazole	Hepatic	360 min	360 min	6 mg/kg IV × 2 doses	100–200 mg oral q 12h	No	None	Normal load and 1/2 maintenance

(continued)

Table 8–7. Use of Antibiotics in Patients with Renal Failure and Hepatic Failure. *(Continued)*

| | Principal Mode of Excretion or Detoxification | Approximate Half-Life in Serum | | Proposed Dosage Regimen in Renal Failure | | Removal of Drugs by Hemodialysis | Dose After Hemodialysis | Dosage in Hepatic Failure[3] |
		Normal	Renal Failure[1]	Initial Dose[2]	Maintenance Dose			
Cefazolin	Renal	90 min		0.5 g	0.5 g qd	Yes	0.5 g	NC
Cefuroxime	Renal	80 min		1–2 g	1–2 g qd	Yes	0.5 g	NC
Cefotetan	Renal	150 min		0.5–1 g	0.5–1 g qd	Yes	0.5 g	NC
Cefoxitin	Renal	60 min		1–2 g	1–2 g qd	Yes	0.5 g	NC
Ceftriaxone	Renal and hepatic	480 min		1–2 g	1–2 g qd	No		NC
Ceftazidime	Renal	120 min		0.5–1 g	0.5–1 g qd	Yes	0.5 g	NC
Cefepime	Renal	120 min	600 min	1–2 g IV	1–2 g IV q12h	Yes	1 g q q 48h	NC

[1]Considered here to be marked by creatinine clearance of 10 mL/min or less.
[2]For a 70-kg adult with a serious systemic infection.
[3]NC = No change.

A. Distinction Between Colonization and Infection with Drug-Resistant Organisms

In community and health care–associated infections, methicillin-resistant *Staphylococcus aureus* (MRSA) and vancomycin-resistant enterococci (VRE) are of notable concern. Most MRSA invasive infections are treated with either vancomycin (dosed to therapeutic trough levels of 15) or linezolid 600 mg intravenously or orally twice daily. Eradication of MRSA nasal carriage begins with a 5-day course of twice-daily intranasal mupirocin. For invasive VRE infections, most people are treated with either linezolid or chloramphenicol. No regimen has been effective in eradicating enteric carriage of VRE.

B. The Emergence and Spread of Extended-Spectrum β-Lactam Resistance

Sequential development and use of β-lactam antibiotics have selected for successive generations of extended-spectrum β-lactamases (ESBLs) such as CTX-M, plasmid-mediated AmpC, KPC carbapenemases, and metallocarbapenemases. In addition to enzyme inhibition, the bacterial-resistance mechanisms of efflux pumps and quorum sensing require a base understanding of prevalent resistance rates in local practice settings to most judiciously select empiric, gram-negative antimicrobial agents.

ANTIMICROBIAL DRUGS USED IN COMBINATION

▶ Indications

Possible reasons for employing two or more antimicrobials simultaneously instead of a single drug are as follows:

1. Prompt treatment in a severely ill patient suspected of having a serious microbial infection. A good guess about the most probable two or three pathogens is made, and drugs are empirically targeted to those organisms. Before such treatment is started, it is essential that adequate specimens be obtained for identifying the etiologic agent in the laboratory.

2. Delay the emergence of antimicrobial resistance to one drug in chronic infections by the use of a second or third non-cross-reacting drug. Treatment of active tuberculosis is a good example.

3. The presence of mixed infections, particularly those following massive trauma.

4. To achieve bactericidal synergism (discussed shortly). In a few infections, eg, enterococcal sepsis, a combination of drugs is more likely to eradicate the infection than either drug used alone. Unfortunately, such synergism is unpredictable, and a given drug pair may be synergistic for only a single microbial strain.

▶ Disadvantages

The following disadvantages of using antimicrobial drugs in combinations must always be considered:

1. Higher chance for adverse drug reactions or drug hypersensitivity.

2. Potentially no greater efficacy than an effective single drug.

3. Empiric, broad-spectrum antimicrobial coverage may compromise the effort to establish a specific etiologic diagnosis.

4. Expense.

5. On rare occasions, drug antagonism with resultant increased rates of illness and death (as noted in bacterial meningitis when a bacteriostatic drug, eg, tetracycline or chloramphenicol was given with or prior to a bactericidal drug, eg, penicillin or ampicillin). Notably, antagonism can usually be overcome by giving a larger dose of one of the drugs in the pair and is therefore an infrequent problem in clinical therapy.

▶ Synergism

Antimicrobial synergism occurs in the situations listed below. Synergistic drug combinations must be selected by specialized laboratory procedures.

1. One drug inhibits a microbial enzyme that might destroy a second drug. For example, clavulanic acid inhibits bacterial β-lactamase and protects simultaneously administered amoxicillin from destruction.

2. Sequential block of a metabolic pathway. Sulfonamides inhibit utilization of extracellular p-aminobenzoic acid by susceptible bacteria. Trimethoprim inhibits the reduction of folates, the next metabolic step. Simultaneous use of sulfamethoxazole and trimethoprim can be strikingly more effective in some bacterial infections than use of either drug alone.

3. One drug enhances greatly the uptake of a second drug. Cell-wall inhibitor (β-lactam) drugs enhance the penetration of various bacteria by aminoglycosides and thus increase the overall bactericidal effect. Eradication of infections by enterococci are enhanced by combinations of a cell wall–active agent and an aminoglycoside. Similarly, the control of sepsis by pseudomonas and other gram-negative rods may be enhanced by combination of a cephalosporin and an aminoglycoside.

▶ Antifungal Therapy

Given the extensive and prolonged use of antimicrobial agents, the increased prevalence of immunocompromised hosts, and the availability of antifungal therapeutic options, there has been an increasing need for the judicious use of antifungal therapeutic agents. The clinical presentations of yeast and mold infections are protean and not pathogen specific. Yeastlike fungi are typically round or oval and reproduce by budding; molds are composed of tubular structures called hyphae that grow by branching and longitudinal extension. Recommendations for treatment will depend upon the characterization of the yeast in the mycology laboratory, perhaps supplemented by in vitro testing of fungi. Assessment of drug, dosage, duration of therapy, and evaluation of adverse events is often best done in consultation with an infectious disease specialist. Drug options include the following.

A. Azoles

There are four fungistatic azoles: ketoconazole, fluconazole, and itraconazole, and voriconazole.

- Ketoconazole is the oldest of these drugs, has the highest frequency of drug interactions, and is markedly hepatotoxic.

- Fluconazole is widely distributed in the body and penetrates readily into the cerebrospinal fluid. It has been effective in the treatment of fungal urinary tract infections, oropharyngeal and esophageal candidiasis, and fungal peritonitis. For most indications, one gives 200 mg orally or intravenously as a loading dose followed by a maintenance dose of 100 mg intravenously or orally daily. Adverse events include headache, gastrointestinal side effects, elevated serum aminotransferases, and rashes.

- Itraconazole is a triazole with a broad antifungal spectrum, approved for the treatment of histoplasmosis and blastomycosis both in immunocompetent and in immunocompromised hosts. Formulations exist both as tablets and as an elixir and are best taken on an empty stomach, with absorption improved by increased gastric acidity. Adverse events include nausea, vomiting, rash, and early hepatitis.

- Voriconazole is approved for the treatment of invasive aspergillosis, where it demonstrates typical response rates of 40–50% and superiority over conventional amphotericin B. It is also recommended for primary treatment of amphotericin B and fluconazole-resistant fungal infections (including *Fusarium* spp and *Scedosporium apiospermum*), invasive fungal infections when patients are intolerant of or refractory to other antifungal therapies, and empiric therapy for neutropenic fever in settings of coprescribed nephrotoxins. It is 96% bioavailable and oral use, when feasible, is recommended.

- New azole compounds are in preclinical and clinical drug development, yet narrow spectrum of activity, susceptibility t efflux pumps, protein binding, and serum inactivation are ongoing challenges.

B. Echinocandins

Caspofungin acetate, the first available drug in this class of antifungal agents, has fungicidal activity against most *Aspergillus* and *Candida* species, including azole-resistant *Candida* strains. It is shown to be at least as effective as and better tolerated than amphotericin formulations for the treatment of esophageal candidiasis, candidemia, invasive candidiasis, and persistent fever in the setting of neutropenia.

C. Amphotericin B

Amphotericin B is a polyene antimicrobial agent that disrupts the fungal cell by binding to ergosterol in the plasma membrane. Historically, it has been the drug of choice for most systemic mycoses except *Pseudallescheria boydii* and some *Fusarium* species. Amphotericin B is poorly absorbed and must be administered intravenously except for topical therapy in azole-resistant oral candidiasis. The initial and total intravenous infusion dose is often determined by the severity of the infection. An initial dose of 0.5–1 mg/kg is usually given over 2–4 hours. In most instances, daily prehydration with 500 mL of normal saline solution will reduce the risk of nephrotoxicity. Recognized adverse events (fever, chills, headache, myalgias, nausea and vomiting) may be reduced by premedication with acetaminophen, 600 mg orally; diphenhydramine, 50 mg orally; plus hydrocortisone, 25–100 mg intravenously. Nephrotoxicity may occur over time via distal renal tubular acidosis, hyperkalemia, hypermagnesemia, or impairment of glomerular filtration.

D. Lipid Preparations of Amphotericin B

These formulations include amphotericin B lipid complex, amphotericin B colloidal dispersion, and liposomal amphotericin B. They alter the pharmacokinetics and distribution of the drug and are often substituted for treatment of infections in patients intolerant of or not responding to regular amphotericin B. Lipid formulations of amphotericin B may be indicated for patients who have documented or suspected severe systemic mycoses that are unsuitable for treatment with azoles or who have baseline renal insufficiency or risk factors for development of renal insufficiency, including a (1) Cr greater than 2.5 mg/dl or Cr clearance (Cl_{Cr}) of less than 40 ml/min, (2) Cr greater than 2 mg/dl or Cl_{Cr} less than 60 ml/min and receipt of a concurrent nephrotoxic medication, or (3) Cr greater than 1.5 mg/dl or Cl_{Cr} less than 75 ml/min and concurrent receipt of at least two nephrotoxic medications. The nephrotoxic medications of most concern are cisplatin, cyclosporin A, aminoglycosides, foscarnet, pentamidine, cidofovir, and scheduled nonsteroidal anti-inflammatory drugs.

E. Flucytosine

Flucytosine, 25–37.5 mg/kg orally every 6 hours, is an effective agent against some isolates of candida species and *Cryptococcus neoformans*. This drug, when used in combination with amphotericin B, will enhance fungicidal activity. Flucytosine is not recommended as monotherapy and is excreted in the kidney, thus requiring alteration of dosage with renal insufficiency. The primary adverse effect is bone marrow suppression, which is dose-related and occurs with peak serum levels greater than 100 µg/mL.

▶ Antiviral Agents

Eleven drugs have been approved by the FDA for the treatment of viral infections (other than those known for HIV infection). Antiviral drugs can be used for prophylaxis, suppression, preemptive therapy, or treatment of overt disease. The goals of treating acute viral infections in immunocompromised patients are to reduce the severity of illness and potential complications and to reduce viral transmission. The goal of antiviral therapy in patients with chronic viral infections is to prevent damage to visceral organs,

especially the liver, lungs, gastrointestinal tract, and central nervous system. Currently, the most commonly used drugs are acyclovir, valacyclovir, and famciclovir.

A. Acyclovir

Acyclovir is active against herpes simplex virus (HSV) and varicella zoster virus (VZV). This drug is used for the treatment of primary and recurrent genital herpes, severe herpes dermatitis, and herpes simplex encephalitis in normal hosts as well as disseminated VZV and herpes zoster ophthalmicus. For severe systemic infections, the dose is 5 mg/kg intravenously every 8 hours for HSV infections and 10 mg/kg intravenously every 8 hours for HSV encephalitis or VZV infections. The oral dose is 400 mg three times daily for HSV infection and 800 mg five times daily for localized herpes zoster infections. Dosage must be adjusted in renal failure. Side effects are uncommon.

B. Valacyclovir

Valacyclovir is an orally administered prodrug of acyclovir approved for treatment of a first herpes zoster infection or for recurring episodes of genital HSV.

C. Famciclovir

Famciclovir is an oral drug that has activity against VZV, HSV, and Epstein-Barr virus (EBV). It is approved for acute herpes zoster and treatment of recurring episodes of genital HSV at a dosage of 500 mg orally every 8 hours for 7 days or, in recurring HSV episodes, 100 mg orally every 12 hours for 5 days. Headache, nausea, and diarrhea have been reported as adverse events.

▶ Antimycobacterial Therapy

Depending on the location of the surgical practice, empiric or pathogen-directed antituberculous therapy may be a concurrent treatment necessity. Effective treatment of *Mycobacterium tuberculosis* infections requires combination chemotherapy, and initial 4-drug regimens are recommended in geographic areas where the prevalence of multidrug-resistant tuberculosis is greater than 4%. Primary treatment regimens include isoniazid, rifampin, ethambutol, and pyrazinamide—with or without streptomycin. Surgical patients suspected of having tuberculosis need to be placed in negative pressure rooms for the protection of health care workers and other patients. Given the public health ramifications, it is often best for the surgical team to include an infectious disease specialist in the initiation and follow-up of patients receiving antituberculous therapy.

Bailey TC et al: A meta-analysis of extended-interval dosing versus multiple daily dosing of aminoglycosides. Clin Infect Dis 1997;24:786.

Balfour HH: Antiviral drugs. N Engl J Med 1999;340:1255.

Cheung AHS, Wong LMF: Surgical infections in patients with chronic renal failure. Infect Dis Clin North Am 2001;15:775.

Eggiman P et al: Invasive candidiasis: comparison of management choices by infectious disease and critical care specialists. Intensive Care Med 2005;31:1514.

Herbrecht R et al: Voriconazole versus amphotericin B for primary therapy of invasive aspergillosis. NEJM 2002;347:408.

Holzheimer RG, Dralle H: Antibiotic therapy in intra-abdominal infections: a review on randomised clinical trials. Eur J Med Res 2001;6:277.

Livermore D, Woodford N: The beta-lactamase threat in Enterobacteriaceae, Pseudomonas and Acinetobacter. Trends Microbiol 2006;14:413.

Pasqualotto AC, Denning DW: Post-operative aspergillosis. Clin Microbiol Infect 2006;12:1060.

Piarrouz R et al: Assessment of preemptive treatment to prevent severe candidiasis in critically ill surgical patients. Crit Care Med 2004;32:2443.

Polk R: Optimal use of modern antibiotics: emerging trends. Clin Infect Dis 1999;29:264.

Recommendations for preventing the spread of vancomycin resistance. Hospital Infection Control Practices Advisory Committee (HICPAC). MMWR Morb Mortal Wkly Rep 1995;44(RR-12):1.

Sayek E: The role of β-lactam/β-lactamase inhibitor combinations in surgical infections. Surg Infect 2001;2:S23.

Stafford RE, Weigelt JA: Surgical infections in the critically ill. Curr Opin Crit Care 2002;8:449.

Sun KO et al: Management of tetanus: a review of 18 cases. J R Soc Med 1994;87:135.

Teppler H et al: Surgical infections with Enterococcus: outcome in patients treated with ertapenem versus piperacillin-tazobactam. Surg Infect 2002;3(4):337.

Walsh TJ et al: Voriconazole compared with liposomal amphotericin B for empirical antifungal therapy in patients with neutropenia and persistent fever. NEJM 2002;346:225.

Fluid & Electrolyte Management

Gerard M. Doherty, MD

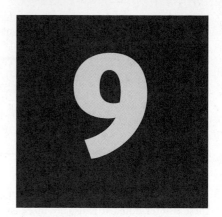

The surgical patient is at risk for several derangements of body fluid volume and composition, some of which may be iatrogenic. Understanding the physiologic mechanisms that regulate the composition and volume of the body fluids and the principles of fluid and electrolyte therapy is essential for optimal patient management.

BODY WATER & ITS DISTRIBUTION

Total body water comprises 45–60% of body weight; the percentage in any individual is influenced by age and the lean body mass, but in healthy individuals it remains remarkably constant from day to day. Table 9–1 lists the average values of total body water as a percentage of body weight for men and women of different ages. Total body water is divided into intracellular fluid (ICF) and extracellular fluid (ECF) compartments. Intracellular water represents about two-thirds of total body water, or 40% of body weight. The remaining one-third of body water is extracellular. ECF is divided into two compartments: (1) plasma water, comprising approximately 25% of ECF, or 5% of body weight; and (2) interstitial fluid, comprising 75% of ECF, or 15% of body weight.

The solute composition of the ICF and ECF compartments differs markedly (Figure 9–1). ECF contains principally sodium, chloride, and bicarbonate, with other ions in much lower concentrations. ICF contains mainly potassium, organic phosphate, sulfate, and various other ions in lower concentrations.

Even though plasma water and interstitial fluid have similar electrolyte compositions, plasma water contains more protein than interstitial fluid. This results in slight differences in electrolyte concentrations, as governed by the Gibbs-Donnan equilibrium. The plasma proteins, chiefly albumin, account for the high colloid osmotic pressure of plasma, which is an important determinant of the distribution of fluid between vascular and interstitial compartments, as defined by the Starling relationships.

The kidneys maintain constant volume and composition of body fluids by two distinct but related mechanisms: (1) filtration and reabsorption of sodium, which adjusts urinary sodium excretion to match changes in dietary intake, and (2) regulation of water excretion in response to changes in secretion of antidiuretic hormone. These two mechanisms allow the kidneys to keep the volume and osmolality of body fluid constant within a few percentage points despite wide variations in intake of salt and water. A corollary is that analysis of the composition and volume of the urine usually provides valuable clues in the diagnosis of disorders of body fluid volume and composition.

Although the movement of certain ions and proteins between the various body fluid compartments is restricted, water is freely diffusible. Consequently, the osmolality (total solute concentration) of all the body compartments is identical—normally, about 290 mosm/kg H_2O. The solutes dissolved in body fluids contribute to total osmolality in proportion to their molar concentration: In ECF, sodium and its salts account for most of the osmolality, whereas in ICF salts of potassium are chiefly responsible. Control of osmolality occurs through regulation of water intake (thirst) and water excretion (urine volume, insensible loss, and stool water), with the kidneys being the chief regulator. If water intake is low, the kidneys can reduce urine volume and raise urine solute concentration fourfold above plasma (ie, to 1200–1400 mosm/kg H_2O). If water intake is high, the kidneys can excrete a large volume of dilute (50 mosm/kg H_2O) urine.

Concentrations of electrolytes are usually expressed as equivalent weights: A 1-molar (M) solution contains 1 gram molecular weight of a compound dissolved in 1 liter (L) of fluid; 1 equivalent (eq) of an ion is equal to 1 mole (mol) multiplied by the valence of the ion. For example, in the case of the monovalent sodium ion, 1 eq is equal to 1 mol. In the case of calcium, which is divalent, 1 eq is equal to 0.5 mol. In the relatively dilute conditions of body fluids, the sum of the molar concentrations of ions is approximately equal to total

Table 9–1. Total Body Water (as Percentage of Body Weight) in Relation to Age and Sex.

Age	Male	Female
10-18	59	57
18-40	61	51
40-60	55	47
Over 60	52	46

fluid osmolality. However, because the chemical activities of these solutes differ, it is usually more accurate to estimate osmolality by multiplying the serum sodium concentration by 2.

The sensitive regulation of salt and water excretion by the kidney produces an intimate relationship between body fluid osmolality and volume. Edelman and his coworkers showed that the osmolality of plasma or any other body fluid can be closely approximated by the sum of exchangeable sodium (Na^+_e) and its anions (A^-) plus exchangeable potassium (K^+_e) and its anions divided by total body water (TBW):

$$Osmolality = \frac{(Na^+_e + A^-) + (K^+_e + A^-)}{TBW} \quad (1)$$

The plasma sodium (P_{Na}) concentration can be determined by the expression shown in equation 2:

$$P_{Na} = \frac{(Na^+_e + (K^+_e)}{TBW} \quad (2)$$

Although it is neither practical nor necessary to measure exchangeable sodium, exchangeable potassium, or total body water routinely, equation 2 illustrates the major factors that affect the serum sodium concentration and are important to the cause and therapy of many fluid and electrolyte disturbances.

In a steady state, the volume and composition of the urine depend upon the intake of water and dietary solutes. An average North American diet generates about 600 mosm of solute daily that must be excreted by the kidneys. Most people ingest more than 5 g of sodium chloride per day, equivalent to about 85 meq of Na^+ (1 g NaCl = 17 meq Na^+). Potassium excretion averages 40–60 meq/d. Water intake is more variable but usually amounts to about 2 L/d; an additional 400 mL of water per day is generated from cellular metabolism. Extrarenal (insensible) water loss amounts to 10 mL/kg body weight/24 h equally divided among losses from the lungs, from the skin, and in the stool. Losses from the lungs and skin may vary under physiologic conditions, but stool water rarely exceeds 200 mL/d in health. Thus, a typical 24-hour urine volume is 1500 mL and has the approximate solute concentrations shown in Table 9–2.

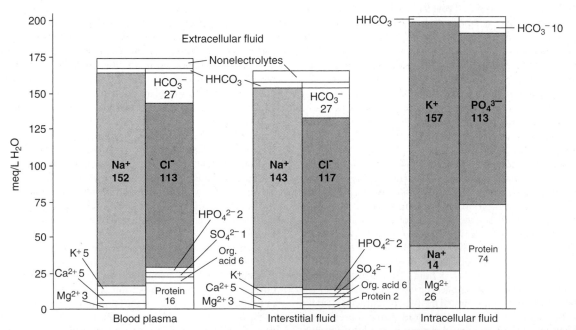

▲ **Figure 9–1.** Electrolyte composition of human body fluids. Note that the values are in meq/L of water, not of body fluid. (From Leaf A, Newburgh LH: *Significance of the Body Fluids in Clinical Medicine,* 2nd ed. Thomas, 1955. Reproduced by permission from Blackwell Publishing.)

Table 9–2. Typical Daily Solute Balances in Normal Subjects.

	Concentration	Total Amount
Intake		
Water		
Ingested	...	2 L
Cell metabolism	...	0.4 L
Total solute	...	600 mosm
Sodium	...	100 meq
Potassium	...	60 meq
Urinary excretion		
Water		1.5 L
Total solute	400 mosm/kg H$_2$O	600 mosm
Sodium	60 meq/L	90 meq[1]
Potassium	36 meq/L	54 meq[1]

[1]Small amounts of sodium and potassium are lost extrarenally (stool, sweat).

VOLUME DISORDERS

RECOGNITION & TREATMENT OF VOLUME DEPLETION

Since volume depletion is common in surgical patients, a general approach to the diagnosis and treatment of volume depletion should be developed and applied to each patient systematically. The clinical manifestations of volume depletion are low blood pressure, narrow pulse pressure, tachycardia, poor skin turgor, and dry mucous membranes. The history may suggest the reason for volume depletion. Records of intake and output, changes in body weight, urine specific gravity, and analysis of the chemical composition of the urine should confirm the clinical impression and be useful when a treatment plan is being devised. Therapy must aim to correct the volume deficit and associated aberrations in electrolyte concentrations.

VOLUME DEPLETION

The simplest form of volume depletion is water deficit without accompanying solute deficit. However, in surgical patients, water and solute deficits more often occur together. Pure water deficits occur in patients who are unable to regulate intake. They may be debilitated or comatose or may have increased insensible water loss from fever. Patients given tube feedings without adequate water supplementation and those with diabetes insipidus may also develop this syndrome. Pure water deficit is reflected biochemically by hypernatremia; the magnitude of the deficit can be estimated from the P_{Na} (equations 2, 3).

Associated findings are an increase in the plasma osmolality, concentrated urine, and a low urine sodium concentration (< 15 meq/L) despite hypernatremia. The clinical manifestations are chiefly caused by hypernatremia, which can depress the central nervous system, resulting in lethargy or coma. Muscle rigidity, tremors, spasticity, and seizures may occur. Since many patients suffering from water deficit have primary neurologic disease, it is often difficult to tell if the symptoms were caused by hypernatremia or by the underlying disease.

Treatment involves replacement of enough water to restore the P_{Na} concentration to normal. The excess sodium for which water must be provided can be estimated from equation 3:

$$\Delta Na = (140 - P_{Na}) \times TBW \qquad (3)$$

The ΔNa represents the total milliequivalents of sodium in excess of water. Divide ΔNa by 140 to obtain the amount of water required to return the serum sodium concentration to 140 meq/L. Because of the dehydration, an estimate of TBW should be used that is somewhat lower than the normal values listed in Table 9–1. In addition to correction of the existing water deficit, ongoing obligatory water losses (due to diabetes insipidus, fever, etc) must be satisfied. Treat the patient with 5% dextrose in water unless hypotension has developed, in which case hypotonic saline should be used. Rarely, isotonic saline may be indicated to treat shock due to dehydration even though the patient is hypernatremic.

VOLUME & ELECTROLYTE DEPLETION

Combined water and electrolyte depletion may occur from gastrointestinal losses due to nasogastric suction, enteric fistulas, enterostomies, or diarrhea. Other causes are excessive diuretic therapy, adrenal insufficiency, profuse sweating, burns, and body fluid sequestration following trauma or surgery. Diagnosis of combined volume and electrolyte deficiency can be made from the history, physical signs, and records of intake and output. The clinical findings are similar to those of pure volume depletion. However, the urine Na^+ concentration is often less than 10 meq/L, a manifestation of renal sodium conservation resulting from the action of aldosterone on the renal tubule. The urine is usually hypertonic (sp gr > 1.020), with an osmolality greater than 450–500 mosm/kg. The decreased blood volume diminishes renal perfusion and often produces prerenal azotemia, reflected by elevated blood urea nitrogen (BUN) and serum creatinine. Prerenal azotemia is characterized by a disproportionate rise of BUN compared to creatinine; the normal BUN/creatinine ratio of 10:1 is exceeded and may go as high as 20–25:1. This relationship helps differentiate prerenal azotemia from acute tubular necrosis, in which the BUN/creatinine ratio remains close to normal as the serum levels of both substances rise.

Combined water-electrolyte deficits are corrected by restoring volume and the deficient electrolytes. The magnitude of the volume deficit can be estimated by serial measurements of body weight, since acute changes in body weight primarily reflect changes in body fluid. Central venous or pulmonary artery pressure may be low in blood volume deficits and may be useful for monitoring replacement therapy.

The composition of the replacement fluid should take into account the P_{Na} concentration: If the P_{Na} is normal, fluid and electrolyte losses are probably isotonic, and the replacement fluid should be isotonic saline or its equivalent. Hyponatremia may result from salt loss exceeding water loss (ie, the decrease in Na^+_e will be greater than the decrease in TBW; equation 2) or from previous administration of hypotonic solutions. In this situation, the magnitude of the salt deficit can be calculated from equation 3.

Replacement therapy should be planned in two steps: (1) The sodium deficit should be calculated, and (2) the volume deficit should be estimated from clinical signs and changes in body weight. From these calculations, a hypothetical replacement solution can be devised in which the sodium deficit is administered as NaCl and the volume deficit as isotonic NaCl solution. Then administer isotonic NaCl solutions and monitor the patient's response (ie, urine volume and composition, serum electrolytes, and clinical signs). With restoration of ECF volume, renal perfusion improves, and excretion of water will occur while Na^+ continues to be reabsorbed. When replacement is adequate, renal function and serum Na^+ and Cl^- concentrations will return to normal.

VOLUME OVERLOAD

Hormonal and circulatory responses to surgery result in postoperative conservation of sodium and water by the kidneys that is independent of the status of the ECF volume. Antidiuretic hormone, released during anesthesia and surgical stress, promotes water conservation by the kidneys. Renal vasoconstriction and increased aldosterone activity reduce sodium excretion. Consequently, if fluid intake is excessive in the immediate postoperative period, circulatory overload may occur. The tendency for water retention may be exaggerated if heart failure, liver disease, renal disease, or hypoalbuminemia is present. Clinical manifestations of volume overload include edema of the sacrum and extremities, jugular venous distention, tachypnea (if pulmonary edema develops), increased body weight, and elevated pulmonary artery and central venous pressure. A gallop rhythm would indicate cardiac failure.

Volume overload may precipitate prerenal azotemia and oliguria. Examination of the urine usually shows low sodium and high potassium concentrations consistent with enhanced tubular reabsorption of Na^+ and water.

Management of volume overload depends upon its severity. For mild overload, sodium restriction will usually be adequate. If hyponatremia is present, water restriction will also be necessary. Diuretics must be used for severe volume overload. If cardiac failure is present, other measures must be employed, and a cardiology consultation may be necessary.

Inappropriate secretion of antidiuretic hormone (which may occur with head injury, some cancers, and burns) will produce a syndrome characterized by hyponatremia, concentrated urine, elevated urine sodium concentration, and a normal or mildly expanded ECF volume. The serum Na^+ values may drop below 110 meq/L and produce confusion and lethargy. In most cases, restriction of water intake alone will be sufficient to correct the abnormality. Occasionally, a potent diuretic (eg, furosemide) should be given and intravenous isotonic saline infused at a rate equal to the urine output; this will rapidly correct the hyponatremia. Patients with intracranial disease may also develop the syndrome of cerebral salt wasting and present with hyponatremia. However, these patients are volume-depleted, and correct treatment is sodium and volume replacement rather than water restriction.

SPECIFIC ELECTROLYTE DISORDERS

SODIUM

Regulation of the sodium concentration in plasma or urine is intimately associated with regulation of TBW (equation 2) and clinically reflects the balance between total body solute and TBW.

Hypernatremia represents chiefly loss of water, discussed earlier in this chapter. Current neurosurgical management of traumatic brain injury utilizes controlled hypernatremia by infusion of hypertonic saline to maintain serum Na^+ between 155 and 160 meq/L.

In addition to dilutional hyponatremia and isotonic dehydration, apparent hyponatremia developed in patients with marked hyperlipidemia or hyperproteinemia due to earlier measurement techniques, since fat and protein contribute to plasma bulk even though they are not dissolved in plasma water. The sodium concentration of plasma water in this situation is usually normal. Current laboratory techniques use ion-specific electrode measurements of the serum electrolytes, so apparent hyponatremia is no longer a clinical concern.

Hyponatremia in severe hyperglycemia results from the osmotic effects of the elevated glucose concentration, which draws water from the intracellular space to dilute ECF sodium. In hyperglycemia, the magnitude of this effect can be estimated by multiplying the blood glucose concentration in mg/dL by 0.016 and adding the result to the existing serum sodium concentration. The sum represents the predicted serum sodium concentration if the hyperglycemia were corrected. This correction factor may be even higher, particularly at very high (> 400 mg/dL) glucose concentrations.

Acute, severe hyponatremia occasionally develops in patients undergoing elective surgery. In these patients, the hyponatremia results from excessive intravenous sodium-free fluid administration coupled with the postsurgical stimulation of antidiuretic hormone release and causes severe permanent brain damage. Premenopausal women are at greater risk for developing this complication. This outcome underscores the need to limit postoperative free water administration and monitor serum electrolytes.

In most cases, hyponatremia can be successfully treated by administering the calculated sodium needs in isotonic solutions. Infusion of hypertonic saline solutions is rarely indicated and could precipitate circulatory overload. Only when severe hyponatremia (usually with $P_{Na} < 120$ meq/L) produces mental obtundation and seizures should the patient be treated with hypertonic sodium solutions. The rate of correction of hyponatremia is a major factor in determining outcome. Rapid correction of severe hyponatremia may cause permanent brain damage due to the osmotic demyelination syndrome. For this reason, serum Na^+ should be increased at a rate not to exceed 10–12 meq/L/h. Hyponatremia with volume overload usually indicates impaired renal ability to excrete sodium.

POTASSIUM

The potassium in extracellular fluids constitutes only 2% of total body potassium (Figure 9–1); the remaining 98% is within body cells.

The serum potassium concentration ($[K^+]$) is thought to be determined primarily by the pH of ECF and the size of the intracellular K^+ pool (Figure 9–2). With extracellular acidosis from administration of inorganic (strong) acids, it has been shown that a large proportion of the excess hydrogen is buffered intracellularly by an exchange of intracellular K^+ for extracellular H^+; this movement of K^+ may produce dangerous hyperkalemia. However, states of clinical metabolic acidosis result from derangements in intracellular metabolism to produce organic acidosis, which may not exert the same effects on the serum K^+. Likewise, simple alkalosis does not regularly result in hypokalemia from movement of K^+ into cells.

In the absence of an acid-base disturbance, serum K^+ reflects the total body pool of potassium (Figure 9–2). With excessive external losses of potassium (eg, from the gastrointestinal tract) (Table 9–3), the serum $[K^+]$ falls: A loss of 10% of total body K^+ drops the serum $[K^+]$ from 4 to 3 meq/L at a normal pH.

Although pH and body composition influence potassium metabolism, measurements of potassium intake and urinary potassium excretion allow the clinician to control potassium balance. Renal excretion of potassium is regulated by mineralocorticoid (aldosterone) levels. Renal failure—particularly acute oliguric renal failure—results in potassium retention and hyperkalemia. Adrenal insufficiency may produce hyper-

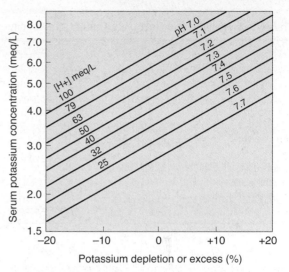

▲ **Figure 9–2.** Relationship of serum potassium to total body potassium stores at different blood pH levels. (Reprinted, with permission, from *University of Washington Teaching Syllabus for the Course on Fluid and Electrolyte Balance.* Edited by Belding Scribner, MD.)

kalemia through impaired renal excretion. Hypokalemia from excessive renal excretion may follow administration of diuretics, adrenal steroid excess, and certain renal tubular disorders associated with potassium wasting. Rarely, potassium deficiency can arise from deficient dietary potassium intake, as in alcoholic patients or in those receiving total parenteral nutrition with inadequate potassium replacement.

1. Hyperkalemia

Hyperkalemia is a treatable problem that may prove fatal if undiagnosed. Blood potassium levels must be closely monitored in susceptible patients such as those with severe trauma, burns, crush injuries, renal insufficiency, or marked catabolism from other causes. Hyperkalemia may also be due to Addison disease. Clinical evidence of significant hyperkalemia is usually not present. Nausea and vomiting, colicky abdominal pain, and diarrhea may occur. The electrocardiographic changes are the most helpful indicators of the severity of the disorder: Early changes include peaking of the T waves, widening of the QRS complex, and depression of the ST segment. With further elevation of the blood potassium level, the QRS widens to such a degree that the tracing resembles a sine wave, a finding that portends imminent cardiac standstill.

A number of factors must be rapidly considered in assessing the hyperkalemic patient. First, one should determine whether the serum potassium level is a true metabolic abnormality or has been elevated by hemolysis, marked

Table 9–3. Volume and Electrolyte Content of Gastrointestinal Fluid Losses.[1]

	Na$^+$(meq/L)	K$^+$(meq/L)	Cl$^-$ (meq/L)	HCO$_3^-$ (meq/L)	Volume (mL)
Gastric juice, high in acid	20 (20–30)	10 (5–40)	120 (80–150)	0	1000–9000
Gastric juice, low in acid	80 (70–140)	15 (5–40)	90 (40–120)	5–25	1000–2500
Pancreatic juice	140 (115–180)	5 (3–8)	75 (55–95)	80 (60–110)	500–1000
Bile	148 (130–160)	5 (3–12)	100 (90–120)	35 (30–40)	300–1000
Small bowel drainage	110 (80–150)	5 (2–8)	105 (60–125)	30 (20–40)	1000–3000
Distal ileum and cecum drainage	80 (40–135)	8 (5–30)	45 (20–90)	30 (20–40)	1000–3000
Diarrheal stools	120 (20–160)	25 (10–40)	90 (30–120)	45 (30–50)	500–17,000

[1]Average values/24 h with range in parentheses.

leukocytosis, or thrombocytosis. Platelet counts greater than 1 million/μL may elevate the serum potassium, since the ion is liberated from platelets as they are consumed during clotting. Second, the acid-base status should be assessed to ascertain its influence (Figure 9–2). Finally, the rapidity with which the elevated serum potassium should be corrected must be determined.

There are five approaches to the emergency treatment of hyperkalemia. Initially, an intravenous infusion of 100 mL of 50% dextrose solution containing 20 units of regular insulin will lower extracellular K$^+$ by promoting its intracellular transport in association with glucose. Intravenous NaHCO$_3$ solutions may lower serum K$^+$ as acidosis is corrected, though this point remains controversial. Calcium antagonizes the tissue effects of potassium; an infusion of calcium gluconate will transiently reverse cardiac depression from hyperkalemia without changing the serum potassium concentration. A slower method of controlling hyperkalemia is to administer the cation exchange resin sodium polystyrene sulfonate (Kayexalate) orally or by enema at a rate of 40–80 g/d. This drug binds potassium in the intestine in exchange for sodium. It is often given with sorbitol to induce osmotic diarrhea and enhance the rate of potassium removal. Finally, when hyperkalemia is a manifestation of renal failure, hemodialysis is often necessary; β-adrenergic stimulation with inhaled albuterol is also helpful in these patients.

2. Hypokalemia

Hypokalemia usually results from renal wasting of potassium; potassium deficiency and hypokalemia from inadequate dietary intake occur only after weeks of a deficient diet. Alcoholics and elderly people with restricted diets are at risk for potassium depletion due to insufficient dietary intake. The clinical manifestations of hypokalemia relate to neuromuscular function: Decreased muscle contractility and muscle cell potential develop, and in extreme cases death may result from paralysis of the muscles of respiration.

When the clinician assesses hypokalemia, the initial goal is to identify the cause. If alkalosis is present, the K$^+$ needs can be estimated from the nomogram in Figure 9–2. If there is no acid-base imbalance, or if hypokalemia persists after alkalosis is corrected, renal losses are probably excessive. Urine potassium excretion of more than 30 meq/24 h associated with a serum [K$^+$] under 3.5 meq/L indicates renal potassium wasting. The primary problem in this situation is usually diuretic therapy, alkalosis, or increased aldosterone activity. If renal potassium excretion is less than 30 meq/24 h, the kidneys are conserving potassium appropriately, and hypokalemia reflects a total body deficit.

Treatment consists of correcting the cause of hypokalemia and administering potassium. If the patient is able to eat, potassium should be given orally; otherwise, it should be given intravenously. Usually, potassium concentrations in intravenous solutions should not exceed 40 meq/L. In moderate to severe hypokalemia ([K$^+$] < 3 meq/L), potassium may be administered at a rate of 20–30 meq/h. With mild hypokalemia ([K$^+$] 3–3.5 meq/L), potassium should be replaced slowly to avoid hyperkalemia. Potassium should usually be administered intravenously as the chloride salt; in metabolic alkalosis, potassium chloride is specific, since it helps to correct the acid-base abnormality as well as the hypokalemia. Occasional patients may have persistent hypokalemia refractory to replacement therapy because of coexistent magnesium deficiency. Therefore, serum magnesium concentration should be measured in hypokalemic patients, particularly since many of the causes of potassium deficiency will also result in magnesium depletion (see section on Magnesium, later).

CALCIUM

Calcium is an important mediator of neuromuscular function and cellular enzyme processes even though most of the body calcium is contained in the skeleton. The usual dietary intake of calcium is 1–3 g/d, most of which is excreted unabsorbed in the feces.

The normal serum calcium concentration (8.5–10.3 mg/dL, 4.2–5.2 meq/L) is maintained by humoral factors, mainly vitamin D, parathyroid hormone, and calcitonin. Acidemia increases and alkalemia decreases the serum ionized calcium concentration. Approximately half of the total serum calcium is bound to plasma proteins, chiefly albumin; a small amount is complexed to plasma anions, such as citrate; and the remainder (approximately 40%) of the total serum calcium is free, or ionized, calcium, which is the fraction responsible for the biologic effects. The ionized calcium usually remains constant when the total serum calcium concentration changes with different serum albumin concentrations. Unless the ionized calcium is measured, the serum calcium can only be reliably assessed if accompanied by measurement of the serum albumin concentration.

Severe disturbances of calcium concentration are uncommon in surgical patients, although transient asymptomatic hypocalcemia is common. After operations on the thyroid or parathyroids, the serum calcium concentration should be measured at regular intervals to detect hypocalcemia early if it appears.

1. Hypocalcemia

Hypocalcemia occurs in hypoparathyroidism, hypomagnesemia, severe pancreatitis, chronic or acute renal failure, severe trauma, crush injuries, and necrotizing fasciitis. The clinical manifestations are neuromuscular: hyperactive deep tendon reflexes, a positive Chvostek sign, muscle and abdominal cramps, carpopedal spasm, and, rarely, convulsions. Hypocalcemia is reflected in the ECG by a prolonged QT interval.

The initial step is to check the whole blood pH; if alkalosis is present, it should be treated. Intravenous calcium, as calcium gluconate or calcium chloride, may be needed for the acute problem (eg, after parathyroidectomy). Chronic hypoparathyroidism requires vitamin D, oral calcium supplements, and often aluminum hydroxide gels to bind dietary phosphate in the intestine.

2. Hypercalcemia

Hypercalcemia most frequently is caused by hyperparathyroidism, cancer with bony metastases, ectopic production of parathyroid hormone, vitamin D intoxication, hyperthyroidism, sarcoidosis, milk-alkali syndrome, or prolonged immobilization (especially in young patients or those with Paget disease). It is also a rare complication of thiazide diuretics.

The symptoms of hypercalcemia are fatigability, muscle weakness, depression, anorexia, nausea, and constipation. Long-standing hypercalcemia may impair renal concentrating mechanisms, resulting in polyuria and polydipsia and in metastatic deposition of calcium. Severe hypercalcemia can cause coma and death. *A serum calcium concentration above 12 mg/dL should be regarded as a medical emergency!*

With severe hypercalcemia ($Ca^{2+} > 14.5$ mg/dL), intravenous isotonic saline should be given to expand ECF, increase urine flow, enhance calcium excretion, and reduce the serum level.

Furosemide and intravenous sodium sulfate are other methods of increasing renal calcium excretion. Plicamycin is particularly useful for hypercalcemia associated with metastatic cancer. Adrenal corticosteroids are useful for hypercalcemia associated with sarcoidosis, vitamin D intoxication, and Addison disease. Calcitonin is indicated in patients with impaired renal and cardiovascular function. When renal failure is present, hemodialysis may be required.

MAGNESIUM

Magnesium is largely present in bone and cells, where it serves an important role in cellular energy metabolism. The normal plasma magnesium concentration is 1.5–2.5 meq/L. Magnesium is excreted primarily by the kidneys. The serum magnesium concentration reflects total body magnesium. Serum magnesium levels may be elevated in hypovolemic shock as magnesium is liberated from cells.

1. Hypomagnesemia

Hypomagnesemia occurs with poor dietary intake, intestinal malabsorption of ingested magnesium, or excessive losses from the gut (eg, severe diarrhea, enteric fistulas, use of purgatives, or nasogastric suction). It may also be caused by excessive urinary losses (eg, from diuretics), chronic alcohol abuse, hyperaldosteronism, and hypercalcemia. Hypomagnesemia occasionally develops in acute pancreatitis, in diabetic acidosis, in burned patients, or after prolonged total parenteral nutrition with insufficient magnesium supplementation. The clinical manifestations resemble those of hypocalcemia: hyperactive tendon reflexes, a positive Chvostek sign, and tremors that may progress to delirium and convulsions.

The diagnosis of hypomagnesemia depends on clinical suspicion with confirmation by measurement of the serum magnesium. Treatment consists of administering magnesium, usually as the sulfate or chloride. In moderate magnesium deficiency, oral replacement is adequate. In more severe deficits, parenteral magnesium must be administered intravenously (40–80 meq of $MgSO_4$ per liter of intravenous fluid). When large doses are infused intravenously, there is a risk of producing hypermagnesemia, with tachycardia and hypotension. The ECG should be inspected for prolongation of the QT interval. Magnesium should be administered cautiously to oliguric patients or those with renal failure and only after magnesium deficiency has been unequivocally documented. Magnesium deficiency may also be accompanied by refractory hypokalemia.

2. Hypermagnesemia

Hypermagnesemia usually occurs in patients with renal disease; it is rare in surgical patients. In patients with renal insufficiency, serum magnesium levels should be monitored closely. Strict attention must be paid to excess magnesium intake, which can occur from a variety of commonly administered antacids and laxatives and which may produce severe and even fatal hypermagnesemia in renal insufficiency.

The initial signs and symptoms of hypermagnesemia are lethargy and weakness. Electrocardiographic changes resemble those in hyperkalemia (widened QRS complex, ST segment depression, and peaked T waves). When the serum level reaches 6 meq/L, deep tendon reflexes are lost; with levels above 10 meq/L, somnolence, coma, and death may ensue.

Treatment of hypermagnesemia consists of giving intravenous isotonic saline to increase the rate of renal magnesium excretion. This may be accompanied by slow intravenous infusion of calcium, since calcium antagonizes some of the neuromuscular actions of magnesium. Patients with hypermagnesemia and severe renal failure may need dialysis.

PHOSPHORUS

Phosphorus is primarily a constituent of bone, but it is also an important intracellular ion with a role in energy metabolism. The serum phosphorus level is only an approximate indicator of total body phosphorus and can be influenced by a number of factors, including the serum calcium concentration and the pH of blood. In urine, phosphorus is an important buffer that facilitates the excretion of acids formed by intermediary metabolism. Urine phosphate buffer is reflected by the excretion of titratable acid.

1. Hypophosphatemia

Clinically important hypophosphatemia may follow poor dietary intake (especially in alcoholics), hyperparathyroidism, and antacid administration (antacids bind phosphate in the intestine). Hypophosphatemia was at one time a frequent complication of total parenteral nutrition until phosphate supplementation became routine. Clinical manifestations appear when the serum phosphorus level falls to 1 mg/dL or less. Neuromuscular manifestations include lassitude, fatigue, weakness, convulsions, and death. Red blood cells hemolyze, oxygen delivery is impaired, and white cell phagocytosis is depressed. Cardiac contractility may be impaired, and rhabdomyolysis can occur. Chronic phosphate depletion has been implicated in the development of osteomalacia.

2. Hyperphosphatemia

Hyperphosphatemia most often develops in severe renal disease, after trauma, or with marked tissue catabolism. It is rarely caused by excessive dietary intake. Hyperphosphatemia is usually asymptomatic. Because it raises the calcium-phosphorus product, the serum calcium concentration is depressed. A high calcium-phosphate product predisposes to metastatic calcification of soft tissues. Treatment of hyperphosphatemia is by diuresis to increase the rate of urinary phosphorus excretion. Administration of phosphate-binding antacids, such as aluminum hydroxide gels, will diminish the gastrointestinal absorption of phosphorus and lower the serum phosphorus concentration. In patients with renal disease, dialysis may be required.

▼ ACID-BASE BALANCE

NORMAL PHYSIOLOGY

During the course of daily metabolism of protein and carbohydrate, approximately 70 meq (or 1 meq/kg of body weight) of hydrogen ion is generated and delivered into the body fluids. In addition, a large amount of carbon dioxide is formed that combines with water to form carbonic acid (H_2CO_3). If efficient mechanisms for buffering and eliminating these acids were not available, the pH of body fluids would fall rapidly. Although mammals have a highly developed system for handling daily acid production, disturbances of acid-base balance are common in disease.

Hydrogen ions generated from metabolism are buffered through two major systems. The first involves intracellular protein, eg, the hemoglobin in red blood cells. More important is the bicarbonate/carbonic acid system, which can be understood from the Henderson-Hasselbalch equation:

$$pH = pK + \log \frac{[HCO_3^-]}{0.03 \times P_{CO_2}}$$

$$\text{where pK for the } \frac{HCO_3^-}{H_2CO_3} \text{ system is 6.1.} \tag{4}$$

Hydrogen ion concentration is related to pH in an inverse logarithmic manner. The following transformation of equation 4 is easier to use, because it eliminates the logarithms:

$$[H^+] = \frac{24 \times P_{CO_2}}{[HCO_e^-]} \tag{5}$$

There is an approximately linear inverse relationship between pH and hydrogen ion concentration over the pH range of 7.9–7.50: For each 0.01 decrease in pH, the hydrogen ion concentration increases 1 nmol. Remembering that a normal blood pH of 7.40 is equal to a hydrogen ion concentration of 40 nmol/L, one can calculate the approximate hydrogen ion concentration for any pH between 7.10 and 7.50. For example, a pH of 7.30 is equal to a hydrogen ion concentration of 50 nmol/L. This estimation introduces an error of approximately 10% at the extremes of this pH range. (See also Figure 9–2.)

A consideration of the right-hand side of equation 5 demonstrates that hydrogen ion concentration is determined by the ratio of the Pa_{CO_2} to the plasma bicarbonate concentration. In body fluids, CO_2 is dissolved and combines with water to form carbonic acid, the acid part of the acid-base pair. If any two of these three variables are known, the third can be calculated using this expression.

Equation 5 also illustrates how the body excretes acid produced through metabolic processes. Blood P_{CO_2} is normally controlled within narrow limits by pulmonary ventilation. The plasma bicarbonate concentration is regulated in the renal tubules by three major processes: (1) Filtered bicarbonate is reabsorbed, mostly in the proximal tubule, to prevent excessive bicarbonate loss in the urine; (2) hydrogen ions are secreted as titratable acid to regenerate the bicarbonate that was buffered when these hydrogen ions were initially produced and to provide a vehicle for excretion of about one-third of the daily acid production; and (3) the kidneys also excrete hydrogen ion in the form of ammonium ion by a process that regenerates bicarbonate initially consumed in the production of these hydrogen ions. Volume depletion, increased Pa_{CO_2}, and hypokalemia all favor enhanced tubular reabsorption of HCO_3^-.

ACID-BASE ABNORMALITIES

The management of clinical acid-base disturbances is facilitated by the use of a nomogram (Figure 9–3) that relates the three variables in equation 5.

Primary respiratory disturbances cause changes in the blood Pa_{CO_2} (the numerator in equation 5) and produce corresponding effects on the blood hydrogen ion concentration. Metabolic disturbances primarily affect the plasma bicarbonate concentration (the denominator in equation 5). Whether the disturbance is primarily respiratory or metabolic, some degree of compensatory change occurs in the reciprocal factor in equation 5 to limit or nullify the magnitude of perturbation of acid-base balance. Thus, changes in blood P_{CO_2} from respiratory disturbances are compensated for by changes in the renal handling of bicarbonate. Conversely, changes in plasma bicarbonate concentration are blunted by appropriate respiratory changes.

Because acute respiratory changes allow insufficient time for compensatory renal mechanisms to respond, the resulting pH disturbances are often great and the abnormalities may be present in pure form. By contrast, chronic respiratory disturbances allow the full range of compensatory mechanisms by the kidneys to come into play, so that blood pH may remain near normal despite wide variations in the blood P_{CO_2}. On the other hand, respiratory compensation for metabolic disturbances occurs almost instantaneously, so that there is little difference in the acid-base variables between acute and chronic disorders.

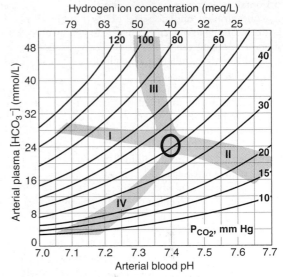

▲ **Figure 9–3.** Acid-base nomogram for use in evaluation of clinical acid-base disorders. Hydrogen ion concentration (top) or blood pH (bottom) is plotted against plasma HCO_3^- concentration; curved lines are isopleths of CO_2 tension (Pa_{CO_2}, mm Hg). Knowing any two of these variables permits estimation of the third. The circle in the center represents the range of normal values; the shaded bands represent the 95% confidence limits of four common acid-base disturbances: I, acute respiratory acidosis; II, acute respiratory alkalosis; III, chronic respiratory acidosis; IV, sustained metabolic acidosis. Points lying outside these shaded areas are mixed disturbances and indicate two primary acid-base disorders. (Courtesy of Anthony Sebastian, MD, University of California Medical Center, San Francisco.)

1. Respiratory Acidosis

Acute respiratory acidosis occurs when respiration suddenly becomes inadequate. CO_2 accumulates in the blood (the numerator in equation 5 increases), and hydrogen ion concentration increases. This occurs most often in acute airway obstruction, aspiration, respiratory arrest, certain pulmonary infections, and pulmonary edema with impaired gas exchange. There is acidemia and an elevated blood P_{CO_2} but little change in the plasma bicarbonate concentration. Over 80% of the carbonic acid resulting from the increased Pa_{CO_2} is buffered by intracellular mechanisms—about 50% by intracellular protein and another 30% by hemoglobin. Because relatively little is buffered by bicarbonate ion, the plasma bicarbonate concentration may be normal. An acute increase in the Pa_{CO_2} from 40 to 80 mm Hg will increase the plasma bicarbonate by only 3 meq/L. This is why the 95% confidence band for acute respiratory acidosis (I in Figure 9–3) is nearly horizontal; ie, increases in $Paco_2$ directly increase hydrogen ion concentration and decrease pH with little change in plasma bicarbonate concentration. Treatment involves restoration of adequate ventilation. If necessary, tracheal intubation and assisted ventilation or controlled ventilation with sedation should be employed.

Chronic respiratory acidosis arises from chronic respiratory failure in which impaired ventilation gives a sustained elevation of blood Pco_2. Renal compensation raises plasma bicarbonate to the extent illustrated by the 95% confidence limits in Figure 9–3 (the area marked by III). Rather marked elevations of $Paco_2$ produce small changes in blood pH, because of the increase in plasma bicarbonate concentration. This is achieved primarily by increased renal excretion of ammonium ion, which enhances acid excretion and regenerates bicarbonate, which is returned to the blood. Chronic respiratory acidosis is generally well tolerated until severe pulmonary insufficiency leads to hypoxia. At this point, the long-term prognosis is very poor. Paradoxically, the patient with chronic respiratory acidosis appears better able to tolerate additional acute increases in blood Pco_2.

Treatment of chronic respiratory acidosis depends largely on attention to pulmonary toilet and ventilatory status. Rapid correction of chronic respiratory acidosis, as may occur if the patient is placed on controlled ventilation, can be dangerous, since the $Paco_2$ is lowered rapidly and the compensated respiratory acidosis may be converted to a severe metabolic alkalosis (posthypercapnic metabolic acidosis).

2. Respiratory Alkalosis

Acute hyperventilation lowers the $Paco_2$ without concomitant changes in the plasma bicarbonate concentration and thereby lowers the hydrogen ion concentration (II in Figure 9–3). The clinical manifestations are paresthesias in the extremities, carpopedal spasm, and a positive Chvostek sign. Acute hyperventilation with respiratory alkalosis may be an early sign of bacterial sepsis.

Chronic respiratory alkalosis occurs in pulmonary and liver disease. The renal response to chronic hypocapnia is to decrease the tubular reabsorption of filtered bicarbonate, increasing bicarbonate excretion, with a consequent lowering of plasma bicarbonate concentration. As the bicarbonate concentration falls, the chloride concentration rises. This is the same pattern seen in hyperchloremic acidosis, and the two can only be distinguished by blood gas and pH measurements. Generally, chronic respiratory alkalosis does not require treatment; if the $Paco_2$ is allowed to return to normal rapidly, posthypocapnic metabolic acidosis with hyperchloremia may occur.

3. Metabolic Acidosis

Metabolic acidosis is caused by increased production of hydrogen ion from metabolic or other causes or from excessive bicarbonate losses. In either case, the plasma bicarbonate concentration is decreased, producing an increase in hydrogen ion concentration (see equation 5). With excessive bicarbonate loss (eg, severe diarrhea, diuretic treatment with acetazolamide or other carbonic anhydrase inhibitors, certain forms of renal tubular disease, and in patients with ureterosigmoidostomies), the decrease in plasma bicarbonate concentration is matched by an increase in the serum chloride, so that the anion gap (the sum of chloride and bicarbonate concentrations subtracted from the serum sodium concentration) remains at the normal level, below 15 meq/L. On the other hand, metabolic acidosis from increased acid production is associated with an anion gap exceeding 15 meq/L. Conditions in which this occurs are renal failure, diabetic ketoacidosis, lactic acidosis, methanol ingestion, salicylate intoxication, and ethylene glycol ingestion. The lungs compensate by hyperventilation, which returns the hydrogen ion concentration toward normal by lowering the blood Pco_2. In long-standing metabolic acidosis, minute ventilation may increase sufficiently to drop the $Paco_2$ to as low as 10–15 mm Hg. The shaded area marked IV on the nomogram (Figure 9–3) represents the confidence limits for sustained metabolic acidosis.

Treatment of metabolic acidosis depends on identifying the underlying cause and correcting it. Often, this is sufficient. In some conditions, particularly when there is an increased anion gap, alkali administration is required. The amount of sodium bicarbonate required to restore the plasma bicarbonate concentration to normal can be estimated by subtracting the existing plasma bicarbonate concentration from the normal value of 24 meq/L and multiplying the resulting number by half the estimated total body water. This is a useful empiric formula. In practice, it is not usually wise to administer enough bicarbonate to return the plasma bicarbonate completely to normal. It is better to raise the plasma bicarbonate concentration by 5 meq/L initially and then reassess the clinical situation. The administration of sodium bicarbonate may cause fluid overload from the large quantity of sodium and may overcorrect the acidosis. The long-term management of patients with metabolic acidosis entails providing adequate alkali, either as supplemental sodium bicarbonate tablets or by dietary manipulation. In all cases, attempts should be made to minimize the magnitude of bicarbonate loss in patients with chronic metabolic acidosis.

4. Metabolic Alkalosis

Metabolic alkalosis is probably the most common acid-base disturbance in surgical patients. In this condition, the blood hydrogen ion concentration is decreased as a result of accumulation of bicarbonate in plasma. The pathogenesis is complex but involves at least three separate factors: (1) loss of hydrogen ion, usually as a result of loss of gastric secretions rich in hydrochloric acid; (2) volume depletion, which is often severe; and (3) potassium depletion, which almost always is present.

HCl secretion by the gastric mucosa returns bicarbonate ion to the blood. Gastric acid, after mixing with ingested food, is subsequently reabsorbed in the small intestine, so that there is no net gain or loss of hydrogen ion in this process. If secreted hydrogen ion is lost through vomiting or drainage, the result is a net delivery of bicarbonate into the circulation. Normally, the kidneys are easily able to excrete the excess bicarbonate load. However, if volume depletion accompanies the loss of hydrogen ion, the kidneys work to preserve volume by increasing tubular reabsorption of sodium and whatever anions are also filtered. Consequently, because of the increased sodium reabsorption, the excess bicarbonate cannot be completely excreted. This perpetuates the metabolic alkalosis. At first, some of the filtered bicarbonate escapes reabsorption in the proximal tubule and reaches the distal tubule. Here it promotes potassium secretion and enhanced potassium loss in the urine. The urine pH will be either neutral or alkaline, because of the presence of bicarbonate. Later, as volume depletion becomes more severe, the reabsorption of filtered bicarbonate in the proximal tubule becomes virtually complete. Now, only small amounts of sodium, with little bicarbonate, reach the distal tubule. If potassium depletion is severe, sodium is reabsorbed in exchange for hydrogen ion. This results in the paradoxically acid urine sometimes observed in patients with advanced metabolic alkalosis.

Assessment should involve examination of the urine electrolytes and urine pH. In the early stages, bicarbonate excretion will obligate excretion of sodium as well as potassium, so the urine sodium concentration will be relatively high for a volume-depleted patient and the urine pH will be alkaline. In this circumstance, the urine chloride will reveal the extent of the volume depletion: A urine chloride of less than 10 meq/L is diagnostic of volume depletion and chloride deficiency. Later, when bicarbonate reabsorption becomes virtually complete, the urine pH will be acid, and urine sodium, potassium, and chloride concentrations will all be low. The ventilatory compensation in metabolic alkalosis is variable, but the maximal extent of compensation can only raise the blood P_{CO_2} to about 55 mm Hg. A Pa_{CO_2} greater than 60 mm Hg in metabolic alkalosis suggests a mixed disturbance also involving respiratory acidosis.

To treat metabolic alkalosis, fluid must be given, usually as saline solution. With adequate volume repletion, the stimulus to tubular sodium reabsorption is diminished, and the kidneys can then excrete the excess bicarbonate. Most of these patients are also substantially potassium-depleted and will require potassium supplementation. This should be administered as KCl, since chloride depletion is another hallmark of this condition and potassium given as citrate or lactate will not correct the potassium deficit.

5. Mixed Acid-Base Disorders

In many situations, mixed disorders of acid-base balance develop. The most common example in surgical patients is metabolic acidosis superimposed on respiratory alkalosis. This problem can arise in patients with septic shock or hepatorenal syndrome. Since the two acid-base disorders tend to cancel each other, the disturbance in hydrogen ion concentration is usually small. The reverse situation, ie, respiratory acidosis combined with metabolic alkalosis, is less common. Combined metabolic and respiratory acidosis occurs in cardiorespiratory arrest and obviously constitutes a medical emergency. Circumstances involving both metabolic and respiratory alkalosis are rare. The clue to the presence of a mixed acid-base disorder can come from plotting the patient's acid-base data on the nomogram in Figure 9–3. If the set of data falls outside one of the confidence bands, then by definition the patient has a mixed disorder. On the other hand, if the acid-base data fall within one of the confidence bands, it suggests (but does not prove) that the acid-base disturbance is pure or uncomplicated.

▼ PRINCIPLES OF FLUID & ELECTROLYTE THERAPY

The development of a rational plan of fluid and electrolyte therapy requires an understanding of the principles developed earlier in this chapter. First, maintenance fluid requirements must be determined. Second, existing deficits of volume or composition should be calculated. This involves the analysis of four aspects of the patient's fluid and electrolyte status based on weight changes, serum electrolyte concentrations, and blood pH and P_{CO_2}: (1) the magnitude of the volume deficit present, (2) the pathogenesis and treatment of abnormal sodium concentration, (3) assessment of any potassium requirement, and (4) management of any coexistent acid-base disturbance. Finally, therapy must also recognize the presence of ongoing obligatory fluid losses and include these losses in the daily plan of treatment.

Normal maintenance requirements can be determined using the guidelines in Table 9–2. Fever or elevated ambient temperature will increase insensible losses and thereby increase these requirements. The normal response to the stress of surgery is to conserve water and electrolytes, so maintenance requirements are decreased in the immediate postoperative period. In addition, increased catabolism will deliver more potassium to the circulation, so that this ion can be omitted from maintenance solutions for several days postoperatively.

Correction of preexisting deficits must be based on the four factors listed above. Volume deficit is best estimated on the basis of acute changes in weight or from clinical estimates; the clinician should remember that deficits less than 5% of body water will not be detectable and that loss of 15% of body water will be associated with severe circulatory compromise. The relationship of net sodium to net fluid deficit is given by the serum sodium concentration according to equation 3. If the serum sodium concentration is normal, fluid losses have been isotonic; if hyponatremia is present, more sodium than water has been lost. In either case, initial replacement should be with isotonic saline solutions. Any potassium excess or deficit must be assessed in the light of the blood pH according to Figure 9–2. If hypokalemia exists at normal pH, the magnitude of the total body potassium deficit can also be estimated using Figure 9–2. For example, a serum potassium concentration of 2.5 meq/L at pH 7.40 suggests a 20% depletion of total body potassium. A normal human has a potassium capacity of 45 meq/kg body weight; a moderately wasted patient, 35 meq/kg. For a normal 70-kg man, total potassium capacity is 45×70, or 3150 meq; the deficit is 20% of this, or 630 meq, and this amount must be considered in therapy calculations. Principles of acid-base therapy have already been outlined.

Two rules of thumb should be applied in prescribing parenteral therapy for fluid and electrolyte deficits. The first is that for most problems, half of the calculated deficits should be replaced in a 24-hour period, with subsequent reassessment of the clinical situation. The second is that a fluid or electrolyte abnormality should take as long to correct as it took to develop. By adherence to these guidelines, overly vigorous replacement will be avoided and, along with it, the production of a different (iatrogenic) electrolyte abnormality.

Ongoing losses must be considered also in the daily fluid therapy plan, with regard to both volume and composition. Characteristic measurements for fluids removed from different segments of the gastrointestinal tract are shown in Table 9–3.

REFERENCES

General

Seldin DW, Giebisch G (editors): *The Kidney: Physiology and Pathophysiology*, 3rd ed. Lippincott Williams & Wilkins, 2000.

Fluid Volume & Sodium Concentration

Adrogue HJ et al: Hypernatremia. N Engl J Med 2000;342:1493.
Adrogue HJ et al: Hyponatremia. N Engl J Med 2000;342:1581.
Ayus JC et al: Chronic hyponatremic encephalopathy in post-menopausal women. Association of therapies with morbidity and mortality. JAMA 1999;281:2342.
Doyle JA et al: The use of hypertonic saline in the treatment of traumatic brain injury. J Trauma 2001;50:367.
Gines P, Cardenas A: The management of ascites and hyponatremia in cirrhosis. Semin Liver Dis 2008;28:43.
Gross P: Treatment of hyponatremia. Intern Med 2008;47:885.
Lien YH, Shapiro JI: Hyponatremia: clinical diagnosis and management. Am J Med 2007;120:653.
Wilcox CS: Metabolic and adverse effects of diuretics. Semin Nephrol 1999;19:557.

Acid-Base Disturbances & Potassium

Adrogue HJ et al: Management of life-threatening acid-base disorders. (Two parts.) N Engl J Med 1998;338:26, 107.
Greenberg A: Hyperkalemia: treatment options. Semin Nephrol 1998;18:46.
Ishihara K et al: Anion gap acidosis. Semin Nephrol 1998;18:83.
Krapf R et al: Chronic respiratory alkalosis. The effect of sustained hyperventilation on renal regulation of acid-base equilibrium. N Engl J Med 1991;324:1394.
Luft FC: Lactic acidosis update for critical care clinicians. J Am Soc Nephrol 2001;12: S 15.

Calcium, Magnesium, & Phosphorus

Aguilera IM et al: Calcium and the anaesthetist. Anaesthesia 2000;55:779.
Body JJ: Current and future directions in medical therapy: hypercalcemia. Cancer 2000;88(12 suppl):3054.
Brown DL et al: Developments in the therapeutic applications of bisphosphonates. J Clin Pharmacol 1999;39:651.
Bugg NC et al: Hypophosphataemia. Pathophysiology, effects and management on the intensive care unit. Anaesthesia 1998;53:895.
Kelepouris E et al: Hypomagnesemia: renal magnesium handling. Semin Nephrol 1998;18:58.
Miller DW et al: Hypophosphatemia in the emergency department therapeutics. Am J Emerg Med 2000;18:457.
Shepard MM, Smith JW 3rd: Hypercalcemia. Am J Med Sci 2007;334:381.
Subramanian R et al: Severe hypophosphatemia. Pathophysiologic implications, clinical presentations, and treatment. Medicine 2000;79:1

Surgical Metabolism & Nutrition

John R. Barbour, MD

English F. Barbour, RD, LD, CNSD

Virginia M. Herrmann, MD

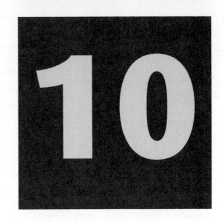

The effects of malnutrition on the surgical patient are well characterized in the literature but are often overlooked in the clinical arena. Between 30% and 50% of hospitalized patients are malnourished. Protein-calorie malnutrition produces a reduction in lean muscle mass, alterations in respiratory mechanics, impaired immune function, and intestinal atrophy. These changes result in diminished wound healing, predisposition to infection, and increased postoperative morbidity. Although most healthy individuals can tolerate up to 7 days of starvation (with adequate glucose and fluid replacement), those subjected to major trauma, the physiologic stress of surgery, sepsis, or cancer-related cachexia require nutritional intervention much sooner. Methods to identify those at greatest need for supplemental nutrition and to adequately address their needs are discussed in this chapter.

NUTRITIONAL ASSESSMENT

Nutrition screening is the process of identifying patients who are either malnourished or at risk for developing malnutrition. Major trauma and surgical stress alter the intake and absorption of nutrients, as well as their utilization and storage by the body. In select patients (eg, those with severe malnutrition as determined below), preoperative nutritional support has been shown to significantly reduce perioperative morbidity and mortality. Although most patients do not require this level of support, nutrition screening is imperative to identify the patient at high risk for malnutrition or its sequelae. A comprehensive nutritional assessment incorporates the initial history, physical examination, and laboratory testing to provide a snapshot of the patient's recent nutritional health.

▶ History & Physical Examination

The history and physical examination are the foundation of nutritional assessment. A complete medical history is essential to identify factors that predispose the patient to alterations in nutritional status (Table 10–1). Chronic illnesses such as alcoholism are commonly associated with protein-calorie malnutrition as well as vitamin and mineral deficiencies. Previous operative procedures such as gastrectomy or ileal resection may predispose to generalized malabsorption or isolated deficiency of iron, vitamin B_{12}, or folate. In most cases, the possibility of malnutrition is suggested by the underlying disease or by a history of recent weight loss. Patients with renal failure who require hemodialysis lose amino acids, vitamins, trace elements, and carnitine in the dialysate. Cirrhotics often suffer from whole-body sodium overload despite being hyponatremic, and they are typically protein-deficient. Patients with inflammatory bowel disease, particularly those with ileal involvement, may develop protein deficiency due to a combination of poor intake, chronic diarrhea, and treatment with corticosteroids. Furthermore, alterations in the enterohepatic circulation of bile salts lead to fat, vitamin, calcium, magnesium, and trace element deficiencies. Approximately 30% of patients with cancer have protein, calorie, and vitamin deficiencies due either to the underlying disease or to antimetabolite chemotherapy (eg, methotrexate). Patients infected with HIV are frequently malnourished and have protein, trace metal (selenium and zinc), mineral, and vitamin deficiencies.

A complete history of current medications is essential to alert caregivers to potential underlying deficiencies and drug-nutrient interactions. Although rarely the sole cause of malnutrition, certain over-the-counter herbal preparations can alter nutrient absorption. Agents containing ephedra and caffeine may be abused to induce excessive weight loss. Ginkgo and other preparations enhance cytochrome p450 metabolism of various drugs. Information about socioeconomic factors and a detailed dietary history may uncover other risk factors.

A careful physical examination begins with an overall assessment of the patient's appearance. Patients with severe malnutrition may appear frankly emaciated, but more subtle signs of malnutrition include temporal muscle wasting, skin pallor, edema, and generalized loss of body fat. Protein status is evaluated from the bulk and strength of the extremity

Table 10–1. Nutritional Assessment.

History (Factors Predisposing to Malnutrition)
  Absorption disorders (eg, celiac sprue)
  AIDS
  Alcoholism
  Chronic renal insufficiency
  Cirrhosis
  Diabetes mellitus
  Enteric obstruction
  Inflammatory bowel disease
  Malignancy
  Past surgical history, especially involving gastrointestinal tract
  Prolonged starvation
  Psychiatric disorders (eg, anorexia nervosa)
  Recent major surgery, trauma, or burn
  Severe cardiopulmonary disease
Physical Examination
  Skin: Quality, texture, rash, follicles, hyperkeratosis, nail deformities
  Hair: Quality, texture, recent loss
  Eyes: Keratoconjunctivitis, night blindness
  Mouth: Cheilosis, glossitis, mucosal atrophy (eg, temporal wasting), dentition
  Heart: Chamber enlargement, murmurs
  Abdomen: Hepatomegaly, abdominal mass, ostomy, fistulas
  Rectum: Stool color, perineal fistula, Guaiac test
  Neurologic: Peripheral neuropathy, dorsolateral column deficit, mental status
  Extremities: Muscle size and strength, pedal edema
Laboratory Tests
  CBC: Hemoglobin, hematocrit, mean corpuscular volume (MCV), white blood cell count and differential, total lymphocyte count, platelet count
  Electrolytes: Sodium, potassium, chloride, calcium, phosphate, magnesium
  Liver function tests: AST (SGOT), ALT (SGPT), alkaline phosphatase, bilirubin, albumin, prealbumin, retinol-binding protein, prothrombin/INR
  Miscellaneous: BUN, creatinine, triglycerides, cholesterol, free fatty acids, ketones, uric acid, calcium, copper, zinc, magnesium, transferrin

muscles and visible evidence of temporal and thenar muscle wasting. Cardiac flow murmurs may result from anemia. Vitamin deficiencies may be indicated by changes in skin texture, the presence of follicular plugging or a skin rash, corneal vascularization, cracks at the corners of the mouth (cheilosis), hyperemia of the oral mucosa (glossitis), cardiac enlargement, altered sensation in the hands and feet, absence of vibration and position sense (dorsal and lateral column deficits), or abnormal quality and texture of the hair. Trace metal deficiencies produce cutaneous and neurologic abnormalities similar to those associated with vitamin deficiency and may cause changes in the mental status of the patient.

▶ Anthropometric Measurements

Anthropometry is the science of assessing body size, weight, and proportions. Anthropometric measurements gauge body weight and composition with the intent of providing specific information about lean body mass and fat stores. Body composition studies may be used to determine total body water, fat, nitrogen, and potassium. Anthropometric measurements that can be easily performed in the clinic or at the bedside include determination of height and weight, with calculation of body mass index (BMI). Additional measurements such as arm span, body part summation, or knee-height measurement can also be used in nutrition assessment. More advanced techniques allow the clinician to assess the patient's visceral and somatic protein mass and fat reserve. Accurate weight is important, as is current weight expressed as a percentage of ideal body weight. Ideal body weight can be obtained from life insurance actuarial tables.

The BMI is used to measure protein-calorie malnutrition as well as overnutrition (eg, obesity). A BMI between 18.5 and 24.9 is considered normal in most Western civilizations. Overweight is defined as a BMI from 25 to 29.9, and a BMI greater than 30 defines obesity. BMI is calculated as follows:

$$BMI = \frac{Weight\ (kg)}{Height\ (m)^2} = 703 \times \frac{Weight\ (lb)}{Height\ (in)^2}$$

Dual-energy x-ray absorptiometry (DEXA) is increasingly available in hospitals and can be used to assess various body compartments (mineral, fat, lean muscle mass). Most protein resides in skeletal muscle. Somatic (skeletal) protein reserve is estimated by measuring the midhumeral circumference. This measurement is corrected to account for subcutaneous tissue, yielding the midhumeral muscle circumference (MHMC). The result is compared with normal values for the patient's age and gender to determine the extent of protein depletion. Fat reserve is commonly estimated from the thickness of the triceps skin fold (TSF). Reliability of anthropometric measurements is dependent on the skill of the person performing the measurement and is subject to error if performed by different caregivers on the same patient.

▶ Laboratory Data

The visceral protein reserve is estimated from various serum protein levels, total lymphocyte count, and antigen skin testing (Table 10–2). The serum albumin level provides a rough estimate of the patient's nutritional status but is a better prognostic indicator than tool for nutritional assessment. Serum albumin less than 3.5 mg/dL correlates with increased perioperative morbidity and mortality and increased length of hospital stay. Because albumin has a relatively long half-life (20 days), other serum proteins with shorter half-lives have greater utility for assessing response to nutritional repletion. Transferrin has a shorter half-life of 8–10 days and is a more sensitive indicator of adequate nutrition repletion than albumin. Prealbumin has a half-life of 2–

Table 10–2. Staging of Malnutrition.

Clinical & Laboratory Parameters	Extent of Malnutrition		
	Mild	Moderate[1]	Severe[1]
Albumin (g/dL)	2.8–3.5	2.1–2.7	< 2.1
Transferrin (mg/dL)	200–250	100–200	< 100
Prealbumin (mg/dL)	10–17	5–10	< 5
Retinol-binding protein (mg/dL)	4.1–6.1 (normal)	< 4.1	
Total lymphocyte count (cells/μL)	1200–2000	800–1200	< 800
Creatinine-height index (%)	60–80	40–60	< 40
Ideal body weight (%)	80–90	70–80	< 70
Weight loss/time	< 5%/month < 7.5%/3 months < 10%/6 months	< 2%/week > 7.5%/3 months > 10%/6 months	> 2%/week
Skin antigen testing (No. reactive/No. placed)	4/4 (normal)	1–2/4 (weak)	0/4 (anergic)
Anthropometric Measurements	Male	Female	
Triceps skin fold (mm)	≤ 12.5	≤ 16.5	
Midhumeral circumference (cm)	> 29	> 28.5	

[1]Nutritional supplementation is indicated.

3 days, and retinol-binding protein has a half-life of 12 hours. Unfortunately, their serum levels are also influenced by other factors, limiting their utility in assessing nutritional status or repletion.

Immune function may be assessed by hypersensitivity skin testing as well as total lymphocytic count, a reflection of T- and B-cell status. Subcutaneous injection of common antigens provides a semiobjective assessment of the antibody-mediated immune response, commonly impaired in malnourished patients. A low total lymphocyte count (TLC) correlates directly with the degree of malnutrition, though the count may be altered by infection, chemotherapy, and other factors, thus limiting its usefulness.

▶ Nutritional Indices

Indices provide a means of risk-stratification and objective comparison among patients (Table 10–3). Additionally, many nutritional indices have been prospectively validated and can provide prognostic information to further guide nutrition support services. Along with the BMI, these indices can assist surgeons in determining the correct timing for intervention and the progress being made toward the goal of adequate nourishment.

A. Creatinine-Height Index (CHI)

CHI may be used to determine the degree of protein malnutrition, although it is less valid in patients who are severely catabolic or have chronic renal disease. A 24-hour urinary creatinine excretion is measured and compared with normal standards. CHI is calculated by the following equation:

$$CHI = \frac{\text{Actual 24-hour urine creatine excretion}}{\text{Predicted creatine excretion}}$$

The urinary excretion of 3-methylhistidine is a more precise measurement of lean body mass and associated protein stores. The amino acid histidine is irreversibly methylated in muscle. During protein turnover, 3-methylhistidine is not reutilized for synthesis, so the urinary excretion of this compound correlates well with muscle protein breakdown. Unfortunately, measurement of 3-methylhistidine is too expensive for use as a routine clinical test.

B. Prognostic Nutrition Index (PNI)

The PNI has been validated in patients undergoing either major cancer or gastrointestinal surgery and found to accurately identify a subset of patients at increased risk for complications. Furthermore, preoperative nutritional repletion has been shown to reduce postoperative morbidity in this patient group. The PNI has been widely adapted to identify patients at risk in nonsurgical populations, who may benefit from nutritional support.

C. Nutrition Risk Index (NRI)

The NRI was used by the VA TPN Cooperative Study Group for determining preoperative malnutrition, and it has since

Table 10–3. Nutritional Indices.

Body Mass Index (BMI)

BMI = weight (kg)/[height (m)]^2 = 703 × weight (lbs)/[height (in)]^2

Normal	18.5–24.9
Overweight	25–29.9
Obese	30–40
Morbid obesity	> 40

Prognostic Nutritional Index (PNI)

PNI = 158 – [16.6 × Alb^1] – [0.78 × TSF^2] – [0.2 × TFN^3] – [5.8 × DH^4]

Note: for DH, > 5 mm induration = 2;

1–5 mm induration = 1;

anergy = 0

Risk for complications:

Low	< 40%
Intermediate	40–49%
High	> 50%

Nutrition Risk Index (NRI)

NRI = [15.19 × Alb] + 41.7 × [actual weight (kg) / ideal weight (kg)]

Well-nourished	> 100
Mild malnutrition	97.5–100
Moderate malnutrition	83.5–97.5
Severe malnutrition	< 83.5

Malnutrition Universal Screening Tool (MUST)

BMI score: weight loss score (unplanned weight loss):

BMI > 20 (> 30 obese) = 0; weight loss < 5% = 0

BMI 18.5–20 = 1; weight loss 5–10% = 1

BMI < 18.5 = 2; weight loss >10% = 2

Acute disease effect: add 2 if there has been or is likely to be no nutritional intake for > 5 days.

Risk of malnutrition: 0 = low risk; 1 = medium risk; ≥ 2 = high risk

Geriatric Nutrition Risk Index (GNRI)

GNRI = [1.489 × albumin (g/L)] + [41.7 × (weight/WLo)]

The GNRI results from replacement of ideal weight in the NRI formula by usual weight as calculated from the Lorentz formula (WLo). Four grades of nutrition-related risk: major risk (GNRI < 82), moderate risk (GNRI 82–91), low risk (GNRI 92 to ≤ 98), no risk (GNRI > 98).

Instant Nutritional Assessment Parameters (INA)

Parameter: abnormal if

Serum albumin < 3.5 g

Total lymphocyte count < 1500/mm^3

---

^{1}Alb, albumin (g/dL).

^{2}TSF, triceps skin fold (mm).

^{3}TFN, transferrin (mg/dL).

^{4}DH, delayed cutaneous hypersensitivity.

been prospectively cross-validated against other nutritional indices with good results. The index successfully stratifies perioperative morbidity and mortality using serum albumin and weight loss as predictors of malnutrition. Of note, the NRI is not a tool for tracking the adequacy of nutritional support, since supplemental nutrition often fails to improve serum albumin levels.

D. Subjective Global Assessment (SGA)

SGA is the only clinical method that has been validated as reproducible and that encompasses the patient's history and physical examination. It is based on five features of the medical history (weight loss in the past 6 months, dietary intake, gastrointestinal symptoms, functional status or energy level, and metabolic demands) along with four features of the physical examination (loss of subcutaneous fat, muscle wasting, edema, and ascites). Limitations of the SGA include its focus on chronic instead of acute nutritional changes and its enhanced specificity at the expense of sensitivity.

E. Mini-Nutritional Assessment (MNA)

The MNA is a rapid and reliable tool for evaluating the nutritional status of the elderly. It is composed of 18 items and takes approximately 15 minutes to complete. The assessment includes an evaluation of a patient's health, mobility, diet, anthropometrics, and a subject self-assessment. An MNA score of 24 or higher indicates no nutritional risk, while a score of 17–23 indicates a potential risk of malnutrition and a score of less than 17 indicates definitive malnutrition.

F. Malnutrition Universal Screening Tool (MUST)

The MUST detects protein-energy malnutrition and identifies individuals at risk of developing malnutrition using three independent criteria: current weight status, unintentional weight loss, and acute disease effect. The patient's current body weight is determined by calculating the BMI (kg/m^2). Weight loss (over past 3–6 months) is determined by looking at the individual's medical record. An acute disease factor is then included if the patient is currently affected by a pathophysiologic condition and there has been no nutritional intake for more than 5 days. A total score is calculated placing the patients in a low, medium, or high category for risk of malnutrition. A major advantage of this screening tool is its applicability to adults of all ages across all health care settings. Additionally, this method provides the user with management guidelines once an overall risk score has been determined. Studies have shown that MUST is quick and easy to use and has good concurrent validity with most other nutrition assessment tools tested.

G. Geriatric Nutritional Risk Index (GNRI)

The GNRI is adapted from the NRI and specifically designed to predict the risk of morbidity and mortality in hospitalized elderly patients. The GNRI is calculated using a formula incorporating both serum albumin and weight loss. After determining the GNRI score, patients are categorized into four grades of nutrition-related risk: major, moderate, low, and no risk. Finally, the GNRI scores are correlated with a severity score that takes into account nutritional status–related complications. The GNRI is not an index of malnutrition but rather a "nutrition-related" risk index.

H. Instant Nutritional Assessment (INA)

The quickest and simplest measure of nutritional status is the INA. Serum albumin level and the TLC form the basis of this evaluation. Significant correlations between depressed levels of these parameters and morbidity and mortality have been noted. Not surprisingly, abnormalities of these same parameters are even more significant in critically ill patients. Although not designed to replace more extensive assessment measures, this technique allows for quick identification and early intervention in those individuals in greatest danger of developing complications of malnutrition.

Determining Energy Requirements

Adult basal energy expenditure (BEE) is calculated using a modification of the Harris-Benedict equation (Table 10–4). This calculation includes four variables: height (cm), weight (kg), gender, and age (yr). Total energy expenditure (TEE) represents the caloric demands of the body under certain physiologic stresses. TEE is determined by multiplying BEE by a disease-specific stress factor. TEE should be used to guide nutritional supplementation.

Indirect calorimetry is the most accurate method for direct measurement of daily caloric requirements. Using a metabolic cart, oxygen consumption ($\dot{V}O_2$) and carbon dioxide production ($\dot{V}CO_2$) are directly measured from the patient's pulmonary gas flow. Based on these measurements and the amount of nitrogen excreted in the urine, the resting energy expenditure (REE) can be derived using the Weir formula as follows:

REE (kcal/min)

$$= 3.9\ (\dot{V}O_2) + 1.1\ (\dot{V}CO_2) - 2.2\ (\text{urine nitrogen})$$

where $\dot{V}O_2$ and ($\dot{V}CO_2$ are expressed in milliliters per minute and urine nitrogen is in grams per minute. The utility of this technique is limited by the expense and cumbersomeness of the metabolic cart.

The respiratory quotient (RQ) is the ratio of carbon dioxide production to oxygen consumption in the metabolism of fuels by the body. When the RQ is 1, pure carbohydrate is being oxidized. Patients metabolizing lipids only will have an RQ of 0.67. Lipogenesis occurs in patients with excess caloric intake (overfeeding). When excessive calories are ingested or administered, the RQ is greater than 1 and can theoretically approach 9. The excess production of CO_2 may impair ventilator weaning in patients with intrinsic lung disease (eg, chronic obstructive pulmonary disease).

NUTRIENT REQUIREMENTS & SUBSTRATES

The body requires an energy source to remain in steady state. About 50% of the basal metabolic rate (BMR) reflects the work of ion pumping, 30% represents protein turnover, and the remainder represents recycling of amino acids, glucose, lactate, and pyruvate. Total energy expenditure is the sum of energy consumed in basal metabolic processes, physical activity, the specific dynamic action of protein, and extra requirements resulting from injury, sepsis, or burns. Energy

Table 10–4. Total Energy Expenditure Equation for Adults.

Basal energy expenditure (BEE) in kcal/day	
Male: 66.4 + [13.7 × weight (kg)] + [5.0 × height (cm)] – [6.8 × age (yrs)]	
Female: 655 + [9.6 × weight (kg)] + [1.7 × height (cm)] – [4.7 × age (yrs)]	
Stress factors	
Starvation	0.80–1.00
Elective surgery	1.00–1.10
Peritonitis	1.05–1.25
Adult respiratory distress syndrome (ARDS) or sepsis	1.30–1.35
Bone marrow transplant	1.20–1.30
Cardiopulmonary disease (uncomplicated)	0.80–1.00
Cardiopulmonary disease with dialysis or sepsis	1.20–1.30
Cardiopulmonary disease with major surgery	1.30–1.55
Acute renal failure	1.30
Liver failure	1.30–1.55
Liver transplantation	1.20–1.50
Pancreatitis or major burns	1.30–1.80
Total energy expenditure (TEE) in kcal/day	
TEE = BEE × stress factor	

consumed in physical activity constitutes 10–50% of the total in normal subjects but decreases to 10–20% for hospitalized patients. Energy expenditure and requirements vary, depending on the illness or trauma. The increase in energy expenditure above basal needs is about 10% for elective operations, 10–30% for trauma, 50–80% for sepsis, and 100–200% for burns (depending on the extent of the wound). Metabolic energy can be derived from carbohydrates, proteins, or fats.

Carbohydrate Metabolism

Carbohydrates are the body's primary fuel source, accounting for 35% of total caloric intake. Each gram of enteric carbohydrate provides 4.0 kilocalories (kcal) of energy. Parenterally administered carbohydrates (eg, intravenous dextrose) yield 3.4 kcal per gram.

Carbohydrate digestion is initiated by salivary amylase, and absorption occurs within the first 150 cm of the small intestine. Salivary and pancreatic amylases cleave starches into oligosaccharides. Surface oligosaccharidases then hydrolyze and transport these molecules across the gastrointestinal tract mucosa. Deficiencies in carbohydrate digestion and absorption are rare in surgical patients. Pancreatic amylase is abundant, and maldigestion of starch is unusual, even in patients with limited pancreatic exocrine function. Patients with diseases such as celiac sprue, Whipple disease, and hypogammaglobulinemia often have generalized intestinal mucosal flattening leading to oligosaccharidase deficiency and diminished carbohydrate uptake.

More than 75% of ingested carbohydrate is broken down and absorbed as glucose. Hyperglycemia stimulates insulin secretion from pancreatic β cells, which stimulates protein synthesis. Intake of 400 kcal of carbohydrate per day minimizes protein breakdown, particularly after adaptation to starvation. Cellular uptake of glucose, stimulated by insulin, inhibits lipolysis and promotes glycogen formation. Conversely, pancreatic glucagon is released in response to starvation or stress; it promotes proteolysis, glycogenolysis, lipolysis, and increased serum glucose. Glucose is vital for wound repair, but excessive carbohydrate intake or repletion with excessive amounts of glucose can cause hepatic steatosis and neutrophil dysfunction.

▶ Protein Metabolism

Proteins are composed of amino acids, and protein metabolism produces 4.0 kcal per gram. Digestion of proteins yields single amino acids and dipeptides, which are actively absorbed by the gastrointestinal tract. Gastric pepsin initiates digestion. Pancreatic proteases, activated by enterokinase in the duodenum, are the principal effectors of protein degradation. Once digested, half of protein absorption occurs in the duodenum, and complete protein absorption is achieved by the midjejunum.

Protein absorption occurs efficiently throughout the small intestine; therefore, protein malabsorption is relatively infrequent even after extensive intestinal resection. Protein balance reflects the sum of protein synthesis and degradation. Because protein turnover is dynamic, the published requirements for protein, amino acids, and nitrogen are only approximations.

Total body protein in a 70-kg person is approximately 10 kg, predominantly in skeletal muscle. Daily protein turnover is 300 g, or roughly 3% of total body protein. The daily protein requirement in healthy adults is 0.8 g/kg body weight. In the United States, the typical daily intake averages twice this amount. Protein synthesis or breakdown can be determined by measuring the nitrogen balance (Table 10–5). Protein intake of 6.25 g is equivalent to 1 gm of nitrogen. Nitrogen intake is the sum of nitrogen delivered from enteric and parenteral feeding. Nitrogen output is the sum of nitrogen excreted in the urine and feces, plus losses from drainage (eg, exudative wounds, fistula). Urea nitrogen losses are determined from a 24-hour urine collection. Fecal nitrogen loss can be approximated by 1 gm per day, and an additional 2–3 gm per day of nonurea nitrogen loss occurs in the urine (eg, ammonia). The accuracy of nitrogen balance calculations can be improved through measurement over several weeks. When losses of nitrogen are large (eg, diarrhea, protein-losing enteropathy, fistula, or burn exudate), measurements of nitrogen balance lose accuracy because of the difficulty in collecting secretions for nitrogen measurement. Despite these shortcomings, 24-hour urine collection is the best practical means of measuring net protein synthesis and breakdown.

Table 10–5. Nitrogen Balance.

$$\text{Nitrogen}_{(balance)} = \text{Nitrogen}_{(intake)} - \text{Nitrogen}_{(output)}$$
$$\text{Nitrogen}_{(intake)} = \text{g protein}_{(intake)} / 6.25$$
$$\text{Nitrogen}_{(output)} = (\text{UUN} \times \text{Vol}) + 3$$

UUN, urine urea nitrogen; Vol, volume of urine produced over the time of measurement.

The 20 amino acids are divided into essential amino acids (EAAs) and nonessential amino acids (NEAAs) depending on whether they can be synthesized de novo in the body. They are further divided into aromatic (AAAs), branched chain (BCAAs), and sulfur-containing amino acids. Only the L-isotype of an amino acid is utilized in human protein. Certain amino acids have unique metabolic functions, particularly during starvation or stress. Alanine and glutamine preserve carbon during starvation; leucine stimulates protein synthesis and inhibits catabolism; and BCAAs are the preferred fuel source during starvation. Specific amino acids are addressed below.

A. Glutamine

As the respiratory fuel for enterocytes, glutamine plays an important role in the metabolically stressed patient. Following injury and other catabolic events, intracellular glutamine stores may decrease by over 50% and plasma levels by 25%. The decline of glutamine associated with injury or stress exceeds that of any other amino acid and persists during recovery after the concentrations of other amino acid have normalized. Supplementation with glutamine maintains intestinal cell integrity, villous height, and mucosal DNA activity and helps minimize reduction in numbers of T and B cells during stress.

Catabolic states are characterized by accelerated skeletal muscle proteolysis and translocation of amino acids from the periphery to the visceral organs. Glutamine accounts for a major portion of the amino acids released by muscle in these states. Supplementation with glutamine may improve neutrophil and macrophage function in burn patients and other critically ill patients. Specially formulated diets that incorporate glutamine show promise for treating patients with short gut syndrome by accelerating intestinal adaptation.

B. Arginine

Arginine is a substrate for the urea cycle and nitric oxide production and a secretagogue for growth hormone, prolactin, and insulin. Arginine has been identified as the sole precursor of nitric oxide (endothelial-derived relaxing factor). The effects of arginine on T cells may be very important in maintaining the gut barrier. Formulas supplemented with arginine have been shown to improve nitrogen balance and wound healing, stimulate T-cell response, and reduce infectious complications. T-cell proliferation and function are stimulated, and albumin synthesis has also been shown to improve in response to arginine.

Lipid Metabolism

Lipids comprise 25–45% of caloric intake in the typical diet. Each gram of lipid provides 9.0 kcal of energy. The introduction of fat to the duodenum results in secretion of cholecystokinin and secretin, leading to gallbladder contraction and pancreatic enzyme release. Reabsorption of bile salts in the terminal ileum (eg, the enterohepatic circulation) is necessary to maintain the bile salt pool. The liver is able to compensate for moderate intestinal bile salt losses by increased synthesis from cholesterol. Ileal resection may lead to depletion of the bile salt pool and subsequent fat malabsorption. Lipolysis is stimulated by steroids, catecholamines, and glucagon but is inhibited by insulin.

The body can synthesize fats from other dietary substrates, but two of the long-chain fatty acids (linoleic and linolenic) are essential. Insufficient intake of these essential fats leads to fatty acid deficiency and can be prevented by supplying a minimum of 3% of the total caloric intake as essential fatty acids.

The polyunsaturated fatty acids (PUFAs) are grouped into two families: ω-6 and ω-3 fatty acids. Linoleic acid is an example of the ω-6 PUFAs; ω-linolenic acid of the ω-3 PUFAs. Both linoleic and linolenic acid can be processed into arachidonic acid, a precursor in the synthesis of eicosanoids.

Eicosanoids are potent biochemical mediators of cell-to-cell communication and are involved in inflammation, infection, tissue injury, and immune system modulation. They also modulate numerous events involving cell-mediated and humoral immunity and can be synthesized in varying amounts by immune cells, particularly macrophages and monocytes. Diets high in ω-6 fatty acids suppress immune function by inhibiting mitogenesis due to increased prostaglandin E_2 synthesis, which inhibits T-cell proliferation. The administration of additional ω-3 PUFAs has been shown to negate this effect.

Medium-chain fatty acids are not components of most oral diets but are widely used in enteral tube feedings. They are easily digested, absorbed, and oxidized and are not precursors to the inflammatory or immunosuppressive eicosanoids. Short-chain fatty acids, such as butyrate and to a lesser extent propionate, are utilized by colonocytes and provide up to 70% of their energy requirements. Since butyrate is not synthesized endogenously, the colonic mucosa relies on intraluminal bacterial fermentation to obtain this fuel.

Nucleotides, Vitamins, & Trace Elements

In addition to the principal sources of metabolic energy (calories), many other substances are necessary to ensure adequate nutrition. Nucleotides are recognized as an important nutritional substrate in critically ill patients. Vitamins are essential for normal metabolism, wound healing, and immune function, and cannot be synthesized de novo. The normal requirements for vitamins are shown in Table 10–6. Vitamin requirements may increase acutely in illness. Trace elements

Table 10–6. Daily Electrolyte, Trace Element, Vitamin, and Mineral Requirements for Adults.

	Enteral	Parenteral
Electrolytes		
Sodium	90–150 meq	90–150 meq
Potassium	60–90 meq	60–90 meq
Trace elements		
Chromium[1]	5–200 μg	10–15 μg
Copper[1]	2–3 mg	0.3–0.5 mg
Manganese[1]	2.5–5 mg	60–100 μg
Zinc	15 mg	2.5–5 mg
Iron	10 mg	2.5 mg
Iodine	150 μg	...
Fluoride[1]	3 mg	...
Selenium[1]	50–200 μg	20–60 μg
Molybdenum[1]	150–500 μg	20–120 μg
Tin[2]	...	...
Vanadium[2]	...	...
Nickel[2]	...	...
Arsenic[2]	...	...
Silicon[2]	...	...
Vitamins		
Ascorbic acid (C)	60 mg	200 mg
Retinol (A)	1000 μg	3300 IU
Vitamin D	5 μg	200 IU
Thiamin (B_1)	1.4 mg	6 mg
Riboflavin (B_2)	1.7 mg	3.6 mg
Pyridoxine (B_6)	2.2 mg	6 mg
Niacin	19 mg	40 mg
Pantothenic acid	4–7 mg	15 mg
Vitamin E	10 mg	10 IU
Biotin	100–200 μg	60 μg
Folic acid[1]	200 μg	600 μg
Cyanocobalamin (B_{12})	2 μg	5.9 μg
Vitamin K[3]	70–149 mg	150 μg
Minerals		
Calcium	1300 mg	0.2–0.3 meq/kg
Phosphorus	800 mg	300–400 meq/kg
Magnesium	350 mg	0.34–0.45 meq/kg
Sulfur	2–3 g	...

[1]Estimated safe and adequate dose.
[2]No available data regarding human requirements.
[3]Weekly requirement.

are integral cofactors for many enzymatic reactions and are generally not stored by the body in excess of requirements.

A. Nucleotides

Nucleic acids are precursors of DNA and RNA and are not normally considered essential for human growth and development. The need for dietary nucleotides increases in severe stress and critical illness. Nucleotides are formed from purines and pyrimidines, and their abundance is especially important for rapidly dividing cells such as enterocytes and immune cells. Immunosuppression has been reported in renal transplant patients being maintained on nucleotide-free diets. Dietary nucleotides are necessary for helper-inducer T-lymphocyte activity. Diets supplemented with RNA or the pyrimidine uracil have been shown to restore delayed hypersensitivity and augment both the lymphoproliferative response and IL-2 receptor expression. Nucleotides may facilitate recovery from infection. These substrates are incorporated into enteral formulas as potential immunomodulators.

B. Fat-Soluble Vitamins

Vitamins A, D, E, and K are fat soluble and are absorbed in the proximal small bowel in association with bile salt micelles and fatty acids. After absorption, they are delivered to the tissues in chylomicrons and stored in the liver (vitamins A and K) or subcutaneous tissue and skin (vitamins D and E). Although rare, there are reports of toxicity from excessive intake of fat-soluble vitamins (eg, hypervitaminosis A from consuming polar bear liver). Fat-soluble vitamins participate in immune function and wound healing. For example, intake of vitamin A 25,000 IU daily counteracts steroid-induced inhibition of wound healing, largely through increases in TBG-β.

C. Water-Soluble Vitamins

Vitamins B_1, B_2, B_6, and B_{12}, vitamin C, niacin, folate, biotin, and pantothenic acid are absorbed in the duodenum and proximal small bowel, transported in portal vein blood, and utilized in the liver and peripherally. Water-soluble vitamins serve as cofactors to facilitate reactions involved in the generation and transfer of energy and in amino acid and nucleic acid metabolism. Water-soluble vitamins have limited storage in the body. Because of their limited storage, water-soluble vitamin deficiencies are relatively common.

D. Trace Elements

The daily requirements for the trace elements (Table 10–6) vary geographically depending on differences in soil composition. There are currently nine identified essential trace minerals (Fe, Zn, Cu, Se, Mn, I, Mb, Cr, Co). Trace elements have important functions in metabolism, immunology, and wound healing. Subclinical trace element deficiencies occur commonly in hospitalized patients and various disease states.

Iron serves as the core of the heme prosthetic group in hemoglobin and in the mitochondrial cytochrome respiratory process. Impaired cerebral, muscular, and immunologic function can occur in patients with iron deficiency before anemia becomes clinically evident. Particular attention should be paid to assessing iron stores in pregnant and lactating women.

Zinc deficiency is characterized by a perioral pustular rash, darkening of skin creases, neuritis, cutaneous anergy, hair loss, and alterations in taste and smell. Copper deficiency is manifested by microcytic anemia (unresponsive to iron), defective keratinization, or pancytopenia. Chromium deficiency presents as glucose intolerance during prolonged parenteral nutrition administration without evidence of sepsis. Selenium deficiency, which can occur in patients receiving parenteral nutrition for a prolonged period, is manifested by proximal neuromuscular weakness or cardiac failure with electrocardiographic changes. Manganese deficiency is associated with weight loss, altered hair pigmentation, nausea, and low plasma levels of phospholipids and triglycerides. Molybdenum deficiency results in elevated plasma methionine levels and depressed uric acid concentrations, producing a syndrome consisting of nausea, vomiting, tachycardia, and central nervous system disturbances.

Iodine is a key component of thyroid hormone. Deficiency is rare in the United States because of the use of iodinated salt. Chronically malnourished patients can become iodine-deficient. Since thyroxine participates in the neuroendocrine response to trauma and sepsis, iodine should be included in parenteral nutrition solutions.

NUTRITIONAL PATHOPHYSIOLOGY

Physiologic processes, immunocompetence, wound healing, and recovery from critical illness all depend upon adequate nutrient intake. A working knowledge of nutritional pathophysiology is essential in planning nutritional regimens.

▶ Starvation

During an overnight fast, liver glycogen is rapidly depleted after a fall in insulin and parallel rise in plasma glucagon levels (Figure 10–1). Carbohydrate stores are depleted after a 24-hour fast. In the first few days of starvation, caloric needs are met by fat and protein degradation. There is an increase in hepatic gluconeogenesis from amino acids derived from the breakdown of muscle protein. Hepatic glucose production must satisfy the energy demands of the hematopoietic and the central nervous systems, particularly the brain, which is dependent on glucose oxidation during acute starvation. The release of amino acids from muscle is regulated by insulin, which signals hepatic amino acid uptake, polyribosome formation, and protein synthesis. The periodic rise and fall of insulin associated with ingestion of nutrients stimulates muscle protein synthesis and breakdown. During starvation, chronically depressed insulin levels result in a net

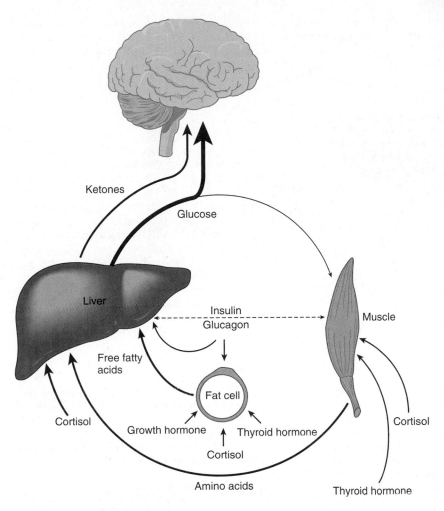

Ketones

Glucose

Liver

Insulin
Glucagon

Muscle

Free fatty
acids

Fat cell

Cortisol

Cortisol

Growth hormone

Thyroid hormone

Cortisol

Amino acids

Thyroid hormone

▲ **Figure 10–1.** The plasma substrate concentrations and hormone levels following an overnight fast. The brain is dependent on glucose, which is supplied predominantly by hepatic glycogenolysis until glycogen supplies are exhausted.

loss of amino acids from muscle. Protein synthesis drops while protein catabolism remains unchanged. Hepatic gluconeogenesis requires energy, which is supplied by the oxidation of unesterified free fatty acid (FFA). The fall in insulin along with a rise in plasma glucagon levels leads to an increase in the concentration of cyclic adenosine monophosphate (cAMP) in adipose tissue, stimulating hormone-sensitive lipase to hydrolyze triglycerides and release FFA. Gluconeogenesis and FFA mobilization require the presence of ambient cortisol and thyroid hormone (a permissive effect).

During starvation, the body attempts to conserve energy substrate by recycling metabolic intermediates. The hematopoietic system utilizes glucose anaerobically, leading to lactate production. Lactate is recycled back to glucose in the liver via the glucogenic (not gluconeogenic) Cori cycle (Figure 10–2). The glycerol released during peripheral triglyceride hydrolysis is converted into glucose via gluconeogenesis. Alanine and glutamine are the preferred substrates for hepatic gluconeo-

genesis from amino acids and contribute 75% of the amino acid–derived carbon for glucose production.

BCAAs are unique because they are secreted rather than taken up by the liver during starvation; they are oxidized by skeletal and cardiac muscle to supply a portion of the energy requirements of these tissues; and they stimulate protein synthesis and inhibit catabolism. The amino groups derived from oxidation of BCAAs or transamination of other amino acids are donated to pyruvate or α-ketoglutarate to form alanine and glutamine. Glutamine is taken up by the small bowel, transaminated to form additional alanine, and released into the portal circulation. Along with glucose, these amino acids participate in the glucose-alanine/glutamine-BCAA cycle, which shuttles amino groups and carbon from muscle to liver for conversion into glucose.

Gluconeogenesis from amino acids results in a urinary nitrogen excretion of 8–12 g per day, predominantly as urea, which is equivalent to a loss of 340 g per day of lean tissue. At

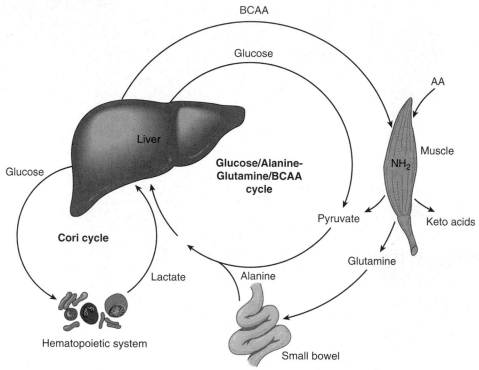

▲ Figure 10–2. The cycles that preserve metabolic intermediates during fasting. Lactate is recycled to glucose via the Cori cycle, while pyruvate is transaminated to alanine in skeletal muscle and converted to glucose by hepatic gluconeogenesis.

this rate, 35% of the lean body mass would be lost in 1 month, a uniformly fatal amount. However, starvation can be survived for 2–3 months as long as water is available. The body adapts to prolonged starvation by decreasing energy expenditures and shifting the substrate preference of the brain to ketones (Figure 10–3). After roughly 10 days of starvation, the brain adapts to use lipid as its primary fuel in the form of ketones. The basal metabolic rate decreases by slowing the heart rate and reducing stroke work, while voluntary activity declines owing to weakness and fatigue. The RQ, which in early starvation is 0.85 (reflecting mixed carbohydrate and fat oxidation), falls to 0.70, indicating near-exclusive fatty acid utilization. Blood ketone levels rise sharply, accompanied by increased cerebral ketone oxidation. Brain glucose utilization drops from 140 g to 60–80 g per day, decreasing the demand for gluconeogenesis. Ketones also inhibit hepatic gluconeogenesis, and urinary nitrogen excretion falls to 2–3 g per day. The main component of urine nitrogen is now ammonia (rather than urea), derived from renal transamination and gluconeogenesis from glutamine, and it buffers the acid urine that results from ketonuria. Acute or chronic starvation is characterized by hormone and fuel alterations orchestrated by changing blood substrate levels and can be conceptualized as a "substrate-driven" process. In summary, the adaptive changes in uncomplicated starvation are a decrease in energy expenditure (as much as a 30% reduction), a change in type of fuel consumed to maximize caloric potential, and preservation of protein.

▶ Elective Operation or Trauma

The metabolic effects of both surgical procedures and trauma (Figure 10–4) differ from those of starvation due to neurohormonal activation, accelerating the loss of lean tissue and inhibiting metabolic adaptation of starvation. Following injury, neural impulses stimulate the hypothalamus. Norepinephrine is released from sympathetic nerve endings, epinephrine from the adrenal medulla, aldosterone from the adrenal cortex, antidiuretic hormone (ADH) from the posterior pituitary; insulin and glucagon from the pancreas; and corticotropin, thyrotropin, and growth hormone from the anterior pituitary. This results in elevation of serum cortisol, thyroid hormone, and somatomedins. The effects of the heightened neuroendocrine secretion include

- peripheral lipolysis from activation of lipase by glucagon, epinephrine, cortisol, and thyroid hormone;

- accelerated catabolism, with a rise in proteolysis stimulated by cortisol;

- decreased peripheral glucose uptake due to insulin antagonism by growth hormone and epinephrine.

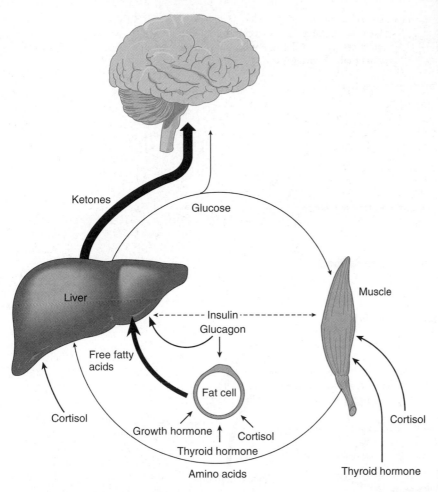

▲ Figure 10–3. The metabolic adaptation to chronic starvation whereby the brain shifts its substrate preference to ketones produced by the liver. Hepatic gluconeogenesis falls and protein breakdown is diminished, thus conserving lean tissue.

These effects result in a rise in plasma FFA, glycerol, glucose, lactate, and amino acids. The liver subsequently increases glucose production, as a result of glucagon-stimulated glycogenolysis and enhanced gluconeogenesis induced by cortisol and glucagon.

Accelerated glucose production, along with inhibited peripheral uptake, produces the glucose intolerance commonly observed in traumatized patients. The kidney retains water and sodium due to increases in ADH and aldosterone. Urinary nitrogen excretion increases up to 15–20 gm per day following severe trauma, equivalent to a daily lean tissue loss of 750 gm. Without exogenous nutrients, the median survival under these circumstances is only 15 days.

In contrast to the substrate dependency of uncomplicated starvation, elective surgical procedures and trauma are "neuroendocrine-driven" processes. In contrast, however, metabolic responses observed following elective procedures are vastly different from those following major trauma. During general anesthesia, the neuroendocrine response is blunted in the operating room through the use of analgesics and immobilization. Sedated patients lack cortical stimulation to the hypothalamus. Careful intraoperative handling of tissues reduces proinflammatory cytokine release. The net result is that the REE rises only 10% in postoperative patients, compared with up to 30% following severe injury or trauma.

▶ Sepsis

The metabolic changes during sepsis differ from those observed after acute injury (Figure 10–5). The REE may increase by 50% to 80%, and urinary nitrogen excretion can reach up to 30 gm per day, predominantly due to profound muscle catabolism and impaired synthesis. Catabolism at this rate results in a median survival of 10 days without nutritional input. The plasma glucose, amino acid, and FFA levels increase more than with trauma. Hepatic protein synthesis is stimulated, with both enhanced secretion of export protein and accumulation of structural protein. The RQ falls to near 0.7, indicative of lipid oxidation. Lipolysis and gluconeogenesis continue despite supplementation with

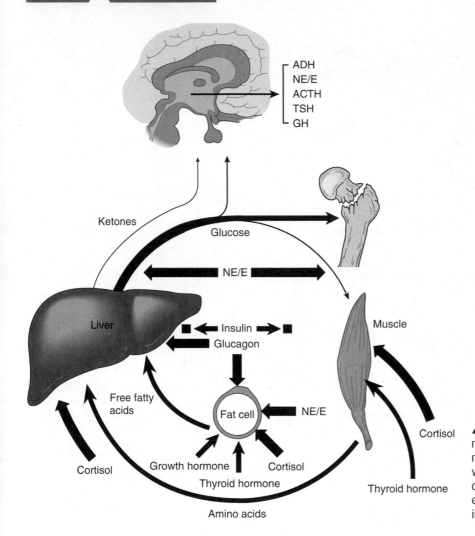

ADH
NE/E
ACTH
TSH
GH

Ketones

Glucose

NE/E

Liver

Insulin

Glucagon

Muscle

Free fatty acids

Fat cell

NE/E

Cortisol

Cortisol

Growth hormone   Cortisol

Thyroid hormone

Thyroid hormone

Amino acids

▲ **Figure 10–4.** The metabolic response to trauma is a result of neuroendocrine stimulation, which accelerates protein breakdown, stimulates gluconeogenesis, and produces glucose intolerance.

carbohydrate or fat, leading to the hyperglycemia and insulin resistance commonly observed in septic patients.

Sepsis results in elaboration of inflammatory cytokines, most notably TNF-α, IL-1, and IL-6. Alteration in hepatic protein synthesis toward production of acute-phase proteins is triggered by IL-6. Septic patients also develop an abnormal plasma amino acid pattern (increased levels of AAAs and decreased levels of BCAAs). In contrast to simple starvation, protein conservation does not occur in sepsis. Terminal sepsis results in further increases in plasma amino acids and a fall in glucose concentration, as hepatic amino acid clearance declines and gluconeogenesis ceases.

Boelens PG et al: Plasma taurine concentrations increase after enteral glutamine supplementation in trauma patients and stressed rats. Am J Clin Nutr 2003;77:250.

Braga M et al: Preoperative oral arginine and n-3 fatty acid supplementation improves the immunometabolic host response and outcome after colorectal resection for cancer. Surgery 2002;132:805.

Gianotti L et al: A prospective, randomized clinical trial on perioperative feeding with an arginine-, omega-3 fatty acid, and RNA-enriched enteral diet: effect on host response and nutritional status. JPEN J Parenter Enteral Nutr 2001;23:314.

Gibbs J et al: Preoperative serum albumin level as a predictor of operative mortality and morbidity. Arch Surg 1999;134:36.

Hambidge M: Biomarkers of trace mineral intake and status. J Nutr 2003;133:948S.

Nagel M: Nutrition screening: identifying patients at risk for malnutrition. Nutr Clin Pract 1998;8:171.

Nathens AB et al: Randomized, prospective trial of antioxidant supplementation in critically ill surgical patients. Ann Surg 2002;236:814.

Sax HC: Effect of immune enhancing formulas (IEF) in general surgery patients. JPEN J Parenter Enteral Nutr 2001;25:519.

Schloerb PR: Immune-enhancing diets: products, components, and their rationales. JPEN J Parenter Enteral Nutr 2001;25:53.

Sungurtekin H et al: Comparison of two nutrition assessment techniques in hospitalized patients. Nutr 2004;20:248.

The Veterans Affairs Total Parenteral Nutrition Cooperative Study Group: Perioperative total parenteral nutrition in surgical patients. N Engl J Med 1991;325:527.

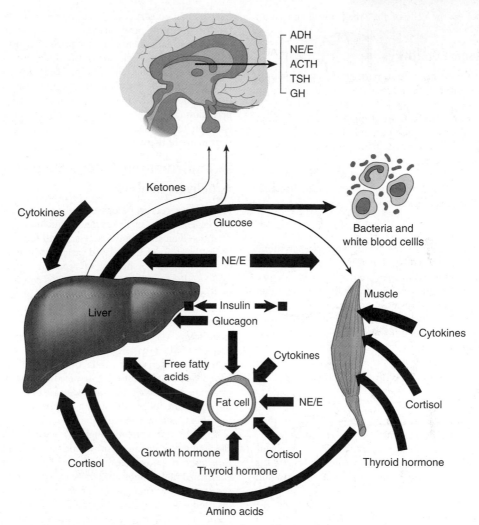

ADH
NE/E
ACTH
TSH
GH

Ketones

Cytokines

Glucose

Bacteria and
white blood cells

NE/E

Liver

Muscle

Insulin

Cytokines

Glucagon

Free fatty
acids

Cytokines

Fat cell

NE/E

Cortisol

Cortisol

Growth hormone

Cortisol

Thyroid hormone

Thyroid hormone

Amino acids

▲ **Figure 10–5.** During sepsis, cytokines (IL-1, IL-2, TNF) released by lymphocytes and macrophages contribute to catabolism of muscle and adipose tissue and amplify the neurohormonal response to antecedent trauma.

ENTERAL NUTRITIONAL THERAPY

▶ Enteral versus Parenteral Nutrition

Enteral nutritional support is safer and less expensive than parenteral nutrition and has the added benefit of preserving gut functionality. Prospective, randomized trials have demonstrated the superiority of enteral nutrition in reducing postoperative complications and length of hospital stay. "Feeding the gut" also results in fewer all-source infectious complications. Parenteral nutrition has a role in the management of surgical patients, but utilizing the gastrointestinal tract should remain the preferred treatment option. Enteral supplementation is not risk-free; physicians must know how to prevent and treat the complications associated with enteral feedings to ensure safe and successful administration.

▶ Benefits of Enteral Feeding

A. Physiologic and Metabolic Benefits

The gastrointestinal tract can be used for administration of complex nutrients, such as intact protein, peptides, and fiber, that cannot be given intravenously. Gut processing of intact nutrients provides a stimulus for hepatic synthetic function of proteins, whereas administration of nutrients directly into the systemic circulation bypasses the portal circulation. In addition to its systemic benefits, enteral feeding has beneficial local effects on gastrointestinal mucosa. These include trophic stimulation and maintenance of absorptive structures by nourishing the enterocytes directly, thus supporting epithelial cell repair and replication. Luminal nutrients such as glutamine and short-chain fatty acids are used as fuel by the cells of the small bowel and colon respectively.

B. Immunologic Benefits

The presence of food in the gut, particularly complex proteins and fats, supports the mucosa's critical function as an immunologic barrier by triggering feeding-dependent neuroendocrine activity. This activity stimulates the production of immunoglobulins in the gut, particularly secretory immunoglobulin A, which is important for preventing bacterial adherence to gut mucosa and bacterial translocation. The presence of nutrients in the gut also helps maintain normal gut pH and flora, thus diminishing opportunistic bacterial overgrowth in the small bowel.

C. Safety Benefits

Enteral feeding is generally considered safer than parenteral feeding. Meta-analysis of prospective trials has demonstrated fewer infectious complications with enteral nutrition compared with parenteral nutrition. Subset analysis suggests that enteral nutrition does not result in a lower risk of infection but rather that parenteral nutrition results in a higher risk. Hyperglycemia, and its resulting inhibition of neutrophil-mediated immunity, also occurs more frequently with parenteral feeding. Enteral nutrition has its own potential complications (discussed shortly).

D. Cost Benefits

The direct costs of enteral feeding are generally less than those with parenteral nutrition. Direct costs include formula, feeding pumps, and tube placement. The cost advantage for enteral feeding is even greater when indirect costs such as central line placement, infection or thrombosis, and home health care are considered.

▶ Indications for Enteral Feeding

Enteral nutrition is the preferred method of nutrition support for malnourished patients or those at risk for developing malnutrition and who have an intact gastrointestinal tract. Patients who are either unable or unwilling to eat to meet their daily needs are candidates for enteral support. Factors influencing the timing of initiation of enteral nutrition include evidence of preexisting malnutrition, expected degree of catabolic activity, duration of the current illness, and anticipated return to intake by mouth. Patients with partially functioning gastrointestinal tracts (eg, short bowel syndrome, proximal enterocutaneous fistula) often can tolerate some enteral feeding but may require a combined regimen of both parenteral and enteral nutrition to meet total caloric needs.

▶ Possible Contraindications to Enteral Feeding

Contraindications to enteral feeding are relative or temporary rather than absolute. Patients with short bowel, gas-trointestinal obstruction, gastrointestinal bleeding, protracted vomiting and diarrhea, fistulas, ileus, or active gastrointestinal ischemia may require a period of bowel rest. In times of physiologic stress, the body shunts blood away from the splanchnic circulation. Feeding a patient who is hemodynamically unstable or requires vasopressors may produce bowel ischemia in the setting of preexisting tenuous perfusion. The choice of an appropriate feeding site, administration technique, formula, and equipment may circumvent many of these contraindications.

▶ Implementing Enteral Supplementation
A. Delivery Methods

Prepyloric access via nasogastric tube is beneficial because it is less expensive, easier to secure and maintain, and less labor-intensive than small bowel access. Contraindications to delivery in the stomach are delayed gastric emptying, gastric outlet obstruction, and a history of repeated aspiration of tube feedings due to reflux. Some physicians consider the inability to protect the airway (eg, in comatose patients) a relative contraindication to gastric feeding. Diabetics and patients with severe head injuries may have profound gastroparesis. Postpyloric access via a duodenal or jejunal nasoenteric tube is preferred when gastric feedings are not tolerated, when patients are at risk for reflux or aspiration, or when early enteral nutrition is desired. A new feeding tube, guided in place by a external magnet, may provide ease of bedside placement of postpyloric tubes. Although a number of bedside methods (eg, auscultation, feeding tube aspirate pH measurements, observation for patient coughing) have been described to check tube placement, these methods can be unreliable. Therefore, tube position below the diaphragm should always be confirmed radiographically before initiating enteral feeding.

Permanent gastrostomy or jejunostomy tubes may be inserted when long-term enteral feeding is indicated. Placement of a feeding tube at the time of the initial operation requires forethought, with consideration given to the patient's expected postoperative course, anticipated ileus, and possible future need for supplementation (eg, during chemoradiation therapy).

B. Formulas

Currently available dietary formulations for enteral feedings may be divided into polymeric commercial formulas, chemically defined formulas, and modular formulas (Table 10–7). Selection of the correct formulation is predicated on patient need, cost, availability and institutional custom.

Nutritionally complete commercial formulas or standard enteral diets vary in protein, carbohydrate, and fat composition. Most formulas use sucrose or glucose as the carbohydrate source and are suitable for lactose-deficient patients. Commercial formulas are convenient, sterile, and affordable. They are recommended for patients experiencing minimal metabolic stress who have normal gut function.

Table 10–7. Enteral Formulas.

Product Name	Cal/mL	Pro g/L	CHO g/L	Fat g/L	Osmolality	mL to meet 100% RDI	Features
Osmolite 1 Cal	1.06	44.3	143.9	34.7	300	1321	Isotonic, low residue
Jevity 1 Cal	1.06	44.3	154.7	34.7	300	1321	14.4 g fiber/L
Jevity 1.5 Cal	1.5	63.8	215.7	49.8	525	1000	22 g fiber/L
Promote	1.0	62.5	130	26	340	1000	High protein
Promote with Fiber	1.0	62.5	138.3	28.2	380	1000	14.4 g fiber /L, high protein
Oxepa	1.5	62.7	105.3	93.8	535	946	Elevated levels of antioxidants
Nepro with Carb Steady	1.8	81	166.8	96	600	948	15.6 g fiber/L; renal-appropriate electrolytes for dialysis
TwoCal HN	2	83.5	218.5	90.5	725	948	Concentrated, low residue
Peptamen AF	1.2	75.6	107	54.8	390	1500	Elemental; high protein; 9.3 g fish oil/L, 5.2 g fiber/L, 50% fat as MCT
Crucial	1.5	94	134	67.6	490	1000	Peptide based; contains arginine, glutamine, DHA, and EPA
Portagen	1	35	115	48	350	Not applicable	87% fat as MCT
Oral Supplements							
Ensure Plus	8 fl oz	Concentrated calories	350	13	50	11	Lactose and gluten free, low residue
Glucerna Shake	8 fl oz	Diabetes	220	9.9	29.3	8.6	Lactose and gluten free
Juven	1 packet (23g)	Wound Care	78	14	7.7	0	Contains arginine and glutamine; lactose and gluten free
Resource Healthshake	4 fl oz	Milk shake	200	6	45	4	Low residue
Resource Breeze	8 fl oz	Clear liquid	250	9	54	0	Fat free, lactose free, low-residue
Modulars							
Pro-Stat 64	2 Tbsp (30 mL)	Protein	60	15	0	0	Liquid protein supplement, sugar free
Resource Benefiber	1 Tbsp	Fiber	16	0	4	0	3 g fiber per serving

All enteral products included are lactose and gluten free.

Chemically defined formulas are commonly called elemental diets. The nutrients are provided in a predigested and readily absorbed form. They contain protein in the form of free amino acids or polypeptides. Amino acid (elemental) and polypeptide diets are efficiently absorbed in the presence of compromised gut function. However, they are more expensive than commercial formulas and are hyperosmolar, which may cause cramping, diarrhea, and fluid losses.

Modular formulations include special formulas used for specific clinical situations such as pulmonary, renal, or hepatic failure or immune dysfunction. The available preparations vary in (1) caloric and protein content; (2) protein, carbohydrate, and fat compositions; (3) nonprotein carbohydrate calorie-to-gram nitrogen ratio; (4) osmolality; (5) content of minor trace metals (selenium, chromium, and molybdenum); and (6) content of various amino acids (glutamine, glutamate, BCAAs).

C. Initiating Feedings

In the past, elaborate protocols for initiating tube feedings were used. It is currently recommended that feedings be started with full-strength formula at a slow rate and steadily advanced. This approach reduces the risk of microbial contamination and achieves full nutrient intake earlier. Formulas are often introduced at full strength at 10–40 mL per hour initially and advanced to the goal rate in increments of 10–20 mL per hour every 4 to 8 hours as tolerated. Conservative initiation and advancement rates are recommended for patients who are critically ill, those who have not been fed for some time, and those who are receiving high-osmolality or calorie-dense formula. In such patients, starting feeding at 10 mL per hour yields the trophic benefit of enteral feeds without unduly stressing the gut. In patients with active lifestyles, gastric feeds can be provided as boluses of up to 400 mL each, delivered at intervals of 4 to 6 hours.

D. Monitoring Feedings

Assessing gastrointestinal tolerance to enteral feeding includes monitoring for abdominal discomfort, nausea and vomiting, abdominal distention, and abnormal bowel sounds or stool patterns. Gastric residual volumes are used to evaluate gastric emptying of enteral feedings. High residuals raise concerns about intolerance to gastric feedings and the potential risk for regurgitation and aspiration. When the gastric residual is greater than 200 mL or is associated with signs or symptoms of intolerance, feedings should be held. If the abdominal examination is unremarkable, feedings should be postponed for at least an hour and the residual volume rechecked. If high residuals persist without associated clinical signs and symptoms, a promotility agent (eg, erythromycin, metoclopramide) may be added to the feeding regimen.

▶ Complications of Enteral Feeding

Technical complications occur in about 5% of enterally fed patients and include clogging of the tube; esophageal, tracheal, bronchial, or duodenal perforation; and tracheobronchial intubation with tube feeding aspiration. Patients with decreased consciousness or impaired gag reflexes or those who have undergone endotracheal intubation are at increased risk for technical complications. The tip of the feeding tube must be positioned and verified radiographically. Other methods to evaluate tube placement are not consistently reliable. Generally, the wire stylet used for positioning should not be reinserted once removed. The incidence of tube clogging can be reduced by periodic water flushes and avoiding administration of syrup-based medications through the tube.

Functional complications occur in up to 25% of tube-fed patients and include nausea, vomiting, abdominal distention, constipation, and diarrhea. Feeding the small bowel instead of the stomach can diminish abdominal symptoms. In the critically injured patient, diarrhea is typically multifactorial; it results from polypharmacy (eg, multiple antibiotics), mechanical gut dysfunction (eg, partial small bowel obstruction), intestinal bacterial overgrowth (eg, *Clostridium difficile*), and protein content or osmolarity of the diet. Treatment consists of stopping any unnecessary medications, correcting gut dysfunction, changing enteral formulation (eg, intact protein versus amino acid or polypeptide

formula), or reducing the osmolarity of the formula. In some circumstances, adding pectin or fiber to the diet or administering antidiarrheal agents can be beneficial.

In the surgical population, *C difficile* is a common cause of diarrhea due to the routine use of perioperative antibiotics. The diagnosis of pseudomembranous colitis is confirmed by *C difficile* toxin assay or sigmoidoscopy. The primary treatment is stopping unnecessary antibiotics. Additionally, either oral metronidazole or vancomycin (oral or retention enema) can be started.

Abnormalities in serum electrolytes, calcium, magnesium, and phosphorus can be minimized through vigilant monitoring. Hyperosmolarity (hypernatremia) may lead to mental lethargy or obtundation. The treatment of hypernatremia includes the administration of free water by giving either D_5W intravenously or additional water flushes. Volume overload and subsequent congestive heart failure may occur as a result of excess sodium administration and is frequently observed in patients with impaired ventricular function or valvular heart disease. Hyperglycemia may occur in any patient but is particularly common in individuals with preexisting diabetes or sepsis. The serum glucose level should be determined frequently and regular insulin administered accordingly.

Alverdy J: Effect of nutrition on gastrointestinal barrier function. Semin Respir Infect 1994;9:248.

Bozetti F et al: Postoperative enteral versus parenteral nutrition in malnourished patients with gastrointestinal cancer: a randomised multicentre trial. Lancet 2001;358:1487.

Braunschweig CL et al: Enteral compared with parenteral nutrition: a meta-analysis. Am J Clin Nutr 2001;74:534.

Cresci GA: The use of probiotics with the treatment of diarrhea. Nutr Clin Pract 2001;16:30.

DeLegge MH: Enteral access—the foundation of feeding. J Parenter Enteral Nutr 2001;25:58.

Heys SD et al: Enteral nutritional supplementation with key nutrients in patients with critical illness and cancer: a meta-analysis of randomized controlled clinical trials. Ann Surg 1999;229:467.

Ibanez J et al: Incidence of gastroesophageal reflux and aspiration in mechanically ventilated patients using small-bore nasogastric tubes. JPEN J Parenter Enteral Nutr 2000;24:103.

McClave SA et al: Use of residual volume as a marker for enteral feeding intolerance: prospective blinded comparison with physical examination and radiographic findings. JPEN J Parenter Enteral Nutr 1992; 16:99.

Metheny NA et al: Bedside methods for detecting aspiration in tube-fed patients. Chest 1997;111:724.

Orlando R: Gastrointestinal motility and tube feeding. Crit Care Med 1998;26:1472.

The Veterans Affairs Total Parenteral Nutrition Cooperative Study Group: perioperative total parenteral nutrition in surgical patients. N Engl J Med 1991;325:527.

Williams MS et al: Diarrhea management in enterally fed patients. Nutr Clin Pract 1998; 13:225.

PARENTERAL NUTRITION THERAPY

The development of parenteral nutritional support in the late 1960s revolutionized care of the surgical patient, particularly those with permanent inability to obtain adequate enteral nourishment. Despite its utility in select patients and circumstances, overuse of parenteral nutrition not only is costly but also poses unnecessary risk to patients. In general, parenteral nutrition should be employed only when the gastrointestinal tract cannot be utilized. Parenteral formulas usually deliver 75–150 nonprotein carbohydrate kcal per gram of nitrogen infused, a ratio that maximizes carbohydrate and protein assimilation and minimizes metabolic complications (aminoaciduria, hyperglycemia, and hepatic glycogenesis). Nonenteral nutrition can be given as peripheral parenteral nutrition (PPN) or total parenteral nutrition via a central line (TPN). In addition to route of administration, the two differ in (1) dextrose and amino acid content of the parenteral solution, (2) primary caloric source (glucose versus fat), (3) frequency of fat administration, (4) infusion schedule, and (5) potential complications.

1. Peripheral Parenteral Nutrition (PPN)

Because PPN avoids the complications associated with central venous access, it is safer to administer than TPN. PPN is indicated for patients with compromised gut function who require supplemental nutrition for less than 14 days. It can be infused via an 18-gauge peripheral IV catheter or via a peripherally inserted central catheter (PICC line). Standard PPN therapy orders should include the administration schedule for the PPN solution and fat supplement, as well as explicit catheter care orders and monitoring guidelines.

▶ PPN Formulation

The osmolarity of the PPN solution is limited to 1000 mOsm to avoid phlebitis. Consequently, unacceptably large volumes of solution, greater than 2.5 L per day, are needed to fulfill the typical patient's total nutritional requirements (Figure 10–6).

2. Total Parenteral Nutrition (TPN)

TPN via a central line is indicated for patients who cannot obtain adequate nourishment via the gastrointestinal tract or, very rarely, as a supplement to oral intake in patients with severe preoperative malnutrition. A minimum duration of treatment of 7–10 days of adequate TPN is needed for preoperative nutritional repletion. Likewise, the use of postoperative TPN for only 2 or 3 days (eg, while awaiting return of bowel function) is discouraged, as the risks outweigh the benefits incurred over this short a period of time.

TPN Formulation

TPN is typically formulated for patients on the basis of their individual nutritional assessment. Most frequently, TPN is prepared in the pharmacy and provided as a 3-in-1 admixture of protein, carbohydrates, and fat. Alternatively, the lipid emulsion can be administered as a separate intravenous pig-

1. TPN components:

Routine additives	Recommended dosage ranges per liter TPN	BAG #___	BAG #___	BAG #___
D$_{50}$W	500 mL	500 mL	500 mL	500 mL
AA 8.5%	500 mL	500 mL	500 mL	500 mL
NaCl	0–140 meq	meq	meq	meq
NaPO$_4$	0–20 mmol	mmol	mmol	mmol
K*Cl	0–40 meq	meq	meq	meq
MgSO$_4$	0–12 meq	meq	meq	meq
Ca gluconate	4.5 or 9 meq	meq	meq	meq
MVI-12®	10 mL/d	10 mL		
Multitrace®	5 mL/d	5mL		
Optional additives				
Na acetate	0–140 meq	meq	meq	meq
K* acetate	0–40 meq	meq	meq	meq
Regular insulin	0–40 units	units	units	units
H$_2$ antagonist**				
25% albumin***	25 g	g	g	g
Nurse's signature				

* Total potassium content per liter of TPN should not exceeed 40 meq.
** Divide the daily dosage equally into each liter of TPN.
*** Only if the serum albumin < 2.5g/dl and enteral diet therapy is anticipated.

Rate:___40___ mL/h via pump.
Final dextrose concentration _25_ %   Final AA concentration _4.25_ %

2. Pharmacy to add vitamin K 10 mg to 1 L of TPN solution every Mon. and Thurs.
3. Fat emulsion 20% 500 mL every Mon., Wed., and Fri. IVPB per pump over 6–8 hours via at least an 18-gauge peripheral IV or via the subclavian catheter.
4. STAT upright and expirational portable chest x-ray to check the position of the subclavian catheter and to rule out a pneumothorax. Notify the physician when the chest x-ray is completed.
5. Heparin lock the TPN catheter with 2 mL of heparin (100 units/mL) until notified by the physician to start the first liter of TPN solution.
6. Strict I/O every shift. Total the I/O every 24 hours.
7. Record the daily weight in kilograms on the vital signs sheet.
8. Check the urine for sugar and acetone every shift and record on the vital signs sheet. If the urine sugar is 4+, request a STAT serum glucose measurement to be drawn by the physician. If the serum glucose is > 160 mg/dL, contact the physician for treatment orders.
9. Notify the physician if the oral temperature is >38C (>100.4F).
10. Routine TPN laboratory tests are to be drawn weekly on the days and times specified below:
   Sun. AM: CBC, SMAC-20
   Tues. AM: Electrolytes, BUN, creatinine, and glucose
   Thurs. AM: CBC, SMAC-20, copper, zinc, magnesium, transferrin, and triglycerides
11. Begin a 24-hour urine collection for urinary urea nitrogen (UUN) at 6:00 AM every Mon. and Thurs. for nitrogen balance determination.
12. TPN catheter dressing and tubing changes per the hospital TPN protocol.
13. Contact the physician for all problems related to TPN.
14. All changes in TPN therapy must be approved by the physician.

▲ **Figure 10–6.** TPN therapy orders.

gyback infusion. Other additives, vitamins, and trace minerals are added to TPN formulations as required (Table 10–8).

▶ Administration

The high osmolarity of TPN solutions necessitates administration via a central vein. The use of multilumen central venous catheters (CVCs) for TPN does not increase the risk of catheter infection; however, a port should be designated for

Table 10–8. TPN Solution Formulation.

Components in 1 L of Standard TPN:	
Routine additives	
$D_{50}W^1$	500 mL
8.5% amino acid[1]	500 mL
Sodium chloride[2]	0–140 meq
Sodium phosphate[3]	0–20 mmol
Potassium chloride[4]	0–40 meq
Magnesium sulfate[5]	0–12 meq
Calcium gluconate[5,6]	4.5–9.0 meq
Trace element-5[7]	1 mL
M.V.I.-13[7]	10 mL
Optional additives	
Sodium acetate[2]	0–140 meq
Potassium acetate[4]	0–40 meq
H_2 antagonist[8]	variable
Regular insulin[9]	0–40 units
Vitamin K[10]	10 mg
Heparin[11]	variable
Fat emulsion schedule:	
Infuse 20–25% fat emulsion intravenously via pump at least 3 times per week	

[1]The solution is formulated to deliver 125 nonprotein kcal per gram of nitrogen infused.
[2]Add sodium chloride if the serum CO_2 > 25 meq/L. Add sodium acetate if the serum CO_2 ≤ 25 meq/L.
[3]The total phosphate dosage should not exceed 20 mmol/L or 60 mmol daily.
[4]Add potassium chloride if the serum CO_2 > 25 meq/L. Add potassium acetate if the serum CO_2 ≤ 25 meq/L. The potassium dosage should not exceed 40 meq/L.
[5]Added to each liter.
[6]Add calcium gluconate 9 meq to each liter if the serum calcium < 8.5 meq/L. Add 4.5 meq if the serum calcium ≥ 8.5 meq/L.
[7]Administered in only 1 L per day.
[8]Dosage depends upon the H_2 antagonist selected. Divide the daily dosage equally in all liters of TPN administered.
[9]Total dosage should not exceed 40 units/L.
[10]Administered only once per week.
[11]Heparin administration in TPN is not required, but it may be added in place of subcutaneous dosing.

exclusive use for TPN infusion to minimize handling of the line. CVC placement in the subclavian vein is ideal and well tolerated by the patient. Furthermore, the rate of catheter infection is lower for catheters placed in the subclavian compared to catheters placed in either the femoral or internal jugular vein. Femoral vein catheterization has a complication rate over 25% and therefore should be avoided if possible. The CVC should be dressed with a sterile, dry gauze and transparent (nonocclusive) dressing, without antibiotic ointment.

If refeeding syndrome is suspected, the introduction of TPN should be gradual, with approximately 1000 kcal provided over the first 24 hours. This amount is increased by 500 kcal per day until the patient's goal is reached. For all patients, additional maintenance IV fluids should be tapered or discontinued accordingly to maintain an even fluid balance.

Standard TPN therapy orders (Figure 10–6) should include the administration schedule for the TPN solution and fat supplement as well as explicit catheter care orders and monitoring guidelines (Figure 10–7). For active patients on long-term TPN, cycling the intravenous nutrition therapy over 8–16 hours at night allows freedom from the infusion pump during the remainder of the day.

Special TPN Solutions

The TPN solution may be concentrated for patients who require fluid restriction (eg, those with pulmonary and cardiac failure). One liter of concentrated TPN solution usually contains a combination of $D_{60}W$ or $D_{70}W$, 500 mL, and 10% or 15% amino acids, 500 mL, plus additives.

Patients in renal failure who cannot be dialyzed and who require fluid restriction should receive low-nitrogen TPN solution. Patients in renal failure who can undergo dialysis may receive the standard or high-nitrogen TPN formulations, with special attention directed toward minimizing potassium and phosphate intake.

COMPLICATIONS OF PARENTERAL NUTRITION

PPN Therapy

Technical complications of PPN are few. The most common problem is maintaining adequate venous access due to frequent incidence of phlebitis. The PPN infusion catheter must be moved frequently to other sites; therefore, prolonged PPN is rarely possible. The addition of fat, heparin, or corticosteroids to PPN solutions has not decreased the incidence of phlebitis. Infectious complications such as catheter site skin infections and septic phlebitis develop in 5% of patients.

TPN Therapy

Technical, infectious, and metabolic complications each occur in approximately 5% of patients, and the overall mortality rate directly attributable to TPN is 0.2% (Table 10–9). Many of the complications originate from the central venous catheter, with more than 15% of patients developing some line-related complication. Other morbidity is attributable to line infection (typically bacterial) or metabolic abnormalities.

A. Technical Complications

The risks of patient injury while placing a CVC are directly related to surgeon experience with the procedure. Arterial puncture (more common in internal jugular or femoral attempts) can occur in up to 15% of patients, while pneumo-

NUTRITION GUIDELINES FOR THE ADULT PATIENT

ADULT PARENTERAL NUTRITION (PN) GUIDELINES

Table 1: INDICATIONS FOR PARENTERAL NUTRITION:
A. Patient has failed enteral nutrition (EN) trial with appropriate tube placement (post-pyloric).
B. Enteral nutrition is contraindicated. Examples include patients with a paralytic ileus, mesenteric ischemia, small bowel obstruction, or GI fistula, except when enterat access can be placed distal to the fistula or the volume of fistula output (< 230 mL/day) justifies a trial of EN.
C. Wound healing would be impaired if PN is not started within 5-10 days postoperatively unable to eat or tolerate EN.

Table 2: BODY WEIGHT CALCULATIONS
Actual body weight (ABW) = pt weight (kg) IF GREATER THAN 125% OF IDEAL. WEIGHT SEE**
Ideal body weight (IBW)   male = 50 kg + (2.3 × # inches > 5 ft)   OR   48 kg + (2 7 × # inches > 5 ft)
                          female = 45 kg + (2.3 × # inches > 5 ft)
                          **Dosing weight (DW) = IBW + 0.25 (ABW − IBW)

Table 3:
A. DAILY CALORIC NEEDS

		CONVERSIONS FOR KCAL TO GRAMS
Maintenance-mild stress:	20-25 kcal/kg/day (15-20 NPC*kg/day)	3.4 kcal = 1 gm dextrose
Mild-moderate stress (routine surgery, minor infection):	26-30 kcal/kg/day (21-25 NPC*/kg/day)	10 kcal = 1 gm lipid
Moderate-severe stress (major surgery, sepsis).	31-35 kcal/kg/day (26-30 NPC*/kg/day)	
	*NPC = nonprotein calories	

B. *HARRIS-BENEDICT (HB) ESTIMATE OF BASAL CALORIES   STRESS FACTOR

Male:	66 + 13.8 (weight in kg) + 5 (height in cm**) − 6.8 (age in year	Maintenance-mild stress :	1-1.2
Female:	655 + 9.6 (weight in kg) + 1.8 (height in cm**) − 4.7 (age in years)	Moderate stress :	1.3 -1.4
		Severe stress:	1.5

*HB × stress factor = total coloric need/day ** height in cm = inches × 2.54

Table 4: DAILY PROTEIN NEEDS   CONVERSIONS FOR KCAL TO GRAMS OF PRO-TEIN

Maintenance-Mild	0.8-1.2 gm/kg/day	4 kcal = 1 gm amino acid
Moderate stress	1.3-1.5 gm/kg/day	
Severe stress	1.6-2 gm/kg/day	
Very high stress	> 2 gm/kg/day	

SUGGESTED LABORATORY TESTS

Baseline: Finger stick blood glucose q 4 hours with correction insulin as written: basic metabolic panel (BMP), magnesium, phosphorus, trigleycerides, hepatic function panel, & prealbumin.
Daily: BMP, magnesium & phosphorus until stabilized, then as clinically indicated.
Weekly: Prealbumin. Triglycerides and hepatic function panel (if clinically indicated).

CALCULATION OF VOLUME OF MAXIMALLY CONCENTRATED PN

1. Amino acid (AA): _____ gm protein/day × 10mL/gm AA =_____ mL 10% AA solution
2. Carbohydrate (CHO): _____ gm/day × 1.43mL/gm = _____ mL 70% dextrose solution
3. Lipid: _____gm/day × 10 kcal/gm = _____ + 2kcal/ml = _____ mL 20% lipids
4. Maximally concentrated volume = _____ mL 10% AA + _____ mL 70% dextrose + _____ mL 20%
        (from 1 above)   (from 2 above)   (from 3 above)
    lipids + 150 mL for additives = _____ mL/day
5. Approximate infusion rate = _____ mL/day + 24 hr/day = _____ mL/hr

▲ **Figure 10–7.** TPN guidelines. (*continued*)

**CONTENT OF STANDARD
MULTIPLE VITAMINS (per 10 mL):**

Vitamin A	3300 international units
Vitamin D	200 international units
Vitamin E	10 international units
Vitamin B_1 (thiamine)	6 mg
Vitamin B_2	3.6 mg
Vitamin B_3	40 mg
Vitamin B_5	15 mg
Vitamin B_6 (pyridoxine HCl)	6 mg
Vitamin B_{12}	5 micrograms
Vitamin C (ascorbic acid)	200 mg
Biotin	60 micrograms
Folic acid	600 micrograms
Vitamin K	150 micrograms

**CONTENT OF STANDARD
TRACE ELEMENTS (per 1 mL):**

Chromium	10 micrograms
Copper	1 mg
Manganese	0.5 mg
Selenium	60 micrograms
Zinc	5 mg

▲ **Figure 10–7.** (*Continued*)

thorax (predominantly during subclavian insertion) can develop in up to 3%. The risk for injury increases dramatically after three failed insertion attempts at the same site.

Air embolism occurs when negative intrathoracic pressure draws air into a catheter or needle into a central vein. This is particularly serious in the presence of pulmonary-systemic shunts (eg, patients with a patent foramen ovale). It is characterized by sudden, severe respiratory distress, hypotension, and a cogwheel cardiac murmur. To reduce this risk, the patient should be placed in the Trendelenburg position (head down) during line insertion. When suspicion of air embolism is high, treatment involves placing the patient in the Durant position (Trendelenburg and left lateral decubitus) to direct the embolus to the apex of the right ventricle. Catheter-based aspiration can then be attempted.

B. Infectious Complications

Infection of the catheter exit site is frequently characterized by mild fever (37.5–38 °C), purulent discharge around the catheter, and erythema/tenderness of the surrounding skin. Late changes include induration of the skin and systemic sepsis. Local wound care and sterile dressing changes every 3 days can reduce site infection rates.

Primary line (catheter) infection may occur in one of every four patients with CVCs. Line infection should be strongly considered in any patient with a CVC who develops fever, new-onset glucose intolerance, leukocytosis, or positive blood cultures. The number of infusion ports does not affect the rate of catheter-related complications; however, the use of antibiotic-impregnated catheters has been shown to reduce colonization rates fourfold. As noted previously, insertion in the subclavian vein reduces the risk of infection. The most common offending organisms are skin flora (*S aureus, S epidermidis*), although gram-negative rods can also colonize an indwelling catheter. Table 10–10 depicts one treatment algorithm for treating suspected CVC infections. Patients with a suspected line infection who have negative blood cultures and no cardiovascular compromise should have the catheter exchanged over a guidewire, and the tip should be sent for bacterial and fungal cultures. If the fever resolves and subsequent cultures are negative, no further therapy is necessary. If the patient remains febrile after catheter exchange or continues to have positive cultures, a new central catheter should be inserted at another site. Antibiotics should be started empirically in patients with sepsis.

C. Metabolic Complications

The refeeding syndrome was first described in prisoners freed from concentration camps after World War II. Similar pathophysiology may develop when initiating TPN in patients with severe malnutrition and weight loss (greater than 30% of their usual weight). In starvation, energy is derived principally from fat metabolism. TPN results in a shift from fat to glucose as the predominant fuel, and rapid anabolism increases the production of phosphorylated intermediates of glycolysis. These intermediates trap phosphate, producing profound hypophosphatemia. Hypokalemia and hypomagnesemia also occur. The lack of phosphate and potassium lead to a relative adenosine triphosphate (ATP) deficiency, resulting in the insidious onset of respiratory failure and reduced cardiac stroke volume. Because of these risks, the rate of TPN administration in a severely malnourished patient should be slowly increased over several days. Twice-daily monitoring of electrolytes is also indicated, with repletion as appropriate.

Hepatic dysfunction is a common manifestation of long-term parenteral nutrition support. The exact etiology is unclear; however, in part it is related to the initial bypassing of the portal circulation when providing intravenous nutrition. Severe hepatic steatosis may progress to cirrhosis. Acalculous

Table 10–9. Complications of Nutritional Therapy.

Enteral Nutrition	Parenteral Nutrition
Technical	*Technical*
Abscess of nasal septum	Air embolus
Acute sinusitis	Arterial laceration
Aspiration pneumonitis	Arteriovenous fistula
Esophagitis (ulceration/ stenosis)	Brachial plexus injury
Gastrointestinal perforation	Cardiac perforation
Hemorrhage (local erosion)	Catheter embolism
Hoarseness	Catheter malposition
Intestinal obstruction	Hemothorax
Intracranial passage	Pneumothorax
Knotting/clogging of tube	Subclavian vein thrombosis
Nasal/alar erosions	Thoracic duct injury
Otitis media	Thromboembolism
Pneumatosis intestinalis	Venous laceration
Skin excoriation	
Tracheoesophageal fistula	
Tube dislodgement	
Variceal rupture	
Functional	*Infectious*
Abdominal distention	Catheter-based bacteremia
Constipation	Catheter colonization
Diarrhea	Exit-site infection/cellulites
Nausea/vomiting	
Metabolic	*Metabolic*
Dehydration	Azotemia
Hypercalcemia	Essential fatty acid deficiency
Hyperglycemia	Fluid overload
Hyperkalemia	Hyperchloremic metabolic acidosis
Hypermagnesemia	Hypercalcemia
Hypernatremia	Hyperglycemia
Hyperphosphatemia	Hyperkalemia
Hypocalcemia	Hypermagnesemia
Hypokalemia	Hypernatremia
Hypomagnesemia	Hyperphosphatemia
Hyponatremia	Hypocalcemia
Hypophosphatemia	Hypokalemia
Hypozincemia	Hypomagnesemia
Overhydration	Hyponatremia
Vitamin deficiency	Hypophosphatemia
	Intrinsic liver disease
	Metabolic bone disease
	Trace element deficiency
	Ventilatory failure
	Vitamin deficiency

cholecystitis can also occur in these patients, likely from biliary stasis and lack of gallbladder contraction. Patients on TPN need weekly liver function tests and lipid panels.

Abrupt discontinuation of TPN can produce rebound hypoglycemia in patients with limited oral intake. Infusion of $D_{10}NS$ may be initiated prior to stopping the TPN. The TPN infusion rate does not need to be tapered if the patient can consume 75% or more of daily caloric requirements, or if receiving less than 1000 kcal per day parenterally.

▶ Home Nutrition Support

Patients requiring home nutrition support (HNS) present clinical challenges different from those in an acute care setting. Route of enteral or parenteral administration must be based on length of therapy, frequency of use, and caregiver/patient ability. Regular physical examinations and frequent lab monitoring (Figure 10–8) should continue as long as patients remain on HNS therapy. Home care services must be established prior to discharge and are vital to the success of these patients.

For patients requiring home parenteral nutrition, weekly lab monitoring continues until electrolytes stabilize. Once stable, laboratory values can often be checked on a monthly basis, and changes can be made to the TPN formula as needed. Electrolyte and hepatic enzymes must be followed to monitor for metabolic derangements and end-organ damage. Parenteral nutrition–associated liver disease is the most devastating complication of long-term parenteral nutrition therapy. Early clinical intervention with a combination of nutritional, medical, hormonal, and surgical therapies is potentially effective in preventing liver disease progression. However, as progression is frequently subtle, it is often not recognized until liver injury is irreversible. Although parenteral nutrition–associated liver failure is hypothesized to be multifactorial in origin, the etiology is poorly understood. When end-stage liver disease (ESLD) develops in these patients, multiorgan transplantation (liver and small bowel) is generally required.

Alverdy JC, Aoys E, Moss GS: Total parenteral nutrition promotes bacterial translocation from the gut. Surgery 1988;104:185.

Buchman A, Iyer K, Fryer J: Parenteral nutrition associated liver disease and the role for isolated intestine and intestine/liver transplantation. Hepatology 2005;43:9.

Dudrick SJ et al: Long-term total parenteral nutrition with growth, development, and positive nitrogen balance. Surgery 1968;64:397.

Fleming CR: Trace element metabolism in adult patients requiring total parenteral nutrition. Am J Clin Nutr 1989;49:573.

Granato D et al: Effects of parenteral lipid emulsions with different fatty acid composition on immune cell functions in vitro. JPEN J Parenter Enteral Nutr 2000;24:113.

McGee DC, Gould MK: Preventing complications of central venous catheterization. N Engl J Med 2003;348:1123.

Seidner DL et al: Parenteral nutrition-associated metabolic bone disease: pathophysiology, evaluation and treatment. Nutr Clin Pract 2000;15:163.

Van Acker BA et al: Response of glutamine metabolism to glutamine-supplemented parenteral nutrition. Am J Clin Nutr 2000;72:79.

Table 10–10 Complications of TPN.

Complication	Treatment
Catheter sepsis	**Algorithms:**
Incidence:	*Negative blood cultures and no cardiovascular signs of sepsis:*
Single-lumen catheter: 3–5%	(1) Aspirate a blood specimen via the TPN catheter and peripherally for bacterial and fungal culture and then sterilely exchange the preexisting TPN catheter for a new catheter over a guidewire; submit the previous catheter tip for bacterial and fungal culture and colony count; and continue the TPN infusion.
Triple-lumen catheter: 10%	
Diagnosis:	*then*
• Unexplained hyperglycemia (> 160 mg/dL)	(2) Monitor the patient's temperature closely. If the patient defervesces, no further therapy is necessary. If the fever continues or recurs, remove the catheter and insert a new one on the contralateral side and continue the TPN infusion.
• "Plateau" temperature elevation (> 38 °C) for several hours or days. (***Note:*** *An isolated spike or "picket fence" temperature pattern is usually not indicative of an infected catheter.*)	
	Positive blood culture or cardiovascular signs of sepsis:
• Leukocytosis (> 10,000/μL)	(1) Aspirate a blood specimen via the TPN catheter and peripherally for bacterial and fungal culture. Then remove the catheter immediately, and submit the catheter tip for bacterial and fungal culture and colony count.
• Exclusion of other potential sources of infection,	
or	*then*
• A positive blood culture (> 15 colony count) aspirated via the TPN catheter or obtained peripherally,	(2) Insert a new TPN infusion catheter on the contralateral side and continue the TPN infusion.
or	*then*
• Catheter site induration, erythema, or purulent drainage.	(3) Initiate appropriate antibiotic therapy.
Hyperglycemia (> 160 mg/dL)	**Algorithms:**
	(1) Maintain the current TPN infusion rate. If the patient is critically ill, initiate intravenous regular insulin infusion. Otherwise initiate a sliding scale with regular insulin and add regular insulin in 10-unit increments to the TPN solution until the serum glucose is maintained at ≤ 140 mg/dL. (***Note:*** *The maximum allowable insulin dosage per liter of TPN is 40 units.*)
	then
	(2) If blood glucose levels remain elevated, consider decreasing the dextrose concentration (eg: decrease the grams of carbohydrate) to 60–80% of the estimated needs until blood glucose levels are within goal range. In addition, either maintain regular insulin infusion or continue to adjust the amount of insulin in the TPN bag based on the amount taken via sliding scale. One half to two-thirds of the previous day's regular insulin requirements can be added to the TPN bag.
	then
	(3) Once goal blood glucose achieved, restart the original TPN solution as in (1) above with adequate insulin to maintain goal blood glucose range.
Hypoglycemia (< 65 mg/dL)	May occur with the sudden discontinuance of TPN infusion. If the TPN infusion administered to either an NPO patient or a patient consuming inadequate oral calories is suddenly discontinued, immediately begin an infusion of D_{10} NS at the previous TPN infusion rate via either the TPN catheter or a peripheral IV to prevent rebound hypoglycemia.
Hypernatremia (> 145 meq/L)	Determine the cause. Hypernatremia secondary to dehydration is treated by administering additional "free water" and providing only the daily maintenance sodium requirements (90–150 meq/L) via the TPN infusion. Hypernatremia secondary to increased sodium intake is treated by reducing or deleting sodium from the TPN solution until the serum sodium ≤ 145 meq/L.
Hyponatremia (< 135 meq/L)	Determine the cause. Hyponatremia secondary to dilution is treated by fluid restriction and by providing only the daily maintenance sodium requirements (90–150 meq/L). Hyponatremia secondary to inadequate sodium intake is treated by increasing the sodium content of the TPN solution until the serum sodium is ≥ 135 meq/L. (***Note:*** *The maximum sodium content per liter of TPN should not exceed 154 meq.*)

(continued)

Table 10–10 Complications of TPN. *(Continued)*

Complication	Treatment
Hyperkalemia (> 5 meq/L)	Immediately discontinue the current TPN infusion containing potassium and begin an infusion of $D_{10}NS$ at the previous TPN infusion rate. Then reorder a new TPN solution without potassium and continue to delete potassium from the TPN solution until the serum potassium $\leq$ 5 meq/L.
Hypokalemia (< 3.5 meq/L)	A TPN solution should not be utilized for the primary treatment of hypokalemia. The potassium content per liter of TPN solution should not exceed 40 meq. If additional potassium is necessary, it should be administered via another route, eg, IV interrupts.
Hyperphosphatemia (> 4.5 mg/dL)	Immediately discontinue the present phosphate-containing TPN infusion and begin an infusion of $D_{10}NS$ at the previous infusion rate. Then reorder a new TPN solution without phosphate and continue to delete phosphate from the TPN solution until the serum phosphate is $\leq$ 4.5 mg/dL.
Hypophosphatemia (< 2.5 mg/dL)	Increase the phosphate content of the TPN solution to a maximum of 20 mmol/L. (**Note:** *The total daily phosphate dosage should not exceed 60 mmol.*) If severe hypophosphatemia exists, carbohydrate infusion or delivery should be restricted.
Hypermagnesemia (> 3 mg/dL)	Immediately discontinue the present magnesium-containing TPN infusion and begin an infusion of $D_{10}NS$ at the previous infusion rate.
Hypomagnesemia (< 1.6 mg/dL)	Increase the magnesium content of the TPN solution to a maximum of 12 meq/L. (**Note:** *The total daily dosage of magnesium should not exceed 36 meq.*)
Hypercalcemia (> 10.5 mg/dL)	Immediately discontinue the present calcium-containing TPN infusion and begin an infusion of $D_{10}NS$ at the previous TPN infusion rate. Then reorder a new TPN solution without calcium and continue to delete calcium from the TPN dilution until the serum calcium is $\leq$ 10.5 mg/dL.
Hypocalcemia (< 8.5 mg/dL)	Increase the calcium content of the TPN solution to a maximum of 9 meq/L. (**Note:** *The total daily calcium dosage should not exceed 27 meq.*)
High serum zinc (> 150 µg/L)	Discontinue the trace metal supplement (Multitrace 5 mL) in the TPN solution until the serum zinc is $\leq$ 150 µg/L.
Low serum zinc (< 55 µg/dL)	Add elemental zinc 2–5 mg daily to 1 L of TPN solution only until the serum zinc is $\geq$ 55 µg/dL. (**Note:** *The elemental zinc is added in addition to the daily supplement.*)
High serum copper (> 140 µg/dL)	Discontinue the trace metal supplement in the TPN solution until the serum copper is $\leq$ 140 µg/dL.
Low serum copper (< 70 µg/dL)	Add elemental copper 2–5 mg daily to 1 L of TPN solution only until the serum copper is $\geq$ 70 µg/dL. (**Note:** *The elemental copper is added in addition to the daily Multitrace 5 mL.*)
Hyperchloremic metabolic acidosis (CO_2 < 22 mmol/L and Cl^- > 110 meq/L)	Reduce the chloride intake by administering the Na^+ and K^+ in the acetate form as either sodium or potassium acetate (or both) until the acidosis resolves (serum $CO_2 \geq$ 22 mmol/L) and the serum chloride level returns to normal (< 110 meq/L).

Van den Berghe G et al: Intensive insulin therapy in critically ill patients. N Engl J Med 2001;345:1359.

The Veterans Affairs Total Parenteral Nutrition Cooperative Study Group: Perioperative total parenteral nutrition in surgical patients. N Engl J Med 1991;325:527.

DIETS

▶ Optimal Diet

The optimal diet should have the following distribution of energy sources: carbohydrate 55–60%, fat 30%, and protein 10–15%. Refined sugar should constitute less than 15% of dietary energy and saturated fats no more than 10%, the latter balanced by 10% monounsaturated and 10% polyunsaturated fats. Cholesterol intake should be limited to about 300 mg per day (one egg yolk contains 250 mg of cholesterol). The amount of salt in the average American diet, 10–18 g daily, far exceeds the recommended 3 g/day. For Western societies to meet the criteria for an optimal diet, consumption of fat must decrease (from 40%) and consumption of complex carbohydrate should increase. Meat is presently overemphasized as a protein source, at the expense of grain, legumes, and nuts. Diets that include substantial fish intake have been associated with a decrease in mortality from cardiovascular disease and are attributed to high concentrations of ω-3 fatty acids, principally eicosapentaenoic and docosahexaenoic acids.

Many adults, particularly those who do not drink milk, consume inadequate amounts of calcium. In women this may result in calcium deficiency and skeletal calcium depletion,

Routine monitoring:

☐ Basic metabolic panel, Magnesium, and Phosphorus dailly Start date:_____ End date:_____

☐ Basic metabolic panel, Magnesium, Phosphorus and weight
    ☐ Weekly   ☐ Bimonthly ☐ Monthly ☐ Quarterly   Start date: _____

☐ Triglyceride
    ☐ Weekly   ☐ Monthly   ☐ Quarterly   Start date: _____

☐ Prealbumin
    ☐ Weekly   ☐ Monthly   ☐ Quarterly   Start date: _____

☐ CBS, AST, ALT, and total Bilirubin
    ☐ Weekly   ☐ Monthly   ☐ Quarterly   Start date: _____

☐ PT/INR, PTT if on Warfarin (Coumadin ®) or multi-vitamin contains Vitamin K
    ☐ Weekly   ☐ Monthly   ☐ Quarterly   Start date: _____

▲ **Figure 10–8.** Lab monitoring form for home nutrition support.

predisposing women to osteoporosis and axial bony fractures. "Fiber" is the generic term for a chemically complex group of indigestible carbohydrate polymers, including cellulose, hemicellulose, lignins, pectins, gums, and mucilages. The amount of fiber in Western diets averages 25 g per day, but some people ingest as little as 10 g daily. Those who consume low-fiber diets are more likely to develop chronic constipation, appendicitis, diverticular disease, and possibly diabetes mellitus and colonic neoplasms. Bran cereals and bread, fruit, potatoes, rice, and leafy vegetables are rich sources of fiber.

Regular Diets

Many concepts regarding diets are archaic and based on currently unaccepted views of illness. For example, the utility of a low-residue diet in diverticular disease is questionable. The "progressive diet," designed for postoperative feeding and consisting of a clear liquid (high in sodium), then a full liquid (high in sucrose), then a regular diet, is based on outmoded concepts. When peristalsis returns after operation, as evidenced by bowel sounds and ability to tolerate water, most patients are able to ingest a regular diet. Regular diets have an unrestricted spectrum of foods and are most attractive to the patient. An average regular hospital diet for 1 day contains 95–110 g of protein, with a total caloric content of 1800–2100 kcal. This composition reflects the nutritional needs of healthy persons of average height and weight and will not meet the increased demands imposed by malnutrition or disease.

Lactose Intolerance & Lactose-Free Diets

A lactose-free diet is indicated for patients who have symptoms such as diarrhea, bloating, or flatulence after the ingestion of milk or milk products. Lactose intolerance is genetically determined and occurs in 5–10% of European Caucasians, 60% of Ashkenazi Jews, and 70% of African Americans. Subclinical lactose intolerance may become unmasked following surgery on gastrointestinal tract (eg, gastrectomy). Similarly, avoid-ance of lactose-containing products is often beneficial advice for patients with Crohn disease, ulcerative colitis, and AIDS. The efficiency of lactose digestion and absorption can be measured by giving 100 g of oral lactose, then measuring the blood glucose concentration at 30-minute intervals over 2 hours. Patients with lactose intolerance exhibit a rise in blood glucose of 20 mg/dL or less. A lactose-free diet may be deficient in calcium, vitamin D, and riboflavin.

Postgastric Bypass Diet

The popularity of gastric bypass surgery for weight loss continues to increase. The diet changes that must occur to ensure safe and appropriate weight loss are quite specific after surgery. Immediately after surgery, only small amounts of liquids (eg, 30mL q3h) should be consumed. After tolerance of liquids is established, pureed foods should be consumed for the 4 weeks after surgery. Food should be consumed as very small meals and snacks throughout the day. Choosing a variety of foods, avoiding concentrated sweets, and consuming adequate protein are essential to the success of these patients. Protein supplements are often required to ensure adequate protein consumption postoperatively.

DISEASE-SPECIFIC NUTRITION SUPPORT

Burns

Thermal injury has a tremendous impact on metabolism because of prolonged, intense neuroendocrine stimulation. Extensive burns can double or triple the REE and urinary nitrogen losses, producing a loss of 1500 g per day of lean tissue and a median survival of 7–10 days without nutritional support. The increase in metabolic demands following thermal injury is proportional to the extent of ungrafted body surface. The principal mediators of burn hypermetabolism are catecholamines, which return to baseline only when skin coverage is complete. Decreasing the intensity of neuroendocrine stimulation by providing adequate analgesia and a thermoneutral environment lowers the accelerated metabolic rate and helps to decrease catabolic protein loss until the burned surface can be grafted. Burned patients are prone to infection, and the cytokines activated by sepsis further augment catabolism.

Because infection often complicates the clinical course of patients with burn injury, and infectious complications are more likely with parenteral nutrition, the enteral route of feeding is preferred whenever tolerated. Enteral feeding may be started within the first 6–12 hours postburn to reduce the hypermetabolic response and improve postburn survival. Gastric ileus can be avoided through the use of a nasojejunal tube.

Patients with burns have increased caloric requirements. In addition to estimated maintenance needs (females, 22 kcal/kg/day; males, 25 kcal/kg/day), these patients require an additional 40 kcal per percentage point of burned total body surface area (TBSA). A 70-kg man with 40% TBSA burns would require 48 kcal/kg/day. Protein requirements are also markedly increased from the normal 0.8 g/kg/day to approximately 2.5 g/kg/day in severely burned patients. Of course, these are initial estimates, and periodic reassessment of nutritional status (eg, prealbumin levels, nitrogen balance) is required in these patients. During the hypermetabolic phase of burn injury (0–14 days), the ability to metabolize fat is restricted, so a diet that derives calories primarily from carbohydrate is preferable. Following the hypermetabolic phase, the metabolism of fat becomes normal. The burn patient should also be given supplemental arginine, nucleotides, and ω-3 polyunsaturated fat to stimulate and maintain immunocompetence.

▶ Diabetes

Glucose intolerance often complicates nutritional supplementation, particularly with parenteral administration. Complications associated with TPN administration occur more frequently during prolonged hyperglycemia. Unopposed glycosuria may lead to osmotic diuresis, loss of electrolytes in the urine, and possibly nonketotic coma. Additionally, it is now evident that strict maintenance of serum glucose levels below 110 mg/dL improves mortality and decreases infectious morbidity in critically ill surgical patients. Factors that may aggravate hyperglycemia include the use of corticosteroids, certain vasopressors (eg, epinephrine), preexisting diabetes mellitus, and occult infection.

Maintaining normoglycemia in injured or postoperative patients may be challenging. Serial serum glucose levels should be monitored regularly. If hyperglycemia does not occur, these measurements can be obtained less frequently once the nutritional goal is reached. Patients may require subcutaneous insulin administered on a sliding scale or continuous intravenous insulin infusions to control their hyperglycemia. For patients who do not require an insulin infusion, the previous day's insulin total from a sliding scale may be determined and half to two-thirds of that amount added to the next TPN order to provide a more uniform administration.

▶ Cancer

Cancer is the second leading cause of death in the United States, and over two-thirds of patients with cancer will develop nutritional depletion and weight loss at some time during the course of the illness. Malnutrition and its sequelae are the direct cause of death in 20–40% of these patients. Weight loss is an ominous presenting sign in many malignancies. Furthermore, antineoplastic treatments, such as chemotherapy, radiation therapy, or operative extirpation, can worsen preexisting malnutrition. Cancer cachexia manifests as progressive involuntary weight loss, fatigue, anemia, wasting, and tissue depletion. It may occur at any stage of the disease. Nutrition support has become an essential adjunct in caring for the cancer patient.

Many studies have evaluated the effectiveness of nutrition support in patients with cancer, with varying results. Klein reported a meta-analysis of 28 prospective, randomized controlled trials evaluating TPN in patients with cancer. Only 1 of 10 surgical trials showed a significant decrease in mortality in the patients receiving TPN, and no other significant benefit was seen in survival, tolerance to treatment, toxicity, or tumor response in patients receiving chemotherapy or radiation therapy. Increasing efforts have been directed toward the use of enteral nutrition because it is simpler, presumably safer, and less costly. Seven prospective, randomized controlled trials of enteral nutrition in patients with cancer who were undergoing surgery showed little if any difference in mortality or morbidity in patients who received enteral feedings. In summary, nutritional supplementation in cancer patients *may* reduce infectious complications or perioperative morbidity, but convincing evidence of improvement in overall survival is lacking.

Patients with cancer may have altered energy expenditure and abnormalities of protein and carbohydrate metabolism. REE increases by 20–30% in certain malignant tumors. The increases in REE can occur even in patients with extreme cachexia in whom a similar degree of uncomplicated starvation would produce profound decreases in REE. Whether the increase in REE correlates with the extent of disease or tumor burden is unknown. Changes in carbohydrate metabolism consist of impaired glucose tolerance, elevated glucose turnover rates, and enhanced Cori cycle activity. Owing to the high rate of anaerobic glucose metabolism in neoplastic tissue, patients with extensive tumors are susceptible to lactic acidosis when given large glucose loads during TPN. These patients also exhibit increased lipolysis, elevated FFA and glycerol turnover, and hyperlipidemia.

Patients with cancer avidly retain nitrogen despite losses in most lean tissue. Animal carcass analysis has shown that the retained nitrogen resides in the tumor, which behaves as a nitrogen trap. Synthesis, catabolism, and turnover of body protein are all increased, but the change in catabolism is greatest.

The utility of enteral supplementation with immune-enhancing agents is unclear. These substances include arginine, glutamine, essential fatty acids, RNA, and BCAAs.

Several studies have attempted to examine outcomes in patients with cancer who are fed with enteral formulas supplemented with immune-enhancing agents, compared to routine enteral feeding alone. The findings were summarized by Heys and coworkers. Meta-analysis of six studies with a total of 487 cancer patients demonstrated a decrease in overall infectious morbidity and hospital stay, but no change in survival, for patients receiving such "targeted therapy." Exactly which elements confer these benefits remains unknown.

Renal Failure

Whether nutritional support improves the outcome from acute renal failure is difficult to determine because of the metabolic complexities of the disease. Patients with acute renal failure may have normal or increased metabolic rates. Renal failure precipitated by x-ray contrast agents, antibiotics, aortic or cardiac surgery, or periods of hypotension is associated with a normal or slightly elevated REE and a moderately negative nitrogen balance (4–8 g per day). When renal failure follows severe trauma, rhabdomyolysis, or sepsis, the REE may be markedly increased and the nitrogen balance sharply negative (15–25 g per day). When dialysis is frequent, losses into the dialysate of amino acids, vitamins, glucose, trace metals, and lipotrophic factors can be substantial.

Patients in renal failure (serum creatinine over 2 mg/dL) with a normal metabolic rate who cannot undergo dialysis should receive a concentrated (minimal volume) enteral or parenteral diet containing protein, fat, dextrose, and limited amounts of sodium, potassium, magnesium, and phosphate.

Hepatic Failure

Most patients with hepatic failure present with acute decompensation superimposed on chronic hepatic insufficiency. Typically, a history of poor dietary intake contributes to the chronic depletion of protein, vitamins, and trace elements. Water-soluble vitamins, including folate, ascorbic acid, niacin, thiamin, and riboflavin, are especially likely to be deficient. Fat-soluble vitamin deficiency may be a result of malabsorption due to bile acid insufficiency (vitamins A, D, K, and E), deficient storage (vitamin A), inefficient utilization (vitamin K), or failure of conversion to active metabolites (vitamin D). Hepatic iron stores may be depleted either from poor intake or as a result of gastrointestinal blood loss. Total body zinc is decreased owing to the above factors plus increased urinary excretion.

The use of BCAA-enriched amino acid formulations for TPN in patients with liver disease is controversial because the results of controlled trials are inconclusive. Therefore, patients with hepatic failure should receive a concentrated enteral or parenteral diet with reduced carbohydrate content, a combination of EFAs and other lipids, a standard mixture of amino acids, and limited amounts of sodium and potassium.

Cardiopulmonary Disease

Malnutrition is associated with myocardial dysfunction, particularly in the late stages, and fatal cardiac failure can develop in extreme cachexia. Cardiac muscle uses FAAs and BCAAs as preferred metabolic fuels instead of glucose. During starvation, the heart rate slows, cardiac size decreases, and the stroke volume and cardiac output decrease. As starvation progresses, cardiac failure ensues, along with chamber enlargement and anasarca.

The profound nutritional depletion that may accompany chronic heart failure, particularly in valvular disease, results from anorexia of chronic disease, passive congestion of the liver, malabsorption due to venous engorgement of the small bowel mucosa, and enhanced peripheral proteolysis due to chronic neuroendocrine secretion. Attempts at aggressive nutritional repletion in patients with cardiac cachexia have produced inconclusive results. Concentrated dextrose and amino acid preparations should be used to avoid fluid overload. Nitrogen balance should be measured to ensure adequate nitrogen intake. Lipid emulsions must be administered cautiously because they can produce myocardial ischemia and negative inotropy. Feeding these patients with either enteral or parenteral nutrition should be undertaken cautiously to avoid refeeding syndrome and hypophosphatemia.

Patients with severe chronic obstructive pulmonary disease may have difficulty weaning from the ventilator if they are overfed. This relates to the RQ, a measure of oxygen consumption and carbon dioxide production by the body in metabolism. An RQ of 1 reflects pure carbohydrate utilization, while an RQ greater than 1 occurs during lipogenesis (energy storage). Although normal lungs can tolerate increased CO_2 production (RQ greater than 1) without adversely affecting respiration, patients with chronic obstructive pulmonary disease may experience CO_2 retention and inability to wean. The treatment is to increase the percentage of calories delivered as lipid and to avoid overfeeding at all costs.

Disease of the Gastrointestinal Tract

Benign gastrointestinal disease (eg, inflammatory bowel disease, fistula, pancreatitis) often leads to nutritional problems due to intestinal obstruction, malabsorption, or anorexia. Chronic involvement of the ileum in inflammatory bowel disease produces malabsorption of fat- and water-soluble vitamins, calcium and magnesium, anions (phosphate), and the trace elements iron, zinc, chromium, and selenium. Protein-losing enteropathy, accentuated by transmural destruction of lymphatics, can add to protein depletion. Treatment with sulfasalazine can produce folate deficiency, and glucocorticoid administration may accelerate breakdown of lean tissue and enhance glucose intolerance owing to stimulation of gluconeogenesis. Patients with inflammatory bowel disease who require elective surgery should be evaluated for malnutrition preoperatively.

Patients with gastrointestinal fistulas can develop electrolyte, protein, fat, vitamin, and trace metal deficiencies; dehydration; and acid-base imbalance. Aggressive fluid replacement is often needed. Patients with fistulas often require nutritional support. The choice of feeding route or formula will depend on the level and length of dysfunctional bowel. Patients with proximal enterocutaneous fistulas (from the stomach to the midileum) should receive TPN with no oral intake. Patients with low fistulas should receive TPN initially, but after infection is brought under control, they can often be switched to an enteral formula or even a low-residue diet.

Pancreatitis

The diagnosis of pancreatitis often mandates strict bowel rest for extended periods of time. Ranson criteria can serve as a rough estimate of the need for nutritional support (see Chapter 26). Patients with acute pancreatitis who present with three or fewer Ranson criteria should be treated with fluid replacement, nasogastric suction, and bowel rest for at least a week before considering parenteral nutrition. Most of these patients can resume an oral diet and do not benefit from TPN. Those with more than three Ranson criteria should receive TPN. Previously, enteral diets, including elemental and polypeptide formulas, were not recommended due to concerns these diets may stimulate the pancreas and aggravate the disease. However, recent data document the successful use of enteral diets, particularly elemental products via jejunal access, in many patients with pancreatitis.

Short Bowel Syndrome

Inadequate intestinal absorptive surface leads to malabsorption, excessive water loss, electrolyte derangements, and malnutrition. The absorptive capacity of the small intestine is highly redundant, and resection of up to half its functional length is reasonably well tolerated. Short bowel syndrome typically occurs when less than 200 cm of anatomic small bowel remain, although the presence of the ileocecal valve may reduce this length to 150 cm. However, short bowel syndrome also may occur from functional abnormalities of the small bowel resulting from severe inflammation or motility disorder. The optimal nutritional therapy for a patient with short bowel syndrome must be tailored individually and depends upon the underlying disease process and the remaining anatomy. Following resection, the remaining bowel undergoes long-term adaptation, with observed increases in villous height, luminal diameter, and mucosal thickness. The estimated minimum length of small bowel required for adult patients to become independent of TPN is 120 cm.

Adaptation to short gut occurs over time, and initial management should be directed at avoiding electrolyte imbalance and dehydration while providing daily caloric requirements through TPN. Some patients may eventually supplement TPN with oral intake. In these patients, dietary management includes consuming frequent small meals, avoiding hyperosmolar foods, restricting fat intake, and limiting consumption of foods high in oxalate (precipitates nephrolithiasis). Uniquely formulated diets containing glutamine and human growth hormone have shown promise for accelerating intestinal adaptation.

AIDS

Patients with AIDS frequently develop protein-calorie malnutrition and weight loss. Many factors contribute to deficiencies of electrolytes (sodium and potassium), trace metals (copper, zinc, and selenium), and vitamins (A, C, E, pyridoxine, and folate). Enteropathy may impair fluid and nutrient absorption and produce a voluminous, life-threatening diarrhea. Standard antidiarrheal agents do not control the diarrhea in AIDS patients, but the synthetic somatostatin analogue octreotide may help. Dehydration occurs as a consequence of refractory diarrhea.

Malnourished AIDS patients require a daily intake of 35–40 kcal and 2.0–2.5 g protein. Those with normal gut function should be given a high-protein, high-calorie, low-fat, lactose-free oral diet. Patients with compromised gut function require an enteral (amino acid or polypeptide) or parenteral nutrition.

Solid Organ Transplant Recipients

Patients who have undergone organ transplantation present unique issues in relation to nutritional management due to both the preexisting disease state and the medications taken to prevent graft rejection. During the acute posttransplant phase, adequate nutrition is required to help prevent infection, promote wound healing, support metabolic demands, replenish lost stores, and mediate the immune response. Organ transplantation complications, including rejection, infection, wound healing, renal insufficiency, hyperglycemia, and surgical complications, require specific nutritional requirements and therapies.

Obesity is associated with both decreased patient survival and decreased graft survival, in part due to a greater incidence of surgical, metabolic, and cardiovascular complications. Patients with BMI greater than 30 kg/m^2 show a higher incidence of steroid-induced posttransplant diabetes mellitus. The first 6 weeks following transplantation is characterized by increased nutritional demands due to a combination of surgical metabolic stress and high doses of immunosuppressive medications. Daily protein intake recommendation in the immediate posttransplant phase, as well as during acute rejection episodes, is 1.5 gm/kg actual body weight.

Long-term immunosuppression is associated with protein hypercatabolism, obesity, dyslipidemia, glucose intolerance, hypertension, hyperkalemia, and alteration of vitamin D metabolism. Approximately 60% of renal recipients develop dyslipidemia posttransplant. Alterations in lipid metabolism may be associated with corticosteroids, cyclosporine, thiazide diuretics, or beta-blockers, as well as with renal insufficiency, nephrotic syndrome, insulin resistance, or obesity. There is evidence that abnormal lipoprotein levels lead to glomerulosclerosis, renal disease progression, and even potential graft failure.

Dietary salt restriction is recommended in transplant patients, as salt intake may play a role in cyclosporine-induced hypertension caused by sodium retention. Sodium intake is recommended not to exceed 3 gm/day. Cyclosporine is associated with hypomagnesemia and hyperkalemia, especially during the immediate posttransplant phase when the dosage is high. Additionally, antihypertensive treatment with beta-blocker agents or with angiotensin-converting enzyme (ACE) inhibitors may exacerbate hyperkalemia. Calcium, phosphorus, and vitamin D metabolism are influenced by prolonged therapy with steroids leading to osteopenia and osteonecrosis. The daily recommendation for dietary calcium is 800–1500 mg, and the recommended intake of phosphorus is 1200–1500 mg/d. Some patients may also require supplementation of active vitamin D. Patients on a low-protein diet often need multivitamin supplements. During the first year, the major nutritional goal is to treat preexisting malnutrition and prevent excessive weight gain.

▶ Major Trauma

In severely injured patients, metabolic changes must be acknowledged early and monitored during the posttraumatic phase. Severe trauma induces alteration of metabolic pathways and activation of the immune system. Depending on the severity of the initial injury, catabolic changes in posttraumatic metabolism can last from several days to weeks. The posttraumatic metabolic changes include hypermetabolism with increased energy expenditure, enhanced protein catabolism, insulin resistance associated with hyperglycemia, failure to tolerate glucose load, and high plasma insulin levels ("traumatic diabetes"). As a general rule, the metabolic demands of the patient can increase by 1.3–1.5 times the normal requirements.

Metabolic changes after trauma are characterized as occurring in two different phases. The first phase is initiated within minutes and persists for several hours after the initial insult. It is characterized by a decline in body temperature and oxygen consumption, aimed at reducing posttraumatic energy depletion. The second phase, which occurs after compensation of the state of traumatic-hemorrhagic shock, is associated with an increased metabolic turnover, activation of the immune system, and induction of the hepatic acute-phase response. This results in increased consumption of energy and oxygen. In addition to the acute hypermetabolic state, the systemic inflammatory cascade is initiated, with the release of proinflammatory cytokines and activation of the complement system. Bacterial translocation from the gut may further aggravate these metabolic sequelae and inflammatory response.

Many severely injured patients require inotropic support, and vasoactive drugs promote catabolism by reducing serum levels of anabolic hormones. In contrast, endogenous catecholamines, cortisol, and glucagon levels are elevated after trauma, leading to increased energy substrate mobilization. Proteinolysis of skeletal muscle and glycolysis are increased to provide the substrates for hepatic gluconeogenesis and biosynthesis of acute-phase proteins. The equilibrium is shifted toward supporting the immune response and wound healing at the cost of enhanced proteinolysis of skeletal muscle. In addition, stimulation of the neuroendocrine axis through stress, pain, inflammation and shock increases the caloric turnover significantly above baseline. This leads to increased serum levels of catabolic hormones, such as cortisol, glucagon and catecholamines, and decreased levels of insulin.

Appropriate immunonutrition should be started in the ICU, preferably by enteral route, in order to counteract the effects of the hypermetabolic state after major trauma. Without absolute contraindications, guidelines clearly favor the concept of early enteral nutrition within 24–48 hours after admission in the ICU. It is important not to overfeed critically injured patients with calories, since this may contribute to adverse outcomes. Early overfeeding of severely injured patients leads to an increase in oxygen consumption, carbon dioxide production, lipogenesis, and hyperglycemia and contributes to secondary immune suppression.

Obese patients are particularly susceptible to the adverse effects of overfeeding. Current feeding recommendations for morbidly obese ICU patients are 20 kcal and 2.0 gm of protein per kg ideal body weight per day. However, a hypocaloric (< 20 kcal/kg/day), high-protein nutrition for critically injured obese patients has been shown to be as effective as hypercaloric feeding (> 20 kcal/kg/day) in the obese patient group.

Barrera R: Nutritional support in cancer patients. JPEN J Parenter Enteral Nutr 2002;26:S63.

Beale RJ, Bryg DJ, Bihari DJ: Immunonutrition in the critically ill: a systematic review of clinical outcome. Crit Care Med 1999; 27:2799.

Bozzetti F et al: Perioperative total parenteral nutrition in malnourished gastrointestinal cancer patients: a randomized, clinical trial. JPEN J Parenter Enteral Nutr 2000;24:7.

Byrne TA et al: Beyond the prescription: optimizing the diet of patients with short bowel syndrome. Nutr Clin Pract 2000;15:306.

Clark RH et al: Nutritional treatment for acquired immunodeficiency virus-associated wasting using beta-hydroxy beta-methylbutyrate, glutamine, and arginine: a randomized, double-blind, placebo-controlled study. JPEN J Parenter Enteral Nutr 2000;24:133.

Curreri PW et al: Dietary requirements of patients with major burns. Nutr Clin Pract 2001;16:169.

Fischer JE: Branched-chain-enriched amino acid solutions in patients with liver failure. JPEN J Parenter Enteral Nutr 1990;14(suppl):226.

Heyland DK et al: Should immunonutrition become routine in critically ill patients? A systematic review of the evidence. JAMA 2001;286:944.

Heys SD et al: Enteral nutritional supplementation with key nutrients in patients with critical illness and cancer: a meta-analysis of randomized controlled clinical trials. Ann Surg 1999;229:467.

Klein S et al: Nutrition support in patients with cancer: what do the data really show? Nutr Clin Pract 1994;9:91.

MacFie J et al: Oral dietary supplements in pre- and postoperative surgical patients: a prospective and randomized clinical trial. Nutr 2000;16:723.

Moore FA: Effects of immune-enhancing diets on infectious morbidity and multiple organ failure. JPEN J Parenter Enteral Nutr 2001;25:536.

Anesthesia

Theodore J. Sanford Jr., MD

Anesthesiology is a "team sport." Providing the best and safest care for patients depends on all members of the team—surgeons, nurses, and anesthesia providers—communicating in a timely, efficient, and patient-focused manner. Anesthesiologists today not only provide patient care in the operating room but also have patient responsibilities in other areas, including preoperative anesthesia clinics (PACs), postanesthesia care units (PACUs), obstetrics, ambulatory surgery centers, endoscopy suites, postoperative pain management, critical care units, and chronic pain management.

Anesthesia is a term derived from the Greek meaning "without sensation" and is commonly used to indicate the condition that allows patients to undergo a variety of surgical or nonsurgical procedures without the pain or distress they would otherwise experience. More importantly, this blocking of pain and/or awareness is reversible. Anesthesiology is the medical practice of providing anesthesia to patients and is most commonly provided by a medical doctor, an anesthesiologist, either alone or in conjunction with a certified registered nurse anesthetist (CRNA), anesthesia assistant, or resident physician-in-training. Anesthesia is most often described as being a general anesthetic, ie, a drug-induced loss of consciousness during which patients are not arousable even by noxious stimulus and often require a controlled airway. Anesthesia can also be provided without inducing unconsciousness by utilizing regional blockade, local anesthesia with monitored anesthesia care (MAC), or conscious sedation.

HISTORY OF ANESTHESIA

One of modern medicine's most important discoveries was that the application of diethyl ether (ether) could provide the classic requirements of anesthesia: analgesia, amnesia, and muscle relaxation in a reversible and safe manner. Crawford Long was the first to use ether in 1842, and William Morton's successful 1846 public demonstration of ether as an anesthetic in the "Ether Dome" of Massachusetts General Hospital ushered in the modern day of anesthesia and surgery. Chloroform was used by Sir James Y. Simpson to provide analgesia to Queen Victoria in 1853 during the birth of Prince Leopold. This royal approval of inhalation agents led to the wide acceptance of their use as surgical anesthesia. Ether (flammability, solubility) and chloroform (liver toxicity) each had significant drawbacks, and over time, inhalation agents were developed with similar anesthetic effects but much safer physiologic and metabolic properties.

Cocaine's ability to produce topical anesthesia for ophthalmic surgery was discovered in the late 1800s. The hypodermic needle was introduced in 1890 and facilitated the injection of cocaine to produce reversible nerve blockade and later the injection of cocaine via a lumbar puncture to produce a spinal anesthetic and the first spinal headache. The chemical properties of cocaine were soon determined and manipulated to synthesize numerous other local anesthetic agents used to achieve what became known as regional anesthesia, which lacks the unconsciousness and amnesia of the general anesthetics but does produce analgesia and lack of motor movement in the "blocked" region.

Underwood EA: Before and after Morton. A historical survey of anaesthesia. Br Med J 1946;2:525.

OVERALL RISK OF ANESTHESIA

Anesthesia is performed over 70 million times per year in the United States and is remarkably safe. The number of anesthesia-related deaths has decreased dramatically in the last 30 years because of intense scrutiny by the American Society of Anesthesiologists. The realization that most problems are related to airway compromise has led to advanced respiratory monitoring utilizing pulse oximetry and capnography for every patient undergoing anesthesia. The Institute of Medicine's *To Err Is Human* complimented the anesthesiology community for its marked decrease in morbidity and mortality from anesthesia. Overall, the risk of anesthesia-related death in the healthy patient is estimated to be as low as 1:100,000–200,000 anesthetics.

The combination of amnesia, with or without unconsciousness, analgesia, and muscle relaxation is purposely induced by an anesthetic caregiver and is achieved either by administering inhalation agents in appropriate doses to affect the central nervous system (CNS) or by using specific intravenous pharmacologic agents to produce the same effects as inhaled vapors. These agents include amnestics, eg, benzodiazepines (midazolam or diazepam); analgesics, eg, the opioids morphine and fentanyl derivatives; the neuromuscular blocking drugs succinylcholine, pancuronium, or vecuronium; and sedative hypnotics, eg, sodium pentothal and propofol. All of the agents have adverse physiologic consequences: respiratory depression, cardiovascular depression, and loss of consciousness. Furthermore, some of these agents may induce allergic reactions. Some have also been known to trigger malignant hyperpyrexia.

The most common problems associated with adverse outcomes today still relate to airway compromise, medication errors, and central venous cannulation. Other concerns are postoperative neurologic complications (eg, nerve injury), ischemic optic neuropathy, coronary ischemia, anesthesia in remote locations (eg, interventional radiology sites), and probably most importantly, inadequate preoperative evaluation and preparation.

The anesthesia provider must be able to (1) achieve a state of anesthesia quickly and safely by choosing the appropriate techniques and agents, taking into consideration the patient's medical condition; (2) maintain and monitor a state of anesthesia throughout the surgical procedure while compensating for the effects of varying degrees of surgical stimulation and blood and fluid losses; (3) reverse the muscle relaxation and amnesia as necessary; (4) return the patient to physiologic homeostasis while maintaining sufficient analgesia to minimize postprocedure pain.

Kohn LT, Corrigan JM, Donaldson MS (editors): *To Err Is Human: Building a Safer Health System*. National Academy Press, 2000.

PREOPERATIVE EVALUATION

A preoperative evaluation is a responsibility of the anesthesiologist and is a basic element of anesthesia care (Table 11–1). This evaluation consists of information gathered from multiple sources, including the patient's medical record, history and physical examinations, and findings from medical tests and consults or other evaluations performed prior to the patient being seen by the anesthesiologist. Improved patient outcome and satisfaction is the result of an adequate, structured, formal presurgical or preprocedure evaluation and preparation performed on all patients.

▶ **Timing**

The timing of the preoperative evaluation depends primarily on the degree of planned surgical invasiveness. For high

Table 11–1. Preoperative Evaluation.

Goals
Optimize patient condition
Understand and control comorbidities and drug therapy
Ensure patient's questions are answered
Timing
High surgical invasiveness: at least 1 day prior
Medium invasiveness: day before or day of surgery
Low invasiveness: day of surgery
Content
Review medical records
Directed history and physical examination: airway, heart, and lungs
Indicated laboratory or additional consultations

surgical invasiveness, the initial assessment should be done at a minimum the day before the planned procedure by the anesthesia staff. Patients undergoing medium surgical invasive procedures can be evaluated the day before or even on the day of surgery, and for low surgical invasiveness, the initial assessment may be done the day of surgery. Time must be allotted to follow up on conditions discovered during the preoperative visit and to answer patient questions. Perioperative complications and deaths are most often a combination of patient comorbidities, surgical complexity, and anesthesia effects. The Physical Status Classification of the American Society of Anesthesiologists is the best known of many perioperative classification schemes (Table 11–2). This classification system does not assign risk but is a common language used to describe patients' preoperative physical status. The system is an alert to the anesthesia practitioner and all members of the patient care team.

Patients should ideally be seen in a PAC staffed by anesthesia personnel who evaluate patients from the anesthetic perspective and who look for physical conditions (airway) and controlled, uncontrolled, or unrecognized medical conditions that can lead to perioperative morbidity and mortality. There must be adequate communication between anesthesiologist and surgeon such that any conditions that may result in patient compromise are optimally addressed. Optimally, a patient's medical status has been adequately addressed by the patient's primary care physician prior to being referred to the PAC. However, in some instances, only a cursory "cleared for anesthesia and surgery" may result in a necessary delay. Any patients other than healthy ASA 1 or 2 patients should be seen in a PAC. Prior to referring patients to the PAC, the surgeon should have already ordered the necessary preoperative labs and in many instances will have already detected uncontrolled medical conditions that require consultations from other specialties in order to recommend and in some instances improve a patient's status.

The optimal preoperative evaluation has the following two elements: (1) **content**—readily accessible medical records, patient interview, a directed preanesthesia examination, indicated preoperative laboratory tests, and additional

Table 11–2. American Society of Anesthesiologists Physical Status Classification.

ASA 1 (PS1): A normal healthy patient
ASA 2 (PS2): A patient with mild systemic disease
ASA 3 (PS3): A patient with severe systemic disease
ASA 4 (PS4): A patient with severe systemic disease that is a constant threat to life
ASA 5 (PS5): A moribund patient who is not expected to survive without the operation
ASA 6 (PS6): A declared brain-dead patient whose organs are being removed for donor purposes
E: Emergency

consultations when indicated; the minimum acceptable examination includes an assessment of the airway, heart, and lungs well in advance of the planned date of surgery; and (2) **preoperative tests**—only as indicated by comorbidities and never as a screen, these tests should be specifically aimed at helping the anesthesiologist formulate an anesthetic plan.

Practice advisory for preanesthesia evaluation: a report by the American Society of Anesthesiologists Task Force on Preanesthesia Evaluation. *Anesthesiology* 2002;96:485.

History and Physical Examination

The anesthesiologist should specifically ask the patient about previous operations, anesthetic type, and any complications, eg, allergic reactions, abnormal bleeding, delayed emergence, prolonged paralysis, difficult airway management, awareness, or jaundice. Each of these describes a possible specific anesthetic morbidity that must be further investigated either by history or specific testing. Medical conditions detected as decreased exercise tolerance, shortness of breath, orthopnea, kidney or liver disease, and metabolic abnormalities, eg, diabetes or thyroid disease, should be ascertained. A comprehensive history seeks to identify serious cardiac conditions, eg, unstable coronary syndromes, angina, myocardial infarctions either recent or past, decompensated congestive heart failure, significant arrhythmias, or severe valvular disease. Any recent changes in cardiac symptoms or other associated diseases, eg, diabetes, renal disease, or cerebrovascular disease symptoms, should be identified.

Any family history of adverse responses to anesthetics (malignant hyperthermia) and social history of smoking, drug use, and alcohol consumption is important. Finally, a comprehensive review of concurrent medications including antihypertensives, insulin, bronchodilators, or any other medications that can interact with anesthetic agents should be documented. Certain medications may result in increased or decreased anesthetic requirements, prolongation of muscle relaxants, abnormal responses to sympathomimetics, delayed or enhanced metabolism of anesthetics, and/or augmentation of the depressant effects of anesthetics. The

patient's use of herbal medicines can have an adverse reaction with some anesthetics (Table 11–3).

Ang-Lee MK, Moss J, Yuan C: Herbal medicines and perioperative care. JAMA 2001;286:208.

Airway Examination and Classification

After the vital signs are obtained, the physical examination begins with the upper airway. Ability to control the airway is mandatory. The focus of the examination is to assess those factors that would make airway control (eg, endotracheal intubation) difficult or impossible. Seven keys to the upper airway examination should be documented:

1. Range of motion of the cervical spine: Patients should be asked to extend and flex their neck to the full range of possible motion so the anesthesiologist may look for any limitations.
2. Thyroid cartilage to mentum distance: ideal is greater than 6 cm.
3. Mouth opening: ideal is greater than 3 cm.
4. Dentition: dentures, loose teeth, poor conservation.
5. Jaw protrusion: ability to protrude the lower incisors past the upper incisors.
6. Presence of a beard.
7. Examination and classification of the upper airway based on the size of patient's tongue and the pharyngeal structures visible on mouth opening with the patient sitting looking forward. This visual description of the airway structures is known as the Mallampati score (Figure 11–1):

   I The soft palate, anterior and posterior tonsillar pillars, and uvula are visible—suggests easy airway intubation.
   II Tonsillar pillars and part of the uvula obscured by the tongue.
   III Only soft palate and hard palate visible.
   IV Only the hard palate is visible—suggests challenging airway.

The physical examination then focuses on heart and lungs, potential intravenous catheter sites, and potential sites for regional anesthesia. Range of motion of limbs must also be noted as this may affect positioning in the operating room. Finally, any neurologic abnormalities must be noted.

When a metabolic or physical finding or symptom is discovered during this visit, the anesthesiologist may believe that a specialty consultation is necessary to suggest ways to optimize the patient for surgery and anesthesia. If this is the case, the anesthesiologist should communicate with the surgeon in order to prevent unnecessary or unexpected delays in the surgical schedule. It is imperative that any consults ordered be completed and the results be available by the day of surgery.

The anesthesiologist can then advise the patient on appropriate options for general anesthesia versus regional techniques

Table 11–3. Perioperative Effects of Common Herbal Medicine.[1]

Name (Other Names)	Alleged Benefits	Perioperative Effects	Recommendations
Echinacea	Stimulates immune system	Allergic reactions; hepatotoxicity; interference with immune suppressive therapy (eg, organ transplants)	Discontinue as far in advance of surgery as possible
Ephedra (ma huang)	Promotes weight loss; increases energy	Ephedrine-like sympathetic stimulation with increased heart rate and blood pressure, arrhythmias, myocardial infarction, stroke	Discontinue at least 24 h prior to surgery; avoid monoamine oxidase inhibitors
Garlic (ajo)	Reduces blood pressure and cholesterol levels	Inhibition of platelet aggregation (irreversible)	Discontinue at least 7 days prior to surgery
Ginkgo (duck foot, maidenhair, silver apricot)	Improves cognitive performance (eg, dementia), increases peripheral perfusion (eg, impotence, macular degeneration)	Inhibition of platelet-activating factor	Discontinue at least 36 h prior to surgery
Ginseng	Protects against "stress" and maintains "homeostasis"	Hypoglycemia; inhibition of platelet aggregation and coagulation cascade	Discontinue at least 7 days prior to surgery
Kava (kawa, awa, intoxicating pepper)	Decreases anxiety	GABA-mediated hypnotic effects my decrease MAC (see Chapter 7); possible risk of acute withdrawal	Discontinue at least 24 h prior to surgery
St. John's wort (amber, goatweed, *Hypericum perforatum*, klamathe-weed)	Reverses mild to moderate depression	Inhibits serotonin, norepinephrine, and dopamine reuptake by neurons; increases drug metabolism by induction of cytochrome P-450	Discontinue at least 5 days prior to surgery
Valerian	Decreases anxiety	GABA-mediated hypnotic effects may decrease MAC; benzodiazepinelike withdrawal syndrome	Taper dose weeks before surgery if possible; treat withdrawal symptoms with benzodiazepines

[1]For more details, see Ang-Lee MK, Moss J, Yuan C: Herbal medicine and perioperative care. JAMA 2001;286:208. GABA, γ-aminobutyric acid; MAC, minimum alveolar concentration.
Reproduced with permission from Morgan GE, Mikhail MS, Murray MJ: *Clinical Anesthesiology*, 4th ed. McGraw Hill, 2006.

based on the patient's history, physical examination, and type of surgery. Although some surgical procedures must always be performed under general anesthesia, the anesthesiologist may discuss other options with the patient. If the referring surgeon has a particular preference for a type of anesthetic, such preferences should be communicated to the anesthesiologist directly rather than through the patient. It is also best if the referring surgeon does not promise any specific agent or technique without first consulting with the anesthesia care givers.

Mallampati SR et al: A clinical sign to predict difficult tracheal intubation: a prospective study. Can Anaesth Soc J 1985;32:429.

Preoperative Fasting

The anesthesiologist must discuss with the patient the requirements for preprocedure fasting and the management of medications up to the time of surgery or procedure. Current guidelines for are as follows: (1) No solid food should be eaten after the evening meal. At the minimum, most anesthesiologists delay an anesthetic so that the last solid food was 6–8

hours prior to nonemergent surgery or procedures involving anesthesia. (2) NPO after midnight except for sips of water to take oral medications. Water may be ingested up to 2 hours before checking in for surgery. Some institutions allow other clear liquids, eg, coffee, a few hours prior to surgery or procedure. However, because surgery schedules can change abruptly and procedure time may be moved forward, NPO after midnight is the best policy. (3) Pediatric fasting guidelines vary among institutions, so practitioners should consult with their particular pediatric anesthesia group.

American Society of Anesthesiologists: Practice guidelines for preoperative fasting and the use of pharmacologic agents to reduce the risk of pulmonary aspiration: application to healthy patients undergoing elective procedures. *Anesthesiology* 1999; 90:896.

Drugs to Continue Preoperatively

Most antihypertensive medications and beta-blocking agents should be continued in the perioperative period. There is some controversy over whether or not certain classes of antihyperten-

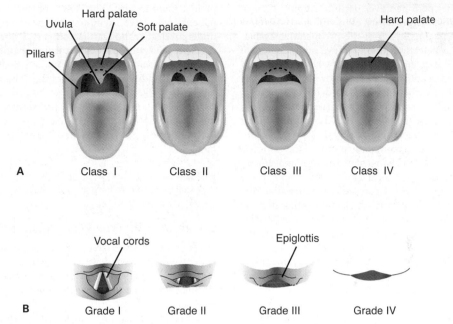

▲ **Figure 11–1.** Mallampati airway classification of oral opening. (Reproduced with permission from Morgan GE, Mikhail MS, Murray MJ: *Clinical Anesthesiology*, 4th ed. McGraw Hill.)

sives, eg, angiotensin II receptor blockers (ARBs) (valsartan, candesartan, losartan) or angiotensin-converting enzyme (ACE) inhibitors, should be continued. Patients taking these medications occasionally experience marked hypotension with induction of general anesthesia and respond poorly to common vasopressors. Some practitioners recommend not taking these drugs on the day of surgery. If the medication is continued, then it is important to know which agents have been used. Smoking should be stopped at least 2 weeks before scheduled surgery.

▶ Comorbidities

Comorbidities should be well controlled in the preoperative period to avoid postprocedure morbidity, and even mortality.

▶ Cardiovascular Disease (Hypertension, Coronary Artery Disease, Congestive Heart Failure)

A. Hypertension

Hypertension is the most common preexisting medical disease identified preoperatively and is a major risk factor for renal, cerebrovascular, peripheral vascular, cardiac ischemia or infarction, and congestive heart failure. The triad of lipid disorders, diabetes, and obesity is classically found in patients with hypertension and should alert the clinician that further evaluation for these conditions is needed. Hypertension has an

association with coronary artery disease, and the preoperative evaluation is a unique opportunity to identify and treat the nonessential causes of hypertension. The literature strongly supports the notion that all hypertensive patients should be treated medically to be as close to normotension as possible before any planned surgical procedure. Diastolic pressures of 110 mm/Hg or higher result in a higher incidence of intraoperative hypotension and myocardial ischemia. However, the literature does not support delaying surgery if the delay would be detrimental to the patient. The introduction of perioperative selective beta-blocking drugs provides a marked benefit in reducing the incidence of significant myocardial ischemia during the perioperative period. Although somewhat controversial, starting patients on beta-blockers immediately preoperatively may have some risk, but any patient already taking beta-blockers should continue taking the drug preoperatively.

Devereaux PJ et al: Rationale, design, and organization of the Perioperative Ischemic Evaluation (POISE) trial: a randomized controlled trial of metoprolol versus placebo in patients undergoing noncardiac surgery. Am Heart J 2006;152:223.
Spahn DR, Priebe HJ. Preoperative hypertension: remain wary? "Yes"—Cancel surgery? "No." Br J Anaesth 2004;92:461.

B. Coronary Artery Disease

Ischemic heart disease is a leading cause of death in the United States and is the leading cause of morbidity and mortality in the perioperative period. About 25% of patients who present for surgery each year have coronary artery disease, and thus much of the preoperative evaluation focuses on detecting the presence and degree of ischemic heart disease and determining whether it is likely to impact anesthesia and surgery. A major goal of preoperative assessment of cardiac status is to determine what, if any, interventions—coronary artery bypass graft (CABG), percutaneous coronary intervention (PCI)—would benefit patients undergoing noncardiac surgery. In general, preoperative cardiac tests are recommended only if the information obtained will lead to changes in patient management. However, certain active clinical conditions (Table 11–4) demand evaluation and treatment before noncardiac surgery. Determining which patient characteristics indicate high perioperative risk is very difficult, but preoperative congestive heart failure, recent myocardial infarction, and unstable angina pose clear, significant clinical risk factors (CRFs). Other CRFs include diabetes mellitus, renal insufficiency, cerebrovascular disease, valvular heart disease, age, and dysrhythmias. Because of the high incidence of silent ischemia, patients over the age of 50 should have an electrocardiogram. A simple exercise tolerance description of the functional capacity of the patient (eg, ability to climb two flights of stairs without stopping) is also a practical screening. This initial history by the surgeon or anesthesiologist may be the first cardiac assessment the patient has ever had. The assessment of functional capacity may be the first indication of the need for further evaluation of potential cardiac pathology.

The American Heart Association (AHA) developed a useful algorithm for all providers (Figure 11–2). This algorithm, updated in 2007, no longer focuses on stress testing but recommends testing only if the results could have an impact on surgery or anesthesia and lead to changes in patient management. The AHA guidelines state that most patients who have asymptomatic heart disease can safely undergo elective noncardiac surgery without performing invasive or even noninvasive cardiac testing. Having three or more CRFs and planning for major vascular surgery may necessitate additional cardiac testing. Those patients with one or two CRFs and who are scheduled for intermediate risk surgery should either undergo additional cardiac testing or proceed with planned surgery, in which case one of the main goals of the anesthesiologist is to control heart rate.

Fleisher LA et al: ACC/AHA 2007 guidelines on perioperative evaluation and care for noncardiac surgery. J Am Coll Cardiol 2007;50:159.

C. Patients with Prior PCI (Angioplasty and Stents)

There is much controversy about the best treatment for patients who have had a PCI procedure, angioplasty without stents, or angioplasty with either a bare metal or drug eluting stent. Because of the risk for thrombosis at the site of intervention, patients are usually placed on a dual antiplatelet therapy of aspirin and clopidogrel for 2–4 weeks following angioplasty, 4–6 weeks for the bare metal stents, and up to 1 year for the drug-eluting stents. Stopping these antiplatelet drugs for a surgical intervention that falls in the therapy period presents a risk for perioperative cardiac events if the stent thromboses. The AHA guidelines recommend that if the procedure is elective, then the operation should be postponed until the case can be done with aspirin as the only antiplatelet drug. If the operation is urgent, then consideration must be given to the timing of the surgery and the risk of surgical bleeding. If the risk of bleeding is low, then a PCI with a stent should be considered and the patient placed on dual antiplatelet therapy.

Table 11–4. Active Cardiac Conditions for Which the Patient Should Undergo Evaluation and Treatment Before Noncardiac Surgery.

Condition	Examples
Unstable coronary syndromes	Unstable or severe angina Recent myocardial infarction (> 7 but < 30 days ago)
Decompensated heart failure (New York Heart Association class IV): worsening or new onset Significant arrhythmias	High-grade atrioventricular block Mobitz II atrioventricular block Third-degree atrioventricular block Symptomatic ventricular arrhythmias Supraventricular arrhythmias (including atrial fibrillation with uncontrolled ventricular rate [> 100] at rest) Symptomatic bradycardia Newly recognized ventricular tachycardia
Severe valvular disease	Severe aortic stenosis (mean pressure gradient > 40 mm Hg or aortic valve area < 1.0 cm² or symptomatic) Symptomatic mitral stenosis (progressive dyspnea on exertion, exertional syncope, or heart failure)

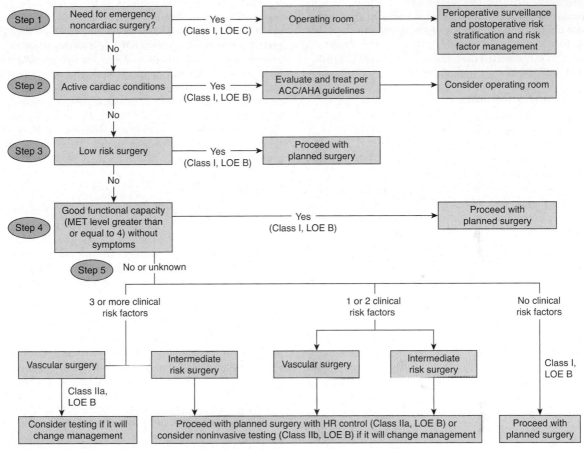

▲ **Figure 11-2.** Cardiac evaluation and care algorithm for noncardiac surgery based on active clinical conditions, known cardiovascular disease or cardiac risk factors for patients 50 years of age or greater. Summary of ACC/AHA 2007 perioperative guideline algorithm on cardiovascular evaluation and care for noncardiac surgery. HR = heart rate, LOE = loss of evidence, MET = metabolic equivalent.

If the bleeding risk is high, the AHA recommends the following based on the timing of surgery: angioplasty for surgery within 14–29 days, bare metal stent for planned surgery within 30–365 days, and drug-eluting stent for surgery that can be delayed 1 year. Truly urgent and/or emergent surgery necessitates angioplasty for a procedure with a high risk of surgical bleeding and stenting for a case with a low risk for bleeding.

The AHA guidelines recommend several other measures: (1) Perioperative beta-blockade is indicated for patients previously on beta-blockers, patients undergoing major vascular surgery, and patients undergoing intermediate-risk surgery with one or more CRFs. Beta-blockade should be started several days to weeks before planned surgery in order to produce a consistent targeted heart rate between 65 and 70 beats per minute. The addition of statin class agents, alpha-2 agonists, and calcium channel blockers may also be

effective. (2) Left ventricular function should be assessed preoperatively for patients with unexplained dyspnea or who have active or a history of compensated heart failure with changing symptoms. (3) Coronary revascularization is suggested for patients with left main disease, symptomatic three-vessel disease and poor ejection fraction (EF), two-vessel disease with left anterior descending coronary artery stenosis, poor EF and a positive stress test, or an acute ST segment elevation myocardial infarction. AHA does not recommend prophylactic CABG surgery in patients with stable coronary artery disease. (4) Blood glucose should be tightly controlled. (5) Patients with pacemakers or implanted defibrillator devices should have them checked 3 to 6 months before major surgery. (6) Patients with drug-eluting cardiac stents should continue aspirin therapy and discontinue other antiplatelet agents for as short a time as possible. (7) Beta-blockers and statin drugs should be continued in the perioperative period. (8) Cardiology consultants should be asked for specific recommendations that would reduce immediate perioperative cardiac risk.

Riddell JW et al: Coronary stents and noncardiac surgery. Circulation 2007;116:378.

D. Pulmonary Disease

The presence of significant pulmonary disease is suspected or confirmed by the history and physical examination. Poor functional capacity may be the first indication that further workup may be necessary. The presence of either obstructive or restrictive lung disease always puts the patient at risk for perioperative complications, eg, pneumonia and prolonged difficulty weaning from the ventilator. In some instances, arterial blood gas analysis or pulmonary function tests are necessary to determine responsiveness to bronchodilators. Asthmatic patients should be asked about the severity of their disease, hospitalizations, responsiveness to inhalers, and steroid usage. There is no value for routine preoperative chest x-rays. Surgical history and physical examination may be the first indication of significant pulmonary disease, and workup may be initiated before sending the patient to the PAC. Optimally, patients who smoke should stop smoking at least 8 weeks before scheduled surgery. Warner demonstrated that the highest rate of pulmonary complications in 200 patients undergoing CABG was in those who had stopped smoking 1 to 8 weeks preoperatively. Recent cessation of cigarette smoking may pose a greater risk of pulmonary complication because of the commonly observed increase in cough and sputum production.

Warner DO: Helping surgical patients quit smoking: why, when, and how. Anesth Analg 2005;101:481.

E. Obesity

The national epidemic of obesity poses particular problems for surgery and anesthesia. The body mass index (BMI), the ratio of weight (kg)/height (meters)^2, gives an idea of the degree of obesity. Normal BMI is about 21.6 kg/m^2, overweight is 25–30 kg/m^2, obese is 30–35 kg/m^2, and extreme obesity is more than 35 kg/m^2. Extreme obesity patients have a variety of perioperative issues and should be evaluated in a PAC. Particular attention should include the upper airway and evaluation of cardiovascular, respiratory, metabolic, and gastrointestinal systems. Abnormal BMI patients have cardiovascular issues with venous access, hypertension, cardiomegaly, decreased left ventricular function, and cor pulmonale, and they have twice the incidence of ischemic heart disease than patients at normal weight. Extreme obesity is associated with significant pulmonary problems, including restrictive lung volumes, obstructive sleep apnea, hypoxemia, increased PaCO_2, increased hematocrit, and

right heart failure. The extremely obese patient's airway is often difficult to maintain with mask ventilation secondary to decreased neck mobility and adiposity and requires careful preoperative evaluation. Almost all the major endocrine problems with extreme obesity involve the effects of diabetes mellitus and require preoperative assessment of glycemic control. Obesity also leads to abnormal fatty deposits in the liver that cause increased metabolism of inhalation anesthetics. Morbidly obese patients may have a higher risk of gastric aspiration and development of aspiration pneumonia. Finally, postoperative pain management must be considered.

F. Diabetes Mellitus

The most common metabolic abnormality is diabetes mellitus, and its presence should cause a high index of suspicion for cardiac problems. Patients on insulin therapy are at higher risk for cardiac morbidity and mortality, including myocardial infarction and heart failure. Glucose control may be very difficult to maintain in the perioperative period, and preoperative assessment of control should always be ascertained through history or laboratory testing. Recent studies show that moderately tight glucose control in the perioperative period is beneficial. Anesthesia providers are responsible for glucose control during the procedure, and the surgical service is typically responsible for this care in the postoperative period.

van den Berghe G et al: Intensive insulin therapy in the critically ill patients. NEJM 2001;345;1359.

G. Patients on Low Molecular Weight Heparin (LMWH)

Patients taking LMWH for deep venous thrombosis prophylaxis present an unusual problem for both surgeon and anesthesiologist. The current guidelines dictate that unless absolutely indicated, neuraxial anesthesia (spinal, epidural) should not be performed unless LMWH has been stopped for at least 12 hours and preferably 24 hours. That means that a substitute anticoagulant should be initiated if neuraxial anesthesia is to be done, or this approach is avoided.

H. Renal Impairment

Acute renal failure (ARF) occurs in approximately 1–5% of all hospitalized patients and is responsible for increased length of stay and mortality. The preoperative visit can help to identify patient risk factors for ARF in those with previously normal renal function undergoing noncardiac surgery. The perioperative onset of ARF in patients with previously normal renal function is associated with increased postoperative mortality, especially significant within 1 year postsurgery. BMI higher than 32 kg/m^2, age, emergency surgery, liver disease, high-risk surgery (intrathoracic, intraperitoneal, suprainguinal vascular, large blood loss), peripheral vascular occlusive disease, and chronic obstructive pulmonary disease necessitating chronic bronchodilator therapy place patients at increased risk for perioperative renal impairment.

Kheterpal S et al: Predictors of postoperative acute renal failure after noncardiac surgery in patients with previously normal renal function. Anesthesiology 2007;107:892.

Preoperative Medications

The use of preoperative medications is hampered by the fact that most patients are not in the medical facility until the day of surgery. Most premedications now consist of an anxiolytic agent (eg, midazolam) and an opiate (eg, fentanyl) given in the immediate preanesthesia period. These premedications are often given because patients have a preconceived notion that they need something to relax. Alternatively, a thorough explanation of what the patient can expect in terms of surgery and anesthesia has a significant calming effect comparable to that of medications given to relieve anxiety. Administration of premedication to prevent pulmonary aspiration syndrome is often considered with the use of agents that increase gastric pH (H$_2$ blockers, proton pump inhibitors, antacids) or agents that lower gastric volume. Occasionally, the use of drugs that stimulate gastric emptying (metoclopramide) is considered. However, metoclopramide has significant neuropsychiatric side effects, and its use should be limited.

Informed Consent

Many institutions and practices obtain a signed informed consent from patients for anesthesia, while other institutions include the anesthesia consent in the surgical consent. Regardless of the particular facility requirements, the anesthesiologist should write a note in the patient chart indicating that the patient has been informed of the issues surrounding anesthesia and understands the risks and complications as described. The informed consent for anesthesia should include a discussion of what to expect from the administration of anesthesia and possible adverse effects and risks. A number of issues should be discussed routinely, including timing of surgery, premedication, risks of dental injury, cardiac risks, sequence of events prior to anesthesia induction, awakening from anesthesia, presence of catheters, duration of time in the PACU, anticipated return to a hospital bed or discharge, postoperative pain management, and the likelihood of nausea and vomiting. Patients may have questions concerning perioperative awareness. Rather than cause undue worry, clinical judgment should dictate how detailed a description of each of these issues should be for each patient.

Choice of Anesthesia

Considerations in choosing an anesthetic technique include the planned surgical procedure, positioning requirements, patient preferences, surgeon preferences, the urgency of the operation, postoperative pain management, and potential for admission to a critical care unit. Some procedures (eg, thoracotomy) cannot be performed under a regional anesthetic or neuraxial blockade and necessitate a general anesthetic. Other procedures (eg, extremity surgery) can be performed under regional, neuraxial, or general anesthesia. Sometimes a combination of an epidural and a general anesthetic may be chosen with continuation of the epidural for postoperative pain management. Emergency surgery for patients with a full stomach may necessitate a rapid-sequence general anesthetic to protect from pulmonary aspiration. Regional anesthesia may provide anesthesia for hip surgery but may not provide much in the way of patient comfort because of the position requirements of a fracture table. Patient age and preference must also be included in the decision of choice of anesthetic technique. However, some regional anesthesia may be contraindicated for patients with the peripheral neuropathy of diabetes. Notation of the proposed type of anesthesia must be entered into record of the preanesthesia evaluation.

Holding Room and Operating Room

The nurse, surgeon, and anesthesiologist have many tasks to perform, starting in the holding area before the surgery can begin. The nurse checks the patient in and records vital signs, checks for a signed consent, and starts an intravenous line if needed. The surgeon should confirm and mark the site of surgery. The anesthesiologist should confirm the preoperative evaluation and type of anesthetic selected.

Wrong Site Surgery

In July 2004, the Joint Commission on the Accreditation of Healthcare Organizations (JCAHO) instituted a patient safety mandate known as the Universal Protocol for Preventing Wrong Site, Wrong Procedure, Wrong Person Surgery. All members of the care team must be familiar with and always participate in and perform the following three steps of this Universal Protocol.

Step 1: Initial verification of the intended patient, procedure, and site of the procedure. This step begins at the time the procedure is scheduled and again at the time of admission into the medical facility, anytime care responsibility is transferred to another caregiver, and before the patient leaves the preoperative area for the operating room.

Step 2: Marking the operative site. An unambiguous mark must be made using a marker that is sufficiently permanent to be visible after surgical prep and draping on or near the intended surgical incision site. This mark should not be an X, as in "X marks the spot," but rather a word or line representing the proposed incision. This mark must be made by the surgeon performing the procedure. If possible, the patient should participate when the site is marked.

Step 3: The time out immediately before starting the procedure. A time out must be conducted in the location where the surgical procedure will be done, and all members of the care team—surgeon, nurses, anesthesiologists—must *actively* participate in verification of correct patient identity, correct side and site of surgery, agreement on the scheduled procedure, and assurance that all of the necessary implants and special equipment are immediately available. This time out must take place before incision. JCAHO requires that the time out be documented in the medical record.

> Joint Commission on the Accreditation of Healthcare Organizations: Universal protocol for preventing wrong site, wrong procedure, wrong person surgery. Available at: www.jointcommission.org/patientsafety/universalprotocol. Accessed November 28, 2008.

▶ The Operating Room

The anesthesiologist must check the equipment in the operating room before helping to transport the patient. Once in the operating room, the patient is transferred to the operating table with the assistance of the nurses and anesthesiologist. It is standard anesthesia practice to apply monitors to measure arterial blood pressure (a-line, blood pressure cuff), heart rate, oxygenation (pulse oximeter), and ventilation (capnography) before induction of anesthesia (Table 11–5).

The anesthesiologist must be certain that a surgeon is present in the room before beginning induction. The final time out should then be performed, confirming site, patient, procedure, and surgical personnel.

▶ General Anesthesia Management

Patients must be preoxygenated before induction of a general anesthetic. General anesthesia is commonly induced by administration of intravenous drugs (eg, propofol or thiopental) and, in cases when cardiovascular status is compromised, etomidate or ketamine. Patients receiving propofol may complain of discomfort at the IV sites, and patients receiving etomidate may have some athetoid movements that appear seizurelike. Almost all anesthetics are preceded by the administration of an opiate (eg, fentanyl) in a dose that is not intended to induce an anesthetic but that helps reduce the amount of induction agent. Most general anesthetics then include a muscle relaxant to facilitate endotracheal intubation. Tracheal intubation is almost always performed during general anesthesia and is especially important for patients presenting for emergent surgery with presumed full stomach or when positive pressure ventilation is required. The laryngeal mask airway (LMA) can also be used to maintain a patent airway. To minimize the time that the trachea is unprotected, a rapid-sequence induction of anesthesia using rapid administration of induction agent and rapid-acting muscle relaxant (eg, succinylcholine) can be utilized. The "crash induction" is a modification of this rapid-sequence technique with the application of cricoid pressure by a caregiver other than the inducing anesthesia personnel.

General anesthesia may also be induced by mask using an inhalation anesthetic (eg, isoflurane or sevoflurane). This method is commonly used for children. Once adequate depth of anesthesia is assured, a muscle relaxant may be administered to help facilitate endotracheal intubation. Inhalation induction takes longer than rapid-sequence induction, and the airway may be unprotected for a longer time. A combination of inhalation agent and intravenous agent can also be used to induce general anesthesia.

Once an adequate depth of anesthesia and adequate muscle relaxation is attained, the trachea is intubated. Ease of endotracheal intubation can usually be predicted from the careful preoperative airway evaluation. However, the anes-

Table 11–5. Standards for Basic Anesthesia Monitoring.

Parameter	Equipment
Oxygenation: ensure patient concentration in inspired gas and blood during all anesthetics	*Oxygen analyzer:* part of anesthesia machine *Pulse oximeter:* continuously audible variable pitch pulse tone
Ventilation: Ensure adequate patient ventilation	*Capnography:* continuous monitoring for the presence of end-tidal CO_2
Circulation: Ensure adequacy of patient circulatory function	*EKG:* Continuously displayed from the beginning until leaving the room *Arterial blood pressure monitor:* measured at least every 5 minutes *Measurement of patient heart rate:* usually from EKG or pulse oximeter
Temperature: Aid in maintenance of appropriate patient temperature	Oral, skin, nasal, or bladder temperature probe

thesiologist occasionally encounters an unexpected difficult intubation and additional maneuvers may be necessary: these can include cricoid manipulation, adjustment of the patient's head position, or use of a long, stiff catheter (eg, a bougie) or a fiberoptic bronchoscope. The American Society of Anesthesiologists provides an algorithm for the management of the difficult airway. If another provider is placing cricoid pressure, the anesthesiologist must directly state what maneuver would be the most helpful. If the airway cannot be secured after multiple attempts, patients can be awakened and a decision made to proceed with an awake fiberoptic intubation or to cancel the anesthetic until further workup can be performed. The most serious complication of endotracheal intubation, and the most common cause of serious anesthesia morbidity and mortality, is the failure to secure the airway. Other common complications are dental injuries, soft tissue injury to the lips, hypertension and tachycardia, and laryngospasm on extubation.

Following anesthetic induction, the patient must be properly positioned for the procedure. It is the responsibility of both surgeon and anesthesiologist to assure that the patient is positioned to avoid physical or physiologic complications. The American Society of Anesthesiologists' closed claims study notes that nerve damage from malpositioning during surgery is the second most common anesthetic complication. Careful attention must be paid to adequately protect all potential pressure and vulnerable areas such as elbows, knees, heels, and eyes. The ulnar nerve is particularly susceptible to injury, as is the brachial plexus when patient's arms are abducted too far. Hemodynamics may also be compromised by position changes that may result in decreased venous return and resultant hypotension.

American Society of Anesthesiologists: Practice guidelines for management of the difficult airway: an updated report by the American Society of Anesthesiologists Task Force on Management of the Difficult Airway. Anesthesiology 2003;98:1269.
Cheney FW et al: Nerve injury associated with anesthesia: a closed claims study. Anesthesiology 1999;90:1062.

▶ Maintenance of General Anesthesia

Once the airway is safely secured, anesthesiologists commonly maintain the anesthetic with a combination of an inhalation agent, nitrous oxide, opiate, and muscle relaxant. This "balanced anesthetic" allows for titration of agents to maintain the requirements of anesthesia: analgesia, amnesia (unconsciousness), skeletal muscle relaxation, and control of the hemodynamic responses to surgical stimulation. Drugs with specific pharmacologic profiles are chosen to help satisfy the anesthetic requirements. Analgesia is provided by opiates and inhalational agents; amnesia is provided by benzodiazepines, nitrous oxide, and inhalation agents; and muscle relaxation is provided by neuromuscular-blocking drugs, inhaled agents, or local anesthetics. The provision of

the right amount of muscle relaxation to facilitate the procedure but not too much to obscure a clinical sign of anesthetic depth or to result in prolonged relaxation postoperatively presents a challenge to the anesthesiologist. A peripheral nerve stimulator can monitor muscle relaxation such that the relaxant is reversible at the end of the case to allow for safe extubation.

▶ Regional Anesthesia for Surgery

Many operations require no general anesthetic. These include almost any procedure done below the waist, on lower abdomen, and on the upper extremities. Spinal or epidural anesthesia provide excellent muscle relaxation, profound analgesia, and avoidance of airway manipulation, and allows the patient to be conscious. Spinal or epidural anesthesia have additional advantages: decreased blood loss during orthopedic procedures, fewer thrombotic complications, less pulmonary compromise, maintenance of vasodilatation for postoperative vascular surgeries, earlier hospital discharge, and avoidance of immune response compromise.

A. Spinal Anesthesia

Most spinal anesthetics are performed in either the lateral position or with the patient sitting on the operating table. Following sterile prep and local skin anesthetic, a small 25-27 gauge spinal needle is introduced in the lower lumbar spine, and the subdural space is identified by the presence of cerebrospinal fluid (CSF). Depending on the planned length of surgery, either lidocaine or bupivacaine (with or without epinephrine or an opiate) is injected. Lidocaine spinal anesthesia provides at most 2 hours of anesthesia, while bupivacaine provides up to 5 hours of anesthesia. However, due to patient discomfort from tourniquet break-through pain, the use of orthopedic tourniquets limits the usefulness of spinals no matter which local anesthetic is used to no more than 2 hours. Once the local agent is injected, patients are placed in the supine position for 5–10 minutes to allow for proper spread of the local anesthetic. During this time, blood pressure and heart rate are monitored; both hypotension and bradycardia can be induced by a sympathectomy due to the cephalad spread of the local. During this 5–10 minute period, patient movement should be limited. Once the block has stabilized, the surgical preparation and positioning can proceed. The anesthesiologist monitors the patient in the same manner as for general anesthesia and administers sedation as needed.

Other than expected hemodynamic changes, the most common complication of spinal anesthesia is postspinal headaches. The incidence is very low when smaller gauge spinal needles are used and are more common in young women. The spinal headache is almost always positional and abates when the patient is recumbent. Severe headaches can result in diplopia because of stretching of the 6th cranial nerve as the brain sinks from loss of CSF. Patients usually complain of the headache a day or two following the operation. Conservative treatment is the maintenance of adequate hydration, remaining recumbent, and an analgesic such as acetaminophen. Severe headache may require a "blood patch" to plug the leak of CSF and is performed by an anesthesiologist.

B. Epidural Anesthesia

Epidural anesthesia has several distinct differences from spinal anesthesia. The epidural space is between the ligamentum flavum and the dural structures; in placing an epidural, the subdural space is not entered, and so no CSF leak is created with the potential for a spinal headache. The epidural anesthetic may be continued by insertion of a small catheter into the epidural space. Additional local anesthetic can be added to move the block to higher spinal levels or to maintain the selected level of anesthesia. This continuous epidural technique can be used for postoperative pain control. The catheter can be placed at spinal levels in the midthoracic region for thoracotomy or lower thoracic or lumbar region for abdominal operations or lower extremity procedures. Epidural anesthesia requires the administration of high volumes of local anesthetics. There is the potential for intravascular injection with resultant cardiovascular compromise or high block. There is also the potential for misplacement of the catheter or epidural needle in the subarachnoid space. Instillation of the larger volumes of local in the subarachnoid space can result in a total spinal or high block with resultant cardiovascular collapse. Therefore, small test doses of local anesthetic are administered to evaluate for signs of intravenous injection or high block. Another potential disadvantage of epidural anesthesia is that the onset is much slower than spinal anesthesia. The same hemodynamic changes observed with epidural can occur with spinals.

A common complication of both spinal and epidural anesthesia is prolonged blockade of parasympathetic fibers that innervate the bladder with resultant urinary retention and the need for a urinary bladder catheter.

C. Peripheral Nerve Block

True regional anesthesia is useful for procedures on the extremities. Useful anesthesia of the upper extremity can be obtained by blockade of the brachial plexus using an interscalene approach, a supraclavicular approach, or an axillary approach. Lower extremity surgery may be performed utilizing blockade of the lumbar plexus and its major branches: femoral nerve, sciatic nerve, lateral femoral cutaneous nerve, obturator nerve, and popliteal nerve. In some instances, a catheter can be placed near the nerve or plexus to allow for continuous blockade and postoperative pain control. The usefulness of these blocks for extremity surgery is limited in time by the use of tourniquets if the patient is to remain awake during the procedure. These blocks are very useful if avoidance of a general anesthetic is desired. Additional advantages of peripheral nerve blocks include earlier discharge from recovery areas and return to home, lack of administration of large doses of opiates, less nausea and vomiting, no instrumentation of patient airway, and earlier ambulation. Intraoperative sedation may be provided, and the anesthesiologist monitors the patient in the standard manner.

▶ Monitored Anesthesia Care (MAC)

MAC was previously termed local anesthesia with standby. The "standby" is an anesthesia caregiver who monitors the patient's status while the surgeon performs a procedure under local anesthesia. The anesthesiologist can also provide sedation and analgesia as needed for the patient. This type of anesthesia is usually requested by the surgeon for patients who may be especially frail in health; it provides the option to convert to a general anesthetic if necessary.

▶ Completion of Surgery

At the end of the procedure, most often patients who have been intubated for the surgery have their muscle relaxation reversed and the anesthetic depth decreased to allow them to return to consciousness. Once the return of muscle function has been assured and the patient is able to respond to commands, the endotracheal tube can be removed and the patient closely observed to ensure adequate ventilation. Patients are then transferred to a stretcher and transported to the PACU, accompanied by a member of the anesthesia care team who monitors the patient's condition during transport. Many institutions require that a member of the surgical team also accompany the patient to the PACU along with the anesthesiologist. Some critically ill patients are transported directly to the intensive care unit (ICU), still intubated, sedated, and ventilated.

▶ Postanesthesia Recovery Room

The PACU, most commonly known as the recovery room, is where most patients are transferred after surgery. The PACU is the designated area in which patients receive postanesthesia monitoring of vital signs as well as the beginning of the nursing care for their surgical recovery. It is the standard of the American Society of Anesthesiologists that all patients, regardless of the type of anesthesia, receive appropriate postanesthesia care, either in a PACU or an equivalent area such as a critical care unit. An exception to this standard can only be made by the anesthesiologist responsible for the patient's care. Once in the PACU, a verbal report is provided to the responsible PACU nurse by a member of the anesthesia care team who is familiar with and who accompanied the patient during transport. The surgeon can also give a report as to the surgical issues that may impact on the patient's recovery.

The PACU is equipped with essentially the same monitors as the operating room and with the drugs and equipment needed for emergency resuscitation. The PACU is a specialized, short-stay ICU. PACUs are staffed with specially trained nurses to monitor patients who are recovering from the anesthetic. Patients are continually monitored in the PACU for approximately 1 hour or until they fulfill specific objective criteria. Discharge from the PACU requires the clinical judgment of the PACU team. Particular attention is focused on the monitoring of oxygenation, ventilation, circulation, level of consciousness, and temperature.

Current literature supports the use of discharge scoring systems (eg, the Aldrete score) describing objective criteria that must be fulfilled before the patient can be discharged from the PACU. These criteria include quantitative analysis of patient's ability to move extremities in response to verbal commands, adequacy of ventilation (pulse oximetry) and circulation (stable vital signs) and level of consciousness, and pain control. After outpatient surgery, patients must have an adult to escort them home. Most institutions have policies requiring that anesthesiologists, in conjunction with the PACU nursing team, discharge patients from PACU.

Aldrete JA, Kroulik D. A postanesthetic recovery score. Anesth Analg 1970;49:924.
Awad JT, Chung F. Factors affecting recovery and discharge following ambulatory surgery. Can J Anaesth 2006;53:858.

COMMON POSTOPERATIVE PROBLEMS

There are many reasons why patients have other than a routine stay in the PACU. The three most common PACU problems are hypothermia, nausea and vomiting, and pain control. Hypotension/hypertension, hypoxemia, hypercapnia/hypoventilation, and agitation can also occur.

▶ Hypothermia

A very common complication of anesthesia and surgery is hypothermia. Every effort should be made in the operating room to avoid patients becoming hypothermic, even if this requires that the operating room temperature is maintained at a warmer-than-comfortable level. Patients who are admitted to the PACU and are hypothermic must be rewarmed to avoid the adverse consequence of shivering (ie, increased oxygen consumption). Hypothermia may also have an adverse effect on coagulation parameters and may delay recovery from anesthesia due to decreased drug metabolism. The most effective methods of rewarming are forced-air warming devices or water-jacket devices. Shivering can be actively treated with small doses of meperidine.

Rajagopalan S et al: The effects of mild perioperative hypothermia on blood loss and transfusion requirement. Anesthesiology 2008;108:71.

▶ Postoperative Nausea and Vomiting (PONV)

According to the Society of Ambulatory Anesthesia (SAMBA), untreated, PONV occurs in 20–30% of the general surgical population and up to 70–80% in the high-risk surgical population. The increased PACU stays and sometimes hospital admission to control PONV adds to patient discomfort and morbidity and adds a financial burden to the health care system. SAMBA's Seven Guidelines have been adopted by many health care facilities for the prevention and treatment of PONV.

1. Identify patients at high risk for PONV. The most consistent independent predictors for PONV are female gender, nonsmoking, and a history of PONV or motion sickness, coupled with the anesthesia-related factors of general anesthesia with volatile anesthetics, nitrous oxide, and postoperative opioids.

2. Reduce baseline risk factors for PONV. The most reliable strategy is to use regional anesthesia when possible. Otherwise, propofol used for induction; minimization of intraoperative volatile agents, opioids, and nitrous oxide; and epidurals for postoperative pain management may be the best strategy to reduce PONV.

3. Administer PONV prophylaxis using one or two interventions in adults at moderate risk for PONV. The 5-HT$_3$ receptor antagonists (ondansetron, dolasetron, granisetron), dexamethasone, and low-dose droperidol are among the most effective first-line antiemetics for PONV prophylaxis: Each independently reduces PONV by 25%. It is recommended that adults who present with moderate risk for PONV receive a combination therapy for prophylaxis with drugs from different classes and different mechanisms. A new drug, aprepitant, a neurokinin-1 (NK-1) receptor antagonist has been shown to significantly reduce PONV given alone or in combination with the 5-HT$_3$s.

4. For patients at high risk for PONV, SAMBA recommends a multimodal approach to prophylaxis that includes using two or more interventions and trying to reduce the baseline factors (eg, anxiolysis), minimizing the anesthetic agents chosen, and using the pharmacologic interventions mentioned above.

5. Administer prophylactic antiemetics to children at high risk for PONV. Use the same combination therapy as in adults.

6. Some patients have no risk factors for PONV and therefore receive no prophylaxis but develop PONV postoperatively. Recommended treatment is to begin with low-dose 5-HT$_3$ antagonist, which is the only class of drugs that has been adequately studied to be effective for the treatment of existing PONV.

7. If rescue therapy for patients who have received prophylaxis is required, it is recommended that the antiemetic(s) chosen should be from a different therapeutic class than the drugs used for prophylaxis.

Gan TJ et al: Society for Ambulatory Anesthesia guidelines for the management of postoperative nausea and vomiting. Anesth Analg 2007;1051:615.

Postoperative Acute Pain Management

The management of postoperative surgical pain is the responsibility of both the anesthesiology and surgery services. Other than PONV, inadequate postoperative pain control is a primary cause of unanticipated hospital admission for outpatient surgery. The severity of the pain is usually site dependent (upper abdominal procedures tend to be more painful than lower abdominal procedures; ie, appendectomy is more painful than inguinal hernia, which is more painful than minor chest wall surgery), but the individual patient's response to the pain and efforts to treat it vary widely. What may appear to be a minor incision to some may be very painful to others. The clinical challenge of providing adequate postoperative pain management is also a major mandate by JCAHO and the national media. Thus, almost every anesthesia department has an acute pain management team that can help with the management of patients in PACU and later in the surgical intensive care or general care unit.

Morphine has been the historical postoperative analgesic, administered either intramuscularly or intravenously. Patient response to a standardized administration protocol is variable, however, and can fail to control pain or cause symptoms of overdosage. Every patient is different in the required serum concentration of drug that results in adequate pain control.

There are four common modalities or approaches to postoperative pain management:

Oral medications. For minor procedures, eg, excision of skin lesions, nonsteroidal analgesics may be sufficient. For more intense levels of pain, oral narcotics in combination with acetaminophen is often effective.

Intravenous opioids. Occasionally, one or two intravenous doses of morphine, hydromorphone, or fentanyl may be sufficient to control postoperative pain. However, a more reliable method is the administration of small doses of narcotic given on demand by the patient. Patient-controlled analgesia (PCA) uses the same or even less total narcotic to control pain and is as safe as intramuscular medications. Patients are instructed on how to use the PCA device to administer narcotic on demand. PCA has widespread acceptance by patients, physicians, and nurses because it provides pain control in a timely manner that more closely matches the patient's requirements. Caution must be used when pain control appears to be inadequate and house staff covering the patient are tempted to give an intravenous "boost" of narcotic.

Epidural opiate analgesia. The application of opioids or narcotics at the neuraxial receptor sites via an epidural catheter is probably the modality of choice for severe acute postoperative pain control. An epidural catheter is preferably placed preoperatively at a spinal dermatome level close to the site of incision: midthoracic level for thoracic surgeries, lower thoracic for upper abdominal surgeries, or lumbar for lower abdominal incisions or lower extremity surgeries. This technique utilizes a continuous infusion of a combined solution of a low concentration of local anesthetic (bupivacaine 0.125 mg/cc) and an opioid (morphine, hydromorphone, or fentanyl). This modality does not require patient cooperation but can be used in a PCA mode. Epidural analgesia can be continued for multiple days; in has beneficial effects for maintaining peripheral vasodilatation after vascular procedures and improving respiratory mechanics due to reduced pain when patients are breathing on their own. Patients must be monitored for respiratory depression while receiving epidural analgesia, as respiratory depression is the major complication from this pain control therapy.

Specific nerve or plexus block. Local anesthesia block of single nerves or continuous catheter infusion of local anesthetic around major nerve plexuses is becoming more popular. Examples include single injection or placement of a continuous catheter around the femoral nerve for controlling pain from knee surgery and continuous catheters around the brachial plexus (usually supraclavicular) for controlling pain from upper extremity surgery.

Complications of Anesthesia

No matter how well patients are prepared for anesthesia and surgery, there is always the possibility of a complication from the delivery of anesthesia. These complications can be minor in nature (eg, intravenous infiltration, hypothermia, or minor ocular injury) or major issues (eg, an unanticipated difficult airway that may result in significant morbidity or death). Many complications are preventable with good preoperative preparation, but some are not preventable (unexpected drug reactions or metabolic crisis, eg, malignant hyperthermia). Four common complications are anesthesia awareness, peripheral nerve injury, malignant hyperthermia, and visual loss.

Awareness

Many patients are concerned about being aware during the surgical procedure. Intraoperative awareness under general anesthesia is rare with a reported incidence of 0.1–0.2%.

Intraoperative awareness does occur and can lead to significant psychological sequelae and extended disability for the patient. Certain types of surgery have a higher incidence of intraoperative awareness, including cardiac surgery, major trauma, and obstetrics. All are associated with critical or life threatening situations of hemodynamic compromise that make awareness unavoidable if the caregiver is to achieve other critical anesthetic goals of maintaining cardiac, respiratory, and vascular homeostasis. The Practice Advisory from the American Board of Anesthesiologists defines intraoperative awareness: "When a patient becomes conscious when a surgical procedure is performed under a general anesthetic and subsequently has (explicit) recall of these events." The Advisory notes that the recall does not include the time before the general anesthetic is induced or the time of intentional emergence and return to consciousness.

Strategies suggested to lessen or eliminate the risk of intraoperative awareness include the following:

1. Preoperative evaluation. Patients with a history of previous intraoperative awareness, substance abuse, chronic use of opioids for pain control, and limited hemodynamic reserve have increased risk for intraoperative awareness. Such patients undergoing high-risk operations should be informed of the potential for awareness. There is no consensus that informing all patients about the possibility of intraoperative awareness leads to higher incidence of awareness.

2. Preanesthesia preparation. A strict preoperative equipment checklist involving the anesthesia machine and its components, eg, the volatile anesthesia vaporizer agent levels, is mandatory. Although this strategy does not prevent human errors, it does provide the anesthesiologist a constant reminder that there are preventable components to the complication of awareness.

3a. Intraoperative monitoring. The currently accepted strategy is to utilize all the standard anesthesia patient monitors (EKG, blood pressure measurements, heart rate monitors, continuous agent analyzers, and capnography) and to intermittently assess for purposeful or reflex movement to detect intraoperative consciousness. There are instances in which there were no reported changes in vital signs in patients who have reported recall.

3b. Monitoring brain electrical activity. Several monitoring devices are claimed to be able to interpret data from the processed, raw electroencephalogram of patients and correlate it to the depth of anesthesia and thus help prevent recall under general anesthesia. The commonest device currently available is known as the bispectral index monitor (BIS; Aspect Medical Systems, Natick, MA). The BIS has engendered discussion among anesthesiologists, surgeons, hospital administrators, and patient advocacy groups. Currently, there is no consensus on the use of BIS for patients undergoing general anesthesia.

In conclusion, when awareness occurs, either reported spontaneously by the patient in the postoperative period or elicited during the postoperative visit by the anesthesiologist, the patient's report must be taken seriously. Telling the patient that recall was impossible or indicating that the patient may be making it up is not acceptable. Some patients will require significant counseling and treatment postoperatively, and caregivers should be sensitive to the potential issue and offer any help requested.

American Board of Anesthesiologists: Practice advisory for intraoperative awareness and brain function monitoring. Anesthesiology 2006;104:847.

Avidan MS et al: Anesthesia awareness and the bispectral index. N Engl J Med 2008;368:1097.

▶ Peripheral Nerve Injury

Peripheral nerve injury is a known complication of anesthesia and can occur under general anesthesia or a regional technique. These injuries are almost always due to patient positioning and the patient's inability to report and respond to abnormal pressure points or awkward position of an extremity. The ulnar nerve at the elbow is the most common injury and occurs even if the patient has had what was felt to be adequate padding provided for protection. Other peripheral nerves that are less commonly injured include the peroneal nerve at the knee and the radial nerve as it passes through the spiral grove of the humerus. The peroneal nerve is typically injured by abnormal position against a lithotomy stirrup, and the radial nerve is injured by a blood pressure cuff or abnormal pressure from surgical towels. Patients usually report numbness along the course of the nerve, but some motor weakness may also occur. These injuries usually resolve in a short time period. Abnormal stretching of the brachial plexus from extreme abduction of the arms, improperly placed shoulder braces, or chest wall retractors during cardiac surgery may result in more serious injuries, including not only sensory but motor loss that may not recover as rapidly or completely as the ulnar, radial, or peroneal nerves. More severe injuries that involve motor loss need to have a baseline examination established and therapy started. Since most of these peripheral nerve injuries are due to malpositioning during surgery, it is the responsibility of surgeons, nurses, and anesthesiologists to adequately position patients and provide sufficient padding or other protection.

Cheney FW et al: Nerve injury associated with anesthesia: a closed claims analysis. Anesthesiology 1999;90:1062.

▶ Malignant Hyperthermia

Malignant hyperthermia is a rare, genetically inherited disease characterized by intense muscle contraction. It results from an uncontrolled release of calcium from the sarcoplasmic reticulum and massive increase of intracellular calcium in skeletal muscle due to the inability of the calcium to be reabsorbed. This intense muscle contraction leads to a hypermetabolic state manifest by hyperthermia, hypercapnia, tachycardia, and metabolic acidosis. It is fatal if untreated. Malignant hyperthermia is commonly triggered by the administration of anesthetic agents; the commonest trigger is the depolarizing muscle relaxant succinylcholine alone or in conjunction with a volatile agent such as halothane. The more modern anesthetic vapors sevoflurane and desflurane are less frequently implicated as triggers. Early clinical manifestations of malignant hyperthermia include unexplained tachycardia and metabolic acidosis, but temperature elevation may be a late finding. Although not always reliable, the earliest sign of malignant hyperthermia is sometimes masseter spasm following the administration of succinylcholine during induction. Careful monitoring must always ensue. Relying on temperature elevation alone is dangerous, and arterial blood gases must be monitored for unexplained metabolic acidosis. In some patients, malignant hyperthermia develops insidiously during the surgery, and temperature elevation can be the first manifestation.

Malignant hyperthermia is treatable and preventable. The treatment of choice is intravenous dantrolene. Every operating room must have a malignant hyperthermia protocol and a kit that includes multiple doses of dantrolene. Dantrolene is supplied as a powder and requires several minutes to mix it into a useable intravenous solution. Malignant hyperthermia is a true anesthesia emergency, and the anesthesiologist will require assistance from the operative team. The surgical procedure may have to be postponed. Successful treatment of malignant hyperthermia is the usual outcome. Patients should be monitored in a critical care unit for 24 hours or until stable and referred for confirmatory testing.

Malignant hyperthermic reactions can be prevented. Any patient with a personal or family history of malignant hyperthermia should be administered a completely nontriggering anesthetic without relying on succinylcholine or volatile agents.

Heggie JE: Malignant hyperthermia: considerations for the general surgeon. Can J Surg 2002;45:369.

▶ Perioperative Visual Loss

A recently described complication of surgical procedures performed in the prone position, associated with large blood losses, is partial or complete visual loss. Vision loss seems to be associated with an ischemic optic neuropathy without any known etiology. The risk of visual loss should be discussed with patients in the preoperative phase of surgery and anesthesia for those operations that require prone positioning.

Ho VT et al: Ischemic Optic neuropathy following spine surgery. J Neurosurg Anesth 2005;17:38.

Lee LA et al: The American Society of Anesthesiologist postoperative visual loss registry: analysis of 93 spine surgery cases with postoperative visual loss. Anesthesiology 2006;105:652.

Shock & Acute Pulmonary Failure in Surgical Patients

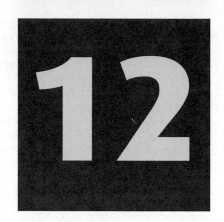

James W. Holcroft, MD

John T. Anderson, MD

Matthew J. Sena, MD

▼ I. INITIAL TREATMENT OF SHOCK

Cardiovascular failure, or shock, can be caused by (1) depletion of the vascular volume, (2) compression of the heart or great veins, (3) intrinsic failure of the heart itself or failure arising from excessive hindrance to ventricular ejection, (4) loss of autonomic control of the vasculature, (5) severe untreated systemic inflammation, and (6) severe but partially compensated systemic inflammation. If the shock is decompensated, the blood pressure or the cardiac output will be inadequate for peripheral perfusion; in compensated shock, the perfusion will be adequate but only at the expense of excessive demands on the heart. Depending on the type and severity of cardiovascular failure and on response to treatment, shock can go on to compromise other organ systems. This chapter discusses the cardiovascular and pulmonary disorders associated with shock.

HYPOVOLEMIC SHOCK

▶ Diagnosis

Hypovolemic shock (shock caused by inadequate circulating blood volume) is most often caused by bleeding but may also be a consequence of protracted vomiting or diarrhea, sequestration of fluid in the gut lumen (eg, bowel obstruction), or loss of plasma into injured or burned tissues. Regardless of the etiology, the compensatory responses, mediated primarily by the adrenergic nervous system, are the same: (1) constriction of the venules and small veins in the skin, fat, skeletal muscle, and viscera with displacement of blood from the peripheral capacitance vessels to the heart; (2) constriction of arterioles in the skin, skeletal muscle, gut, pancreas, spleen, and liver (but not the brain or heart); (3) improved cardiac performance through an increase in heart rate and contractility; and (4) increased sodium and water reabsorption through renin-angiotensin-aldosterone as well as vasopressin release. The result is improved cardiac filling, increased cardiac output (both directly by the increase in contractility and indirectly through increased end-diastolic volumes), and increased blood flow to organs with no or limited tolerance for ischemia (brain and heart).

The symptoms and signs of hypovolemic shock are many and can be caused either by the inadequate blood volume or by the compensatory responses. Some manifest themselves early, some late. One of the earliest signs is that of postural hypotension—a fall in the systolic blood pressure of more than 10 mm Hg that persists for more than 1 minute when the patient sits up. It can be very useful in patients who are suspected of being hypovolemic from either dehydration or occult internal blood loss (eg, in a patient who might have gastrointestinal bleeding). Other signs will have to be used, however, in very ill patients and in injured patients, who might not tolerate changes in position.

Another early sign can make itself known when the physician has difficulty in establishing intravenous access. In addition, the skin might be cold and pale. The pallor, which can be detected in all patients, including those with deeply pigmented skin, is best detected by compressing a toe to produce blanching on its plantar surface and then releasing the compression and watching for color return. In a normovolemic patient without peripheral vascular disease, the color should return within 2 seconds; in a hypovolemic patient, the refill takes longer. The test is usually done with the foot at the level of the heart, but if the patient is not badly injured, it is more sensitive if it can be done with the foot raised above the level of the heart, to a height of perhaps 30 cm.

Low filling pressures in the right atrium are always present in hypovolemic shock, even in cases of mild shock, assuming there is no accompanying cardiac compression, and can sometimes be detected by observation of the neck veins. Looking for collapsed neck veins is best done with the patient's head, neck, and torso elevated 30 degrees. A normal right atrial pressure will distend the neck veins to about 2 cm above the manubrium. Failure to see the veins suggests hypovolemia.

Oliguria is another consistent finding in early shock. A bladder catheter should be inserted in any patient suspected of being hypovolemic. Urine output is considered to be potentially inadequate if it is less than 0.5 mL/kg/h in an adult, less than 1 mL/kg/h in a child, or less than 2 mL/kg/h in an infant.

A decrease in hematocrit, as a result of blood loss, is delayed in the absence of exogenous fluid administration. Full restitution of the intravascular volume from the interstitium requires 1 or 2 days, in the absence of fluid administration. Intravascular volume expansion with blood-free fluids, such as isotonic crystalloid or plasma, results in a rapid drop in the hematocrit (within minutes) with the change proportional to the blood loss. For example, a hematocrit fall of 3–4% indicates that the blood volume was depleted by about 10%; a fall of 6–8% indicates a depletion of about 20% (or 1 L in an average adult). These calculations assume that the patient has been given enough fluid to correct the hypovolemia. It should also be noted that in the setting of dehydration, the hematocrit may be elevated and the proportional change in fluid loss is less predictable.

Hypovolemic shock is easier to recognize when it becomes more severe. In moderate cases (a deficit of 20–30% of the blood volume), the patient can be thirsty. Hypotension can be present, even in the supine position. A metabolic acidemia, usually with a compensatory rapid respiratory rate, can develop after initial resuscitation. (The acidemia is usually not present before resuscitation. The products of anaerobic metabolism in the ischemic tissues are only flushed into the circulating blood volume once some degree of reperfusion has been achieved.)

In profound hypovolemic shock (a deficit of more than 30% of blood volume), the blood pressure will always be low, even in the supine position. Cerebral and cardiac perfusion can become inadequate. Signs of the former include changes in mental status, restlessness, agitation, confusion, lethargy, or the appearance of inebriation; signs of the latter include an irregular heartbeat or electrocardiographic evidence of myocardial ischemia, such as ST–T segment depression and, over time, the appearance of Q waves. A metabolic acidemia will always be present, after initial resuscitation.

There are many pitfalls in making the diagnosis of hypovolemic shock, and every clinician will miss the diagnosis on occasion. In some patients, especially children and young adults, strong compensatory mechanisms can maintain the blood pressure at normal levels in the setting of mild to moderate shock. In other patients, one might not know if the observed pressure is abnormally low—a young patient might normally have systolic pressures in the low 100s; the same pressure in a chronically hypertensive patient might precede catastrophe. Pain-producing injuries in the absence of blood loss should produce hypertension; a normal pressure in a patient with a pain-producing injury suggests hypovolemia. Administration of a sedative or narcotic in the face of hypovolemia can produce hypotension but usually has no effect on the pressure in a normovolemic subject—one

should not ascribe hypotension to sedatives or narcotics until the possibility of hypovolemia has been ruled out.

The heart rate is notoriously unreliable as a sign of hypovolemic shock. Although the heart rate in anesthetized animals increases in response to graded hemorrhage, the correlation between hypovolemia and heart rate in unanesthetized human beings is poor. Unanesthetized hypovolemic human beings often have normal heart rates. Severe hypovolemia can even produce bradycardia, as the cardiovascular system makes a last attempt to allow filling of the ventricles during diastole. A normal heart rate provides no assurance that the patient is not in shock.

As last examples of pitfalls, the vasoconstriction of hypovolemic shock can be ablated by the vasodilation induced by alcohol or other pharmacologic agents, both therapeutic and recreational; the patient might have well-perfused skin even when hypovolemic. The oliguria of shock can be overcome by an osmotic diuresis induced by high blood alcohol or glucose levels. One should not ascribe alterations in mental status to possible drug use or alcoholic inebriation until one is certain there is no other problem; the alterations might be caused by inadequate cerebral blood flow, a preterminal event in the patient's response to shock.

▶ Treatment

A. Airway, Ventilation, Bleeding

Resuscitation of patients in hypovolemic shock, either hemorrhagic or nonhemorrhagic, begins with ensuring that the airway is secure, by demonstrating that ventilation and oxygenation are adequate, and, in the case of hemorrhagic shock, by controlling bleeding.

With regard to the airway, if there is any question, intubate. The physician cannot let uncertainty about the airway interfere with evaluation and resuscitation of other problems in the often confusing picture of shock. A patient who later turns out to need no support for the airway or ventilation can easily be extubated; failure to intubate a patient who later loses control of an airway or who can no longer ventilate means, at the least, an emergency intubation under difficult conditions and, at the worse, anoxic brain damage or death.

If the patient requires mechanical ventilation, and almost all patients intubated for shock do, volume control ventilation, or some variant thereof, is preferable. The ventilator is set up to minimize the mean airway pressure. The tidal volume is set at 7 mL/kg ideal body weight (IBW); the inspiratory time, at 1 second; the respiratory rate, at 15 breaths/min; and the end expiratory pressure, at 0 cm H_2O. To maintain adequate arterial oxygen saturation, the inspired oxygen concentration is set at 1.00. (The oxygen concentrations can be decreased later, after blood gases come back and the patient is more stable.)

Initial control of external bleeding is accomplished through the use of direct pressure or, in some cases, by tourniquet. Surgical control or direct clamping should not be attempted except in rare circumstances. Blind clamping can result in target vessel injury or, worse, adjacent venous laceration with increased bleeding. Commercially available tourniquets or improvised pneumatic tourniquets are easy to apply and are usually safe for periods of up to 2 hours, with the caveat that bleeding should be controlled quickly so as to minimize tourniquet time. In addition, several commercially available hemostatic agents ore approved for temporary control of external bleeding. Although experience has primarily been in prehospital and combat environments, they can be very effective in the hospital setting as well.

Cavitary hemorrhage from the chest or abdomen and bleeding from major musculoskeletal injuries require special consideration. Blood in the pleural cavities should be drained to stop further bleeding from the pulmonary parenchyma through apposition of the visceral and parietal pleurae and to reestablish ventilation through the compressed lung. Bleeding from pelvic fractures may require temporary binder placement. More definitive control can come later, with angiographic embolization or surgical control. Patients with intra-abdominal or intractable intrathoracic bleeding should be prepared for the operating room. Major long bone fractures should be immobilized.

B. Initial Fluid Resuscitation

Vascular access is best obtained with percutaneously placed, large-bore (ideally 14-gauge or larger) venous catheters. The catheters can be placed in superficial veins in the upper extremities, in central veins at the thoracic outlet, or in the femoral veins; catheters can also by placed in the saphenous veins, by cutdown, or directly into interosseus sites (sternum or tibia) using specially designed needle introducer systems (FAST-1, EZ IO). The major advantage of the later is the minimal training required to achieve successful access. Choice of access depends on severity of the shock, pattern of injury, and experience of the provider gaining the access. Patients in shock are at high risk for complications during central venous catheter placement because of venous collapse; the urgency of placement also predisposes to errors in technique. A pneumothorax or an unintentional arterial puncture in the unstable patient might prove fatal. If veins in the lower extremities are to be used, they must be decannulated within 24 hours to minimize the risk of thrombosis and infection.

Initial fluid resuscitation begins with a warmed crystalloid solution. Either normal saline or lactated Ringer solution can be used. Use of lactate in the resuscitative fluid is reasonable if the shock seems to be severe and if the arterial pH is likely to be less than 7.20. The lactate will buffer the hydrogen ions that are released into the central circulation with the initiation of resuscitation. The resultant lactic acid is then oxidized in the liver to carbon dioxide and water, which are excreted by the lungs and kidneys.

If the arterial pH is not likely to be excessively low, normal saline can be used as the initial resuscitative fluid. A modest hyperchloremic acidemia in the immediate postresuscitative state might favorably change the confirmation of albumin molecules, decreasing movement of plasma into the interstitium. The acidemia might also increase myocardial contractility.

Blood flow to the liver is not a factor in deciding on lactated Ringer versus normal saline. Even minimal flow, as in severe shock, will be enough to deliver the buffered hydrogen ion to the liver parenchyma. Lactated Ringer should not be used, however, if the patient has preexisting liver disease. Adequate oxidation requires functioning liver cells.

The rate at which the initial crystalloid resuscitation should be given depends on two factors: the severity of the shock and the presence of uncontrolled bleeding. When bleeding has been controlled (direct pressure or surgical control), resuscitation to normovolemia is the goal, and 2 L is given as fast as possible, followed by a third liter infused over 10 minutes if necessary. This amount of fluid will resuscitate most patients in whom hemorrhage has been arrested. If the patient is not resuscitated with this amount of fluid, one should renew the search for bleeding, which might be into the chest, abdomen, or retroperitoneum. In addition, one should begin to use blood products.

There is no general agreement about how much fluid should be given after the initial 3 L, especially in the patient who may have ongoing blood loss. Giving excessive amounts of crystalloid in an effort to restore the blood pressure to normal or supranormal levels will create edema. Edema in the gut can create an abdominal compartment syndrome, with compression of the inferior vena cava, displacement of the diaphragm into the chest, and compression of the heart and lungs; edema in the liver can lead to compression of biliary ductules and inability to excrete bilirubin into the gut; edema in the lungs can hinder ventilation and oxygenation; and edema in wounded tissues can hinder healing and the ability to fight off infection. Unnecessarily high pressures can also potentially exacerbate bleeding. On the other hand, inadequate resuscitation can leave the patient exposed to the many adverse late effects of prolonged shock, such as multiorgan failure.

The primary goal in fluid resuscitation for all forms of shock is the same: restoration of adequate end organ perfusion. Resuscitating to a brachial systolic pressure of 80 mm Hg or a radial pulse in the bleeding patient is reasonable until hemorrhage has been controlled. After the bleeding is controlled, a systolic pressure of 90 mm Hg might be reasonable. One must keep in mind, however, that using the blood pressure to define severity of shock or to assess the adequacy of resuscitation is hazardous. Young patients have a tremendous capacity to constrict their arterioles, especially in the skin and muscles. They can often maintain a normal pressure even in the face of continued shock. In the very old, the blood pressure goal should be higher to ensure a cushion of perfusion for the brain, heart, and other viscera that might be supplied by arteries obstructed by atherosclerosis. One must consider other variables, besides the blood pressure, in assessing restoration of adequate end-organ perfusion and should aim for normal peripheral perfusion, urine output, mental status, and acid base balance and for resolution of any signs of myocardial ischemia.

C. Blood Products

Transfusion therapy can be life saving, but it is not without risk. Transfusion reactions, transmission of bloodborne pathogens, acute lung injury, and immunomodulation can all arise from the administration of blood products. In the acutely bleeding patient, allogeneic packed red cells should be used when the estimated blood loss exceeds 1.5 L (30% of the blood volume), especially if there is the potential for ongoing bleeding or if the patient is at risk for having coronary artery disease (see Table 12–1). If blood has to be given and there is no time for a full crossmatch, type-specific uncrossmatched cells, which can usually be obtained within 10 minutes, are used. In treating mass casualties, type O, Rh-negative universal donor cells have the advantage of minimizing the chance of giving the wrong type of blood to a misidentified patient. Universal donor cells can also be used if there is not even enough time to type the patient's blood.

The volume of red blood cells to be transfused to a patient in hemorrhage depends on the indication for transfusion and on the clinical condition of the patient. In the case of a good response to the initial resuscitation with nonsanguineous fluids, one can withhold transfusion of red cells until hemorrhage has been controlled. On the other hand, red cells should be given promptly to any patient in hemorrhagic shock who does not respond to the initial 3 liters of crystalloid. In the case of profound shock with continued bleeding, 6 units or more should be given rapidly along with plasma, platelets, and cryoprecipitate, while obtaining control of the bleeding.

D. Correction of Coagulation Abnormalities

After severe trauma or major sepsis, many patients will demonstrate signs of intravascular coagulation, with prolonged clotting times, low platelet counts, decreased fibrinogen levels, and production of fibrin degradation products or fibrin monomers. Correction requires administration of fresh-frozen plasma and platelets, especially to patients who continue to bleed and to those with severe head injuries, in whom intracranial bleeding could be devastating. If the patient is not bleeding and is not at risk for a devastating consequence of rebleeding, one should not give procoagulant factors—they will only fuel the fire of systemic inflammation and coagulation.

Recombinant activated Factor VII for treatment of bleeding from trauma-induced coagulopathies and for control or prevention of intracranial bleeding has now become commonplace. Administration of doses between 80 and 100 mcg/kg is generally recommended for coagulopathy in trauma patients. Smaller doses may be useful for warfarin reversal in the setting of intracranial hemorrhage. Due to the mechanism of action, platelet and fibrinogen levels should be adequate at the time of administration.

E. Modalities to Be Avoided

There is no role for using colloid solutions in the setting of hypovolemic shock except when size and weight of the crystalloid solutions limit their availability, as in treating mass casualties or under wartime conditions. Under these circumstances, solutions containing hetastarch or hypertonic saline and dextran (HSD) can be used. Otherwise, colloids provide no benefit over crystalloid solutions, and they add to cost. Vasopressors should not be used in resuscitating neurologically intact hypovolemic patients, except in desperate situations for short periods while the vascular volume is reexpanded. The idea that vasopressors divert flow from nonessential organs to essential

Table 12–1. Hematocrit Triggers for Transfusion: Influence of Coronary Artery Disease (CAD), Environment in Which the Patient Is Being Treated (Emergency Department versus Intensive Care Unit), and Likelihood of Bleeding.

Coronary Artery Disease (CAD)	Environment	Likelihood of Bleeding	Desired Hematocrit
No	ICU	Unlikely	21%
No	ICU	Possible	21%
No	ED	Unlikely	24%
No	ED	Possible	27%
Yes	ICU	Unlikely	30%[1]
Yes	ICU	Possible	33%[2]
Yes	ED	Unlikely	36%[2]
Yes	ED	Possible	39%[2]

[1]Hematocrit values less than 30 may be sufficient in some patients with treated CAD when there is no risk of bleeding.
[2]Hematocrit values greater than 30 generally serve as a buffer for unanticipated or unmeasurable bleeding. They are not necessary in all patients with CAD.

organs is ill-conceived. Although some organs can withstand ischemia for longer periods of time than others, there are very few parts of the body that are not essential. Patients given vasopressors in shock are at risk for ischemic gangrene of the limbs, gut necrosis, liver failure, and acute tubular necrosis. Vasopressors, however, are often indicated in patients in neurogenic shock, because those patients may have lost critical physiological compensatory responses.

Elevation of the lower extremities above the level of the heart (Trendelenburg position) in a normovolemic subject shifts blood to the heart and increases ventricular end-diastolic volumes. In the hypovolemic patient, however, adrenergically mediated venoconstriction has likely already achieved this shift. Thus the position is of little value in treating hypovolemic shock, and its awkwardness can make evaluation and treatment of other problems more complicated. The position, however, is useful for the treatment of neurogenic shock.

In trauma patients, the pneumatic antishock garment can be useful for temporary compression of bleeding sites that cannot be controlled by other means, for temporary stabilization of pelvic fractures, and as a temporary expedient to increase the blood pressure during transport in patients in neurogenic shock. It has no other uses. It limits the physical examination. It precludes use of the veins in the lower part of the body as sites for venous access. It can hinder filling of the ventricles by compressing the inferior vena cava and the renal and hepatic veins. It can hinder left ventricular ejection by compressing the arterioles in the lower body. It can push the diaphragm into the chest and interfere with ventilation. It is of no use in displacing blood from the periphery to the heart in neurologically intact patients—discharge of the adrenergic system will already have achieved that goal.

CARDIAC COMPRESSIVE SHOCK

Diagnosis

Cardiac compressive shock can arise from any condition that compresses the heart or great veins, including pericardial tamponade, tension pneumothorax, massive hemothorax, rupture of the diaphragm with encroachment of abdominal viscera into the chest, and distention of the abdomen with compression of the intra-abdominal great veins and elevation of the diaphragm into the chest. All of these conditions are worsened if the patient has to be mechanically ventilated.

The signs of compressive shock are similar to those of hypovolemic shock—postural hypotension, poor cutaneous perfusion, oliguria, hypotension in the supine position, mental status changes, electrocardiographic signs of myocardial ischemia, metabolic acidemia, and hyperventilation—combined with distended neck veins. The only other type of shock that can produce the combination of poor perfusion associated with distended neck veins is cardiogenic shock, which rarely poses a problem in differential diagnosis. Cardiogenic shock usually develops against a background of evident disease that predisposes to primary myocardial dys-

function. Cardiac compression usually follows trauma or occurs in a setting where mechanical compromise of the heart or great veins can arise from imposition of external pressure (as in a possible pericardial tamponade).

The so-called paradoxic pulse is occasionally helpful in diagnosis. A spontaneous breath in a normovolemic subject without cardiac compression produces little effect on systemic blood pressure. If the heart is compressed, the systolic pressure can fall by more than 10 mm Hg. (In contrast, a fall in the blood pressure with positive-pressure ventilation is common and nonspecific, especially in hypovolemic patients; the concept of a paradoxic pulse applies only to patients who are breathing on their own.)

The diagnosis of cardiac compression is facilitated if the patient can be monitored in an intensive care unit (ICU) with a pulmonary artery catheter, when small stroke volumes in the face of high filling pressures can be documented by direct measurement. In addition, the catheter can be used to compare pressures in the left and right atria. Under normal circumstances, the pressure in the left atrium is about 5 mm Hg higher than in the right. In tamponade, the pressures are the same.

Treatment

Infusion of fluid can transiently overcome some of the ill effects of cardiac compression, but the cause of shock in these patients is mechanical, and definitive treatment must correct the mechanical abnormality. Pericardial tamponade, tension pneumothorax, massive hemothorax, intra-abdominal hypertension, and ruptured diaphragm are discussed in Chapter 13. Treatment of compressive shock caused by large-volume, high-pressure mechanical ventilation is discussed later in this chapter in the section on mechanical ventilation.

CARDIOGENIC SHOCK

Diagnosis

Cardiogenic shock can arise from several causes, including arrhythmias, ischemia-induced myocardial failure, valvular or septal defects, systemic or pulmonary hypertension, myocarditis, and myocardiopathies. Of all the forms of shock, it can be the most resistant to treatment. If the heart cannot pump, there may be nothing that can be done. On the other hand, in less severe cases, it is possible to improve the efficiency of the pumping capability that remains.

The diagnosis of cardiogenic shock usually depends on recognizing an underlying medical condition predisposing the heart to dysfunction in conjunction with an abnormal electrocardiogram. Given the relative oxygen demands of the left and right ventricles, shock caused by left ventricular failure is much more common in patients with ischemic heart disease and typically presents with chest pain, a third heart sound, rales, ST segment elevation on a 12-lead electrocardiogram, and, on chest film, an enlarged heart or pulmonary edema. Cardiogenic shock may be associated with distended neck veins if the right ventricle has failed, unless the patient is also hypovolemic, as in a bleeding patient with a recent myocardial infarction. In many cases, patients with recent shock or trauma may have mild to moderate forms of right ventricular dysfunction related primarily to the heart's response to systemic inflammation or markedly elevated ventilator pressures. Right-sided dysfunction can be associated with peripheral edema, an enlarged and tender liver, and, on chest film, an enlarged heart. The diagnosis is usually easy, but two common situations may pose a problem.

The first is a ruptured abdominal aortic aneurysm in a patient with coronary artery disease. The patient might have abdominal pain consistent with a myocardial infarction and electrocardiographic signs of ischemia—the ischemia being caused by hypovolemia and shock. The key is to observe the neck veins.

The second is to ascribe shock to myocardial contusion in a patient who has just suffered a blunt injury to the chest. Although blunt chest trauma can damage the heart, the damage is usually either fatal, with death at the scene of the injury, or, more often, of no clinical significance. A contusion that produces failure but not death is rare. Shock after blunt trauma in a patient who survives to reach the hospital is almost never caused by contusion—it is far more likely to be caused by hypovolemia or by a mechanical problem.

▶ Treatment

A. Arrhythmias

Hypotension in a patient with a heart rate less than 50 beats/min deserves treatment, even if the ventricular contractions are well coordinated. One should begin with the intravenous administration of atropine, at a dose of 0.5 mg, repeated at 2-minute intervals for a maximum dose of 2 mg. If the rate remains slow and the patient is still unstable, the heart should be paced by transvenous or external means.

Several factors must be considered when deciding on treatment for tachycardia. Maximal ventricular rate declines with age (220 age in years), and the maximal aerobic rate is 60–80% of this value depending on the physical condition of the patient and the presence or absence of ischemic heart disease. For example, a healthy 20-year-old man in good condition should be able to tolerate and sustain a heart rate of 160 (80% of 200) without difficulty (although one should search for the cause of the tachycardia). On the other hand, a 65-year-old man with known coronary stenosis may have a myocardial aerobic threshold of 93 beats/min: $(220\ 65) \times 0.6$. Too rapid rates put the patient at risk for ischemia regardless of origin (sinus vs. nonsinus) or etiology (hypovolemic or cardiogenic shock).

Moribund patients with a tachyarrhythmia should undergo synchronized cardioversion using a monophasic or newer biphasic defibrillator. This should be distinguished from unsynchronized defibrillation indicated in the setting of ventricular fibrillation or pulseless ventricular tachycardia. One hundred joules should be used initially. If unsuccessful, the energy should be rapidly escalated to 360 J. The cardioversion takes precedence over securing the airway, and it takes precedence over obtaining vascular access; it even takes precedence over making a precise diagnosis of the arrhythmia.

Cardioversion in the moribund patient can result in full cardiac function with normal blood supply to the brain in a matter of seconds. No other treatment has this potential. It is the treatment of choice for coarse ventricular fibrillation, ventricular tachycardia, and for supraventricular arrhythmias with unsustainably rapid ventricular responses.

Cardioversion is of no value if it turns out that the patient was in asystole or had a fine ventricular fibrillation. But then no treatment for these arrhythmias has a chance of achieving resuscitation with full neurological function. Nothing will be gained with cardioversion in these patients, but nothing will have been lost.

Treatment of any nonmoribund patient with a tachycardia begins with ensuring euvolemia and treating other possible extracardiac causes of a tachycardia (such as fever, stress, pain, and anxiety) followed by pharmacologic rate control or pharmacological cardioversion, the latter decision depending on ventricular conduction.

The nonmoribund patient with a tachyarrhythmia associated with abnormal ventricular conduction should be cardioverted. Treatment after successful cardioversion will usually require consultation.

In the nonmoribund patient with normal ventricular conduction but not atrial fibrillation, the rate can be controlled with a calcium channel blocker and, as needed, a beta-blocker.

If ventricular conduction is normal and the patient is in atrial fibrillation, and if it is thought that the fibrillation is going to be of long duration, and if the patient needs an atrial kick, conversion can be attempted with amiodarone, which can be used to keep the rate in a desirable range. It is preferable, however, to avoid the use of amiodarone if the patient does not need an atrial kick. The drug depresses myocardial contractility and has a long half-life. Its effects can last for weeks. In most patients in atrial fibrillation, rate control, rather than conversion of the rhythm to a sinus rhythm, is the critical issue. In these circumstances, initial treatment can be with diltiazem, a short-acting calcium channel blocker, which can be given as a bolus followed by a continuous infusion. Alternatively, verapamil can be used if a longer acting agent is desired. The major side effect of these agents is depression of myocardial contractility. Digoxin, a sodium potassium ATPase inhibitor, slows atrioventricular (AV) conduction and may increase contractility. It should be considered for rate control if ventricular systolic function is compromised. It is administered as a loading dose of 0.5 g intravenously, followed by 0.25 g every 6 hours for two additional doses (total of 1.0 g). Daily maintenance doses are needed, and the serum levels should be measured along with serum electrolyte monitoring. Beta-adrenergic blocking agents are another class of antiarrhythmics that can be used for short-term and long-term rate control. All three classes of drugs slow AV nodal conduction. Their use in combination should be done in a closely monitored setting. Complete heart block is a potentially disastrous side effect.

B. Opioids

Opioids can be especially effective in treating cardiac failure after myocardial infarction. They relieve pain, provide sedation, block adrenergic discharge to the arterioles, block discharge to the venules and small veins, redistribute the blood from the atria and ventricles to the venous capacitance vessels in the periphery, and decrease myocardial oxygen requirements.

C. Diuretics

Diuretics are the keystone of therapy in congestive heart failure with large ventricular end-diastolic volumes. By decreasing vascular volume, diuretics decrease atrial pressures and mobilize peripheral and pulmonary edema. Pulmonary vascular pressures and volumes decrease; effectiveness of right ventricular contraction increases. Coronary blood flow increases as coronary sinus pressure drops. Decreasing pressures in the ventricles during diastole, when the ventricular muscle receives its nutrient blood flow, alleviates compression of the coronary vasculature in the endocardium. Decreasing pressures in the right atrium decreases the stiffness of the coronary vasculature, which decreases the stiffness of the ventricles during diastole (the garden hose effect). The ventricular end-diastolic volumes potentially can increase without much of an associated increase in the end-diastolic pressures.

D. Beta-Blockers

Almost all patients in cardiac failure with ischemia and a rapid heart rate will benefit from a beta-adrenergic blocking agent (eg, esmolol or metoprolol). Decreasing the rate and reducing ventricular stiffness during systole decreases myocardial oxygen requirements. Increasing time in diastole and decreasing ventricular stiffness during diastole augments ventricular filling and increases efficiency of ventricular contraction. All of these effects reduce myocardial oxygen consumption and potentially salvage marginal myocardium. In many patients, the reduced oxygen requirements can be achieved with only minimal loss of energy output from the ventricles. The only contraindication to the use of beta-blockers, beyond the rare development of bronchospasm with administration of the drugs, is hypotension. This latter problem is easily monitored.

E. Vasodilators

Hypertension is unusual but not unheard of in patients with cardiogenic shock. The hypertension is usually associated with inefficient delivery of energy into the aortic root. Treatment should begin with opioids, if the patient is in pain, and then diuresis, if the ventricular end-diastolic volumes are large. Nitroprusside and nitroglycerin are the most useful short-term vasodilators in surgical patients in heart failure (besides opioids). Both drugs act quickly and are easy to monitor; both dilate the systemic arterioles; nitroglycerin also dilates the systemic venules and small veins. For long-term control of pressure, angiotensin-converting enzyme (ACE) inhibitors and calcium channel blockers should be used in place of the nitrates. If the patient has a tachycardia or, as may well be the case, if the patient is at risk for having coronary artery disease or myocardial ischemia, beta-blockade can be used.

Beneficial consequences of controlling the pressure include mobilization of edema, both pulmonary and systemic; enhanced perfusion of the myocardium; reduction of ventricular work and oxygen requirements and, consequently, relief of myocardial ischemia. On the other hand, excessive venous dilation can decrease cardiac filling enough so that stroke volumes and blood pressures fall; excessive arteriolar dilation can make the pressures fall further.

F. Inotropic Agents

Inotropic agents, such as dobutamine or milrinone, can increase cardiac output in some, but not all, patients in cardiogenic shock. Inotropic agents almost always result in increased myocardial oxygen requirements, but this is not usually a problem. Patients receiving the agents should be monitored in an ICU. Development of chest pain or ischemic electrocardiogram changes suggest that oxygen demand is exceeding supply. If it is necessary to use inotropic agents for more than 1 hour, a pulmonary artery catheter should be inserted. Systemic arterial pressures, atrial filling pressures, and cardiac output should be determined at different infusion rates. If any question remains about the adequacy of volume resuscitation, cardiovascular parameters should be measured before and after a fluid bolus is given.

Digitalis compounds should not be used in acute cardiac failure except to control ventricular rates in patients with supraventricular tachydysrhythmias. Toxicity may develop, especially when pH and electrolyte changes are unpredictable. The inotropic actions of digitalis are no different from those of dopamine and milrinone.

G. Chronotropic Agents

Although uncommon in the surgical setting, patients with cardiac failure and a low heart rate (< 70) may temporarily benefit from the administration of a chronotropic agent, such as dopamine. (Isoproterenol is almost never used nowadays.) When using dopamine, the heart rate should be increased only to levels that can be tolerated comfortably. A

60-year-old patient with normal coronary arteries gains little with a heart rate that exceeds 120 beats/min; the limit is about 90 beats/min in the presence of coronary artery disease. In most cases, however, the price to be paid for using a chronotropic agent exceeds the potential benefit. Chronotropic agents increase myocardial work and oxygen requirements and shorten the time during diastole for coronary blood flow and ventricular filling. They should be used only as a temporary expedient. If they are used for more than 30 minutes, a pulmonary arterial catheter should be inserted. The goal of therapy is a normal or slightly supranormal cardiac output that provides adequate end-organ perfusion and reverses shock. Trying to achieve more than that only increases the risk of myocardial ischemia.

H. Vasoconstrictors

A vasoconstrictor is occasionally useful to increase coronary perfusion pressure in the setting of coronary stenoses. To be effective, the agent must increase aortic pressure enough so that the increased myocardial perfusion compensates for the increase in the myocardial oxygen requirements.

The major untoward effect of these agents is ischemic necrosis of noncardiac organs, such as the extremities or intestine. They will not increase perfusion to the brain in the setting of cardiogenic shock, assuming that the carotid arteries are open and that the patient has a functioning adrenergic nervous system. The endogenous adrenergic nervous system is ideally suited for ensuring adequate blood flow to the brain. Constrictors should be used only when absolutely necessary and for no more than 60 minutes unless a pulmonary arterial catheter is in place.

I. Transaortic Balloon Pump

The transaortic balloon pump decreases the hindrance that the left ventricle faces when it ejects its blood into the aortic root and can be very effective in resuscitating selected patients with severe reversible left ventricular dysfunction (eg, after cardiopulmonary bypass or acute myocardial infarction). It should be used only if a pulmonary arterial catheter is in place.

J. Extracorporeal Membrane Oxygenation

Extracorporeal membrane oxygenation is most often used in conditions in which one can expect cardiac function to recover within a matter of a few days. Bleeding complications make it impractical for periods exceeding that time.

K. Operative Correction

Although listed last, surgically correctable cardiac conditions should be identified and corrected early, prior to the development of irreversible organ dysfunction. Ruptured valves, occluded arteries, aneurysmal ventricular walls, and certain arrhythmias are examples of potentially correctable lesions.

In these cases, early cardiac surgical consultation should be the rule.

NEUROGENIC SHOCK

▶ Diagnosis

Shock caused by failure of the autonomic nervous system can arise from regional or general anesthetics, injuries to the spinal cord, or administration of autonomic blocking agents. The venules and small veins lose tone, worsened by paralysis of surrounding skeletal muscles. Blood pools in the periphery, ventricular end-diastolic volumes decrease, and stroke volumes and blood pressure fall. Loss of arteriolar tone in the denervated areas makes the pressure fall further. If the lesion is below the midthoracic sympathetic outflow (approximately T6), activation of the cardiac adrenergic nerves will increase the heart rate and augment ventricular systolic function; if the lesion is more cephalad, the heart will not be able to compensate. Cardiovascular decompensation in neurogenic shock can be profound.

The diagnosis rests on knowledge of the circumstances preceding the onset of shock and on the physical examination. The patient will always be hypotensive, and the skin will be warm and flushed in the denervated areas. The cause is usually obvious.

Nonfatal head injury—in contrast to spinal cord injury—does not produce neurogenic shock or any other kind of shock. In fact, increased intracranial pressure typically increases blood pressure and slows the heart rate (Cushing reflex). Hypotension and tachycardia should never be attributed to head injury—even severe head injury with cerebral dysfunction—until hypovolemia has been ruled out. It is a tragedy to ascribe shock to a head injury when the problem is bleeding from a ruptured spleen.

▶ Treatment

Trendelenburg position, if it does not complicate other aspects of care, is useful. Intravenous fluids to fill the dilated venules and small veins should be given. Vasoconstrictors should be used if fluids and Trendelenburg position are not enough. Norepinephrine and phenylephrine are good choices if the heart rate is rapid. Dopamine is a good choice if the heart rate is slow.

The primary purpose of vasoconstricting agents in this setting is to restore tone in the venules and small veins; a secondary goal is to constrict dilated arterioles. The blood pressure should be increased to the point that coronary perfusion is sustained—as judged by normal ST–T segments on electrocardiography and absence of chest pain—and to the point that perfusion to the brain and spinal cord is supported. The pressure also has to be high enough to perfuse organs with preexisting obstructing proximal arterial lesions. These patients should be placed in the ICU for both neurologic and hemodynamic monitoring. If vasoconstrictors are used for more than several hours, or if the patient is at high risk for bleeding from multisystem trauma, central venous pressure monitoring or a pulmonary arterial catheter should be employed.

LOW-OUTPUT INFLAMMATORY SHOCK

▶ Diagnosis

Bowel perforation, intestinal necrosis, abscesses, gangrene, and soft tissue infections can produce low-output inflammatory shock, as can ischemia-reperfusion and inadequate resuscitation of massive injuries or large burns. The cytokinemia arising from the systemic inflammation can disrupt the microvascular endothelium and prompt the loss of plasma into the interstitium. The shock mimics the clinical picture of severe hypovolemic shock, with signs of adrenergic discharge, oliguria, obtundation, and metabolic acidemia. The EKG may show signs of ischemia. Hyperthermia or hypothermia may be present. The diagnosis is usually clear from the clinical circumstances.

▶ Treatment

Treatment consists of administration of intravenous fluids and antibiotics, correction of gastrointestinal leaks, debridement of dead tissue, and drainage of pus. The patient should be transferred to an ICU. Vasoconstrictors can be given for very short periods of time if the hypotension is so profound that it threatens the brain, the heart, or an organ with an obstructed arterial supply. Inotropes can be used more liberally, while the vascular volume is being replenished, but even then they should not be given for more than an hour unless the patient has a Swan-Ganz catheter in place. Successful volume expansion will convert the low-output inflammatory shock into a high-output state.

HIGH-OUTPUT INFLAMMATORY SHOCK

▶ Diagnosis

High-output inflammatory shock can precede low-output inflammatory shock or can be the result of successful treatment of low-output shock. The shock usually, but not always, is associated with a fever. The patient is hypotensive with warm, well-perfused extremities, as the body attempts to control its core temperature by off-loading heat to the environment. If a pulmonary arterial catheter is placed, the cardiac output is found to be high, assuming that the ventricular end-diastolic volumes have been brought back to normal levels. The outputs will remain high, occasionally as high as twice normal, as long as the inflammatory state persists. The oxygen consumption may be increased by a factor of 1.5.

▶ Treatment

Treatment consists of control of the underlying cause and fluid administration. Inotropes may be useful. If large amounts of fluids are necessary for the resuscitation and if inotropes are being considered, a Swan-Ganz catheter should be inserted. The goal is to perfuse the inflamed tissues with adequate power so that the product of the cardiac output and the mean arterial pressure is normal. In many patients, the result will be a cardiac output that is increased by a factor of 1.5 with a blood pressure that is decreased to a value that is two thirds of normal. As in other forms of shock, the pressure has to be high enough to perfuse the heart and brain and organs with potentially obstructed arteries, but it does not have to be normal. Vasoconstrictors can be dangerous, potentially leading to necrosis of the limbs, the gut, and the kidneys, especially if there is any degree of hypovolemia. They should not be used unless the clinician is positive that both the right and left ventricular end-diastolic volumes are normally expanded.

American College of Surgeons: *ATLS: Advanced Trauma Life Support Student Manual*. American College of Surgeons, 2004.

Beekley AC, Starnes BW, Sebesta JA: Lessons learned from modern military surgery. Surg Clin North Am 2007;87:57.

Bernard GR, Vincent JL, Laterre PF: Efficacy and safety of recombinant human activated protein C for severe sepsis. N Engl J Med 2001;344:699.

Bickell WH et al: Immediate versus delayed fluid resuscitation for hypotensive patients with penetrating torso injuries. N Engl J Med 1994;331:1105.

Brown MA, Daya MR, Worley JA: Experience with Chitosan dressings in a civilian EMS System. J Emerg Med 2007;Epub ahead of print.

Calkins MD et al: Intraosseous infusion devices: a comparison for potential use in special operations. J Trauma 2000;48:1068.

Carson JL et al: Mortality and morbidity in patients with very low postoperative Hb levels who decline blood transfusion. Transfusion 2002;42:812.

Chan PS et al, American Heart Association National Registry of Cardiopulmonary Resuscitation Investigators: Delayed time to defibrillation after in-hospital cardiac arrest. N Engl J Med 2008;358:9.

Chang MC et al: Effects of abdominal decompression on cardiopulmonary function and visceral perfusion in patients with intra-abdominal hypertension. J Trauma 1998;44:440.

Chang MC et al: Maintaining survivors' values of left ventricular power output during shock resuscitation: a prospective pilot study. J Trauma 2000;49:26.

Chang MC et al: Redefining cardiovascular performance during resuscitation: ventricular stroke work, power, and the pressure-volume diagram. J Trauma 1998;45:470.

Ciesla DJ et al: Hypertonic saline attenuation of polymorphonuclear neutrophil cytotoxicity: timing is everything. J Trauma 2000;48:388.

Cotton BA et al: The cellular, metabolic, and systemic consequences of aggressive fluid resuscitation strategies. Shock 2006;26:115.

Croce MA et al: Emergent pelvic fixation in patients with exsanguinating pelvic fractures. J Am Coll Surg 2007;204:935.

Demetriades D et al: Relative bradycardia in patients with traumatic hypotension. J Trauma 1998;45:534.

Diebel LN, Tyburski JG, Dulchavsky SA: Effect of acute hemodilution on intestinal perfusion and intramucosal pH after shock. J Trauma 2000;49:800.

Doyle, GS, Taillac PP: Tourniquets: a review of current use with proposals for expanded prehospital use. Prehosp Emerg Care 2008;12:241.

Eastridge BJ et al: Hypotension begins at 110 mm Hg: redefining "hypotension" with data. J Trauma 2007;63:291.

Finfer S et al: A comparison of albumin and saline for fluid resuscitation in the intensive care unit. N Engl J Med 2004;350:2247.

Fleisher LA, Eagle KA: Clinical practice. Lowering cardiac risk in noncardiac surgery. N Engl J Med 2001;345:1677.

Forsythe SM, Schmidt GA: Sodium bicarbonate for the treatment of lactic acidosis. Chest 2000;117:260.

Gattinoni L et al: A trial of goal-oriented hemodynamic therapy in critically ill patients. SvO$_2$ Collaborative Group. N Engl J Med 1995;333:1025.

Gore DC et al: Influence of glucose kinetics on plasma lactate concentration and energy expenditure in severely burned patients. J Trauma 2000;49:673.

Gunst, MA, Minei JP: Transfusion of blood products and nosocomial infection in surgical patients. Curr Opin Crit Care 2007;13:428.

Hébert PC et al: A multicenter, randomized, controlled clinical trial of transfusion requirements in critical care. Transfusion Requirements in Critical Care Investigators, Canadian Critical Care Trials Group. N Engl J Med 1999;340:409.

Heughan C, Grislis G, Hunt TK: The effect of anemia on wound healing. Ann Surg 1974;179:163.

Ho HS, Liu H, Cala PM, Anderson SE: Hypertonic perfusion inhibits intracellular Na and Ca accumulation in hypoxic myocardium. Am J Physiol Cell Physiol 2000;278:C953.

Holcomb JB: Use of recombinant activated factor VII to treat the acquired coagulopathy of trauma. J Trauma 2005;58:1298.

Human albumin administration in critically ill patients: systematic review of randomised controlled trials. Cochrane Injuries Group Albumin Reviewers. BMJ 1998;317:235.

Jonsson K et al: Tissue oxygenation, anemia, and perfusion in relation to wound healing in surgical patients. Ann Surg 1991;214:605.

Kraut EJ et al: Right ventricular volumes overestimate left ventricular preload in critically ill patients. J Trauma 1997;42:839.

Macnab A et al: A new system for sternal intraosseous infusion in adults. Prehosp Emerg Care 2000;4:173.

Martin MJ et al: Discordance between lactate and base deficit in the surgical intensive care unit: which one do you trust? Am J Surg 2006;191:625.

Miller PR, JW Meredith, MC Chang: Randomized, prospective comparison of increased preload versus inotropes in the resuscitation of trauma patients: effects on cardiopulmonary function and visceral perfusion. J Trauma 1998;44:107.

Perdue PW et al: "Renal dose" dopamine in surgical patients: dogma or science? Ann Surg 1998;227:470.

Rivers E et al: Early goal-directed therapy in the treatment of severe sepsis and septic shock. N Engl J Med 2001;345:1368.

Shenkin HA et al: On the diagnosis of hemorrhage in man: a study of volunteers bled large amounts. Amer J Med 1944;208:421.

Sibbald WJ et al: The Trendelenburg position: hemodynamic effects in hypotensive and normotensive patients. Crit Care Med 1979;7:218.

Spinella PC et al: The effect of recombinant activated factor VII on mortality in combat-related casualties with severe trauma and massive transfusion. J Trauma 2008;64:286.

Ursic C, Harken HA: Critical care: acute cardiac dysrhythmia. ACS Surgery: Principles & Practice, pp. 1462-1475.WebMed Inc., 2006.

Velmahos GC et al: Endpoints of resuscitation of critically injured patients: normal or supranormal? A prospective randomized trial. Ann Surg 2000;232:409.

Victorino GP, Battistella FD, Wisner DH: Does tachycardia correlate with hypotension after trauma? J Am Coll Surg 2003;196:679.

Wade CE et al: Individual patient cohort analysis of the efficacy of hypertonic saline/dextran in patients with traumatic brain injury and hypotension. J Trauma 1997;42(5 Suppl):S61.

Wakai A et al: Pneumatic tourniquets in extremity surgery. J Am Acad Orthop Surg 2001;9:345.

Wedmore I et al: A special report on the chitosan-based hemostatic dressing: experience in current combat operations. J Trauma 2006;60:655.

II. INITIAL TREATMENT OF ACUTE PULMONARY FAILURE

DIAGNOSIS OF PULMONARY FAILURE IN SURGICAL PATIENTS

Most causes of pulmonary failure in the surgical patient can be ascribed to one or more of nine causes: the pulmonary failure of shock, trauma, and sepsis; mechanical failure caused by deranged respiratory system mechanics; atelectasis; aspiration; pulmonary contusion; pneumonia; pulmonary embolism; cardiogenic pulmonary edema; and, rarely, neurogenic pulmonary edema.

The pulmonary failure of shock, trauma, and sepsis arises from extrapulmonary trauma, infection, or ischemia-reperfusion in the setting of shock. Products of coagulation and inflammation are washed out from the damaged tissues and carried to the lungs (or to the liver, in the case of the splanchnic circulation, and from there to the lungs), where they set up an acute inflammatory reaction. The extrapulmonary causes are many and range from necrotizing infections to noninfective inflammatory responses (such as pancreatitis) to reperfusion of ischemic limbs to soft tissue injury to broken bones (and embolism of fat and clot from the bone marrow—the so-called fat embolism syndrome, now an outdated term). Nothing is gained by making a distinction between it and the more general concept of pulmonary failure of shock and trauma.

The concept of pulmonary failure secondary to extrapulmonary ischemia-reperfusion, coagulation, and inflammation, which is common in surgical patients, can be subsumed into a broader category of pulmonary failure, known as the **acute respiratory distress syndrome** (ARDS). ARDS is defined by the sudden onset of hypoxemia with bilateral infiltrates, a PaO$_2$:FIO$_2$ less than 200 and the absence of left atrial hypertension (a pulmonary arterial wedge pressure < 18 if measured). A less severe form, acute lung injury (ALI) requires a PaO$_2$:FIO$_2$ less than 300 with the other criteria.

The causes of ARDS include those that are responsible for pulmonary failure of shock, trauma, and sepsis and also include severe pneumonia and aspiration. The end result in all of these conditions is activation of macrophages and other inflammatory cells in the lungs. The mediators disrupt the microvascular endothelium, and plasma extravasates into the interstitium and, in the case of the lungs, into the alveoli. The resultant pulmonary edema impairs both ventilation and oxygenation; the microembolization to the lungs impairs perfusion. Arterial oxygen saturation decreases and carbon dioxide content increases—assuming that no compensatory mechanisms come into play. Lastly, to make things worse, the inflammatory process in the lungs releases mediators into the systemic circulation that can lead to inflammation and dysfunction in the liver, gut, and kidneys.

A number of different mediators of coagulation and inflammation have been implicated as causes of the increased permeability. Proteases, kinins, complement, oxygen radicals, prostaglandins, thromboxanes, leukotrienes, lysosomal enzymes, and other mediators are released from aggregates of platelets and white cells or from the endothelium or plasma as a consequence of the interaction between the aggregates and the vessel wall. Some of these substances are chemoattractants of more platelets and white blood cells, and a vicious cycle of inflammation develops that worsens the disruption of the vascular endothelium.

Pathologically, ARDS (and the pulmonary failure of shock, trauma, and sepsis) is characterized by diffuse alveolar damage and a nonspecific inflammatory reaction, with the loss of alveolar epithelium and hyaline membrane formation. Monocytes and neutrophils invade the interstitium. Edema appears within a few hours, alveolar flooding is florid within 1 day, and fibrosis begins in 1–2 weeks. If the process is unchecked, the lungs become sodden and resemble liver tissue on gross inspection; scar tissue appears within a week, and function-limiting fibrosis begins to develop within 2 weeks. If early treatment is effective, the lungs return to normal, both grossly and microscopically.

Mechanical failure can arise from chest wall trauma, pain and weakness after surgery and anesthesia, debility caused by the catabolic metabolism of long-term illness, or bronchopleural fistula. Massive trauma to the chest with multiple fractures of multiple ribs or bilateral disruption of the costochondral junctions can result in a free-floating segment of chest wall known as a **flail chest.** Expansion and relaxation of the chest wall during spontaneous breathing results in paradoxic motion of the free segment in response to changes in intrathoracic pressure; ventilation becomes compromised; and the partial pressure of arterial carbon dioxide ($PaCO_2$) increases. In addition, hypoventilation leads to progressive atelectasis and hypoxemia. Lesser degrees of chest wall injury can lead to hypoventilation secondary to pain with similar results. Prolonged mechanical ventilation with loss of muscle mass and power in the diaphragm and the accessory muscles of respiration can require ventilatory support until muscle function returns to normal. A bronchopleural fistula—a communication from the airway to the pleural cavity to the atmosphere, either through a chest tube or through a hole in the chest wall—can develop after pulmonary surgery, trauma, or infection. Large air leaks can compromise ventilation to the uninvolved lung as well as to the diseased side because insufflated air preferentially goes to the side with the fistula.

Atelectasis—localized collapse of alveoli—can develop with prolonged immobilization, as during anesthesia or in association with bed rest. The problem is usually full blown within a few hours after the initiating event. Only mechanical failure (to which it is related), aspiration, cardiogenic pulmonary edema, and pulmonary embolism can produce equivalent levels of hypoxemia so soon, and no other cause of hypoxemia can respond so quickly to therapy. The diagnosis is supported by auscultation of bronchial breath sounds at dependent portions of the lung and occasionally, if severe enough, by x-ray confirmation of platelike collapse of pulmonary parenchyma. The most reliable confirmation of the diagnosis, however, comes with response to therapy, which can include encouragement of deep breathing and coughing, ambulation, bronchoscopy, and intubation and mechanical ventilation. Atelectasis should respond within a few hours.

Aspiration of gastric contents or blood can occur in any patient who cannot protect the airway. Shock, severe brain injury, or pharmacologic depression (anesthesia, narcotics, or benzodiazepines) can result in a depressed level of consciousness and loss of airway protective reflexes. Gastric acid or particulate matter in the airways leads to disruption of the alveolar and microvascular membranes, causing interstitial and alveolar edema. The resultant hypoxemia is usually evident within a few hours and is associated with a localized infiltrate on x-ray. Recovery of gastric contents by suctioning from the endotracheal tree confirms the diagnosis.

Pulmonary contusion arises from direct trauma to the chest wall and the underlying lung parenchyma. Hypoxemia associated with a localized infiltrate on x-ray develops over 24 hours as the injured lung becomes edematous.

Pneumonia can arise primarily or may be superimposed on aspiration, pulmonary contusion, or the pulmonary failure of shock, trauma, and sepsis. The diagnosis is made by recovery of bacteria and purulent material from the endotracheal tree, hypoxemia, signs of systemic inflammation, and a localized infiltrate on x-ray. The Clinical Pulmonary Infection Score (CPIS), which is derived from these parameters, can be used to quantify the clinical, radiographic, and laboratory findings of pneumonia. It is useful both for diagnosis and for determining length of treatment. Bronchoalveolar lavage and quantitative culture may occasionally be used to assist in distinguishing pneumonia from ARDS and other causes of pulmonary inflammation.

Pulmonary embolism typically presents with sudden deterioration of pulmonary function 3 days or more after an event—such as an operation, injury, or the beginning of immobilization—that can stimulate deposition of clot in a large systemic vein. Patients with cancer are at particularly high risk, and in any patient the greater the magnitude of operation or injury, the greater the chance of venous thrombosis and embolization. Clot emboli must be organized to be clinically significant; embolism to the lung of fresh soft clot rarely causes any difficulty. The pulmonary endothelium contains potent fibrinolysins that can break up any poorly organized embolus. Sudden deterioration in pulmonary function sooner than 3 days after an event that stimulates clot formation is unlikely to be caused by an embolus; the deterioration is more likely to be caused by mechanical failure, atelectasis, aspiration, or pneumonia.

The chest film is usually nonspecific. A fairly definite diagnosis can often be made by high-definition contrast enhanced computed tomograms of the pulmonary vasculature. The study requires transfer to the radiology suite and the use of large amounts of radiographic contrast material. Pulmonary arteriography carries the same risks—transfer to the radiology suite and use of contrast—and requires right-heart catheterization, but it does have advantages. It gives a definitive diagnosis with one test. At the end of the diagnostic study, an indwelling catheter can be placed proximal to the clot and used for infusion of lytic agents. If needed, a filter can be placed in the inferior vena at the end of the study, before the patient leaves the angiography suite.

Cardiogenic pulmonary edema arises from high left atrial and pulmonary microvascular hydrostatic pressures. Patients who have suffered an acute myocardial infarction can present this way, as can patients with underlying myocardial or coronary artery disease when faced with fluid shifts and surgical stress. Occasionally, the rapid administration of intravenous fluid—especially in elderly patients with poor myocardial performance—will outstrip the heart's ability to pump, and pulmonary edema will result. Acute valvular disease, though rare after injury or cardiac surgery, is another possible cause of inability of the left heart to pump effectively.

The diagnosis is made on the basis of hypoxemia, rales, a third heart sound, perihilar infiltrates, Kerley lines, and cephalization of blood flow on x-ray along with elevated pulmonary arterial wedge pressures on pulmonary arterial catheterization. A wedge (or left atrial) pressure of 24 mm Hg can produce cardiogenic pulmonary edema even in the presence of an intact endothelium in the pulmonary microvasculature. Pulmonary arterial wedge pressures less than 24 mm Hg will generally not produce edema if the pulmonary vascular endothelium is intact; pressures exceeding 16 mm Hg can worsen the edema associated with increased permeability (such as ARDS). The goal for the wedge pressure in a patient with uncomplicated cardiogenic pulmonary edema in the absence of an inflammatory process in the lungs should be 20 mm Hg or less; the goal in a patient with an inflammatory process should be 12–16 mm Hg.

Neurogenic pulmonary edema is associated both experimentally and clinically with head injury and increased intracranial pressure. The exact mechanism by which this occurs is unknown, but it is probably related to sympathetic discharge with postmicrovascular vasoconstriction in the lungs and a resultant increase in pulmonary microvascular hydrostatic pressure. This form of pulmonary edema and oxygenation defect is rare. In the great majority of patients with a head injury and pulmonary edema, the edema will be caused by some other mechanism, such as ARDS.

INDICATIONS FOR INTUBATION & USE OF MECHANICAL VENTILATION

The indications for intubation and mechanical ventilation are related but often assessed separately. Patients who have primary airway compromise—caused by stridor, maxillofacial trauma, facial and airway burns with edema, or a depressed mental status—may need intubation to protect the airway. In these cases, early intervention is the rule as rapid clinical deterioration can convert a semiurgent procedure into an emergency. In some cases, intubation should be performed before the patient shows evidence of airway compromise. In severe cases, such as massive facial edema, early cricothyroidostomy should be performed.

Intubation of the airway is also indicated if mechanical ventilation is needed for the treatment of established pulmonary failure or for prophylaxis against potential failure or for pulmonary toilet in the face of aspiration. The decision to intubate and initiate mechanical ventilation should be made on the basis of clinical criteria. A respiratory rate exceeding 36 breaths/min, labored ventilation, use of accessory muscles of ventilation, and tachycardia are all indications for intervention. Finally, intubation and mechanical ventilation should be performed in anticipation of treatment that can compromise the airway or worsen the pulmonary status. These include the need for excessive sedation or narcotics, massive fluid resuscitation, and the manipulation of fractures.

Arterial blood gas (ABG) measurements are of no value in making decisions about intubation and mechanical ventilation in patients in extremis. These patients should be intubated regardless of the blood gas results. ABG measurements, however, can assist in the decision to intubate less severely stressed patients. In the setting of hypoxemia, intubation should be considered if the PaO_2 is less than 60 mm Hg and the patient's supplemental oxygen exceeds an O_2 concentration of 50%. For hypercapneic patients, a $PaCO_2$ greater than 45 mm Hg in the setting of acidemia should prompt intubation, especially if serial measurements demonstrate a worsening respiratory acidosis. Regardless of the laboratory values, these guidelines should always be put in the clinical context. A $PaCO_2$ of 40 mm Hg in a patient breathing 40 breaths/min is as alarming as a $PaCO_2$ of 60 mm Hg in a patient with a respiratory rate of 10 breaths/min. A PaO_2 of 60 mm Hg on room air in a patient with chronic lung disease may be acceptable; the same value in a patient who is tensing the sternocleidomastoid and intercostal muscles with each breath, making excessive or dyscoordinated use of the abdominal musculature, and who seems to be struggling to draw in enough air, mandates immediate intubation.

The indications for intubation should be more liberal for a surgical patient than for a medical patient. The medical patient with an exacerbation of chronic obstructive lung disease can be poorly served by placement of a foreign body in the trachea. Airway resistance increases, coughing becomes less effective, and opportunistic organisms obtain a foothold on and near the tube. The benefit from intubation may be minimal and noninvasive ventilation techniques, such as bilevel positive airway pressure (BiPAP), may be all that is needed. This support can be given simultaneously with other treatments—such as administration of bronchodilators, antibiotics, and diuretics—in order to avoid intubation and its potential complications.

Circumstances for the seriously ill surgical patient are usually different. The patient who has multiple injuries, for example, can temporarily tolerate the increased airway resistance, loss of cough, and increased likelihood of tracheobronchial infection. What cannot be tolerated is respiratory arrest during trauma resuscitation or during preparation for an operation.

The indications for intubation in the patient with a suspected or known injury to the cervical spine are the same as those in patients with no likelihood of injury. Under no circumstances should concern about the cervical spine lead to procrastination about securing the airway. The consequences of respiratory arrest and anoxic brain damage are as tragic as those of exacerbating a cervical spine injury.

▶ Types of Intubation

The trachea can be intubated via the mouth, the nose, the cricothyroid membrane (cricothyroidostomy), or directly (tracheostomy). The tubes used for intubation come with either of two different types of cuffs. Tubes with high-pressure, low-volume cuffs are easy to insert and are useful for short-term intubation and ventilation. The high cuff pressure, however, can interfere with tracheal blood supply and lead to tracheomalacia, erosion into the innominate artery (tracheoinnominate fistula), erosion into the esophagus (tracheoesophageal fistula), or airway stenosis. Tubes with low-pressure, high-volume cuffs are more difficult to insert but should be used for intubation if the intubation is expected to be longer than 24 hours.

Of the four methods available for intubation, the orotracheal route is usually the easiest. Nasotracheal intubation requires the presence of spontaneous ventilation in order to guide tube placement; cricothyroidostomy and tracheostomy require surgical exposure. Orotracheal intubation allows for passage of a larger tube than the nasotracheal route and avoids the problems of sinusitis and necrosis of the nares, which can occur with nasotracheal intubation. On the other hand, nasotracheal intubation can be accomplished in the awake patient with minimal sedation, and some patients seem to find long-term presence of a nasotracheal tube more comfortable than that of an orotracheal tube. Neither nasotracheal nor orotracheal intubation requires neck flexion or axial rotation. Either approach can be used in patients with suspected injuries to the cervical spine, assuming that axial traction is maintained during the intubation.

Cricothyroidostomy is indicated when an urgent surgical airway is needed. Extensive maxillofacial trauma can make intubation by the orotracheal or nasotracheal route impossi-

ble. Translaryngeal intubation can also be difficult because of poor patient cooperation, altered anatomy, or airway or laryngeal swelling. If the patient is in extremis and respiratory collapse is imminent, attempts at orotracheal or nasotracheal intubation should not be prolonged. As a rule, if transpharyngeal intubation is not successful after one or two attempts, cricothyroidostomy should be done. The cricothyroid membrane in the midline is bounded superiorly by the lower border of the thyroid cartilage. It is located by palpation and is incised by a stab incision. After the hole has been enlarged with the knife handle, a No. 4 or No. 6 tracheostomy tube should be inserted into the trachea. The patient can then be supported with mechanical ventilation and supplemental oxygen as necessary. Cricothyroidostomies maintained for longer than 2 or 3 days may produce glottic and subglottic stenosis; tracheostomies are less likely to do so. Cricothyroidostomies should be converted to tracheostomies as soon as is safe and practical, assuming that continued intubation is needed.

Conversion to tracheostomy should be done under controlled conditions. A transverse incision overlying the upper trachea is developed by separating the strap muscles of the neck in the midline. Often the thyroid isthmus must be either displaced or divided to allow for adequate exposure of the anterior surface of the trachea. The tracheostomy tube is placed through the second or third tracheal ring.

For long-term care, translaryngeal intubation has three major advantages over a tracheostomy. First, a tube passed through the larynx can be repositioned, distributing pressure on the tracheal mucosa over a larger area, compared with the balloon on the end of a tracheostomy tube, which is fixed in place. The result is a much lower incidence of late tracheal stenosis and tracheoinnominate artery and tracheoesophageal fistulas, compared with a tracheostomy. Second, because the opening of a translaryngeal tube is well away from the neck and chest, intravenous catheters in these areas can be kept sterile. Third, the cuffs on translaryngeal tubes usually lie in a more axial position in the trachea than those on a tracheostomy tube and are better able to maintain a seal in patients with poor pulmonary compliance and high inspiratory pressures.

On the other hand, for long-term care, airway resistance with a tracheostomy is lower, nursing care is simpler, suctioning is more direct, and the tubes do not damage the vocal cords or larynx. In addition and perhaps most importantly, accidental extubation is less serious—a well-established tracheostomy tract can be easily reintubated while the patient continues to breathe through the stoma. Tracheostomy is also of benefit when weaning from mechanical ventilation is slow and the patient has failed extubation on multiple occasions. The presence of a tracheostomy allows for prolonged periods off the ventilator without the need for reintubation. If the patient develops respiratory distress off the ventilator and a tracheostomy is present, the ventilator can simply be reconnected to the tracheostomy tube.

The timing of conversion from a translaryngeal intubation to a tracheostomy is controversial. Recommendations as short as 3 days have been made, but large numbers of patients have been intubated for months by the orotracheal or nasotracheal route without serious sequelae. Patients should be converted when airway protection, pulmonary toilet, or any of the other indications outlined above are present. If, in addition, the need for more than 2–3 weeks of intubation is obvious, the threshold for performing tracheostomy should be lowered.

▶ Modes of Mechanical Ventilation

Once the airway is controlled, the ventilator should be set up beginning with the mode of ventilation. There are three primary variables used to describe the mode of mechanical ventilation: trigger, limit, and cycle (see Table 12–2). The **trigger** can be patient or time triggered with the latter often referred to as "machine triggered." This is the variable that determines when a patient receives a breath (starts inspiration). The second is the **limit** variable and refers to the setting that, when reached, is maintained constant throughout the inspiratory cycle (ie, the "upper limit"). Limit variables are either pressure or flow. When flow is the limit variable, the ventilator is said to be in **volume control** or **volume limited** because of the relationship *flow × time = volume.* Finally, the **cycle** variable is that which, once reached, terminates the inspiratory cycle and allows passive expiration. Using these three variables, different modes of ventilation have been created. Some are mostly of historical interest, and others are newer, combination modes designed to maximize patient physiology, safety, and comfort.

Machine triggers are time functions based on the set rate, inspiratory time, and inspiratory to expiratory ratio (I:E ratio). Two of the three can be set, and the third is determined. A rate of 20 breaths/min and an inspiratory time of 1 second results in an I:E ratio of 1:2 (1 s inspiration + 2 s expiration = 3 s for a complete cycle; 20 cycles/min).

Patient triggers for delivery of an assisted breath can be either pressure-based or "flow by" depending on the ventilator model. A pressure trigger requires the patient to generate negative pressure at the onset of inspiration—the pressure in the ventilator tubing falls below a preset value and the ventilator detects this fall in pressure and responds by delivering a breath. The time involved in generating and delivering the breath to the patient, however, can make this form of breathing uncomfortable for the patient. Modern ventilators avoid this problem of triggering by using a flow-by circuit. The ventilator delivers a constant flow of air through the ventilator tubing during expiration, usually at a low level of approximately 5 L/min. The ventilator compares the expiratory and inspiratory flow rates. If the patient is making no inspiratory effort, the flow rates will be the same. If the patient begins to take a breath, the expiratory rate will fall below the inspiratory rate. The ventilator is programmed to trigger a breath when the difference in the flow rates reaches a preset value, usually around 2 L/min, or when the expiratory flow rate falls to 3 L/min. The patient is rewarded with the free flow of at least some air as soon as the effort is initiated. The great majority of patients prefer flow-by over pressure triggering.

Table 12–2. Characteristics of Five Commonly Used Modes of Mechanical Ventilation.

Mode	Trigger	Limit	Cycle	Notes
Intermittent Mandatory Ventilation (IMV)	Time (machine)	Flow (volume) or pressure	Time	Volume Control IMV or Pressure control IMV Can be synchronized to patients effort (SIMV) and/or used in conjunction with pressure support
Assist control (AC)	Patient and/or time	Flow (volume) or pressure	Time	Assist control volume control (AC VC) or Assist control pressure control (AC PC)
Pressure support (PS)	Patient	Pressure	Flow	Purely spontaneous mode and often referred to as a form of continuous positive airway pressure (CPAP) on the ventilator controls
Inverse ratio	Time	Pressure	Time	PC IMV mode with prolonged inspiratory phase to increase mean airway pressure and functional residual capacity
Pressure-regulated volume control	Patient and/or time	Pressure	Time	Variation of pressure control that limits pressure but adjusts between breaths to ensure preset tidal volume

A. Volume Control Ventilation

Volume control ventilation is most often used today in situations in which the ventilation needs to be kept simple and the efforts made by the patient need to be minimized, as in the acutely injured or ill patient. The assist-control mode is the most commonly used mode of volume ventilation. It is designed to assist any ventilatory effort made by the patient by delivering a machine breath. Whenever the patient begins to inspire, the ventilator is triggered and the preset machine tidal volume is given. A machine backup rate is also set to ensure a minimal number of machine breaths in the absence of spontaneous ventilatory efforts.

B. Pressure Control Ventilation & Pressure Support Ventilation

In **pressure control ventilation,** the inspiratory pressure, inspiratory time, and I:E ratio are selected, and the ventilator automatically adjusts the gas flow rate to maintain a constant pressure during inspiration. The main advantage of this over volume control is that gas flow more closely matches the change in lung compliance that occurs during inspiration. This has the theoretical benefit of a more even distribution of inspired gas and possibly a lower risk of regional alveolar overdistention. It is also more comfortable for the awake patient. Although this can be achieved through manipulating the flow pattern in more advanced volume control ventilators, it is automatic in pressure control ventilation. Physiologic inspiratory times and I:E ratios are usually chosen to improve patient comfort. An inspiratory time of 1 second with an expiratory time of 2 or 3 seconds is typical. Longer inspiratory times with shorter expiratory times (**inverse ratio ventilation**) can be used if the physiologic times prove inadequate to provide enough support. The long inspiratory times, along with the short expiratory times, result in air trapping and increase the mean airway pressure. The net result is an increase in functional residual capacity (FRC), similar to that accomplished with high positive end-expiratory pressure (PEEP) levels.

Pressure support ventilation is also a pressure-limited form of ventilation and in most cases, can be considered a distinct mode of ventilation (see Table 12–2). It differs from pressure control in that it is always patient triggered and the inspiratory time is determined by the patient and not set by the ventilator. As in pressure control ventilation, the ventilator adjusts the flow to maintain a constant pressure during inspiration. The inspiratory time, however, is determined by the interaction of the gas flow with the patient's inspiratory effort. To do this, the ventilator measures the peak inspiratory flow rate during inspiration. The flow rate usually reaches a maximum value early in the inspiration and then tapers off as the patient's inspiratory effort decreases. When the flow rate decreases to a predetermined fraction of the maximal flow (generally 25% of maximum), gas flow is terminated, and the patient is allowed to exhale. Pressure support can also be used in conjunction with the intermittent mandatory ventilation mode (see next section).

The level of the pressure support is set so that the patient breathes comfortably at a reasonable rate, usually less than 24 breaths/min. The goal of the support is to ensure adequate oxygenation and a pH greater than 7.30. The tidal volume generated under these circumstances is generally unimportant.

The mode has many advantages. It is usually comfortable for the patient. It overcomes resistance to inspiratory flow in the endotracheal tube and in the ventilatory apparatus and decreases the work of breathing. It makes it impossible for the ventilator to deliver excessively high pressures. The flow is maintained for as long as the patient continues to make an inspiratory effort, so the patient can sigh at will. This minimizes the development of atelectasis. It is also ideally suited for preparing the patient for weaning and extubation.

C. Intermittent Mandatory Ventilation & Assist Control Ventilation

With **intermittent mandatory ventilation** (IMV), all aspects of breathing are controlled including the rate, inspiratory time, and expiratory time (and as a result, I:E ratio). The limit variable can be either pressure (PC IMV) or volume (VC IMV). The breaths are generally synchronized (SIMV) if the patient has spontaneous respiratory effort. In this mode, any attempt to breathe at a greater frequency than the set rate is unsupported unless additional pressure support is added. In this case, the patient receives two different modes during mechanical ventilation. The first is the mandatory, machine-triggered breath at the set rate and inspiratory time. The second is a spontaneous, patient-triggered breath at a rate equal to the total minus the set rate with an inspiratory time determined by the patient (see previous discussion of pressure support ventilation). These two breaths will have different waveform characteristics on the ventilator display.

Assist control mode was originally set up to "assist" the patient's spontaneous effort with a completely supported mechanical breath. It can be used with a volume or pressure limit (VC or PC) and set up with a backup rate when spontaneous effort is minimal or absent. The main distinction from SIMV is that all of the patient's inspiratory efforts are completely supported (not just those at the set rate). This has the small disadvantage of air trapping when the patient's respiratory rate is excessively high (> 30–35 breaths per minute) and should be used with caution in patients at risk for hyperinflation (severe emphysema). There is no role for pressure support ventilation in this mode as all breaths are completely assisted.

D. Hybrid Modes

Over the past 15 years, it has become possible to ventilate patients with even more sophisticated hybrid modes. Some ventilators can be set up to deliver constant pressure during the inspiration in such a way that the tidal volume delivered falls in a preset range (**pressure-regulated volume control, PRVC**). Some ventilators can be set up to deliver a preset tidal volume but without exceeding a preset pressure. Some ventilators can be set up with gradually decreasing ventilatory support with algorithms built into the system to minimize the need for physician adjustment of the ventilator during weaning.

▶ Setting Up the Ventilator

After choosing the mode (AC, SIMV, or PS; PC or VC), five parameters remain to be determined: the backup ventilatory rate, the goal tidal volume of the machine-delivered breaths, the inspiratory time, the inspired oxygen concentration (FIO_2), and the PEEP level. The first two of these parameters determine ventilation; the latter three are important in determining oxygenation.

Ventilation has three components: minute ventilation (V_E), alveolar ventilation (V_A), and dead space ventilation (V_D). Although V_A is most closely related to $PaCO_2$, at steady state, the relationship with V_E and V_D is roughly constant, and therefore, V_E, which is easily quantified, can be used as a surrogate. In patients with uncomplicated pulmonary failure, the respiratory rate can be set at 12–15 breaths/min and the tidal volume set to 7 mL/kg IBW. This produces a V_E of 6–7.5 L/min and a V_A of 4–5 L/min (assuming V_D of 33% in a 70 kg patient). In the absence of significant pulmonary dysfunction, this will result in a $PaCO_2$ of approximately 40 mm Hg and is a good starting point from which adjustments can be made.

If the $PaCO_2$ is elevated, increases in the respiratory rate will often correct the problem. Although this is less efficient than increasing the tidal volume (due to the increased dead space ventilation that occurs with higher respiratory rates), it is a reasonable first step when the respiratory rate is less than 25. Excessively high respiratory rates (> 30 breaths/min) can result in air trapping, especially in patients with expiratory air flow obstruction (chronic obstructive pulmonary disease or severe asthma). On the other hand, excessively high volumes may be associated with elevated airway pressures and can result in barotrauma (pneumothorax), volutrauma (alveolar overdistention), or both. Except in certain circumstances (intracranial hypertension), it is better to accept a mild respiratory acidosis than to ventilate the patient using excessively large tidal volumes (greater than 10 mL/kg IBW) or excessively high airway pressures (plateau pressure greater than 30 cm H_2O). When the pH is less than 7.20, very high rates or volumes may be necessary until the pH can be brought into the normal range either through renal compensatory mechanisms or administered bicarbonate. Very high rates or volumes may also be necessary when a bronchopleural fistula is present, to compensate for the volume lost through the fistula.

The inspired oxygen concentration should be kept high enough so that, in most cases, the oxygen saturation of arterial blood exceeds 92%. Patients with chronic obstructive pulmonary disease and long-standing CO_2 retention are an exception. Such patients have lost the ability to increase their respiratory drive in response to increases in $PaCO_2$ and rely instead on their response to hypoxemia. Increasing the arterial oxygen saturation by adding exogenous oxygen takes away this hypoxic ventilatory stimulus and makes weaning from ventilatory support more difficult.

All of the nonoxygen volume of ventilator gas is made up of nitrogen, which, unlike oxygen, is not absorbed from alveoli. Nitrogen can be of great value in stenting open the alveoli. When it is replaced by increasing concentrations of oxygen, increased atelectasis caused by oxygen absorption can occur. In addition, high concentrations of oxygen can cause chronic pulmonary fibrosis. Ideally, the inspired oxygen concentration should be kept at 0.50 or less.

Keeping the inspired oxygen levels at acceptably low levels is frequently facilitated by the use of PEEP. The pressure is generated by closure of a valve in the expiratory circuit of the ventilator to keep the airway pressure above a preset level during expiration and to minimize alveolar collapse. Placement of an endotracheal tube bypasses the normal physiologic PEEP present during spontaneous ventilation from closure of the glottis at the end of expiration. In addition, supine patients may have a lower functional residual capacity due to increased intra-abdominal pressure and cephalad displacement of the diaphragm into the chest. This can be overcome through the use of low levels of "physiologic" PEEP (5 cm H_2O). Increasing the PEEP should be considered when the respiratory system compliance is low or when adequate oxygenation requires an FIO_2 that exceeds 0.50.

Low levels of PEEP (< 10 cm H_2O) are well tolerated by most patients. The consequences of excessive PEEP are barotrauma and decreased cardiac output. First, the high pressure can compress the superior and inferior vena cava and the pulmonary veins, compromising diastolic filling of the ventricles (in contrast with a spontaneous inspiration, which augments filling). Second, the high pressures can compress the thin-walled atria and right ventricle, further compromising end-diastolic volumes (also in contrast with a spontaneous inspiration). Finally, the high pressures can compress the pulmonary microvasculature, making it difficult for the right ventricle to push blood through the pulmonary vasculature. The remedy for the decreased cardiac output is usually fluid infusion. The potential problem with this remedy is worsening of the pulmonary failure that prompted the use of the PEEP in the first place. Accounting for all of these factors, PEEP levels greater than 10–12 cm H_2O should generally be used with a pulmonary arterial catheter in place. Titrating to the optimal oxygen delivery, and not arterial PaO_2, will ensure a balance between the risks and benefits of high PEEP levels. Monitoring the mixed venous oxygen saturation serves as a reasonable method to achieve this goal. Even with invasive monitoring, PEEP levels greater than 15–20 cm H_2O are rarely of benefit.

Ventilator Safety & Alarms

As can be inferred, modern ventilators are complex, and they should, in general, be used only in the setting of continuous cardiopulmonary monitoring to include electrocardiography and pulse oximetry. In addition, the ventilators themselves have alarms for early warning of apnea, changes in tidal volume or minute ventilation, and excessive inspiratory pressures. These should be individualized to each patient so that nurses, respiratory therapists, and physicians are notified early in the course of the physiologic derangement. In many cases, the ventilator alarm will precede changes in the pulse oximeter or electrocardiogram. All personnel taking care of the patient should be knowledgeable with both the equipment and the mode of ventilation.

Discontinuing Mechanical Ventilation

Patients who seem to be doing well and who have required mechanical ventilation for less than 24 hours can frequently be extubated quickly after undergoing a trial of spontaneous ventilation. Patients must be able to maintain their own airway, and their acute illness should be resolving. They should be able to maintain adequate oxygenation with an inspired oxygen concentration of 0.40 or less and with a PEEP of 8 cm water or less.

The majority of ventilated patients are most effectively weaned with daily spontaneous breathing trials. The breathing trial can be given with T-piece ventilation in which the endotracheal tube is attached to a length of tubing connected to a blow-by oxygen source. Alternatively, the trial can be accomplished with a low level (typically 5 cm of water) of pressure support with PEEP or with PEEP alone. In either case, the patient is asked to support his or her own breathing for 30 minutes. If the patient is breathing comfortably at the end of the trial, the patient can be extubated. If a question arises as to the degree of comfort, arterial blood should be drawn for gases, and the patient should be put back on the ventilator while waiting for the results of the blood gas analysis. If the patient was reasonably comfortable at the end of the 30-minute trial and if the pH comes back at a normal value, the patient can be extubated. Note that at the conclusion of the 30-minute trial, full ventilator support should be resumed pending the laboratory results. The patient needs to be well rested when the endotracheal tube is removed. If the patient fails the 30 minute trial, full support is resumed for the remainder of the day, and the trial is repeated the following day.

Weaning from mechanical ventilation can also be achieved with IMV. Although generally inferior to the once-daily spontaneous breathing trial, patients who are severely debilitated and have required mechanical ventilation for prolonged periods (> 2–3 weeks) can be successfully weaned using this technique when combined with a gradual reduction in pressure support. The IMV rate is gradually decreased, requiring the patient to contribute increasingly to the maintenance of adequate minute ventilation. The patient's overall clinical status, respiratory rate, and arterial PCO_2 are used as guidelines to determine the rate of weaning. When an IMV of 4/min or less is well tolerated for long periods, the patient is placed on pressure support, which is weaned daily until mechanical support is no longer needed. Patients who repeatedly fail extubation or are severely deconditioned benefit from a more deliberate and gradual weaning of the ventilator. Frequently, these patients benefit from tracheostomy and optimization of nutritional status as adjuncts to weaning. Factors that increase the work of breathing—such as reactive airway disease, large pleural effusions, and chest wall or visceral edema—should be treated and minimized.

Extubation

The decision to extubate the patient depends both on the assessment for the need for airway protection as well as the need for mechanical ventilation. As mentioned previously, the latter can be determined based on the result of a 30-minute trial of spontaneous breathing. The former should be based on several factors, including the patient's level of consciousness, the presence of airway injury or edema, the need for ongoing endotracheal suctioning, and the possible need for further operative procedures within the next 24 hours. Finally, a subjective determination of a patient's ability to tolerate extubation and spontaneous ventilation should be made. An alert and communicative patient who can lift her head off the pillow is a good candidate for extubation; a lethargic, diaphoretic patient is not. For patients who require continued airway protection but no longer require mechanical ventilatory support, a tracheostomy should be considered.

ADJUVANT DIAGNOSTIC & THERAPEUTIC MEASURES

Chest Radiographs

Chest x-rays should be obtained daily in patients being treated with mechanical ventilation. A review of the film should confirm the placement of all lines and tubes, including the endotracheal tube, central venous catheters, pleural tubes (thoracostomies), and nasogastric or nasoenteric tubes. A search for specific pulmonary and pleural processes should be performed. Local infiltrates such as pneumonia or patchy/diffuse processes such as the acute respiratory distress syndrome should be identified.

In addition to a daily chest radiograph, a stat chest x-ray should be obtained whenever a patient's cardiopulmonary status rapidly deteriorates. Tubes or lines might be displaced; new problems with a reversible etiology—such a pneumothorax, a lobar collapse, or a new infiltrate suggesting aspiration—might be identified.

Sedation & Muscle Relaxants

Mechanically ventilated patients frequently require sedatives and/or analgesia to ameliorate the agitation and pain associated with their disease and treatment. Narcotic analgesia in the form of intermittent or continuous opiate infusion may be sufficient. Narcotics, however, should not be used to treat agitation and anxiety that is thought to be caused by the ventilator. Sedating agents, including propofol and benzodiazepines, should be used instead. In addition, haloperidol and risperidone may be useful adjuncts, either alone or in combination with benzodiazepines. As a general rule, intermittent dosing is preferred to continuous infusions. When the latter is used, the agent should be stopped at least once daily—giving the patient a so-called sedation holiday—to assess neurologic status and determine the need for continuing sedation.

Neuromuscular blocking agents add an additional level of patient control and can greatly simplify ventilatory management in patients with severe pulmonary insufficiency. These agents should be reserved for severe patient-ventilator dyssynchrony, a situation in which the patient's spontaneous respiratory efforts result in dyscoordinated and inadequate ventilation by the mechanical ventilator. This may have the untoward effect of life-threatening hypoxemia in a patient with little physiologic reserve.

Nonphysiologic ventilatory methods, such as inverse ratio or high-frequency oscillatory ventilation, may also require the use of neuromuscular blocking agents. Major side effects include a potential increased risk of ventilator-associated pneumonia (VAP), through loss of cough mechanism, and an association with late polyneuromyopathy of critical illness. As a result, they should be used only when absolutely necessary and for the shortest possible time.

Antibiotics

VAP is the most common nosocomial infection in the intensive care unit. The risk of acquiring VAP is directly related to the duration of mechanical ventilation. There is no gold standard for VAP diagnosis. Possible criteria include a new or progressive infiltrate on chest radiograph, worsening hypoxemia, increased sputum quantity, new onset of purulent sputum associated with abundant white cells and organisms on Gram-stained smears, or positive sputum cultures with known pathogenic organisms. Signs of systemic sepsis with increased temperature, leukocytosis, increasing fluid requirements, and glucose intolerance are also common findings in VAP.

If all of these are present, antibiotics should be started. If only one or two are present, antibiotics are probably best withheld to avoid overgrowth of resistant organisms that could later cause fatal pneumonia. Exceptions to this approach include older, severely debilitated patients, immunocompromised patients, and those who are critically ill in whom delayed antibiotic therapy might result in irretrievable deterioration. Thus, an 80-year-old patient with flail chest and a new infiltrate should probably be given antibi-

otics early; a 20-year-old patient who was hospitalized for a gunshot wound involving the colon and who develops questionable pneumonia 2 weeks later is more likely to tolerate a delay in the initiation of antibiotics until the diagnosis is more definite. In addition, the latter patient may have an alternative explanation for his fever and leukocytosis, such as an intra-abdominal abscess. In this case, the wrong diagnosis might delay appropriate source control (abscess drainage). The CPIS can be useful to guide the diagnosis. The goal is to avoid overtreatment with the risk of antimicrobial resistance and superinfection. Antibiotics can safely be discontinued in patients empirically started on antibiotics for suspected pneumonia who have a CPIS value of 6 or less at 72 hours.

The Acute Respiratory Distress Syndrome Network: Ventilation with lower tidal volumes as compared with traditional tidal volumes for acute lung injury and the acute respiratory distress syndrome. N Engl J Med 2000;342:1301.

Aldrich TK et al: Weaning from mechanical ventilation: adjunctive use of inspiratory muscle resistive training. Crit Care Med. 1989;17:143.

Amato MB, Barbas CS, Medeiros DM: Effect of a protective-ventilation strategy on mortality in the acute respiratory distress syndrome. N Engl J Med 1998;338:347.

Bernard GR et al: The American-European Consensus Conference on ARDS. Definitions, mechanisms, relevant outcomes, and clinical trial coordination. Am J Respir Crit Care Med 1994; 149:818.

Bidani A et al: Permissive hypercapnia in acute respiratory failure. JAMA 1994;272:957.

Blaisdell FW et al: Pulmonary microembolism. A cause of morbidity and death after major vascular surgery. Arch Surg 1966;93:776.

Brochard L et al: Inspiratory pressure support prevents diaphragmatic fatigue during weaning from mechanical ventilation. Am Rev Respir Dis 1989;139:513.

Brochard L et al: Noninvasive ventilation for acute exacerbations of chronic obstructive pulmonary disease. N Engl J Med 1995;333:817.

Chastre J et al: Comparison of 8 vs 15 days of antibiotic therapy for ventilator-associated pneumonia in adults: a randomized trial. JAMA 2003;290:2588.

Esteban A et al: A comparison of four methods of weaning patients from mechanical ventilation. Spanish Lung Failure Collaborative Group. N Engl J Med 1995;332:345.

Esteban A et al: Effect of spontaneous breathing trial duration on outcome of attempts to discontinue mechanical ventilation. Spanish Lung Failure Collaborative Group. Am J Respir Crit Care Med 1999;159:512.

Fu Z et al: High lung volume increases stress failure in pulmonary capillaries. J Appl Physiol 1992;73:123.

Gattinoni L et al: Regional effects and mechanism of positive end-expiratory pressure in early adult respiratory distress syndrome. JAMA 1993;269:2122.

Gausche M et al: Effect of out-of-hospital pediatric endotracheal intubation on survival and neurological outcome: a controlled clinical trial. JAMA 2000;283:783.

Heyland DK et al: The attributable morbidity and mortality of ventilator-associated pneumonia in the critically ill patient. The Canadian Critical Trials Group. Am J Respir Crit Care Med 1999;159:1249.

Hickling KG, Henderson SJ, Jackson R: Low mortality associated with low volume pressure limited ventilation with permissive hypercapnia in severe adult respiratory distress syndrome. Intensive Care Med 1990;16:372.

Iregui M et al: Clinical importance of delays in the initiation of appropriate antibiotic treatment for ventilator-associated pneumonia. Chest 2002;122:262.

Kress JP et al: Daily interruption of sedative infusions in critically ill patients undergoing mechanical ventilation. N Engl J Med 2000;342:1471.

Leone M et al: Risk factors for late-onset ventilator-associated pneumonia in trauma patients receiving selective digestive decontamination. Intensive Care Med 2005;31:64.

MacIntyre NR: Respiratory function during pressure support ventilation. Chest 1986;89:677.

MacIntyre NR et al: Evidence-based guidelines for weaning and discontinuing ventilatory support: a collective task force facilitated by the American College of Chest Physicians; the American Association for Respiratory Care; and the American College of Critical Care Medicine. Chest 2001;120(6 Suppl):375S.

Marelich GP et al: Protocol weaning of mechanical ventilation in medical and surgical patients by respiratory care practitioners and nurses: effect on weaning time and incidence of ventilator-associated pneumonia. Chest 2000;118:459.

Maziak DE, MO Meade, TR Todd: The timing of tracheotomy: a systematic review. Chest 1998;114:605.

Minei JP et al: Alternative case definitions of ventilator-associated pneumonia identify different patients in a surgical intensive care unit. Shock 2000;14:331.

Plant PK, Owen JL, Elliott MW: Early use of non-invasive ventilation for acute exacerbations of chronic obstructive pulmonary disease on general respiratory wards: a multicentre randomised controlled trial. Lancet 2000;355:1931.

Pugin J et al: Diagnosis of ventilator-associated pneumonia by bacteriologic analysis of bronchoscopic and nonbronchoscopic "blind" bronchoalveolar lavage fluid. Am Rev Respir Dis 1991;143:1121.

Ranieri VM et al: Effect of mechanical ventilation on inflammatory mediators in patients with acute respiratory distress syndrome: a randomized controlled trial. JAMA 1999;282:54.

Saito S, Tokioka H, Kosaka F: Efficacy of flow-by during continuous positive airway pressure ventilation. Crit Care Med. 1990;18:654.

Sassoon CS et al: Inspiratory work of breathing on flow-by and demand-flow continuous positive airway pressure. Crit Care Med 1989;17:1108.

Schweickert WD et al: Daily interruption of sedative infusions and complications of critical illness in mechanically ventilated patients. Crit Care Med 2004;32:1272.

Schweickert, WD, Hall J: ICU-acquired weakness. Chest 2007;131:1541.

Singh N et al: Short-course empiric antibiotic therapy for patients with pulmonary infiltrates in the intensive care unit. A proposed solution for indiscriminate antibiotic prescription. Am J Respir Crit Care Med 2000;162:505.

Stewart TE et al: Evaluation of a ventilation strategy to prevent barotrauma in patients at high risk for acute respiratory distress syndrome. Pressure- and Volume-Limited Ventilation Strategy Group. N Engl J Med 1998;338:355.

III. TREATMENT OF THE MORE CHALLENGING PATIENT

So far, the discussion of shock and pulmonary failure in the surgical patient has concentrated on making a clinical diagnosis and directing treatment on the basis of that diagnosis. This approach works well in many patients, but in some it is not enough. Effective treatment in the more seriously ill patient frequently has to take into account the underlying physiological abnormalities if the treatment is to work. With this approach, the clinical diagnosis becomes less important. Dealing with the underlying physiological problem becomes paramount.

COMMON PHYSIOLOGICAL RESPONSES TO SEVERE SHOCK

The body responds to the shock state with compensatory responses. These responses help the patient deal with the initial abnormalities of the shock but can contribute to the later consequences of cardiac and pulmonary failure. Understanding these responses can help the physician in managing the consequences.

▶ Neurohumoral Responses

The neurohumoral responses to shock include discharge of the cardiovascular nerves and release of vasoactive, metabolically active, and volume-conserving hormones. The responses can be lifesaving before therapy begins and serve to maintain homeostasis once therapy has started.

Adrenergic discharge constricts the arterioles, venules, and small veins in all parts of the body except the brain and heart and augments myocardial systolic function. The result is increased cardiac output and blood pressure and diversion of flow to the brain and heart.

The vasoactive hormones angiotensin II and vasopressin act in concert with discharge of the cardiovascular adrenergic nerves. Angiotensin II constricts the vasculature in the skin, kidneys, and splanchnic organs and diverts blood flow to the heart and brain. It also stimulates the adrenal medulla to release aldosterone, resulting in reabsorption of sodium ions from the glomerular filtrate. Vasopressin, like adrenergic discharge and angiotensin II, constricts the vascular sphincters in the skin and splanchnic organs (it does not constrict the renal vasculature) and diverts blood flow to the heart and brain. It also stimulates reabsorption of water from the distal tubules.

▶ Metabolic Responses

In all severe shock states, intracellular hydrogen ion concentrations increase. To compensate, extracellular sodium flows down its electrochemical gradient into the cells, along with chloride and water, in exchange for intracellular hydrogen ion. Intracellular pH increases back toward normal, but the cells swell, with perhaps an increase of 3 L in the intracellular volume.

Hypovolemia, hypotension, pain, and other stresses of critical illness stimulate the release of cortisol, glucagon, and epinephrine—all of which increase extracellular glucose concentrations. Thus, glucose should not be used in the initial fluid resuscitation of the patient in shock—it is not necessary and can even induce an osmotic diuresis, worsening hypovolemia and confusing the clinical picture. Glucose-containing solutions should be reserved for those patients who might be in insulin shock.

On the other hand, the endogenously produced glucose generated by the physiological release of the counterregulatory hormones provides fuel for nervous system function, metabolism of blood cells, and wound healing. The modest increase in extracellular osmolality also helps to replenish vascular volume by drawing water out of the cells and by increasing the interstitial hydrostatic pressure. The increased pressure drives interstitial protein into the lymphatics and from there into the vascular space. Interstitial oncotic pressure falls, and plasma oncotic pressure rises. The augmented oncotic gradient between the vascular and interstitial spaces draws water, sodium, and chloride into the vascular space from the interstitial space. This replenishment of vascular volume will continue as long as interstitial hydrostatic pressures are maintained and as long as interstitial protein stores, which constitute more than half of the total extracellular protein content, can be recruited. A certain degree of hyperglycemia might be beneficial in the postresuscitative phase. Once the patient has recovered, however, it appears that it is best to aggressively keep the blood glucose levels low, at 120 mg/dL or less.

Other hormones with potential metabolic actions, including insulin and growth hormone, are also released during critical illnesses. They have little effect, however, compared with cortisol, glucagon, and epinephrine. Indeed, infusion of cortisol, glucagon, and epinephrine in normal subjects can produce most of the metabolic changes of critical illness.

▶ Microvascular Responses

In severely ill patients, three responses—dilation of systemic arterioles, failure of cell membrane function, and disruption of the vascular endothelium—serve to worsen the patient's condition. In decompensated shock, the systemic arterioles lose their ability to constrict, while the postcapillary sphincters remain constricted. Microvascular hydrostatic pressure rises. Water, sodium, and chloride are driven out of the vascular space and into the interstitium. The process is limited, however, because the oncotic gradient, which increases as fluid is lost from plasma, prevents further fluid losses.

Trauma and sepsis activate coagulation and inflammation, which can disrupt microvascular endothelial integrity in severely ill patients. Platelet and white cell microaggregates that form in injured or infected tissues embolize to the lungs or liver, where they lodge in the microvasculature. The microaggregates, endothelium, and plasma in the regions of embolization release kinins, platelet-activating factors, fibrin degradation products, thromboxanes, prostacyclin, prostaglandins, complement, leukotrienes, lysoso-

mal enzymes, oxygen radicals, and other toxic factors, which damage the endothelium and dilate the vasculature in the region of the emboli and distally. Protein, water, sodium, and chloride extravasate into the interstitium. The amount of extravasation is limited by the increases in interstitial hydrostatic pressure that arise from interstitial flooding and by dilution of interstitial protein concentrations. The edema that results can be massive and can involve any tissue in the body.

PULMONARY ARTERY CATHETER (SWAN-GANZ CATHETER)

The pulmonary arterial catheter can be useful in evaluating the cardiovascular consequences associated with the physiological responses described above, and it can be invaluable in directing treatment in selected, seriously ill patients. The modern pulmonary arterial catheter is equipped with a thermistor and an oximeter on its tip. It permits measurement of the cardiac output; right atrial, pulmonary arterial, and pulmonary arterial wedge pressures; and mixed venous oxygen contents. Knowledge of the cardiac output and filling pressures can be used to assess ventricular function as fluid is administered or withheld. The mixed venous oxygen saturation reflects the adequacy of oxygen delivery to the periphery; a value less than 60% indicates inadequate peripheral oxygenation and can be used to evaluate adequacy of the cardiac output and of systemic arterial oxygen content. It can also be used to determine oxygen consumption, which is calculated as the cardiac output multiplied by the difference of the oxygen contents of blood in the systemic and pulmonary arteries. Oxygen consumption can fall in severely ill patients, and measurements of consumption can help assess the patient's response to resuscitation. All of this information can help in dealing with the physiological abnormalities of the shock state and the pulmonary failure that can arise from the shock.

The catheter is particularly useful when treatment of one organ system might harm another. For example, fluid administration might be needed to treat septic shock, but excess fluid might contribute to pulmonary failure; a diuretic might be indicated in an oliguric patient in congestive heart failure, but excessive diuresis might decrease the cardiac output to the point that the kidneys fail; and fluid might be needed for cardiovascular resuscitation in a patient with multiple injuries, but too much fluid might exacerbate cerebral edema. The pulmonary arterial catheter can be extremely helpful in these situations.

Data obtained from the Swan-Ganz catheter can be misleading, however, if mistakes are made in performing the measurements. The cardiac output, as measured by thermodilution, is obtained by creating a temperature differential in the blood in the right atrium and analyzing the change in temperature in the blood over time as it flows past a thermistor on the end of the pulmonary arterial catheter.

The greater the area under the temperature curve, the smaller the flow through the right heart. If injections of cold saline are used to create the temperature differential, they should be made at random times during the respiratory cycle to give the best indication of the output available to the patient, but some prefer to make the injections at a consistent time in the cycle to minimize variability in the cardiac output–associated heart-lung interactions. If a heater coil in the catheter is used to create the temperature differential, the changes are made randomly by a program in the equipment used with the catheter. All calculations are made by a computer in the equipment.

When one is obtaining pulmonary arterial or mixed venous blood, the balloon on the end of the catheter should be deflated, and the blood should be withdrawn slowly. If the blood is withdrawn too quickly, the walls of the pulmonary artery will collapse around the end of the catheter, and the specimen will be contaminated by blood that is pulled back, in a retrograde manner, past ventilated and nonperfused alveoli. The oximeter on the tip of the catheter has to be calibrated frequently by comparing the oxygen saturations of blood obtained from the pulmonary artery with the saturations readout by the oximeter. One must be certain that the blood that is to be used for calibration is truly representative.

The pressures measured with the pulmonary arterial catheter are displayed on an oscilloscope and include a mean pressure that is calculated by computer circuitry in the monitoring equipment. These mean pressures can be used in patient management. They have the advantage that they represent the pressures throughout the respiratory cycle and thus average in the variability associated with heart-lung interactions. Some clinicians prefer to read the end-expiratory pressures from the oscilloscope screen and use those values in patient management. Those pressures are relatively independent of heart-lung interactions, but they can be difficult to interpret, even by the most experienced ICU nurse or physician.

Of the five pressures obtained from the catheter, only two—the right atrial and the mean pulmonary arterial pressures—can be taken at face value; the other three—the pulmonary arterial systolic, diastolic, and wedge pressures—are subject to errors of measurement and interpretation. The pulmonary arterial wedge pressure usually is the same as the left atrial pressure. The wedge pressure will not reflect left atrial pressure, however, if the catheter is in a portion of the vasculature occluded by inflated alveoli. If the wedge pressure varies by more than 10 mm Hg with cycles of mechanical ventilation, one should assume that the tip of the catheter is facing the pressure in the alveoli rather than the pressure in the left atrium.

To account for variations in size of the patient, the cardiac output can be indexed to the calculated body surface area. Alternatively, however, one can use the patient's desirable body weight, calculated on the assumption that a desirable weight is one that is associated with longevity and freedom from diabetes. A body mass index of 21 is convenient to use for both men and women. Making a rough approximation of the patient's height, to the nearest half-foot, the desirable weights associated with that height, assuming a body mass index of 21, are indicated in Table 12–3. The cardiac outputs associated with that weight are also indicated, assuming that the subjects are supine, nonstressed, resting, fasting, and in a thermoneutral environment. The resting oxygen consumptions under these conditions are 3.5 mL $\times$ weight(-1) $\times$ min(-1). The outputs and the consumptions for patients older than 50 years are adjusted with the assumption that metabolic activity decreases by 10% per decade after age 50. Thus, for a 70-year-old person who is 6 feet tall, a normal cardiac output is 7 L/min multiplied by 0.8, or 5.6 L/min. The oxygen consumption is 245 mL/min multiplied by 0.8 or 195 mL/min.

OXYHEMOGLOBIN DISSOCIATION

The amount of oxygen contained in the blood and the amount of oxygen available to be delivered to the tissues can be expressed as a concentration, a saturation, or a partial pressure. All three have their value. Understanding their relationships can help in understanding the cardiac and pulmonary pathophysiology of the critically ill surgical patient.

Table 12–3. Approximate Desirable Weight, Cardiac Output, and Oxygen Consumption in Young Resting, Supine, Fasting Individuals of Varying Heights, in a Thermoneutral Environment.

Height (ft, in)	Desirable Weight[1] (kg)	Cardiac Output[2] (L/min)	Oxygen Consumption[3] (mL/min)
5'0"	49	5	170
5'6"	59	6	205
6'0"	70	7	245
6'6"	83	8	290

[1]Calculated with assumption that the desirable weight is that which gives a body mass index of 21.
[2]Calculated as 100 mL·kg^{-1}·min^{-1}.
[3]Calculated as 3.5 mL·kg^{-1}·min^{-1}.

The concentration of oxygen in the blood, or oxygen content, is expressed as milliliters of O_2/dL of blood, or vol%. The oxygen content can be measured directly, but the measurement is time-consuming, and the content is usually calculated on the basis of the other two measures of blood oxygenation, the oxygen saturation (So_2) and the Po_2. The oxygen content is related to these other quantities by the following formula:

$$Co_2 = 1.34 \times [Hb] \times So_2 + 0.0031 \times Po_2 \qquad (1)$$

where [Hb] is expressed as g/dL and the Po_2 as mm Hg. Thus, for example, the oxygen content of a blood specimen with a [Hb] of 12 g/dL, an So_2 of 90%, and a Po_2 of 60 mm Hg is 14.7 vol%.

The first term in the equation represents the O_2 carried by the hemoglobin molecule; the second, the O_2 dissolved in the blood water. This second term is small compared with the first as long as the [Hb] is greater than, say, 7 g/dL and the Po_2 is less than, say, 100 mm Hg. Omitting the second term then simplifies the formula to read as follows:

$$Co_2 = 1.34 \times [Hb] \times So_2 \qquad (2)$$

For the previous set of blood gases, this would give a Co_2 of 14.5 vol%.

The formula can be made even simpler by substituting the fraction $^4/_3$ for the decimal 1.34:

$$Co_2 = \frac{4}{3} \times [Hb] \times So_2 \qquad (3)$$

Because [Hb] and the So_2 can usually be approximated by integers with little loss of accuracy, the calculation frequently allows cancellation of the three and can be done mentally. For the previous example, the oxygen content would be 14.4 vol%.

Calculation of the oxygen content requires knowledge of the So_2. Many pulmonary arterial catheters are now equipped with sensors mounted on their tips that directly measure the saturation of the blood in the pulmonary artery. Alternatively, blood can be withdrawn from the tip of the catheter and sent to the laboratory, where the So_2 can be easily measured by an instrument known as a co-oximeter. Most laboratories will make this measurement by specific request, but some will calculate the So_2 from the Po_2. This calculation is frequently inaccurate for mixed venous specimens but is usually accurate for arterial blood. The calculation is made from equations that are based on the oxyhemoglobin dissociation curve (Figure 12–1), an empirically derived relationship between the So_2 of nonfetal human blood and its Po_2. The saturation for a given Po_2 depends on blood temperature, [H$^+$], and Pco_2 and on the red cell concentration of 2,3-diphosphoglycerate (2,3-DPG). The laboratory should be told the temperature, and it will measure the [H$^+$] and Pco_2.

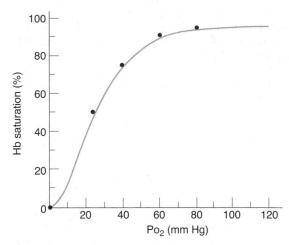

▲ **Figure 12–1.** Oxyhemoglobin dissociation curve for human blood at 37 °C with a Pco_2 of 40 mm Hg, a pH of 7.40, and a normal 2,3-DPG red cell concentration. Approximate values from Table 12–4 fall close to the idealized curve.

It will then calculate the So_2 from the Po_2 with the assumption that the 2,3-DPG concentration is normal.

It is helpful, however, to have some guidelines for converting back and forth between So_2 and Po_2. Five approximations for points on the dissociation curve for a patient with normal temperature, [H$^+$], Pco_2, and 2,3-DPG levels are given in Table 12–4. The P_{50} of human hemoglobin—the Po_2 at which the molecule is half-saturated—is 27 mm Hg (approximated as 25 mm Hg in the table). The Po_2 and So_2 for mixed venous blood in a person with a [Hb] of 15 g/dL and a normal O_2 consumption and cardiac output are 40 mm Hg and 75%, respectively. A Po_2 of 60 mm Hg—a value that should be exceeded by most patients in an intensive care unit—corresponds to a So_2 of 90%. A Po_2 of 80 mm Hg corresponds to a So_2 of 95%. Remembering the values in the table allows construction of a dissociation curve and facilitates conversion from one measure of oxygenation to the

Table 12–4. Approximate Correlations for Partial Pressures of Oxygen and Oxygen Saturation in Blood at 37 °C with a pH of 7.4, a Pco_2 of 40 mm Hg, and a Normal 2,3-DPG Red Cell Concentration.

Po_2	So_2
0 mm Hg	0%
25 mm Hg	50%
40 mm Hg	75%
60 mm Hg	90%
80 mm Hg	95%

other. For example, in a patient with a normal temperature, [H+], P_{CO_2}, and 2,3-DPG, and a [Hb] of 10 g/dL, a P_{O_2} of 60 mm Hg in the systemic arterial blood would create an oxygen content of 12 vol% (from Equation 1), a value that would be adequate if the patient had normal coronary arteries and a good heart. Such a value would be inadequate, however, in the face of underlying heart disease.

CAUSES OF ELEVATED Pa_{CO_2}

The patient in pulmonary failure will frequently have an elevated arterial carbon dioxide tension. The arterial P_{CO_2} is proportionate to CO_2 production divided by alveolar ventilation—defined as the volume of air exchanged per unit time in functioning alveoli. Since CO_2 production is usually fairly constant in adequately perfused patients, the P_{CO_2} comes to be inversely proportionate to alveolar ventilation. An elevated P_{CO_2} in the presence of normal CO_2 production means inadequate alveolar ventilation. Ventilation should be assessed with respect to how much work is required to generate the P_{CO_2}. In the case of spontaneous ventilation, this assessment involves the frequency and depth of breathing; in the case of mechanical ventilation, the frequency of the machine-generated breaths and the tidal volume of those breaths.

The P_{CO_2} also gives an indication of dead space ventilation—the ventilation of nonperfused airways. Since minute or total ventilation is dead space ventilation plus alveolar ventilation, a normal P_{CO_2} combined with a normal minute ventilation implies a normal dead space ventilation. A normal P_{CO_2} that must be generated by a supranormal minute ventilation implies increased dead space ventilation. Normal dead space ventilation is one-third of total ventilation, but many critically ill surgical patients will have a dead space ventilation that is up to two-thirds of total ventilation. Increased dead space ventilation can be caused by hypovolemia with poor perfusion of nondependent alveoli, ARDS, pulmonary emboli, pulmonary vasoconstriction, and mechanical ventilation-induced compression of the pulmonary vasculature. Hypovolemia should be treated by expansion of the vascular volume. Emboli should be treated by anticoagulation or by elimination of their source. Dead space generated by mechanical ventilation should be minimized by adjustment of the ventilator, usually by decreasing tidal volumes or end-expiratory pressures, while at the same time maintaining enough mechanical support to generate a normal P_{CO_2} and alveolar ventilation.

CAUSES OF LOW Pa_{O_2}

Almost all surgical patients with pulmonary failure will have systemic arterial hypoxemia. There are five physiological causes: low inspired O_2 concentration, diffusion block between alveolar gas and capillary blood, subnormal alveolar ventilation, shunting of blood through completely nonventilated portions of the lung or bypassing of blood past the

lung, and perfusion of parts of the lung that have low ventilation/perfusion ratios. In addition, any process that decreases the mixed venous oxygen content in the presence of any of the above can lower the arterial P_{O_2} even further. Low mixed venous oxygen content can be caused by a low arterial oxygen content, low cardiac output, or high O_2 consumption.

Arterial hypoxemia in the surgical patient is usually caused by shunting, low ventilation/perfusion ratios, low mixed venous oxygen content, or a combination of these factors. Low inspired O_2 concentrations at sea level are impossible so long as the ventilator is functioning properly. (This must be checked, however, as the first step in diagnosing and correcting the cause of a low P_{O_2}.) Diffusion block is exceedingly rare in surgical patients. Subnormal alveolar ventilation can be ruled out with a normal arterial P_{CO_2} assuming CO_2 production is not depressed. Thus, shunting and areas of low ventilation/perfusion ratios, along with low mixed venous oxygen content, remain as causes for almost all cases of hypoxemia in the surgical patient. Shunting and low ventilation/perfusion ratios do not need to be distinguished from each other very often, but the distinction can be made by increasing the inspired O_2 concentration to 100%: Hypoxemia caused by areas of low ventilation/perfusion ratios will be at least partially corrected by 100% O_2; hypoxemia caused by shunting will not. The mixed venous oxygen content can be measured with the pulmonary arterial catheter.

ACID-BASE BALANCE

Acid-base abnormalities can arise from the hypoventilation of pulmonary insufficiency or from the metabolic abnormalities of shock. The former has already been discussed. The latter can become more involved.

The hydrogen ion, carbon dioxide gas, and bicarbonate equilibrate with one another in the plasma water, and if two of the quantities are known, the third can be calculated. In practice, the P_{CO_2} and [H+], which are measured directly with the blood gas apparatus, will be known. The [HCO_3^-] can then be calculated by the Henderson-Hasselbalch equation, which can be written in the following form:

$$[HCO_3^-] = \frac{24 \times P_{CO_2}}{[H^+]} \qquad (4)$$

where [HCO_3^-] is expressed as mmol/L, P_{CO_2} as mm Hg, and [H+] as nmol/L. This form of the equation requires conversion of pH, the more common expression of [H+], into nmol/L, the more logical expression, but the conversion is not difficult (Table 12–5). The values in the table are easy to remember if one notes that each value in the column under [H+] is 80% of the value immediately above, with the exception of 80 and 63, which are off by 1. Thus, by Equation 4, if the P_{CO_2} is 60 mm Hg and the pH is 7.30, the [HCO_3^-] is 29 mmol/L.

Table 12–5. Conversion of pH to Hydrogen Ion Concentration.

pH	Hydrogen Ion Concentration (mol/L)
7.0	100
7.1	$100 \times 0.8 = 80$
7.2	$80 \times 0.8 = 63$
7.3	$63 \times 0.8 = 50$
7.4	$50 \times 0.8 = 40$
7.5	$40 \times 0.8 = 32$
7.6	$32 \times 0.8 = 25$

Note: Values not indicated in the table can be derived by interpolation. For example, a pH of 7.35 corresponds to a hydrogen ion concentration of approximately 45.

The $[HCO_3^-]$ calculated by this equation is the amount of bicarbonate ion dissolved in the plasma water and can be obtained only from a specimen of blood that is obtained and processed without exposure to the atmosphere. The "CO_2 combining power" that is typically measured along with electrolyte concentrations in blood that is not processed anaerobically includes not only the $[HCO_3^-]$ but any CO_2 gas and carbonic acid that is dissolved in the plasma as well. The CO_2 combining power is usually about 2 mmol/L greater than the calculated (and actual) $[HCO_3^-]$.

The base deficit or excess is determined by comparing the calculated $[HCO_3^-]$ with the $[HCO_3^-]$ that might be expected in a patient with a given P_{CO_2} and $[H^+]$. These expected values have been determined by analyzing blood obtained from patients with a wide variety of pulmonary disorders. For example, the kidneys in a patient with chronic respiratory acidemia can usually compensate to the extent that a chronic elevation in P_{CO_2} of 10 mm Hg will generate an increase in $[HCO_3^-]$ of 3 mmol/L. A patient with chronic obstructive lung disease and a chronically elevated P_{CO_2} of 60 mm Hg would be expected to have a $[HCO_3^-]$ of 30 mmol/L— 6 mmol/L more than a normal value of 24. If such a patient had a pH of 7.30, the actual $[HCO_3^-]$ would be 29 mmol/L (from Equation 4; see the example in the preceding paragraph). That is, the observed value would be 1 mmol/L less than predicted, and the patient would be said to have a base deficit of 1 mmol/L.

The difficulty with the concept of base deficit and excess is that it rests on historically determined values, which may not be applicable to the patient at hand. For example, if a surgical patient with previously normal lungs lost his or her airway after an operation and began to hypoventilate, one would expect the $[HCO_3^-]$ to be normal—24 mmol/L—because the kidneys would not have had time to compensate for the hypercapnia. If the P_{CO_2} was 60 mm Hg and the pH 7.30, the physician should be concerned because the $[HCO_3^-]$ is 29 mmol/L (these values are the same as in the preceding paragraphs). A value of 29 mmol/L should alert the physician to the fact that the $[HCO_3^-]$ is too high, perhaps because $NaHCO_3$ had been given unnecessarily. The base deficit, however, would be 1 mmol/L, suggesting that the patient's $[HCO_3^-]$ was appropriate. The base deficit would be misleading.

The use of base deficit and excess is ensconced in the literature, and the terms are used in this chapter. However, the concept of $[HCO_3^-]$ may be preferable. Errors in patient evaluation are more likely to be minimized if the physician interprets that value in the light of a particular patient's situation. If a chronically ill patient in the intensive care unit has severe ARDS and a P_{CO_2} of 60 mm Hg with a pH of 7.30, no attempt should be made to change the accompanying $[HCO_3^-]$ of 29 mmol/L—that value represents the expected renal compensation for such a chronic hypercapnia (though the impaired alveolar ventilation should be of concern). Alternatively, if the patient's P_{CO_2} is 60 mm Hg and the pH is 7.45, the patient has an inappropriately high $[HCO_3^-]$ of approximately 40 mmol/L (calculated from Equation 4), perhaps because of unreplaced losses of hydrogen ion from the stomach, chronic use of a loop diuretic, or administration of excessive amounts of acetate in the patient's parenteral nutrition. In this situation, the $[HCO_3^-]$ should be brought down into the low 30s. The excessively high $[HCO_3^-]$ and its resultant alkalemia may be blunting the patient's ventilatory drive.

Thus, in dealing with acid-base disorders, the calculation of the bicarbonate concentration in arterial plasma can be taken from the blood gas laboratory or calculated by the clinician. In the case of a metabolic acidemia, the underlying abnormality should be corrected and then, if the pH remains less than 7.20, sodium bicarbonate can be used, but only after resuscitation has been initiated. The bicarbonate produces carbon dioxide and water locally, in the interstitial fluid at the sites where the hydrogen ions are being produced. In the absence of resuscitation, the locally generated carbon dioxide can cross back into the cell, worsening intracellular acidosis. There is no problem with bicarbonate if it is given after some local flow has been achieved. The generated carbon dioxide will be washed centrally into the pulmonary vasculature, where it will be eliminated by the lungs.

Metabolic alkalemia in the surgical patient is usually easy to recognize and treat. Contraction alkalemia is treated with fluid expansion. Hypokalemic, hypochloremic metabolic alkalemia caused by unreplaced loss of gastric fluid (continuous nasogastric suction or protracted vomiting), is treated with normal saline supplemented with potassium chloride. Hypokalemic hypochloremic alkalemia caused by use of loop diuretics is treated by withholding diuresis. In situations where continued diuresis is warranted, the addition of acetazolamide to the diuretic regimen is helpful. Although the administration of 0.1 N hydrochloric acid can reverse severe alkalemia, it is rarely necessary and should only be given as a slow central intravenous drip over a period of 48 hours. The amount of acid to be given is calculated on the basis of the presumed extracellular chloride deficit, with the assumption that the interstitial chloride concentration is the same as the plasma concentration, that is, with the assumption that the Donnan factor for chloride is 1.

IV. RISK ASSESSMENT

Predicting the likelihood of survival in critically ill surgical patients is best accomplished by evaluating clinical and laboratory findings. Computation of a severity of illness score is usually unnecessary. Nonetheless, several scoring systems have been developed with the intention of increasing the precision of the estimate. All such systems assign a mathematical probability for survival in groups of patients, and many are useful for research purposes because they allow comparisons of patients among different institutions. None of them, however, are accurate enough to predict survival for an individual patient, though some are still clinically useful for assessing the effects of therapy.

The APACHE II score, in which clinical data and 14 measured variables are entered into a formula to assess the probability of survival, takes about 30 minutes to calculate by hand—less by computer. The score can predict survival in critically ill medical patients; it has not been found to be of value in the usual surgical patient, and in any case, it is too cumbersome unless one has a particular interest in this kind of methodology.

Methods for predicting survival in trauma patients are well established, though most trauma systems are designed to evaluate all trauma patients and not the specific subset of critically ill trauma patients. The Injury Severity Score, the Revised Trauma Score, and the ASCOT score have proved to be most reliable. The Glasgow Coma Score is quite accurate for predicting survival in patients with head injuries. Combining the Glasgow Coma Score with a simple measurement of fluid requirement has also proved to be accurate in critically injured trauma patients.

Barie PS, Hydo LJ, Fischer E: Comparison of APACHE II and III scoring systems for mortality prediction in critical surgical illness. Arch Surg 1995;130:77.

Bessey PQ: Critical care: metabolic response to critical illness. *ACS Surgery: Principles & Practice*, WebMed Inc., 2006. Available exclusively online at www.acssurgery.com.

Griffiths RD, Jones C, Palmer TE: Six-month outcome of critically ill patients given glutamine-supplemented parenteral nutrition. Nutrition 1997;13:295.

Horan TC et al: Nosocomial infections in surgical patients in the United States, January 1986–June 1992. National Nosocomial Infections Surveillance (NNIS) System. Infect Control Hosp Epidemiol 1993;14:73.

Houdijk AP et al: Randomised trial of glutamine-enriched enteral nutrition on infectious morbidity in patients with multiple trauma. Lancet 1998;352:772.

O'Quin R, Marini JJ: Pulmonary artery occlusion pressure: clinical physiology, measurement, and interpretation. Am Rev Respir Dis 1983;128:319.

Vassar MJ et al: Comparison of APACHE II, TRISS, and a proposed 24-hour ICU point system for prediction of outcome in ICU trauma patients. J Trauma 1992;32:490.

Vassar MJ et al: Prediction of outcome in intensive care unit trauma patients: a multicenter study of Acute Physiology and Chronic Health Evaluation (APACHE), Trauma and Injury Severity Score (TRISS), and a 24-hour intensive care unit (ICU) point system. J Trauma 1999;47:324.

Wilmore DW: Metabolic response to severe surgical illness: overview. World J Surg 2000;24:705.

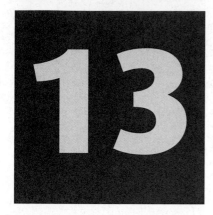

Management of the Injured Patient

Mark R. Hemmila, MD
Wendy L. Wahl, MD

EPIDEMIOLOGY OF TRAUMA

As a "disease," trauma is a major public health problem. In the United States, it is the leading cause of death among people aged 1–45 and the fifth leading cause of death for all age groups. For persons under age 30, trauma is responsible for more deaths than all other diseases combined. Each year, 160,000 lives are lost because of injuries and homicide. Because trauma adversely affects a young population, it results in the loss of more working years than all other causes of death. Presence of alcohol is a significant contributor to trauma fatalities, and 41% of all traffic deaths in 2006 were alcohol related. The financial costs of injury are staggering and exceed $500 billion annually. Regrettably, nearly 40% of all trauma deaths could be avoided by injury prevention measures (55% of passenger vehicle occupants killed were unrestrained), alcohol cessation, and by the establishment of regional trauma systems that would expedite the evaluation and treatment of seriously injured patients.

Trauma deaths have been classically described as having a trimodal distribution (Figure 13–1), with peaks that correspond to the types of intervention that would be most effective in reducing mortality. The first peak, the **immediate deaths,** represents patients who die of their injuries before reaching the hospital. The injuries accounting for these deaths include major brain or spinal cord trauma and those resulting in rapid exsanguination. Few of these patients would have any chance of survival even with access to immediate care because almost 60% of these deaths occur at the same time as the injury. Prevention remains the major strategy to reduce these deaths.

The second peak, the **early deaths,** are those that occur within the first few hours after injury. Half are caused by internal hemorrhage, and the other half, by central nervous system injuries. Almost all of these injuries are potentially treatable. However, in most cases, salvage requires prompt and definitive care of the sort available at a trauma center, which is a specialized institution that can provide immediate resuscitation, identification of injuries, and access to a ready operating room 24 hours a day. Development of well-organized trauma systems with rapid transport and protocol-driven care can reduce the mortality in this time period from 30% to less than 10%.

The third peak, the **late deaths,** consists of patients who die days or weeks after injury. Ten percent to 20% of all trauma deaths occur during this period. Mortality for this period has traditionally been attributed to infection and multiple organ failure. However, development of trauma systems has changed the epidemiology of these deaths. During the first week, refractory intracranial hypertension following severe head injury is now responsible for a significant number of these deaths. Improvements in critical care management continue to be essential in reducing deaths during this phase. It is paramount that surgeons caring for trauma patients have genuine expertise in surgical critical care.

TRAUMA SYSTEMS

The terrorist events of September 11, 2001, highlighted the need for national and state trauma systems that can handle both routine events and mass casualty situations. The purpose of a trauma system is to provide timely, organized care in order to minimize preventable morbidity and mortality following injury. The system includes prehospital care designed to identify, triage, treat, and transport victims with serious injuries. Criteria for staging patients with major trauma consist of standardized scoring systems based on readily discernible anatomic and physiologic variables. The criteria are designed to identify not only the more severe and complex single injuries but also combinations of injuries that require tertiary care.

Trauma centers that are part of a larger trauma system are already organized to respond to unexpected multiple casualty events. These centers have established links with emergency medical service providers and participate in systemwide patient triage and quality improvement. Gaps remain, how-

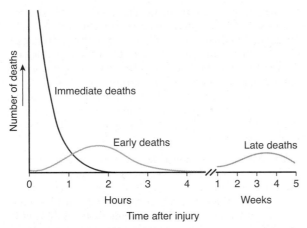

▲ **Figure 13–1.** Periods of peak mortality after injury. (Modified from Hoyt DB, Coimbra R: Trauma: Introduction. In: Greenfield LJ, Mulholland MW, Oldham KT, et al: *Surgery, Scientific Principles and Practice*, 3rd ed. Lippincott Williams & Wilkins, 2001; p. 271.)

ever, in areas of the country not served by trauma systems, and a wide range in the degree of disaster preparedness exists at all levels of trauma care.

The American College of Surgeons (ACS) defines four levels of institutional trauma care. **Level I** is the highest designation a trauma center can receive. It indicates that the hospital has committed itself to the care of trauma patients and offers the highest level of skill available in trauma care. A level I trauma center is directed by a board-certified surgeon specializing in trauma care and is staffed by a team of board-certified trauma care specialists available 24 hours a day—including emergency room physicians, trauma surgeons, neurosurgeons and neurologists, orthopedic surgeons, plastic surgeons, anesthesiologists, and radiologists. The level I center maintains a quality improvement program including a trauma registry and has an active commitment to research, teaching, and community outreach/injury prevention. **Level II** trauma centers provide 24-hour care by in-hospital and on-call physicians. They can deliver the same quality of care as a level I center but without the same teaching and research obligations. Immediate operating room capability must be maintained 24 hours a day in level II centers. The **level III** trauma center provides prompt assessment, resuscitation, and stabilization followed by surgical treatment or interhospital transfer as appropriate. Although they may not be able to provide definitive care in all circumstances, level III centers serve a valuable function in less populated areas where resuscitation and stabilization before transport may be lifesaving. **Level IV** centers are designed to provide advanced trauma life support prior to patient transfer in remote areas in which no higher level of care is available.

PREHOSPITAL CARE & IMMEDIATE MEASURES AT THE SCENE OF AN ACCIDENT

At first glance, the victim of an accident may not appear to be badly injured. Sometimes there may be little external evidence of injury; however, when the mechanism of trauma is sufficient to produce severe injury, the victim must be handled as if a severe injury has occurred. It is critical at the scene that the injured person be protected from further trauma; likewise, rescue personnel need to take precautions to avoid injury to themselves. First aid at the scene of an accident should be administered by trained personnel whenever possible.

Whether the patient is first seen on the battlefield, beside a road, in the emergency ward, or in the hospital, the basic principles of initial management are the same:

1. Is the victim breathing? If not, provide an airway and establish bag-mask ventilation.
2. Is there a pulse or heartbeat? If not, begin closed-chest compression.
3. Is there gross external bleeding? If so, elevate the part if possible and apply enough external pressure to stop the bleeding. A tourniquet when utilized by trained providers is acceptable in circumstances of extreme bleeding.
4. Is there any question of injury to the spine? If so, protect the neck and spine before moving the patient.
5. Splint obvious fractures.

As soon as these steps have been taken, the patient can be safely transported.

EVALUATION OF THE TRAUMA PATIENT

In most situations, a brief history is obtained from prehospital personnel via radio communication or when the patient arrives at the hospital. In the case of motor vehicle accidents, for example, it is important to determine the circumstances of the injury, including the speed of impact, the condition of the vehicle, the position of the patient at the scene, type of restraint systems present, evidence of blood loss, and the condition of other passengers. The time that the injury occurred and the treatment rendered while en route is recorded. Knowing the mechanism of injury often gives a clue to concealed trauma. Information regarding serious underlying medical problems should be sought from Medic Alert bracelets or wallet cards. If the patient is conscious and stable, the examiner should obtain a complete history and use this information to direct the examination in order to avoid unnecessary tests.

Trauma victims require a precise, rapid, systematic approach to initial evaluation in order to ensure their survival. The Advanced Trauma Life Support (ATLS) system developed by the ACS Committee on Trauma represents the best current approach to the severely injured patient. The sequence of evaluation includes primary survey, resuscitation, secondary survey, and definitive management. The primary survey attempts to identify and treat immediate life-threatening conditions. Resuscitation is performed, and the response to therapy is evaluated. The secondary survey includes a comprehensive physical examination designed to detect all injuries and establish a treatment priority for potentially life-threatening and/or limb-threatening ones. During the primary and secondary surveys, appropriate laboratory and imaging studies are performed to aid in the identification of injuries and prepare the patient for definitive care.

1. Primary Survey

The ATLS manual and provider course published by the ACS Committee on Trauma is the accepted guideline for the primary survey. The primary survey is a rapid assessment to detect life-threatening injuries following the ABCDE: airway, breathing, circulation, disability, and exposure/environment.

AIRWAY

The establishment of an adequate airway has the highest priority in the primary survey. Oxygen by high-flow nasal cannula (10–12 L/min), 100% nonrebreather mask, or bag-mask ventilation with pulse oximetry should be started if not already in place. Maneuvers used in the trauma patient to establish an airway must consider a possible cervical spine injury. Any patient with multisystem trauma, especially those with an altered level of consciousness or blunt trauma above the clavicles, should be assumed to have a cervical spine injury. The rapid assessment for signs of airway obstruction should include inspection for foreign bodies and facial, jaw, or tracheal/laryngeal fractures that may result in acute loss of airway patency. Techniques that can be used to establish a patent airway while protecting the cervical spine include the chin lift or jaw thrust maneuvers (Figure 13–2).

Patients who can communicate verbally without difficulty are unlikely to have an impaired airway. Repeated assessment of airway patency is always prudent. Those patients with severe head injury, an altered level of consciousness, or a Glasgow Coma Scale (GCS) score of 8 or less usually require placement of a definitive airway. Orotracheal or nasotracheal intubation can be attempted with cervical spine precautions if a second person maintains axial immobilization of the head to prevent destabilization of the spine (Figure 13–3). If ventilatory failure occurs and an adequate airway cannot be obtained readily by orotracheal or nasotracheal intubation, surgical cricothyroidotomy should be performed as rapidly as possible (Figure 13–4).

BREATHING

Once the airway has been established, it is necessary to make certain that oxygenation and ventilation is adequate. Examine the patient to determine the degree of chest expansion, breath sounds, tachypnea, crepitus from rib fractures, subcutaneous emphysema, and the presence of penetrating or open wounds. Immediately life-threatening pulmonary injuries that must be detected and treated promptly include tension pneumothorax, open pneumothorax, flail chest, and massive hemothorax. Chest injury has the second highest case fatality rate in the trauma patient. The following are examples of life-threatening pulmonary injuries and their treatment:

1. **Tension pneumothorax:** This condition occurs when air becomes trapped in the pleural space under pressure. The harmful effects result primarily from shift of the mediastinum, impairment of venous return, and potential occlusion of the airway. Tension pneumothorax is difficult to diagnose even when the patient reaches the hospital. The clinical findings consist of hypotension in the presence of distended neck veins, decreased or absent breath sounds on the affected side, hyperresonance to percussion, and tracheal shift away from the affected side. These signs may be difficult to detect in a hypovolemic patient with a cervical collar in place. Cyanosis may be a late manifestation. Emergency treatment consists of insertion of a large-

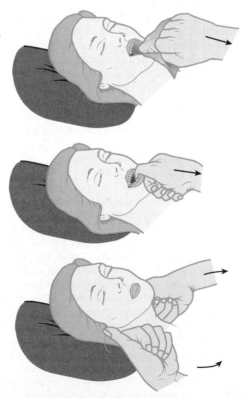

▲ **Figure 13–2.** Relief of airway obstruction.

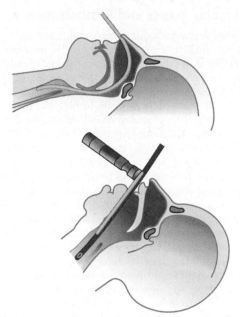

▲ Figure 13–3. *Top:* Nasotracheal intubation. *Bottom:* Orotracheal intubation.

bore needle or plastic intravenous cannula (angiocath) through the chest wall into the pleural space in the second intercostal space along the midclavicular line to relieve the pressure and convert the tension pneumothorax to a simple pneumothorax. The needle or cannula should be left in place until a thoracostomy tube is inserted for definitive management (Figure 13–5).

2. **Open pneumothorax:** This condition results from an open wound of the chest wall with free communication between the pleural space and the atmosphere. The resulting impairment of the thoracic bellows, and its ability to expand the lung results in inadequate ventilation. With chest expansion during a breath, air moves in and out of the chest wall opening instead of through the trachea, producing hypoventilation that can be rapidly fatal. Emergency treatment consists of sealing the wound with an occlusive sterile dressing taped on three sides to act as a flutter-type valve or with any material if nothing sterile is available. Definitive treatment requires placement of a chest tube to reexpand the lung and surgical closure of the defect. Airway intubation with positive-pressure mechanical ventilation can be helpful in massive open pneumothorax.

3. **Flail chest:** Multiple rib fractures resulting in a free-floating segment of chest wall may produce paradoxical motion that impairs lung expansion (Figure 13–6). In patients with flail chest, injury-associated pulmonary contusion is common and is often the major cause of respiratory failure. The injury is identified by careful inspection and palpation during physical examination. Patients with large flail segments will almost always require endotracheal intubation and mechanical ventilation both to stabilize the flail segment and to optimize gas exchange. Smaller flail segments may be well tolerated if supplemental oxygen and adequate analgesia are provided. The work of breathing is increased considerably, and many patients who initially appear to be compensating well may suddenly deteriorate a few hours later. Therefore, most patients with flail chest require monitoring in an intensive care unit.

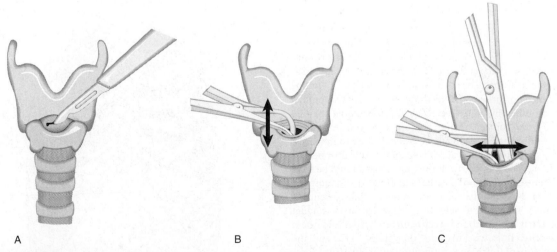

A   B   C

▲ Figure 13–4. Surgical cricothyroidotomy.

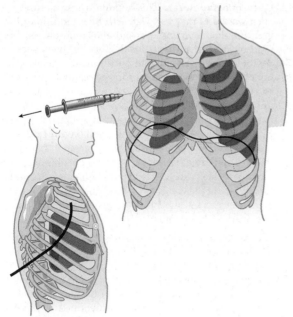

▲ **Figure 13–5.** Relief of pneumothorax. Tension pneumothorax must be immediately decompressed by a needle introduced through the second anterior intercostal space. A chest tube is usually inserted in the midaxillary line at the level of the nipple and is directed posteriorly and superiorly toward the apex of the thorax. The tube is attached to a "three-bottle" suction device, and the rate of escape of air is indicated by the appearance of bubbles in the second of the three bottles. Cessation of bubbling suggests that the air leak has become sealed.

CIRCULATION

Hemorrhage

Free hemorrhage from accessible surface wounds is usually obvious and can be controlled in most cases by local pressure and elevation of the bleeding point. Firm and precise pressure on the major artery in the axilla, antecubital space, wrist, groin, popliteal space, or at the ankle may suffice for temporary control of arterial hemorrhage distal to these points. When all other measures have failed, a tourniquet may be necessary to control major hemorrhage from extensive wounds or major vessels in an extremity. Failure to manage a tourniquet properly may cause irreparable vascular or neurologic damage. For this reason, the tourniquet should be used only when necessary and must be kept exposed and loosened at least every 20 minutes for 1 or 2 minutes while the patient is in transit. Transport to definitive care where the tourniquet can be safely removed and treatment rendered should be a top priority. It is wise to write the letters "TK" and the military time of tourniquet application on the patient's forehead with a skin-marking pen or on adhesive tape.

Vascular Access and Resuscitation

All patients with significant trauma should have large-caliber peripheral intravenous catheters inserted immediately for administration of crystalloid fluids as needed. If any degree of shock is present, at least two 14–16 gauge peripheral intravenous lines should be established usually in the antecubital fossa. If venous access cannot be obtained by percutaneous peripheral or central venous cannulation, a venous cutdown of the saphenous vein at the ankle using an angiocath or intravenous extension tubing with the tip cut off can be performed. A blood sample for type and crossmatch should be sent from the venous line, if not already drawn.

As soon as the first intravenous line is inserted, rapid crystalloid infusion should begin. Adult patients should be given 2 L of Ringer lactate or normal saline. For children, the initial administered crystalloid volume should be 20 mL/kg. Patients who experience a transient response should receive an additional infusion of 2 L of crystalloid. For patients in whom there is no improvement in blood pressure from the initial crystalloid or who transiently respond but fail, the second crystalloid bolus should rapidly be switched to infusion of blood products. Beyond the administration of the first two units of packed red blood cells (PRBC), it is important to also administer fresh plasma or thawed fresh frozen plasma (FFP) to avoid coagulopathy in the massively transfused patient. Massive transfusion is defined as at least 10 units of PRBC. The exact ratio of FFP to PRBC is still under investigation, but a target range of 1:1 or 2:3 is considered acceptable. Military data has shown that the early use of plasma can reduce mortality by up to 50% in the massively transfused trauma patient. Giving platelets as part of the massive transfusion protocol is also supported by military data demonstrating a 20% reduction in mortality for patients who received platelets as fresh whole blood or

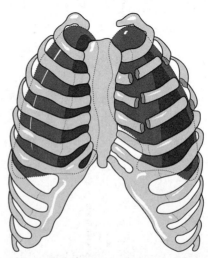

▲ **Figure 13–6.** Flail chest.

apheresis platelets in conjunction with PRBC. The exact platelet-to-PRBC ratio for optimal treatment of the hemorrhaging trauma patient is not known, but giving a unit of platelets for every 5 units of PRBC is a reasonable ratio. Type O, Rh-negative PRBC should be immediately available in the emergency department for any patient with impending cardiac arrest or massive hemorrhage. Some high-volume centers now also stock fresh or "prethawed" AB plasma as well. Type-specific blood should be available within 15–20 minutes of patient arrival to the hospital.

Transfusion of blood products is not without risk. Despite rigorous screening programs, transmission of viral bloodborne diseases can occur. The current incidence of bloodborne pathogen transmission following red blood cell transfusion are hepatitis A, 1:1 million; hepatitis B, 1:250,000; hepatitis C 1:150,000; and HIV, 1:2 million. Transfusion of blood products is also associated with transfusion-related immunomodulation and transfusion-related acute lung injury. Both of these problems can increase morbidity and mortality. The age of blood transfused can also contribute to problems. Transfusion of a patient with older units of PRBC has been shown to cause generation of systemic proinflammatory mediators and increase the risk of wound infection.

Recombinant activated factor VII is a new drug approved by the Food and Drug Administration for treatment of hemophilia and factor VII deficiencies. It has been used off-label with success in reducing the need for PRBC transfusion in severely injured patients. Concerns have arisen about the use of activated factor VII in trauma patients with regard to cost and risk of thromboembolic events. Use of the drug in acidotic patients with a pH less than 7.1 or a platelet count under 50,000 cells/μL is considered ineffective. Recommendations for use of activated factor VII in trauma patients suggest using it in only those who are in a massive transfusion circumstance with active bleeding or in patients with known intracranial hemorrhage and coagulopathy. The dosage is 100 mcg/kg, rounded to the nearest 1200 mcg, given as an intravenous bolus over 2–5 minutes.

▶ Monitoring

As intravenous access is obtained, electrocardiogram leads for continuous cardiac monitoring should be placed. Noninvasive blood pressure measurements should be obtained with a time-cycled blood pressure cuff. Pulse oximetry is valuable in ensuring that adequate hemoglobin oxygen saturation is present in the injured patient. Temperature is a crucial vital sign, and it should be measured and recorded along with the first pulse and blood pressure in the emergency department.

NEUROLOGIC DISABILITY

A brief neurologic examination should be documented to assess patients' degree of neurologic impairment. Many factors may contribute to altered levels of consciousness and should be considered in addition to central nervous system injury in all trauma patients. Other than the direct trauma, the most common contributing causes of altered mental status for trauma patients are alcohol intoxication, other central nervous system stimulants or depressants, diabetic ketoacidosis, cerebrovascular accident, and hypovolemic shock. Less common causes are epilepsy, eclampsia, electrolyte imbalances associated with metabolic and systemic diseases, anaphylaxis, heavy metal poisoning, electric shock, tumors, severe systemic infections, hypercalcemia, asphyxia, heat stroke, severe heart failure, and hysteria. These uncommon causes of coma or diminished mental status should be considered if routine testing such as blood alcohol and glucose level, urine toxicology, and head computerized tomography (CT) scanning are unrevealing as to the etiology of mental impairment. In such cases, further laboratory and diagnostic testing may be warranted.

The differential diagnosis depends upon a careful history and complete physical examination, with particular attention to the neurologic examination with documentation of the patient's GCS score (Table 13–1), and an urgent head CT scan. The GCS score is useful in monitoring acute changes in neurologic function and is used for prognosticating outcomes after severe head injury. The motor component of the GCS score is the most accurate for predicting outcome and has a linear relationship with mortality. Lateralizing signs

Table 13–1. Glasgow Coma Scale Score.

Parameter	Score
Best motor response	
Normal	6
Localizes	5
Withdraws	4
Flexion	3
Extension	2
None	1
Best verbal response	
Oriented	5
Confused	4
Verbalizes	3
Vocalizes	2
None	1
Eye opening	
Spontaneous	4
To command	3
To pain	2
None	1

may also suggest evidence of an intracranial mass effect or carotid or vertebral artery injury, while loss of distal motor and/or sensory function may help localize potential spinal cord injuries.

EXPOSURE/ENVIRONMENT

All clothing should be removed at once (cut off with trauma shears, usually) from the seriously injured patient, with care taken to avoid unnecessary movement. The removal of helmets or other protective clothing may require additional personnel to stabilize the patient and prevent further injury. All skin surfaces should be examined to identify injuries that may not be readily apparent, such as posterior penetrating trauma or open fractures. After inspecting all surfaces, warm blankets or warming devices should be placed to avoid hypothermia in the seriously injured patient.

EMERGENCY ROOM THORACOTOMY

Certain injuries are so critical that operative treatment must be undertaken as soon as the diagnosis is made. In these cases, resuscitation is continued as the patient is being operated on. For cardiopulmonary arrest that occurs in the emergency room as a direct result of trauma, external cardiac compression is rarely successful in maintaining effective perfusion of vital organs. An emergency left anterolateral thoracotomy should be performed in the fourth or fifth intercostal space, and the pericardium should be opened anterior to the phrenic nerve (Figure 13–7). Open cardiac massage, cross-clamping of the descending thoracic aorta, repair of cardiac injuries, and internal defibrillation can be performed as appropriate. Wounds of the lung producing severe hemorrhage or systemic air embolus may require pulmonary hilar cross-clamping.

Emergency room thoracotomy is most useful for cardiac arrest due to penetrating thoracic trauma, particularly in patients with pericardial tamponade from stab wounds. This extreme procedure is ineffective for most patients with cardiac arrest due to blunt trauma and for all patients who have no detectable vital signs in the field (< 1%

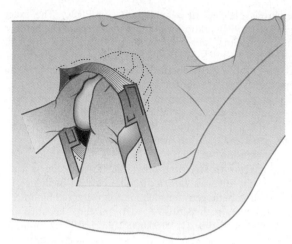

▲ **Figure 13–7.** Emergency thoracotomy and open cardiac massage.

survival). If vital signs are present in the emergency room but arrest appears imminent, the patient should be transferred rapidly to the operating room if at all possible, since conditions in the operating room are optimal for surgical intervention.

RESUSCITATION PHASE

▶ Shock

Shock is defined as inadequate end-organ tissue perfusion. Some degree of shock accompanies most severe injuries and is manifested initially by pallor, cold sweat, weakness, light-headedness, tachycardia, hypotension, thirst, air hunger, and, eventually, loss of consciousness. Patients with any of these signs should be presumed to be in shock and evaluated thoroughly. All patients determined to be in any degree of shock should be reexamined at regular intervals. The degree of shock has been categorized to guide resuscitation and help caregivers recognize the severity of symptoms (Table 13–2).

Table 13–2. Classification of Hypovolemic Shock.

	Class I	Class II	Class III	Class IV
Blood loss (mL)	Up to 750	750–1500	1500–2000	> 2000
Blood loss (% BV)	Up to 15%	15–30%	30–40%	> 40%
Pulse rate (beats/min)	< 100	> 100	> 120	> 140
Blood pressure	Normal	Minimal decrease	Decreased	Significantly decreased
Pulse pressure	Normal	Narrowed	Narrowed	Unobtainable or very narrow
Hourly urine output	≥ 0.5 mL/Kg	≥ 0.5 mL/Kg	< 0.5 cc/Kg	Minimal
CNS/mental status	Slightly anxious	Mildly anxious	Anxious & confused	Confused or lethargic

A. Hypovolemic Shock

Hypovolemic shock is due to loss of whole blood or plasma. Blood pressure may be maintained initially by vasoconstriction. Tissue hypoxia increases when hypotension ensues, and shock may become irreversible if irreparable damage occurs to the vital organs. Massive or prolonged hemorrhage, severe crush injuries, major fractures, and extensive burns are the most common causes. The presence of any of these conditions is an indication for prompt intravenous fluid infusion.

The most reliable clinical guide in assessing hypovolemic shock is skin perfusion. In mild or class 1 shock (< 15% blood volume loss), compensatory mechanisms may preserve adequate perfusion, and no skin or physiologic changes may be apparent. In moderate or class 2 shock (15–30% blood loss), the skin on the extremities becomes pale, cool, and moist as a result of vasoconstriction and release of epinephrine. Systolic blood pressure is often maintained at near-normal levels, but urine output will usually decrease. With severe or class 3 shock (30–40% blood volume loss), these changes—particularly diaphoresis—become more marked, and urine output declines significantly. Hypotension ensues. In addition, changes in cerebral function become evident consisting chiefly of agitation, disorientation, and memory loss. A common error is to attribute uncooperative behavior to intoxication, drug use, or brain injury when in fact it may be due to cerebral ischemia from blood loss. With class 4 shock (> 40% blood volume loss), profound hypotension is typically accompanied by loss of consciousness and anuria. In this situation, rapid resuscitation with crystalloid and blood products is necessary to prevent imminent death.

With any degree of shock, intravenous balanced salt solution (eg, lactated Ringer solution) should be given rapidly until the signs of shock abate and urine output returns to normal. If shock appears to be due to blood loss, blood transfusion should be given, starting with 2 units of uncrossmatched O-negative blood if crossmatched blood is unavailable. Additional resuscitation with crystalloid and/or blood products is guided by the cause of volume loss and response to fluid administration. Successful resuscitation is indicated by warm, dry, well-perfused skin, a urine output of 30–60 mL/h, and an alert sensorium. Improvement in pH toward normal and minimization of base deficit as measured on an arterial blood gas sample are also indicators of successful resuscitation.

As a general principle, measurements of blood pressure and pulse are less reliable than changes in urine output in assessing the severity of shock. Young patients and athletic older ones have compensatory mechanisms that often maintain adequate blood pressure even with moderate volume loss. Older patients and those taking cardiac or blood pressure medications often do not exhibit tachycardia even with extreme volume loss. Therefore, a Foley catheter should be inserted into the bladder to monitor urine output in any patient with major injuries or shock. Oliguria is the most reliable sign of moderate shock, and successful resuscitation is indicated by a return of urine output to 0.5–1 mL/kg/h. Absence of oliguria is an unreliable index of the absence of shock if the patient has an osmotic diuresis due to alcohol, glucose, mannitol, or intravenous contrast material.

A patient who is receiving intravenous fluids at a high rate may not exhibit signs of shock even in the setting of ongoing hemorrhage. If a patient continues to require high volumes of fluid after initial resuscitation in order to maintain urine output, mental status, and blood pressure, further investigation must be performed to rule out occult hemorrhage. The patient must be kept recumbent and given reassurance and analgesics as necessary. If opioids are necessary for pain relief, they are best administered intravenously in small doses.

B. Neurogenic Shock

Neurogenic shock is due to the pooling of blood in autonomically denervated venules and small veins and is usually due to spinal cord injury. Neurogenic shock is not caused by an isolated head injury, and in those patients, other causes of shock should be sought. A patient exhibiting signs of neurogenic shock (warm and well-perfused distal extremities in the presence of hypotension) should be given a 2 L crystalloid fluid bolus—followed by an additional bolus if the response is suboptimal. If neurogenic shock persists with fluid resuscitation, phenylephrine or another vasopressor should be given as a drip with the dosage adjusted until the blood pressure is maintained at a satisfactory level. If the patient does not improve quickly, other kinds of shock must be considered. Patients with neurogenic shock may require central venous pressure monitoring to ensure an optimal volume status.

C. Cardiac Compressive Shock

Cardiac compressive shock is caused by compression of the thin-walled chambers of the heart—the atria and the right ventricle—or by compression or distortion of the great veins entering the heart. The usual causes of this type of shock in the trauma patient are pericardial tamponade, tension pneumothorax, massive hemothorax, diaphragmatic rupture with herniation of abdominal contents into the chest, and an elevated diaphragm from massive abdominal hemorrhage. Treatment consists of urgent decompression depending on the specific cause. In severe cases, emergency thoracotomy may be necessary to restore adequate cardiac function.

D. Cardiogenic Shock

Cardiogenic shock is caused by decreased myocardial contractility and is most commonly caused by myocardial infarction or arrhythmia. Older trauma patients may develop a myocardial infarction as a complication of their injuries. On occasion an acute myocardial infarction may preclude a traumatic event and be a cause of injury or loss of consciousness. Rarely, a severe myocardial contusion may lead to cardiogenic shock. Treatment is supportive, with volume replacement guided by hemodynamic monitoring and administration of inotropic agents to augment cardiac output as necessary to maintain adequate end-organ perfusion. Unfortunately, patients with traumatic injuries are not usually candidates for anticoagulant or lytic therapy, and treatment of their acute myocardial ischemia is sometimes hindered by concerns about bleeding.

▶ Laboratory Studies

Immediately after intravenous catheters are placed, blood should be drawn for blood typing and crossmatching. If the patient has a history of renal, hepatic, or cardiac disease or is taking diuretics or anticoagulants, serum electrolytes and coagulation parameters should be measured. In most patients with serious injuries, an arterial blood gas provides rapid data about acidosis and base deficit, both of which are markers of under-resuscitation in addition to oxygenation (Po_2) and ventilation (Pco_2). Gross blood in the urine indicates the need for further diagnostic testing with abdominal CT scan or, in selected cases, a cystogram and urethrogram. Patients with obvious severe head injury, where intracranial pressure monitoring may be indicated, should have coagulation studies and a platelet count performed. Measurement of blood alcohol level and urine toxicology screen may be useful in patients with altered mental status.

▶ Imaging Studies

Radiographic plain films of the chest and pelvis are required in all major injuries. Lateral C-spine films have largely been supplanted by formal CT scanning of the neck in patients with suspicion of or mechanism for cervical spine injury. Bedside focused assessment with sonography for trauma (FAST) is the preferred triage method for determining the presence of hemoperitoneum in blunt trauma patients or cardiac tamponade in blunt and penetrating trauma patients. The presence of hemoperitoneum in an unstable patient on FAST may be an indication for exploratory laparotomy. Presence of hemoperitoneum in a stable patient or a negative FAST in a patient with abdominal pain is indication for further evaluation with abdominal CT scan.

Patients who have an abnormal chest radiograph with a mechanism for blunt aortic injury should undergo further screening with either helical chest CT done at the time of abdominal imaging or with aortography, if necessary. Cervical spine CT scans should be obtained for patients who are unconscious, have pain in the cervical region, have neurologic deficits, or have painful or distracting injuries. CT scanning of the head should be performed in all patients with loss of consciousness or more serious neurologic impairment. Radiographs of the long bones and noncervical spine can usually be deferred until the more critical injuries of the thorax and abdomen have been delineated and stabilized.

2. Secondary Survey & Patterns of Injury

A rapid and complete history and physical examination are essential for patients with serious or multiple injuries. Progressive changes in clinical findings are often the key to correct diagnosis, and negative findings that change to positive may be of great importance in revising an initial clinical evaluation. This is particularly true in the case of abdominal, thoracic, and intracranial injuries, which frequently do not become manifest until hours after the trauma.

Recognition of injury patterns is also important in identifying all injuries. For example, fractures of the calcaneus resulting from a fall from a great height are often associated with central dislocation of the hip and fractures of the spine and of the skull base. A crushed pelvis is often combined with laceration of the posterior urethra or bladder, vagina or rectum. Crush injuries of the chest are often associated with lacerations or rupture of the spleen, liver, or diaphragm. Penetrating wounds of the chest may involve not only the thoracic contents but also the abdominal viscera. These combinations occur frequently and should always be suspected.

TREATMENT PRIORITIES

In all cases of patients with multiple injuries, there must be a "captain of the team" who directs the resuscitation, decides which x-rays or special diagnostic tests should be obtained, and establishes priority for care by continuous consultation with other surgical specialists and anesthesiologists. A trauma surgeon or a general surgeon experienced in the care of injured patients usually has this role.

After controlling the airway if necessary, resuscitation and blood volume replacement have first priority. Deepening stupor in patients under observation should arouse suspicion of an expanding intracranial lesion requiring serial neurologic examinations and head CT. Too often, obvious signs of acute alcohol intoxication have been assumed to be the cause of unconsciousness, and intracranial hemorrhage has been overlooked.

Cerebral injuries take precedence in care only when there is rapidly deepening coma. Extradural bleeding is a critical emergency, requiring operation for control of bleeding and cerebral decompression. Subdural bleeding may produce a similar emergency. If the patient's condition permits, CT scanning should be performed for localization of the bleeding within the cranium prior to other operative interventions being initiated. In many cases of combined cerebral and abdominal injury with massive bleeding, laparotomy and craniotomy should be performed simultaneously.

Most urologic injuries are managed at the same time as associated intra-abdominal injuries. Pelvic fractures present special problems and are discussed in Chapter 40. Unless there is associated vascular injury with threatened ischemia of the limb, fractures of the long bones can be splinted and treated on an urgent basis. Open contaminated fractures should be cleansed and debrided as soon as possible. Injuries of the hand run the risk of infection that may result in a lifelong handicap without early effective treatment. Early treatment of the hand at the same time as treatment of any life-threatening injuries avoids infection and preserves the means of livelihood. Tetanus prophylaxis should be given in all instances of open contaminated wounds, puncture wounds, and burns.

Patients with a severe burden of trauma and shock may not be candidates for definitive treatment of all injuries in the immediate setting. Three physiological derangements comprise the "lethal triad" in the trauma literature: hypothermia, acidosis, and coagulopathy. These are boundaries of a patient's physiologic envelope beyond which the patient will develop irreversible shock and eventual death. Bailing out of the abdomen with damage control maneuvers in a patient headed for the lethal triad is not a sign of defeat; instead it is usually the intelligent option. Early warning signs of physiologic compromise that could lead to the lethal triad are edema of the small bowel, midgut distension, dusky serosal surfaces, tissue that is cool to the touch, noncompliant swollen abdominal wall, diffuse oozing from surgical or raw surfaces, and lack of obvious clot formation. Successful packing relies on clot formation, so employing a strategy of early packing is recommended rather than turning to it as a last resort.

Details of definitive management of injuries are discussed in the sections on trauma that follow and in the various organ system chapters of this book.

NECK INJURIES

All injuries to the neck are potentially life threatening because of the many vital structures in this area. Injuries to the neck are classified as blunt or penetrating, and the treatment is different for each. The patient must be examined closely for associated head and chest injuries. The initial level of consciousness is of paramount importance; progressive depression of the sensorium may signify intracranial bleeding or cerebral ischemia and requires neurosurgical evaluation. Trauma to the base of the neck may lacerate major blood vessels or have associated pneumothorax. Hemorrhage into the pleural cavity may occur suddenly as contained hematomas rupture.

▶ Clinical Findings

Injuries to the larynx and trachea can be asymptomatic or may cause hoarseness, laryngeal stridor, or dyspnea secondary to airway compression or aspiration of blood. Subcutaneous emphysema in the neck can be present if the wall of the larynx or trachea has been disrupted.

Esophageal injuries are rarely isolated and by themselves may not cause immediate symptoms. Severe chest pain and dysphagia are characteristic of esophageal perforation. Hours later, as mediastinitis develops, progressive sepsis may occur. Mediastinitis results because the deep cervical space is in direct continuity with the mediastinum. Esophageal injuries can be recognized promptly if the surgeon is alert to the possibility and seeks out early diagnosis. Exploration of the neck, radiographic examination of the esophagus with contrast medium, and in selected cases flexible esophagoscopy confirms the diagnosis.

Cervical spine fractures and spinal cord injuries should always be suspected in deceleration injuries or following direct trauma to the neck. If the patient complains of cervical pain or tenderness or if the level of consciousness is depressed, the head and neck should be immobilized (eg, with a rigid cervical collar or sandbags) until cervical radiographs can be taken to rule out a cervical fracture or ligamentous injury.

Injury to the great vessels (subclavian, common carotid, internal carotid, and external carotid arteries; subclavian, internal jugular, and external jugular veins) may follow blunt or penetrating trauma. Fractures of the clavicle or first rib may lacerate the subclavian artery and vein. With vascular injuries, the patient typically presents with visible external blood loss, neck hematoma formation, and in varying degrees of shock. Occasionally, bleeding may be contained and the injury may go undetected for a short time. Auscultation may reveal bruits that suggest arterial injury.

▶ Types of Injuries

A. Penetrating Neck Injuries

Penetrating injuries of the neck are divided into three anatomic zones (Figure 13–8). Zone I injuries occur at the thoracic outlet, which extends from the level of the cricoid cartilage to the clavicles. Included in this area are the proximal carotid arteries, the subclavian vessels, and the major vessels of the chest. Proximal control of injuries to vascular structures in this zone often requires a thoracotomy or sternotomy. Zone II injuries occur in the area between the cricoid and the angle of the mandible. Injuries here are the easiest to expose and evaluate. Zone III injuries are between the angle of the mandible and the base of the skull. Exposure is much more difficult in this zone and in some cases may require disarticulation of the mandible. High injuries can be inaccessible, and control of hemorrhage may require ligation of major proximal vessels or angiographic embolization.

Penetrating trauma to the posterior neck may injure the vertebral column, the cervical spinal cord, the interosseous portion of the vertebral artery, and the neck musculature. Penetrating trauma to the anterior and lateral neck may injure the larynx, trachea, esophagus, thyroid, carotid arteries, subclavian arteries, jugular veins, subclavian veins, phrenic and vagus nerves, and thoracic duct.

With any penetrating cervical trauma, the likelihood of significant injury is high because there are so many vital structures in such a small space. Any patient with shock, expanding hematoma, or uncontrolled hemorrhage should be taken to the operating room for emergency exploration.

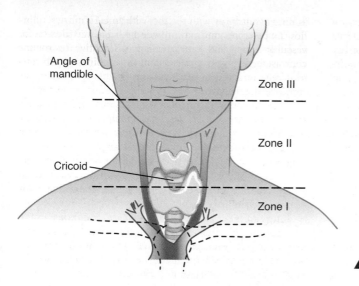

▲ **Figure 13–8.** Zones of the neck.

The location of the injury suggests which structures may be involved. Vascular injuries at the base of the neck require thoracotomy to obtain proximal control of injured blood vessels before the site of probable injury is exposed. If the patient is stable after resuscitation, additional diagnostic testing may be considered.

Arteriography is usually recommended for patients with stable injuries in zones I and III because precise identification of the location and extent of injury may alter the operative approach. If possible, arteriography should be performed before exploration of any injury in which blood vessels may be damaged below the level of the cricoid cartilage or above a line connecting the mastoid process with the angle of the jaw. Arterial injuries above this line are practically inaccessible. If injury to the carotid artery at the base of the skull is confirmed by arteriography, repair may not be possible and ligation may be required to control bleeding, or angiographic intervention may be required. Injured carotid arteries that have produced a neurologic deficit should be repaired if possible. The morbidity and mortality of patients undergoing carotid artery repair are significantly lower than those who have ligation of the carotid artery (15% versus 50%). Carotid artery ligation is indicated in the patient who presents with uncontrollable hemorrhage or coma with no prograde flow in the carotid artery.

Since exposure of injuries in zone II is relatively easy to obtain, a policy of mandatory exploration was the traditional recommendation for all injuries penetrating the platysma muscle. Although this approach is safe, reliable, and time-tested, recent studies have demonstrated that a selective approach is as safe provided that diagnostic testing does not detect a major injury and the patient is stable. High-resolution helical CT scanning of the neck has been used recently to guide surgical decision making in zone II penetrating injuries. Invasive studies such as endoscopy and arteriography can often be eliminated if CT demonstrates a trajectory remote from vital structures such as vessels or the aerodigestive tract.

In the absence of an obvious vascular injury on clinical examination, ultrasound with color-flow Doppler has been demonstrated to be reliable in ruling out carotid artery injuries. Arteriography can also be used in this setting and may offer the advantage of identifying an unsuspected vertebral artery injury. Vertebral artery injuries should also be suspected when bleeding from a posterior or lateral neck wound cannot be controlled by pressure on the carotid artery or when there is bleeding from a posterolateral wound associated with fracture of a cervical transverse process. Flexible or rigid endoscopy can be used to evaluate the trachea and esophagus. A contrast study of the upper esophagus should be performed to identify esophageal injuries that might not be readily apparent on endoscopy. These injuries can be difficult to detect and are occasionally missed on surgical exploration. In either case, repeated, careful examinations should be performed.

B. Blunt Neck Injuries

Blunt cervical trauma may cause fracture or dislocation of the cervical vertebrae (with the risk of spinal cord injury), traumatic occlusion or dissection of the carotid arteries, cerebrospinal fluid cysts, or laryngeal and tracheal injuries complicated by hemorrhage and airway obstruction. Fractures of the cervical spine can be confirmed by plain radiographs or CT scan.

The most important injuries resulting from blunt cervical trauma are (1) cervical fracture, (2) cervical spinal cord injury, (3) vascular injury, and (4) laryngeal and tracheal injury. Radiographs of the cervical spine and soft tissues are essential. Careful neurologic examination can differentiate between injuries to the spinal cord, brachial plexus, and brain.

Blunt trauma to the neck rarely requires direct surgical treatment. Cervical fractures are managed with external immobilization using rigid collars or a halo/vest apparatus. In some cases, unstable cervical spine fractures require reduction and internal fixation. Vascular injuries may occur in cases of severe or localized blunt neck trauma. The common or internal carotid arteries can be torn or sustain intimal disruption and require intervention. Imaging of the cervical vessels is recommended in blunt trauma patients with lateralizing neurologic symptoms or GCS less than 8 with head CT findings that do not explain the neurologic symptoms, Horner syndrome, significant contusions overlying the neck, fractures involving the vertebral canal, and multiple severe facial fractures. While four-vessel arteriography of bilateral carotid and vertebral arteries was the gold standard, newer imaging techniques with dedicated cervical CT-angiogram or MR-angiogram are acceptable screening tools. Formal arteriograms are reserved for patients who may have injuries amenable to angiographic intervention or if the diagnosis cannot be made by other means and would alter treatment. Most blunt carotid injuries are not amenable to operative intervention due to the location or extent of injury. The use of endovascular stent techniques to repair or control blunt carotid artery injuries is in evolution. Patients with blunt carotid or vertebral artery injuries should be considered for anticoagulation or antiplatelet therapy. The value of anticoagulation continues to be debated due to associated bleeding complications, and antiplatelet therapy is a reasonable alternative to full systemic anticoagulation.

▶ Complications

The complications of untreated neck trauma are related to the individual structures injured. Injuries to the larynx and trachea can result in acute airway obstruction, late tracheal stenosis, and sepsis. Cervicomediastinal sepsis can result from esophageal injuries. Carotid artery injuries can produce death from hemorrhage, stroke or cerebral ischemia, and arteriovenous fistula with cardiac decompensation. Major venous injury can result in exsanguination, air embolism, and arteriovenous fistula formation if there is concomitant arterial injury. Cervical fracture can result in paraplegia, quadriplegia, or death.

Prevention of these complications depends upon immediate resuscitation by intubation of the airway, prompt control of external hemorrhage and blood replacement, protection of the head and neck when cervical fracture is possible, accurate and rapid diagnosis, and prompt operative treatment when indicated.

▶ Treatment

Control of the airway with early intubation is the first key maneuver to successful management of severe neck injuries. Any wound of the neck that penetrates the platysma requires prompt surgical exploration or diagnostic workup to rule out major vascular injury. In patients with zone II injuries, color-flow Doppler imaging may provide a reliable way to assess for vascular injury and can be a safe alternative to routine contrast angiography. Arteries damaged by high-velocity missiles require debridement. End-to-end anastomosis of the mobilized vessels is preferred, but if a significant segment is lost, an autogenous vein graft can be used. Vertebral artery injury presents a formidable technical problem because of the interosseous course of the artery shortly after it arises from the subclavian artery. Although unilateral vertebral artery ligation has been followed by fatal midbrain or cerebellar necrosis, because of inadequate communication to the basilar artery, only 3% of patients with left vertebral ligation and 2% of patients with right vertebral ligation develop these complications. Therefore, in the face of massive hemorrhage from a partially severed vertebral artery, ligation with surgical clips applied to the vessel between the transverse processes above and below the laceration is accepted.

Subclavian artery injuries are best approached through a combined cervicothoracic incision. Proper exposure is the key to success in the management of these difficult and too-often fatal injuries. Ligation of the subclavian artery is relatively safe, but primary repair is preferable. Care should be taken to avoid phrenic nerve and thoracic duct injury when operating in this region of the neck. If the patient is stable and a subclavian injury is identified at arteriography, an endovascular stent is another therapeutic option.

Venous injuries are best managed by ligation. The possibility of air embolism must be kept constantly in mind. A simple means of preventing this complication is to lower the patient's head using the Trendelenburg position until bleeding is controlled.

Esophageal injuries should be sutured closed primarily and drained. Use of muscle flaps using omohyoid or sternocleidomastoid muscles to cover the repair can be helpful. Drainage is the mainstay of treatment. Extensive injury to the esophagus is often immediately fatal because of associated injuries to the spinal cord. Systemic antibiotics should be administered routinely to patients with esophageal injuries.

Minor laryngeal and tracheal injuries do not require treatment, but immediate tracheostomy should be performed when airway obstruction exists. If there has been significant injury to the thyroid cartilage, a temporary laryngeal stent (Silastic) should be employed to provide support. Mucosal lacerations should be approximated before insertion of the stent. Conveniently located small perforations of the trachea can be utilized for tracheostomy. Otherwise, the wounds can be closed after they are debrided and a distal tracheostomy performed. Extensive circumferential tracheal injuries may require resection and anastomosis or reconstruction using synthetic materials.

Cervical spinal cord injury should be managed in such a way as to prevent further damage. When there is cervical cord compression from hematoma, vertebral fractures, or foreign bodies, decompression laminectomy is necessary.

Prognosis

Severe laceration of the cervical spinal cord often results in paralysis. Injuries to the soft tissues of the neck, trachea, and esophagus have a good to excellent prognosis if promptly treated. Major vascular injuries have a good prognosis if promptly treated before the onset of irreversible shock or neurologic deficit. The overall death rate for major cervical injuries is about 10%.

Barba CA et al: A new cervical spine clearance protocol using computed tomography. J Trauma 2001;51:652.

Biffl WL et al: Sixteen-slice computed tomographic angiography is a reliable noninvasive screening test for clinically significant blunt cerebrovascular injuries. J Trauma 2006;60:745.

Cothren CC et al: Anticoagulation is the gold standard therapy for blunt carotid injuries to reduce stroke rate. Arch Surg 2004;139:540.

Demetriades D et al: Penetrating injuries of the neck in patients in stable condition. Physical examination, angiography, or color flow Doppler imaging. Arch Surg 1995;130:971.

Eddy VA and the Zone 1 Penetrating Neck Injury Study Group: Is routine arteriography mandatory for penetrating injury to zone 1 of the neck? J Trauma 2000;48:208.

Gonzalez RP et al: Penetrating zone II neck injury: does dynamic computed tomographic scan contribute to the diagnostic sensitivity of physical examination for surgically significant injury? A prospective blinded study. J Trauma 2003;54:61.

Gracias VH et al: Computed tomography in the evaluation of penetrating neck trauma. Arch Surg 2001;136:1231.

Irish JC et al: Penetrating and blunt neck trauma: 10-year review of a Canadian experience. Can J Surg 1997;40:33.

Liekweg WG, Greenfield LJ: Management of penetrating carotid arterial injury. Ann of Surg 1978;188:587.

Mazolewski PJ et al: Computed tomographic scan can be used for surgical decision making in zone II penetrating neck injuries. J Trauma 2001;51:315.

Schenarts P et al: Prospective comparison of admission CT scan and plain films of the upper cervical spine in trauma patients with altered mental status. J Trauma 2000;49:1163.

Sofianos C et al: Selective surgical management of zone II gunshot injuries of the neck: a prospective study. Surgery 1996;120:785.

Wahl WL et al: Antiplatelet therapy: an alternative to heparin for blunt carotid injury. J Trauma 52:896.

THORACIC INJURIES

Thoracic trauma accounts directly for or is a contributing factor in 50% of deaths due to trauma. Early deaths are commonly due to (1) airway obstruction, (2) flail chest, (3) open pneumothorax, (4) massive hemothorax, (5) tension pneumothorax, and (6) cardiac tamponade. Later deaths are due to respiratory failure, sepsis, and unrecognized injuries. The majority of blunt thoracic injuries are the result of automobile accidents. Even what appears to be a minor blunt thoracic injury leading to rib fractures and pulmonary contusions can have a profound effect on patients. Near-side collisions are responsible for a higher incidence of blunt aortic injury among older adults and are associated with lower delta V forces compared to those in younger patients. Penetrating chest injuries from knives, bullets, etc, are deadly and can result in complex patterns of injury. The mortality rate in hospitalized patients with isolated chest injury is 4–8%; it is 10–15% when one other organ system is involved and rises to 35% if multiple additional organs are injured.

Combined injuries of multiple intrathoracic structures are typical. There are often other injuries to the abdomen, head, or skeletal system. When performing an operation on the chest for trauma, it is often necessary to operate on the abdomen as well. Therefore, when trauma patients are brought to the operating room for a laparotomy or thoracotomy, both body regions should be prepped into the operative field. Eighty-five percent of chest injuries do not require open thoracotomy, but immediate use of lifesaving measures is often necessary and should be within the competence of all surgeons.

A rapid estimate of cardiorespiratory status and possible associated injuries from the physical examination gives the physician a valuable overview a patient who has sustained thoracic injuries. For example, patients with upper airway obstruction appear cyanotic, ashen, or gray; examination reveals stridor or gurgling sounds, ineffective respiratory excursion, constriction of cervical muscles, and retraction of the suprasternal, supraclavicular, intercostal, or epigastric regions. The character of chest wall excursions and the presence or absence of penetrating wounds should be observed. If respiratory excursions are not visible, ventilation is probably inadequate. Severe paradoxic chest wall movement in flail chest is usually located anteriorly and can be seen immediately. Sucking wounds of the chest wall should be obvious. A large hemothorax may be detected by percussion, and subcutaneous emphysema is easily detected on palpation. Both massive hemothorax and tension pneumothorax may produce absent or diminished breath sounds and a shift of the trachea to the opposite side, but in massive hemothorax the neck veins are usually collapsed. If the patient has a thready or absent pulse and distended neck veins, the main differential diagnosis is between cardiac tamponade and tension pneumothorax.

In moribund patients, diagnosis must be immediate, and treatment may require chest tube placement, pericardiocentesis, or thoracotomy in the emergency room. The first priority of management should be to provide an airway and restore circulation. One can then reassess the patient and outline definitive measures. A cuffed endotracheal tube and assisted ventilation are required for apnea, ineffectual breathing, severe shock, deep coma, airway obstruction, flail chest, or open sucking chest wounds. Persistent shock or hypoxia due to thoracic trauma may be caused by any of the following: massive hemopneumothorax, cardiac tamponade, tension pneumothorax or massive air leak, or air embolism. If hemorrhagic shock is not explained readily by findings on chest x-ray or external losses, it is almost certainly due to intra-abdominal bleeding.

Tube Thoracostomy

If time permits, the chest is prepared and draped in a sterile fashion. In awake patients, local anesthetic (1% lidocaine) is injected in the skin and surrounding tissues at the planned site of tube insertion. In an unconscious patient, this step is usually unnecessary. The location of the chest tube insertion site is the interspace between the fourth and fifth ribs in the midaxillary line. A 2–3 cm skin incision is created with a #10 scalpel and carried down into the subcutaneous tissue. Using a large hemostat, a soft tissue tunnel is created just superior to the cephalad edge of the fifth rib. A finger or blunt clamp is used to penetrate the parietal pleura and enter the pleural space. The wound is explored with an index finger to confirm entry into the pleural cavity and check for pulmonary adhesions. A 36F straight thoracostomy tube is inserted and directed posteriorly toward the apex of the lung. The tube is anchored to the skin with stitches and connected to a Pleur-Evac device set at 20 cm H_2O suction with a water seal.

▶ Types of Injuries

A. Chest Wall

Rib fracture, the most common chest injury, varies across a spectrum from simple fracture to fracture with hemopneumothorax to severe multiple fractures with flail chest, pulmonary contusion, and internal injuries. With simple fractures, pain on inspiration is the principal symptom; treatment consists of providing adequate analgesia. In cases of multiple fractures, intercostal nerve blocks or epidural analgesia may be required to ensure adequate ventilation. The use of transdermal lidocaine patches for local analgesia is under investigation and could prove useful. Multiple fractures can be associated with voluntarily decreased ventilation and subsequent pneumonitis, particularly in the elderly patient.

Flail chest occurs when a portion of the chest wall becomes isolated by multiple fractures and paradoxically moves in and out with inspiration and expiration with a potentially severe reduction in ventilatory efficiency. The magnitude of the effect is determined by the size of the flail segment and the amount of pain with breathing. The rib fractures are usually anterior, and there are at least two fractures of the same rib. Bilateral costochondral separation and sternal fractures can also cause a flail segment. An associated lung contusion may produce a decrease in lung compliance not fully manifest until 12–48 hours after injury. Increased negative intrapleural pressure is then required for ventilation, and chest wall instability becomes apparent. If ventilation becomes inadequate, atelectasis, hypercapnia, hypoxia, accumulation of secretions, and ineffective cough occur. Arterial P_{O_2} is often low before clinical findings appear. Serial blood gas analysis is the best way to determine if a treatment regimen is adequate. For less severe cases, intercostal nerve block or continuous epidural analgesia may be adequate treatment. However, most cases require ventilatory assistance for variable periods of time with a cuffed endotracheal tube and a mechanical ventilator.

Most rib or sternal fractures will heal without treatment. In selected patients, internal fixation may be useful; however, determining the patient population who would most benefit is still under investigation. A commercially produced rib and sternal fracture plating system is now available, and a system with bioabsorbable plates has been described in the literature. Patients who would potentially benefit from an open reduction internal fixation procedure are those with nonunion, severely displaced rib fractures with overriding fragments, severe pain with respiratory compromise (eg, difficulty in being weaned off the mechanical ventilator), multiple unstable rib fractures, and those undergoing thoracotomy for other intrathoracic indication. Because of the peristomal bacterial burden associated with a tracheostomy, this procedure should be used with caution, if at all, in patients with a prior tracheostomy.

B. Trachea and Bronchus

Blunt tracheobronchial injuries are often due to compression of the airway between the sternum and the vertebral column in decelerating or high velocity crush accidents. The distal trachea or main stem bronchi are usually involved, and 80% of all injuries are located within 2.5 cm from the carina. Penetrating tracheobronchial injuries may occur at any location. Most patients have pneumothorax, subcutaneous emphysema, pneumomediastinum, and hemoptysis. Cervicofacial emphysema may be dramatic. Tracheobronchial injury should be suspected when there is a massive air leak or when the lung does not readily reexpand after chest tube placement. In penetrating injuries of the trachea or main stem bronchi, there is usually massive hemorrhage and hemoptysis. Systemic air embolism resulting in cardiopulmonary arrest may occur if a bronchovenous fistula is present. If air embolism is suspected, emergency thoracotomy should be performed with cross-clamping of the pulmonary hilum on the affected side. The diagnosis is confirmed by aspiration of air from the heart. In blunt injuries, the tracheobronchial injury may not be obvious and may be suspected only after major atelectasis develops several days later. Diagnosis may require flexible or rigid bronchoscopy. Immediate primary repair with absorbable sutures is indicated for all tracheobronchial lacerations.

C. Pleural Space

Hemothorax (blood within the pleural cavity) is classified according to the amount of blood: minimal, 350 mL; moderate, 350–1500 mL; or massive, 1500 mL or more. The rate of bleeding after evacuation of the hemothorax is clinically even more important. If air is also present, the condition is called hemopneumothorax.

Hemothorax should be suspected with penetrating or severe blunt thoracic injury. There may be decreased breath sounds and dullness to percussion, and a chest x-ray should be promptly obtained. In experienced hands, ultrasound can diagnose pneumothorax and hemothorax, but this technique is not widely employed at this time. Tube thoracostomy should be performed expeditiously for all hemothoraces or pneumothoraces. In 85% of cases, tube thoracostomy is the only treatment required. If bleeding is persistent, as noted by continued output from the chest tubes, it is more likely to be from a systemic (eg, intercostal) rather than a pulmonary artery. The use of positive end-expiratory pressure (PEEP) can help tamponade pulmonary parenchymal bleeding in trauma patients who are intubated. When the rate of bleeding shows a steady trend of greater than 200 mL/h or the total hemorrhagic output exceeds 1500 mL, thoracoscopy or thoracotomy should usually be performed. The trend and rate of thoracic bleeding is probably more important than the absolute numbers in deciding to perform surgical intervention. Thoracoscopy has been shown to be effective in controlling chest tube bleeding in 82% of cases. This technique has also been shown to be 90% effective in evacuating retained hemothoraces. In most of these cases, the chest wall is the source of hemorrhage. Thoracotomy is required for management of injuries to the lungs, heart, pericardium, and great vessels.

Pneumothorax occurs in lacerations of the lung or chest wall following penetrating or blunt chest trauma. Hyperinflation (eg, blast injuries, diving accidents) can also rupture the lungs. After penetrating injury, 80% of patients with pneumothorax also have blood in the pleural cavity. Most cases of pneumothorax are readily diagnosed on chest x-ray. In some cases, an occult pneumothorax will be identified on a chest or abdominal CT scan. Pneumothorax or hemothorax may be identified on the lateral scans performed as part of the FAST examination of the abdomen for trauma (see section on abdominal trauma). Most cases of traumatic pneumothorax should be treated with immediate tube thoracostomy; however, small occult pneumothoraces in stable patients can sometimes be observed.

Tension pneumothorax develops when a flap-valve leak allows air to enter the pleural space but prevents its escape; intrapleural pressure rises, causing total collapse of the lung and a shift of the mediastinal viscera to the opposite side, interfering with venous return to the heart. It must be relieved immediately to avoid impairment of cardiac function. Immediate treatment involves placement of a large-bore needle or plastic angiocath in the pleural space with care being taken to avoid injury to the intercostal vessels. After this emergency measure has been instituted, tension pneumothorax should be treated definitively by tube thoracostomy.

Sucking chest wounds, which allow air to pass in and out of the pleural cavity, should be promptly treated by a three-sided occlusive dressing and tube thoracostomy. The pathologic physiology resembles flail chest except that the extent of associated lung injury is usually less. Definitive management includes surgical closure of the defect in the chest wall.

D. Lung Injury

Pulmonary contusion due to sudden parenchymal concussion occurs after blunt trauma or wounding with a high-velocity missile. Pulmonary contusion occurs in 75% of patients with flail chest but can also occur following blunt trauma without rib fracture. Alveolar rupture with fluid transudation and extravasation of blood are early findings. Fluid and blood from ruptured alveoli enter alveolar spaces and bronchi and produce localized airway obstruction and atelectasis. Increased mucous secretions and overzealous intravenous fluid therapy may combine to produce copious secretions and further atelectasis. The patient's ability to cough and clear secretions effectively is weakened because of chest wall pain or mechanical inefficiency from fractures. Elasticity of the lungs is decreased, resistance to air flow increases, and as the work of breathing increases, blood oxygenation and pH drop and Pco_2 rises. The cardiac compensatory response may be compromised, because as many as 35% of these patients have an associated myocardial contusion.

Treatment is often delayed because clinical and x-ray findings may not appear until 12–48 hours after injury. The clinical findings are copious, thin, blood-tinged secretions; chest pain;, restlessness; apprehensiveness; and labored respirations. Eventually, dyspnea, cyanosis, tachypnea, and tachycardia develop. X-ray changes consist of patchy parenchymal opacification or diffuse linear peribronchial densities that may progress to diffuse opacification ("white-out") characteristic for acute respiratory distress syndrome.

Mechanical ventilatory support permits adequate alveolar ventilation and reduces the work of breathing. Blood gases should be monitored and arterial saturation adequately maintained. There is some controversy over the best regimen for fluid management, but excessive hydration or blood transfusion should be avoided. Optimal management may require placement of a pulmonary artery catheter, preferably with a thermistor tip for measurement of continuous cardiac output by thermodilution. Serial measurement of central venous pressure, pulmonary arterial pressure, wedge pressures, mixed venous oxygen saturation, and cardiac output help to avoid either undertransfusion or overtransfusion. Despite optimal therapy, about 15% of patients with pulmonary contusion die. Use of protective mechanical ventilator strategies is essential in these patients to avoid progressive ventilator induced lung injury. Use of low-tidal volumes (6 mL/kg) and avoidance of plateau pressures greater than 35 cm H_2O are recommended.

Most lung lacerations are caused by penetrating injuries, and hemopneumothorax is usually present. Tube thoracostomy is indicated to evacuate pleural air or blood and to monitor continuing leaks. Since expansion of the lung tamponades the laceration, most lung lacerations do not produce massive hemorrhage or persistent air leaks. Should a pulmonary laceration require operative intervention, lung-sparing techniques rather than formal anatomic lung resection should be employed when feasible to reduce morbidity and mortality.

Lung hematomas are the result of local parenchymal destruction and hemorrhage. The x-ray appearance is initially a poorly defined density that becomes more circumscribed a few days to 2 weeks after injury. Cystic cavities occasionally develop if damage is extensive. Most hematomas resolve adequately with expectant treatment.

E. Heart and Pericardium

Blunt injury to the heart occurs most often from compression against the steering wheel in auto accidents. This injury is in decline with the increasing prevalence of airbag technology in motor vehicles. The injury varies from localized contusion to cardiac rupture. Autopsy studies of victims of immediately fatal accidents show that as many as 65% have rupture of one or more cardiac chambers, and 45% have pericardial lacerations. The incidence of blunt myocardial injury in patients who reach the hospital is unknown but is probably higher than generally suspected. The clinical relevance of this diagnosis is widely debated. Most trauma surgeons advocate the diagnosis and treatment of the actual clinical problem such as acute heart failure, valvular injury, cardiac rupture, or dysrhythmia.

Early clinical findings include friction rubs, chest pain, tachycardia, murmurs, dysrhythmias, or signs of low cardiac output. Patients with risk factors for blunt myocardial injury should undergo evaluation with a 12-lead electrocardiogram (ECG). If the ECG is normal and the patient is asymptomatic, the work up is complete. An abnormal ECG should prompt further evaluation with an echocardiogram. Patients with proven injury on echocardiogram and/or hemodynamic instability should be admitted to the intensive care unit and managed appropriately for the diagnosed injury. An abnormal ECG with a normal echocardiogram merits at least 24 hours of monitoring in a telemetry unit and daily repeat ECGs until stable or the dysrhythmia resolves. Standard measurement of cardiac enzymes is not useful and has no role in the diagnosis of blunt myocardial injury. If the patient is suspected of having a myocardial infarction or acute myocardial ischemia, then cardiac enzymes should be obtained and a cardiology consultation arranged.

Management of symptomatic blunt myocardial injury should be the same as for acute myocardial infarction. Hemopericardium may occur without tamponade and can be treated by pericardiocentesis. Tamponade in blunt cardiac trauma is often due to myocardial rupture or coronary artery laceration. Tamponade produces distended neck veins, shock, and cyanosis. Immediate thoracotomy and control of the injury are indicated. If cardiopulmonary arrest occurs before the patient can be transported to the operating room, emergency room thoracotomy with relief of tamponade should be performed. Treatment of injuries to the valves, papillary muscles, and septum must be individualized; and when tolerated, delayed repair is usually recommended.

Pericardial lacerations from stab wounds tend to seal and cause tamponade, whereas gunshot wounds frequently leave a sufficient pericardial opening for drainage. Gunshot wounds produce more extensive myocardial damage, multiple perforations, and massive bleeding into the pleural space. Hemothorax, shock, and exsanguination occur in nearly all cases of cardiac gunshot wounds. The clinical findings are those of tamponade or acute blood loss. Use of ultrasound and the FAST examination technique can reveal the presence of clinically significant blood in the pericardial space.

Treatment of penetrating cardiac injuries requires prompt thoracotomy, pericardial decompression, and control of hemorrhage. Most patients do not require cardiopulmonary bypass. The standard approach has been to repair the laceration using mattress sutures with pledgets while controlling hemorrhage with a finger on the heart. Suture control of cardiac lacerations may be technically difficult when working with a beating heart or in patients with large or multiple lacerations. Several studies have demonstrated that in most cases, emergency temporary control of hemorrhage from cardiac lacerations can be achieved with the use of a skin stapler (Figure 13–9). Following stabilization of the patient, the staples can be removed after definitive suture repair is performed in the operating room. Hemostatic sealants such as FloSeal offer significant promise as additional tools in the surgical armamentarium when dealing with lacerations to the heart or great vessels. Regardless of the approach utilized, care must be taken to avoid injury to the coronary arteries.

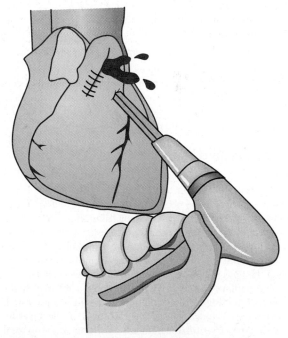

▲ **Figure 13–9.** Technique of cardiac stapling. Finger pressure (not shown) is used to maintain hemostasis during stapling. (Reproduced, with permission, from Macho JR, Markison RE, Schecter WP: Cardiac stapling in the management of penetrating injuries of the heart: rapid control of hemorrhage and decreased risk of personal contamination. J Trauma 1993;34:711.)

Pericardiocentesis or creation of a pericardial window is reserved for selected cases when the diagnosis is uncertain or in preparation for thoracotomy. In approximately 75% of cases of stab wounds and 35% of cases of gunshot cardiac wounds, the patient survives the operation. However, it is estimated that 80–90% of patients with gunshot wounds of the heart do not reach the hospital.

F. Esophagus

Anatomically, the esophagus is well protected, and perforation from external penetrating trauma is relatively infrequent. Blunt injuries are exceedingly rare. The most common symptom of esophageal perforation is pain; fever develops within hours in most patients. Hematemesis, hoarseness, dysphagia, or respiratory distress may also be present. Physical findings include shock, local tenderness, subcutaneous emphysema, or Hamman sign (pericardial or mediastinal "crunch" synchronous with cardiac sounds). Leukocytosis occurs soon after injury. X-ray findings on plain chest films include evidence of a foreign body or missile and mediastinal air or widening. Pleural effusion or hydropneumothorax is frequently seen, usually on the left side. Contrast x-rays of the esophagus should be performed but are positive in only about 70% of proven perforations.

A nasogastric tube should be passed to evacuate gastric contents. If recognized within 24–48 hours after injury, the esophageal perforation should be closed and pleural drainage instituted with large-bore catheters. Repair of these perforations requires special techniques that include buttressing of the esophageal closure with pleural or pericardial flaps; pedicles of intercostal, diaphragmatic, or cervical strap muscles; and serosal patches from stomach or jejunum. Illness and death are due to mediastinal and pleural infection.

G. Thoracic Duct

Chylothorax and chylopericardium are rare complications of trauma but are difficult to manage when they occur. Penetrating injuries of the neck, thorax, or upper abdomen can injure the thoracic duct or its major tributaries.

Symptoms are due to mechanical effects of the accumulations (eg, shortness of breath from lung collapse or low cardiac output from tamponade). The diagnosis is established when the fluid is shown to have characteristics of chyle.

The patient should be maintained on a fat-free, high-carbohydrate, high-protein diet and the effusion aspirated. Chest tube drainage should be instituted if the effusion recurs. Lipid-free total parenteral nutrition with no oral intake may be effective in treating persistent leaks. Three or 4 weeks of conservative treatment usually are curative. If daily chyle loss exceeds 1500 mL for 5 successive days or persists after 2–3 weeks of conservative treatment, the thoracic duct should be ligated via a right thoracotomy. Intraoperative identification of the leak may be facilitated by preoperative administration of fat-containing a lipophilic dye.

H. Diaphragm

Penetrating injuries of the diaphragm outnumber blunt diaphragmatic injuries by a ratio of at least 6:1. Diaphragmatic lacerations occur in 10–15% of cases of penetrating wounds to the chest and in as many as 40% of cases of penetrating trauma to the left chest. Injuries to the right diaphragm are more common than previously thought. The injury is rarely obvious. Wounds of the diaphragm must not be overlooked because they rarely heal spontaneously and because herniation of abdominal viscera into the chest can occur with catastrophic complications either immediately or years after the injuries.

Associated injuries are usually present, and as many as 25% of patients are in shock when first seen. There may be abdominal tenderness, dyspnea, shoulder pain, or unilateral breath sounds. The diagnosis is often missed. Although chest radiography is a sensitive diagnostic tool, it may be entirely normal in 40% of cases. The most common finding is ipsilateral hemothorax, which is present in about 50% of patients. Occasionally, a distended, herniated stomach is confused with a pneumothorax. Passage of a nasogastric tube before x-rays will help to identify an intrathoracic stomach. CT scan or contrast x-rays may be necessary to establish the diagnosis in some cases. Newer generation helical CT scanners that allow sagittal reformatting can be helpful in definitively diagnosing diaphragmatic injury. Laparoscopy is a useful but invasive technique for detecting occult diaphragmatic injuries in patients who have no other indications for formal laparotomy.

Once the diagnosis is made, a transabdominal surgical approach should be used in cases of acute rupture. Laparoscopic suturing for repair of the injury may be possible in selected cases. The diaphragm should be reapproximated and closed with interrupted or running nonabsorbable sutures. Chronic herniation is associated with adhesions of the affected viscera to the thoracic structures and should be approached via thoracotomy, with the addition of a separate laparotomy when indicated. These cases can be quite challenging and appropriate preoperative planning is recommended.

Asensio JA et al: Penetrating cardiac injuries: a prospective study of variables predicting outcomes. J Am Coll Surg 1998;186:24.

Bergeron E et al: Elderly trauma patients with rib fractures are at greater risk of death and pneumonia. J Trauma 2003;54:478.

Brasel KJ et al: Treatment of occult pneumothoraces from blunt trauma. J Trauma 1999;46:987.

Cothren C et al: Lung-sparing techniques are associated with improved outcome compared with anatomic resection for severe lung injuries. J Trauma 2002;53:483.

Dulchavsky SA et al: Prospective evaluation of thoracic ultrasound in the detection of pneumothorax. J Trauma 2001;50:201.

Feliciano DV, Rozycki GS: Advances in the diagnosis and treatment of thoracic trauma. Surg Clin North Am 1999;79:1417.

Gasparri M et al: Pulmonary tractotomy versus lung resection: viable options in penetrating lung injury. J Trauma 2001;51:1092.

Karmy-Jones R et al: Timing of urgent thoracotomy for hemorrhage after trauma. Arch Surg 2001;136:513.

Karmy-Jones R et al: Urgent and emergent thoracotomy for penetrating chest trauma. J Trauma 2004;56:664.

Lowdermilk GA, Naunheim KS: Thoracoscopic evaluation and treatment of thoracic trauma. Surg Clin North Am 2000;80:1535.

Macho JR, Markison RE, Schecter WP: Cardiac stapling in the management of penetrating injuries of the heart: rapid control of hemorrhage and decreased risk of personal contamination. J Trauma 1993;34:711.

Mayberry JC et al: Absorbable plates for rib fracture repair: preliminary experience. J Trauma 2003;55:835.

Meredith JW, Hoth JJ: Thoracic trauma: when and how to intervene. Surg Clin N Am 2007;87:95.

Miller PR et al: ARDS after pulmonary contusion: accurate measurement of contusion volume identifies high-risk patients. J Trauma 2001;51:223.

Richardson JD et al: Operative fixation of chest wall fractures and underused procedure? Am Surg 2007;73:591.

Rozycki GS et al: The role of ultrasound in patients with possible penetrating cardiac wounds: a prospective multicenter study. J Trauma 1999;46:543.

Schultz JM, Trunkey DD: Blunt cardiac injury. Crit Care Clin 2004;20:57.

Stassen NA et al: Reevaluation of diagnostic procedures for transmediastinal gunshot wounds. J Trauma 2002;53:635.

ABDOMINAL INJURIES

The specific type of abdominal injury varies according to whether the trauma is penetrating or blunt. Blunt injuries predominate in rural areas, while penetrating injuries are more common in urban areas. The mechanism of injury in blunt trauma is rapid deceleration, and noncompliant organs such as the liver, spleen, pancreas, and kidneys are at greater risk of injury due to parenchymal fracture. Occasionally, hollow viscous organs may be injured, with the duodenum and urinary bladder being particularly susceptible. The small bowel occupies a large portion of the total abdominal volume and is more likely to be injured by penetrating trauma. Most blunt abdominal injuries are related to motor vehicle accidents. Although the use of restraints has been associated with a decrease in the incidence of head, chest, and solid organ injuries, their use may be associated with pancreatic, mesenteric, and intestinal injuries due to compression against the spinal column. These injuries should be considered in the evaluation of patients who have signs of seat belt–related contusions of the abdominal wall. Internal injury may be present in as many as 30% of these cases. In any abdominal trauma, hemoperitoneum may not manifest clinical signs of peritoneal irritation, particularly in patients with other distracting injuries or depressed mental status. Retroperitoneal injury may be more subtle and difficult to diagnose during the initial evaluation.

Deaths from abdominal trauma result largely from early severe hemorrhage and coagulopathy or from later sepsis. Most deaths from abdominal trauma are preventable. Patients at risk of abdominal injury should undergo prompt and thorough evaluation. In most trauma centers, after physical examination, the initial diagnostic evaluation includes bedside FAST and portable radiographs of the pelvis

and chest to assess for other potential sites of bleeding. In unstable patients who cannot be adequately evaluated with FAST due to size, technical problems, or subcutaneous air, diagnostic peritoneal lavage is warranted. After the initial FAST exam, patients who are stable or who respond to initial fluid resuscitation should have a CT scan of the abdomen and pelvis to evaluate for intraabdominal and retroperitoneal injuries. Patients with persistent hypotension requiring fluid and blood resuscitation in the face of a positive FAST or diagnostic peritoneal lavage should be transported to the operating room emergently for exploratory laparotomy.

In some cases, dramatic physical findings may be due to abdominal wall injury in the absence of intraperitoneal injury. If the results of diagnostic studies are equivocal, diagnostic laparoscopy or exploratory laparotomy should be considered, since they may be lifesaving if serious injuries are identified early. Evaluation always includes comprehensive physical examination with pelvic and rectal examinations and may require specific laboratory and radiologic tests (eg, retrograde urethrogram or cystogram, rigid sigmoidoscopy, abdominal CT). Serial physical examinations may be necessary to detect subtle findings.

▶ Types of Injuries

A. Penetrating Trauma

Penetrating injuries to the abdomen that present with shock or ongoing resuscitation require prompt exploration. Lacerations of major blood vessels or the liver can cause severe and early shock. Penetrating injuries of the spleen, pancreas, or kidneys usually do not bleed massively unless a major vessel to the organ (eg, the renal artery) is damaged. Bleeding must be controlled promptly with packing and appropriate clamping for vascular control. A patient in shock with a penetrating injury of the abdomen who does not respond to 2 L of fluid resuscitation should be operated on immediately following chest x-ray.

Patients with hollow visceral injuries may have very few physical signs initially but may progress to sepsis if the injuries are not recognized. Increasing abdominal tenderness demands surgical exploration. White blood cell count elevations and fever appearing several hours following injury are keys to early diagnosis.

The treatment of hemodynamically stable patients with penetrating injuries to the lower chest or abdomen varies. All surgeons agree that patients with signs of peritonitis or hypovolemia should undergo surgical exploration, but treatment is less certain for patients with no signs of peritonitis or sepsis who are cardiovascularly stable.

Most stab wounds of the lower chest or abdomen should be explored, since a delay in treatment of a hollow viscous perforation can result in severe sepsis. Some surgeons recommend a selective policy in the management of these patients. When the depth of injury is in doubt, local wound exploration may rule out peritoneal penetration. Laparoscopy may ultimately have a role in the evaluation of penetrating injuries. All gunshot wounds of the lower chest and abdomen should be explored, because the incidence of injury to major intra-abdominal structures exceeds 90% in such cases.

B. Blunt Trauma

A major advance in management of blunt trauma has been the FAST examination. Ultrasound has proven to be an ideal modality in the immediate evaluation of the trauma patient because it is rapid and accurate for the detection of intra-abdominal fluid or blood and is readily repeatable. It provides valuable information that augments the surgeon's diagnostic capabilities. Since its introduction in North America in 1989, ultrasonography has become commonplace, and a recent survey reports that 78% of United States trauma centers routinely use the FAST examination in the evaluation of patients.

The goal of the FAST examination is the identification of abnormal collections of blood or fluid. In this regard, it obviates the need for diagnostic peritoneal lavage. The primary focus is on the peritoneal cavity, but attention is directed also to the pericardium and to the pleural space. Unclotted blood or fluid allows transmission of ultrasound waves without echoes and thus appears black (Figure 13–10). In the standard FAST examination, four areas are scanned: the right upper quadrant, the subxiphoid area, the left upper quadrant, and the pelvis (Figure 13–11). Most surgeons recommend scanning initially in the right upper quadrant because more than half of the positive tests will reveal blood or fluid in this area. Unstable patients with a positive FAST examination should undergo urgent exploratory laparotomy.

The other diagnostic procedures most commonly used in patients without obvious indications for immediate laparotomy include peritoneal lavage, CT scanning, and diagnostic laparoscopy.

▶ Diagnostic Peritoneal Lavage

Diagnostic peritoneal lavage is designed to detect the presence of intraperitoneal blood. Although its use has decreased significantly at many centers with the use of the FAST examination, it is still an important test in certain circumstances because of its high sensitivity for the presence of blood. Additional determinations of leukocytes, Gram stain, particulate matter, or amylase in the lavage fluid may indicate the presence of a bowel injury. Drainage of lavage fluid from a chest tube or urinary catheter may indicate a lacerated diaphragm or bladder. Lavage can be performed easily and rapidly, with minimal cost and morbidity. It is an invasive procedure that will affect the findings on physical examination and should be performed by a surgeon.

The procedure is neither qualitative nor quantitative. It cannot identify the source of hemorrhage, and relatively small amounts of intraperitoneal bleeding may result in a positive study. It may not detect small and large injuries to

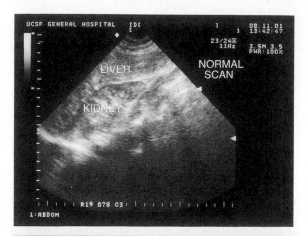

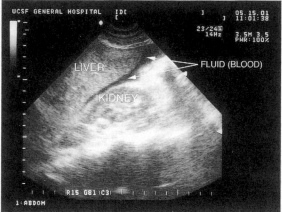

▲ **Figure 13–10.** *Top:* Normal ultrasound of the right upper quadrant. *Bottom:* Right upper quadrant ultrasound revealing blood between the liver and the kidney and between the liver and the diaphragm. (Courtesy of San Francisco General Hospital.)

the diaphragm and cannot rule out injury to the bowel or retroperitoneal organs. The overall indications for diagnostic peritoneal lavage include abdominal pain or tenderness, low abdominal rib fractures, unexplained hypotension, spinal or pelvic fractures, paraplegia or quadriplegia, and assessment hampered by altered mental status due to neurologic injury or intoxication. Despite the many potential indications, FAST followed by abdominal pelvic CT scanning has replaced the need for most diagnostic peritoneal lavages. The only contraindication is a need for emergency laparotomy.

The procedure may be performed with careful technique on patients with prior abdominal surgery and in pregnant patients. It should usually be performed through a small infraumbilical incision with placement of the catheter under direct vision (Figure 13–12). In pregnant patients and those with pelvic fractures, a supraumbilical approach is indicated.

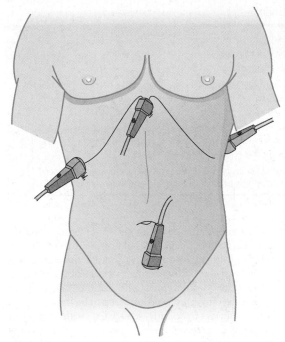

▲ **Figure 13–11.** Transducer positions for FAST. Pericardial area, right and left upper quadrants, and pelvis. (Reproduced, with permission, from Rozycki GS et al: Surgeon-performed ultrasound for the assessment of truncal injuries: lessons learned from 1540 patients. Ann Surg 1998;228:557.)

Closed techniques of catheter placement utilizing trocars or guidewires have been shown to be almost as safe as the open technique, but the rate of failure with the closed technique is higher, thus eliminating most of the potential advantage. After placement of the catheter, 1 L of normal saline solution is instilled into the peritoneal cavity and then allowed to drain by gravity. At least 200 mL of lavage fluid should be recovered to allow for accurate interpretation. A portion of the recovered fluid is sent for laboratory analysis of cell counts, the presence of particulate matter, and amylase. Criteria for evaluation of results are summarized in Table 13–3.

▶ Computed Tomography

CT is noninvasive, qualitative, sensitive, and accurate for the diagnosis of intra-abdominal and retroperitoneal injuries. Modern spiral scanners have greatly decreased the time required for obtaining high-quality images. However, CT scanning remains expensive, involves the use of intravenous contrast administration, exposes the patient to radiation, and requires an experienced radiologist for proper interpretation of the scans. CT scanning also involves transport from the acute care area and should not be attempted in the unstable patient.

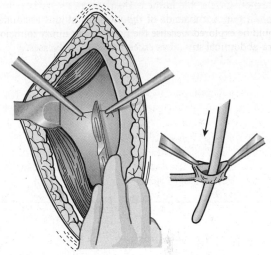

▲ **Figure 13–12.** Diagnostic peritoneal lavage.

CT scanning has a primary role in defining the location and magnitude of intra-abdominal injuries related to blunt trauma. It has the advantage of detecting most retroperitoneal injuries, but it may not identify all gastrointestinal injuries. The information provided on the magnitude of injury allows for nonoperative management of patients with solid organ injuries. Nonsurgical therapy is now used in more than 80% of blunt liver and spleen injuries. Detection of high-grade solid organ injuries or bleeding pelvic fractures by CT in relatively stable patients can also lead to other potential interventions, such as angiographic embolization, which increases the success of nonoperative management. Table 13–4 compares the time, costs, advantages, and disadvantages of nonoperative methods used for evaluation of the injured abdomen.

Table 13–3. Criteria for Evaluation of Peritoneal Lavage Fluid.

Positive
= 100,000 red cells/µL
= 500 white cells/µL
= 175 units amylase/dL
Bacteria on Gram-stained smear
Bile
Food particles
Intermediate
Pink fluid on free aspiration
50,000–100,000 red cells/µL in blunt trauma
100–500 white cells/µL
75–175 units amylase/dL
Negative
Clear aspirate
< 100 white cells/µL
< 75 units amylase/dL

Table 13–4. Comparison of Diagnostic Methods for Abdominal Trauma.

Methods	Time/Cost	Advantages/Disadvantages
Physical examination	Quick/no cost	Useful for serial examinations, very limited by other injuries, coma, drug intoxication, poor sensitivity and specificity.
Diagnostic peritoneal lavage (DPL)	Quick/inexpensive	Rapid results in unstable patient but invasive and may be overly sensitive for blood and not specific for site of injury; requires experience and may be limited if previous surgery.
Focused assessment with sonography for trauma (FAST)	Quick/inexpensive	Rapid detection of intra-abdominal fluid and pericardial tamponade; may be limited by operator experience, large body habitus, subcutaneous air; poor for detection of bowel injury. Fairly sensitive but not highly specific.
Helical computerized abdominal tomography (CT)	Slower/expensive	Most specific for site of injury and can evaluate retroperitoneum; very good sensitivity but may miss bowel injury; risk of reaction to contrast dye.

▶ Diagnostic Laparoscopy

Laparoscopy has an important diagnostic role in stable patients with penetrating abdominal trauma. It can quickly establish whether peritoneal penetration has occurred and thus reduce the number of negative and nontherapeutic trauma laparotomies performed. In selected patients, therapeutic laparoscopy has been used to repair injuries to the bowel and diaphragm. This approach offers all the advantages and disadvantages of minimally invasive surgery. Laparoscopy has also been applied safely and effectively as a screening tool in stable patients with blunt abdominal trauma. However, its use in this context requires further study. Concerns regarding the use of laparoscopy in trauma include the possibility of missed injuries, air embolism, hemodynamic instability related to the pneumoperitoneum, and complications related to trocar placement.

▶ Exploratory Laparotomy

The three main indications for exploration of the abdomen following blunt trauma are peritonitis, ongoing intra-abdominal hemorrhage, and the presence of other injuries known to be frequently associated with intra-abdominal injuries. Peritonitis after blunt abdominal trauma is rare and can arise from rupture of a hollow organ, such as the duodenum, bladder, intestine, or gallbladder; from pancreatic injury; or occasionally from the presence of retroperitoneal blood.

Emergency abdominal exploration should be considered for patients with profound hypovolemic shock and a normal chest x-ray unless extra-abdominal blood loss is sufficient to account for the hypovolemia. In most cases, a rapidly performed FAST examination or peritoneal lavage will confirm the diagnosis of intraperitoneal hemorrhage. Patients with blunt trauma and hypovolemia should be examined first for intra-abdominal bleeding even if there is no overt evidence of abdominal trauma. For example, hypovolemia may be due to loss of blood from a large scalp laceration, but it may also be due to unsuspected rupture of the spleen. Hemoperitoneum may present with no signs except hypovolemia. The abdomen

may be flat and nontender. Patients whose extra-abdominal bleeding has been controlled should respond to initial fluid resuscitation with an adequate urine output and stabilization of vital signs. If signs of hypovolemia (tachycardia, hypotension, low urine output, metabolic acidosis) recur, intra-abdominal bleeding must be considered to be the cause.

Other injuries frequently associated with abdominal trauma are rib fractures, pelvic fractures, abdominal wall injuries, and fractures of the thoracolumbar spine (eg, 20% of patients with fractures of the left lower ribs have a splenic laceration).

▶ Treatment

A. Splenic Injuries

The spleen is the most commonly injured organ in cases of blunt abdominal trauma. Splenic injuries in children have been managed traditionally without surgery. Currently, 50–88% of adults with blunt splenic injuries are treated nonoperatively. Patients must be monitored closely in the intensive care unit, and immediate availability of an operating room is essential. Patients should be evaluated frequently for the possibility of other missed injuries or recurrent bleeding. Stable patients who have high-grade splenic injuries on CT scan or have evidence of ongoing bleeding on CT scan may be candidates for angiographic embolization. Unstable patients with splenic injuries should undergo splenectomy or attempts at splenic repair if appropriate.

Associated injuries are uncommon for patients in whom nonoperative management is attempted. In unstable patients, emergent celiotomy should be performed. Splenic salvage procedures such as splenorrhaphy, partial resection, wrapping with Vicryl mesh, or topical therapy with hemostatic agents should be attempted if the patient's condition permits and there are a limited number of concomitant abdominal injuries. In the face of multiple injuries, ongoing cardiovascular compromise, or vascular avulsion of the spleen, total splenectomy is indicated. Following splenectomy, immunizations against *Pneumococcus* species, *Menin-*

gococcus species, and *Haemophilus influenzae* are recommended postoperatively to reduce the risk of overwhelming postsplenectomy sepsis.

B. Liver Injuries

Approximately 85% of all patients with blunt hepatic trauma are stable following resuscitation. In this group, nonoperative management has been shown to be superior to open operation in avoiding complications and decreasing mortality. The primary requirement for nonoperative therapy is continued hemodynamic stability. Patients are monitored in the intensive care unit with frequent assessment of vital signs and serial hematocrits. If transfusion with more than two units of PRBC is required, arteriography with possible embolization of bleeding vessels should be considered

Nonoperative management of blunt hepatic trauma is successful in more than 90% of cases. With more severe injuries, repeat CT scanning may be necessary to evaluate for possible complications such as parenchymal infarction, hematoma, or biloma. Extrahepatic bile collections should generally be drained percutaneously. Intrahepatic collections of blood and bile usually resolve spontaneously over the course of several months. Patients with high-grade liver injuries have up to a 40% chance of developing bile leaks from the injured liver bed. Nuclear medicine scanning to delineate biliary flow with derivatives of iminodiacetic acid is useful in detection of bile leaks and should be done in the first few days after injury to reduce complications. In addition, 1–4% of patients with blunt liver injury will have injuries to other abdominal organs, which should prompt the clinician to consider the possibility of missed injury in patients who develop abdominal sepsis after injury.

Severe liver injury may result in exsanguinating hemorrhage with hypotension that does not respond to fluid resuscitation. For these patients, exploration is warranted. At laparotomy, immediate efforts should be directed to control of hemorrhage and stabilization of the patient by restoration of circulating blood volume. The initial techniques for the control of hepatic hemorrhage include manual compression, perihepatic packing, and the Pringle maneuver. Manual compression or perihepatic packing with laparotomy pads will control hemorrhage in most cases. The Pringle maneuver—clamping of the hepatic pedicle—should be performed when life-threatening hemorrhage is unresponsive to packing; it will control all hepatic bleeding except that from the hepatic veins or the intrahepatic vena cava. In most cases, the Pringle maneuver should not be maintained for more than 1 hour in order to prevent ischemic damage to the liver. Hepatic bleeding can be controlled by suture ligation or application of surgical clips directly to the bleeding vessels. Electrocautery or the argon beam coagulator can be used to control bleeding from raw surfaces of the liver. Microfibrillar collagen or hemostatic gelatin foam sponges soaked in thrombin can be applied to bleeding areas with pressure to control diffuse capillary bleeding. Fibrin glue has been used

in treating both superficial and deep lacerations and appears to be the most effective topical agent but reports of fatal anaphylactic reactions have limited its use. When injury has already resulted in massive blood loss, packing of the abdomen with laparotomy pads and planned reexploration should be considered. Avoidance of hypothermia, acidosis, and coagulopathy are paramount to successful surgical treatment of a major liver injury and may require further resuscitation in the intensive care unit prior to return to the operating room. At the time of reexploration in 24–48 hours, hemorrhage is usually well controlled and can be managed with individual vessel ligation and debridement. Evidence of persistent hemorrhage should prompt earlier reexploration. Angiographic embolization may be a useful adjunct to surgical packing if arterial hemorrhage is still present or not well controlled. Rarely, selective hepatic artery ligation, resectional debridement, or hepatic lobectomy may be required to control hemorrhage. The raw surface of the liver may then be covered with omentum. Drains should always be used. Decompression of the biliary system is contraindicated, though sutures or clips should be used to control intraparenchymal bile ducts.

Hepatic vein injuries frequently bleed massively. Hepatic venous or intrahepatic vena caval injury should be suspected immediately when the Pringle maneuver fails to control bleeding. Several techniques have been described for isolation of the intrahepatic cava prior to attempted repair of these injuries. Unfortunately, even with the use of these techniques, mortality remains very high.

C. Biliary Tract Injuries

Biliary tract injuries are relatively uncommon, particularly for blunt trauma. Injury to the gallbladder should be treated in most cases by cholecystectomy. Minor injuries to the common bile duct can be treated by suture closure and insertion of a T-tube. Avulsion of the common bile duct or in combination with duodenal or ampullary trauma may require choledochojejunostomy in conjunction with total or partial pancreatectomy, duodenectomy, or other diversion procedures. Segmental loss of the common bile duct is best treated by choledochojejunostomy and drainage.

D. Pancreatic Injuries

Pancreatic injuries may present with few clinical manifestations. Injury should be suspected whenever the upper abdomen has been traumatized, especially when serum amylase levels remain persistently elevated. The best diagnostic study for pancreatic injury (other than exploratory celiotomy) is CT scan of the abdomen. Peritoneal lavage is usually not helpful. Upper gastrointestinal studies with water-soluble contrast material may suggest pancreatic injury by demonstrating widening of the duodenal C-loop. Endoscopic retrograde cholangiopancreatography may be used in selected cases to evaluate for injuries to the major ducts.

The treatment of pancreatic injury depends on its grade and extent. Minor injuries not involving a major duct may be treated nonoperatively. Moderate injuries usually require operative exploration, debridement, and the placement of external drains. More severe injuries, including those with major duct injury or transection of the gland, may require distal resection or external drainage. Traumatic injuries to the head of the pancreas often include associated vascular injuries and carry a high mortality rate. Efforts should be directed at controlling hemorrhage, and drains can be placed in the area of the pancreatic injury. In most cases, pancreaticoduodenectomy should not be attempted in the setting of an unstable patient with multiple injuries.

The late complications of pancreatic injuries include pseudocyst, pancreatic fistula, and pancreatic abscess. Patients treated without resection may require reoperation for resection or Roux-en-Y internal gastrointestinal drainage.

E. Gastrointestinal Tract Injuries

Most injuries of the stomach can be repaired. Large injuries, such as those from shotgun blasts, may require subtotal or total resection. Failure to identify posterior stomach wall injuries by opening the lesser space is a pitfall to guard against.

Duodenal injuries may not be evident from the initial physical examination or x-ray studies. Abdominal films will reveal retroperitoneal gas within 6 hours after injury in most patients. CT performed with a contrast agent will frequently identify the site of perforation. Most duodenal injuries can be treated with lateral repair. Some may require resection with end-to-end anastomosis. Occasionally, pancreaticoduodenectomy or duodenal diversion with gastrojejunostomy and pyloric closure is required to manage a severe injury. A duodenostomy tube is useful in decompressing the duodenum and can be used to control a fistula caused by an injury. Jejunal or omental patches may also aid in preventing a suture line leak. A distal jejunostomy feeding tube is helpful in the long-term recovery from these injuries.

Duodenal hematomas causing high-grade obstruction usually resolve with nonoperative management. Patients may require total parenteral nutrition. In some cases, a small-bore enteral feeding tube can be passed beyond the area of obstruction utilizing interventional radiology techniques. Large hematomas may require operative evacuation, particularly when the obstruction lasts for more than 10–14 days and a persistent hematoma is seen on CT scan.

Most small bowel injuries can be treated with a two-layer sutured closure, though mesenteric injuries leading to devascularized segments of small bowel will require resection. The underlying principle is to preserve as much small bowel as possible.

For injuries to the colon, the past approach has been to divert the fecal stream or exteriorize the injury. However, more recent studies have shown a higher complication rate with colostomy formation than with primary repair. Wounds should be considered for primary repair if the blood supply is not compromised. Primary repair is more likely to be associated with complications in patients with ongoing shock, in those requiring multiple transfusions, if more than 6 hours elapse between injury and operation, or if there is gross contamination or peritonitis. Small, clean rectal injuries may be closed primarily if conditions are favorable. The treatment of larger rectal wounds involving pelvic fracture should include proximal diversion. Insertion of presacral drains is optional. In this latter case, direct repair of the rectal injury is not mandatory but should be performed if it can be readily exposed. Irrigation of the distal stump should be performed in most cases unless it would further contaminate the pelvic space.

F. Abdominal Wall Injuries

Abdominal wall injuries from blunt trauma are most often due to shear forces, such as being run over by the wheels of a tractor or bus. The shearing often devitalizes the subcutaneous tissue and skin, and if debridement is delayed, a serious necrotizing anaerobic infection may develop. The management of penetrating abdominal wall injuries is usually straightforward. Debridement and irrigation are appropriate surgical treatment. Every effort must be made to remove foreign material, shreds of clothing, necrotic muscle, and soft tissue. Abdominal wall defects may require insertion of absorbable mesh or coverage with a myocutaneous flap.

G. Genitourinary Tract Injuries

The most commonly injured genitourinary tract organs are the male genitalia, the uterus, the urethra, the bladder, the ureters, and the kidneys. The workup for these injuries consists primarily of radiologic examinations, which may include abdominal CT scan, cystogram, or retrograde urethrogram. In unstable patients with associated injuries, it may not be possible to obtain these studies prior to emergency laparotomy. In these patients, an intraoperative single-shot intravenous urogram is safe and of high quality in most cases. This study often provides important information that facilitates rapid and accurate decision making. It can confirm function in the noninjured kidney and help in identifying blunt renal injuries that may be safely observed.

1. Bladder injuries—Rupture of the bladder, like urethral disruption, is frequently associated with pelvic fractures. Seventy-five percent of ruptures are extraperitoneal and 25% intraperitoneal. Bladder ruptures should be repaired through a midline abdominal incision. Rupture of the anterior wall of the bladder can be repaired by direct suture; rupture of the posterior wall can be repaired from inside the bladder after an opening has been made in the anterior wall. Care should be taken to avoid entering a pelvic hematoma. Postoperatively, urine should be diverted for at least 7 days.

2. Urethral injuries—Membranous prostatic urethral disruption is often associated with pelvic fractures or deceleration injuries. Blood at the urethral meatus associated with scrotal hematoma and high-riding prostate on digital rectal examination are the classic signs of injury to the male urethra. The prostate may be elevated superiorly by the pelvic hematoma and will be free-riding and high on rectal examination. If these signs are present, a retrograde urethrogram should be performed before attempts at catheter placement, which may convert an incomplete injury to a complete disruption. If an injury is present, urethrography will demonstrate free extravasation of contrast from the urethra into the preperitoneal space.

Penetrating injuries are best treated with primary repair. Suprapubic bladder drainage and delayed reconstruction of blunt urethral disruption injuries are safe and effective in most cases. Immediate realignment with cystourethroscopy and placement of a urethral catheter is an attractive, minimally invasive alternative. In cases of partial disruption, it has been shown to result in stricture-free outcomes.

Major injuries to the bulbous or penile urethra should be managed by suprapubic urinary diversion. A voiding cystourethrogram may later reveal a stricture, but operative correction or dilation is usually not necessary.

3. Renal injuries—Advances in the imaging and staging of renal trauma as well as in treatment strategies have decreased the need for operation and increased renal preservation. More than half of renal injuries can be treated nonoperatively. Management criteria are based on radiographic, laboratory, and clinical findings. Nonoperative treatment of penetrating renal lacerations is appropriate in hemodynamically stable patients without other injuries. Small to moderate injuries can be treated nonoperatively, but severe injuries are associated with a significant risk of delayed bleeding if treated expectantly. Stable patients may be candidates for angiographic procedures to control bleeding or revascularize dissection or injuries leading to vessel thrombosis. Renal exploration should be considered if laparotomy is indicated for associated injuries. A midline transabdominal approach is preferred. The renal artery and vein are secured before the Gerota fascia is opened. The injury should be managed by suture repair, partial nephrectomy, or, rarely, total nephrectomy. Pedicle grafts of omentum or free peritoneal patch grafts can be used to cover defects. Renal vascular injuries require immediate operation to save the kidney. Meticulous attention to reconstructive techniques in renal exploration can ensure an excellent renal salvage rate. Adherence to the principles of early proximal vascular control, debridement of devitalized tissue, hemostasis, closure of the collecting system, and coverage of the defect will maximize the salvage of renal function while minimizing potential complications.

Perirenal hematomas found incidentally at celiotomy should be explored if they are expanding, pulsatile, or not contained by retroperitoneal tissues or if a preexploration urogram shows extensive urinary extravasation.

4. Injuries to the male genitalia—Injuries to the male genitalia usually result in skin loss only; the penis, penile

urethra, and testes are usually spared. Skin loss from the penis should be treated with a primary skin graft. Scrotal skin loss should be treated by delayed reconstruction; an exposed testis can be temporarily protected by placing it in a subcutaneous tissue pocket in the thigh.

5. Uterine injuries—Injuries of the female reproductive organs are infrequent except in combination with genitourinary or rectal trauma. Injuries to the uterine fundus usually can be repaired with absorbable sutures; drainage is not necessary. In more extensive injuries, hysterectomy may be preferable. The vaginal cuff may be left open for drainage, particularly if there is an associated urinary tract or rectal injury. Injuries involving the uterus in a pregnant woman usually result in death of the fetus. Bleeding may be massive in such patients, particularly in women approaching parturition. Cesarean section plus hysterectomy may be the only alternative.

6. Ureteral injuries—Ureteral injuries are easily missed because urinalysis and imaging studies can be unreliable. Most such injuries can be successfully reconstructed by primary repair over stents, ureteral reimplantations, or ureteroureterostomy depending on the level of injury.

Armenakas NA, Duckett CP, McAninch: Indications for nonoperative management of renal stab wounds. J Urol 1999;161:768.

Asensio JA et al: Approach to the management of complex hepatic injuries. J Trauma 2000;48:66.

Asensio JA et al: Operative management and outcomes in 103 AAST-OIS grades IV and V complex hepatic injuries: trauma surgeons still need to operate, but angioembolization helps. J Trauma 2003;54:647.

Bee TK et al. Failures of splenic nonoperative management: is the glass half empty or half full? J Trauma 2000;39:177.

Bradley EL 3rd et al: Diagnosis and initial management of blunt pancreatic trauma: guidelines for a multiinstitutional review. Ann Surg 1998;227:861.

Brandes SB, McAninch JW: Reconstructive surgery for trauma of the upper urinary tract. Urol Clin North Am 1999;26:183.

Carrillo EH et al: Evolution in the treatment of complex blunt liver injuries. Curr Probl Surg 2001;38:1.

Chappuis CW et al: Management of penetrating colon injuries. A prospective randomized trial. Ann Surg 1991;213:492.

Chen RJ et al: Surgical management of juxtahepatic venous injuries in blunt hepatic trauma. J Trauma 1995;38:886.

Croce MA et al: Nonoperative management of blunt hepatic trauma is the treatment of choice for hemodynamically stable patients. Results of a prospective trial. Ann Surg 1995;221:744.

Curran TJ, Borzotta AP: Complications of primary repair of colon injury: literature review of 2,964 cases. Am J Surg 1999;177:42.

Fakhry SM et al: Relatively short diagnostic delays (<8 hours) produce morbidity and mortality in blunt small bowel injury: an analysis of time to operative intervention in 198 patients from a multicenter experience. J Trauma 1999;47:207.

Fulcher AS et al: Magnetic resonance cholangiopancreatography in the assessment of pancreatic duct trauma and its sequelae: preliminary findings. J Trauma 2000;48:1001.

Jacobs IA et al: Nonoperative management of blunt splenic and hepatic trauma in the pediatric population: significant differences between adult and pediatric surgeons? Am Surg 2001;67:149.

Kielb SJ, Voeltz ZL, Wolf JS Jr: Evaluation and management of traumatic posterior urethral disruption with flexible cystourethroscopy. J Trauma 2001;50:36.

Malhotra AK et al: Blunt bowel and mesenteric injuries: the role of screening computed tomography. J Trauma 2000;48:991.

Miller PR et al: Associated injuries in blunt solid organ trauma: implications for missed injury in nonoperative management. J Trauma 2002;52:238.

Mohr AM et al: Angiographic embolization for liver injuries: low mortality, high morbidity. J Trauma 2003;55:1077.

Nicholas JM et al: Changing patterns in the management of penetrating abdominal trauma: the more things change, the more they stay the same. J Trauma 2003;55:1095.

Patton JH et al: Pancreatic trauma: a simplified management guideline. J Trauma 1997;43:234.

Peitzman AB et al: Blunt splenic injury in adults: multi-institutional study of the eastern association for the surgery of trauma. J Trauma 2000;49:177.

Rozycki GS, Newman PG: Surgeon-performed ultrasound for the assessment of abdominal injuries. Adv Surg 1999;33:243.

Sartorelli KH et al: Nonoperative management of hepatic, splenic, and renal injuries in adults with multiple injuries. J Trauma 2000;49:56.

Shapiro MB et al: Damage control: collective review. J Trauma 2000;49:969.

Takishima T et al: Serum amylase level on admission in the diagnosis of blunt injury to the pancreas: its significance and limitations. Ann Surg 1997;226:70.

Udobi KF et al: Role of ultrasonography in penetrating abdominal trauma: a prospective clinical study. J Trauma 200;150:475.

Wahl WL et al: Diagnosis and management of bile leaks after blunt liver injury. Surgery 2005;138:742.

Wei B et al: Angioembolization reduces operative intervention for blunt splenic injury. J Trauma 2008;64:1472.

Zantut LF et al: Diagnostic and therapeutic laparoscopy for penetrating abdominal trauma: a multicenter experience. J Trauma 1997;42:825.

VASCULAR INJURIES

Historical Perspective

Much of our knowledge of blood vessel injuries was developed during the course of military conflicts in the 20th century. Although techniques for the management of vascular injuries were in use prior to World War I, arterial ligation to save a life rather than arterial repair to salvage a limb was generally employed, and amputation frequently resulted after vascular injury.

During World War II, only 33% of arterial injuries were repaired. The amputation rate was 49% following arterial ligation and 36% following arterial repair. In the Korean and Vietnam wars, with the advent of antibiotics and advanced vascular surgical techniques, the amputation rate decreased to 13% of cases. The amputation rate associated with vascular injuries during the Iraq War is 20% and is likely higher due to the combined bone, soft-tissue, and vascular extremity injuries created from improvised explosive devices.

The mortality rate for lower extremity arterial injury is low in both civilian and recent military series: 2–6%. Limb salvage rates in civilian series are 85–90%, with best results

obtained for interposition vein grafts. Ligation, need for reoperation, and failed revascularization are associated with worse outcomes and higher amputation rates. Low mortality and improved limb salvage is a result of more rapid transport of injured people, improved blood volume replacement, selective use of arteriography and shunts, and better operative techniques.

The Epidemiology of Vascular Trauma

The epidemiology of vascular trauma has been studied in three different settings: military conflicts, large urban locations, and, to a lesser extent, rural areas. The types of injuries seen in civilian vascular trauma, once much different from military settings, are now more similar to military wounds, and the incidence is increasing as a result of the rise in urban violence, motor vehicle crashes, and iatrogenic injuries owing to more frequent use of minimally invasive diagnostic and therapeutic procedures.

Peripheral vascular trauma typically occurs in young men between the ages of 20 and 40 years. In both urban and rural environments, penetrating mechanisms dominate, accounting for 50–90% of vascular injuries. Because many vascular injuries of the head, neck, and torso are immediately fatal, most patients with vascular injuries surviving transport have extremity trauma. This is especially true in the military experience—in Vietnam, extremity vascular injuries accounted for approximately 90% of all arterial trauma. In the urban civilian experience, extremity vascular injuries comprise about 50% of arterial injuries. In rural vascular trauma, blunt injuries occur more frequently than in urban populations.

Mortality and utilization of medical resources is higher among patients with vascular injuries than among patients who do not have blood vessel injuries. Vascular injuries from automobile accidents or falls from heights and crush injuries account for up to half of all noniatrogenic vascular injuries in US hospitals. The likelihood of vascular injury after blunt trauma correlates with the overall severity of the injury and the presence of specific orthopedic injuries. For example, up to 45% of patients with posterior knee dislocations or severe instability from high-velocity blunt trauma sustain popliteal artery injury.

The number of iatrogenic vascular injuries has risen dramatically in recent decades. Most involve diagnostic and therapeutic procedures utilizing the femoral (less frequently the brachial or axillary) vessels, which serve as access routes. In order of decreasing frequency, injuries include hemorrhage and hematoma, pseudoaneurysm, arteriovenous fistula formation, vessel thrombosis, and embolization. Rates of injury range from 0.5% for diagnostic procedures to as high as 10% for therapeutic procedures involving large catheters. Increasing age, female gender, use of anticoagulation, and the presence of atherosclerosis increase the risk of these complications. Complications remote from the puncture site include vessel rupture and dissection. Operative procedures (especially hepatic and pancreaticobiliary surgery) are associated with iatrogenic vascular trauma. In addition, anterior and retroperitoneal approaches to the lumbar spine and other orthopedic procedures such as total joint replacement and arthroscopy can produce vascular injuries.

► Types of Injuries

A. Penetrating Trauma

The local and regional effects of penetrating wounds are determined by the mechanism of vessel injury. Stab wounds, low-velocity (< 2000 ft/s) bullet wounds, iatrogenic injuries from percutaneous catheterization, and inadvertent intra-arterial injection of drugs produce less soft tissue injury and disrupt collateral circulation less than injuries from sources with greater kinetic energy. The high-velocity missiles responsible for war wounds produce more extensive vascular injuries, which involve massive destruction and contamination of surrounding tissues. The temporary cavitational effect of high-velocity missiles causes additional trauma to the ends of severed arteries and may produce arterial thrombosis due to disrupted intima even when the artery has not been directly hit. This blast effect can also draw material such as clothing, dirt, or pieces of skin along the wound tract, which contributes to the risk of infection. Associated injuries are often major determinants of the eventual outcome.

Shotgun blasts present special problems. Although muzzle velocity is low (about 1200 ft/s), the multiple pellets produce widespread damage, and shotgun wadding entering the wound enhances the likelihood of infection. Similar to high-velocity injuries, the damage is often much greater than might be anticipated from inspection of the entry wound. Moreover, the multiplicity of potential sites of arterial damage often mandates diagnostic arteriography even in the presence of obvious arterial insufficiency.

B. Blunt Trauma

Motor vehicle accidents are a major cause of blunt vascular trauma. Multiple injuries include fractures and dislocations; and while direct vascular injury may occur, in most instances the damage is indirect due to fractures. This is especially likely to occur with fractures near joints, where vessels are relatively fixed and vulnerable to shear forces. For example, the popliteal artery and vein are frequently injured in association with posterior dislocation of the knee. Fractures of large heavy bones such as the femur or tibia transmit forces that have cavitation effects similar to those caused by high-velocity bullets. There is extensive damage to soft tissues and neurovascular structures, and edema formation interferes with evaluation of pulses. Delay in diagnosis and the presence of associated injuries decrease the chances of limb salvage. Contusions or crush injuries may result in complete or partial disruption of arteries, producing intimal flaps or intramural hematomas that impede blood flow.

Blunt thoracic aortic injury (BTAI) is a serious traumatic injury that continues to have a high initial mortality and is associated with modern high-speed methods of transportation or significant falls. Autopsy data from cases of fatal BTAI demonstrated that 57% of patients were dead at the scene or on arrival to the hospital, 37% died during the first 4 hours at the hospital, and only 6% died after 4 hours in the hospital. The disruption generally occurs at the aortic isthmus (between the left subclavian artery and the ligamentum arteriosum) due to a deceleration injury in which the heart, the ascending aorta, and the transverse arch continue to move forward while movement of the isthmus and the descending aorta is limited by their posterior attachments. Clinical findings associated with traumatic rupture of the thoracic aorta are listed in Table 13–5 and radiographic findings in Table 13–6. Blunt traumatic injury to the abdominal aorta is uncommon, but it has been reported from lap seat belt trauma.

Almost any vessel can be injured by blunt trauma, including the extracranial cerebral and visceral arteries. Blunt carotid arterial injuries are associated with mortality rates of 20–30%, with over 50% of survivors having permanent, severe neurologic deficits. Whereas in the past vertebral artery injuries were considered innocuous, recent studies have reported devastating complications related to these injuries, including a 70% incidence of coexistent cervical spine injuries. Traumatic injury to the superior mesenteric artery is associated with a 50% mortality rate. The brachial and popliteal arteries, which cross joints and are exposed to direct trauma, are particularly susceptible to injury as a result of fractures and dislocations.

► Clinical Findings

A. Hemorrhage

When pulsatile external hemorrhage is present, the diagnosis of arterial injury is obvious, but when blood accumulates in deep tissues of the extremity, the thorax, abdomen, or retroperitoneum, the only manifestation may be shock. Peripheral vasoconstriction may make evaluation of peripheral pulses difficult until blood volume is restored. If the artery is completely severed, thrombus may form at the contracted vessel ends and a major vascular injury may not be suspected. The presence of arterial pulses distal to a

Table 13–5. Clinical Features of Traumatic Aortic Rupture.

History of high-speed deceleration injury
Flail chest
Fractured sternum
Superior vena cava syndrome
Multiple or first or second rib fractures
Upper extremity hypertension or pulse deficits
Hematoma in the carotid sheaths
Interscapular bruits
Hoarseness with normal larynx

Table 13–6. Radiographic Features of Traumatic Aortic Rupture.

Widening of mediastinum
Fractured sternum
Multiple or first rib or second rib fractures
Esophageal deviation to the right
Tracheal deviation to the right
Apical cap
Depression of left main stem bronchus
Obliteration of the aortic knob
Obliteration of the descending aorta
Obliteration of the aortopulmonary window
Obliteration of the medial left upper lobe
Widened paravertebral stripe

penetrating wound does not preclude arterial injury; as many as 20% of patients with injuries of major arteries in an extremity have palpable pulses distal to the injury, either because the vessel has not thrombosed or because pulse waves are transmitted through soft clot. Conversely, the absence of a palpable pulse in an adequately resuscitated patient is a sensitive indicator of arterial injury.

B. Ischemia

Acute arterial insufficiency must be diagnosed promptly to prevent tissue loss. Ischemia should be suspected when the patient has one or more of the "five Ps": pain, pallor, paralysis, paresthesia, or pulselessness. The susceptibility of different cells to hypoxia varies (eg, sudden occlusion of the carotid artery results in brain damage within minutes unless collateral circulation can maintain adequate perfusion, but a kidney can survive severe ischemia for up to an hour). Peripheral nerves are quite vulnerable to ischemia because they have a high basal energy requirement to maintain ion gradients over large membrane surfaces and because they have few glycogen stores. Hence, interruption of arterial flow for relatively short periods can result in nerve damage due to interrupted substrate delivery. In contrast, skeletal muscle is more tolerant of decreased arterial flow. Muscle can be ischemic for up to 4 hours without developing histologic changes. In general, complete interruption of all arterial inflow (including collateral blood supply) results in neuromuscular ischemic damage after 4–6 hours. Restoration of flow can actually worsen this damage as part of the reperfusion syndrome and can increase the severity of the original ischemic insult.

Prolonged ischemia can produce muscle necrosis and rhabdomyolysis, which releases potassium and myoglobin into the circulation. Myoglobin is an oxygen-transporting protein similar in structure to hemoglobin; it is innocuous unless it dissociates into hematin, which is nephrotoxic in an acidic milieu. Precipitation of hematin pigment also occurs when urine flow is reduced by hypotension or hypovolemia, obstructing renal tubules and worsening nephrotoxicity.

Myoglobinemia can lead to acute tubular necrosis and renal failure, hyperkalemia, and a risk of life-threatening arrhythmias. Thus, in addition to limb loss, acute arterial ischemia can produce organ failure and death.

C. False Aneurysm

Disruption of an arterial wall as a result of trauma may lead to formation of a false aneurysm. The wall of a false aneurysm is composed primarily of fibrous tissue derived from nearby tissues, not arterial tissue. Because blood continues to flow past the fistulous opening, the extremity is seldom ischemic. False aneurysms may rupture at any time. They continue to expand because they lack vascular wall integrity. Spontaneous resolution of pseudoaneurysms larger than 3 cm is unlikely, and operative repair becomes increasingly difficult as the aneurysms increase in size and complexity with time. Symptoms gradually appear as a result of compression of adjacent nerves or collateral vessels or from rupture of the aneurysm—or as a result of thrombosis with ischemic symptoms. Iatrogenic false aneurysms after arterial puncture thrombose spontaneously within 4 weeks when they are less than 3 cm in diameter. Simple ultrasound follow-up rather than operative therapy is indicated. Color-flow duplex-guided compression of iatrogenic pseudoaneurysms is successful in 70–90% of attempts, but the procedure is uncomfortable and may take hours of probe pressure. Ultrasound-guided thrombin injection has been effective for thrombosis of large false aneurysms in a matter of seconds, but distal arterial thrombosis has also been described using this technique.

D. Arteriovenous Fistula

With simultaneous injury of an adjacent artery and vein, a fistula may form that allows blood from the artery to enter the vein. Because venous pressure is lower than arterial pressure, flow through an arteriovenous fistula is continuous; accentuation of the bruit and thrill can be detected over the fistula during systole. Traumatic arteriovenous fistulas may occur as operative complications (eg, aortocaval fistula following removal of a herniated intervertebral disk). Iatrogenic femoral arteriovenous fistulas after arteriograms and cardiac catheterization are seen with increasing frequency. Long-standing large arteriovenous fistulas may result in high-output cardiac failure. Similar to iatrogenic pseudoaneurysms occurring after arteriography, spontaneous resolution of acute arteriovenous fistulas usually occurs.

▶ Diagnosis

Arterial injury must be considered in any injured patient. Patients who present in shock following penetrating injury or blunt trauma should be assumed to have vascular injury until proven otherwise. Any injury near a major artery should arouse suspicion. A plain film may be helpful in demonstrating a fracture whose fragments could jeopardize an adjacent vessel or a bullet fragment that could have passed near to a major vessel. Before the x-ray is taken, entrance and exit wounds should be marked with radiopaque objects such as a paper clip.

Diagnosis is usually established on the basis of physical examination looking for signs of injury (Table 13–7). In addition to checking for obvious hemorrhage and the five Ps, the physician should listen for a bruit, palpate for a thrill (eg, of an arteriovenous fistula), and look for an expanding hematoma (eg, of a false aneurysm). Secondary hemorrhage from a wound is an ominous sign that may herald massive hemorrhage. The finding of these "hard" signs reliably reflects the presence of a vascular injury; hard signs mandate immediate exploration in most instances. The presence of "soft" signs (history of bleeding, diminished but palpable pulse, injury in proximity to a major artery, neurapraxia) requires further tests or serial observation.

Doppler flow studies have gained importance in the diagnosis of arterial trauma. An ankle brachial index (ABI), determined by dividing the systolic pressure in the injured limb by the systolic pressure in an uninjured arm, is highly reliable for excluding arterial injury after both blunt and penetrating trauma. An ABI less than 0.9 has sensitivity of 95%, specificity of 97%, and negative predictive value of 99% for determining the presence of clinically significant arterial injury. Thus, only patients with soft signs and an ABI less than 0.9 require arteriography.

Color-flow duplex ultrasonography combines real-time B mode (brightness modulation) ultrasound imaging with a steerable pulsed Doppler flow detector. This technology can provide images of vessels and velocity spectral analysis. Color-flow duplex scanning of an area of injury is noninvasive, painless, portable, and easily repeated for follow-up examinations. When compared with arteriography and performed by experienced examiners, duplex ultrasound identifies nearly all major injuries that require treatment, potentially at considerable cost savings. In addition to screening for arterial trauma, duplex scanning has been used to detect pseudoaneurysms, arteriovenous fistulas, and intimal flaps. However, potential logistical and resource problems exist. The technology is sophisticated and requires skill in operation and interpretation, which is not always immediately available.

Arteriography is the most accurate diagnostic procedure for identifying vascular injuries (Figure 13–13). Arteriography to exclude vascular injury for soft signs results in a negative exploration rate of 20–35% and an arteriography-related complication rate of 2–4%. Proximity as the sole indication for arteriography has an extremely low yield, ranging from 0% to 10%. Patients with unequivocal signs of arterial injury on physical examination or plain films should have urgent operation. The false-negative rate of arteriography is low, and a normal arteriogram precludes the need for surgical exploration. Virtually all arteriographic errors are due to false-positives, which occur in 2–8% of patients. Technical considerations in performing arteriography include the following: (1) entrance and exit wounds should be marked with a radiopaque marker; (2) the injection site should not be near the suspected injury; (3) an area 10–15 cm proximal and distal to the suspected injury should be included in the arteriographic field; (4) sequential films should be obtained to detect early venous filling; (5) any abnormality should be considered an indication of arterial injury unless it is obviously the result of preexisting disease; and (6) two different projections should be obtained.

Emergency center arteriography using micropuncture Seldinger technique or cannulating the artery to be studied with an 18-gauge catheter (antegrade in the lower extremity and prograde in the upper extremity arteries) is quick and accurate. The use of fluoroscopy, especially if equipped with subtraction capability, simplifies the timing of contrast injection and x-ray exposure. Fluoroscopy is particularly helpful to visualize distal arteries and minimize the amount of contrast media needed. Arteriography may be particularly useful in differentiating arterial injury from spasm. In general, it is risky to attribute abnormal physical findings in an injured patient to arterial spasm; an arteriogram is indicated in such patients.

Arteriography is also valuable when arterial injuries may have occurred at multiple sites or to localize an injury when a long parallel penetration makes this determination difficult. Complications of arteriography include groin hemato-

Table 13–7. Signs of Extremity Vascular Injury.

Hard signs
Expanding or pulsatile hematoma
Limb ischemia
Bruit or thrill
Absence of distal pulse
Soft signs
History of hemorrhage at scene, now stopped
Deficit of nerve associated with vessel
Stable, nonexpanding hematoma
Proximity of wound to major extremity blood vessel
Ankle brachial index < 0.9

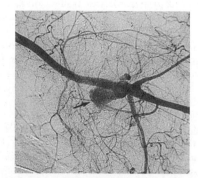

▲ **Figure 13–13.** Arteriogram showing traumatic pseudo-aneurysm of subclavian/axillary artery from penetrating injury.

mas, iatrogenic pseudoaneurysms, arteriovenous fistulas, embolic occlusions, and delays in diagnosis that may lead to irreversible ischemia in marginally perfused limbs. The availability of CT angiograms with latest generation multidetector contrast-enhanced spiral scanners is a viable alternative to traditional angiography. CT angiograms can diagnose intimal dissections, pseudoaneurysms, arteriovenous fistulas, thrombosis or occlusion, and active bleeding. Metallic foreign bodies can create artifacts that interfere with generation of optimal CT angiogram studies.

For patients suspected of having BTAI based on mechanism of injury, the chest x-ray is a good screening tool to determine the need for further investigation. The most significant radiographic findings for possible BTAI include widened mediastinum, obscured aortic knob, deviation of the left mainstem bronchus or nasogastric tube, and opacification of the aortopulmonary window. Helical chest CT scanning is a useful diagnostic tool for screening and diagnosis of BTAI (Figure 13–14). A negative chest CT scan can obviate the need for further evaluation with a contrast aortogram. Patients with indeterminate CT scans or positive scans should have confirmation and delineation of the extent of BTAI with arteriography or a CT angiogram. In selected instances, cardiothoracic and/or trauma surgeons may consider helical CT scanning alone to be an adequate and complete work-up for BTAI. In addition, a helical CT angiogram with 3D reconstruction guides potential endovascular approach for treatment of BTAI. The use of either transesophageal echocardiography or intraluminal ultrasound in the diagnosis of BTAI continues to evolve, but they are not considered standard diagnostic modalities.

▶ Management

A. Initial Treatment

A rapid but thorough examination should be performed to determine the complete extent of injury. The physician must establish the priority of arterial injury in the overall management of the patient and should remember that delay in arterial repair decreases chances of a favorable outcome. When repair is performed within 12 hours after injury, amputation is rarely necessary; if repair is performed later, the incidence of amputation is about 50%. Depending on the degree of ischemia, delay in arterial repair will lead to lasting neuromuscular damage after as short a period as 4–6 hours.

Restoration of blood volume and control of hemorrhage are done simultaneously. If exsanguinating hemorrhage precludes resuscitation in the emergency room, the patient should be moved directly to the operating room. External bleeding is best controlled by firm direct pressure or packing. Probes or fingers should not be inserted into the wound because a clot may be dislodged, causing profuse bleeding. Tourniquets occlude venous return, disturb collateral flow, and further compromise circulation and should not be employed unless exsanguinating hemorrhage cannot be controlled by other

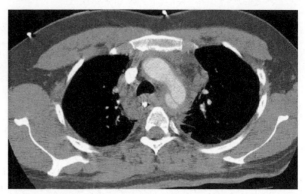

▲ **Figure 13–14.** Computed tomography scan of the chest showing traumatic disruption of the aorta from blunt injury.

means. Atraumatic vascular clamps may be applied to accessible vessels by trained surgeons, but blind clamping can increase damage and injure adjacent nerves and veins.

After hemorrhage has been controlled and general resuscitation accomplished, further assessment is possible. The extent of associated injuries is determined and a plan of management made. Large-bore intravenous catheters should be placed in extremities with no potential venous injuries. It is prudent to preserve the saphenous or cephalic vein in an uninjured extremity for use as a venous autograft for vascular repair.

B. Nonoperative Treatment

Some arterial injuries remain asymptomatic and heal. Data supporting the practice of observation of small or asymptomatic arterial injuries have emerged from experimental animal studies and clinical reports showing resolution, improvement, or stabilization of arterial injuries. In well-defined settings, this strategy has proved safe in follow-up reports covering periods of up to 10 years. Thus, a nonoperative approach may be appropriate for compliant patients willing to return for follow-up who have (1) no active hemorrhage, (2) low-velocity injuries (particularly stab wounds or iatrogenic punctures), (3) minimal arterial wall disruptions (< 5 mm), (4) small (< 5 mm) intimal defects, and (5) intact distal circulation.

Follow-up must include frequent physical examinations and carefully performed noninvasive studies, and patients should be asymptomatic—and the strategy must be reconsidered if symptoms develop. Adjuvant therapy with antiplatelet agents is usually recommended to improve patency in patients with intimal flaps.

Endovascular management has assumed a greater role in the treatment of arterial trauma in recent years. Transcatheter embolization with coils or balloons has been successful in managing selected arterial injuries such as pseudoaneurysms, arteriovenous fistulas, and active bleeding from nonessential arteries. Coils are made of stainless steel with wool or polyester tufts. They are extruded at the site of vessel injury through 5F or 7F catheters. After deployment, the coils expand and lodge at the extrusion site and the tufts promote thrombosis. Catheter-based intra-arterial infusion of vasodilators has also been used to treat vasospasm in small distal arteries.

The recent popularity of endovascular grafting in elective vascular surgery (see Chapter 34) has been applied to the treatment of arterial trauma. A fixation device such as a stent is attached to a graft, and the Stent graft is inserted endoluminally from a remote site and deployed at the site of injury to repair false aneurysms or arteriovenous fistulas. The indications for endovascular grafting are likely to change as technology advances, but the most frequent application currently is in stable patients with delayed presentations who have complex false aneurysms or arteriovenous fistulas. Use of Stent grafts in the acute setting requires the availability of a wide variety of sizes and lengths of grafts and advanced catheter skills.

Endovascular repair of BTAI can be performed either electively or even emergently (Figure 13–15). In a recent American Association for the Surgery of Trauma (AAST) multicenter study, two-thirds of patients underwent endovascular Stent graph repair as compared to one-third who underwent traditional open repair. When adjusted for confounding variables, the endovascular approach was associated with reduced mortality (odds ratio 8.42, 95% confidence interval 2.76–25.69) and fewer blood transfusions. Further study is needed to determine the long-term outcome using endovascular techniques to repair BTAI. Commercial grafts have yielded better results than the noncommercial "homemade" grafts. Thoracic aorta lacerations of more than 1.5 cm resulting in graft apposition length less than 2 cm or those near or in the curvature of the aortic arch are associated with an increased risk of endoleak. Endoleak occurred in 14% of the AAST BTAI trial patients, with half being successfully managed with the deployment of additional stent grafts.

In selected cases of BTAI repair, whether it is operative or endovascular, treatment is delayed because treatment and recovery from other more life-threatening injuries has priority (eg, severe pulmonary contusion, brain injury). This is acceptable, and the incidence of aortic rupture after 4 hours in the hospital is low. Systemic blood pressure and heart rate should be controlled with a beta-blocker and other pharmacologic agents as necessary to minimize the risk of rupture while waiting for definitive repair of the injured aorta.

C. Operative Treatment

General anesthesia is preferable to spinal or regional anesthesia. When vascular injuries involve the neck or thoracic outlet, endotracheal intubation must be performed carefully to avoid dislodging a clot and to protect the airway. Moreover, care is necessary to avoid neurologic damage in patients with associated cervical spine injuries. At least one

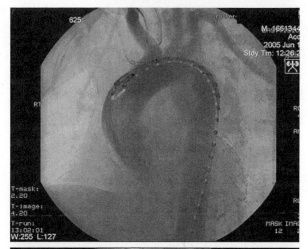
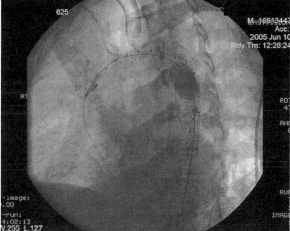

▲ **Figure 13–15.** Aortogram and placement of aortic stent graft to repair a blunt aortic disruption.

uninjured extremity should also be prepared for surgery so that saphenous or cephalic vein conduit may be obtained if a vein graft is required. Provision should also be made for operative arteriography.

Incisions should be generous and parallel to the injured vessel. Meticulous care in handling incisions is essential to avoid secondary infections; all undamaged tissue should be conserved for use in covering repaired vessels. Preservation of all arterial branches is important in order to maintain collateral circulation. Atraumatic control of the vessel should be achieved proximal and distal to the injury so that the injured area may be dissected free of other tissues and inspected without risk of further bleeding. When large hematomas and multiple wounds make exposure and clamping of vessels difficult, it is wise to place a sterile orthopedic tourniquet proximal to the injury that can be inflated temporarily if needed.

The extent of arterial injury must be accurately determined. Arterial spasm generally responds to gentle hydraulic or mechanical dilation. Local application of warm saline or drugs such as papaverine, tolazoline, lidocaine, or nitroglycerin is occasionally effective in relieving spasm. Intra-arterial injection of nitroglycerin or papaverine is also very effective in alleviating spasm. If spasm persists, however, it is best to assume that it is caused by an intramural injury, and the vessel should be opened for direct inspection. An old adage is that spasm is spelled "c-l-o-t."

All devitalized tissue, including damaged portions of the artery, must be debrided. One should resect only the grossly injured portion of the vessel. The method of reconstruction depends on the degree of arterial damage. In selected instances, the ends of injured vessels can be approximated and an end-to-end anastomosis created. If the vessels cannot be mobilized well enough to provide a tension-free anastomosis, an interposition graft should be used. Early experience with prosthetic interposition grafts was disappointing since postoperative infection, thrombosis, and anastomotic disruption were common. These problems have decreased considerably with the use of grafts made of expanded polytetrafluoroethylene (PTFE). Proponents of synthetic grafts focus on the fact that they fail well (eg, infected pseudoaneurysm), whereas a vein graft will disintegrate and result in a sudden blow-out type hemorrhage. Nevertheless, most surgeons still prefer to use an autogenous graft (ie, vein or artery) in severely contaminated wounds. Saphenous vein grafts should be obtained from the *noninjured* leg to avoid impairment of venous return on the side of the injury. Patch angioplasty using saphenous vein is performed when closure of a partially transected vessel would result in narrowing. Suturing should be done with fine 5-0 or 6-0 monofilament material.

In the unusual circumstance of isolated vascular injury, 5,000–10,000 units of intravenous heparin can be given to prevent thrombosis. Otherwise, a small amount of dilute heparin solution (100 units/mL) may be gently injected into the proximal and distal lumen of the injured vessel before clamps are applied. Proximal and distal thrombi are removed with a Fogarty embolectomy catheter. Back-bleeding from the distal artery is not a sure indication that thrombus is absent. A completion operative arteriogram is indicated to determine distal patency and to check on the adequacy of the reconstruction—even when distal pulses are palpable.

It was formerly taught that fractures should be stabilized before vascular injuries were repaired so that manipulation of bones would not jeopardize vascular repair. The disadvantages of this dictum were delay in restoration of flow to ischemic tissue and interference with vascular reconstruction and subsequent arteriographic study of the completed repair by the fixation device. It is currently recommended that vascular repair be performed first, followed by careful application of external traction devices that allow easy access to the wound for observation and dressing changes. Another alternative is to place an intraluminal shunt temporarily across the vascular injury to decrease ischemia while fractures or other injuries are treated. Improved outcomes similar to civilian lower extremity vascular trauma have been attributed to the use of temporary vascular shunts and damage control techniques in the current Iraq War.

Repaired vessels must be covered with healthy tissue. If left exposed, they invariably desiccate and rupture. Skin alone is inadequate, because subsequent necrosis of the skin would leave the vessels exposed, greatly endangering the reconstruction. Generally, an adjacent muscle (eg, sartorius muscle for coverage of the common femoral artery) can be mobilized and placed over the repair. Musculocutaneous flaps can be constructed by plastic surgeons to cover almost any site. In an extensive or severely contaminated wound, a remote bypass may be routed through clean tissue planes to circumvent difficult soft tissue coverage problems.

D. Venous Injuries

Venous injuries commonly accompany arterial injuries. In order of decreasing frequency, the most common extremity venous injuries are the superficial femoral vein, the popliteal vein, and the common femoral vein. The relative importance and timing of venous repair in an injured extremity is controversial. Advocates of routine venous repair contend that ligation is associated with significant postoperative morbidity, including more frequent failure of arterial repairs due to compromised outflow, venous insufficiency, compartment syndrome, and limb loss. Proponents of venous ligation argue that venous repairs are difficult (requiring interposition, compilation, and spiral grafting), time consuming (dangerous in the multiply-injured patient), and likely to cause occlusion (patency rates are only about 50%). The presence of postoperative edema after combined arterial and venous injuries is not reliably reduced by attempted venous repair. It seems reasonable to recommend repair of venous injuries when the repair is not too technically difficult (lateral venorrhaphy) and the patient is hemodynamically stable. Complex repair with autologous vein or ringed PTFE can yield good short-term patency in experienced hands (77% primary repair, 67% vein graft, 74% PTFE). Thus, the decision to repair the vein depends on the condition of the patient and the condition of the vein. When venous ligation is necessary, postoperative edema can be controlled by elevation of the extremity and use of compression stockings or wraps. In patients undergoing venous repair, patency should be monitored using duplex scanning. If thrombosis of the repair is detected and there are no contraindications, anticoagulation should be instituted and maintained for at least 3 months postoperatively.

E. Fasciotomy

Fasciotomy is an important adjunctive treatment in many cases of arterial trauma. Indications include the following: (1) combined arterial and venous injury, (2) massive soft tissue damage, (3) delay between injury and repair (4–6 hours), (4) prolonged hypotension, and (5) excessive swelling or high tissue pressure measured by one of several techniques. Whenever compartment pressures (measured with a needle and manometer) approach 25–30 mm Hg, fasciotomy should be considered. Fasciotomies must be performed through adequate skin incisions because when edema is massive, the skin envelope itself can compromise neurovascular function.

Fasciotomies are not benign procedures. They create large open wounds, and chronic venous insufficiency is a recognized late complication even in the absence of venous reflux or obstruction. The chronic swelling is thought to be related to loss of integrity of the ensheathing fascia of the calf muscles, reducing the efficiency of the calf muscle pump. Thus, some authorities recommend against routine use of fasciotomies at the initial operation. This approach is dependent on the ability to conduct frequent serial physical examinations and the ready availability of an operating room should problems arise. In the postoperative period, compartmental pressures can be measured using a handheld solid-state transducer as often as clinically indicated. Normal intracompartment pressure is less than 10 mm Hg. In general, a pressure of 25–30 mm Hg requires either fasciotomy or continuous monitoring. When the pressure exceeds 30 mm Hg, fasciotomy is mandatory. In patients who are obtunded or who cannot cooperate with serial physical examination, earlier fasciotomy should be considered.

F. Immediate Amputation

High-energy or crush injuries of the extremities are associated with high morbidity and a poor prognosis for useful limb function—there is a high late amputation rate despite initial limb salvage. Vascular injuries are now repaired with a high rate of success, but associated orthopedic, soft tissue, and nerve injuries are the critical factors that determine long-term function. A number of scoring systems or indices have been proposed to help determine when to amputate immediately and thus reduce the number of protracted reconstructive procedures that ultimately fail. Management of the mangled extremity is particularly difficult, and none of the scoring systems are universally accepted. Evaluation and management of these patients should be multidisciplinary, and the decision to amputate emergently should be made by two independent surgeons whenever possible.

Asensio JA et al: Visceral vascular injuries. Surg Clin North Am 2002;82:1.

Brandt MM, Kazanjian S, Wahl WL: The utility of endovascular stents in the treatment of blunt arterial injuries. J Trauma 2001; 51:901.

Brinker MR et al: Tibial shaft fractures with an associated infrapopliteal arterial injury: a survey of vascular surgeons opinions on the need for vascular repair. J Orthop Trauma 2000;14:194.

Brown KR et al: Determinants of functional disability after complex upper extremity trauma. Ann Vasc Surg 2001;15:43.

Buckman RF Jr, Miraliakbari R, Badellino MM: Juxtahepatic venous injuries: a critical review of reported management strategies. J Trauma 2000;48:978.

Cox CS Jr et al: Blunt versus penetrating subclavian artery injury: presentation, injury pattern, and outcome. J Trauma 1999;46:445.

Demetriades D et al: Penetrating injuries to the subclavian and axillary vessels. J Am Coll Surg 1999;188:290.

Demetriades D et al and the American Association for the Surgery of Trauma Thoracic Aortic Injury Study Group: Operative repair or endovascular stent graft in blunt traumatic thoracic aortic injuries: results of an American Association for the Surgery of Trauma Multicenter Study. J Trauma 2008;64:561.

Dennis JW et al: Validation of nonoperative management of occult vascular injuries and accuracy of physical examination alone in penetrating extremity trauma: 5- to 10-year follow-up. J trauma 1998;44:243.

Fox CJ et al: Contemporary management of wartime vascular trauma. J Vasc Surg 2005;41:638.

Fox CJ et al: Damage control resuscitation for vascular surgery in a combat support hospital. J Trauma 2008;65:1.

Fujikawa T et al: Endovascular stent grafting for the treatment of blunt thoracic aortic injury. j trauma 2001;50:223.

Gasparri MG et al: Physical examination plus chest radiography in penetrating periclavicular trauma: the appropriate trigger for angiography. J Trauma 2000;49:1029.

Gonzalez RP, Falimirski ME: The utility of physical examination in proximity penetrating extremity trauma. Am Surg 1999; 65:784.

Granchi T et al: Prolonged use of intraluminal arterial shunts without systemic anticoagulation. Am J Surg 2000;180:493.

Hafez HM, Woolgar J, Robbs JV: Lower extremity arterial injury: results of 550 cases and review of risk factors associated with limb loss. J Vasc Surg 2001;33:1212.

Hemmila MR et al: Delayed repair for blunt thoracic aortic injury: is it really equivalent to early repair? J Trauma 2004;56:13.

Kalakuntla V et al: Six-year experience with management of subclavian artery injuries. Am Surg 2000;66:927.

Kang SS et al: Percutaneous ultrasound guided thrombin injections: a new method for treating postcatheterization femoral pseudoaneurysms. J Vasc Surg 1998;27:1032.

Knudson MM et al: Outcome after major renovascular injuries: a Western Trauma Association multicenter report. J Trauma 2000; 49:1116.

Lyden SP et al: Common iliac artery dissection after blunt trauma: case report of endovascular repair and literature review. J Trauma 2001;50:339.

Martinez D et al: Popliteal artery injury associated with knee dislocations. Am Surg 2001;67:165.

McKinley AG, Carrim AT, Robbs JV: Management of proximal axillary and subclavian artery injuries. Br J Surg 2000;87:79.

McQueen MM et al: Acute compartment syndrome. Who is at risk? J Bone Joint Surg Br 2000;82:200.

Nagy K et al: Guidelines for the diagnosis and management of blunt aortic injury: and EAST practice management guidelines work group. J Trauma 2000;48:1128.

Naidoo NM et al: Angiographic embolisation in arterial trauma. Eur J Vasc Endovasc Surg 2000;19:77.

Nehler MR et al: Iatrogenic vascular injuries from percutaneous vascular suturing devices. J Vasc Surg 2001;33:943.

Nehler MR, Taylor LM, Porter JM: Iatrogenic vascular trauma. Semin Vasc Surg 1998;11:283.

Ofer A et al: CT angiography of the carotid arteries in trauma to the neck. Eur J Vasc Endovasc Surg 2001;21:401.

Parry NG et al: Management and short-term patency of lower extremity venous injuries with various repairs. Am J Surg 2003;186:631.

Rasmussen TE et al: The use of temporary vascular shunts in the management of wartime vascular injury. J Trauma 2006;61:8.

Rozycki GS et al: Blunt vascular trauma in the extremity: diagnosis, management, and outcome. J Trauma 2003;55:814.

Sohn VY et al: Demographics, treatment, and early outcomes in penetrating vascular combat trauma. Arch Surg 2008;143:783.

Sparks SR, DeLaRosa J, Bergan JJ: Arterial injury in uncomplicated upper extremity dislocations. Ann Vasc Surg 2000;14:110.

Subramanian A et al: A decade's experience with temporary intravascular shunts at a civilian level I trauma center. J Trauma 2008;65:316.

Velmahos GC, Toutouzas KG: Vascular trauma and compartment syndromes. Surg Clin North Am 2002;82:125.

Velmahos GC et al: Angiographic embolization for arrest of bleeding after penetrating trauma to the abdomen. Am J Surg 1999;178:367.

Wahl WL et al: Blunt thoracic aortic injury: delayed or early repair? J Trauma 1999;47:254.

Woodward EB et al: Penetrating femoropopliteal injury during modern warfare: experience of the Balad Vascular Registry. J Vasc Surg 2008;47:1259.

BLAST INJURY

Blast injuries in civilian populations occur as a result of fireworks, household explosions, or industrial accidents. Urban guerrilla warfare or terrorist tactics may take the form of letter bombs, suitcase bombs, vehicle bombs, and suicide bombers. Injuries occur from the effects of the blast itself, propelled foreign bodies, or, in large blasts, from falling objects. Military blast injuries may also involve personnel submerged in water. Water increases energy transmission and the possibility of injury to the viscera of the thorax or abdomen. The pathophysiology of blast injuries involves two mechanisms. Crush injury results from rapid displacement of the body wall and may result in laceration and contusion of underlying structures. Minor displacements may produce serious injury if the body wall velocity is high. In addition, the motion of the body wall generates waves that propagate within the body and transfer energy to internal sites.

▶ Clinical Findings

A. Symptoms and Signs

The injury is dependent upon proximity to the blast, space confinement, and detonation size. Large explosions cause multiple foreign body impregnations, bruises, abrasions, and lacerations. Gross soilage of wounds from clothing, flying debris, or explosive powder is usual. About 10% of all casualties have deep injuries to the chest or abdomen. Blast-induced circulatory shock may be caused by immediate myocardial depression without a compensatory vasoconstriction. Lung damage usually involves rupture of the alveolus with hemorrhage. Air embolism from bronchovenous fistula may cause sudden death. The mechanisms of lung injury are thought to be due to spalling effects (splintering

forces produced when a pressure wave hits a fluid-air interface), implosion effects, and pressure differentials. Hypoxia may result from a ventilation-perfusion mismatch caused by the pulmonary hemorrhage. Patients with pulmonary blast injury may die despite intensive respiratory support.

Blast injury causing pneumatic disruption of the esophagus or bowel has been reported. Tension pneumoperitoneum is a known although rare complication of barotrauma. Letter bombs cause predominantly hand, face, eye, and ear injuries. Energy transmission within the fluid media of the eye can cause globe rupture, dialysis of the iris, hyphema of the anterior chamber, lens capsule tears, retinal rupture, or macular pucker. Ear injuries may consist of drum rupture or cochlear damage. There may be nerve or conduction hearing deficit or deafness. Tinnitus, vertigo, and anosmia are also seen in letter bomb casualties.

B. Imaging Studies

Chest x-ray may initially be normal or may show pneumothorax, pneumomediastinum, or parenchymal infiltrates. In mass casualty situations it may be necessary to reserve the use of CT scans for those patients with acute changing neurologic exams during the immediate intake period. Patients with multiple penetrating injuries from shrapnel may benefit from full-body CT scanning following initial stabilization and evaluation. Correlation of radiologic imaging studies with clinical examination is useful in guiding which injuries may need operative intervention when the number of skin surface wounds is high and it is impractical to explore all of these wounds.

▶ Treatment

Severe injuries with shock from blood loss or hypoxia require resuscitative measures to restore perfusion and oxygenation. The usual criteria for exploring penetrating wounds of the thorax or abdomen are employed. Perforation of hollow organs should be suspected in patients with appropriate histories, particularly those who were submerged at the time of injury. Respiratory insufficiency may result from pulmonary injury or may be secondary to shock, fat embolism, or other causes. Tracheal intubation and prolonged respiratory care with mechanical ventilation may be necessary. In cases of tension pneumoperitoneum, surgical decompression may dramatically improve respiratory and hemodynamic functions. Surgical treatment of extremity injuries requires wide debridement of devitalized muscle, thorough cleansing of wounds, and removal of foreign materials. The possibility of gas gangrene in contaminated muscle injuries may warrant open treatment. Eye injuries may require immediate repair. Ear injuries are usually treated expectantly.

Cernak I et al: Blast injury from explosive munitions. J Trauma 1999;47:96.

Coupland RM, Meddings DR: Mortality associated with the use of weapons in armed conflicts, wartime atrocities, and civilian mass shootings: literature review. BMJ 1999;319:407.

Davis TP et al: Distribution and care of shipboard blast injuries (USS Cole DDG-67). J Trauma 2003;55:1022.

Frykberg ER: Medical management of disasters and mass casualties from terrorist bombings: how can we cope? J Trauma 202;53:201.

Guy RJ et al: Physiologic responses to primary blast. J Trauma 1998;45:983.

Irwin RJ et al: Shock after blast wave injury is caused by a vagally mediated reflex. J Trauma 1999;47:105.

Leibovici D, Gofit ON, Shapira SC: Eardrum perforation in explosion survivors: is it a marker of pulmonary blast injury? Ann Emerg Med 1999;34:168.

Mallonee S et al: Physical injuries and fatalities resulting from the Oklahoma City bombing. JAMA 1996;276:382.

Oppenheim A et al: Tension pneumoperitoneum after blast injury: dramatic improvement in ventilatory and hemodynamic parameters after surgical decompression. J Trauma 1998;44:915.

Shaham D, et al: The role of radiology in terror injuries. Isr Med Assoc J 2002;4:564.

Stein M, Hirshberg A: Medical consequences of terrorism. The conventional weapon threat. Surg Clin North Am 1999;79:1537.

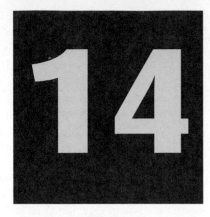

Burns & Other Thermal Injuries

Robert H. Demling, MD

BURNS

A severe thermal injury is one of the most devastating physical and psychological injuries a person can suffer. Over 2 million injuries due to burns require medical attention each year in the United States, with 14,000 deaths resulting. Fires in the home are responsible for only 5% of burn injuries but for 50% of burn deaths—most due to smoke inhalation. About 75,000 patients require hospitalization every year, and 25,000 of those remain hospitalized for over 2 months—evidence of the severity of illness associated with this injury.

ANATOMY & PHYSIOLOGY OF THE SKIN

The skin is the largest organ of the body, ranging in area from 0.25 m² in the newborn to 1.8 m² in the adult. It consists of two layers: the epidermis and the dermis (corium). The outermost cells of the epidermis are dead cornified cells that act as a tough protective barrier against the environment, including bacterial invasion and chemical exposure. The inner cells of the epidermis are metabolically active, producing compounds like growth factor, which help the ongoing replication process every 2 weeks. The second, thicker layer, the dermis (0.06–0.12 mm), is composed chiefly of fibrous connective tissue. The dermis contains the blood vessels and nerves to the skin and the epithelial appendages of specialized function like sweat glands. The nerve endings that mediate pain are found in the dermis.

The dermis is a barrier that prevents loss of body fluids by evaporation and loss of excess body heat. Sweat glands help maintain body temperature by controlling the amount of water that evaporates. The dermis is also interlaced with sensory nerve endings that mediate the sensations of touch, pressure, pain, heat, and cold. This is a protective mechanism that allows an individual to adapt to changes in the physical environment.

The skin produces vitamin D, which is synthesized by the action of sunlight on certain intradermal cholesterol compounds.

DEPTH OF BURNS

The depth of the burn (Figure 14–1) significantly affects all subsequent clinical events. The depth may be difficult to determine and in some cases is not known until after spontaneous healing has occurred or when the eschar is surgically removed or separates, exposing the wound bed.

Traditionally, burns have been classified as first-, second-, and third-degree, but the current emphasis on burn healing has led to classification as partial-thickness burns, which can heal spontaneously, and full-thickness burns, which require skin grafting, although deep partial-thickness burns are usually excised and grafted as well.

A **first-degree burn** involves only the epidermis and is characterized by erythema and minor microscopic changes; tissue damage is minimal, protective functions of the skin are intact, skin edema is minimal, and systemic effects are rare. Pain, the chief symptom, usually resolves in 48–72 hours, and healing takes place uneventfully. In 5–10 days, the damaged epithelium peels off in small scales, leaving no residual scarring. The most common causes of first-degree burns are overexposure to sunlight and brief scalding.

Second-degree or partial-thickness burns are deeper, involving all of the epidermis and some of the corium or dermis. The systemic severity of the burn and the quality of subsequent healing are directly related to the amount of undamaged dermis. Superficial burns are often characterized by blister formation, while deeper partial-thickness burns have a reddish appearance or a layer of whitish, nonviable dermis firmly adherent to the remaining viable tissue. Blisters, when present, continue to increase in size in the postburn period as the osmotically active particles in the blister fluid attract water. Complications from superficial second-degree burns are mainly severe pain related. These burns usually heal with minimal scarring in 10–14 days unless they become infected.

Deep dermal burns heal over a period of 4–8 weeks with only a fragile epithelial covering developing that arises from

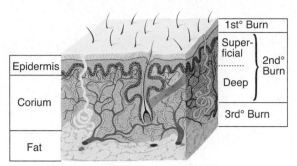

▲ Figure 14–1. Layers of the skin showing depth of first-degree, second-degree, and third-degree burns.

the residual uninjured epithelium of the deep dermal sweat glands and hair follicles. Severe hypertrophic scarring occurs when such an injury heals; the resulting epithelial covering is prone to blistering and breakdown. Evaporative losses after healing remain high compared with losses in normal skin. Conversion to a full-thickness burn by bacteria is common. Skin grafting of deep dermal burns, when feasible, improves the biologic quality and appearance of the skin cover.

Full-thickness (third-degree) burns have a characteristic white, dry, waxy appearance and may appear to the untrained eye as unburned skin. Burns caused by prolonged exposure to heat, with involvement of fat and underlying tissue, may be brown, dark red, or black. The diagnostic findings of full-thickness burns are lack of sensation in the burned skin, lack of capillary refill, and a leathery texture that is unlike normal skin. All dermal epithelial elements are destroyed, leaving no potential for reepithelialization.

DETERMINATION OF SEVERITY OF INJURY

Illness and death are related to the size (surface area) and depth of the burn, the age and prior state of health of the victim, the location of the burn wound, and the severity of associated injuries, particularly lung injuries caused by smoke inhalation.

The total body surface area involved in the burn is most accurately determined by using the age-related charts designed by Lund and Browder (Figure 14–2). A set of these charts should be filled out for every burn patient on admission and when resuscitation is begun.

A careful calculation of the percentage of total body burn is useful for several reasons. First, there is a general clinical tendency to both underestimate and overestimate the size of the burn and thus its severity. The American Burn Association has adopted a severity index for burn injury (Table 14–1). Second, prognosis is directly related to the extent of injury both size and depth. Third, the decision about who should be treated in a specialized burn facility or managed as an outpatient is based on the estimate of burn size and depth.

Patients under age 2 years and over age 60 years have a significantly higher death rate for any given extent of burn. The higher death rate in infants results from a number of factors. First, the body surface area in children relative to body weight is much greater than in adults. Therefore, a burn of comparable surface area has a greater physiologic impact on a child. Second, immature kidneys and liver do not allow for removal of a high solute load from injured tissue or the rapid restoration of adequate nutritional support. Third, the incompletely developed immune system increases susceptibility to infection. Associated conditions such as cardiac disease, diabetes, or chronic obstructive pulmonary disease significantly worsen the prognosis in elderly patients.

Burns involving the hands, face, feet, or perineum are at risk for severe complications if not properly treated. Patients with such burns should always be admitted to the hospital, preferably to a burn center. Chemical and electrical burns or those involving the respiratory tract are invariably far more extensive than is evident on initial inspection. Therefore, hospital admission is also necessary in these cases.

PATHOLOGY & PATHOPHYSIOLOGY OF THERMAL INJURIES

The microscopic pathologic feature of the burn wound is principally surface coagulation necrosis. Burned tissue has three distinct zones. The first is the zone of "coagulation," or necrosis with irreversible cell death and no capillary blood flow. Surrounding this is a zone of injury or stasis, characterized by sluggish capillary blood flow and injured cells. Although damaged, the tissue is still viable. Further tissue injury can be caused by products of inflammation such as oxidants and vasoconstrictor mediators. Environmental insults such as hypoperfusion, desiccation, or infection can also cause the injured tissue to become necrotic. This process is called **wound conversion**. The third zone is that of "hyperemia," which is the usual inflammatory response of healthy tissue to nonlethal injury. Vasodilatation and increased capillary permeability is typically present.

A rapid loss of intravascular fluid and protein occurs through the heat-injured capillaries. The volume loss is greatest in the first 6–8 hours, with capillary integrity returning toward normal by 36–48 hours. A transient increase in vascular permeability also occurs in nonburned tissues, probably as a result of the initial release of vasoactive mediators. However, the edema that develops in nonburned tissues during resuscitation appears to be due in large part to the marked hypoproteinemia caused by protein loss into the burn itself. A systemic inflammatory response occurs in response to a large body burn, resulting in the release of oxidants and other inflammatory mediators into unburned tissues. A generalized decrease in cell energy and membrane potential occurs as a result. This leads to a shift of extracellular sodium and water into the intracellular space. This process

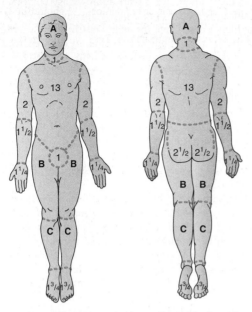

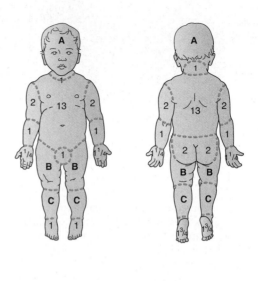

Relative percentages of areas affected by growth

Area	Age		
	10	15	Adult
A = half of head	5 1/2	4 1/2	3 1/2
B = half of one thigh	4 1/4	4 1/2	4 3/4
C = half of one leg	3	3 1/4	3 1/2

Relative percentages of areas affected by growth

Area	Age		
	0	1	5
A = half of head	9 1/2	8 1/2	6 1/2
B = half of one thigh	2 3/4	3 1/4	4
C = half of one leg	2 1/2	2 1/2	2 3/4

▲ **Figure 14-2.** Table for estimating extent of burns. In adults, a reasonable system for calculating the percentage of body surface burned is the "rule of nines": Each arm equals 9%, the head equals 9%, the anterior and posterior trunk each equal 18%, and each leg equals 18%; the sum of these percentages is 99%.

Table 14-1. Summary of American Burn Association Burn Severity Categorization.

Major burn injury
Second-degree burn of > 25% body surface area in adults
Second-degree burn of > 20% body surface area in children
Third-degree burn of > 10% body surface area
Most burns involving hands, face, eyes, ears, feet, or perineum
Most patients with the following:
    Inhalation injury
    Electrical injury
    Burn injury complicated by other major trauma
    Poor-risk patients with burns
Moderate uncomplicated burn injury
Second-degree burn of 15-25% body surface area in adults
Second-degree burn of 10-20% body surface area in children
Third-degree burn of < 10% body surface area
Minor burn injury
Second-degree burn of < 15% body surface area in adults
Second-degree burn of < 10% body surface area in children
Third-degree burn of < 2% body surface area

is also corrected as hemodynamic stability is restored but will return if the systemic inflammation is amplified. Smoke inhalation markedly increases the hemodynamic instability, fluid requirements, and mortality rates by adding another source of intense inflammation leading to local lung and systemic tissue damage.

METABOLIC RESPONSE TO BURNS & METABOLIC SUPPORT

The initial metabolic response appears to be activated by proinflammatory cytokines and in turn oxidants. The secretion of catecholamines, cortisol, glucagon, renin-angiotensin, antidiuretic hormone, and aldosterone is also increased. Early in the response, energy is supplied by the breakdown of stored glycogen and by the process of anaerobic glycolysis.

Profound hypermetabolism and catabolism occur in the postburn period, characterized by an increase in metabolic rate that approaches doubling of the basal rate in severe burns and a rapid loss of the components of lean body mass with muscle loss exceeding a pound a day. The degree of response is proportionate to the degree of injury, with a plateau occurring when the burn involves about 70% of total body surface. The initiating and perpetuating factors are the mediators of inflammation, especially the cytokines and endotoxin. Added environmental stresses such as pain, cooling, and sepsis syndrome increase the obligatory hypermetabolism and catabolism.

During the first postburn week, the metabolic rate (or heat production) and oxygen consumption rise progressively from the normal level present during resuscitation and remain elevated until the wound is covered and no other sources of inflammation remain. The specific pathophysiologic mechanism remains undefined, but increased and persistent catecholamine and cortisol secretion are major factors, as is increased circulating endotoxin absorbed from wound or gut and proinflammatory cytokines.

The evaporative water loss from the wound may reach 300 mL/m^2/h (normal is about 15 mL/m^2/h). This produces a heat loss of about 580 kcal/L of water evaporated. Covering the burn with an impermeable membrane, such as skin substitute, reduces the heat loss. Similarly, placing the burn patient in a warm environment, where convection and radiant loss of heat are minimized, also modestly reduces the heat loss and the metabolic rate. The persistently elevated circulating levels of catecholamines and cortisol stimulate an exaggerated degree of gluconeogenesis and protein breakdown. Protein catabolism, glucose intolerance, and marked total body weight loss result.

Aggressive nutritional support along with rapid wound closure and control of pain, stress, and sepsis will help control the hypermetabolic catabolic state. Controlled use of a beta-blocker has been shown to decrease catabolism. In addition, insulin, growth hormones, and testosterone analogues have been shown to both decrease catabolism and increase anabolism.

IMMUNOLOGIC FACTORS IN BURNS

A number of immunologic abnormalities in burn patients predispose to infection. Serum IgA, IgM, and IgG are frequently depressed, reflecting depressed B cell function. Cell-mediated immunity or T cell function is also impaired, as demonstrated by prolonged survival of homografts and xenografts.

Polymorphonuclear (PMN) chemotactic activity is suppressed. A decrease in chemotaxis predates evidence of clinical sepsis by several days. Decreased oxygen consumption and impaired bacterial killing have also been demonstrated in PMNs. Depressed killing is probably due to decreased production of hydrogen peroxide and superoxide; this has been demonstrated by decreased PMN chemiluminescent activity in burn patients.

ACUTE RESUSCITATION

The burn patient should be assessed and treated like any patient with major trauma. The first priority is to ensure an adequate airway. If there is a possibility that smoke inhalation has occurred—as suggested by exposure to a fire in an enclosed space or burns of the face, nares, or upper torso—arterial blood gases and arterial oxygen saturation of hemoglobin and carboxyhemoglobin CoHgb levels should be measured, and 100% oxygen should be administered. If CoHgb is elevated, 100% oxygen should be administered until levels return to normal.

Endotracheal intubation is indicated if the patient is semicomatose, has deep burns to the face and neck, or is otherwise critically injured. Intubation should be done early in all doubtful cases, because delayed intubation will be difficult to achieve in cases associated with facial and pharyngeal edema or upper airway injury, and an emergency tracheostomy may become necessary later under difficult circumstances. Respiratory support is necessary for severe smoke damage to the lower airways. If the burn exceeds 20% of body surface area, a urinary catheter should be inserted to monitor urine output. A large-bore intravenous catheter should be inserted, preferably into a large peripheral vein. There is a significant complication rate with the use of central lines in burn patients owing to the increased risk of infection.

Severe burns are characterized by large losses of intravascular fluid, which are greatest during the first 8–12 hours. Fluid loss occurs as a result of the altered capillary permeability, severe hypoproteinemia, and the shift of sodium into the cells. Both fluid shifts diminish significantly by 24 hours postburn. The lung appears to be reasonably well protected from the early edema process, and pulmonary edema is uncommon during the resuscitation period unless there is a superimposed inhalation injury. Increasing perfusion rather than infusion of bicarbonates is the appropriate approach.

Initially, an isotonic crystalloid salt solution is infused to counterbalance the loss of plasma volume into the extravascular space and the further loss of extracellular fluid into the intracellular space. Lactated Ringer solution is commonly used, the rate being dictated by urine output, pulse (character and rate), state of consciousness, and, to a lesser extent, blood pressure. Urine output should be maintained at 0.5 mL/kg/h and the pulse at 120 beats/min or slower. Base deficit has been shown to be an excellent marker, with an increasing deficit indicating inadequate perfusion.

Swan-Ganz catheters and central venous pressure lines are seldom needed except in the case of severe smoke inhalation injury or unless the patient has sufficient cardiopulmonary disease that accurate monitoring of volume status would be difficult without measurement of filling pressures or unless a persistent base deficit is present, indicating continued impaired perfusion. The amount of lactated

Ringer necessary in the first 24 hours for adequate resuscitation is approximately 3–4 mL/kg of body weight per percent of body burn, which is the amount of fluid needed to restore the estimated sodium deficit. At least half of the fluid is given in the first 8 hours because of the greater initial volume loss. Dextrose-containing solutions are not used initially because of early stress-induced glucose intolerance.

Although the importance of restoring colloid osmotic pressure and plasma proteins is well recognized, the timing of colloid infusion remains somewhat varied. Plasma proteins are ordinarily not infused until after the initial plasma leak begins to decrease. This usually occurs about 4–8 hours postburn. The addition of a protein infusion to the treatment regimen after this period will decrease the fluid requirements and—in very young or elderly patients and in patients with massive burns (in excess of 50% of body surface)—will improve hemodynamic stability.

After intravenous fluids are started and vital signs stabilized, the wound should be debrided of all loose skin and dirt. To avoid severe hypothermia, debridement is best done by completing one body area before exposing a second. An alternative is to use an overhead radiant heater, which will decrease net heat loss. Cool water is a very good analgesic on a small superficial burn; however, it should not be used for larger burns because of the risk of hypothermia. Pain is best controlled with the use of intravenous rather than intramuscular narcotics. Tetanus toxoid, 0.5 mL, should be administered to patients with any significant burn injury.

POSTRESUSCITATION PERIOD

Treatment should aim to decrease excessive catecholamine stimulation and provide enough calories to offset the effects of the hypermetabolism. Hypothermia, pain, and anxiety all need to be aggressively controlled. Hypovolemia should be prevented by giving enough fluid to make up for the body losses.

Ongoing management of any smoke inhalation injury will be necessary using vigorous pulmonary toilet to avoid airway plugging and hypoxia. Nutritional support should begin as early as possible in the postburn period to maximize wound healing and minimize immune deficiency. Patients with moderate body burns may be able to meet nutritional needs by voluntary oral intake. Patients with large burns invariably require calorie and protein supplementation to reach a goal of 30 cal/Kg body weight for calories and 1.5 g/kg body weight for protein. This can usually be accomplished by administering a formula diet through a small feeding tube. Parenteral nutrition is also occasionally required, but the intestinal route is preferred if needs can be met this way. Early restoration of gut function will also decrease gut bacterial translocation and endotoxin leak.

Vitamins A, E, and C and zinc should be given until the burn wound is closed. Low-dose heparin therapy may be beneficial, as with other immobilized patients with soft tissue injury.

CARE OF THE BURN WOUND

In the management of superficial partial or second-degree burns, one must provide as aseptic an environment as possible to prevent infection. However, superficial burns generally do not require the use of topical antibiotics. Occlusive dressings are used to minimize exposure to air, increase the rate of reepithelialization, and decrease pain. The exception is the face, which can be treated open with an antibacterial ointment. If there is no infection, burns will heal spontaneously.

The goals in managing deep partial-thickness or full-thickness (third-degree) burns are to prevent invasive infection (ie, burn wound sepsis), to remove dead tissue, and to cover the wound with skin or skin substitutes as soon as possible.

All topical antibiotics retard wound healing to some degree and therefore should be used only on deep second- or third-degree burns or wounds, which have a high risk of infection.

▶ Topical Antibacterial Agents

Topical agents have definitely advanced the care of burn patients. Although burn wound sepsis is still a major problem, the incidence is lower and the death rate has been markedly reduced, particularly in burns of less than 50% of body surface area. A silver-containing product is the treatment of choice because silver has superior antimicrobial properties. Silver sulfadiazine is the most widely used preparation. Mafenide, silver nitrate, povidone-iodine, and gentamicin ointments are also used. Silver release dressings are now very popular. A secondary dressing is placed over the top to retain heat and optimize the wound environment.

Silver sulfadiazine, a cream that is effective against a wide spectrum of gram-positive and gram-negative organisms, is only moderately effective in penetrating the burn eschar. A transient leukopenia secondary to bone marrow suppression often occurs with use of silver sulfadiazine in large burns, but the process is usually self-limiting, and the agent does not have to be discontinued.

Silver release dressings are available in a slow-release form that release silver ions for several days, decreasing dressing changes and improving patient comfort.

▶ Exposure versus Closed Management

There are two methods of management of the burn wound with topical agents. In **exposure therapy,** no dressings are applied over the wound after application of the agent to the wound twice or three times daily. This approach is typically used on the face and head. Disadvantages are increased pain and heat loss as a result of the exposed wound and an increased risk of cross-contamination.

In the **closed method,** an occlusive dressing is applied over the agent and is usually changed twice daily. The disadvantage of this method is the potential increase in bacterial growth if the dressing is not changed twice daily, particularly when thick eschar is present. The advantages are less pain, less heat loss, and less cross-contamination. The closed method is generally preferred.

Temporary Skin Substitutes

Skin substitutes are another alternative to topical agents for the partial-thickness burn or the clean excised wound. A number of synthetic and biologically active temporary skin substitutes are in use. Reepithelialization is accelerated. Also, pain is better controlled. **Homografts (human skin)** work better for this purpose on large excised wounds but are difficult to obtain. Other alternatives include a number of tissue engineered skin substitutes, which contain bioactive matrix components.

Hydrotherapy

The use of immersion hydrotherapy for wound management has substantially decreased. A number of studies have shown that the infection rate is actually increased when patients are immersed in a tub because of the generalized inoculation of burn wounds with bacteria from what was previously a localized infection. Hydrotherapy, on a slant board, is a very useful approach once the wounds are in the process of being debrided and closed. Showering is also effective for wound cleansing in the more stable patient.

Debridement & Grafting

Burn wound inflammation, even in the absence of infection, can result in multiple organ dysfunction and perpetuation of the hypermetabolic catabolic state. Early wound closure would be expected to control this process more effectively. Surgical management of burn wounds has now become much more aggressive, with operative debridement beginning within the first several days postburn rather than after eschar has sloughed. More rapid closure of burn wounds clearly decreases the rate of sepsis and significantly decreases the death rate. The approach to operative debridement varies from an extensive burn excision and grafting within several days of injury to a more moderate approach of limiting debridements to less than 15% of the burned area. Excision can be carried down to fascia or to viable remaining dermis or fat. Excision to fascia is more commonly used when the burn extends well into the fat. A meshed skin graft can be covered with a biologic dressing to avoid desiccation of the uncovered wound. Excision to viable tissue, referred to as tangential excision, is advantageous because it provides a vascular base for grafting while preserving remaining viable tissue, especially dermis. Tourniquets can be used to decrease blood loss. Blood loss is substantial in view of the vascularity of the dermis.

A number of **permanent skin substitutes** could further facilitate wound closure, particularly in large burns with insufficient donor sites. Autologous cultures of epithelium

have been applied with some success. Permanent skin substitutes composed of both dermis and epidermis have been designed to maintain coverage and improve skin function.

Maintenance of Function

The maintenance of functional motion during evolution of the burn wound is necessary to avoid loss of motion at joints. Wound contraction, a normal event during healing, may result in extremity contracture. Immobilization will produce joint stiffness. Contracture of the scar, muscles, and tendons across a joint causes loss of motion, which can be diminished by traction and early motion.

The scar is a metabolically active tissue, continually undergoing reorganization. The extensive scarring that frequently occurs after burns can lead to disfiguring and disabling contractures, but it may be avoided by the use of splints and elevation to maintain a functional position. Following application of the skin graft, maintenance of proper positioning with splints is indicated along with active motion exercises.

If reinjury does not occur, the amount of collagen in the scar tends to decrease with time (usually over a year). Stiff collagen becomes softer, and on flat surfaces of the body, where reinjury and inflammation are prevented, remodeling may totally eliminate contracture. However, around joints or the neck, contractures can persist, and surgical reconstruction is necessary. The sooner the burn wound can be covered with skin grafts, the less likely is contracture formation.

MANAGEMENT OF COMPLICATIONS

Infection remains a critical problem in burns, though the incidence has been reduced by modern therapy with the combination of early excision and grafting along with topical antibacterial agents. An infection is present when a quantitative culture of the burn indicates a concentration of 10^5 organisms; a semiquantitative swab culture is used more commonly. The cultures also show the sensitivity of the bacteria, and when the bacterial concentration passes 10^5 organisms per gram, systemic administration of specific antibiotics should be instituted (Tables 14–2 and 14–3).

Sepsis syndrome occurs in all major burns. Fever, hypermetabolism, catabolism, and often leukocytosis are typical characteristics, the result of local burn and total body inflammation. Infection is often not present as this process can be attributed to an autodestructive response to inflammation. This intense inflammatory response can lead to death from multisystem organ failure and hemodynamic parameters comparable to sepsis shock.

Any significant infection can further perpetuate this response. Continued deterioration of a wound is likely due to invasive infection. A more common cause of infection today is a pulmonary complication: either a chemical or bacterial insult leading to pneumonia. Catheter sepsis is the third most common cause of infection. If infection is found,

Table 14–2. Diagnosis of Burn Wound Infection.

Systemic Changes	Colonized or Clean	Wound Infection
Body temperature	Increased	Variable
White blood cell count	Increased Mild left shift	High or low Severe left shift
Wound appearance	Variable—may appear purulent or benign	Purulence may be present, or wound surface may appear dry and pale
Bacterial content		
Surface	Scant to large amount	Variable
Quantitative	Usually $< 10^5/g$	Usually $> 10^5/g$
Biopsy	No invasion of normal tissue	Invasion of normal tissue by organisms

an aggressive antibiotics regime is indicated. Early excision and wound closure is the best way to avoid later development of burn wound sepsis.

Circumferential burns of an extremity or of the trunk pose special problems. Swelling beneath the unyielding eschar may act as a tourniquet to blood and lymph flow, and the distal extremity may become swollen and tense. More extensive swelling may compromise the arterial supply. Escharotomy, or excision of the eschar, may be required. To avoid permanent damage, escharotomy must be performed before arterial ischemia develops. Constriction involving the chest or abdomen may severely restrict ventilation and may require longitudinal escharotomies. Anesthetics are rarely required, and the procedure can usually be performed in the patient's room.

Acute gastroduodenal (Curling) ulcers were at one time a frequent complication of severe burns, but the incidence is now extremely low, largely as a result of the early and routine institution of antacid and nutritional therapy and the decrease in the rate of sepsis.

A complication unique to children is seizures, which may result from electrolyte imbalance, hypoxemia, infection, or drugs; in one-third of cases, the cause is unknown. Hyponatremia is the most frequent cause. Systemic hypertension occurs in about 10% of cases in the postresuscitation period.

RESPIRATORY INJURY IN BURNS

Today the major cause of death after burns is respiratory failure or complications in the respiratory tract. The problems include inhalation injury, aspiration in unconscious patients, bacterial pneumonia, pulmonary edema, and posttraumatic pulmonary insufficiency. Smoke inhalation markedly increases mortality from burn injury.

Smoke inhalation injuries, caused by incomplete products of combustion and which predispose to other complications, are divided into three categories: carbon monoxide poisoning (Table 14–4), upper airways injury, and inhalation of noxious compounds in the lower airways (Table 14–5).

Carbon monoxide poisoning must be considered in every patient suspected of having inhalation injury on the basis of having been burned in a closed space and physical evidence of inhalation. Arterial blood gases and carboxyhemoglobin levels must be determined. Levels of carboxyhemoglobin above 5% in nonsmokers and above 10% in smokers indicate carbon monoxide poisoning. Carbon monoxide has an affinity for hemoglobin 200 times that of oxygen, displaces oxygen, and produces a leftward shift in the oxyhemoglobin dissociation curve (P_{50}, the oxygen tension at which half the hemoglobin is saturated with oxygen, is lowered). Calculations of oxyhemoglobin saturation may be misleading because the hemoglobin combined with carbon monoxide is not detected and the percentage saturation of oxyhemoglobin may appear normal.

Mild carbon monoxide poisoning (< 20% carboxyhemoglobin) is manifested by headache, slight dyspnea, mild confusion, and diminished visual acuity. Moderate poisoning (20–40% carboxyhemoglobin) leads to irritability, impairment of judgment, dim vision, nausea, and fatigability. Severe poisoning (40–60% carboxyhemoglobin) produces hallucinations, confusion, ataxia, collapse, and coma. Levels in excess of 60% carboxyhemoglobin are usually fatal.

Table 14–3. Most Common Pathogens in Burn Infections.

	S aureus	*P aeruginosa*	*C albicans*
Wound appearance	Loss of wound granulation	Surface necrosis; patchy, black	Minimal exudate
Course	Slow onset over 2–5 days	Rapid onset over 12–36 hours	Slow (days)
CNS signs	Disorientation	Modest changes	Often no change
Temperature	Marked increase	High or low	Modest changes
White blood count	Marked increase	High or low	Modest changes
Hypotension	Modest	Often severe	Minimal change
Mortality rate	5%	20–30%	30–50%

Table 14–4. Carbon Monoxide Poisoning.

Carboxyhemoglobin Level	Severity	Symptoms
< 20%	Mild	Headache, mild dyspnea, visual changes, confusion
20–40%	Moderate	Irritability, diminished judgment, dim vision, nausea, easy fatigability
40–60%	Severe	Hallucinations, confusion, ataxia, collapse, coma
> 60%	Fatal	

Various **toxic chemicals** in inspired smoke produce tracheo bronchial respiratory injuries. Inhalation of kerosene smoke, for example, is relatively innocuous. Smoke from a wood fire is extremely irritating because it contains aldehyde gases, particularly acrolein. Direct inhalation of acrolein, even in low concentrations, irritates mucous membranes and causes severe airway damage. Smoke from some plastic compounds, such as polyurethane, is the most serious kind of toxic irritant, and some plastics give off poisonous gases such as chlorine, sulfuric acid, and cyanides. Cyanide absorption can be lethal. Oxidants are released after all smoke exposures, causing mucosal and alveolar injury.

Inhalation injury causes severe mucosal edema followed soon by sloughing of the mucosa. The destroyed mucosa in the larger airways is replaced by a mucopurulent membrane. The edema fluid enters the airway and, when mixed with the pus in the lumen, may form casts and plugs in the smaller bronchioles. Terminal bronchioles and alveoli contain carbonaceous material. Acute bronchiolitis and bronchopneumonia commonly develop within a few days. Sputum smears should be examined daily to detect early bacterial tracheobronchial infection.

When inhalation injury is suspected, early endoscopic examination of the airway with fiberoptic bronchoscopy is helpful in determining the area of injury (ie, the extent of upper and lower airway involvement). Unfortunately, the severity of the injury cannot be accurately quantified by bronchoscopy—it can only be shown that an injury is present. Direct laryngoscopy probably gives as much information.

After several days, small bronchi become obstructed by inflammation and mucin plugs, leading to severe atelectasis and resulting hypoxia. This process is typically confined to the airways; in severe cases, alveolar edema will be present.

The most common cause of respiratory failure is a chemical tracheobronchitis due to the inhalation injury. Airway clearance is impeded due to ciliary damage and denuded airways. Alteration of oropharyngeal normal flora with colonization by pathogens then leads to bronchopneumonia.

Pulmonary insufficiency is associated with systemic sepsis. Differentiating acute respiratory distress syndrome (ARDS) from bacterial pneumonia may be difficult in severe cases of inhalation of sepsis. There is damage to the pulmonary capillaries and leakage of fluid and protein into the interstitial spaces of the lung, resulting in loss of compliance and difficulty in oxygenation of the blood. Modern methods of ventilatory support and vigorous pulmonary toilet have significantly reduced the death rate from pulmonary insufficiency.

▶ Treatment

Management of a burn patient should include frequent evaluation of the lungs throughout the hospital course. All patients who initially have evidence of smoke inhalation should receive humidified oxygen in high concentrations. If carbon monoxide poisoning has occurred, 100% oxygen should be given until the carboxyhemoglobin content returns to normal levels and symptoms of carbon monoxide toxicity resolve. With severe exposures, carbon monoxide may still be bound to the cytochrome enzymes, leading to cell hypoxia even after carboxyhemoglobin levels have returned to near normal. Continued oxygen administration will also reverse this process. Hyperbaric oxygen is often used in these cases.

The use of corticosteroids for inhalation injuries is no longer controversial and is clearly contraindicated with the exception of chronic bronchiolitis obliterans. The exception is the patient with a relative steroid insufficiency.

Bronchodilators by aerosol or aminophylline given intravenously may help if wheezing is due to the reflex bronchospasm typically present. Chest physical therapy is also required.

When endotracheal intubation is used without mechanical ventilation (eg, for upper airway obstruction), mist and continuous positive pressure ventilatory assistance should be included. The humidity will help loosen the secretions and prevent drying of the airway; the continuous positive pressure will help prevent atelectasis and closure of lung units distal to the swollen airways. Tracheostomy is indicated in the first several days for patients who are expected to require ventilatory support for a few weeks or more. If the neck is burned, excision and grafting followed by tracheostomy is indicated in order to improve pulmonary toilet.

Table 14–5. Sources of Toxic Chemicals in Smoke.

Wood, cotton	Aldehydes (acrolein), nitrogen dioxide, CO
Polyvinylchloride	Hydrochloric acid, phosgene, CO
Rubber	Sulfur dioxide, hydrogen sulfide, CO
Polystyrene	Copious black smoke and soot—CO_2, H_2O, and some CO
Acrylonitrile, polyurethane, nitrogenous compounds	Hydrogen cyanide
Fire retardants may produce toxic fumes	Halogens (F_2, Cl_2, Br_2), ammonia, hydrogen cyanide, CO

Mechanical ventilation should be instituted early if a significant pulmonary injury is anticipated. A large body burn with chest wall involvement will result in decreased chest wall compliance, increased work of breathing, and subsequent atelectasis. Tracheobronchial injury from inhaled chemicals is accentuated by the presence of a body burn, with a resultant increase in the potential for atelectasis and infection. Controlled ventilation along with sedation will diminish the degree of injury and also conserve energy expenditure. Early excision of the deep chest wall burn will help remove the constricting component. Wound closure in turn will decrease the excessive CO_2 production caused by the hypermetabolic state.

REHABILITATION OF THE BURNED PATIENT

Plastic surgical revisions of scars are often necessary after the initial grafting, particularly to release contractures over joints and for cosmetic reasons. The physician must be realistic in defining an acceptable result, and the patient should be told that it may take years to achieve. Burn scars are often unsightly, and—although hope should be extended that improvement can be made—total resolution is not possible in many cases.

Skin expansion techniques utilizing a subdermal Silastic bag that is gradually expanded have greatly improved scar revision management. The ability to enlarge the available skin to be used for replacement of scar improves both cosmetic appearance and function. Advances in microvascular flap surgery have also resulted in substantial improvements in outcome.

The patient must take special care of the skin of the burn scar. Prolonged exposure to sunlight should be avoided, and when the wound involves areas such as the face and hands, which are frequently exposed to the sun, ultraviolet screening agents should be used. Hypertrophic scars and keloids are particularly bothersome and can be diminished with the use of pressure garments, which must be worn until the scar matures—approximately 12 months. Since the skin appendages are often destroyed by full-thickness burns, creams and lotions are required to prevent drying and cracking and to reduce itching. Substances such as lanolin, vitamin A and D ointment, and Eucerin cream are all effective.

Fraburg C: Effects of differences in percent total surface burn surface area estimation on fluid resuscitation of transferred burn patients. J Burn Care Res 2007;28:42.

Garrel D et al: Decreased mortality and infectious morbidity in adult burn patients given enteral glutamine supplements: A prospective, controlled, randomized clinical trial. Crit Care Med 2003;31:2444.

Hagstrom M et al: The review of emergency department fluid resuscitation of burn patients transferred to a regional verified burn center. Ann Plast Surg 2003;51:173.

Hall JJ: Use of high frequency percussive ventilation in inhalation injury. J Burn Care Res 2007;3:396.

Ipaktchi K: Attenuating burn wound inflammation improves pulmonary function and survival in a burn pneumonia model. Crit Care Med 2007;35:2139.

Jeschke M: Effect of insulin on the inflammatory and acute phase response after burn injury. Crit Care Med 2007;9:519.

Palmieri T: Inhalation injury research progress and needs. J Burn Care 2007;4:594.

Pereira C: Post burn muscle wasting and the effects of treatment. Int Biochem Cell Biol 2005;37:1948.

Rubino C: Total upper and low eyelid replacement following thermal injury using an ALT flap. J Plast Reconstruct Aesthet Surg 2007;20:215.

Tenenhaus M: Burn surgery. Clin Plast Surg 2007;34:697.

Wascak J: Early versus later internal nutritional support in adults with burn injury: a systemic review. J Hum Nutr Diet 2007;20:25.

ELECTRICAL INJURY

There are three kinds of electrical injuries: electrical current injury, electrothermal burns from arcing current, and flame burns caused by ignition of clothing. Occasionally, all three are present in the same victim.

Electrical current injury, or "hidden injury," results from the passage of electrical current through the body. Flash or arc burns are thermal injuries to the skin caused by a high-tension electrical current creating local heat and damaging skin. The thermal injury to the skin is intense and deep, because the electrical arc has a temperature of about 2500 °C (high enough to melt bone). Flame burns from ignited clothing are often the most serious part of the injury. Treatment is the same as for any thermal injury.

Once current enters the body, its pathway depends on the resistances it encounters in the various organs. The following are listed in descending order of resistance: bone, fat, tendon, skin, muscle, blood, and nerve. The pathway of the current determines immediate survival; for example, if the current passes through the heart or the brain stem, death may be immediate from ventricular fibrillation or apnea. Current passing through muscles may cause spasms severe enough to produce long-bone fractures or dislocations.

The type of current is also related to the severity of injury with low-voltage (150 v) current. The usual 60-cycle alternating current that causes most injuries in the home is particularly severe. Alternating current causes tetanic contractions, and the victim may become "locked" to the contact. Cardiac arrest is common from contact with low-voltage house current.

High-voltage electrical current injuries are more than just burns. Focal deep burns occur at the points of entrance and exit through the skin. These burns often extend through local muscle, resulting in fourth-degree burn. Once inside the body, the current travels through muscles, causing an injury more like a crush than a thermal burn. This leads to blood and fluid extravasation, increasing interstitial pressure in the muscle compartments. A fasciotomy is often necessary, opening all the muscle compartments involved. Early action is necessary to avoid severe vascular insufficiency or nerve damage. Thrombosis frequently occurs in vessels deep in an extremity, causing a greater depth of tissue necrosis than is evident at the initial examination. The greatest muscle injury is usually closest to the bone, where the highest heat of resistance is generated. The treatment of electrical injuries depends on the extent of deep muscle and nerve destruction more than on any other factor.

Severe myoglobinuria may develop with the risk of acute tubular necrosis as the muscle pigment is released from muscle and precipitates in renal tubules. The urine output must be kept two to three times normal with intravenous fluids. Alkalinization of the urine and osmotic diuretics may be indicated if myoglobinuria is present to more rapidly clear the pigment.

A rapid drop in hematocrit sometimes follows as sudden destruction of red blood cells by the electrical energy occurs. Bleeding into deep tissues may occur as a result of disruption of blood vessels and tissue planes. In some cases, thrombosed vessels disintegrate later and cause massive interstitial hemorrhage. Increased fluid infusion is required for initial resuscitation compared to extent of external thermal burns alone.

The skin burn at the entrance and exit sites is usually a depressed gray or yellow area of full-thickness destruction surrounded by a sharply defined zone of hyperemia. Charring may be present. The lesion should be debrided to underlying healthy tissue. Frequently, there is deep destruction not initially evident, especially to muscles beneath the skin surface. This dead and devitalized tissue must also be excised as soon as possible. Amputation rate for extremity involved is still high but decreasing. A second debridement is usually indicated 24–48 hours after the injury, because the necrosis is found to be more extensive than originally thought. The strategy of obtaining skin covering for these burns can tax ingenuity because of the extent and depth of the wounds. Microvascular flaps are now used routinely to replace large tissue losses.

In general, the treatment of electrical injuries is complex at every step, and these patients are referred to specialized centers. There are no formulas for determining severity and outcome of high-voltage electrical injuries.

Edlich R: Modern concepts of treatment and prevention of electrical burns. J Long Term Eff Med Implants 2005;15:511.

Moughsoudi H: Electrical and lightning injuries. J Burn Care Res 2007;28:255.

▼ HEAT STROKE & RELATED INJURIES

Heat stroke occurs when core body temperature exceeds 40 °C and produces severe central nervous system dysfunction. Two related syndromes induced by exposure to heat are heat cramps and heat exhaustion.

In humans, heat is dissipated from the skin by radiation, conduction, convection, and evaporation. When the ambient temperature rises, heat loss by the first three is impaired; loss by evaporation is hindered by a high relative humidity. Predisposing factors to heat accumulation are dermatitis; use of phenothiazines, beta-blockers, diuretics, or anticholinergics; intercurrent fever from other disease; obesity; alcoholism; and heavy clothing. Cocaine and amphetamines may increase metabolic heat production.

Heat cramps—muscle pain after exertion in a hot environment—are usually attributed to salt deficit. It is probable, however, that many cases are really examples of **exertional rhabdomyolysis**. This condition, which may also be a complicating factor in heat stroke, involves acute muscle injury due to severe exertional efforts beyond the limits for which the individual has trained. It often produces myoglobinuria, which rarely affects kidney function except when it occurs in patients also suffering from heat stroke. Complete recovery is the rule after uncomplicated heat cramps.

Heat exhaustion consists of fatigue, muscular weakness, tachycardia, postural syncope, nausea, vomiting, and an urge to defecate caused by dehydration and hypovolemia from heat stress. Temperature usually exceeds 39 °C. Although body temperature is normal in heat exhaustion, there is a continuum between this syndrome and heat stroke.

Heat stroke, a result of imbalance between heat production and heat dissipation, kills about 4000 persons yearly in the United States. Exercise-induced heat stroke most often affects young people (eg, athletes, military recruits, laborers) who are exercising strenuously in a hot environment, usually without adequate training. Heat production exceeds the ability to dissipate the heat; core temperature then rises and hypovolemia is evident. Sedentary heat stroke is a disease of elderly or infirm people whose cardiovascular systems are unable to adapt to the stress of a hot environment and release sufficient heat such that body temperature rises. Epidemics of heat stroke in elderly people can be predicted when the ambient temperature surpasses 32.2 °C and the relative humidity reaches 50–76%.

The mechanism of injury is direct damage by heat to the parenchyma and vasculature of the organs. In addition, there is a marked cytokine-induced activation of inflammation similar to sepsis, leading to inflammation-induced organ damage. The central nervous system is particularly vulnerable, and cellular necrosis is found in the brains of those who die of heat stroke. Hepatocellular and renal tubular damage are apparent in severe cases. Subendocardial damage and occasionally transmural infarcts are discovered in fatal cases even in young persons without previous cardiac disease. Disseminated intravascular coagulation may develop, aggravating injury in all organ systems and predisposing to bleeding complications.

▶ Clinical Findings

A. Symptoms and Signs

Heat stroke should be suspected in anyone who develops sudden neurological changes in a hot environment. If the patient's temperature is above 40 °C (range: 40–43 °C), the diagnosis of heat stroke is definitive. Measurements of body temperature must be made rectally. A prodrome including dizziness, headache, nausea, chills, and goose-flesh of the chest and arms is seen occasionally but is not common. In most cases, the patient recalls having experienced no warning symptoms except weakness, tiredness, or dizziness. Confusion, belligerent behavior, or stupor may precede coma. Convulsions may occur.

The skin is pink or ashen and sometimes, paradoxically, dry and hot; dry skin in the presence of hyperpyrexia is virtually pathognomonic of heat stroke. Profuse sweating is usually present in runners and other athletes who have heat stroke. The heart rate ranges from 140 beats/min to 170 beats/min; central venous or pulmonary wedge pressure is high; and in some cases the blood pressure is low. Hyperventilation may reach 60 breaths/min and may give rise to respiratory alkalosis. Pulmonary edema and bloody sputum may develop in severe cases. Jaundice is frequent within the first few days after onset of symptoms.

Dehydration, which may produce the same central nervous system symptoms as heat stroke, is an aggravating factor in about 50% of cases.

B. Laboratory Findings

There is no characteristic pattern to the electrolyte changes: The serum sodium concentration may be normal or high, and the potassium concentration is usually low on admission or at some point during resuscitation. In the first few days, the aspartate aminotransferase (AST), lactate dehydrogenase (LDH), and creatine kinase (CK) may be elevated, especially in exertional heat stroke. Proteinuria and granular and red cell casts are seen in urine specimens collected immediately after diagnosis. If the urine is dark red or brown, it probably contains myoglobin. The blood urea nitrogen and serum creatinine rise transiently in most patients and continue to climb if renal failure develops. Hematologic findings may be normal or may be typical of disseminated intravascular coagulation (ie, low fibrinogen, increased fibrin split products, slow prothrombin and partial thromboplastin times, and decreased platelet count).

C. Prevention

For the most part, heat stroke in military recruits and athletes in training is preventable by adhering to a graduated schedule of increasing performance requirements that allows acclimatization over 2–3 weeks and increasing fluid replacement using water and some electrolytes, especially sodium. Heat produced by exercise is dissipated by increased cardiac output, vasodilation in the skin, and increased sweating. With acclimatization, there is increased efficiency for muscular work, increased myocardial performance, expanded extracellular fluid volume if hydration is maintained, greater output of sweat for a given amount of work (releasing more heat), a lower salt content of sweat, and a lower central temperature for a given amount of work.

Access to drinking water should be unrestricted during vigorous physical activity in a hot environment. Free water is preferable to electrolyte-containing solutions. Clothing and protective gear should be lightened as heat production and air temperature rise, and heavy exercise should not be scheduled at the hottest times of day, especially at the beginning of a training schedule.

▶ Treatment

The patient should be cooled rapidly. The most efficient method is to induce evaporative heat loss by spraying the patient with water at 15 °C and fanning with cool air. Immersion in an ice water bath or use of ice packs is also effective but causes cutaneous vasoconstriction and shivering and makes patient monitoring more difficult. Monitor the rectal temperature frequently. To avoid overshooting the end point, vigorous cooling should be stopped when the temperature reaches 38.9 °C. Shivering should be controlled with parenteral phenothiazines. Oxygen should be administered, and if the Pao_2 drops below 65 mm Hg, tracheal intubation should be performed to control ventilation. Fluid, electrolyte, and acid-base balance must be controlled by frequent monitoring. Intravenous fluid administration should be based on the central venous or pulmonary artery wedge pressure, blood pressure, and urine output; overhydration must be avoided. Intravenous mannitol (12.5 g) may be given early if myoglobinuria is present to avoid renal dysfunction. Disseminated intravascular coagulation may require treatment with heparin. Occasionally, inotropic agents (eg, isoproterenol, dopamine) may be indicated for cardiac insufficiency, which should be suspected if hypotension persists after hypovolemia has been corrected.

▶ Prognosis

Bad prognostic signs are temperature of 42.2 °C or more, coma lasting over 2 hours, shock, hyperkalemia, and an AST greater than 1000 units/L during the first 24 hours. The death rate is about 10% in patients who are correctly diagnosed and treated promptly. Deaths in the first few days are usually due to cerebral damage; later deaths may be from bleeding or may be due to cardiac, renal, or hepatic failure.

Bouchama A, DeVol EB: Acid-base alterations in heatstroke. Intensive Care Med 2001;27:680.
Jardine DS: Heat illness and heat stroke. Pediatr Rev 2007;28:249.
Leon LR: Heat stroke and cytokines. Prog Brain Res 2007;162:481.

▼ FROSTBITE

Frostbite involves freezing of tissues. Ice crystals form between and in the cells and grow at the expense of intracellular water. The resulting ischemia due to vasoconstriction and increased blood viscosity is the mechanism of tissue injury. Skin and muscle are considerably more susceptible than tendons and bones to freezing damage due to a lower oxygen requirement, which explains why the patient may still be able to move severely frostbitten digits.

Frostbite is caused by cold exposure, the effects of which can be magnified by moisture or wind. For example, the chilling effects on skin are the same with an air temperature of 6.7 °C and a 40-mph wind as with an air temperature of −40 °C and only a 2-mph wind. Contact with metal or gasoline in very cold weather can cause virtually instantaneous freezing; skin will often stick to metal and be lost. The risk of frostbite is increased by generalized hypothermia, which produces peripheral vasoconstriction as part of the mechanism for preservation of core body temperature.

Two related injuries, trench foot and immersion foot, involve prolonged exposure to wet cold above freezing (eg, 10 °C). The resulting tissue damage is produced by tissue ischemia.

▶ Clinical Findings

Frostnip, a minor variant of this syndrome, is a transient blanching and numbness of exposed parts that may progress to frostbite if not immediately detected and treated. It often appears on the tips of fingers, ears, nose, chin, or cheeks and should be managed by rewarming through contact with warm parts of the body or warm air.

Frostbitten parts are numb, painless, and of a white or waxy appearance. With **superficial frostbite,** only the skin and subcutaneous tissues are frozen, so the tissues beneath are still compressible with pressure. **Deep frostbite** involves freezing of underlying tissues, which imparts a wooden consistency to the extremity.

After rewarming, the frostbitten area becomes mottled blue or purple and painful and tender. Blisters appear that may take several weeks to resolve. The part becomes edematous and to a varying degree painful.

▶ Treatment

The frostbitten part should be rewarmed (thawed) in a water bath at 40–42.2 °C for 20–30 minutes. Thawing should not be attempted until the victim can be kept permanently warm and at rest. It is far better to continue walking on frostbitten feet even for many hours than to thaw them in a remote cold area where definitive care cannot be provided. If a thermometer is unavailable, the temperature of the water should be adjusted to be warm but not hot to a normal hand. Never use the frozen part to test the water temperature or expose it to a source of direct heat such as a fire. The risk of seriously compounding the injury is great with any method of thawing other than immersion in warm water.

After thawing has been completed, the patient should be kept recumbent and the injured part left open to the air,

protected from direct contact with sheets, clothing, or other material. Blisters should be left intact and the skin gently debrided by immersing the part in a whirlpool bath for about 20 minutes twice daily. No scrubbing or massaging of the injured part should be allowed, and topical ointments, antiseptics, and so on, are of no value. Vasodilating agents and surgical sympathectomy do not appear to improve healing.

The tissue will heal gradually, and any dead tissue will become demarcated and usually slough spontaneously. Early in the course, it is nearly impossible, even for someone with considerable experience in the treatment of frostbite, to judge the depth of injury; most early assessments tend to overestimate the extent of permanent damage. Therefore, expectant treatment is the rule, and surgical debridement should be avoided even if evolution of the injury requires many months. Surgery may be indicated to release constricting circumferential eschars, but rarely should the process of spontaneous separation of gangrenous tissue be surgically facilitated. Even in severe injuries, amputation is rarely indicated before 2 months unless invasive infection supervenes. Nuclear scans may be useful to delineate tissue viability.

Concomitant fractures or dislocations create challenging and complex problems. Dislocations should be reduced immediately after thawing. Open fractures require operative reduction, but closed fractures should be managed with a posterior plastic splint. Anterior tibial compartment syndrome, which may develop in patients with associated fractures, may be diagnosed by arteriography and treated by fasciotomy.

After the eschar separates, the skin is noted to be thin, shiny, tender, and sensitive to cold; occasionally it exhibits a tendency to perspire more readily. Gradually, it returns toward normal, but pain on exposure to cold may persist indefinitely.

▶ Prognosis

The prognosis for normal function is excellent if appropriate treatment is provided. Individuals who have recovered from frostbite have increased susceptibility to another frostbite injury on exposure to cold.

Affleck DG et al: Assessment of tissue viability in complex extremity injuries: utility of the pyrophosphate nuclear scan. J Trauma 2001;50:263.

Murphy JV et al: Frostbite: pathogenesis and treatment. J Trauma 2000;48:171.

▼ ACCIDENTAL HYPOTHERMIA

Accidental hypothermia consists of the uncontrolled lowering of core body temperature below 35 °C by exposure to cold. The syndrome may be seen, for example, in elderly people living alone in inadequately heated homes, in alcoholics exposed to the cold during a binge, in those engaged in winter sports, and in people who become lost in cold weather. Alcohol facilitates the induction of hypothermia by producing sedation (inhibiting shivering) and cutaneous dilation. Other sedatives, tranquilizers, and antidepressants are occasionally implicated. Diseases that predispose to hypothermia include myxedema, hypopituitarism, adrenal insufficiency, cerebral vascular insufficiency, mental impairment, and cardiovascular disorders.

The heart is the organ most sensitive to cooling and is subject to ventricular fibrillation or asystole when the temperature drops to 21–24 °C. Hypothermia affects the oxyhemoglobin dissociation curve, so less oxygen is released to the tissues. Cardiac standstill may cause death in less than 1 hour in shipwreck victims immersed in cold water (6.7 °C). Increased capillary permeability, manifested by generalized edema and pulmonary, hepatic, and renal dysfunction, may develop as the patient is rewarmed. Coagulopathies and disseminated intravascular coagulation are seen occasionally. Pancreatitis and acute renal failure are common in patients whose temperature on admission is below 32 °C.

▶ Clinical Findings

A. Symptoms and Signs

The patient is mentally depressed (somnolent, stuporous, or comatose), cold, and pale to cyanotic. The clinical findings are not always striking and may be mistaken for the effects of alcohol. The core temperature ranges from 21 to 35 °C. Shivering is absent when the temperature is below 32 °C. Respirations are slow and shallow. The blood pressure is usually normal and the heart rate slow. When the core temperature drops below 32 °C, the patient may appear to be dead. The extremities may be frostbitten or frozen.

B. Laboratory Findings

Dehydration may increase the concentration of various blood constituents. Severe hypoglycemia is common, and unless detected and treated immediately, it may become dangerously worse as rewarming produces shivering. The serum amylase is elevated in about half of cases, but autopsy studies show that it does not always reflect pancreatitis. Diabetic ketoacidosis becomes a management problem in some patients whose amylase values are elevated on entry. The AST, LDH, and CK enzymes are usually elevated but are of no predictive significance. The electrocardiogram shows lengthening of the PR interval, delay in interventricular conduction, and a pathognomonic J wave at the junction of the QRS complex and ST segment.

▶ Treatment

Hypothermic patients should never be considered dead until all measures for resuscitation have failed, because cardiopulmonary arrest in severe hypothermia is still compatible with some recovery.

Mild hypothermia (body temperature 32–35 °C) can be treated in most cases by passive rewarming (heavy clothing and blankets in a warm environment) for a few hours—especially when the patient is shivering. The patient's temperature should be continuously monitored with a rectal or esophageal probe until body temperature reaches normal. Since the volume of intravenous fluids required for resuscitation is often substantial, their temperature can affect the outcome. Consequently, intravenous fluids should be warmed with a heat exchanger during administration.

Active rewarming is indicated for temperature below 32 °C, cardiovascular instability, or failure of passive rewarming. The methods include immersion in a warm water bath, inhalation of heated air, pleural lavage, and blood warming with an extracorporeal bypass machine. Active external rewarming is most often performed by immersion in a warm (40–42 °C) water bath, which will raise body temperature at a rate of 1–2 degrees per hour. A disadvantage of this method is that the core temperature may continue to decline after initiation of the rewarming efforts (known as afterdrop), which is associated with worsening cardiovascular function.

Closed pleural irrigation should be performed by flushing the right hemithorax with warm (40–42 °C) saline solution through two large thoracostomy tubes, one anterior and the other posterior. Rewarming by peritoneal lavage involves giving warm (40–45 °C) crystalloid solutions, 6 L/h, which raises core temperature by 2–4 degrees per hour.

Active core rewarming with partial cardiopulmonary bypass, the most efficient technique, is indicated for patients with ventricular fibrillation and severe hypothermia or those with frozen extremities. At a flow rate of 6–7 L/min, core temperature can be raised by 1–2 °C every 3–5 minutes.

In severe cases, endotracheal intubation should be used for better management of ventilation and protection against aspiration, a common lethal complication. Arterial blood gases should be monitored frequently. Bretylium tosylate in an initial dose of 10 mg/kg is the best drug for ventricular fibrillation. Antibiotics are often indicated for coexisting pneumonitis. Serious infections are often unsuspected upon admission, and delay in appropriate therapy may contribute to the severity of the illness. Hypoglycemia calls for intravenous administration of 50% glucose solution. Fluid administration must be gauged by central venous or pulmonary artery wedge pressures, urine output, and other circulatory parameters. Increased capillary permeability following rewarming predisposes to the development of pulmonary edema and compartment syndromes in the extremities. To minimize these complications, the central venous or wedge pressure should be kept below 12–14 cm water. Drugs should not be injected into peripheral tissues, because absorption will not take place while the patient is cold and because drugs may accumulate to produce serious toxicity as rewarming occurs.

As rewarming proceeds, the patient should be continually reassessed for signs of concomitant disease that may have been masked by hypothermia, especially myxedema and hypoglycemia. Any inexplicable failure to respond should suggest adrenal insufficiency.

▶ Prognosis

Survival can be expected in only 50% of patients whose core temperature drops below 32.2 °C. Coexisting diseases (eg, stroke, neoplasm, myocardial infarction) are common and increase the death rate to 75% or more. Survival does not correlate closely with the lowest absolute temperature reached. Death may result from brain damage pneumonitis, heart failure, or renal insufficiency.

Brunette DD, McVaney K: Hypothermic cardiac arrest: an 11-year review of ED management and outcome. Am J Emerg Med 2000;18:418.

Farstad M et al: Recovering from accidental hypothermia by extra-corporeal circulation: a retrospective study. Eur J Cardiothorac Surg 2001;20:58.

Light TD: Real time metabolic monitors, ischemia perfusion, titration endpoints and ultraprecise burn resuscitation. J Burn Care Rehab 2004;25:33.

Peng RY, Bongard FS: Hypothermia in trauma patients. J Am Coll Surg 1999;188:685.

Punja K et al: Continuous infusion of epidermal morphine in frostbite. J Burn Care Rehabil 1998;19:142.

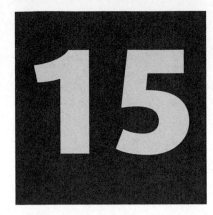

Otolaryngology—Head & Neck Surgery

Paul M. Weinberger, MD
David J. Terris, MD

INTRODUCTION

Otolaryngology/head and neck surgery is a surgical subspecialty that focuses on the management of a wide range of disorders of the head and neck, from hearing loss or nasal hemorrhage (epistaxis) to endocrine surgery and expert management of acute airway emergencies. This chapter presents an overview of selected disease processes in otolaryngology that are of importance to the general surgeon in training.

DISORDERS OF THE EAR, AUDITORY & VESTIBULAR SYSTEMS, & TEMPORAL BONE

▶ Anatomy & Physiology

The external ear consists of two parts, the auricle (projecting from the lateral aspect of the head) and the external auditory canal (EAC) projecting medially to the tympanic membrane. Functioning as resonant amplifiers of sound energy, the concha of the auricle (Figure 15–1) has a resonance frequency of approximately 5 KHz, and the EAC has a resonance frequency of approximately 3.5 KHz. Combined, the external ear amplifies sound by approximately 10–15 dB in the 2–5 KHz range.

The tympanic membrane is positioned in an oblique plane, separating the external auditory canal from the middle ear. It functions in transforming acoustic energy from sound waves to mechanical energy, which is transmitted via the ossicles, malleus, incus, and stapes to the oval window of the cochlea. The mechanics of the middle ear further amplify sound energy using two methods. First, the tympanic membrane is approximately 17 times larger than the footplate of the stapes; second, the ossicles act as a lever, providing a mechanical advantage of 1:1.3 from the tympanic membrane to the oval window. Combined, the result in a 25 to 30 dB gain in amplification.

The temporal bone houses the bony portion of the external auditory canal, the middle, and the inner ear. The otic capsule of the inner ear is the hardest bone in the human body. Other important structures passing through or adjacent to the temporal bone include the carotid artery, the jugular vein, and the facial nerve (seventh cranial nerve). All of these structures are at risk for injury from temporal bone trauma.

The inner ear consists of the cochlea, which is both the auditory and vestibular sense organ. The vestibular system senses both linear acceleration (gravity) and angular acceleration (rotation). The hearing portion of the cochlea is a coiled tube that resembles a snail. The cochlea has separate chambers: The scala vestibule and the scala tympani are filled with perilymph (similar in composition to extracellular fluid), and the scala media is filled with endolymph (similar in composition to intracellular fluid). The endolymph composition is maintained by Na^+/K^+ ATPase pumps within the stria vascularis found on the lateral walls of the scala media. These different chambers thus have different electrolyte composition, creating an electrical potential between the compartments. The sound energy, once transferred through the ossicles to the oval window of the cochlea, is coupled directly to the perilymph of the scala vestibule.

The resulting traveling wave is in the form of mechanical energy, which is then converted to electrical (neural) impulses within the scala media by the organ of Corti. The organ of Corti consists of inner hair cells (which are the sensory cells) and outer hair cells (which function as modulators of the inner hair cells), support cells, and tectorial membrane. The nerve impulses produced by the inner hair cells are transmitted to the brainstem by the eighth cranial nerve, which travels from the cochlea through the internal auditory canal.

The vestibular system consists of the utricle, saccule, and three semicircular canals. Enveloped within the endolymphatic membrane, which is filled with endolymph, they are surrounded by perilymph, and then the very hard bone of the otic capsule. The utricle detects horizontal acceleration, while the saccule detects vertical acceleration. The three semicircular canals, situated at right angles to each other and paired with a semicircular canal on the opposite side of the head, detect angular acceleration.

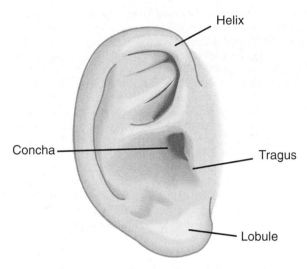

▲ Figure 15–1. Normal external ear anatomy.

Simplified, linear, or angular motion causes their respective sensory cells to deflect and the sensory cell body to depolarize. Depending on the direction, each vestibular apparatus will either increase or decrease the discharge rate relative to the basal rate, providing both direction and speed of acceleration. Vestibular information is transmitted to the brainstem by the vestibular branch of the eighth cranial nerve.

Donaldson JA: Normal anatomy of the inner ear. Otolaryngol Clin North Am 1975;8:267.

Hudspeth AJ: How hearing happens. Neuron 1997;19:947.

Proctor B: Surgical anatomy and embryology of the middle ear. Trans Am Acad Ophthalmol Otolaryngol 1963;67:801.

Mills JH et al: (2006). Anatomy and physiology of hearing. In: Bailey BJ, Johnson JT, Newlands SD, *Head and Neck Surgery: Otolaryngology* 4th ed. Lippincott Williams & Wilkins, 2006; 1883.

▶ Urgencies & Emergencies

A. Sudden Sensorineural Hearing Loss (SSHL)

The sudden onset of unilateral (or more uncommonly bilateral) hearing loss occurs at an annual incidence of 5–20 cases per 100,000 persons and can be an extremely unsettling experience for a patient. Most experts use a definition based on at least a 30 dB hearing loss occurring over 3 days or less. The causes of SSHL include viral infection (particularly herpes-family viruses), trauma, vascular compromise from thromboembolic phenomena or vasospasm, autoimmune disease, ototoxic (from chemotherapy, antibiotics, or salicylates), and congenital anatomic defects.

Prompt evaluation and initiation of treatment is critical and may improve the prognosis for hearing improvement.

Because of the multitude of potential mechanisms, a careful history should be obtained. Often, the cause remains unknown. Patients may report an antecedent loud noise exposure, such as an explosion (suggesting traumatic perilymphatic fistula), or an upper respiratory tract infection symptoms (suggesting possible viral mechanism). Recent heart surgery or thromboembolic phenomenon could suggest a vascular etiology. Patients should be questioned about coincident imbalance or vertiginous symptoms and tinnitus (ringing in the ears), indicative of vestibular as well as auditory pathology.

Formal pure-tone audiometry testing should be performed. If the patient reports vestibular or balance symptoms, investigation of the vestibular system should be performed. Dix-Hallpike and Baranay maneuvers test for vertigo in response to specific position changes with respect to gravity. Simple tests of the auditory system (Weber and Rinne tests) can also be performed at the bedside using a 512 KHz tuning fork (Table 15–1). Pneumatic otoscopy should be performed to evaluate for fistula sign (vertigo on pneumatoscopy insufflation).

Workup should include evaluation for a vestibular schwannoma, which represents approximately 1–3% of SSHL. This evaluation can be done by auditory-evoked brainstem response (ABR) or magnetic resonance imaging (MRI) with contrast using internal auditory canal (IAC) protocols. Some authors advocate a less expensive screening MRI without contrast as an acceptable first step, followed by more definitive evaluations if any abnormalities are present. Laboratory studies should include a complete blood cell count (CBC) with differential, erythrocyte sedimentation rate (ESR), prothrombin time/partial thrombo-

Table 15–1. Weber and Rinne Tuning Fork Tests.

Condition	Weber	Rinne
Left sensorineural hearing loss	Louder on *right*	A > B bilaterally
Left conductive hearing loss	Louder on *left*	A > B on right A = B or A < B on left
Normal hearing	Midline/no difference	A > B bilaterally

In the Weber test, the tuning fork is struck and applied in the midline to the skull or teeth. This stimulates both cochlea by direct bone conduction. The patient is asked whether they hear the sound the same on both sides or louder on one side.

In the Rinne test, a tuning fork is struck and held by the auricle (condition A, air conduction). Sound is conducted through the ossicular chain and to the cochlea. The fork is then applied to the mastoid tip, and acoustic energy is transmitted to the cochlea by direct bone conduction (condition B, bone conduction). The patient is then asked which is louder, A or B. In a normal hearing ear, A (air) is greater than B (bone). In sensorineural hearing loss, A will still be greater than B. In conductive hearing loss, A = B or even B > A.

plastin time (PT/PTT), and cochlear antibodies. Additional studies that may be helpful include syphilis testing (either microhemagglutination-Treponema pallidum or fluorescent treponemal antibody absorption) and thyroid function tests. If there is a family history of sudden hearing loss, a computerized tomography (CT) scan looking for enlarged vestibular aqueduct can be obtained.

If the workup reveals a cause for the SSHL, this should be addressed. Unfortunately, most incidents of SSHL remain idiopathic. In this case, unless contraindicated due to comorbidities, initial treatment should be started empirically. Oral corticosteroids, such as a prednisone taper (60 mg daily for 9 days then tapering over 5 days), and antiviral medication, such as acyclovir, should be administered for a minimum of 2 weeks. Other treatments such as hyperbaric oxygen, carbogen inhalation, anticoagulation, and diuretics have been proposed for the treatment of SSHL, but results of these therapies have been inconclusive.

The prognosis for spontaneous recovery of function is hopeful, and approximately 60% of patients will recover full or partial hearing. With corticosteroid treatment, this percentage may increase to 80%, according to some studies. The addition of acyclovir has not been shown to be effective, but some authors recommend it due to low side effects and a plausible mechanism of action; further studies in this area are obviously warranted.

Aslan A et al: Clinical observations on coexistence of sudden hearing loss and vestibular schwannoma. Otolaryngol Head Neck Surg 1997;117:580.

Byl FM Jr: Sudden hearing loss: eight years' experience and suggested prognostic table. Laryngoscope 1984;94:647.

Fisch U: Management of sudden deafness. Otolaryngol Head Neck Surg 1983;913.

Mattox DE, Simmons FB: Natural history of sudden sensorineural hearing loss. Ann Otol Rhinol Laryngol 1977;86:463.

Veldman J: Immune-mediated sensorineural hearing loss. Auris Nasus Larynx 1998;25:309.

Wilson WR, Byl FM, Laird N. The efficacy of steroids in the treatment of idiopathic sudden hearing loss. A double-blind clinical study. Arch Otolaryngol 1980;106:772.

B. Acute Facial Nerve Paralysis

The seventh cranial nerve (facial nerve) innervates the muscles of facial expression (as well as special motor afferents to the parotid and lacrimal glands). A careful history will help define the onset of paralysis (eg, acute deterioration over less than 2–3 days, or gradual decline). Antecedent events (temporal bone trauma, acute otitis media, hearing loss or imbalance, recent viral illness) should be elicited and can help guide further workup and management.

Potential causes of acute facial nerve paralysis are numerous, however over 50% are idiopathic and termed Bell palsy. Note that Bell palsy is a diagnosis of exclusion, and therefore a focused but complete workup must be performed. Fully 20% of facial nerve paralyses are caused by trauma. Other common causes (but by no means an inclusive list) include herpes zoster oticus (Ramsey Hunt syndrome), complications from otitis media and mastoiditis, Lyme disease, cholesteatoma, and neoplasm.

A complete physical exam with emphasis on the neurologic system and cranial nerves is critical. An important consideration in evaluating the patient with acute facial nerve paralysis is distinguishing between central and peripheral lesions. In central lesions, there is sparing of forehead elevation on the affected side due to decussating fibers from the contralateral side. In peripheral lesions, the fibers have already crossed and there is no forehead sparing. The degree of facial nerve functional loss should be documented and has important bearing on prognosis. Several grading systems have been proposed; the House-Brackmann scale, presented in Table 15–2, is the most widely used. Facial nerve function is graded from I (normal) to VI (total paralysis) for each side.

Evaluation should include pure-tone audiometry and electrophysiological testing. A high-resolution CT of the temporal bone is the imaging study of choice for evaluating bone changes (from mastoiditis, temporal bone trauma, cholesteatoma, or neoplasm), whereas MRI with contrast is helpful when inflammation (eg, herpes zoster oticus) or neoplasm affecting the nerve is suspected. Laboratory studies should include a CBC with differential and ESR or C-reactive protein (CRP). If clinically suspected, autoimmune serologies and Lyme titers can be obtained.

If the facial nerve paralysis was caused by traumatic injury, management depends on the onset of paralysis; immediate and complete paralysis will often benefit from surgical decompression. In delayed or partial dysfunction, spontaneous recovery is likely, and surgical intervention may not be beneficial. For idiopathic paralysis (Bell palsy), initial medical therapy focuses on reducing inflammation and targeting a possible viral etiology. A corticosteroid course should be initiated, either prednisone or prednisolone. Previous recommendations for the use of acyclovir (or similar antiherpetic analog) have recently been questioned. A recent large-scale, randomized double-blind study demonstrated no benefit for acyclovir but significant benefit for prednisolone in the treatment of Bell palsy. If the paralysis progresses, surgical decompression may be beneficial. Another study demonstrated a significant benefit to performing surgical decompression for progression to severe paralysis if performed within 14 days of the onset of paralysis. Severe injury was defined as developing greater than 90% degeneration on electroneuronography (ENoG) and lacking voluntary motor potentials on electromyogram (EMG). Of note, this study also demonstrated that after 14 days, surgical decompression offered no benefit. Therefore, close follow-up of these patients is warranted.

Brodie HA, Thompson TC: Management of complications from 820 temporal bone fractures. Am J Otol 1997;18:188.

Table 15–2. House-Brackmann Facial Nerve Paralysis Scale.

Grade	Characteristics
I (normal)	Normal function in all branches
II (mild dysfunction)	Slight weakness to visual inspection
	Normal symmetry and tone at rest
	Forehead: moderate to good function
	Eye: complete closure, minimal effort
	Mouth: slight asymmetry
III (moderate dysfunction)	Mild difference to gross inspection between sides
	Normal symmetry and tone at rest
	Forehead: slight to moderate movement
	Eye: compete closure, requires effort
	Mouth: slightly weak, requires effort
IV (moderately severe dysfunction)	Obvious weakness to gross inspection between sides
	Normal symmetry and tone at rest
	Forehead: no motion even with effort
	Eye: incomplete closure even with effort
	Mouth: asymmetric with maximum effort
V (severe dysfunction)	Only barely perceptible motion to gross inspection
	Asymmetry at rest
	Forehead: no motion even with effort
	Eye: incomplete closure even with effort
	Mouth: slight movement even with maximum effort
VI (total paralysis)	No movement

Chang CY, Cass SP: Management of facial nerve injury due to temporal bone trauma. Am J Otol 1999;20:96.

Fisch U: Prognostic value of electrical tests in acute facial paralysis. Am J Otol 1984;5:494.

Gantz BJ et al: Surgical management of Bell's palsy. Laryngoscope 1999;109:1177.

Ramsey MJ et al: Corticosteroid treatment for idiopathic facial nerve paralysis: a meta-analysis. Laryngoscope 2000;110:335.

Sullivan FM et al: Early treatment with prednisolone or acyclovir in Bell's palsy. N Engl J Med 2007;357:1598.

C. Foreign Body in the External Auditory Canal

The vast majority of cases of foreign bodies in the external auditory canal occur in children or mentally impaired adults. Many otologic foreign bodies are actually amenable to removal under direct visualization in an emergency department or primary care office setting. A large series of over 600 cases of ear foreign bodies showed an overall 77% success rate for removal under direct visualization by emergency physicians. It is important to note that most foreign bodies successfully removed in this manner fit the category of "soft, irregular" material, such as paper or cotton, and "pliable or rubberlike," such as silly putty or erasers. Success with hard objects, especially spherical objects such as plastic beads, was markedly lower. Thus, an argument can be made for a single attempt by the pediatrician or emergency physician under direct visualization if the object meets the former criteria. This should be tempered, however, with the understanding that complication rates are much higher with removal under direct vision. Complications of foreign body removal most commonly include canal wall lacerations (47%), with tympanic membrane perforations less common (4%). More serious complications, such as ossicular chain injury and oval window perforation, are possible but rare. When initial foreign body removal is performed instead by the otolaryngologist using binocular otomicroscopy either in the office or operative setting, the complication rate is quite low (6.3%).

Foreign body removal using binocular otomicroscopy is the primary method used by most otolaryngologists. Specific techniques depend on the characteristics of the foreign body. Objects with sharp edges can often be grasped with alligator or duck-bill forceps. Soft objects are often amenable to removal with otologic suction. Removal of spherical and hard, irregular objects requires more finesse. In these cases, a 90-degree probe is invaluable. The probe is carefully guided behind the object under binocular otomicroscopic visualization. Then the probe is rotated along its axis to bring the end behind the object. The object is then guided out of the external auditory canal. Another special case is an insect within the external auditory canal, most commonly cockroaches. This can be quite alarming to the patient if the insect is still alive. The proximity of the insect to the tympanic membrane translates movement of the insect to distressingly loud perceived sound levels. In such cases, the external ear canal can be gently irrigated with either mineral oil or lidocaine to suffocate the insect before removal.

Some nonotolaryngologists advocate the use of gentle irrigation to attempt dislodgement of external auditory canal foreign bodies. This technique can be used successfully but requires caution. If there is any suspicion of tympanic membrane perforation, irrigation is contraindicated because it could flush debris into the middle ear space. If the foreign body is composed of vegetable material (such as a popcorn kernel), irrigation should also be avoided: If the object is not successfully flushed out, subsequent swelling of the vegetable foreign body can result in extreme pain as the external auditory canal skin is compressed against the bony canal. Removal of swollen matter can be problematic and may require general anesthesia and the use of an operating microscope. Otologic medications are also contraindicated in vegetable material otologic foreign bodies for the same reason. A third condition in which irrigation and otologic medications are specifically contraindicated is in the case of external auditory canal button batteries.

While the previously described foreign bodies can be managed on an outpatient basis, the finding of a button battery in the external auditory canal is considered an emergent situation, requiring urgent removal by an otolaryngologist. If left in place for any length of time, batteries in the external auditory canal can result in severe complications. In an early description of this problem, 100% of patients experienced multiple, serious sequelae, including tympanic membrane perforation or total destruction (75%), marked dermal destruction with bone exposure (88%), impairment of hearing (38%), ossicular chain erosion (25%), and even facial nerve paralysis (13%). Both leakage of corrosive battery acid and electrical current discharge resulting in chlorine gas and sodium hydroxide by electrolysis have been hypothesized to contribute to the destructive effects of button batteries. Removal is accomplished under binocular otomicroscopy in the operating room and sometimes requires piecemeal removal of the battery. Following removal of the battery, the external auditory canal should be flushed with copious amounts of saline, and careful inspection of the external canal and tympanic membrane should be performed.

Kavanagh KT, Litovitz T: Miniature battery foreign bodies in auditory and nasal cavities. JAMA 1986;255:1470.

Schulze SL et al: Pediatric external auditory canal foreign bodies: a review of 698 cases. Otolaryngol Head Neck Surg 2002;127:73.

▶ Disorders & Diseases

A. Otitis Externa

Otitis externa is an infection of the external auditory canal, usually from bacterial species such as *Pseudomonas*, *Proteus*, *Klebsiella*, *Streptococcus*, and *Enterobacter*. Evaluation and management of a patient with suspected otitis externa includes a complete history and physical examination with emphasis on the otologic examination. Patients will often give a history of recent water exposure to the external ear, such as from swimming, or other predisposing factors such as chronic hearing aid use. The external pinna should be manipulated gently. In otitis media, manipulation should not elicit pain, whereas for patients with otitis externa, movement of the pinna is extremely painful. On handheld otoscopy, the canal wall will appear edematous and erythematous. Sometimes the edema is severe enough that the tympanic membrane cannot be seen. In this case, insertion of a Pope otowick is indicated to carry ototopical medications the length of the external ear canal past the obstructed site. Severe cases may require frequent suction debridement under microscopic visualization. Patients should be placed on ototopical antibiotic drops containing a topical corticosteroid, such as ciprofloxacin 0.3%/dexamethasone 0.1% suspension (Ciprodex). Some (largely nonotolaryngologist) physicians allow use of hydrocortisone 1%/polymyxin/neomycin (Cortisporin) as an

alternative. This is not recommended for several reasons: First, several authors have demonstrated up to 10% risk of contact dermatitis with polymyxin/neomycin ototopical drops. Second, if a possibility of tympanic membrane perforation exists, these drops carry the possibility of ototoxicity, according to laboratory studies in animals; they are not approved for middle ear use (unlike fluoroquinolones). Additionally, some studies have demonstrated faster pain relief with Ciprodex than with Cortisporin. It is essential to note that failure to respond to appropriate therapy within 48 to 72 hours should prompt the clinician to reassess the patient to confirm a diagnosis of otitis externa.

Of note, patients with a history of diabetes (or any immunocompromising condition) should demand more aggressive therapy targeted toward *Pseudomonas*. This will usually involve an ototopical fluoroquinolone, ototopical corticosteroid, and oral or intravenous fluoroquinolone therapy. In the past, this subset of otitis externa carried the misnomer "malignant otitis externa" because of the high mortality rate even with surgical debridement and antibiotics. Modern antibiotic therapy and earlier diagnoses and intervention have dramatically improved outcomes, and mortality from this disease is now relatively rare.

Otomycosis is otitis externa due to a fungal infection, usually *Aspergillus* or *Candida* species. On otoscopy, there is usually far less edema and erythema than with bacterial infection. The use of ototopical antibiotic solutions will not improve these patients and usually worsens their condition. Otomycosis can be notoriously difficult to treat, but many cases respond to suction debridement followed by acidic ear drops and a topical corticosteroid. A commonly used topical preparation is acetic acid 2% with hydrocortisone 1% (Vosol HC). Topical antifungals such as nystatin or amphotericin B are also available but their use should be reserved for difficult cases under the care of an otolaryngologist.

Roland PS et al: A comparison of ciprofloxacin/dexamethasone with neomycin/polymyxin/hydrocortisone for otitis externa pain. Adv Ther 2007;24:671.

Rosenfeld RM et al: Clinical practice guideline: acute otitis externa. Otolaryngol Head Neck Surg 2006;134(4 Suppl):S4.

B. Otitis Media

Classification of common middle ear pathology is often poorly understood by nonotolaryngologists. There are multiple disease processes of the middle ear that include the root term *otitis media*. Additionally, the acronyms used to represent diseases of abnormal middle ear fluid are quite similar.

The first condition, acute otitis media (AOM), represents what is commonly called a "middle ear infection." The typical patient is a young child with history of upper respiratory tract symptoms, fever, and pulling at one ear. Handheld otoscopy will reveal a bulging, erythematous tympanic membrane. Unlike otitis externa, there is no pain with manipulation of the auricle. Several studies from Europe have demonstrated that the majority of AOM cases resolve spontaneously without intervention. Nevertheless, in the United States, most parents would be unhappy with a decision not to treat, and antibiotic therapy for AOM is routine. Usual pathogens include bacteria such as *Streptococcus, Haemophilus,* and *Moraxella.* The latter two are often resistant to penicillins, so treatment with amoxicillin may not clear the infection; many practitioners thus recommend a second-generation cephalosporin. Failure to respond to these agents often necessitates a second-line antibiotic such as amoxicillin-clavulanic acid (Augmentin).

Otitis media with effusion (OME) is defined as fluid in the middle ear but no active signs of an infection. OME often results from eustachian tube dysfunction, which predisposes to accumulation of a sterile serous fluid in the middle ear cleft that does not clear. OME is common in young children, with a prevalence approaching 30% according to some reports. Patients with otitis media with effusion present with complaints of muffled or decreased hearing. Examination will reveal fluid in the middle ear cleft. Chronic serous otitis media (CSOM) results when middle ear fluid, after an episode of AOM, fails to clear after a reasonable time span (4–6 weeks).

The most common surgical intervention to treat these problems is myringotomy and tympanostomy (M&T), or "ventilation tube" placement. Basic indications for M&T include multiple episodes of AOM (4 episodes in 6 months or 6 episodes in 12 months), CSOM with hearing impairment present for 3 months or longer, or presence of complications of AOM. Some authors advocate a more stratified approach to indications, where patients presenting with problems at an early age warrant surgical intervention with less stringent criteria.

Higgins TS et al: Medical decision analysis: indications for tympanostomy tubes in RAOM by age at first episode. Otolaryngol Head Neck Surg 2008;138:50.

Lous J et al: Grommets (ventilation tubes) for hearing loss associated with otitis media with effusion in children. Cochrane Database Syst Rev 2005;1:CD001801.

C. Vestibular Schwannoma

Vestibular schwannomas (sometimes referred to by the misnomer "acoustic neuromas") represent a nonmalignant but neoplastic proliferation of schwann cells ensheathing the eighth cranial nerve. These tumors represent nearly 10% of all intracranial tumors and usually present with a unilateral high-frequency sensorineural hearing loss followed later by development of imbalance symptoms. Even a mild degree of hearing loss may be misleading because sensory processing (as evidenced by speech discrimination scores) are often more impaired than pure-tone averages would predict. Tinnitus and true vertigo are less common symptoms. Interestingly, these tumors arise more often from the vestibular division than from the auditory division of cranial nerve eight. The symptoms associated with vestibular schwannomas are associated with compressive effects from the neoplastic growth. In the case of larger tumors, patients can sometimes present with facial nerve weakness. One important syndrome associated with vestibular schwannomas is neurofibromatosis type 2. Patients with type 2 neurofibromatosis can present with bilateral vestibular schwannomas, and consideration of hearing preservation strategies thus is extremely important for these patients.

Definitive diagnosis of vestibular schwannoma is usually made by MRI with gadolinium. Schwannomas enhance brightly on T1 or T2 weighted images with gadolinium. Other diagnostic tests can include ABR and electronystagmography (ENG). All patients with suspected vestibular schwannomas should have audiometric testing (pure-tone averages and speech discrimination scores) performed.

Management of vestibular schwannomas remains controversial. Many authors watching small schwannomas confined to the internal auditory canal via serial imaging. Tumors demonstrating no growth (< 2 mm) can continue to be watched, while most authors would argue for intervention if more than 2 mm of growth occurs. A recent study of 123 patients with small schwannomas who underwent serial observations demonstrated 65% had less than 2 mm of growth over a mean follow-up time of almost 5 years. If intervention is elected, treatment can be microsurgical (often involving combined neurosurgical and otologist collaboration) or by stereotactic radiosurgery (gamma knife) for small tumors. The goal of treatment is eradication of the tumor while preserving hearing and facial nerve function when possible. Preservation of facial nerve function is generally successful, regardless of surgical approach used. In a large series of 400 patients, 71% of patients had mild to no facial nerve impairment at 1 year following surgery (House-Brackmann grade 2 or better).

Bennett M, Haynes DS: Surgical approaches and complications in the removal of vestibular schwannomas. Otolaryngol Clin North Am 2007;40:589.

Darrouzet V et al: Vestibular schwannoma surgery outcomes: our multidisciplinary experience in 400 cases over 17 years. Laryngoscope 2004;114:681.

Ferri GG et al: Conservative management of vestibular schwannomas: an effective strategy. Laryngoscope 2008;118:951.

Slattery WH 3rd et al: Hearing preservation surgery for neurofibromatosis Type 2-related vestibular schwannoma in pediatric patients. J Neurosurg 2007;106(4 Suppl):255.

D. Benign Paroxysmal Positional Vertigo

Dizziness is an extremely common phenomenon estimated to affect as many as 30% of patients. Important distinctions exist among the various sensations commonly described by patients as "dizziness," so the practitioner should always attempt to elicit an accurate description of the patient's dizziness symptoms. Vertigo is defined as the illusion of rotation and should be distinguished from sensations of imbalance or unsteadiness or of almost losing consciousness (presyncope).

Benign paroxysmal positional vertigo (BPPV) is the most common cause of acute-onset vertigo. Patients describe sudden onset of intense vertigo lasting seconds rather than minutes, usually brought on by changes in head or body position relative to gravity. There is sometimes an associated history of head trauma. The etiology is thought to be due to dislocation of microcrystals of calcium hydroxyapatite (otoconia) from the vestibule into the posterior semicircular canal. Certain head movements cause the otoconia to abnormally trigger copular deflection and thus elicit unbalanced vestibular input to the brainstem, triggering intense vertigo. Diagnosis of BPPV can be made by positional testing, such as the Dix-Hallpike maneuver. In this test, the patient's head is turned to one side, and the patient is laid into a recumbent position with the head maintained in the rotated position. Elicitation of vertigo, often accompanied by the expected rotatory nystagmus, essentially confirms the diagnosis. Treatment consists of directed repositioning techniques such as the Epley maneuver. These maneuvers are designed to rotate the otoconia through the semicircular canal, depositing them back in a more physiologic location within the vestibule. Often, several treatments are required, and patients can be instructed in the self-application of these maneuvers.

White J et al: Canalith repositioning for benign paroxysmal positional vertigo. Otol Neurotol 2005;26:704.

E. Ménière Disease

Ménière disease is characterized by waxing and waning sensorineural hearing loss (typically low frequency more than high), episodes of vertigo, sensation of aural fullness, and tinnitus. Hearing loss typically follows an episodic but slowly progressive course, with times of worse hearing followed by partial recovery. The hearing loss (and vestibular dysfunction) are most commonly unilateral, although bilateral disease can develop. The vertigo attacks associated with Ménière disease can be debilitating and are often accompanied by nausea, vomiting, and inability to perform normal activities.

Diagnosis of Ménière disease is made on the basis of clinical presence of the tetrad of symptoms combined with evidence of hearing loss and vestibular dysfunction. The episodic nature of the disease is an important characteristic; a single episode of hearing loss and vertigo should not prompt a diagnosis of Ménière disease. In this case, viral labyrinthitis is a more likely culprit.

First described in 1861 by Prosper Ménière, the pathogenesis of Ménière disease remains essentially unknown. It is thought to relate to dilation of the membranous labyrinth, possibly from dysfunction within the endolymphatic sac. Anatomic cadaver studies have demonstrated endolymphatic hydrops (swelling of the scala media and endolymphatic sac) in patients with Ménière disease. Unfortunately, these anatomic changes have also been demonstrated in presumably healthy (or at least asymptomatic) patients.

The mainstay of treatment for Ménière disease remains medical therapy. Patients are typically begun on a low-salt diet initially. Patients are also instructed to avoid caffeine, nicotine, and alcohol. Diuretics can be added, along with vestibular suppressants such as diazepam. Antihistamines (meclizine, dimenhydrinate, etc) have also demonstrated benefit in ameliorating vertigo symptoms associated with Ménière disease.

Patients suffering from severe, incapacitating vertigo and failing medical therapy can be offered several surgical interventions. Many authors advocate unilateral chemical ablation of the vestibular system. This is most often accomplished by transtympanic injection of gentamycin and is associated with sensorineural hearing loss in up to 25% of patients. For patients with intact hearing, endolymphatic sac decompression and shunting can offer significant relief with preservation of hearing. Similarly, selective sectioning of the vestibular branch of the eighth cranial nerve (vestibular neurectomy) may conserve hearing. For patients with severe hearing loss and vertigo, a total transmastoid labyrinthectomy relieves vertigo in over 90% of patients at the cost of complete hearing loss on the affected side.

Coelho DH, Lalwani AK: Medical management of Ménière's disease. Laryngoscope 2008;118:1099.
Gordon AG: Ménière's disease. Lancet 2006;367:984.
Kaylie DM et al: Surgical management of Ménière's disease in the era of gentamycin. Otolaryngol Head Neck Surg 2005;132:443.

F. Cholesteatoma

A cholesteatoma is a cystlike, expansile lesion of the temporal bone consisting of stratified squamous epithelium and trapped desquamated keratin. It occurs in the pneumatized temporal bone, most commonly the middle ear and mastoid (Figure 15–2). There are two types of cholesteatoma, acquired and congenital. Acquired cholesteatomas, the most common type, arise from either retraction pockets within the tympanic membrane or secondarily from a tympanic membrane perforation. Congenital cholesteatomas are thought to arise from epithelial cell rests that fail to undergo apoptosis during development. Whatever the origin, once formed, cholesteatomas behave in a locally destructive manner. Bone erosion is common, especially of the ossicular chain but also potentially the bone surrounding the inner ear (the otic capsule). If left untreated, cholesteatomas can even invade intracranially.

Early cholesteatomas have few if any symptoms and usually start with a slowly progressive hearing loss. If an infection develops in a cholesteatoma, a foul otorrhea will develop, and this sometimes is the presenting symptom. If a cholesteatoma is suspected, careful inspection under binocular otomicroscopy is essential. All debris must be removed to allow full visualization of the entire visible portion of the tympanic membrane. Cholesteatomas will appear as a whitish keratin mass. A pneumatic otoscopy test is essential; if vertigo is elicited the surgeon must suspect erosion into the inner ear structures.

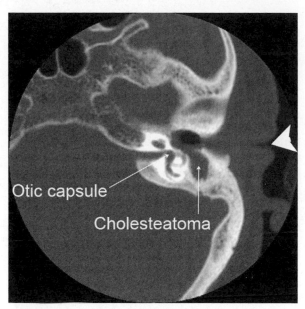

▲ **Figure 15–2.** Cholesteatoma of the left middle ear. Large arrowhead indicates the external ear canal. Note the soft tissue density (cholesteatoma) in the middle ear space and the absence of any visible ossicular chain. Part of the bony covering of the inner ear semicircular canal (the otic capsule) has also been eroded.

The treatment for cholesteatoma is surgery, usually involving removal of the mastoid air cell septations by otologic drill, exposing the middle ear space. This treatment accomplishes two goals: safe visualization and access and removal of all cholesteatoma tissue. This procedure is performed under careful microscopic visualization because many important structures (such as the facial nerve and the inner ear) should be preserved. The primary goal of surgery is creation of a safe, dry ear. All other considerations, including preservation of hearing, take second place.

Michaels L: Biology of cholesteatoma. Otolaryngol Clin North Am 1989;22:869.

Parisier SC: Management of cholesteatoma. Otolaryngol Clin North Am 1989;22:927.

DISORDERS OF THE NOSE & PARANASAL SINUSES

▶ Anatomy & Physiology

The nose and paranasal sinuses serve to warm, filter, and humidify inspired air; modulate vocalizations and speech; and provide for the sense of smell. The external nose consists of soft tissue and skin resting on a largely cartilaginous framework. The internal nose (nasal cavity) begins at the nasal vestibule anteriorly and extends posteriorly to the

choana (which forms the boundary between the nasal cavity and the nasopharynx).

The nasal cavity (Figure 15–3) is divided in the sagittal plane into largely symmetric halves by the nasal septum. These cavities are partially filled by the three turbinates (superior, middle, and inferior), and occasionally by a fourth supreme turbinate, which arise from the lateral nasal wall. The spaces below each turbinate are called meatus (superior meatus, middle meatus, inferior meatus). These meatus are important for localizing the outflow tracts of the various paranasal sinuses, which drain in a characteristic pattern. The nasolacrimal duct drains into the inferior meatus. The maxillary, frontal, and anterior ethmoid sinuses all drain into the middle meatus. The sphenoid sinus and posterior ethmoids drain into the superior meatus. Additionally, the olfactory nerve endings (the end organ for the sense of smell) are located on the superior nasal septum and superior turbinate mucosa.

The paranasal sinuses consist of hollow cavities that derive from pneumatization into the frontal, ethmoid, sphenoid, and maxillary bones of the craniofacial skeleton. They are lined with respiratory epithelium (pseudostratified ciliated columnar epithelium), which serves to circulate and drain mucous along with entrapped particulate matter. They are normally air filled but can become fluid filled if the ostia becomes obstructed by inflammation, anatomic problems, or disease process.

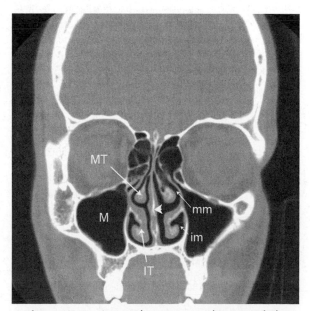

▲ **Figure 15–3.** Sinonasal anatomy. In this coronal plane CT scan, several key sinonasal landmarks can be seen. M, maxillary sinus; IT, inferior turbinate; MT, middle turbinate; im, inferior meatus; mm, middle meatus; arrowhead indicates nasal septum.

Baroody FM: Nasal and paranasal sinus anatomy and physiology. Clin Allergy Immunol 2007;19:1.

Bridger MW, van Nostrand AW: The nose and paranasal sinuses—applied surgical anatomy. A histologic study of whole organ sections in three planes. J Otolaryngol 1978;6:1.

▶ Urgencies & Emergencies

A. Nasal Foreign Body

As is the case for foreign bodies of the external ear, nasal foreign bodies are typically encountered in children. Typical presentation is a young child with several day history of *unilateral* foul rhinorrhea. Often, the offending foreign body was inserted days to weeks before symptom onset, and the patient or parents may not recall a specific event precipitating the symptoms.

Offending foreign bodies can include vegetative, inert (plastic/metal) material, and button batteries. Unlike external ear foreign bodies, nasal foreign bodies should always be treated as relative urgencies, regardless of the type of object present, because of the anatomic relationship of the nose to the upper airway: If the object becomes dislodged, it could easily become an airway foreign body (a true emergency).

For this reason, many otolaryngologists recommend removal of all but the most anteriorly placed nasal foreign bodies under general anesthesia using endoscopic visualization. The threshold for performing retrieval under sedation should likewise be low. In our practice, nasal foreign bodies confined to the nasal vestibule or easily visible by anterior rhinoscopy can be safely removed without sedation *in a cooperative patient*. Young children, superior or posterior location, or difficult visualization all result in removal in the operating room with endoscopic visualization. Another advantage to removing nasal foreign bodies in this manner is that postremoval inspection of the nasal cavity is easily performed. Often, the nasal mucosa can be significantly inflamed and placement of absorbable material can prevent unwanted adhesions between opposing mucosal surfaces.

Nasal button batteries present a similar situation to external ear button batteries (see earlier section on foreign body in the external auditory canal). The potential for extensive tissue damage from leakage of acid and electrical current discharge usually necessitates removal under general anesthesia. Following removal, extensive flushing with normal saline and careful inspection of the nasal cavity should be performed.

Brown L et al: Procedural sedation use in the ED: management of pediatric ear and nose foreign bodies. Am J Emerg Med 2004;22:310.

Loh WS et al: Hazardous foreign bodies: complications and management of button batteries in nose. Ann Otol Rhinol Laryngol 2003;112:379.

B. Invasive Fungal Sinusitis

Invasive fungal sinusitis is almost always encountered in immunocompromised patients, most often patients undergoing chemotherapy for malignancy, or in patients with poorly controlled diabetes. It is caused by uncontrolled infiltrative growth of usually nonpathogenic fungal organisms. Offending agents are ubiquitous in the environment and are commonly found in the nasal secretions of healthy normal patients. The two most common fungi are *Aspergillus* and *Rhizopus* species. The latter is more aggressive and is termed mucormycosis. *Rhizopus* tends to preferentially grow in acidic environments and is thus found more often in the setting of diabetic ketoacidosis. Even with early diagnosis and maximal surgical therapy, and with modern antifungal agents, the disease carries a significant mortality rate. The mortality rate varies depending on causative agent, from approximately 10% (*Aspergillus*) to 30% (*Rhizopus*).

The index of suspicion for invasive fungal sinusitis must be high for any immunocompromised patient because the symptoms can be subtle and the disease rapidly progressive. Patients usually appear ill and complain of facial pain, headache, nasal discharge, and may have mental status changes. Careful inspection of the face, oral cavity, and nasal cavity is mandatory. Dark ulcers (Figure 15–4) may be noted on the anterior face of the middle turbinate, inferior turbinate, lateral nasal wall, septum, or palate. Cranial nerve deficits may be noted in later stages of the disease.

If invasive fungal sinusitis is suspected, biopsies should be taken of the suspicious areas and sent for immediate pathologic examination. The pathologist should be alerted that invasive fungal sinusitis is suspected so that special fungal

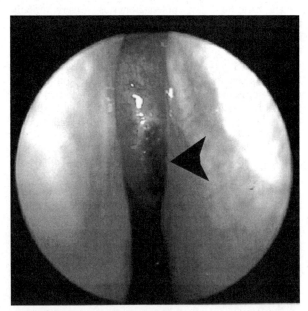

▲ **Figure 15–4.** Invasive fungal sinusitis. In this patient with invasive fungal sinusitis, the initial finding was a dark area (arrowhead) on the inferior face of the middle turbinate found on bedside nasal endoscopy.

stains can be performed. A worrisome finding is lack of bleeding at the biopsy site, which may signify retrograde tissue infarction secondary to angioinvasive fungus.

Once invasive fungal sinusitis is confirmed, therapy consists of rapid reversal of immunosuppression followed by aggressive surgical debridement of all necrotic tissue (down to healthy, bleeding tissue) and systemic antifungal therapy. Two commonly used agents are voriconazole (Vfend) and amphotericin B. Usually, multiple surgical debridements are required. Typically, patients do not recover unless the underlying immunosuppression is resolved (eg, absolute neutrophil counts > 500) or diabetic ketoacidosis is rapidly reversed. Patients should be very closely followed by a multidisciplinary team, including otolaryngology, hematology/oncology, and infectious disease specialists. Many patients develop metastatic fungal infections and can develop necrotic cavitation at distant sites. This often occurs as the patient's immune system recovers and can result in lethal pulmonary hemorrhage, strokes, and other serious systemic sequelae.

Invasive fungal sinusitis should not be confused with other forms of fungal disease of the paranasal sinuses. In allergic fungal sinusitis, chronic host immunologic/inflammatory response to noninvasive fungal elements result in tissue eosinophilia, nasal polyps (hyperplastic growth that obstructs normal drainage and airflow), and bony remodeling.

Gillespie MB, O'Malley BW: An algorithmic approach to the diagnosis and management of invasive fungal rhinosinusitis in the immunocompromised patient. Otolaryngol Clin North Am 2000;33:323.

Parikh SL et al: Invasive fungal sinusitis: a 15-year review from a single institution. Am J Rhinol 2004;18:75.

C. Epistaxis

Epistaxis most commonly arises from the anterior portion of the nasal septum called Little area. In this region, blood vessels derived from both the internal and external carotid anastomose to form the Kiesselbach plexus. This rich blood supply can result in quite dramatic amounts of bleeding, which can be distressing for the patient. Fortunately, many of these episodes respond to simple external pressure (pinching the anterior external nose) for 10 minutes.

The etiology of epistaxis is primarily related to disruption of nasal mucosa, thus exposing small blood vessels, which can rupture. In children, this often relates to nose picking. In adults, the etiology often relates to turbulent nasal airflow, such as from a deviated nasal septum. Other predisposing factors include drying of the nasal mucosa and hypertension. The latter is particularly important in the acute management of epistaxis; often, the bleeding will not be controllable until the accompanying hypertension is dealt with.

Epistaxis not responding to conservative management may require intranasal tamponade. Several different packing devices, including petrolatum gauze, thrombin-containing collagen products, sponges, and inflatable balloons, can be used to perform anterior packing. Anterior bleeding from Little area can also sometimes be controlled with topical silver nitrate chemical cauterization, usually under endoscopic visualization.

Another common source of epistaxis is bleeding from branches of the anterior ethmoid or sphenopalatine artery. Epistaxis from these sources often requires posterior packing (such as with Foley catheter occlusion of the choanae and complete obliteration of the nasal airspace with gauze packing). Patients requiring posterior packing should be hospitalized and placed on pulse oximetry. Of note, nasal packing materials should be covered with topical antibiotics before placement, and all patients with intranasal packing should be placed on antistaphylococcal antibiotics to prevent possible toxic shock syndrome. Epistaxis recalcitrant to anterior and posterior packing can be managed by surgical ligation of the offending arterial supply (internal maxillary, sphenopalatine, anterior ethmoid) or by arterial embolization by an interventional radiologist.

Chronic medical management of patients predisposed to epistaxis includes management of hypertension and promoting moist nasal mucosa. Patients are commonly placed on two to three times daily application of nasal saline spray and topical petroleum jelly or antibiotic ointment to the anterior septum. Patients with severe, recurrent epistaxis should be evaluated for possible systemic disease (eg, hereditary hemorrhagic telangiectasia, Wegener granulomatosis).

Douglas R, Wormald PJ: Update on epistaxis. Curr Opin Otolaryngol Head Neck Surg 2007;15:180.

Gifford TO, Orlandi RR: Epistaxis. Otolaryngol Clin North Am 2008;41:525.

▶ Disorders & Diseases

A. Acute Rhinosinusitis

Rhinosinusitis refers to inflammation of the mucosal lining of the nose and paranasal sinuses. Acute rhinosinusitis is present for less than 3 weeks and is usually precipitated by a viral upper respiratory tract infection. It is important to emphasize that only a minority of cases of acute rhinosinusitis (0.5–2%) become complicated by bacterial superinfection. Similarly, change in color of nasal discharge is not a specific sign of bacterial rhinosinusitis.

Symptoms initially reflect the precipitating upper respiratory viral infection (cough, sneezing, fever, nasal congestion, facial pain/pressure, rhinorrhea, sore throat) followed by development of rhinosinusitis symptoms. A set of diagnostic symptoms for rhinosinusitis (both acute and chronic) have been established. Patients must have two major or one major and two minor criteria, outlined in Table 15–3.

Acute bacterial rhinosinusitis should be suspected if symptoms persist after 10 days or worsen within 10 days after an initial improvement. Physical examination may reveal purulent nasal secretions, nasal mucosal erythema, and tenderness overlying the sinuses. Nasal endoscopy (with

Table 15–3. Major and Minor Criteria for Diagnoses of Rhinosinusitis.

Major Criteria	Minor Criteria
Facial pain or pressure	Headache
Nasal obstruction	Fever (for chronic rhinosinusitis)
Nasal discharge or purulence	Halitosis
Purulence in nasal cavity	Fatigue
Anosmia or hyposmia	Dental pain
Fever (for acute rhinosinusitis)	Cough
	Ear pain/pressure/fullness

Adapted with permission from Lanza DC, Kennedy DW: Adult rhinosinusitis defined. Otolaryngol Head Neck Surg 1997;117:S1.

middle meatal cultures) can be very useful, and visualization of purulent secretions emanating from the osteomeatal complex should increase suspicion for bacterial rhinosinusitis.

Treatment of acute rhinosinusitis is largely conservative in nature. Nasal saline lavage helps to eliminate excess mucous and inflammatory mediators and restore mucociliary clearance. Topical decongestants (such as oxymetazoline) can help reduce mucosal edema and restore sinus ostia drainage. Use should be restricted to 3 days, because tachyphylaxis and dependence can result from overuse of topical decongestants. Mucolytics such as guaifenesin can help thin mucous secretions, allowing easier mucociliary transport. The only therapy tested and confirmed by placebo-controlled trials is intranasal topical steroids (such as mometasone or flunisolide). Topical steroids have been demonstrated to reduce time to symptom resolution for both bacterial and nonbacterial acute rhinosinusitis. It is important to note that antihistamines have no proven benefit in acute rhinosinusitis and may actually cause symptom exacerbation by drying mucous secretions. Antibiotics should be reserved for patients suspected of having acute bacterial rhinosinusitis. Current recommendations specify first-line antibiotic therapy should consist of amoxicillin. After 7 days, if a patient fails to improve clinically, a broader spectrum antibiotic such as a fluoroquinolone, trimethoprim/sulfamethoxazole, azithromycin, or amoxicillin/clavulanic acid can be tried. All of these have greater than 80% efficacy in clearing acute bacterial rhinosinusitis.

Patients experiencing multiple episodes of acute rhinosinusitis should be evaluated carefully for predisposing conditions. These may include anatomic obstruction (which may be relieved by septoplasty and/or functional endoscopic sinus surgery), underlying impairment of mucociliary clearance (such as from immotile cilia/Kartagener syndrome, or cystic fibrosis), or immune system dysfunction. Complications of acute bacterial rhinosinusitis can include orbital cellulitis and subperiosteal abscess formation, meningitis, and cavernous sinus thrombosis.

Brook I, Frazier EH: Microbiology of recurrent acute rhinosinusitis. Laryngoscope 2004;114:129.

Lanza DC, Kennedy DW: Adult rhinosinusitis defined. Otolaryngol Head Neck Surg 1997;117:S1.

Rosenfeld RM: Clinical practice guideline on adult sinusitis. Otolaryngol Head Neck Surg 2007;137:365.

Zalmanovici A, Yaphe J: Steroids for acute sinusitis. Cochrane Database Syst Rev 2007;2:CD005149.

B. Chronic Rhinosinusitis

Chronic rhinosinusitis is extremely common and affects 2–15% of people in the United States. It is defined as presence of rhinosinusitis symptoms for more than 12 weeks (major criteria listed in Table 15–3) combined with evidence of inflammation. The latter can include findings of purulent mucous in the middle meatus or ethmoid region, nasal polyps, or polypoid degeneration of the nasal mucosa. Radiographic findings (Figure 15–5) can also document inflammation, most commonly by CT. Findings can include diffuse mucosal thickening, chronic bony remodeling, and sinus opacification.

Management of chronic rhinosinusitis is primarily by topical and systemic medication. Most otolaryngologists place chronic rhinosinusitis patients on topical nasal steroids for at least 1 month. If symptoms persist, a CT scan may be useful in demonstrating any anatomic abnormalities that may be amenable to surgical correction. Surgery is aimed at removing the obstruction to allow natural mucous flow from the paranasal sinuses, and most patients will continue to require medication after surgery to prevent return of symptoms.

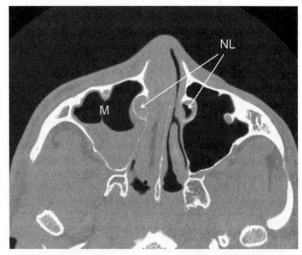

▲ **Figure 15–5.** Chronic sinusitis. In this axial plane CT of a patient with chronic sinusitis, radiographic evidence of inflammation can be seen. The right nasolacrimal duct (NL) mucosa is edematous. There is an air-fluid level and opacification of the right maxillary sinus (M).

The etiology of chronic rhinosinusitis is not fully elucidated. Most otolaryngologists feel that there are several disease processes currently described together under the generic heading chronic rhinosinusitis. Tissue eosinophilia may play an important role in differentiating these groups; current molecular evidence supports this distinction. Future research will undoubtedly change our understanding of these disease processes and how they are managed.

Benninger MS et al: Adult chronic rhinosinusitis: definitions, diagnosis, epidemiology, and pathophysiology. Otolaryngol Head Neck Surg 2003;129(3 Suppl):S1.
Kountakis SE et al: Molecular and cellular staging for the severity of chronic rhinosinusitis. Laryngoscope 2004;114:1895.
Rosenfeld RM: Clinical practice guideline on adult sinusitis. Otolaryngol Head Neck Surg 2007;137:365.

C. Rhinitis Medicamentosa

As previously mentioned, extended use of topical nasal decongestants (such as oxymetazoline) or other vasoconstrictors (such as intranasal cocaine) can lead to tachyphylaxis and mucosal dependence. The resulting severe mucosal edema, hyperemia, and nasal obstruction is termed *rhinitis medicamentosa*. Patients report daily topical vasoconstrictor/ decongestant use and absolute dependence on these medications for any appreciable nasal airflow. It is not unusual for patients suffering from rhinitis medicamentosa to carry their topical vasoconstrictor medication with them due to their frequent use. This is often a telltale sign of dependence. On physical examination, the nasal mucosa will be thickened, erythematous, and edematous and will lack appreciable decongestion on topical decongestant application.

Treatment requires complete cessation of the offending agent. Patients should be started on nasal saline lavage and nasal topical steroids. Oral decongestants and a course of oral corticosteroids may help hasten symptom resolution and increase patient compliance. Resolution usually takes 3– 4 weeks and may require much more time in the case of long-term vasoconstrictor use or intranasal cocaine abuse.

Complications of untreated rhinitis medicamentosa include poor healing after nasal surgery, septal perforation, and formation of synechiae. It is therefore important to recognize and treat rhinitis medicamentosa preoperatively before embarking on any nasal surgical treatment.

Toohill RJ et al: Rhinitis medicamentosa. Laryngoscope 1981; 91:1614.

DISORDERS OF THE ORAL CAVITY & PHARYNX

▶ Anatomy & Physiology

The oral cavity is bounded anteriorly by the vermillion border of the lips and posteriorly by the anterior pillars of the palatine tonsils. The superior aspect of the oral cavity includes the hard and soft palates and inferiorly includes the lingual mucosa and the anterior two thirds of the tongue. This region of the tongue is bounded by the circumvallate papilla, which lie along the sulcus terminalis and separate the oral tongue from the base of tongue (part of the oropharynx).

The pharynx connects the nasal and oral cavities to the esophagus and larynx. It consists of three segments: the nasopharynx, the oropharynx, and the hypopharynx (Figure 15–6). The nasopharynx begins as an extension from the posterior aspect of the nasal cavity and extends from the nasal choana to the soft palate. The oropharynx extends from the soft palate to the level of the hyoid bone and is bounded laterally by the tonsillar pillars (the palatoglossal and palatopharyngeal arches). It includes the base of tongue, lateral/posterior pharyngeal wall, and tonsillar fossae. The hypopharynx extends from the level of the hyoid bone to the inferior aspect of the cricoid cartilage and includes the pyriform sinuses, postcricoid region, and posterior hypopharyngeal wall.

The primary functions of the oral cavity are related to chewing and swallowing (mastication and deglutition) and shaping of phonatory vibrations to produce intelligible speech. Taste buds on the dorsum of the tongue are responsible for basic taste perception: sweet, salty, bitter, and sour. This sensory information is transmitted to the facial nerve via the chorda tympani nerve for the anterior two thirds of the tongue. General sensation of the tongue is carried by the lingual nerve. All sensory information from the posterior one third of the tongue is carried by the glossopharyngeal nerve. Complex nuances of taste are mediated by olfactory receptors in the superiormost aspect of the nasal cavity and are not directly related to the tongue or oral cavity.

The tongue has four pairs of intrinsic muscles, which interdigitate throughout the tongue. These muscles act to lengthen or shorten the tongue, curl the apex and edges, and flatten or round the dorsal surface. The intrinsic tongue muscles originate and insert within the tongue itself. Extrinsic tongue muscles (genioglossus, hyoglossus, styloglossus, and palatoglossus) also act to protrude, depress, elevate, and retract the tongue. All motor function of the tongue is mediated by the twelfth cranial nerve (the hypoglossal nerve).

The act of swallowing, or deglutition, is complex and consists of three main phases: oral, pharyngeal, and esophageal. The oral phase is under voluntary control; the pharyngeal and esophageal phases proceed under reflex control. The oral phase of swallowing consists of preparation of the food bolus by mastication to soften and shape the bolus. Oral transport then ensues, and the food bolus is transported to the posterior tongue. The anterior tongue then elevates against the hard palate, contracts, and propels the bolus to the oropharynx. Simultaneously, the nasopharynx is sealed off, preventing nasal regurgitation. In the pharyngeal phase, several complex actions occur, which elevate the larynx, temporarily halt respirations and protect the airway from aspiration, and relax the cricopharyngeus muscle to allow passage of the food bolus. The esophageal phase then propels

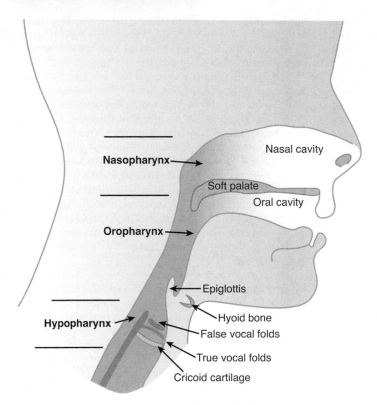

Nasal cavity

Nasopharynx

Soft palate

Oral cavity

Oropharynx

Epiglottis

Hypopharynx

Hyoid bone

False vocal folds

True vocal folds

Cricoid cartilage

▲ **Figure 15–6.** Relationship of the three sections of the pharynx. The nasopharynx extends from the nasal choanae to the soft palate. The oropharynx then extends from the soft palate to the level of the hyoid bone. The hypopharynx extends from the level of the hyoid bone to the level of the cricoid cartilage.

the food bolus distally by means of sequential peristaltic contractions. Alteration of the timing or execution of any of these phases can result in dysphagia, or difficulty swallowing.

Dodds WJ: Physiology of swallowing. Dysphagia 1989;3:171.

▶ Urgencies & Emergencies

A. Acute Angioedema & Ludwig Angina

Acute angioedema is characterized by localized swelling of subcutaneous and submucosal tissue of the head and neck. The swelling may begin with mild facial involvement but may progress to involve the oral cavity, tongue, pharynx, and larynx. It is often self-limited but may present as a medical emergency. Tongue or laryngeal involvement may rapidly lead to airway obstruction and asphyxiation. Angioedema has a rapid onset and with proper medical treatment usually resolves within 24–48 hours. The underlying pathophysiology of angioedema involves vasoactive mediators such as bradykinin and histamine, causing interstitial edema through endothelial-mediated vasodilatation of arterioles with subsequent capillary and venule leakage. The three major etiologies are drug-induced, hereditary, and allergic angioedema. Drug-induced and hereditary angioedema appear to be mediated by the kallikrein-kinin system, while allergic angioedema appears to be mast cell mediated.

Initial management of acute angioedema is focused on airway maintenance. Depending on clinical presentation, this may include nebulized epinephrine inhalation, intubation (either oral or transnasal fiberoptic), or tracheotomy. Due to the potentially rapid progression of this disease process, there should be a low threshold for securing an airway by the latter two methods. Many authors advocate the use of glucocorticoids (10 mg dexamethasone intravenously every 8 hours) combined with histamine receptor antagonists (both an H1 antagonist, such as diphenhydramine 25 mg intravenously every 6 hours, and an H2 antagonist, such as ranitidine 50 mg intravenously every 6 hours) for 24 hours. Recent evidence has shown that the latter therapies may not be beneficial in drug-induced or hereditary angioedema. This should be balanced with the understanding that in clinical practice, rapid differentiation of the exact subtype of angioedema may not be as practical as empiric therapy given the relatively benign nature of these medications compared to potentially life-threatening airway obstruction.

Drug-induced angioedema has classically been associated with the use of angiotensin-converting enzyme inhibitors (ACE inhibitors), although many other medications can also (less commonly) cause this phenomenon. The incidence of angioedema secondary to ACE inhibitor use has been noted to be 0.4–0.7%. The pathophysiology of ACE inhibitor–induced angioedema appears to be secondary to a localized increase in bradykinin levels related to the inhibition of ACE. Studies have shown that half of all cases of ACE inhibitor–induced angioedema occur within the first week of initiating treatment. However, some patients undergo years of ACE inhibitors therapy without incident before their first attack of acute angioedema. Treatment should begin with emergent airway maintenance and discontinuation of any possible drugs that may be inducing the edema. Other drugs with known complications of angioedema include rituximab, alteplase, fluoxetine, laronidase, lepirudin, and tacrolimus. Studies involving angiotensin II receptor antagonists have revealed a much decreased incidence of angioedema in comparison to ACE inhibitors therapy. However, clinicians should still use caution when initiating an angiotensin II receptor antagonist in a patient with known ACE inhibitor–induced angioedema.

Hereditary angioedema involves a deficiency or dysfunction of C1-esterase inhibitor, which leads to increased levels of vasoactive bradykinin. It is autosomally dominant in inheritance, and the defect has been mapped to chromosome 11q. Clinically, hereditary angioedema often presents with recurrent episodes of facial and oral swelling as well as abdominal pain secondary to intestinal wall edema. Studies have revealed that certain drugs (estrogen, ACE inhibitors, angiotensin II receptor antagonists), surgery, and infections may elicit acute angioedema attacks in hereditary angioedema patients. After airway maintenance has been ensured, intravenous C1-esterase inhibitor is the treatment modality of choice. The synthetic steroid danazol has also been used prophylactically to help prevent future acute episodes by increasing the functional levels of C1-esterase inhibitor.

Allergic angioedema is mast cell mediated, and histamine plays the major role in its pathophysiology. In contrast to drug-induced and hereditary angioedema, skin changes including urticaria and pruritus are commonly seen in allergic angioedema. Clinically, the pruritic wheals are spread by scratching, and lesions are usually limited to the lips and periorbital areas and less commonly to the extremities and genitalia. This form of angioedema is frequently seen in patients who also suffer from atopic dermatitis, allergic rhinitis, and asthma. Triggers of acute attacks of allergic angioedema include certain drugs, infections, and food and plant products.

Ludwig angina is an uncommon, life-threatening condition characterized by cellulitis involving the submental, sublingual, and submandibular spaces. The source of the infection is odontogenic and spreads rapidly. The infection is usually polymicrobial with aerobic and anaerobic gram-positive cocci and gram-negative rods. Prior to antibiotics, the mortality rate exceeded 50%. Clinically, patients present with painful neck swelling and edema of the floor of mouth, often leading to elevation and displacement of the tongue. Patients will have a prominent "hot potato" voice and palpation of the floor of mouth reveals woody edema. The

most common cause of death in these patients is airway compromise, and therefore, primary treatment should be centered on airway maintenance with early involvement of anesthesiology and otolaryngology physicians. Intubation is often anatomically difficult, and tracheotomy under local anesthesia is often the preferred method of ensuring a patent airway. Recent case studies have shown the benefit of intravenous dexamethasone and nebulized epinephrine to aid with temporizing the airway and transnasal intubation. Airway observation in the intensive care unit may be an option for less severe cases. After the airway has been secured, proper systemic antibiotic therapy should be initiated and immediately followed by incision and drainage for most cases. Major complications include extension of the infection posteriorly to involve the parapharyngeal and retropharyngeal spaces as well as the superior mediastinum. The diagnosis is clinical, but CT may be used to assess the retropharyngeal extension of the infection.

Bas M et al: Evaluation and management of angioedema of the head and neck. Curr Opin Otolaryngol Head Neck Surg 2006;14:170.
Fritsch DE, Klein DG: Ludwig's angina. Heart Lung 1992;21:39.

B. Peritonsillar Abscess

Peritonsillar abscess is a common infection of the peritonsillar space around the palatine tonsil, tonsillar pillars, and the superior pharyngeal constrictor muscle. Its prevalence in the United Stated has been estimated at 30 per 100,000 people annually. The infection is suppurative in nature and thought to be secondary to either extension of adjacent acute tonsillitis or obstruction of Weber glands (minor salivary glands) at the tonsillar pole. Peritonsillar abscess is seen in both children and adults. The typical patient presents complaining of a 4–5 day history of sore throat and fever with worsening trismus, odynophagia, dysphagia, and inability to tolerate secretions. Peritonsillar abscess should be managed acutely because the infection may progress and spread to the deep neck tissue and compromise the airway.

The gold standard in diagnosis of peritonsillar abscess is physical examination, which reveals bulging soft tissue, tonsillar erythema and exudate, and possible uvular deviation. Needle aspiration or incision and drainage confirms the diagnosis. Recent studies have revealed the benefit of intraoral ultrasound in the diagnosis of peritonsillar abscess. CT may be necessary in patients with severe trismus or in young, uncooperative patients and can aid in differentiating peritonsillar abscess from retropharyngeal abscess.

The management of peritonsillar abscess is dependent on the patient characteristics. Needle aspiration can be performed quickly, is relatively safe, and can be both diagnostic and therapeutic. Incision and drainage should be performed only by physicians with an understanding of the relevant pharyngeal anatomy because multiple vital structures, including cranial nerves and the carotid artery, potentially lie within the surgical field. In cooperative adults, incision and drainage can usually be performed using local anesthesia, but patients with severe trismus may require general anesthesia. Preprocedure administration of 900 mg clindamycin, 10 mg dexamethasone, intravenous fluid hydration, and intravenous morphine for analgesia can greatly facilitate the procedure by reducing trismus and promoting patient comfort and cooperation. After instillation of local anesthetic, a needle aspiration can be used to confirm the site of incision. A limited mucosal incision is made with a scalpel, taking care not to penetrate the underlying muscular layer. Blunt dissection is then used to penetrate the abscess cavity. Oral suction should be in place before penetration of the abscess cavity to prevent possible aspiration of purulence. Studies have shown both needle aspiration and incision and drainage to be greater than 90% effective, but both carry a 10–15% risk of recurrent peritonsillar abscess. The pediatric patient usually will not tolerate either needle aspiration or incision and drainage under local anesthesia, and general anesthesia is often necessary. Antibiotic therapy against *Streptococcus pyogenes* and oral anaerobes with either penicillin or clindamycin should follow abscess drainage. Most patients with peritonsillar abscess can be treated as outpatients.

Emergent tonsillectomy in the setting of acute infection (Quincy tonsillectomy) is usually reserved for cases of peritonsillar abscess that are not successfully drained by simple incision and drainage. While some authors advocate this as a first-line therapeutic option, the increased operative difficulty secondary to acute inflammation and the increased incidence of postoperative hemorrhage make this a less attractive option. It requires general anesthesia, and most otolaryngologists would advocate overnight hospitalization postoperatively for observation.

If needle aspiration or incision and drainage of a peritonsillar abscess is performed, it is important to counsel the patient that future risk of peritonsillar abscess is increased. Many otolaryngologists therefore recommend an elective tonsillectomy be performed two to three months following a peritonsillar abscess.

Johnson RF, Stewart MG: The contemporary approach to diagnosis and management of peritonsillar abscess. Curr Opin Otolaryngol Head Neck Surg 2005;13:157.

C. Deep Neck Space Infections

Although greatly decreased in incidence since the advent of modern antibiotics, deep neck space infections remain a potentially life-threatening condition and require acute recognition and treatment. The source of deep neck space infection is most commonly odontogenic. Other sources of infection include adjacent tonsillar, upper respiratory, and salivary infections as well as instrumentation and foreign bodies. These infections are usually polymicrobial, composed predominantly of anaerobes mixed with various *Streptococcal* and *Staphylococcal* species. Drug-resistant bacteria are commonly seen in intravenous drug users who present with deep neck space infections secondary to needle injection disruption of the cervical fascia. Presenting symptoms depend on the exact location of the abscess, but patients commonly present with fever, painful sore throat, decreased neck range of motion, dysphagia, and odynophagia. Physical examination can reveal trismus, a toxic appearance with facial and neck edema, cervical lymphadenopathy, and purulent oral secretions. It is not uncommon for patients to present several days after being discharged on antibiotics for a less severe, local infection. It is important to note that patients on antibiotic or immunosuppression therapy may have more subtle signs of infection, and systemic toxicity may be masked.

A thorough understanding of the anatomy of the cervical fascia and deep spaces of the neck is paramount in diagnosing and managing these rapidly spreading infections. The cervical fascia is divided into two layers, the superficial cervical fascia and the deep cervical fascia. The deep cervical fascia is further divided into three layers: the superficial, middle, and deep layers of deep cervical fascia. Furthermore, the middle layer of deep cervical fascia is subdivided into muscular and visceral divisions, and the deep layer of deep cervical fascia is subdivided into alar and prevertebral layers.

These divisions of the deep cervical fascia separate the neck into numerous potential spaces that may harbor these life-threatening infections. One easy way of categorizing these spaces is by their relationship to the hyoid bone. Potential spaces that exist entirely above the hyoid bone include the submandibular space and the parapharyngeal space. The pretracheal space exists entirely below the hyoid bone. The prevertebral space, danger space, and retropharyngeal space extend along the entire length of the neck.

Parapharyngeal abscess must be differentiated from peritonsillar abscess because the former requires external drainage via the submaxillary fossa while the latter is best drained intraorally. Retropharyngeal abscesses are most commonly seen in children and are located between the visceral layer of the middle layer of deep cervical fascia and the alar division of the deep layer of deep cervical fascia. Because of the smaller caliber airway in children, retropharyngeal abscess represents a potential source of airway obstruction and should be managed accordingly. The danger space is the region between the alar and prevertebral layers of the deep cervical fascia, which extends from the base of the skull to the diaphragm. Infection of the danger space usually arises from contiguous spread from retropharyngeal, prevertebral, or pharyngomaxillary infections. The lack of definitive anatomic barriers in the danger space offers very little resistance to spread of infection. The prevertebral space is directly posterior to the danger space. Infection of prevertebral space is usually secondary to penetrating trauma or tuberculosis.

Lateral and anteroposterior neck films have traditionally been used to help localize an abscess, although CT has now largely replaced films. Recent studies have shown a potential benefit of MRI in delineating soft tissue and vascular spread of infection, although the time required for MRI makes its use of questionable value. Deep neck space infections can progress rapidly, and patients usually require hospitalization under close supervision.

Initial treatment should focus on an evaluation of need for securing an airway with either endotracheal intubation or tracheotomy. Once airway patency has been verified or secured, needle aspiration can sometimes be performed (in the case of easily accessible abscesses) to obtain culture and Gram stain. Intravenous antibiotics are started immediately and should cover both aerobic and anaerobic organisms. Ampicillin-sulbactam or clindamycin are commonly used. If methicillin-resistant *Staphylococcus aureus* is suspected, vancomycin should also be initiated. If the patient does not improve clinically on antibiotic therapy after 48 hours, open surgical drainage of the abscess may be necessary. Major complications of deep neck space infections include mediastinitis, osteomyelitis, Horner syndrome, and cranial nerve deficits. Involvement of the carotid sheath may also lead to suppurative jugular thrombophlebitis (Lemierre syndrome). Early diagnosis and proper treatment may help limit these serious complications.

Brook I: Microbiology and management of peritonsillar, retropharyngeal, and parapharyngeal abscesses. J Oral Maxillofac Surg 2004;62:1545.
Lalakea M, Messner AH: Retropharyngeal abscess management in children: current practices. Otolaryngol Head Neck Surg 1999;121:398.

▶ Disorders & Diseases

A. Oral Cavity Lesions

Inspection and palpation of the oral cavity is an essential part of the head and neck examination. Numerous types of lesions may affect the oral cavity, and this review focuses on those which may predispose patients to oral cavity neoplasms. Approximately half of all head and neck cancers occur in the oral cavity.

Leukoplakia is actually a descriptive term rather than a true pathologic term. It represents an asymptomatic white plaque that cannot be scraped off. It is frequently found on the oral and buccal mucosa as well as the tongue. Its prevalence has been estimated at 1–5% of the population. Some studies have linked leukoplakia to tobacco use, although the true etiology is still uncertain. Leukoplakia represents the clinically evident result of hyperplastic epithelial growth. Many authors recommend a short, 1–2 week trial of oral topical steroid preparation (Kenalog in Orabase) for initial management. Leukoplakia is associated with a malignant transformation rate of approximately 5%, and persistent lesions should be biopsied to assess for premalignant dysplasia or malignancy. The rates of dysplasia are highest for lesions found on the floor of mouth, tongue, and lower lip. Treatment is aimed at preventing malignant transforma-

tion to oral cavity squamous cell carcinoma (OCSCC). Surgical excision, KTP (K [potassium] titanyl phosphate) laser, and CO_2 laser excision have all been shown to be effective. Recent studies have also revealed potential efficacy of medical treatment with both topical bleomycin in dimethyl sulfoxide and retinoid compounds.

Erythroplakia is categorized as a nonhomogenous leukoplakia and is described as a velvety red plaque that cannot be removed. It is found in similar regions of the oral cavity as leukoplakia and is also usually asymptomatic at presentation. It is less common than traditional homogenous white leukoplakia with a prevalence estimated at 0.2%–0.8%. However, it has a higher degree of premalignant dysplasia than leukoplakia, with over half of cases having in situ or overtly invasive squamous cell carcinoma on histologic examination.

Lichen planus is a common dermatologic lesion that may present in the oral cavity. The skin lesions are classically described as pruritic, planar, purple, polygonal papules, while the oral lesions have several different phenotypic subtypes. Reticular, plaquelike, atrophic, erosive, and bullous forms are all described in the literature. The oral lesions have a questionable capacity for malignant transformation. The data is controversial, but one study estimated the rate of malignant transformation to OCSCC between 1% and 5%. The lesions require biopsy to confirm the diagnosis. Treatment includes vigorous oral hygiene, topical steroids, and immunosuppressive agents.

Greer RO: Pathology of malignant and premalignant oral epithelial lesions. Otolaryngol Clin North Am 2006;39:249.

B. Sialadenitis & Sialolithiasis

There are several nonneoplastic and inflammatory conditions that may affect the major and minor salivary glands. Infection of the salivary glands may be either viral or bacterial in etiology. Viral sialadenitis is most commonly secondary to mumps, which presents with a flulike prodrome followed by parotid gland swelling. Mumps normally affects children and may be complicated by orchitis, oophoritis, aseptic meningitis, and encephalitis. The incidence of mumps has declined significantly since routine vaccination has been instituted. Other viruses known to cause sialadenitis include cytomegalovirus, coxsackievirus A and B, echovirus, Epstein-Barr virus, and influenza A.

Bacterial sialadenitis may be acute or chronic. Acute suppurative sialadenitis occurs most commonly in dehydrated patients who are postoperative, elderly, or on diuretic therapy. The parotid gland is affected in most cases secondary to the diminished bacteriostatic activity of its serous saliva. Salivary stasis, ductal obstruction, and decreased saliva production appear to be predisposing conditions to acute sialadenitis. Patients usually present with fever, systemic toxicity, and tender swelling and enlargement of the affected glands. The most common organism isolated is

S aureus, though culture may reveal a polymicrobial infection with both aerobic and anaerobic organisms. Treatment involves ample hydration, warm facial compresses, and sialogogues (such as lemon wedges) to stimulate saliva secretion in the affected gland. Antibiotics targeted against *S aureus* should be started immediately and continued for 7–10 days. CT may be necessary to rule out abscess formation or stone (sialolithiasis) in patients who do not improve clinically after several days of appropriate therapy.

Sialolithiasis may occur in the setting of acute or chronic sialadenitis, or it may be an incidental finding on routine imaging studies. Salivary calculi affect males more than females and are seen most frequently between ages 30 and 60. In contrast to sialadenitis, sialolithiasis preferentially affects the submandibular glands because of their alkaline, high-calcium, mucus-rich environment. Large, solitary, radiopaque stones are usually found in the submandibular glands, while the parotid glands are more likely to have multiple smaller, radiolucent stones. Calculus formation is believed to be secondary to partial obstruction of the salivary duct combined with calcium-rich stagnant saliva. Salts composed of calcium phosphate, magnesium, ammonium, and carbonate precipitate in this environment. Contributing factors to the development of salivary calculi include underlying acute or chronic sialadenitis, dehydration, and anticholinergic medications. Uric acid salivary calculi may also be seen in the setting of gout.

Patients with sialolithiasis frequently present with pain and swelling of the affected gland, although many patients have asymptomatic calculi discovered incidentally. The pain is usually exacerbated by eating. Physical examination may reveal the location of the calculi by simple palpation. Obstruction of the flow of saliva can be analyzed by massaging the gland. It is important to note that stones are more commonly found in the salivary ductal structures than in their associated glands. CT is the preferred method of imaging if sialolithiasis is suspected, but a calculus is unable to be palpated on physical examination. CT has a 10-fold greater sensitivity than plain films in detecting salivary calculi. Ultrasound may also have benefit in locating calculi when CT is unavailable. Sialography is no longer routinely used and is contraindicated in patients with acute sialadenitis.

Treatment of sialolithiasis should begin conservatively with hydration, salivary gland massage, heating pads applied to the affected gland, and sialogogues. Anticholinergic medications should be discontinued and antibiotics should be initiated if there is concern for acute suppurative sialadenitis. There are several options for more invasive therapy for patients who do not respond to conservative management. Transoral removal of submandibular stones, sialadenectomy, lithotripsy, wire-basket removal, and sialoendoscopy have all been shown to be effective in the appropriate patient.

Brook I: Diagnosis and management of parotitis. Arch Otolaryngol Head Neck Surg 1992;118:469.

C. Acute & Chronic (Recurrent) Tonsillitis

Tonsillitis is one of the most common problems encountered by the otolaryngologist. In general, tonsillitis refers to inflammation of the palatine tonsils located on the lateral walls of the oropharynx between the palatoglossal and palatopharyngeal folds. The pharyngeal tonsils or adenoids, while part of the Waldeyer ring of lymphatic tissue are anatomically separate from the palatine tonsils. The adenoids are located on the posterior wall of the nasopharynx in close proximity to the eustachian tube opening.

Acute tonsillitis is primarily a pediatric disease that tends to affect children aged 5–15. It is most commonly caused by group A beta-hemolytic streptococcal species, although anaerobes, *Haemophilus influenzae*, and viruses can also be causative agents. Patients usually present with fever, painful sore throat, halitosis, and dysphagia. It is important to note the distinctions in clinical presentation of acute tonsillitis, viral pharyngitis, and infectious mononucleosis (caused by the Epstein-Barr virus). Viral pharyngitis commonly presents with a triad of cough, coryza, and conjunctivitis, while patients with mononucleosis typically present with anterior and posterior cervical lymphadenopathy, odynophagia, and a grayish tonsillar exudate. On physical examination, the acute tonsillitis patient has erythematous tonsils, purulent tonsillar exudate, and anterior cervical lymphadenopathy.

Tonsillar hyperplasia is measured in the medial-to-lateral plane of the oropharynx and helps in the assessment of upper airway obstruction. It is traditionally rated on a 1–4 scale, with 1+ being confined below the level of the tonsillar pillars, 2+ at the pillars, 3+ extending past the pillars, and 4+ meeting in the midline. Tonsillar hypertrophy in the pediatric population may predispose to the development of sleep disordered breathing. Patients typically present with heroic snoring, voice changes, observed episodes of sleep apnea, and daytime somnolence. In these cases, elective tonsillectomy (usually combined with adenoidectomy) can often provide resolution of obstructive symptoms.

The diagnosis of acute tonsillitis is clinical, although many practitioners rely on a positive streptococcal test or culture. The mainstay in treatment of acute tonsillitis continues to be a 7–10 day course of penicillin or a comparable cephalosporin. However, it is now estimated that failure with penicillin therapy occurs in up to 30% of cases. Following up culture results and adjusting the antibiotic therapy has therefore become an important step in management. Complications from acute tonsillitis include the formation of peritonsillar abscess and neck abscess. Antibiotic use has greatly decreased the incidence of rarer systemic complications like poststreptococcal glomerulonephritis and rheumatic fever.

Many patients have a solitary episode of acute tonsillitis that responds favorably to antibiotic treatment, while some patients have recurrent acute tonsillitis with multiple infections over the course of years. Chronic tonsillitis is a state of persistent tonsillar inflammation for more than 3 months following an episode of acute infection. It is characterized by chronic sore throat and odynophagia with tonsillar enlargement, tonsillolithic debris, and cervical lymphadenitis present on physical examination. Recent studies have suggested that polymicrobial infections, drug-resistant organisms, *H influenzae, S aureus,* anaerobes, and actinomycetes may play a role in chronic tonsillar disease. Treatment of chronic tonsillitis, therefore, should begin with the use of broader spectrum antibiotics like amoxicillin-clavulanate or clindamycin, which may target these offending organisms.

The critical question in the treatment of both acute and chronic tonsillitis is whether or not to perform a tonsillectomy. Medical management with antibiotics is always the first-line therapy for acute tonsillitis. Tonsillectomy for acute episodes (Quincy tonsillectomy) is usually considered only when complications such as deep neck-space abscess or acute airway obstruction are concurrently present. Tonsillectomy is generally performed for patients with recurrent acute tonsillitis, defined as 7 episodes within 1 year, 5 episodes each year for the past 2 years, or 3 episodes per year for 3 successive years.

Smith SL, Pereira KD: Tonsillectomy in children: indications, diagnosis and complications. ORL J Otorhinolaryngol Relat Spec 2007;69:336.

D. Obstructive Sleep Apnea

Obstructive sleep apnea is an intrinsic dyssomnia that affects roughly 15–20 million people in the United States. It is classically described as the presence of hypopneic episodes, apneic episodes, and respiratory effort–related arousals that occur during sleep. An apneic event requires 10 or more seconds of cessation of airflow, followed by arousal with restoration of normal ventilation. The definition of hypopnea varies among sleep laboratories but generally refers to an episode of decreased airflow (> 50% reduction) for longer than 10 seconds, associated with decreased oxygen saturation or arousal. Patients usually present with nighttime snoring, daytime hypersomnolence, irritability, morning headaches, cognitive impairment, and often witnessed apneic events with cessation of airflow followed by choking or gasping. When taking a history, it is important to confer with the patient's bed partner because the patient may be unaware of his or her nighttime symptoms. Cardiovascular disease, hypertension, metabolic dysfunction, respiratory failure, and cor pulmonale are among the serious long-term effects of obstructive sleep apnea.

The pathophysiology of obstructive sleep apnea appears to be a combination of upper airway collapse and decreased neural output from the respiratory center in the brainstem. During normal inspiration, the pharyngeal muscles are stimulated via a central nervous system reflex pathway to help maintain pharyngeal airway patency. During sleep, however, these neural reflexes are attenuated, and the airway becomes more susceptible to collapse. Patients who are predisposed to airway obstruction due to anatomic reasons are at high risk

for developing obstructive sleep apnea. Documented anatomic risk factors for obstructive sleep apnea include macroglossia, adenotonsillar hypertrophy, elongation of the soft palate, and retrognathia.

Obstructive sleep apnea is more common in men, and the overall incidence appears to increase with age. The most significant risk factor is obesity, and the recent increase in prevalence is thought to be related to the current obesity epidemic. Other known risk factors include nasal obstruction, smoking, diabetes mellitus, alcohol consumption, and the previously mentioned anatomic abnormalities. Physical examination may reveal obesity with an increased neck circumference. A thorough head and neck examination should be performed to fully assess airway patency. Oral cavity examination may reveal tonsillar hyperplasia. The nasal cavity and nasopharynx should be examined using a flexible fiberoptic endoscope to rule out nasal obstruction secondary to deviated septum, nasal polyps, or turbinate hyperplasia. The modified Müller maneuver should be performed to assess for site of upper airway collapse during inspiration. Patients are asked to inspire against a closed mouth while their nose is pinched shut, thus creating a column of negative pressure within the upper airway. The airway at the level of the soft palate, lateral pharyngeal wall, and base of tongue are then observed for luminal collapse and graded on a 1–3 scale.

Polysomnography remains the gold standard in diagnosing obstructive sleep apnea, which can be defined by either the apnea-hypopnea index (AHI) or the respiratory disturbance index (RDI). The AHI includes the number of hypopnea and apnea episodes that occur per hour of sleep, while RDI is the number of hypopnea and apnea episodes and respiratory effort–related arousals per hour of sleep. The generally accepted guidelines for diagnosis of obstructive sleep apnea are an AHI of 15 or greater in an asymptomatic patient or an AHI of greater than 5 in a symptomatic patient. Imaging studies are usually not required to diagnose obstructive sleep apnea, although they may help assess for upper airway anatomic abnormalities.

Treatment of obstructive sleep apnea should begin with the identification and prevention of risk factors. Behavior modifications such as weight loss, smoking and alcohol cessation, and discontinuation of any central nervous system depressants may help improve the patient's apneic index. Safety precautions related to daytime hypersomnolence need to be discussed for high-risk patients like pilots and commercial truck drivers.

Continuous positive airway pressure (CPAP) is considered first-line therapy after behavioral modifications. The positive pressure helps keep the airway patent and has been shown to be highly effective in reducing obstructive sleep apnea symptoms. Some patients experience difficulty tolerating CPAP therapy. Breathing against the positive pressure airflow can be difficult to adjust to, and this difficulty must be considered when treating the obstructive sleep apnea patient. Bilevel positive airway pressure (BiPAP) is another system that employs a higher inspiratory pressure with a lower expiratory pressure to allow for easier expiration. There are numerous oral appliances that may help adjust the airway during sleep to improve patency, although studies have shown these appliances to be less effective than CPAP in improving the apneic index.

Several surgical options are available for patients who do not respond well to initial treatment. Routine adenoidectomy and tonsillectomy has been shown to be effective in pediatric patients with isolated adenotonsillar hypertrophy contributing to their obstructive sleep apnea symptoms. For adult patients, more extensive surgery is usually required. Uvulopalatopharyngoplasty (UP3) is the first-line surgical therapy in which the uvula, a small amount of soft palate, and the palatine tonsils are removed. The concept of "multilevel sleep surgery" is important, as UP3 alone is associated with a significant (> 50%) failure rate. Most commonly, UP3 is combined with additional procedures to address other areas of obstruction. Septoplasty and inferior turbinate reduction can improve nasal airflow. The tongue base can be advanced by suture suspension, hyoid suspension, or genioglossus advancement. Other more invasive surgical interventions include maxillomandibular advancement. Some authors advocate less invasive therapy, including palatal stiffening implants and radiofrequency ablation, but long-term data is lacking. Life-threatening obstructive sleep apnea that does not respond to CPAP/BiPAP or surgical intervention may require permanent tracheostomy. A repeat polysomnography should be performed in surgical patients 1–3 months postoperatively to monitor for improvements.

Lin HC et al: The efficacy of multilevel surgery of the upper airway in adults with obstructive sleep apnea/hypopnea syndrome. Laryngoscope 2008;118:902.

Terris DJ et al: Reliability of the Müller maneuver and its association with sleep-disordered breathing. Laryngoscope 2000;110:1819.

DISORDERS OF THE LARYNX & TRACHEA

▶ Anatomy & Physiology

The anatomy of the larynx (Figures 15–7 and 15–8) is best understood in the context of its function. The primary function of the larynx is to protect the airway from aspiration during swallowing. The epiglottis and aryepiglottic folds help direct food and liquids laterally into the pyriform sinuses and away from the midline laryngeal inlet. The paired arytenoid cartilages act as attachment points for most of the intrinsic muscles of the larynx, serving to move the vocal folds together (adduction) and apart (abduction). The false vocal folds and true vocal folds adduct to prevent entry of food or liquids into the airway.

The larynx also functions in respiration. Owing to reflex pathways in the brainstem, the glottis opens just prior to inspiration. Other laryngeal reflexes respond to subglottic

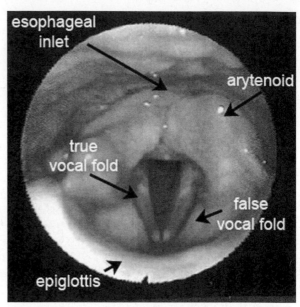

▲ **Figure 15–7.** Internal anatomy of the larynx as seen on endoscopy.

pressure and hypercapnia. Additionally, initiation of swallowing causes a reflex period of involuntary apnea.

Phonation is the most uniquely human of the three functions of the larynx. At its most basic description, the glottic

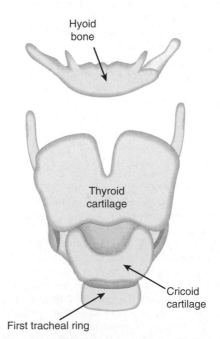

▲ **Figure 15–8.** Cartilaginous and bony laryngeal framework.

larynx produces a fundamental tone by the vibration of the free edge of the true vocal folds. This vibration is due to passive vibration of the vocal folds from air moving past the opposed free edges. Changing the tension within the vocal fold changes the pitch at which the vocal fold vibrates.

Several cartilages comprise the framework of the larynx (Figure 15–8). The thyroid cartilage is the largest laryngeal cartilage. This shield-shaped cartilage is responsible for the anterior neck prominence, sometimes called the "Adam's apple" in lay terminology, and it provides protection to the internal components of the larynx. The cricoid cartilage lies inferior to the thyroid cartilage and serves as the major support for the larynx. It is the only complete cartilaginous ring within the upper airway. Internally, the paired arytenoid cartilages articulate with the cricoid cartilage and attach to the vocal folds. Movement of the arytenoids results in abduction or adduction of the vocal folds. The epiglottis is a flexible cartilage located above the larynx. It is not involved in structural support of the larynx but assists in protecting the airway during deglutition (swallowing).

Innervation to the larynx is provided by the vagus nerve (tenth cranial nerve). The vagus nerve originates from three nuclei located within the medulla: the nucleus ambiguous, the dorsal nucleus, and the solitary tract nucleus. All motor fibers (and thus laryngeal motor innervation) originate from the nucleus ambiguous. The dorsal (parasympathetic) nucleus is the origination for efferents to involuntary muscles of the bronchi, esophagus, heart, stomach, and intestine. Sensory innervation from the pharynx, larynx, and esophagus terminates in the solitary tract nucleus. The vagus nerve exits the skull base through the jugular foramen. It descends in the neck behind the jugular vein and carotid artery and sends pharyngeal branches to the muscles of the pharynx and soft palate. The superior laryngeal nerve arises directly from the vagus and has an internal and external branch. The internal superior laryngeal nerve enters the larynx through the thyrohyoid membrane and supplies sensation to the larynx above the true vocal cords. The external superior laryngeal nerve innervates the cricothyroid muscle, the only muscle of the larynx not innervated by the recurrent laryngeal nerve. The right recurrent laryngeal nerve arises from the vagus and loops around the subclavian artery. The left recurrent laryngeal nerve arises more distally in the thorax and loops around the aortic arch. Both recurrent laryngeal nerves then ascend in the tracheoesophageal grooves and enter the larynx near the cricothyroid joint. The recurrent laryngeal nerves provide motor innervation to all of the intrinsic muscles of the larynx except the cricothyroid. A summary of the laryngeal muscles is provided in Table 15–4.

Armstrong WB, Netterville JL: Anatomy of the larynx, trachea, and bronchi. Otolaryngol Clin North Am 1995;28:685.

Sasaki CT, Isaacson G: Functional anatomy of the larynx. Otolaryngol Clin North Am 1988;21:595.

Sataloff RT et al: Clinical anatomy and physiology of the voice. Otolaryngol Clin North Am 2007;40:909.

▶ **Urgencies & Emergencies**

A. Pediatric Airway Obstruction

The rapid and accurate evaluation of a child in respiratory distress is one of the most critical skills an otolaryngologist must master. Noisy breathing and respiratory distress have multiple etiologies, and differentiation between acute emergencies and chronic conditions is essential. An important point to learn early on is that not all noisy breathing is stridor.

True stridor may represent an impending airway failure and thus must be distinguished from other upper airway noises that are sometimes mistakenly referred to as stridor. Airway obstruction at the level of the nasopharynx produces snoring sounds, or stertor. Tracheobronchitis can produce a wheezy, barking cough characteristic of croup. Asthma, tracheobronchial foreign bodies, and bronchomalacia can produce wheezing. Stridor specifically refers to the noise produced by air movement through a partially obstructed airway. Inspiratory stridor usually signifies an obstruction above the level of the vocal cords, while expiratory stridor most often occurs with subglottic obstruction. Biphasic stridor usually signifies an obstruction at the level of the vocal cords or subglottis.

Table 15–4. Major Muscles of the Larynx.

Muscle	Function	Innervation	Key Point
Posterior cricoarytenoid	Abducts, tenses vocal folds	Recurrent laryngeal nerve	*Only* abductor of vocal folds
Lateral cricoarytenoid	Adducts true vocal folds	Recurrent laryngeal nerve	
Interarytenoid	Adducts posterior glottis	Recurrent laryngeal nerve	*Only* laryngeal muscle receiving bilateral innervation
Oblique arytenoids	Closes laryngeal inlet during swallowing	Recurrent laryngeal nerve	
Thyroarytenoid	Adducts, tenses vocal fold	Recurrent laryngeal nerve	
Cricothyroid	Increases vocal fold tension, especially at higher pitches	External branch of superior laryngeal nerve	*Only* muscle not innervated by recurrent laryngeal nerve

The immediate concern in evaluating a child with stridor is verifying or establishing a stable airway. The initial evaluation should consist of noninvasive examination to avoid exacerbating a potentially unstable airway. If the child is in acute respiratory distress, evaluations such as flexible fiberoptic laryngoscopy should not routinely be performed.

A careful history should be obtained, including the duration of the stridor and relationship to feedings. Parents should be questioned about any change in symptoms with position changes. Presence of any birth or intrauterine complications, history of intubation, as well as congenital anomalies should be determined.

If the child is not in acute distress, flexible fiberoptic laryngoscopy may provide valuable diagnostic information. This can be done with the child awake and restrained, or under general anesthesia with spontaneous ventilations. This allows determination of nasopharyngeal and supraglottic anatomy, as well as vocal cord motion. If recording equipment is available, the examination may be recorded to allow playback and review because real-time examination can be problematic in an often uncooperative child.

Other investigations should be based on the presence of suggestive symptoms. Swallowing function is often impaired in children with stridor and should be evaluated. Vascular rings may produce extrinsic compression of the esophagus and trachea leading to stridor, feeding difficulties, and failure to thrive. An altered, weak, or absent cry from birth can suggest neurologic impairment. Recurrent pneumonia or excessive cough with feeding may be present with vocal cord impairment, severe reflux, or tracheoesophageal fistula.

One of the most common causes of pediatric stridor is laryngotracheobronchitis, or croup, an acute viral illness most commonly caused by the parainfluenza virus. The typical patient is an infant or young child with low grade fever, seallike barking cough, and occasionally biphasic stridor. The classic radiographic finding is a "steeple" sign visible on AP views, indicative of the characteristic narrowed subglottic airway from edema. The typical course for most patients is resolution over several days, and few patients require hospitalization. Signs of respiratory distress, including tachypnea, retractions, and cyanosis, may necessitate closer observation such as hospitalization. For these more severe cases, treatment with humidified air, nebulized racemic epinephrine, and systemic steroids may be indicated. Manipulation of the airway may exacerbate the clinical situation and should be avoided unless clearly indicated.

Epiglottitis is fortunately becoming rare in most industrialized countries, owing to nearly universal vaccination of children against H influenzae type B. If recognized and managed appropriately (with aggressive airway control), outcomes are usually excellent. If managed conservatively, epiglottitis is associated with up to 6–10% mortality. Patients present with high fever, drooling, and odynophagia and are usually toxic in appearance. Of note, epiglottitis tends to progress quite rapidly; patients can decompensate clinically in a matter of hours. Patients with epiglottitis characteristically lean forward to maximize their marginal airway opening. Even oral cavity examination with a tongue blade can precipitate an airway crisis; therefore, evaluation and treatment ideally consists of immediate control of the airway in the operating room under general inhalational anesthesia. A cherry-red epiglottis will be visible on endoscopic exam. Pharyngeal and blood cultures should be obtained and the child started on broad spectrum intravenous antibiotics such as ceftriaxone. Once definitive identification of the culprit organism is made, antibiotic selection can be narrowed appropriately. Children are left intubated until air leak around the endotracheal tube is evident.

Chronic pediatric stridor is most often due to laryngomalacia. Parents will usually report onset of symptoms shortly after birth. It often worsens initially, but in the vast majority of cases, it resolves without the need for intervention, usually by 12–18 months. A variety of factors are hypothesized to contribute to laryngomalacia, including neurologic, muscular, and reflux-induced inflammation. The stridor is worsened while crying or in an excited state and is usually relieved by placement in the prone position. Flexible fiberoptic laryngoscopy reveals collapse of floppy supraglottic structures such as the epiglottis and aryepiglottic folds. There is a strong association of laryngomalacia with reflux, and presumptive treatment with an acid-blocking medication (such as ranitidine) may be beneficial. Surgical treatment of the supraglottis is reserved for severe cases such as patients with cyanosis or failure to thrive. The most common procedure is aryepiglottiplasty, where cold knife or carbon dioxide laser is used to excise redundant mucosa over the arytenoid cartilages. Rarely, tracheostomy may be necessary.

Subglottic stenosis is the second-most common cause of chronic pediatric stridor. It may be either congenital or acquired (most often from prolonged intubation). Typically, patients have recurrent "croup" and biphasic stridor. If present in older children, the patient may become symptomatic only periodically, in association with upper respiratory tract infections. Diagnosis requires endoscopic evaluation and can be defined as a subglottic airway diameter of less than 4 mm in full-term infants and less than 3 mm in premature infants. Pediatric subglottic stenosis is traditionally graded according to the Cotton scale (Table 15–5). Tracheotomy may be required in moderate to severe cases. Treatment of subglottic stenosis can consist of tracheal dilatation (either by rigid serial dilation or controlled radial expansion balloon), debridement by microdebrider or carbon dioxide laser, cricoid split, or laryngotracheoplasty.

Cotton RT, Richardson MA: Congenital laryngeal anomalies. Otolaryngol Clin North Am 1981;14:203.

Myer CM 3rd: Evaluation and management of stridor in the newborn. Clin Pediatr (Phila) 1993;32:511.

Myer CM 3rd et al: Proposed grading system for subglottic stenosis based on endotracheal tube sizes. Ann Otol Rhinol Laryngol 1994;103:319.

Table 15–5. Summary of the Cotton Grading System for Subglottic Stenosis.

Grade	Degree of subglottic obstruction
Grade 1	Less than 50% obstruction
Grade 2	50–70% obstruction
Grade 3	71–99% obstruction
Grade 4	100% obstruction

B. Foreign Body Aspiration

Airway foreign body typically involves children between 1 and 4 years of age but can occur in any age group. Children in this age range tend to place objects in their mouths and lack molars for grinding food. Objects can range from peanuts (most common) to coins, marbles, and toy products. Adult foreign body aspiration is usually associated with food, typically meat. Foreign body aspiration is potentially life threatening and is recognized as the fifth-most common cause of unintentional injury–related mortality in the United States. Pharyngeal foreign body (most commonly in the vallecula) represents a potential impending airway foreign body and should be treated as such.

The clinical presentation of patients with airway foreign body depends on the anatomic location. Patients with pharyngeal or hypopharyngeal foreign bodies typically present with dysphagia, odynophagia, and occasionally drooling from inability to tolerate secretions. If large objects become lodged in the larynx, patients may present with pain, dysphonia, inspiratory stridor, and dyspnea. Tracheal foreign bodies produce both inspiratory and expiratory stridor. Distally located foreign bodies (Figure 15–9) often lodge in the right bronchus (especially in adults) because of the angles at which the left and right mainstem bronchi branch off the trachea, with the right being a less acute angle. Distal foreign bodies typically produce unilateral wheezing and decreased breath sounds. A history of acute choking episode is very common and is 76–92% sensitive in diagnosing foreign body aspiration.

Acute management of airway foreign body is dictated by patient condition. In a conscious patient who is able to exchange air and cough, an attempt at foreign body removal should not be made immediately. Unconscious patients or victims unable to cough or move air require immediate intervention. If the means for performing a cricothyrotomy or tracheotomy are not available, the Heimlich maneuver can be performed as three manual abdominal thrusts to compress the lungs and potentially produce enough airway pressure to dislodge the foreign body. For patients without impending loss of airway, anteroposterior and lateral radiographs of the airway, including larynx and chest, can be helpful. While only radiopaque foreign bodies can be visualized, radiographs may demonstrate obstructive emphysema,

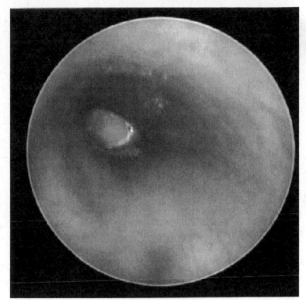

▲ **Figure 15–9.** Airway foreign body in a 4 year old. The patient in question had a history of brief choking while eating dinner three nights earlier, followed by intermittent nonproductive cough. He had a normal chest x-ray and slight wheezing heard on one side only. On rigid bronchoscopy, a soft green bean was found in a right distal bronchus.

atelectasis, or consolidation. Additionally, they can provide a baseline study for future comparison.

Definitive removal of an airway foreign body requires general anesthesia and direct laryngoscopy. Distally located foreign bodies are best addressed with rigid bronchoscopy for removal. A clear history consistent with aspiration often should prompt operative evaluation even if specific symptoms (stridor, unilateral wheezing, decreased breath sounds) are lacking, as these symptoms may be absent in up to 40% of cases. Suspected nut aspiration (common in children) should be treated aggressively. Local tissue reactions to the nut oils and proteins are common and can be robust. Postremoval, patients with peanut aspiration may require intensive care unit observation and ventilatory support while the inflammatory reaction resolves.

Zaytoun GM et al: Endoscopic management of foreign bodies in the tracheobronchial tree: predictive factors for complications. Otolaryngol Head Neck Surg 2000;123:311.
Zerella JT et al: Foreign body aspiration in children: value of radiography and complications of bronchoscopy. J Pediatr Surg 1998;33:1651.

C. Laryngeal Trauma

Laryngeal trauma is rare, representing 1 out of every 14,000–42,000 emergency room visits. Quick recognition of laryngeal trauma is essential because it can rapidly lead to death. Up to one third of laryngeal trauma victims die before reaching a hospital setting.

Laryngeal trauma can be classified as blunt or penetrating. Blunt laryngeal trauma results from crushing of the laryngeal framework against the cervical spine and usually results from motor vehicle accidents. Other common etiologies include strangulation type injuries and clothesline injuries. Penetrating laryngeal trauma usually results from projectile injury, such as a gunshot or knife wounds to the neck.

Every patient with trauma to the neck should be evaluated for potential laryngeal trauma. Patients may report dyspnea, hoarseness, or aphonia. Less common symptoms include dysphagia, anterior neck pain, and odynophagia. Evaluation should begin with the ABCs of trauma: airway, breathing, circulation. Severe laryngeal trauma (particularly clothesline-type injuries) can result in loss of airway and may necessitate immediate tracheotomy. Physical findings common in patients with laryngeal trauma include stridor, subcutaneous crepitus (emphysema), bruising or edema to the anterior neck, loss of palpable landmarks, and hemoptysis. As outlined in the section on pediatric airway obstruction, the type of stridor can often give an indication of the site of airflow obstruction.

Further evaluation of laryngeal trauma is dictated by the patient's condition. If an adult patient's airway is unstable, most experts advocate awake tracheostomy or cricothyrotomy under local anesthesia because endotracheal intubation in the setting of laryngeal trauma can be problematic. For unstable pediatric laryngeal trauma, inhalational anesthetic followed by rigid endoscopic intubation is recommended by many experts. Once a stable airway has been determined or secured, evaluation can proceed.

Flexible fiberoptic laryngoscopy is advocated for awake, stable patients. The airway should be evaluated for vocal cord mobility, edema, and laryngeal lacerations and hematomas. Because the underlying mechanism of injury often results in damage to other adjacent structures, laryngeal trauma patients should undergo complete cervical spine radiography, and evaluation for esophageal or vascular injury should be considered. Some authors recommend fine-cut CT imaging of the larynx to help guide treatment planning. CT scanning rarely provides useful information regarding the immediate airway management for patients suspected of having laryngeal trauma but often provide helpful information regarding surgical planning for repair.

Management of the patient with laryngeal trauma depends on the severity of injury. Patients with small laryngeal hematomas, small lacerations not involving the vocal fold edge or anterior commissure, and nondisplaced stable thyroid cartilage fractures can often be managed without tracheostomy. Most such patients should be hospitalized for 24 hours of airway observation and placed on systemic steroids, humidified air, and proton pump inhibitor (PPI) therapy. If mucosal disruption is present, antibiotics should be initiated.

More severe laryngeal traumas often require tracheotomy and direct laryngoscopy or even open laryngeal exploration and repair. This should ideally be performed within 24 hours of the initial injury. Open laryngeal exploration is performed via a midline thyrotomy approach. A horizontal skin incision is made at the level of the cricothyroid membrane. Subplatysmal flaps are elevated, and the strap muscles are divided at the midline. The airway is then entered in the midline of the cricothyroid membrane, and a vertical incision through the midline thyroid cartilage extended superiorly. Care must be taken to avoid injury to the underlying endolaryngeal mucosa. The mucosa is then incised, allowing inspection of the endolarynx. Once the endolarynx is exposed, all mucosal lacerations should be repaired to cover all exposed cartilage. If the anterior commissure is disrupted, a laryngeal stent may need to be placed, although placement of a stent itself leads to some degree of laryngeal injury. If placed, stents should be removed as soon as possible, usually around 2 weeks.

Outcomes for laryngeal trauma patients are fairly good once initial control of the airway is obtained. Most patients usually achieve a stable airway and undergo decannulation, which may take 1–6 months or longer depending on the extent of injury. Overall, greater than 90% of patients will recover a satisfactory vocal quality if managed appropriately.

Hwang SY, Yeak SC: Management dilemmas in laryngeal trauma. J Laryngol Otol 2004;118:325.

Kennedy KS, Harley EH: Diagnosis and treatment of acute laryngeal trauma. Ear Nose Throat J 1988;67:584.

Schaefer SD: The acute management of external laryngeal trauma. A 27-year experience. Arch Otolaryngol Head Neck Surg 1992;118:598.

▶ Disorders & Diseases

A. Hoarseness

Hoarseness or dysphonia is an alteration in the quality or character of phonation. Patients may describe their voice as breathy, harsh, or rough. Common etiologies of hoarseness include viral illness, vocal fold paralysis, laryngopharyngeal reflux, laryngeal polyps, allergy, vocal abuse, dysplasia, and cancer.

Patients should be questioned about onset, frequency, and nature of the hoarseness. As previously discussed, the larynx is an essential part of swallowing, and any history of coughing or choking after eating should be elicited. Likewise, the patient should be questioned about recurrent episodes of pneumonia. Any history of intubation, head and neck trauma, or previous head and neck surgery should be sought. Patients should be questioned about smoking and alcohol use.

Physical examination begins with a full head and neck examination. It is important to visualize the larynx. Methods of visualization include indirect mirror exam, rigid endoscopy, or transnasal flexible fiberoptic laryngoscopy. Videostroboscopy offers invaluable information about vocal fold motion and can identify adynamic segments and altered areas of mucosal wave propagation.

One common benign cause of hoarseness is vocal polyps, which are due to local tissue inflammation. Vocal nodules are distinct from polyps and always occur bilaterally. They are most often a result of vocal abuse or misuse and usually respond dramatically to voice therapy. Vocal fold granulomas are usually due to extraesophageal acid reflux damage.

Hoarseness can also be the presenting symptom for cancer, most often for cancer of the true vocal folds. The vast majority of laryngeal cancer is squamous cell cancer, and smoking is the biggest risk factor for its development. Laryngeal cancer is discussed further in the section head and neck cancer. While early-stage laryngeal cancer is highly curable, advanced stage carries a dramatically reduced prognosis. Thus, any patient with hoarseness lasting longer than 2 weeks should be evaluated and undergo visualization of their larynx.

Koufman JA: The otolaryngologic manifestations of gastroesophageal reflux disease (GERD): a clinical investigation of 225 patients using ambulatory 24-hour pH monitoring and an experimental investigation of the role of acid and pepsin in the development of laryngeal injury. Laryngoscope 1991;101(4 Pt 2 Suppl 53):1.
Sataloff RT et al: Clinical anatomy and physiology of the voice. Otolaryngol Clin North Am 2007;40:909.

B. Laryngopharyngeal Reflux

Laryngopharyngeal reflux (LPR) impacts hundreds of thousands of patients annually, with some studies estimating as many as 30% of Americans may suffer from some degree of LPR. It is increasingly clear that LPR is a disease separate and distinct from classic gastroesophageal reflux (GERD). Patients with LPR typically present with frequent throat clearing, globus sensation, cough and hoarseness (as opposed to postprandial heartburn with GERD).

Physical examination of patients suspected of having LPR should include an examination of the larynx, most commonly by flexible transnasal fiberoptic laryngoscopy. Hoarseness is not pathognomonic for LPR and can also be present in more serious disorders. Several laryngeal findings are common in patients with LPR. Presence of vocal cord granuloma or pseudosulcus vocalis, although uncommon, are highly suggestive of LPR. Other common laryngoscopic findings consistent with LPR include posterior laryngeal hypertrophy, laryngeal edema and erythema, cobblestoning, or posterior commissure bar.

The diagnosis of LPR relies on a combination of symptoms and physical findings rather than one isolated factor being pathognomonic. Several studies have demonstrated the presence of many of the above symptoms and laryngeal findings in healthy, normal control patients. Many clinicians advocate the use of a metric scale that combines multiple common symptoms or physical findings. Two such instruments are the reflux finding score (RFS) and the reflux symptom index (RSI). In general, an RFS of greater than 8

suggests LPR, and a score of greater than 13 on the RSI likewise indicates LPR.

Treatment for laryngopharyngeal reflux currently consists of PPIs as a first-line therapy with surgery (eg, Nissen fundoplication) for selected treatment failures. Although multiple uncontrolled studies have demonstrated benefit of PPIs for the treatment of LPR, the majority of randomized controlled trials have failed to confirm this. Possible confounding factors include lack of a clear gold standard for the diagnosis of LPR and differing treatment regimens. Our current practice is to place patients with LPR on once-daily PPI therapy for 3–6 months, after which response to treatment is assessed. The extended length of time is critical, as studies have shown that resolution of laryngeal findings can take up to 6 months to resolve once PPI therapy is initiated. If there is no response to once-daily PPI therapy, the patient can be advanced to twice-daily PPI therapy. Disease severity can prompt initiation of PPI therapy at twice-daily dosing; severe laryngeal edema or presence of subglottic stenosis would be two such indications.

If a patient is diagnosed with LPR, some form of evaluation of the esophagus should be undertaken. There is up to a 20% incidence of unsuspected esophageal abnormalities in patients with LPR. This evaluation can take the form of imaging modalities such as barium swallow or endoscopic examination such as esophagoscopy.

Belafsky PC et al: The validity and reliability of the reflux finding score (RFS). Laryngoscope 2001;111:1313.
Belafsky PC et al: Validity and reliability of the reflux symptom index (RSI). J Voice 2002;16:274.
Koufman JA: The otolaryngologic manifestations of gastroesophageal reflux disease (GERD): a clinical investigation of 225 patients using ambulatory 24-hour pH monitoring and an experimental investigation of the role of acid and pepsin in the development of laryngeal injury. Laryngoscope 1991;101(4 Pt 2 Suppl 53):1.

C. Vocal Cord Immobility & Paralysis

Vocal cord mobility problems represent a wide range of etiologies characterized by diverse patient presentation and prognostic outcomes. The distinction between unilateral and bilateral and between paretic (hypomobile) and paralyzed cords is imperative.

Patients with unilateral vocal cord paralysis may be asymptomatic but often present with a hoarse, breathy voice. Their voice often starts out stronger in the morning and worsens throughout the day as they develop vocal fatigue. Accompanying symptoms can include frequent throat clearing, cough, vague globus sensation, and aspiration. Often, patients will report subjective shortness of breath or a feeling of "running out of air" despite normal pulmonary function. This is secondary to glottal incompetence (lack of apposition of the vocal folds) resulting in escaped air during phonation. Thus, a patient with unilateral vocal fold paralysis may be able to climb a flight of stairs without difficulty yet feel short of breath when attempting to carry on a telephone conversation.

Patients should be questioned specifically about swallowing, weight loss, recent illnesses or intubations, and surgeries (especially cardiac, cervical spine, and thyroid procedures).

The etiologies of vocal cord paralysis reflect the diverse nature of illnesses and injuries that can result in the final common pathway of vocal cord immobility or paralysis. The vocal cords derive their innervation from the vagus nerve, and any injury along the course of this nerve may result in vocal cord paralysis. Unilateral vocal cord paresis is by far the most common, with bilateral representing less than 20% of all paralysis. Historically, the most common cause of unilateral vocal cord paralysis was malignancy (such as lung cancer or skull base tumors). More recent studies show that iatrogenic surgical injury is now the most common cause. Non-thyroid surgical procedures (including anterior approaches to the cervical spine and carotid endarterectomy) now account for the majority of these iatrogenic injuries. Thyroid surgery remains the most common cause of bilateral vocal cord paralysis. Table 15–6 summarizes the most common causes of vocal fold paralysis. Laryngeal manifestations of rheumatoid arthritis can rarely mimic vocal cord paralysis, although the underlying problem in this case is vocal cord immobility secondary to fixation of the arytenoid cartilages.

Vocal cord immobility or paralysis is a *sign of pathology* and not a diagnosis. Thus, the first concern when evaluating a patient with vocal cord paralysis should be investigation of the etiology. Often, the cause is not identifiable, and the vocal cord paralysis is deemed idiopathic. A thorough head and neck examination should be performed, including endoscopic evaluation of the larynx. This most often is by flexible fiberoptic laryngoscopy, with most laryngologists recommending videostroboscopy as well. For unilateral recurrent laryngeal nerve injury, the affected immobile cord will usually lie in a paramedian position because of lack of abduction, with some retained adduction (due to the cricothyroid muscle, which is innervated by the superior laryngeal nerve). For more proximal vagal lesions, the affected cord will usually rest in intermediate position because of loss of both abduction and adduction innervation. There is also loss of sensation to the affected hemilarynx, and aspiration is common.

Diagnostic testing should include a chest radiograph and CT scan following the entire vagus nerve course (ie, neck and chest, from skull base to the midchest). More esoteric tests are likely to be low yield and poorly cost-effective, and should be reserved for more selective use. Many laryngologists advocate the use of laryngeal EMG. This test is performed percutaneously and tests the superior laryngeal nerve and recurrent laryngeal nerve by evaluating motor unit electrical activity in the cricothyroid and thyroarytenoid muscles respectively. Laryngeal EMG can provide useful information regarding the degree and likely site of injury (central versus peripheral), as well as the potential for spontaneous recovery. It is most predictive if performed 6 weeks to 6 months after initial injury.

Initial therapy for unilateral vocal cord paralysis consists of observation and speech therapy. Often, the opposing vocal cord can compensate by crossing the midline and closing the glottal gap. This can produce an acceptable vocal quality, usually occurring within 3–6 months. Patients not obtaining a good result using these conservative measures can be treated by a variety of surgical interventions. The goal of surgical treatment for unilateral vocal cord paralysis is medialization of the affected cord. This reduces the glottic gap and allows the opposing, innervated cord to contact the other vocal fold with less effort. Treatment selection for unilateral vocal cord paralysis depends on the potential for recovery. In cases such as iatrogenic surgical injury with little chance of spontaneous recovery, definitive therapy can be initiated early. For idiopathic causes, a more conservative approach is usually advocated. Overall, up to 60% of patients with idiopathic unilateral vocal cord paralysis will recover to a near-normal voice within 8–12 months. Thus, most experts recommend waiting at least 1 year before proceeding with definitive therapy. Clear indications for earlier intervention include significant dysphagia and aspiration from glottic incompetence.

Definitive surgical procedures for unilateral vocal fold paralysis include laryngeal framework surgery, injection of longer-lasting material, and reinnervation techniques. The thyroplasty technique (a laryngeal framework surgical procedure) is performed through an external skin incision. After exposing the thyroid cartilage, a window is cut in the thyroid ala overlying the position of the vocal fold on the affected side. An implant is then placed in a subperichondrial win-

Table 15–6. Most Common Causes of Vocal Cord Paralysis.

Unilateral vocal cord paralysis	
Surgical injury	37%
Cardiovascular, anterior cervical spine procedures	(51%)
Thyroid surgery	(33%)
Idiopathic (viral, inflammatory)	19%
Malignancy	18%
Intubation-related injury	6%
Trauma	6%
Bilateral vocal cord paralysis	
Surgical injury	37%
Cardiovascular, anterior cervical spine procedures	(10%)
Thyroid/parathyroid surgery	(90%)
Malignancy	14%
Intubation	13%
Idiopathic (viral, inflammatory)	11%
Neurologic (Wallenberg syndrome, Parkinson disease, multiple sclerosis, Guillain-Barré syndrome, others)	11%
Trauma	7%

dow, thus pushing the vocal fold toward the midline. Implants can include Silastic, autologous cartilage, and Gore-Tex. Most laryngologists perform this procedure with the patient lightly sedated. A flexible fiberoptic laryngoscope can be suspended in position, and the patient is asked to phonate periodically so that the surgical effects can be evaluated in real time and adjusted accordingly.

Another common surgical intervention is injection medialization. This can be performed as an office-based procedure using only local anesthesia or in the operating room under general anesthesia. In either case, a variety of injectable materials are placed within the vocal fold lateral to the vocal process to medialize the cord. In the past, Teflon was commonly used for this purpose, but it has now largely fallen out of favor secondary to a high rate of complications. An alternative, long-lasting (but not permanent) injectable is calcium hydroxyapatite microspheres in methylcarboxycellulose carrier gel (RADIESSE Voice). Temporary injectables include Gelfoam paste, hyaluronic acid, micronized cadaveric dermis (Cymetra), crosslinked collagen (Zyderm), and methylcarboxycellulose gel (RADIESSE Voice Gel).

Surgical reinnervation for unilateral vocal cord paralysis is gaining utilization. Approaches can include nerve-muscle pedicle (using the omohyoid and ansa hypoglossi nerve) and direct nerve-nerve reinnervation (ansa cervicalis to recurrent laryngeal nerve). Results from these techniques are generally good but can take 6 months or longer to be realized. Many surgeons therefore combine reinnervation with injection medialization using a temporary substance.

For bilateral vocal cord paralysis, treatment approaches have a different perspective. Whereas restoration of voice is the primary goal for unilateral paralysis, resolution of potential or actual airway compromise is of tantamount importance in cases of bilateral paralysis. Most patients are initially treated with a tracheotomy to bypass the glottic obstruction. One common surgical procedure is lateralization of the vocal folds by arytenoidectomy. While this procedure usually provides a patent airway and allows decannulation (reversal of the tracheotomy), the patient's vocal quality usually suffers significantly.

Another surgical approach, partial posterior cordectomy, can often preserve vocal quality to some degree, while providing improved airway. This approach uses a laser through a surgical laryngoscope to remove a C-shaped wedge from the posterior portion of one vocal cord. This preserves a bilateral vibratory margin anteriorly while providing an airway posteriorly. The technique is often best performed as multiple, less-aggressive procedures to fine tune vocal quality versus airway rather than as a single definitive procedure.

Koufman JA et al: Diagnostic laryngeal electromyography: The Wake Forest experience 1995–1999. Otolaryngol Head Neck Surg 2001;124:603.

Rosenthal LH et al: Vocal fold immobility: a longitudinal analysis of etiology over 20 years. Laryngoscope 2007;117:1864.

Terris DJ et al: Contemporary evaluation of unilateral vocal cord paralysis. Otolaryngol Head Neck Surg 1992;107:84.

D. Recurrent Respiratory Papillomatosis

Recurrent respiratory papillomatosis is caused by the HPV, specifically types 6 and 11. HPV is a small, nonenveloped virus that infects the nuclei of host cells for replication. Papillomaviruses show a preference for infection of epithelial tissues and are very common in humans. HPV is responsible for a variety of disease, including skin warts, recurrent respiratory papillomatosis, and invasive cancers such as cervical or oropharyngeal carcinoma. Transmission is hypothesized to involve vertical transmission during childbirth; maternal presence of condylomata during the perinatal period confers a 200-fold increase in relative risk for developing respiratory papillomatosis.

Benign, recurrent hyperplastic tissue growth of the upper airway characterizes this disease. It has a bimodal age distribution, with incidence peaks in children (infants to 12 years old) and in adults (30–40 years old). Patients typically present with dysphonia or aphonia, although advanced disease can cause stridor from impending airway obstruction.

The primary site affected is the larynx, with the glottis being the most common area followed by the supraglottic larynx (Figure 15–10). Respiratory papillomatosis generally remains confined to the larynx but can spread distally to affect the trachea, bronchi, and lungs. Disease recurrence is frequent, and reports of children requiring more than 100 surgical procedures are not uncommon.

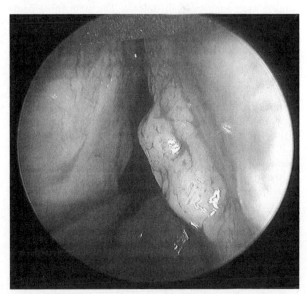

▲ **Figure 15–10.** Adult recurrent respiratory papillomatosis. The right true vocal fold is involved with respiratory papillomatosis. In this patient, the disease was confined mostly to the single true vocal fold, although some disease was also present in the anterior portion of the contralateral vocal fold.

The primary therapy for respiratory papillomatosis remains surgical debulking, primarily by microdebrider or carbon dioxide laser ablation. Adjuvant medical treatments include cidofovir, indole-3-carbinol, ribavirin, mumps vaccine, and photodynamic therapy. The role for these adjuvant therapies in the treatment of respiratory papillomatosis is still being elucidated. Many otolaryngologists advocate avoidance of tracheotomy if possible, because this has been epidemiologically associated with increased risk of spread of papillomas to the lower respiratory tract. It is possible this is because patients with inherently more aggressive disease are also those who are more likely to require tracheostomy.

Goon P et al: Recurrent respiratory papillomatosis: an overview of current thinking and treatment. Eur Arch Otorhinolaryngol 2007;265:147.

Silverberg MJ et al: Condyloma in pregnancy is strongly predictive of juvenile-onset recurrent respiratory papillomatosis. Obstet Gynecol 2003;101:645.

Stamataki S et al: Juvenile recurrent respiratory papillomatosis: still a mystery disease with difficult management. Head Neck 2007;29:155.

HEAD & NECK CANCER

▶ Pathophysiology of Head & Neck Squamous Cell Carcinoma

Excluding skin cancer, the vast majority of head and neck cancers are squamous cell cancers. The sixth most common malignancy, head and neck squamous cell carcinoma is diagnosed in over 500,000 patients worldwide each year. Head and neck squamous cell carcinoma is a potentially curable malignancy when diagnosed at an early stage. Unfortunately, patients often present with locally advanced disease. Overall, the prognosis is poor in this latter group of patients. For patients with advanced disease, between 60 to 70% will develop locoregional recurrences within 2 years.

Despite numerous advances in our understanding of this disease and in development of improved medical and surgical therapies, mortality rates have not changed significantly over the last two decades. Additionally, current therapies (both surgical and nonsurgical) carry a high level of treatment related morbidity; patients with advanced-stage disease often suffer significant speech and swallowing impairment following treatment.

Development of head and neck squamous cell carcinoma is traditionally attributed to the synergistic carcinogenic effects of tobacco and alcohol. Other factors, such as poor oral dentition, gastroesophageal reflux, betel nut chewing, and viral infection may also be important contributors to the development of head and neck squamous cell carcinoma. Mounting evidence points toward association of high-risk types (eg, 16, 18, and 31) of HPV with the development of some head and neck squamous cell carcinomas, particularly cancers of the oropharynx. While as many as 50% of oropharyngeal cancers have detectable HPV-16 DNA, only 25–30% of all oropharyngeal cancers are thought to have a viral etiology (as opposed to the usual insults of tobacco and alcohol). In HPV-mediated transformation, oncoproteins (primarily E6 and E7) encoded by the HPV genome are transcribed by infected human epithelial cells, resulting in the degradation and inactivation of host tumor suppressor genes *TP53* (p53) and *RB* (Rb protein, or p105-RB). This is thought to allow unchecked cell cycle progression and development of genetic instability. Head and neck squamous cell carcinomas with active (eg, transcribed) HPV share a common molecular phenotype, similar to that of HPV-caused cervical cancer. Head and neck squamous cell carcinomas with inactive HPV appear to share a molecular phenotype in common with HPV-negative head and neck squamous cell carcinomas. The role, if any, of HPV in these cancers is under investigation.

Head and neck cancers are thought to progress through characteristic stages of premalignancy (dysplasia, carcinoma in situ) until finally reaching invasive carcinoma. This progression reflects the accumulation of multiple genetic changes from mutation, gene silencing (via methylation), chromosomal rearrangements, deletions and duplications. Common changes include mutational inactivation of p53 and Rb tumor suppressors, abrogation of the tumor suppressor p16 axis, amplification of the CCND1 locus (the gene encoding the cell cycle mediator cyclin D1), and various changes resulting in overexpression of epidermal growth factor receptor (EGFR), c-Met, and transforming growth factor alpha (TGF-α).

Another important concept in head and neck cancer biology is that of *field cancerization*. According to this theory, first described in 1953, the entire mucosa of the upper aerodigestive tract is exposed to the same carcinogenic insults. Thus, premalignant changes are likely in a wide field, not just at the site of the original cancer. Even if that cancer is successfully treated, the patient remains at high risk for developing subsequent malignancies throughout the upper aerodigestive tract. Recent molecular-based investigations have provided strong support for this concept, and multiple studies have demonstrated genetic alterations in histologically normal tissue from high-risk individuals. For this reason, patients with a history of head and neck squamous cell carcinoma should be closely followed with yearly screening examinations for life.

Carvalho AL et al: Trends in incidence and prognosis for head and neck cancer in the United States: a site-specific analysis of the SEER database. Int J Cancer 2005;114:806.

Sidransky D: Molecular biology of head and neck tumors. In: *Cancer, principles and practice of oncology.* Hellman S, Rosenberg SA, De Vita VT (editors). Lippincott-Raven, 1997.

Weinberger PM et al: Molecular classification identifies a subset of human papillomavirus-associated oropharyngeal cancers with favorable prognosis. J Clin Oncol 2006;24:736.

▶ Evaluation of the Patient with Head & Neck Cancer

A. History & Physical Examination

Any patient with a significant history of alcohol and tobacco use who presents with complaints related to the upper aerodigestive system should be evaluated with an index of suspicion for head and neck squamous cell carcinoma. Common symptoms of head and neck cancer can be quite subtle. Mechanical obstruction and dysfunction from tumor mass can produce dysphagia. Head and neck cancers are often associated with significant pain, and odynophagia is common for cancers of the oral cavity and oropharynx. Referred pain from neck metastases can result in otalgia, as can cancers arising in the nasopharynx or those affecting the external auditory canal. Cancers of the true vocal cords often produce significant hoarseness early in the course of disease progression. Other symptoms can include hemoptysis, globus sensation, trismus, and weight loss. Sometimes the presenting symptom is a neck mass representing nodal metastases from an asymptomatic primary source.

Patients should be asked about family history of cancers and personal risk factors such as alcohol use and all forms of tobacco (cigarettes, cigars, chewing tobacco, etc). Certain ethnic populations (specifically emigrants from India) may give a history of betel nut chewing. This nut has been found, like tobacco, to have synergistic carcinogenic risk when present in combination with alcohol consumption.

Physical examination should include a comprehensive evaluation of all sites of the head and neck. Inspection of the face and scalp for skin lesions, masses, and asymmetry should be performed. Otoscopy and anterior rhinoscopy allow evaluation of the external auditory canal, tympanic membrane, and nasal cavity. Unilateral serous fluid in the middle ear space in an adult should raise suspicion for a nasopharyngeal lesion. The entire oral cavity should be evaluated, including each gingivobuccal sulcus. The floor of mouth and base of tongue should be manually palpated for induration, pain on palpation, and asymmetry. Evaluation of the larynx and base of tongue can be performed by head lamp and mirror examination (indirect laryngoscopy). Flexible fiberoptic evaluation often provides additional detail, and visualization not possible with the former method. Additionally, the nasal cavity and nasopharynx can easily be evaluated during the same procedure. A complete evaluation of the cranial nerves should be performed. This can often give insight into nerves affected by tumor mass effect (compression) or direct nerve invasion (perineural spread).

The neck should be carefully palpated for cervical lymphadenopathy. This is most easily accomplished by standing behind the patient and palpating each area of the neck symmetrically using both hands. This allows tactile comparison between sides. The pads of the fingers and thumbs are the most sensitive parts of the hands and should be used instead of the tips of the digits.

B. Imaging

Imaging is an important part of the diagnostic evaluation of a patient with head and neck cancer. Goals of imaging include preoperative identification of site and extent of tumor infiltration, presence of suspicious lymph nodes, and presence of anatomic variations. The imaging modality of choice for most suspected head and neck tumors is CT scan with intravenous contrast, which allows adequate soft tissue and bony detail. Most head and neck cancers will demonstrate enhancement on intravenous contrast administration, and the contrast additionally makes delineation of soft tissue structures much easier. In some cases, contrasted MRI may offer additional information. These cases include evaluation of the skull base, parapharyngeal space and orbit, and evaluation of cranial nerves for signs of perineural spread.

Increasingly, evaluation of head and neck squamous cell carcinoma patients for distant metastases and monitoring for posttreatment disease recurrence or persistence involves the use of tumor imaging by 18F-flourodeoxyglucose positron emission tomography (FDG-PET) (Figure 15–11). The use of FDG-PET and combined PET-CT modalities is extremely important because early identification of persistent or recurrent disease may impact survival, especially for patients with advanced nodal disease. While CT and MRI rely on contrast enhancement patterns and differences in tissue attenuation, FDG-PET works somewhat independently of these criteria. FDG follows a cellular uptake pathway similar to glucose and becomes concentrated in cells with elevated glucose utilization. Because changes in tumor metabolism often precede changes discernible on clinical examination, FDG-PET is potentially valuable in discovering clinically nondetectable tumor spread or recurrence. PET-CT results are generally reported as standardized uptake values (SUV). This is a ratio of tissue FDG uptake normalized to injected dose of FDG, patient body weight, and serum glucose levels. Higher SUV indicates increased FDG uptake. Multiple tissue metabolic changes can lead to increased FDG uptake, including inflammation, infection, radiation response, and malignancy. While still a matter of debate, general consensus is that SUV greater than 2.5–3.5 should be considered suspicious for malignancy.

Alberico RA et al: Imaging in head and neck oncology. Surg Oncol Clin North Am 2004;13:13.
Goerres GW et al: Assessment of clinical utility of 18F-FDG PET in patients with head and neck cancer: a probability analysis. Eur J Nucl Med Mol Imaging 2003;30:562.

C. Staging of Head & Neck Squamous Cell Carcinoma: TNM Staging

Staging for head and neck squamous cell carcinoma in the United States uses a TNM system. Staging is important because it allows estimation of prognosis, treatment planning, and expected response to treatment. The TNM system classifies cancers by primary tumor size (T), locoregional for malignancy with the exception of the postcricoid region and subglottis. Transnasal esophagoscopy has the advantage of being able to be performed as an office-based procedure without the need for sedation.

Cancers of the Waldeyer ring, which includes the palatine tonsil and base of tongue (lingual tonsil), while usually squamous cell cancer, can also be lymphoid in origin (such as lymphoma). If there is a suspicion for lymphoma, biopsy specimens should be sent as fresh material and not placed into formaldehyde. Often, flow cytometry and other pathologic tests useful for evaluation of lymphomas cannot be performed on formaldehyde-fixed specimens.

N-stage is determined by the presence of clinically evident regional lymph node metastases. It is important to point out that for head and neck cancer, suspicious lymphadenopathy identified only on CT or MRI scan is included in the clinical staging. Radiologic findings suspicious for malignant lymph node metastases include lymph nodes that are round, heterogeneously enhancing, and larger than 1 cm. Table 15–7 summarizes the current criteria for N-staging (for subsites other than nasopharynx).

M-stage is determined by the presence of distant metastatic disease. The most common sites of metastases for head and neck squamous cell carcinoma are the liver and the lungs. Therefore, part of the initial staging workup for a patient with head and neck cancer includes some method of evaluating these structures. This most commonly consists of liver function blood tests and a chest roentgenogram, although at some institutions whole-body CT-PET scan is becoming more prevalent. M-stage is reported as Mx (cannot be determined), M0 (no distant metastases), or M1 (distant metastatic disease).

Overall staging is achieved by combining the T, N, and M stages to yield four broad stages (stages I–IV, with I carrying the best prognosis and IV the worst). Stage IV is further split into IVa (simplified, denoting a surgically treatable cancer) and IVb and IVc (surgically unresectable). The overall staging system (based on the *AJCC Cancer Staging Manual*, 6th edition) for sites other than nasopharynx is summarized in Table 15–8 and Figure 15–12.

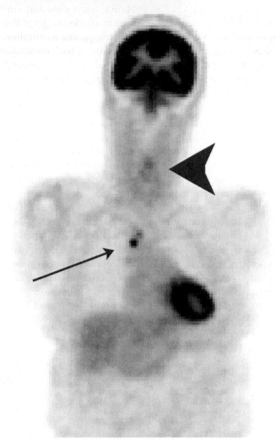

▲ **Figure 15–11.** Positron-emission tomography (PET scan). PET scan showing uptake in the original primary site (palate, indicated by large arrowhead) as well as new mediastinal uptake indicative of nodal metastases (thin arrow). Note the normal physiologic uptake in the liver (moderate intensity) and heart and brain (high intensity) demonstrating the relatively high glucose utilization of these organs.

nodal metastases (N), and distant metastatic spread (M). The rules for classification vary by subsite within the head and neck. In general, cancers of subsites that can be seen directly (oral cavity, oropharynx, etc) are T-staged by size. By comparison, cancers of subsites not visible directly (larynx, hypopharynx, sinonasal, etc) are T-staged by anatomic spread of disease.

Initial evaluation of the primary site and T-staging is best accomplished by operative direct laryngoscopy and esophagoscopy. This allows examination of the primary site and evaluation of the entire upper aerodigestive tract for simultaneous second primary tumors and biopsy of suspicious areas. Some authors propose transnasal esophagoscopy as an acceptable alternative to operative endoscopy. This method allows evaluation (and biopsy) of the most common areas

Table 15–7. Determination of N Stage for Cancers of the Oral Cavity, Oropharynx, Hypopharynx, and Larynx.

Nx	Regional lymph nodes cannot be assessed
N0	No regional lymph node metastases
N1	Metastases in a single ipsilateral lymph node, 3 cm or less
N2 N2a	Metastases in a single ipsilateral lymph node, > 3 cm but not more than 6 cm
N2b	Metastases in multiple ipsilateral lymph nodes < 6 cm
N2c	Metastases in bilateral or contralateral lymph nodes < 6 cm
N3	Metastases in lymph node(s) > 6 cm

Table 15–8. Summary of TNM Staging for Cancers of the Oral Cavity, Oropharynx, Hypopharynx and Larynx.

Stage	T	N	M
0	T-is (in situ)	N0	M0
I	T1	N0	M0
II	T2	N0	M0
III	T3	N0	M0
	T1–T3	N1	
IVa	T4a	N0–N1	M0
	T1–T4a	N2	
IVb	T4b	N0–N2	M0
	Any T	N3	
IVc	Any T	Any N	M1

Greene FL: *AJCC Cancer Staging Manual*, 6th ed. Springer-Verlag, 2003.
Postma GN et al: The role of transnasal esophagoscopy in head and neck oncology. Laryngoscope 2002;112:2242.

▶ Therapy

Traditional therapy for head and neck squamous cell carcinoma depends on the stage of the cancer and varies by subsite. Simplified, early-stage cancers are usually treated with single modality therapy, either surgical excision or radiation therapy. Advanced-stage (stages III and IV) cancers are best treated by combined modality therapy, either surgery followed by radiotherapy or surgery followed by chemotherapy and radiation therapy. Current research has shown that the latter is best delivered as concurrent chemoradiotherapy.

One new modality being investigated for head and neck squamous cell carcinoma includes molecularly targeted therapy. These therapies are designed to be specific for cancer cells and include monoclonal antibodies and small molecule protein inhibitors. The most studied targeted therapy in head and neck squamous cell carcinoma is cetuximab. In the initial randomized controlled clinical trial, researchers found that concurrent cetuximab and radiotherapy improved survival and locoregional disease control compared to radiotherapy alone. Interpretation of this study is hampered by the lack of a comparison arm using combined modality chemoradiotherapy. Studies have also demonstrated improvement in survival when cetuximab is combined with traditional chemotherapy. The EXTREME (Erbitux in First-Line Treatment of Recurrent or Metastatic Head and Neck Cancer) trial randomized 442 patients from 17 countries to either chemotherapy (5-fluorouracil plus either cisplatin or carboplatin) or the same chemotherapy plus cetuximab. Patients in the cetuximab arm had 20% reduction in risk of death, and overall survival was increased from a median 7.4 months to 10.1 months. Other targeted therapies currently being studied include bevacizumab (an inhibitor of the vascular endothelial growth factor [VEGF] receptor involved in angiogenesis) and erlotinib (an orally administered inhibitor of the epidermal growth factor [EGF] receptor).

▶ Cancers of the Oral Cavity

Patients with oral cavity cancer typically present with a painful mass of the tongue, buccal mucosa, floor of mouth, or alveolar ridge. Appearance to visual examination alone can be misleading. While most cancers have either an ulcerative or an exophytic appearance, many can have only subtle visually detectable changes. On palpation, the involved area is usually firm and indurated. A bimanual examination of the floor of mouth is mandatory for a complete exam. The mass should be manipulated to discern mobility. Oral cavity cancers can invade the mandible quite readily, and immobility should raise concern for bone invasion.

As with other head and neck subsites where the primary tumor can be directly visualized, T-staging is assessed by tumor size (summarized in Table 15–9). Cancers that invade

	N0	N1	N2	N3
T1	Stage I			
T2	Stage II			
T3	Stage III			
T4a			Stage IVa	
T4b				Stage IVb

▲ **Figure 15–12.** Summary of staging criteria for cancers of the oral cavity, oropharynx, hypopharynx, and larynx. Carcinoma in situ is stage 0, and presence of distant metastases (M1) is staged as stage IVc regardless of T or N stage.

Table 15–9. T Stage for Cancers of the Oral Cavity.

T1	Tumor ≤ 2 cm in greatest dimension
T2	Tumor > 2 cm but not > 4 cm in greatest dimension
T3	Tumor > 4 cm in greatest dimension
T4	Tumor invades through adjacent structures
T4a	Lip: cortical bone, floor of mouth, facial skin of chin or nose
	Oral cavity proper: cortical bone, deep muscles of tongue (genioglossus, palatoglossus, hyoglossus, styloglossus), skin
T4b	Tumor invades masticator space, pterygoid plates, skull base, and/or encases carotid artery

adjacent structures are, in general, upstaged to T4 regardless of size. Note that superficial erosion of the bony tooth socket by a gingival primary tumor is not sufficient to upstage to T4.

The nodal drainage patterns of oral cavity cancers are of particular concern, because the incidence of occult metastases can approach 30% depending on T-stage and depth of invasion. Cancers of the upper lip can drain to the parotid bed in addition to the submandibular region (level I). When planning treatment of occult metastases, it is important to remember that midline cancers of the oral cavity often drain bilaterally.

Treatment for oral cavity cancer is primarily surgical. Cancers of the lip can often be addressed with simple wedge excision, with 5 mm borders of surrounding normal tissue. If less than one third of the lip is excised, a reasonable result can be obtained with simple closure. Larger excisions require a reconstructive procedure, often involving transfer of lip tissue from the contralateral lip. Cancers of the tongue, floor of mouth, and buccal mucosa are excised with a margin of 1 cm normal-appearing tissue. Primary closure, with or without a split-thickness skin graft, often will provide acceptable functional outcomes. Large resections usually require a flap reconstruction, especially if bone is involved, and a segmental mandibulectomy must be performed. The flap reconstruction can be either a pedicled flap (such as pectoralis major flap) or a free flap (radial forearm and fibular being common flap harvest sites).

Assuming appropriate treatment, outcomes for patients with oral cavity cancer are generally good. The prognosis for squamous cell carcinoma of the lip is excellent, with 5-year survival of 91% for stages I–II, 83% for stages III–IVb, and 52% for stage IVc. Squamous cell carcinoma of the oral cavity proper carries a reduced yet still relatively good prognosis. Five-year survival rates are 72% for stages I–II, 44% for stages III–IVb, and 35% for stage IVc.

Carvalho AL et al: Trends in incidence and prognosis for head and neck cancer in the United States: a site-specific analysis of the SEER database. Int J Cancer 2005;114:806.

Mashberg A, Samit AM: Early detection, diagnosis, and management of oral and oropharyngeal cancer. CA Cancer J Clin 1989;39:67.

Palme CE et al: Current treatment options in squamous cell carcinoma of the oral cavity. Surg Oncol Clin North Am 2004;13:47.

▶ Cancers of the Oropharynx

The oropharynx consists of the soft palate, base of tongue, palatine tonsils, and posterior and lateral oropharyngeal walls. Patients with cancer of the soft palate usually present with relatively early-stage lesions, which typically remain fairly superficial. They usually arise on the anterior aspect of the palate, and patients may report noticing a lump in the palate while swallowing. This contrasts with cancers of the tongue base, tonsillar region, and pharyngeal walls, which typically present at advanced stage. These anatomic regions lack the rich supply of pain nerve fibers typical of the oral cavity and soft palate, and cancers can spread significantly before being noticed. Typical presenting symptoms usually are attributable to sequelae from invasion of adjacent structures and can include dysphagia, cranial nerve defects, referred otalgia, trismus (from pterygoid muscle invasion), or neck mass (from nodal metastases). Because early-stage oropharyngeal cancers often are asymptomatic, any erythroplastic or suspicious lesion in these areas should be biopsied even if no associated symptoms are present.

As is the case for oral cavity cancer, T-staging for squamous cell cancer of the oropharynx is generally determined by tumor size (summarized in Table 15–10). Again, invasion of adjacent structures results in classification as T4 regardless of size. Oropharyngeal cancer N-staging is the same as other head and neck squamous cell carcinoma subsites (except nasopharynx). Nodal metastases from oropharyngeal cancers are common, with 70% of patients with oropharyngeal cancer having ipsilateral cervical nodal metastases at time of presentation. Bilateral cervical nodal metastases are also relatively common, up to 30–50%, depending on size and subsite of the primary tumor.

Treatment for oropharyngeal cancer, especially the tongue base and soft palate, is often weighted toward nonsurgical therapy because surgical resection can result in extensive morbidity in terms of velopharyngeal insufficiency (for palate) and dysphagia (for tongue base). Because of interruption of the blood supply to the remainder of the tongue, large base of tongue cancers usually require total glossectomy even if the anterior tongue is spared. Surgical resections of all but the smallest oropharyngeal cancers usually require flap reconstruction; in the modern era, this is most often in the form of a free flap with microvascular anastomoses. A tracheotomy is usually performed during the initial surgical resection for maintenance of adequate airway. As with other head and neck squamous cell carcinomas, early-stage (I–II) cancers are treated with single-modality therapy, and advanced stage (III–IV) cancers require multiple modalities. Nonsurgical modalities have their own set of consequences, and there is some evidence demonstrating

Table 15–10. T Stage for Cancers of the Oropharynx.

T1	Tumor ≤ 2 cm in greatest dimension
T2	Tumor > 2 cm but not > 4 cm in greatest dimension
T3	Tumor > 4 cm in greatest dimension
T4 T4a	Tumor invades through adjacent structures (larynx; deep muscles of tongue such as genioglossus, palatoglossus, hyoglossus, styloglossus; medial pterygoid; hard palate; mandible)
T4b	Tumor invades masticator space, pterygoid plates, lateral nasopharynx, skull base, and/or encases carotid artery

worse swallowing outcomes following chemoradiotherapy compared to surgery and postoperative radiotherapy for advanced-stage oropharyngeal lesions.

The association between HPV and oropharyngeal cancers deserves special mention. HPV is the accepted etiologic cause of greater than 95% of cervical cancer. Our understanding of its role in head and neck squamous cell carcinoma is still evolving, but it appears to play a causative role in at least a subset of these cancers. Since the first demonstration of HPV in a head and neck squamous cell carcinoma tumor in 1985, numerous studies have found HPV DNA in head and neck squamous cell carcinomas from various subsites, most commonly the oropharynx. It now appears that of oropharyngeal squamous cell carcinomas, approximately 50% have no association with HPV, 25% are likely to be caused by HPV (similar to cervical cancer), and 25% have HPV DNA but an unclear relationship between the virus and the cancer. Future studies assessing the role of HPV in this latter group are currently being developed.

Survival for oropharyngeal cancer is generally worse than that for oral cavity cancer. Five-year survival for stages I–II oropharyngeal cancer is 58%, for stages III–IVb is 41%, and for stage IVc is only 20%.

Carvalho AL et al: Trends in incidence and prognosis for head and neck cancer in the United States: a site-specific analysis of the SEER database. Int J Cancer 2005;114:806.
Lin DT et al: Squamous cell carcinoma of the oropharynx and hypopharynx. Otolaryngol Clin North Am 2005;38:59.
Psyrri A, DiMaio D: Human papillomavirus in cervical and head-and-neck cancer. Nat Clin Pract Oncol 2008;5:24.

▶ Cancers of the Larynx

Laryngeal cancer was an extremely rare disease until the 20th century. Mass-produced cigarettes came into vogue in the 1900s; soon afterward, a dramatic rise in the incidence of laryngeal cancer began to be noted. Tobacco exposure is now accepted as the primary etiologic agent responsible for laryngeal cancer. Other possible additive factors include laryngopharyngeal reflux and possibly certain viruses such as herpes simplex or HPV.

Laryngeal cancers can arise from above the true vocal folds (supraglottic region), below the true vocal folds (subglottic region), or from the true vocal folds (glottic region). The latter represents greater than 75% of all laryngeal cancers. For patients with glottic laryngeal cancer, dysphonia (hoarseness) is the most common presenting symptom. Any hoarseness that persists longer than 2 weeks, especially in a patient with associated risk factors of tobacco or alcohol use, should undergo laryngeal examination. Patients with hoarseness, however, are more likely to have a nonmalignant cause of their symptoms than to have laryngeal cancer.

Laryngeal cancers arising from the subglottis or supraglottis usually present at a later stage than do glottic cancers, as hoarseness does not develop until late in the disease process. Often, the presenting symptom can be life-threatening stridor from an obstructive mass. Emergent awake tracheotomy is sometimes required to secure a stable patent airway in these cases. Other symptoms can include globus sensation ("lump in throat") and dysphagia. Evaluation for preexisting swallowing dysfunction is emerging as an essential part of the diagnostic workup for laryngeal cancers. Because of the emphasis on organ-preservation strategies, identification of patients likely to end up with a nonfunctioning larynx may alter treatment planning. Currently, this is an area of active investigation.

Unlike oral cavity and oropharyngeal cancer (T-staged by tumor size), cancers of the larynx are T-staged by anatomic spread of disease (Table 15–11). One important factor is determination of vocal cord fixation. This can be reliably determined with greater than 90% accuracy based on in-office flexible fiberoptic evaluation combined with high-resolution CT imaging of the larynx. Laryngeal cancer N-staging follows the convention for other head and neck subsites (except nasopharynx).

Therapy for early (T1–T2) glottic cancer has traditionally been radiation therapy, especially for early, diffuse disease involving both true vocal folds and the anterior commissure. In these cases, surgical resection would result in significant disruption of the normal vocal fold architecture and function. This should be balanced with the knowledge that radiation therapy is essentially a one-time treatment modality, which carries its own spectrum of side effects and sequelae.

The goal of organ preservation (ie, preserving a functional ability to phonate and protect the airway during deglutition) should be kept in mind when planning treatment options. In the now-famous "fireman's study," McNeil and colleagues found that many people would accept a 20% decrease in survival rather than lose their larynx. Surgical organ preservation strategies include endoscopic microsurgical excision, supracricoid laryngectomy, and vertical partial laryngectomy. Endoscopic microsurgical excision can allow maximal preservation of vocal function in selected T1 glottic cancers, while maintaining a sound oncologic outcome. In this approach, dissection is meticulously performed just deep to the most involved layer of the true vocal fold (epithelium, superficial lamina propria, deep lamina propria or vocal ligament, vocalis muscle). Partial laryngectomies (vertical partial and supracricoid) can yield satisfactory voice and swallowing function but require extensive patient cooperation in the postoperative period. Supracricoid laryngectomy involves removal of the supraglottis, false and true vocal cords, and thyroid cartilage. The hyoid bone, cricoid cartilage, and at least one arytenoid are preserved. The movement of the remaining arytenoid against the tongue base allows phonation and (eventual) preservation of swallowing function. Postoperatively, aspiration is to be expected, and patients with poor preoperative pulmonary function should not be offered this option. Total laryngectomy is the treatment of choice for salvage of organ-preservation failures as well as for most advanced glottic (T3–T4) cancers.

Table 15–11. T Stage for Cancers of the Larynx.

	Supraglottis
T1	Tumor limited to one subsite of the supraglottis; normal vocal cord mobility
T2	Tumor invades mucosa of more than one subsite of the supraglottis, glottis, or adjacent structure (tongue base, vallecula, medial wall of pyriform); normal vocal cord mobility
T3	Tumor limited to the larynx but presence of vocal cord fixation and/or invades postcricoid, preepiglottic tissues, paraglottic space, *inner cortex only* invasion of thyroid cartilage
T4a	Tumor invades through thyroid cartilage and/or extends to other tissues beyond the larynx (eg, trachea, deep extrinsic tongue muscles, strap muscles, thyroid, esophagus)
T4b	Tumor invades prevertebral space, encases carotid artery, or invades mediastinal structures
	Glottis
T1a	Tumor limited to unilateral true vocal cord with normal mobility (may involve anterior or posterior commissure)
T1b	Tumor limited to bilateral true vocal cords with normal mobility (may involve anterior or posterior commissure)
T2	Tumor extends to supraglottis and/or subglottis and/or impaired vocal cord mobility
T3	Tumor limited to larynx with vocal cord fixation and/or invades paraglottic space, and/or minor thyroid cartilage invasion (*inner cortex only*)
T4a	Tumor invades through the thyroid cartilage and/or invades tissues beyond the larynx (trachea, soft tissues of the neck including deep extrinsic tongue muscles, strap muscles, thyroid, esophagus)
T4b	Tumor invades prevertebral space, encases carotid artery, or invades mediastinal structures
	Subglottis
T1	Tumor limited to subglottis
T2	Tumor extends to true vocal cord(s) with normal or impaired mobility (but no fixation)
T3	Tumor limited to larynx with vocal cord fixation
T4a	Tumor invades cricoid or thyroid cartilage and/or invades tissues beyond larynx (trachea, soft tissues of the neck including deep extrinsic tongue muscles, strap muscles, thyroid, esophagus)
T4b	Tumor invades prevertebral space, encases carotid artery, or invades mediastinal structures

Outcomes for patients with laryngeal cancer can be excellent. For early stage I glottic carcinoma (tumor limited to the true vocal folds), 5-year overall survival rates of 90% can be expected. Overall, laryngeal cancer carries a 5-year survival of 79% for stages I–II disease. With invasion of adjacent structures characteristic of stages III–IVb disease, 5-year survival decreases to 55%, and with distant metastases (stage IVc) the 5-year survival is 35%.

Carvalho AL et al: Trends in incidence and prognosis for head and neck cancer in the United States: a site-specific analysis of the SEER database. Int J Cancer 2005;114:806.

Jalisi M, Jalisi S: Advanced laryngeal carcinoma: surgical and non-surgical management options. Otolaryngol Clin North Am 2005;38:47.

Laccourreye O et al: Vertical partial laryngectomy versus supracricoid partial laryngectomy for selected carcinomas of the true vocal cord classified as T2N0. Ann Otol Rhinol Laryngol 2000;109:965.

McNeil EJ et al. Speech and survival: tradeoffs between quality and quantity of life in laryngeal cancer. N Engl J Med 1981;305:982.

▶ Cancers of the Hypopharynx

The hypopharynx is a continuation of the oropharynx and extends superiorly from the level of the hyoid bone to the level of the inferior aspect of the cricoid cartilage. It consists of the pyriform sinuses (the most common subsite for hypopharyngeal cancer), the posterior pharyngeal wall, and postcricoid regions. The hypopharynx is lined with stratified squamous epithelium and is invested with an abundant lymphatic drainage network. Patients with hypopharyngeal cancer typically present with advanced stage disease, stage III or worse. There are several contributing factors, including lack of specific symptoms for small lesions in this region and lack of anatomic boundaries to prevent spread of disease. Typical presenting symptoms can include referred otalgia, odynophagia, and dysphagia. Other symptoms can include a neck mass (from nodal metastases), hoarseness (due to laryngeal involvement), and weight loss. Like laryngeal cancer, hypopharyngeal cancer is chiefly related to excessive alcohol and tobacco exposure. There is also some evidence for a possible contribution of GERD to hypopharyngeal cancer, which may explain the increased likelihood for patients with Plummer-Vinson syndrome to develop hypopharyngeal cancer regardless of tobacco or alcohol exposure. In Plummer-Vinson syndrome, patients develop esophageal webs, and chronic acid exposure above the site of webbing is thought to possibly result in chronic inflammation predisposing to malignancy.

Hypopharyngeal cancer T-staging is somewhat unique, as it is a combination of tumor size (as for oral cavity and oropharyngeal tumors) and anatomic spread (as for laryngeal cancer). The T-staging criteria for hypopharyngeal cancer are summarized in Table 15–12. N-staging and M-staging are the same as for the majority of head and neck sites (except nasopharynx).

Early stage (T1–T2 tumors) hypopharyngeal cancer is often treated with primary radiotherapy. Surgical resection is more likely in these instances to lead to dysphagia and aspiration. Alternatively, laryngeal conservation surgery may be a reasonable option for some of these early-stage cancers. More

Table 15-12. T Stage for Cancers of the Hypopharynx.

T1	Tumor limited to 1 subsite *and* ≤ 2 cm in greatest dimension
T2	No fixation of hemilarynx, and tumor: • invades more than subsite or an adjacent area (larynx, oropharynx) *and/or* • > 2 cm but not > 4 cm in greatest dimension
T3	Tumor > 4 cm in greatest dimension *or* fixation of hemilarynx
T4 T4a	Tumor invades through adjacent structures (thyroid/cricoid cartilage, hyoid bone, thyroid gland, esophagus, central compartment)
T4b	Tumor involves prevertebral fascia, mediastinal structures, and/or encases carotid artery

advanced (T3–T4) tumors can be treated by surgical resection with postoperative radiotherapy or chemoradiotherapy therapy. The standard surgical procedure is total laryngectomy with partial pharyngectomy. Tumor extension into the esophagus requires a cervical esophagectomy. The resulting alimentary tract defects require repair by various methods, including microvascular jejunal free flap, gastric pull up, or microvascular myocutaneous flap (most often tubed radial forearm or anterolateral thigh). Organ-preservation surgical strategies can achieve laryngeal preservation rates of up to 40% for highly selected cases, but these remain somewhat controversial. As previously described for laryngeal cancer, preoperative evaluation of a patient's pulmonary function status is critical, as significant postoperative aspiration can be expected. Because of the high incidence of occult nodal metastases, treatment of the neck lymphatics should be included in any therapeutic plan. For clinically evident neck disease, neck dissection is indicated. For patients with a clinically negative neck, optimal management is still being elucidated. Elective neck dissection represents one option for the clinically negative neck. Alternatively, if radiation therapy is planned for treatment of the primary site, the radiation fields can be adjusted to include treatment doses to the neck lymphatics.

Hypopharyngeal cancer carries the worst prognosis of any head and neck subsite. The underlying reasons for this poor prognosis are still unclear, and several hypotheses have been suggested. A distinctive pathologic feature of hypopharyngeal cancer is the propensity for submucosal spread of disease, often resulting in clinically understaging disease extent. The abundant lymphatic drainage of the hypopharynx may also predispose the patient to early nodal metastases. It has also been suggested that the lack of definitive anatomic boundaries may allow early spread of disease. Given all of these factors, 5-year survival for stages I–II hypopharyngeal cancer is 47%, stages III–IVb is 30%, and stage IVc is only 16%.

Carvalho AL et al: Trends in incidence and prognosis for head and neck cancer in the United States: a site-specific analysis of the SEER database. Int J Cancer 2005;114:806.

Clayman GL et al: Laryngeal preservation for advanced laryngeal and hypopharyngeal cancers. Arch Otolaryngol Head Neck Surg 1995;121:219.

Lin DT et al: Squamous cell carcinoma of the oropharynx and hypopharynx. Otolaryngol Clin North Am 2005;38:59.

▶ Salivary Gland Neoplasms

Neoplasms (both benign and malignant) of the salivary glands are relatively uncommon, representing approximately 2% of all head and neck neoplasms. In general, the larger the salivary gland, the higher the overall incidence of neoplasms—but these neoplasms are also less likely to be malignant. Major salivary glands include the parotid, submandibular, and sublingual glands. The minor salivary glands are scattered mainly throughout the mucosa of the lips and oral cavity, and to a lesser extent, the entire upper aerodigestive tract. For these smaller glands, the incidence of neoplasms is lower, but if one does occur, it is more likely to be malignant. The parotid gland accounts for 80% of all neoplasms, while 15% arise from the submandibular glands and 5% from the sublingual and minor salivary glands. For any given tumor, the incidence of malignancy is 20% for parotid tumors, 60% for submandibular tumors, and 80% for sublingual and minor salivary gland tumors. Unlike squamous cell carcinoma, tobacco and alcohol exposure do not appear to play an etiologic role in salivary gland malignancy. The parotid gland contains lymph nodes that drain the preauricular and temporal skin; any parotid mass should raise suspicion for a skin cancer with intraparotid nodal metastases, and a complete examination of the scalp and preauricular skin is indicated.

The most common benign salivary gland tumor is pleomorphic adenoma (also called benign mixed tumor), representing 60% of all salivary gland neoplasms. Patients typically present with a slowly enlarging, painless firm mass (most often in the parotid gland). Facial nerve paralysis is exceedingly rare, even with very large tumors, due to the slow-growing nature of these neoplasms. Malignant transformation of pleomorphic adenoma is rare but does occur; the resultant malignancy is highly aggressive. Treatment for pleomorphic adenoma is complete surgical excision including a surrounding margin of normal tissue. Due to microscopic transcapsular tumor infiltration, simple enucleation is insufficient for these benign neoplasms.

The second-most common benign salivary neoplasm is papillary cystadenoma lymphomatosum (also known as Warthin tumor). This benign tumor is responsible for 10% of parotid neoplasms but is rare outside of the parotid gland. Bilateral tumors are present in up to 10% of patients, so careful palpation and/or imaging of both parotid beds is important if this tumor is suspected. Patients typically present with a slowly enlarging parotid mass, which is painless and rubbery upon palpation. Standard treatment is complete surgical excision (such as superficial parotidectomy with facial nerve preservation), although some authors advocate that enucleation of these tumors may be adequate therapy.

The most common salivary gland malignancy is mucoepidermoid carcinoma. Despite the propensity of the smaller salivary gland neoplasms to be malignant, the most common site for mucoepidermoid carcinoma is still the parotid gland. Approximately 45–70% of mucoepidermoid carcinomas arise from the parotid gland, while 20% occur in minor salivary glands of the palate. Typical symptoms at presentation can be quite similar to those of benign salivary neoplasms, with a painless enlarging mass. Symptoms such as pain or facial paralysis are uncommon but when present should raise suspicion for a high-grade aggressive lesion. Mucoepidermoid cancers are graded as low grade (mostly mucus cells), intermediate grade, and high grade (characterized by a hypercellular solid tumor). The latter can be difficult to distinguish from squamous cell carcinoma without immunohistochemical staining. Treatment is tailored to the extent of disease, tumor grade, and location. Localized disease is usually amenable to surgical excision (parotidectomy with facial nerve preservation, submandibular gland excision, or wide local excision for minor salivary gland origin). Advanced disease requires extensive resection, often combined with neck dissection and/or postoperative radiotherapy.

The second-most common salivary gland malignancy is adenoid cystic carcinoma. It is most common in the submandibular, sublingual, and minor salivary glands. Of all parotid neoplasms, adenoid cystic carcinoma is more likely to present with pain or paresthesias, although an asymptomatic mass is still the more common presentation. Adenoid cystic carcinoma is characterized by a propensity for perineural spread. Thus, preoperative imaging with gadolinium-enhanced MRI is often helpful in therapeutic planning. Treatment consists of complete surgical resection (sometimes requiring facial nerve sacrifice) and postoperative radiation therapy. There is some evidence that postoperative proton-beam therapy offers improved outcomes compared to traditional radiation therapy, although the former is available at only a few centers in the United States. Adenoid cystic carcinoma rarely spreads to cervical lymphatics, so neck dissection is not routinely advocated. It does, however, have a propensity for distant metastases—especially the lung. The disease is also characterized by frequent local recurrence, up to 40% even after adequate local excision. Because of the relatively slow-growing nature of this disease, survival for adenoid cystic carcinoma at 5 years is favorable, approximately 65% for all stages. Due to the propensities for local recurrence and distant metastases, however, this statistic decreases to 12–15% at 15 years.

Table 15–13. T Stage for Major Salivary Gland Cancer.

T1	Tumor ≤ 2 cm in greatest dimension, no extraparenchymal extension
T2	Tumor > 2 cm but not > 4 cm in greatest dimension, no extraparenchymal extension
T3	Tumor > 4 cm in greatest dimension and/or extraparenchymal extension
T4a	Tumor invades through adjacent structures (skin, mandible, external auditory canal, and/or facial nerve involvement)
T4b	Tumor invades skull base, pterygoid plates, and/or encases carotid artery

As mentioned previously, malignant degeneration of pleomorphic adenomas can occur, although it is uncommon. Some authors have estimated the risk of malignant degeneration at 1.5% for the first 5 years, increasing to 9.5% by 15 years or longer. The resulting malignant tumor is termed *carcinoma ex-pleomorphic adenoma* and is characterized by an aggressive natural history and poor clinical outcome. The most common presentation is sudden, rapid growth of a previously stable parotid mass. Histologically, the malignant cells can take the form of any epithelial malignancy except acinic cell. Carcinoma ex-pleomorphic adenoma is characterized by frequent lymph node metastases, and up to 25% of patients will have clinically evident cervical lymphadenopathy on presentation. Treatment includes radical surgical resection, often combined with neck dissection and/or postoperative radiotherapy.

The prognosis of salivary gland malignancies varies according to histologic type, location, extent of disease, and grade. The criteria for T-staging are similar to other head and neck sites with directly measurable tumor size and is summarized in Table 15–13. Overall, early-stage (stages I–II) salivary gland cancers carry an excellent prognosis, greater than 80% at 5 years. Advanced (stage III–IV) salivary gland cancers, on the other hand, have overall 5-year survival rates ranging from 23% to 56% depending on type and grade.

Califano J, Eisele DW: Benign salivary gland neoplasms. Otolaryngol Clin North Am 1999;32:861.
Rice DH: Malignant salivary gland neoplasms. Otolaryngol Clin North Am 1999;32:875.
Witt RL: Major salivary gland cancer. Surg Oncol Clin North Am 2004;13:113.

Thyroid & Parathyroid

Orlo H. Clark, MD

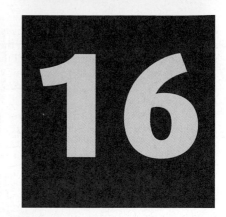

▼ I. THE THYROID GLAND

EMBRYOLOGY & ANATOMY

See Figure 16–1. The main anlage of the thyroid gland develops as a median endodermal downgrowth from the first and second pharyngeal pouches. During its migration caudally, it contacts the ultimobranchial bodies developing from the fourth pharyngeal pouches. When it reaches the position it occupies in the adult, with the isthmus situated just below the cricoid cartilage, the thyroid divides into two lobes. The site from which it originated persists as the foramen cecum at the base of the tongue. The path the gland follows may result in thyroglossal remnants (cysts) or ectopic thyroid tissue (lingual thyroid). A pyramidal lobe is frequently present. Agenesis of one thyroid lobe, almost always the left, may occur.

The normal thyroid weighs 15–25 g and is attached to the trachea by loose connective tissue. It is a highly vascularized organ that derives its blood supply principally from the superior and inferior thyroid arteries. A thyroid ima artery may also be present.

PHYSIOLOGY

The function of the thyroid gland is to synthesize, store, and secrete the hormones thyroxine (T_4) and triiodothyronine (T_3). Iodide is absorbed from the gastrointestinal tract and actively trapped by the acinar cells of the thyroid gland. It is then oxidized and combined with tyrosine in thyroglobulin to form monoiodotyrosine (MIT) and diiodotyrosine (DIT). These are coupled to form the active hormones T_4 and T_3, which initially are stored in the colloid of the gland. Following hydrolysis of the thyroglobulin, T_4 and T_3 are secreted into the plasma, becoming almost instantaneously bound to plasma proteins. Most T_3 in euthyroid individuals, however, is produced by extrathyroidal conversion of T_4 to T_3.

The function of the thyroid gland is regulated by a feedback mechanism that involves the hypothalamus and pituitary. Thyrotropin-releasing factor (TRF), a tripeptide amide, is formed in the hypothalamus and stimulates the release of the thyroid-stimulating hormone (TSH) thyrotropin, a glycoprotein, from the pituitary. Thyrotropin binds to TSH receptors on the thyroid plasma membrane, stimulating increased adenylyl cyclase activity; this increases cyclic adenosine monophosphate (cAMP) production and thyroid cellular function. Thyrotropin also stimulates the phosphoinositide pathway and—along with cAMP—stimulates thyroid growth.

De Felice M, Di Lauro R: Thyroid development and its disorders: genetics and molecular mechanisms. Endocr Rev 2004;25:722.

EVALUATION OF THE THYROID

In a patient with enlargement of the thyroid (goiter), the history (including local and systemic systems and family history) and examination of the gland are most important and are complemented by the selective use of thyroid function tests. The surgeon must develop a systematic method of palpating the gland to determine its size, contour, consistency, nodularity, and fixation and to examine for displacement of the trachea and the presence of palpable cervical lymph nodes. The thyroid gland moves cephalad with deglutition, whereas adjacent lymph nodes do not. The isthmus of the thyroid gland is situated immediately caudal to the cricoid cartilage.

Thyroid function is assessed by highly sensitive TSH assays that can differentiate among patients with hypothyroidism (increased TSH levels), euthyroidism, and hyperthyroidism (decreased TSH levels). In most cases, therefore, serum T_3, T_4, and other variables need not be measured. A free T_4 level is helpful in patients after treatment for Graves disease because the TSH level may remain suppressed despite the patient being euthyroid. A serum T_3

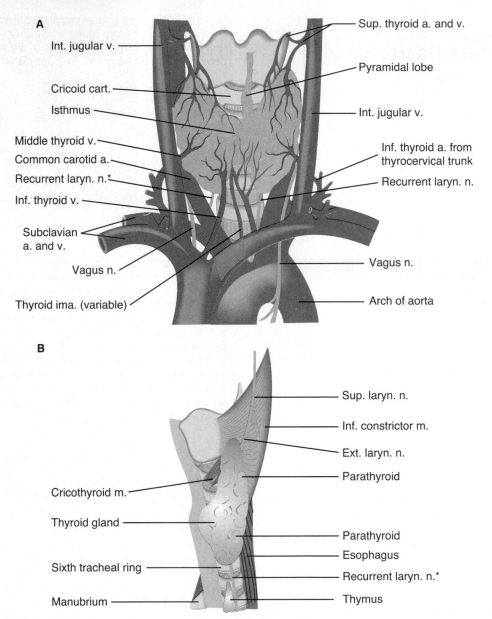

A

Int. jugular v.

Sup. thyroid a. and v.

Pyramidal lobe

Cricoid cart.

Isthmus

Int. jugular v.

Middle thyroid v.

Common carotid a.

Recurrent laryn. n.*

Inf. thyroid v.

Inf. thyroid a. from thyrocervical trunk

Recurrent laryn. n.

Subclavian a. and v.

Vagus n.

Vagus n.

Thyroid ima. (variable)

Arch of aorta

B

Sup. laryn. n.

Inf. constrictor m.

Ext. laryn. n.

Parathyroid

Cricothyroid m.

Thyroid gland

Parathyroid

Esophagus

Sixth tracheal ring

Recurrent laryn. n.*

Manubrium

Thymus

▲ **Figure 16–1.** Thyroid anatomy. *The recurrent laryngeal nerve runs in the tracheoesophageal groove on the left and has a slightly more oblique course on the right before it enters the larynx just posterior to the cricothyroid muscle at the level of the cricoid cartilage.

level is useful for diagnosing T_3 toxicosis (high T_3 and low TSH), or the euthyroid sick, low T_3 syndrome (low T_3 and normal or slightly increased TSH).

Radioactive iodine (RAI) uptake is useful for differentiating between hyperthyroidism and increased secretion of thyroid hormone (low TSH and increased radioactive iodine uptake) on the one hand and subacute thyroiditis (low TSH and low radioactive iodine uptake) on the other. Patients with the latter "leak" thyroid hormone from the gland, which suppresses serum TSH levels and, consequently, iodine uptake by the thyroid. Patients with Graves disease have increased levels of thyroid-stimulating immunoglobulins that increase iodine uptake despite low TSH levels.

DISEASES OF THE THYROID

HYPERTHYROIDISM (THYROTOXICOSIS)

 ESSENTIALS OF DIAGNOSIS

▶ Nervousness, weight loss with increased appetite, heat intolerance, increased sweating, muscular weakness and fatigue, increased bowel frequency, polyuria, menstrual irregularities, infertility.

▶ Goiter, tachycardia, atrial fibrillation, warm moist skin, thyroid thrill and bruit, cardiac flow murmur; gynecomastia.

▶ Eye signs: stare, lid lag, exophthalmos.

▶ TSH low or absent; TSI, iodine uptake, T_3, and T_4 increased; T_3 suppression test abnormal (failure to suppress radioiodine uptake).

General Considerations

Hyperthyroidism is caused by the increased secretion of thyroid hormone (**Graves disease, Plummer disease,** iodine-induced [**jodbasedow effect**], amiodarone toxicity, TSH-secreting pituitary tumors, human chorionic gonadotropin [hCG]-secreting tumors) or by other disorders that increase thyroid hormone levels without increasing thyroid gland secretion (factitious hyperthyroidism, subacute thyroiditis, struma ovarii, and, rarely, metastatic thyroid cancers that secrete excess thyroid hormone). The most common causes of hyperthyroidism are diffusely hypersecretory goiter (Graves disease) and nodular toxic goiter (Plummer disease).

In all forms, the symptoms of hyperthyroidism are due to increased levels of thyroid hormone in the blood stream. The clinical manifestations of thyrotoxicosis may be subtle or marked and tend to go through periods of exacerbation and remission. Some patients ultimately develop hypothyroidism spontaneously (about 15%) or as a result of treatment. Graves disease is an autoimmune disease—often with a familial predisposition—whereas the etiology of Plummer disease is unknown. Most cases of hyperthyroidism are easily diagnosed on the basis of the signs and symptoms; others (eg, mild or **apathetic hyperthyroidism**—which occurs most commonly in the elderly) may be recognized only with laboratory testing for a suppressed TSH level.

Thyrotoxicosis has been described with a normal T_4 concentration, normal or elevated radioiodine uptake, and normal protein binding but with increased serum T_3 by RIA (T_3 toxicosis). T_4 pseudothyrotoxicosis is occasionally seen in critically ill patients and is characterized by increased levels of T_4 and decreased levels of T_3 due to failure to convert T_4 to T_3. Thyrotoxicosis associated with toxic nodular goiter is usually less severe than that associated with Graves disease and is only rarely if ever associated with the extrathyroidal manifestations of Graves disease such as exophthalmos, pretibial myxedema, thyroid acropathy, or periodic hypocalcemic paralysis.

If left untreated, thyrotoxicosis causes progressive and profound catabolic disturbances and cardiac damage. Death may occur in thyroid storm or because of heart failure or severe cachexia.

Clinical Findings

A. Symptoms and Signs

The clinical findings are those of hyperthyroidism as well as those related to the underlying cause (Table 16–1). Nervousness, increased diaphoresis, heat intolerance, tachycardia, palpitations, fatigue, and weight loss in association with a nodular, multinodular, or diffuse goiter are the classic findings in hyperthyroidism. The patient may have a flushed and staring appearance. The skin is warm, thin, and moist, and the hair is fine.

In Graves disease, there may be exophthalmos, pretibial myxedema, or vitiligo, virtually never seen in single or multinodular toxic goiter. The Achilles reflex time is shortened in hyperthyroidism and prolonged in hypothyroidism. The patient on the verge of thyroid storm has accentuated symptoms and signs of thyrotoxicosis, with hyperpyrexia, tachycardia, cardiac failure, neuromuscular excitation, delirium, or jaundice.

Table 16–1. Clinical Findings in Thyrotoxicosis.*

Clinical Manifestations	Percent	Clinical Manifestations	Percent
Tachycardia	100	Weakness	70
Nervousness	99	Increased appetite	65
Goiter	98	Eye complaints	54
Skin changes	97	Leg swelling	35
Tremor	97	Hyperdefecation (without diarrhea)	33
Increased sweating	91		
Hypersensitivity to heat	89	Diarrhea	23
		Atrial fibrillation	10
Palpitations	89	Splenomegaly	10
Fatigue	88	Gynecomastia	10
Weight loss	85	Anorexia	9
Bruit over thyroid	77	Liver palms	8
Dyspnea	75	Constipation	4
Eye signs	71	Weight gain	2

*Data from Williams RH: *J Clin Endocrinol Metab* 1946:6:1.

B. Laboratory Findings

Laboratory tests reveal a suppressed TSH and an elevation of T_3, free T_4, and radioactive iodine. A history of medications is important, since certain drugs and organic iodinated compounds affect some thyroid function tests, and iodide excess may result in either iodide-induced hypothyroidism or iodine-induced hyperthyroidism (jodbasedow effect). In mild forms of hyperthyroidism, the usual diagnostic laboratory tests are likely to be only slightly abnormal. In these difficult to diagnose cases, two additional tests are helpful: the T_3 suppression test and the thyrotropin-releasing hormone (TRH) test. In the T_3 suppression test, hyperthyroid patients fail to suppress the thyroidal uptake of radioiodine when given exogenous T_3. In the TRH test, serum TSH levels fail to rise in response to administration of TRH in hyperthyroid patients.

Other findings include a high thyroid-stimulating immunoglobulin (TSI) level, low serum cholesterol, lymphocytosis, and occasionally hypercalcemia, hypercalciuria, or glycosuria.

▶ Differential Diagnosis

Anxiety neurosis, heart disease, anemia, gastrointestinal disease, cirrhosis, tuberculosis, myasthenia and other muscular disorders, menopausal syndrome, pheochromocytoma, primary ophthalmopathy, and thyrotoxicosis factitia may be clinically difficult to differentiate from hyperthyroidism. Differentiation is especially difficult when the thyrotoxic patient presents with minimal or no thyroid enlargement. Patients may also have painless or spontaneously resolving thyroiditis and are hyperthyroid because of increased release of thyroid hormone from the thyroid gland. This condition, however, is self-limited, and treatment with antithyroid drugs, radioactive iodine, or surgery is rarely necessary.

Anxiety neurosis is perhaps the condition most frequently confused with hyperthyroidism. Anxiety is characterized by persistent fatigue usually unrelieved by rest, clammy palms, a normal sleeping pulse rate, and normal laboratory tests of thyroid function. The fatigue of hyperthyroidism is often relieved by rest, the palms are warm and moist, tachycardia persists during sleep, and thyroid function tests are abnormal.

Organic disease of nonthyroidal origin that may be confused with hyperthyroidism must be differentiated largely on the basis of evidence of specific organ system involvement and normal thyroid function tests.

Other causes of exophthalmos (eg, orbital tumors) or ophthalmoplegia (eg, myasthenia) must be ruled out by ophthalmologic, ultrasonographic, computer tomography (CT) or magnetic resonance imaging (MRI) scans, and neurologic examinations.

▶ Treatment

Hyperthyroidism may be effectively treated by antithyroid drugs, radioactive iodine, or thyroidectomy. Treatment must be individualized and depends on the patient's age and general state of health, the size of the goiter, the underlying pathologic process, and the patient's ability to obtain follow-up care.

A. Antithyroid Drugs

The principal antithyroid drugs used in the United States are propylthiouracil (PTU), 300–1000 mg orally daily, and methimazole, 30–100 mg orally daily. These agents interfere with organic binding of iodine and prevent coupling of iodotyrosines in the thyroid gland. One advantage over thyroidectomy and radioiodine in the treatment of Graves disease is that drugs inhibit the function of the gland without destroying tissue; therefore, there is a lower incidence of subsequent hypothyroidism. This form of treatment is usually used in preparation for surgery or radioactive iodine treatment but may be used as definitive treatment. When propylthiouracil is given as definitive treatment, the goal is to maintain the patient in a euthyroid state until a natural remission occurs. Reliable patients with small goiters are good candidates for this regimen. A prolonged remission after 18 months of treatment occurs in 30% of patients, some of whom eventually become hypothyroid. Side effects include rashes and fever (3–4%), agranulocytosis (0.1–0.4%), and, rarely, liver failure. Patients must be warned to immediately stop the drug, see a physician, and have a white blood cell count if sore throat or fever develops.

B. Radioiodine

Radioiodine (^{131}I) may be given safely after the patient has been treated with antithyroid medications and has become euthyroid. Radioiodine is indicated for patients who are over 40 or are poor risks for surgery and for patients with recurrent hyperthyroidism. It is less expensive than operative treatment and is effective. Radioiodine treatment at doses necessary to treat hyperthyroidism does not increase the risk of leukemia or of congenital anomalies. However, an increased incidence of benign thyroid tumors and, rarely, thyroid cancer has been noted to follow treatment of hyperthyroidism with radioiodine. In young patients, the radiation hazard is certainly increased, and the chance of developing hypothyroidism is virtually 100%. After the first year of treatment with radioiodine, the incidence of hypothyroidism increases about 3% per year. In patients with Graves ophthalmopathy, steroids should be given when radioiodine therapy is used.

Hyperthyroid children and pregnant women should not be treated with radioiodine.

C. Surgery

1. Indications for subtotal thyroidectomy—The main advantages of subtotal thyroidectomy are rapid control of the disease and a lower incidence of hypothyroidism than can be achieved with radioiodine treatment. Surgery is often the preferred treatment (1) in the presence of a very large goiter or a multinodular goiter with relatively low radioactive iodine uptake, (2) if there is a suspicious or malignant thyroid nodule, (3) for patients with ophthalmopathy, (4) for the treatment of pregnant patients or children, (5) for the treatment of women who wish to become pregnant within 1 year after treatment, (6) for patients with amiodarone-induced hyperthyroidism, and (7) for the treatment of psychologically or mentally incompetent patients or patients who are for any reason unable to maintain adequate long-term follow-up evaluation.

2. Preparation for surgery—The risk of thyroidectomy for toxic goiter is small since the introduction of the combined preoperative use of iodides and antithyroid drugs. Propylthiouracil or another antithyroid drug is administered until the patient becomes euthyroid and is continued until the time of operation. Three drops of potassium iodide solution or Lugol iodine solution are then given for about 10 days before surgery in conjunction with the propylthiouracil to decrease the friability and vascularity of the thyroid, thereby technically facilitating thyroidectomy.

An occasional untreated or inadequately treated hyperthyroid patient may require an emergency operation for some unrelated problem such as acute appendicitis and thus require immediate control of the hyperthyroidism. Such a patient should be treated in a manner similar to one in thyroid storm, since **thyroid storm** or hyperthyroid crises may be precipitated by surgical stress or trauma. Treatment of hyperthyroid patients requiring an emergency operation or those in thyroid storm is as follows: Prevent release of preformed thyroid hormone by administration of Lugol iodine solution or with ipodate sodium; give the β-adrenergic blocking agent propranolol to antagonize the peripheral manifestations of thyrotoxicosis; and decrease thyroid hormone production and extrathyroidal conversion of T_4 to T_3 by giving propylthiouracil. The combined use of propranolol and iodide has been demonstrated to lower serum thyroid hormone levels. Other important considerations are to treat precipitating causes (eg, infection, drug reactions); to support vital functions by giving oxygen, sedatives, intravenous fluids, and corticosteroids; and to reduce fever. Reserpine may be useful in the patient in whom nervousness is a prominent symptom, and a cooling blanket—not aspirin—should be used in patients requiring an operation.

3. Subtotal thyroidectomy—The treatment of hyperthyroidism by subtotal, near total, or total thyroidectomy eliminates both the hyperthyroidism and the goiter. As a rule, all but about 5 g of thyroid are removed, sparing the parathyroid glands and the recurrent laryngeal nerves. Total thyroidectomy is generally indicated for patients with Graves ophthalmopathy.

The death rate associated with these procedures is extremely low—less than 0.1% in a recent collected review.

Thyroidectomy thus provides safe and rapid correction of the thyrotoxic state. The frequency of recurrent hyperthyroidism and hypothyroidism depends on the amount of thyroid remaining and on the natural history of the hyperthyroidism. Given an accomplished surgeon and good preoperative preparation, injuries to the recurrent laryngeal nerves and parathyroid glands occur in less than 2% of cases. Adequate exposure and avoidance of injury to the recurrent laryngeal nerves and parathyroid glands are essential.

▶ Ocular Manifestations of Graves Disease

The pathogenesis of the ocular problems in Graves disease remains unclear. Evidence originally supporting the role of either long-acting thyroid stimulator (LATS) or exophthalmos-producing substance (EPS) has not been authenticated.

The eye complications of Graves disease may begin before there is any evidence of thyroid dysfunction or after the hyperthyroidism has been appropriately treated. Usually, however, the ocular manifestations develop concomitantly with the hyperthyroidism. Relief of the eye problems is often difficult to accomplish until coexisting hyperthyroidism or hypothyroidism is controlled.

The eye changes of Graves disease vary from no signs or symptoms to loss of sight. Mild cases are characterized by upper lid retraction and stare with or without lid lag or proptosis. These cases present only minor cosmetic problems and require no treatment. When moderate to severe eye changes occur, there is retroorbital soft tissue involvement with proptosis, extraocular muscle involvement, and finally optic nerve involvement. Some cases may have marked chemosis, periorbital edema, conjunctivitis, keratitis, diplopia, ophthalmoplegia, and impaired vision. Ophthalmologic consultation is required.

Treatment of the ocular problems of Graves disease includes maintaining the patient in a euthyroid state without increase in TSH secretion, protecting the eyes from light and dust with dark glasses and eye shields, elevating the head of the bed, using diuretics to decrease periorbital and retrobulbar edema, and giving methylcellulose or guanethidine eye drops. High doses of glucocorticoids are beneficial in certain patients, but their effectiveness is variable and unpredictable. If exophthalmos progresses despite medical treatment, lateral tarsorrhaphy, retrobulbar irradiation, or surgical decompression of the orbit may be necessary. Total thyroid, as mentioned, is the treatment of choice when it can be done with a low risk of complications. Graves disease is more likely to worsen after radioiodine treatment than after thyroidectomy. It is important that patients with ophthalmopathy be made aware of the natural history of the disease and also that they be kept euthyroid, since hyperthyroidism and hypothyroidism may produce visual deterioration. Operations to correct diplopia should be deferred until after the ophthalmopathy has stabilized.

Franklyn JA et al: Mortality after the treatment of hyperthyroidism with radioactive iodine. N Engl J Med 1998;338:712.

Grodski S et al: Surgery versus radioiodine therapy as definitive management for Graves' disease: the role of patient preference. Thyroid 2007;17:157.

Lal G et al: Should total thyroidectomy become the preferred procedure for surgical management of Graves' disease? Thyroid 2005;15:569.

Lee JA, Grumbach MM, Clark OH: The optimal treatment for pediatric Graves' disease is surgery. J Clin Endocrinol Metab 2007;92:801.

Ljunggren JG et al: Quality of life aspects and costs in treatment of Graves' hyperthyroidism with antithyroid drugs, surgery, or radioiodine: results from a prospective, randomized study. Thyroid 1998;8:653.

McLachlan SM, Nagayama Y, Rapoport B: Insight into Graves' hyperthyroidism from animal models. Endocr Rev 2005;26:800.

Metso S et al: Increased cancer incidence after radioiodine treatment for hyperthyroidism. Cancer 2007;109:1972.

Moleti M, et al: Effects of thyroidectomy alone or followed by radioiodine ablation of thyroid remnants on the outcome of Graves' ophthalmopathy. Thyroid 2003;13:653.

EVALUATION OF THYROID NODULES & GOITERS

▶ Thyroid Nodules

The clinician should determine whether a nodular goiter or thyroid nodule is causing localized or systemic symptoms and whether it is benign or malignant. The differential diagnosis includes benign goiter, intrathyroidal cysts, thyroiditis, benign and malignant tumors, and, rarely, metastatic tumors to the thyroid. The history should specifically emphasize the duration of swelling, recent growth, local symptoms (dysphagia, pain, or voice changes), and systemic symptoms (hyperthyroidism, hypothyroidism, or those from possible tumors metastatic to the thyroid). The patient's age, sex, place of birth, family history, and history of radiation to the neck are most important. Low-dose therapeutic radiation (6.5–2000 cGy) in infancy or childhood is associated with an increased incidence of benign goiter (about 35%) or thyroid cancer (about 13%) in later life. A thyroid nodule is more likely to be a cancer in a man than in a woman and in young (under 20 years) and older (over 60 years) patients rather than in others. In certain geographic areas, endemic goiter is common, making benign nodules more common. Thyroid cancer is familial in about 25% of patients with medullary thyroid cancer (familial medullary thyroid cancer, multiple endocrine neoplasia [MEN] types 2a and 2b) and in about 7% of patients with papillary or Hürthle cell cancer. Papillary thyroid cancer occurs more often in patients with Cowden syndrome, Gardner syndrome, or Carney syndrome.

The clinician must systematically palpate the thyroid to determine whether there is a solitary thyroid nodule or if it is a multinodular gland and whether there are palpable lymph nodes. A solitary hard thyroid nodule is likely to be malignant, whereas most multinodular goiters are benign. Ultrasound evaluation helps document the number of nodules, whether a nodule is suspicious for cancer, and whether there are coexistent suspicious lymph nodes.

In many patients, the possibility of cancer is difficult to exclude without microscopic examination of the gland itself. Percutaneous needle biopsy is the most cost-effective diagnostic test and, along with ultrasound, has replaced radioiodine scanning. Cytologic results are classified as malignant, benign, indeterminate or suspicious, and inadequate specimen (Figure 16–2). False-positive diagnoses of cancer are rare, but about 20% of biopsy specimens reported as indeterminate and 5% of those reported as benign are actually malignant. If the specimen is reported as inadequate, biopsy should be repeated. Needle biopsy is not as helpful in patients with a history of irradiation to the neck or familial thyroid cancer because radiation-induced tumors are often multifocal, and a negative biopsy may therefore be unreliable. About 40% of these patients will have thyroid cancer. Radioiodine scanning is used selectively to determine whether a follicular neoplasm by cytologic examination is functioning (warm or hot) or nonfunctioning (cold). Hot solitary thyroid nodules may cause hyperthyroidism but are rarely malignant, whereas cold solitary thyroid nodules have an incidence of cancer of about 20% and should be removed. Thyroid carcinoma is uncommon (about 3%) in multinodular goiters, but if there is a dominant nodule or one that enlarges, it should be biopsied or removed. Thyroid cancer occurs in nearly 40% of the children with solitary thyroid nodules; therefore, fine-needle biopsy or thyroidectomy is indicated. Ultrasound differentiates solid and cystic lesions and, as mentioned, may detect enlarged lymph nodes. About 15% of cold solitary lesions are cystic. A chest x-ray including the neck is helpful in demonstrating tracheal displacement, calcification of the thyroid nodule, or the presence of pulmonary metastases. CT or MRI scans are usually not necessary but are helpful when the limits of the tumor cannot be defined, such as in patients with large, invasive, or substernal goiters or tumors.

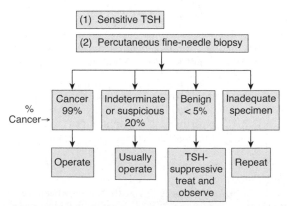

▲ **Figure 16–2.** Evaluation of thyroid nodule.

The principal indications for surgical removal of a nodular goiter are (1) suspicion of or documented cancer, (2) symptoms of pressure, (3) hyperthyroidism, (4) substernal extension, and (5) cosmetic deformity. Incidentally discovered thyroid nodules by ultrasonography, CT, MRI, or positron emission tomography (PET) scans should be evaluated by fine-needle aspiration biopsy and ultrasound. About 50% of thyroid nodules discovered on PET scanning are malignant. Nonoperative treatment is indicated in patients with small or moderately sized multinodular goiters and Hashimoto thyroiditis unless there is a clinically suspicious area that is growing or if the patient was exposed to radiation or has a family history of thyroid carcinoma.

▶ Simple or Nontoxic Goiter (Diffuse & Multinodular Goiter)

Simple goiter may be physiologic, occurring during puberty or pregnancy, or it may occur in patients from endemic (iodine-poor) regions or as a result of prolonged exposure to goitrogenic foods or drugs. As the goiter persists, there is a tendency to form nodules. Goiter may also occur early in life as a consequence of a congenital defect in thyroid hormone production or in patients with Hashimoto thyroiditis. It is generally assumed that nontoxic goiter represents a compensatory response to inadequate thyroid hormone production, although thyroid growth immunoglobulins may also be important. Nontoxic diffuse goiter usually responds favorably to thyroid hormone administration.

Symptoms are usually awareness of a neck mass and dyspnea, dysphagia, or symptoms caused by interference with venous obstruction. In diffuse goiter, the thyroid is symmetrically enlarged and has a smooth surface without areas of encapsulation. However, most patients have multinodular glands by the time they seek medical care. Thyroid function is usually normal, though the sensitive TSH may be suppressed and the radioiodine uptake increased. Surgery is indicated to relieve the pressure symptoms of a large goiter for substernal goiter or to rule out cancer when there are localized areas of hardness or rapid growth. Aspiration biopsy cytology is helpful in these patients.

Bellantone R et al: Management of cystic or predominantly cystic thyroid nodules: the role of ultrasound-guided fine-needle aspiration biopsy. Thyroid 2004;14:43.

Brenta G et al: Comparative efficacy and side effects of the treatment of euthyroid goiter with levo-thyroxine or triiodothyroacetic acid. J Clin Endocrinol Metab 2003;88:5287.

Brunaud L et al: Incision length for standard thyroidectomy and parathyroidectomy: when is it minimally invasive? Arch Surg 2003;138:1140.

Frates MC et al: Management of thyroid nodules detected at US: Society of Radiologists in Ultrasound consensus conference statement. Radiology 2005;237:794.

Kang HW et al: Prevalence, clinical and ultrasonographic characteristics of thyroid incidentalomas. Thyroid 2004;14:29.

Ogilvie JB, Piatigorsky EJ, Clark OH: Current status of fine needle aspiration for thyroid nodules. Adv Surg 2006;40:223.

Sippel RS et al: Does the presence of additional thyroid nodules on ultrasound alter the risk of malignancy in patients with a follicular neoplasm of the thyroid? Surgery 2007;142:851.

INFLAMMATORY THYROID DISEASE

The inflammatory diseases of the thyroid are termed acute, subacute, or chronic thyroiditis, which can be either suppurative or nonsuppurative.

Acute suppurative thyroiditis is uncommon and is characterized by the sudden onset of severe neck pain accompanied by dysphagia, fever, and chills. It usually follows an acute upper respiratory tract infection; can be diagnosed by percutaneous aspiration, smear, and culture; and is treated by surgical drainage. The organisms are most often streptococci, staphylococci, pneumococci, or coliforms. It may also be associated with a piriform sinus fistula. A barium swallow is therefore recommended in persistent or recurrent cases.

Subacute thyroiditis, a noninfectious disorder, is characterized by thyroid swelling, head and chest pain, fever, weakness, malaise, palpitations, and weight loss. Some patients with subacute thyroiditis have no pain (silent thyroiditis), in which case the condition must be distinguished from Graves disease. In subacute thyroiditis, the erythrocyte sedimentation rate and serum gamma globulin are almost always elevated, and radioiodine uptake is very low or absent with increased or normal thyroid hormone levels. The illness is usually self-limited, and aspirin and corticosteroids relieve symptoms. Most of these patients eventually become euthyroid.

Hashimoto thyroiditis, the most common form of thyroiditis, is usually characterized by enlargement of the thyroid with or without pain and tenderness. It is much more common in women (about 15% of U.S. women) and occasionally causes dysphagia or hypothyroidism.

Hashimoto thyroiditis is an autoimmune disease. Serum titers of antimicrosomal and antithyroglobulin antibodies are elevated. Appropriate treatment for most patients consists of giving small doses of thyroid hormone. Operation is indicated for marked pressure symptoms, for suspected malignant tumor, and for cosmetic reasons. In patients with pressure or choking symptoms, surgical division of the isthmus provides relief. If the thyroid is large or asymmetric and fails to regress after treatment with exogenous thyroid hormone, or if it contains a discrete nodule, or grows rapidly, percutaneous needle biopsy or thyroidectomy is recommended. Thyroid lymphoma can rarely occur in patients with Hashimoto thyroiditis.

Riedel thyroiditis is a rare condition that presents as a hard woody mass in the thyroid region with marked fibrosis and chronic inflammation in and around the gland. The inflammatory process infiltrates muscles and causes symptoms of tracheal compression. Hypothyroidism is usually present, and hypoparathyroid may develop. Surgical treatment is required to relieve tracheal or esophageal obstruction.

Kon YC, DeGroot LJ: Painful Hashimoto's thyroiditis as an indication for thyroidectomy: clinical characteristics and outcome in seven patients. J Clin Endocrinol Metab 2003;88:2667.
Mezosi E et al: Aberrant apoptosis in thyroid epithelial cells from goiter nodules. J Clin Endocrinol Metab 2002;87:4264.

BENIGN TUMORS OF THE THYROID

Benign thyroid tumors are adenomas, involutionary nodules, cysts, or localized thyroiditis. Most adenomas are of the follicular type. Adenomas are usually solitary and encapsulated and compress the adjacent thyroid. The major reasons for removal are a suspicion of cancer, functional overactivity producing hyperthyroidism, and cosmetic disfigurement.

MALIGNANT TUMORS OF THE THYROID

 ESSENTIALS OF DIAGNOSIS

▸ History of irradiation to the neck in some patients.

▸ Painless or enlarging nodule, dysphagia, or hoarseness.

▸ Firm or hard, fixed thyroid nodule; ipsilateral cervical lymphadenopathy.

▸ Normal thyroid function; nodule stippled with microcalcifications and solid (ultrasound), cold (radioiodine scan); positive or suspicious cytology.

▸ Family history of thyroid cancer.

▸ General Considerations

An appreciation of the classification of malignant tumors of the thyroid is important, because thyroid tumors demonstrate a wide range of growth and malignant behavior. At one end of the spectrum is **papillary adenocarcinoma,** which usually occurs in young adults, grows very slowly, metastasizes through lymphatics, and is compatible with long life even in the presence of metastases (Figure 16–3). At the other extreme is **undifferentiated carcinoma,** which appears late in life and is nonencapsulated and invasive, forming large infiltrating tumors composed of small or large anaplastic cells. Most patients with anaplastic thyroid carcinoma succumb as a consequence of local recurrence, pulmonary metastasis, or both within 6 months. Between these two extremes are follicular, Hürthle cell, and medullary carcinomas, sarcomas, lymphomas, and metastatic tumors. The prognosis depends on the histologic pattern, the age and sex of the patient, the extent of tumor spread at the time of diagnosis, whether the tumor takes up radioiodine, and other factors. On average, 5% of patients with papillary, 10% of those with follicular, 15% of those with Hürthle cell, and 20% of those with medullary thyroid cancer will die within 10 years from these tumors.

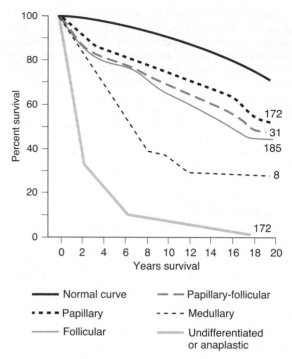

▲ **Figure 16–3.** Survival rates after thyroidectomy for papillary, mixed papillary-follicular, follicular, medullary, and undifferentiated thyroid cancer.

The cause of most cases of thyroid carcinoma is unknown, although persons who received low-dose (6.5–2000 cGy) therapeutic radiation to the thymus, tonsils, scalp, and skin in infancy, childhood, and adolescence have an increased risk of developing thyroid tumors. Children are most susceptible to radiation exposure such as occurred with the Chernobyl nuclear accident, but adults up to 50 years of age who were exposed to the atomic blast at Hiroshima had an increased incidence of benign and malignant thyroid tumors. The incidence of thyroid cancer increases for at least 30 years after irradiation. *RET/PTC* rearrangements occur in about 80% of radiation associated papillary thyroid cancers.

▸ Types of Thyroid Cancer

A. Papillary Adenocarcinoma

Papillary adenocarcinoma accounts for 85% of cancers of the thyroid gland. The tumor usually appears in early adult life and presents as a solitary nodule. It then spreads via intraglandular lymphatics within the thyroid gland and then to the subcapsular and pericapsular lymph nodes. Fifty percent of children and 20% of adults present with palpable lymph nodes. The tumor may metastasize to lungs or bone. Microscopically, it is composed of papillary projections of columnar epithelium. Psammoma bodies are present in about 60% of cases. Mixed papillary-follicular, follicular variants of papillary carcinoma, and poorly differentiated cancers including tall cell and columnar cell papillary thyroid cancers are sometimes found. The rate of growth may be stimulated by TSH. A *BRAF* mutation is the most common mutation in papillary thyroid cancer and is associated with lymph node metastases and a higher recurrence rate.

B. Follicular Adenocarcinoma

Follicular adenocarcinoma accounts for approximately 10% of malignant thyroid tumors. It appears later in life than the papillary form and may be rubbery or even soft on palpation. Follicular tumors are encapsulated. Microscopically, follicular carcinoma may be difficult to distinguish from normal thyroid tissue. Capsular (invasion through the capsule) and vascular invasion distinguish follicular carcinomas from follicular adenomas. Follicular thyroid cancers only occasionally (6%) metastasize to the regional lymph nodes, but they have a greater tendency to spread by the hematogenous route to the lungs, the skeleton, and, rarely, the liver. Metastases from this tumor often demonstrate an avidity for radioactive iodine after total thyroidectomy. Skeletal metastases may appear years after resection of the primary lesion. Hürthle cell carcinoma is considered to be a variant of follicular carcinoma. It is more likely to be multifocal and involve lymph nodes than follicular carcinoma. Like follicular carcinoma, it makes thyroglobulin, but it does not usually take up radioiodine. The prognosis is not as good for either follicular or Hürthle cell cancers as with the papillary type (Figure 16–3).

C. Medullary Carcinoma

Medullary carcinoma accounts for approximately 7% of malignant tumors of the thyroid and 15% of thyroid cancer deaths. It contains amyloid and is a solid, hard, nodular tumor that does not take up radioiodine and secretes calcitonin. Medullary carcinomas arise from parafollicular cells of the ultimobranchial bodies or C cells. Familial medullary carcinoma occurs in about 25% of patients. It may be isolated or occur with pheochromocytomas (often bilateral), lichen planus amyloidosis, and hyperparathyroidism (MEN 2a). It may also occur with or without pheochromocytomas (usually bilateral), marfanoid habitus, multiple neuromas, and ganglioneuromatosis (MEN 2b). Hirschsprung disease occurs more frequently in patients with familial medullary cancer. All patients with medullary thyroid cancer should be screened for an *RET* point mutation on chromosome 10 because 10% of patients without a positive family history have de novo mutations. For patients detected by family genetic screening, most experts recommend prophylactic total thyroidectomy prior to age 6. Isolated familial medullary thyroid cancer is the least aggressive form, whereas this cancer is most aggressive in MEN 2b patients.

D. Undifferentiated Carcinoma

This rapidly growing tumor occurs principally in women beyond middle life and accounts for 1% of all thyroid cancers. This tumor usually evolves from a papillary or follicular neoplasm. It is a solid, quickly enlarging, hard, irregular mass diffusely involving the gland and often invades the trachea, muscles, and neurovascular structures. The tumor may be painful and somewhat tender, may be fixed on swallowing, and may cause laryngeal or esophageal obstructive symptoms. Microscopically, there are three major types: giant cell, spindle cell, and small cell. Mitoses are frequent. Cervical lymphadenopathy and pulmonary metastases are common. Local recurrence after surgical treatment is the rule. Combination treatment with external radiation therapy, chemotherapy, and surgery offers palliation to some patients but is rarely curative (Figure 16–3).

▶ Treatment

The treatment of differentiated thyroid carcinoma is operative removal. For papillary carcinoma over 1 cm, acceptable operations are near-total or total thyroidectomy. For solitary papillary carcinomas less than 1 cm, thyroid lobectomy is adequate treatment. Subtotal or partial lobectomy is contraindicated because the incidence of tumor recurrence is greater and survival is shorter. Total thyroidectomy is recommended by the author and many others for papillary (> 1.0 cm), follicular, Hürthle cell, and medullary carcinomas if the operation can be done without producing permanent hypoparathyroidism or injury to the recurrent laryngeal nerves. Total thyroidectomy is preferred over other operations because of the high incidence of multifocal tumor within the gland, a clinical recurrence rate of about 7% in the contralateral lobe if it is spared, and the ease of assessment for recurrence by serum thyroglobulin assay and neck ultrasound examinations during follow-up examinations. It also allows one to treat with radioiodine. Preoperative ultrasound is essential in patients with papillary cancer, and all abnormal central and lateral neck should be removed. Whether an ipsilated prophylactic central neck dissection should be done is controversial.

A functional modified radical neck dissection preserving the sternocleidomastoid muscle, spinal accessory nerve, and sensory nerve is performed if lymph nodes in the lateral neck are clinically involved.

Medullary carcinoma is associated with such a high incidence of nodal involvement that a bilateral central neck node cleanout should be done in all patients as well as concomitant ipsilateral and contralateral modified radical neck dissection for primary tumors more than 1.5 cm in diameter and when the central neck nodes are involved. When serum calcitonin or carcinoembryonic antigen (CEA) levels remain elevated after thyroidectomy, ultrasound or MRI examination of the neck and MRI of the mediastinum should be done. Laparoscopic evaluation of the liver for the common miliary metastases is recommended for patients with markedly elevated calcitonin levels. If there is no metastatic in the liver, then central neck dissection and bilateral functional neck dissections should be done, if not already done, including removal of nodes from the superior mediastinum.

Isolated distant metastatic deposits of differentiated thyroid carcinoma should be removed surgically and treated with ^{131}I after total thyroidectomy or thyroid ablation with radioactive iodine. All patients with thyroid cancer should be maintained indefinitely on suppressive doses of thyroid hormone (mild suppression for low-risk patients). For follow-up, it is helpful to measure basal and TSH-stimulated serum levels of thyroglobulin (a tumor marker for differentiated thyroid cancer), which are usually increased (> 2 ng/mL) in patients with residual tumor after total thyroidectomy. For **undifferentiated carcinoma, malignant lymphoma,** or **sarcoma,** the tumor should be excised as completely as possible and then treated by radiation and chemotherapy. Doxorubicin (Adriamycin), vincristine, and chlorambucil are the most effective agents. Carcinomas of the kidney, breast, and lung and other tumors sometimes metastasize to the thyroid, but they rarely present as a solitary nodule.

Bilimoria KY et al: Extent of surgery affects survival for papillary thyroid cancer. Ann Surg 2007;246:375.

Caron NR, Clark OH: Well differentiated thyroid cancer. Scand J Surg 2004;93:261.

Caron NR, Clark OH: Papillary thyroid cancer. Curr Treat Options Oncol 2006;7:309.

Cooper DS et al: Management guidelines for patients with thyroid nodules and differentiated thyroid cancer. Thyroid 2006; 16:109.

Elaraj DM, Clark OH: Changing management in patients with papillary thyroid cancer. Curr Treat Options Oncol 2007;8:305.

Hay ID: Management of patients with low-risk papillary thyroid carcinoma. Endocr Pract 2007;13:521.

Kebebew E et al: Medullary thyroid carcinoma: clinical characteristics, treatment, prognostic factors, and a comparison of staging systems. Cancer 2000;88:1139.

Kebebew E, Clark OH: Differentiated thyroid cancer: "complete" rational approach. World J Surg 2000;24:942.

Kebebew E et al: Anaplastic thyroid carcinoma. Treatment outcome and prognostic factors. Cancer 2005;103:1330.

Mazzaferri EL: Management of low-risk differentiated thyroid cancer. Endocr Pract 2007;13:498.

Moley JF, Fialkowski EA: Evidence-based approach to the management of sporadic medullary thyroid carcinoma. World J Surg 2007;31:946.

Schlosser K et al: Laryngoscopy in thyroid surgery—essential standard or unnecessary routine? Surgery 2007;142:858.

Sherman SI et al: Thyroid carcinoma. J Natl Compr Canc Netw 2005;3:404.

Sippel RS, Caron NR, Clark OH: An evidence-based approach to familial nonmedullary thyroid cancer: screening, clinical management, and follow-up. World J Surg 2007;31:924.

Triponez F et al: Does familial non-medullary thyroid cancer adversely affect survival? World J Surg 2006;30:787.

White ML, Gauger PG, Doherty GM: Central lymph node dissection in differentiated thyroid cancer. World J Surg 2007;31:895.

▼ II. THE PARATHYROID GLANDS

EMBRYOLOGY & ANATOMY

Phylogenetically, the parathyroids appear rather late, being first seen in Amphibia. They arise from pharyngeal pouches III and IV and may be arrested as high as the level of the hyoid bone during their descent to the posterior capsule of the thyroid gland. Four parathyroid glands are present in 85% of the population, and 85% are situated on the posterior lateral surface of the thyroid gland. About 15% have more than four glands. Occasionally, one or more may be incorporated into the thyroid gland or thymus and hence are intrathyroidal or intrathymic in location. Parathyroid III, which normally assumes the inferior position, may be found in the anterior mediastinum, usually in the thymus. The upper parathyroids (parathyroid IV) usually remain in close association with the upper portion of the lateral thyroid lobes at the level of the cricoid cartilage but may be loosely attached by a long vascular pedicle and migrate caudally in the tracheo esophageal groove into the posterior mediastinum. About 85% of parathyroid glands lie within 1 cm of where the inferior thyroid artery and recurrent laryngeal nerve cross.

The normal parathyroid gland has a distinct yellowish-brown color, is ovoid, tongue-shaped, polypoid, or spherical, and averages $2 \times 3 \times 7$ mm. The total mean weight of four normal parathyroids is about 150 mg. These encapsulated glands are usually supplied by a branch of the inferior thyroid artery but may be supplied by the superior thyroid artery. The vessels can be seen entering a hilumlike structure, a feature that differentiates parathyroid glands from fat.

Maret A et al: Expression of GCMB by intrathymic parathyroid hormone-secreting adenomas indicates their parathyroid cell origin. J Clin Endocrinol Metab 2004;89:8.

PHYSIOLOGY

Parathyroid hormone (PTH), vitamin D, and calcitonin play vital roles in calcium and phosphorus metabolism in bone, kidney, and gut. Specific radioimmunoassays are available to measure PTH, vitamin D, and calcitonin. Ionized calcium, the physiologically important fraction, can now be accurately measured. Total serum calcium concentration is composed of approximately 48% ionized calcium, 46% protein-bound calcium, and 6% calcium complexed to organic anions. Total serum calcium varies directly with plasma protein concentrations, but calcium ion concentrations are unaffected.

PTH and calcitonin work in concert to modulate fluctuations in plasma levels of ionized calcium. When the ionized calcium level falls, the parathyroids secrete more PTH, and the parafollicular cells within the thyroid secrete less calcitonin. The rise in PTH and fall in calcitonin produce increased bone resorption and increased resorption of calcium in the renal tubules. More calcium enters the blood, and ionized calcium levels return to normal.

In the circulation, immunoreactive PTH is heterogeneous, consisting of the intact hormone and several hormonal fragments. The amino terminal (N-terminal) fragment is biologically active, whereas the carboxyl terminal (C-terminal) fragment is biologically inert. Measurement of intact PTH by immunoassay is best for screening for hyperparathyroidism and for selective venous catheterization to localize the source of PTH production. PTH-related peptide (PTHrP) that is secreted by nonparathyroid malignant tumors does not cross-react with intact PTH assays.

Because PTH levels rise in normal subjects if ionized calcium levels are low, calcium and PTH must be determined from samples drawn simultaneously to diagnose hyperparathyroidism. The combination of increased PTH levels and hypercalcemia without hypocalciuria is almost always pathognomonic of hyperparathyroidism.

Shattuck TM et al: Somatic and germ-line mutations of the HRPT2 gene in sporadic parathyroid carcinoma. N Engl J Med 2003;349:1722.

▼ DISEASES OF THE PARATHYROIDS

PRIMARY HYPERPARATHYROIDISM

 ESSENTIALS OF DIAGNOSIS

► Increased fatigue, weakness, arthralgias, nausea, vomiting, dyspepsia, constipation, polydipsia, polyuria, nocturia, psychiatric disturbances, renal colic, bone pain, and joint pain. ("Stones, bones, abdominal groans, psychic moans, and fatigue overtones.") Some patients are asymptomatic.

► Nephrolithiasis and nephrocalcinosis, osteopenia, osteoporosis, osteitis fibrosa cystica, peptic ulcer disease, renal dysfunction, gout, pseudogout, chondrocalcinosis, pancreatitis.

► Hypertension, band keratopathy, neck masses.

► Serum calcium, PTH, chloride, usually increased; serum phosphate low or normal; uric acid and alkaline phosphatase sometimes increased; urine calcium increased, normal, or, rarely, decreased; urine phosphate increased; tubular reabsorption of phosphate decreased, osteocalcin and deoxypyridinoline cross-links increased.

► X-rays: subperiosteal resorption of phalanges, demineralization of the skeleton (osteopenia or osteoporosis), bone cysts, and nephrocalcinosis or nephrolithiasis.

► General Considerations

Primary hyperparathyroidism is due to excess PTH secretion from a single parathyroid adenoma (83%), multiple adenomas (6%), hyperplasia (10%), or carcinoma (1%). Fewer abnormal parathyroid glands are identified at scan-directed (sestamibi/ultrasound) focal exploration. Once thought to be rare, primary hyperparathyroidism is now found in 0.1–0.3% of the general population and is the most common cause of hypercalcemia in unselected patients. It is uncommon before puberty; its peak incidence is between the third and fifth decades, and it is two to three times more common in women than in men.

Overproduction of parathyroid hormone results in mobilization of calcium from bone and inhibition of the renal reabsorption of phosphate, thereby producing hypercalcemia and hypophosphatemia. This causes a wasting of calcium and phosphorus, with osseous mineral loss and osteopenia or **osteoporosis.** Other associated or related conditions that offer clues to the diagnosis of hyperparathyroidism are nephrolithiasis, nephrocalcinosis, osteitis fibrosa cystica, peptic ulcer, pancreatitis, hypertension, and gout or pseudogout. Hyperparathyroidism also occurs in both MEN 1, known as **Werner syndrome**, and MEN 2, known as **Sipple syndrome.** The former is characterized by tumors of the parathyroid, pituitary, and pancreas (hyperparathyroidism, pituitary tumors, and functioning or nonfunctioning islet cell pancreatic tumors) that may cause Zollinger-Ellison syndrome (gastrinoma), hypoglycemia (insulinoma), glucagonoma, somatostatinoma, and pancreatic polypeptide tumors (PPomas). Other tumors in MEN 1 syndrome include adrenocortical tumors, carcinoid tumors, multiple lipomas, and cutaneous angiomas. MEN 2a consists of hyperparathyroidism (20%) in association with medullary carcinoma of the thyroid (98%), pheochromocytoma (50%), and lichen planus amyloidosis. MEN 2b patients have a marfanoid habitus, multiple neuromas, and pheochromocytomas but rarely have hyperparathyroidism. Familial hyperparathyroidism can also occur alone or in the presence of jaw tumor syndrome.

Parathyroid adenomas range in weight from 65 mg to over 35 g, and the size usually parallels the degree of hypercalcemia. Microscopically, these tumors may be of chief cell, water cell, or, rarely, oxyphil cell type.

Primary parathyroid hyperplasia involves all of the parathyroid glands. Microscopically, there are two types: chief cell hyperplasia and water-clear cell (wasserhelle) hyperplasia. Hyperplastic glands vary considerably in size but are usually larger than normal (65 mg).

Parathyroid carcinoma is rare but is more common in patients with profound hypercalcemia and in patients with familial hyperparathyroidism and jaw tumor syndrome. Parathyroid cancers are palpable in half the patients and should be suspected in patients at operation when the parathyroid gland is hard, has a whitish or irregular capsule, or is invasive. Parathyromatosis is a rare condition causing hypercalcemia due to multiple embryologic rests or, more commonly, due to seeding when a parathyroid tumor has ruptured or the tumor capsule has been disrupted.

▶ Clinical Findings

A. Symptoms and Signs

Historically, the clinical manifestations of hyperparathyroidism have changed. Forty years ago, the diagnosis was based on bone pain and deformity (osteitis fibrosa cystica), and in later years on the renal complications (nephrolithiasis and nephrocalcinosis). At present, over two thirds of patients are detected by routine screening, or because of osteopenia or osteoporosis, and some are asymptomatic. Patients with even mild primary hyperparathyroidism are predisposed to cardiovascular events and fractures. After successful surgical treatment, many patients thought to be asymptomatic become aware of improvement in unrecognized preoperative symptoms such as fatigue, mild depression, weakness, constipation, polydipsia and polyuria, and bone and joint pain. Hyperparathyroidism should be suspected in all patients with hypercalcemia and the above symptoms, especially if associated with nephrolithiasis, nephrocalcinosis, hypertension, left ventricular hypertrophy, peptic ulcer, pancreatitis, or gout. Patients with primary hyperparathyroidism appear to have a shortened life expectancy that improves after successful parathyroidectomy. Younger patients and those with less severe hypercalcemia after parathyroidectomy have the best prognosis.

B. Laboratory Findings, Imaging Studies, and Differential Diagnosis (Approach to the Hypercalcemic Patient)

1. Laboratory findings—See Table 16–2. Hyperparathyroidism and cancer are responsible for about 90% of all cases of hypercalcemia. Hyperparathyroidism is the most common cause of hypercalcemia detected by undirected methods such as routine screening, whereas cancer is the most common cause of hypercalcemia in hospitalized patients. Other causes of hypercalcemia are listed in Table 16–3. In many patients the diagnosis is obvious, while in others it may be difficult. At times, more than one reason for hypercalcemia may exist in the same patient, such as cancer or sarcoidosis plus hyperparathyroidism. A careful history must be obtained documenting (1) the duration of any symptoms possibly related to hypercalcemia; (2) symptoms related to malignant disease; (3) conditions associated with hyperparathyroidism, such as renal colic, peptic ulcer disease, pancreatitis, hypertension, or gout; and (4) possible excess use of milk products, antacids, baking soda, or vitamins. In patients with a recent cough, wheeze, or hemoptysis, epidermoid carcinoma of the lung should be considered. Hematuria might suggest hypernephroma, bladder tumor, or renal lithiasis. A long history of renal stones or peptic ulcer disease suggests that hyperparathyroidism is likely.

Table 16–2. Laboratory Evaluation of Hypercalcemia.

Essential	Selective
Blood tests	
Calcium	Creatine and BUN
Phosphate	Chloride
PTH (intact or two-site assay)	Uric acid
Alkaline phosphatase	pH
	Protein electrophoresis or albumin: globulin ratio
	25-Dihydroxyvitamin D and 1,25-dihydroxyvitamin D
Radiographic or nuclear medicine procedures	
Chest x-ray	Sestamibi scan of neck and ultrasound of neck
Abdominal plain films	
Ultrasound of kidneys	
Bone density (hip, lumbar spine, wrist)	
Urine tests	
24-hour urinary calcium[1]	Urinalysis
	Deoxypyridinoline cross-links
	Osteocalcin

[1]When urine calcium is < 100 mg/24 h, a diagnosis of benign familial hypocalciuric hypercalcemia must be considered.

The most important tests for the evaluation of hypercalcemia are, in order of importance, serum calcium, parathyroid hormone, phosphate, chloride, alkaline phosphatase, creatinine; uric acid and urea nitrogen; urinary calcium; blood hematocrit and pH; serum magnesium; and erythrocyte sedimentation rate. Measurement of 25-hydroxy and 1,25-hydroxy vitamin D levels, and serum protein electrophoresis are helpful in selected patients when other tests are equivocal.

A high serum calcium and a low serum phosphate suggest hyperparathyroidism, but about half of patients with hyperparathyroidism have normal serum phosphate concentrations. Patients with vitamin D intoxication, sarcoidosis, malignant disease without metastasis, and hyperthyroidism may also be hypophosphatemic, but patients with breast cancer and hypercalcemia are only rarely so. In fact, if hypophosphatemia and hypercalcemia are present in association with breast cancer, concomitant hyperparathyroidism is probable. Measurement of **serum parathyroid hormone** has its greatest value in this situation, since the PTH level is low or nil in patients with hypercalcemia due to *all* causes other than primary or ectopic hyperparathyroidism or familial hypocalciuric hypercalcemia. In general, serum PTH levels should be measured in all patients with persistent hyper-

Table 16–3. Causes of Hypercalcemia.

	Approximate Frequency (%)
Cancer	45
Breast cancer	
Metastatic	
PTH-related peptide secreting (lung, kidney)	
Multiple myeloma	
Leukemias	
Others	
Endocrine disorders	46
Hyperparathyroidism	
Hyperthyroidism	
Addison disease, pheochromocytoma	
Hypothyroidism, VIPoma	
Increased intake	4
Milk-alkali syndrome	
Vitamin D and A overdosage	
Thiazides, lithium, aluminum	
Granulomatous diseases	3
Sarcoidosis, tuberculosis, etc	
Benign familial hypocalciuric hypercalcemia and other disorders	2
Paget disease	
Immobilization	
Idiopathic hypercalcemia of infancy	
Aluminum intoxication	
Dysproteinemias	
Rhabdomyolysis	

calcemia without an obvious cause and in normocalcemic patients who are suspected of having hyperparathyroidism. Determination of intact serum PTH levels is best because it is sensitive and is not influenced by tumors that secrete parathyroid-related peptide. Nonparathyroid tumors that secrete pure PTH are extremely rare.

An elevated serum chloride concentration is a useful diagnostic clue found in about 40% of hyperparathyroid patients. PTH acts directly on the proximal renal tubule to decrease the resorption of bicarbonate, which leads to increased resorption of chloride and mild hyperchloremic renal tubular acidosis. An increased serum chloride is not found in other causes of hypercalcemia. Calculation of the **serum chloride to phosphate ratio** takes advantage of slight increases in serum chloride and slight decreases in serum phosphate concentrations. A ratio above 33 suggests hyperparathyroidism.

Serum protein electrophoretic patterns are helpful for excluding multiple myeloma and sarcoidosis. Hypergammaglobulinemia is rare in hyperparathyroidism but is not uncommon in patients with multiple myeloma and sarcoidosis. Roentgenograms of the skull or site of bone pain in patients with elevated alkaline phosphatase levels will often reveal typical "punched-out" bony lesions, and the diagnosis of myeloma can be firmly established by bone marrow examination. Sarcoidosis can be difficult to diagnose, because it may exist for several years with few clinical findings. A chest x-ray revealing a diffuse fibronodular infiltrate and prominent hilar adenopathy is suggestive, and the demonstration of noncaseating granuloma in lymph nodes is diagnostic. The **hydrocortisone suppression test** (150 mg of hydrocortisone per day for 10 days) reduces the serum calcium concentration in most cases of sarcoidosis and vitamin D intoxication and in many patients with carcinoma and multiple myeloma but only rarely in patients with hyperparathyroidism. It is therefore a useful diagnostic maneuver if these conditions are considered. Hydrocortisone suppression is used to treat the hypercalcemic crises that may occur with these disorders.

Serum alkaline phosphate levels are elevated in about 10% of patients with primary hyperparathyroidism and may also be increased in patients with Paget disease and cancer. When the serum alkaline phosphatase level is elevated, serum 5'-nucleotidase, which parallels liver alkaline phosphatase, should be measured to determine if the increase is from bone, which suggests parathyroid disease, or liver. A 24-hour urine calcium level is helpful for diagnosing hypercalcemic patients who have low urinary calcium levels resulting from benign familial hypocalciuric hypercalcemia (BFHH) and for patients with marked hypercalciuria (> 400 mg/24 h). Patients with BFHH do not benefit from parathyroidectomy.

2. Bone studies—Bone densitometry and radiographic examination of bone frequently reveals osteopenia (1 standard deviation) or osteoporosis (2.5 standard deviations from normal), but overt skeletal changes such as subperiosteal resorption or brown tumor are found in only 10% of patients with hyperparathyroidism. Dual photon bone density studies of the femur, lumbar spine, and radius help document osteopenia that occurs in about 70% of female patients with hyperparathyroidism. Bone changes of osteitis fibrosa cystica are rare on x-ray unless the serum alkaline phosphatase concentration is increased. Primary and secondary hyperparathyroidism produce subperiosteal resorption of the phalanges and bone cysts (Figure 16–4). A ground-glass appearance of the skull with loss of definition of the tables and demineralization of the outer aspects of the clavicles are less frequently seen. In patients with markedly elevated serum alkaline phosphatase levels without subperiosteal resorption on x-ray, Paget disease or cancer must be suspected. A 24-hour urine test for deoxypyridinoline crosslink assay or osteocalcin detects increased bone loss.

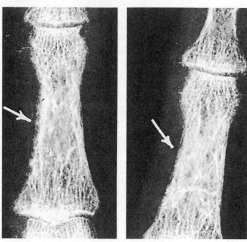

▲ **Figure 16–4.** Subperiosteal resorption of radial side of second phalanges.

3. Differential diagnosis—The differentiation between hyperparathyroidism due to primary parathyroid disease and that due to ectopic hyperparathyroidism or nonparathyroid cancer can now almost always be determined by measuring intact PTH (increased in primary hyperparathyroidism) and PTHrP (increased in nonparathyroid malignant tumors). The most common tumors causing ectopic hyperparathyroidism are squamous cell carcinoma of the lung, renal cell carcinoma, and bladder cancer. Less commonly it is due to hepatoma or to cancer of the ovary, stomach, pancreas, parotid gland, or colon. Recent onset of symptoms, increased sedimentation rate, anemia, serum calcium greater than 14 mg/dL, and increased alkaline phosphatase activity without osteitis fibrosa cystica suggest **malignancy-associated hypercalcemia;** mild hypercalcemia with a long history of nephrolithiasis or peptic ulcer suggests primary hyperthyroidism. Documented hypercalcemia of 6 months or longer essentially rules out malignancy-associated hypercalcemia.

In **milk-alkali syndrome,** a history of excessive ingestion of milk products, calcium-containing antacids, and baking soda is often obtained. These patients become normocalcemic after discontinuing these habits. Patients with milk-alkali syndrome usually have renal insufficiency and low urinary calcium concentrations and are usually alkalotic rather than acidotic. Because of the high incidence of ulcer disease in hyperparathyroidism, milk-alkali syndrome may occasionally coexist with that disorder.

Hyperthyroidism, another cause of hypercalcemia and hypercalciuria, can usually be differentiated because manifestations of thyrotoxicosis rather than hypercalcemia bring the patient to the physician. Occasionally, an elderly patient with apathetic hyperthyroidism may be hypercalcemic. A sensitive TSH test should be evaluated in hypercalcemic patients whose PTH levels are not increased. Treatment of hyperthyroidism with antithyroid medications causes serum calcium to return to normal levels within 8 weeks.

Normal subjects taking **thiazide diuretics** may develop a transient increase in serum calcium levels, usually less than 1 mg/dL. Larger rises in serum calcium induced by thiazides have been reported in patients with primary hyperparathyroidism and idiopathic juvenile osteoporosis. Most patients who have hypercalcemia while taking thiazides have another reason for the increase. The best way to evaluate these patients is to switch them to a nonthiazide antihypertensive agent or diuretic and to measure the PTH level. Thiazide-induced hypercalcemia is not associated with increased serum PTH in patients without hyperparathyroidism.

Benign familial hypocalciuric hypercalcemia is one of the few conditions that causes chronic hypercalcemia and mildly elevated PTH levels. It can be difficult to distinguish from primary hyperparathyroidism. The best way to diagnose this disorder is to document a low urinary calcium and a family history of hypercalcemia, especially in children.

Other miscellaneous causes of hypercalcemia are Paget disease, immobilization (especially in Paget disease or in young patients), dysproteinemias, idiopathic hypercalcemia of infancy, aluminum intoxication, and rhabdomyolysis (Table 16–3).

C. Approach to the Normocalcemic Patient with Possible Hyperparathyroidism

Renal failure, hypoalbuminemia, pancreatitis, deficiency of vitamin D or magnesium, and excess phosphate intake may cause serum calcium levels to be normal in hyperparathyroidism. Correction of these disorders results in hypercalcemia if hyperparathyroidism is present. The incidence of normocalcemic hyperparathyroidism in patients with hypercalciuria and recurrent nephrolithiasis (idiopathic hypercalciuria) is not known. Because the serum calcium concentration may fluctuate, it should be measured on more than three separate occasions. The serum calcium should be determined the day the sample is obtained, because the calcium level decreases with refrigeration or freezing. Determination of serum ionized calcium is also useful, since it may be increased in patients with normal total serum calcium levels.

If a patient has elevated serum levels of ionized calcium and PTH, the diagnosis of normocalcemic hyperparathyroidism has been confirmed. There are three major causes of hypercalciuria and nephrolithiasis: (1) increased absorption of calcium from the gastrointestinal tract (absorptive hypercalciuria), (2) increased renal leakage of calcium (renal hypercalciuria), and (3) primary hyperparathyroidism. Patients with absorptive hypercalcemia absorb too much calcium from the gastrointestinal tract and therefore have low serum PTH levels. Patients with renal hypercalciuria lose calcium from leaky renal tubules and have increased PTH levels. They can be distinguished from patients with normocalcemic hyperparathyroidism by their response to treatment with thiazides. In renal leak hypercalcemia, serum PTH levels become normal because thiazides correct the excessive loss of calcium, whereas in primary hyperparathyroidism increased serum PTH levels persist and the patient often becomes hypercalcemic.

▶ Natural History of Untreated & Treated Hyperparathyroidism

Patients with untreated hyperparathyroidism have an increased risk of dying prematurely, mainly from cardiovascular and malignant disease. There is decreased respiratory muscular capacity and increased frequency of hypertrophic cardiomyopathy with left ventricular hypertrophy and decreased vascular compliance even in hyperparathyroid patients without hypertension. Hyperparathyroid patients have more hypertension, nephrolithiasis, osteopenia, peptic ulcer disease, gout, renal dysfunction, and pancreatitis. After successful parathyroidectomy, previously hyperparathyroid patients still have an increased risk of premature death, however, younger patients and those with less severe disease return to a normal survival curve sooner than do older patients or those with more severe hyperparathyroidism. Most patients with hyperparathyroidism—even those with normocalcemic hyperparathyroidism—have symptoms and associated conditions. In 80% of patients, these clinical manifestations improve or disappear after parathyroidectomy.

▶ Treatment

The only curative treatment of primary hyperparathyroidism is parathyroidectomy. The author believes that virtually all patients with either asymptomatic or symptomatic hyperparathyroidism benefit from the operation both symptomatically and metabolically as well as with improved survival. There are no convincing data to support a plan of medical observation, and considerable data support a surgical approach. Once associated conditions such as hypertension and renal dysfunction become well established, they seem to progress despite correction of the primary hyperparathyroidism. Thus, it appears to be better to intervene early while it is still possible to correct these problems. In all patients, however, the diagnosis should be established, and short delays to clarify the diagnosis are justified.

A. Marked Hypercalcemia (Hypercalcemic Crisis)

The initial treatment in patients with marked hypercalcemia and acute symptoms is hydration and correction of hypokalemia and hyponatremia. While the patient is being hydrated, assessment of the underlying problem is essential so that more specific therapy may be started. Milk and alkaline products, estrogens, thiazides, and vitamins A and D should be immediately discontinued. Furosemide is useful to increase calcium excretion in the rehydrated patient. Etidronate, plicamycin, and calcitonin are usually effective for short periods in treating hypercalcemia regardless of cause. Glucocorticoids are very effective in vitamin D intoxication, hyperthyroidism, and sarcoidosis and in many patients with cancer, including those with peptide-secreting tumors, but are less effective when there is extensive bone disease. As mentioned previously, hyperparathyroid patients only occasionally respond to glucocorticoid administration.

In patients with marked hypercalcemia, once the diagnosis of hyperparathyroidism is established, localization studies, cervical exploration, and parathyroidectomy should be performed in a vigorously hydrated patient, since this is the most rapid and effective method of reducing serum calcium.

B. Localization

Preoperative localization of parathyroid tumors can now be accomplished in about 75% of patients with ultrasonography and 85% with sestamibi scans. These studies, however, are helpful in only about 35% of patients with parathyroid hyperplasia (Figure 16–5). Localization studies are essential in patients with persistent or recurrent hyperparathyroidism and can direct a focused exploration in patients with sporadic primary hyperparathyroidism. An experienced surgeon can find the tumors in about 95% of patients who have not had previous parathyroid or thyroid surgery without preoperative tests. Selective venous catheterization with parathyroid hormone immunoassay is also recommended for patients who have had an unsuccessful previous operation when the noninvasive localization tests are negative or equivocal. This study helps localize the tumor in about 80% of patients. Digital subtraction angiography is useful, while arteriography is now rarely used.

C. Operation

Three approaches are now acceptable for patients with sporadic primary hyperparathyroidism. The bilateral approach is safe and does not require preoperative tests or intraoperative PTH testing. A unilateral approach can be elected when one or more localization tests identify a solitary parathyroid tumor. At operation, a normal and abnormal parathyroid should be identified on the side of the localized tumor. A focal operation can be done in similar patients and the operation completed when the intraoperative PTH level decreases by more than 50% from the highest pre-removed value 10 minutes after the parathyroid tumor is removed. When the sestamibi and ultrasound scans both independently identify the same tumor, a successful operation occurs in approximately 96% of patients. Endoscopic parathyroidectomy is recommended by a minority of surgeons.

In over 80% of cases, the parathyroid tumor is found attached to the posterior capsule of the thyroid gland. The parathyroid glands are usually symmetrically placed, and lower parathyroid glands are situated anterior to the recurrent laryngeal nerve, whereas the upper parathyroid glands lie posterior to the recurrent laryngeal nerve, where it enters

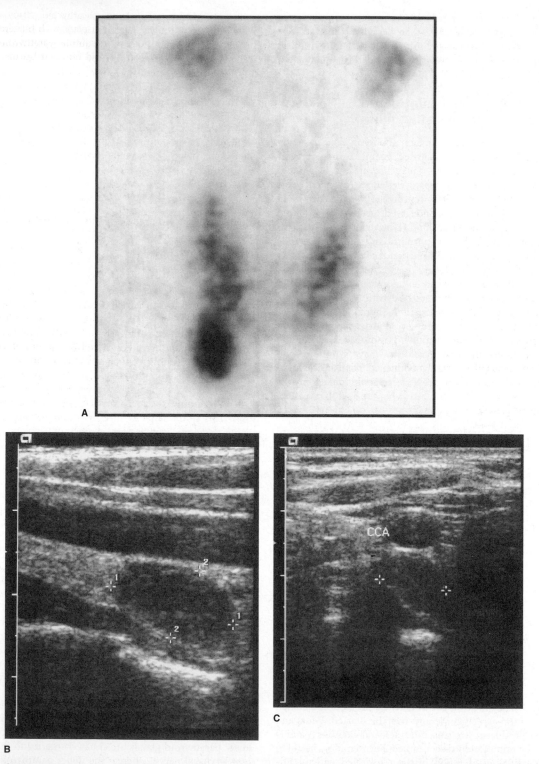

▲ **Figure 16–5.** Parathyroid adenomas. **A:** Sestamibi scan of right lower parathyroid adenoma. **B:** Longitudinal ultrasound scan of left lower parathyroid adenoma. **C:** Transverse ultrasound scan of left lower parathyroid adenoma.

the cricothyroid muscle. Parathyroid tumors may also lie cephalad to the superior pole of the thyroid gland, along the great vessels of the neck in the tracheoesophageal area, in thymic tissue, in the substance of the thyroid gland itself, or in the mediastinum. Care must be taken to avoid bleeding and not to traumatize the parathyroid gland or tumors, since color is useful in distinguishing them from surrounding thyroid, thymus, lymph node, and fat. Furthermore, rupture of the parathyroid gland may result in parathyromatosis (seeding of parathyroid tissue) and possible recurrent hyperparathyroidism. Two helpful maneuvers for localizing parathyroid tumors at operation are following the course of a branch of the inferior thyroid artery and gently palpating for the parathyroid tumor. One should attempt to identify four parathyroid glands when a bilateral approach is elected, though there may be more than four or fewer than four.

If a probable parathyroid adenoma is found, it is removed and the diagnosis confirmed by frozen section or by a greater than 50% decrease in PTH. It seems unwise to remove a grossly normal parathyroid gland intentionally, both because this has no beneficial effect and because the gland may be needed to maintain normal function after all the hyperfunctioning tissue is removed. If two adenomas are found, both are removed, and both normal glands are marked and biopsied but not removed.

The presence of a normal parathyroid gland at operation indicates that the tumor removed is an adenoma rather than parathyroid hyperplasia, since in hyperplasia all the parathyroid glands are involved. A compressed rim of normal parathyroid tissue is also suggestive of an adenoma. When all parathyroid glands are hyperplastic, the most normal gland should be subtotally resected, leaving a 50 mg remnant, and confirmed histologically before removal of the remaining glands. The upper thymus and perithymic tract should be removed in patients with hyperplasia, because a fifth parathyroid gland is present in 15% of cases.

If exploration fails to reveal a parathyroid tumor, a missing lower gland is often in the thymus (anterior mediastinum), whereas a missing upper gland is usually paraesophageal (or in the posterior mediastinum). One should therefore perform a thymectomy, thyroid lobectomy, or partial thyroidectomy on the side that has only one parathyroid gland, since tumors may be found within the thymus or intrathyroidally. If thyroid nodules are present and suspicious on ultrasound, a fine needle biopsy for cytological examination is useful. Differentiated thyroid carcinoma occurs in 3% of patients with hyperparathyroidism and more frequently in patients with a history of radiation exposure.

The recurrence rate of hyperparathyroidism after the removal of a single adenoma in patients with sporadic hyperparathyroidism is 2% or less. In patients with multiple endocrine neoplasia and familial hyperparathyroidism, recurrent hyperparathyroidism is more common (approximately 33%); therefore, extra care should be taken to remove all abnormal parathyroid tissue by subtotal parathyroidectomy or total parathyroidectomy and auto transplant with bilateral upper thymectomy. The author prefers subtotal parathyroidectomy leaving a well-marked parathyroid remnant because not all parathyroid autografts function effectively.

Exploration of the mediastinum via a sternal split at the initial operation is necessary in only 1–2% of cases and is only recommended in patients with a serum calcium level above 13.5 mg/dL. If cervical exploration was nonproductive or if localization studies suggest a mediastinal tumor, the patient should be allowed to recover from the initial operation and return in 6–8 weeks for mediastinal exploration. Preoperative localization tests are essential before reoperation. Angiographic ablation is possible for poor-risk patients with mediastinal parathyroid adenomas not easily removed via a cervical incision.

D. Postoperative Care

Following removal of a parathyroid adenoma or hyperplastic glands, the serum calcium concentration falls to normal or below normal in 24–48 hours. Patients with severe skeletal depletion ("hungry bones"), long-standing hyperparathyroidism, or high calcium levels may develop profound hypocalcemia with paresthesias, carpopedal spasm, or even seizures. If the symptoms are mild and serum calcium falls slowly, oral supplementation with calcium is all that is required. When marked symptoms develop, it is necessary to give calcium gluconate intravenously. If the response is not rapid, the serum magnesium concentration should be determined and magnesium given if low. Treatment with calcitriol, 0.5 micrograms twice daily is sometimes required. (See section on Hypoparathyroidism.)

E. Reoperation

Reexploration for persistent or recurrent hyperparathyroidism or after a previous thyroidectomy presents formidable problems and an increased risk of complications. First ascertain that the diagnosis is correct and that the patient does not have benign familial hypocalciuric hypercalcemia or hypercalcemia due to another cause such as a malignant tumor. Ultrasound, CT or MRI, and sestamibi scanning should be done first. If these studies are unsuccessful or equivocal, digital subtraction angiography and highly selective venous catheterization with parathyroid hormone immunoassay are recommended. Most such patients have a parathyroid tumor that can be removed through a cervical incision, making mediastinal exploration unnecessary. The success rate of parathyroidectomy performed by experienced surgeons is 95% or better at an initial operation versus a success rate of about 75% with surgeons less experienced at this procedure. The success rate for patients requiring reoperation is about 90%. This success rate is lower in patients with negative or equivocal localization tests and in patients with parathyromatosis and parathyroid cancer.

The American Association of Clinical Endocrinologists and the American Association of Endocrine Surgeons position statement on the diagnosis and management of primary hyperparathyroidism. Endocr Pract 2005;11:49.

Brunaud L et al: Incision length for standard thyroidectomy and parathyroidectomy: when is it minimally invasive? Arch Surg 2003;138:1140.

Clark OH: How should patients with primary hyperparathyroidism be treated? J Clin Endocrinol Metab 2003;88:3011.

Eigelberger MS et al: The NIH criteria for parathyroidectomy in asymptomatic primary hyperparathyroidism: are they too limited? Ann Surg 2004;239:528.

Genc H et al: Differing histologic findings after bilateral and focused parathyroidectomy. J Am Coll Surg 2003;196:535.

Haciyanli M et al: Accuracy of preoperative localization studies and intraoperative parathyroid hormone assay in patients with primary hyperparathyroidism and double adenoma. J Am Coll Surg 2003;197:739.

Karakousis GC et al: Interpretation of intra-operative PTH changes in patients with multi-glandular primary hyperparathyroidism (pHPT). Surgery 2007;142:845.

Kebebew E et al: Predictors of single-gland vs multigland parathyroid disease in primary hyperparathyroidism: a simple and accurate scoring model. Arch Surg 2006;141:777.

Lal G, Clark OH: Primary hyperparathyroidism: controversies in surgical management. Trends Endocrinol Metab 2003;14:417.

Miccoli P et al: Minimally invasive video assisted parathyroidectomy (MIVAP). Eur J Surg Oncol 2003;29:188.

Ogilvie JB, Clark OH: Parathyroid surgery: we still need traditional and selective approaches. J Endocrinol Invest 2005;28:566.

Peacock M et al: Cinacalcet hydrochloride maintains long-term normocalcemia in patients with primary hyperparathyroidism. J Clin Endocrinol Metab 2005;90:135.

Siilin H et al: Disturbances of calcium homeostasis consistent with mild primary hyperparathyroidism in premenopausal women and associated morbidity. J Clin Endocrinol Metab 2008;93:47.

Stavrakis AI et al: Surgeon volume as a predictor of outcomes in inpatient and outpatient endocrine surgery. Surgery 2007;142:887.

Utiger RD: Treatment of primary hyperparathyroidism. N Engl J Med 1999;341:1301.

SECONDARY & TERTIARY HYPERPARATHYROIDISM

In secondary hyperparathyroidism, there is an increase in parathyroid hormone secretion in response to low plasma concentrations of ionized calcium, usually owing to renal disease and malabsorption. This results in chief cell hyperplasia. When secondary hyperparathyroidism occurs as a complication of renal disease, the serum phosphorus level is usually high, whereas in malabsorption, osteomalacia, or rickets it is frequently low or normal. Secondary hyperparathyroidism with renal osteodystrophy is a frequent if not universal complication of hemodialysis and peritoneal dialysis. Factors that play a role in renal osteodystrophy are (1) phosphate retention secondary to a decrease in the number of nephrons; (2) failure of the diseased or absent kidneys to hydroxylate 25-dihydroxyvitamin D to the biologically active metabolite 1,25-dihydroxyvitamin D, with decreased intestinal absorption of calcium; (3) resistance of the bone to the action of parathyroid hormone; and (4) increased serum calcitonin concentrations. The resulting skeletal changes are identical with those of primary hyperparathyroidism but are often more severe.

Most patients with secondary hyperparathyroidism may be treated medically. Maintaining relatively normal serum concentrations of calcium and phosphorus during hemodialysis and treatment with calcitriol (orally or intravenously) have decreased the incidence of bone disease.

Occasionally, a patient with secondary hyperparathyroidism develops relatively autonomous hyperplastic parathyroid glands. In most patients after successful renal transplantation, the serum calcium concentration returns to normal, and the hyperplastic parathyroid glands regress. One should therefore wait at least 6 months after surgery before considering parathyroidectomy for persistent mild hypercalcemia. In some patients, however, profound hypercalcemia develops (**tertiary hyperparathyroidism**). In general, surgical therapy for so-called tertiary hyperparathyroidism should be delayed until all medical approaches, including treatment with vitamin D, calcium supplementation, and phosphate binders, have been exhausted. Indications for operation in patients with secondary hyperparathyroidism include (1) a calcium × phosphate product > 70, (2) severe bone disease and pain, (3) pruritus, (4) extensive soft tissue calcification with tumoral calcinosis, and (5) calciphylaxis. Most patients with secondary hyperparathyroidism requiring parathyroidectomy have very high serum PTH levels, whereas patients with aluminum bone disease who do not warrant parathyroidectomy may be hypercalcemic with bone pain, but PTH levels are normal or only slightly increased. In the patient with secondary hyperparathyroidism in whom subtotal parathyroidectomy or total parathyroidectomy with autotransplantation is indicated, all but about 50 mg of the most normal parathyroid gland should be removed, or fifteen 1-mm slices of parathyroid tissue should be transplanted into individual muscle pockets in the forearm. Some parathyroid tissue should also be cryopreserved in case the autotransplanted tissue does not function. Patients, following parathyroidectomy, usually respond with dramatic relief of bone and joint pain and pruritus. Profound hypocalcemia frequently results following subtotal or total parathyroidectomy with autotransplantation for renal osteodystrophy, both because of "hungry bones" and because of decreased parathyroid hormone secretion. Hypocalcemia due to hungry bones can be anticipated in patients with markedly elevated alkaline phosphatase levels and hand films documenting subperiosteal resorption.

Pasieka JL, Parsons LL: A prospective surgical outcome study assessing the impact of parathyroidectomy on symptoms in patients with secondary and tertiary hyperparathyroidism. Surgery 2000;128:531.

Savio RM et al: Parathyroidectomy for tertiary hyperparathyroidism associated with X-linked dominant hypophosphatemic rickets. Arch Surg 2004;139:218.

Schlosser K, Zielke A, Rothmund M: Medical and surgical treatment for secondary and tertiary hyperparathyroidism. Scand J Surg 2004;93:288.

Triponez F et al: Less-than-subtotal parathyroidectomy increases the risk of persistent/recurrent hyperparathyroidism after parathyroidectomy in tertiary hyperparathyroidism after renal transplantation. Surgery 2006;140:990.

HYPOPARATHYROIDISM

 ESSENTIALS OF DIAGNOSIS

▶ Paresthesias, muscle cramps, carpopedal spasm, laryngeal stridor, convulsions, malaise, muscle and abdominal cramps, tetany, urinary frequency, lethargy, anxiety, psychoneurosis, depression, and psychosis.

▶ Surgical neck scar. Positive Chvostek and Trousseau signs.

▶ Brittle and atrophied nails, defective teeth, cataracts.

▶ Hypocalcemia and hyperphosphatemia, low or absent urinary calcium, low or absent circulating parathyroid hormone.

▶ Calcification of basal ganglia, cartilage, and arteries as seen on x-ray.

General Considerations

Hypoparathyroidism, although uncommon, occurs most often as a complication of thyroidectomy, especially when performed for carcinoma or recurrent goiter. Idiopathic hypoparathyroidism, an autoimmune process associated with autoimmune adrenocortical insufficiency, is also unusual, and hypoparathyroidism after ^{131}I therapy for Graves disease is rare. Neonatal tetany may be associated with maternal hyperparathyroidism. Hypothyroidism as well as hypoparathyroidism may occur in patients with Riedel struma.

Clinical Findings

A. Symptoms and Signs

The manifestations of acute hypoparathyroidism are due to hypocalcemia. Low serum calcium levels precipitate tetany. Latent tetany may be indicated by mild or moderate paresthesias with a positive Chvostek or Trousseau sign. The initial manifestations are paresthesias, circumoral numbness, muscle cramps, irritability, carpopedal spasm, convulsions, opisthotonos, and marked anxiety. Dry skin, brittleness of the nails, and spotty alopecia including loss of the eyebrows are common. Since primary hypoparathyroidism is rare, a history of thyroidectomy is almost always present. Generally speaking, the sooner the clinical manifestations appear postoperatively, the more serious the prognosis. After many years, some patients become adapted to a low serum calcium concentration, so that tetany is no longer evident.

B. Laboratory Findings

Hypocalcemia and hyperphosphatemia are demonstrable. The urine phosphate is low or absent, tubular resorption of phosphate is high, and the urine calcium is low.

C. Imaging Studies

In chronic hypoparathyroidism, x-rays may show calcification of the basal ganglia, arteries, and external ear.

Differential Diagnosis

A good history is most important in the differential diagnosis of hypocalcemic tetany. Occasionally, tetany occurs with alkalosis and hyperventilation. Symptomatic hypocalcemia occurring after thyroid or parathyroid surgery is due to parathyroid removal or injury by trauma or devascularization or is secondary to hungry bones. Other major causes of hypocalcemic tetany are intestinal malabsorption and renal insufficiency. These conditions may also be suggested by a history of diarrhea, pancreatitis, steatorrhea, or renal disease. Laboratory abnormalities include decreased concentrations of serum proteins, cholesterol, and carotene and increased concentrations of stool fat in malabsorption and an increased blood urea nitrogen and creatinine in renal failure. Serum parathyroid hormone concentrations are low in hypocalcemia secondary to idiopathic or iatrogenic hypoparathyroidism. Consequently, serum calcium concentrations and urinary calcium, phosphorus, and hydroxyproline levels are decreased, whereas serum phosphate concentrations are increased. In hypocalcemia secondary to malabsorption and renal failure, serum PTH concentrations are elevated and the serum alkaline phosphatase concentration is normal or increased.

Treatment

The aim of treatment is to raise the serum calcium concentration, to bring the patient out of tetany, and to lower the serum phosphate level so as to prevent metastatic calcification. Most postoperative hypocalcemia is transient; if it persists longer than 2–3 weeks or if treatment with calcitriol (1,25-dihydroxyvitamin D) is required, the hypoparathyroidism may be permanent.

A. Acute Hypoparathyroid Tetany

Acute hypoparathyroid tetany requires emergency treatment. Make certain an adequate airway exists. Reassure the anxious patient to avoid hyperventilation and resulting alkalosis. Give calcium gluconate, 10–20 mL of 10% solution slowly intravenously, until tetany disappears. Fifty milliliters of 10% calcium gluconate may then be added to 500 mL of 5% dextrose solution and administered by intravenous drip at a rate of 1 mL/kg/h. Adjust the rate of infusion so that hourly determinations of serum calcium are normal. Calcitriol (1,25-dihydroxyvitamin D), 0.25–0.5 μg twice daily, is very helpful for managing acute hypocalcemia because of its rapid onset of action (compared to other vitamin D preparations) and its short duration of action. Hypomagnesemia is present in some cases of tetany not responding to calcium treatment. In such cases, magnesium (as magnesium sulfate) should be given in a dosage of 4–8 g/d intramuscularly or 2–4 g/d intravenously.

B. Chronic Hypoparathyroidism

Once tetany has responded to intravenous calcium, change to oral calcium (citrate, gluconate, lactate, or carbonate) three times daily or as necessary. The management of the hypoparathyroid patient is difficult, because the difference between the controlling and intoxicating dose of vitamin D may be quite small. Episodes of hypercalcemia in treated patients are often unpredictable and may occur in the absence of symptoms. Vitamin D intoxication may develop after months or years of good control on a given therapeutic regimen. Dihydrotachysterol is useful in the exceptional case to supplement treatment with calcium, 1,25-dihydroxyvitamin D, when the usual measures fail to control the hypocalcemia. Frequent serum calcium determinations are necessary to regulate the proper dosage of vitamin D and to avoid vitamin D intoxication. The dose of vitamin D required to correct hypocalcemia may vary from 25,000 to 200,000 IU/d. Phosphorus should also be limited in the diet; in most patients, simple elimination of dairy products is sufficient. In some patients, aluminum hydroxide gel may be necessary to bind phosphorus in the gut to increase fecal losses.

PSEUDOHYPOPARATHYROIDISM & PSEUDOPSEUDOHYPOPARATHYROIDISM

Pseudohypoparathyroidism is an X-linked autosomal syndrome due to a defective renal adenylyl cyclase system. It is characterized by the clinical and chemical features of hypoparathyroidism associated with a round face; a short, thick body; stubby fingers with short metacarpal and metatarsal bones; mental deficiency; and x-ray evidence of calcification. It is also associated with thyroid and ovarian dysfunction. There is evidence of increased bone resorption and osteitis fibrosa cystica despite the hypocalcemia that accompanies the syndrome. Patients with pseudohypoparathyroidism do not respond to intravenous administration of 200 units of parathyroid hormone with phosphaturia (Ellsworth-Howard test) and have increased serum concentrations of PTH. This condition is usually controlled with smaller amounts of vitamin D than idiopathic hypoparathyroidism, and resistance to therapy is uncommon.

Pseudopseudohypoparathyroidism is also a genetically transmitted disease with the same physical findings of pseudohypoparathyroidism but with normal serum calcium and phosphorus concentrations. Patients with this condition may become hypocalcemic during periods of stress, such as pregnancy and rapid growth; this suggests that a genetic defect is common with pseudohypoparathyroidism.

Long DN et al: Body mass index differences in pseudohypoparathyroidism type 1a versus pseudopseudohypoparathyroidism may implicate paternal imprinting of Galpha(s) in the development of human obesity. J Clin Endocrinol Metab 2007;92:1073.
Savio RM et al: Parathyroidectomy for tertiary hyperparathyroidism associated with X-linked dominant hypophosphatemic rickets. Arch Surg 2004;139:218.

Breast Disorders

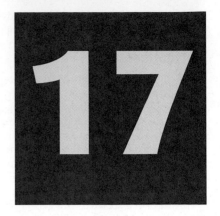

Armando E. Giuliano, MD

BENIGN BREAST DISORDERS

FIBROCYSTIC CONDITION

ESSENTIALS OF DIAGNOSIS

- Painful, often multiple, usually bilateral masses in the breast.
- Rapid fluctuation in the size of the masses is common.
- Frequently, pain occurs or worsens and size increases during premenstrual phase of cycle.
- Most common age is 30–50. Rare in postmenopausal women not receiving hormonal replacement.

▶ General Considerations

Fibrocystic condition is the most frequent lesion of the breast. Although commonly referred to as "fibrocystic disease," it does not, in fact, represent a pathologic or anatomic disorder. It is common in women 30–50 years of age but rare in postmenopausal women who are not taking hormonal replacement. Estrogen is considered a causative factor. There may be an increased risk in women who drink alcohol, especially women between 18 and 22 years of age. Fibrocystic condition encompasses a wide variety of benign histologic changes in the breast epithelium, some of which are found so commonly in normal breasts that they are probably variants of normal but have nonetheless been termed a "condition" or "disease."

The microscopic findings of fibrocystic condition include cysts (gross and microscopic), papillomatosis, adenosis, fibrosis, and ductal epithelial hyperplasia. Although fibrocystic condition has generally been considered to increase the risk of subsequent breast cancer, only the variants with a component of epithelial proliferation (especially with atypia) represent true risk factors.

▶ Clinical Findings

A. Symptoms and Signs

Fibrocystic condition may produce an asymptomatic mass in the breast that is discovered by accident, but pain or tenderness often calls attention to it. Discomfort often occurs or worsens during the premenstrual phase of the cycle, at which time the cysts tend to enlarge. Fluctuations in size and rapid appearance or disappearance of a breast mass are common with this condition as are multiple or bilateral masses and serous nipple discharge. Patients will give a history of a transient lump in the breast or cyclic breast pain.

B. Diagnostic Tests

Mammography and ultrasonography should be used to evaluate a mass in a patient with fibrocystic condition. Ultrasonography alone may be used in women under 30 years of age. Because a mass due to fibrocystic condition is difficult to distinguish from carcinoma on the basis of clinical findings, suspicious lesions should be biopsied. Fine-needle aspiration (FNA) cytology may be used, but if a suspicious mass that is nonmalignant on cytologic examination does not resolve over several months, it should be excised. Surgery should be conservative, since the primary objective is to exclude cancer. Occasionally, core needle biopsy or FNA cytology will suffice. Simple mastectomy or extensive removal of breast tissue is rarely, if ever, indicated for fibrocystic condition.

▶ Differential Diagnosis

Pain, fluctuation in size, and multiplicity of lesions are the features most helpful in differentiating fibrocystic condition from carcinoma. If a dominant mass is present, the diagnosis of cancer should be assumed until disproved by biopsy. Mammography may be helpful, but the breast tissue in these young women is usually too radiodense to permit a worthwhile study. Sonography is useful in differentiating a cystic mass from a solid mass, especially in women with dense breasts. Final diagnosis, however, depends on analysis of the excisional biopsy specimen or needle biopsy.

Treatment

When the diagnosis of fibrocystic condition has been established by previous biopsy or is likely because the history is classic, aspiration of a discrete mass suggestive of a cyst is indicated to alleviate pain and, more importantly, to confirm the cystic nature of the mass. The patient is reexamined at intervals thereafter. If no fluid is obtained by aspiration, if fluid is bloody, if a mass persists after aspiration, or if at any time during follow-up a persistent or recurrent mass is noted, biopsy should be performed.

Breast pain associated with generalized fibrocystic condition is best treated by avoiding trauma and by wearing a good, supportive brassiere during the night and day. Hormone therapy is not advisable, because it does not cure the condition and has undesirable side effects. Danazol (100–200 mg orally twice daily), a synthetic androgen and only treatment approved by the US Food and Drug Administration (FDA), has been used for patients with severe pain. This treatment suppresses pituitary gonadotropins, but androgenic effects (acne, edema, hirsutism) usually make this treatment intolerable; in practice, it is rarely used. Similarly, tamoxifen reduces some symptoms of fibrocystic condition, but because of its side effects, it is not useful for young women unless it is given to reduce the risk of cancer. Postmenopausal women receiving hormone replacement therapy may stop or change doses of hormones to reduce pain. Oil of evening primrose (OEP), a natural form of gamolenic acid, has been shown to decrease pain in 44–58% of users. The dosage of gamolenic acid is 6 capsules of 500 mg orally twice daily. Studies have also demonstrated a low-fat diet or decreasing dietary fat intake may reduce the painful symptoms associated with fibrocystic condition. Further research is being done to determine the effects of topical treatments such as nonsteroidal anti-inflammatory drugs as well as topical hormonal drugs such as tamoxifen.

The role of caffeine consumption in the development and treatment of fibrocystic condition is controversial. Some studies suggest that eliminating caffeine from the diet is associated with improvement, while other studies refute the benefit entirely. Many patients are aware of these studies and report relief of symptoms after giving up coffee, tea, and chocolate. Similarly, many women find vitamin E (400 international units daily) helpful; however, these observations remain anecdotal.

Prognosis

Exacerbations of pain, tenderness, and cyst formation may occur at any time until menopause, when symptoms usually subside, except in patients receiving hormonal replacement. The patient should be advised to examine her own breasts regularly just after menstruation and to inform her practitioner if a mass appears. The risk of breast cancer developing in women with fibrocystic condition with a proliferative or atypical component in the epithelium is higher than that of the general population. These women should be monitored carefully with physical examinations and imaging studies.

Guray M et al: Benign breast diseases: classification, diagnosis, and management. Oncologist 2006;11:435.

Mannello F et al: Human gross cyst breast disease and cystic fluid: bio-molecular, morphological, and clinical studies. Breast Cancer Res Treat 2006;97:115.

Qureshi S et al: Topical nonsteroidal anti-inflammatory drugs versus oil of evening primrose in the treatment of mastalgia. Surgeon 2005;3:7.

Rosolowich V et al. Mastalgia. J Obstet Gynaecol Can 2006;28:49.

FIBROADENOMA OF THE BREAST

This common benign neoplasm occurs most frequently in young women, usually within 20 years after puberty. It is somewhat more frequent and tends to occur at an earlier age in black women. Multiple tumors are found in 10–15% of patients.

The typical fibroadenoma is a round or ovoid, rubbery, discrete, relatively movable, nontender mass 1–5 cm in diameter. It is usually discovered accidentally. Clinical diagnosis in young patients is generally not difficult. In women over 30 years, fibrocystic condition of the breast and carcinoma of the breast must be considered. Cysts can be identified by aspiration or ultrasonography. Fibroadenoma does not normally occur after menopause but may occasionally develop after administration of hormones.

No treatment is usually necessary if the diagnosis can be made by needle biopsy or cytologic examination. Excision or vacuum-assisted core needle removal with pathologic examination of the specimen is performed if the diagnosis is uncertain. In a 2005 study, cryoablation, or freezing of the fibroadenoma, appears to be a safe procedure if the lesion is consistent with fibroadenoma on histology prior to ablation. Cryoablation is not appropriate for all fibroadenomas because some are too large to freeze or the diagnosis may not be certain. The advantages of cryoablation over observation are not clear. It is usually not possible to distinguish a large fibroadenoma from a phyllodes tumor on the basis of needle biopsy results or imaging alone.

Phyllodes tumor is a fibroadenoma-like tumor with cellular stroma that grows rapidly. It may reach a large size and, if inadequately excised, will recur locally. The lesion can be benign or malignant. If benign, phyllodes tumor is treated by local excision with a margin of surrounding breast tissue. The treatment of malignant phyllodes tumor is more controversial, but complete removal of the tumor with a rim of normal tissue avoids recurrence. Because these tumors may be large, simple mastectomy is sometimes necessary. Lymph node dissection is not performed, since the sarcomatous portion of the tumor metastasizes to the lungs and not the lymph nodes.

Bode MK et al: Ultrasonography and core needle biopsy in the differential diagnosis of fibroadenoma and tumor phyllodes. Acta Radiol 2007;48:708.
Jacklin RK et al: Optimising preoperative diagnosis in phyllodes tumour of the breast. J Clin Pathol 2006;59:454.
Lee AH et al: Histological features useful in the distinction of phyllodes tumour and fibroadenoma on needle core biopsy of the breast. Histopathology 2007;51:336.
Telli ML et al: Phyllodes tumors of the breast: natural history, diagnosis, and treatment. J Natl Compr Canc Netw 2007;5:324.

NIPPLE DISCHARGE

In order of decreasing frequency, the following are the most common causes of nipple discharge in the nonlactating breast: duct ectasia, intraductal papilloma, and carcinoma. The important characteristics of the discharge and some other factors to be evaluated by history and physical examination are as follows:

1. Nature of the discharge (serous, bloody, or other).
2. Association with a mass.
3. Unilateral or bilateral.
4. Single or multiple duct discharge.
5. Discharge is spontaneous (persistent or intermittent) or must be expressed.
6. Discharge is produced by pressure at a single site or by general pressure on the breast.
7. Relation to menses.
8. Premenopausal or postmenopausal.
9. Patient is taking contraceptive pills or estrogen.

Spontaneous, unilateral, serous, or serosanguineous discharge from a single duct is usually caused by an intraductal papilloma or, rarely, by an intraductal cancer. A mass may not be palpable. The involved duct may be identified by pressure at different sites around the nipple at the margin of the areola. Bloody discharge is suggestive of cancer but is more often caused by a benign papilloma in the duct. Cytologic examination may identify malignant cells, but negative findings do not rule out cancer, which is more likely in women over age 50 years. In any case, the involved duct—and a mass if present—should be excised. A ductogram (a mammogram of a duct after radiopaque dye has been injected) is of limited value, since excision of the suspicious ductal system is indicated regardless of findings. Ductoscopy, evaluation of the ductal system with a small scope inserted through the nipple, has been attempted but is not effective management.

In premenopausal women, spontaneous multiple duct discharge, unilateral or bilateral, most noticeable just before menstruation, is often due to fibrocystic condition. Discharge may be green or brownish. Papillomatosis and ductal ectasia are usually detected only by biopsy. If a mass is present, it should be removed.

A milky discharge from multiple ducts in the nonlactating breast may occur from hyperprolactinemia. Serum prolactin levels should be obtained to search for a pituitary tumor. Thyroid-stimulating hormone (TSH) helps exclude causative hypothyroidism. Numerous antipsychotic drugs and other drugs may also cause a milky discharge that ceases on discontinuance of the medication.

Oral contraceptive agents or estrogen replacement therapy may cause clear, serous, or milky discharge from a single duct, but multiple duct discharge is more common. In the premenopausal woman, the discharge is more evident just before menstruation and disappears on stopping the medication. If it does not stop, is from a single duct, and is copious, exploration should be performed, since this may be a sign of cancer.

A purulent discharge may originate in a subareolar abscess and require removal of the abscess and the related lactiferous sinus.

When localization is not possible, no mass is palpable, and the discharge is nonbloody, the patient should be reexamined every 3 or 4 months for a year, and a mammogram and an ultrasound should be performed. Although most discharge is from a benign process, patients may find it annoying or disconcerting. Cytologic examination of the nipple discharge for exfoliated cancer cells is rarely helpful in determining a diagnosis. To eliminate the discharge, proximal duct excision can be performed both for treatment and diagnosis.

Barghav RK et al: The value of clinical characteristics and breast imaging studies in predicting a histopathologic diagnosis of cancer or high-risk lesion in patients with spontaneous nipple discharge. Am J Surg 2007;193:141.
Escobar PF et al: The clinical applications of mammary ductoscopy. Am J Surg 2006;191:211.
Hussain AN et al: Evaluating nipple discharge. Obstet Gynecol Surv 2006;61:278.
Louie LD et al: Identification of breast cancer in patients with pathologic nipple discharge: does ductoscopy predict malignancy? Am J Surg 2006;192:530.

FAT NECROSIS

Fat necrosis is a rare lesion of the breast but is of clinical importance because it produces a mass (often accompanied by skin or nipple retraction) that is indistinguishable from carcinoma even with imaging studies. Trauma is presumed to be the cause, though only about 50% of patients give a history of injury. Ecchymosis is occasionally present. If untreated, the mass effect gradually disappears. The safest course is to obtain a biopsy. Needle biopsy is often adequate, but frequently the entire mass must be excised, primarily to exclude carcinoma. Fat necrosis is common after segmental resection, radiation therapy, or flap reconstruction after mastectomy.

Li S et al: Surgical management of recurrent subareolar breast abscesses: Mayo Clinic experience. Am J Surg 2006;192: 528.
Tan PH et al: Fat necrosis of the breast—a review. Breast 2006;15:313.

BREAST ABSCESS

During nursing, an area of redness, tenderness, and induration may develop in the breast. The organism most commonly found in these abscesses is *Staphylococcus aureus*.

Infection in the nonlactating breast is rare. A subareolar abscess may develop in young or middle-aged women who are not lactating. These infections tend to recur after incision and drainage unless the area is explored during a quiescent interval, with excision of the involved lactiferous duct or ducts at the base of the nipple. In the nonlactating breast, inflammatory carcinoma must always be considered. Thus, incision and biopsy of any indurated tissue with a small piece of erythematous skin is indicated when suspected abscess or cellulitis in the nonlactating breast does not resolve promptly with antibiotics. Often, needle or catheter drainage is adequate to treat an abscess, but surgical incision and drainage may be necessary.

Scott BG et al: Rate of malignancies in breast abscesses and argument for ultrasound drainage. Am J Surg 2006;192:869.

DISORDERS OF THE AUGMENTED BREAST

At least 4 million American women have had breast implants. Breast augmentation is performed by placing implants under the pectoralis muscle or, less desirably, in the subcutaneous tissue of the breast. Most implants are made of an outer silicone shell filled with a silicone gel, saline, or some combination of the two. Capsule contraction or scarring around the implant develops in about 15–25% of patients, leading to a firmness and distortion of the breast that can be painful. Some require removal of the implant and surrounding capsule. In 2006, the FDA reapproved silicone implants for augmentation cosmetic surgery.

Implant rupture may occur in as many as 5–10% of women, and bleeding of gel through the capsule is noted even more commonly. Although silicone gel may be an immunologic stimulant, there is no increase in autoimmune disorders in patients with such implants. The FDA has advised symptomatic women with ruptured implants to discuss possible surgical removal with their clinicians. However, women who are asymptomatic and have no evidence of rupture of a silicone gel prosthesis should probably not undergo removal of the implant. Women with symptoms of autoimmune illnesses should consider removal.

Studies have failed to show any association between implants and an increased incidence of breast cancer. However, breast cancer may develop in a patient with an augmentation prosthesis, as it does in women without them. Detection in patients with implants is more difficult because mammography is less able to detect early lesions. Mammography is better if the implant is subpectoral rather than subcutaneous. The prosthesis should be placed retropectorally after mastectomy to facilitate detection of a local recurrence of cancer, which is usually cutaneous or subcutaneous and is easily detected by palpation.

If a cancer develops in a patient with implants, it should be treated in the same manner as in women without implants. Such women should be offered the option of mastectomy or breast-conserving therapy, which may require removal or replacement of the implant. Radiotherapy of the augmented breast often results in marked capsular contracture. Adjuvant treatments should be given for the same indications as for women who have no implants.

Fryzek JP et al: Silicone breast implants. J Rheumatol 2005;32:201.
McCarthy CM et al: Breast cancer in the previously augmented breast. Plast Reconstr Surg 2007;119:49.
McIntosh SA et al: Breast cancer following augmentation mammoplasty—a review of its impact on prognosis and management. J Plast Reconstr Aesthet Surg 2007;60:1127.

CARCINOMA OF THE FEMALE BREAST

 ESSENTIALS OF DIAGNOSIS

▶ Most women with breast cancer do not have identifiable risk factors.

▶ Risk factors include delayed childbearing, positive family history of breast cancer or genetic mutations (*BRCA1, BRCA2*), and personal history of breast cancer or some types of proliferative conditions.

▶ *Early findings:* Single, nontender, firm to hard mass with ill-defined margins; mammographic abnormalities and no palpable mass.

▶ *Later findings:* Skin or nipple retraction; axillary lymphadenopathy; breast enlargement, erythema, edema, pain; fixation of mass to skin or chest wall.

▶ Incidence & Risk Factors

Breast cancer will develop in one of eight American women. Next to skin cancer, breast cancer is the most common cancer in women; it is second only to lung cancer as a cause of death. The probability of developing breast cancer increases throughout life. The mean age and the median age of women with breast cancer are between 60 and 61 years.

There are about 178,000 new cases of breast cancer annually and about 41,000 deaths from this disease in women in the United States. An additional 62,000 cases of ductal carcinoma in situ (DCIS) will be detected, principally by screening mammography. The incidence of breast cancer has slightly decreased, presumably because of decreased use of postmenopausal hormone replacement therapy. Mortality has also decreased slightly due to early detection and increased use of systemic therapy.

Although more than 75% of women in whom breast cancer has been diagnosed do not have an obvious risk factor, there are several that play a role in breast cancer development. Breast cancer is three to four times more likely to develop in women with a first-degree relative (mother, daughter, or sister) who had breast cancer than in those without a family history. Risk is further increased in patients whose mothers' or sisters' breast cancers occurred before menopause or were bilateral and in those with a family history of breast cancer in two or more first-degree relatives as well as in women of Ashkenazi Jewish descent. Nulliparous women and women whose first full-term pregnancy was after age 35 have a 1.5 times higher incidence of breast cancer than multiparous women. Late menarche and artificial menopause are associated with a lower incidence, whereas early menarche (under age 12) and late natural menopause (after age 50) are associated with a slight increase in risk. Fibrocystic condition, when accompanied by proliferative changes, papillomatosis, or atypical epithelial hyperplasia, and increased breast density on mammogram are also associated with an increased incidence. A woman who had cancer in one breast is at increased risk for cancer developing in the other breast. In these women, a contralateral cancer develops at the rate of 1% or 2% per year. Women with cancer of the uterine corpus have a risk of breast cancer significantly higher than that of the general population, and women with breast cancer have a comparably increased risk for endometrial cancer. In the United States, breast cancer is more common in white women. The incidence of the disease among nonwhite (mostly black) women is increasing, especially in younger women. In general, rates reported from developing countries are low, whereas rates are high in developed countries, with the notable exception of Japan. Some of the variability may be due to underreporting in the developing countries, but a real difference probably exists. Dietary factors, particularly increased fat consumption, may account for some differences in incidence. Oral contraceptives do not appear to increase the risk of breast cancer. There is evidence that administration of estrogens to postmenopausal women may result in a slightly increased risk of breast cancer, but only with higher, long-term doses of estrogens. Concomitant administration of progesterone and estrogen may markedly increase the incidence of breast cancer compared with the use of estrogen alone. The Women's Health Initiative prospective randomized study of hormone replacement therapy stopped treatment with estrogen and progesterone early because of an increased risk of breast cancer compared with untreated controls or women treated with estrogen alone. With decreasing use of these hormones, breast cancer rates may continue to decrease. Alcohol consumption increases the risk very slightly.

Some inherited breast cancers have been found to be associated with a gene on chromosome 17. This gene, BRCA1, is mutated in families with early-onset breast and ovarian cancer. Breast cancer will develop in approximately 85% of women with BRCA1 gene mutations during their lifetime. Other genes are associated with increased risk of breast and other cancers, such as BRCA2 (associated with a gene on chromosome 13), ataxia-telangiectasia mutation, and mutation of TP53, the tumor suppressor gene. Mutations to TP53 have been found in approximately 1% of breast cancers in women under 40 years of age. Genetic testing is commercially available for women at high risk for breast cancer. Women with genetic mutations in whom breast cancer develops may be treated in the same way as women who do not have mutations (ie, lumpectomy), though there is an increased ipsilateral and contralateral recurrence rate after lumpectomy for these women. Such women with mutations often elect bilateral mastectomy as treatment. Some states have enacted legislation to prevent insurance companies from considering mutations as "preexisting conditions," preventing insurability.

Women at greater than normal risk for developing breast cancer (Table 17–1) should be identified by their practitioners and monitored carefully. Those with an exceptional family history should be counseled about the option of genetic testing. Some of these high-risk women may consider prophylactic mastectomy, oophorectomy, or tamoxifen, an FDA-approved preventive agent.

▶ Prevention

The National Surgical Adjuvant Breast Project (NSABP) conducted the first Breast Cancer Prevention Trial (BCPT) P-1, which evaluated tamoxifen as a preventive agent in women with no personal history of breast cancer but at high risk for developing the disease. Women who received tamoxifen for 5 years had about a 50% reduction in noninvasive and invasive cancers compared with women taking placebo. However, women over age 50 who received the drug had an increased incidence of endometrial cancer and deep venous thrombosis. Unfortunately, no survival data will be produced from this trial because it was stopped.

The selective estrogen receptor modulator (SERM) raloxifene, effective in preventing osteoporosis, is also effective in

Table 17–1. Factors Associated with Increased Risk of Breast Cancer.

Race	White
Age	Older
Family history	Breast cancer in mother, sister, or daughter (especially bilateral or premenopausal)
Genetics	BRCA1 or BRCA2 mutation
Previous medical history	Endometrial cancer Proliferative forms of fibrocystic disease Cancer in other breast
Menstrual history	Early menarche (under age 12) Late menopause (after age 50)
Reproductive history	Nulliparous or late first pregnancy

preventing breast cancer. The initial study, Multiple Outcomes of Raloxifene Evaluations (MORE) trial, aimed at determining the effect of raloxifene on bone, demonstrated that raloxifene also reduced breast cancer risk in women being given the drug. After 8 years, raloxifene demonstrated an overall reduction of invasive breast cancer of 66%. Because this study was designed to determine the effect of raloxifene on bone density, it was conducted in women at lower risk for breast cancer. To better understand the preventive effect of raloxifene in the high-risk population, a randomized study comparing raloxifene with tamoxifen was conducted.

The Study of Tamoxifen and Raloxifene (STAR) P-2 trial, conducted by the National Surgical Adjuvant Breast and Bowel Project (NSABP) and completed in 2006, demonstrated that raloxifene and tamoxifen are equivalent in preventing invasive breast cancer in the high-risk population. Many of the side effects of raloxifene are the same as tamoxifen with a slight decrease in cataracts and thromboembolic events in the raloxifene group. Surprisingly, noninvasive cancer (DCIS) occurred more commonly in women treated with raloxifene.

Similar to SERMs, aromatase inhibitors (AIs) have shown great success in treating breast cancer with fewer side effects, although bone loss is a significant side effect of this long-term treatment. Several large multicenter studies (eg, International Breast Cancer Intervention Study II [IBIS-II] and National Cancer Institute of Canada Clinical Trials Group [NCIC CTG]) are underway to determine whether AIs have a role in preventing breast cancer.

In addition to pharmaceutical therapy, patients continue to seek a way to prevent breast cancer. There has been considerable research on incorporating diet and exercise into the lifestyle of women who may be at risk for cancer. The Women's Intervention Nutrition Study was conducted to determine whether decreasing dietary fat intake would reduce the incidence of breast cancer recurrence after initial treatment. Although the trial demonstrated a decrease in recurrence in the follow-up period, it did not reach statistical significance.

Bao T et al: Chemoprevention of breast cancer: tamoxifen, raloxifene, and beyond. Am J Ther 2006;13:337.

Boyd NF et al: Mammographic density and the risk and detection of breast cancer. N Engl J Med 2007;356:227.

Chan K et al: Chemoprevention of breast cancer for women at high risk. Semin Oncol 2006;33:642.

Chlebowski RT et al: Dietary fat reduction and breast cancer outcome: interim efficacy results from the Women's Intervention Nutrition Study. J Natl Cancer Inst 2006;98:1767.

Jemal A et al: Cancer Statistics, 2007. CA Cancer J Clin 2007;57:43.

Jordan VC: Chemoprevention of breast cancer with selective estrogen-receptor modulators. Nat Rev Cancer 2007;7:46.

Linos E et al: Diet and breast cancer. Curr Oncol Rep 2007;9:31.

Lynch HT et al: Hereditary breast cancer: part I. Diagnosing hereditary breast cancer syndromes. Breast J 2008;14:3.

Newman LA et al: Breast cancer risk assessment and risk reduction. Surg Clin North Am 2007;87:307.

Palma M et al: BRCA1 and BRCA2: the genetic testing and the current management options for mutation carriers. Crit Rev Oncol Hematol 2006;57:1.

Patel RR et al: Optimizing the antihormonal treatment and prevention of breast cancer. Breast Cancer 2007;14:113.

Prentice RL et al: Low-fat dietary pattern and risk of invasive breast cancer: the Women's Health Initiative Randomized Controlled Dietary Modification Trial. JAMA 2006;295:629.

Pruthi S et al: A multidisciplinary approach to the management of breast cancer, part 1: prevention and diagnosis. Mayo Clin Proc 2007;82:999.

Vogel VG et al; National Surgical Adjuvant Breast and Bowel Project (NSABP): Effects of tamoxifen vs raloxifene on the risk of developing invasive breast cancer and other disease outcomes: the NSABP Study of Tamoxifen and Raloxifene (STAR) P-2 trial. JAMA 2006;295:2727.

▶ Early Detection of Breast Cancer

A. Screening Programs

A number of large screening programs have been conducted over the years. Such programs, consisting of physical and mammographic examination of asymptomatic women, identify about 10 cancers per 1000 women over the age of 50 and about 2 cancers per 1000 women under the age of 50. These studies show the increased survival benefit of screening programs, as screening detects cancer before it has spread to the lymph nodes in about 80% of the women evaluated. This increases the chance of survival to about 85% at 5 years.

Both physical examination and mammography are necessary for maximum yield in screening programs, since about 35–50% of early breast cancers can be discovered only by mammography and another 40% can be detected only by palpation. About one third of the abnormalities detected on screening mammograms will be found to be malignant when biopsy is performed. The probability of cancer on a screening mammogram is directly related to the Breast Imaging and Reporting Data System (BIRADS) assessment, and workup should be performed based on this classification. Women 20–40 years of age should have a breast examination as part of routine medical care every 2–3 years. Women over age 40 years should have annual breast examinations. The sensitivity of mammography varies from approximately 60% to 90%. This sensitivity depends on several factors, including patient age (breast density) and tumor size, location, and mammographic appearance. In young women with dense breasts, mammography is less sensitive than in older women with fatty breasts, in whom mammography can detect at least 90% of malignancies. Smaller tumors, particularly those without calcifications, are more difficult to detect, especially in dense breasts. The lack of sensitivity and the low incidence of breast cancer in young women have led to questions concerning the value of mammography for screening in women 40–50 years of age. The specificity of mammography in women under 50 years varies from about 30% to 40% for nonpalpable mammographic abnormalities to 85% to 90% for clinically evident malignancies.

Screening recommendations for women in their 40s are based, in part, on trials from Sweden. Two trials showed a statistical advantage for screening women in their 40s, and a meta-analysis similarly revealed a statistical survival advantage for screened women with longer follow-up. The National Cancer Advisory Board recommended that women in their 40s with average risk factors have screening mammography every 1–2 years and that women at higher risk seek medical advice on when to begin screening. Studies continue to support the value of screening mammography in women over 40 years. Such women should have annual mammography and physical examination.

The beneficial effect of screening in women aged 50–69 years is undisputed and has been confirmed by all clinical trials. The efficacy of screening in older women—those older than 70 years—is inconclusive and is difficult to determine because few studies have examined this population.

B. Self-Examination

Breast self-exam (BSE) has not been shown to improve survival. Because of the lack of strong evidence demonstrating value, the American Cancer Society no longer recommends monthly BSE beginning at age 20 years. The recommendation is that patients be made aware of the potential benefits, limitations, and harms (increased biopsies or false-positive results) associated with BSE. Women who choose to perform BSE should be advised regarding the proper technique. Premenopausal women should perform the examination 7–8 days after the start of the menstrual period. First, breasts should be inspected before a mirror with the hands at the sides, overhead, and pressed firmly on the hips to contract the pectoralis muscles causing masses, asymmetry of breasts, and slight dimpling of the skin to become apparent. Next, in a supine position, each breast should be carefully palpated with the fingers of the opposite hand. Some women discover small breast lumps more readily when their skin is moist while bathing or showering. While BSE is not a recommended practice, patients should recognize and report any breast changes to their practitioners as it remains an important facet of proactive care.

C. Imaging

Mammography is the most reliable means of detecting breast cancer before a mass can be palpated. Slowly growing cancers can be identified by mammography at least 2 years before reaching a size detectable by palpation. Film screen mammography delivers less than 0.4 cGy to the midbreast per view. Although full-field digital mammography provides an easier method to maintain and review mammograms, it has not been proven that it provides better images or increases detection rates more than film mammography. In subset analysis of a large study, digital mammography seemed slightly superior in women with dense breasts. Computer-assisted detection (CAD) has not shown any increase in detection of cancers and is not routinely performed at centers with experienced mammographers.

Calcifications are the most easily recognized mammographic abnormality. The most common findings associated with carcinoma of the breast are clustered polymorphic microcalcifications. Such calcifications are usually at least five to eight in number, aggregated in one part of the breast and differing from each other in size and shape, often including branched or V- or Y-shaped configurations. There may be an associated mammographic mass density or, at times, only a mass density with no calcifications. Such a density usually has irregular or ill-defined borders and may lead to architectural distortion within the breast but may be subtle and difficult to detect.

Indications for mammography are as follows: (1) to screen at regular intervals asymptomatic women at high risk for developing breast cancer (see above); (2) to evaluate each breast when a diagnosis of potentially curable breast cancer has been made and at yearly intervals thereafter; (3) to evaluate a questionable or ill-defined breast mass or other suspicious change in the breast; (4) to search for an occult breast cancer in a woman with metastatic disease in axillary nodes or elsewhere from an unknown primary; (5) to screen women prior to cosmetic operations or prior to biopsy of a mass, to examine for an unsuspected cancer; (6) to monitor those women with breast cancer who have been treated with breast-conserving surgery and radiation; and (7) to monitor the contralateral breast in those women with breast cancer treated with mastectomy.

Patients with a dominant or suspicious mass must undergo biopsy despite mammographic findings. The mammogram should be obtained prior to biopsy so that other suspicious areas can be noted and the contralateral breast can be evaluated. Mammography is never a substitute for biopsy because it may not reveal clinical cancer, especially in a very dense breast, as may be seen in young women with fibrocystic changes, and may not reveal medullary cancers.

Communication and documentation among the patient, the referring practitioner, and the interpreting physician are critical for high-quality screening and diagnostic mammography. The patient should be told about *how* she will receive timely results of her mammogram, that mammography does not "rule out" cancer, and that she may receive a correlative examination such as ultrasound at the mammography facility if referred for a suspicious lesion. She should also be aware of the technique and need for breast compression and that this may be uncomfortable. The mammography facility should be informed *in writing by the clinician* of abnormal physical examination findings. The Agency for Health Care Policy and Research (AHCPR) Clinical Practice Guidelines strongly recommend that all mammography reports be communicated in writing to the patient and referring practitioner. MRI and ultrasound may be useful screening modalities in women who are at high risk for breast cancer but not for the general population. The sensitivity of MRI is much higher than mammography; however, the specificity is significantly lower, which results in multiple unnecessary biopsies. The increased sensitivity despite decreased specificity may be considered a reasonable trade-off for those at increased risk for developing breast cancer but not for normal-risk population. MRI is useful in women with breast implants to determine the character of a lesion present in the breast and to search for implant rupture and at times is helpful in patients with prior lumpectomy and radiation. In addition, positron emission tomography (PET) may play a role in imaging atypical lesions but is less sensitive for early breast cancer than is MRI or mammography. The primary role remains evaluation of metastatic deposits.

Armstrong K et al: Screening mammography in women 40 to 49 years of age: a systematic review for the American College of Physicians. Ann Intern Med 2007;146:516.

Bartella L et al: Imaging breast cancer. Radiol Clin North Am 2007;45:45.

Budakoglu II et al: The effectiveness of training for breast cancer and breast self-examination in women aged 40 and over. J Cancer Educ 2007;22:108.

Elmore JG et al: Screening for breast cancer. JAMA 2005;293:1245.

Knutson D et al: Screening for breast cancer: current recommendations and future directions. Am Fam Physician 2007;75:1660.

Kuhl C: The current status of breast MR imaging. Part I. Choice of technique, image interpretation, diagnostic accuracy, and transfer to clinical practice. Radiology 2007;244:356.

Pisano ED et al; Digital Mammographic Imaging Screening Trial (DMIST) Investigators Group: Diagnostic performance of digital versus film mammography for breast cancer screening. N Engl J Med 2005;353:1773.

Reddy DH et al: Incorporating new imaging models in breast cancer management. Curr Treat Options Oncol 2005;6:135.

Smith RA et al: American Cancer Society guidelines for the early detection of cancer, 2005. CA Cancer J Clin 2005;55:31.

Terry MB et al: Lifetime alcohol intake and breast cancer risk. Ann Epidemiol 2006;16:230.

Weaver DL et al: Pathologic findings from the Breast Cancer Surveillance Consortium: population-based outcomes in women undergoing biopsy after screening mammography. Cancer 2006;106:732.

Van Ongeval Ch: Digital mammography for screening and diagnosis of breast cancer: an overview. JBR-BTR 2007;90:163.

▶ Clinical Findings Associated with Early Detection of Breast Cancer

A. Symptoms and Signs

The presenting complaint in about 70% of patients with breast cancer is a lump (usually painless) in the breast. About 90% of these breast masses are discovered by the patient. Less frequent symptoms are breast pain; nipple discharge; erosion, retraction, enlargement, or itching of the nipple; and redness, generalized hardness, enlargement, or shrinking of the breast. Rarely, an axillary mass or swelling of the arm may be the first symptom. Back or bone pain, jaundice, or weight loss may be the result of systemic metastases, but these symptoms are rarely seen on initial presentation.

The relative frequency of carcinoma in various anatomic sites in the breast is shown in Figure 17–1.

Inspection of the breast is the first step in physical examination and should be carried out with the patient sitting, arms at her sides and then overhead. Abnormal variations in breast size and contour, minimal nipple retraction, and slight edema, redness, or retraction of the skin can be identified. Asymmetry of the breasts and retraction or dimpling of the skin can often be accentuated by having the patient raise her arms overhead or press her hands on her hips to contract the pectoralis muscles. Axillary and supraclavicular areas should be thoroughly palpated for enlarged nodes with the patient sitting (Figure 17–2). Palpation of the breast for masses or other changes should be performed with the patient both seated and supine with the arm abducted (Figure 17–3). Palpation with a rotary motion of the examiner's fingers as well as a horizontal stripping motion has been recommended.

Breast cancer usually consists of a nontender, firm or hard mass with poorly delineated margins (caused by local infiltration). Very small (1–2 mm) erosions of the nipple epithelium may be the only manifestation of Paget carcinoma. Watery, serous, or bloody discharge from the nipple is an occasional early sign but is more often associated with benign disease.

A small lesion, less than 1 cm in diameter, may be difficult or impossible for the examiner to feel but may be discovered by the patient. She should always be asked to demonstrate the location of the mass; if the practitioner fails to confirm the patient's suspicions and imaging studies are normal, the examination should be repeated in 2–3 months, preferably 1–2 weeks after the onset of menses. During the premenstrual phase of the cycle, increased innocuous nodularity may suggest neoplasm or may obscure an underlying

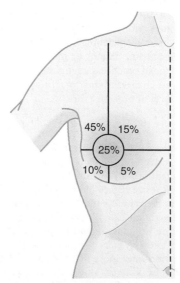

▲ **Figure 17–1.** Frequency of breast carcinoma at various anatomic sites.

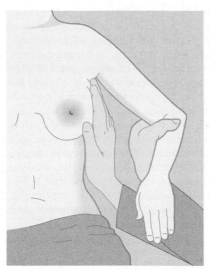

▲ **Figure 17–2.** Palpation of axillary region for enlarged lymph nodes.

lesion. If there is any question regarding the nature of an abnormality under these circumstances, the patient should be asked to return after her period. Ultrasound is often valuable and mammography essential when an area is felt by the patient to be abnormal but the physician feels no mass. MRI may be considered, but the lack of specificity should be discussed by the practitioner and the patient. MRI should not be used to rule out cancer because MRI has a false-negative rate of about 3–5%. Although lower than mammography, this false-negative rate cannot permit safe elimination of the possibility of cancer. False negatives are more likely seen in infiltrating lobular carcinomas and DCIS.

Metastases tend to involve regional lymph nodes, which may be palpable. One or two movable, nontender, not particularly firm axillary lymph nodes 5 mm or less in diameter are

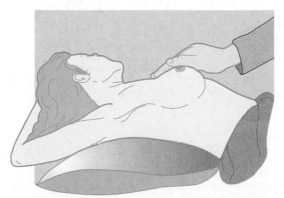

▲ **Figure 17–3.** Palpation of breasts. Palpation is performed with the patient supine and arm abducted.

frequently present and are generally of no significance. Firm or hard nodes larger than 1 cm are typical of metastases. Axillary nodes that are matted or fixed to skin or deep structures indicate advanced disease (at least stage III). On the other hand, if the examiner thinks that the axillary nodes are involved, that impression will be borne out by histologic section in about 85% of cases. The incidence of positive axillary nodes increases with the size of the primary tumor. Noninvasive cancers (in situ) do not metastasize. Metastases are present in about 30% of patients with clinically negative nodes.

In most cases, no nodes are palpable in the supraclavicular fossa. Firm or hard nodes of any size in this location or just beneath the clavicle are suggestive of metastatic cancer and should be biopsied. Ipsilateral supraclavicular or infraclavicular nodes containing cancer indicate that the tumor is in an advanced stage (stage III or IV). Edema of the ipsilateral arm, commonly caused by metastatic infiltration of regional lymphatics, is also a sign of advanced cancer.

B. Laboratory Findings

A consistently elevated sedimentation rate may be the result of disseminated cancer. Liver or bone metastases may be associated with elevation of serum alkaline phosphatase. Hypercalcemia is an occasional important finding in advanced cancer of the breast. Carcinoembryonic antigen (CEA) and CA 15-3 or CA 27-29 may be used as markers for recurrent breast cancer but are not helpful in diagnosing early lesions. Many scientists are further investigating breast cancer markers through proteomics and hormone assays. These studies are ongoing and may prove to be helpful in early detection or evaluation of prognosis.

C. Imaging for Metastases

Chest radiographs may show pulmonary metastases. CT scanning of the liver and brain is of value only when metastases are suspected in these areas. Bone scans utilizing ^{99m}Tc-labeled phosphates or phosphonates are more sensitive than skeletal radiographs in detecting metastatic breast cancer. Bone scanning has not proved to be of clinical value as a routine preoperative test in the absence of symptoms, physical findings, or abnormal alkaline phosphatase or calcium levels. The frequency of abnormal findings on bone scan parallels the status of the axillary lymph nodes on pathologic examination. PET scanning is less useful than a bone scan to identify metastatic bone lesions. It is effective in soft tissue or visceral metastases in patients with signs or symptoms of metastatic disease. PET scanning combined with CT (PET-CT) is an effective screening method for detecting soft tissue metastases and is replacing CT scans.

D. Diagnostic Tests

1. Biopsy—The diagnosis of breast cancer depends ultimately on examination of tissue or cells removed by biopsy. Treatment should never be undertaken without an unequivocal histologic or cytologic diagnosis of cancer. The safest course is biopsy examination of all suspicious lesions found on physical examination or mammography, or both. About 60% of lesions clinically thought to be cancer prove on biopsy to be benign, while about 30% of clinically benign lesions are found to be malignant. These findings demonstrate the fallibility of clinical judgment and the necessity for biopsy.

All breast masses require a histologic diagnosis with one probable exception, a nonsuspicious, presumably fibrocystic mass, in a premenopausal woman. Rather, these masses can be observed through one or two menstrual cycles. However, if the mass is not cystic and does not completely resolve during this time, it must be biopsied. Figures 17–4 and 17–5 present algorithms for management of breast masses in premenopausal and postmenopausal patients.

The simplest biopsy method is needle biopsy, either by aspiration of tumor cells (FNA cytology) or by obtaining a small core of tissue with a hollow needle (core biopsy).

FNA cytology is a useful technique whereby cells are aspirated with a small needle and examined cytologically. This technique can be performed easily with virtually no morbidity and is much less expensive than excisional or open biopsy. The main disadvantages are that it requires a pathologist skilled in the cytologic diagnosis of breast cancer and that it is subject to sampling problems, particularly because deep lesions may be missed. Furthermore, noninvasive cancers usually cannot be distinguished from invasive cancers. The incidence of false-positive diagnoses is extremely low, perhaps 1–2%. The false-negative rate is as high as 10%. Most experienced clinicians would not leave a suspicious dominant mass in the breast even

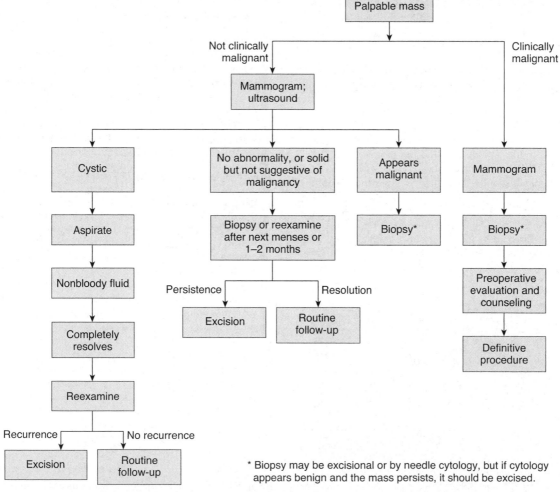

* Biopsy may be excisional or by needle cytology, but if cytology appears benign and the mass persists, it should be excised.

▲ **Figure 17–4.** Evaluation of breast masses in premenopausal women. (Adapted, with permission, from Giuliano AE: Breast disease. In: *Practical Gynecologic Oncology,* 3rd ed. Berek JS, Hacker NF [editors], Lippincott Williams & Wilkins, 2000.)

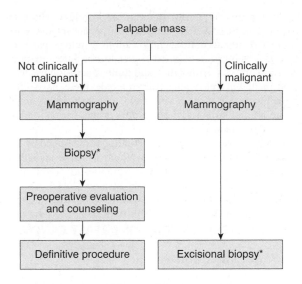

Palpable mass

Not clinically malignant → Mammography → Biopsy* → Preoperative evaluation and counseling → Definitive procedure

Clinically malignant → Mammography → Excisional biopsy*

* Biopsy may be excisional or by needle cytology, but if cytology appears benign and the mass persists, it should be excised.

▲ **Figure 17–5.** Evaluation of breast masses in post-menopausal women. (Adapted, with permission, from Giuliano AE: Breast disease. In: *Practical Gynecologic Oncology*, 3rd ed. Berek JS, Hacker NF [editors], Lippincott Williams & Wilkins, 2000.)

when FNA cytology is negative unless the clinical diagnosis, breast imaging studies, and cytologic studies were all in agreement, such as a fibrocystic lesion or fibroadenoma.

Large-needle (core needle) biopsy removes a core of tissue with a large cutting needle. Handheld biopsy devices make large-core needle biopsy of a palpable mass easy and cost effective in the office with local anesthesia. As in the case of any needle biopsy, the main problem is sampling error due to improper positioning of the needle, giving rise to a false-negative test result. Core biopsy has the advantage that tumor markers, such as estrogen receptor (ER), progesterone receptor (PR), and HER-2/*neu* overexpression can be performed on cores of tissue.

Open biopsy under local anesthesia as a separate procedure prior to deciding upon definitive treatment is the most reliable means of diagnosis. Needle biopsy or aspiration, when positive, offers a more rapid approach with less expense and morbidity, but when nondiagnostic it must be followed by open biopsy. It generally consists of an excisional biopsy, which is done through an incision with the intent to remove the entire abnormality, not simply a sample. Additional evaluation for metastatic disease and therapeutic options can be discussed with the patient after the histologic or cytologic diagnosis of cancer has been established. In situ cancers are not easily diagnosed cytologically and usually require excisional biopsy.

As an alternative in highly suspicious circumstances, the diagnosis may be made on frozen section of tissue obtained by open biopsy under general anesthesia. If the frozen section is positive, the surgeon can proceed immediately with the definitive operation. This one-step method is rarely used today except when a cytologic study has suggested cancer but is not diagnostic and there is a high clinical suspicion of malignancy in a patient well prepared for the diagnosis of cancer and its treatment options.

In general, the two-step approach—outpatient biopsy followed by definitive operation at a later date—is preferred in the diagnosis and treatment of breast cancer, because patients can be given time to adjust to the diagnosis of cancer, can consider alternative forms of therapy, and can seek a second opinion if they wish. There is no adverse effect from the short delay of the two-step procedure.

2. Ultrasonography—Ultrasonography is performed primarily to differentiate cystic from solid lesions but may show signs suggestive of carcinoma. Ultrasonography may show an irregular mass within a cyst in the rare case of intracystic carcinoma. If a tumor is palpable and feels like a cyst, an 18-gauge needle can be used to aspirate the fluid and make the diagnosis of cyst. If a cyst is aspirated and the fluid is nonbloody, it does not have to be examined cytologically. If the mass does not recur, no further diagnostic test is necessary. Nonpalpable mammographic densities that appear benign should be investigated with ultrasound to determine whether the lesion is cystic or solid. These may even be needle biopsied with ultrasound guidance.

3. Mammography—When a suspicious abnormality is identified by mammography alone and cannot be palpated by the clinician, the lesion should be biopsied under mammographic guidance. In the **computerized stereotactic guided core needle** technique, a biopsy needle is inserted into the lesion with mammographic guidance, and a core of tissue for histologic examination can then be examined. Vacuum assistance increases the amount of tissue obtained and improves diagnosis.

Mammographic localization biopsy is performed by obtaining a mammogram in two perpendicular views and placing a needle or hook-wire near the abnormality so that the surgeon can use the metal needle or wire as a guide during operation to locate the lesion. After mammography confirms the position of the needle in relation to the lesion, an incision is made and the subcutaneous tissue is dissected until the needle is identified. Often, the abnormality cannot even be palpated through the incision—as is the case with microcalcifications—and thus it is essential to obtain a mammogram of the specimen to document that the lesion was excised. At that time, a second marker needle can further localize the lesion for the pathologist. Stereotactic core needle biopsies have proved equivalent to mammographic localization biopsies. Core biopsy is preferable to mammographic localization for accessible lesions, since an operation can be avoided. A metal clip should be placed after any image-guided core biopsy to facilitate finding the site of the lesion if subsequent treatment is necessary.

4. Other imaging modalities—Other modalities of breast imaging have been investigated for diagnostic purposes. Automated breast ultrasonography is useful in distinguishing cystic from solid lesions but should be used only as a supplement to physical examination and mammography. Ductography may be useful to define the site of a lesion causing a bloody discharge, but since biopsy is almost always indicated, ductography may be omitted and the blood-filled nipple system excised. Ductoscopy has shown some promise in identifying intraductal lesions, especially in the case of pathologic nipple discharge, but in practice, this technique is rarely used. MRI is highly sensitive but not specific and should not be used for screening except in highly selective cases. For example, MRI is useful in differentiating scar from recurrence postlumpectomy and may be valuable to screen high-risk women (eg, women with *BRCA* mutations). It may also be of value to examine for multicentricity when there is a known primary cancer; to examine the contralateral breast in women with cancer; to examine the extent of cancer, especially lobular carcinomas; or to determine the response to neoadjuvant chemotherapy. PET scanning does not appear useful in evaluating the breast itself but is valuable to examine regional lymphatics and distant metastases.

5. Cytology—Cytologic examination of nipple discharge or cyst fluid may be helpful on rare occasions. As a rule, mammography (or ductography) and breast biopsy are required when nipple discharge or cyst fluid is bloody or cytologically questionable. Ductal lavage, a technique that washes individual duct systems with saline and loosens epithelial cells for cytologic evaluation, is being evaluated as a risk assessment tool but appears to be of little value.

▶ Differential Diagnosis

The lesions to be considered most often in the differential diagnosis of breast cancer are the following, in descending order of frequency: fibrocystic condition of the breast, fibroadenoma, intraductal papilloma, lipoma, and fat necrosis.

▶ Staging

The American Joint Committee on Cancer and the International Union Against Cancer have agreed on a TNM (tumor, regional lymph nodes, distant metastases) staging system for breast cancer. Using the TNM staging system enhances communication between researchers and clinicians. Table 17–2 outlines the TNM classification.

▶ Pathologic Types

Numerous pathologic subtypes of breast cancer can be identified histologically (Table 17–3).

Except for the in situ cancers, the histologic subtypes have only a slight bearing on prognosis when outcomes are compared after accurate staging. Various histologic parameters, such as invasion of blood vessels, tumor differentiation, invasion of breast lymphatics, and tumor necrosis have been examined, but other than tumor grade these have little prognostic value. Genetic analysis for certain high-risk genes in the primary tumor appears to offer prognostic and therapeutic information.

The noninvasive cancers by definition are confined by the basement membrane of the ducts and lack the ability to spread. However, in patients whose biopsies show noninvasive intraductal cancer, associated invasive ductal cancers metastasize to lymph nodes in about 1–3% of cases.

SPECIAL CLINICAL FORMS OF BREAST CANCER

▶ Paget Carcinoma

Paget carcinoma is not common (about 1% of all breast cancers). It affects the nipple and may or may not be associated with a breast mass. The basic lesion is usually a well-differentiated infiltrating ductal carcinoma or a DCIS. The ducts of the nipple epithelium are infiltrated, but gross nipple changes are often minimal, and a tumor mass may not be palpable.

Because the nipple changes appear innocuous, the diagnosis is frequently missed. The first symptom is often itching or burning of the nipple, with superficial erosion or ulceration. These are often diagnosed and treated as dermatitis or bacterial infection, leading to delay or failure in detection. The diagnosis is established by biopsy of the area of erosion. When the lesion consists of nipple changes only, the incidence of axillary metastases is less than 5%, and the prognosis is excellent. When a breast mass is also present, the incidence of axillary metastases rises, with an associated marked decrease in prospects for cure by surgical or other treatment.

▶ Inflammatory Carcinoma

This is the most malignant form of breast cancer and constitutes less than 3% of all cases. The clinical findings consist of a rapidly growing, sometimes painful mass that enlarges the breast. The overlying skin becomes erythematous, edematous, and warm. Often, there is no distinct mass, since the tumor infiltrates the involved breast diffusely. The inflammatory changes, often mistaken for an infection, are caused by carcinomatous invasion of the subdermal lymphatics, with resulting edema and hyperemia. If the practitioner suspects infection but the lesion does not respond rapidly (1–2 weeks) to antibiotics, biopsy should be performed. The diagnosis should be made when the redness involves more than one-third of the skin over the breast and biopsy shows infiltrating carcinoma with invasion of the subdermal lymphatics. Metastases tend to occur early and widely, and for this reason, inflammatory carcinoma is rarely curable. Radiation, hormone therapy, and chemotherapy are the measures most likely to be of value rather than operation. Mastectomy is indicated when chemotherapy and radiation have resulted in clinical remission with no evidence of distant metastases. In these cases, residual disease in the breast may be eradicated.

▶ Breast Cancer Occurring during Pregnancy or Lactation

Breast cancer complicates approximately one in 3000 pregnancies. The diagnosis is frequently delayed, because physio-logic changes in the breast may obscure the lesion. When the cancer is confined to the breast, the 5-year survival rate is about 70%. In 60–70% of patients, axillary metastases are already present, conferring a 5-year survival rate of 30–40%. Pregnancy (or lactation) is not a contraindication to operation or treatment, and therapy should be based on the stage of the disease as in the nonpregnant (or nonlactating) woman. Overall survival rates have improved, since cancers are now diagnosed in pregnant women earlier than in the past and treatment has improved. Breast-conserving surgery may be performed—and radiation and chemotherapy given—even during the pregnancy.

Table 17–2. TNM Staging for Breast Cancer.

Primary Tumor (T)

Definitions for classifying the primary tumor (T) are the same for clinical and for pathologic classification. If the measurement is made by physical examination, the examiner will use the major headings (T1, T2, or T3). If other measurements, such as mammographic or pathologic measurements, are used, the subsets of T1 can be used. Tumors should be measured to the nearest 0.1 cm increment.	
TX	Primary tumor cannot be assessed
T0	No evidence of primary tumor
Tis	Carcinoma in situ
Tis (DCIS)	Ductal carcinoma in situ
Tis (LCIS)	Lobular carcinoma in situ
Tis (Paget)	Paget disease of the nipple with no tumor
Note: Paget disease associated with a tumor is classified according to the size of the tumor.	
T1	Tumor < 2 cm in greatest dimension
T1mic	Microinvasion $\leq$ 0.1 cm in greatest dimension
T1a	Tumor > 0.1 cm but not > 0.5 cm in greatest dimension
T1b	Tumor > 0.5 cm but not > 1 cm in greatest dimension
T1c	Tumor > 1 cm but not > 2 cm in greatest dimension
T2	Tumor > 2 cm but not > 5 cm in greatest dimension
T3	Tumor > 5 cm in greatest dimension
T4	Tumor of any size with direct extension to (a) chest wall or (b) skin, only as described below
T4a	Extension to chest wall, not including pectoralis muscle
T4b	Edema (including peau d'orange) or ulceration of the skin of the breast, or satellite skin nodules confined to the same breast
T4c	Both T4a and T4b
T4d	Inflammatory carcinoma

N2a	Metastasis in ipsilateral axillary lymph nodes fixed to one another (matted) or to other structures
N2b	Metastasis only in clinically apparent[1] ipsilateral internal mammary nodes and in the *absence* of clinically evident axillary lymph node metastasis
N3	Metastasis in ipsilateral infraclavicular lymph node(s) with or without axillary lymph node involvement, or in clinically apparent[1] ipsilateral internal mammary lymph node(s) and in the *presence* of clinically evident axillary lymph node metastasis; or metastasis in ipsilateral supraclavicular lymph node(s) with or without axillary or internal mammary lymph node involvement
N3a	Metastasis in ipsilateral infraclavicular lymph node(s)
N3b	Metastasis in ipsilateral internal mammary lymph node(s) and axillary lymph node(s)
N3c	Metastasis in ipsilateral supraclavicular lymph node(s)
Pathologic (pN)[2]	
pNX	Regional lymph nodes cannot be assessed (eg, previously removed, or not removed for pathologic study)
pN0	No regional lymph node metastasis histologically, no additional examination for isolated tumor cells
Note: Isolated tumor cells (ITC) are defined as single tumor cells or small cell clusters not greater than 0.2 mm, usually detected only by immunohistochemical (IHC) or molecular methods but which may be verified on hematoxylin and eosin stains. ITCs do not usually show evidence of malignant activity, (eg, proliferation or stromal reaction).	
pN0(i–)	No regional lymph node metastasis histologically, negative IHC
pN0(i+)	No regional lymph node metastasis histologically, positive IHC, no IHC cluster > 0.2 mm
pN0(mol–)	No regional lymph node metastasis histologically, negative molecular findings (RT-PCR)
pN0(mol+)	No regional lymph node metastasis histologically, positive molecular findings (RT-PCR)

(continued)

Table 17–2. TNM Staging for Breast Cancer. *(Continued)*

Regional lymph nodes (N)				
Clinical				
NX	Regional lymph nodes cannot be assessed (eg, previously removed)			
N0	No regional lymph node metastasis			
N1	Metastasis to movable ipsilateral axillary lymph node(s)			
N2	Metastases in ipsilateral axillary lymph nodes fixed or matted, or in clinically apparent ipsilateral internal mammary nodes in the *absence* of clinically evident axillary lymph node metastasis			
pN2	Metastasis in 4 to 9 axillary lymph nodes, or in clinically apparent[1] internal mammary lymph nodes in the *absence* of axillary lymph node metastasis			
pN2a	Metastasis in 4 to 9 axillary lymph nodes (at least one tumor deposit > 2.0 mm)			
pN2b	Metastasis in clinically apparent[1] internal mammary lymph nodes in the *absence* of axillary lymph node metastasis			
pN3	Metastasis in 10 or more axillary lymph nodes, or in infraclavicular lymph nodes, or in clinically apparent[1] ipsilateral internal mammary lymph nodes in the *presence* of 1 or more positive axillary lymph nodes; or in more than 3 axillary lymph nodes with clinically negative microscopic metastasis in internal mammary lymph nodes; or in ipsilateral supraclavicular lymph nodes			
pN3a	Metastasis in 10 or more axillary lymph nodes (at least one tumor deposit > 2.0 mm), or metastasis to the infraclavicular lymph nodes			
pN3b	Metastasis in clinically apparent[1] ipsilateral internal mammary lymph nodes in the *presence* of 1 or more positive axillary lymph nodes; or in more than 3 axillary lymph nodes and in internal mammary lymph nodes with microscopic disease detected by sentinel lymph node dissection but not clinically apparent[1]			
pN3c	Metastasis in ipsilateral supraclavicular lymph nodes			

pN1	Metastasis in one to three axillary lymph nodes and/or in internal mammary nodes with microscopic disease detected by sentinel lymph node dissection but not clinically apparent[1]
pN1mi	Micrometastasis (> 0.2 mm, none > 2.0 mm)
pN1a	Metastasis in 1 to 3 axillary lymph nodes
pN1b	Metastasis in internal mammary nodes with microscopic disease detected by sentinel lymph node dissection but not clinically apparent[1]
pN1c	Metastasis in 1 to 3 axillary lymph nodes and in internal mammary lymph nodes with microscopic disease detected by sentinel lymph node dissection but not clinically apparent.[1] (If associated with > 3 positive axillary lymph nodes, the internal mammary nodes are classified as pN3b to reflect increased tumor burden)

Distant metastasis (M)	
MX	Distant metastasis cannot be assessed
M0	No distant metastasis
M1	Distant metastasis

Stage grouping			
Stage 0	Tis	N0	M0
Stage 1	T1[3]	N0	M0
Stage IIA	T0	N1	M0
	T1[3]	N1	M0
	T2	N0	M0
Stage IIB	T2	N1	M0
	T3	N0	M0
Stage IIIA	T0	N2	M0
	T1[3]	N2	M0
	T2	N2	M0
	T3	N1	M0
	T3	N2	M0
Stage IIIB	T4	N0	M0
	T4	N1	M0
	T4	N2	M0
Stage IIIC	Any T	N3	M0
Stage IV	Any T	Any N	M1

Note: Stage designation may be changed if postsurgical imaging studies reveal the presence of distant metastases, provided that the studies are carried out within 4 months of diagnosis in the absence of disease progression and provided that the patient has not received neoadjuvant therapy.

(continued)

Table 17-2. TNM Staging for Breast Cancer. *(Continued)*

[1]*Clinically apparent* is defined as detected by imaging studies (excluding lymphoscintigraphy) or by clinical examination or grossly visible pathologically. *Not clinically apparent* is defined as not detected by imaging studies (excluding lymphoscintigraphy) or by clinical examination.

[2]Classification is based on axillary lymph node dissection with or without sentinel lymph node dissection. Classification based solely on sentinel lymph node dissection without subsequent axillary lymph node dissection is designated (sn) for "sentinel node," eg, pN0(i+)(sn).

[3]T1 includes T1mic.

RT-PCR, reverse transcriptase/polymerase chain reaction.

Reproduced, with permission, of the American Joint Committee on Cancer (AJCC), Chicago, Illinois. *AJCC Cancer Staging Manual*, 6th edition, Springer-Verlag, 2002. www.springeronline.com.

▶ Bilateral Breast Cancer

Bilateral breast cancer occurs in less than 5% of cases, but there is as high as a 20–25% incidence of later occurrence of cancer in the second breast. Bilaterality occurs more often in familial breast cancer, in women under age 50 years, and when the tumor in the primary breast is lobular. The incidence of second breast cancers increases directly with the length of time the patient is alive after her first cancer—about 1–2% per year.

In patients with breast cancer, mammography should be performed before primary treatment and at regular intervals thereafter, to search for occult cancer in the opposite breast or conserved ipsilateral breast. MRI may be useful in this high-risk group.

▶ Noninvasive Cancer

Noninvasive cancer can occur within the ducts (DCIS) or lobules (lobular carcinoma in situ, LCIS). LCIS, although thought to be a premalignant lesion or a risk factor for breast cancer, in fact may behave like DCIS. In a 2004 analysis of multiple NSABP studies, invasive lobular breast cancer not only developed in patients with LCIS but it developed in the same breast and indexed location as the original LCIS. Although more research needs to be done in this area, the invasive potential of LCIS is being reconsidered. The subtype pleomorphic LCIS may behave more like DCIS. DCIS tends to be unilateral and most often progresses to invasive cancer if untreated. In approximately 40–60% of women who have DCIS treated with biopsy alone, invasive cancer develops within the same breast.

The treatment of intraductal lesions is controversial. DCIS can be treated by wide excision with or without radiation therapy or with total mastectomy. Conservative management is advised in patients with small lesions amenable to lumpectomy. Although research is defining the malignant potential of LCIS, it can be managed with observation. Patients unwilling to accept the increased risk of breast cancer may be offered surgical excision of the area in question or bilateral total mastectomy. Currently, the accepted standard of care offers the alternative of chemoprevention, which is effective in preventing invasive breast cancer in both LCIS and DCIS that has been completely excised. Axillary metastases from in situ cancers should not occur unless there is an occult invasive cancer. Sentinel node biopsy may be indicated in large DCIS treated with mastectomy.

Table 17-3. Histologic Types of Breast Cancer.

Type	Frequency of Occurrence
Infiltrating ductal (not otherwise specified)	80–90%
Medullary	5–8%
Colloid (mucinous)	2–4%
Tubular	1–2%
Papillary	1–2%
Invasive lobular	6–8%
Noninvasive	4–6%
Intraductal	2–3%
Lobular in situ	2–3%
Rare cancers	< 1%
Juvenile (secretory)	
Adenoid cystic	
Epidermoid	
Sudoriferous	

Barnes DM et al: Pregnancy-associated breast cancer: a literature review. Surg Clin North Am 2007;87:417.

Barni S et al: Locally advanced breast cancer. Curr Opin Obstet Gynecol 2006;18:47.

Bodner-Adler B et al: Breast cancer diagnosed during pregnancy. Anticancer Res 2007;27:1705.

Chen CY et al: Paget disease of the breast: changing patterns of incidence, clinical presentation, and treatment in the U.S. Cancer 2006;107:1448.

Cristofanilli M et al: Inflammatory breast cancer (IBC) and patterns of recurrence: understanding the biology of a unique disease. Cancer 2007;110:1436.

Daly MB: Tamoxifen in ductal carcinoma in situ. Semin Oncol 2006;33:647.

Dawood S et al: What progress have we made in managing inflammatory breast cancer? Oncology (Williston Park) 2007;21:673.

Erbas B et al: The natural history of ductal carcinoma in situ of the breast: a review. Breast Cancer Res Treat 2006;97:135.

Habel KL et al: A population-based study of tumor gene expression and risk of breast cancer death among lymph node-negative patients. Breast Cancer Res 2006;8:R25.

Hansen NM et al: Breast cancer: pre- and postoperative imaging for staging. Surg Oncol Clin N Am 2007;16:447.

Irvine T et al: Biology and treatment of ductal carcinoma in situ. Expert Rev Anticancer Ther 2007;7:135.

Lakhani SR et al: The management of lobular carcinoma in situ (LCIS). Is LCIS the same as ductal carcinoma in situ (DCIS)? Eur J Cancer 2006;42:2205.

Ring AE et al: Breast cancer and pregnancy. Ann Oncol 2005; 16:1855.

Schirrmeister H: Detection of bone metastases in breast cancer by positron emission tomography. Radiol Clin North Am 2007;45:669.

Theriault R et al: Management of breast cancer in pregnancy. Curr Oncol Rep 2007;9:17.

West JG et al: Multidisciplinary management of ductal carcinoma in situ: a 10-year experience. Am J Surg 2007;194:532.

BIOMARKERS

The ER and PR status and HER-2/*neu* status of the tumor should be determined at the time of initial biopsy. Other studies such as proliferation indices may be performed. These markers may be obtained on core biopsy specimens, which will be necessary to institute neoadjuvant therapy.

The presence or absence of ER and PR is a critical element of breast cancer management. Patients whose primary tumors are receptor-positive have a more favorable course than those whose tumors are receptor-negative. Up to 60% of patients with metastatic breast cancer will respond to hormonal manipulation if their tumors are ER-positive. Fewer than 5% of patients with metastatic, ER-negative tumors can be treated successfully in this fashion. Adjuvant hormonal therapy, with or without chemotherapy, in receptor-positive tumors and adjuvant chemotherapy alone in receptor-negative tumors improve survival rates even in the absence of lymph node metastases. Hormone receptors have no relationship to response to chemotherapy (see discussion on adjuvant therapy later in chapter).

PR status may be more sensitive than ER status in determining which patients are likely to respond to hormonal manipulation. Up to 80% of patients with metastatic PR-positive tumors improve with hormonal manipulation.

In addition to ER status and PR status, the rate at which tumor divides and the differentiation of the cells (proliferative indices) are important. In order to establish the rate of growth and differentiation, the amount and type of DNA is measured with flow cytometry.

Another key element in determining treatment and prognosis is the amount of the HER-2/*neu* oncogene present in the cancer. HER-2/*neu* overexpression is scored using a numerical system: 1+ is not an overexpressor, 2+ is borderline, and 3+ is an overexpressor. In the case of 2+ expression, fluorescence in situ hybridization (FISH) is recommended to more accurately assess HER-2/*neu* amplification and provide better prognostic information. The presence of HER-2/*neu* amplification predicts the response to trastuzumab.

While individually these biomarkers provide insight to appropriate adjuvant therapy, when combined they provide a great deal of information regarding risk of recurrence. Several tests now predict relapse rates for patients treated with tamoxifen or chemotherapy. Oncotype DX combines 21 genetic markers, including ER, PR, and HER-2/*neu* expression, in a tumor specimen to categorize risk of recurrence into three groups: high risk, intermediate risk, and low risk. The test is able to identify that the high-risk group is more likely to benefit from chemotherapy in addition to tamoxifen while the low-risk group does not. This type of test is quite helpful when the survival advantage of therapy is difficult to determine. It has been most used for ER-positive node-negative tumors but now may apply to node-positive tumors as well.

Another promising biomarker being studied is vascular endothelial growth factor (VEGF), a protein that stimulates the growth of blood vessels. Elevated levels of VEGF may be a marker for a tumor that is more aggressive because of its ability to develop blood vessels and grow. While researchers look for more specific markers to determine the presence of breast cancer, these markers also provide insight to targeted methods of treatment. Other markers being evaluated are p53, nm23, DNA 5c exceeding rate (DNA 5cER), G-actin, urokinase-type plasminogen activator (u-PA), and its type-1 inhibitor (PAI-1).

Ferretti G et al: sHER2/*neu* role in breast cancer: from a prognostic foe to a predictive friend. Curr Opin Obstet Gynecol 2007; 19:56.

Luadido J et al: HER2 testing: a review of detection methodologies and their clinical performance. Expert Rev Mol Diagn 2007;7:53.

Nicolini A et al: Biomolecular markers of breast cancer. Front Biosci 2006;11:1818.

Paik S et al: A multigene assay to predict recurrence of tamoxifen treated, node-negative breast cancer. N Engl J Med 2004;351:2817.

▶ Treatment: Curative

Clearly, not all breast cancer is systemic at the time of diagnosis. A pessimistic attitude concerning the management of breast cancer is therefore unwarranted. Most patients with early breast cancer can be cured.

Treatment may be curative or palliative. Curative treatment is advised for clinical stage I, II, and III disease (see Table 17–2). Patients with locally advanced (T3, T4) and even inflammatory tumors may be cured with multimodality therapy, but in most, palliation is all that can be expected. Palliative treatment is appropriate for all patients with stage IV disease and for previously treated patients in whom distant metastases develop or who have unresectable local cancers (see Treatment: Palliative section later in chapter).

A. Choice of Primary Therapy

The extent of disease and its biologic aggressiveness are the principal determinants of the outcome of primary therapy.

Clinical and pathologic staging help in assessing extent of disease (see Table 17–2), but each is to some extent imprecise. Other factors, such as DNA flow cytometry, tumor grade, hormone receptor assays, and oncogene amplification, may be of prognostic value but are not important in determining the type of local therapy.

Controversy has surrounded the choice of primary therapy of stages I, II, and III breast carcinoma. A number of states require physicians to inform patients of alternative treatment methods in the management of breast cancer. Currently, the standard of care for stage I, stage II, and most stage III cancer is surgical resection followed by adjuvant radiation or systemic therapy when indicated. Neoadjuvant therapy is becoming more popular, since large tumors may be shrunk by chemotherapy prior to surgery, making some patients who require mastectomy candidates for lumpectomy.

B. Surgical Resection

1. Breast-conserving therapy

—Multiple, large, randomized studies, including the Milan and NSABP trials, show that disease-free and overall survival rates are similar for patients treated with partial mastectomy plus axillary dissection followed by radiation therapy and for those treated by modified radical mastectomy (total mastectomy plus axillary dissection).

Twenty years of follow-up of the NSABP trial has shown that lumpectomy with axillary dissection followed by postoperative radiation therapy is as effective as modified radical mastectomy for the management of patients with stage I and stage II breast cancer.

Tumor size is a major consideration in determining the feasibility of breast conservation. The lumpectomy trial of the NSABP randomized patients with tumors as large as 4 cm. To achieve an acceptable cosmetic result, the patient must have a breast of sufficient size to enable excision of a 4-cm tumor without considerable deformity. Therefore, large size is only a relative contraindication. Subareolar tumors, also difficult to excise without deformity, are not contraindications to breast conservation. Clinically detectable multifocality is a relative contraindication to breast-conserving surgery, as is fixation to the chest wall or skin or involvement of the nipple or overlying skin. The patient—not the surgeon—should be the judge of what is cosmetically acceptable.

Axillary dissection is valuable in preventing axillary recurrences, in staging cancer, and in planning therapy. Intraoperative lymphatic mapping and sentinel node biopsy identify lymph nodes most likely to harbor metastases if present in the axillary nodes. Sentinel node biopsy is a reasonable alternative to axillary dissection in selected patients with invasive cancer.

Breast-conserving surgery with radiation is the preferred form of treatment for patients with **early-stage breast cancer.** Despite the numerous randomized trials showing no survival benefit of mastectomy over breast-conserving par-

tial mastectomy and irradiation, breast-conserving surgery still appears underutilized.

2. Mastectomy

—Modified radical mastectomy was the standard therapy for most patients with early-stage breast cancer. This operation removes the entire breast, overlying skin, nipple, and areolar complex as well as the underlying pectoralis fascia with the axillary lymph nodes in continuity. The major advantage of modified radical mastectomy is that radiation therapy may not be necessary, although radiation may be used when multiple lymph nodes are involved with cancer. The disadvantage of mastectomy is the cosmetic and psychological impact associated with breast loss. Radical mastectomy, which removes the underlying pectoralis muscle, should be performed rarely, if at all. Axillary node dissection is not indicated for noninfiltrating cancers because nodal metastases are rarely present. Skin-sparing mastectomy is currently gaining favor but is not appropriate for all patients. Breast-conserving surgery and radiation should be offered whenever possible, since most patients would prefer to save the breast. Breast reconstruction, immediate or delayed, should be discussed with patients who choose or require mastectomy. Patients should have an interview with a reconstructive plastic surgeon to discuss options prior to making a decision regarding reconstruction. Time is well spent preoperatively in educating the patient and family about these matters.

Radiotherapy after partial mastectomy consists of 5–7 weeks of five daily fractions to a total dose of 5000–6000 cGy. Most radiation oncologists use a boost dose to the cancer location. Several studies are underway examining the utility and recurrence rates after intraoperative radiation or dose dense radiation in which the time course of radiation is shortened. Accelerated partial breast irradiation, in which only the portion of the breast from which the tumor was resected is irradiated for 1–2 weeks, appears effective in achieving local control. A prospective randomized trial to examine the efficacy of this technique is underway. Accrual should be completed this year, but long-term follow-up will be necessary. Current studies suggest that radiotherapy after mastectomy may improve survival in a subset of patients and is being further researched in a large cooperative trial to better identify which subgroups will benefit. Researchers are also examining the utility of axillary irradiation as an alternative to axillary dissection in the clinically node-negative patient with sentinel node micrometastases.

C. Adjuvant Systemic Therapy

In practice, most medical oncologists are currently using systemic adjuvant therapy for patients with either node-negative or node-positive breast cancer. Prognostic factors other than nodal status being used to determine the patient's risks are tumor size, ER and PR status, nuclear grade, histologic type, proliferative rate, and oncogene expression

(Table 17–4). The assumption is made that all patients with node-negative aggressive tumors should receive adjuvant therapy except those who have serious coexistent medical problems. In general, systemic chemotherapy decreases the chance of recurrence by about 30%. Most patients tolerate at least tamoxifen.

1. Chemotherapy—Following surgery and possible radiation therapy, systemic therapy improves survival and is advocated for most patients with curable breast cancer. In addition, chemotherapy may decrease local recurrence in patients treated with breast conservation, whereas hormonal manipulation decreases contralateral breast cancer occurrence as well as ipsilateral recurrence.

On the basis of the superiority of anthracycline-containing regimens in metastatic breast cancer, both doxorubicin and epirubicin have been studied extensively in the adjuvant setting. Studies comparing Adriamycin (generic name: doxorubicin) and cyclophosphamide (AC) or epirubicin and cyclophosphamide (EC) with cyclophosphamide methotrexate fluorouracil (CMF) have shown that treatments with anthracycline-containing regimens are at least as effective as, and perhaps more effective than, treatment with CMF. The NSABP B-23 compared four cycles of AC with six cycles of CMF and demonstrated the equivalence of these two regimens in node-negative, ER-negative disease. Whereas four cycles of AC or EC have not demonstrated improved survival compared with CMF, the use of six cycles of fluorouracil plus AC (FAC) or fluorouracil plus EC (FEC) has shown improved survival compared with CMF alone. For node-negative patients, the results of clinical trials support the use of four cycles of AC or six cycles of CMF in the adjuvant setting.

For **node-positive patients** and recently selected node-negative patients, taxanes (paclitaxel and docetaxel) are fre-quently combined with anthracycline-based regimens. Initial studies demonstrated a 20% proportional reduction in recurrence and a 4% absolute improvement in disease-free survival with the addition of paclitaxel to an AC regimen. Paclitaxel is FDA-approved for and increasingly used as adjuvant therapy in node-positive breast cancer. Taxanes are commonly added to AC for node-positive women. A trial comparing six cycles of FAC to six cycles of Docetaxel, doxorubicin, and cyclophosphamide (TAC) showed an improvement in disease-free survival for patients receiving the addition of docetaxel. This benefit was most marked for patients with positive nodes and was seen in both ER-negative and ER-positive tumors. High-risk node-negative patients are also treated with taxanes. A large study from the Breast Cancer International Research Group, presented at the San Antonio Breast Cancer Symposium in December 2007, suggests that anthracyclines may only be effective in patients with HER-2/*neu* overexpression. This remains to be confirmed.

Chemotherapy side effects are now well controlled. Nausea and vomiting are abated with drugs that directly affect the central nervous system, such as ondansetron and granisetron. Growth factors such as erythropoietin (epoetin alfa), which stimulates red blood cell production and mimics the effect of erythropoietin, and filgrastim (granulocyte colony-stimulating factor [G-CSF]), which stimulates proliferation and differentiation of hematopoietic cells, prevent life-threatening anemia and neutropenia seen commonly with high doses of chemotherapy. These agents greatly diminish the incidence of infections that may complicate the use of myelosuppressive chemotherapy.

The overall duration of adjuvant chemotherapy still remains uncertain. However, based on the meta-analysis performed in the Oxford Overview (Early Breast Cancer Trialists' Collaborative Group), the current recommendation is for 3–6 months of the commonly used regimens. The addition of taxanes required an additional duration of therapy of up to 6 months. Increasing the frequency of chemotherapy administration (dose dense chemotherapy) has been shown to be superior to standard dosing. It is often used when there is a greater risk of recurrence or in the younger patient, since it is a difficult regimen to tolerate physically. Although it is clear that dose intensity to a specific threshold is essential, there are little to no data supporting the benefit to high-dose therapy with stem cell support.

2. Targeted therapy

A. HER-2/NEU OVEREXPRESSION—Controversy exists about whether patients whose tumors overexpress the HER-2/*neu* oncogene benefit more from anthracycline regimens than from CMF regimens. Trastuzumab (Herceptin), a monoclonal antibody that binds to the HER-2/*neu* receptors, when studied in the metastatic setting, has proved effective in combination with chemotherapy in patients with HER-2/*neu* overexpression. A second monoclonal antibody lapa-

Table 17–4. Prognostic Factors in Node-Negative Breast Cancer.

Prognostic Factors	Increased Recurrence	Decreased Recurrence
Size	T3, T2	T1, T0
Hormone receptors	Negative	Positive
DNA flow cytometry	Aneuploid	Diploid
Histologic grade	High	Low
Tumor labeling index	< 3%	> 3%
S phase fraction	> 5%	< 5%
Lymphatic or vascular invasion	Present	Absent
Cathepsin D	High	Low
HER-2/*neu* oncogene	High	Low
Epidermal growth factor receptor	High	Low

tinib (Tykerb) is effective for metastatic breast cancer in patients who have received trastuzumab. Cardiac toxicity is seen from these antibodies. A multicenter trial from Finland, by the Fin-Her collaborative group, studied the use of trastuzumab in combination with docetaxel or vinorelbine for patients with early breast cancer that demonstrated HER-2/*neu* overexpression. The 3-year recurrence-free survival was better in those who took trastuzumab than in those who did not receive the antibody, 89% versus 78%, respectively. In another study, the HERA trial, a similar disease-free survival at interim analysis was demonstrated when giving trastuzumab subsequent to adjuvant chemotherapy in early breast cancer. In several trials, trastuzumab appears to decrease recurrence by nearly 50% when used as an adjuvant. It is currently given for 1 year postoperatively.

B. VASCULAR ENDOTHELIAL GROWTH FACTOR (VEGF)—Bevacizumab (Avastin) is a monoclonal antibody directed against VEGF. This growth factor stimulates endothelial proliferation and neoangiogenesis in cancer. A phase-three randomized trial showed increased effectiveness of a combination of bevacizumab and paclitaxel over paclitaxel alone. This antibody is being tested in other phase-three studies, adjuvant studies, and neoadjuvant studies. Results are promising.

C. HORMONAL THERAPY—Adjuvant hormonal therapy is highly effective in decreasing recurrence and mortality by 25% in women with ER-positive tumors regardless of menopausal status. The standard regimen has been tamoxifen for 5 years. AIs are also effective in the adjuvant setting for postmenopausal women. The large Arimidex, Tamoxifen, Alone or in Combination (ATAC) trial in postmenopausal women with ER-positive disease showed improved disease-free survival in patients treated with anastrozole compared with those treated with tamoxifen alone or with the combination of tamoxifen and anastrozole. In addition, anastrozole has shown a greater than 50% reduction in contralateral breast tumors with fewer side effects such as endometrial cancers, hot flushes, and thromboembolic events. However, anastrozole did have an increase in fractures due to bone loss. Anastrozole is used in the adjuvant setting in postmenopausal women. Because of the extensive long-term data supporting the use of tamoxifen, the American Society of Clinical Oncology, while recommending the use of AI in the appropriate populations, still encourages the use of tamoxifen for adjuvant hormonal therapy in the absence of significant contraindications. Tamoxifen should be used as a systemic agent in all women whose tumors are hormone receptor–positive, regardless of age, menopausal status, or other prognostic factors. HER-2/*neu* status should not affect the choice of cytotoxic agents or the use of hormone therapy. Furthermore, anastrozole is being used after completion of tamoxifen therapy or prior to completing therapy (year 2 or 3) to further decrease recurrences.

The long-term advantage of systemic therapy has been well established. Selection of patients for adjuvant treatment should be based on the patient's axillary nodal status, tumor size and grade, receptor status, HER-2/*neu,* and age. The value of *TP53,* angiogenesis factors, and vascular invasion is being investigated, but they remain to be proven prognostic factors. The use of anthracyclines is superior to combinations without anthracyclines. Ovarian ablation in premenopausal patients with ER-positive tumors may produce a benefit similar to that of adjuvant systemic chemotherapy. Taxanes have demonstrated benefit in patients with metastatic cancer and are being used in node-negative patients. Adjuvant systemic therapy should not be given to women who have small node-negative breast cancers with favorable histologic findings and tumor markers such as mucinous or tubular carcinoma, ER-positive, low grade, HER-2/*neu* non-amplified.

D. Neoadjuvant Therapy

The use of chemotherapy or hormonal therapy prior to resection of the primary tumor (neoadjuvant) is gaining popularity. This enables the assessment of in vivo chemosensitivity. A complete tumor response in vivo prior to operation is associated with improvement in survival. Neoadjuvant chemotherapy also permits breast conservation by shrinking the primary tumor in women who would otherwise need mastectomy for local control. Survival after neoadjuvant chemotherapy has not been shown to be superior to that seen with postoperative adjuvant chemotherapy but is certainly no worse. There is considerable concern as to the timing of sentinel lymph node biopsy (SLNB), since the chemotherapy may affect any cancer present in the lymph nodes. Several studies have shown that sentinel node biopsy can be done after neoadjuvant therapy. However, a large multicenter study, NSABP B-27, demonstrated a false-negative rate as high as 10.7%, well above the false-negative rate outside the neoadjuvant setting (< 1–5%). Many physicians recommend performing SLNB before administering the chemotherapy in order to avoid a false-negative result and to aid in planning subsequent radiation therapy. If a complete dissection is necessary, this can be performed at the time of the definitive breast surgery.

Important questions remaining to be answered are the timing and duration of adjuvant and neoadjuvant chemotherapy, which chemotherapeutic agents should be applied for which subgroups of patients, the use of combinations of hormonal therapy and chemotherapy as well as possibly targeted therapy, and the value of prognostic factors other than hormone receptors in predicting response to therapy. Adjuvant systemic therapy is not generally used in patients with small tumors and those with negative lymph nodes who have favorable tumor markers. However, a small disease-free survival benefit, even in patients with small favorable tumors, is seen. It appears that adjuvant systemic therapy benefits all breast cancer patients, but the clinician and patient must decide if the benefits outweigh the risks, complications, and expense.

▶ Treatment: Palliative

A. Radiotherapy

Palliative radiotherapy may be advised for primary treatment of locally advanced cancers with distant metastases to control ulceration, pain, and other manifestations in the breast and regional nodes. Irradiation of the breast and chest wall and the axillary, internal mammary, and supraclavicular nodes should be undertaken in an attempt to cure locally advanced and inoperable lesions when there is no evidence of distant metastases. A small number of patients in this group are cured in spite of extensive breast and regional node involvement.

Palliative irradiation is of value also in the treatment of certain bone or soft-tissue metastases to control pain or avoid fracture. Radiotherapy is especially useful in the treatment of isolated bony metastases, chest wall recurrences, brain metastases, and acute spinal cord compression.

B. Targeted Therapy

Disseminated disease may shrink—or grow less rapidly—after endocrine therapy such as administration of hormones (eg, estrogens, androgens, progestins; see Table 17–5); ablation of the ovaries, adrenals, or pituitary; or administration of drugs that block hormone receptor sites (eg, antiestrogens) or drugs that block the synthesis of hormones (eg, AIs). Hormonal manipulation is usually more successful in postmenopausal women even if they have received estrogen replacement therapy. Treatment should be based on the ER status of the primary tumor or metastases. The rate of response is nearly equal in premenopausal and postmenopausal women with ER-positive tumors. A favorable response to hormonal manipulation occurs in about one third of patients with metastatic breast cancer. Of those whose tumors contain ER, the response is about 60% and perhaps as high as 80% for patients whose tumors contain PR as well. In addition, women with ER-positive tumors who do not respond to hormone therapy or experience progression should be placed on a different form of hormonal manipulation. Because only 5–10% of women with ER-negative tumors do respond, they should not receive hormonal therapy except in unusual circumstances (eg, in an older patient who cannot tolerate chemotherapy). Because the quality of life during a remission induced by endocrine manipulation is usually superior to a remission following cytotoxic chemotherapy, it is usually best to try endocrine manipulation whenever possible. Women who do not respond to tamoxifen may try a third-generation AI and have an equal if not better response than those who responded to tamoxifen. However, when receptor status is unknown and the disease is progressing rapidly or involves visceral organs, endocrine therapy is rarely successful, and introducing it may waste valuable time.

In addition to radiotherapy, bisphosphonate therapy has shown excellent results in delaying and reducing skeletal events in women with bony metastases. Bisphosphonates are also sometimes used in conjunction with AIs to decrease the potential bony events associated with AIs. Bisphosphonates are routinely given with AIs to patients with bone metastases.

In general, only one type of therapy should be given at a time unless it is necessary to irradiate a destructive lesion of weight-bearing bone while the patient is receiving another regimen. The regimen should be changed only if the disease is clearly progressing. This is especially important for patients with destructive bone metastases, since changes in

Table 17–5. Agents Commonly Used for Hormonal Management of Metastatic Breast Cancer.

Drug	Action	Dose, Route, Frequency	Major Side Effects
Tamoxifen citrate (Nolvadex)	SERM	20 mg orally daily	Hot flushes, uterine bleeding, thrombophlebitis, rash
Fulvestrant (Faslodex)	Steroidal estrogen receptor antagonist	250 mg intramuscularly monthly	Gastrointestinal upset, headache, back pain, hot flushes, pharyngitis
Toremifene citrate (Fareston)	SERM	40 mg orally daily	Hot flushes, sweating, nausea, vaginal discharge, dry eyes, dizziness
Diethylstilbestrol (DES)	Estrogen	5 mg orally three times daily	Fluid retention, uterine bleeding, thrombophlebitis, nausea
Goserelin (Zoladex)	Synthetic luteinizing hormone-releasing analogue	3.6 mg subcutaneously monthly	Arthralgias, blood pressure changes, hot flushes, headaches, vaginal dryness
Megestrol acetate (Megace)	Progestin	40 mg orally four times daily	Fluid retention
Letrozole (Femara)	AI	2.5 mg orally daily	Hot flushes, arthralgia/arthritis, myalgia
Anastrozole (Arimidex)	AI	1 mg orally daily	Hot flushes, skin rashes, nausea and vomiting
Exemestane (Aromasin)	AI	25 mg orally daily	Hot flushes, increased arthralgia/arthritis, myalgia, and alopecia

SERM, selective estrogen receptor modulator; AI, aromatase inhibitor.

the status of these lesions are difficult to determine radiographically. A plan of therapy that would simultaneously minimize toxicity and maximize benefits is often best achieved by hormonal manipulation.

The choice of endocrine therapy depends on the menopausal status of the patient. Women within 1 year of their last menstrual period are arbitrarily considered to be premenopausal, whereas women whose menstruation ceased more than a year ago are postmenopausal. If endocrine therapy is the initial choice, it is referred to as primary hormonal manipulation; subsequent endocrine treatment is called secondary or tertiary hormonal manipulation. In metastatic disease, for patients with HER-2/*neu* oncogene overexpression, trastuzumab has been shown to increase survival.

In addition, the use of an antiangiogenesis drug bevacizumab in the treatment of metastatic disease is effective to improve survival. Based on the amount of VEGF detected in the primary tumor, bevacizumab can increase overall survival and disease-free survival when used in combination with chemotherapy when metastases are present.

1. The Premenopausal Patient

A. PRIMARY HORMONAL THERAPY—The potent SERM tamoxifen is by far the most common and preferred method of hormonal manipulation in the premenopausal patient. Tamoxifen is usually given orally in a dose of 20 mg daily. There is no significant difference in survival or response between tamoxifen therapy and bilateral oophorectomy. The average remission is about 12 months. Tamoxifen can be given with little morbidity and few side effects. Toremifene, a tamoxifen analog, has similar side effects but is less likely to cause uterine cancer. The response to tamoxifen is predictive of probable success with other forms of endocrine manipulation in premenopausal women.

Bilateral oophorectomy is less desirable than tamoxifen in premenopausal women because tamoxifen is so well tolerated. However, oophorectomy can be achieved rapidly and safely by surgery or by irradiation of the ovaries if the patient is a poor surgical candidate. Chemical ovarian ablation using a gonadotropin-releasing hormone (GnRH) analog can also be used. Oophorectomy presumably works by eliminating estrogens, progestins, and androgens, which stimulate growth of the tumor. AIs should not be used in a patient with functioning ovaries since they do not block ovarian functions.

B. SECONDARY OR TERTIARY HORMONAL THERAPY—Although patients who do not respond to tamoxifen or oophorectomy should be treated with cytotoxic drugs, those who respond and then relapse may subsequently respond to another form of endocrine treatment (Table 17–5). The initial choice for secondary endocrine manipulation has not been clearly defined.

Patients who improve after oophorectomy but subsequently relapse should receive tamoxifen or an AI; if one fails, the other may be tried but is not likely to succeed. Megestrol acetate, a progesterone agent, may be considered. These drugs cause less morbidity and mortality than surgical adrenalectomy, can be discontinued once the patient improves, and are not associated with the many problems of postsurgical hypoadrenalism, so that patients who require chemotherapy are more easily managed. Adrenalectomy or hypophysectomy, procedures rarely done today, induced regression in 30–50% of patients who previously responded to oophorectomy. Pharmacologic hormonal manipulation has replaced these invasive procedures. AIs are of value when a tumor responded to tamoxifen or oophorectomy but then progresses.

2. The Postmenopausal Patient

A. PRIMARY HORMONAL THERAPY—Tamoxifen, 20 mg orally daily, or anastrozole, 1 mg orally daily, is the initial therapy of choice for postmenopausal women with metastatic breast cancer amenable to endocrine manipulation. Anastrozole (an AI) has fewer side effects than tamoxifen and may be more effective. The main side effects of tamoxifen are nausea, vomiting, skin rash, and hot flushes. Rarely, it may induce hypercalcemia in patients with bony metastases. The main side effects of anastrozole are similar but lower in incidence; however, osteoporosis and bone fractures are significantly higher than tamoxifen. Other AIs are letrozole or exemestane. They have similar efficacy and side-effect profiles.

B. SECONDARY OR TERTIARY HORMONAL THERAPY—AIs are also available for the treatment of advanced breast cancer in postmenopausal women after tamoxifen treatment. In the event that the patient responds to AI but then has progression of disease, an antiestrogen, fulvestrant, has shown efficacy with about 20–30% of women benefiting from use. Postmenopausal patients who do not respond to SERM or AI should be given cytotoxic drugs. Postmenopausal women who respond initially to a SERM or AI but later manifest progressive disease may be crossed over to another hormonal therapy. If they do not respond, they should receive cytotoxic drugs. Androgens have many toxicities and should rarely be used. As in premenopausal patients, neither hypophysectomy nor adrenalectomy should be performed.

C. Chemotherapy

Cytotoxic drugs should be considered for the treatment of metastatic breast cancer (1) if visceral metastases are present (especially brain or lymphangitic pulmonary), (2) if hormonal treatment is unsuccessful or the disease has progressed after an initial response to hormonal manipulation, or (3) if the tumor is ER-negative. Prior adjuvant chemotherapy does not seem to alter response rates in patients who relapse. The most useful single chemotherapeutic agent to date is doxorubicin, with a response rate of 40–50%.

Combination chemotherapy with multiple agents is more effective, with objectively observed favorable responses achieved in 60–80% of patients with stage IV disease. Doxorubicin (40 mg/m^2 intravenously on day 1) and cyclophosphamide (200 mg/m² orally on days 3–6) produce an objective response in about 85% of patients so treated. Various combinations of drugs have been used, and clinical trials are always ongoing to identify a combination to increase survival and reduce side effects. Other chemotherapeutic regimens have consisted of various combinations of drugs, including cyclophosphamide, vincristine, methotrexate, fluorouracil, and taxanes with response rates ranging up to 60–70%. Researchers continue to study new drugs and combinations of chemotherapy agents, such as capecitabine, mitoxantrone, vinorelbine, gemcitabine, irinotecan, cisplatin, and carboplatin. Many of these agents or combinations are available to patients in a clinical trial setting or by physician's choice. For patients whose tumors have progressed after many therapies and who are considering additional therapy, clinical trial participation with experimental drugs in phase I, II, or III testing should be encouraged.

Although infrequent, single-agent use with taxanes (paclitaxel and docetaxel) has been shown to be very effective for patients with metastatic breast cancer, with a response rate of 30–40%. They have usually been given after failure of combination chemotherapy for metastatic disease or relapse shortly after completion of adjuvant chemotherapy. They may be especially valuable in treating anthracycline-resistant tumors. High-dose chemotherapy and autologous bone marrow or stem cell transplantation aroused widespread interest for the treatment of metastatic breast cancer. With this technique, the patient receives high doses of cytotoxic agents, eradicating the marrow, for which the patient subsequently undergoes autologous bone marrow or stem cell transplantation. Most randomized trials, however, comparing high-dose chemotherapy with stem cell support showed no improvement in survival over conventional chemotherapy. Enthusiasm for high-dose chemotherapy with stem cell support has waned, and the procedure is rarely performed. The technique is extremely costly, and the treatment itself is associated with a mortality rate of about 3–7%.

American College of Radiology: Practice guideline for the breast conservation therapy in the management of invasive breast carcinoma. J Am Coll Surg 2007;205:362.

Arimidex, Tamoxifen, Alone or in Combination (ATAC) Trialists' Group et al: Effect of anastrozole and tamoxifen as adjuvant treatment for early-stage breast cancer: 100-month analysis of the ATAC trial. Lancet Oncol 2008;9:45.

Bhatnagar AS: Review of the development of letrozole and its use in advanced breast cancer and in the neoadjuvant setting. Breast 2006;15(Suppl 1):S3.

Carlson RW et al: NCCN Task Force report: adjuvant therapy for breast cancer. J Natl Compr Canc Netw 2006;4(Suppl 1):S1.

Chu QD et al: Adjuvant therapy for patients who have node-positive breast cancer. Adv Surg 2006;40:77.

Dienstmann R et al: Evidence-based neoadjuvant endocrine therapy for breast cancer. Clin Breast Cancer 2006;7:315.

Fitzal F et al: Breast conservation: evolution of surgical strategies. Breast J 2006;12(5 Suppl 2):S165.

Gould RE et al: Update on aromatase inhibitors in breast cancer. Curr Opin Obstet Gynecol 2006;18:41.

Howell A et al; ATAC Trialists' Group: Results of the ATAC (Arimidex, Tamoxifen, Alone or in Combination) trial after completion of 5 years' adjuvant treatment for breast cancer. Lancet 2005;365:60.

Ingle JN et al; North Central Cancer Treatment Group Trial N0032: Fulvestrant in women with advanced breast cancer after progression on prior aromatase inhibitor therapy: North Central Cancer Treatment Group Trial N0032. J Clin Oncol 2006;24:1052.

Joensuu H et al; FinHer Study Investigators: Adjuvant docetaxel or vinorelbine with or without trastuzumab for breast cancer. N Engl J Med 2006;354:809.

Kaasa S et al: Prospective randomised multicenter trial on single fraction radiotherapy (8 Gy × 1) versus multiple fractions (3 Gy × 10) in the treatment of painful bone metastases. Radiother Oncol 2006;79:278.

Kim T et al: Lymphatic mapping and sentinel lymph node biopsy in early-stage breast carcinoma: a metaanalysis. Cancer 2006;106:4.

Lee MC et al: Management of patients with locally advanced breast cancer. Surg Clin North Am 2007;87:379.

Leonard C et al: Prospective trial of accelerated partial breast intensity-modulated radiotherapy. Int J Radiat Oncol Biol Phys 2007;67:1291.

Mamounas EP et al: Sentinel node biopsy after neoadjuvant chemotherapy in breast cancer: results from National Surgical Adjuvant Breast and Bowel Project Protocol B-27. J Clin Oncol 2005;23:2694.

Mieog JS et al: Preoperative chemotherapy for women with operable breast cancer. Cochrane Database Syst Rev 2007;2:CD005002.

Miller K et al: Paclitaxel plus bevacizumab versus paclitaxel alone for metastatic breast cancer. N Engl J Med 2007;357:2666.

Orlando L et al: Management of advanced breast cancer. Ann Oncol 2007;18(Suppl 6):vi74.

The National Institutes of Health Consensus Development Conference: Adjuvant Therapy for Breast Cancer: Bethesda, Maryland, USA. November 1–3, 2000. Proceedings. J Natl Cancer Inst Monogr 2001;30:1.

Piccart-Gebhart MJ et al; Herceptin Adjuvant (HERA) Trial Study Team: Trastuzumab after adjuvant chemotherapy in HER2-positive breast cancer. N Engl J Med 2005;353:1659.

Posther KE et al: Sentinel node skills verification and surgeon performance: data from a multicenter clinical trial for early-stage breast cancer. Ann Surg 2005;242:593.

Pruthi S et al: A multidisciplinary approach to the management of breast cancer, part 2: therapeutic considerations. Mayo Clin Proc 2007;82:1131.

Romond EH et al: Trastuzumab plus adjuvant chemotherapy for operable HER2-positive breast cancer. N Engl J Med 2005;353:1673.

Seidman AD: Systemic treatment of breast cancer. Two decades of progress. Oncology (Williston Park) 2006;20:983.

Slamon DJ et al: Advances in adjuvant therapy for breast cancer. Clin Adv Hematol Oncol 2006;4(Suppl 1):4.

Slamon DJ et al: Use of chemotherapy plus a monoclonal antibody against HER2 for metastatic breast cancer that overexpresses HER2. N Engl J Med 2001;344:783.

Smith I: Goals of treatment for patients with metastatic breast cancer. Semin Oncol 2006;33(1 Suppl 2):S2.

Smith I et al: 2-year follow-up of trastuzumab after adjuvant chemotherapy in HER2-positive breast cancer: a randomised controlled trial. Lancet 2007;369:29.

Stolier AJ et al: Postlumpectomy insertion of the MammoSite brachytherapy device using the scar entry technique: initial experience and technical considerations. Breast J 2005;11:199.

Veronesi U et al: Lessons from the initial adjuvant cyclophosphamide, methotrexate, and fluorouracil studies in operable breast cancer. J Clin Oncol 2008;26:342.

Veronesi U et al: Breast conservation: current results and future perspectives at the European Institute of Oncology. Int J Cancer 2007;120:1381.

Voogd AC et al: Prognosis of patients with locally recurrent breast cancer. Am J Surg 2007;193:138.

Waljee JF et al: Neoadjuvant systemic therapy and the surgical management of breast cancer. Surg Clin North Am 2007; 87:399.

▶ Prognosis

Stage of breast cancer is the most reliable indicator of prognosis (Table 17–6). Patients with disease localized to the breast with no evidence of pathologic involvement of the lymph nodes have the most favorable prognosis. Axillary lymph node status is the best-analyzed prognostic factor and correlates with survival at all tumor sizes. In addition, increased number of axillary nodes involved correlates directly with lower survival rates. Biologic marker status, such as ER, PR, grade, HER-2/*neu*, aides in determining the aggressiveness of a tumor and are important prognostic variables, but no markers are as significant as lymph node metastases in predicting outcome (see Biomarkers). The histologic subtype of breast cancer (eg, medullary, lobular, colloid) seems to have little significance in prognosis of invasive carcinomas. Flow cytometry of tumor cells to analyze DNA index and S-phase frequency aid in prognosis. Tumors with marked aneuploidy have a poor prognosis (see Table 17–4). Gene analysis studies, such as Oncotype DX, can predict survival for some subsets of patients.

The mortality rate of breast cancer patients exceeds that of age-matched normal controls for nearly 20 years. Thereafter, the mortality rates are equal, though deaths that occur among breast cancer patients are often directly the result of tumor. Five-year statistics do not accurately reflect the final outcome of therapy.

When cancer is localized to the breast, with no evidence of regional spread after pathologic examination, the clinical cure rate with most accepted methods of therapy is 75% to greater than 90%. Variations to this generalization may be related to the hormonal receptor content of the tumor, genetic markers, tumor size, host resistance, or associated illness. Patients with small mammographically detected biologically favorable tumors and no evidence of axillary spread have a 5-year survival rate greater than 95%. When the axillary lymph nodes are involved with tumor, the survival rate drops to 50–70% at 5 years and probably around 25–40% at 10 years. In general, breast cancer appears to be somewhat more malignant in younger than in older women, and this may be related to the fact that fewer younger women have ER-positive tumors. Adjuvant systemic chemotherapy, in general, improves survival by about 30% and adjuvant hormonal therapy by about 25%.

For those patients whose disease progresses despite treatment, studies suggest supportive group therapy may improve survival. As they approach the end of life, such patients will require meticulous efforts at palliative care.

Stuart K et al: Life after breast cancer. Aust Fam Physician 2006;35:219.

▶ Follow-up Care

After primary therapy, patients with breast cancer should be monitored for life in order to detect recurrences and to observe the opposite breast for a second primary carcinoma. Local and distant recurrences occur most frequently within the first 2–5 years. During the first 2 years, most patients should be examined every 6 months, then annually thereafter. The patient should examine her own breasts monthly, and a mammogram should be obtained annually. Special attention is paid to the contralateral breast because a new primary breast malignancy will develop in 20–25% of patients. In some cases, metastases are dormant for long periods and may appear 10–15 years or longer after removal of the primary tumor. Although studies have failed to show an adverse effect of hormonal replacement in disease-free patients, it is rarely used after breast cancer treatment, particularly if the tumor was hormone receptor positive. Even pregnancy has not been clearly associated with shortened survival of patients rendered disease free—yet most oncologists are reluctant to advise a young patient with breast cancer that she may become pregnant, and most are less than enthusiastic about prescribing hormone replacement for the postmenopausal breast cancer patient. The use of estrogen replacement for conditions such as osteoporosis and hot flushes may be considered for a woman with a history of breast cancer after discussion of the benefits and risks, but it is not recommended.

A. Local Recurrence

The incidence of local recurrence correlates with tumor size, the presence and number of involved axillary nodes, the histologic type of tumor, the presence of skin edema or skin

Table 17–6. Approximate Survival (%) of Patients with Breast Cancer by TNM Stage.

TNM Stage	5 Years	10 Years
0	95	90
I	85	70
IIA	70	50
IIB	60	40
IIIA	55	30
IIIB	30	20
IV	5–10	2
All	65	30

and fascia fixation with the primary tumor, and the type of definitive surgery and local irradiation. Local recurrence on the chest wall after total mastectomy and axillary dissection develops in as many as 8% of patients. When the axillary nodes are not involved, the local recurrence rate is less than 5%, but the rate is as high as 25% when they are heavily involved. A similar difference in local recurrence rate was noted between small and large tumors. Factors such as multifocal cancer, in situ tumors, positive resection margins, chemotherapy, and radiotherapy have an effect on local recurrence in patients treated with breast-conserving surgery.

Chest wall recurrences usually appear within the first several years but may occur as late as 15 or more years after mastectomy. All suspicious nodules and skin lesions should be biopsied. Local excision or localized radiotherapy may be feasible if an isolated nodule is present. If lesions are multiple or accompanied by evidence of regional involvement in the internal mammary or supraclavicular nodes, the disease is best managed by radiation treatment of the entire chest wall including the parasternal, supraclavicular, and axillary areas and usually by systemic therapy.

Local recurrence after mastectomy usually signals the presence of widespread disease and is an indication for studies to search for evidence of metastases. Distant metastases will develop within a few years in most patients with locally recurrent tumor after mastectomy. When there is no evidence of metastases beyond the chest wall and regional nodes, irradiation for cure after complete local excision should be attempted. Patients with local recurrence may be cured with local resection and radiation. After partial mastectomy, local recurrence does not have as serious a prognostic significance as after mastectomy. However, those patients in whom a recurrence develops have a worse prognosis than those who do not. It is speculated that the ability of a cancer to recur locally after radiotherapy is a sign of aggressiveness and resistance to therapy. Completion of the mastectomy should be done for local recurrence after partial mastectomy; some of these patients will survive for prolonged periods, especially if the breast recurrence is DCIS or occurs more than 5 years after initial treatment. Systemic chemotherapy or hormonal treatment should be used for women in whom disseminated disease develops or those in whom local recurrence occurs.

B. Edema of the Arm

Significant edema of the arm occurs in about 10–30% of patients after axillary dissection with or without mastectomy. It occurs more commonly if radiotherapy has been given or if there was postoperative infection. Partial mastectomy with radiation to the axillary lymph nodes is followed by chronic edema of the arm in 10–20% of patients. Sentinel lymph node dissection has proved to be a more accurate form of axillary staging without the side effects of edema or infection. It does not replace axillary dissection if the sentinel lymph nodes are involved with metastases. Judicious use of radiotherapy, with treatment fields carefully planned to spare the axilla as much as possible, can greatly diminish the incidence of edema, which will occur in only 5% of patients if no radiotherapy is given to the axilla after a partial mastectomy and lymph node dissection.

Late or secondary edema of the arm may develop years after treatment, as a result of axillary recurrence or infection in the hand or arm, with obliteration of lymphatic channels. When edema develops, a careful examination of the axilla for recurrence or infection is performed. Infection in the arm or hand on the dissected side should be treated with antibiotics, rest, and elevation. If there is no sign of recurrence or infection, the swollen extremity should be treated with rest and elevation. A mild diuretic may be helpful. If there is no improvement, a compressor pump or manual compression decreases the swelling, and the patient is then fitted with an elastic glove or sleeve. Most patients are not bothered enough by mild edema to wear an uncomfortable glove or sleeve and will treat themselves with elevation or manual compression alone. Benzopyrones have been reported to decrease lymphedema but are not approved for this use in the United States. Rarely, edema may be severe enough to interfere with use of the limb.

C. Breast Reconstruction

Breast reconstruction is usually feasible after total or modified radical mastectomy. Reconstruction should be discussed with patients prior to mastectomy, because it offers an important psychological focal point for recovery. Reconstruction is not an obstacle to the diagnosis of recurrent cancer. The most common breast reconstruction has been implantation of a silicone gel or saline prosthesis in the subpectoral plane between the pectoralis minor and pectoralis major muscles. Alternatively, autologous tissue can be used for reconstruction.

Autologous tissue flaps are aesthetically superior to implant reconstruction in most patients. They also have the advantage of not feeling like a foreign body to the patient. The most popular autologous technique currently is the transrectus abdominis muscle flap (TRAM flap), which is done by rotating the rectus abdominis muscle with attached fat and skin cephalad to make a breast mound. The free TRAM flap is done by completely removing a small portion of the rectus with overlying fat and skin and using microvascular surgical techniques to reconstruct the vascular supply on the chest wall. A latissimus dorsi flap can be swung from the back but offers less fullness than the TRAM flap and is therefore less acceptable cosmetically. An implant often is used to increase the fullness with a latissimus dorsi flap. Reconstruction may be performed immediately (at the time of initial mastectomy) or may be delayed until later, usually when the patient has completed adjuvant therapy. When considering reconstructive options, concomitant illnesses should be considered, since the ability of an autologous flap to survive depends on medical comorbidities. In addition, the need for radiotherapy may affect the choice of reconstruction, as radiation may increase fibrosis around an implant or decrease the volume of a flap.

D. Risks of Pregnancy

Data are insufficient to determine whether interruption of pregnancy improves the prognosis of patients who are identified to have potentially curable breast cancer and who receive definitive treatment during pregnancy. Theoretically, the increasingly high levels of estrogen produced by the placenta as the pregnancy progresses could be detrimental to the patient with occult metastases of hormone-sensitive breast cancer. Moreover, occult metastases are present in most patients with positive axillary nodes, and treatment by adjuvant chemotherapy could be potentially harmful to the fetus early in gestation, although chemotherapy may be given to pregnant women later. Under these circumstances, interruption of early pregnancy seems reasonable, with progressively less rationale for the procedure as term approaches. The decision is affected by many factors, including the patient's desire to have the baby and the prognosis especially when axillary nodes are involved.

Equally important is the advice regarding future pregnancy (or abortion in case of pregnancy) to be given to women of child-bearing age who have had definitive treatment for breast cancer. It is assumed that pregnancy will be harmful if occult metastases are present, though this has not been demonstrated. Patients whose tumors are ER negative (most younger women) may not be affected by pregnancy. To date, no adverse effect of pregnancy on survival of pregnant women who have had breast cancer has been demonstrated, though most oncologists advise against it.

In patients with inoperable or metastatic cancer (stage IV disease), induced abortion is usually advisable because of the possible adverse effects of hormonal treatment, radiotherapy, or chemotherapy upon the fetus.

Banks E et al: Pregnancy in women with a history of breast cancer. BMJ 2007;334:166.

Dian D et al: Quality of life among breast cancer patients undergoing autologous breast reconstruction versus breast conserving therapy. J Cancer Res Clin Oncol 2007;133:247.

Hayes DF: Prognostic and predictive factors for breast cancer: translating technology to oncology. J Clin Oncol 2005;23:1596.

Hu E et al: Breast reconstruction. Surg Clin North Am 2007;87:453.

Kronowitz SJ et al: Advances and surgical decision-making for breast reconstruction. Cancer 2006;107:893.

Moseley AL et al: A systematic review of common conservative therapies for arm lymphoedema secondary to breast cancer treatment. Ann Oncol 2007;18:639.

Pomahac B et al: New trends in breast cancer management: is the era of immediate breast reconstruction changing? Ann Surg 2006;244:282.

Sakorafas GH et al: Lymphedema following axillary lymph node dissection for breast cancer. Surg Oncol 2006;15:153.

Salhab M et al: Skin-sparing mastectomy and immediate breast reconstruction: patient satisfaction and clinical outcome. Int J Clin Oncol 2006;11:51.

Soran A et al: Breast cancer-related lymphedema—what are the significant predictors and how they affect the severity of lymphedema? Breast J 2006;12:536.

CARCINOMA OF THE MALE BREAST

 ESSENTIALS OF DIAGNOSIS

▶ A painless lump beneath the areola in a man usually over 50 years of age.

▶ Nipple discharge, retraction, or ulceration may be present.

▶ Generally poorer prognosis than in women.

General Considerations

Breast cancer in men is a rare disease; the incidence is only about 1% of that in women. The average age at occurrence is about 60—somewhat older than the most common presenting age in women. There may be an increased incidence of breast cancer in men with prostate cancer. As in women, hormonal influences are probably related to the development of male breast cancer. There is a high incidence of both breast cancer and gynecomastia in Bantu men, theoretically owing to failure of estrogen inactivation by a liver damaged by associated liver disease. It is important to note that first-degree relatives of men with breast cancer are considered to be at high risk. This risk should be taken into account when discussing options with the patient and family. In addition, *BRCA2* mutations are common in men with breast cancer. Men with breast cancer, especially with a history of prostate cancer, should receive genetic counseling. The prognosis, even in stage I cases, is worse in men than in women. Blood-borne metastases are commonly present when the male patient appears for initial treatment. These metastases may be latent and may not become manifest for many years.

Clinical Findings

A painless lump, occasionally associated with nipple discharge, retraction, erosion, or ulceration, is the primary complaint. Examination usually shows a hard, ill-defined, nontender mass beneath the nipple or areola. Gynecomastia not uncommonly precedes or accompanies breast cancer in men. Nipple discharge is an uncommon presentation for breast cancer in men but is an ominous finding associated with carcinoma in nearly 75% of cases.

Breast cancer staging is the same in men as in women. Gynecomastia and metastatic cancer from another site (eg, prostate) must be considered in the differential diagnosis. Benign tumors are rare, and biopsy should be performed on all males with a defined breast mass.

▶ Treatment

Treatment consists of modified radical mastectomy in operable patients, who should be chosen by the same criteria as women with the disease. Breast-conserving therapy is rarely performed. Irradiation is the first step in treating localized metastases in the skin, lymph nodes, or skeleton that are causing symptoms. Examination of the cancer for hormone receptor proteins is of value in predicting response to endocrine ablation. Men commonly have ER-positive tumors. Adjuvant systemic therapy and radiation is used for the same indications as in breast cancer in women.

Because breast cancer in men is frequently a disseminated disease, endocrine therapy is of considerable importance in its management. Tamoxifen is the main drug for management of advanced breast cancer in men. Tamoxifen (20 mg orally daily) should be the initial treatment. There is little experience with AIs, though they should be effective. Castration in advanced breast cancer is a successful measure and more beneficial than the same procedure in women but is rarely used. Objective evidence of regression may be seen in 60–70% of men with hormonal therapy for metastatic disease—approximately twice the proportion in women. The average duration of tumor growth remission is about 30 months, and life is prolonged. Bone is the most frequent site of metastases from breast cancer in men (as in women), and hormonal therapy relieves bone pain in most patients so treated. The longer the interval between mastectomy and recurrence, the longer the remission following treatment is likely. As in women, there is correlation between ERs of the tumor and the likelihood of remission following hormonal therapy.

AIs should replace adrenalectomy in men as it has in women. Corticosteroid therapy alone has been considered to be efficacious but probably has no value when compared with major endocrine ablation. Either tamoxifen or AIs may be primary or secondary hormonal manipulation.

Estrogen therapy—5 mg of diethylstilbestrol three times daily orally—may be effective hormonal manipulation after others have been successful and failed, just as in women. Androgen therapy may exacerbate bone pain. Chemotherapy should be administered for the same indications and using the same dosage schedules as for women with metastatic disease or for adjuvant treatment.

▶ Prognosis

The prognosis of breast cancer is poorer in men than in women. The crude 5-year and 10-year survival rates for clinical stage I breast cancer in men are about 58% and 38%, respectively. For clinical stage II disease, the 5-year and 10-year survival rates are approximately 38% and 10%. The survival rates for all stages at 5 and 10 years are 36% and 17%. For those patients whose disease progresses despite treatment, meticulous efforts at palliative care are essential.

Agrawal A et al: Male breast cancer: a review of clinical management. Breast Cancer Res Treat 2007;103:11.
Fentiman IS et al: Male breast cancer. Lancet 2006;367:595.
Karhu R et al: Large genomic BRCA2 rearrangements and male breast cancer. Cancer Detect Prev 2006;30:530.
Nahleh ZA: Hormonal therapy for male breast cancer: A different approach for a different disease. Cancer Treat Rev 2006;32:101.

Thoracic Wall, Pleura, Mediastinum, & Lung

Pierre R. Theodore, MD
David Jablons, MD

▼ ANATOMY & PHYSIOLOGY

ANATOMY OF THE CHEST WALL & PLEURA

The chest wall is an airtight, expandable, cone-shaped cage. Lung ventilation occurs by generation of negative pressure within the thorax due to simultaneous expansion of the rib cage and downward diaphragmatic excursion.

The ventral wall of the bony thorax is the shortest dimension. It extends from the suprasternal notch to the xiphoid—a distance of approximately 18 cm in the adult. It is formed by the vertically aligned manubrium, sternum, and xiphoid process. The first seven pairs of ribs articulate directly with the sternum, the next three pairs connect to the lower border of the preceding rib, and the last two terminate in the wall of the abdomen. The sides of the chest wall consist of the upper ten ribs, which slope obliquely downward from their posterior attachments. The posterior chest wall is formed by the 12 thoracic vertebrae, their transverse processes, and the 12 ribs (Figure 18–1). The upper ventral portion of the thoracic cage is covered by the clavicle and the subclavian vessels. Laterally, it is covered by the shoulder girdle and axillary nerves and vessels; dorsally, it is covered in part by the scapula.

The superior aperture of the thorax (also called either the thoracic inlet or the thoracic outlet) is a downwardly slanted 5- to 10-cm kidney-shaped opening bounded by the first costal cartilages and ribs laterally, the manubrium anteriorly, and the body of the first thoracic vertebra posteriorly. The inferior aperture of the thorax is bounded by the 12th vertebra and ribs posteriorly and the cartilages of the 7th to 10th ribs and the xiphisternal joint anteriorly. It is much wider than the superior aperture and is occupied by the diaphragm.

The blood supply and innervation of the chest wall are via the intercostal vessels and nerves (Figures 18–2 and 18–3), and the upper thorax also receives vessels and nerves from the cervical and axillary regions. The underside of the ster-

num's blood supply derives from the internal thoracic artery branches, which anastomose with the intercostal vessels along the lateral aspect of the chest wall.

The parietal pleura is the innermost lining of the chest wall and is divided into four parts: the cervical pleura (cupula), costal pleura, mediastinal pleura, and diaphragmatic pleura. The visceral pleura is a mesodermal layer investing the lungs and is continuous with the parietal pleura, joining it at the hilum of the lung. The potential pleural space is a capillary gap that normally contains only a few drops of serous fluid. However, this space may be enlarged when fluid (hydrothorax), blood (hemothorax), pus (pyothorax or empyema), lymphatic fluid (chylothorax), or air (pneumothorax) is present.

PHYSIOLOGY OF THE CHEST WALL & PLEURA

▶ Mechanics of Respiration

Breathing entails expansion of thoracic volume by elevation of the rib cage and descent of the diaphragm. Infants, in whom the ribs have not yet assumed their oblique contour, are dependent on diaphragmatic breathing. Furthermore, accessory muscles of respiration contribute to the conformational change in the thoracic cage during periods of intense exercise or respiratory distress (Figure 18–4).

Expiration is mainly passive and depends upon elastic recoil of the lungs except with deep breathing, when the abdominal musculature contracts, pulling the rib cage downward and simultaneously elevating the diaphragm by compressing the abdominal viscera against it.

▶ Physiology of the Pleural Space

A. Pressure

The pleural cavity pressure is normally negative, owing to the opposing forces of elastic recoil of the lung and active expansion of the space by the chest wall. During quiet

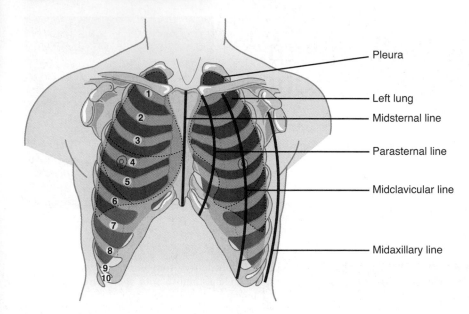

▲ **Figure 18–1.** The thorax, showing rib cage, pleura, and lung fields.

respiration, it varies from −15 cm H_2O with inspiration to 0–2 cm H_2O during expiration. Deep breathing may cause large pressure changes (eg, −60 cm H_2O during forced inspiration to +30 cm H_2O during vigorous expiration). Because of gravity, pleural pressure at the apex is more negative when the body is erect and changes about 0.2 cm H_2O per centimeter of vertical height.

B. Fluid Formation & Reabsorption

Transudation and absorption of fluid within the pleural space normally follow the Starling equation, which depends on hydrostatic, colloid, and tissue pressures in addition to permeability of the pleural membrane. In health, fluid is formed by the parietal pleura and absorbed by the visceral

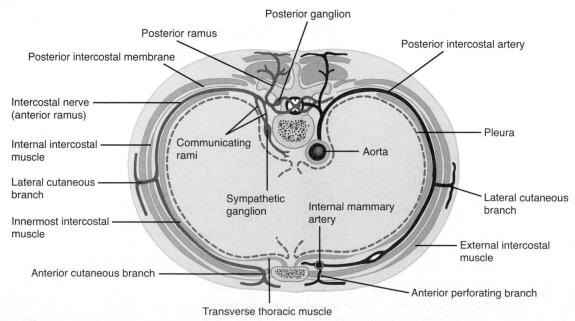

▲ **Figure 18–2.** Transverse section of thorax.

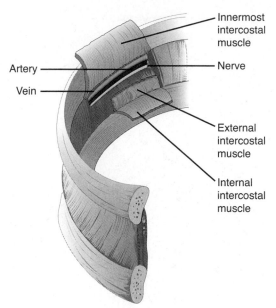

Artery

Vein

Innermost intercostal muscle

Nerve

External intercostal muscle

Internal intercostal muscle

▲ **Figure 18–3.** Intercostal muscles, vessels, and nerves.

pleura (Figure 18–5). Systemic capillary hydrostatic pressure is 30 cm H_2O, and intrapleural negative pressure averages –5 cm H_2O. Together, these give a net hydrostatic pressure of 35 cm H_2O that causes fluid transudation from the parietal pleura. The colloid osmotic pressure of the systemic capillaries is 34 cm H_2O; this is opposed by 8 cm H_2O of pleural space osmotic pressure. Thus, a net 26 cm H_2O osmotic pressure draws fluid back into systemic capillaries. Systemic hydrostatic pressure (35 cm H_2O) exceeds osmotic capillary pressure (26 cm H_2O) by 9 cm H_2O; thus, there is a 9 cm H_2O net drive of fluid into the pleural space by systemic capillaries in the chest wall. Similar calculations for the visceral pleura involving the low-pressure pulmonary circulation will show that there is a resulting net drive of 10 cm H_2O that attracts pleural fluid into pulmonary capillaries.

In health, pleural fluid is low in protein (<100 mg/dL). When it increases in disease to about 1 g/dL, the net colloid osmotic pressure of the visceral pleural capillaries is equaled and pleural fluid reabsorption becomes dependent on lymphatic drainage. Thus, abnormal amounts of pleural fluid may accumulate (1) when hydrostatic pressure is increased, such as in heart failure; (2) when capillary permeability is increased, as in inflammatory or neoplastic disease; or (3) when colloid osmotic pressure is decreased.

ANATOMY OF THE MEDIASTINUM

The mediastinum is the compartment between the pleural cavities. It extends anteriorly from the suprasternal notch to the xiphoid process and posteriorly from the 1st to the 11th thoracic vertebrae. Superiorly, fascial planes in the neck are in direct communication; inferiorly, the mediastinum is limited by the diaphragm. Apertures through the inferior extent of the mediastinum are traversed by the aorta, inferior vena cava, esophagus, and vagus nerve.

In the Burkell classification (Figure 18–6), the anterior mediastinum contains the thymus gland, the lymph nodes, the ascending aorta and transverse aorta, the great vessels, and areolar tissue. The **middle mediastinum** contains the heart, the pericardium, the trachea, the hila of the lungs, the phrenic nerves, lymph nodes, and areolar tissue. The **posterior mediastinum** contains the sympathetic chains, the vagus nerves, the esophagus, the thoracic duct, lymph nodes, and the descending aorta.

Congenital abnormalities within the mediastinum are numerous. A defect in the anterior mediastinal pleura with communication of the right and left hemithorax is rare in humans. This retrosternal part of the anterior mediastinum is normally thin, and overexpansion of one pleural space may cause "mediastinal herniation" or a bulge of mediastinal pleura toward the opposite side.

Displacements of the mediastinum occur from masses or from accumulations of air, fluid, blood, or chyle interfering with vital functions. Tracheal compression, vena caval obstruction, and esophageal obstructions cause clinical symptoms. The mediastinum can also be displaced laterally when pathologic processes of one hemithorax cause mediastinal shift. Fibrosis and lung volume loss can shift the mediastinum toward the affected side. Open pneumothorax and massive hemothorax shift the mediastinum away from the affected side. Open pneumothorax produces alternating paradoxic mediastinal shifts with respiration and will adversely affect ventilation. Acute mediastinal displacement may produce hypoxia or reduced venous return and cause dysrhythmias, hypotension, or cardiac arrest.

ANATOMY OF THE LUNG

See Figure 18–7 for lung anatomy.

The lobes of the lung comprise multiple bronchopulmonary segments. The right lung has three lobes: upper, middle, and lower. The left lung consists of two lobes: upper and lower. On the left, the lingular segments of the upper lobe are the homolog of the right middle lobe. Two fissures of varying completeness separate the lobes on the right side. The major, or oblique, fissure divides the upper and middle lobes from the lower lobe. The minor, or horizontal, fissure separates the middle from the upper lobe. On the left side, the single oblique fissure separates the upper and lower lobes. These are the normal anatomic segments; congenital defects such as situs inversus reverse this arrangement, and bilateral right-sided anatomy (asplenia) or bilateral left-sided anatomy (polysplenia) can also occur. The parenchymal anatomy can be seen by studying the sequential division of the bronchopulmonary tree down to the smallest unit of ventilation, the alveolus. The trachea and main stem bronchi and

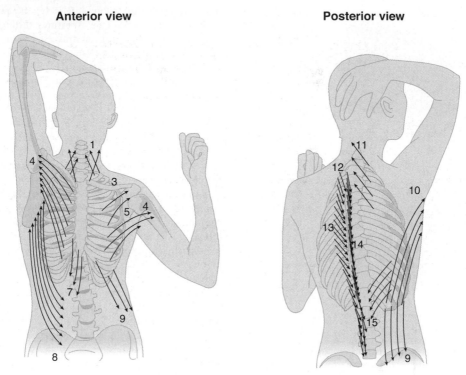

Secondary muscles of inspiration
(1) sternocleidomastoideus (3) scalenes (4) pectoralis major (5) pectoralis minor
(10) serratus anterior (11) serratus posterior superior (12) upper iliocostalis

Secondary muscles of expiration
(8) external oblique (9) internal oblique (7) rectus abdominus (13) lower iliocostalis
(14) lower longissimus (15) serratus posterior inferior

▲ **Figure 18–4.** Accessory muscles of respiration. (From Kapandji IA: Functional components of the vertebral column. In: *The Physiology of the Joints:* Vol. 3. *The Trunk and the Vertebral Column.* Kapandji IA (editor). Churchill Livingstone, 1974.)

their branches contain a posterior membranous area and are prevented from collapsing by horseshoe-shaped anterior segments of cartilage in their walls. The cartilaginous reinforcement of the airway gradually becomes less complete as the branches become smaller, and reinforcement ceases with bronchi of 1–2 mm. The bronchopulmonary segmental anatomy is designated by numbers (Boyden) or by name (Jackson and Huber). The segmental bronchial anatomy is most constant with the pulmonary vascular structures showing more variability.

The lungs have a dual blood supply: the pulmonary and the bronchial arterial systems. The pulmonary arteries transmit venous blood from the right ventricle for oxygenation. They closely accompany the bronchi. The bronchial arteries usually arise directly from the aorta or nearby intercostal arteries and are variable in number. They transmit oxygenated blood at systemic arterial pressure to the bronchial wall to the level of the terminal bronchioles.

The pulmonary veins travel in the interlobar septa and do not correspond to the distribution of the bronchi or the pulmonary arteries.

THE LYMPHATIC SYSTEM

The lymphatics travel in intersegmental septa centrally as well as to the parenchymal surface to form subpleural networks. Drainage continues toward the hilum in channels that follow the bronchi and pulmonary arteries. The lymphatics eventually enter lymph nodes in the major fissures of the lungs, the hilum, and the paratracheal regions.

The direction of lymphatic drainage—irrespective of the primary site—is cephalad and usually ipsilateral, but contralateral flow may occur from any lobe. The lymphatics from the left lower lobe may be almost equally distributed to the left and right. From the left upper lobe, distribution is often to the anterior mediastinal group (A-P window and para-

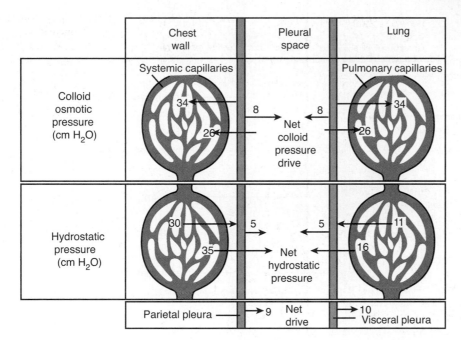

▲ **Figure 18–5.** Movement of fluid across the pleural space, showing production and absorption of pleural fluid.

aortic lymph nodes). Otherwise, the usual sequence of lymphatic spread of pulmonary cancer is first to the regional parabronchial nodes and then to the ipsilateral paratracheal, subcarinal, scalene, or inferior deep cervical nodes.

DIAGNOSTIC STUDIES

Skin Tests

Skin tests are used in the diagnosis of tuberculosis, histoplasmosis, and coccidioidomycosis. Tuberculin testing is usually done with purified protein derivative (PPD) injected intradermally. Intermediate-strength PPD should be used in patients who seem likely to have active disease. Induration of 10 mm or more at the injection site after 48–72 hours is called positive and indicates either active or arrested disease. Because false-negative reactions are rare, a negative test fairly reliably rules out tuberculosis. Mumps antigen is usually placed on the opposite forearm to test for anergy. Skin tests for histoplasmosis and coccidioidomycosis are performed in a similar way, but skin tests for fungal infections are unreliable and serologic tests should be performed instead.

Endoscopy

A. Laryngoscopy

Indirect laryngoscopy is used to assess vocal cord mobility in patients suspected of having lung carcinoma, especially when there has been a voice change. It should be performed also to search for an otherwise occult source for malignant cells in sputum or metastases in cervical lymph nodes.

B. Bronchoscopy

Roentgenographic evidence of bronchial obstruction, unresolved pneumonia, foreign body, suspected carcinoma, hemoptysis, aspiration pneumonia, and lung abscess are only a few of the indications for bronchoscopy. The procedure can be done using either the standard hollow metal (rigid) or the flexible fiberoptic bronchoscope under local or general anesthesia. Rigid bronchoscopy must be done under general anesthesia and is most often used for clearing major airways of bulky obstructing lesions such as tumors, foreign bodies, or blood clots. Traditionally, the CO_2 laser required use of the rigid bronchoscope, though more recently developed technology (Nd:YAG) can be applied with flexible bronchoscopy.

Flexible bronchoscopy is a highly effective diagnostic and therapeutic tool. It can be performed under local and intravenous sedation. Washings are usually obtained for bacterial or fungal culture and cytologic examination. Visible lesions are biopsied directly, and biopsy specimens are sometimes taken from the carina even though it appears normal. Brush biopsies are obtained from specific bronchopulmonary segments. Occasionally, transcarinal needle biopsy of a subcarinal node is obtained. Bronchoscopically, 30–50% of lung tumors are visible. Brushing, random biopsies, and sputum cytology may still yield a positive diagnosis of cancer or tuberculosis in the absence of a visible lesion. The yield is influenced by size, location, and histologic cell type of the lesion.

Mediastinoscopy

Cervical mediastinoscopy remains a mainstay of evaluation of the mediastinum despite advances in imaging. Properly

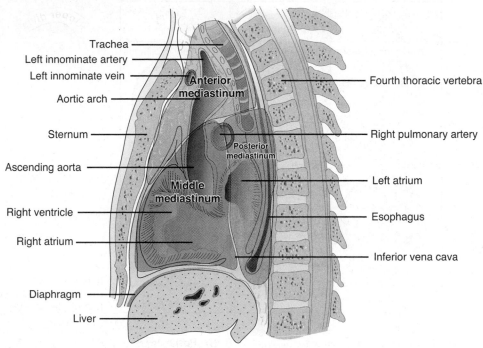

▲ Figure 18-6. Divisions of the mediastinum (Burkell classification). Light screening: anterior mediastinum; lower dark screening: middle mediastinum; dotted area at right: posterior mediastinum.

performed mediastinoscopy samples nodes from at least three stations, including ipsilateral and contralateral paratracheal levels 2, 3, and 4 and subcarinal level 7. Cervical mediastinoscopy is performed through a 3- to 4-cm incision one fingerbreadth above the sternal notch. Dissection proceeds beneath the pretracheal fascia, allowing safe access to mediastinal nodes and avoiding major vascular structures. After palpation, the mediastinoscope can be inserted and nodes biopsied under direct vision. Unclear structures care aspirated prior to attempted biopsy.

Enlarged lymph nodes in the aorticopulmonary window are technically inaccessible by means of standard cervical mediastinoscopy. Extended cervical mediastinoscopy, however, is a technique that provides access to these aorticopulmonary window nodes. It is performed through the same small neck incision as standard mediastinoscopy except the dissection is carried laterally beside the left carotid artery toward and then over the aorta into the aorticopulmonary space. In older patients with densely calcific aortas, extended mediastinoscopy is contraindicated because of the risk of embolic phenomena and stroke from aortic manipulation.

In experienced hands, the complications of mediastinoscopy are minimal (< 1–2%). Major bleeding complications requiring sternotomy or thoracotomy for repair are infrequent (1–2%). Other possible complications include pneumothorax, recurrent nerve injury, infection, and esophageal injury.

Mediastinoscopy is almost invariably accurate in the diagnosis of sarcoidosis. It is also useful to diagnose tuberculosis, histoplasmosis, Castleman silicosis, metastatic carcinoma, lymphoma, and carcinoma of the esophagus. It should not be used in the investigation of primary mediastinal tumors, which should be approached by an incision permitting definitive excision.

▶ Chamberlain Procedure

Anterior mediastinotomy (the Chamberlain procedure) is used to sample nodes and biopsy tissue in the anterior mediastinum and most commonly in the aorticopulmonary window. A small (3- to 4-cm) incision is made over the second or third interspace on the appropriate side of the lesion. Alternatively, the procedure can be performed with videoscopic guidance (VATS). The mediastinum is approached through the interspace directly or after excising the costochondral cartilage using either the mediastinoscope or open technique. Careful attention is paid to preserving the mammary vessels encountered in the dissection. The mediastinum is approached extrapleurally unless lesions specifically within the thorax—effusions, tumors invading the hilum or chest wall—need to be investigated. Furthermore, if additional access is required to facilitate the dissection or to treat a complication, the incision can be converted easily to a larger anterior thoracotomy.

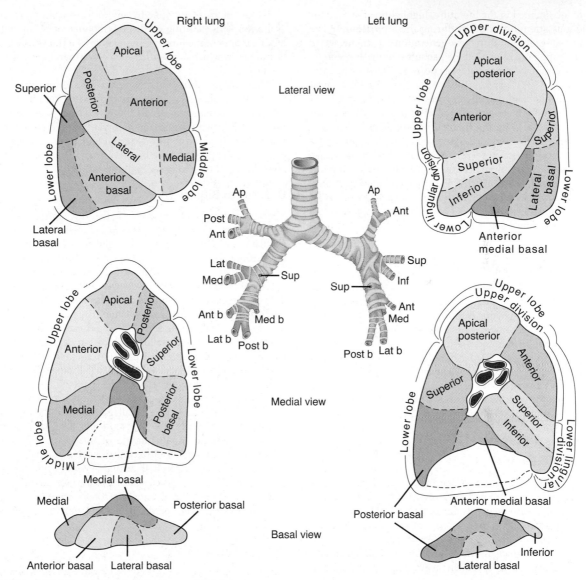

▲ **Figure 18–7.** Segmental anatomy of the lungs.

Complications resulting from anterior mediastinotomy are similar to those encountered with cervical mediastinoscopy and include bleeding, recurrent nerve injury, and infection. Major morbidity should be less than 1–2%.

▶ **Video-Assisted Thoracoscopic Surgery (VATS)**

With the advent of sophisticated video technology and optics, VATS has evolved as an important tool in thoracic surgery. While thoracoscopic procedures have been used for many years, newer technical advances as well as increasing

surgeon familiarity with minimally invasive surgery have made VATS increasingly popular and useful.

VATS plays an important role in the diagnosis and staging of thoracic malignancies (lung cancer, mesothelioma, etc) as well as in the resection of isolated peripheral pulmonary nodules and bullous lung disease. Furthermore, it has been an advance in lung biopsy and pleurodesis procedures.

However, despite gaining popularity, many thoracic surgeons consider the approach suboptimal for lung cancers. Full mediastinal lymph node dissections are not generally obtainable with standard VATS. Even for metastasectomy, concerns over pleural and chest wall seeding with VATS have been documented in the literature, highlighting the need for assiduous attention to detail during these procedures. The improved resolution from new-generation CT scanners have in part supplanted the need for palpation of the entire lung, and increasingly advanced resections are now being performed via VATS approaches. At present VATS is most commonly applied to benign processes, including spontaneous pneumothoraces and pleural effusions, as well for thoracic sympathectomy and thoracic vertebral discectomy.

As instruments and techniques have evolved, complications from VATS procedures (persistent air leaks, hemorrhage, tumor seeding, etc) have decreased. Overall, major complication rates of 1–2% are reported. Faster patient recovery, shorter hospital stays, decreased pain are major advantages of VATS, although long-term differences between videoscopic and formal thoracotomy using muscle-sparing incisions are yet to be demonstrated.

▶ Scalene Lymph Node Biopsy

Scalene lymph node biopsy has been largely replaced by mediastinoscopy in the evaluation of pulmonary disease because it offers the same information but is less reliable and does not evaluate nodes within the mediastinum. Furthermore, scalene lymph nodes are accessible via cervical mediastinoscopy using the mediastinoscope. In the evaluation of lung cancer, about 15% of scalene node biopsies are positive when the cervical nodes are not palpable compared with 85% when the nodes are palpable. The risk of major complications is about 5%. Deaths are rare.

▶ Pleural Biopsy

A. Needle Biopsy

This procedure is indicated when the cause of a pleural effusion cannot be determined by analysis of the fluid or when tuberculosis is suspected. Any one of three needles can be used: Vim-Silverman, Cope, or Abrams (Harefield). A definitive diagnosis can be obtained in 60–80% of cases of tuberculosis or cancer. The principal complication is pneumothorax. Five to 10 percent of biopsy specimens are inadequate for diagnosis.

B. Surgical Biopsy

Biopsy of the pleura can be performed via videoscopic or open technique with minimal morbidity, providing the pathologist with a specimen superior to that of needle biopsy.

▶ Lung Biopsy

A. Needle Biopsy

The indications for percutaneous needle biopsy are not well established. It may be indicated in diffuse parenchymal disease and in some patients with localized lesions. The diagnosis of interstitial pneumonia, carcinoma, sarcoidosis, hypersensitivity lung disease, lymphoma, pulmonary alveolar proteinosis, and miliary tuberculosis has been established by this method.

Needle biopsies are done by any of three techniques: by aspiration with a cutting needle, by trephine, or by air drill. Needle biopsy of the lung is also possible by a transbronchial technique in which a modified Vim-Silverman or ultrathin needle is used.

There is controversy concerning the risks of spreading the tumor by needle biopsy in localized disease. Complications following percutaneous needle biopsy include pneumothorax (5–30%), hemothorax, hemoptysis, and air embolism. Pulmonary hypertension or cysts and bullae are contraindications. Several deaths have been reported. There is about a 60% chance of obtaining useful information.

B. Surgical Biopsy

Thoracoscopy or VATS has become the procedure of choice for open lung biopsy in patients who can tolerate single lung ventilation. A single anterior axillary line incision can be used for introduction of a stapler and operating thoracoscope. For open biopsies a limited intercostal or anterior parasternal incision is used to remove a 3- to 4-cm wedge of lung tissue in diffuse parenchymal lung disease. The site of incision is selected for accessibility and potential diagnostic value. The incision is generally made at the fifth interspace on the right at the anterior axillary line to allow for access to all three lobes for biopsy—or at the lower lobes bilaterally. The middle lobe and lingula are selected in specific cases when pathology exists only in these areas, as they generally yield results of the poorest quality. Open lung biopsy is associated with a lower death rate, fewer complications, and greater diagnostic yield than needle biopsy. It is especially useful in critically ill, immunosuppressed patients for differentiation of infectious infiltrative lesions from neoplastic infiltrative lesions. Open lung biopsy can be performed in the ICU setting and does not require single lung ventilation. When a focal lesion is biopsied, a larger incision is used. Peripheral lesions are totally excised by wedge or segmental resection, and deeply placed lesions are removed by lobectomy in suitable candidates.

▶ Sputum Analysis

Exfoliative sputum cytology is most valuable for detection of lung cancer. Specimens are obtained by deep coughing or by abrasion with a brush, or bronchial washings are obtained by either bronchoscopic or percutaneous transtracheal washing techniques. Specimens should be collected in the morning and delivered to the laboratory promptly. Centrifugation or filtration can be used to concentrate the cellular elements.

In primary lung cancer, sputum cytology is positive in 30–60% of cases. Repeated sputum examination improves the diagnostic return. Examination of the first bronchoscopic washing material yields a diagnosis in 60% of cases. Postbronchoscopy sputum analysis should always be made at 6–12 and 24 hours, as findings may be positive at these times when previous tests were negative.

Newer technologies, including better sputum-inducing agents, are currently in clinical trials and appear effective.

Also, more sophisticated cytologic analysis using immuno-histochemistry to molecular markers (cytokeratins, hnRNP, etc) has improved accuracy and sensitivity and the ability to detect premalignant lesions.

Computed Tomography (CT) Scan

Computed tomography is a cornerstone of evaluation of chest pathology. CT scanning is critical in the staging of carcinoma, and has value in defining the extent of metastatic disease. Mediastinoscopy remains the gold standard for evaluation of the mediastinum in lung cancer.

Magnetic Resonance Imaging (MRI)

Although the major value of MRI in the thorax has been in cardiovascular imaging, it has been moderately helpful in showing invasion of lung cancer into the chest wall, vertebrae, and spinal cord as well as mediastinal structures. MRI has a particular niche in the evaluation of superior sulcus (Pancoast) tumors to establish involvement of the brachial plexus, subclavian vessel, or bony chest wall.

Positron Emission Tomography (PET)

PET has become an important tool in staging and workup of the cancer patient. PET scanners are more widely available, and current data suggest that PET scanning identifies unsuspected regional or distant disease in 20–30% of patients with lung cancer or esophageal cancer compared with conventional imaging methods (CT, bone scan). PET scanning is more accurate than CT scan in detection of cancer spread to mediastinal lymph nodes. Because of the high negative predictive value of PET scanning, a negative PET scan in the mediastinum permits direct progression to thoracotomy. The presence of a positive PET scan in the mediastinum mandates either mediastinoscopy or, more recently, endoscopic evaluation of mediastinal lymph nodes because of false-positive PET scan results.

The combined PET/CT is highly accurate (> 90%), but by itself it has a 10–20% false-positive rate in the mediastinum. Therefore, interpretations of PET results must be accepted with caution and must be confirmed by surgical staging when inconsistent with the overall clinical picture.

DISEASES OF THE CHEST WALL

LUNG HERNIA

A lung hernia results from a defect in the chest wall caused by abnormal development, trauma, or surgery. Most lung hernias are thoracic in location, but cervical (defects of Sibson fascia) or diaphragmatic herniation may occur occasionally. Lung hernias are usually asymptomatic, but some patients experience local tenderness, pain, or mild dyspnea. Operative repair rather than external support produces optimal results if symptoms are present.

CHEST WALL INFECTIONS

Infections that appear to involve only the skin and soft tissues may actually represent outward extensions of deeper infection of the ribs, cartilage, sternum, or even the pleural space (empyema necessitatis). Inadequate drainage of superficial infection can lead to inward extension into the pleural space, causing empyema.

Subpectoral abscess is caused by suppurative adenitis of the axillary lymph nodes, rib or pleural infection, or posterior extension of a breast abscess—or it may occur as a complication of chest wall surgery (eg, mastectomy, pacemaker placement). Symptoms include systemic sepsis, erythema, induration of the pectoral region, and obliteration of the normal infraclavicular depression. Shoulder movement is painful. Organisms most commonly involved include hemolytic streptococci and *Staphylococcus aureus*. Treatment involves incisional drainage along the lateral border of the pectoralis major muscle and administration of systemic antibiotics.

Subscapular abscess may arise from osteomyelitis of the scapula but most commonly follows thoracic operations such as thoracotomy or thoracoplasty. Winging of the scapula or paravertebral induration of the trapezius muscle is usually present. A pleural communication is suggested if a cough impulse is present or if the size of the mass varies with position or direct pressure. The diagnosis is established by needle aspiration. Open drainage is indicated for pyogenic infections not involving the pleural space. Tubercular lesions should be treated by chemotherapy and needle aspiration, if possible.

Osteomyelitis of the Ribs

In the past, osteomyelitis of the ribs was often caused by typhoid fever and tuberculosis. Except in children, hematogenous osteomyelitis is a rare problem today. Thoracotomy incisions may result in osteomyelitis.

Sternal Osteomyelitis

Infection of the sternum most commonly follows median sternotomy incisions, particularly in diabetics. It presents as a postoperative wound infection or mediastinitis with drainage, fever, leukocytosis, and instability of the sternal closure. Treatment consists of open drainage, resection of the involved sternum, and reconstruction of the defect with pectoralis muscle, serratus muscle, or omental coverage. Recently success has been achieved through use of vacuum-assisted closure systems following debridement.

Occasionally, sternal osteomyelitis will be due to tuberculosis.

Infection of the Costal Cartilages & Xiphoid

Costal cartilage infections are relatively unresponsive to antibiotic therapy. Once devascularized, perichondral tissue necroses and remains as a foreign body to perpetuate the infection and sinus tract formation. The infection may be established during the course of septicemia, but the most common cause is direct extension of other surgical infections (eg, wound infection, subphrenic abscess). Surgical division of costal cartilages, as in a thoracoabdominal incision, may predispose to cartilage infection postoperatively if local sepsis develops. A wide variety of organisms have been implicated.

Erythema and induration with fluctuance and often spontaneous drainage can occur. The course can be fulminant or may be indolent over months or years, with periodic exacerbations. Associated osteomyelitis of the sternum, ribs, or clavicle may occur.

The differential diagnosis includes local bone or cartilage tumors, Tietze syndrome, chest wall metastasis, eroding aortic aneurysm, and bronchocutaneous fistula.

The treatment of choice includes resection of the involved cartilage and adjacent involved bony structures. Recurrence is due to underestimation of the extent of disease and inadequate resection.

Reconstruction of the Chest Wall

Chest wall reconstruction may be necessary following trauma, surgical resection, or infectious processes. Recent advances in the use of musculocutaneous flaps and the supportive use of methyl methacrylate and Marlex mesh to produce solidity below these muscular flaps have facilitated repairs. In massive chest wall defects, vascularization of the area is essential and can be accomplished by use of omental flaps as well as pectoralis, latissimus dorsi, and rectus flaps. Microsurgical techniques for repair of such defects have greatly expanded the ability of plastic surgeons to deal with extensive resectional and infective processes.

Adler BD, Padley SP, Muller NL: Tuberculosis of the chest wall: CT findings. J Comput Assist Tomogr 1993;17:271.

Mansour KA, Anderson TM, Hester TR: Sternal resection and reconstruction. Ann Thorac Surg 1993;55:838.

Pairolero PC, Arnold PG, Harris JB: Long-term results of pectoralis major muscle transposition for infected sternotomy wounds. Ann Surg 1991;213:583.

TIETZE SYNDROME

Tietze syndrome is a painful, nonsuppurative inflammation of the costochondral cartilages and is of unknown cause. Recent evidence suggests that costochondritis may represent a manifestation of seronegative rheumatic disease. Local swelling and tenderness are the only symptoms; they usually disappear without therapy. The syndrome may recur.

Several recent reports have suggested the use of bone scintigraphy and chest CT for diagnosis of infected costochondritis. Bone scanning was effective in localizing and identifying inflamed costochondral junctions. Chest CT was less sensitive in one study. Furthermore, in a small study of patients with Tietze syndrome, transthoracic echo was able to demonstrate a dishomogeneous increase in echogenicity in the pathologically involved cartilage. Treatment is sympto-matic and may include analgesics (NSAIDs) and local or systemic corticosteroids. When symptoms persist longer than 3 weeks and tumefaction suggests neoplasm, excision of the involved cartilage may be indicated and is usually curative.

Jensen S. Musculoskeletal causes of chest pain. Australian Family Physician 2001;30:834.

MONDOR DISEASE (THROMBOPHLEBITIS OF THE THORACOEPIGASTRIC VEIN)

Mondor disease consists of localized thrombophlebitis of the anterolateral chest wall. It is more prominent in women than in men and occasionally follows radical mastectomy. There are few symptoms other than the presence of a localized tender, cordlike structure in the subcutaneous tissues of the abdomen, thorax, or axilla. The disease is self-limited and devoid of complications such as thromboembolism. The possibility of an infective origin or stasis of the interrupted venous return due to neoplasm must be ruled out.

Bejanga BI: Mondor's disease: analysis of 30 cases. J R Coll Surg Edinb 1992;37:322.

CHEST WALL TUMORS

Chest wall tumors may be simulated by enlarged costal cartilages, chest wall infection, fractures, rickets, scurvy, hyperparathyroidism, and other conditions. Most commonly, chest wall lesions present as a mass with localized or referred pain; less than 25% are asymptomatic. Approximately 60% of all chest wall masses prove to be malignant. Lesions arise from one of the three components of the chest wall, including soft tissues (muscle, nerve, fascia), bone, and cartilage.

The majority of tumors arise from bone or cartilage. Rib involvement is more common than sternal presentation. Chest CT offers the most information for diagnosis and staging. In particular, chest wall sarcomas are associated with pulmonary metastasis. Simple chest x-rays may initially identify a mass, especially if it is calcified. Bone scans should be obtained in all cases.

Initial diagnosis is obtained by limited incisional biopsy (transverse) if the mass is large (> 4 cm). Smaller lesions are excised en bloc, ensuring negative margins, with full knowledge that a malignancy is present in many cases. Classic teaching has been to perform en bloc wide local excisions with immediate reconstruction for all lesions at initial presentations. Progress with adjuvant multimodality therapy, however, for tumors such as rhabdomyosarcomas and Ewing sarcoma supports the use of initial limited biopsy for tissue diagnosis to guide treatment planning.

Specific Neoplasms

A. Benign Soft Tissue Tumors

1. Lipomas—Lipomas are the most common benign tumors of the chest wall. Occasionally, they are very large and lobulated, and they may have dumbbell-shaped extensions that indent the endothoracic fascia beneath the sternum through an intercostal space. They may communicate with a large mediastinal or supraclavicular component.

2. Neurogenic tumors—These may arise from intercostal or superficial nerves. Solitary neurofibromas are most common, followed by neurolemmomas.

3. Cavernous hemangiomas—Hemangiomas of the thoracic wall are usually painful and occur in children. Tumors may be isolated or may involve other tissues (eg, lung), as in Rendu-Osler-Weber syndrome.

4. Lymphangiomas—This rare lesion is seen most often in children. It may have poorly defined borders that make complete excision difficult.

B. Malignant Soft Tissue Tumors

Roughly 50% of all chest wall masses are sarcomas, yet overall they represent only a small percentage (5%) of all malignant soft tissue sarcomas. Survival is determined by the histologic grade, the completeness of resection, and the presence and development of metastases (synchronous or metachronous). Low-grade tumors have 5-year and 10-year survivals approaching 90% and 82%, respectively. With high-grade lesions, however, 5-year survival rates are only 30–50%. The development of metastasis greatly reduces the chances of survival.

Treatment is directed at complete resection with emphasis on achieving negative margins (1–2 cm). En bloc resection techniques include raising skin flaps and reconstruction with soft tissue flaps, Marlex mesh, and methyl methacrylate to correct chest wall deformity and prevent paradoxic chest movement.

Various histologic subtypes of soft tissue sarcoma are encountered. Typically, low-grade sarcomas include desmoids or liposarcomas with low-grade features. Next most frequently seen are malignant fibrosarcoma, rhabdomyosarcoma, and malignant fibrous histiocytoma, which are usually high-grade lesions.

Individual histologic subtype is not by itself a significant prognostic variable, but histologic grade does have that role. Metastases—either synchronous or metachronous—are commonly to the lungs (75%) and should be resected if negative margins can be achieved and adequate lung function preserved. Therapy for low-grade lesions should consist of complete resection. Incompletely resected lesions can be treated with external beam radiation therapy. High-grade lesions should be resected and patients enrolled into clinical trials evaluating the efficacy of systemic adjuvant chemotherapy. Postoperative radiotherapy is often helpful in the setting of close margins or tumor spillage.

1. Fibrosarcomas—Fibrosarcoma is the most common primary soft tissue cancer of the chest wall. It occurs most frequently in young adults.

2. Liposarcomas—These tumors account for approximately one third of all primary cancers of the chest wall. They occur more often in men.

3. Neurofibrosarcomas—These uncommon tumors involve the thoracic wall almost twice as often as other parts of the body. They often occur in patients with Recklinghausen disease and usually originate from intercostal nerves.

C. Benign Skeletal Tumors

1. Chondromas, osteochondromas, and myxochondromas—The combined frequency of these three cartilaginous tumors is about 30–45% of all benign skeletal tumors. Cartilaginous tumors are usually single and occur with equal frequency in males and females between childhood and the fourth decade. The tumors are usually painless and tend to occur anteriorly along the costal margin or in the parasternal area. Wide local excision is curative.

2. Fibrous dysplasia—Fibrous dysplasia (bone cyst, osteofibroma, fibrous osteoma, fibrosis ossificans) accounts for a third or more of benign skeletal tumors of the chest wall. This cystic bone tumor can occur in any portion of the skeletal system, but approximately half involve the ribs. The differential diagnosis includes cystic bone lesions associated with hyperparathyroidism. The tumor is usually single and may be trauma related. Some patients complain of swelling, tenderness, or vague discomfort, but the lesion is usually silent and is detected on routine chest x-ray. Treatment consists of local excision.

3. Eosinophilic granuloma—Eosinophilic granuloma may occur in the clavicle, the scapula, or (rarely) the sternum. Coexisting infiltrates of the lung are often present. This condition often represents a more benign form of Letterer-Siwe disease or Hand-Schüller-Christian disease. Fever, malaise, leukocytosis, eosinophilia, or bone pain may be present. Rib involvement presents as a swelling with cortical bone destruction and periosteal new growth. The clinical picture can resemble osteomyelitis or Ewing sarcoma. When the disease is localized, excision will result in cure.

4. Hemangioma—Cavernous hemangioma of the ribs presents as a painful mass in infancy or childhood. The tumor appears on chest x-ray either as multiple radiolucent areas or as a single trabeculated cyst.

5. Miscellaneous—Fibromas, lipomas, osteomas, and aneurysmal bone cysts are all relatively rare lesions of the chest wall. The diagnosis is established after excisional biopsy.

D. Malignant Skeletal Tumors

1. Chondrosarcomas—Chondrosarcomas are the most common primary malignant tumor of the chest wall (20–40%). They can involve the sternum but more commonly develop from the costochondral junctions of the first four ribs. About 15–20% of all skeletal chondrosarcomas occur in the ribs or sternum. Most appear in patients 20–40 years of age. Local involvement of pleura, adjacent ribs, muscle, diaphragm, or other soft tissue may develop. Pain is rare, however, and most patients complain only of the mass. Chest x-ray shows destroyed cortical bone, usually with diffuse mottled calcification, and the border of the tumor is indistinct. Successful treatment necessitates wide local excision and en bloc resection to achieve negative margins. Incomplete excision carries a significantly worse prognosis. Overall survival, as in all soft tissue sarcomas, is heavily dependent on the histologic grade. Completely resected low-grade chondrosarcoma has a 60–80% 5-year survival rate. Patients with high-grade lesions who subsequently develop distant metastasis have only 20–30% 5-year survival.

Local recurrence portends future metastatic disease and poor survival. Yet complete resection can often be curative. Therefore, even in the setting of large tumors (> 15–20 cm), resection should be considered even when it necessitates removal of more than six to eight ribs. With advances in epidural pain control and immediate reconstruction techniques, most patients will do surprisingly well. Despite large chest wall resections, most patients can be immediately extubated and will not suffer drastic changes in pulmonary function or chest wall dynamics.

2. Osteogenic sarcoma (osteosarcoma)—Osteosarcoma

occurs in the second and third decades, and 60% of cases occur in men. It is more malignant than chondrosarcoma. X-ray findings consist of bone destruction and recalcification at right angles to the bony cortex, which gives the characteristic "sunburst" appearance. Osteogenic sarcoma presents commonly as an extremity lesion, with only a small percentage of cases being truncal primaries. Overall, less than 5% of all osteogenic sarcomas arise in the chest wall. Osteogenic sarcoma occurs in the second to fourth decades of life, half-again more commonly in men than in women. Typically, they are more aggressive tumors with a propensity for early metastasis to lung and bone.

Osteogenic sarcoma should be considered a systemic disease upon presentation, and treatment should consist of wide local excision and postoperative chemotherapy. The number of primary osteogenic sarcomas of the chest wall is small, and it is therefore difficult to draw conclusions about definitive therapy. In the series with the most patients ($n = 38$), overall 5-year survival after complete resection and postoperative chemotherapy was only 15%.

As in all sarcomas, development of metastasis markedly decreases survival. In osteogenic sarcoma, 60–70% of resected primary cancers will ultimately develop metastasis. While prospective randomized trials of adjuvant chemotherapy are needed, most investigators agree that the current best therapy for osteogenic sarcoma of the chest wall includes resection followed by postoperative chemotherapy.

3. Myeloma (solitary plasmacytoma)—Solitary plasma-

cytomas of the chest wall are comparatively rare lesions. They constitute 5–20% of all chest wall tumors. Radiologically, they present as classic "punched-out" lytic lesions without evidence of new bone formation. They are more

common in men than in women and typically present in the fifth to seventh decades of life.

Over three fourths of the time, solitary chest wall plasmacytomas are harbingers of diffuse multiple myeloma. Survival is based on the development of systemic disease. Surgery plays a role in diagnosis. Incisional biopsy is performed unless the lesion is small (< 3 cm) and can be full excised. Local control and relief of pain are achieved with radiation therapy (usually 3000–4600 cGy). Once systemic disease is diagnosed, treatment consists of chemotherapy. Overall, 5-year and 10-year survivals for solitary plasmacytomas of the chest wall are 35–40% and 15–20%, respectively. Typical median survivals after treatment with radiation therapy and chemotherapy average 56 months.

4. Ewing sarcoma (hemangioendothelioma, endothelioma)—Ewing sarcoma accounts for 10–15% of all primary

chest wall tumors. Presentation as a primary chest lesion is not common (< 15%). Typically, Ewing sarcoma presents as a large, warm, painful soft tissue mass usually associated with pleural effusion. Systemic symptoms such as fever, malaise, and weight loss are common. Radiologic studies demonstrate the classic "onion skin" appearance caused by widening and sclerosis of the cortex as multiple layers of new bone are produced.

Diagnosis can be made usually by fine-needle aspirate or incisional biopsy. Histologically, these tumors are unique and consist of broad sheets of small polyhedral cells with pale cytoplasm and small hyperchromatic nuclei. They stain periodic acid-Schiff-positive.

Ewing sarcoma is commonly a disease of childhood and adolescence, although in several studies, age and gender were not significant prognostic indicators. The most important prognostic indicator for survival was development of distant metastases. Current therapy after diagnosis by needle or incisional biopsy consists of chemotherapy (including cyclophosphamide, dactinomycin, doxorubicin, vincristine) followed by local radiation (5000 cGy) or surgical resection. Some data suggest that better long-term survival may be achieved by resection following chemotherapy. Overall, 5-year survivals range from 15% to 48%. Long-term survivals (10 years) are achievable by patients who do not develop metastases.

E. Metastatic Chest Wall Tumors

Metastases to bones of the thorax are often multiple and are usually from tumors of the kidney, thyroid, lung, breast, prostate, stomach, uterus, or colon. Renal cell and thyroid malignancies have a high propensity for metastasizing to the sternum. Occasionally, they present as a pulsatile mass due to the excessive vascularity of the metastasis. An aneurysm of the ascending thoracic aorta, while rare, must be considered in the differential diagnosis and ruled out prior to attempts at excisional biopsy. Involvement by direct extension occurs in carcinoma of the breast and lung. Primary lung cancer with direct extension to chest wall without nodal involvement (T3 N0) carries a reasonable 5-year survival (40–50%) when treated with radical en bloc resection. Lung metastasis with direct chest wall extension should be treated with radical en bloc resection of the chest wall and underlying lung.

Brodsky JT et al: Desmoid tumors of the chest wall: a locally recurrent problem. J Thorac Cardiovasc Surg 1992;104:900.

Burt M: Primary malignant tumors of the chest wall. The Memorial Sloan-Kettering Cancer Center experience. Chest Surg Clin N Am 1994;4:137.

Burt M et al: Medical tumors of the chest wall. Solitary plasmacytoma and Ewing's sarcoma. J Thorac Cardiovasc Surg 1993;105:89.

Burt M et al: Primary bony and cartilaginous sarcomas of chest wall: results of therapy. Ann Thorac Surg 1992;54:226.

Perry RR et al: Survival after surgical resection for high-grade chest wall sarcomas. Ann Thorac Surg 1990;49:363.

▼ DISEASES OF THE PLEURA

The pleura can be the site of both benign and malignant diseases that may represent primary pleural processes, localized extrapleural diseases, or systemic illnesses. Perhaps the most common pleural problem is the presence of air (pneumothorax) within the pleural space. Pleural effusions—accumulations of fluid—result from benign sterile fluid, malignant fluid, pus, chyle, or blood. Although primary pleural tumors are uncommon, involvement of the pleura with metastatic cancer is common.

Pain and dyspnea are the most common symptoms of pleural disease. The pain most commonly is described as sharp, and it is characteristically worsened by respiratory movements, often inhibiting inspiration. Pleural pain is mediated through somatic intercostal nerves of the chest wall (cervical and costal pleura) and through the phrenic nerve (diaphragmatic and mediastinal pleura), causing chest wall or back pain and pain referred to the shoulder, respectively. The visceral pleura contains only sympathetic and parasympathetic nerve fibers and therefore is insensate; however, extension of visceral processes to involve the parietal pleura can produce typical pleuritic chest pain.

PLEURAL EFFUSION

Pleural effusion is the presence of fluid within the pleural space. More specific terminology may be used when the nature of the fluid is known. **Hydrothorax** is a collection of serous (most often transudative but also exudative) fluid, while pus in the pleural cavity is referred to as a **pyothorax** or **empyema**. Additional terms are used for blood (**hemothorax**) and chyle (**chylothorax**). Abnormal pleural fluid accumulates as a result of one or more of the following mechanisms: (1) increase in the pulmonary vascular hydrostatic pressure (congestive heart failure, mitral stenosis), (2) decrease in the vascular colloidal osmotic pressure (hypoproteinemia), (3) increase in the capillary permeability due to inflammation (pneumonia, pancreatitis, sepsis), (4) decrease in the intrapleural pressure (atelectasis), (5) decrease in the lymphatic drainage (carcinomatosis), (6) transdiaphragmatic movement of abdominal fluid through lymphatics or physical defects (ascites, pancreatic pseudocyst rupture), and (7) rupture of a vascular or lymphatic structure (traumatic injury).

Decreased respiratory excursion, diminished breath sounds (often with a bronchial quality due to compression of underlying lung), dullness to percussion, a pleural friction rub, and local tenderness are signs that indicate the presence of pleural effusion. With long-standing and advanced disease, contraction of the hemithorax with narrowed intercostal spaces and localized bulging, swelling, or redness may occur. Chest radiographs demonstrate varying degrees of opacification of the ipsilateral hemithorax. Accumulation of 300–500 mL fluid causes blunting of the costophrenic angle on x-ray. If the entire hemithorax is opacified, 2000–2500 mL may be present. The mediastinum may be shifted to the contralateral side in the presence of a large effusion, or it may remain in the midline—particularly if proximal bronchial obstruction results in lobar or total lung atelectasis, if the mediastinum is fixed from fibrosis or tumor infiltration, if the ipsilateral lung is infiltrated with tumor, or if malignant mesothelioma is present. CT scanning may be required to evaluate complex, loculated, or recurrent pleural fluid collections. Interventional radiology services are useful for loculated pleural effusions that may be managed by percutaneous drain placement under CT guidance.

Generally, serous effusions are separated into two broad categories—transudates and exudates—based on the physical and cellular characteristics of the pleural fluid. Identification of the specific type of effusion aids in determination of the cause and most often depends on examination of at least 20 mL of fluid obtained by thoracentesis. Basic tests should include total protein, lactate dehydrogenase (LDH), total and differential cell counts, glucose, pH, cytology, and Gram stain with culture. Furthermore, simultaneous serum total protein, LDH, and glucose should be measured. Effusions with total protein content less than 3 g/dL (or a fluid-serum ratio lower than 0.5), an LDH level less than 200 units/dL (or a fluid-serum ratio < 0.6), and a specific gravity below 1.016 represent transudates, while all other effusions are classified as exudates. The results of these basic tests frequently allow the underlying pathologic process to be elucidated (see Table 18–1).

Specific disease processes associated with pleural effusions are described in the following paragraphs.

1. Hydrothorax

▶ Malignancy

More than 25% of all pleural effusions are secondary to cancer, and 35% of patients with lung cancer, 23% of patients with breast cancer (12% of patients with adenocarcinomas of unknown primary site), and 10% of patients with lymphoma develop malignant pleural effusions during the course of their disease. Approximately 10% of malignant effusions are secondary to primary pleural tumors (mostly mesotheliomas). The mechanism (as noted above) is primarily through lymphatic obstruction in either the peripheral lung or central lymph node channels of the mediastinum. Malignant pleural

Table 18–1. Differential Diagnosis of Pleural Effusions.[1]

	Tuberculosis	Cancer	Congestive Heart Failure	Pneumonia and Other Nontuberculous Infections	Rheumatoid Arthritis and Collagen Disease	Pulmonary Embolism
Clinical context	Younger patient with history of exposure to tuberculosis.	Older patient in poor general health.	Presence of congestive heart failure.	Presence of respiratory infection.	History of joint involvement; subcutaneous nodules.	Postoperative immobilized, or venous disease.
Gross appearance	Usually serous; often sanguineous.	Often sanguineous.	Serous.	Serous.	Turbid or yellow-green.	Often sanguineous.
Microscopic examination	May be positive for acid-fast bacilli; cholesterol crystals.	Cytology positive in 50%.	—	May be positive for bacilli.	—	—
Cell count	Few have > 10,000 erythrocytes; most have > 1000 leukocytes, mostly lymphocytes.	Two-thirds bloody; 40% >1000 leukocytes, mostly lymphocytes.	Few have > 10,000 erythrocytes or > 1000 leukocytes.	Polymorphonuclears predominate.	Lymphocytes predominate.	Erythrocytes predominate.
Culture	May have positive pleural effusion; few have positive sputum or gastric washings.	—	—	May be positive.	—	—
Specific gravity	Most > 1.016.	Most > 1.016.	Most > 1.016.	> 1.016.	> 1.016.	> 1.016.
Protein	90% 3 g/dL or more.	90% 3 g/dL or more.	75% > 3 g/dL.	3 g/dL or more.	3 g/dL or more.	3 g/dL or more.
Sugar	60% < 60 mg/dL.	Rarely < 60 mg/dL.	—	Occasionally < 60 mg/dL.	5–17 g/dL (rheumatoid arthritis).	—
Other	No mesothelial cells on cytology. Tuberculin test usually positive. pleural biopsy positive.	If hemorrhagic fluid, 65% will be due to tumor; tends to recur after removal.	Right-sided in 55-70%.	Associated with infiltrate on x-ray.	Rapid clotting time; LE cell or rheumatoid factor may be present.	Source of emboli may be noted.

Other exudates: spgr > 1.016

Fungal infection: Exposure in endemic area. Source fluid. Microscopy and culture may be positive for fungi. Protein 3 g/dL or more. Skin and serologic tests may be helpful.

Trauma: Serosanguineous fluid. Protein 3 g/dL or more.

Chylothorax: History of injury or cancer. Chylous fluid with no protein but with fat droplets.

[1]Modified from: Therapy of pleural effusion: A statement by the Committee on Therapy of the American Thoracic Society. Am Rev Respir Dis 1968;97:479.

effusions can be serous, serosanguineous, or frankly bloody and are diagnosed primarily by demonstrating malignant cells in the fluid. Cytologic confirmation is successful 50%, 65%, and 70% of the time after one, two, or three thoracenteses, respectively. Closed pleural biopsy alone is successful in only 50% of cases, but coupled with thoracentesis it can increase the diagnostic yield to 80%. Thoracoscopy with direct pleural biopsy, however, is successful in 97% of patients and should be considered in any patient with a suspicious effusion after two negative thoracenteses.

Treatment of malignant effusions is strictly palliative: Most patients die within 3–6 months of developing a malignant pleural effusion, so prompt diagnosis and therapy are essential. The goals of treatment are lung reexpansion and pleural symphysis. This is most readily accomplished with placement of a chest tube (20–28F) and closed-tube drainage for 24–48 hours. Generally, no more than 1 L is allowed to drain initially. Subsequently, 200–500 mL is allowed to drain every 1–2 hours until the effusion is fully drained. This controlled draining avoids the rare complication of reexpansion pulmonary edema.

Once full lung expansion is obtained (regardless of the ongoing drainage), pleurodesis should be performed with an appropriate agent before loculations have formed. Different chemical, radioactive, and infectious agents have been used in the past with varying success rates, including mechlorethamine (success rate 48–57%), thiotepa (nil to 63%), fluorouracil (66%), bleomycin (50–100%), quinacrine (50–83%), tetracycline (83–100%), doxorubicin (80%), mitoxantrone (76%), talc (87–100% insufflation; 83—100% slurry), radioactive colloidal gold and chromium phosphate (50%), and *Corynebacterium parvum* (81%). Finally, mechanical pleurectomy without chemical instillation can control pleural effusions in over 99% of patients, but this requires an operative procedure (although usually only thoracoscopy). Previously, tetracycline was the most popular agent, but this option is no longer available. Doxycycline, bleomycin, and talc are now the most frequently used. Talc is inexpensive, highly effective, and easily administered either as a powder insufflated into the open chest or as a slurry instilled through a chest tube. The other two agents are less successful and are expensive (bleomycin costs $1000 per 30-unit vial). In addition, two randomized trials have proved talc to be superior to both bleomycin and tetracycline. Some hesitancy to use talc has been expressed because of the associated patient discomfort, but there have been no reports of unmanageable pain similar to that seen previously with tetracycline instillation. Furthermore, talc no longer contains asbestos, and the induction of fibrothorax, which is a long-term theoretical concern, is not a problem in these short-lived patients. Talc is a foreign body, however, and use of antibiotics during pleurodesis for empyema prophylaxis may be prudent.

Complications following pleurodesis include pneumothorax, loculated hydrothorax, fever, infection (empyema), acute respiratory distress syndrome (particularly following bilateral simultaneous pleurodeses, which for this reason alone are contraindicated), and recurrence. Fortunately, problems are uncommon, and most patients can have their chest tubes removed within 48–72 hours following talc pleurodesis.

Cardiovascular Disease

Pleural effusions are common findings in patients with moderate to severe congestive heart failure. The heart failure may be secondary to ischemia (coronary artery disease), valvular heart disease (mitral stenosis, mitral regurgitation, etc), viral myocarditis, congenital heart disease, and other less common lesions. The effusion may be bilateral or unilateral. When unilateral, the right hemithorax is most often affected. Fluid frequently involves the interlobar fissures (most commonly the minor fissure on the right) and can form localized collections simulating mass lesions known as "pseudotumors." Other cardiovascular causes of pleural effusions include constrictive pericarditis and pulmonary venous obstruction.

Renal Disease

Hydronephrosis, nephrotic syndrome, and acute glomerulonephritis are on occasion associated with pleural effusions.

Rupture of the collecting system into the pleural space can also produce a hydrothorax. In this latter case, the pleural fluid creatinine will be elevated (fluid-serum creatinine ratio significantly > 1.0).

Pancreatitis

Moderate to severe pancreatitis is associated with a pleural effusion that characteristically occurs on the left and contains fluid with an amylase concentration substantially higher than that in the serum. Rarely pseudocysts of the capsule of the pancreas may communicate with the pleural space, resulting in high-volume pleural effusions.

Cirrhosis

Approximately 5% of patients with cirrhosis and ascites will develop a pleural effusion. In contrast to pancreatitis, nearly all of these effusions occur on the right side.

Thromboembolism

Pulmonary thromboemboli are sometimes accompanied by a pleural effusion. These effusions are typically serosanguineous and small, but they may be frankly bloody and massive. Characteristic x-ray findings are almost always present in the lung. Since the fluid is usually reabsorbed in a short period of time, drainage is seldom necessary.

2. Thoracic Empyema

Pyothorax (empyema thoracis) is the accumulation of pus within the pleural cavity. The pus is usually thick, creamy, and malodorous. If empyema occurs in the setting of underlying suppurative lung disease (ie, pneumonia, lung abscess, or bronchiectasis), it is referred to as a parapneumonic empyema (60% of cases). Other causes of thoracic empyema are surgery (20%), trauma (10%), esophageal rupture, other chest wall or mediastinal infections, bronchopleural fistula, extension of a subphrenic or hepatic abscess, instrumentation of the pleural space (thoracentesis, chest tube placement, etc), and, rarely, hematogenous seeding from a distant site of infection.

Empyemas are divided into three phases based on their natural history: acute exudative, fibrinopurulent, and chronic organizing. The acute exudative phase is characterized by the outpouring of sterile pleural fluid (incited by pleural inflammation), which has a low viscosity, white blood cell count, and LDH concentration as well as normal glucose level and normal pH. The pleura remains mobile during this phase. A transitional or fibrinopurulent phase develops subsequently, marked by an increase in the turbidity, white content, and LDH levels of the fluid. In addition, the glucose levels and pH of the fluid decrease progressively and fibrin is deposited on both pleural surfaces, thereby limiting the empyema but also fixing (trapping) the lung. The chronic organizing phase begins 7–28 days after the onset of the disease and is characterized by a pleural fluid glucose level less than 40 mg/dL and a pH less than 7.0. The pleural exudate becomes quite thick, and the pleural fibrin deposits thicken and begin to organize, further immobilizing the lung. In patients with inadequately treated chronic empyema, erosion through the chest wall (empyema necessitatis), chondritis, osteomyelitis of the ribs or vertebral bodies, pericarditis, and mediastinal abscesses may occur.

The bacteriology of thoracic empyema has evolved over the years. Prior to the discovery of penicillin in the 1940s, most empyemas were caused by pneumococci and streptococci. With modern antibiotics and improved anaerobic culture techniques, however, the most common isolates from adult empyemas are now anaerobic bacteria, particularly bacteroides species as well as fusobacterium and *Peptococcus* species.

Staphylococcus is the most common organism causing empyema (92% in children under 2 years old), and staphylococcal empyema is one of the most common complications of staphylococcal pneumonias in both adults and children (Table 18–2). Gram-negative bacteria also continue to be significant pathogens, particularly in parapneumonic empyemas. *Escherichia coli* and pseudomonas species account for 66% of aerobic gram-negative empyemas, and other organisms include *Klebsiella pneumoniae,* proteus species, *Enterobacter aerogenes,* and salmonella. Rarely, fungi (aspergillus, *Coccidioides immitis,* blastomyces, and *Histoplasma capsulatum*) and parasites such as *Entamoeba histolytica* can cause empyemas. In a recent review, empyemas were found to contain anaerobic bacteria in only 35% of cases, aerobic bacteria in only 24%, and a combination in 41%. In addition, the average number of bacterial species isolated was 3.2 per patient. Aspiration of oropharyngeal flora may represent a source of polymicrobial infection.

Although patients may rarely be completely asymptomatic, most patients with thoracic empyemas present with varying symptoms depending on the underlying disease process, the extent of the pleural involvement, and the immunologic state of the patient. Patients typically complain of fever, pleuritic chest pain or a sense of chest heaviness, dyspnea, hemoptysis, and a cough usually productive of purulent sputum. Signs of thoracic empyema include anemia, tachycardia, tachypnea, diminished breath sounds with dullness to percussion on the involved side, clubbing of fingertips, and occasionally pulmonary osteoarthropathy.

Although the medical history and physical examination often suggest the presence of thoracic empyema, the plain chest radiograph is the most important noninvasive diagnostic test. Empyemas can have almost any appearance and may be associated with an underlying pneumonia, lung abscess, or pleural effusion, but most commonly they appear as posterolateral D-shaped densities on x-ray. In large empyemas, the mediastinum may be shifted away from the affected side. Bronchoscopy should be performed on all patients to exclude the presence of endobronchial obstruction. CT scanning provides critical anatomic detail regarding loculations and can assist in differentiation of empyema from lung abscess. Thoracentesis, however, is the procedure of choice for the diagnosis of thoracic empyema. Aspiration of pus establishes the diagnosis, permitting identification of the offending organisms. In early empyemas—particularly those partially treated with antibiotics—the pleural fluid may not be frankly purulent. In these cases, a pleural fluid pH less than 7.0, glucose less than 40 mg/dL, and an LDH level greater than 1000 units/L strongly suggests an evolving empyema even if Gram stain and cultures fail to identify organisms.

Goals for the treatment of thoracic empyemas include (1) control of the infection, (2) removal of the purulent material with obliteration and sterilization of the pleural space and reexpansion of the lung, and (3) elimination of the underlying disease process. Options for treatment include repeated thoracentesis, closed tube thoracostomy, rib resection and open drainage, decortication and empyemectomy, thoracoplasty, and muscle flap closure. Adjunctive maneuvers reported to aid in the disruption and drainage of loculated empyemas include instillation of fibrinolytic enzymes, placement of high (100 cm H_2O) suction, and video-assisted thoracoscopic debridement. A rational approach to empyema management is outlined in Figure 18–8. Initially, an intercostal catheter of adequate size is carefully inserted into the most dependent portion of the empyema cavity. If after 24–72 hours sepsis persists—or if there is any question as to the adequacy of drainage—a CT scan should be obtained. If, on the other hand, complete drainage and reexpansion of the lung are achieved, no further drainage procedures are necessary.

Patients with residual spaces that are inadequately drained, patients with continued sepsis, and patients thought to require prolonged tube drainage are candidates for open drainage procedures. These can usually be safely performed 10–14 days after closed-tube drainage, since the pleurae fuse by that time and the risk of pneumothorax and lung collapse is eliminated. Options for open drainage include simple rib resection and open flap drainage (Eloesser procedure). Simple rib resection involves the removal of short segments (3–6 cm) of one, two, or three ribs at the most dependent portion of the empyema cavity (at or anterior to the poster-

Table 18–2. Incidence of Various Complications of Staphylococcal Pneumonia in Adults and Children (in %).

	Adults	Children
Abscess	25	50
Empyema	15	15
Pneumatocele	1	35
Effusion	30	55
Bronchopleural fistula	2	5

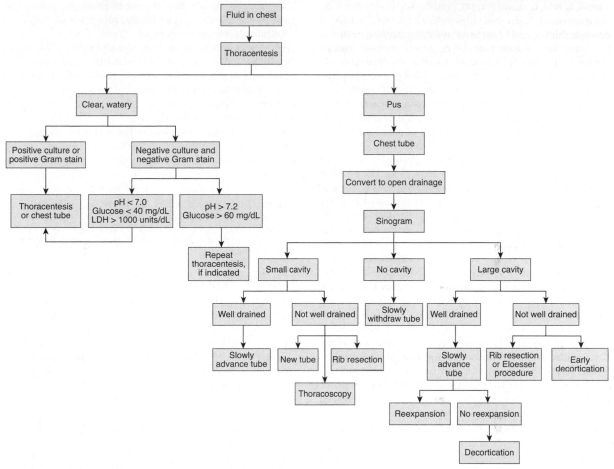

▲ **Figure 18–8.** Management of empyema. (Modified and reproduced, with permission, from Shields TW: *General Thoracic Surgery,* 3rd ed. Williams & Wilkins, 1989.)

ior axillary line). A tube can be placed through this opening and effective drainage established. A second approach involves the creation of a U-shaped flap of chest wall that is sewn to the parietal pleura after resection of short segments (3–6 cm) of one, two, or three ribs. This creates an epithelialized tract for long-term tubeless drainage of empyema cavities. The flap also acts as a one-way valve allowing fluid and air to escape during exhalation but sealing during inspiration to prevent the ingress of air. Symbas later modified the original Eloesser procedure by changing the flap to an inverted U-shaped flap with the base of the flap placed parallel to and at the level of the inferiormost aspect of the empyema cavity. This type of open drainage allows the empyema cavity to drain reliably and to be easily debrided, irrigated, and cleaned. Ultimately, through lung reexpansion, wound contraction, and granulation, the cavity often completely disappears.

Another option is early decortication and empyemectomy. This has been increasingly advocated in good-risk patients with early loculated empyemas and inadequate tube drainage or lung expansion. Furthermore, if performed early in the course of the process, resection of both parietal and visceral pleural peels (decortication) can be performed via minimally invasive technique without the need for rib spreading. More advanced or chronic disease involves a thoracotomy with decortication with resection of the intact empyema itself (empyemectomy), if possible. The best results with this approach are obtained when the underlying lung is entirely normal and reexpands fully. Posttraumatic empyema, in particular, has been amenable to this treatment.

Empyemas that occur following pulmonary resection often are more difficult to manage. If residual lung is present (resections less than pneumonectomy), the general principles outlined above still apply, although a complicating bronchopleural fistula is often present (Figure 18–9). Simple tube drainage is instituted initially followed by open drainage if necessary. Empyemas following pneumonectomy, however, pose a special problem because there is no longer any lung to obliterate the infected space. In addition, postpneumonectomy empyemas frequently are associated with bronchopleural fistulas. In these patients, specific surgical procedures designed to obliterate residual intrathoracic spaces and in many cases close remaining bronchopleural fistulas may be required (Figure 18–10). In the absence of a bronchopleural fistula, sterilization and closure of a postpneumonectomy space (without obliteration) may be attempted using an irrigation catheter inserted into the apex of the chest cavity. An antibiotic solution specific for the organisms present is then infused into the chest. The solution is allowed to drain through a dependent tube or opening created by simple rib resection. After 2–8 weeks, the catheters are removed and the cavity is closed. The success rate with this technique is quite variable and is reported to be 20–88%. For patients who fail this approach and for those patients with bronchopleural fistulas, the main goal of therapy is to obliterate the residual space and close any bronchopleural fistulas. This is most readily accomplished by the transposition of muscle with or without omentum into the empyema cavity. Multiple muscles may be required, including pectoralis major, latissimus dorsi, serratus anterior, intercostal muscle, and rectus abdominis (Figure 18–11). Use of these muscles is highly successful in closing any remaining bronchopleural fistulas and in completely obliterating the remaining intrathoracic space.

The success of muscle flap closure of empyema spaces has made thoracoplasty (once a common procedure for reducing empyema spaces) a rare operation.

Antibiotics are an important adjunct in the treatment of empyemas, but it must be emphasized that drainage is the primary treatment modality. Although antibiotic therapy is always instituted early in the course of therapy when signs of systemic infection generally are present, they need not be continued once effective drainage is established. In fact, overuse of antibiotics may lead to the generation of resistant bacteria and therefore compromise the success of any subsequent procedures designed to obliterate residual intrathoracic space.

Alfageme I et al: Empyema of the thorax in adults: etiology, microbiologic findings, and management. Chest 1993;103:839.
Arnold PG, Pairolero PC: Intrathoracic muscle flaps: an account of their use in the management of 100 consecutive patients. Ann Surg 1990;211:656.

3. Hemothorax

Blood in the pleural space usually occurs secondary to trauma, surgery, diagnostic or therapeutic procedures, neoplasms, pulmonary infarction, and infections (tuberculosis). Most hemothoraces can be treated effectively with large-bore (32–36F) closed chest tube drainage, particularly since small amounts of blood (occupying less than one third of the hemithorax) are readily reabsorbed by the body. However, if significant blood clot has formed (occupying more than one

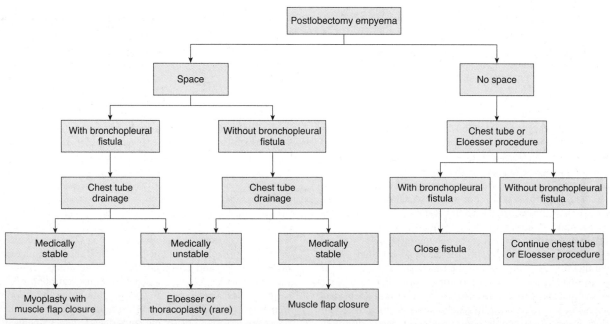

▲ **Figure 18–9.** Postlobectomy empyema. (Modified and reproduced, with permission, from Shields TW: *General Thoracic Surgery*, 3rd ed. Williams & Wilkins, 1989.)

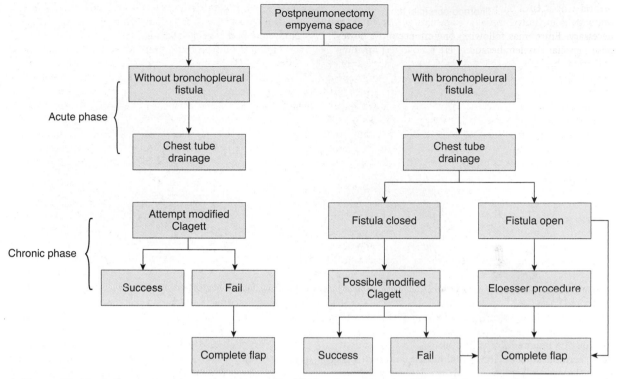

▲ **Figure 18–10.** Postpneumonectomy empyema. (Modified and reproduced, with permission, from Shields TW: *General Thoracic Surgery,* 3rd ed. Williams & Wilkins, 1989.)

third of the hemithorax) or if secondary infection occurs, further measures must be taken to avoid the development of an empyema or fibrothorax with pulmonary compromise. Currently, most hemothoraces requiring more than simple tube drainage can be managed with VATS procedures. Rarely, open thoracotomy may be required for complete decortication and evacuation.

4. Chylothorax

Accumulation of chyle within the pleural space is most often due to surgical procedures, particularly cardiothoracic and esophageal operations. Trauma, malignancy, central venous catheterization, congenital lymphatic malformations, thoracic aortic aneurysms, filariasis, and cirrhosis may also rarely cause chylothorax. Penetrating thoracic trauma can lacerate the thoracic duct at any level, but blunt thoracic trauma usually causes a shearing of the duct at the right crus of the diaphragm. This may also occur with violent coughing or hyperextension of the spine. The initial treatment of chylothorax is similar to that of a malignant pleural effusion. Closed chest tube drainage is instituted; the lung is fully reexpanded; and a low-fat diet is started. In some cases, intravenous hyperalimentation (either peripheral or central)

may greatly improve the patient's condition. Some evidence supports the use of somatostatin to decrease the output from chylous effusions. The irritating nature of chyle promotes pleurodesis, and in half of patients the leak will stop spontaneously. The instillation of sclerosing agents (see section on pleural effusion, above) has also been advocated to increase the chances of success. If chyle continues to drain for more than 7 days or if significant drainage continues for even a shorter period of time, serious consideration should be given to operation since patients quickly become malnourished from the large associated protein losses. Video-assisted thoracoscopic techniques are usually ideal, making open thoracotomy rarely necessary. The standard approach is via the right chest, where the thoracic duct may be identified as it emerges from beneath the diaphragm between the aorta and the azygos vein. Ligation of the tissues in this area is usually all that is needed.

PNEUMOTHORAX

Air in the pleural space (pneumothorax) can occur as a result of a breach in either the parietal (trauma, esophageal perforation, surgery, etc) or visceral pleura (bulla, fine-needle aspirations, etc). Rarely, infections of the pleural space with gas-

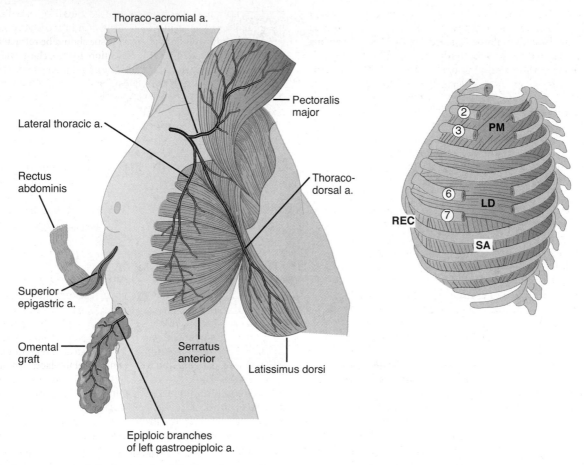

Figure 18–11. Extrathoracic muscle flap closure of a postpneumonectomy empyema cavity.

forming organisms may produce a pneumothorax. Since a chest radiograph is only a two-dimensional representation of a three-dimensional space, a relatively small separation of the pleural surfaces (eg, 1 cm) on a chest x-ray can translate into a relatively large pneumothorax. A large amount of intrapleural air that causes a shift of the mediastinum toward the contralateral lung is referred to as a tension pneumothorax. A pneumothorax associated with an open chest wound may be termed an open pneumothorax or sometimes a "sucking chest wound." *Tension and open pneumothoraces are surgical emergencies because both ventilation and venous return of blood to the heart are compromised.* Intrapleural air may mix with blood, as frequently occurs after trauma (hemopneumothorax) or esophageal perforation (pyopneumothorax).

Pneumothoraces usually are classified as either spontaneous or acquired (those caused by a specific event such as trauma, invasive procedures, etc). Spontaneous pneumothoraces sometimes are divided into "primary" and "secondary" categories; however, all spontaneous pneumothoraces are

secondary to some underlying pathologic process, and such a division is therefore strictly artificial. Most commonly, spontaneous pneumothoraces are caused by rupture of small subpleural blebs due to increased transpulmonary pressure most pronounced at the apex of the lung (apex of the upper lobe and superior segment of the lower lobe). Coughing, rapid falls in atmospheric pressure (> 10 millibars/24 h), rapid decompression (scuba divers), and high altitudes (jet pilots) all are associated with increased transpulmonary pressures and spontaneous pneumothorax. In addition, normal transpulmonary pressures can cause rupture of blebs in patients with connective tissue disorders such as Marfan syndrome. Other causes of spontaneous pneumothorax include apical bullae (patients with COPD), *Pneumocystis* pneumonia (patients with AIDS), metastatic cancer (particularly sarcomas), lymphangioleiomyomatosis, eosinophilic granuloma, rupture of the esophagus or of a lung abscess, cystic fibrosis, and menstruation (catamenial pneumothorax). Classically, however, spontaneous pneumothoraces occur in asthenic males (male-to-female ratio 6:1) between the ages of 16 and 24, often with a history of smoking. The true incidence is unknown, since up to 20% of patients remain asymptomatic and do not seek medical attention.

Patients with pneumothoraces complain of pleuritic chest pain and dyspnea. If severe underlying cardiopulmonary disease exists or if a tension pneumothorax develops, symptoms become much more dramatic and include diaphoresis, cyanosis, weakness, and symptoms of hypotension and cardiovascular collapse. Physical examination reveals tachypnea, tachycardia, deviation of the trachea away from the involved side (tension pneumothorax), decreased breath sounds, hyperresonance, and diminished vocal fremitus on the involved side. Arterial blood gases may demonstrate hypoxia and occasionally hypocapnia from hyperventilation, and the ECG may show axis deviations, nonspecific ST segment changes, and T wave inversion. The standard test for the diagnosis of pneumothoraces is the posteroanterior (PA) and lateral chest radiograph. Exhalation accentuates the contrast between the collapsed lung and the intrapleural air as well as the magnitude of the collapse. Rarely, a CT scan may be necessary to differentiate a pneumothorax from a large bulla in patients with severe emphysema. In 5–10% of patients, a small pleural effusion may be present and can be hemorrhagic.

The treatment of spontaneous pneumothoraces varies depending on the patient's symptoms and condition, the degree of collapse, the cause, and the estimate of the chance of recurrence. Small (< 20–25%), stable, asymptomatic pneumothoraces in otherwise healthy patients can be followed (often on an outpatient basis) with the expectation of complete resolution within several weeks, since air is normally reabsorbed at a rate of 1–1.25% per day. Larger asymptomatic pneumothoraces taking longer than 2–3 weeks to resolve place the patient at risk for developing trapped lung as a result of deposition of fibrin on the visceral pleura. These patients—as well as patients with symptoms, increasing pneumothoraces, or pneumothoraces associated with pleural effusions—should have them evacuated. In highly selected patients, this can be accomplished with simple aspiration as long as the immediate and 2-hour delayed chest radiographs document reexpansion. It should be emphasized, however, that some small breaks in the visceral pleural seal once the lung collapses and can reopen with reexpansion. The chance of recurrence is 20–50% with this method, and follow-up x-ray is therefore mandatory after 24 hours.

Most patients with significant pneumothoraces (> 30%) require placement of a closed-chest catheter (8–20F) for acceptable reexpansion. This catheter then can be placed either to underwater suction drainage or to a Heimlich (one-way) valve. If a Heimlich valve maintains full expansion, the patient may be treated as an outpatient; however, if a Heimlich valve fails to reexpand the lung fully or if the patient's condition is not optimal, admission to hospital and underwater chest tube suction drainage is required. Unless some contraindication exists, chest tubes should be placed in the midaxillary line at the level of the fifth intercostal space (nipple line). In women, the breast tissue should be retracted medially and avoided in the dissection to the chest wall. Placement with the use of blunt clamp dissection avoids the dangers of trocar insertion and should almost always be used. Following resolution of any air leakage, the tube may be taken off suction (water seal) and removed if the lung remains fully inflated. In patients with classic spontaneous pneumothoraces, the chance of recurrence increases with each episode. Following a single episode, the risk of a recurrent pneumothorax is 40–50%. After two episodes, the risk increases to 50–75%, and with three previous episodes, the risk is in excess of 80%. Currently, most first-time patients are treated initially with simple chest tube drainage; however, with subsequent recurrences, additional therapy generally is indicated. Furthermore, with the development of VATS, some feel that a more aggressive approach should be taken even for first-time pneumothoraces.

Patients with air leaks lasting longer than 7 days, patients who do not fully reexpand their lungs, patients in high-risk occupations (scuba divers, airline pilots, etc), patients with large bullae or poor pulmonary function, and patients with bilateral or recurrent pneumothoraces are candidates for additional medical (pleurodesis) or surgical intervention. Furthermore, patients who frequently travel to places distant from medical care are offered early surgical intervention. Previously, tetracycline pleurodesis was used to decrease the incidence of recurrent pneumothoraces. The use of this substance, however, was associated with significant pain and controversy. It is currently no longer available. The use of talc slurry or powder in this setting is also controversial due to the potential for long-term fibrothorax and restrictive lung disease but has been shown to reduce the recurrence rate to as low as 2%. Many other chemical agents have been used in the past, including mechlorethamine, doxycycline, iodoform, guaiacol, urea, and hypertonic glucose, with varying success rates. Since pleurodesis can make subsequent surgical procedures more difficult, the use of this treatment option continues to generate controversy.

Medically fit patients who are candidates for pleurodesis are also candidates for operation. The procedures used to prevent recurrent pneumothoraces include (1) axillary thoracotomy with apical bullectomy, mechanical pleurodesis, and partial pleurectomy; and (2) complete parietal pleurectomy. Both procedures can be performed with either open or VATS techniques. Complete parietal pleurectomy generally is avoided, since some patients may require future thoracic surgical procedures that are extremely difficult in the face of total parietal pleurectomy. Apical bullectomy, mechanical pleurodesis, and partial apical pleurectomy have been shown to reduce the recurrence rate to near zero. In addition, this procedure is easily accomplished either with VATS techniques or through a small transaxillary thoracotomy, both of which are well tolerated.

Several special situations exist that require particular expertise in treatment decisions. Patients with cystic fibrosis and severe chronic obstructive pulmonary disease (COPD) may be candidates for lung transplantation, and both pleurodesis and operation may make subsequent transplantation more dangerous. Therefore, consultation with a transplant surgeon is advisable prior to considering these therapies. AIDS patients with *Pneumocystis* pneumonia and pneumothorax are extremely difficult to manage, having a high rate of persistent bronchopleural fistula, treatment failure, and death. For optimal management, the pulmonary surgeon should have extensive experience in the management of chest catheters.

PRIMARY PLEURAL TUMORS

Primary pleural tumors are uncommon neoplasms of two main types: diffuse malignant pleural mesotheliomas and localized fibrous tumors of the pleura (previously referred to as localized mesotheliomas). Although diffuse malignant pleural mesothelioma is the most common primary pleural tumor, involvement of the pleura with metastatic disease is more frequent and represents the most likely cause of any newly diagnosed pleural malignancy.

1. Localized Fibrous Tumors of the Pleura

Localized fibrous tumors of the pleura arise from subpleural fibroblasts than produce an array of lesions varying from peripheral pulmonary nodules to sessile subpleural masses to the more typical large pedunculated neoplasms. The visceral pleura is involved more often than the parietal pleural, and both benign (70%) and malignant (30%) variations exist. Histologically, benign tumors can exhibit three patterns— fibrous, cellular, and mixed—while malignant ones also have three distinct appearances: tubulopapillary, fibrous, and dimorphic. These tumors behave more like sarcomas of the pleura than diffuse malignant mesotheliomas. Most localized fibrous tumors of the pleura are asymptomatic, discovered only incidentally on chest radiography. Extremely large tumors, however, may produce symptoms of bronchial compression with dyspnea, cough, and chest heaviness—and, rarely, symptoms of hypoglycemia from the production of an insulinlike peptide (4% of patients). On physical examination, signs of clubbing and hypertrophic pulmonary osteoarthropathy (20–35%) may be present. Chest radiography most often demonstrates a well-circumscribed mass that may move with changes in position if the tumor is pedunculated. A pleural effusion is present in 15% of cases and can be bloody, though this does not indicate unresectability. Fine-needle aspiration cytology may be suggestive; however, the diagnosis generally can be established with certainty only at surgery.

The treatment of these lesions is complete resection. Although lobectomy is usually not required for lesions involving the visceral pleura, wedge resection of the pulmonary parenchyma in the area of the tumor is recommended.

For neoplasms arising from the parietal pleura, chest wall resection is prudent. Following complete surgical excision, no further therapy is indicated and the prognosis is good, with some patients surviving for over 10 years without recurrence; however, if the resection is incomplete, radiation therapy should be contemplated because the prognosis is poor, with a median survival of only 7 months.

2. Diffuse Malignant Pleural Mesothelioma

Diffuse malignant pleural mesothelioma is the most common primary tumor of the pleura. Since 1960, the disorder has been strongly linked to the use of asbestos. Thick serpentine asbestos fibers (chrysotile) generally are deposited in the proximal airways and are easily cleared with less risk of the development of tumors; however, thin needlelike amphibole fibers (crocidolite, amosite, actinolite, anthophyllite, and tremolite) and the soil silicate zeolite, found in the Anatolia region of Turkey, usually lodge in the terminal airways and migrate to the pleura, thereby increasing the risk of diffuse malignant pleural mesothelioma to more than 300 times that of the general population. The increased incidence of mesothelioma in shipbuilders exposed to asbestos-laden insulation from World War II–era ships further implicates asbestosis in the pathophysiology of the disease. The latency period after exposure ranges from 15 years to 50 years. Recent research suggests that the generation of free radicals (including nitric oxide), depression of the immune system (both cellular and humoral), induction of cytokines (tumor necrosis factor [TNF]-α, interleukin [IL]-1α, IL-1β, and IL-6), and the production of genetic defects, such as abnormalities of chromosomes 1, 3, 4, 6, 7, 9, 11, 17 (p53), and 22 (involves c-*sis*, which encodes for one chain of platelet-derived growth factor) all may play a role in the mechanism of asbestos-related disease.

Histologically, diffuse malignant pleural mesotheliomas are divided into four categories: (1) epithelial or tubopapillary (35–40%), which are associated with pleural effusions and a slightly better prognosis; (2) fibrosarcomatous or mesenchymal (20%), which are often "dry" mesotheliomas; (3) mixed (35–40%); and (4) undifferentiated (5–10%). The right hemithorax (60%) is affected more often than the left (35%), and 5% are bilateral.

Most patients with diffuse malignant pleural mesotheliomas complain of dyspnea on exertion and chest wall discomfort, but other symptoms, such as cough, fever (paraneoplastic), malaise, weight loss, and dysphagia, also occur. Complaints of severe chest wall pain, abdominal distention, pericardial tamponade, and superior vena cava syndrome suggest advanced disease. Although most patients develop distant metastases at some time during the course of their disease, these lesions rarely become symptomatic. Chest radiographs are distinctly abnormal, showing pleural thickening, effusion (75%), and narrowing of intercostal spaces. CT often suggests the diagnosis because of diffuse irregular pleural thickening. The diagnosis generally requires substantial tissue samples and is not generally obtainable from fine-needle aspiration cytology. Tissue can be easily acquired with VATS techniques. Immunohistochemical stains for carcinoembryonic antigen (CEA), LeuM1, B72.3, and BerEP4 are usually negative, while those for vimentin and keratin are generally positive. Calretinin stain, which is specific for cells of mesothelial origin, has recently become available. This immunohistochemical marker can with near certainty determine whether an epithelial malignant tumor is either metastatic to pleura—for example, an adenocarcinoma (calretinin-negative)—or a primary malignant mesothelioma (calretinin-positive). This stain has become an important clinical tool and should be performed on all suspected cases of diffuse malignant pleural mesothelioma. Electron microscopy may also be helpful in distinguishing this disorder from metastatic adenocarcinoma, with which it is often confused. Pathologic staging of diffuse malignant pleural mesothelioma, like its treatment (see below), has been controversial. The original Butchart staging system and a more recently promulgated tumor, node, metastases (TNM) staging system are set forth in the Table 18–3; however, neither is widely accepted or utilized.

The treatment of diffuse malignant pleural mesothelioma also remains variable. Owing to the low incidence of this disease, its natural history has not been carefully defined with regard to various prognostic factors, and few randomized trials have been conducted to compare treatment strategies. The reported median survival for all patients ranges from 7 months to 16 months. Recent randomized prospective trials have demonstrated benefit of platinum-based chemotherapy in combination with the antifolates pemetrexed or raltitrexed. Voglezang and coworkers randomized 448 patients with unresectable pleural mesothelioma to receive cisplatin versus cisplatin in combination with pemetrexed. Patients treated with pemetrexed in addition to cisplatin demonstrated improved median survival (12.1 versus 9.3 months) and progression-free survival. The improved survival came at a cost of increased bone marrow–related toxicity (neutropenia and leukopenia). van Meerbeeck and coworkers demonstrated similar findings in a randomized sample of patients comparing cisplatin and combination cisplatin and raltitrexed. Mean survival in the cohort receiving combination cisplatinum and raltitrexed was 11.2 months versus 8.8 months in patients receiving cisplatin alone. Newer chemotherapeutic agents under active investigation include Rampirinase, intrapleural IL-2, and vascular endothelial-derived growth factor antagonists (bevacizumab).

Surgery alone has also been used in attempts to improve survival, and two major approaches have been utilized: radical pleuropneumonectomy or parietal pleurectomy with decortication. The initial experience with radical pleuropneumonectomy demonstrated only a higher associated morbidity but not better long-term survival when compared to less radical pleurectomy and decortication. When combined with postoperative chest wall irradiation, the latter procedure results in a median survival of up to 25 months. Other approaches have

Table 18–3. Staging Systems for Malignant Mesothelioma.

BUTCHART STAGING SYSTEM

Stage I: Tumor is confined within the "capsule" of the parietal pleura–ie, involving the ipsilateral pleura, lung, diaphragm, and external surface of the pericardium within the pleural reflection only.

Stage II: Tumor invades the chest wall or mediastinum (esophagus, trachea, or great vessels). Alternatively, lymph nodes within the chest are involved with metastatic disease.

Stage III: Tumor penetrates the diaphragmatic muscle to involve the peritoneum or retroperitoneum, the pericardium to involve the internal surface or heart, and the mediastinum to involve the contralateral pleura. Alternatively, lymph nodes outside the chest are involved with metastatic disease.

Stage IV: Distant hematogenous metastatic.

TNM STAGING SYSTEM

Tumor stage

TX: The primary tumor cannot be assessed.

T0: No evidence of primary tumor exists.

T1: The primary tumor is limited to the ipsilateral parietal or visceral pleura.

T2: Tumor invades any of the following: ipsilateral lung, endothoracic fascia, diaphragm, pericardium.

T3: Tumor invades any of the following: ipsilateral chest wall muscles, ribs, mediastinal organs or tissues.

T4: Tumor extends to any of the following: contralateral pleura or lung by direct extension, peritoneum or intra-abdominal organs by direct extension, cervical tissues.

Lymph node stage

NX: Regional lymph nodes cannot be assessed.

N0: No regional lymph node metastases are present.

N1: Metastases are present in ipsilateral bronchopulmonary or hilar lymph nodes.

N2: Metastases are present in ipsilateral mediastinal lymph nodes.

N3: Metastases are present in contralateral mediastinal, internal mammary, supraclavicular, or scalene lymph nodes.

Metastatic stage

MX: The presence of distant metastases cannot be assessed.

M0: No distant metastases exist.

M1: Distant metastases are present.

STAGE GROUPINGS

Stage I: T1–2, N0, M0

Stage II: T1–2, N1, M0

Stage III: T3, N0–1, M0; T1–3, N2, M0

Stage IV: T4, any N, M0; any T, N3, M0; any T, any N, M1

combined preoperative chemotherapy (MD Anderson), intraoperative and postoperative chemotherapy (Lung Cancer Study Group, Cleveland Clinic), photodynamic therapy (NCI), and immunotherapy with TNF-α as well as interferon (IFN)-α and IFN-γ (NCI, SWOG) with limited success. Currently, the use of intraoperative radiation therapy (UCSF, MSKCC) and gene therapy are also being investigated. Although the general impression is that multimodality therapy is superior to any one therapy alone, the exact combination of treatment options for this disease is yet to be defined. It is clear, however, that new therapies are needed.

Antman KH: Natural history and epidemiology of malignant mesothelioma. Chest 1993;103:373S.

Cheng AY: Neoplasms in the mediastinum, chest wall, and pleura. Curr Opin Oncol 1999;6:17.

Patz EF Jr et al: Malignant pleural mesothelioma: value of CT and MR imaging in predicting resectability. AJR Am J Roentgenol 1992;159:961.

Rusch VW, Piantadosi S, Holmes EC: The role of extrapleural pneumonectomy in malignant pleural mesothelioma: a Lung Cancer Study Group trial. J Thorac Cardiovasc Surg 1991;102:1.

Steele JP, Klabatsa A: Chemotherapy options and new advances in malignant pleural mesothelioma Ann Oncol 2005; 16:345.

van Meerbeeck JP et al: A randomized phase II study of cisplatin with or without raltitrexed in patients (pts) with malignant pleural mesothelioma (MPM): an intergroup study of the EORTC Lung Cancer Group and NCIC. Proc Am Soc Clin Oncol 2004;(Abstr 7021).

Voefelzang NJ, Porta C, Mutti L: Phase III study of pemetrexed in combination with cisplatin versus cisplatin alone in patients with malignant pleural mesothelioma (MPM). J Clin Oncol 2003;21:2696.

DISEASES OF THE MEDIASTINUM

MEDIASTINITIS

Mediastinitis may be acute or chronic. There are four sources of mediastinal infection: direct contamination, hematogenous or lymphatic spread, extension of infection from the neck or retroperitoneum, and extension from the lung or pleura. The most common direct contamination is esophageal perforation. Acute mediastinitis may follow esophageal, cardiac, and other mediastinal operations. Rarely, the mediastinum is directly infected by suppurative conditions involving the ribs or vertebrae. Most direct mediastinal infections are caused by pyogenic organisms. Most mediastinal infections that invade via the hematogenous and lymphatic routes are granulomatous. Contiguous involvement of the mediastinum along fascial planes from cervical infection is frequent; this occurs less commonly from the retroperitoneum because of the influence of the diaphragm. Empyema often loculates to form a paramediastinal abscess, but extension to form a true mediastinal abscess is uncommon. Extension of mediastinal infections to involve the pleura is common.

1. Acute Mediastinitis

Esophageal perforation, the source of 90% of acute mediastinal infections, can be caused by vomiting (Boerhaave syndrome), iatrogenic trauma (endoscopy, dilation, operation), external trauma (penetrating or blunt), cuffed endotracheal tubes, ingestion of corrosives, carcinoma, or other esophageal disease. Mediastinal infection secondary to cervical disease may follow oral surgery; cellulitis; external trauma involving the pharynx, esophagus, or trachea; and cervical operative procedures such as tracheostomy, mediastinoscopy, and thyroidectomy.

▶ Clinical Findings

Emetogenic esophageal perforation (Boerhaave syndrome) is usually associated with a history of vomiting but in some cases is insidious in onset. Severe boring pain located in the substernal, left or right chest, or epigastric regions is the chief complaint in over 90% of cases. One third of patients have radiation to the back, and in some cases pain in the back may predominate. Low thoracic mediastinitis can sometimes be confused with acute abdominal diseases or pericarditis. Acute mediastinitis is often associated with chills, fever, or shock. If pleural extension develops, breathing may aggravate the pain or cause radiation to the shoulder. Swallowing increases the pain, and dysphagia may be present. The patient is febrile, and tachycardia is noted. About 60% of patients have subcutaneous emphysema or pneumomediastinum. A pericardial crunching sound with systole (Hamman sign) is often a late sign. Fifty percent of patients with esophageal perforation have pleural effusion or hydropneumothorax. Pneumomediastinum or pneumothorax following esophageal endoscopy are sine qua non of esophageal perforation. Neck tenderness and crepitation are more often found in cervical perforations.

The diagnosis may be confirmed by contrast x-ray examination of the esophagus, preferably using water-soluble media. Endoscopic visualization of the perforation is not recommended as an initial diagnostic maneuver as this may inadvertently extend the perforation. Chest CT scan with oral and intravenous contrast is helpful in determining the level of the perforation and the degree of mediastinal soilage as well as possible underlying esophageal or pulmonary pathology. The patient, however, must be clinically stable to be subjected to the rigors of these tests. For more critically ill patients, simple oral administration (or administration through a proximally placed nasogastric tube) of contrast and a simultaneous portable chest x-ray in an intensive care setting can often confirm the diagnosis. Myocardial infarction is sometimes mistakenly diagnosed in patients with esophageal perforation when a predisposing cause of pneumomediastinum is not apparent.

▶ Treatment

Surgical management of intrathoracic esophageal perforation depends on the underlying cause (iatrogenic, tumor, stricture, etc) and the amount of elapsed time from leak to diagnosis. All intrathoracic leaks should be surgically explored. Initial management includes immediate drainage of associated pleural contamination by large-bore chest tubes and decompression of the occasional pneumothorax. Broad-spectrum antibiotics, including antifungal therapy, are initiated and vigorous fluid hydration administered.

Typically, a right thoracotomy offers the most access to the intrathoracic esophagus and should be used through the sixth interspace. Even distal left-sided perforations can be managed from the right side. A left thoracotomy, however, is useful when a perforated esophagus from a distal esophageal stricture is encountered.

Treatment of an immediately recognized (< 24 hours) iatrogenic esophageal perforation in an otherwise normal esophagus includes primary two-layer closure with careful attention to complete mucosal closure by interrupted absorbable sutures. Esophageal muscle is then closed over the mucosal injury and buttressed with either a flap of parietal pleura, diaphragm, or intercostal muscle. Copious irrigation and wide drainage is performed. Occasionally, closure over a T-tube drain has been successful.

Esophageal perforations more than 48 hours old are widely drained and the esophagus either defunctionalized or resected. This depends on the degree of mediastinal soilage discovered upon exploration, the extent of sepsis, and the patient's performance status. When perforation occurs secondary to esophageal cancer or manipulation for severe reflux stricture, achalasia, or an otherwise abnormal esophagus, different surgical options exist. If the perforation is recognized immediately and the patient is not floridly septic, esophageal resection is preferred. Reconstruction (usually with a gastric pull-up) can be done at the same setting but only if the patient is stable and the degree of contamination minimal. Otherwise, reconstruction is performed at a later date when the patient has fully recovered from the septic event.

The mortality associated with esophageal perforation remains high (30–60%) despite advances in critical care, nutritional support, and operative management. The specific surgical approach—repair versus diversion or resection—must be tailored to the individual circumstances (mechanism of perforation, underlying pathology, time to diagnosis, and patient performance status) in order to achieve optimal results.

2. Chronic Mediastinitis

Chronic mediastinitis usually involves specific granulomatous processes with associated mediastinal fibrosis and chronic abscesses. Histoplasmosis, tuberculosis, actinomycosis, nocardiosis, blastomycosis, and syphilis have been incriminated. Amebic abscesses and parasitic disease such as echinococcal cysts are rare causes. The infectious process is usually due to histoplasmosis or tuberculosis and involves the mediastinal lymph nodes. Esophageal obstructions may occur. Adjacent mediastinal structures may become secondarily infected. Granulomatous mediastinitis and fibrosing mediastinitis are different manifestations of the same disease. Mediastinal fibrosis is a term used synonymously with idiopathic, fibrous, collagenous, or sclerosing mediastinitis. Eighty or more cases of mediastinal fibrosis have been reported, but the cause has been determined in only 16%, and of these over 90% were due to histoplasmosis. In only 25% of 103 cases of granulomatous mediastinitis has the cause been identified. Histoplasmosis was the most common known cause (60%) and tuberculosis the second-most common (25%).

About 85% of patients with mediastinal fibrosis have symptoms from entrapment of mediastinal structures as follows: superior vena caval obstruction in 82%; tracheobronchial obstruction, 9%; pulmonary vein obstruction, 6%; pulmonary artery occlusion, 6%; and esophageal obstruction, 3%. Rarely, inferior vena caval obstruction or involvement of the thoracic duct, atrium, recurrent laryngeal nerve, or stellate ganglion is found. Multiple structures may be simultaneously involved.

Seventy-five percent of patients with granulomatous mediastinitis have no symptoms, and disease is discovered by chest x-ray, which shows a mediastinal mass. The mass is in the right paratracheal region in 75% of cases. In the 25% of patients with symptoms, about half have superior vena caval obstruction and one third have esophageal obstruction. Occasional patients have bronchial obstruction, bronchoesophageal fistula, or pulmonary venous obstruction.

A mediastinal tuberculous or fungal abscess occasionally dissects long distances to present on the chest wall paravertebrally or parasternally. Secondary rib or costal cartilage infections with multiple draining sinus tracts occur.

▶ Clinical Findings

A. Symptoms and Signs

Granulomatous and fibrosing mediastinitis affects women two to three times more commonly than men. Women aged 20–30 years are most typically affected, though the disorder may present in the fourth to fifth decades. Esophageal involvement results in dysphagia or hematemesis. Tracheobronchial involvement may cause severe cough, hemoptysis, dyspnea, wheezing, and episodes of obstructive pneumonitis. Pulmonary vein obstruction—the most common serious manifestation—produces congestive heart failure resembling advanced mitral stenosis and is usually fatal. Although not diagnostic, the respective skin tests in cases due to histoplasmosis or tuberculosis are strongly positive.

B. Imaging Studies

X-ray findings demonstrate a right paratracheal or anterior mediastinal mass. There may be spotty or subcapsular calcifications. Classically, histoplasmosis presents with hilar node calcification or so-called popcorn granuloma appearance. Calcification can also occur in thymoma or teratoma located in the anterior mediastinum. Chest CT (with intravenous and oral contrast) is most effective in defining the extent of mediastinal fibrosis and impingement on vital structures.

▶ Treatment

Specific antimicrobial therapy is indicated when an infecting organism is identified. Patients with symptomatic mediastinal masses and fibrosis can require resection for relief of obstruction.

Prognosis

The prognosis following surgical excision of granulomatous mediastinal masses is good. Operative procedures do not appear to activate fibrosing mediastinitis, but success in treatment has been unpredictable. Most patients with fibrosing mediastinitis—whether treated or not—survive but have persistent symptoms.

Cherveniakov A, Cherveniakov P: Surgical treatment of acute purulent mediastinitis. Eur J Cardiothorac Surg 1992;6:407.

Gottlieb LJ et al: Rigid internal fixation of the sternum in postoperative mediastinitis. Arch Surg 1994;129:489.

Karworde SV et al: Mediastinitis in heart transplantation. Ann Thorac Surg 1992;54:1034.

Marty-Ane CH et al: Descending neurotizing mediastinitis. Advantage of mediastinal drainage with thoracotomy. J Thorac Cardiovasc Surg 1994;57:55.

Ringelman PR et al: Long-term results of flap reconstruction in median sternotomy wound infection. Plast Reconstr Surg 1994;93:1208.

SUPERIOR VENA CAVAL SYNDROME

Superior vena caval obstruction produces a distinctive clinical syndrome. Malignant tumors are the cause in 80–90% of cases; lung cancer accounts for about 90%. The incidence of superior vena caval syndrome in lung cancer patients is 3–5%. The male-to-female ratio is about 5:1. Other primary mediastinal tumors that may cause superior vena caval obstruction include thymoma, Hodgkin disease, and lymphosarcoma. Metastatic tumors from the breast or thyroid or from melanoma also occasionally cause superior vena caval obstruction. Benign tumors are an unusual cause, but substernal goiter, any large benign mediastinal masses, and atrial myxoma have been implicated. Thrombotic conditions, either idiopathic or associated with polycythemia, mediastinal infection, or indwelling catheters, are unusual causes. The association of superior vena caval obstruction with chronic mediastinitis is discussed in the preceding section. Trauma may produce acute venous obstruction (eg, traumatic asphyxia, mediastinal hematoma).

The clinical manifestations depend on the abruptness of onset, the location of the obstruction, the completeness of occlusion, and the availability of collateral pathways. Venous pressure measured in the arms or head varies from 200 to 500 mm H_2O, and severity of symptoms is correlated with the pressure. Fatal cerebral edema can occur within minutes of an acute complete obstruction, whereas a slowly evolving one permits development of collaterals and may be only mildly symptomatic. Symptoms are milder when the azygos vein is patent. Azygous blood flow—normally about 11% of the total venous return—can increase to 35% of the venous return from the head, neck, and upper extremities. Thus, the most severe cases occur when occlusion is complete and the azygos vein is involved. The thrombus may propagate proximally to occlude the innominate and axillary veins.

Clinical Findings

Symptoms include puffiness of the face, arms, and shoulders and a blue or purple discoloration of the skin. Central nervous system symptoms include headache, nausea, dizziness, vomiting, distortion of vision, drowsiness, stupor, and convulsions. Respiratory symptoms include cough, hoarseness, and dyspnea, often due to edema of the vocal cords or trachea. Nasal congestion is often an early presenting symptom. These symptoms are made worse when the patient lies flat or bends over. In long-standing cases, esophageal varices may develop and produce gastrointestinal bleeding. The veins of the neck and upper extremities are visibly distended, and in long-standing cases there are marked collateral venous channels over the anterior chest and abdomen. Chronic pleural effusions may develop as a result of impaired lymphatic drainage. Onset of symptoms in fibrosing mediastinitis may be insidious, consisting initially of early morning edema of the face and hands. Occasionally, symptoms and findings are localized to one side when the level of obstruction is above the vena cava and only the innominate vein is blocked. In this situation, symptoms are mild because communicating veins in the neck usually decompress the affected side.

The diagnosis is confirmed by measuring upper extremity venous pressure; in patients with severe symptoms, a pressure of 350 mm H_2O or more is usual. The location and extent of obstruction are best determined by venography. When patients with malignant vena caval obstruction are studied by venography, 35% have thrombosis involving the innominate or axillary veins, 15% have complete caval obstruction without thrombosis, and 50% have partial superior vena caval obstruction. If patency of the azygos vein is in question, interosseous azygography may be useful. Chest x-ray may show a right upper lobe lung lesion or right paratracheal mass. Aortography is occasionally required to exclude aortic aneurysm, though CT scan with contrast enhancement for such lesions is increasingly diagnostic. The differential diagnosis may include angioneurotic edema, congestive heart failure, constrictive pericarditis, and fibrosing mediastinitis. Effort thrombosis of the axillary vein and innominate vein obstruction from elongation and buckling of the innominate artery can be considered in unilateral cases.

Complications

In patients with partial superior vena caval obstruction, thrombosis may suddenly change mild symptoms to marked venous distention, cyanotic swelling, vocal cord edema, and impaired cerebration. Bleeding from esophageal varices is rare except in severe long-standing cases.

Treatment

Superior vena caval obstruction caused by cancer should be treated with diuretics, restriction, avoidance of upper extremity intravenous lines, head elevation, and prompt radiation therapy. Cases of superior vena cava obstruction due to tumor begin to subside by 7–10 days of treatment. Because of the possibility of thrombosis in malignant cases, the use of fibrinolytic agents has been suggested. Caution must be advised in using anticoagulants, however, because many patients have advanced disease and may harbor occult cerebral metastases. Therefore, before starting therapy, patients should undergo CT or MRI brain scanning to prevent the occurrence of intracerebral hemorrhage. Recently, the use of intravascular expansile stents has been pioneered. Limited early experience suggests that the lumen can be reopened and that good venous drainage and decompression can be achieved by minimally invasive interventional radiologic techniques. Long-term results have not been reported, and disadvantages include the need for anticoagulation to prevent recurrent thrombosis. Chemotherapy is sometimes used alone or with radiotherapy. Most cases of malignant superior vena caval obstruction are not remediable by operation. Tissue diagnosis is important for diagnosis and for guiding therapy. Invasive procedures, however, must be tailored to the individual patient and the severity of the caval obstruction. Patients with new, severe, or rapidly progressive symptoms should receive immediate palliative radiation therapy. Patients with subacute presentations can better tolerate the time required to make the diagnosis.

Fine-needle aspiration, bronchoscopy, cervical mediastinoscopy, and anterior mediastinotomy—and even, occasionally, thoracotomy—offer possible approaches for obtaining tissue. Caution must be advised, however, in the setting of acute fulminant superior vena caval obstruction because any invasive procedure will carry a significantly higher morbidity due to bleeding from venous obstruction. In this case, attempts at invasive techniques for tissue diagnosis should be avoided. Most frequently, the disease process has been previously histologically confirmed because superior vena caval obstruction presents typically as a complication of locally advanced disease. In benign incomplete superior vena caval obstruction, surgical excision of the compressing mass can provide an excellent result. In total obstruction, such as occurs in fibrosing mediastinitis, most patients will gradually improve without treatment. There are numerous surgical procedures designed to bypass caval obstruction, replace the superior vena cava, or recanalize the vena caval lumen. These procedures have been dramatically effective in some cases, but only recently have they been sufficiently successful to warrant consideration.

▶ Prognosis

Radiotherapy is most effective when superior vena caval obstruction is incomplete. Mean survival of patients with malignant caval obstruction from lung cancer is 6–8 months. The death rate from causes related to vena caval obstruction itself is only 1–2%.

Doty DB, Doty JR, Jones KW: Bypass of superior vena cava: fifteen years' experience with spiral vein graft for obstruction of superior vena cava caused by benign disease. J Thorac Cardiovasc Surg 1990;99:889.

Kistler AM et al: Superior vena cava obstruction in fibrosing mediastinitis: demonstration of right-to-left shunt and venous collaterals. Nucl Med Commun 1991;12:1067.

Stea B, Kinsella T: Superior vena caval syndrome: clinical features, diagnosis, and treatment. In: *Mediastinal Surgery*. Shields T (editor). Lea & Febiger, 1991.

MEDIASTINAL MASS LESIONS

Lesions within the mediastinum represent an interesting variety of masses, both malignant and benign, that arise from the diverse organs and tissues which occupy the central thorax. Overall, the incidence of all mediastinal masses is low, especially compared with the frequency of lesions arising within the lung (bronchogenic cancer, etc). Mediastinal malignancies constitute less than 20% of all thoracic tumors.

Mediastinal masses arise from specific structures that reside in relatively constant anatomic arrangement. The mediastinum itself is defined laterally by the mediastinal pleura of each lung; superiorly and inferiorly by the thoracic inlet and diaphragm, respectively; anteriorly by the sternum; and posteriorly by the vertebral bodies. For purposes of definition, the mediastinum is divided loosely into three main compartments: anterior (or anterosuperior), middle, and posterior. The great vessels and heart, pericardium, trachea, and esophagus define and occupy the middle compartment, which separates anterior from posterior areas. The posterior compartment extends to both sides of the vertebrae to incorporate the paravertebral sulci bilaterally. The distribution and origin of mediastinal masses are summarized in Table 18–4.

Table 18–4. Distribution of Tumors and Other Mass Lesions in the Mediastinum.

All parts of mediastinum
Lymph node lesions
Middle mediastinum
Aneurysms, vascular lesions
Lipoma
Myxoma
Bronchogenic cysts
Pericardial cysts
Esophageal lesions
Pheochromocytomas
Anterior mediastinum
Thymoma
Lymphoma
Teratoma
Stem cell tumor
Thyroid
Parathyroid
Lipoma

The most common mediastinal masses in children are neurogenic tumors (50–60%). In young children (< 4 years of age), they are invariably malignant (neuroblastomas). In adults, neurogenic tumors are the most common mediastinal mass. They arise in the posterior compartment (typically from nerve sheaths) and are usually benign, occasionally calcified, and well circumscribed. Anterior mediastinal masses are more frequently malignant. The most common anterior mediastinal mass is a thymoma, though lymphoma is a close second in prevalence.

Complete resection is the treatment of choice for all neurogenic tumors. A standard posterolateral thoracotomy offers optimal exposure; however, more limited incisions, including thoracoscopy, can be effective for resection of clinically benign small (< 6 cm) lesions. For lesions that cannot be completely excised, postoperative radiation may decrease local recurrence and symptoms. Incompletely excised or especially large or infiltrative neuroblastomas should receive combination radiation and chemotherapy in conjunction with surgery.

Although classically in adults the majority of mediastinal masses tend to be benign (cysts, neurogenic tumors, etc), recent series have demonstrated a shift toward malignant processes being more prevalent. Whether this represents a true change in tumor incidence or enhanced detection secondary to improved imaging techniques is unclear. Some general rules remain valid, however.

An extensive workup of a mediastinal lesion is usually not required for diagnosis, since surgery is usually required both to establish the diagnosis and provide effective treatment. Standard posteroanterior and especially lateral chest films will often provide much useful information; however, contrast CT scanning has become the diagnostic test of choice. MRI, while helpful for assessing vascular or spinal cord extension, has not proved to be more effective than dynamic CT scanning.

Oblique or overpenetrating x-rays are sometimes helpful. Fluoroscopy may show pulsation or variation of shape or location with change of position and respiration. Tomography may reveal calcification or air-fluid levels. Barium swallow is used to evaluate intrinsic esophageal lesions or esophageal displacement by extrinsic masses. Contrast studies of the intestinal tract may reveal the stomach, colon, or small bowel in a hernia. Myelography can be of crucial importance in neurogenic tumors to explain symptoms or plan operative management. Computerized tomographic reconstructed images (virtual bronchography) may be useful to differentiate lung tumors mimicking a mediastinal mass.

CT angiography help to identify aneurysms or displacement. Pulmonary arteriography may be useful to distinguish mediastinal and pulmonary tumors.

Scintiscan is important in evaluating possible substernal goiter in anterior mediastinal lesions, since goiters can generally be removed by the standard cervical approach. Skin tests and serologic studies may be used in suspected granulomatous disease. Bone marrow examination, hormone assays, and serum tumor markers (α-fetoprotein [AFP], β-human chorionic gonadotropin [β-HCG], LDH) are important adjuncts.

Bronchoscopy and esophagoscopy are occasionally useful to identify primary lung lesions or lesions of the esophagus. Mediastinoscopy and mediastinal biopsy must be used cautiously in mediastinal tumors that are potentially curable. Excisional biopsy is imperative in lesions (eg, thymomas) that are histologically difficult to evaluate since a curable cancer might be dispersed. Mediastinoscopy is useful for the diagnosis of sarcoidosis, Castleman disease, or disseminated lymphoma.

When substernal goiter is excluded, neurogenic tumors constitute 26% of mediastinal masses, cysts 21%, teratodermoids 16%, thymomas 12%, lymphomas 12%, and all other lesions 12%. About 25% are malignant. In children, the incidence of cancer is about the same, but teratodermoids and vascular tumors are more common.

▶ Clinical Findings

Symptoms are more frequent in malignant than benign lesions. About one third of patients have no symptoms. Fifty percent of patients have respiratory symptoms such as cough, wheezing, dyspnea, and recurrent pneumonias. Hemoptysis and, rarely, expectoration of cyst contents may occur. Chest pain, weight loss, and dysphagia are found with equal frequency, each in about 10% of patients. Myasthenia (15–20% with thymoma), fever, and superior vena caval obstruction are each found in about 5% of patients.

The following symptoms suggest cancer: hoarseness, Horner syndrome, severe pain, and superior vena caval obstruction. Malignant tumors, especially lymphomas, may produce chylothorax. Fever may be intermittent in Hodgkin disease. Thymoma causes myasthenia, hypogammaglobulinemia, Whipple disease, red blood cell aplasia, and Cushing disease. Hypoglycemia is a rare complication of mesotheliomas, teratomas, and fibromas. Hypertension and diarrhea occur with pheochromocytoma and ganglioneuroma. Neurogenic tumors may produce specific neurologic findings from cord pressure or may be associated with hypertrophic osteoarthropathy and peptic ulcer disease.

A. Neurogenic Tumors

Neurogenic tumors almost always occur in the posterior mediastinum—often the superior portion—arising from intercostal or sympathetic nerves. Rarely, the vagus or phrenic nerve is involved. The most common variety of tumors (40–65%) arises from the nerve sheath (schwannoma and neurofibroma) and is usually benign. Ten percent of neurogenic tumors are malignant. Malignant tumors occur more frequently in children. Most malignant tumors (neuroblastoma, etc) arise from the nerve cells. Neurogenic tumors may be multiple or dumbbell in type, with widening of the intervertebral foramen. In these cases, MRI is necessary to determine if the mass extends within the spinal canal. Dumbbell tumors have been removed in the past by a two-stage approach, though a single-stage approach is now extensively used.

Pheochromocytomas of the middle mediastinum can be localized using ^{123}I metaiodobenzylguanidine.

B. Mediastinal Cystic Lesions

Cysts of the mediastinum may arise from the pericardium, bronchi, esophagus, or thymus. Pericardial cysts are also called springwater or mesothelial cysts. Seventy-five percent are located near the cardiophrenic angles, and 75% of these are on the right side. Ten percent are actually diverticula of the pericardial sac that communicate with the pericardial space. Bronchogenic cysts arise close to the main stem bronchus or trachea, often just below the carina. Histologically, they contain elements found in bronchi, such as cartilage, and are lined by respiratory epithelium. Enterogenous cysts are known by several names, including esophageal cyst, enteric cyst, or duplication of the alimentary tract. They arise along the surface of the esophagus and may be embedded within its wall. They may be lined by squamous epithelium similar to the esophagus or gastric mucosa. Enterogenous cysts are occasionally associated with congenital abnormalities of the vertebrae. About 10% of cysts in the mediastinum are nonspecific, without a recognizable lining.

C. Germ Cell Tumors

Germ cell tumors are common mass lesions of the anterior mediastinum. Historically, they are both solid and cystic, and the more differentiated ones may contain hair or teeth. Microscopically, ectodermal, endodermal, and mesodermal elements are present. These tumors occasionally rupture into the pleural space, lung, pericardium, or vascular structures.

Most germ cell tumors of the mediastinum are metastatic and present with concomitant retroperitoneal disease. Primary mediastinal extragonadal germ cell malignancies are rare, representing less than 5% of all mediastinal germ cell cancers and less than 5% of all primary mediastinal tumors. Men—particularly white males in their 20s and 30s—are most commonly affected, though extragonadal germ cell tumors can arise in women.

Because germ cells are pluripotent cells, they can give rise to several histologically distinct malignancies, including seminoma (40%), embryonal carcinomas and nongestational choriocarcinomas (20%), and yolk sac tumors (20%). Teratomas (20%) can have both benign and malignant components.

Almost all of these tumors (> 90%) produce tumor markers, including β-HCG and AFP. LDH—a nonspecific tumor marker—is produced by most bulky mediastinal germ cell tumors and is often an effective indicator of tumor burden.

Much progress in treating these tumors has been made with combination therapy (surgery, radiation therapy, and chemotherapy). Currently, over 50% 5-year survival is achievable for nonseminomatous, and over 90% 5-year survival is typical for seminomatous mediastinal germ cell cancer. Patients should be screened and followed with AFP, β-HCG, and LDH markers. Surgical resection should be offered after combination chemotherapy has been administered and only after all elevated tumor markers have normalized.

Residual mediastinal masses following chemotherapy and normalization of tumor markers should be resected. At surgery, approximately 40% will be mature teratomas (with the potential for malignant degeneration), 40% necrotic tumors, and 20% residual tumors (requiring postoperative salvage chemotherapy). Rarely is palliative debulking surgery indicated if tumor markers remain elevated after several cycles of chemotherapy. Instead, alternative chemotherapy or investigational therapy should be offered.

D. Lymphoma

Lymphoma is usually associated with disseminated disease metastatic to the mediastinum. It is typically identified in the anterior compartment but can present anywhere through the mediastinum. This is the second-most common mass in the anterior mediastinum. Occasionally, lymphosarcoma, Hodgkin disease, or reticulum cell sarcoma arises as a primary mediastinal lesion.

▶ Treatment

Treatment is tailored to the specific disease process causing the mediastinal mass. In almost all cases, tissue diagnosis is imperative for guiding appropriate therapy. Minimally invasive techniques (fine-needle aspiration or core-needle biopsy) or mediastinoscopy and mediastinotomy are appropriate for diagnosis of a mediastinal mass that is secondary to metastatic disease (eg, lymphomas, germ cell tumors). Mediastinal masses, however, that represent primary malignancies (thymoma, neurogenic tumors, etc) are treated usually with initial surgical resection. Surgical approaches include median sternotomy (anterior masses), posterolateral thoracotomy (posterior and middle mediastinal masses) as well as VATS or bilateral anterior thoracotomy (all mediastinal compartments). Adjuvant chemotherapy is important for malignant germ cell lesions, malignant neurogenic tumors, and bulky or advanced thymomas. Postoperative radiation therapy decreases local recurrence in higher-stage thymoma and in other incompletely resected lesions. Radiation and chemotherapy constitutes the principal therapy for primary mediastinal lymphoma.

▶ Prognosis

Overall, the outlook for patients with mediastinal masses has improved, with advances in combined chemotherapy and multimodality therapy. Surgical morbidity and mortality remain low (1–4%). Patients with benign mediastinal lesions do significantly better (> 95% cure rates) than those who have malignant mediastinal masses (< 50% overall survival).

Golbey RB: Mediastinal germ cell tumors. A continuing odyssey. Chest Surg Clin N Am 1994;4:195.

Gossot D et al: Thoracoscopy or CT-guided biopsy for residual intrathoracic masses after treatment of lymphoma. Chest 2001;120:289.

Hagberg H et al: Value of transsternal core biopsy in patients with a newly diagnosed mediastinal mass. Acta Oncol 2000;39:195.

TUMORS OF THE THYMUS & MYASTHENIA GRAVIS

The thymic gland is the site of many neoplasms—thymomas, lymphomas, Hodgkin granulomas, and other less common tumors. Thymoma, the most common type, may be difficult to differentiate from lymphoma even with an adequate biopsy. About 30% of patients with thymoma have myasthenia gravis, and about 15% of patients with myasthenia develop a thymoma.

Besides myasthenia, thymomas can produce a variety of paraneoplastic syndromes. These include cytopenias, red cell aplasias, and hypogammaglobulinemias as well as autoimmune disorders such as rheumatoid arthritis, lupus erythematosus, and polymyositis.

The relationship of myasthenia gravis to thymoma is interesting and incompletely understood. Myasthenia gravis is a neuromuscular disorder characterized by weakness and fatigability of voluntary muscles owing to decreased numbers of acetylcholine receptors at neuromuscular junctions. Because of the high incidence of thymic abnormalities, improvement after thymectomy, association with other autoimmune disorders, and presence in the serum of 90% of patients of an antibody against acetylcholine receptors, myasthenia gravis is thought to be the result of autoimmune processes. The disease has been induced in several species of laboratory animals by immunization with specific acetylcholine receptors. About 85% of patients with myasthenia gravis have thymic abnormalities consisting of germinal center formation in 70% and thymoma in 15%.

Thymoma may be classified according to predominant cell type into lymphocytic (25%), epithelial (25%), and lymphoepithelial (50%) varieties. Spindle cell tumor, which is sometimes associated with red cell aplasia, is considered among the epithelial tumors. Histologic subtypes, however, classically have not had prognostic significance. Recent reports demonstrate that aneuploidy and the presence of epithelial cells resembling thymic carcinoma have adverse prognostic implications. The histologic classification of thymomas is currently being revised.

Myasthenia gravis may occur in association with tumors of any cell type but is more common with the lymphocytic variety.

Malignant thymoma cannot be determined by the histologic appearance of the tumor alone. Evidence of local invasion grossly or microscopically defines thymoma as malignant. Thymoma is staged according to the Masaoka staging system as set forth in the accompanying box.

STAGE	DESCRIPTION
I	Macroscopically, completely encapsulated; microscopically, no capsular invasion.
IIa	Macroscopic invasion into surrounding fatty tissues or mediastinal pleura (without microscopic invasion).
IIb	Microscopic evidence of capsular invasion or microscopic invasion of surrounding fatty tissues or mediastinal pleura.
III	Macroscopic invasion into a neighboring organ (pericardium, great vessels, or lung).
IVa	Pleural or pericardial dissemination.
IVb	Lymphatic or hematogenous distant metastases.

▶ Clinical Findings

Fifty percent of thymomas are first identified in an asymptomatic patient on a chest x-ray obtained for another purpose. Symptomatic patients may present with chest pain, dysphagia, myasthenia gravis, dyspnea, or superior vena caval syndrome.

CT scans are useful in making the diagnosis in equivocal cases and in assessing the extent of the lesion. MRI is occasionally helpful to assess vascular invasion.

The diagnosis of myasthenia gravis can be made from the patient's history of easy fatigability and associated decremental response in muscular contraction to repeated stimulation of the motor nerve or from improvement in these abnormalities in response to edrophonium (Tensilon), a short-acting anticholinesterase drug.

Definitive diagnosis of thymoma is based on histologic study of a tissue sample usually after excisional biopsy or complete resection has been performed. Small, well-encapsulated anterior mediastinal masses should not be biopsied, as the procedure penetrates the tumor's capsule and can lead to tumor seeding and recurrence and may jeopardize the chance of cure of an early-stage thymoma.

▶ Treatment

The treatment of choice for thymoma is total thymectomy. The operation is usually performed through a median sternotomy. Posterior lateral thoracotomy, as well as "clamshell" (bilateral anterior thoracotomy) or "trapdoor" incisions, offers excellent exposure for resection of locally advanced thymomas. Cervical incisions, while useful for thymectomy for benign conditions (myasthenia, etc), have a limited role in the surgical treatment of malignant thymoma. A careful but aggressive resection should be performed for stage III lesions when they can be removed completely without sacrificing vital structures. Postoperative radiotherapy is indicated for invasive thymoma (stage II and stage III).

En bloc resection of the thymoma and associated pericardium, pleura, or lung (including lobectomy or extrapleural pneumonectomy) or great vessel (aorta, superior vena cava) reconstruction is warranted when complete resection is possible. Incomplete resections or debulking procedures do not benefit patients. Administration of neoadjuvant therapy with platinum-based chemotherapy will frequently shrink the tumor and allow subsequent complete resection. Recently, larger thymomas (> 5–6 cm) with evidence of probable invasion are being treated with combined-agent induction chemotherapy. Response rates exceed 70%, and complete resection rates are facilitated.

Large, bulky lesions with clinically apparent gross invasion of local structures, pleura, or lung should be biopsied to confirm histologically the diagnosis of thymoma. Neoadjuvant chemotherapy with platinum-based regimens has been effective in shrinking bulky high-grade thymomas, thus allowing for complete resection and greater chances of cure.

Anticholinesterase drugs (eg, neostigmine bromide) are given as initial treatment to patients with myasthenia gravis. Corticosteroids may be given in selected cases, but a high incidence of side effects makes them unsuitable for more liberal use. Early thymectomy is now recommended for all patients with symptomatic myasthenia gravis whether or not a thymoma is suspected. The course of the disease is usually improved, and subsequent development of a malignant thymoma is eliminated. Thymectomy may be postponed in the occasional patient with mild disease well controlled by anticholinesterase therapy.

Following thymectomy, about 75% of patients with myasthenia gravis are improved and 30% achieve complete remission. Younger patients benefit more from thymectomy than do those over age 40 years, but a positive effect also accrues to the latter group. Recently, video-assisted thymectomy for myasthenia patients has resulted in reduced length of stay, decreased blood loss, and decreased pain in comparison with more traditional partial sternal splitting procedures.

▶ Prognosis

The rates of complication and death with thymectomy are low except when there are extensive tumors. Respiratory care of patients with myasthenia gravis in the immediate postoperative period now presents little difficulty because of the availability of anticholinesterase drugs.

The stage and histologic type of the tumor are the main determinants of survival after thymectomy, though the presence of myasthenia no longer has an adverse effect.

Overall survival rates are extremely good for early-stage thymomas, and 10-year survival rates are excellent. Stage I lesions approach 100% 10-year survival rates. Stage II tumors with resection and postoperative radiation therapy have approximately 75% 10-year survival rates. Patients with locally advanced stage III thymomas, however, have long-term survival rates of less than 25%. Outcomes with multimodality therapy (neoadjuvant chemotherapy, surgery followed by chemotherapy and radiation therapy) are improving, as marked by significant tumor responses and enhanced resectability rates. Long-term survival data with these patients have not yet been reported.

THYMIC CARCINOMA

This tumor is a rare variant (< 15%) of thymic lesions and is histologically and biologically quite different from invasive or malignant thymoma. Thymic carcinomas tend to be very invasive and difficult to resect completely. Unfortunately, even in the setting of complete resection, recurrence is common both locally and at distant sites. Still, when at all possible, an aggressive combined-modality approach (induction chemotherapy, resection, and postoperative chemoradiotherapy) should be employed. Typically, these are young men (< age 50 years) with an otherwise excellent performance status. While a good response to induction therapy and complete resection will provide a significant disease-free interval, long-term survival is still unlikely. Better systemic agents and a molecular understanding of this cancer holds hope for significant improvements in cure rates.

Cooper JD: Current therapy for thymoma. Chest 1993;103(4 Suppl):3345. (Review.)

Maggi G et al: Thymoma: results of 241 operated cases. Ann Thorac Surg 1991;51:152.

Park HS et al: Thymoma. A retrospective study of 87 cases. Cancer 1994;73:2491.

Rea F et al: Chemotherapy and operation for invasive thymoma. J Thorac Cardiovasc Surg 1993;106:543.

Toker et al: Comparison of early postoperative results of thymectomy: partial sternotomy vs. videothoracoscopy. Thorac Cardiovasc Surg 2005;53:110.

▼ DISEASES OF THE LUNGS

CONGENITAL CYSTIC ANOMALIES OF THE LUNG

Congenital lesions of the lung include primarily tracheobronchial atresia, bronchogenic cysts, pulmonary dysplasia, pulmonary sequestration, congenital cystic adenomatoid malformations, and congenital lobar emphysema. Although many of these lesions present early in life with dramatic symptoms and physical findings, most remain occult until late childhood and even into adult life. These uncommon lesions arise from aberrations in normal aerodigestive tract development, which begins during the fourth week of fetal life when the lung bud forms at the caudal end of a groove in the primordial pharynx. An initial phase of sequential airway branching occurs until as many as 20–25 generations are reached by the 16th week of fetal life. These branches are divided into three zones: a proximal conductive zone (branches 1–16), an intermediate transitional zone (branches 17–19), and a distal respiratory zone (branches 20–25). A second canalicular phase is then entered as capillaries develop in the distal air passages. Finally, the alveolar phase begins at approximately 26 weeks of fetal life as prototype alveolar air sacs appear complete with both type I and type II pneumocytes. The number and size of alveoli continue to increase until the total alveolar surface reaches the adult size of nearly 100 m^2.

1. Tracheobronchial Atresia

Atresia of the tracheobronchial tree can occur at any level and may involve an isolated segment or multiple diffuse areas of the airway. Tracheal atresia is associated with polyhydramnios, prematurity, esophageal atresia, and tracheoesophageal fistula. Typically, neonates present with intractable cyanosis and despite a normal-appearing larynx are unable to be intubated. Emergency tracheostomy can be life-sustaining in babies with isolated subglottic atresia; in other infants with more diffuse disease, mask ventilation can achieve some palliation through anomalous esophagobronchial connections. Diffuse airway involvement, however, is invariably fatal.

Isolated bronchial atresia results in a bronchus that ends in a blind pouch. A mucocele develops distal to the obstruction and, as a result of compression of neighboring normal bronchial structures, causes emphysematous changes in the surrounding lung. Since children frequently develop wheezing, stridor, and pulmonary infections in the involved segments, resection is almost always indicated. Like bronchial atresia, true congenital bronchial stenosis is rare, although right main stem bronchial stenosis occurs not infrequently from iatrogenic airway trauma in chronically ventilated patients.

Related anomalies of the tracheobronchial tree include anomalous tracheal or esophageal bronchi and tracheal diverticula. These rare lesions often present with symptoms of bronchial obstruction and in many cases require resection of involved lung tissue due to chronic infection and the development of bronchiectasis (see section on Bronchiectasis). Similar to pulmonary sequestration, these lesions can have a dominant systemic arterial blood supply that must be kept in mind if operation is contemplated.

2. Bronchogenic Cysts

Abnormal budding of the foregut during development can result in the formation of bronchogenic cysts. These occur most commonly in the pulmonary hilum or mediastinum (primarily in the paratracheal and subcarinal areas) but can also arise in the pulmonary parenchyma. The cysts are usually single, are lined by cuboidal respiratory epithelium, and occur preferentially in the lower lobes. The cyst wall is generally thin, occasionally containing cartilage, and except for mediastinal cysts they frequently communicate with the tracheobronchial tree. Radiographically, these cysts appear as discrete round densities that often are sharply defined and air-filled. They may also present as a solitary pulmonary nodule (if completely fluid-filled) or as a pulmonary abscess with an air-fluid level (see below). In general, mediastinal bronchogenic cysts present with airway compression and parenchymal cysts are manifested by pulmonary infection. Some cysts have been noted to enlarge rapidly and rupture into the pleural space, causing tension pneumothorax. All bronchogenic cysts—regardless of location—are best treated with either simple or segmental resection. Rarely, lobectomy is required.

3. Bronchopulmonary Dysplasia

Bronchopulmonary dysplasia includes pulmonary agenesis and aplasia as well as primary and secondary pulmonary hypoplasia. Unilateral pulmonary agenesis occurs when one lung and the associated vascular structures fail to develop. Neonates with pulmonary agenesis may present with tachypnea and cyanosis, particularly if associated cardiac anomalies exist (50% of cases). Some patients, however, remain asymptomatic until childhood, when they complain of dyspnea and wheezing suggestive of asthma. Physical examination in these patients reveals marked tracheal deviation toward the side of the agenesis, and chest x-ray, barium esophagography, and chest CT may be required to exclude other diagnostic possibilities such as total lung atelectasis from foreign body aspiration, total lung sequestration, and esophageal bronchus. Once bronchopulmonary dysplasia is diagnosed, treatment is limited to supportive care. The prognosis is guarded because only one half to two thirds of patients survive for longer than 5 years—succumbing in part from the coexisting cardiac disease. Pulmonary aplasia is essentially identical to pulmonary agenesis except that a blind bronchial tumor stump of varying length exists and can chronically soil the normal lung with infected pooled secretions. This problem necessitates resection of the bronchial stump to prevent this potentially fatal complication.

Pulmonary hypoplasia is defined pathologically as an abnormally low radial alveolus count and low ratio of lung weight to body weight and is considered primary if no inciting cause can be identified. These neonates present with tachypnea and hypoxemia resistant to administration of supplemental oxygen due to abnormal thickening of the pulmonary arteriolar wall. Persistent fetal circulation, hypoxemia, hypercapnia, and acidosis lead to early death in over 75% of patients. Secondary pulmonary hypoplasia results from numerous fetal and maternal abnormalities that physically restrict lung growth and development. The most common of these abnormalities is congenital diaphragmatic hernia (see Chapter 43). Other conditions associated with secondary pulmonary hypoplasia include those that produce oligohydramnios and direct chest compression (eg, bilateral renal agenesis [Potter syndrome], renal dysplasia, and amniotic fluid leaks); those with abnormal bone development and small rigid chest walls (eg, achondroplasia, chondrodystrophia fetalis calcificans, osteogenesis imperfecta, and spondyloepiphyseal dysplasia); those with decreased fetal respiratory movements (eg, phrenic nerve agenesis, abdominal masses or ascites with elevation of the diaphragm, arthrogryposis multiplex congenita, camptodactyly, and congenial myotonic dystrophy); those with intrathoracic mass lesions (eg, congenital cystic adenomatoid malformation, cystic hygroma, and esophageal duplication cysts); and those with pulmonary vascular abnormalities (eg, scimitar syndrome and pulmonary artery agenesis).

dell'Agnola CA et al: Prenatal ultrasonography and early surgery for congenital cystic disease of the lung. J Pediatr Surg 1992;27:1414.

Eber E, Zach MS: Long term sequelae of bronchopulmonary dysplasia (chronic lung disease of infancy). Thorax 2001; 56:317.

4. Pulmonary Sequestration

Pulmonary sequestrations are masses of lung parenchyma that arise through abnormal budding of the caudal embryonic foregut and consequently have *no bronchial communication* with the otherwise normal tracheobronchial tree. Sequestrations may occur either within normal lung tissue, termed intralobar sequestrations; or as separate masses with their own visceral pleura, referred to as extralobar sequestrations. The majority (85%) of sequestrations are of the intralobar type. Both types, however, occur in or around the right (42%) or left (58%) lower lobes and have an abnormal systemic blood supply, often from the abdominal aorta. The venous drainage of intralobar sequestrations is through the pulmonary venous system in 96%, and in some cases this may be associated with anomalous venous drainage of the normal lung. The venous drainage of extralobar sequestrations, however, is to the systemic (hemiazygos or azygos) veins. Although some sequestrations (particularly extralobar) present as asymptomatic lower lobe masses, many present with recurrent lower lobe infections due to bacterial seeding that occurs through communications with the remaining normal lung known as the pores of Kohn. In rare instances, patients may present with hemoptysis or congestive heart failure from large left-to-right shunts through the sequestration. The diagnosis is usually suspected on chest x-ray and confirmed with a CT scan of the chest. Although angiography was formerly used to confirm the diagnosis, currently it is indicated only if questions regarding the diagnosis, arterial blood supply, or venous drainage exist despite CT. Treatment consists of segmental resection or, if necessary, lobectomy. Great care must be taken to identify the nature of both the arterial blood supply and the venous drainage to avoid exsanguinating hemorrhage from division of an unrecognized systemic artery or venous infarction of the normal lung from ligation of the common draining vein. Following successful resection, the prognosis is favorable.

Campbell RE et al: Image interpretation session: 1993. Intralobar pulmonary sequestration. Radiographics 1994;14:199.

Dolkart LA et al: Antenatal diagnosis of pulmonary sequestration: a review. Obstet Gynecol Surv 1992;47:515.

Javaid A, Aamir AU: Pulmonary sequestration: a case report and review. Respir Med 1994;88:65.

Louie HW, Martin SM, Mulder DG: Pulmonary sequestration: 17-year experience at UCLA. Am Surg 1993;59:801.

Nicolette LA et al: Intralobar pulmonary sequestration: a clinical and pathological spectrum. J Pediatr Surg 1993;28:802.

5. Congenital Cystic Adenomatoid Malformation

Congenital cystic adenomatoid malformation results from an overgrowth of terminal bronchiolar structures that are lined by typical respiratory epithelium and are associated with disorganized elastic connective tissue and smooth muscle. These "solid" structures are interspersed with cysts that resemble immature alveoli with bronchial-type epithelium, polypoid luminal projections, an absence of mucoserous glands and cartilage, and occasional "intestinal" mucus-secreting cells. These lesions are classified into one of three categories based on their presentation and pathologic features. Some lesions present with a predominantly solid lung mass, occur primarily in stillborn or premature neonates, and are associated with fetal anasarca, ascites, and polyhydramnios. Intermediate lesions with mixed solid and cystic components often present at birth with severe respiratory distress secondary to a large space-occupying mass and the resulting ipsilateral and occasional contralateral pulmonary hypoplasia. Many cystic adenomatoid malformations are detected antenatally, though predominantly cystic lesions frequently escape detection at birth and may present in the older infant, child, or adult with chronic pulmonary infection. The radiographic diagnosis of congenital cystic adenomatoid malformation can be difficult, especially in the newborn, when it can be confused with congenital diaphragmatic hernia and, less frequently, congenital lobar emphysema. A radiograph demonstrating a paucity of intestinal air in the abdomen favors the diagnosis of diaphragmatic hernia, while a chest CT scan may be required in some patients to make a correct diagnosis. The treatment of essentially all lesions is surgical resection, which may be required emergently in neonates who present with severe respiratory distress. The prognosis for the intermediate and predominantly cystic types is good following resection.

6. Congenital Lobar Emphysema

Congenital lobar emphysema is associated with hypoplastic or dysplastic bronchial cartilage in 25–79% of patients and with an increased number of alveoli ("polyalveoli") in up to 37% of affected children. The left upper lobe is most commonly involved, and the right middle lobe is next in frequency. In addition, neonates who require prolonged mechanical ventilation (eg, those with hyaline membrane disease) may develop lobar emphysema from a combination of suction catheter trauma and barotrauma. The right lower lobe is most frequently affected in these patients. Most infants present within the first 6 months of life with respiratory distress. In some patients, severe respiratory distress may occur in the neonatal period, requiring emergent evaluation and treatment. Almost all infants present with tracheal and mediastinal deviation away from the affected side, hyperresonance and decreased breath sounds on the affected side, and a chest x-ray demonstrating hyperlucency in the area of the affected lobe with compression of adjacent lung. A chest x-ray often is all that is necessary prior to operation; however, occasional patients, particularly older children, may require chest CT scans to exclude other pathology (eg, bronchogenic cysts, anomalous pulmonary vessels, and hilar lymphadenopathy). Bronchoscopy also may be necessary to rule out the presence of a foreign body acting as a ball valve. Successful therapy in all patients requires surgical resection, which almost uniformly consists of lobectomy. Great care is necessary with airway management at the time of induction of general anesthesia in these patients as positive-pressure ventilation may result in further shifting of the mediastinum resulting in impaired venous return.

Kennedy CD et al: Lobar emphysema: long-term imaging follow-up. Radiology 1991;180:189.

Stigers KB, Woodring JH, Kanga JF: The clinical and imaging spectrum of findings in patients with congenital lobar emphysema. Pediatr Pulmonol 1992;14:160.

CONGENITAL VASCULAR LESIONS OF THE LUNG

Vascular diseases of the lung include two main processes: arteriovenous malformations and vascular rings. Arteriovenous malformations are uncommon congenital lesions that develop as a result of abnormal capillary formation during the canalicular phase of development. Most arise from the pulmonary artery, but occasionally a systemic arterial source may be involved similar to that in pulmonary sequestration. Rarely, the coronary arteries may be the origin of arteriovenous malformations, with the right coronary artery involved 55% of the time. Coronary arteriovenous fistulas drain into the right ventricle (40%), right atrium (25%), pulmonary artery (20%), coronary sinus (7%), superior vena cava (1%), or left-sided heart chambers (7%). Patients are either asymptomatic or develop signs of congestive heart failure. Myocardial infarction is rare. A continuous murmur and signs of reduced left ventricular afterload may be present. Though the diagnosis often can be established with echocardiography and color Doppler imaging, the definitive diagnosis, shunt fraction, and complete preoperative planning require catheterization and angiography. Operation is indicated for symptomatic patients and for those asymptomatic patients with large shunts.

Vascular rings occur from abnormal development of the aortic arches and major branches, with resulting compression of the trachea and esophagus. In normal fetal development, a dual system of six aortic arches regresses in such a way that the left fourth arch becomes the main left-sided aorta, the left sixth arch develops as the ductus arteriosus, and the right fourth arch persists as the right innominate artery and subclavian artery. Most vascular rings, however, are associated with a right-sided aortic arch and may be classified as complete vascular rings or incomplete rings (arterial slings). Complete vascular rings include a double aortic arch (67%, the most common complete ring), a right aortic arch with a left subclavian and left ductus arteriosus (30%), a right aortic arch with mirror-image branching and a left ductus arteriosus (rare), and a left aortic arch with an aberrant right subclavian and right ductus arteriosus (very rare). Incomplete rings consist of an aberrant right subclavian artery that originates on the left side and passes poster-

ior to the esophagus (most common incomplete ring) and an anomalous left pulmonary artery arising from the right pulmonary artery and passing between the trachea and the esophagus (pulmonary artery sling).

Most patients present with symptoms of tracheal or esophageal compression. Patients with an anomalous right subclavian artery may present later in life with swallowing symptoms (dysphagia lusoria), while those with complete vascular rings and pulmonary artery slings typically present early in life (within 6 months) with symptoms of respiratory distress (often frank stridor), particularly with neck flexion and poor feeding. The diagnosis is often suggested by characteristic findings on barium esophagraphy. Bilateral indentations imply double aortic arch. A posterior indentation points to an aberrant right subclavian artery, large right-sided indentations suggest complete rings associated with a right aortic arch, and an anterior impression is typical of a pulmonary artery sling. Often, the diagnosis can be confirmed by echocardiography. MRI/MRA often provides useful anatomic details. Surgical repair of these lesions is indicated once the diagnosis is established and is accomplished by dividing the vascular ring usually through a left thoracotomy. With double aortic arches, the smaller of the two arches is divided distal to the subclavian artery, while other complete rings generally are treated by division of the ligamentum arteriosum. Aberrant right subclavian arteries may be simply divided or, if necessary, reimplanted on the right side. Pulmonary artery slings require reimplantation of the left pulmonary artery and often resection of the compressed trachea, which often has severe tracheomalacia and stenosis. Rarely, tracheomalacia secondary to vascular ring compression necessitates suspension of the aortic arch from the sternum.

Anend R et al: Follow-up of surgical correction of vascular anomalies causing tracheobronchial compression. Pediatr Cardiol 1994; 51:58.

Lowe GM, Donaldson JS, Backer CL: Vascular rings: 10-year review of imaging. Radiographics 1996,11:637.

van Son JA et al: Surgical treatment of vascular rings: the Mayo Clinic Experience. Mayo Clin Proc 1993;68:1056.

SUPPURATIVE DISEASES OF THE LUNG

1. Lung Abscess

A lung abscess is a localized collection of pus contained within a cavity formed by the disintegration of the surrounding tissues. The pus consists of leukocytes and a thin fluid referred to as "liquor puris." Arbitrarily, abscesses are termed acute if the duration is less than 6 weeks and chronic if more than 6 weeks. Although the incidence of lung abscesses fell dramatically following the introduction of effective antibiotics in the 1940s and 1950s, a recent increase in the number of immunocompromised individuals secondary to organ transplantation, chemotherapy, and AIDS has resulted in a resurgence in the numbers of lung abscesses requiring treatment.

Lung abscesses may be divided into two major categories based on etiology: primary and secondary. Primary lung abscesses occur because of aspiration of oropharyngeal contents (most common), acute necrotizing pneumonia (due to S aureus, K pneumoniae), chronic pneumonia (due to fungi, tubercle bacilli), and opportunistic infection in an immunodeficient host. Conditions that predispose to aspiration include anesthesia (both general and monitored), neurologic disorders (cerebrovascular accidents, seizures, diabetic coma, head trauma, etc), drug ingestion (alcohol, narcotics, etc), normal sleep, poor oral hygiene (increases bacterial load), and esophageal disease (gastroesophageal reflux, achalasia, cancer, tracheoesophageal fistula). Secondary causes of lung abscesses include bronchial obstruction (cancer, foreign body, hilar lymphadenopathy), cavitating lesions (cancer, pulmonary infarct), direct extension (amebiasis, subphrenic abscess), and hematogenous dissemination (S aureus, E coli, etc). It should be noted that secondary infections of congenital or acquired cystic lesions, such as bronchogenic cysts, bullae, tuberculous cavities, and hydatid cysts, are not true pulmonary abscesses because they occur in a preformed spaced. The bacteriologic findings of lung abscesses depend somewhat on the underlying cause and the thoroughness of the laboratory. Classically, aerobic grampositive cocci (S aureus, Streptococcus pyogenes) and facilitative gram-negative bacilli (K pneumoniae, E coli, pseudomonas species) have been incriminated; however, with more fastidious culture techniques, anaerobic bacteria (bacteroides species, Clostridium ramosum, Peptostreptococci, Peptococci) are now isolated in over 85% of cultures. In immunocompromised patients, more unusual organisms predominate (eg, Candida albicans, Legionella micdadei and L pneumophila, and Pneumocystis carinii).

Clinical Findings & Diagnosis

Patients with lung abscesses typically complain of cough, fever, dyspnea, and occasionally pleuritic chest pain. The symptoms are often insidious in onset and associated with malaise and weight loss if chronic. Complications include rupture into a bronchus, with initial hemoptysis followed by the production of foul-smelling, purulent sputum (and the potential for life-threatening pneumonia from aspiration of pus into normal lung); rupture into the pleural space with resulting pyopneumothorax, sepsis, and possibly empyema necessitatis; and, rarely, massive hemoptysis requiring emergent pulmonary resection. On physical examination, signs of lobar consolidation predominate; but clubbing, signs of pleural effusion, cachexia, and rarely a draining chest wound (empyema necessitatis) can be present. Laboratory studies should include a differential white blood cell count and sputum culture. Chest radiography may demonstrate an area of intense consolidation or a rounded density with or without an air-fluid level. In unusual cases, a CT scan may be required for better radiographic visualization, and in cases of suspected bronchial obstruction or in all patients with unexplained lung abscesses, bronchoscopy is indicated. Fineneedle aspiration of the abscess cavity for diagnostic culture has been shown to isolate the offending pathogens in 94% of patients compared with only 11% and 3% from sputum culture and bronchoalveolar lavage, respectively. Early fineneedle aspiration also has been reported to change the antibiotic regimen in 43% of cases and can be life-saving in immunocompromised patients with unusual organisms.

Treatment

Antibiotic administration has been the mainstay of therapy following general resuscitation measures. The selection of antibiotics varies and depends on the underlying cause, but penicillin and clindamycin are commonly used. In immunocompromised individuals, trimethoprim-sulfamethoxazole, pentamidine, erythromycin, and amphotericin B are often indicated. Once the acute sepsis subsides (after up to 2 weeks), therapy can frequently be changed to an oral outpatient regimen and continued until complete resolution of the abscess occurs (3–5 months). Important adjuncts to antibiotic administration include chest physiotherapy, bronchoscopy (may require repeated examinations to maintain bronchial drainage), and health maintenance measures (general nutrition, dental hygiene, etc). In patients who do not respond to this initial regimen and who do not have surgical indications (see below), early percutaneous drainage has been shown to be a safe and effective procedure (mortality rate, 1.5%; morbidity rate, 10%). Specific proposed indications for percutaneous drainage include (1) an abscess under tension as evidenced by mediastinal shift, displacement of fissures, or downward movement of the diaphragm; (2) radiographic verification of contralateral lung contamination; (3) unremitting signs of sepsis after 72 hours of adequate antibiotic therapy; (4) abscess size larger than 4 cm or increasing abscess size; (5) rising fluid level; and (6) persistent ventilatory dependency. Thoracotomy today is rarely indicated in the management of lung abscess but continues to be indicated in patients with massive hemoptysis, empyema, bronchial obstruction (particularly if secondary to resectable cancer), and failure of medical therapy. Furthermore, acute rupture into the pleural space (pyopneumothorax) is still a surgical emergency. When surgery is indicated, lobectomy generally is the preferred procedure.

Prognosis

Since the appearance of effective antibiotics, the mortality rate from lung abscesses has declined from 30–50% down to 5–20%. Medical therapy alone is successful in 75–88% of patients, and those requiring operation are cured 90% of the time with a mortality rate of only 1%. In the growing population of intensive care and immunocompromised patients, however, the mortality rate remains high (approximately 28%).

Bartlett JG: Antibiotics in lung abscess. Semin Respir Infect 1991;
6:103.

Groskin SA et al: Bacterial lung abscess: a review of the radiographic and clinical features of 50 cases. J Thorac Imaging 1991;6:62.

Lambiase RE et al: Percutaneous drainage of 335 consecutive abscesses: results of primary drainage with 1-year follow-up. Radiology 1992;184:167.

vanSonnenberg E et al: Lung abscess: CT-guided drainage. Radiology 1991;178:347.

2. Bronchiectasis

Bronchiectasis strictly defined is abnormal dilation of the bronchi, but common usage expands the definition to denote the clinical syndrome marked by chronic dilation of bronchi, a paroxysmal cough that produces variable amounts of fetid, mucopurulent sputum, and recurrent pulmonary infections. Bronchiectasis was at one time a common problem frequently complicated by hemoptysis, lung and brain abscesses, empyema, respiratory failure, and death. Since the introduction of vaccination programs, antibiotics, and antituberculous medications, however, it is reported commonly only in isolated geographic locations.

Although congenital diseases (Kartagener syndrome, cystic fibrosis, Williams-Campbell syndrome, Mounier-Kuhn syndrome, immunoglobulin deficiencies, and α_1-antitrypsin deficiency) can lead to the development of bronchiectasis, most cases are related to acquired disorders and are caused by two factors: infection and bronchial obstruction. Viral and bacterial pneumonias in infancy and childhood—eg, pertussis, measles, influenza, tuberculosis, and bronchopneumonia—were common predisposing conditions that led to bronchiectasis in the past. Either a single severe bout of pneumonia or repeated moderate infections can cause progressive destruction of bronchial cilia, mucosa, musculoelastic tissue, and even cartilage. Healing with fibrosis and contraction of the peribronchial tissues subsequently produces bronchial dilation. Retention of secretions resulting from destruction of normal mucociliary action leads to repeated bouts of infection and progressive scarring and bronchial dilation. Aspirated foreign bodies, endobronchial neoplasms, and hilar lymphadenopathy (see section on Middle Lobe Syndrome, later) also can cause retention of secretions, infections, and progressive bronchiectasis. The presence of true established bronchiectasis, however, must be distinguished from pseudobronchiectasis, which is a cylindric bronchial dilation that is associated with acute bronchopneumonia. When left untreated, true bronchiectasis progresses, while pseudobronchiectasis reverses completely after weeks to months.

Since the original description of bronchiectasis by Laennec in 1826, the disorder has been divided into two main types based on pathologic appearance: saccular and cylindric. Saccular bronchiectasis follows most infections and bronchial obstruction, while the cylindric variety is associated with posttuberculosis bronchiectasis. A third type of bronchiectasis, mixed or varicose bronchiectasis, is distinguished by alternating saccular and cylindric areas. In general, bronchiectasis involves the second-order to fourth-order branches of the segmental bronchi, and its distribution is largely characteristic of the underlying pathology. Congenital disorders, for example, are associated with diffuse bilateral bronchiectasis, while tuberculosis and granulomatous diseases are characterized by unilateral or bilateral disease, most commonly limited to the upper lobes and superior segments of the lower lobes. Furthermore, bronchiectasis following pyogenic and viral pneumonias usually involves only the lower lobes, middle lobe, and lingula, and postobstructive bronchiectasis is generally limited to the obstructed segments (see also Middle Lobe Syndrome, later). Common pathogens in patients with bronchiectasis include *H influenzae, S aureus, K pneumoniae, E coli*, and, in the chronic setting, pseudomonas species. Mycobacteria, fungi, and legionella should also be cultured.

▶ Clinical Findings & Diagnosis

Patients with a history of recurrent febrile episodes often complain of a chronic or intermittent cough that produces variable amounts of foul-smelling sputum (up to 500 mL/d). Hemoptysis occurs in 41–66%, but rarely is it massive. Bronchiectasis associated with granulomatous disease may not be associated with a productive cough (so-called dry bronchiectasis). Exacerbations and advanced disease are manifested by increased sputum production, fever, dyspnea, anorexia, fatigue, and weight loss. A history of sinus problems, infertility, or a family history of similar problems suggests the presence of an inherited disorder associated with bronchiectasis. Physical examination may reveal cyanosis, clubbing, pulmonary osteoarthropathy, evidence of malnutrition, and, in advanced disease, signs of cor pulmonale. Although bronchiectasis is suspected, an imaging study is usually required for confirmation. Bronchograms were at one time required, but high-resolution, fine-cut (1.5–5 mm) CT scans are now the imaging procedure of choice to document bronchial dilation, particularly with saccular disease. Even with the diagnosis of bronchiectasis, however, endobronchial neoplasm or foreign body must be excluded by flexible fiberoptic bronchoscopy.

▶ Treatment

In nearly all patients, conservative medical therapy is indicated and generally is sufficient. This includes broad-spectrum antibiotics, bronchodilators, humidification, expectorants, mucolytics, and effective routine postural drainage. In patients with continued infection, bronchoscopy with bronchoalveolar lavage should be considered to obtain more accurate culture results. Other adjunctive therapies include influenza and pneumococcal vaccines and, in some patients, chronic "prophylactic" antibiotic administration with trimethoprim-sulfamethoxazole, erythromycin, or ciprofloxacin. A recent advance in controlling underlying bacterial (especially pseudomonas) infection and symptoms associated with bronchiectasis has been the use of inhaled antibiotics. In the cystic fibrosis and chronic bronchiectasis population, nebulized tobramycin or gentamicin has proved effective in controlling infection, sputum production, and symptoms in a significant proportion of patients.

Patients who fail intensive medical therapy may be candidates for surgical resection if the following criteria are met: (1) the disease must be localized and completely resectable, (2) pulmonary reserve must be adequate, (3) the process must be irreversible (ie, not pseudobronchiectasis, bronchial stricture, foreign body, etc), and (4) significant symptoms must persist. Preoperative assessment requires a high-resolution, fine-cut CT scan, though some surgeons still prefer a bronchogram as a "road map." Pulmonary function studies generally are not necessary, since the involved segments do not function. The goals of surgery are to remove all active disease and to preserve as much functioning lung parenchyma as possible. The surgical approach includes complete segmental resection of the involved areas. Partial resection almost always ends in recurrence. Resection most commonly involves all basal segments (unilaterally or bilaterally) along with the middle lobe or lingula. With tuberculosis, however, removal of the upper lobe or lobes with or without the superior segment of the lower lobes is more likely. During surgery, meticulous maintenance of a clear airway devoid of mucopurulent secretions and blood is essential. Careful dissection of the bronchovascular structures is difficult in patients with chronic inflammation and scarring but is essential to avoid complications.

▶ Prognosis

Although most patients are successfully treated with medical therapy, some require surgery. The results of surgical resection depend on the cause and type of pulmonary involvement. Success with elimination of symptoms occurs in up to 80% of patients with limited localized disease but only 36% of those with diffuse disease. Prognostic factors include (1) unilateral disease restricted to the basal segments, (2) young age, (3) absence of sinusitis and rhinitis, (4) history of pneumonia, and (5) no major airway obstruction. Overall morbidity and mortality rates are surprisingly low at 3–5% and less than 1%, respectively.

Ip M et al: Multivariate analysis of factors affecting pulmonary function in bronchiectasis. Respiration 1993;60:45.
McGuinness G et al: Bronchiectasis: CT evaluation. AJR Am J Roentgenol 1993;160:253.
Trucksis M, Swartz MN: Bronchiectasis: a current view. Curr Clin Top Infect Dis 1991;11:170.

3. Middle Lobe Syndrome

Relapsing lateral pneumonia of the middle pulmonary lobe is typically caused by intermittent obstruction, most often extrinsic. In a patient with repeated episodes of right-sided pneumonia, this diagnosis should be entertained, but only after other causes of obstruction (bronchogenic cancer, foreign body, etc), have been ruled out.

Broncholithiasis (see section on Broncholithiasis, later) and middle lobe syndrome have been considered to be caused by compression or erosion of the bronchus by adjacent diseased lymph nodes. Other factors, such as poor natural drainage and lack of collateral ventilation, probably explain the frequency of middle lobe.

Endobronchial tumors and foreign bodies must be excluded by bronchoscopy.

Most patients respond to intensive medical therapy, and surgery is rarely required. Indications for surgery, which usually involves middle lobectomy, include bronchiectasis, fibrosis (bronchostenosis), abscess, unresolved or intractable recurrent pneumonia, and suspicion of neoplasm.

Ring-Mrozik E et al: Clinical findings in middle lobe syndrome and other processes of pulmonary shrinkage in children (atelectasis syndrome). Eur J Pediatr Surg 1991;1:266.

4. Broncholithiasis

Broncholithiasis is defined as the presence of calculi (broncholiths) within the tracheobronchial tree. In most cases, a calcified parabronchial lymph node erodes through the bronchial wall into the lumen; however, severely inspissated mucus may calcify. Calcified lymph nodes may remain attached to the bronchial wall, lodge in a bronchus, or be expectorated (lithoptysis). The most common cause of broncholithiasis in the United States is histoplasmosis. Tuberculosis is another frequent cause in some parts of the world.

Patients with broncholithiasis often complain of hemoptysis, lithoptysis (30%), cough, sputum production, fever, chills, and pleuritic chest pain. The hemoptysis is characteristically sudden and self-limited, though rarely it may be massive. Symptoms of pneumonia may indicate bronchial obstruction from an impacted broncholith. Signs suggesting broncholithiasis include localized wheezing on physical examination, evidence of hilar calcifications or segmental atelectasis and pneumonia on chest x-ray, and bronchoscopic evidence of peribronchial disease. The diagnosis is confirmed by documentation of lithoptysis or the presence of an endobronchial "lung stone."

The complications of broncholithiasis include hemoptysis, which on occasion can be massive and life threatening; suppurative lung diseases (eg, pneumonia and bronchiectasis); midesophageal traction diverticula; and, rarely, tracheobronchoesophageal fistula. In addition to instituting appropriate therapy for underlying pulmonary diseases, treatment is primarily directed at removal of endobronchial stones. This can be accomplished at the time of bronchoscopy if the broncholith is freely floating within the tracheobronchial tree or if it extends well into the bronchial lumen and can be removed without excessive force or traction (20% of cases). The main danger of transbronchoscopic removal of broncholiths is the real possibility of massive hemorrhage. This results during inappropriate removal of broncholiths that remain substantially attached to the parabronchial tissues. Because of intense peribronchial fibrosis in this situation, the broncholith not infrequently becomes adherent to vascular structures such as the pulmonary artery, which may be torn with vigorous attempts at broncholith removal. Nearly 80% of patients with broncholiths that remain in situ require surgical removal. The goal of surgery in this disease is preservation of lung function. The broncholith may be removed safely with bronchotomy; however, most patients require segmentectomy or lobectomy, particularly if destruction of lung parenchyma has occurred from postobstruction suppurative lung disease. Fistulas between the airway and the esophagus should be repaired with interposition of normal tissue (intercostal muscle flap, etc) between the two structures to prevent recurrence. Following surgery, the prognosis is excellent.

Conces DJ Jr, Tarver RD, Vix VA: Broncholithiasis: CT features in 15 patients. AJR Am J Roentgenol 1991;157:249.

Galdermans D et al: Broncholithiasis: present clinical spectrum. Respir Med 1990;84:155.

Igoe D, Lynch V, McNicholas WT: Broncholithiasis: bronchoscopic vs. surgical management. Respir Med 1990; 84:163.

McLean TR, Beall AC Jr, Jones JW: Massive hemoptysis due to broncholithiasis. Ann Thorac Surg 1991;52:1173.

5. Cystic Fibrosis & Mucoid Impaction of the Bronchi

Cystic fibrosis is a serious congenital disorder that may lead to bronchitis, bronchiectasis, pulmonary fibrosis, emphysema, and lung abscess. Mucoid impaction occurs in patients with asthma and bronchitis. Mucoid plugs are rubbery, semisolid, gray to greenish-yellow in color, and round, oval, or elongated in shape. There is often a history of recurrent upper respiratory infection, fever, and chest pain. Expectoration of hard mucus plugs or hemoptysis may occur.

Bronchogenic carcinoma, fungal infection, tuberculosis, bronchiectasis, abscess, bacterial pneumonia, lipoid pneumonia, pulmonary eosinophilic granuloma, and Löffler syndrome must be ruled out.

Treatment is with expectorants, detergents, bronchodilators, antibiotics, and aerosol inhalation. The availability of acetylcysteine has largely converted this condition to a purely medical disease. Surgery is indicated when cancer cannot be ruled out, for destroyed lung, or in the treatment of abscess.

Double lung transplantation is a consideration for advanced cystic fibrosis patients with end-stage pulmonary function. Overall, survivals have improved (85% at 1 year, 50% at 5 years) due to improvements in surgical technique (bronchial anastomosis) and immunosuppressive regimens. Still, chronic bronchitis obliterans remains a major obstacle after several years and is the leading cause of eventual transplant failure. Limited donor organ availability prevents the many eligible cystic fibrosis patients from being transplanted.

Fiel SB: Clinical management of pulmonary disease in cystic fibrosis. Lancet 1993;341:1070.

Shennib H et al: Double-lung transplantation for cystic fibrosis. The Cystic Fibrosis Transplant Study Group. Ann Thorac Surg 1992;54:27.

6. Tuberculosis

Tuberculosis markedly declined as a cause of death between 1953 and 1984, but since 1985, this disease has experienced a resurgence due to increased immigration of infected individuals and HIV infection. A reservoir of about 5000–8000 clinical cases exists, and an additional 25,000 new cases occur annually. Less than 20% of the United States population are tuberculin-positive, but tuberculosis remains a common infectious cause of death worldwide.

Several species of the genus mycobacterium may cause lung disease, but 95% of cases of lung disease are due to *Mycobacterium tuberculosis. Mycobacterium bovis* and *Mycobacterium avium* are seldom found in humans. Several "atypical" species of mycobacterium that are chiefly soil-dwellers have become clinically more important in recent years because they are less responsive to preventive and therapeutic measures. Mycobacteria are nonmotile, nonsporulating, weakly gram-positive rods classified in the order Actinomycetales. Dormant organisms remain alive for the life of the host.

The initial infection often involves pulmonary parenchyma in the midzone of the lungs. When hypersensitivity develops after several weeks, the typical caseation appears. Regional hilar lymph nodes become enlarged. Most cases arrest spontaneously at this stage. If the infection progresses, caseation necrosis develops and giant cells produce a typical tubercle. A cause of latent disease in the elderly or debilitated patient is dormant reactivation tubercles. Sites in the apical and posterior segments of the upper lobes and superior segments of the lower lobes are the usual areas of infection.

▶ Clinical Findings

A. Symptoms and Signs

Patients may present with minimal symptoms, including fever, cough, anorexia, weight loss, night sweats, excessive perspiration, chest pain, lethargy, and dyspnea. Extrapulmonary disease may be associated with more severe symptoms, such as involvement of the pericardium, bones, joints, urinary tract, meninges, lymph nodes, or pleural space. Erythema nodosum is seen occasionally in patients with active disease.

B. Laboratory Findings

False-negative tests with intermediate-strength PPD are usually due to anergy, improper testing, or outdated tuberculin. Anergy is sometimes associated with disseminated tuberculosis, measles, sarcoidosis, lymphomas, or recent vaccination with live viruses (eg, poliomyelitis, measles, rubella, mumps, influenza, or yellow fever). Immunosuppressive drugs (eg, corticosteroids, azathioprine) and disease states (eg, AIDS, organ transplantation) may also cause false-negative responses. Mumps skin tests are negative in patients taking immunosuppressive drugs.

Culture of sputum, gastric aspirates, and tracheal washings as well as pleural fluid and pleural and lung biopsies may establish the diagnosis.

C. Imaging Studies

X-ray findings include involvement of the apical and posterior segments of the upper lobes (85%) or the superior segments of the lower lobes (10%). Seldom is the anterior segment of the upper lobe solely involved, as in other granulomatous diseases such as histoplasmosis. Involvement of the basal segments of the lower lobes is uncommon except in women, blacks, and diabetics, but endobronchial disease usually involves the lower lobes, producing atelectasis or consolidation. Differing x-ray patterns correspond to the pathologic variations of the disease: the local exudative lesion, the local productive lesion, cavitation, acute tuberculous pneumonia, miliary tuberculosis, Rasmussen aneurysm, bronchiectasis, bronchostenosis, and tuberculoma.

▶ Differential Diagnosis

It is critical to distinguish the x-ray findings from bronchogenic carcinoma, particularly when there is tuberculoma without calcification.

▶ Treatment
A. Medical Treatment

Active disease should be treated with one of the chemotherapeutic regimens that have recently been shown to shorten the period of treatment while maintaining their potency. Such drugs include isoniazid, streptomycin, rifampin, and ethambutol (Table 18–5). These multiple-drug regimens are designed to prevent the emergence of resistant strains and minimize toxicity.

B. Surgical Treatment

The role of surgery in treatment of tuberculosis has diminished dramatically since chemotherapy became available. It is now confined to the following indications: (1) failure of chemotherapy, (2) performance of diagnostic procedures, (3) destroyed lung, (4) postsurgical complications, (5) persistent bronchopleural fistula, and (6) intractable hemorrhage.

Surgical resection for diagnosis may be necessary to rule out other diseases, such as cancer, or to obtain material for cultures. Patients with destroyed lobes or cavitary tuberculosis of the right upper lobe containing large infected foci may sometimes be candidates for resection.

The disease becomes reactivated in some patients who have had thoracoplasty, plombage, or resection, and a few

will require reoperation. The most common indications for surgery after plombage therapy are pleural infection (pyogenic or tuberculous) and migration of the plombage material, causing pain or compression of other organs. Following pulmonary resection, tuberculous empyema may develop in the postpneumonectomy space, sometimes associated with a bronchopleural fistula or bony sequestration. Persistent bronchopleural fistula after chemotherapy and closed tube drainage may require direct operative closure. Use of muscle flaps (intercostal, etc) is highly recommended to cover any bronchial stumps, especially in the setting of pneumonectomy.

Tuberculous empyema poses unique problems of management. Treatment depends upon whether the empyema is (1) associated with parenchymal disease, (2) mixed tuberculous and pyogenic or purely tuberculous, and (3) associated with bronchopleural fistula. The ultimate objective is complete expansion of the lung and obliteration of the empyema space. Pulmonary decortication or resection may be used for tuberculosis, but open or closed drainage is necessary when the process is complicated by pyogenic infection or bronchopleural fistula.

▶ Prognosis

The prognosis is excellent in most cases treated medically; the death rate decreased from 25% in 1945 to less than 10% currently. Perioperative mortality for pulmonary resections for tuberculosis ranges from 10% for pneumonectomy to 3% for lobectomy and 1% for segmentectomy and subsegmental resections.

The relapse rate following modern chemotherapy is about 4%.

Horowitz MD et al: Late complications of plombage. Ann Thorac Surg 1992;53:803.
Langston HT: Thoracoplasty: the how and the why. Ann Thorac Surg 1991;52:1351.
Nolan CM: Failure of therapy for tuberculosis in human immunodeficiency virus infection. Am J Med Sci 1992;304:168.
Pomerantz M et al: Surgical management of resistant mycobacterial tuberculosis and other mycobacterial pulmonary infections. Ann Thorac Surg 1991;52:1108.

FUNGAL INFECTIONS OF THE LUNG

Pulmonary fungal infections are increasing due to the widespread use of broad-spectrum antibiotics, the use of corticosteroids and other immunosuppressive drugs, and the spread of HIV infection. However, infection can occur in immunocompetent hosts. Fungal infections frequently involve the respiratory tract and include histoplasmosis, coccidioidomycosis, blastomycosis, cryptococcosis, aspergillosis, mucormycosis, and candidiasis. Fungal infections, though ubiquitous, are notable for several characteristic endemic areas. Candidiasis rarely if ever requires operative treatment and thus will not be discussed here.

Table 18–5. Antituberculosis Drugs and Their Side Effects.[1]

Drug	Dosage (Adult Daily)	Side Effects (Usual)	Monitoring	Remarks
Isoniazid	5–10 mg/kg; 300–600 mg.	Peripheral neuritis, hepatitis, hypersensitivity, convulsions.	SGOT (AST)/SGPT (ALT) (not as routine).	To prevent neuritis, give pyridoxine, 25–50 mg/d orally.
Ethambutol	15–25 mg/kg/d for 60 days, then 15 mg/kg/d.	Optic neuritis (very rare at 15 mg/kg/d).	Visual acuity, red-green color discrimination.	Ocular history and funduscopic examination before use; contraindicated with optic neuritis.
Rifampin	600 mg once daily (children, 10–20 mg/kg to a maximum of 600 mg).	Hepatotoxicity (rare under age 20; 2.5% of cases over age 50). Occasionally, thrombocytopenia, anemia, nephritis.	SGOT (AST)/SGPT (ALT).	Harmless orange staining of urine, sweat, contact lenses, etc. "Flu syndrome" if rifampin given less than twice weekly.
Streptomycin	0.5–1.5 g/d IM (children, 20–40 mg/kg/d IM).	Ototoxicity, nephrotoxicity.	Gross hearing (ticking of watch); if abnormal audiograms, BUN and creatinine.	Used mainly in very ill patients as part of triple-drug regimen.
Aminosalicylic acid	10–12 g/d.	Gastrointestinal intolerance, skin rashes, hypersensitivity.	SGOT (AST)/SGPT (ALT).	Because of poor tolerance, rarely used now.
Pyrazinamide[2]	20–35 mg/kg/d, up to 3 g/d.	Hyperuricemia, hepatotoxicity, arthralgia.	Uric acid, SGOT (AST)/SGPT (ALT).	Sometimes given as first-line drug in short-course regimen (50 mg/kg twice weekly); inexpensive.
Ethionamide[2]	0.5–1 g/d.	Gastrointestinal, hepatotoxicity, hypersensitivity (rash).	SGOT (AST)/SGPT (ALT).	Temporarily stop or reduce dose with gastrointestinal irritation and hepatotoxicity.
Cycloserine[2]	0.5–1 g/d.	Psychosis, personality changes, convulsions, rash.	Drug blood levels if poor renal function.	CNS reactions sometimes controlled by phenytoin.
Capreomycin[2]	20 mg/kg/d IM (up to 1 g/d)	Nephrotoxicity, ototoxicity, hepatotoxicity.	Same as streptomycin with SGOT (AST)/SGPT (ALT) in addition.	Sometimes given as 1 g 2 or 3 times weekly.
Viomycin[2]	1 g twice daily IM 2 or 3 times weekly.	Nephrotoxicity, ototoxicity.	As for streptomycin, plus urinalysis.	As for streptomycin.
Kanamycin[2]	0.5–1 g IM.	See streptomycin.	As for streptomycin, plus urinalysis.	Used mainly for atypical mycobacterial infections.

[1]See also Chambers HF: Antimycobacterial drugs. in: *Basic and Clinical Pharmacology,* 8th ed. Katzung BG (editor). McGraw-Hill, 2001.
[2]Used only as second-line drug in *M tuberculosis* infections, mainly for retreatment or in drug-resistant cases. Used as first-line drug, in combinations, in atypical mycobacterial infections.

1. Histoplasmosis

Histoplasma capsulatum is a dimorphic soil fungus frequently found in fowl and bat excreta, pigeon roosts, chicken houses, caves, hollow trees, attics, and lofts. It is endemic in fertile river valleys, such as the Mississippi, Missouri, Ohio, St. Lawrence, and Rio Grande. Infection occurs almost exclusively after inhalation of a large number of spores and occurs with a male-to-female ratio of 3:1. Once in the lungs, the fungus germinates in yeast form, resulting in caseation, necrosis, fibrosis, and calcification. The diagnosis of histoplasmosis relies on high or rising serum antibody complement fixation titers (> 1:32 or fourfold rise) in the appropriate clinical setting. The histoplasmin skin test, which becomes positive 2–6 weeks following infection, is useful only for epidemiologic studies and not for the diagnosis of acute disease. Sputum culture is positive in less than 10%, but tissue cultures may be more reliable.

Most infections in immunocompetent individuals are asymptomatic. Infections are classified as acute, chronic, or disseminated. Acute infections are manifested (1) as a flulike syndrome with fever, chills, dry cough, headache, retrosternal discomfort, arthralgias, and a rash suggesting erythema nodosum; (2) with symptoms similar to a flulike syndrome but limited to the lungs and occasionally accompanied by a productive cough; or (3) as an acute diffuse nodular disease with mild symptoms. Radiographic findings in these three acute syndromes typically demonstrate ill-defined upper lobe nonsegmental opacities; nonsegmental areas of consolidation that tend to change; and diffuse, discrete 3- to 4-mm nodules, respectively. Hilar adenopathy on chest x-ray is common. Physical examination can be normal or may reveal signs of pneumonia.

In contrast, chronic infections include (1) an asymptomatic solitary, discrete nodule less than 3 cm in diameter known as a histoplasmoma (most common), often with central and concentric calcifications ("target lesion") and frequently located in the lower lobes; (2) chronic cavitary histoplasmosis, which typically occurs in patients with underlying obstructive disease, characteristically mild symptoms, fibronodular upper lobe infiltrates, and centrilobular emphysematous spaces; (3) mediastinal granulomas that may result in broncholithiasis, esophageal traction diverticula, superior vena cava compression, and tracheobronchoesophageal fistulas; and (4) fibrosing mediastinitis, which can produce compression of the superior vena cava, tracheobronchial tree, or esophagus.

Disseminated disease includes an acute, subacute, and chronic form.

These infections occur in children (acute and subacute) as well as adults (subacute and chronic). Fever and abdominal pain are common. Other findings include hepatosplenomegaly, pancytopenia, meningitis, endocarditis, adrenocortical insufficiency, and oropharyngeal ulceration (chronic form).

Radiographic imaging in disseminated disease may demonstrate diffuse interstitial pneumonitis (25%) or minimal findings.

The symptoms and roentgenographic findings of histoplasmosis resemble those of tuberculosis, although the disease appears to progress more slowly. There may be cough, malaise, hemoptysis, low-grade fever, and weight loss. As many as 30% of cases coexist with tuberculosis. Pulmonary fibrosis, bulla formation, and pulmonary insufficiency occur in advanced cases of histoplasmosis. Mediastinal involvement is quite frequent and may take the form of granuloma formation, or dysphagia. Furthermore, mediastinal fibrosis is among the most common benign causes of superior vena caval syndrome (discussed earlier in the chapter). Erosion of inflammatory lymph nodes into bronchi may cause expectoration of broncholiths, hemoptysis, wheezing, or bronchiectasis. Traction diverticula of the esophagus may lead to development of tracheoesophageal fistula. Pericardial involvement may lead to constrictive pericarditis.

In lesions that present as solitary pulmonary nodules, histoplasmosis is diagnosed in about 15–20% of cases. Radiologically, early infections appear as diffuse mottled parenchymal infiltrations surrounding the hila, with enlargement of hilar lymph nodes. Cavitation indicates advanced infection and is the complication about which the surgeon is most often consulted. The diagnosis rests upon finding a positive skin test or complement fixation test and culturing the fungus from sputum or a bronchial aspirate.

Medical therapy of histoplasmosis is indicated only in cavitary and severe disease and for most infections in immunocompromised hosts. Ketoconazole (400 mg/d for 6 months)

or itraconazole (200–400 mg/d for 6 months) is useful in cavitary disease, while amphotericin B (1–2 g total dose) is reserved for patients with more serious infections and infections in immunocompromised patients. Surgery is reserved for treatment of complications and to rule out neoplastic disease in the case of suspicious pulmonary nodules. Broncholithectomy with or without pulmonary resection, repair of tracheobronchoesophageal fistulas, decompression of mediastinal granulomas, and spiral saphenous vein bypass of severe symptomatic superior vena cava obstruction are typical examples.

2. Coccidioidomycosis

Coccidioides immitis is a dimorphic soil fungus endemic to the Sonoran life zone (Utah, Arizona, California, Nevada, and New Mexico) and is associated with creosote brush. Dry heat with brief intense rain is essential for this fungus, which is spread by strong winds. Infection occurs through inhalation of as few as 1 to 10 arthrospores, which then germinate as parasitic spherules. Spherules have a double refractile cell wall and produce endospores that cause the spherule to rupture, spreading the infection into the surrounding tissues. Caseation, suppuration, abscess formation, and fibrosis follow. The diagnosis of coccidioidomycosis relies on the detection of acutely elevated titers of immunoglobulin M (IgM) antibodies (by latex agglutination and confirmed by immunodiffusion tube precipitin tests) or rising serum immunoglobulin G (IgG) antibody complement fixation titers (seroconversion or fourfold rise) in the appropriate clinical context. The coccidioidin and Spherulin skin tests, which become positive 3–21 days following infection, are generally useful only for epidemiologic studies and not for the diagnosis of acute disease. *C immitis* grows well in culture, but it is extremely hazardous to handle and requires a laminar flow hood due to the highly infectious nature of the arthrospores. Identification of the spherules in tissue, lavage samples, and fine-needle aspirates is helpful in making the diagnosis in some patients. Although many stains can be used, including routine fungal (potassium hydroxide, KOH) preparations, Pap staining is most sensitive. Gram stains, however, fail to demonstrate spherules.

Primary infection is asymptomatic in 60% of patients, while most others develop **desert fever,** with fever, productive cough, pleuritic chest pain, pneumonitis, and a rash typical of erythema nodosum or erythema multiforme. Disease that includes arthralgias is known as **desert rheumatism.** Radiographic findings demonstrate segmental or nonsegmental, homogeneous or mottled infiltrates with a predilection for the lower lobes. Physical examination is often unrevealing, but rales and rhonchi may be present. Other findings include eosinophilia (66%), hilar adenopathy (20%), and small exudative pleural effusions (2–20%). Symptomatic persistent infection associated with chest x-ray findings 6–8 weeks after primary infection is classified as one of five types: persistent pneumonia, chronic progressive pneumonia, miliary coccidioidomycosis, coccidioidal nodules, or pulmonary cavities. Persistent pneumonia manifests with symptoms of fever, productive cough, and pleuritic chest pain in association with protracted infiltrates and consolidation on chest x-ray generally resolving within 8 months. Patients with chronic progressive pneumonia complain of fever, cough, dyspnea, hemoptysis, and weight loss, with bilateral apical nodular densities and multiple cavities lasting years. This presentation closely resembles tuberculosis and chronic histoplasmosis. Miliary coccidioidomycosis occurs early and rapidly, associated with bilateral diffuse infiltrates. This form of disease implies the presence of impaired immunity and has an associated mortality rate of 50%. Nearly half of patients with coccidioidal nodules are asymptomatic. These nodular densities (coccidiomas) appear in the middle and upper lung fields, often within 5 cm of the hilum; range from 1 cm to 4 cm in size; and do not calcify, making it hard to distinguish them from malignancy. In endemic areas, 30–50% of all nodules are coccidiomas. Patients develop pulmonary cavities in 10–15% of cases of coccidioidomycosis. Typically, these are solitary (90%), thin-walled, located in the upper lobes (70%), less than 6 cm in size (90%), and close spontaneously within 2 years (50%). Some cavities, however, cross fissures; cause hemoptysis (25–50%), usually mild; rupture, producing a pyopneumothorax with a bronchopleural fistula; or become infected with aspergillus. Uncommonly, dissemination can occur, particularly in immunocompromised individuals, in pregnancy (third trimester), and in non-Caucasian individuals. Although pulmonary symptoms in disseminated disease are mild, meningeal involvement is common and the mortality rate is high (50%).

Medical therapy is not indicated in asymptomatic, immunocompetent individuals. Patients with persistent or chronic pneumonia, miliary disease, and those at risk for dissemination should be treated with antifungal therapy. Amphotericin B (0.5–2.5 g intravenously as total dose) is the standard treatment, though the newer azole compounds (fluconazole, ketoconazole, and itraconazole) may be used for long-term maintenance therapy, since the relapse rate may be as high as 25–50%. Surgery is reserved for patients with coccidiomas when cancer is a concern and in patients with cavities that have an associated radiographic abnormality suggesting carcinoma (ie, thick wall) or that develop a complication (eg, hemoptysis and pyopneumothorax from rupture). Resection should include all diseased tissue and most often requires lobectomy.

3. Blastomycosis

Blastomyces dermatitidis is a dimorphic soil fungus found in warm, wet, nitrogen-rich soil in an endemic area that extends east of a line from the Texas Gulf coast to the border between Minnesota and North Dakota (except Florida and New England). Infection occurs characteristically in males (male-to-female ratio 6:1–15:1) from 30–60 years of age through inhalation of conidia (asexual spores). At 37 °C the conidia germinate as yeasts, producing caseation in a manner similar to tuberculosis. Rarely, infection may develop through direct skin inoculation. Risk factors include poor hygiene, exposure to dust and wood, manual labor, and poor housing conditions. Since no accurate skin or serologic tests exist, the diagnosis depends on culture or histologic identification of the yeast form. Culture of the mycelial form can be hazardous. *B dermatitidis* grows as white to tan colonies of septate hyphae at room temperature but changes to budding yeast at 37 °C. This temperature-dependent change reflects the uncoupling of oxidative phosphorylation. The yeast form can be found in sputum (33%), bronchoalveolar lavage specimens (38%), lung biopsies (21%), and fine-needle aspirates (7%) and can be demonstrated with standard KOH preparations or many other histologic stains (but not Gram stain). The yeast, however, does not have a large capsule (distinguishes it from *Cryptococcus neoformans*) and does not grow intracellularly (differentiates it from *Histoplasma capsulatum*).

Manifestations of blastomycosis can occur in many organ systems, including the lungs, skin, bone, genitourinary tract (prostatitis and epididymoorchitis), and central nervous system. Pulmonary infection can be asymptomatic or may present with flulike symptoms, evidence of pneumonia, or pleurisy. Cough (36%), weight loss (20%), pleuritic pain (26%), fever (23%), hemoptysis (21%), erythema nodosum, and ulcerative bronchitis are common. Radiographic findings include homogeneous or patchy consolidation in a nonsegmental distribution with pleural effusions or thickening or cavitation (15–35%). In some patients, the appearance of pulmonary masses may mimic carcinoma. A predilection for the upper lobes has been noted; however, unlike histoplasmosis and coccidioidomycosis, in blastomycosis, hilar and mediastinal adenopathy is unusual.

Limited disease in asymptomatic immunocompetent patients requires no specific therapy. Itraconazole, 100–200 mg/d orally for at least 2–3 months, is now the therapy of choice for nonmeningeal disease, with a response rate of over 80%. Amphotericin B (0.5–2 g), however, is indicated in patients with meningeal disease or failed therapy. Surgical resection is rarely necessary except when the possibility of malignancy cannot be excluded.

4. Cryptococcosis

Cryptococcus neoformans is an encapsulated yeastlike budding fungus. It is a saprophyte existing on the skin, nasopharynx, gastrointestinal tract, and vagina of humans as well as in pigeon excreta, grasses, trees, plants, fruits, bees, wasps, insects (cockroaches), birds, milk products, pickle brine, and soil. Cryptococcal infection generally indicates the presence of an underlying debilitating disease in an immunocompromised host. Infection occurs from inhalation of the yeast form. The diagnosis can be established by the detection of serum antigen (via complement fixation tests) in patients with appropriate clinical and radiographic findings. More commonly, however, histologic identification with India ink stains is used; routine cultures are not performed because they are extremely time-consuming and require multiple biochemical tests for differentiation of cryptococcus from other fungi. No accurate skin test exists for cryptococcosis.

The most common sites of infection are the lungs and central nervous system. Pulmonary infection may remain asymptomatic, or patients may complain of cough, pleuritic chest pain, and fever. Radiographically, cryptococcus can appear as a localized, well-defined 3- to 10-cm pleural-based mass without smooth borders; as single or multiple areas of consolidation, usually within one lobe but in nonsegmental distribution; or as a disseminated miliary nodular infiltrate. A predilection for the lower lobes has been noted. Central nervous system infection usually follows an asymptomatic pulmonary infection. Central nervous system symptoms are highly variable, since many patients are severely immunocompromised and do not manifest the usual signs and symptoms of meningitis or cerebritis.

Medical therapy is indicated in most cases of pulmonary infection except for rare cases of limited localized disease. Amphotericin B (0.5–2 g) remains the treatment of choice and is often combined with flucytosine (150/mg/kg per day) for synergy. New azole compounds (eg, fluconazole, itraconazole, and voriconazole) have been used with increasing frequency as first-line therapy both as single agents and in combination. Surgery is rarely indicated and is useful only to exclude the possibility of malignancy or to determine the etiology of an undiagnosed diffuse pulmonary infiltrate by open lung biopsy.

5. Aspergillosis

Aspergillus species are ubiquitous dimorphic soil fungi found in soil and decaying organic matter. The most common pathogenic species include A fumigatus (most common), A niger, A flavus, and A glaucus. In culture, these fungi resemble an aspergillum, which is a brush used to sprinkle holy water. Aspergillosis represents the second-most common (after candidiasis) opportunistic fungal infection in immunocompromised hosts and the third-most common systemic fungal infection requiring hospital care. Infection occurs almost exclusively through inhalation of conidia into areas of lung with impaired mucociliary function (eg, tuberculous cavities). Although the diagnosis is supported by demonstrating immediate and delayed-type hypersensitivity skin reactions, by culturing uniform septate hyphae with dichotomous branching at 45 degrees, and by detecting specific IgG and IgE antibodies, a definitive diagnosis requires demonstration of hyphal tissue invasion or documentation of hyphae on methenamine silver stain in a suspected aspergilloma. Galactomannan enzyme-linked immunosorbent assays have recently become available and serve as a sensitive serum measure of invasive infection.

Infection with aspergillus species usually takes one of three forms: allergic bronchopulmonary aspergillosis, invasive aspergillosis, and aspergilloma. Allergic bronchopulmonary aspergillosis occurs in patients who are atopic (asthmatics) and in patients with cystic fibrosis. Endobronchial fungal growth leads to dilated airways filled with mucus and fungus. Continuous exposure to fungal antigens results in precipitating antibodies, increased IgE levels (which correlate with disease activity), and both immediate and delayed-type hypersensitivity. Patients complain of cough, fever, wheezing, dyspnea, pleuritic pain, and hemoptysis. Chest x-ray shows homogeneous densities in a "gloved-finger," inverted Y, or "cluster of grapes" pattern. Five stages have been defined depending on disease activity and steroid dependency: Stage 1 includes acute infection with characteristic x-ray and laboratory evidence of disease; stage 2 occurs with steroid-induced remission; stage 3 is characterized by asymptomatic exacerbations of laboratory and x-ray findings; steroid-dependent asthma with worsening laboratory tests (total IgE, precipitins, etc) is indicative of stage 4 disease; and end-stage fibrosis, bronchiectasis, and obstruction define stage 5.

Invasive aspergillosis is found exclusively in immunocompromised patients, particularly in patients with leukemia (50–70% of cases). Dissemination occurs frequently, and three types of pulmonary disease have been described: tracheobronchitis (uncommon), necrotizing bronchopneumonia, and hemorrhagic infarction (most common). In tracheobronchitis, disease is usually limited to the larger airways (bronchus more so than trachea) with little parenchymal involvement. Focal or diffuse mucosal ulceration, pseudomembranes, and intraluminal fungal plugs are common. Patients often present with cough, dyspnea, wheezing, and hemoptysis. Occasionally, patchy areas of atelectasis secondary to bronchial obstruction can be seen on chest x-ray. Necrotizing bronchopneumonia should be suspected in patients with unremitting fever, dyspnea, tachypnea, radiologic evidence of bronchopneumonia, and a poor response to standard antibiotic therapy. Finally, hemorrhagic infarction due to vascular permeation with nonthrombotic occlusion of small to medium-sized arteries and necrosis typically results in either a well-defined nodule or a wedge-shaped, pleura-based density. Symptoms are nonspecific and include fever, dyspnea, dry cough, pleuritic chest pain, and hemoptysis. Cavitation is common, and radiologic examination may reveal "round" pneumonia or "air crescents" of a mycotic lung sequestrum.

Aspergillomas ("fungus balls" or mycetomas) are divided into two types: simple, thin-walled cysts lined with ciliated epithelium and surrounded by normal parenchyma; and complex cavities associated with markedly abnormal surrounding lung tissue. Aspergillomas most often occur in the upper lobes and in the superior segments of the lower lobes. Although they may be multiple (22%), calcification and air-fluid levels are rare. Most aspergillomas—particularly complex ones—are associated with cavitary lung disease, ie, tuberculosis (most common), histoplasmosis, sarcoidosis, bronchiectasis, and others. Hemoptysis occurs in 50–80% and can present with frequent minor episodes (30% subsequently have massive bleeding), repeated moderate episodes, or a single episode of massive hemoptysis. Chest x-ray may reveal a 3- to 6-cm round, mobile density with a crescent of air.

Corticosteroids are indicated in patients with allergic bronchopulmonary aspergillosis in addition to measures to relieve bronchospasm (inhaled β-agonists or anticholinergics). In invasive aspergillosis, amphotericin B (0.5–2 g intravenously as total dose) has been standard therapy despite a mortality of 90%. In addition, some patients with complex aspergillomas and severe pulmonary disease are not candidates for surgical resection, and intracavitary amphotericin has been used with modest success. Surgery is indicated for complications of aspergillus infection. Hemoptysis due to aspergillomas is usually best treated by surgical resection. Furthermore, hemoptysis associated with localized invasive aspergillosis (particularly once cavitation has occurred) can be treated by resection and amphotericin B. Generally, wide excision (lobectomy) is required; however, in some high-risk patients with aspergillomas, cavernostomy and muscle flap closure is an alternative.

6. Mucormycosis

Infection with *Rhizopus arrhizus*, Absidia species, and Rhizomucor species of the class Zygomycetes and the order Mucorales occurs in certain distinct immunosuppressed patient populations: people with poorly controlled diabetes and leukemia patients. These fungi are ubiquitous organisms that are found in decaying fruit, vegetable matter, soil, and manure. Infection occurs following inhalation of sporangiospores, which germinate in a hyphal form. The diagnosis is made by demonstrating the organism in symptomatic patients. No accurate skin or serologic tests exist. Although the fungi do grow in culture as broad, irregular nonseptate hyphae that branch at angles up to 90 degrees (occasionally being confused with aspergillus species), most commonly the diagnosis is made on histologic examination. The sine qua non for mucormycosis is hyphal vascular invasion between the internal elastic membrane and the media of blood vessels, causing thrombosis, infarction, and necrosis.

In addition to pulmonary infections, mucormycosis manifests as distinct clinical syndromes such as rhinocerebral infection (direct extension into the central nervous system from paranasal sinus infection), cutaneous infection (burn patients), gastrointestinal infection (children with protein-calorie malnutrition), and disseminated infection (uremic patients receiving deferoxamine therapy). Patients with pulmonary infection complain of fever, cough, pleuritic chest pain, and hemoptysis. Frequently, this type of infection occurs in immunocompromised hosts and follows a fulminant course. Three patterns of infection are noted on chest x-ray: limited disease with involvement of a single lobe or segment, diffuse or disseminated disease with involvement of both

lungs and the mediastinum, and endobronchial disease with bronchial obstruction and secondary bacterial infection. Characteristic CT findings include a halo sign (area of low attenuation around a dense infiltrate), ring enhancement, and an air-crescent sign (area of contrast between normal lung and a radiodense cavitating lesion). Amphotericin B is standard treatment. In nonneutropenic patients, the newer azole compounds may be useful; however, infection with these fungi remains highly lethal, with a mortality of 90%. The cause of death in these patients is often fungal sepsis, progressive pulmonary dysfunction, and hemoptysis. In the small group of patients with limited disease, aggressive surgical resection in combination with amphotericin B has lowered the mortality to only 50%. In contrast, the endobronchial form can be effectively treated with transbronchoscopic resection (using the Nd:YAG laser) in a large proportion of patients.

7. Pneumocystosis

Pneumocystis carinii is a fungal organism that has been found in the lungs of a variety of domesticated and wild mammals and is distributed worldwide in humans. Pulmonary involvement leads to progressive pneumonia and respiratory insufficiency. Disease has been seen with increasing frequency in recipients of organ transplants who are undergoing immunosuppressive therapy. Diagnosis is made by open lung biopsy. Without treatment with trimethoprim-sulfamethoxazole, pentamidine, or inhaled antimicrobial therapy, the course is one of relentless progression. With improved antiviral therapy for HIV infections, the incidence of pneumocystosis has been declining.

Benfield TL et al: Prognostic markers of short-term mortality in AIDS-associated *Pneumocystis carinii* pneumonia. Chest 2001; 119:844.

Boyars MC, Zwischenberger JB, Cox CS Jr: Clinical manifestations of pulmonary fungal infections. J Thorac Imaging 1992;7:12.

Johnson P, Sarosi G: Current therapy of major fungal diseases of the lung. Infect Dis Clin North Am 1991;5:635.

Ledergerber B et al: Discontinuation of secondary prophylaxis against *Pneumocystis carinii* pneumonia in patients with HIV infection who have a response to antiretroviral therapy. Eight European Study Groups. N Engl J Med 2001;344:168.

Lopez Bernaldo de Quiros JC et al: A randomized trial of the discontinuation of primary and secondary prophylaxis against *Pneumocystis carinii* pneumonia after highly active antiretroviral therapy in patients with HIV infection. Grupo de Estudio del SIDA 04/98. N Engl J Med 2001;344:159.

Russian DA, Levine SJ: *Pneumocystis carinii* pneumonia in patients without HIV infection. Am J Med Sci 2001;321:56.

SARCOIDOSIS (BOECK SARCOID, BENIGN LYMPHOGRANULOMATOSIS)

Sarcoidosis is a noncaseating granulomatous disease of unknown cause involving the lungs, liver, spleen, lymph nodes, skin, and bones. The highest incidence is reported in Scandinavia, England, and the United States. The incidence in blacks is 10–17 times that in whites. Half of patients are between ages 20 and 40 years, with women more frequently affected than men.

Clinical Findings

A. Symptoms and Signs

Sarcoidosis may present with symptoms of pulmonary infection, but usually these are insidious and nonspecific. Erythema nodosum may herald the onset, and weight loss, fatigue, weakness, and malaise may appear later. Fever occurs in approximately 15% of cases. Pulmonary symptoms occur in 20–30% and include dry cough and dyspnea. Hemoptysis is rare. One fifth of patients with sarcoidosis have myocardial involvement, and heart block or failure may occur. Peripheral lymph nodes are enlarged in 75%, scalene lymph nodes are microscopically involved in 80% and mediastinal nodes in 90%, and cutaneous involvement is present in 30%. Hepatic and splenic involvement can be shown by biopsy in 70% of cases. There may be migratory or persistent polyarthritis, and central nervous involvement occurs in a few patients.

B. Imaging Studies

The x-ray findings in sarcoidosis are classified into five descriptive categories or stages (Table 18–6). Pulmonary disease can manifest as a reticulonodular infiltrate, an acinar pattern of opacities, or large nodules with or without mediastinal adenopathy. Mediastinal lymph node involvement characteristically includes bilateral symmetric hilar and paratracheal lymphadenopathy. Anterior or posterior mediastinal adenopathy or asymmetric hilar involvement should prompt a suspicion of other diseases, particularly Hodgkin disease and non-Hodgkin lymphomas. Pleural effusions and cavitation are rare and, if present, necessitate an evaluation for tuberculosis, congestive heart failure, and coincidental pneumonia.

Diagnosis

Although no single test exists to confirm absolutely the diagnosis of sarcoidosis (the diagnosis remains one of exclusion), it may be suggested by the characteristic radiographic appearance of bilateral hilar and mediastinal lymphadenopathy, by gallium 67 scanning, and by elevated serum and bronchoalveolar fluid levels of angiotensin-converting enzyme and lysozyme. Pathologic documentation of noncaseating granulomas should normally be obtained either via transbronchial biopsy or mediastinoscopy (more reliable, with > 95% success rate). Culture for mycobacteria, fungi, and other atypical infections must also be negative.

Treatment

Asymptomatic patients and those with minimal clinical disease may require no therapy. Corticosteroids have been used in patients with pulmonary impairment and symptomatic disease with good success. Despite the indolent nature of the

Table 18–6. Radiographic Stages of Sarcoidosis.

Stage 0: No x-ray abnormality
Stage 1: Hilar and mediastinal lymph node enlargement without pulmonary abnormalities
Stage 2: Hilar and mediastinal lymph node enlargement with pulmonary abnormalities
Stage 3: Diffuse pulmonary disease without adenopathy
Stage 4: Pulmonary fibrosis

disease and steroid therapy, long-term mortality is reported as high as 10%. Lung transplantation has been utilized with success in patients refractory to medical management.

NEOPLASMS OF THE LUNG

PRIMARY LUNG CANCER

Lung cancer is the most common cause of cancer-related deaths in both men and women in the United States. In 2004, it is estimated that 165,500 new cases and 155,000 deaths will occur due to pulmonary malignancies. This represents 15% of all new cancer cases and 28% of all cancer-related deaths. In addition, although the incidence in males appears to have stabilized, the incidence continues to rise rapidly in females.

Tobacco smoking accounts for 85% of all lung cancer cases. The effect is greatest for cigarettes and least for pipe smoking and is directly related to the amount of tobacco smoked. Following 5–6 years of smoking cessation, the risk exponentially declines, and after 15 years approaches, but never reaches, that of nonsmokers. "Passive" exposure to cigarette smoke, on the other hand, increases the risk in nonsmokers by two to three times. Exposure to all forms of asbestos (amosite, chrysotile, and crocidolite) has been implicated in as many as 23% of lung cancers, accounting for the high incidence among shipyard workers, insulators, cement makers, truck drivers, and plumbers. The effect is particularly pronounced in smokers and is most commonly associated with squamous cell and small cell carcinoma. Recently, exposure to radon and its alpha-emitting daughter isotopes have been implicated in the increased incidence of lung cancer in both uranium miners and populations living in geographic areas naturally contaminated with high levels of radon gas. Although it has been known for some time that people with high activity of 4-debrisoquine hydroxylase, the so-called debrisoquine metabolic phenotype, have a 10-fold increased risk of lung cancer, only recently has the role of genetic factors been appreciated. Chromosome deletions (particularly 11p, 13q, 17p, and 3p), tumor suppressor gene mutations (p53, Hap-1, ErbAb, etc), and constitutive, high-level expression of both growth factor genes (insulinlike and transferrinlike growth factors), epidermal growth factor receptors (HER2/neu, EGFR1, etc), and protooncogenes (c-, N- and

L-*myc*; H-, N-, and K-*ras*; and c-*myb*) have all been implicated in the pathogenesis of lung cancer. Other factors such as vitamin A deficiency, air pollution; exposure to arsenic, cadmium, chromium, ether, and formaldehyde; and employment as bakers, cooks, construction workers, cosmetologists, leather workers, pitchblende miners, printers, rubber workers, and pottery workers have also been incriminated. Finally, certain diseases (eg, progressive systemic sclerosis [scleroderma]) have a defined predisposition for the development of lung cancer. Silencing of genes by aberrant promoter hypermethylation is viewed as a crucial component in lung cancer pathobiology. Newer polymerase chain reaction (PCR) assays for specific methylation events have permitted identification of genes implicated in the progression of lung cancers.

▶ Pathology

Lung cancer occurs more commonly in the right lung than the left, and the upper lobes are involved more commonly than the lower lobes or the right middle lobe. Synchronous primary lung cancers occur in up to 7% of patients, and 10% of patients will develop a metachronous new tumor (2% per year risk postresection of early stage disease). Furthermore, patients with lung cancer are at higher risk of developing cancers of the upper respiratory tract, oral cavity, esophagus, bladder, and kidney presumably related to the "field effect" of smoking. Lung cancers typically spread by local extension to involve the visceral and parietal pleura, chest wall, great vessels, pericardium, diaphragm, esophagus, and vertebral column. Common sites of metastatic involvement include the ipsilateral pulmonary and hilar lymph nodes, the mediastinal lymph nodes, the lung, liver, bone, brain, adrenal glands, pancreas, kidney, soft tissues, and myocardium. The exact pathologic classification of lung cancer has not been uniform despite attempts at standardization by the World Health Organization. Functionally, however, squamous cell carcinoma, large cell carcinoma, and adenocarcinoma are grouped together under the designation of non–small cell carcinomas and constitute 80% of all lung tumors. Small cell carcinoma represents 15–20%, while bronchial gland adenomas, including carcinoids, comprise the remaining 5%. The differential locations of some of these neoplasms are summarized in Table 18–7.

A. Squamous Cell Carcinoma

The major pathologic features of squamous cell carcinoma are keratinization, cellular stratification, and intercellular bridges. Squamous cell carcinomas account for about 20% of all cases of lung cancer and 70% of non–small cell tumors. Two thirds are located centrally near the hilum and one third peripherally. The growth rate and the rate of metastasis tend to be slower than those of other lung tumors.

B. Adenocarcinoma

Adenocarcinomas, which constitute 30% of lung cancers and 60% of non–small cell tumors, are characterized as acinar,

Table 18–7. Location of Lung Cancer by Histologic Type.[1]

Histology	Central (%)	Peripheral (%)
Squamous cell carcinoma	64–81	19–36
Adenocarcinoma	5–29	71–95
Large cell carcinoma	42–49	51–58
Small cell carcinoma	74–83	17–26
Overall	63	37

[1]From Cameron RB: Malignancies of the lung. In: *Practical Oncology*. Cameron RB (editor). Originally published by Appleton & Lange. Copyright © 1994 by The McGraw-Hill Companies, Inc.

papillary, and bronchoalveolar. Acinar adenocarcinoma is composed of glands lined by columnar cells that secrete mucin. Bronchoalveolar carcinoma is characterized by intraluminal papillary fragments that appear in alveoli or small bronchioles. Bronchoalveolar carcinoma may be spread by aerosol transmission. The incidence of adenocarcinoma of the lung is increasing relative to squamous cell carcinoma, perhaps as a consequence of the rise in lung cancer among women, although the exact cause remains unclear.

C. Small Cell Carcinoma

Small cell (oat cell) carcinomas have small, round nuclei with nuclear chromatin and cytoplasm. They are so biologically and clinically distinct from all other cell types that the term non–small cell lung cancer (NSCLC) often is applied to all other cell types. Small cell carcinomas comprise 15–20% of all lung cancers. They occur centrally, metastasize early, and are the most resistant to combined-modality treatment.

D. Large Cell Carcinoma

Large cell carcinomas are composed of large polygonal spindle or oval cells arranged in sheets, nests, or clusters. Multinucleated giant cells, intracellular hyalin droplets, glycogen, and acidophilic nuclear inclusions may be present. These tumors are seen peripherally and are less common.

E. Adenosquamous Tumors

Adenosquamous tumors show both cellular features and are more biologically aggressive than other non–small cell lung cancers. Survival percentages of patients with adenosquamous tumors are significantly lower than what is reported for adenocarcinoma or squamous cell cancer.

F. Bronchial Gland Adenomas

Bronchial gland adenoma is a misnomer, since the vast majority of these tumors are malignant. Included in this group are carcinoid tumors, adenoid cystic carcinomas, mucoepidermoid carcinoma, mixed tumors of the salivary gland type, and mucous gland adenoma. Carcinoid tumors are derived from Kulchitsky cells, have a vascular stroma, and tend to be located centrally in proximal airways. Although they are slow-growing, they can metastasize widely. Carcinoid syndrome is rarely associated with bronchial carcinoids, as opposed to intestinal carcinoids that metastasize to the liver. Adenoid cystic carcinomas—also referred to as cylindromas—feature groups of epithelial cells that form ductlike structures interspersed with cystic spaces. These neoplasms are locally aggressive and often extend beyond apparent gross pathologic margins. Metastases from adenoid cystic carcinomas often involve the lung, are slow growing, and are amenable to surgical excision. Mucoepidermoid carcinomas are rare tumors characterized by the presence of squamous cells, mucus-secreting cells, and an intermediate cell type. The cells are bland and less aggressive than those of adenosquamous carcinomas. Mixed tumors of the salivary type are extremely rare infiltrating tumors that are curable with wide local excision. Finally, mucus gland adenomas (papillary or bronchial cyst adenomas) are the only true benign "adenomas" of this group with no metastatic potential. These neoplasms are rare tumors of the major bronchi and consist of numerous mucus-filled cysts lined by a well-differentiated epithelium. Generally, bronchoscopic removal can be accomplished and results in long-term cure.

Clinical Presentation

Nearly 94% of patients present with symptoms from the effects of the primary tumor, regional spread, or metastatic disease. Local effects of the primary tumor account for 27% of presenting symptoms and vary depending on the location of the tumor. Central tumors are associated with cough, hemoptysis, respiratory difficulty (wheezing, stridor, or dyspnea), pain, and pneumonia. Peripheral tumors can cause cough, chest wall pain, pleural effusions, pulmonary abscess, Horner syndrome (ipsilateral miosis, ptosis, and anhidrosis), and Pancoast syndrome (ipsilateral shoulder and arm pain in the C8–T1 nerve root distribution, Horner syndrome, and a superior sulcus—usually squamous—lung cancer). Symptoms due to the effect of regional spread include hoarseness from recurrent nerve paralysis, dyspnea due to phrenic nerve paralysis, dysphagia from compression of the esophagus, superior vena cava syndrome from compression or invasion of the superior vena cava, and pericardial tamponade from invasion of the pericardium. Metastatic disease may present with symptoms of systemic illness (anorexia, weight loss, weakness, and malaise), local manifestations of distant metastases (jaundice, abdominal mass, bony pain or fracture, neurologic deficits, mental status changes, seizures, and soft tissue masses). A number of paraneoplastic syndromes associated with lung cancer have been identified (Table 18–8).

Table 18–8. Paraneoplastic Syndromes Associated with Lung Cancer.

Cardiovascular
Thrombophlebitis
Nonbacterial thrombotic endocarditis
Neuromuscular
Subacute cerebellar degeneration
Dementia
Limbic encephalitis
Optic neuritis, retinopathy
Subacute necrotic myelopathy
Autonomic neuropathy (small cell)
Myasthenic (Eaton-Lambert) syndrome (small cell)
Polymyositis
Gastrointestinal
Carcinoid syndrome (carcinoid and small cell)
Anorexia, cachexia
Hematologic
Erythrocytosis
Leukocytosis
Metabolic
Inappropriate adrenocorticotropic hormone (ACTH) (small cell)
Inappropriate antidiuretic hormone (ADH) (small cell)
Hypercalcemia (squamous cell carcinoma)
Inappropriate gonadotropins
Dermatologic
Acanthosis nigricans (adenocarcinoma)
Dermatomyositis
Erythema gyratum
Ichthyosis
Other
Hypertrophic pulmonary osteoarthropathy (squamous cell, large cell, and adenocarcinoma)
Nephrotic syndrome
Fever

Diagnosis & Workup

Lung cancer is usually suspected from abnormal findings on a chest x-ray obtained in the course of a routine physical examination or, more commonly, after a complaint of pulmonary symptoms (see previous discussion). Findings vary from a small peripheral nodule to an unresolving infiltrate or even total lung atelectasis. Occasionally, the location of the abnormality may suggest certain cell types (Table 18–7). Despite the utility of chest x-rays in the diagnosis of lung cancer, prospective randomized trials at three major institutions have failed to demonstrate a survival benefit from mass screening programs incorporating chest x-rays with or without the addition of sputum cytologic examinations. Newer PCR assays of sputum seeking methylation events in expectorated bronchial epithelial cells show promise as a screening tool but are yet to be widely applied or vigorously studied. Once the diagnosis of lung cancer is suspected, a definitive diagnosis can be obtained in over 90% of patients with either bronchoscopy for proximal lesions or fine-needle aspiration cytology for peripheral lesions.

Currently, CT scanning is an integral part of the assessment of patients with lung cancer. Chest CT scans should also include the upper abdomen to assess two of the most common sites of metastases (liver and adrenal glands). Injection of intravenous contrast while the scan is obtained facilitates evaluation of the mediastinum. Additional radiographic workup includes tests to evaluate other common sites of metastases, such as bone and brain. A serum alkaline phosphatase is essential, and a bone scan and brain CT scan (or preferably MRI) should be obtained if indicated by elevated alkaline phosphatase levels, neurologic symptoms, or bone pain or if advanced-stage disease (stage III or beyond) is present. Fluorodeoxyglucose (FDG) PET has evolved into a critical staging test. It is most effective at assay for distant occult disease. It can be helpful for assessing mediastinal node involvement, but it is not definitive. False-positive rates as high as 15–20% have been reported. Furthermore, nodules less than 1 cm in diameter are generally not reliably imaged by PET scanning. Combination high-resolution CT scan and PET scan assessment permits improved correlation of abnormal CT findings with FDG uptake suggestive of tumor. Thoracentesis or thoracoscopy (or both) should be performed in any patient with evidence of a pleural effusion to exclude diffuse involvement of the pleura (T4 or stage IIIB disease), which makes the lesion incurable with surgery. Despite increasing reliance on PET scan to stage the mediastinum, patients with non–small cell lung cancer but without metastatic disease should be evaluated with cervical mediastinoscopy and parasternal mediastinotomy (Chamberlain) if necessary to document the status of the mediastinal nodes in equivocal cases. PET scanning is informative but less accurate than mediastinoscopy. With small cell lung cancer, however, this usually is not necessary. The use of CT scans alone is inaccurate in 40–60% of patients with enlarged lymph nodes over 1 cm (false positive) and 15% of patients without "significant" lymphadenopathy (false negative). Once all the information from these staging procedures is in hand, the patient with non–small cell lung cancer can be classified into one of three categories: (1) early lung cancer without mediastinal involvement, or stage I/II (see next section); (2) locally advanced lung cancer, or stage IIIA/B; and (3) metastatic lung cancer, or stage IV. Therapy is determined by disease stage. Patients with small cell lung cancer are usually grouped into two categories: disease limited to the ipsilateral hemithorax, including supraclavicular nodes (limited disease), or disease extending beyond the thorax (extensive disease, ie, below the diaphragm or brain metastases).

▶ Staging

By 1987, the American Joint Committee on Cancer (AJCC) and the Union Internationale Contre le Cancer (UICC) had developed a joint staging system for lung carcinoma based on data gathered primarily by Clifford Mountain of the MD Anderson Cancer Center. The lung cancer staging system is based on the tumor (T), the status of regional lymph nodes (N), and the presence or absence of distant metastases (M), as outlined in Table 18–9.

Table 18–9. TNM Stage Groupings.

Primary tumor	
TX	Primary tumor cannot be assessed, or cytologic evidence of malignant cells in sputum or bronchial washings but not visualized by imaging or bronchoscopy
T0	No evidence of primary tumor
Tis	Carcinoma in situ
T1	Tumor ≤ 3 cm in greatest diameter, completely surrounded by lung or visceral pleura, and without bronchoscopic evidence of involvement of more proximal than a lobar bronchus
T2	Tumor > 3 cm in greatest diameter, invading the visceral pleura, involving the main stem bronchus but > 2 cm distal to the carina, or tumor associated with atelectasis or obstructive pneumonitis extending to the hilum but not involving the entire lung
T3	Tumor of any size invading the chest wall, diaphragm, mediastinal pleura, parietal pericardium; tumor involving the main stem bronchus within 2 cm of but not involving the carina; or tumor associated with atelectasis or obstructive pneumonitis of the entire lung
T4	Tumor of any size invading the mediastinum, heart, great vessels, trachea, esophagus, vertebral body, or carina or tumor associated with a malignant pleural effusion

Regional lymph nodes (N stage)	
NX	Regional lymph nodes cannot be assessed
N0	No evidence of regional lymph node metastases
N1	Metastases in ipsilateral peribronchial or hilar lymph nodes, including by direct extension
N2	Metastases in ipsilateral mediastinal or subcarinal lymph nodes
N3	Metastases in contralateral mediastinal or hilar lymph nodes or ipsilateral or contralateral scalene or supraclavicular nodes

Distant metastases (M stage)	
MX	Presence of distant metastases cannot be assessed
M0	No evidence of distant metastases
M1	Distant metastases are present

Stage grouping	
Occult disease	TX, N0, M0
Stage 0	Tis, N0, M0
Stage IA	T1, N0, M0
Stage IB	T2 N0 M0
Stage IIA	T1 N1 M0
Stage IIB	T2 N1 M0
	T3 N0 M0
Stage IIIA	T1-2, N2, M0, or T3, N0-2, M0
Stage IIIB	T4, any N, M0, or any T, N3, M0
Stage IV	Any T, Any N, M1

Treatment

Treatment for small cell carcinoma consists primarily of chemotherapy and radiation, though recent data indicate that for early disease (T1–T2 lesions and limited hilar adenopathy) resection may improve local control and result in increased long-term survival (as high as 50%), particularly when combined with postoperative chemotherapy. Treatment for non–small cell lung cancer, however, varies with stage. Early-stage disease (stage I/II) has historically been treated with surgery alone. However, the results of several randomized prospective trials involving adjuvant chemotherapy for early (Ib and higher) non–small cell lung cancer suggest benefit. Locally advanced but surgically resectable disease (stage IIIA) is currently best treated with combined-modality therapy utilizing induction chemotherapy or chemoradiotherapy followed by surgery and, if necessary, postoperative radiotherapy. Locally advanced and surgically unresectable disease (stage IIIB) is best managed with concurrent platinum-based chemotherapy and fractionated radiation therapy. Metastatic disease (stage IV) is only poorly treated with chemotherapy. Radiotherapy in this case is reserved for symptomatic lesions. Combined-agent chemotherapy offers 2–3 months (20%) survival extension to advanced-stage patients. It has been shown to be cost-effective and improve quality of life and is generally well tolerated by patients with reasonable performance status. New biologic agents—so-called targeted therapies—are showing activity in clinical trials and should improve overall survival statistics. It is hoped that with advances in targeted and conventional therapies, the current overall survival (< 15% at 5 years) of patients with lung cancer can be improved.

Induction Chemotherapy

Recently completed clinical trials and several ongoing clinical trials suggest survival benefit of treatment with platinum-based chemotherapy prior to definitive resection. Induction chemotherapy has been standard for locally advanced surgically resectable disease, but evidence is accumulating to support induction therapy in early stage non–small cell lung cancer.

A. Surgical Treatment

1. Surgical staging—As noted earlier, almost all patients with non–small cell lung cancer limited to the thorax should undergo cervical mediastinoscopy to exclude involvement of N2 mediastinal lymph nodes (N2 or N3 disease). A possible exception is a small peripheral (T1) nodule, especially of squamous cell histology without any evidence for mediastinal adenopathy on chest CT scan. PET scan is used with increasing frequency to stage the mediastinum. Surgical staging with cervical mediastinoscopy remains the most accurate staging maneuver. Adenocarcinomas with negative mediastinal nodes by CT have an 18–25% false-negative rate. For left-sided lesions, left parasternal mediastinotomy

(Chamberlain) may be required to assess the status of the aorticopulmonary lymph nodes. Without pathologic confirmation of the status of mediastinal lymph nodes, CT scans have been associated with high false-positive and false-negative rates. A surgical assessment of the proximal airways is also required even if this means repeating this invasive procedure, often previously performed by the pulmonologist. Because treatment decisions are based on accurate staging and treatment of early-stage disease (stage I/II) differs significantly from locally advanced disease (stage IIIA/B), this approach is essential. The importance of accurate staging for patients with non–small cell lung cancer cannot be overstated.

2. Indications and preoperative assessment—Surgical resection is indicated for early-stage lung cancer (stage I/II) and in combination with chemotherapy and radiation in locally advanced resectable disease (stage IIIA or resectable T4, IIIb). In addition, surgery may be indicated for patients with a single site of metastatic disease, such as a solitary brain or adrenal gland metastasis. Both relative and absolute contraindications to surgical resection are listed in Table 18–10.

Preoperative assessment is aimed at evaluating both cardiopulmonary reserve and overall patient fitness. The patient's general performance status or functional classification is probably the most accurate factor in predicting a successful outcome following surgery. Advanced age, by itself, is not a contraindication to surgery. It is the physiologic age, as manifested by functional status—not the

Table 18–10. Medical and Surgical Contraindications to Pulmonary Resection.

Absolute	Relative
Myocardial infarction within previous 3 months	Myocardial infarction within previous 6 months
SVC syndrome (due to metastatic tumor)	SVC syndrome (due to primary tumor)
Bilateral endobronchial tumor	Recurrent laryngeal nerve paralysis (due to primary tumor in aortico-pulmonary window)
Contralateral lymph node metastases (N3)	Horner syndrome
Malignant pleural effusion	Small cell histology
Distant metastases (except solitary brain and adrenal metastases)	Metastases higher than the midtracheal lymph nodes
	Pericardial involvement
	FEV_1 < 0.8 L (< 50%)
	FEV_1 0.9–2.4 and insufficient pulmonary reserve for planned resection
	Main pulmonary artery involvement

chronologic age—that is important. A thorough cardiac evaluation is also necessary, since lung cancer and cardiac disease share common risk factors (eg, smoking). Patients with cardiac symptoms, an abnormal ECG, or other findings suggestive of ischemic heart disease should be screened by a stress test (exercise treadmill, dipyridamole- or adenosine-thallium study, dobutamine echocardiogram). Significant left main coronary artery disease should be treated with coronary artery bypass prior to any contemplated pulmonary resection, and other significant disease should be individually assessed for possible bypass or angioplasty. Furthermore, significant pulmonary hypertension and myocardial infarction within 3 months are associated with up to 20% perioperative mortality and constitute absolute contraindications to surgery. Other high-risk findings include myocardial infarction within 6 months, ventricular arrhythmias, and heart block, particularly left posterior fascicular hemiblock. Finally, the patient's pulmonary function and ability to tolerate the required pulmonary resection need to be assessed. This is accomplished with pulmonary function tests (spirometry, diffusing capacity, exercise oximetry) and with differential (quantitative) ventilation-perfusion scanning when appropriate. In a 70 kg patient, the following preoperative studies indicate high morbidity risk and are relative contraindications to resection: forced expiratory volume in 1 second (FEV_1) below 0.8 L, a predicted postoperative FEV_1 below 0.8, a predicted maximum voluntary ventilation under 50%, a $PaCO_2$ higher than 45 mm Hg, and a PaO_2 less than 50 mm Hg. A diffusion limitation capacity of carbon monoxide (DLCO) under 60% predicted is correlated with an increase in perioperative mortality.

3. Surgical resection

A. EARLY AND LOCALLY ADVANCED NON–SMALL CELL LUNG CANCER—The extent of pulmonary resection is dictated by the location of the primary tumor and the presence or absence of involved hilar (interlobar) lymph nodes. Limited segmental resection for stage I/II non–small cell lung cancer has been evaluated by the Lung Cancer Study Group and found to result in an increased local recurrence rate (15% versus 3%) and lower overall survival. Segmental resections, therefore, are viewed as compromise procedures indicated only in patients who cannot tolerate lobectomy. Lobectomy continues to be the standard of care for resection for non–small cell lung cancer. This should include a 1-cm margin of normal proximal bronchus. Samples of interlobar (hilar) lymph nodes are submitted for immediate pathologic examination to exclude involvement that would require pneumonectomy. A "sleeve" resection of main stem bronchus can also be included in the resection, particularly with the right upper lobe. Pneumonectomy is required for proximal lesions involving the main stem bronchus or the interlobar (hilar) lymph nodes. In addition, techniques are available for more extensive resection such as intrapericardial pneumonectomy

and tracheal sleeve pneumonectomy. The overall mortality rates following segmental resection, lobectomy, and pneumonectomy are 1.4%, 2.9%, and 6.2%, respectively, in centers with large experience. Complications following pulmonary resection include cardiac arrhythmias, hemorrhage, infection (empyema), bronchopleural fistula, respiratory insufficiency, and pulmonary embolism.

B. ADVANCED (METASTATIC) NON–SMALL CELL LUNG CANCER—Patients with solitary brain and adrenal metastases, especially if metachronous, are still candidates for surgical resection and have benefited by prolonged survival in a few small retrospective studies in comparison with historical controls. Systemic preoperative (induction) chemotherapy and radiotherapy, however, should be administered initially. In addition, transbronchial Nd:YAG laser resection of tumors obstructing the proximal airways can significantly palliate selected patients. In addition, improvements in the design and deployment techniques of expansile stents have been a significant advance for palliation of proximal airway obstruction. Finally, photodynamic laser therapy with photosensitizers can alleviate airway obstruction from tumors, albeit not as quickly as Nd:YAG laser ablation.

C. SMALL CELL LUNG CANCER—Resection for small peripheral tumors followed by aggressive postoperative chemotherapy may increase the local control rate and potentially the overall survival rate in the early small cell lung cancer. Survival rates as high as 50% with this approach have been reported.

B. Radiation Therapy

1. Non–small cell lung cancer—Radiation therapy can be administered with curative intent in stage I/II disease in patients who refuse or are not medically suitable candidates for surgery. The 5-year survival rate with this approach, however, is only 22–33%. With locally advanced disease (stage IIIA/B), radiation therapy (5500–6000 cGy) until recently has been the treatment of choice. Although local or nodal recurrence rates are less than 30%, long-term survival is less than 10% in these patients, and the type of fractionation scheme has not altered the outcome. Adjuvant radiation therapy following surgical resection has been extensively studied by the Lung Cancer Study Group and has been found to decrease local or nodal recurrences but not to prolong overall survival. A much-disputed meta-analysis (the PORT study) showed a decrease in survival for stage II patients treated with postoperative radiation. Differences in radiotherapy techniques within the analysis may account for the worse outcomes. Preoperative radiation has been used with T3 lesions, particularly Pancoast tumors, with improved survival; however, there is no objective evidence that radiation must be given preoperatively. Recently, a multicenter intergroup trial (SWOG) showed a significant survival advantage for combined chemoradiotherapy (etoposide, platinum, and 4500 cGy) prior to resection for Pancoast (superior sulcus) tumors that were N1 or less. Complete resection rates were improved, 20–25% complete pathologic responses were achieved, and survival was significantly improved (45–50% at 3 years) over surgery alone or preoperative radiotherapy and surgery. Intraoperative radiation has been investigated but to date has been associated with unacceptably high morbidity. Finally, in patients with metastatic disease, therapeutic radiation is indicated in patients with symptoms of pain, neurologic symptoms, and symptoms of superior vena cava compression.

2. Small cell lung cancer—Multiple randomized trials comparing the combination of radiation and chemotherapy to chemotherapy alone in limited-stage small cell lung cancer have been conducted. The majority show improved local control and modest (3–4 months) prolonged survival with the combination. This was at the cost of increased morbidity, however. In extensive disease, no benefit has been demonstrated for radiation therapy outside of palliative radiation of symptomatic metastases. Prophylactic cranial irradiation may be beneficial but can cause significant cognitive deficits.

C. Chemotherapy

1. Non–small cell lung cancer—Although chemotherapy alone has not generally been used in the treatment of early or locally advanced non–small cell lung cancer, combinations of chemotherapy and radiotherapy have been evaluated in locally advanced unresectable disease. In some instances, no benefit to the combination was demonstrated, particularly when only single agents were used; however, improved results with both radiation and combined-agent chemotherapy have recently been documented. In the presence of metastatic disease, multiple trials of combination chemotherapy have demonstrated a modest improvement in overall survival (14 weeks or 25% improved survival) but not without some toxicity. Even so, quality of life assessments and cost analyses support the use of outpatient combined-agent chemotherapy over palliative care alone.

A. POSTOPERATIVE ADJUVANT THERAPY—A progressive trend in lung cancer therapy has evolved in favor of far more widespread use of adjuvant chemotherapy. Three large mul-

ticenter randomized trials in Europe and North America have served as a basis for the increased application of postoperative platinum-based chemotherapy (Italian Stage IB, the International Adjuvant Lung Cancer Trial [IALT], Cancer and Leukemia Group B [CALGB] 9633, and National Cancer Institute of Canada [NCIC] BR10). The benefit of chemotherapy appears to vary based on patient selection but is estimated to be an increase of 5–15% survival measured at 5 years from diagnosis (Table 18–11).

2. Small cell lung cancer—Combination chemotherapy currently produces 85–95% and 75–85% response rates in limited-stage and extensive-stage disease, respectively. Furthermore, median survival is 12–16 months and 7–11 months in each group. Three or four drugs have been shown to be optimal. One of the most effective regimens combines cyclophosphamide, doxorubicin, and vincristine. In addition, a regimen of cisplatin and etoposide has been active in salvage. The optimal duration of therapy has not been defined, but the majority of the effect appears to occur within the first four cycles.

D. Immunotherapy

Immunotherapy using bacillus Calmette-Guérin (BCG), levamisole, IL-2, TNF-α, lymphokine-activated killer (LAK) cells, and tumor-infiltrating lymphocytes has not proved beneficial in any clinical studies to date.

E. Targeted Therapies

Molecular-based therapies targeting overexpressed growth receptors (*EGFR1*, HER-2/*neu*) by monoclonal antibody or small molecules are beginning to show clinical effectiveness. Additional agents targeting signal transduction pathways (eg, farnesyl transferase inhibitors) for the *ras* pathway as well as antisense oligonucleotide and gene therapies are all in advanced clinical testing stages and in combination with standard cytotoxic chemotherapy appear to enhance response rates. A current prospective randomized trial from Canada (CAN-NCIC-BR19) is aimed at addressing the effectiveness of EGF inhibition in conjunction with platinum-based chemotherapeutics in the adjuvant setting.

Table 18–11. Adjuvant Trials Favoring Use of Chemotherapy in Completely Resected Non–Small Cell Lung Cancer.[1]

Study	CT Regimen	Radiation Therapy	5-year Survival CT vs. Control
Italian Stage IB Study	Cis/Etoposide × 6	No	63% vs. 45%
IALT LeChevalier	Various platinum	Yes ±	44.5% vs. 40.4%
CALGB 9633 Strauss	Carbo/Taxol × 4	No	69% vs. 54%
JBR.10 Alam	Vin/P × 4	No	71% vs. 59%[2]

[1]CT, Carbo/Taxol, carboplatin paclitaxel; Vin/P, vinorelbine cisplatin; Cis, cisplatin.
[2]4-year survival statistics.

Prognosis

A. Non–Small Cell Lung Cancer

The survival of patients with non–small cell lung cancer is highly dependent on the pathologic stage. Overall, the 5-year survival of patients with stages I, II, IIIA, IIIB, and IV is 43–64%, 20–40%, 15–25%, 5–7%, and less than 2%, respectively. A breakdown of survival by TNM classification is set forth in Table 18–12. Improved survival will likely depend on earlier diagnosis and further coordinated efforts among surgeons, medical oncologists, and radiation oncologists.

B. Small Cell Lung Cancer

Patients with limited-stage disease achieve a median survival of 12–16 months with 5–25% 2-year survival, while those with extensive-stage disease have a median survival of only 7–11 months, with only 1–3% surviving 2 years.

Albain KS et al: Long-term survival after concurrent cisplatin/etoposide (PE) plus chest radiotherapy (RT) followed by surgery in bulky stages IIIA N2 and IIIB non-small cell lung cancer (NSCLC): 6-year outcomes from Southwest Oncology Group study 8805. Proc Am Soc Clin Oncol 1999;18:467a (abst.)

Albain KS et al: Concurrent cisplatin/etoposide plus chest radiotherapy followed by surgery for stages IIIA N2 and IIIB non-small cell lung cancer: mature results of Southwest Oncology Group Phase II study 8805. J Clin Oncol 1995;13:1880.

Friedel G et al: Neoadjuvant chemoradiotherapy of stage III non-small cell lung cancer. Lung Cancer 2000;30:175.

Grunenwald DH et al: Benefit of surgery after chemoradiotherapy in stage IIIB (T4 and/or N3) non-small cell lung cancer. J Thorac Cardiovasc Surg 2001;122:796.

Table 18–12. Survival in Non–Small Cell Lung Cancer.

Stage	TNM Description	Five-Year Survival
I		70–76%
a	T1, N0	80–83%
b	T2, N0	60–65%
II		30–40%
a	T1, N1	32–40%
b	T2, N1	28–35%
	T3, N0	
IIIA		10–30%
	T3, N1	30–45%
	T1–2, N2	7–30%
	T3, N2	0–5%
IIIB		<10%
	T4, any N	<10%
	Any T, N3	<10%
IV	M1	<5%
Overall		14.5%

Le Chevalier et al: Should adjuvant chemotherapy become standard treatment in all patients with resected non-small-cell lung cancer? Lancet Oncol 2005;6:182.

Pisters KMW, Le Chevalier T: Adjuvant chemotherapy in completely resected non-small-cell lung cancer. J Clin Oncol 2005;23:3270.

Rosell R et al: A randomized trial comparing preoperative chemotherapy plus surgery with surgery alone in patients with non-small cell lung cancer. N Engl J Med 1994;330:153.

Roth JA et al: A randomized trial comparing perioperative chemotherapy and surgery with surgery alone in resectable stage IIIA non-small cell lung cancer. J Natl Cancer Inst 1994;86:673.

Schiller JH et al: Comparison of four chemotherapy regimens for advanced non-small-cell lung cancer. N Engl J Med 2002;346:92.

Sugarbaker DJ et al: Results of Cancer and Leukemia Group B protocol 8935: a multiinstitutional phase II trimodality trial for IIIA N2 non-small-cell lung cancer. J Thorac Cardiovasc Surg 1995;109:473.

Voltolini L et al: Results of induction chemotherapy followed by surgical resection in patients with stage IIIA (N2) non-small cell lung cancer: the importance of the nodal downstaging after chemotherapy. Eur J Cardiothorac Surg 2001;20:1106.

UNUSUAL PULMONARY NEOPLASMS

Malignant Neoplasms

Bronchial adenomas are a group of low-grade malignancies arising from the bronchial tree. Carcinoid tumors constitute 85–90% of these neoplasms, with adenoid cystic carcinoma (10%) and mucoepidermoid carcinoma (< 5%) accounting for most of the remainder. Carcinoid tumors are classified as either typical or atypical, with markedly different histologic characteristics (Table 18–13). Adenoid cystic carcinomas occur in the lower trachea; infiltrate locally along submucosal and perineural tissue planes, often far beyond the boundaries of gross tumor; and metastasize late. Mucoepidermoid carcinomas resemble salivary tumors, with varying numbers of three distinct cell types: mucous, squamous, and intermediate. Patients with bronchial adenomas complain of cough, recurrent pulmonary infections, hemoptysis, pain, and wheezing. Only 15% of patients are completely asymptomatic. Carcinoid syndrome is rare with pulmonary carcinoid tumors. Most bronchial adenomas are diagnosed with a combination of plain chest radiography, CT, and bronchoscopy. Biopsy at the time of bronchoscopy can be associated with significant bleeding, and measures to control this must be readily available.

Surgical resection is indicated for these tumors, with lobectomy being the most common procedure. Sleeve and bronchoplastic resections are particularly useful to preserve pulmonary function in these patients and make standard pneumonectomy rare. Removal of adenoid cystic carcinomas requires generous margins and frozen section examination of the margins at the time of surgery. Up to 8 cm of trachea can be removed with primary anastomosis. In addition, postoperative radiation may be indicated for close margins. With the possible exception of atypical carcinoid,

Table 18–13. Characteristics of Typical and Atypical Carcinoid Tumors.

	Typical	Atypical
Incidence	90%	10%
Central location	80%	50%
Peripheral location	20%	50%
Metastases	10–15%	50–70%

chemotherapy is generally not indicated in the treatment of these neoplasms.

The long-term outlook is good for patients with metastatic disease. Even patients with adenoid cystic carcinoma and distant metastases may do well for extended periods due to the slow-growing nature of this malignancy; however, lymph node and distant metastases in patients with carcinoid tumors generally carry a poor prognosis.

▶ Benign Neoplasms

Benign neoplasms of the lung are uncommon, accounting for less than 1% of all pulmonary tumors. Most are hamartomas, but fibromas, leiomyomas, neurofibromas, myoblastomas, and benign metastasizing leiomyomas also occur. Most lesions are peripheral and asymptomatic; however, central lesions can produce symptoms of cough, wheezing, hemoptysis, and recurrent pneumonia. Typically, the lesions are discovered on routine chest radiographs and appear as a 1- to 2-cm well-circumscribed, bosselated lower lung nodule with calcifications in 10–30%. Central lesions may require bronchoscopy for diagnosis, but a pathologic diagnosis is most often obtained by fine-needle aspiration biopsy or surgery. Surgical resection should be conservative and limited to wedge excision unless the lesion occupies the proximal bronchial airway and is associated with recurrent distal infections or bronchiectasis. In such cases, lobectomy is indicated.

Following resection, the prognosis is excellent.

SPECIAL PROBLEM: THE SOLITARY PULMONARY NODULE

With the frequent use of chest radiography, solitary pulmonary nodules ("coin lesions") are frequently found in patients without pulmonary symptoms. These lesions pose a diagnostic problem for clinicians because they may represent something as benign as a nipple shadow or as malignant as lung cancer. The overall incidence of cancer in coin lesions is as low as 10%. Other diagnostic possibilities include (1) infections due to mycobacteria (tuberculosis), fungi (histoplasmosis, coccidioidomycosis), and helminths (echinococcosis); (2) inflammatory nodules from rheumatoid arthritis, focal pneumonitis, and Wegener granuloma-

tosis; (3) congenital anomalies, such as bronchogenic cysts and arteriovenous malformations; (4) benign neoplasms such as hamartomas, hemangiomas, papillary tumors, fibrous tumors of the pleura; (5) malignant neoplasms of the lung; and (6) miscellaneous processes such as hematomas, pulmonary infarcts, pleural plaques, loculated effusions, chest wall masses, and mucoid impaction. Although certain radiographic findings may suggest malignancy or benignity, solid pathologic proof that the nodule does not represent a malignancy rests with the clinician. In general, malignant neoplasms are larger and grow rapidly, appear spiculated, often with surface umbilication or notching and eccentric excavation. In addition, cancers often occur in smokers (or former smokers) over the age of 40 with negative skin tests for tuberculosis, histoplasmosis, or coccidioidomycosis (although positive tests do not exclude cancer), and in nodules that lack calcium (CT Hounsfield units < 175). In contrast, benign lesions are small (< 1 cm), stable (> 2 years), and calcified ("target" or "popcorn" distribution; CT Hounsfield units > 175) and are associated with positive skin tests in 70–90% of patients. Evaluation of these patients usually includes chest CT scan, but sputum cytology, cultures, bronchoscopy, and mediastinoscopy are sometimes helpful. FDG-PET scanning plays an important role in the evaluation of tumors that are suspicious for malignancy. PET scan can often differentiate among lesions suspicious for malignancy.

With the advent of spiral CT scanning, the incidence of asymptomatic pulmonary nodules can vary from 25% to 70%. The vast majority of these lesions now identified are less than 1 cm and often as small as 2–3 mm. In one series, the incidence of lung cancer in the asymptomatic 10 pack-year smoking history population over the age of 50 years was 27% of all lesions identified, followed, and treated. Ongoing trials are assessing the efficacy and cost-effectiveness of CT screening for lung cancer. In the properly selected high-risk patient population (eg, over 60 years of age, moderate COPD, FEV_1 < 70%), and an over 20 pack-year smoking history), spiral CT may prove to be cost-effective and will save lives.

Ultimately, a pathologic diagnosis must be made. In some instances, fine-needle aspiration cytology may be helpful, particularly if a tissue diagnosis of hamartoma can be made or if cultures demonstrating infectious organisms are obtained. The vast majority of solitary pulmonary nodules, however, require surgical excisional biopsy to exclude the possibility of malignancy. Currently, this is accomplished with video-assisted techniques in most patients, particularly if the lesion is in the periphery of the lung. If a benign lesion is encountered, nothing further is warranted; but if a lung cancer is diagnosed, immediate lobectomy is indicated. The prognosis following resection of a coin lesion that turns out to be a bronchogenic carcinoma is good, with a 5-year survival of as high as 80–90% for lesions smaller than 1 cm.

Baaklini WA et al: Diagnostic yield of fiberoptic bronchoscopy in evaluating solitary pulmonary nodules. Chest 2000;117:1049.

Gould MK et al: Accuracy of positron emission tomography for diagnosis of pulmonary nodules and mass lesions: a meta-analysis. JAMA 2001;285:914.

Midthun DE, Swensen SJ, Jett JR: Approach to the solitary pulmonary nodule. Mayo Clin Proc 1993;68:378.

Midthun DE, Swensen SJ, Jett JR: Clinical strategies for solitary pulmonary nodule. Annu Rev Med 1992;43:195.

Swanson SJ et al: Management of the solitary pulmonary nodule: role of thoracoscopy in diagnosis and therapy. Chest 1999;116(6 Suppl):523S.

SECONDARY LUNG CANCER

Autopsy studies have demonstrated that 30% of all patients with malignancies develop pulmonary metastases, and 12% have been shown to have isolated lung disease that is totally resectable. In addition, 10% of these latter patients (1.2% of all patients) have solitary lung metastases. Most pulmonary metastases occur through hematogenous spread from the primary site; lymphatic or transbronchial spread is extremely rare. Secondary metastatic spread to the pulmonary and mediastinal lymph nodes, however, can also occur. In patients with known extrathoracic primary cancers, multiple pulmonary lesions almost always represent metastatic disease. Solitary lesions, however, may be due to benign disease (18%) or new primary lung cancer (18%) as well as metastatic disease (64%). Most patients with pulmonary metastases are asymptomatic even with extensive disease. If symptoms do develop, cough, hemoptysis, fever, dyspnea, and pain are common. The diagnosis is generally initially suggested by routine chest radiography, and CT of the chest should always be ordered to assess the lungs for other nodules. Although CT scans are more sensitive, detecting nodules as small as 3 mm, they are also less specific (false-positive rate of 55%) than plain x-rays. Pathologic confirmation of the diagnosis is essential and usually is obtained at the time of resection. For patients who are not surgical candidates, fine-needle aspiration cytology is useful for peripheral lesions, while central lesions may require bronchoscopy for tissue diagnosis.

Medically fit patients with resectable disease are surgical candidates as long as the following criteria are fulfilled: (1) the primary tumor must be controlled or imminently controllable, (2) no other sites of disease may exist, (3) no other therapy can offer comparable results, and (4) the operative risk must be low. Since adenocarcinomas (especially breast cancer) commonly involve multiple organs, it is imperative that with this histology a full evaluation be performed, including bone scan and head CT or MRI. Solitary squamous cell nodules, however—even in the presence of a previous squamous cell carcinoma (eg, head and neck tumors)—should be addressed as a new primary (lung)

cancer. Surgical resection can be accomplished through a standard posterolateral thoracotomy, median sternotomy, or bilateral anterior thoracotomies. The latter approach is particularly beneficial for bilateral disease involving the lower lobes. Video-assisted thoracoscopy is increasingly applied to metastatic disease in an attempt to reduce the morbidity of multiple resections. On occasion, during open operations for metastatic disease, several unsuspected nodules are found by direct palpation that may be missed with thoracoscopy. Wedge resection is the treatment of choice unless the lesion is a solitary squamous cell carcinoma or adenocarcinoma. These latter lesions cannot be distinguished from primary lung cancer on frozen section pathologic examination, and they must therefore be treated as primary lung cancers with lobectomy and mediastinal lymph node dissection. Occasionally, other malignant tumors identified by histologic examination may require lobectomy or, rarely, even pneumonectomy because of involvement of the proximal pulmonary artery or bronchus.

The success rate with surgical removal of pulmonary metastases has been greatest with testicular (51% 5-year survival) and head-neck cancers (47% 5-year survival). Other types of tumors, such as osteogenic and soft tissue sarcomas, renal cell carcinoma, and colon carcinoma, are all associated with prolonged survival in 20–35% of patients. Results of resection for melanoma are less favorable (10–15% survival benefit). Isolated, resectable pulmonary metastases from rectal cancer can have as high as a 55% 5-year survival with metastasectomy alone.

Furthermore, multiple thoracotomies over periods in excess of 10 years are not unusual with the sarcomas. Numerous studies have been conducted in attempts to identify prognostic factors that could aid in the selection of patients for resection Adverse prognostic factors have included (1) multiple or bilateral lesions, (2) more than four lesions seen on CT scan, (3) tumor doubling time less than 40 days, (4) a short disease-free interval, and (5) advanced age.

Although no consensus has developed regarding the selection of candidates for surgical exploration, it is generally agreed that no single criterion should be used to exclude patients from surgical resection. In all series, long-term benefit and survival hinges on complete resection. If complete resection is not deemed possible, resection should not be offered.

LaQuaglia MP: The surgical management of metastases in pediatric cancer. Semin Pediatr Surg 1993;2:75.

Pogrebniak HW, Pass HI: Initial and reoperative pulmonary metastasectomy: indications, technique, and results. Semin Surg Oncol 1993;9:142.

Todd TR: Pulmonary metastectomy: current indications for removing lung metastases. Chest 1993;103(4 Suppl):401S.

The Heart: I. Surgical Treatment of Acquired Cardiac Disease

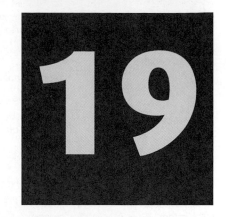

Jonathan W. Haft, MD

CORONARY ARTERY DISEASE

▶ Pathophysiology

The heart has the highest metabolic demands when compared to other organs. The vast majority of the energy substrate utilization is expended during unrelenting periodic contraction of the myocardium. Blood flow is delivered at a rate of 1 mL per gram of cardiac tissue per minute at rest. Increases in myocardial oxygen consumption, via adenosine diphosphate and adenosine mediated arteriolar vasodilation, can result in a reciprocal increase in blood flow, up to five times normal. This increased blood flow is accommodated by recruitment of an extensive capillary bed within the myocardium, with nearly 1 capillary per myocyte. Between 70% and 80% of available oxygen is extracted from coronary blood flow at rest. Thus, the metabolic needs of the heart are tightly coupled to the availability of coronary blood flow, since additional extraction is limited. In addition, blood flow through the left ventricular epicardial arteries is phasic. During myocardial contraction, extravascular compression of intramyocardial capillaries prevents forward flow during systole, limiting flow to the diastolic phase of the cardiac cycle. This is even more pronounced in the subendocardial region where myocardial oxygen demands are greatest as a result of increased wall tension and greater sarcomere shortening. Because of the elevated and insistent myocardial oxygen consumption, the restriction of blood flow to diastole, and the high basal level of oxygen consumption, the heart is particularly susceptible to ischemic injury related to stenosis of the epicardial coronary arteries.

The heart receives its blood supply from the left and right coronary arteries (Figure 19–1). These epicardial vessels originate as the first branches off of the aortic root, in their respective sinuses of Valsalva. The coronary circulation is traditionally divided into three territories or regions: the left anterior descending and the circumflex (arising from the left coronary artery) and the right (from the right coronary artery). The dominance of the heart refers to which major

artery terminates as the posterior descending branch. Ninety percent of individuals are right dominant, as the right coronary artery supplies the posterior descending artery. The remaining 10% are left dominant, as the terminal branch of the circumflex artery supplies the posterior descending artery.

The left coronary artery is referred to as the left main coronary artery. After its origin in the left sinus of Valsalva, it courses between the left atrial appendage and the pulmonary artery. The left main coronary artery varies in length but is typically less than 2 cm long. It terminates in 2 branches: the left anterior descending (LAD) and the circumflex coronary arteries. In less than 1% of patients, the left main artery is absent, with the LAD and circumflex originating as separate ostia from the left sinus of Valsalva.

The LAD, or anterior interventricular artery, courses anteriorly and inferiorly in the interventricular groove toward the apex of the heart. Several branches of the LAD travel along the anterolateral surface of the left ventricle and are known as diagonal arteries. Their number and size are highly variable. Branches to the interventricular septum take off perpendicularly, the first of which is often sizable. Occasionally, additional branches traverse toward the right, supplying a portion of the anterior surface of the right ventricle. Often, the LAD wraps around the cardiac apex and supplies the distal segment of the posterior interventricular septum. The LAD is the most prominent of the three coronary territories and carries approximately 50% of myocardial blood flow.

After arising from the left main, the circumflex coronary artery dives posteriorly along the atrioventricular groove. Several obtuse marginal branches supply the lateral wall of the left ventricle; these branches vary in both size and number. In 10% of patients, the circumflex continues posteriorly and gives rise in its terminal branch to the posterior descending coronary artery, running from the posterior atrioventricular groove toward the posterior apex in the interventricular groove. This occurs in patients characterized

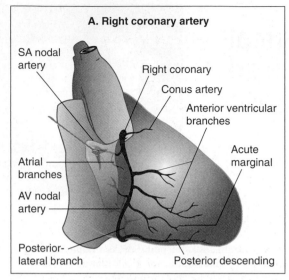
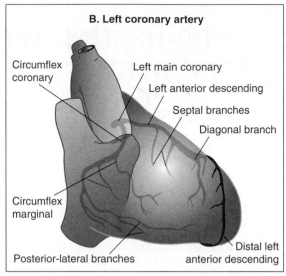

▲ **Figure 19–1.** Anatomy of the coronary circulation.

as left dominant. Some patients have a third branch of the left main referred to as the ramus intermedius. If present, this branch is often large and supplies the anterolateral wall of the left ventricle.

The right coronary artery originates from the right sinus of Valsalva in the aortic root. It courses anteriorly and rightward until reaching the right atrioventricular groove. The vessel then descends around the acute margin of the heart, giving rise to one or more branches supplying the right ventricle. In 90% of patients, the right coronary artery continues posteriorly, terminating as the posterior descending coronary artery and the posterolateral artery.

Atherosclerosis, a progressive multifocal disease of medium and large muscular arteries of the systemic circulation, tends to occur predominantly at vessel bifurcations, sharp curvatures, and other regions creating pressure wave reflections and recirculation. Because of these flow-related considerations, atherosclerotic stenotic lesions are generally restricted to the proximal regions of the large epicardial coronary arteries. In particular, stenosis found in the LAD and circumflex vessels are frequently isolated, short, and in the proximal segments. The right coronary artery, however, develops diffuse obstructions, although rarely extending into the posterior descending or intramural branches.

The pathologic mechanism of coronary atheroma formation is identical to the lesions found elsewhere in the vascular tree. Endothelial injury from cigarette smoke, hypercholesterolemia, hyperglycemia, hypertension, or other causes of inflammation initiate a cascade of events. These include endothelial dysfunction with reduced nitric oxide production, monocyte adhesion and migration, lipid accumulation, and smooth muscle cell proliferation. The end result is an enlarging plaque encroaching on the arterial lumen, sepa-

rated from the blood stream by a collagen-rich fibrous plaque. The lesion can cause flow limitations, particularly when the luminal cross-sectional area is reduced by at least 75%. With this degree of obstruction, the vasodilatory reserve required during increased myocardial demand is restricted, resulting in transient myocardial ischemia until demand returns to baseline. The atherosclerotic plaque also causes coronary ischemia when the lesion becomes unstable. The fibrous plaque can fracture, causing rupture of the plaque contents and complete epicardial thrombosis, the presumed mechanism of ST-segment elevation myocardial infarction (STEMI). Additionally, subtotal plaque disruption can cause vasoconstriction, platelet activation, and embolization, resulting in ischemia without total occlusion of the epicardial vessel. This is the presumed mechanism of unstable angina and non-ST-segment elevation myocardial infarction (NSTEMI).

▶ Patient Presentation

Patients with coronary atherosclerosis can present with a variety of symptoms depending on the severity and nature of their occlusive lesions as well as on their other medical comorbidities. Chronic stable angina is the most frequent complaint of the patient with coronary artery disease. At rest, coronary blood flow is adequate to meet myocardial demand, and patients are without symptoms. However, during exercise or stress, as myocardial oxygen demand increases, autoregulatory mechanisms vasodilate to increase myocardial blood flow fivefold to sixfold. Stable coronary obstructions become flow limiting, resulting in an imbalance of oxygen demand and supply. Chest pain develops rapidly and builds up quickly. It is typically described as tightness, squeezing, constricting, or aching. It is usually midsternal and radiates to the left shoulder, arm, or neck. The classically described Levine sign with a clenched fist over the sternum is a common finding. Some patients, however, describe symptoms that are collectively referred to as "anginal equivalents." These include dyspnea, diaphoresis, nausea, heartburn, and dizziness or presyncope. Although the clinical manifestations of angina are variable, the pathognomonic feature of chronic stable angina is that the symptoms occur predictably with exertion and are always relieved with rest.

Acute coronary syndrome (ACS) encompasses a spectrum of conditions related to coronary occlusive disease, including unstable angina, NSTEMI, and STEMI. Patients with unstable angina experience chest pain or an anginal equivalent that is new, occurs at rest, or occurs with increasing severity from their baseline chronic stable symptoms, also called crescendo angina. Patients who develop NSTEMI have evidence of myocardial injury with elevated blood levels of myocardial enzymes (troponin and the myoglobin [Mb] fraction of creatine kinase). Unstable angina and NSTEMI are important prognostic indicators, as 10% of patients will die of cardiovascular causes within 6 months.

STEMI represents the consequences of large epicardial vessel occlusion typically associated with plaque rupture. Patients usually describe severe retrosternal chest pain that persists for more than 30 minutes. Patients with previous chronic stable angina will report that the current pain does not resolve with rest or nitroglycerine and is more intense in quality. Patients often describe additional symptoms such as diaphoresis, nausea, and dizziness. Although improvements in health systems have drastically increased survival from myocardial infarction, mortality for STEMI remains near 10%.

▶ Diagnostic Evaluation

Patients with suspected coronary artery disease should undergo a resting electrocardiogram. Although most patients with chronic stable angina have a normal electrocardiogram pattern, evidence of previous myocardial infarctions may be identified with the presence of either Q waves or conduction abnormalities. The most widely used diagnostic test to evaluate for coronary artery disease is exercise electrocardiography. Using standardized protocols, patients are exercised on a treadmill or bicycle ergometer while a 12-lead electrocardiogram is continuously recorded. The test is continued until the patient's symptoms are noted or until the development of significant ST segment shifts suggesting myocardial ischemia. The diagnostic accuracy of exercise stress electrocardiogram testing can be enhanced with myocardial perfusion imaging. Several radioactive tracers are used clinically, the most frequent of which is thallium-201. Because of its similarities to potassium ions, it is taken up preferentially by the viable cardiac myocytes. Its distribution within the myocardium is proportional to the rate of perfusion. In some cases, patients are unable to exercise because of additional physical or psychological limitations. Pharmacologic agents can substi-

tute for exercise by increasing myocardial oxygen demand (dobutamine) or by directly vasodilating coronary arteries (adenosine), thus demonstrating regions with fixed restrictions in myocardial blood flow. Echocardiography can be used as an alternative to nuclear perfusion imaging to increase the accuracy of exercise electrocardiogram testing. Echocardiography demonstrates regional changes in wall motion that can be observed during myocardial ischemia. It can also identify valvular abnormalities or other conditions that may influence treatment choices.

Coronary angiography, also known as cardiac catheterization, is indicated in symptomatic patients with suspected coronary occlusive lesions. After percutaneous access is obtained in the arterial system, preformed catheters of varying sizes are advanced fluoroscopically to selectively engage the ostia of the left and right coronary arteries. Radiopaque contrast is injected with imaging of the opacified coronary artery. Standardized views are obtained of both the right and left coronary systems to provide different special projections to clearly define the vascular anatomy and to quantify the severity of occlusive lesions (Figure 19–2). Automated computer analysis systems can calculate area reduction, improving interobserver consistency. Additionally, catheters can be inserted across the aortic valve into the left ventricular cavity. Contrast injection for ventriculography can provide information about ventricular systolic function, cavity size, and the presence of left-sided valvular abnormalities. During cardiac catheterization, stenotic lesions in the epicardial vessels can be treated using percutaneous techniques, described in the section on Percutaneous Intervention. Newer imaging techniques using high-resolution multislice CT scanning with 3D reconstruction and magnetic resonance imaging (MRI) are increasingly utilized. These noninvasive approaches have the potential to improve the safety and convenience of coronary imaging; however, resolution remains inferior to standard coronary angiography.

▶ Medical Treatment

Medical therapy of coronary artery disease begins with controlling risk factors that contribute to formation and destabilization of the atherosclerotic plaque. The most important intervention is cessation of cigarette smoking. Other interventions include control of hypertension, diabetes, and hypercholesterolemia. Dietary modifications and exercise can improve all of these conditions, but pharmacologic treatment is often necessary.

Statins can improve cholesterol levels and improve the ratio of low-density to high-density lipoproteins, and they have been demonstrated to reduce rates of myocardial infarction and death. Angiotensin-converting inhibitors have been shown to reduce mortality and myocardial infarction in patients with coronary artery disease coupled with hypertension, diabetes, or left ventricular dysfunction. Aspirin, by inhibiting platelet activity, reduces death and myocardial infarctions in patients with coronary artery disease and

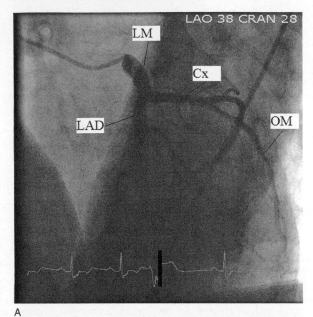

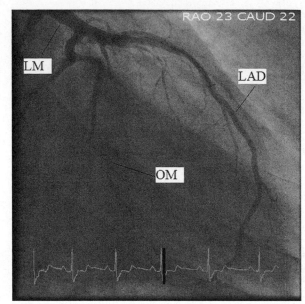

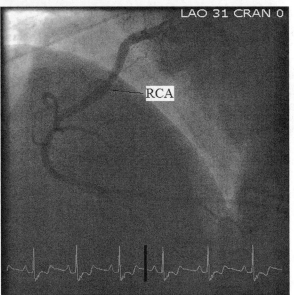

▲ **Figure 19–2. A:** Left anterior oblique (LAO) view of the left coronary artery. **B:** Right anterior oblique (RAO) view of the left coronary artery. **C:** LAO view of the right coronary artery. LM, left main; LAD, left anterior descending; Cx, circumflex; RCA, right coronary artery; OM, obtuse marginal.

should be prescribed to all patients unless significant contra-indications exist. Beta-blocking agents reduce myocardial oxygen consumption by reducing heart rate and wall tension, and they increase oxygen delivery by increasing the diastolic phase and thus subendocardial perfusion. Despite these perceived benefits, beta-blockers have not been shown to reduce cardiovascular mortality or morbidity in patients without left ventricular dysfunction or hypertension. Nitrates also decrease myocardial oxygen consumption via venodilation, reducing cardiac preload and wall tension, and vasodilation,

reducing afterload. Some epicardial vasodilation will occur, improving coronary blood flow. Nitrates can control symptoms, either immediately when given sublingually or prophylactically when used as an oral long-acting agent. Headaches are notable side effects, and the vasodilatory properties of nitrates can be exaggerated by phosphodiesterase inhibitors frequently used for the treatment of erectile dysfunction. Medical treatment alone is appropriate for patients with coronary artery disease affecting one or two epicardial vessel territories and satisfactory symptom control.

Percutaneous Intervention

In 1977, Dr. Andreas Gruentzig performed the first percutaneous intervention with balloon angioplasty on a stenotic lesion in the LAD. This pioneer laid the foundation for a revolution in the treatment of coronary artery disease worldwide. Percutaneous coronary intervention is among the most frequently performed medical procedures in the world, and its use continues to expand. These interventions include balloon angioplasty, intracoronary stent implantation, as well as rotational and laser atherectomies. Using the same techniques described for cardiac catheterization, small, highly flexible and steerable guidewires can be advanced percutaneously down the lumen of stenotic epicardial coronary arteries. Over this guidewire, balloon tipped-catheters can be advanced across the stenosis and inflated to supra-atmospheric pressures. This stretches and dilates the affected vessel, restoring the lumen to its predisease dimensions. Restenosis was common, occurring in nearly 40% of patients. The use of nitinol scaffolding stents has greatly reduced restenosis rates to nearly 15%; they are used in nearly 90% of percutaneous procedures in the United States. The latest addition in the armamentarium of percutaneous coronary interventions is the drug-eluting stent. The drugs impregnated into the walls of the stent are antiproliferative, similar to agents used to prevent replication of immune cells in transplant recipients. The sirolimus-eluting and paclitaxel-eluting stents have further reduced the rate of target vessel restenosis and the need for repeat interventions. However, reports of late stent thrombosis have raised concerns, and indefinite use of antiplatelet regimens has been recommended.

Surgical Treatment

Although alternative surgical approaches to myocardial ischemia had been attempted previously, René Favaloro is credited with creation of the coronary bypass procedure from his work at the Cleveland Clinic. Since its inception in 1967, coronary artery bypass grafting (CABG) has increased in volume until the last decade, with minimal growth, presumably from improved percutaneous and medical treatments (Figure 19–3). Despite the recent trends, CABG continues to be among the most frequent, successful, and well-studied procedures performed in medicine.

A. Indications

Three large prospective multicenter randomized clinical trials evaluating CABG versus medical therapy are widely quoted and should be understood when considering the indications for coronary bypass grafting. Despite the historical nature of these studies and the enormous differences in both surgical technique and medical treatment, these trials continue to provide important information about the benefits of surgical revascularization in patients with advanced coronary atherosclerosis.

The Veterans Administration Cooperative Study enrolled 1000 patients between 1970 and 1974. Patients had chronic

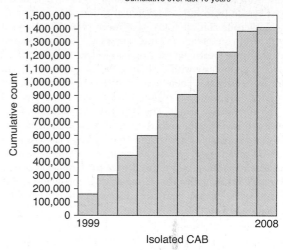

▲ **Figure 19–3.** Trend in reduction of coronary bypass graft procedures in United States.

anginal complaints and were free of myocardial infarction within 6 months. Medical treatment consisted largely of nitrates and aspirin, and surgical mortality was extremely high when compared to contemporary results. A statistically significant survival advantage was seen in the surgical group versus the medical group at 7 years (77% vs 72%), despite 38% of medical patients crossing over to surgical treatment. Subgroup analysis demonstrated more pronounced survival advantages for patients with three-vessel disease, patients with left ventricular dysfunction, and patients with significant stenosis of the left main coronary artery.

The European Coronary Surgery Study recruited 767 men with chronic angina from 1973 to 1976. Only patients with preserved left ventricular function were included. A survival advantage for the surgical group was seen in the overall cohort, but particularly in patients with three-vessel disease and those with proximal LAD stenosis. There were also advantages demonstrated in reduction of angina and exercise capacity.

The Coronary Artery Surgery Study enrolled patients from a nonrandomized registry of patients who underwent coronary angiography from 1974 to 1979 at 15 centers. Patients with mild angina were randomized to medical treatment and CABG. There was no survival advantage in the 790 randomized patients; however, the cohort with left ventricular dysfunction had better survival with surgery, particularly those with left ventricular dysfunction and three-vessel disease. Evaluation of the nonrandomized patients in the registry also found survival advantages for surgically treated patients with left main stenosis or left main equivalent stenosis. Although these three landmark studies are nearly 30 years old, some important principles continue to apply: Patients with more advanced coronary atherosclerosis, particularly those with left ventricular dysfunction, stand to achieve the most benefit from surgical revascularization.

Numerous clinical trials have more recently compared CABG with percutaneous interventions. The Randomized Intervention Treatment of Angina (RITA) trial compared balloon angioplasty with CABG for patients with single and multivessel disease. There was no difference in survival, but repeat intervention was required five times more frequently in the angioplasty group. The Bypass Angioplasty Revascularization Investigation (BARI) enrolled 1829 patients with chronic or unstable angina from 1988 to 1991. There was no survival advantage at 5 years; however, 31% of the patients in the percutaneous group crossed over for CABG. The need for repeat revascularization was again five times higher in the percutaneous group, and the subgroup of patients with diabetes had improved survival at 5 years (81% vs 66%).

Several additional randomized trials continue to evaluate the relative merits of surgical, percutaneous, or medical treatment across the spectrum of patients with coronary artery disease. As technology and pharmacology continue to evolve, additional studies will be required. However, CABG offers survival and quality-of-life advantages in selected patients with coronary artery disease. The most recent recommendations from the American Heart Association and the American College of Cardiology regarding the indications for coronary bypass surgery are presented in Table 19–1.

B. Techniques

The principles of coronary bypass surgery are to restore normal myocardial perfusion by creating alternative routes for blood to reach the jeopardized territories. This strategy has several advantages, including the large-caliber conduits, their extramyocardial location in avoiding the compressive forces during systole, and their attachment at strategic locations to maximize return of normal blood flow. The most important aspect of the procedure is construction of a technically sound and strategically well-created bypass graft.

A variety of conduits may be chosen; the most traditional and still most frequently utilized is the saphenous vein. The vessel is easily harvested with minimal morbidity, and it is technically easy to create the precise anastomosis. Minimally invasive approaches using endoscopic techniques now reduce the impact on the patient during the saphenectomy. Limitations of the saphenous vein are primarily based on its tendency to develop accelerated atherosclerotic lesions. The vein graft plaque is more frequently circumferential and diffuse, with a weaker fibrous cap and a higher predilection for distal embolization. Patency of saphenous vein grafts is approximately 50% at 10 years. In addition, suitable vein conduit may not be available, either harvested for previous coronary or peripheral bypass procedures or unusable from varicosities or sclerosis.

The internal mammary artery can be mobilized from its pedicle on the left subclavian artery and anastomosed to the

Table 19–1. American Heart Association Guidelines for Coronary Bypass Graft Surgery.*

Asymptomatic
- Left main coronary artery disease or left main equivalent (proximal LAD, proximal circumflex) (class I)
- Three-vessel coronary artery disease (class I)
- Proximal LAD disease and one- or two-vessel disease (class IIa, particularly if there is decreased LV function or extensive ischemia on noninvasive study

Symptomatic
  Stable angina
- Left main coronary artery disease or left main equivalent (class I)
- Three-vessel coronary artery disease (class I)
- Two-vessel coronary artery disease and proximal LAD with decreased LV function or significant ischemia on noninvasive study (class I)
- One- or two-vessel disease not involving the proximal LAD but with high-risk findings on noninvasive study (class I)
  One-vessel disease involving the proximal LAD (class IIa)
  Unstable angina/NSTEMI
- Left main coronary artery disease or left main equivalent (class I)
- Three-vessel coronary artery disease (class I)
- One- or two-vessel disease with ongoing ischemia; vessels are not amenable to percutaneous therapy (class I)
- One- or two-vessel disease not involving the proximal LAD (class IIa)

STEMI
- Ongoing chest pain or hemodynamic instability with lesions not amenable to percutaneous treatment (class I)
- Surgical complications of myocardial infarction, such as ruptured papillary muscle or postinfarct ventricular septal defect (class I)
- Cardiogenic shock (class I)
- Recurrent malignant arrhythmias (class I)

Decreased LV function
- Left main, left main equivalent, or three-vessel coronary artery disease (class I)
- Two-vessel coronary artery disease (class I)
- Proximal LAD disease (class IIa)

Failed PTCA
- Ongoing ischemia with adequate distal target (class I)
- Hemodynamic instability (class I)

*Evidence class I: Evidence of or general agreement that the treatment is effective. Class IIa: Conflicting evidence or diverging opinion, but evidence favors treatment. Class IIb: Conflicting evidence or diverging opinion, but efficacy is less well established. Class III: Evidence suggests the treatment is *not* helpful.

LAD, left anterior descending; LV, left ventricular; NSTEMI, non-ST-segment elevation myocardial infarction; STEMI, ST-segment elevation myocardial infarction.

anterior or lateral epicardial vessels of the heart, most frequently to the LAD. This strategy has several well-described advantages owing to the improved patency rate of the internal mammary graft when compared to saphenous vein grafts. The right internal mammary artery can also serve as a bypass conduit; however, harvesting of both internal mammary vessels increases the risk of sternal ischemia and surgical wound-healing complications. Because of the improved patency of arterial grafts as compared to saphenous vein grafts, the radial and gastroepiploic artery have been explored as alternatives to vein grafts. However, improved long-term patency has not been reliably established, and morbidity from harvesting has slowed widespread adoption of this approach.

The standard approach for coronary bypass grafting is via the median sternotomy, where the sternum is divided longitudinally, exposing the heart and great vessels. The left thoracotomy could be alternatively used, particularly after previous heart surgery where sternal reentry could hazard injury to adhesed cardiac structures or patent grafts. Preparation is then made to institute cardiopulmonary bypass (CPB). Anticoagulation with 300 IU heparin per kilogram is infused to achieve an activated clotting time of greater than 400 seconds. Typically, the ascending aorta is used for arterial inflow, and venous return is accomplished via a cannula in the right atrial appendage (Figure 19–4). CPB is commenced, evacuating venous blood into the cardiotomy reservoir. Mechanical ventilation can be discontinued. Using a heat exchanger, the blood is actively cooled to 28–32 °C to reduce tissue oxygen requirements and organ injury. Shed mediastinal blood can be scavenged and returned to the CPB system, reducing blood loss during the extensive anticoagulation period. Cardioplegic arrest is then initiated by cross-clamping the ascending aorta and infusing cold blood cardioplegia solution into the aortic root. The makeup of cardioplegia solutions differs among centers and even among surgeons; however, most centers combine autologous blood obtained from the CPB system with crystalloid solution cooled to 12 °C containing citrate to bind ionic calcium, dextrose, pH buffers, and potassium (approximately 30 mM/L) to arrest all cardiac activity. Cardioplegia is administered intermittently to maintain myocardial temperature and diastolic arrest during the cross-clamp period.

With the arrested heart, a dry and motionless surgical field is created, allowing creation of precise surgical anastomoses on even the smallest of epicardial coronary arteries. The targets are identified on the epicardial surface, and the sites for anastomotic reconstruction are determined on the basis of information from the preoperative cardiac catheterization and suitability of the native vessel. An arteriotomy is created on the exposed vessel, and it is extended for approximately 5 mm. The conduit is fashioned with an appropriately sized bevel or spatulation, and the anastomosis is created, typically in running fashion with fine polypropylene suture. The conduits are tested for patency and hemostasis, and they are cut to the appropriate size, avoiding tension or kinking. Saphenous vein or free arterial conduits are typically connected to the ascending aorta. A 4–5 mm punch device is used to create a circular aortotomy. The anastomoses are constructed in running fashion with polypropylene suture. If conduit length is limited, the proximal anastomoses can be created as Y grafts off of other vein grafts or off of the pedicled internal mammary artery graft.

After completion of all anastomoses, weaning from CPB is prepared. The patient is warmed to normothermia. As the heart begins to warm, ventricular fibrillation often occurs, requiring electrical defibrillation. Temporary conduction abnormalities may require epicardial pacing, but it is often transient. Mechanical ventilation is resumed, and the patient is gradually weaned from CPB. Pharmacologic inotropic support may be required but is often unnecessary if ventricular function was preserved preoperatively. An appropriate dose of protamine is infused to reverse the effects of heparin, and cannulae for bypass are removed. Once hemostasis is adequate, chest closure is performed with stainless steel wires. The pericardium is typically left open to avoid constriction of the atria or kinking of the bypass grafts. The pedicled left internal mammary artery graft is positioned posterior to the anterior surface of the left lung to protect it from injury should sternal reentry be required in the future.

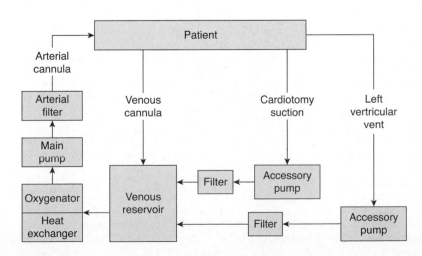

▲ **Figure 19–4.** Schematic of cardiopulmonary bypass (CPB). (From Morgan GE, Mikhail MS, Murray MJ. *Clinical Anesthesiology*, 4th ed. McGraw-Hill, 2006.)

Recently, attempts to reduce the invasive nature of coronary bypass grafting and the potential complications of CPB have been introduced. Techniques to perform bypass grafting without CPB have improved and are promoted by its advocates. Off-pump coronary bypass grafting (OPCAB) have potential advantages in reducing neurologic complications associated with air and atheroemboli, as well as reducing blood transfusion requirements and cost. The procedure involves manipulation and stabilization of the beating heart to expose the epicardial targets. Particularly for vessels on the posterior and posterolateral surfaces, hemodynamic instability can result while the heart is elevated and rotated for optimal exposure. The anesthesiologist must be capable of responding to these rapid changes, and the surgeon must have the judgment and ability to immediately abandon off-pump attempts and institute CPB before significant organ injury occurs. The anastomoses are more challenging, with blood in the moving operative field. Although several single-center reports have demonstrated satisfactory short-term results and mid-term graft patency rates, multicenter randomized and observation studies have suggested that OPCAB techniques may offer some benefits but at the expense of reduced graft patency rates. As a result, OPCAB penetrance has not markedly increased over the last several years.

C. Results

Since the creation of the Society of Thoracic Surgeons voluntary reporting database in 1989, short-term outcomes of coronary bypass grafting are widely available to the public, providing information for patients, referring physicians, and practicing surgeons to compare their results to national averages. The Society also provides a validated risk assessment scoring system, creating mortality estimates based on an individual patient's clinical data. Overall, risk of perioperative death remains at 1–3%. Multivariate predictors of death include advanced age, recent myocardial infarction, decreased ventricular function, renal insufficiency, and female gender. Conduit patency is determined from clinical trials that included angiographic assessments at varying time intervals in the absence of symptoms. Data are largely historical and are subject to biases of patient selection but are largely considered to be reliable. Saphenous vein grafts occlude 20–30% by 1 year. Early graft loss is felt to be attributable to anastomotic imperfections or graft kinking, endothelial injury during harvest, limited native coronary runoff, or progression of native occlusive disease. Late failures appear to occur at a rate of 5% per year, with 10-year patency approximately 40–50%. Late failures are primarily attributed to accelerated atherosclerosis of the vein conduit. The pedicled internal mammary artery has far superior patency, particularly when anastomosed to the LAD. With adequate target vessel runoff, 10-year patency rates of 90–95% have been reported in multiple independent studies. Radial arteries and free mammary artery conduits appear to have patency rates intermediate to saphenous vein and pedicled mammary arteries and are more frequently utilized in younger patients.

ACC/AHA 2004 guideline update for coronary artery bypass graft surgery. Circulation 2004;110:1168.

Alderman EL et al: Ten-year follow-up of survival and myocardial infarction in the randomized Coronary Artery Surgery Study. Circulation 1990;82:1629.

Barter P et al: HDL cholesterol, very low levels of LDL cholesterol, and cardiovascular events. Treating to New Targets Investigators. New Eng J Med 2007;357:1301.

Bypass Angioplasty Revascularization Investigation (BARI) Investigators: Comparison of coronary bypass surgery with angioplasty in patients with multivessel disease. New Eng J Med 1996;335:217.

Cleveland JC et al: Off-pump coronary artery bypass grafting decreases risk-adjusted mortality and morbidity. Ann Thorac Surg 2001;72:1282.

Davi G, Patrono C: Platelet activation and atherothrombosis. New Eng J Med 2007;357:2482.

Favaloro RG: Saphenous vein graft in the surgical treatment of coronary artery disease. Operative technique. J Thorac Cardiovasc Surg 1969;58:178.

Fox KA et al: Management of acute coronary syndromes. Variations in practice and outcomes: findings from Global Registry of Acute Coronary Events (GRACE). Eur Heart J 2002;23:117.

Henderson RA et al: Long-term results of RITA-1 trial: clinical and cost comparisons of coronary angioplasty and coronary-artery bypass grafting. Randomised Intervention Treatment of Angina. Lancet 1998;352:1419.

Kelbaek H et al: Drug-eluting versus bare metal stents in patients with st-segment-elevation myocardial infarction: eight-month follow-up in the Drug Elution and Distal Protection in Acute Myocardial Infarction (DEDICATION) trial. DEDICATION Investigators. Circulation 2008;118:1155.

Loop FD et al: Influence of the internal-mammary-artery graft on 10-year survival and other cardiac events. New Eng J Med 1986;314:1.

Malenka DJ et al: Comparing long-term survival of patients with multivessel coronary disease after CABG or PCI: analysis of BARI-like patients in northern New England. Northern New England Cardiovascular Disease Study Group. Circulation 2005;112:I371.

Puskas JD et al: Off-pump coronary bypass provides reduced mortality and morbidity and equivalent 10-year survival. Ann Thorac Surg 2008;86:1139.

Reddy GP et al: MR imaging of ischemic heart disease. Magn Reson Imaging Clin N Am 2008;16:201.

Schmieder RE et al: Renin-angiotensin system and cardiovascular risk. Lancet 2007;369:1208.

Schroeder S et al: Cardiac computed tomography: indications, applications, limitations, and training requirements. Working Group Nuclear Cardiology and Cardiac CT. Eur Heart J 2008;29:531.

Society of Thoracic Surgeons. 2008 adult cardiac surgery database executive summary. Available at: http://www.sts.org/sections/stsnationaldatabase/publications/executive/article.html. Accessed November 12, 2008.

Takagi H et al: Off-pump coronary artery bypass sacrifices graft patency: meta-analysis of randomized trials. J Thorac Cardiovasc Surg 2007;133:e2.

Varnauskas E: Twelve-year follow-up of survival in the randomized European Coronary Surgery Study. New Eng J Med 1988;319:332.

Veterans Administration Coronary Artery Bypass Surgery Cooperative Study Group: Eleven-year survival in the Veterans
Administration randomized trial of coronary bypass surgery for
stable angina. New Eng J Med 1984;311:1333.

Wenaweser P et al: Incidence and correlates of drug-eluting stent
thrombosis in routine clinical practice. 4-year results from a
large 2-institutional cohort study. J Am Col Cardiol
2008;52:1134.

▼ VALVULAR HEART DISEASE

MITRAL REGURGITATION

▶ Pathophysiology

A. Anatomy

The mitral valve separates the left atrium from the left
ventricle. It should be considered as the sum of its three
components: the leaflets, the annulus to which the leaflets
attach, and the subvalvar apparatus, consisting of the cords
and papillary muscles. The mitral valve has two leaflets,
anterior and posterior (Figure 19–5). The anterior leaflet is
larger in surface area, but its attachment to the annulus
represents only one third of the circumference. The anterior
portion of the mitral valve annulus is in direct continuity
with the annulus of the left and noncoronary cusps of the
aortic valve, also known as the aortomitral continuity. The
posterior leaflet is shorter, but its annular attachments cover
two thirds of the circumference. The posterior leaflet often
can be separated into three distinct scallops, although the
prominence of these separations varies among individuals.
The anterior and posterior leaflets are separated from each
other by the anterolateral and posteromedial commissures,
which mark the location of the right and left fibrous trigones
respectively. The trigones are dense collagenous structures
within the annulus representing a portion of the fibrous

skeleton of the heart. The mitral annulus is elliptical in
shape, and its dimensions change dynamically during cardiac contraction, reducing its cross-sectional area by as
much as 40%. The anterolateral and posteromedial papillary
muscles are vertically oriented bundles of cardiac myocytes.
Chordae tendineae originate from the heads of the papillary
muscles and span the distance to both the anterior and
posterior mitral valve leaflets. Chords are designated as
primary if they attach to the leading edge of the leaflet,
secondary if they attach to the ventricular surface of the
leaflets, or tertiary if they attach to the ventricular surface of
the mitral annulus. The chords play an important role in
preventing leaflet prolapse. The posteromedial papillary
muscle is prone to ischemic injury, since it relies on a single
right coronary artery for circulation. In contrast, the anterolateral papillary muscle gains its blood supply from the LAD
and circumflex branches and tends to be more resistant to
ischemic injury.

B. Classification of Mitral Regurgitation

Regurgitation through the mitral valve can result from a
variety of pathologic conditions. Alain Carpentier developed
a simplified classification scheme based on leaflet motion
(Table 19–2) to organize the different disease processes that
can cause mitral regurgitation. In Carpentier type I mitral
regurgitation, the leaflet motion is normal. The regurgitation
is a result of either dilation of the annulus, as can be seen in
cardiomyopathy with progressive ventricular enlargement,
or of leaflet perforation, as can be seen with destructive
endocarditis. Type II is associated with excessive leaflet
motion. Patients with type II mitral regurgitation have ruptured chordae or papillary muscles from ischemia or endocarditis, or they have with pathologically redundant mitral
leaflet tissue. Redundant, prolapsing, or myxomatous mitral
leaflets can be either acquired from fibroelastic deficiency or
hereditary from weak connective tissue. In either case, the
excessive leaflet motion prevents proper coaptation of the
anterior and posterior leaflets. Patients with type III have
restricted leaflet motion. Type III is often associated with
rheumatic heart disease, where leaflets can become calcified,
and the chords are thickened and foreshortened. The leaflets
do not adequately rise in systole, and coaptation is impaired.

Table 19–2. Carpentier Classification
of Mitral Regurgitation.

I	Normal leaflet motion
	Annular dilation, leaflet perforation
II	Excessive leaflet motion
	Prolapsed or myxomatous leaflet, ruptured chord
III	Restricted leaflet motion
	Rheumatic disease, ischemic mitral regurgitation

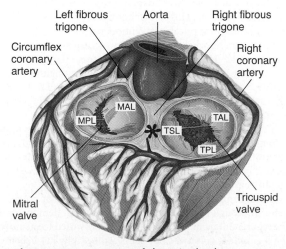

▲ **Figure 19–5.** Anatomy of the mitral valve.

Alternatively, some patients develop severe mitral regurgitation owing to ischemic injury. Typically, a previous myocardial infarction has resulted in ventricular remodeling, resulting in dilation and retraction of the papillary muscles. As a result, the leaflets are tethered into the ventricle, limiting mobility and preventing proper coaptation.

Mitral regurgitation is always pathologic but can be tolerated surprisingly well when the onset is gradual, allowing for a series of physiologic adaptations. On the other hand, acute mitral regurgitation, as can be associated with infective endocarditis or ischemic papillary muscle rupture, results in immediate pulmonary congestion because the unprepared left atrium is incapable of handling the additional volume load. Several compensatory mechanisms occur as mitral regurgitation develops and progressively worsens. The left atrium and pulmonary venous system gradually dilates, thus increasing compliance to better accommodate the excess volume. The backwards flow of mitral regurgitation reduces ventricular afterload, reducing myocardial wall tension. The reduction in forward flow is accounted for by increased diastolic filling, increasing preload. This maintains cardiac output and can delay onset of symptoms for significant time. Gradually, left ventricular end diastolic volume continues to rise, resulting in pathologic remodeling, creating a dilated and more spherical ventricular cavity. Systolic function is progressively and inexorably impaired as a result of both mechanical considerations owing to the altered shape and molecular mechanisms both intracellular and extracellular. A vicious cycle ensues, with deteriorating systolic function and rising end diastolic volume promoting further ventricular remodeling and dilation and worsening mitral regurgitation. Longstanding mitral regurgitation will result in sustained elevation in left atrial pressure and volume, resulting in pulmonary vascular changes, pulmonary hypertension, and eventually, right ventricular dysfunction.

C. Symptoms

Acute mitral regurgitation is poorly tolerated and is typically associated with pulmonary congestion and low cardiac output. Patients describe dyspnea, poor exercise tolerance, and fatigue. Often, the etiology of the mitral regurgitation is more dominant in the clinical presentation. Patients with acute endocarditis patients may have fever, shaking chills, and manifestations of septic embolization such as stroke and intestinal or extremity ischemia. Patients suffering from acute myocardial infarction with a ruptured papillary muscle complain of chest pain and diaphoresis.

Chronic mitral regurgitation can be asymptomatic for many years as a result of progressive atrial and ventricular adaptation. Eventually, patients develop symptoms of heart failure, including dyspnea, fatigue, and lower extremity edema. When left atrial dilation results in atrial fibrillation, patients may describe heart palpitations. Often, the onset of atrial fibrillation is the initial presentation of symptoms, as

rapid ventricular response decreases diastolic filling time and creates a sudden reduction in cardiac output. As ventricular function deteriorates and pulmonary vascular changes occur, signs of right sided heart failure develop, such as lower extremity edema and ascites.

▶ Diagnostic Testing

The physical findings of mitral regurgitation vary depending on the duration and the degree of compensation. For patients with longstanding mitral regurgitation, ventricular dilation displaces the point of maximal impulse (PMI) laterally. On auscultation, an S3 gallop is often heard, resulting from increased diastolic flow. The systolic murmur is characteristically described as blowing, best heard over the cardiac apex and radiating to the axilla. In acute mitral regurgitation, the murmur tends to be limited to early in systole. With more chronicity, the murmur is progressively holosystolic.

The chest radiograph often demonstrates cardiomegaly from ventricular dilation. With severe uncompensated heart failure, pulmonary edema may be evident; however, this is more commonly seen with acute mitral regurgitation. The electrocardiogram is often nonspecific but may demonstrate evidence of previous myocardial infarction and will confirm the presence of atrial fibrillation.

Echocardiography is the mainstay in the diagnosis of mitral regurgitation; it provides information about the mechanism of the disease, which is essential in planning surgical intervention. Images of the leaflets can determine if the leaflet motion is normal, restricted, or excessive. Information about annular size and mobility can be obtained. Using color, the size and direction of the regurgitant jet can quantify the severity and give clues as to the mechanism (Figure 19–6). The severity of the regurgitation is determined by the width and length of the regurgitant jet or the presence of reversed flow within the pulmonary veins. Echocardiography also provides information about the chronicity of the disease and can document progressive adaptation such as left atrial and ventricular dilation. This information is often used in determining timing of surgical intervention, particularly in asymptomatic patients. Echocardiography is usually performed transthoracic. However, in some patients, the views are obscured by body habitus or emphysema, limiting the image quality. Transesophageal echocardiography (TEE) can improve the resolution of images and better clarify the severity and mechanism of the mitral valve pathology.

Cardiac catheterization is an important adjunctive tool, helping to identify additional cardiac pathology, and can determine the adequacy of preoperative medical optimization. Coronary angiography is performed preoperatively to identify coronary arterial occlusive lesions that may require bypass grafting at the time of mitral valve repair or replacement. Although contrast ventriculography can demonstrate the regurgitant jet, it is no longer necessarily used to quantify the regurgitant volume, since echocardiography has become the standard technique. Right heart catheterization will dem-

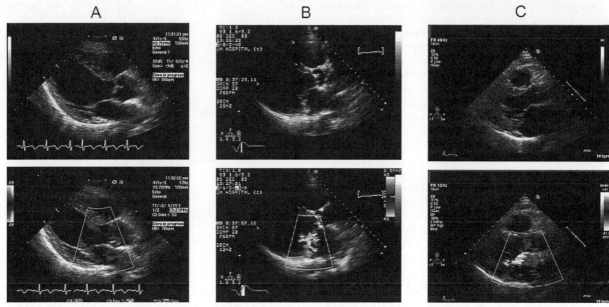

▲ **Figure 19–6.** Echocardiographic view of the mitral valve. **A:** Normal valve. **B:** Dilated annulus with central regurgitation. **C:** Prolapsing posterior leaflet with eccentric regurgitation.

onstrate intravascular volume overload and low cardiac output. It may also be helpful in diagnosing pulmonary vascular changes in patients who deny symptoms.

▶ Surgical Treatment

A. Indications

The indications for operation on the mitral valve depend on the specific pathology as well as clinical symptoms. In addition, the indications have evolved in recent years owing to improved outcomes related to better surgical techniques, anesthetic considerations, myocardial protection, and postoperative care. Furthermore, intervention on the mitral valve may be performed for less severe disease if operation is indicated for coronary artery disease or aortic valve pathology.

Certainly, among patients who represent reasonable operative risks, those with severe mitral regurgitation and heart failure symptoms should be offered an operation. In addition, those with severe mitral regurgitation and signs of left ventricular dysfunction should undergo operation because myocardial decompensation can progress rapidly without corrective action. There is insufficient evidence that operative intervention for asymptomatic severe mitral regurgitation and normal ventricular function improves survival. Historically, these patients were observed with close clinical follow-up and serial echocardiography. Signs of left ventricular dilation, dysfunction, or new-onset symptoms prompted surgical referral. Some have argued that the presence of pulmonary hypertension should indicate maladaptive changes and suggests surgical correction.

Surgical techniques of addressing the mitral valve have changed dramatically in recent years. Increasingly, operations have focused on repair rather than prosthetic replacement of the mitral valve. Valve preservation has several advantages. The interaction of the mitral valve and the left ventricle goes beyond just competence and the handling of blood volume. A complex interdependence exists between ventricle and valve, and long-term ventricular function depends on its relationship with the mitral annulus, papillary muscles, and chordae tendineae. Surgical techniques to correct mitral regurgitation that preserve these relationships are more likely to maintain normal ventricular function. In addition to the effects on ventricular function, prosthetic mitral valves carry limitations. Bioprosthetic devices (porcine or bovine) have limited durability because of structural valvular degeneration. The rate of bioprosthetic valve failure is proportional to age, with faster deterioration in younger patients. Mechanical valves are more durable but require lifelong systemic anticoagulation with warfarin. Because of the limitations imposed by prosthetic valves (durability and anticoagulation), surgical referral for mitral regurgitation is often delayed if there is a high likelihood of valve replacement. If valve repair is more likely because of mitral pathology and surgeon experience, earlier operation for mitral regurgitation is often considered, particularly in the absence of symptoms or ventricular dilation.

Surgical indications for operation in endocarditis of the mitral valve are different than for other pathologies. Certainly, valvular destruction with severe mitral regurgitation, heart failure, and ventricular dilation requires operative intervention. However, there are other specific indications for valve replacement. A history of systemic embolization or the presence of large, highly mobile vegetations at risk of embolization necessitates urgent surgical intervention. In addition, ongoing bacteremia despite appropriate antibiotic treatment coverage mandates early operation. The presence of certain organisms, such as highly resistant bacteria or fungal endocarditis warrants surgical treatment. Surgery is required for the presence of mitral annular abscess with incipient cardiac conduction abnormalities or creation of an intracardiac fistula. Prior to surgery, attempts at controlling the original source of infection should be made, including dental extractions and drainage of abscesses.

B. Techniques

Approach to the mitral valve is best accomplished via a median sternotomy. Although the mitral valve can be exposed via a right or left thoracotomy, the median sternotomy offers the best access for initiation of CPB as well as the ability to perform other cardiac procedures if necessary, such as coronary bypass grafting or aortic valve replacement. CPB is initiated, typically draining the superior and inferior vena cavae separately, and infusing into the ascending aorta. The heart is arrested using cold cardioplegia delivered into the aortic root. The left ventricle is vented, typically using the right superior pulmonary vein.

A variety of incisions can be used to expose the mitral valve, and the quality of exposure is essential in obtaining a good surgical result. The most frequent approach is by an incision directly into the left atrium. The interatrial groove of Sondergaard can be developed using sharp technique, lifting the right atrium anteriorly off of the left atrium (Figure 19–7). A vertical incision is made in the left atrium, just medial to the confluence of the right-sided pulmonary veins. Self-retaining retractors are available to elevate the atriotomy and provide visualization. Often, rotation of the table to the left away from the surgeon improves the exposure. Alternatively, an approach across the interatrial septum can be chosen. The superior and inferior vena cavae are controlled with snares, and the right atrium is opened. The fossa ovalis is identified and incised vertically. This incision is extended superiorly toward the superior vena cava through the muscular portion of the interatrial septum. The septal incision can also be extended medially along the dome of the left atrium, the so-called superior septal approach. While exposure of the mitral valve is excellent, there is a risk of injury to the sinus node, requiring implantation of a permanent pacemaker.

Once the valve has been exposed, assessment of the mitral valve is performed to determine the mechanism of mitral regurgitation and the technique for repair or replacement.

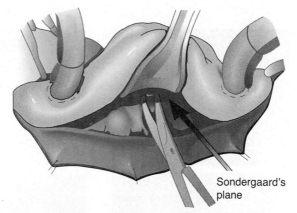

Sondergaard's plane

▲ **Figure 19–7.** Exposure of the mitral valve via the interatrial groove. (From Cohn LH. *Cardiac Surgery in the Adult,* 3rd ed. McGraw-Hill, 2007.)

Injection of cold saline into the left ventricle will identify the location of regurgitation and the presence of flail or significantly prolapsed leaflets. The leaflets are inspected for their mobility and the presence of calcifications or perforations. The annulus is inspected for dilation and calcium. Once the mechanism of regurgitation is clear, a plan is made for repair or replacement. The strategy used depends on the pathologic mechanism (Figure 19–8).

When the mitral regurgitation is purely a result of annular dilation or posterior leaflet restriction from a previous myocardial infarction, mitral annuloplasty alone often adequately alleviates the leak. Horizontal sutures are placed along the mitral annulus, including the fibrous trigones. Care must be taken to avoid injury to underlying structures, such as the circumflex coronary artery, the coronary sinus, and the atrioventricular node. Annuloplasty is typically performed with the assistance of prosthetic rings or bands of varying degrees of rigidity. Some of the rings completely encircle the entire annulus, and some are incomplete, designed to extend posteriorly from trigone to trigone (Figure 19–9). The annular mattress sutures are brought up through the sewing cuff of the ring and tied down. The size of the ring is selected to match the area of the anterior leaflet and the distance between the trigones. Competence is tested with saline injection, and the cardiac chambers are closed. After weaning from CPB, the valve is inspected using transesophageal echocardiography. An adequate repair must demonstrate both competence and low resistance, as evidenced by low pressure gradients across the valve.

Myxomatous degeneration of the mitral valve typically involves the posterior leaflet, particularly the P2 scallop. This lesion can be reproducibly repaired using techniques with the potential for indefinite durability. After exposure of the mitral valve, the point of prolapse is identified. A quadrangular portion of the prolapsing section is excised to the

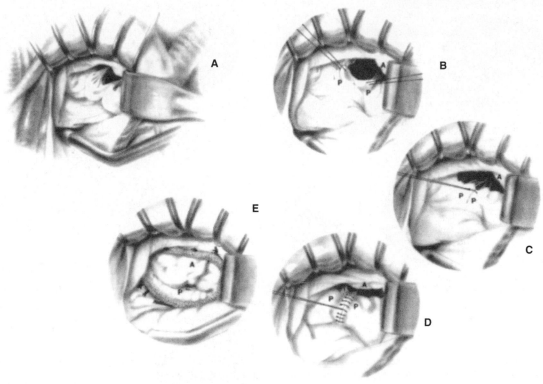

▲ **Figure 19–8.** Panels **A–E** represent atrial views of posterior leaflet reconstruction for isolated posterior leaflet prolapse and insertion of a Carpentier annuloplasty ring.

annulus. The gap is bridged by undercutting the annular attachments of the adjacent portion of the posterior leaflet. The mobilized edge of the posterior leaflet is sewn back to the annulus with running suture (Figure 19–10), reducing its effective height. An annuloplasty can be performed to address any annular dilation as well as to provide reinforcement to the posterior annular reconstruction.

When prolapse or chordal rupture involve the anterior leaflet, repair is more difficult. A variety of approaches have been described, but the likelihood of durable repair is far less when compared to the more common posterior leaflet prolapse. One approach involves the creation of artificial cords. Typically, polytetrafluoroethylene is used to create neochords from the papillary muscle to the edge of the leaflet. The challenge is to create the precise length to allow coaptation without prolapse. Alternatively, the flail anterior segment can be removed and is replaced with a resected portion of the posterior leaflet, including its attached chords. A simpler approach is the edge-to-edge technique, in which the opposing edges of the anterior and posterior leaflets are sewn together with a single suture, creating a double-orifice mitral valve. Popularized by Alfieri and colleagues, this approach

has been applied using catheter-based techniques, obviating the need for open surgery.

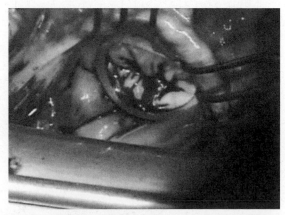

▲ **Figure 19–9.** Operative photograph of semiflexible mitral ring annuloplasty for ischemic mitral regurgitation. The ring plicates the posterior annulus to restore leaflet coaptation.

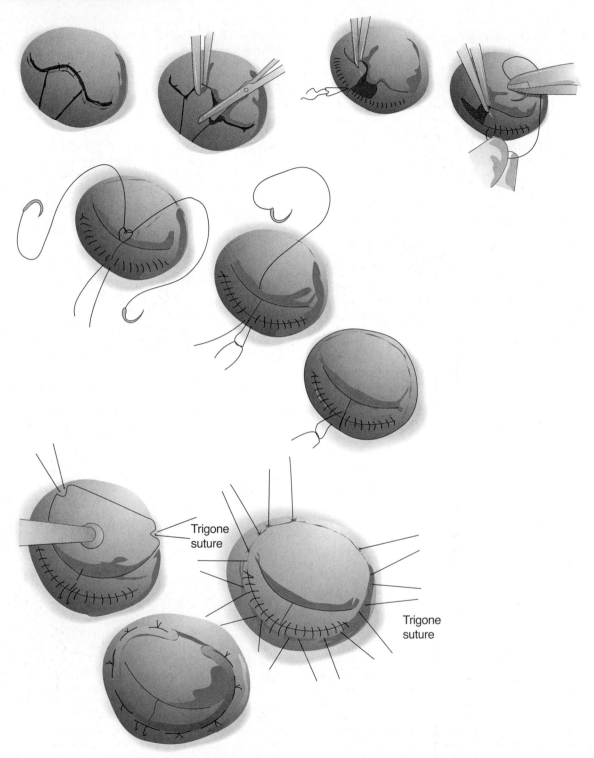

Figure 19–10. Quadrangular resection and sliding annuloplasty for prolapse of the posterior mitral valve leaflet. (From Cohn LH. *Cardiac Surgery in the Adult,* 3rd ed. McGraw-Hill, 2007.)

Often, the regurgitant mitral valve cannot be repaired, such as when there is severe valvular destruction from infective endocarditis or extensive calcifications as can be seen with rheumatic mitral valve disease. The mitral valve is exposed, and the leaflets are excised. Attempts are made to preserve chordal attachments to the annulus, and portions of the posterior leaflet can be plicated to the annulus to preserve secondary chords. This is typically not possible with rheumatic disease because the calcified annulus will require extensive debridement. Annular mattress sutures with felt or Teflon pledgets are placed circumferentially. For mechanical prostheses, the pledgets are oriented on the atrial side to avoid interference with the actuation of the disk. For bioprosthetic implants, the pledgets can be placed on the ventricular side, which allows for a slightly larger prosthetic (Figure 19–11). After sutures are placed, the annulus is sized and an appropriate prosthetic is chosen. The sutures are driven through the sewing ring of the valve and tied down. After weaning from CPB, the valve is carefully inspected using transesophageal echocardiography for signs of paravalvular leak, normal motion of the leaflets or disks, and a low pressure gradient across the valve.

C. Results

Repair or replacement of the mitral valve for regurgitation preserves ventricular function and allows some remodeling by eliminating the volume overload and its associated incipient changes. However, loss of myocardial contractility, as a result of longstanding mitral regurgitation or otherwise, typically does not recover. Only its progressive decline can be halted. This reinforces the need to intervene before severe ventricular dilation has occurred, even in asymptomatic patients.

Mitral regurgitation associated with prolapsing myxomatous leaflets carries low perioperative mortality, and the freedom from degeneration of a repaired valve is greater than 90% at 10 years. Some of the low periprocedural mortality is related to the young age and low incidence of comorbidities in this patient population. Mitral valve repair associated with coronary bypass grafting carries a perioperative mortality of approximately 5%, with ejection fraction, renal function, and age being independent predictors of death. Although mortality after coronary bypass grafting is associated with the severity of preoperative mitral regurgitation, there is no evidence that mitral repair reduces this mortality. Repairing the mitral valve, however, is associated with improved long-term survival, as compared to replacing the valve.

MITRAL VALVE STENOSIS

▶ Pathophysiology

Rheumatic heart disease is the most common cause of mitral valve stenosis. Although nearly 20 million people are affected with rheumatic fever in underdeveloped countries, the incidence in the United States and Western Europe has declined markedly, largely a result of advanced medical care and use of antibiotics to treat infections caused by group A streptococci. Untreated infection results in an immunologic response to bacterial antigens that resemble cardiac tissue. The degree of the immunologic response and the severity of ongoing valvular destruction appear to be related to genetic factors. Although the damage can affect the entire endocardium and even the pericardium, the mitral valve is the most commonly involved, with 40% of patients having only mitral valve disease. Mitral and aortic valve disease is also

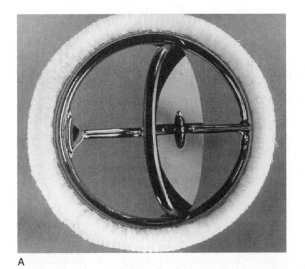

A

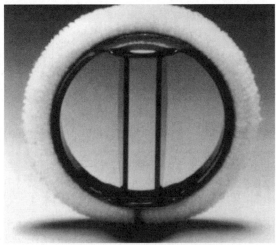

B

▲ **Figure 19–11. A:** Medtronic-Hall tilting-disk mechanical valve. **B:** St. Jude Medical bileaflet mechanical valve.

frequently seen, and rarely patients will have isolated aortic valve involvement. It remains unclear why right-sided valves are rarely affected.

The characteristic features of rheumatic mitral valve disease include leaflet and chordal thickening and retraction (Figure 19–12). Commissural fusion is also apparent, and a late feature is dense calcification of the annulus and leaflets. Turbulence created by impaired leaflet mobility exacerbates the valve destruction, accelerating further fibrosis and calcification.

Mitral valve stenosis can also be caused by mitral annular calcification, which can become quite bulky, protruding into the valve orifice. The posterior leaflet can become contracted and fixed, while the anterior leaflet thickens and becomes less mobile. Structural valvular degeneration of bioprosthetic mitral valves can cause mitral valve stenosis as well as thrombosis or pannus formation in mechanical prostheses. Advanced endocarditis can result in effective mitral valve stenosis, as bulky vegetations obstruct the inflow path. Congenital abnormalities, such as the parachute mitral valve with a single papillary muscle, can become stenotic, requiring intervention.

The stenotic mitral valve results in a pressure gradient between the left atrium and ventricle. This fixed resistance increases the left atrial pressure even further during exercise, as cardiac output increases, but resistance across the valve is unchanged. Severe mitral valve stenosis is associated with a mean transvalvular gradient of 10–15 mm Hg at rest. Cardiac output is dependent on ventricular filling, and left ventricular end diastolic pressure and volume are typically low. Exercise-induced tachycardia decreases diastolic filling time, producing a paradoxical reduction in cardiac output. Left ventricular function is typically normal or hyperdynamic, but some patients have combined mitral valve stenosis and mitral regurgitation, as well as significant aortic valve insufficiency, and will develop chronic left ventricular volume overload and dysfunction. Thus, the hemodynamic consequences of mitral valve stenosis depend to a certain degree on the presence of mitral regurgitation and other associated valvular pathology.

As the mitral transvalvular gradient worsens, the left atrial wall hypertrophies. The a-wave on the atrial pressure tracing is accentuated during atrial contraction. Progressively, the left atrium dilates, creating disorganized electrical conduction pathways. Reentry pathways lead to frequent premature atrial contractions and eventually to atrial fibrillation. The onset of atrial fibrillation often is the inciting clinical event, with the reduced diastolic filling time from rapid ventricular response and the loss of atrial contraction both resulting in reduced left ventricular filling and a drop in cardiac output. The sustained elevation in left atrial pressure results in pulmonary vascular changes producing pulmonary hypertension. These changes can lead to right ventricular pressure overload with tricuspid valve insufficiency and to right ventricular volume overload.

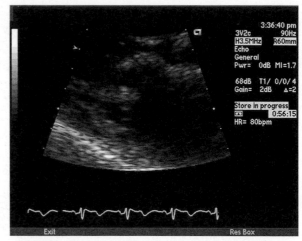

▲ **Figure 19–12.** Echocardiographic image of a rheumatic mitral valve with thickened leaflet and chord.

Symptoms of mitral valve stenosis often do not develop until the disease is advanced, owing to ventricular and atrial adaptive responses. Patients describe dyspnea from pulmonary congestion or reduced cardiac output, initially limited to exertion. Onset of atrial fibrillation often prompts urgent evaluation, as the loss of atrial contraction and tachycardia cause a precipitous drop in cardiac output and pulmonary congestion. Late findings include signs of right-sided heart failure such as ascites and lower extremity edema. Cerebrovascular events or other thromboembolic complications from an intracardiac thrombus are not uncommon with longstanding mitral valve stenosis, as the dilated left atrium and left atrial appendage have regions of stagnation and thrombus formation, particularly in the setting of atrial fibrillation. Since two thirds of the patients with mitral valve stenosis are women, symptoms often present during later stages of pregnancy as the increased cardiac output results in higher left atrial pressures and pulmonary congestion.

▶ Diagnostic Evaluation

Because presentation tends to be late, many patients present with signs of longstanding heart failure, including cachexia, ascites, and lower extremity edema. On auscultation, the low diastolic rumble is best heard over the cardiac apex. An opening snap can be heard in the early stages of the disease, and the systolic murmur of tricuspid regurgitation is a late finding, as is a parasternal heave from right ventricular hypertrophy.

The electrocardiogram will diagnose atrial fibrillation, and right axis deviation may be present, suggesting advanced pulmonary hypertension. Otherwise, the electrocardiogram can be nonspecific or normal. The chest radiograph is often normal but may demonstrate straightening of the left heart border caused by dilation of the pulmonary arteries. Pulmonary edema may be present on initial evaluation when atrial fibrillation is the inciting event. Cardiac catheterization is important in identifying associated coronary arterial pathology and can confirm the severity of the mitral stenosis using simultaneous left and right heart catheterization with pressure measurements. The degree of pulmonary hypertension and its reversibility with provocative agents may be assistive in determining surgical candidacy in advanced cases.

Echocardiography is the mainstay in diagnosis of mitral valve stenosis. Surface, or transthoracic echocardiography is preferred because it is noninvasive, and can usually provide images demonstrating the characteristic thickening and restricted mobility of the mitral leaflets. If images are obscured by patient body habitus or obstructive lung disease, a transesophageal echocardiogram can be performed. The proximity of the esophagus with the left atrium provides excellent visualization and can easily demonstrate the thickened mitral subvalvar apparatus typical of rheumatic disease. Color Doppler can be used to show turbulent flow across the valve orifice, and the pressure gradients can be estimated by measuring the peak and mean velocity of blood through the valve.

▶ Treatment

Medical treatment is limited to control of symptoms. Recurrent episodes of infection must be prevented, as accelerated progression of the disease can be seen. Prompt initiation of antibiotics for suspected infections is prudent. Complications of mitral valve stenosis should be addressed and controlled. Rapid ventricular response to atrial fibrillation can be treated with a number of pharmacologic agents, and attempts at cardioversion should be made once the presence of intracardiac thrombus has been excluded. It is often difficult to maintain sinus rhythm in the mitral valve stenosis patient with a significantly dilated left atrium in whom rate control alone may be acceptable. Systemic anticoagulation with warfarin should be initiated if there has been a history of atrial fibrillation. Once the patient describes symptoms of heart failure, intervention on the mitral valve should be considered. For symptomatic patients not candidates for catheter-based or surgical intervention, diuretics and oral sodium restriction to control heart failure symptoms is all that is available.

Catheter-based balloon mitral valvotomy can reduce the obstructing pressure gradient and improve symptoms in selected patients. Patients with severe mitral valve stenosis and symptoms and asymptomatic patients with severe mitral valve stenosis and pulmonary hypertension are eligible if there is no mitral regurgitation, no left atrial thrombus, and favorable valve morphology, such as absence of extensive subvalvular fibrosis and calcification. The procedure is performed by femoral venous puncture and transseptal access to the mitral valve across the interatrial septum. A 25-mm hourglass Inoue balloon is advanced across the valve orifice and inflated.

Significant improvement in hemodynamics is seen immediately, with reduction in transvalvular pressure gradients by as much as 15 mm Hg. The incidence of restenosis in selected patients is approximately 25% at 4 years.

Indications for surgical treatment are the same as for balloon valvuloplasty, including symptomatic patients with moderate or severe mitral valve stenosis and asymptomatic patients with pulmonary hypertension. Valve repair can be performed in carefully selected patients with reasonable long-term results. CPB is initiated in the same manner as for mitral repair for mitral regurgitation. After cardioplegic arrest, the mitral valve is exposed. Any thrombus within the atrium or atrial appendage is removed. The left atrial appendage can be transected and oversewn at its base to remove its future embolic potential. The areas of commissural fusion are cut, and the leaflets are decalcified. Occasionally, fused chords are divided to increase leaflet mobility. In carefully selected patients, recurrent mitral valve stenosis is less than 20% in up to 15 years.

In most cases, however, severe leaflet and subvalvular calcification has made the valve unreconstructable, requiring valve replacement. Overaggressive debridement of the posterior mitral annulus can result in perforation and atrioventricular separation and should be avoided. The selection of valve prosthetic depends on the unique clinical circumstances. Bioprosthetic valves are minimally thrombogenic and do not require lifelong anticoagulation with warfarin. However, they are prone to structural valvular degeneration resulting in recurrent mitral valve stenosis or mitral regurgitation. Valve prosthetics are improving, and freedom from structural valvular degeneration is as high as 85% at 10 years. Mechanical valves are thrombogenic and require lifelong anticoagulation, such as warfarin, which is associated with a 1–2% annual incidence of major bleeding complications. They are more durable and reduce the need for reoperation. In general, patients younger than 60 years of age or those already requiring warfarin for atrial fibrillation should be considered for a mechanical valve.

AORTIC VALVE DISEASE

The aortic valve separates the outflow tract of the left ventricle with the ascending aorta. It is a trileaflet structure, with three semilunar cusps named for the coronary arteries that arise within the underlying sinuses. The left and right coronary arteries originate within these respective sinuses, with no coronary artery arising within the *non*coronary sinus. The free edges of the cusps are thickened at regions called the nodules of Arantius. The valve leaflets attach to the wall of the aorta at the annulus, and the locations where two adjacent cusps meet are the commissures. Important structures can be identified under these triangular-shaped zones (Figure 19–13). The commissure between the right and noncoronary cusp serves as the superior border to the membranous interventricular septum and the atrioventricular

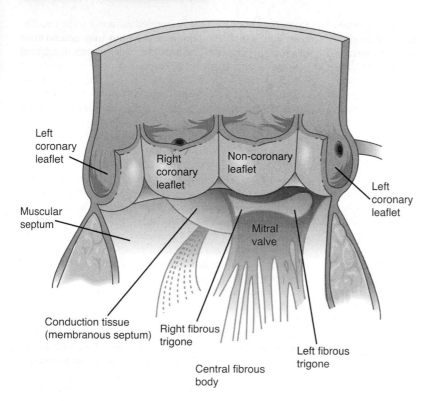

Left coronary leaflet

Right coronary leaflet

Non-coronary leaflet

Left coronary leaflet

Muscular septum

Mitral valve

Conduction tissue (membranous septum)

Right fibrous trigone

Left fibrous trigone

Central fibrous body

▲ **Figure 19–13.** Anatomic relationships of the aortic root. (From Cohn LH. *Cardiac Surgery in the Adult,* 3rd ed. McGraw-Hill, 2007.)

conduction center. The nonleft commissure guards the aortomitral curtain and the center of the anterior leaflet of the mitral valve. The left-right commissure overlies the muscular interventricular septum and the medial border of the right ventricular outflow tract. These intimate intracardiac relationships are no more apparent than within the left ventricular outflow tract.

The thin-walled aortic valve leaflets easily open and close during the cardiac cycle, purely following the pressure changes and blood flow path. Under normal circumstances, opening offers very little resistance to flow. The aortic sinuses have an important role during valve closure, as the volume of blood within the space between the opened valve cusp and the aortic wall develop vortices as blood velocity falls. These vortices exert central pressure and initiates valve closure. The sudden reversal of flow from deceleration completes the diastolic closure.

AORTIC STENOSIS

▶ Pathophysiology

The most common cause of aortic stenosis is senile calcific aortic stenosis. It is believed to represent degenerative changes at the cellular level, including lipid accumulation and inflammatory infiltrates, similar to atherosclerotic changes seen in the medium-sized arterial tree. Not surpris-

ingly, it is associated with elevated cholesterol, hypertension, cigarette smoking, diabetes, and other risk factors for atherosclerosis. It is most common in the seventh and eighth decades of life and occurs in patients whose valves previously appeared normal. The cusps become progressively immobilized and calcified, starting at the flexion points and extending both along the leaflets and into the wall of the aortic root.

Congenital bicuspid aortic valve represents the most common congenital cardiac lesion, occurring in 2% of the general population. Turbulent flow across the valve causes trauma, leading to fibrosis and calcium deposition, further increasing turbulence, and accelerating the process. Significant stenosis typically occurs in the fifth and sixth decades of life, although they can present earlier. Patients with congenital bicuspid aortic valves often have dilation or aneurysmal degeneration of the ascending aorta. Some evidence suggests a genetic etiology, with presence of abnormal microfibrils causing premature cystic medial necrosis.

Rheumatic heart disease can affect the aortic valve, although it is unusual for the disease to be limited to the aorta, with mitral involvement far more common. As with rheumatic mitral stenosis, fusion of the commissures tends to be the initial feature, followed by progressive thickening and retraction of the leaflets. The reduced leaflet mobility results in a clinical picture of combined aortic valve stenosis and insufficiency.

Aortic stenosis develops gradually, allowing adaptive changes to maintain cardiac output. The left ventricle gradually hypertrophies in response to the severity of the outflow tract obstruction, often resulting in pressure gradients exceeding 100 mm Hg. As a result, patients can remain asymptomatic until severely advanced disease is present. While concentric left ventricular hypertrophy maintains systolic function in the face of severe outflow obstruction, diastolic function of the thickened and noncompliant ventricle is progressively impaired. Diastolic dysfunction can be overcome to a certain degree with atrial hypertrophy and enhanced atrial kick. In addition, as left ventricular end diastolic pressure rises, intravascular volume status and peripheral vascular resistance adjust to maintain the required preload. Certain triggers can disrupt this delicate balance, including loss of atrial contribution from atrial fibrillation or reduced diastolic filling time from increased heart rate, as might be seen during exercise. These triggers can create sudden clinical decompensation, producing markedly reduced cardiac output and pulmonary edema, even in a previously asymptomatic patient.

The most common clinical presentation in a patient with aortic stenosis is gradual decrease in exercise tolerance. The fixed outflow obstruction prevents an increase in stroke volume typically seen in exercise with elevated circulating catecholamines. Any change in cardiac output is limited to an increase in heart rate, decreasing diastolic filling time for the stiff and noncompliant ventricle. As a result, there is limited boost in cardiac output during exercise, producing premature exertional fatigue and dyspnea. Some patients describe angina, as myocardial oxygen demand exceeds supply. The hypertrophied heart consumes more oxygen without reciprocal increase in epicardial delivery. In addition, the outflow obstruction prolongs systole, further increasing oxygen demand. Symptoms are typically exertional, as the increased heart rate reduces diastolic coronary perfusion time. Syncope or presyncope is occasionally described in patients with aortic stenosis, presumable related to systemic vasodilation during exercise without a reciprocal increase in cardiac output. Advanced heart failure with symptoms at rest or with minimal activity suggest a decrease in systolic function, likely a result of longstanding disease with alterations within the myocardium at the cellular level.

▶ Diagnostic Evaluation

Physical examination of the patient reveals several findings specific for aortic stenosis. There is a characteristic systolic crescendo/decrescendo murmur heard best over the base of the heart and radiating up the carotid arteries. The murmur becomes harsher and peaks later in systole as the severity worsens. Palpation of the carotid pulses reveals parvus and tardus, or a late peaking and low-amplitude pulse. A palpable thrill may be felt over the right second intercostal space.

The electrocardiogram demonstrates left ventricular hypertrophy in the majority of patients. Conduction or rhythm abnormalities is identified in some patients. The chest radiograph typically is normal but may demonstrate dilation of the ascending aorta in patients with congenital bicuspid valve. Cardiac catheterization provides important information about associated cardiac pathology, particularly coronary occlusive disease. In addition, hemodynamic assessment can confirm the severity of the aortic valve stenosis and quantify the degree of pulmonary hypertension.

The standard evaluation of patients with suspected aortic stenosis is echocardiography. Images of the valve reveal the severity of the stiffness and calcifications. Images also differentiate bicuspid from tricuspid anatomy and identify associated dilation of the ascending aorta. Ventricular function and additional valvular pathology, particularly in patients with rheumatic heart disease, is essential. Doppler echocardiography can measure the velocity of the aortic jet, allowing reliable estimates of the pressure gradients using the modified Bernoulli equation.

▶ Treatment

A. Medical Therapy

Because aortic stenosis can progress over 10–15 years, patients with mild to moderate disease and without symptoms can be followed without intervention. Serial echocardiography should be performed annually or every other year to assess for disease progression. The most important aspect of medical therapy is education of the patient about potential symptoms. Since symptoms can develop gradually, many patients will unconsciously alter their lifestyles and activity levels without recognizing the presence of limitations. Although there is some suggestion that cholesterol reduction with statins can reduce the calcifications, there is little evidence that medications can adequately palliate the symptomatic patient or can alter the timing of surgical intervention in asymptomatic patients.

B. Indications for Surgery

The indications for surgery on the stenotic aortic valve have been largely determined by the presence of symptoms. Numerous studies have demonstrated reasonably good prognosis in asymptomatic patients managed without surgery. However, symptoms may be equivocal, particularly in the elderly population. Exercise stress testing under the observation of a physician can help elucidate significant limitations that may not be apparent by merely questioning the patient. Surgery is also indicated for patients with moderate to severe aortic stenosis who are undergoing cardiac surgery for other indications, such as coronary bypass grafting or mitral valve replacement.

Handling of the asymptomatic patient with severe aortic stenosis is under some controversy. The severity of aortic stenosis can be quantified using Doppler echocardiography to estimate the pressure gradient across the aortic valve using the velocity of the outflow jet and the modified Bernoulli equation.

Severe aortic stenosis is present when the mean gradient exceeds 40 mm Hg in the normal ventricle. Although some have described an increase in the rate of sudden death in patients with severe aortic stenosis, there remains no evidence to justify aortic valve replacement in the absence of symptoms.

AORTIC INSUFFICIENCY

▶ Pathophysiology

Several conditions can cause incompetence of the aortic valve. Any of the disease processes that cause aortic stenosis can also cause some degree of aortic valve insufficiency, including senile calcific aortic stenosis, degenerated bicuspid aortic valve, and rheumatic aortic valve disease. Aortic valve endocarditis is another common cause of aortic valve insufficiency. The most common cause of incompetence of the aortic valve is related to pathology within the aortic root and ascending aorta. Aneurysmal dilation of the ascending aorta, either from congenital conditions such as Marfan disease, from degenerative age-related changes, or from changes associated with a bicuspid aortic valve, can cause aortic valve insufficiency. As the wall of the aorta enlarges, the aortic valve annulus dilates and the leaflets separate, causing incompetence.

As with mitral valve regurgitation, aortic valve insufficiency is best tolerated when it occurs gradually. As the volume of regurgitation worsens, the ventricle adapts by dilating to accommodate the increased preload, and it hypertrophies to maintain the same level of systolic pressure at larger volumes. Despite progressive dilation, ventricular output and systolic function are maintained for long periods of time, leaving many patients asymptomatic for years. While end diastolic volume is elevated, end systolic volume is normal. With severe degrees of chronic aortic insufficiency, the heart can require ejecting as much as two to three times the circulating cardiac output, resulting in longstanding volume overload. Eventually, systolic function declines, resulting in a rapid and progressive rise in end diastolic volume, and heart failure symptoms ensue.

Most patients with chronic aortic insufficiency do not develop symptoms of heart failure until there is severe left ventricular dilation. Some patients describe palpitations or the sensation of ventricular heave, particularly when lying down. Acute aortic valve insufficiency, as can occur with aortic valve endocarditis, can present with cardiogenic shock because the relatively noncompliant ventricle is unprepared for the excess volume during both systole and diastole. There is a combination of high intracardiac filling pressures and low cardiac output. Patients are tachycardic and hypotensive as well as acutely dyspneic at rest. The patient with endocarditis may also be febrile with signs of embolization of vegetations, causing stroke or extremity or intestinal ischemia.

▶ Diagnostic Testing

Certain characteristic physical examination findings are pathognomonic for chronic aortic valve insufficiency. The water-hammer pulse can be appreciated, with accentuated systole and abrupt collapse. Patients may have a head bob with each heart beat, or a pulse may be seen in the uvula. A systolic thrill is also described over the femoral artery from the augmented forward flow. The apical impulse is displaced laterally and inferiorly from cardiomegaly, and diastolic blood pressure is low. Auscultation will reveal a high-pitched diastolic murmur heard immediately after the second heart sound. The severity of the valvular lesion usually correlates with the duration of the murmur, not the intensity. The murmur is best heard with the patient leaning forward during a breath hold.

Echocardiography will establish the etiology of the aortic valve insufficiency, visualizing the motion of the leaflets and dilation of the aorta or the presence of vegetations or leaflet perforations. In addition, the ventricular size can be followed, as elevated end systolic volumes or reduced ejection fraction are indications for surgery. Reversal of flow seen in the descending aorta is a sign of severe aortic valve insufficiency. More sophisticated techniques can quantify the regurgitant volume, such as evaluating the regurgitant jet velocity/time integral.

▶ Treatment

For asymptomatic patients with moderate aortic insufficiency and normal ventricular dimensions, no treatment is necessary. Patients with severe aortic valve insufficiency and normal ventricular size should be followed every 6 months with assessment of symptoms and echocardiography. Some advocate the use of afterload reduction agents to reduce the volume of regurgitant blood, but no evidence demonstrates reduced need for surgery. Symptomatic patients who are not candidates for surgery should be treated with afterload reduction agents, such as calcium channel blockers or inhibitors of angiotensin-converting enzyme. Diuretics and salt restrictions may help in alleviating heart failure symptoms.

For operative candidates, development of heart failure symptoms is an indication for surgery. Asymptomatic patients with decreased left ventricular systolic function or elevated left ventricular end systolic volumes should also undergo operative treatment. Because ventricular dilation is associated with irreversible changes at the cellular level, intervention is best performed before these permanent changes occur.

▶ Surgical Techniques

As with most other cardiac surgical procedures, median sternotomy is the standard incision utilized for access to the aortic valve. The pericardium is opened longitudinally, and the reflection is mobilized off of the great vessels. The pulmonary artery and aorta are separated as they emanate from the heart, taking care to avoid injury to the takeoff of the right pulmonary artery or the left main coronary artery. The patient is anticoagulated with 300 IU heparin, and an activated clotting time of at least 400 seconds is confirmed. Cannulation for CPB is performed, using the distal ascending aorta or the transverse aortic arch to maximize the distance between the aortic cross-clamp and the aortotomy. Venous return is via the right atrial appendage. CPB is initiated, and the left ventricle is vented via a catheter advanced from the right superior pulmonary vein. The patient is cooled systemically to 32 °C. An aortic cross-clamp is applied to the distal ascending aorta just proximal to the CPB cannula. The heart is arrested with cold blood cardioplegia solution with dextrose, phosphate, and potassium at 8 °C. The cardioplegia is delivered antegrade down the coronary arteries using a catheter in the aortic root. Cardioplegia is also delivered retrograde via a balloon-tipped catheter in the coronary sinus. If severe aortic valve insufficiency is present, only retrograde cardioplegia can be delivered. Once diastolic cardiac arrest is achieved, the ascending aorta is opened transversely approximately 1–2 cm above the takeoff of the right coronary artery. The aortotomy is extended two thirds of the circumference of the aorta, providing excellent visualization of the valve, the coronary ostia, and the ventricular outflow tract (Figure 19–14).

Excision of the stenotic aortic valve can be time consuming and requires meticulous attention to detail. The extensive calcifications can extend deep into the annulus and up the wall of the aortic root or down along the anterior leaflet of the mitral valve. The calcium buildup must be debrided aggressively enough to allow proper seating of the valve prosthesis without a paravalvular leak while avoiding residual outflow tract obstruction. However, overaggressive debridement can result in perforations of the aortic wall, ventricular septal defect, or unhinging of the mitral leaflet with resultant severe mitral regurgitation. In cases of endocarditis, any granulation tissue or residual vegetations must be removed and debrided to avoid recurrent infection of the implanted prosthetic. The outflow tract and aortic root is thoroughly irrigated to ensure removal of loose deposits and debris.

Once the native valve has been removed and the annulus satisfactorily debrided, the outflow tract is sized using tools provided by each manufacturer of valve prostheses. The appropriately sized valve is selected and secured in place. Mechanical valve prosthetics are implanted using a pledgeted mattress technique, leaving the pledgets on the aortic side. This eliminates the likelihood of the bulky pledgets interfering with the disk mechanisms on the ventricular surface. Alternatively, if a bioprosthetic valve is selected, the pledgets can be oriented on the ventricular side of the annulus. This allows supra-annular seating of the bioprosthetic and implantation of a slightly larger valve. The sutures are then placed through the sewing cuff of the prosthetic, and the valve is lowered into the surgical field. The sutures are tied, ensuring that the valve has seated properly to the annulus. The ostia of the coronary arteries should be inspected and clearly free of impingement by the prosthetic valve. The aortotomy is then closed with running polypropylene suture, occasionally reinforced with Teflon felt in the older patient with a thin aortic wall.

The patient is then gradually weaned from CPB, thoroughly deairing with gentle suction applied using the left ventricular vent and the aortic root catheter. The valve is carefully inspected using the transesophageal echocardiogram for competency and adequacy of the size. There should be no paravalvular leak, and the gradients across the valve should be low. Elevated pulmonary artery pressures or reduced cardiac output should alert the surgeon of the possibility of an unrecognized paravalvular leak.

Occasionally, the aortic annulus and aortic root are small, allowing implantation of an undersized valve, creating postoperative pressure gradients and leaving the patient with residual left ventricular outflow tract obstruction. A variety of maneuvers can be performed to enlarge the aortic root. A Nicks procedure involves extending the aortotomy obliquely down the noncoronary sinus and across the aortic annulus into the anterior leaflet of the mitral valve. The defect is closed with a small diamond-shaped patch of Dacron or pericardium. The reconstructed annulus is now increased in size approximately 2–4 mm, allowing upsizing of the chosen prosthetic. A Konno procedure involves creating an anterior longitudinal aortotomy, extending into the right coronary sinus and across the right ventricular outflow tract. The muscular interventricular septum is opened below the annulus, allowing expansion of the annulus beyond 4 mm. This procedure is typically performed in children to allow insertion of a prosthetic for congenital stenosis, which will allow for increased flow with the child's growth.

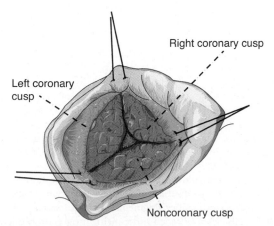

▲ Figure 19–14. Surgeon's view of the stenotic trileaflet aortic valve. (From Cohn LH. *Cardiac Surgery in the Adult*, 3rd ed. McGraw-Hill, 2007.)

Right coronary cusp

Left coronary cusp

Noncoronary cusp

Aortic valve endocarditis also poses unique surgical challenges. The infective process often results in abscess formation and occasionally intracardiac fistulas. The most important first step in addressing these problems is aggressive debridement of infected and devitalized tissue. Not only will residual infection colonize the implanted prosthetic but inadequate debridement with securing of the prosthetic to infected and devitalized tissue will lead to dehiscence with need for early reoperation. Abscesses are common within the intervalvular fibrous body. The annular defect should be covered with a pericardial patch. Often, the entire root requires excision, requiring replacement with a valved conduit and reimplantation of the coronary ostia. Results for endocarditis are dependent on the clinical status of the patient at the time of surgery as well as the etiology of the infection. Intravenous drug users carry the worst prognosis, in large part related to recurrence of their addiction with subsequent reinfection.

Alfieri O et al: The double-orifice technique in mitral valve repair: a simple solution for complex problems. J Thorac Cardiovasc Surg 2001;122:674.

Bonow RO et al: ACC/AHA 2006 guidelines for the management of patients with valvular heart disease: a report of the American College of Cardiology/American Heart Association Task Force on Practice Guidelines Circulation. J Am Coll Cardiol 2006;48:e1.

Carabello BA: Evaluation and management of patients with aortic stenosis. Circulation 2002;105:1746.

Cohn LH et al: Long-term results of mitral valve reconstruction for regurgitation of the myxomatous mitral valve. J Thorac Cardiovasc Surg 1994;107:143.

Cotrufo M et al: Percutaneous mitral commissurotomy versus open mitral commissurotomy: a comparative study. Eur J Cardiothorac Surg 1999;15:646.

Essop MR, Nkomo VT: Rheumatic and nonrheumatic valvular heart disease: epidemiology, management, and prevention in Africa. Circulation 2005;112:3584.

Fredak PWM et al: Clinical and pathophysiological implications of a bicuspid aortic valve. Circulation 2002;106:900.

Mihaljevic T et al: Impact of mitral valve annuloplasty combined with revascularization in patients with functional ischemic mitral regurgitation. J Am Coll Cardiol 2007;49:2191.

Moura LM et al: Rosuvastatin affecting aortic valve endothelium to slow the progression of aortic stenosis. J Am Coll Cardiol 2007;49:554.

Otto CM et al: Prospective study of asymptomatic valvular aortic stenosis. Clinical, echocardiographic, and exercise predictors of outcome. Circulation 1997;95:2262.

Palacios IF et al: Which patients benefit from percutaneous mitral balloon valvuloplasty? Prevalvuloplasty and postvalvuloplasty variables that predict long-term outcome. Circulation 2002;105:1465.

Roberts WC et al: Causes of pure aortic regurgitation in patients having isolated aortic valve replacement at a single US tertiary hospital (1993-2005). Circulation 2006;114:442.

Thompson ME, Shaver JA, Leon DF: Effect of tachycardia on atrial transport in mitral stenosis. Am Heart J 1977;94:297.

Wu AH et al: Impact of mitral valve annuloplasty on mortality risk in patients with mitral regurgitation and left ventricular systolic dysfunction. J Am Coll Cardiol 2005;46:381.

▼ THORACIC AORTA

The ascending aorta represents a continuation of the aortic root at the sinotubular junction. The aortic arch extends from the ascending aorta, traveling posteriorly and to the left as it gives off the three "head vessels" superiorly: the innominate, left carotid, and left subclavian arteries. The thoracic aorta continues from the aortic arch into the descending thoracic aorta beyond the left subclavian artery. The descending thoracic aorta continues until the level of the diaphragm, where it becomes the abdominal aorta. The only branches originating from the descending thoracic aorta are the bronchial and esophageal arteries and multiple intercostal vessels that contribute important sources of blood flow to the spinal cord.

Some common variants are seen in the branch pattern of the thoracic aorta. The most common is the "bovine arch" in which the left carotid originates from the innominate artery. An aberrant right subclavian artery originates from the distal aortic arch on the lesser curvature and travels posterior to the esophagus from left to right. It has been associated with unusual causes of dysphagia from mechanical compression of the esophagus. Other abnormal variants of the aortic arch include a right-sided arch and double ligamentum arteriosum, which can cause tracheal or esophageal compression early in life and are discussed in the second part of this chapter, Congenital Heart Disease.

THORACIC AORTIC ANEURYSMS

▶ Pathophysiology

During systole, kinetic energy imparted by ventricular ejection is absorbed in the compliance of the aorta, resulting in transient expansion and recoil. The amount of energy absorption is proportional to the proximity to the left ventricle. As such, the ascending, descending, and abdominal aortae have different cellular features to accommodate their unique fluid-mechanical environments. Elastin fiber content is typically higher in the ascending aorta. These fibers are synthesized and degraded continuously by the smooth muscle cells, and a progressive fragmentation of these fibers is associated with aging, which is the reason for gradual dilation of the ascending aorta in the elderly. However, certain acquired conditions can accelerate the process, producing the pathologically enlarged aorta resulting in aneurysms. Aortic atherosclerosis is associated with aneurysm formation, predominantly in the descending thoracic aorta. The inflammatory process extends from the intima to the media, causing elastin fiber breakdown. Cystic medial degeneration is the end result of any of the acquired degenerative processes, resulting in elastin fiber fragmentation and loss of smooth muscle cells. The weakened aortic media progressively dilates and can become prone to rupture or dissection. Infection, inflammatory conditions, and trauma can also cause localized medial degeneration and aneurysm formation.

Certain heritable conditions are also associated with aneurysmal disease of the thoracic aorta. Most notable is Marfan syndrome, an autosomal dominant abnormality of fibrillin, an important component in elastin. Patients with Marfan syndrome present with aneurysmal degeneration of the thoracic aorta at any level, most notably in the ascending aorta, in the second and third decades of life. Patients with bicuspid aortic valves are prone to develop aneurysms of the ascending aorta, likely related to abnormalities of their aortic smooth muscle.

The natural history of unresected thoracic aortic aneurysms is dependent on the size and the etiology. The larger the aneurysm, the greater the wall tension and thus the risk of rupture or dissection. Beyond 5.5 cm in maximal diameter, there is a significant increase in the risk of rupture, dissection, or death. Although it varies with age and etiology, there is a reasonably predictable growth rate, estimated at approximately 0.1–0.2 cm per year. Marfan syndrome and other genetic causes of thoracic aortic pathology tend to have a higher likelihood of rupture at smaller aneurysm sizes, and the growth rate is faster than in acquired thoracic aneurysms.

Most patients with thoracic aortic aneurysms are asymptomatic. The diagnosis is often established on screening chest radiograph, CT, or echocardiography performed for other indications. Occasionally, patients with unruptured aneurysms describe chest pain presumably related to rapid enlargement or encroachment on adjacent structures. Unfortunately, many patients are not diagnosed with a thoracic aortic aneurysm until the time of rupture or dissection. Rupture of ascending aneurysms typically presents with crushing chest pain, whereas descending aneurysms cause tearing back or flank pain.

▶ Diagnostic Testing

In a patient presenting with a thoracic aneurysm without rupture, the physical examination is typically unremarkable. Chest radiograph may demonstrate a widened mediastinum. The electrocardiogram is helpful only for associated cardiac pathology. An echocardiogram demonstrates enlargement of the ascending aorta or descending aorta. The aortic arch is typically obscured from view by the trachea and the lungs.

Contrast-enhanced CT scanning is the most widely used test for aneurysms of the thoracic aorta (Figure 19–15). The CT scan can diagnose the aneurysm and accurately describe its size and extent, can be used for direct comparison for patients managed expectantly, and can differentiate isolated aneurysmal disease from an aortic dissection. Three-dimensional reconstruction is helpful in accurately assessing size and location of branch vessels. The limitation of CT scanning is the need for intravenous iodinated contrast, with its inherent nephrotoxic properties.

MRI provides quality resolution similar to CT scanning but can provide dynamic imaging for cardiac assessment and does not require iodinated contrast material. MRI, however, is more time consuming and less available in many centers. Cardiac catheterization and aortography are performed only in planning operative intervention to exclude coronary artery disease or pulmonary hypertension.

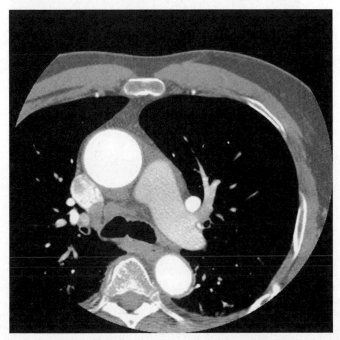

▲ **Figure 19–15.** CT scan of a dilated ascending aorta.

Surgical Therapy

The most frequent indication for operation on the aneurysmal ascending aorta is incidental to other cardiac pathology. It is generally agreed that an asymptomatic ascending aorta greater than 4.5–5 cm in size should be replaced at the time of aortic valve replacement or coronary bypass surgery, assuming the risk of the procedure would not be significantly altered. Any patient with a symptomatic ascending aneurysm should receive urgent surgery, although it is unusual for patients with ruptured ascending aortas to survive long enough to be given this opportunity. For asymptomatic patients without associated cardiac pathology, the indication for surgery is when the maximal diameter of the ascending aorta is greater than 5.5 cm. For patients with Marfan syndrome, surgery is indicated for lesser degrees of dilation. Additionally, for patients followed with serial CT scans, interval enlargement of the ascending aorta by a least 1 cm warrants consideration for surgical resection.

Sudden rupture or dissection is less frequent in the descending aorta, and thus the indications for operation are less stringent. In general, operation should be considered when the aneurysm reaches 6 cm in maximal diameter or if there is interval enlargement by at least 1 cm over 1 year. Patients with Marfan syndrome require surgery at smaller aortic sizes to prevent catastrophic complications.

Medical treatment of small ascending or descending aneurysms involves aggressive blood pressure control using beta-blocking agents to reduce the forceful contraction against the weakened aortic wall, activity restriction to avoid straining, cessation of cigarette smoking, and weight loss. Patients followed with ascending or descending aortic aneurysms should receive repeat imaging for signs of interval growth prompting surgical intervention.

AORTIC DISSECTION

Pathophysiology

Dissection of the thoracic aorta is among the most feared entities in all of medicine because of the exceedingly high mortality and the speed with which its injuries become irreversible. An intimal tear of the aorta allows blood flow to exit the lumen and travel a variable distance within the media. Depending on the location of the intimal tear and the direction in which blood travels, aortic dissections can be categorized using two prominent classification schemes. The DeBakey classification describes the location and the extent, whereas the more simplified Stanford classification looks at location alone. A Stanford type A dissection involves the ascending aorta; a Stanford type B involves the arch or descending aorta (Figure 19–16).

The precise etiology of aortic dissections is unclear, but there is an unambiguous association with a variety of conditions, including aortic aneurysms, hypertension, smoking, pregnancy, and recent intravascular trauma. Once blood

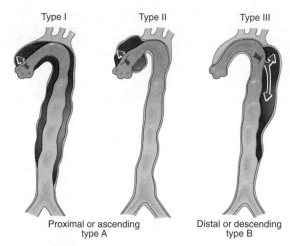

| Type I | Type II | Type III |

Proximal or ascending type A   Distal or descending type B

▲ **Figure 19–16.** DeBakey and Stanford Classifications of aortic dissection.

enters the medial plane, the intima "floats" within the aortic lumen and has a characteristic appearance on CT scans. (Figure 19–17). The blood within the false lumen reenters the true lumen through any number of naturally created fenestrations or holes, either from disruption of the side branches or from reentry at the termination of the false lumen. Blood flow to any of the side branches off of the aorta

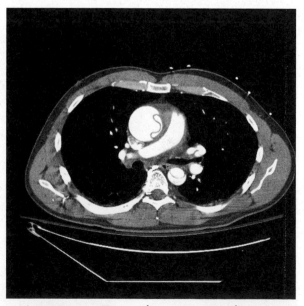

▲ **Figure 19–17.** CT scan of an acute aortic dissection. This Stanford type A dissection involves both the ascending and descending aortae. The large false lumen is nearly obstructing the true lumen.

can be compromised by the intimal flap, causing ischemia, a condition referred to as malperfusion. Malperfusion can involve the coronary arteries, branches of the aortic arch to the brain, the renal arteries, the mesenteric arteries, or branches to the lower extremities or the spinal cord. Blood can also exit the false lumen pathway into the adventitial space, causing free rupture. Rupture is more likely in Stanford type A dissections because of the intrapericardial location of the ascending aorta and the increased mechanical forces related to the proximity to the left ventricular outflow tract. Type B dissections in the descending aorta do not experience the same mechanical forces, because the more proximal aorta absorbs a significant amount of the kinetic energy. In addition, the extrapleural tissue helps reinforce the weakened adventitia, containing potential ruptures.

In addition to the free intrapericardial rupture of type A dissections, there are two other modes of early death responsible for the nearly 50% mortality associated with type A dissections. Malperfusion of the coronary ostia, typically the right coronary artery, causes acute myocardial infarction resulting in ventricular arrhythmias and myocardial dysfunction with shock. In addition, proximal migration of the dissection flap can disrupt the attachments of the aortic valve to the wall of the aortic root. The unsupported valve tissue prolapses into the ventricle during diastole, producing massive aortic valve insufficiency.

Patients with aortic dissections complain of tearing back pain or crushing chest pain. They are often hypertensive and tachycardic. The diagnosis can often be confused with acute myocardial infarction, ureterolithiasis, cholelithiasis, or pancreatitis. Patients with malperfusion can present with flank or abdominal pain from renal or mesenteric ischemia, lower extremity pain or paresthesias from iliac occlusion, stroke from carotid occlusion, or acute paralysis from occlusion of the multiple branches to the spinal cord. These symptoms of malperfusion can often overwhelm the chest or back pain from the dissection, clouding the diagnostic evaluation. Delay in diagnosis is exceedingly common in acute aortic dissection.

▶ Diagnostic Testing

On physical examination, patients appear acutely ill and are tachycardic and hypertensive. Hypotension should warrant suspicion of pericardial tamponade, myocardial infarction, aortic valve insufficiency, or free rupture. Blood pressure should be assessed in all four extremities to document perfusion abnormalities from the dissection flap. Abdominal pain should prompt evaluation of possible mesenteric or renal malperfusion. Neurologic deficits suggest either cerebral embolization or spinal ischemia.

Chest radiographs are often performed as the initial diagnostic test. They may reveal widening of the mediastinum, a left pleural effusion, or cardiomegaly if pericardial tamponade is present. CT is the standard imaging modality used to diagnose aortic dissection and should be obtained promptly in a patient with new-onset tearing back or chest pain. The CT scan diagnoses the dissection and identifies associated aneurysmal disease as well as organs at risk for malperfusion. Transesophageal echocardiography has a critical role in patients with aortic dissection. TEE excludes involvement of the ascending aorta in cases that are equivocal on CT scan. In addition, TEE identifies cardiac dysfunction and, most importantly, aortic valve insufficiency from extension of the dissection into the aortic root.

▶ Treatment

A. Medical Therapy

Initial management of the patient with an acute aortic dissection is immediate control of elevated blood pressure. Narcotic agents can be given initially to control pain and reduce the catecholamine surge. Beta-blocking agents are particularly critical not only to reduce blood pressure but also to lower the force of contraction and the sheer stress directly impacting the weakened aortic tissue. Esmolol is a short-acting agent that can be administered as a continuous infusion to obtain fine control of blood pressure, avoiding excessive bradycardia or hypotension. If high blood pressure persists, an arterial vasodilator can be given, such as nitroprusside, with a goal of maintaining systolic blood pressure of 100–120 mm Hg.

Patients with type B aortic dissections are frequently treated with medical therapy only, consisting of pain and blood pressure control, as well as observation for signs of malperfusion or rupture. Most patients with type B dissections can be safely discharged from the hospital once blood pressure control is adequate and the pain has resolved. They are carefully followed for good antihypertensive control as well as surveillance CT scanning to assess for interval growth in the size of the descending aorta. The indications for operative intervention in an acute type B aortic dissection is ongoing chest pain despite adequate blood pressure control, aneurysmal enlargement of the descending aorta greater than 6 cm, or evidence of impending rupture on CT scanning.

B. Surgical Therapy

1. Indications—Patients with type A aortic dissections should undergo emergency surgery to avoid one of the three fatal complications associated with 95% of patients with untreated dissections. These complications include intrapericardial rupture with tamponade, aortic valve insufficiency, or acute myocardial infarction. Once the diagnosis of a type A dissection has been established, either by CT scan or TEE, the patient should be taken emergently to the operating room in preparation for emergency surgery. The only exception to immediate emergency surgery is when signs of malperfusion of the abdominal viscera exist. Although this strategy remains controversial, some advocate angiographic investigation for signs of malperfusion. Using a combination of contrast fluoroscopy, intravascular ultrasound, and selective cannulation of all branches from the aorta with pressure measurements, the extent of the dissection can be evaluated and areas of definite malperfusion can be identified. If the intimal flap is obstructing blood flow to any of the aortic branches, fenestration using balloon catheters can restore flow from the false to the true lumen, reperfusing ischemic organs. While patients with severe visceral malperfusion can have mortality rates of nearly 80%, more recent series adopting a strategy of initial catheter-based fenestration followed by surgical repair show estimated mortality rates in selected patients of less than 20%. Since catheter-based techniques are becoming more universally available, this strategy of delayed surgical repair may become more widespread.

2. Techniques—Once a patient with a type A dissection has been diagnosed, emergency surgery is usually indicated. The femoral or axillary artery is exposed for arterial cannulation for CPB. A median sternotomy is performed, exposing the dilated and dissected ascending aorta. After administration of 300 IU/kg of heparin, the patient is cannulated for CPB, using the right atrium for venous drainage. The patient is cooled aggressively to 18 °C in preparation for hypothermic circulatory arrest. A catheter is placed in the coronary sinus to deliver retrograde cardioplegia for myocardial protection. A left ventricular vent is placed in the right superior pulmonary vein. Once the patient has reached 18 °C, CPB is discontinued, and the ascending aorta can be opened. The dissected aorta is removed, typically extending along the lesser curvature of the aortic arch. The remaining arch is carefully inspected for additional intimal tears. An appropriately sized and spatulated Dacron graft is anastomosed to the aortic arch using running polypropylene suture buttressed with Teflon felt. CPB can be reinstituted, flushing air and debris out of the open anastomosis. The aortic cross-clamp can then be applied to the graft material. The proximal ascending aorta is resected to the sinotubular junction, and the Dacron graft is trimmed to size. The proximal anastomosis is performed in a similar fashion using running polypropylene suture buttressed with felt. A deairing needle is placed in the graft, and the aortic cross-clamp is removed. The patient is rewarmed and weaned from CPB.

Occasionally, the pathology extends proximally into the aortic root, requiring reconstruction or resection. If the root is not significantly enlarged, the dissection flap can be obliterated by inserting Teflon felt into the false lumen and reapproximating the intima to the adventitia using polypropylene suture. The aortic valve commissures can be resuspended to the aortic wall with pledgeted sutures from intima to adventitia. If the aortic root is dilated, the sinuses and valve tissue can be excised and replaced with a mechanical valve conduit, reattaching the coronary ostia using the Bentall technique (Figure 19–18). Under certain scenarios, the entire aortic arch must be removed and replaced with Dacron graft material. When the aortic arch is significantly aneurysmal, if the intimal tear is within the aortic arch, or in a patient with Marfan syndrome, the entire arch should be replaced. Each branch of the arch can be individually reimplanted to the graft, the three vessels can be

attached as an island, or a multibranch graft of Dacron with side branches preattached can be anastomosed to the individual arch branches. When the arch is reconstructed, a longer duration of hypothermic circulatory arrest will be required. Cerebral perfusion can be initiated using balloon-tipped catheters inserted directly into the innominate and left carotid arteries. Blood flow at a rate of 600 cc/min at 18 °C is generally considered adequate to prevent neurologic compromise.

3. Results—As previously described, the mortality of acute aortic dissection may be as high as 50%, since many patients will rupture before arrival at a qualified hospital. Operative mortality is in the range of 10–20%, which includes consideration of the selection bias of choosing operative candidates. Cause of death is primarily related to malperfusion syndrome, resulting in neurologic, intestinal, or extremity ischemia. Cerebral injury related to hypothermic circulatory arrest is limited and should result in clinically significant stroke in less than 5% of patients. Long-term survival following repair of acute aortic dissection is good, approximately 50–60% at 10 years.

Davies RR et al: Yearly rupture or dissection rates for thoracic aortic aneurysms: Simple prediction based on size. Ann Thorac Surg 2002;73:17.
Driever R et al: Long-term effectiveness of operative procedures for Stanford type A aortic dissections. Cardiovasc Surg 2003;11:265.
Patel HJ et al: Operative delay for peripheral malperfusion syndrome in acute type A aortic dissection: a long-term analysis. J Thorac Cardiovasc Surg 2008;135:1288.

▼ SURGICAL TREATMENT OF HEART FAILURE

HEART TRANSPLANTATION

▶ Indications

The incidence of congestive heart failure (CHF) is steadily rising, owing to the increase in the aging population and the reduced mortality of myocardial infarction. Nearly 5 million Americans live with heart failure, and 500,000 new cases are diagnosed annually. Causes are multifactorial, but by far the most frequent etiology is related to coronary occlusive disease, with repeated ischemic insults and loss of viable myocardial contractility. Chronic ventricular volume overload from conditions such as undiagnosed valvular pathology or intracardiac septal defects can result in cardiomyopathy and advanced heart failure. Other causes of heart failure include viral myocarditis, peripartum cardiomyopathy, and idiopathic dilated cardiomyopathy.

All of these processes lead to the same result: loss of myocardial contractility with decreased cardiac output, elevated diastolic cardiac filling pressures, and pathologic neurohormonal adaptive responses. This results in increased sympathetic tone, elevated peripheral vascular resistance, and salt and water retention, creating a vicious cycle with

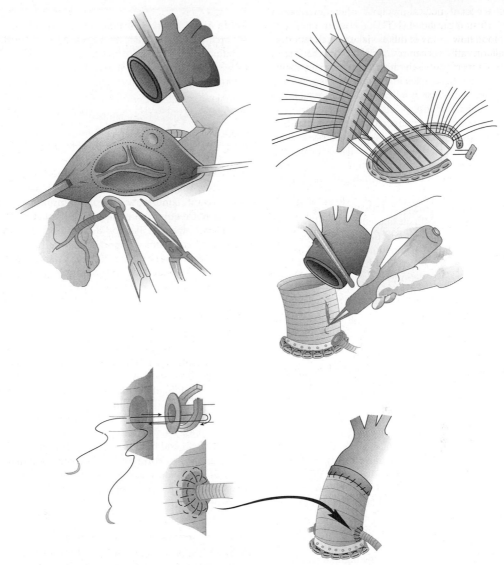

▲ **Figure 19–18.** Aortic root replacement with a mechanical valve conduit using the Bentall technique. (From Cohn LH. *Cardiac Surgery in the Adult,* 3rd ed. McGraw-Hill, 2007.)

further reduction in cardiac output, edema, and pulmonary congestion. Medical therapy includes reduction in salt intake and modest exercise to reduce sympathetic activation. Diuretics and aldosterone inhibitors counteract the inappropriately activated renin-angiotensin system. Angiotensin-converting enzyme inhibitors decrease peripheral vascular resistance and alter the myocardial intercellular matrix, allowing opportunities for reverse cardiac remodeling. The inotropic properties of digitalis glycosides have been demonstrated to reduce hospital admission for heart failure exacerbations, although at higher levels can increase mortality because of its proarrhythmic properties. Beta-blocking

agents reduce sympathetic tone, allow upregulation of β-receptors, and significantly reduce mortality in advanced heart failure patients. As the left ventricle dilates, electrical reentry pathways are generated, predisposing to malignant ventricular arrhythmias and sudden cardiac death. Strong evidence now demonstrates that implantation of automated internal cardiac defibrillators reduces mortality, and their use has become standard practice in heart failure management. In addition, selected patients with conduction system disturbances may benefit from cardiac resynchronization therapy by insertion of biventricular pacemakers that stimulate both the left and right ventricles simultaneously.

The effectiveness of medical therapy is often described by the New York Heart Association (NYHA) classification (Table 19–3). As a patient's NYHA functional class deteriorates despite adequate medical therapy, consideration for transplantation should be made. Because heart transplantation remains a scarce resource, selection of patients is crucial to maximize outcomes. Exclusion criteria have been established on the basis of solid evidence of increased perioperative or reduced long-term survival; criteria are listed in Table 19–4. The most frequently applied exclusion criteria include advanced age, end-organ injury from diabetes mellitus, chronic renal insufficiency (serum creatinine > 2.5), poor medical compliance or psychosocial instability, and morbid obesity (body mass index > 35).

Creation of concrete inclusion criteria has been more elusive because it is often difficult to predict mortality in this population. Historically, patient selection has relied on exercise stress evaluation and determination of maximal oxygen consumption (VO_2 max). Patients with a VO_2 max of less than 10 mL/kg/min have a definite survival advantage with transplantation, and those with a peak VO_2 of less than 14 mL/kg/min with NYHA class III or IV limitations appear to have a survival advantage. Recently, several scoring models have allowed more accurate risk stratification of mortality for ambulatory patients with advanced heart failure. These models have proven helpful for those patients in whom exercise testing appears intermediate in risk assessment, such as those with peak VO_2 between 10 and 14 mL/kg/min. The Heart Failure Survival Score (HFSS) uses seven independent predictors of mortality and creates high-, medium-, and low-risk groups for 1 year mortality. These variables include peak VO_2, QRS interval, ejection fraction, serum sodium, resting heart rate, ischemic versus nonischemic etiology, and mean blood pressure. Patients with intermediate peak VO_2 scores should be considered for transplantation if scoring models such as the HFSS predict high or medium risk for mortality.

Heart transplants are allocated according to a protocol prioritizing based on need and geographic distribution. Patients are assigned within a classification system as listed in Table 19–5. Status 1A patients receive the highest priority, as they require mechanical circulatory support with a device that will not allow discharge from the hospital, are supported by a device that is failing, or require infusion of inotropic agents at high doses and require pulmonary artery catheters to continuously monitor intracardiac filling pressures. Patients are

assigned status 1B if they are supported with implantable circulatory support devices that allow ambulatory support or if they require continuous inotropic infusions at modest doses and do not require pulmonary artery catheters. Patients are considered status 2 if they do not require inotropes or mechanical circulatory support. Patients are designated status 7 if they are temporarily unsuited for a transplant. Organs are allocated with a complex algorithm that considers patient status, size, blood type compatibility, and geography.

▶ Technique

Patients are briefly evaluated to ensure that there have been no interval changes in their health status since their transplant evaluation. In particular, anticoagulation status is assessed and reversed if necessary, renal function should be reasonably stable, and a pulmonary artery catheter should be inserted to ensure that pulmonary vascular resistance has not changed appreciably since the most recent evaluation. Potential concerns should be discussed between the transplant surgeon and heart failure cardiologist.

Upon confirmation by the procuring team that the donor heart is visibly suitable, the recipient is anesthetized and prepared. A median sternotomy is performed. In the current era, the majority of recipients have undergone previous

Table 19–4. Heart Transplant Exclusion Criteria.

Severe renal insufficiency
Recent malignancy
Advanced age
Obesity
Elevated pulmonary vascular resistance
Medication noncompliance

Table 19–3. New York Heart Association Classification of Heart Failure Symptoms.

I	No limitations
II	Dyspnea with ordinary activity
III	Dyspnea with less than ordinary activity
IV	Dyspnea

Table 19–5. United Network for Organ Sharing Listing Status for Heart Transplantation.

Listing Status	Clinical Criteria
1A	Dependent on extracorporeal membrane oxygenation, intra-aortic balloon pump, total artificial heart, mechanical ventilation, or ventricular assist device with evidence of device malfunction or device-related complications
	Dependent on 2 inotropic infusions or 1 high-dose inotrope (7.5 mcg/kg/min dobutamine, dopamine, or 0.5 mcg/kg/min milrinone) with pulmonary artery catheter in place
1B	Dependent on ventricular assist device or inotropic infusion
2	Eligible for transplant but not dependent on inotropes or mechanical circulatory support
7	Hold; temporarily medically unsuitable for transplant

cardiac surgery, often including insertion of ventricular assist devices. As such, significant time may be required for dissection and identification of cardiac structures, and appropriate time should be allowed. The patient is heparinized to achieve an activated clotting time of at least 450 seconds. Arterial cannulation is preferred high on the lesser curvature of the aortic arch to allow for significant aortic removal, particularly if the recipient has a ventricular assist device. Venous cannulation is in the superior and inferior vena cavae, and CPB is initiated. The cavae are controlled with snares, and an aortic cross-clamp is applied when the donor heart is within 20–30 minutes of arrival. Recipient cardiectomy is performed initially along the right atrioventricular groove and extending down into the coronary sinus. The aorta is transected just above the coronary arteries, avoiding entry into the dome of the left atrium or injury to the right pulmonary artery. The pulmonary artery is transected at the level of the pulmonary valve, limiting the tendency to bevel the posterior wall distally, which reduces length for the anastomosis. The interatrial septum is opened, and the left atrium is divided along the mitral valve annulus. Once the recipient heart is removed, the left atrium is trimmed, removing the appendage and a portion of the interatrial septum.

The donor heart is carefully inspected for abnormalities, including a patent foramen ovale. The atrial cuff is trimmed to size-match the recipient. The left atrial anastomosis is performed with polypropylene in running fashion, everting the edges to minimize incorporation of epicardial tissue within the atria. Before completion of the anastomosis, the left ventricular vent is inserted via the right superior pulmonary vein through the mitral valve. This facilitates deairing and prevents premature rewarming from pulmonary effluent. The donor and recipient ascending aortas are trimmed appropriately, and the anastomosis is performed with running polypropylene suture. At the completion of this suture line, the aortic cross-clamp can be removed, thus terminating the period of cold ischemia. The ascending aorta and left ventricle are vented of residual air. Spontaneous resumption of cardiac activity typically occurs. The inferior vena cava anastomosis is completed with running polypropylene suture. A flexible cardiotomy suction catheter is placed through the donor superior vena cava and advanced into the coronary sinus to improve visualization. The superior vena cava is anastomosed with running polypropylene suture, and the caval snares can be removed. The pulmonary artery anastomosis is performed with running polypropylene, typically imbricating the posterior wall for greater strength. Care must be taken to avoid excess length and potential kinking of the pulmonary artery. Several laparotomy pads can be placed behind the heart to reduce tension on the suture line until the anastomosis is complete. The technique just described is for a *bicaval* implant. With a *biatrial* technique, the recipient cardiectomy preserves the superior and inferior vena caval attachments, instead creating an atriotomy along the lateral wall of the right atrium. The donor superior vena cava is ligated, and an incision in the inferior vena cava is extended several centimeters along the posterolateral atrial wall. This older technique is technically easier but is associated with more tricuspid valve regurgitation and atrial arrhythmias, and thus is infrequently performed.

The patient is rewarmed, ventilated, and then weaned off of CPB. If sinus rhythm is less than 100–110 beats per minute, atrial pacing is initiated. Inotropic support is typically required in light of the cold ischemic time, even for young and vigorous donor hearts. Right ventricular dysfunction is the most frequently seen complication, attributed to recipient pulmonary hypertension in the "untrained" heart and the inherent sensitivity of the right ventricle to preservation injury. This can be exacerbated by postoperative bleeding necessitating large volumes of blood product transfusions with volume overload and worsening of pulmonary vascular resistance. Judicious volume administration, rapid pacing, and catecholamine infusions can overcome right ventricular dysfunction. Inhaled nitric oxide or prostacycline can selectively reduce pulmonary vascular resistance and improve hemodynamic stability.

Immunosuppression after heart transplantation is similar to that for other solid organs and includes antimetabolite agents such as mycophenolate, calcineurin inhibitors such as cyclosporine or tacrolimus, and corticosteroids. Because of their nephrotoxicity, initiation of calcineurin inhibitors is often delayed during the immediate postoperative period. As an alternative, induction therapy with either monoclonal or polyclonal antibodies against specific immune cells can be administered. Although routine use of induction therapy has not been demonstrated to improve outcomes, selected use for patients with perioperative renal insufficiency may be beneficial.

▶ Outcomes

Despite the absence of any prospective randomized evidence, heart transplantation offers long-term survival advantages of medical therapy for appropriately selected patients with advanced heart failure. Survival rates have improved since the introduction of the procedure in 1967, with 1 year survival now approximately 85%. Most early deaths are attributable to perioperative complications or severe rejection. After this early period of attrition, there continues to be a linear decrement in survival, at a rate of approximately 3–4% per year, and this rate has not decreased over the last 20 years. Causes of late mortality are variable but include transplant vasculopathy, opportunistic infections, immunosuppressive related malignancies, and rejection. Transplant vasculopathy is an accelerated coronary artery disease unique to the heart transplant recipient and is a result of repetitive vascular injury and sustained inflammatory response. Statins and vitamin supplements appear to slow the progression of vasculopathy, but the diffuse nature makes the disease unamenable to percutaneous or surgical revascularization. Median survival after heart transplant is estimated to be between 10 and 11 years (Figure 19–19).

MECHANICAL CIRCULATORY SUPPORT

▶ Indications

Although heart transplantation has long been considered the gold standard treatment for advanced heart failure, the limited availability of suitable donors affords support for only a small percentage of those in need. Mechanical circulatory support to assist or replace the failing heart has made enormous progress over the last 40 years. Since the introduction of CPB by Gibbon in 1953, the engineering of mechanical blood pumps has become more sophisticated, allowing treatment of an increasing population of patients on an ambulatory basis with better blood biocompatibility and improved pump durability. As this rapid evolution continues, the indications, techniques, and expected results will change dramatically. More than any other aspect of cardiac surgery, the treatment of today will likely be remarkably different only a few years in the future.

The indications for implantable circulatory support are severe cardiac dysfunction despite maximal medical therapy. However, there are three distinct goals of support that represent vastly different patient populations and clinical scenarios: bridge to recovery, bridge to transplant, and destination therapy. Cardiogenic shock may have reversible causes, such as viral or peripartum cardiomyopathy, acute myocardial infarction, and postcardiotomy shock. Initiation of temporary mechanical circulatory support can restore hemodynamics, unload the ventricle, and allow time for myocardial recovery. Chronic heart failure patients felt to be suitable candidates for heart transplantation can rapidly deteriorate, causing end-organ dysfunction and closing their window of opportunity. Implantable circulatory support can reverse acute organ injury and allow functional rehabilitation, improving their candidacy for and potentially their outcomes after heart transplantation. Patients with advanced heart failure and contraindications for transplantation, such as older age, chronic renal insufficiency, obesity, or fixed pulmonary hypertension, may benefit from implantable circulatory support as destination therapy, as evidenced by the REMATCH trial.

▶ Pumps

A variety of devices are available for mechanical circulatory support to satisfy each of the goals, and many more are currently in clinical trials or preclinical testing. Device selection depends on the clinical circumstances, with considerations including ease of implantation, adequacy and flexibility of support, patient quality of life, durability, and cost. The available devices are discussed in the context of their most frequently used application.

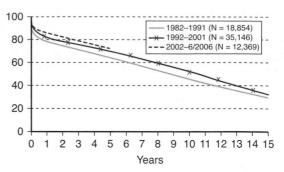

▲ **Figure 19–19.** Kaplan-Meier survival for adult heart transplants performed between January 1982 and June 2006 by era. All comparisons are significant at $p < 0.0001$. (Reproduced with permission from Taylor DO et al. Registry of the International Society for Heart and Lung Transplantation: Twenty-fifth official adult heart transplant report—2008. J Heart Lung Transplant 2008;27:943.)

A. Short-term Devices

Depending on the clinical circumstances, acute-onset heart failure is often reversible. When circulatory support is provided, it is often with the intention of recovering the native heart. Intra-aortic balloon pumps provide counterpulsation during diastole, increasing coronary perfusion and reducing afterload and myocardial oxygen consumption. They are typically inserted percutaneously via the femoral artery and advanced into the descending thoracic aorta. Balloon timing automatically coincides with the electrocardiogram tracing or the arterial pressure waveform. They can be easily removed and have few complications. Intra-aortic balloon pump support is limited, improving cardiac output by as much as 20%. The Abiomed BVS 5000 is a pneumatically driven extracorporeal blood pump capable of up to 6 L/min of blood flow (Figure 19–20). The device can be connected to the circulation to provide support for the failing left or right ventricle in a variety of configurations. This system remains one of the most frequently used circulatory support devices worldwide. Abiomed has introduced the recently approved AB5000 pumps, also pneumatically driven extracorporeal blood pumps. The newer design boasts improved blood biocompatibility and better patient mobility. Both of the Abiomed devices are designed for patients with acute-onset heart failure with the intention of providing hemodynamic support until cardiac recovery. As such, they are not approved for ambulatory use outside of the hospital setting. The CentriMag is a centrifugal blood pump with a magnetically levitated rotor to improve biocompatibility. It is currently in clinical trials as a short-term extracorporeal ventricular assist device (VAD) to serve either as a bridge to recovery or a bridge to long-term VAD implantation.

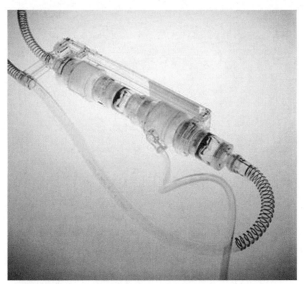

▲ **Figure 19–20.** Abiomed BVS ventricular assist device. (Reproduced with permission from Abiomed, Inc., Danvers, MA.)

B. Long-term Devices

When heart failure is felt to be irreversible and refractory to medical therapy, heart transplantation is considered. The lack of available suitable donor organs makes transplantation unfeasible for many patients in whom treatment is urgently required. Implantable mechanical circulatory support, such as left ventricular assist devices (LVADs) have allowed stabilization of hemodynamic parameters, restoration of renal and hepatic function, and rehabilitation of critically ill patients. Stabilization allows time for a suitable donor to become available and appears to improve outcomes after transplant, when compared to a strategy of using inotropes or balloon counterpulsation for heart transplant candidates.

A variety of LVADs are available in the United States. The most frequently used device is the HeartMate XVE (Figure 19–21). The device is connected to the apex of the left ventricle, and a rotary motor actuates a pusher plate diaphragm, which ejects blood into a graft connected to the ascending aorta. Valved conduits in the inflow and outflow regions allow only unidirectional flow. The device is placed infradiaphragmatically in the preperitoneal position, with a percutaneous driveline exiting the abdominal wall and connected to an external controller and wearable batteries. The patient can remain untethered to the power source for periods up to 6 hours. The unique feature of the HeartMate XVE is its sintered titanium surface, which creates adherence of cellular blood elements, producing a "neointimal" lining, reducing thromboembolic complications, and minimizing

the requirements for anticoagulation to aspirin alone. Its large size restricts its use to patients with a body surface area of at least 1.5 m^2, and bearing wear and valvular failure limit durability of the device to approximately 1.5 years.

The Thoratec Intracorporeal VAD, or IVAD, represents a modification to a similar device called the Paracorporeal VAD, allowing implantation and discharge from the hospital to await transplantation from home. The device is pneumatically driven by a large extracorporeal console containing the required air compressor, electronics for synchronized drive and feedback, and a battery for untethered support. Tilting-disk mechanical inflow and outflow valves direct flow, and the untextured internal surface requires systemic anticoagulation with heparin or coumadin. The unique features of this device are the small size, allowing use in smaller patients or insertion of two pumps for right and left ventricular support.

A new generation of circulatory support devices has appeared on the US market. These are valveless continuous-flow pumps using axial design impellers to generate blood flow. Since there is no displacement chamber to generate the

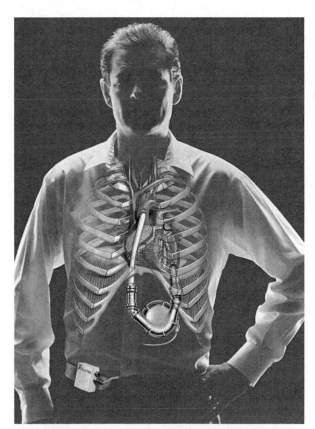

▲ **Figure 19–21.** HeartMate XVE left ventricular assist device. (Reproduced with permission from Thoratec, Inc., Pleasanton, CA.)

flow pulse, the devices are smaller and silent, allowing support to smaller patients and improved patient satisfaction. In addition, the continuous nature of the mechanical load on a single bearing has the important advantage of improved durability, with theoretical support for up to 10 years. The first of these pumps to gain FDA approval is the HeartMate II (Figure 19–22). Early experience demonstrates improved success as a bridge to heart transplant with a reduction in complication rates. Despite the size and durability advantages, concerns remain about the long-term implications of nonpulsatile blood flow, although early evidence suggests preserved renal, neurologic, and hepatic function. Reports of gastrointestinal bleeding suggest a possible association with nonpulsatile blood flow, but the extent of these problems appears limited. In addition, unlike pulsatile pumps, which automatically increase beat rate with increased pump filling, valveless continuous-flow pumps currently have no mechanism to automatically regulate flow with varying preload. Reductions of flow during exercise have been reported, and excessive pump rate during conditions of relative underfilling can result in collapse of the left ventricular cavity, hazarding arrhythmias, hemolysis, and distortion of the interventricular septum causing right ventricular dysfunction.

The next generation of LVADs are continuous-flow pumps with centrifugal design, utilizing magnetically levitated rotors. These LVADs eliminate entirely the need for contacting bearings, creating the potential for indefinite support without mechanical failure. Several of these devices

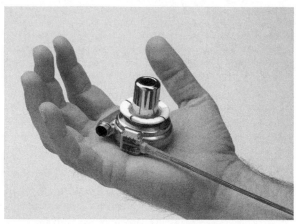

▲ **Figure 19–23.** HeartWare HVAD left ventricular assist device. (Reproduced with permission from HeartWare International, Inc., Framingham, MA.)

have begun clinical trials in the United States. Devices are being miniaturized, allowing implantation directly in the pericardium, obviating the need for the preperitoneal pocket and division of the diaphragm (Figure 19–23). Additionally, some devices are designed to be placed outside of the chest cavity, eliminating the need for sternotomy (Figure 19–24). How effective and safe these devices are remains to be seen, but the significant technological progress will likely have an enormous impact on the nature of surgical treatment of heart failure in the near future.

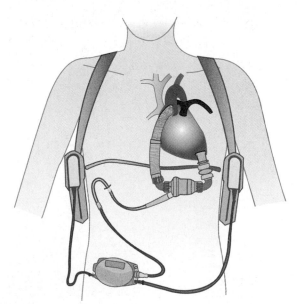

▲ **Figure 19–22.** HeartMate II left ventricular assist device. (Reproduced with permission from Thoratec, Inc., Pleasanton, CA.)

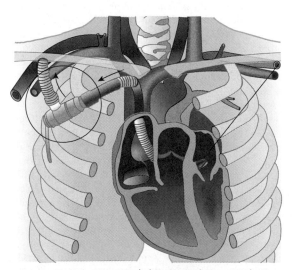

▲ **Figure 19–24.** Synergy left ventricular assist device. (Reproduced with permission from CircuLite, Inc., Saddle Brook, NJ.)

Aaronson KD et al: Left ventricular assist device therapy improves utilization of donor hearts. J Am Coll Cardiol 2002;39:1247.

Bardy GH et al: Amiodarone or an implantable cardioverter-defibrillator for congestive heart failure. N Engl J Med 2005;352:225.

Cleland JG et al: The effect of cardiac resynchronization on morbidity and mortality in heart failure. N Engl J Med 2005;352:1539.

Dargie HJ: Effect of carvedilol on outcome after myocardial infarction in patients with left-ventricular dysfunction: The CAPRICORN randomised trial. Lancet 2001;357:1385.

Drews T et al: Differences in pulsatile and non-pulsatile mechanical circulatory support in long-term use. J Heart Lung Transplant 2008;27:1096.

Flather MD et al: Long-term ACE-inhibitor therapy in patients with heart failure or left-ventricular dysfunction: a systematic overview of data from individual patients. ACE-Inhibitor Myocardial Infarction Collaborative Group. Lancet 2000;355:1575.

Gheorghiade M, Adams KF Jr, Colucci WS: Digoxin in the management of cardiovascular disorders. Circulation 2004;109:2959.

Haft J et al: Hemodynamic and exercise performance with pulsatile and continuous-flow left ventricular assist devices. Circulation 2007;116:I8.

Hunt SA et al: ACC/AHA 2005 guideline update for the diagnosis and management of chronic heart failure in the adult—summary article. Circulation 2005;112:1825.

Lund LH, Aaronson KD, Mancini DM: Validation of peak exercise oxygen consumption and the Heart Failure Survival Score for serial risk stratification in advanced heart failure. Am J Cardiol 2005;95:734.

Miller LW et al: Use of a continuous-flow device in patients awaiting heart transplantation. HeartMate II Clinical Investigators. New Eng J Med 2007;357:885.

Rose EA et al: Long-term mechanical left ventricular assistance for end-stage heart failure. Randomized Evaluation of Mechanical Assistance for the Treatment of Congestive Heart Failure (REMATCH) Study Group. New Eng J Med 2001;345:1435.

Taylor DO et al: Registry of the International Society for Heart and Lung Transplantation: Twenty-fifth official adult heart transplant report—2008. J Heart Lung Transplant 2008;27:943.

19

II. Congenital Heart Disease

Jennifer C. Hirsch, MD, MS
Eric J. Devaney, MD
Richard G. Ohye, MD
Edward L. Bove, MD

DIAGNOSIS

Congenital heart disease encompasses a wide range of anomalies that result from abnormal fetal development of the heart. Defects can range from simple to complex. The age of presentation of these defects depends primarily on the physiologic impact of the anomaly. With improvements in ultrasound imaging, an increasing number of cardiac anomalies are being identified on prenatal examination. After birth, patients can present within minutes to hours with profound hypoxemia or hemodynamic collapse or may present weeks to months later with evidence of a new murmur or signs of congestive heart failure. Relatively asymptomatic lesions can go undetected until children are school age or adolescents.

Early and accurate diagnosis of congenital heart disease requires careful identification of signs and symptoms of heart disease. Classification of heart murmurs can be highly suggestive of underlying cardiac anomalies. Early signs of heart disease include cyanosis, tachypnea, unequal pulses, and failure to thrive. Key symptoms of congenital heart disease in the patient's history include feeding difficulties, irritability, and frequent respiratory infections.

The initial workup for suspected congenital heart disease begins with a focused history and physical examination. Standard studies include a chest radiograph and electrocardiography. Chest radiography can identify cardiomegaly, increased or decreased pulmonary markings, aortic arch sidedness, and situs abnormalities (the heart located in the mid- or right chest rather than the typical location in the left chest). There are some cardiac defects with pathognomonic findings on chest radiograph. Electrocardiography can identify rhythm disturbances, axis deviation, atrial enlargement, and ventricular hypertrophy. Two-dimensional color-flow Doppler echocardiography is usually the first and often only noninvasive diagnostic test required to provide adequate anatomic definition of the defect to allow for surgical planning. Cardiac catheterization, cardiac magnetic resonance imaging (MRI), and computed tomography (CT) angiogra-

phy are used as adjunct diagnostic tests when additional information on flow, pressure, resistance, or anatomic detail is required.

PREOPERATIVE MANAGEMENT

For the majority of congenital heart defects, surgical correction or catheter-based intervention is necessary for definitive treatment. Certain defects such as atrial septal defects, ventricular septal defects (VSDs), and patent ductus arteriosus (PDA) may resolve spontaneously over the first several years of life. The remainder require intervention when the risk of surgery is reasonable, when symptoms can no longer be managed medically, and prior to the onset of irreversible complications.

Neonates presenting with ductal-dependent lesions require ductal blood flow to maintain systemic or pulmonary perfusion. Ductal patency is achieved with intravenous prostaglandin E_1 therapy. Supplemental oxygen is supplied as necessary for cyanosis; however, newborns tolerate relative cyanosis (oxygen saturations > 70%) quite well, so the use of oxygen is minimized. The remainder of therapy is directed toward managing congestive heart failure symptoms with diuretics, afterload reduction, and maximal caloric intake.

The care of congenital heart disease patients requires a collaborative effort of a multidisciplinary team of cardiologists, surgeons, interventionalists, echocardiographers, and radiologists. Careful timing and planning of operative and catheter-based interventions along with highly skilled preoperative and postoperative care are essential to a successful outcome.

OPERATIVE MANAGEMENT

For most congenital heart defects, surgical correction is possible. Staged repair with early palliation as well as staged palliation remain options for more complex defects. The anticipated somatic growth of the child must be considered when determining the surgical approach. Invasive monitoring lines are essential for monitoring patients during surgery and postoperatively. All patients have arterial and central venous catheters placed along with 2 peripheral intravenous catheters and a Foley catheter. For neonates, the umbilical vessels are the desired venous and arterial access. Avoidance of long-standing and repeated femoral lines is important because patency of these vessels is often essential for diagnostic and interventional catheter procedures later life. Temperature probes are placed in the nasopharynx, the rectum, and on the skin to allow for accurate temperature monitoring. Due to variable blood flow with perfusion techniques and underlying cardiac anomalies, it is possible to have differential cooling and rewarming.

Most surgical repairs require cardiopulmonary bypass. This involves drainage of venous blood from the patient via cannulae placed in the superior and inferior vena cava (for intracardiac repairs) or a single cannula in the right atrium. Blood passes through the bypass circuit, which warms or cools the blood to the desired temperature, adds oxygen and removes carbon dioxide, and pumps the blood back into the body via an arterial cannula, usually in the ascending aorta. Hypothermia may be employed to decrease the metabolic demands of the body and heart, which provides additional protection against ischemia. The degree of hypothermia, 18–32 °C, depends on the complexity and time needed to complete the procedure. The heart can be arrested with high-potassium cardioplegic solution delivered antegrade (through a cannula proximal to an aortic cross-clamp in the aorta) or retrograde (through a cannula placed in the coronary sinus). Arresting the heart allows the surgeon to operate safely with a still and bloodless field. An additional vent can be placed via the right superior pulmonary vein to capture pulmonary venous return and to assist in deairing of the heart.

Hypothermic circulatory arrest is required for complex aortic arch reconstructions. This involves cooling the patient to 18 °C for a minimum of 20 minutes to ensure even cooling of the brain and body. The head is packed in ice, the patient's blood is drained into the venous reservoir, and the pump is turned off. The cannulae can then be removed from the field to aid in visualization and repair of the arch. No absolute safe duration of hypothermic circulatory arrest has been determined, but it is generally felt that it should be limited to no more than 45 minutes. Alternative techniques, such as regional cerebral perfusion and intermittent low-flow perfusion, have been suggested to minimize the need for hypothermic circulatory arrest. To date, however, there is no literature to support that these techniques have additional benefit without additional risk.

POSTOPERATIVE MANAGEMENT

Patients are brought to the intensive care unit intubated and mechanically ventilated. All patients have temporary pacing wires in place for management of bradyarrhythmias and tachyarrhythmias. Many patients have additional intracardiac lines in place for pulmonary artery and left atrial pressure monitoring. Drainage catheters are placed within the mediastinum to prevent accumulation of blood and fluid. These are usually removed 2–4 days following surgery. Prophylactic antibiotics are given preoperatively as well as postoperatively when drainage tubes are in place.

Cardiopulmonary bypass produces a significant inflammatory response due to activation of cytokines. Patients exhibit fluid retention and pulmonary dysfunction as a result, requiring aggressive use of diuretics and mechanical ventilation as needed. Bleeding is a common complication following cardiac surgery and infrequently requires surgical exploration (< 2%). Postoperative coagulopathy results from a multitude of factors, including hemodilution, platelet damage, factor consumption, immature hepatic production of clotting factors, and incomplete reversal of heparin with protamine sulfate. Approximately 30% of all patients will have some arrhythmia after surgery, ranging from simple premature ventricular contractions to malignant tachyarrhythmias. The risk for long-term arrhythmias requiring chronic medication or heart block requiring a permanent pacemaker is approximately 1%. Most patients require hemodynamic support with vasopressors along with afterload reduction as necessary for ventricular dysfunction. Dopamine, epinephrine, and vasopressin are the first-line vasopressors for pediatric patients. Milrinone is used primarily for afterload reduction. Critically ill neonates may have thyroid and adrenal hypofunction, which can further exacerbate postoperative hemodynamic instability. Profound hemodynamic compromise occasionally requires additional mechanical assistance. Extracorporeal membrane oxygenation (ECMO) is the most widely and acutely available mechanical support for the pediatric population. The survival for congenital heart disease patients requiring ECMO support is approximately 50%. For patients in low cardiac output state, it is essential to rule out residual defects or repair failures that could be readdressed surgically or in the catheterization laboratory.

The pediatric population has highly reactive pulmonary vasculature that is unique from the adult cardiac surgery population. Postoperative pulmonary hypertensive crises can occur commonly in the newborn and infant population. Crises can be initiated with agitation such as endotracheal suctioning. Maneuvers to minimize and treat pulmonary hypertensive crises include high-dose opioid anesthesia with fentanyl, paralysis, respiratory alkalosis, high fraction of inspired oxygen, and inhaled nitric oxide. Chronic agents to treat persistent pulmonary hypertension include phosphodiesterase inhibitors (eg, sildenafil) and prostacyclin (eg, Flolan).

CYANOTIC HEART DEFECTS

Cyanotic heart defects result from shunting of deoxygenated blood from the right side of the heart to the oxygenated left side of the heart or inadequate pulmonary blood flow. The relative mixing of deoxygenated and oxygenated blood produces desaturation of the arterial blood. The majority of cyanotic heart defects are diagnosed within the first few weeks to months of life. Cyanotic heart defects represent approximately 25% of all congenital heart defects.

The classic 5 T's of cyanotic heart defects—(1) tetralogy of Fallot, (2) transposition of the great arteries, (3) truncus arteriosus, (4) total anomalous pulmonary venous return, and (5) tricuspid atresia—are presented in this chapter along with hypoplastic left heart syndrome.

▶ Tetralogy of Fallot

ESSENTIALS OF DIAGNOSIS

▶ History of hypoxic spells associated with pulling the legs to the chest or squatting.

▶ Progressive cyanosis.

▶ Prominent right ventricular impulse.

▶ Single S2 with a grade 1–3/6 ejection murmur over the right ventricular outflow tract along the mid- to upper left sternal border.

▶ Chest radiograph demonstrates the classic coeur en sabot, boot-shaped heart with decreased pulmonary vascular markings.

▶ Echocardiographic evidence of right ventricular hypertrophy, with right ventricular outflow tract obstruction with or without pulmonary stenosis/atresia, and malalignment ventricular septal defect with aortic override.

A. General Considerations

Tetralogy of Fallot (TOF) is the most common cyanotic congenital heart defect. It occurs in 0.6 per 1000 live births and has a prevalence of about 4% among all patients with congenital heart disease. The pathologic anatomy is frequently described as having four components: VSD, overriding aorta, pulmonary stenosis, and right ventricular hypertrophy (Figure 19–25). Embryologically, the anatomy of TOF is thought to result from a single defect: anterior malalignment of the infundibular septum. The infundibular septum normally separates the primitive outflow tracts and fuses with the ventricular septum. Anterior malalignment of the infundibular septum creates a VSD due to failure of fusion with the ventricular septum and also displaces the aorta over the VSD and right ventricle. Infundibular malalignment also crowds the right ventricular outflow tract, causing pulmonary stenosis and, secondarily, right ventricular hypertrophy. Prominent muscle bands also extend from the septal insertion of the infundibular septum to the right ventricular free wall and contribute to the obstruction of the right ventricular outflow tract. The pulmonary valve is usually stenotic and is bicuspid in 58% of cases. Pulmonary atresia occurs in about 7% of cases of TOF. The branch pulmonary arteries in TOF may exhibit mild diffuse hypoplasia or discrete stenosis (most frequently of the left pulmonary artery at the site of ductal insertion). Coronary artery anomalies are frequently present. The origin of the left anterior descending artery from the right coronary artery, which occurs in 5% of cases, is clinically important because the vessel crosses the right ventricular infundibulum and is vulnerable to injury at the time of surgery. A right aortic arch is present in 25% of patients with TOF. Associated defects include atrial septal defect (ASD), complete atrioventricular septal defect (AVSD), PDA, or multiple VSDs.

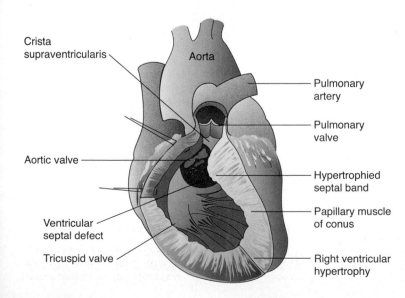

▲ **Figure 19–25.** Tetralogy of Fallot. The aorta overrides the ventricular septum. A large ventricular septal defect is present, and the hypoplastic infundibulum with hypertrophied muscle bands obstructs blood to the pulmonary arteries.

Labels: Crista supraventricularis, Aorta, Pulmonary artery, Pulmonary valve, Aortic valve, Hypertrophied septal band, Papillary muscle of conus, Ventricular septal defect, Tricuspid valve, Right ventricular hypertrophy

B. Clinical Findings

Patients with TOF develop cyanosis due to right-to-left shunting across the VSD. The degree of cyanosis depends on the severity of obstruction of the right ventricular outflow tract. Frequently, cyanosis is mild at birth and may remain undetected for weeks or months. Neonates with severe infundibular obstruction or pulmonary atresia will develop symptoms shortly after birth and require a prostaglandin infusion to maintain ductal patency to ensure adequate pulmonary blood flow. In other patients, the right ventricular outflow tract obstruction is minor, and the predominant physiology is that of a large VSD with left-to-right shunting and congestive heart failure.

The occurrence of intermittent cyanotic spells is a well-known feature of tetralogy. The etiology of spelling is still controversial but is clearly related to a transient imbalance between pulmonary and systemic blood flow. A spell may be triggered by hypovolemia or peripheral vasodilation (eg, after a bath or vigorous physical exertion). Spells may occur in neonates but are most frequently reported in infants between the ages of 3 and 18 months. Most spells resolve spontaneously within a few minutes, but some spells may be fatal. Older children have been observed to spontaneously squat to terminate spells. The squatting position is thought to increase systemic vascular resistance, which thereby favors pulmonary blood flow.

Cyanosis is the most frequent physical finding in TOF. Auscultation reveals a normal first heart sound and a single second heart sound. A systolic ejection murmur is present at the left upper sternal border. Older children may develop clubbing of the fingers and toes. Chest radiography typically demonstrates a boot-shaped heart due to elevation of the cardiac apex from right ventricular hypertrophy. Pulmonary vascular markings are usually reduced. A right aortic arch may be present. An electrocardiogram shows right ventricular hypertrophy. Echocardiography is definitive, and catheterization is not necessary in most cases.

C. Treatment

The medical management of TOF is directed toward the treatment and prevention of cyanotic spells. The immediate treatment of the spelling patient includes administration of oxygen, narcotics for sedation, and correction of acidosis. Transfusion is indicated for anemic infants. Alpha-agonists are useful for increasing systemic vascular resistance (which favors pulmonary blood flow). Some centers have used beta-blockers as a form of long-term therapy to suppress the incidence of spells. Long-term complications of untreated TOF include clubbing of the fingers and toes, severe dyspnea on exertion, brain abscesses (secondary to right-to-left shunting), paradoxical embolization, and polycythemia (which may lead to cerebral thrombosis). Long-term survival is unlikely for most patients with untreated TOF.

All patients with TOF should undergo surgical repair. Asymptomatic patients should be repaired electively between 4 and 6 months of age. Early repair is indicated for neonates with severe cyanosis and for infants who have had a documented spell or worsening cyanosis.

Classically, the repair of TOF was accomplished in two stages. During the first stage, pulmonary blood flow was augmented by creating a connection (or shunt) between a systemic artery and the pulmonary artery. At the second stage, the shunt was taken down, and a complete repair was performed. The first shunt procedure was the Blalock-Taussig shunt, in which the subclavian artery was mobilized and divided distally, and an end-to-side anastomosis was created between the inferiorly deflected subclavian and the ipsilateral pulmonary artery. The modified Blalock-Taussig shunt is the most common type of shunt used today and consists of an interposition graft (polytetrafluoroethylene) between the innominate or subclavian artery and the ipsilateral pulmonary artery. Creation of a shunt may be accomplished with or without the use of cardiopulmonary bypass.

Currently, one-stage repair of TOF is preferred by most centers. Initial palliation with a shunt is still indicated for some patients who present a high risk for complete repair, such as those with multiple congenital anomalies, severe concurrent illness, or an anomalous coronary artery crossing a hypoplastic infundibulum.

Complete repair of TOF is performed using a median sternotomy and cardiopulmonary bypass with bicaval venous cannulation. By a transatrial approach, the right ventricular outflow tract can be examined through the tricuspid valve. Muscle bundles obstructing the right ventricular outflow tract are divided or resected. The VSD is closed with a patch. Pulmonary valvotomy is performed, when indicated, via a vertical incision in the main pulmonary artery. When the pulmonary valve annulus or infundibulum is severely hypoplastic, a transannular outflow tract patch may be necessary to relieve the obstruction. When an anomalous coronary artery crosses the infundibulum, a transannular incision may be contraindicated. In these cases, and in patients with pulmonary atresia, placement of a conduit (cryopreserved homograft or bioprosthetic heterograft) between the right ventricle (via a separate ventriculotomy) and main pulmonary artery will be necessary. Patients who undergo construction of a transannular patch develop pulmonary insufficiency as a consequence. This is surprisingly well tolerated in most infants, as long as the tricuspid valve is competent. As these patients grow older, some will develop right ventricular failure due to chronic pulmonary insufficiency, and pulmonary valve implantation may be necessary.

D. Prognosis and Complications

The early mortality following repair of TOF is between 1% and 5%. The results are worse for patients with TOF and pulmonary atresia. Long-term complications include recurrent obstruction of the right ventricular outflow tract and development of right ventricular dysfunction due to chronic pulmonary insufficiency. Actuarial survival at 20 years is 90% with excellent functional status.

Bacha EA et al: Long-term results after early primary repair of tetralogy of Fallot. J Thorac Cardiovasc Surg 2001;122:154.

de Ruijter FT et al: Right ventricular dysfunction and pulmonary valve replacement after correction of tetralogy of Fallot. Ann Thorac Surg 2002;73:1794.

Discigil B et al: Late pulmonary valve replacement after repair of tetralogy of Fallot. J Thorac Cardiovasc Surg 2001;121:344.

Hirsch JC, Mosca RS, Bove EL. Complete repair of tetralogy of Fallot in the neonate: results in the modern era. Ann Surg 2000;232:508.

Shinebourne EA, Babu-Narayan SV, Carvalho JS. Tetralogy of Fallot: from fetus to adult. Heart 2006;92:1353.

▶ Transposition of Great Arteries

 ESSENTIALS OF DIAGNOSIS

▶ Cyanosis shortly after birth.

▶ Symptoms of congestive heart failure.

▶ Variable murmurs.

▶ Chest radiograph with the classic "egg-on-a-string" appearance.

▶ Echocardiographic confirmation of ventriculoarterial discordance (aorta arising from the right ventricle and pulmonary artery arising from the left ventricle).

A. General Considerations

Transposition of the great arteries (TGA) is a congenital cardiac anomaly in which the aorta arises from the right ventricle and the pulmonary artery originates from the left ventricle (Figure 19–26). TGA is divided into *dextro*-looped (d-TGA) and *levo*-looped (l-TGA). The looping refers to the right or left looping of the primitive heart tube during fetal development, which determines whether the atria and ventricles are concordant (right atrium attaches to right ventricle and left atrium attaches to left ventricle) or discordant. L-transposition of the great arteries is associated with atrioventricular discordance (right atrium attaches to left ventricle and left atrium attaches to right ventricle) and is also termed congenitally corrected TGA. L-transposition of the great arteries is a rare variant of TGA and is beyond the scope of this chapter, which focuses on d-TGA. The defect can be subdivided into d-TGA with intact ventricular septum (IVS) (55–60%) and d-TGA with VSD (40–45%), one third of which are hemodynamically insignificant. Pulmonic stenosis, causing significant left ventricular outflow tract obstruction, occurs rarely with an IVS and in approximately 10% of d-TGA/VSD.

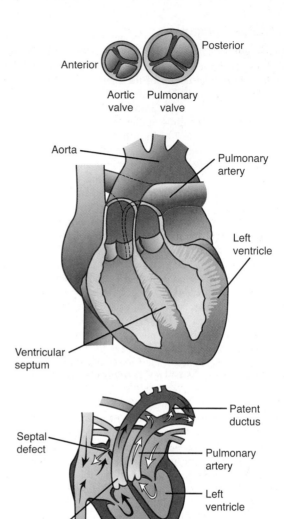

▲ **Figure 19–26.** Typical transposition of the great arteries. The aorta arises from the morphologic right ventricle and is anterior to and slightly to the right of the pulmonary artery, which originates from the morphologic left ventricle. Inset at bottom illustrates the independent systemic and pulmonary circulations, which may be connected by a patent ductus arteriosus or atrial septal defect. Inset at top illustrates a common relationship of the two great arteries in typical transposition.

B. Clinical Findings

D-TGA is a relatively common cardiac anomaly and is the most common form of congenital heart disease presenting as cyanosis in the first week of life. The malformation accounts for approximately 10% of all congenital cardiovascular malformations in infants. The degree of cyanosis depends on the amount of mixing between the pulmonary and systemic circulations. In TGA, oxygenated pulmonary venous blood is returned to the lungs, and desaturated systemic blood is returned to the body. Because the two circulations exist in parallel, some mixing between them must occur to allow oxygenated blood to reach the systemic circulation and the desaturated blood to reach the lungs. Mixing may occur at a number of levels, most commonly at the atrial level through an ASD or a patent foramen ovale. Generally, two levels of mixing are necessary to maintain adequate systemic oxygen delivery with a VSD or PDA serving as an additional site for cardiac mixing. In TGA, there can be no fixed shunt in one direction without an equal amount of blood passing in the other direction; otherwise, one circulation would eventually empty into the other. Therefore, the amount of desaturated blood reaching the lungs (effective pulmonary blood flow) must equal the amount of saturated blood reaching the aorta (effective systemic blood flow). Clinical characteristics are dependent on the degree of mixing and the amount of pulmonary blood flow. These factors relate to the specific anatomic subtype of d-TGA. Neonates with d-TGA with IVS (or small VSD) have mixing limited to the atrial level and PDA. The ASD may be restrictive, and the PDA generally will close over the first days to week of life. As the degree of mixing decreases, the patient becomes increasingly cyanotic and will eventually suffer cardiovascular collapse. Fortunately, the majority of these neonates will manifest cyanosis early in life, which is recognized by a nurse or physician within the first hour in 56% and in the first day in 92%. In d-TGA with a large VSD, there is additional opportunity for mixing and increased pulmonary blood flow. The neonate with d-TGA/VSD may manifest only mild cyanosis, which may be initially overlooked. However, generally within 2–6 weeks, signs and symptoms of congestive heart failure will emerge. Tachypnea and tachycardia become prominent, while cyanosis may remain mild. Auscultatory findings are consistent with congestive heart failure with increased pulmonary blood flow, including a pansystolic murmur, third heart sound, middiastolic rumble, gallop, and narrowly split second heart sound with an increased pulmonary component. Neonates with d-TGA and significant pulmonic stenosis present with severe cyanosis at birth. Lesser degrees of pulmonic stenosis will result in varying levels of cyanosis.

In cases of TGA, the electrocardiogram is normal at birth, demonstrating the typical pattern of right ventricular dominance. Although the classic chest radiographic appearance of an egg-shaped heart with a narrow superior mediastinum may be seen, this finding is often obscured by an enlarged thymic shadow. The abnormal ventriculoarterial connection is clearly seen on echocardiography, which demonstrates that the posterior great vessel arising from the left ventricle is a pulmonary artery that bifurcates soon after its origin. The anterior great vessel is the aorta and arises from the right ventricle. Associated lesions, including VSD, left ventricular outflow tract obstruction, and coarctation, may also be

diagnosed. Although used less frequently for diagnosis, cardiac catheterization may be helpful to improve cardiac mixing by means of balloon atrial septostomy.

C. Treatment

The infant with TGA and severe cyanosis requires prompt diagnosis and treatment to improve mixing and increase the arterial oxygen saturation. The first intervention to improve mixing in a cyanotic newborn suspected of having TGA is to insure ductal patency by beginning an infusion of prostaglandin E_1. In the presence of a restrictive ASD, a balloon atrial septostomy, a technique developed by William Rashkind in 1966, is performed. The procedure involves inserting a balloon-tipped catheter across the foramen ovale into the left atrium. Inflation and forcible withdrawal of the catheter tears the septum primum and enlarges the ASD. Mixing generally increases immediately, with a substantial increase in arterial oxygen saturation. Without intervention, d-TGA is universally fatal. Untreated, 30% of neonates will die in the first week of life, 50% by the first month, 70% within 6 months, and 90% by 1 year. The definitive surgical treatment of patients with TGA has changed dramatically with the advent of the arterial switch operation. Historically, definitive repair was achieved by redirecting venous inflow at the atrial level with either a Senning or Mustard procedure. In both techniques, the atrial septum is repositioned such that superior and inferior vena caval blood is rerouted to the mitral valve and then to the left ventricle and pulmonary artery. Pulmonary venous blood is redirected to the tricuspid valve and right ventricle. The right ventricle then ejects the oxygenated blood to the systemic circulation. Although physiologic repair at the atrial level is associated with a low operative mortality rate (< 5%), even in infants, a number of late problems have occurred. Obstruction to vena caval inflow, particularly at the junction of the superior vena cava and the right atrium, still occurs in about 5% of patients and may be more common when the procedure is performed in an infant. Additionally, pulmonary venous obstruction may develop and is often difficult to repair. Perhaps because of the complex atrial suture lines, atrial dysrhythmias are common and occur in more than half of patients observed on a long-term basis. The most serious long-term complication of repair by either the Senning or Mustard technique has been right ventricular dysfunction. Right ventricular failure with an enlarged, poorly contractile chamber and secondary tricuspid regurgitation has been found in a significant number of these patients in long-term follow-up studies.

The arterial switch operation, first successfully performed by Jatene in 1975, has become the optimal surgical procedure for infants with this condition. Current techniques have reduced the operative mortality to 2–10%. The operative technique involves transection of both great vessels and direct reanastomosis to reestablish ventriculoarterial concordance. Additionally, the coronary arteries are removed from the anterior aorta and relocated to the posterior great vessel (neoaorta). The extensive experience gained with this procedure has confirmed that any variant of coronary artery anatomy can be successfully repaired, although certain unusual forms clearly impose a higher risk. Because many patients with TGA have an IVS, left ventricular pressure falls early in life as pulmonary vascular resistance (PVR) decreases. In this situation, it is essential that the arterial repair be performed within the first 2–3 weeks of life, while the left ventricle is still able to meet systemic workloads. In patients presenting later, the left ventricle can be retrained with a preliminary pulmonary artery band and aortopulmonary shunt followed by the definitive arterial repair. Although patients with large VSDs do not require early repair because of their decreased left ventricular pressure, experience has indicated that even in this subgroup, the operation is best performed within the first month of life, before secondary complications such as pulmonary hypertension, congestive heart failure, or infection develop.

Patients with fixed left ventricular outflow tract obstruction are not candidates for the arterial repair because correction would result in systemic ventricular outflow tract obstruction. Most of these patients also have large VSDs. Palliation early in life with systemic-to-pulmonary artery shunting is an option, with definitive repair postponed until somatic growth results in cyanosis as the shunt is outgrown. At that time, the Rastelli procedure is performed, in which left ventricular blood is redirected through the VSD to the anterior aorta by placement of an intraventricular patch. The pulmonary artery is ligated, and right ventricle-to-distal pulmonary artery continuity is reestablished with a valve-bearing conduit. An increasing number of experienced centers currently recommend early complete repair in the neonatal period using a Rastelli procedure. Early repair eliminates the interim morbidity and mortality associated with a systemic-to-pulmonary artery shunt and chronic cyanosis.

D. Prognosis

Current hospital survival for the arterial switch operation is 90–95%. D-TGA/IVS generally has a lower mortality than d-TGA/VSD or d-TGA/VSD/PS. Hospital mortality for d-TGA/IVS is 3.5–7.6%, compared to 9.4–13.1% for d-TGA/VSD. Recent studies have neutralized the increased risk of the additional VSD closure. Long-term survivals at 5–10 years and 15 years are 87.9–93% and 86–88%, respectively. The most common cause for reintervention is supravalvar pulmonic stenosis, occurring in 4–16%. A recent study of 101 patients undergoing a Rastelli operation over a 25-year period revealed a hospital mortality of 7%, with no deaths in the last 7 years of the study. Actuarial survival at 5, 10, 15, and 20 years was 82%, 80%, 68%, and 52%.

Brown JW, Park HJ, Turrentine MW: Arterial switch operation: factors impacting survival in the current era. Ann Thorac Surg 2001;71:1978.

Haas F et al: Long-term survival and functional follow-up in patients after the arterial switch operation. Ann Thorac Surg 1999;68:1692.
Kreutzer C et al: Twenty-five-year experience with Rastelli repair for transposition of the great arteries. J Thorac Cardiovasc Surg. 2000;120:211.
Qamar ZA et al: Current risk factors and outcomes for the arterial switch operation. Ann Thorac Surg 2007;84:871.
Warnes CA: Transposition of the great arteries. Circulation 2006; 114:2699.

▶ Truncus Arteriosus

 ESSENTIALS OF DIAGNOSIS

▶ Early signs of congestive heart failure and collapsing peripheral pulses.

▶ Often associated with interrupted aortic arch and DiGeorge syndrome.

▶ Chest radiograph with cardiomegaly, pulmonary plethora, and a small thymic shadow.

▶ Echocardiography confirms a common semilunar (truncal) valve rather than a separate aortic and pulmonary valve with the pulmonary arteries originated off the ascending aorta.

A. General Considerations

Truncus arteriosus is a rare anomaly that accounts for 0.4–4% of all cases of congenital heart disease. A single arterial vessel arises from the heart, overriding the ventricular septum, and gives rise to the systemic, coronary, and pulmonary circulations. The Collett and Edwards classification of truncus arteriosus focuses on the origin of the pulmonary arteries from the common arterial trunk, as follows:

Type I: Common arterial trunk gives rise to a main pulmonary artery and the aorta.

Type II: Right and left pulmonary arteries arise directly from and in close proximity to the posterior wall of the truncus.

Type III: Right and left pulmonary arteries arise from more widely separated orifices on the posterior truncal wall.

Type IV: Branch pulmonary arteries are absent. Pulmonary blood flow is derived from aortopulmonary collaterals.

Persistent truncus arteriosus is the result of failed development of the aortopulmonary septum and subpulmonary infundibulum (conal septum). Normal septation leads to the development of both pulmonary and systemic outflow tracts, division of the semilunar valves, and formation of the aorta and pulmonary arteries. Failure of septation results in a VSD (absence of the infundibular septum), a single semi-lunar valve, and a single arterial trunk. Most cases are associated with a VSD reminiscent of the VSD associated with TOF. However, in this anomaly, the superior margin of the defect is formed by the truncal valve. The truncal valve leaflets are generally dysmorphic, and their motion may be restricted. Leaflet number is highly variable, with about 65% tricuspid, 22% quadricuspid, 9% bicuspid, and rarely unicuspid or pentacuspid. As a result of these abnormally developed valve leaflets, a moderate or greater degree of truncal insufficiency is present in 20–26% of patients. The pulmonary arteries are usually of normal size and most often arise from the left posterolateral aspect of the truncal artery, often in close proximity to the truncal valve and ostium of the left coronary artery.

Other cardiac anomalies are common and include an ASD (9–20%), an interrupted aortic arch (10–20%), and coronary ostial abnormalities (37–49%) with the left coronary artery frequently noted to have a high origin, not uncommonly near the takeoff of the pulmonary arteries. Extracardiac anomalies are reported in approximately 28% of patients with truncus arteriosus. Described abnormalities include skeletal, genitourinary, gastrointestinal deformities, and DiGeorge syndrome (11%).

B. Clinical Findings

The anatomy of truncus arteriosus results in the obligatory mixing of systemic and pulmonary venous blood at the level of the VSD and truncal valve, which produces arterial saturations of 85–90%. The systemic arterial saturation depends on the volume of pulmonary blood flow, which in turn is determined by the PVR. As the PVR begins to fall, excessive pulmonary circulation ensues and leads to pulmonary congestion and signs and symptoms of congestive heart failure. This nonrestrictive left-to-right shunt may cause early development of irreversible pulmonary vascular obstructive disease.

The presence of truncal valve abnormalities poses further hemodynamic burdens. Truncal valve regurgitation leads to ventricular dilatation and low diastolic coronary perfusion pressures that can result in myocardial ischemia. Truncal valve stenosis promotes ventricular hypertrophy, increases the myocardial oxygen demand, and limits coronary and systemic perfusion, especially with the large volume of run-off into the pulmonary vascular bed.

Neonates with truncus arteriosus present with signs of congestive heart failure and collapsing peripheral pulses. Chest radiography shows marked cardiomegaly, pulmonary plethora, often with minimal thymus shadow, and a right aortic arch. The electrocardiogram most often depicts biventricular hypertrophy. Echocardiography is the diagnostic procedure of choice and can demonstrate the truncal vessel, the structure and function of the truncal valve, associated lesions such as interrupted aortic arch, and often the pulmonary arterial anatomy. Cardiac catheterization is not performed unless the anatomy is unclear, further information is needed about the status of the truncal valve, or the status of the pulmonary vasculature is unclear (ie, infants older than 3 months at diagnosis).

C. Treatment

The natural history of patients born with truncus arteriosus is early demise. Approximately 40% of infants are dead within 1 month, 70% by 3 months, and 90% by 1 year. Early death is caused by congestive heart failure. Survivors may do well for a period of time until the development of pulmonary vascular obstructive disease and Eisenmenger syndrome. The ultimate treatment of truncus arteriosus is surgical correction in the neonatal period. Medical treatment is palliative and directed toward controlling congestive heart failure with fluid restriction, diuretics, and afterload reduction. Complete repair entails separating the pulmonary arteries from the truncus, repairing the resulting defect in the aorta, closing the VSD, and restoring the continuity of the right ventricular outflow tract with an extracardiac conduit (Figure 19–27). Severe truncal valve regurgitation requires truncal valve repair or replacement. An associated interrupted aortic arch is repaired by constructing a primary end-to-end anastomosis of the distal ascending aorta with proximal augmentation if necessary.

D. Prognosis

The results of truncus arteriosus repair have improved greatly during the last two decades. Before the importance of early operation to avoid irreversible pulmonary vascular disease was appreciated, patients underwent repair at most institutions at an average age of 2–5 years with high mortality rates. Current hospital mortality for the neonatal repair of truncus arteriosus ranges between 4.3% and 17%, with the majority of deaths occurring in complex truncus arteriosus or in truncus arteriosus with associated severe truncal valve regurgitation. All patients will ultimately require reoperation for replacement of the right ventricle to pulmonary artery conduit with only 36% being free from reoperation at 10 years.

Brown JW et al: Truncus arteriosus repair: outcomes, risk factors, reoperation and management. Eur J Cardiothorac Surg 2001; 20:221.

Henaine R et al: Fate of the truncal valve in truncus arteriosus. Ann Thorac Surg 2008;85:172.

Konstantinov IE et al: Truncus arteriosus associated with interrupted aortic arch in 50 neonates: a Congenital Heart Surgeons Society study. Ann Thorac Surg 2006;81:214.

Rodefeld MD, Hanley FL. Neonatal truncus arteriosus repair: surgical techniques and clinical management. Semin Thorac Cardiovasc Surg Pediatr Card Surg Annu 2002;5:212.

Thompson LD et al: Neonatal repair of truncus arteriosus: continuing improvement in outcomes. Ann Thorac Surg 2001;72:391.

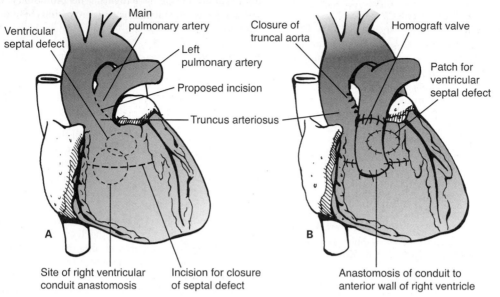

▲ Figure 19–27. Type 1 truncus arteriosus. **A:** The main pulmonary artery arises from the truncus arteriosus downstream to the truncal valve. A ventricular septal defect is present. **B:** The main pulmonary artery is incised from the truncus. The ventricular septal defect is closed with a patch. A conduit of Dacron that contains a homograft aortic valve is sutured to the anterior wall of the right ventricle and the distal pulmonary artery. A conduit between the right ventricle and pulmonary artery was successfully introduced by J. W. Kirklin in 1964 during correction of severe tetralogy of Fallot.

▶ Total Anomalous Pulmonary Venous Connection

ESSENTIALS OF DIAGNOSIS

▶ One of the few remaining pediatric cardiac surgical emergencies.

▶ Variable cyanosis, may be profound with obstructed total anomalous pulmonary venous connection and associated with cardiovascular collapse.

▶ High risk for pulmonary hypertension.

▶ Chest radiograph with pulmonary congestion with enlarged right atrium and ventricle.

▶ Echocardiogram demonstrates the pulmonary veins draining into a systemic vein.

▶ Equalization of saturation in all of the heart chambers (pathognomonic).

A. General Considerations

Total anomalous pulmonary venous connection (TAPVC) is a relatively uncommon congenital defect representing approximately 2% of all congenital heart anomalies. TAPVC encompasses a group of anomalies in which the pulmonary veins connect directly to the systemic venous circulation via persistent splanchnic connections. This abnormality results from failed transfer, in the normal developmental sequence, of pulmonary venous drainage from the splanchnic plexus to the left atrium. The most common classification system consists of four types: supracardiac (type 1), cardiac (type 2), infracardiac (type 3), and mixed (Figure 19–28). Partial anomalous pulmonary venous connection defines patients in whom some but not all venous drainage enters the left atrium, while the remaining veins connect to one or more persistent splanchnic veins.

TAPVC can also be classified by the presence of obstruction. Impingement from surrounding structures or inadequate caliber of the draining pulmonary vein(s) can result in varying degrees of obstruction. Obstruction in supracardiac TAPVC can occur by compression of the ascending vertical vein between the left main stem bronchus and left pulmonary artery or by narrowing at the insertion of the vertical vein into the innominate vein. Obstruction is always present in the infracardiac type because the pulmonary venous blood must pass through the sinusoids of the liver. Obstruction is uncommon in the cardiac type.

Supracardiac occurs in approximately 45% of patients. The common pulmonary vein drains superiorly into the innominate vein, superior vena cava, or azygous vein via

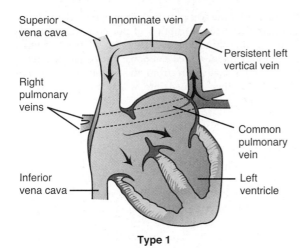

Type 1

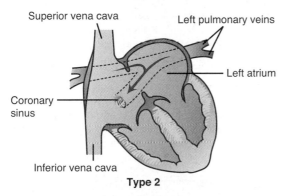

Type 2

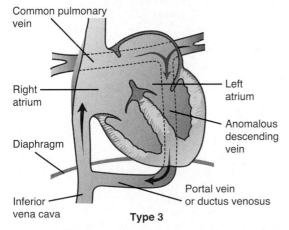

Type 3

▲ **Figure 19–28.** Common types of total anomalous pulmonary venous connection. Type 1: The pulmonary veins connect to a persistent left vertical vein, the innominate vein, and the right superior vena cava. Type 2: The pulmonary veins connect to the coronary sinus and the right atrium. Type 3: The pulmonary veins connect to an anomalous descending vein, a portal vein or persistent ductus venosus, and eventually the inferior vena cava.

an ascending vertical vein. Cardiac TAPVC occurs in approximately 25% of patients. The pulmonary venous confluence drains into the coronary sinus or, on rare occasions, individual pulmonary veins will connect directly into the right atrium. Infracardiac TAPVC occurs in approximately 25% of patients. The pulmonary venous confluence drains into a descending vertical vein through the diaphragm into the portal vein or ductus venosus. Finally, a mixed type of TAPVC occurs in approximately 5% of patients and can involve any or all components of the previous three types.

B. Clinical Findings

TAPVC produces a mixing lesion because oxygenated blood from the pulmonary system drains back into the systemic venous circulation. The size of the ASD dictates the distribution of blood flow. Most patients with unobstructed TAPVC have few or no symptoms in infancy and present with signs and symptoms similar to an ASD. In the neonate with obstructed TAPVC, venous drainage from the pulmonary vasculature is impaired, leading to pulmonary venous hypertension and pulmonary edema. In severe cases, this increased pressure will lead to reflexive vasoconstriction of the pulmonary vasculature with pulmonary hypertension. Patients with obstruction present early in life with profound cyanosis from pulmonary edema.

The diagnosis can be made with echocardiographic identification of the anomalous connection of the pulmonary venous confluence to the systemic venous system. The ASD and other associated anomalies can be delineated. Cardiac catheterization is rarely necessary unless accurate measurement of PVR is needed.

The management of TAPVC is surgical repair. In patients with obstruction, medical management for stabilization may be employed but is often unsuccessful and should not delay surgical intervention.

C. Treatment

The principle of operative repair is to establish an unobstructed communication between the pulmonary venous confluence and the left atrium, interrupt the connections with the systemic venous circulation, and close the ASD. The specific repair is dependent on the type of anomalous connection.

Supracardiac TAPVC—The repair of supracardiac TAPVC may be performed with moderate hypothermia and bicaval cannulation or with a brief period of hypothermic circulatory arrest. The optimal approach is to retract the ascending aorta to the left and the superior vena cava to the right to expose the pulmonary venous confluence. This approach provides excellent exposure without distortion of the heart or venous structures. The vertical vein can be identified and ligated (just prior to opening the confluence) outside the pericardium at the level of the innominate vein. A transverse incision is made in the pulmonary venous confluence, and a parallel incision is placed in the dome of the left atrium beginning at the base of the left atrial appendage. The common pulmonary vein is then anastomosed to the left atrium, taking care to construct an unrestrictive connection. A right atriotomy is made to close the ASD.

Cardiac TAPVC—The repair of cardiac TAPVC can be performed with bicaval cannulation and moderate hypothermia (28–32 °C) with the use of a vent or a cardiotomy sucker to capture the pulmonary venous return. A right atriotomy is performed with identification of the ASD and the orifice of the coronary sinus. The roof of the coronary sinus is excised into the left atrium. A patch of pericardium or prosthetic material is then placed to close the enlarged ASD, effectively channeling the pulmonary venous return into the left atrium. The conduction system travels in proximity to the coronary sinus, and care must be taken while suturing the patch in this area to avoid heart block.

Infracardiac TAPVC—For infracardiac connections, a brief period of hypothermic circulatory arrest is often required. The heart is rotated superiorly. The descending vertical vein is identified by opening the posterior pericardium. The connection to the descending vertical vein is ligated at the level of the diaphragm. An incision is made along the length of the pulmonary venous confluence with a parallel incision on the posterior wall of the left atrium. The pulmonary venous confluence is then anastomosed to the left atrium, taking care not to narrow the connection. Tissue from the descending vertical vein can be used in the anastomosis. A right atriotomy is performed through which the ASD is closed.

Recurrent Pulmonary Venous Obstruction—The approach to recurrent pulmonary venous obstruction is dependent upon the level of obstruction. Obstruction can develop at the anastomosis or within the individual pulmonary veins. The latter may initially present as an anastomotic constriction, as the true extent of obstruction is not always apparent at first. Isolated narrowing of the anastomosis between the common pulmonary vein and left atrium often can be repaired with revision or patch augmentation of the anastomosis.

Obstruction of the individual pulmonary venous ostia is the greater challenge. Although the obstruction may initially appear to be limited to the ostium, progressive narrowing along the entire length of the vein into the hilum of the lung will occur with time. Repair of this lesion is technically challenging, and recurrent early obstruction is common. A new approach to recurrent pulmonary vein stenosis employs a sutureless technique utilizing in situ pericardium to create a neoatrium. The theory behind this repair is based on the concept that pulmonary venous obstruction results from inflammation induced locally by suture placement. Repair involves wide unroofing of the narrowed portion of each involved pulmonary vein from the left atrial anastomosis to

the hilum. A wide flap of pericardium is then elevated with care taken to avoid disruption of posterior adhesions and injury to the phrenic nerve. This flap of pericardium is rotated over the unroofed pulmonary veins and sutured to the left atrial wall away from the venous ostia. A large neoatrium is then created into which pulmonary venous return can drain.

D. Prognosis

Early mortality in patients undergoing repair of TAPVC is associated with the initial degree of obstruction present. Early diagnosis and repair as well as optimal postoperative management, including aggressive treatment of pulmonary hypertension, have resulted in a dramatic reduction in operative risk. For patients surviving the perioperative period, the long-term survival and functional status are excellent.

Recurrent venous obstruction develops in 5–15% of patients. Results following balloon angioplasty and/or stent insertion have been disappointing, and recurrent stenoses are the rule. Individual patch angioplasty of the ostia has also been utilized with poor long-term results. Lung transplantation has been considered in severe cases of extensive, bilateral disease. The mortality associated with reoperation for obstruction can be up to 50% when bilateral stenoses are present. The use of the sutureless technique for recurrent pulmonary vein obstruction has demonstrated improved survival and decreased recurrence.

Devaney EJ, Ohye RG, Bove EL: Pulmonary vein stenosis following repair of total anomalous pulmonary venous connection. Semin Thorac Cardiovasc Surg Pediatr Card Surg Ann 2006;9:51.

Hancock Friesen CL et al: Total anomalous pulmonary venous connection: an analysis of current management strategies in a single institution. Ann Thorac Surg 2005;79:596.

Kanter KR: Surgical repair of total anomalous pulmonary venous connection. Semin Thorac Cardiovasc Surg Pediatr Card Surg Ann 2006;9:40.

Lacour-Gayet F: Surgery for pulmonary venous obstruction after repair of total anomalous pulmonary venous return. Semin Thorac Cardiovasc Surg Pediatr Card Surg Ann 2006;9:45.

Michielon G et al: Total anomalous pulmonary venous connection: long-term appraisal with evolving technical solutions. Eur J Cardiothorac Surg 2002;22:184.

▶ Tricuspid Atresia

ESSENTIALS OF DIAGNOSIS

▶ Variable cyanosis.

▶ Usually no obstruction to systemic output.

▶ Echocardiography confirms absence of a tricuspid valve with a hypoplastic right ventricle.

A. General Considerations

Tricuspid atresia refers to single-ventricle hearts that lack a communication between the right atrium and right ventricle. The only outlet for the right atrium is the ASD. If present, aneurysmal tissue of the septum primum may prolapse into the left atrium The left atrium is normal in morphology but is often dilated. A normal communication with a mitral valve between the left atrium and left ventricle is present. The right ventricle is diminutive in size without an inlet portion. It is connected to the left ventricle by a VSD surrounded completely by muscle. The anatomic subtypes of tricuspid atresia are based on the relationship of the great arteries. Type I defects (70%) have normally related great vessels, type II (30%) have transposed great arteries, and type III (rare) have congenitally corrected transposition of the great arteries. These types are further subclassified by the degree of obstruction to pulmonary blood flow, which is present in 45–75% of patients. Aortic valve (10%) and aortic arch (25%) obstruction may also be present. Patients with tricuspid atresia are at increased risk for Wolff-Parkinson-White syndrome due to congenital and surgically acquired pathways.

B. Clinical Findings

The clinical presentation depends on the relationship of the great vessels and degree of restriction at the level of the atrial and ventricular septum. Most infants present with some degree of cyanosis. Systemic output is usually unobstructed. Prostaglandins may be necessary to maintain ductal patency in infants with severe obstruction to pulmonary blood flow.

C. Treatment

The initial palliation for most patients is the placement of a modified Blalock-Taussig shunt to maintain adequate pulmonary blood flow. A more complex initial palliation with a Norwood procedure may be necessary in the case of transposed great vessels. The remainder of the palliation involves a hemi-Fontan and Fontan procedure (discussed in the section on Hypoplastic Left Heart Syndrome).

D. Prognosis

The overall survival for tricuspid atresia is similar to that reported for other single-ventricle lesions palliated with a Fontan procedure. The survival is 83% at 1 year, 70% at 10 years, and 60% at 20 years.

Hager A et al: Congenital and surgically acquired Wolff-Parkinson-White syndrome in patients with tricuspid atresia. J Thorac Cardiovasc Surg 2005;130:48.

Rao PS: Tricuspid atresia. Curr Treat Options Cardiovasc Med 2000;2:507.

Sittiwangkul R et al: Outcomes of tricuspid atresia in the Fontan era. Ann Thorac Surg 2004;77:889.

Wald RM et al: Outcome after prenatal diagnosis of tricuspid atresia: a multicenter experience. Am Heart J 2007;153:772.

▶ Hypoplastic Left Heart Syndrome

ESSENTIALS OF DIAGNOSIS

▶ Increasingly diagnosed prenatally.

▶ Male predominance.

▶ Newborn respiratory distress with cyanosis and hemodynamic collapse as the duct closes.

▶ Echocardiographic evidence of aortic and mitral atresia or stenosis with a hypoplastic left ventricle and ascending aorta.

A. General Considerations

A variety of congenital cardiovascular malformations may result in a functional single-ventricle anatomy, most commonly tricuspid atresia, pulmonary atresia, unbalanced AVSD, and hypoplastic left heart syndrome (HLHS). The most common lesion is HLHS. Approximately 1000 infants with HLHS are born in the United States each year. It is the most common severe congenital heart defect, comprising 7–9% of all anomalies diagnosed within the first year of life. All single-ventricle lesions share the common physiology of only a single ventricle capable of supporting cardiac output. HLHS refers to a constellation of congenital cardiac anomalies characterized by marked hypoplasia or absence of the left ventricle and severe hypoplasia of the ascending aorta. The systemic circulation is dependent upon the right ventricle via a PDA, and there is obligatory mixing of pulmonary and systemic venous blood in the right atrium. There is associated aortic valve stenosis or atresia and mitral valve stenosis or atresia. The descending aorta is essentially a continuation of the ductus arteriosus, and the ascending aorta and aortic arch are a diminutive branch from this vessel. Initial management includes a prostaglandin infusion to maintain ductal patency and correction of metabolic acidosis. The patient may require intubation and ventilator adjustment to reduce supplemental oxygen and maintain a Pco_2 of about 40 mm Hg to avoid excessive pulmonary flow.

B. Treatment

Alternative approaches to the treatment of this problem include cardiac transplantation and staged reconstructive surgery. In the context of improving results for staged reconstruction, risks of immunosuppression, and limited donor availability, competing risk analysis favors staged repair, and most centers pursue this option as primary therapy for HLHS. Transplantation is generally reserved for very high-risk patients, such as those with depressed right ventricular function of severe tricuspid regurgitation.

The first successful palliation of HLHS was reported by Norwood on a series of infants operated on between 1979 and 1981. This procedure has been technically refined over the years, but three essential components remain: atrial septectomy, anastomosis of the proximal pulmonary artery to the aorta with homograft augmentation of the aortic arch, and aortopulmonary shunt. The ultimate goal of surgical correction in patients with a univentricular heart is the total diversion of all vena caval blood directly into the pulmonary arteries. The Fontan procedure was first successfully performed in a patient with tricuspid atresia but has since evolved as an excellent way to establish physiologic repair for patients with more complex forms of univentricular heart. The superior vena caval blood returns directly via an end-to-side anastomosis with the pulmonary artery (bidirectional Glenn) or through a right atrial-pulmonary artery connection (hemi-Fontan) performed at 4–6 months of age. The inferior vena caval flow is directed to the pulmonary artery with an intra-atrial baffle (lateral tunnel technique) or an extracardiac conduit at 2–4 years of age. All oxygenated pulmonary venous flow empties into the ventricular chamber through the atrioventricular (A-V) valves to be ejected to the systemic circulation, while superior and inferior vena caval blood flows directly to the lungs to acquire oxygen prior to returning to the heart. For the Fontan procedure to be performed with a low operative mortality and an acceptable functional result, certain criteria must be met. Normal pulmonary artery pressure (< 20 mm Hg) and PVR (< 2 Woods units·m^2) are the most important prerequisites. Additionally, it is essential that ventricular function and A-V valve function be normal. Although the Fontan procedure cannot be considered a truly corrective operation, it offers benefits that cannot be equaled by those of any of the other palliative procedures. The major advantages include restoration of normal systemic oxygen saturation and reduction of ventricular volume overload.

C. Prognosis

Universally fatal only two decades ago, tremendous strides have been made in improving the outcomes for patients with HLHS. Of the three stages, the highest-risk stage of the repair remains the Norwood operation. During the 1990s, the hospital survival for the Norwood procedure across the United States was approximately 40%. Currently, select centers have reported hospital survivals of 90% or greater. Reported survivals for the hemi-Fontan and Fontan procedures have also been excellent at 98% for both operations. Overall, 75% of patients diagnosed with HLHS will survive through the Fontan procedure.

The current results for the Fontan procedure are excellent with hospital mortality ranging from 2% to 9%. The condition of survivors is generally good, and most attain a functional status of New York Heart Association class I or II. The long-term results have been reported with a 93% 5-year survival and a 91% 10-year survival. Although long-term results are encouraging, late complications may be seen. Continued surveillance for arrhythmias, congenital heart failure, protein-losing enteropathy, and hepatic dysfunction remains important.

Bove EL, Ohye RG, Devaney EJ: Hypoplastic left heart syndrome: conventional surgical management. Semin Thorac Cardiovasc Surg Pediatr Card Surg Annu 2004;7:3.

Bove EL et al: Tricuspid valve repair for hypoplastic left heart syndrome and the failing right ventricle. Semin Thorac Cardiovasc Surg Pediatr Card Surg Annu 2007;10:101.

Hirsch JC et al: The lateral tunnel Fontan procedure for hypoplastic left heart syndrome: results of 100 consecutive patients. Pediatr Cardiol 2007;28:426.

Pizarro C et al: Right ventricle to pulmonary artery conduit improves outcome after stage I Norwood for hypoplastic left heart syndrome. Circulation 2003;108(Suppl 1):II155.

Stasik CN et al: Current outcomes and risk factors for the Norwood procedure. J Thorac Cardiovasc Surg 2006;131:412.

ACYANOTIC HEART DEFECTS

1. Left-to-Right Shunting

▷ Atrial Septal Defect

 ESSENTIALS OF DIAGNOSIS

▶ Asymptomatic in childhood; may develop late atrial dysrhythmias.

▶ Cyanosis may develop with Eisenmenger syndrome.

▶ Widely split and fixed S2 with 1–3/6 systolic ejection murmur at lower left sternal border.

▶ Cardiomegaly on chest radiograph.

▶ Echocardiogram demonstrates an atrial level shunt.

A. General Considerations

Cardiac septation occurs between the third and sixth weeks of fetal development. The septum primum, which arises from the roof of the common atrium and descends inferiorly, initially divides the common atrium. The ostium primum is the opening below the inferior edge of the septum primum, which is obliterated as the septum primum fuses with the endocardial cushions. The ostium secundum forms in the midportion of the septum primum prior to closure of the ostium primum. The septum secundum also arises from the roof of the atrium and descends along the right side of the septum primum and covers the ostium secundum. This creates a flap valve whereby blood from the inferior vena cava may preferentially stream beneath the edge of the septum secundum and through the ostium secundum into the left atrium. After birth, the increase in left atrial pressure usually closes this pathway.

An ASD is a hole in the atrial septum (Figure 19–29). ASDs are the third-most common congenital heart defect, occurring in 1 out of 1000 live births and representing 10% of

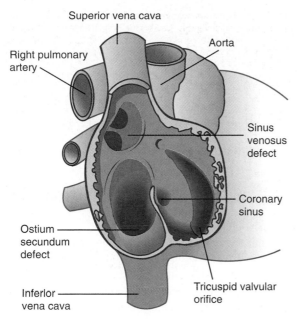

▲ **Figure 19–29.** Sinus venosus and ostium secundum defects in the atrial septum as viewed from the opened right atrium.

congenital heart defects. The most common ASD is the secundum defect, which occurs when the ostium secundum is too large for complete coverage by the septum secundum. Ostium secundum defects account for about 80% of ASDs. An ostium primum ASD, representing 10% of ASDs, occurs as a result of failure of fusion of the septum primum with the endocardial cushions (ostium primum defect is discussed later in the section on Atrioventricular Septal Defects). A third type of ASD is the sinus venosus defect, seen in about 10% of cases. Sinus venosus ASDs are caused by abnormal fusion of the venous pathways with the atrium and are characterized by defects high in the atrial septum near the orifice of the superior vena cava or, less commonly, low in the atrial septum near the inferior vena cava. Sinus venosus defects are frequently associated with partial anomalous pulmonary venous connection, usually with the right upper pulmonary vein draining into the superior vena cava near the cavoatrial junction. The rarest type of ASD is the unroofed coronary sinus septal defect. This occurs when there is loss of the common wall between the coronary sinus and the left atrium adjacent to the atrial septum. This unroofing of the coronary sinus leads to a communication between the right and left atria at the site of the coronary sinus.

Failure of postnatal fusion of the septum secundum to the septum primum results in a persistent slitlike communication known as a patent foramen ovale (PFO). PFOs are extremely common in the general population, and autopsy studies have demonstrated a prevalence of 27%. PFOs are generally considered separate from other ASDs because of the absence of significant shunting, but they remain important clinically because of the occurrence of paradoxical embolization. A paradoxical embolus is usually a blood clot arising from a systemic vein, which would normally pass to the lungs, but in the presence of a septal defect may instead cross into the systemic circulation.

B. Clinical Findings

ASDs lead to increased pulmonary blood flow secondary to left-to-right shunting. Shunting at the atrial level is determined by the size of the defect and by the relative ventricular compliance (ie, blood preferentially fills the more compliant ventricle). At birth, both chambers are equally compliant, but as PVR falls, the right ventricle remodels and becomes more compliant. Shunting across the atrial septum causes a volume load on the right heart. A volume load is created by additional venous return to a chamber during diastole.

The volume overload from an ASD is usually well tolerated, and patients are frequently asymptomatic. Symptoms tend to develop when the ratio of pulmonary to systemic blood flow (Q_p/Q_s) exceeds two. The most common symptoms are fatigue, shortness of breath, exercise intolerance, and recurrent respiratory infections. Older patients with untreated ASDs tend to develop atrial dysrhythmias, and adults may develop congestive heart failure and right ventricular dysfunction. Pulmonary vascular obstructive disease may develop rarely as a late complication of untreated ASD. Paradoxical embolization is also an important potential complication of ASD.

The classic physical findings in patients with ASDs include fixed splitting of the second heart sound and a systolic ejection murmur at the left upper sternal border due to relative pulmonary stenosis (increased flow across a normal pulmonary valve). A diastolic flow murmur across the tricuspid valve is occasionally audible. A prominent right ventricular lift and increased intensity of the pulmonary component of the second heart sound may occur with pulmonary hypertension. Chest radiography shows cardiomegaly, with enlargement of the right atrium, right ventricle, and pulmonary artery. Electrocardiography frequently demonstrates right axis deviation and an incomplete right bundle branch block. When right bundle branch block occurs with a leftward or superior axis, the diagnosis of AVSD should be considered. Echocardiography confirms the diagnosis of ASD and defines the anatomy. Cardiac catheterization is important in selected cases to assess PVR in older patients, but it is used more frequently with therapeutic intent for device closure of ASDs.

C. Treatment

Because of the long-term complications associated with ASD, repair is recommended for all patients with symptomatic defects and in asymptomatic patients in whom the Q_p/Q_s is greater than 1.5. Repair is usually performed in children prior to school age. Closure of ASDs may be performed surgically or using a device deployed in the cardiac catheterization lab.

Surgical repair is usually recommended for large secundum defects and for most other types of ASDs. The heart is usually exposed by median sternotomy. Other surgical approaches have been proposed, including minimally invasive techniques, but there are technical drawbacks associated with each of the alternative approaches. In most cases, a limited midline incision with a partial lower sternal split provides adequate exposure and a cosmetically acceptable scar. The atrial septum is exposed through a right atriotomy. Small secundum defects or PFOs may sometimes be closed primarily by suturing the edge of septum primum to the edge of septum secundum. More commonly, larger defects are closed using a patch (polytetrafluoroethylene or autologous pericardium) and a running polypropylene suture. When anomalous pulmonary venous drainage is present, a baffle is created to redirect the flow across the ASD. In all cases, care is taken to deair the left atrium to avoid the complication of air embolization.

The first transcatheter device closure of an ASD was performed in 1976. A number of devices are currently available for percutaneous closure of secundum ASD, and success rates for device deployment are greater than 90%. Device closure has the advantages of fewer complications and a shorter hospitalization. Device closure of small to moderate secundum ASDs and PFOs has now become the standard of care at most large centers.

Occasionally, adults will present with a newly diagnosed ASD. Many studies have confirmed that ASD closure in adults over the age of 40 increases survival and limits the development of heart failure. When the Q_p/Q_s is less than 1.5 and the ratio of pulmonary to systemic vascular resistance (R_p/R_s) is greater than 0.7, significant pulmonary vascular obstructive disease is usually present. A PVR in excess of 10–12 Woods units·m^2 represents a contraindication to ASD closure.

D. Prognosis

Operative mortality for ASD repair is close to 0%. Atrial arrhythmias (1.2%) and postpericardiotomy syndrome (4.7%) are the most common postoperative complications. The long-term survival for patients undergoing ASD repair in childhood is normal. The major long-term complication following surgical closure of ASD is the development of supraventricular arrhythmias, although the risk is lowered when the ASD is closed in childhood. The persistence of this risk despite relief of right-sided volume overload is thought to be related to incomplete atrial remodeling or due to the presence of the atriotomy scar. Longer follow-up is required to determine whether device closure alters the risk of atrial dysrhythmias.

Christensen DD, Vincent RN, Campbell RM: Presentation of atrial septal defect in the pediatric population. Pediatr Cardiol 2005; 26:812.

Cowley CG et al: Comparison of results of closure of secundum atrial septal defect by surgery versus Amplatzer septal occluder. Am J Cardiol 2001;88:589.
Hopkins RA et al: Surgical patch closure of atrial septal defects. Ann Thorac Surg 2004;77:2144.
Krasuski RA: When and how to fix a "hole in the heart": approach to ASD and PFO. Cleve Clin J Med 2007;74:137.
Purcell IF, Brecker SJ, Ward DE: Closure of defects of the atrial septum in adults using the Amplatzer device: 100 consecutive patients in a single center. Clin Cardiol 2004;27:509.

▶ Ventricular Septal Defect

 ESSENTIALS OF DIAGNOSIS

- ▶ Asymptomatic if small.
- ▶ Significant congestive heart failure with failure to thrive develops in the first few months of life if large.
- ▶ Most VSDs close spontaneously.
- ▶ 2–6/6 pansystolic murmur greatest at the left sternal border with an active precordium.
- ▶ Chest radiograph with cardiomegaly and increased pulmonary vascular markings.
- ▶ Echocardiogram demonstrates ventricular level shunting, delineates anatomic type, and defines the relation to the great vessels.

A. General Considerations

Ventricular septation is a complex process that requires accurate development and alignment of a number of structures including the muscular interventricular septum, the atrioventricular septum (arising from the endocardial cushions), and the infundibular septum (which divides the outflow tracts of the right and left ventricles). The membranous septum is a fibrous portion of the ventricular septum, which is adjacent to the central fibrous body (where the mitral, tricuspid, and aortic valve annuli make contact).

VSDs are the most common congenital heart anomalies (with the exception of bicuspid aortic valve, which occurs in about 1.3% of the population). VSDs are present in about 4 of 1000 live births and represent about 40% of congenital heart defects. VSDs are classified based on their location in the ventricular septum (Figure 19–30). The most common defects are perimembranous (80%), which are located in the area of the membranous septum. Inlet defects (5%) are located beneath the septal leaflet of the tricuspid valve and are sometimes called atrioventricular (A-V) canal-type defects. Defects located high in the ventricular septum are outlet defects (10%). Outlet VSDs are typically adjacent to both the pulmonary and aortic valves. Outlet defects are also known by several other names, including supracristal, infundibular, or doubly committed subarterial. Outlet defects

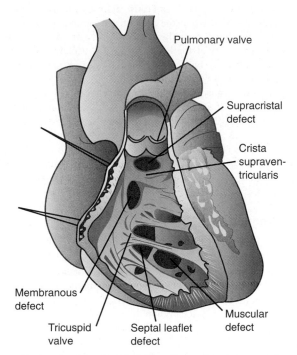

Pulmonary valve

Supracristal
defect

Crista
supraven-
tricularis

Membranous
defect

Tricuspid
valve

Septal leaflet
defect

Muscular
defect

▲ **Figure 19–30.** Anatomic locations of various ventricular septal defects. The wall of the right ventricle has been excised to expose the ventricular septum.

are more common in the Asian population. Trabecular (or muscular) VSDs (5%) are completely bordered by muscle. Trabecular VSDs are frequently multiple and may be associated with perimembranous or outlet defects. The size of VSDs varies. By definition, a VSD is nonrestrictive when its size (or the cumulative size of multiple defects) is greater than or equal to the size of the aortic annulus.

B. Clinical Findings

A VSD causes increased pulmonary blood flow due to left-to-right shunting primarily during systole. This creates a volume load on the left heart (the left atrium and ventricle receive the increased venous return during diastole). The right ventricle is not volume loaded (blood is ejected from the left ventricle through the VSD and directly into the pulmonary circulation), but it does experience a pressure load. The volume of shunt flow is determined by the size of the defect and by the ratio of R_p/R_s. After birth, the PVR is still high, and shunting across a VSD is sometimes minimal. Over the first several weeks of life, shunting tends to increase as the PVR normally falls. Therefore, a patient with a large VSD may be asymptomatic at birth but eventually develop severe congestive heart failure.

The natural history for patients with isolated VSDs is highly variable. Most VSDs are restrictive and tend to close

spontaneously during the first year of life. Large VSDs are nonrestrictive, resulting in right ventricular and pulmonary pressures that are systemic or nearly systemic, and high pulmonary blood flow with Q_p/Q_s ratios greater than 2.5–3. Moderate VSDs are restrictive, with pulmonary pressures that are one-half systemic (or less) and Q_p/Q_s ratios of 1.5–2.5. Small VSDs are highly restrictive; right ventricular pressures remain normal, and the Q_p/Q_s is less than 1.5. Patients with large VSDs tend to develop symptoms of congestive heart failure by 2 months of age. Untreated, excessive pulmonary blood flow leads to pulmonary vascular obstructive disease by the second year of life. Patients with smaller VSDs may remain asymptomatic. In patients with outlet VSDs, prolapse of the aortic valve may occur, producing aortic insufficiency.

Signs of heart failure in infants with large VSDs include tachypnea, hepatomegaly, poor feeding, and failure to thrive. On physical examination, there is a pansystolic murmur at the left sternal border. Usually, the murmur is louder with smaller defects. The precordium is active. The pulmonary component of the second heart sound is accentuated in the presence of pulmonary hypertension. Chest radiography shows increased pulmonary vascular markings and cardiomegaly. Electrocardiography is significant for right ventricular hypertrophy.

Patients with small VSDs have little shunting and are usually asymptomatic, having only a pansystolic murmur. Patients with moderate VSDs manifest symptoms and signs proportional to the degree of shunting.

In patients who have developed significant pulmonary vascular obstructive disease, the volume of left-to-right shunting is decreased, and the murmur may disappear. Eisenmenger physiology results when the shunt flow reverses to right-to-left, creating cyanosis.

The diagnosis of VSD is confirmed by echocardiography, which accurately defines the anatomy and excludes the presence of associated defects. Cardiac catheterization is used selectively in older children and adults in whom elevated PVR is suspected. PVR is calculated by the following formula: $PVR = (PA_{mean} - LA)/Q_p$, where PA_{mean} is the mean pulmonary artery pressure and LA is the left atrial pressure. The units of resistance by this formulation (using pressures in millimeters of mercury and pulmonary flow in liters per minute) are Woods units (which can be expressed in dynes·sec/cm⁵ by multiplying by 80). PVR may be fixed or reactive, and at the time of cardiac catheterization, response to various pulmonary vasodilators may be assessed.

C. Treatment

The management of a patient with a VSD depends on the size of the defect, the type of the defect, the shunt volume, and the PVR. In general, patients with large defects who have intractable congestive heart failure or failure to thrive should undergo early surgical repair. If the congestive symptoms can be moderated by medical therapy, then surgery may be deferred until 6 months of age. Patients with moderate VSDs may be safely followed. If closure has not occurred by school age, then surgical closure is indicated. Small VSDs with Q_p/Q_s of less than 1.5 do not require closure. There is a small long-term risk of endocarditis for these patients, but this can be minimized with the appropriate use of prophylactic antibiotics. Patients with outlet VSDs have a significant risk of developing aortic insufficiency due to leaflet prolapse, and, therefore, all of these patients should undergo surgical closure. Older children and adults must undergo catheterization to assess the pulmonary circulation. When there is a fixed PVR greater than 8–10 Woods units·m^2, then surgery is contraindicated.

Exposure of the ventricular septum is most often achieved by making a right atriotomy and retracting the leaflets of the tricuspid valve. This provides access to perimembranous, inlet, and most trabecular VSDs. Outlet VSDs are frequently best exposed via a pulmonary arteriotomy because the defect lies just beneath the valve. Trabecular VSDs located near the ventricular apex can be very difficult to expose, and an apical ventriculotomy may be necessary. Once the defect is exposed, it is closed using a polytetrafluoroethylene patch and a running polypropylene suture, although some centers may prefer other patch material or interrupted suture technique. It is important to understand the anatomy of the conduction tissue when closing VSDs. The AV node is an atrial structure that lies at the apex of an anatomic triangle (known as the triangle of Koch) formed by the coronary sinus, the tendon of Todaro (a prominent band leading from the inferior vena cava and inserting in the atrial septum), and the septal attachment of the tricuspid valve. The node then gives rise to the bundle of His, which penetrates the A-V junction beneath the membranous septum. The bundle of His then bifurcates into right and left bundle branches, which pass along either side of the muscular ventricular septum. In the presence of a perimembranous VSD, the bundle of His passes along the posterior and inferior rim of the defect, generally on the left ventricular side. In this critical area, sutures must be placed superficially on the right ventricular side a few millimeters from the edge of the defect. The bundle of His tends to run along the posterior and inferior margin of inlet VSDs as well. The conduction tissue is usually remote from outlet and trabecular VSDs.

Pulmonary artery banding is a palliative maneuver used to protect the pulmonary circulation from excessive blood flow. Pulmonary artery banding is currently performed only in patients who are felt to be poor candidates for VSD closure because of either associated illness or anatomic complexity, such as multiple trabecular VSDs ("Swiss cheese" septum). A band is placed around the main pulmonary artery and tightened to achieve a distal pulmonary artery pressure of about one-half systemic. The band is secured to the adventitia of the pulmonary artery to prevent its migration. Distal migration may result in narrowing and poor growth of one or both branch pulmonary arteries,

while proximal migration can cause deformity of the pulmonary valve. Later, when the patient is a candidate for VSD closure, the band must be removed. Repair of the main pulmonary artery at the band site is also usually necessary and can typically be accomplished by scar resection and primary closure or patch repair.

Recently, transcatheter devices have been developed to allow closure of some VSDs in the cardiac catheterization lab. For specific VSDs, such as muscular, device closure may be preferable. Complications with device closure include complete heart block (3.8%), device embolization (0.01%), and aortic insufficiency (0.03%). For simple perimembranous VSDs, the risk of device closure is in excess of traditional surgical closure.

D. Prognosis

Surgical closure of a VSD is associated with a mortality of less than 1%. Potential complications include injury to the conduction tissue and injury to the tricuspid or aortic valves. Transient heart block may result from tissue swelling or injury from retraction, but permanent heart block occurs in less than 1% of cases. When heart block develops after surgery, patients are usually observed for a period of 7–10 days prior to permanent pacemaker implantation. Tricuspid insufficiency may be precipitated by annular distortion or chordal restriction by the VSD patch or sutures. The aortic valve may also be injured by inaccurate suturing (especially in perimembranous and outlet defects). A residual VSD is seen in about 5% of cases, and reoperation is indicated when significant shunting persists ($Q_p/Q_s > 1.5$) or the residual defect is larger than 2 mm in size. The Q_p/Q_s ratio can be calculated by measuring oxygen saturations and using the following formula derived from the Fick equation: $Q_p/Q_s = (Ao – SVC)/(PV – PA)$, where Ao is the aortic (or systemic) saturation, SVC is the saturation in the superior vena cava, PV is the saturation in the pulmonary veins (which is usually estimated to be 95–100%), and PA is the saturation in the pulmonary arteries. Intraoperative echocardiography is used routinely to identify residual defects, which can then be repaired before the patient leaves the operating room.

Anderson H et al: Is complete heart block after surgical closure of ventricular septal defects still an issue? Ann Thorac Surg 2006;82:948.

Carminati M et al: Transcatheter closure of congenital ventricular septal defects: results of the European registry. Eur Heart J 2007;28:2361.

Dodge-Khatami A et al: Spontaneous closure of small residual ventricular septal defects after surgical repair. Ann Thorac Surg 2007;83:902.

McDaniel NL: Ventricular and atrial septal defects. Pediatr Rev 2001;22:265.

Tweddell JS, Pelech AN, Frommelt PC: Ventricular septal defect and aortic valve regurgitation: pathophysiology and indications for surgery. Semin Thorac Cardiovasc Surg Pediatr Card Surg Annu 2006;9:147.

▶ Atrioventricular Septal Defect

ESSENTIALS OF DIAGNOSIS

▶ Common defect in patients with trisomy 21.

▶ Significant congestive heart failure develops in early infancy.

▶ Chest radiograph with cardiomegaly and increased pulmonary vascular markings.

▶ Electrocardiography shows left axis deviation.

▶ Echocardiogram demonstrates the right and left atrioventricular valves to be present on the same plane with a common orifice along with associated atrial and/or ventricular septal defects.

A. General Considerations

The embryological abnormality in AVSDs is the failure of the proper development of the endocardial cushions, which results in variable deficiency of the atrial and ventricular septa and malformation of the A-V valves. AVSDs represent a group of congenital abnormalities bound by a variable deficiency of the atrioventricular septum immediately above and below the A-V valves. Other terms commonly applied to an AVSD include atrioventricular canal defects, endocardial cushion defects, and atrioventricular communis. Complete AVSDs have a single common A-V valve orifice resulting in a single 5-leaflet valve overlying both the right and left ventricles. Incomplete AVSDs have two separate A-V valve orifices (tricuspid and mitral) with the mitral valve invariably having a cleft in the anterior leaflet. While most incomplete AVSDs have no ventricular level shunting, the classification of AVSDs as complete and incomplete depends only on the valve anatomy, not on the presence or absence of a VSD. Incomplete defects without associated ventricular level shunting have also been termed ostium primum ASDs, while those with a VSD have been described as intermediate or transitional AVSDs. AVSDs represent approximately 4% of congenital cardiac anomalies and are frequently associated with other cardiac malformations. AVSDs comprise 30–40% of the cardiac abnormalities seen in patients with Down syndrome.

Complete AVSD is characterized by a common atrioventricular orifice, rather than separate mitral and tricuspid orifices, and a deficiency of endocardial cushion tissue, which results in an ASD and an inlet type of VSD (Figure 19–31). AVSDs were subclassified by Rastelli into the following three types according to the morphology of the anterior leaflet of the common A-V valve:

Type A: The anterior bridging leaflet is divided and attached to the septum by multiple chordae.

Type B: The anterior bridging leaflet is attached to a papillary muscle in the right ventricle.

Type C: The anterior bridging leaflet is free-floating with no attachments except to the valve annulus.

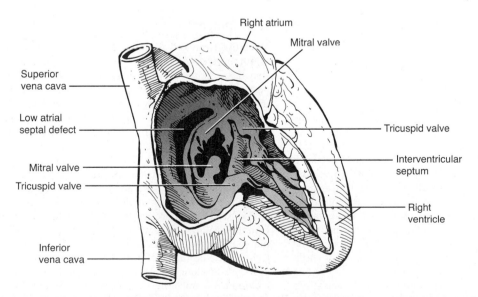

▲ **Figure 19–31.** Complete atrioventricular canal. The most common type has a divided anterior bridging leaflet. Both the left and right valvular components are attached to the interventricular septum with long, nonfused chordae. The left and right components of the posterior bridging leaflet are not separated.

When both left and right A-V valves equally share the common A-V valve orifice, the AVSD is termed balanced. Occasionally, the orifice may favor the right A-V valve (right dominance) or the left A-V valve (left dominance). In marked right dominance, the left A-V valve and left ventricle are hypoplastic and frequently coexist with other left-sided abnormalities, including aortic stenosis, hypoplasia of the aorta, and coarctation. Conversely, marked left dominance results in a deficient right A-V valve with associated hypoplasia of the right ventricle, pulmonary stenosis or atresia, and TOF. Patients with severe imbalance require staged single-ventricle reconstruction.

The conduction tissue is displaced in an ASVD and is at risk during the surgical repair. The AV node is located posteriorly and inferiorly of its normal position toward the coronary sinus in the triangle of Koch. This triangle is bounded by the coronary sinus, the posterior attachment of the inferior bridging leaflet, and the rim of the ASD. The bundle of His courses anteriorly and superiorly to run along the leftward aspect of the crest of the VSD, giving off the left bundle branch and continuing as the right bundle branch.

Cardiac anomalies are associated with AVSDs, including PDA (10%) and TOF (10%). Important abnormalities of the left A-V valve include single papillary muscle (parachute mitral valve) (2–6%) and double orifice mitral valve (8–14%). A persistent left superior vena cava with or without an unroofed coronary sinus is encountered in 3% of patients with an AVSD. Double-outlet right ventricle (2%) significantly complicates or may even preclude complete surgical correction. As mentioned previously, left ventricular outflow tract obstruction from subaortic stenosis or redundant A-V valve tissue occurs in 4–7%. Associated transposition of the great arteries and left ventricular inflow obstruction have been rarely reported.

B. Clinical Findings

The predominant hemodynamic features of an AVSD are the result of left-to-right shunting at the atrial and ventricular levels. In the absence of ventricular level shunting, the hemodynamics and clinical presentation of a patient with an incomplete AVSD resemble that of a typical secundum ASD with right atrial and right ventricular volume overload. Patients with a complete AVSD with both atrial-level and ventricular-level shunting generally present early in infancy with signs and symptoms of congestive heart failure. In addition, moderate or severe left A-V valve regurgitation occurs in approximately 10% of patients with an AVSD worsening the clinical picture. On physical examination, the precordium is hyperactive, often with a prominent thrill. Auscultatory findings include a systolic murmur along the left sternal border, a high-pitched murmur at the apex from left A-V valve regurgitation, and a middiastolic flow murmur across the common A-V valve. In the presence of elevated PVR, there may be a split first heart sound. Significant cardiomegaly and pulmonary overcirculation are found on the chest radiograph. Electrocardiogram reveals biventricular hypertrophy, atrial enlargement, prolonged PR interval, leftward axis, and counterclockwise frontal plane loop. Doppler/echocardiography is diagnostic, defining the atrial and ventricular level shunting, valvular anatomy, and any associated anomalies. Up to 90% of untreated individuals with a complete AVSD develop pulmonary vascular disease by 1 year of age due to the large left-to-right shunt, potentially exacerbated by the associated A-V valve regurgitation. Patients with trisomy 21 tend to develop pulmonary vascular obstructive disease earlier than chromosomally normal infants due to small airway disease, chronic hypoventilation, and elevated P_{CO_2}. Initial aggressive medical management is undertaken to relieve the symptoms of congestive heart failure. Elective surgical correction should be performed by age 3–6 months. Earlier intervention is indicated for failure of medical management.

Cardiac catheterization should be performed for patients over the age of 1 year, for patients with signs or symptoms of increased PVR, or in some cases to further evaluate other associated major cardiac anomalies. If the PVR is high, it is important to remeasure it while the child is breathing 100% oxygen with and without nitric oxide. If the pulmonary resistance falls, it implies that much of the elevated resistance is dynamic and can be managed in the perioperative period by ventilatory manipulation, supplemental oxygen, and nitric oxide. More recently, sildenafil has been shown to decrease elevation in PVR in children with congenital heart disease. Markedly elevated PVR (greater than 10 Woods units·m^2) that does not respond to oxygen administration is generally considered a contraindication to repair.

C. Treatment

Operative treatment is almost always necessary as soon as symptoms are observed to prevent further clinical deterioration. Even in the absence of symptoms, operation is best performed before 6 months of age. Pulmonary artery banding, which permits delaying the repair until the child is larger, is no longer used today except in select complex or single-ventricle cases, extremely low birth weight or prematurity, and very poor clinical condition. This approach exposes the child to the risks of two operations, and the overall mortality exceeds that of primary repair in infancy. Patients with incomplete AVSDs usually require repair within the first few years of life.

Two techniques are widely employed for the repair of complete AVSDs: a 1-patch technique and a 2-patch technique. Incomplete AVSDs are repaired with the single-patch technique. Regardless of which approach is selected, the goals are to close the ASD and VSD and to separate the common A-V valve into 2 nonstenotic, competent valves. The cleft in the anterior leaflet of the mitral valve is generally closed to lessen the risks of long-term mitral regurgitation. For the 2-patch technique, separate patches are used for the ASD and VSD. For the 1-patch technique, the superior and inferior bridging leaflets are divided along a line separating them into right and left components. A single patch is utilized to close both the ventricular and ASDs. The cut edges of the leaflets are then resuspended to the patch. For defects with a small VSD component, a modified single-patch technique may be employed. For this method, a single patch is sewn directly to the rim of the VSD, sandwiching the bridging leaflets between the patch and the crest of the VSD.

The short-term and long-term success of the operation is highly dependent on the status of the PVR and the surgeon's ability to maintain competence of the mitral valve. In developed countries, it is fortunately relatively uncommon for patients to present late in the course of an AVSD with refractory PVR elevations. Although earlier reports recommend that the cleft in the left A-V valve should not be closed and the valve should be treated as a trileaflet structure, most authors now believe that closure of the cleft is an important mechanism in preventing postoperative left A-V valve regurgitation. Significant A-V valve regurgitation at the conclusion of surgery, severe dysplasia of the left A-V valve, and failure to close the cleft of the left A-V valve have been identified as important risk factors for reoperation. Significant postoperative left A-V valve regurgitation is also a risk factor for operative and long-term mortality. The cleft should not be completely closed in the presence of a single papillary muscle to avoid causing left A-V valve stenosis. In the case of a double-orifice valve, the bridging tissue should not be divided to create a single opening in the valve.

D. Prognosis

Operative mortality is related largely to associated cardiac anomalies and left A-V valve regurgitation. Mortality for repair of uncomplicated incomplete AVSDs is 0–0.6%, while the addition of left A-V valve regurgitation increases mortality to 4–6%. For complete AVSDs, the mortality without left A-V valve regurgitation is approximately 5%, compared with 13% when significant degrees of regurgitation are present. The difference in operative mortality between patients with and without regurgitation underscores the importance of careful management of the left A-V valve.

The majority of reoperations after repair of AVSD are due to left A-V valve regurgitation or the development of subaortic stenosis. Significant postoperative A-V valve regurgitation occurs in 10–15% of patients, necessitating reoperation for valve repair or replacement in 7–12%. The incidence of permanent complete heart block is approximately 1%. Heart block encountered in the immediate postoperative period may be transient due to edema of or trauma to the AV node or bundle of His. However, right bundle branch block is common (22%).

Backer CL, Stewart RD, Mavroudis C: What is the best technique for repair of complete atrioventricular canal? Semin Thorac Cardiovasc Surg 2007;19:249.

Boening A et al: Long-term results after surgical correction of atrioventricular septal defects. Eur J Cardiothorac Surg 2002; 22:167.

Dunlop KA et al: A ten year review of atrioventricular septal defects. Cardiol Young 2004;14:15.

Singh RR et al: Early repair of complete atrioventricular septal defect is safe and effective. Ann Thorac Surg 2006;82:1598.

Welke KF et al: Population-base perspective of long-term outcomes after surgical repair of partial atrioventricular septal defect. Ann Thorac Surg 2007;82:624.

▶ Patent Ductus Arteriosus

 ESSENTIALS OF DIAGNOSIS

▶ Widened pulse pressure.

▶ Continuous "machinery" murmur heard over the left upper sternal border radiating into the back.

▶ Very common in premature infants.

▶ May cause hypoperfusion due to diastolic run off.

▶ Older patients are asymptomatic with a continuous murmur heard in the back and radiating into both lung fields.

A. General Considerations

The ductus arteriosus is a normal fetal vascular structure that allows blood from the right ventricle to bypass the high resistance pulmonary vascular bed and pass directly to the systemic circulation. The ductus communicates between the main pulmonary artery (or proximal left pulmonary artery) and the proximal descending thoracic aorta. Histologically, the media of the ductus contains a predominance of smooth muscle cells, while the media of the aorta and pulmonary artery contain well-developed elastic fibers. Vasocontrol of the ductus is mediated by two important mechanisms: oxygen tension and prostaglandin levels. During fetal development, low oxygen tension and high levels of circulating prostaglandin maintain ductal patency. During the final trimester, the ductus becomes less sensitive to prostaglandins and more sensitive to the effects of oxygen tension. Following birth, the rise in oxygen tension and a fall in prostaglandins (which were previously supplied principally by the placenta) lead to ductal closure, which is usually complete by 12–24 hours. After closure, the ductus becomes a fibrous cord known as the ligamentum arteriosum. Failure of closure of the ductus leads to the condition called patent ductus arteriosus. PDA occurs in about 1 out of 1200 live births and accounts for 7% of congenital heart defect. The incidence is much higher in premature infants (greater than 20%). This elevated incidence is thought to be related to immaturity of the ductal wall resulting in impaired sensitivity to oxygen tension.

PDA may occur as an isolated defect, or it may occur in association with a number of other anomalies. Patency of the ductus arteriosus is desirable in a number of defects in which there is either inadequate pulmonary blood flow (such as pulmonary atresia) or inadequate systemic blood flow (as in severe coarctation of the aorta). The discovery that extrinsic delivery of prostaglandins can maintain ductal patency has played a critical role in improving the survival of these patients.

B. Clinical Findings

The physiologic manifestation of PDA is shunting of blood across the ductus. The shunt volume is determined by the size of the ductus and by the ratio of pulmonary to systemic vascular resistance. At birth, the PVR drops dramatically and continues to decline over the first several weeks of life. As a result, shunting across a PDA is from left-to-right. Excessive pulmonary blood flow can lead to congestive heart failure. In extreme cases, hypotension and systemic malperfusion may result. Patients with a large PDA who survive infancy tend to develop pulmonary vascular obstructive disease. Eisenmenger physiology results when the PVR exceeds the systemic vascular resistance, producing a reversal of shunting across the ductus to right-to-left. This leads to cyanosis and, eventually, right ventricular failure. Small PDAs may persist to adulthood without producing any symptoms or physiologic derangement. Endocarditis and endarteritis have been reported as long-term complications of PDA.

In patients with PDA, symptoms are proportional to the shunt volume and the presence of associated defects. Left-to-right shunting produces volume overload of the left heart. Infants with congestive heart failure demonstrate symptoms of tachypnea, tachycardia, and poor feeding. Older children may present with recurrent respiratory infections, fatigue, and failure to thrive. Physical findings include a widened pulse pressure and a continuous "machinery" murmur heard best along the left upper sternal border. Chest radiography shows increased pulmonary vascular markings and left heart enlargement. Left ventricular hypertrophy and left atrial enlargement may be evident on the electrocardiogram. Echocardiography is the diagnostic method of choice. Diagnostic cardiac catheterization is performed only in older patients with suspected pulmonary hypertension to evaluate for pulmonary vascular obstructive disease. More frequently, catheterization is utilized for transcatheter occlusion of the ductus in selected cases.

C. Treatment

PDA closure is performed for all symptomatic patients. Closure is also recommended for asymptomatic patients due to the risk of heart failure, pulmonary hypertension, and endocarditis. Closure of the ductus may be accomplished by one of three approaches: pharmacologic, surgical, and endovascular. Indomethacin, which is a prostaglandin inhibitor, stimulates PDA closure in premature infants. It is rarely effective in full-term infants. The dosing regimen is 0.1–0.2 mg/kg intravenously at 12-hour or 24-hour intervals for a total of three doses. This is effective in about 80% of premature babies. Due to its side effects, indomethacin is contraindicated in patients with sepsis, renal insufficiency, intracranial hemorrhage, or bleeding disorders. Failure of indomethacin after two complete courses results in referral for surgical closure.

The surgical approach to PDA is through a left posterolateral thoracotomy via the third or fourth intercostal space. The pleura is incised over the proximal descending thoracic aorta, which allows medial retraction of the vagus nerve. The recurrent laryngeal nerve curves behind the ductus and should be protected throughout the procedure. Dissection is then performed to demonstrate the pertinent anatomy. In many cases, the ductus is the largest vascular structure present, and it must not be confused with the aorta. Ductal tissue is extremely friable, so direct manipulation is minimized. In premature infants, the ductus is controlled with a single surgical clip; this procedure is commonly performed in the neonatal intensive care unit, thereby avoiding problems associated with patient transfer. In older patients, occlusion of the ductus is achieved with simple silk ligature or, preferably, by division between ligatures to minimize recurrence.

Recently, thoracoscopic techniques have been developed to perform PDA ligation. This approach has the potential benefits of decreased pain and quicker recovery. Disadvantages include a substantial learning curve and increased operating time.

A number of endovascular devices have been developed for the purpose of transcatheter occlusion of the PDA. This approach is very successful in older infants, children, and adults with small and moderate sized PDAs and has become the treatment of choice at many centers. Surgical therapy is reserved for PDAs having a large diameter or very short length.

Rarely, an adult will present with a significant PDA. These patients must be carefully evaluated for the presence of pulmonary vascular obstructive disease prior to ductal closure. If the patient is not a candidate for device closure, surgical closure can be problematic. Calcification of the ductal wall is common in adults, which makes ligation hazardous. In some cases, cardiopulmonary bypass may be required with closure of the ductus from within the pulmonary artery.

D. Prognosis

Closure of the ductus by surgical or transcatheter techniques is achieved with a mortality that approaches zero. Potential complications include pneumothorax, recurrent laryngeal nerve injury, and chylothorax (from injury to the thoracic duct). Long-term survival should be normal following PDA ligation in most patients. Survival in premature infants depends primarily on the extent of prematurity with its attendant complications.

Burke RP et al: Video-assisted thoracoscopic surgery for patent ductus arteriosus in low birth weight neonates and infants. Pediatrics 1999;104(2 Pt 1):227.

Cowley CG, Lloyd TR: Interventional cardiac catheterization advances in nonsurgical approaches to congenital heart disease. Curr Opin Pediatr 1999;11:425.

Giroud JM, Jacobs JP: Evolution of strategies for management of the patent arterial duct. Cardiol Young 2007;17:68.

Malviya M, Ohlsson A, Shah S: Surgical versus medical treatment with cyclooxygenase inhibitors for symptomatic patent ductus arteriosus in preterm infants. Cochrane Database Syst Rev 2008;1.

2. Right-Sided Anomalies

► Pulmonary Stenosis

ESSENTIALS OF DIAGNOSIS

► Mild to moderate lesions are asymptomatic.

► Right heart failure and cyanosis with severe lesions.

► Systolic ejection murmur on the left upper sternal border with a delayed, soft S2.

► Ejection click is often present.

► Increased right ventricular impulse.

A. General Considerations

Isolated pulmonary stenosis occurs in 5–8% of all congenital cardiac anomalies. The pulmonary valve is usually trileaflet with fusion of the commissures. The valve can appear thickened and domed on echocardiography. Most patients have an associated PFO or a secundum ASD. Pulmonary stenosis may be valvar or subvalvar due to muscular narrowing of the infundibulum (Figure 19–32).

B. Clinical Findings

Young infants with severe pulmonary stenosis present with failure to thrive, right heart failure, and possible hypoxic spells. Older children tend to have mild to moderate stenosis that is asymptomatic. They may, however, complain of shortness of breath with exertion or arrhythmias. The murmur of pulmonary stenosis tends to be prominent and therefore is not missed on routine exam. The presence of a systolic ejection murmur should prompt further workup, including an echocardiogram, which is diagnostic. Patients may be followed symptomatically with mild to moderate pulmonary stenosis. Surgical or catheter-based intervention should be considered for a gradient higher than 50 mm Hg, progressive ventricular hypertrophy, or new tricuspid regurgitation.

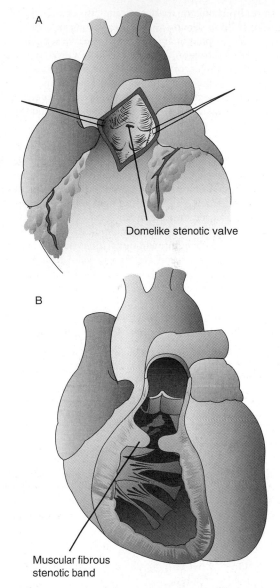

▲ **Figure 19-32.** Pulmonary stenosis. **A:** Valvular pulmonary stenosis. **B:** Infundibular pulmonary stenosis.

C. Treatment

Neonates presenting with profound cyanosis from severe pulmonary stenosis need to be placed on PE_1 to maintain ductal patency. The ductus will maintain adequate pulmonary blood flow so that the patient can be stabilized. For isolated pulmonary stenosis, balloon valvuloplasty by the interventional cardiologists is highly successful and has replaced surgical intervention for the majority of patients. Asymptomatic infants with systemic right ventricular pressures from pulmonary stenosis are also excellent candidates for balloon dilation. Surgical valvotomy or a transannular patch for pulmonary stenosis is reserved for patients who have failed balloon dilation, who have a severely hypoplastic valve annulus, or who have other associated anomalies including muscular infundibular narrowing. Older patients with progressive isolated pulmonary stenosis are excellent candidates for elective balloon dilation when they develop elevated right ventricular pressures.

D. Prognosis

Early mortality for patients with critical pulmonary stenosis is 3–10%. Restenosis occurs in 10–25% of patients. Once the outflow obstruction is relieved, the right ventricular hypertrophy and tricuspid insufficiency regress. Although overall survival is excellent for isolated pulmonary stenosis, over 50% of patients will require additional interventions, including repeat balloon dilation, pulmonary valve replacement, and ASD closure. Late atrial and ventricular arrhythmias occur in 38% of patients.

Earing MG et al: Long-term follow-up of patients after surgical treatment for isolated pulmonary stenosis. Mayo Clin Proc 2005;80:871.

Peterson C et al: Comparative long-term results of surgery versus balloon valvuloplasty for pulmonary valve stenosis in infants and children. Ann Thorac Surg 2003;76:1078.

Poon LK, Menaham S: Pulmonary regurgitation after percutaneous balloon valvoplasty for isolated pulmonary valvar stenosis in childhood. Cardiol Young 2003;13:444.

▶ Ebstein's Anomaly

 ESSENTIALS OF DIAGNOSIS

▶ Timing of presentation and degree of symptoms are highly variable.

▶ Cyanosis and heart failure in infants.

▶ New-onset atrial arrhythmias and reentrant tachycardia in older children.

▶ Poorest prognosis in symptomatic infants.

▶ Chest radiograph with the classic "wall-to-wall" heart in infants.

▶ Electrocardiogram demonstrates a right bundle branch block, right axis deviation, and ventricular preexcitation.

A. General Considerations

Ebstein's malformation was first described by Wilhelm Ebstein in 1866 as a constellation of clinical findings resulting from an abnormality of the tricuspid valve. It has become evident over time that the malformation is a disease of the entire right ventricle and the development of the tricuspid valve. It involves a spectrum of anatomical abnormalities of variable severity, which include apical displacement of the septal and mural leaflets of the tricuspid valve, which have failed to dilaminate from the underlying myocardium; thinning or atrialization of the inlet component of the right ventricle, with variable dilation; and malformation of the anterosuperior leaflet, with anomalous attachments, redundancy, and fenestrations. Several other cardiac anomalies are often associated with the right ventricular changes, such as atrial and ventricular septal defects, obstruction of the outlet from the right ventricle, and Wolff-Parkinson-White syndrome. Ebstein malformation can also afflict the left-sided systemic atrioventricular valve in the setting of congenitally corrected transposition.

B. Clinical Findings

The malformation is rare, accounting for no more than 1% of all congenital cardiac anomalies. Due to the significant anatomic variability in the abnormalities of the tricuspid valve and right ventricle, the age at presentation and severity of symptoms can also be highly variable. Patients who present in infancy have the poorest prognosis. There is a high rate of fetal death, hydrops, and pulmonary hypoplasia when the diagnosis is made during fetal life. Cyanosis is the most common presentation in infancy. These patients have severe tricuspid regurgitation with a poorly functioning right ventricle in the face of elevated pulmonary arterial resistance. The result is a state of low cardiac output dependent upon right-to-left shunting across the oval fossa.

With less severe derangements of the tricuspid valve and preserved ventricular function, patients tend to present later in adolescence or early adulthood. Many patients are asymptomatic and present with a murmur noted on physical examination. In symptomatic patients, a common presentation involves the new onset of atrial arrhythmias or reentrant tachycardia. Exercise tolerance may be diminished, with cyanosis during extreme exertion if an ASD is present. Those patients with an intact atrial septum will often progress to congestive heart failure with increasing cardiomegaly.

Echocardiography is usually sufficient for accurate diagnosis and anatomic evaluation. The degree of displacement, tethering, and dysplasia of the valvar leaflets, as well as the amount of regurgitation, can be determined. Ventricular function and the extent of atrialization of the right ventricle can also be evaluated. Additional abnormalities, including the presence and direction of a shunt at the atrial level, can be assessed. Electrocardiographic findings include incomplete right bundle branch block, right axis deviation, ventricular preexcitation, and atrial arrhythmias. The chest radiograph can vary from normal, in patients with mild anatomic abnormalities, to the classic "wall-to-wall" heart. Cardiac catheterization is rarely necessary.

C. Treatment

As noted previously, neonates often present with profound cyanosis and may require prostaglandins to maintain adequate flow of blood to the lungs during the early neonatal period when pulmonary resistance is high. It is important to distinguish functional from anatomic pulmonary atresia. In patients with functional atresia, it may be possible to wean them from the infusion of prostaglandins while maintaining adequate saturations of oxygen as pulmonary resistance falls. These patients can then be followed for development of further symptoms.

In neonates who cannot be weaned from prostaglandins due to unacceptable levels of hypoxemia, or in those with anatomic pulmonary atresia, it is necessary to construct a systemic-to-pulmonary shunt to maintain adequate pulmonary blood flow. For neonates who also develop significant symptoms of congestive heart failure while on prostaglandin, it is necessary to address the underlying valvar pathology. The options include closure of the tricuspid valve, with or without fenestration, along with construction of a modified Blalock-Taussig shunt, repair of the tricuspid valve if ventricular function is reasonable, or cardiac transplantation.

In the older patient with progressive symptoms, a variety of surgical options exist to address the malformed tricuspid valve. Most are based on techniques designed to mobilize the leading edge of the anterosuperior leaflet, aiming to create a competent monocusp valve with or without plication of the atrialized portion of the right ventricle. There is ongoing debate as to the necessity of obliterating the atrialized portion of the right ventricle. Historically, plication of this portion of the ventricle has been an integral part of most repairs, albeit that no clear physiologic benefit with regards to improved ventricular function has been demonstrated. In addition, the potential exists for injury to the right coronary artery as a result of the plication, which may adversely impact late outcomes and contribute to ventricular arrhythmias.

Replacement of the tricuspid valve is a final option. The late survival free from reoperation, however, has been equivalent to valvar repair. If replacement is required, heterografts are preferred over mechanical valves due to risks of thrombosis. Other options using tissue valves include the insertion of pulmonary autografts, mitral valve homografts, and "top hat" mounted pulmonary or aortic homografts. When replacing the valve, the sutures should be brought around the coronary sinus, leaving it to drain into the right ventricle so as to minimize potential injury to the atrioventricular node.

D. Prognosis

Ebstein malformation is a rare but challenging congenital cardiac defect. The high degree of anatomic variability makes it difficult to have a standardized approach to these children. The symptomatic neonate carries a very grave prognosis. The presence of associated cardiac and other congenital anomalies often make survival impossible. Surgical options are limited at this age and often still result in a poor outcome. Medical management, if possible, is the best, as surgical success improves with age. If surgery is required, conversion to functional tricuspid atresia often offers the best survival, as the ventricle in the severely symptomatic neonate functions poorly. Transplantation remains an option, but the availability of organs limits its utility.

Patients who are not symptomatic in the neonatal period will often remain free from symptoms well into adolescence. Electrophysiologic symptoms usually precede symptoms of congestive heart failure. Indications for repair at these ages include symptoms, cyanosis, and progressive cardiomegaly.

Boston US et al: Tricuspid valve repair for Ebstein's anomaly in young children: a 30-year experience. Ann Thorac Surg 2006; 81:690.

Dearani JA, Danielson GK: Tricuspid valve repair for Ebstein's anomaly. Operat Tech Thorac Cardiovasc Surg 2004;8:188.

Jaquiss RD, Imamura M: Management of Ebstein's anomaly and pure tricuspid insufficiency in the neonate. Semin Thorac Cardiovasc Surg 2007;19:258.

Paranon S, Acar P: Ebstein's anomaly of the tricuspid valve: from fetus to adult: congenital heart disease. Heart 2008;94:237.

Ullmann MV et al: Ventricularization of the atrialized chamber: A concept of Ebstein's anomaly repair. Ann Thorac Surg 2004;78:918.

3. Left-Sided Anomalies
► Aortic Stenosis

 ESSENTIALS OF DIAGNOSIS

► Infants present with significant heart failure and hemodynamic collapse.

► Sudden cardiac death is the most common cause of mortality.

► Narrow and delayed pulse pressure.

► Classic crescendo-decrescendo murmur at the upper sternal border that radiates into the neck with a prominent left ventricular impulse.

A. General Considerations

Aortic stenosis is a form of left ventricular outflow tract obstruction that may occur at a valvar (70%), subvalvar (25%), or supravalvar (5%) level. Aortic stenosis occurs in about 4% of patients with congenital heart disease. The severity of aortic stenosis may be graded as mild (peak pressure gradient less than 50 mm Hg), moderate (50 to 75 mm Hg), or severe (greater than 75 mm Hg).

Valvar aortic stenosis occurs secondary to maldevelopment of the aortic valve. Most commonly, a bicuspid valve is present, although tricuspid and unicuspid valves are also represented. In valvar aortic stenosis, the leaflets are thickened and frequently dysmorphic, and there is a variable degree of leaflet fusion along the commissures. The aortic annulus may be hypoplastic. In 20% of cases, valvar aortic stenosis is associated with other cardiac defects, most commonly coarctation of the aorta, PDA, VSD, or mitral stenosis. Males with valvar aortic stenosis outnumber females by a ratio of 4:1. There is a wide spectrum of clinical presentation of valvar aortic stenosis, but patients tend to present in one of two groups: neonates and infants with severe aortic stenosis develop symptoms of rapidly progressive congestive heart failure, while older children generally have less severe obstruction and a more slowly progressive course.

Subvalvar aortic stenosis occurs below the level of the aortic valve and may be discrete (80%) or diffuse (20%). Discrete (or membranous) subaortic stenosis is rarely seen in infants and tends to progress over time. This lesion consists of a crescentic or circumferential fibrous or fibromuscular membrane that protrudes into the left ventricular outflow tract. The pathogenesis of discrete subaortic stenosis is unknown, but it is thought to be an acquired lesion that develops secondary to a congenital abnormality of the left ventricular outflow tract in which abnormal flow patterns lead to endocardial injury with resultant fibrosis. Although the aortic valve leaflets are usually normal in discrete subaortic stenosis, the turbulent flow created by the obstruction can cause leaflet thickening and progressive aortic insufficiency. Diffuse subaortic stenosis is a more severe form of stenosis that creates a long, tunnellike obstruction. Diffuse subaortic stenosis should be distinguished from hypertrophic cardiomyopathy. Both forms of subaortic stenosis are associated with a high risk of endocarditis.

Supravalvar aortic stenosis is characterized by thickening of the wall of the ascending aorta. The lesion may be localized (80%) to the region of the sinotubular ridge (at the level of the valve commissures), creating an hourglass deformity, or it may be more diffuse (20%), extending into the aortic arch and its branches. In both varieties, the aortic valve leaflets may be abnormal. The free edges of the aortic valve leaflets may adhere to the aortic wall in the region of intraluminal thickening, and this may lead to reduced coronary blood flow during diastole. Aortic wall thickening may also extend into the coronary ostia and further impair coronary blood flow. Associated cardiac lesions are common, particularly branch pulmonary artery stenoses. A genetic basis for supravalvar aortic stenosis has been established. About 50% of cases of supravalvar aortic stenosis are associated with Williams syndrome, in which a partial deletion of chromosome 7 (including the elastin gene) leads to the triad of supravalvar stenosis, mental retardation, and a characteristic "elfin" facies. Isolated mutations in the elastin gene have also been shown to produce familial supravalvar aortic stenosis with an autosomal dominant pattern of transmission. There is a significant incidence of endocarditis in patients with supravalvar aortic stenosis. Sudden death is frequently reported and is probably related to coronary obstruction.

B. Clinical Findings

Severe aortic stenosis is usually well-tolerated during fetal development. Although left ventricular output and antegrade flow across the aortic valve are decreased, the right ventricle compensates with increased output, and systemic perfusion is maintained by flow across the ductus. After birth, there is increased venous return to the left heart, and this exacerbates the pressure load created by the stenotic aortic valve, leading to left ventricular dysfunction. As the ductus closes during postnatal life, systemic malperfusion may develop with resulting hypotension, acidosis, and oliguria. Coronary perfusion is also impaired due to the combination of systemic hypotension and elevated left ventricular end-diastolic pressures. Patients with critical aortic stenosis typically exhibit severe left ventricular dysfunction. These patients usually show signs of distress soon after birth. On examination, there is impaired distal perfusion with poor capillary refill and diminished, thready pulses. A systolic ejection murmur may be absent if the cardiac output is severely diminished. Differential cyanosis may be observed due to perfusion of the lower body with desaturated blood shunting through the ductus. The electrocardiogram shows left ventricular hypertrophy, and the chest radiograph displays cardiomegaly and pulmonary congestion. Echocardiography establishes the diagnosis.

In contrast to infants with critical aortic stenosis, older children with valvar aortic stenosis usually present with less severe stenosis (mild or moderate), and most are asymptomatic. Symptoms of angina, syncope, and congestive heart failure are not commonly reported. Congenital valvar aortic stenosis is a progressive lesion, however, and survival is dependent on the severity of stenosis and its rate of progression. Sudden cardiac death is the most common cause of mortality. Endocarditis occurs in less than 1% of patients. The diagnosis of valvar aortic stenosis in older children can frequently be made on physical exam. There is a classic systolic crescendo-decrescendo murmur at the upper sternal border, which radiates to the neck. An ejection click is often present. A visible apical impulse is suggestive of significant left ventricular hypertrophy. In severe cases, the pulse may be weak and delayed (pulsus tardus et parvus). The electrocardiogram shows left ventricular hypertrophy. The chest radiograph is usually normal. Echocardiography accurately defines the level of stenosis and its severity. Using Doppler techniques, the pressure gradient across the stenotic valve may be estimated using a simplified form of the Bernoulli equation $P = 4V^2$, where P is the pressure gradient and V is the peak flow velocity. Cardiac catheterization is generally reserved for therapeutic intervention.

The clinical findings in subvalvar aortic stenosis are similar to those for valvar stenosis. The signs and symptoms of supravalvar aortic stenosis are similar to those in other forms of left ventricular outflow tract obstruction. The diagnosis is made by echocardiography, but cardiac catheterization (and more recently MRI) is essential to define the aortic, coronary, and pulmonary arterial anatomy prior to surgical intervention.

C. Treatment

The neonate or infant with critical aortic stenosis represents a true emergency. Endotracheal intubation and inotropic support is routine. Ductal patency is maintained with prostaglandins, and acidosis is corrected. All patients with critical aortic stenosis require some form of urgent intervention. The approach is determined by the valve morphology and by the presence of associated defects. In its most extreme form, critical aortic stenosis may be associated with underdeveloped left-sided cardiac chambers and therefore may represent a form of HLHS. In these cases, single-ventricle palliation must be undertaken. For patients with adequate left-sided chambers, relief of aortic stenosis may be achieved by one of the following three approaches: percutaneous balloon valvuloplasty, surgical valvotomy, or aortic valve replacement. Balloon valvuloplasty is generally considered the procedure of choice when the aortic valve annulus is adequate and there are no associated cardiac defects. Alternatively, surgical valvotomy may be accomplished by closed or open techniques. The closed approach is performed using cardiopulmonary bypass but without aortic cross-clamping. Dilators of increasing size are passed through a ventriculotomy in the left ventricular apex and advanced across the aortic valve. Some centers prefer open surgical valvotomy, which allows a precise valvotomy under direct vision, although aortic cross-clamping with cardioplegia is necessary. In all cases, the goal of therapy is to relieve stenosis without creating excessive aortic insufficiency. Dramatic clinical improvement is expected following balloon or surgical valve valvotomy, and early survivals of greater than 80% have been reported. The incidence of aortic insufficiency is slightly higher following balloon valvotomy. In most cases, however, stenosis will recur and repeat valvotomy or aortic valve replacement will eventually be required. Aortic valve replacement is problematic in the neonate due to small patient size. In these cases, many consider the best valve replacement to be a pulmonary autograft (Ross procedure) with enlargement of the aortic annulus (Konno aortoventriculoplasty). The Ross-Konno procedure has been used successfully for neonates with critical aortic stenosis in whom the aortic annulus is hypoplastic and for selected patients in whom valvuloplasty was unsuccessful. Survival following the Ross-Konno procedure in infants has been shown to be excellent. Growth of the pulmonary autograft has been documented, thereby making it an ideal valve replacement for children. Unfortunately, as part of the Ross procedure, the pulmonary valve must be replaced using a cryopreserved homograft, which does not grow, and homograft replacement must be anticipated at intervals as the patient grows.

All patients with severe valvar aortic stenosis should undergo intervention, as should all symptomatic patients with moderate stenosis. Asymptomatic patients with mild or moderate stenosis are generally observed. As described for critical aortic stenosis, the techniques used to relieve aortic stenosis in older patients include percutaneous balloon valvuloplasty, surgical valvulotomy, and valve replacement. Balloon valvuloplasty is usually performed as the primary intervention and is associated with a success rate of nearly 90% and a mortality of less than 1%. Open surgical valvotomy is an alternative approach with similar results. For valves that are severely dysplastic, develop restenosis after intervention, or become insufficient as a result of prior intervention, valve replacement may be necessary. For older children, there are more options for valve replacement. The choices include mechanical prostheses, bioprosthetic valves, and tissue substitutes, such as porcine xenografts, cryopreserved human allografts, and pulmonary autografts (Ross procedure). The mechanical valves are the most durable but require chronic anticoagulation. The bioprosthetic and tissue valves do not require long-term anticoagulation but tend to deteriorate over time (with the exception of the pulmonary autograft). The pulmonary autograft has the potential advantage of growth, but the homograft used to replace the pulmonary valve will require replacement. Selection of the appropriate replacement valve is a complex decision requiring input from all involved parties.

Intervention for discrete subvalvar stenosis is usually undertaken when the gradient exceeds 30–50 mm Hg or when aortic insufficiency is present. In these patients, resection of the membrane is readily performed by a transaortic approach. In order to reduce the incidence of restenosis, many centers advocate concurrent performance of a septal myomectomy to alter the geometry of the left ventricular outflow tract.

When diffuse subaortic stenosis is associated with hypoplasia of the aortic annulus, repair is best achieved with a Konno aortoventriculoplasty, whereby an incision is carried across the aortic annulus and subjacent ventricular septum, the opening patched, and an aortic valve implanted. Patients with an adequate aortic annulus may undergo a septoplasty (modified Konno), in which the septal incision is confined to the immediate subvalvar area and a patch is used to widen the left ventricular outflow tract without replacing the aortic valve.

Operative intervention is indicated for patients with supravalvar aortic stenosis in whom the gradient exceeds 50 mm Hg. A number of operations have been proposed for the treatment of localized supravalvar stenosis. The classical repair involves a longitudinal incision across the obstruction in the ascending aorta, which is extended into the noncoronary sinus. The thickened, hypertrophic ridge is resected by endarterectomy, and the aortotomy is augmented with an elliptical patch. A variation of this repair involves creation of an inverted-Y aortotomy with one limb of the Y extended into the noncoronary sinus and the other into the right coronary sinus. A Y-shaped patch is then used to augment the aortotomy. Finally, the Brom repair is performed by transection of the ascending aorta beyond the supravalvar ridge. Separate incisions are then made through the supravalvar ridge into each sinus of Valsalva. Triangular patches are placed to augment each of these incisions, thereby relieving the supravalvar obstruction. Reconnection of the aortic root to the ascending aorta completes the repair. The repair of the diffuse type of supravalvar stenosis is performed under circulatory arrest with extensive patching of the ascending aorta, transverse arch, and involved arch arteries. Branch pulmonary stenoses are best managed using transcatheter techniques.

D. Prognosis

Operative mortality approaches zero for resection of discrete subaortic stenosis. The recurrence rate of discrete stenosis following membrane resection and myomectomy has been reported to be as low as 4%. Despite the technical complexity of repair of diffuse subaortic stenosis, excellent results have been reported with high survival and freedom from reoperation. The results of surgery for localized supravalvar aortic stenosis are generally good with low operative mortality and excellent long-term survival. The diffuse form is more difficult to treat, and recurrence is more likely. Overall results are much worse when severe bilateral pulmonary artery stenoses are present. The mortality for aortic valve replacement regardless of valve choice is 2–5%. The need for reoperation is dependent on valve choice and patient size. Early and late ventricular arrhythmias may occur commonly in patients with significant left ventricular hypertrophy.

Aboulhosn J, Child JS: Left ventricular outflow obstruction: subaortic stenosis, bicuspid aortic valve, supravalvar aortic stenosis, and coarctation of the aorta. Circulation 2006;114:2412.

Brown JW et al: The Ross-Konno procedure in children: outcomes, autograft and allograft function, and reoperations. Ann Thorac Surg 2006;82:301.

Cowley CG et al: Balloon valvuloplasty versus transventricular dilation for neonatal critical aortic stenosis. Am J Cardiol 2001; 87:1125.

Ohye RG et al: The Ross/Konno procedure in neonates and infants: intermediate-term survival and autograft function. Ann Thorac Surg 2001;72:823.

▶ Aortic Coarctation

ESSENTIALS OF DIAGNOSIS

- ▶ Absent or weak femoral pulses.
- ▶ Systolic pressure higher in the upper extremities than in the lower extremities with similar diastolic pressures.
- ▶ Neonates present with hemodynamic collapse, while older children are usually asymptomatic.
- ▶ Rib notching on chest radiograph.
- ▶ Commonly associated with a bicuspid aortic valve.
- ▶ Patients with Turner syndrome have a high incidence of aortic coarctation.

A. General Considerations

Coarctation of the aorta is a narrowing of the proximal descending thoracic aorta distal to the origin of the left subclavian artery, near the insertion of the ductus arteriosus (or ligamentum arteriosum). The severity of luminal narrowing and the length of the aorta affected are variable. Coarctation is thought to occur as a result of ectopic tissue from the ductus arteriosus that migrates into the wall of the adjacent aorta. After birth, as the ductus closes, the ectopic tissue in the aorta also constricts. Frequently, a posterior shelf of tissue is present at the point of most severe obstruction. The aortic obstruction caused by coarctation creates a pressure load on the left ventricle.

The incidence of coarctation is about 0.5 per 1000 live births, and its prevalence is 5% of congenital heart defects. Coarctation is commonly associated with other heart defects, including bicuspid aortic valve (in more than 50% of cases), PDA, and VSD. Other left-sided obstructive lesions may also be present, such as aortic arch hypoplasia, aortic stenosis, mitral stenosis, and left ventricular hypoplasia. Coarctation is also recognized to occur in association with Turner syndrome.

B. Clinical Findings

Patients with severe coarctation present in the newborn period. Aortic obstruction is so significant that perfusion of the lower body is dependent upon flow from the ductus arteriosus. Spontaneous ductal closure typically worsens the aortic obstruction and may lead to malperfusion of tissues distal to the coarctation. The pressure load on the left ventricle may precipitate congestive heart failure. Patients may develop shock with severe acidosis, oliguria, and diminished distal pulses. Infants with severe coarctation will generally not survive without intervention.

Older children with coarctation are usually asymptomatic. The diagnosis is commonly made on the basis of hypertension in the upper extremities with decreased pulses in the lower extremities. Noninvasive blood pressure measurements in all four extremities help to quantify the severity of aortic obstruction. These older patients tend to develop extensive collateral arteries that bypass the obstruction. Life expectancy for these patients is limited due to the development of heart failure later in life. Other long-term complications of coarctation include endocarditis (frequently involving a bicuspid aortic valve), endarteritis (in the poststenotic area of the aorta at the site of the jet of turbulent flow), aortic dissection, aortic aneurysm, and intracranial hemorrhage (from Berry aneurysms, which occur more commonly in patients with coarctation).

The diagnosis of coarctation can usually be made clinically. The infant with significant coarctation is frequently asymptomatic at birth but following closure of the ductus develops signs of heart failure such as irritability, tachypnea, and poor feeding. Lower extremity pulses are absent, and upper extremity pulses may be weak. Chest radiography shows cardiomegaly and pulmonary venous congestion. There is a left ventricular strain pattern on the electrocardiogram. Echocardiography is usually diagnostic, demonstrating narrowing of the aorta at the coarctation site with a loss of pulsatility in the descending aorta.

In older children and adults with coarctation, a pressure gradient between the arms and legs usually can be demonstrated by measuring cuff pressures in all four extremities. On chest radiography, rib notching may be evident, secondary to erosion of the inferior rib borders from the development of large intercostal collateral vessels. Echocardiography usually confirms the diagnosis. Anatomic details may also be clarified with CT and MRI. Cardiac catheterization is usually not necessary.

C. Treatment

Generally, all patients with coarctation should undergo surgical repair. For neonates, the acute medical management includes initiation of PE_1 for the purpose of reopening the ductus; this maneuver partially relieves the aortic obstruction and augments perfusion of the lower body due to improved antegrade flow across the arch as well as right-to-left flow across the ductus. Prostaglandins are usually effective for reopening the ductus when initiated within 7–10 days of life but are less successful thereafter.

Surgical repair of coarctation is usually performed through a left posterolateral thoracotomy via the third or fourth intercostal space. The descending thoracic aorta, ductus (or ligamentum), transverse aortic arch, and brachiocephalic vessels are mobilized. Care is taken to preserve the vagus nerve and its recurrent laryngeal branch.

The coarctation is usually evident externally by narrowing or posterior indentation; however, the degree of internal narrowing is usually much more severe. A dose of heparin (100 units/kg) may be given intravenously for patients younger than 2 years. Proximal and distal control of the aorta is achieved using clamps. Usually, the proximal clamp is positioned on the transverse arch between the innominate and left carotid vessels with concomitant occlusion of the left carotid and left subclavian. In infants and children, the preferred surgical approach to coarctation is resection with extended end-to-end repair. A generous resection of the coarctation segment is performed. The proximal aorta is then spatulated along the lesser curvature and the distal aorta along the greater curvature. An extended end-to-end anastomosis is then performed.

In older children and adults, it may not be possible to perform a resection with primary repair without creating excessive tension on the anastomosis, which may lead to hemorrhage or scarring with recurrent coarctation. An alternative strategy is necessary in these cases. Patch aortoplasty may be performed in children in whom further growth is anticipated. The subclavian flap repair augments the narrowed aorta using native arterial tissue. Blood flow to the left arm is maintained by collateral vessels, although long-term

studies have demonstrated a slight discrepancy in limb length in some patients. Prosthetic patch material may also be used. By avoiding circumferential prosthetic material, growth potential of the native aorta is preserved. The disadvantage of patch repair is a high risk of aneurysm formation. In adults, where growth is no longer an issue, resection of the coarctation may be performed with subsequent placement of a prosthetic interposition graft (either Dacron or polytetrafluoroethylene).

One of the principal concerns during coarctation repair is interruption of distal aortic blood flow, especially to the spinal cord. The anterior spinal artery is fed by major radicular branches from intercostal arteries. In patients without well-formed collaterals, ischemia of the spinal cord may be precipitated by aortic cross-clamping, and paraplegia may result. Protective measures include induction of mild hypothermia, maintenance of a high proximal aortic pressure, and minimization of cross-clamp time. In older patients, distal aortic perfusion may be maintained by the technique of left heart bypass, where oxygenated blood is taken from the left atrium and delivered to the femoral artery or distal aorta using a centrifugal pump. Overall, the incidence of paraplegia following coarctation repair is less than 1%.

Transcatheter therapy has been proposed for the primary therapy of coarctation, but this approach is controversial due to the incidence of recurrent coarctation, need for multiple interventions, injury to the femoral vasculature (for access), and aneurysm formation. Improved results have been achieved with balloon angioplasty with concurrent stent placement in older children and adults in whom further aortic growth is not anticipated. Balloon angioplasty is widely accepted for the treatment of recurrent coarctation following surgery, in which the success rate is on the order of 90%.

D. Prognosis

The early mortality following repair of coarctation in neonates is 2–10%, while the risk in older children and adults is about 1%. The incidence of recurrent coarctation following resection and end-to-end repair is about 5%. The long-term survival following repair of coarctation is determined by the presence of associated defects and the persistence of hypertension.

Following repair, patients may develop severe hypertension. This can be managed using intravenous beta-blockers (eg, as esmolol) or vasodilators (eg, sodium nitroprusside). Uncontrolled hypertension can lead to the complication of mesenteric arteritis. Hypertension usually resolves within days to weeks after repair, although older children and adults may require lifelong antihypertensive therapy. Repair of coarctation during infancy is thought to minimize the risk of late hypertension.

Golden AB, Hellenbrand WE: Coarctation of the aorta: stenting in children and adults. Catheter Cardiovasc Interv 2007;69:289.

Ovaert C et al: Balloon angioplasty of native coarctation: clinical outcomes and predictors of success. J Am Coll Cardiol 2000;35:988.

Thomson JD et al: Outcome after extended arch repair for aortic coarctation. Heart 2006;92:90.

Wong CH, Watson B, Smith J: The use of left heart bypass in adult and recurrent coarctation repair. Eur J Cardiothorac Surg 2001;20:1199.

Wright GE et al: Extended resection and end-to-end anastomosis for aortic coarctation in infants: results of a tailored surgical approach. Ann Thorac Surg 2005;80:1453.

▶ Vascular Ring

ESSENTIALS OF DIAGNOSIS

▶ Varying degree of tracheoesophageal compression.

▶ Patients present with frequent respiratory infections and upper airway symptoms.

▶ "Seal bark" or brassy cough.

▶ Often misdiagnosed.

▶ Pulmonary artery slings are associated with complete tracheal rings.

A. General Considerations

Vascular rings comprise a spectrum of vascular anomalies of the aortic arch, pulmonary artery, and brachiocephalic vessels. The clinically significant manifestation of these lesions is a varying degree of tracheoesophageal compression. These vascular anomalies can be divided into complete vascular rings and partial vascular rings. Complete vascular rings can be divided into double aortic arch and right aortic arch with left ligamentum arteriosum. These two categories can be further subdivided on the basis of the specific anatomy. Incomplete vascular rings include aberrant right subclavian artery, innominate artery compression, and pulmonary artery sling. Other rare variations, which have been described, include left aortic arch with right descending aorta and right ligamentum, and left aortic arch with aberrant right subclavian artery and right ligamentum. The incidence of clinically significant vascular rings is 1–2% of all congenital heart defects.

Vascular rings and pulmonary slings have been described in conjunction with other cardiac defects, including, TOF, ASD, branch pulmonary artery stenosis, coarctation, AVSD, VSD, interrupted aortic arch, and aortopulmonary window. Significant associated cardiac anomalies occur in 11–20% of patients with a vascular ring. A right aortic arch is generally associated with a greater incidence of coexisting anomalies.

By the end of the fourth week of embryonic development, the 6 aortic or branchial arches have formed between the dorsal aortae and ventral roots. Subsequent involution and migration of the arches results in the anatomically normal or abnormal development of the aorta and its branches. The majority of the first, second, and fifth arches regress. The third arch forms the common carotid artery and proximal internal carotid artery. The right fourth arch forms the proximal right subclavian artery. The left fourth arch contributes to the portion of the aortic arch from left carotid to left subclavian arteries. The proximal portion of the right sixth arch becomes the proximal portion of the right pulmonary artery, while the distal segment involutes. Similarly, the proximal left sixth arch contributes to the proximal left pulmonary artery, and the distal sixth arch becomes the ductus arteriosus.

The pulmonary artery is formed from 2 vascular precursors as well as through a combination of angiogenesis, the de novo development of new blood vessels, and vasculogenesis, the budding and migration of existing vessels. As stated previously, the proximal pulmonary arteries are based on the sixth arches, whereas the primitive lung buds initially derive their blood supply from the splanchnic plexus. Ultimately, these two segments of the pulmonary artery join to form the vascular network of the lung parenchyma.

B. Clinical Findings

Children with a complete vascular ring generally present within the first weeks to months of life. Typically, children with a double aortic arch present earlier in life than those with a right arch and retroesophageal left ligamentum. In the younger age group, respiratory symptoms predominate, as liquids are generally well tolerated. Respiratory symptoms may include stridor, nonproductive cough, apnea, or frequent respiratory infections. The cough is classically described as "seal bark," or brassy." These symptoms may mimic asthma, respiratory infection, or reflux, and children with vascular rings are often initially misdiagnosed. With the transition to solid food, dysphagia becomes more apparent.

The presentation of a patient with an incomplete vascular ring is variable. Children with innominate artery compression usually present within the first 1 to 2 years of life with respiratory symptoms. Although, aberrant right subclavian artery is the most common arch abnormality, occurring in approximately 0.5–1% of the population, it rarely causes symptoms. Classically, when symptoms do occur, they present in the seventh and eighth decade, as the aberrant vessel becomes ectatic and calcified, causing dysphagia lusoria due to impingement of the artery on the posterior esophagus. An aberrant right subclavian rarely causes symptoms except when it is of an abnormally large caliber or associated with tracheomalacia.

Children with pulmonary artery slings generally present with respiratory symptoms within the first few weeks to months of life. As with complete rings, respiratory symptoms may include stridor, nonproductive cough, apnea, or frequent respiratory infections and may mimic other conditions leading to misdiagnosis. Pulmonary artery slings are associated with complete tracheal rings in 30–40% of patients, leading to focal or diffuse tracheal stenosis.

The methods for diagnosing a vascular ring are variable because of the variability in presentation and the spectrum of diagnostic tests available. A child with a presumptive diagnosis of asthma or tracheomalacia may be referred to a pulmonologist and a diagnosis of vascular ring made or suspected initially by chest radiograph and bronchoscopy. In some situations, the diagnosis is made by echocardiography during evaluation for concurrent cardiac defects. Regardless, the diagnosis generally begins with a chest radiograph. Complementary studies may include barium esophagogram, CT, MRI, and bronchoscopy. CT, MRI, or bronchoscopy are important modalities to define the tracheal anatomy in a patient with a pulmonary artery sling. Echocardiography may be diagnostic and may be used to rule out other cardiac anomalies. Tracheograms and cardiac catheterizations, which have been used extensively in the past, are rarely currently indicated.

C. Treatment

A double aortic arch occurs when the distal portion of the right dorsal aorta fails to regress. The two arches form a complete ring, encircling the trachea and esophagus. The right arch is dominant in the majority of the cases, followed by left dominant, with codominant arches being the least common. The left and right carotid and subclavian arteries generally arise from their respective arches. The ligamentum arteriosum and descending aorta usually remain on the left.

The approach to repair of a double aortic arch is via a left posterolateral thoracotomy. The procedure can easily be accomplished through a limited, muscle sparing incision through the third or fourth intercostal space. The pleura is incised, after identifying the vagus and phrenic nerves. The ligamentum or ductus arteriosum is divided while preserving the recurrent laryngeal nerve. The nondominant arch is then divided between two vascular clamps at the point where brachiocephalic flow is optimally preserved. If there is concern regarding the location for division, the arches can be temporarily occluded at various points while monitoring pulse and blood pressure in each limb. If there is an atretic segment, the division is done at the point of the atresia. Dissection around the esophagus and trachea in the regions of the ligamentum/ductus and nondominant arch allows for retraction of the vascular structures and lysis of any residual obstructing adhesions.

There are three anatomic variations for a right arch with a left ligamentum, which cause a complete vascular ring. If the left fourth arch regresses between the aorta and left subclavian, a right aortic arch with aberrant left subclavian artery results. The ligamentum arteriosum is retroesophageal, bridging the left pulmonary artery and aberrant left subclavian, forming a complete vascular ring. If the left fourth arch regresses after the origin of the left subclavian artery but before the arch reaches the dorsal aorta to communicate with the left sixth arch (which becomes the ductus arteriosus), there is mirror-image branching. The ligamentum arteriosum arises directly from the descending aorta, or from a Kommerell diverticulum off of the descending aorta, forming

the complete ring. If communication is maintained between the left fourth and sixth arches, there is mirror-image branching with the ligamentum arising from the anterior, mirror-image left subclavian, and a ring is not formed.

The surgical approach for a right aortic arch with retroesophageal left ligamentum arteriosum is the same as for a double arch. The ligamentum is divided, and any adhesions around the esophagus and trachea are lysed. Rarely, the Kommerell diverticulum has been reported to cause compression even after division of the ligamentum. As such, it may be prudent to resect or suspend the diverticulum posteriorly.

In innominate artery compression syndrome, the aortic arch and ligamentum are in their normal leftward position. However, the innominate artery arises partially or totally to the left of midline. As the artery courses from left to right anterior to the trachea, it causes tracheal compression. The symptoms of innominate artery compression may be mild to severe. With mild symptoms and minimal tracheal compression on bronchoscopy, children can be observed expectantly because the symptoms may resolve with growth. Indications for surgery include apnea, severe respiratory distress, significant stridor, or recurrent respiratory tract infection. Several approaches for the correction of innominate artery compression syndrome have been described. These include simple division, division with reimplantation into the right side of the ascending aorta, and suspension to the overlying sternum.

An aberrant right subclavian artery occurs when there is regression of the right fourth arch between the right common carotid and right subclavian arteries. The right subclavian then arises from the leftward descending aorta, laying posterior to the esophagus as it crosses from left to right. Although the artery can compress the esophagus posteriorly, it is rarely the cause of symptoms in children. Surgical treatment involves simple division via a left posterolateral thoracotomy. Rarely, reimplantation or grafting from the right carotid or aortic arch may be necessary.

Normally, the right and left sixth aortic arches contribute to the proximal portions of their respective pulmonary arteries. If the proximal left sixth arch involutes and the bud from the left lung migrates rightward to meet the right pulmonary artery, a pulmonary artery sling is formed. Pulmonary artery slings are associated with complete tracheal rings and tracheal stenosis in 30–40% of patients. Origin of the right upper lobe bronchus from the trachea has been reported in frequent association with pulmonary artery sling.

Initial attempts at the repair of a pulmonary artery sling involved reimplantation after division of the left pulmonary artery and translocation of the trachea without cardiopulmonary bypass. These early reports had a high incidence of left pulmonary artery thrombosis. This has led some authors to advocate division of the trachea and translocation of the left pulmonary artery. This approach would seem sensible if the trachea were being divided in the course of tracheal reconstruction. However, currently most authors advocate the reimplantation of the left pulmonary artery, which has resulted in excellent results. The procedure is done via a median sternotomy on cardiopulmonary bypass to insure optimal visualization of the repair. Aortic cross-clamping is not necessary. The left pulmonary artery is divided off of the right pulmonary artery, translocated anterior to the trachea, and reimplanted into the main pulmonary artery.

Any necessary reconstruction of the trachea is done concurrently with bronchoscopic assistance. Many techniques for tracheal reconstruction have been described, the most common of which are resection with primary reanastomosis and sliding tracheoplasty for short segment stenosis, and rib cartilage or pericardial patch for long areas of narrowing.

Over 95% of vascular rings without concurrent cardiac defects can be performed through a left thoracotomy. A right thoracotomy is indicated for the rare cases where there is a right ligamentum arteriosum. A right ligamentum occurs in the setting of a left aortic arch with right descending aorta, where the ligamentum bridges from the descending aorta to the right pulmonary artery forming a complete ring. Right ligamentum arteriosum has also been described with a left aortic arch with aberrant right subclavian artery. In this case, the ligamentum may arise from the aberrant subclavian artery, from a diverticulum off of the arch, or directly from the left arch to the right pulmonary artery. In addition, a double aortic arch with an atretic segment proximal to the right carotid artery is more easily divided through a right thoracotomy. The approach to these anomalies is the same as for a left-sided ring division, with the caveat that the right recurrent laryngeal nerve will loop around the right ligamentum.

Repair of vascular rings has been described using video-assisted thoracoscopic surgery (VATS) both with and without robotic assistance. Candidates for thoracoscopic division are limited to those patients requiring only the division of nonpatent vascular structures. In general, VATS is used for patients weighing more than15 kg due to current size limitations of the instruments.

D. Prognosis

Mortality for the repair of a vascular ring is 0.5–7.6%, with improved survival occurring in more recent series. The majority of deaths are related to other cardiac defects or respiratory infection and failure. Backer and colleagues reported a series of 16 patients repaired utilizing left pulmonary artery division and reimplantation for pulmonary artery sling, all of whom also required tracheal reconstruction. There were no operative mortalities and one late death due to respiratory complications. The major source of morbidity, as well as mortality, in this and other series is related to the tracheal reconstruction.

Alsenaidi K et al: Management and outcomes of double aortic arch in 81 patients. Pediatrics 2006;118:e1336.

Backer CL et al: Pulmonary artery sling: results with median sternotomy, cardiopulmonary bypass, and reimplantation. Ann Thorac Surg 1999;67:1738.

Backer CL et al: Trends in vascular ring surgery. J Thorac Cardiovasc Surg 2005;129:1339.

Humphrey C, Duncan K, Fletcher S: Decade of experience with vascular rings at a single institution. Pediatrics 2006;117:e903.

Woods RK et al: Vascular anomalies and tracheoesophageal compression: a single institution's 25-year experience. Ann Thorac Surg 2001;72:434.

▶ Coronary Anomalies

 ESSENTIALS OF DIAGNOSIS

▶ Variable symptoms include congestive heart failure, angina, and sudden death.

▶ Electrocardiogram often demonstrates ischemia or prior infarction.

▶ Mitral regurgitation is commonly present along with significantly depressed ventricular function; the mitral regurgitation usually returns to normal following surgical intervention.

▶ Cardiac catheterization or cardiac MRI is often helpful to delineate the coronary anatomy.

A. General Considerations

Coronary artery anomalies occur in between 0.3 and 1.3% of the population. They can be classified as minor, secondary, or major on the basis of their clinical significance. Minor defects have no functional significance and are usually detected as incidental findings at cardiac catheterization. Secondary defects have no intrinsic significance but alter surgical management when they are present. An example of a secondary defect is an anomalous origin of the left anterior descending from the right coronary artery, which crosses the hypoplastic infundibulum in a patient with TOF. The presence of this vessel may prevent the safe performance of a transannular incision and thereby mandate the use of a conduit. Major defects are the most important form of coronary anomaly because they exert an intrinsically adverse effect on the myocardium. Major anomalies can be subdivided based on anatomy: coronary arteriovenous fistula, anomalous pulmonary origin of a coronary artery, anomalous aortic origin of a coronary artery, myocardial bridging, or coronary artery aneurysm.

Coronary arteriovenous fistula is the most common major coronary anomaly. An abnormal connection exists between a coronary artery (usually the right) and another vascular structure (usually one of the right heart chambers). Most fistulas are isolated and solitary. The fistula leads to left-to-right shunting, which can produce congestive heart failure. Other symptoms include angina, endocarditis, myocardial infarction, arrhythmia, and sudden death. The diagnosis is suggested by echocardiography and confirmed by catheterization.

The second-most common major coronary anomaly is the origin of a coronary artery from the pulmonary artery. The most common manifestation is the anomalous left coronary artery arising from the pulmonary artery (ALCAPA). The right coronary (or both coronaries) may also arise anomalously from the pulmonary artery but only in very rare cases. ALCAPA is usually well tolerated during fetal development, but after birth, the pulmonary systolic pressure usually drops (following ductal closure and decline in PVR) and the anomalous coronary is perfused with desaturated blood at low pressure. Collateral vessels develop between the normal right coronary artery and the abnormal left coronary, but the benefit is negated due to the development of coronary steal, whereby the collateral blood shunts left to right by retrograde flow in the anomalous coronary into the low-pressure pulmonary artery. Most patients will present between 6 weeks and 3 months of life. Typical symptoms include irritability, difficulty in feeding, and other signs of congestive heart failure. Untreated, ALCAPA is nearly always fatal. Rarely, patients will survive to adulthood and present with symptoms of angina or sudden death. On examination, patients with ALCAPA frequently have a holosystolic murmur of ischemic mitral regurgitation. The pulmonary component of the second heart sound may be pronounced because of pulmonary hypertension. Chest radiography is significant for cardiomegaly and pulmonary edema. Electrocardiographic evidence of ischemia and infarction is usually present. Echocardiography is usually diagnostic and is useful for assessing the severity of left ventricular dysfunction and ischemic mitral regurgitation that are commonly present. Catheterization is occasionally necessary to clarify the anatomy, but this technique is used less frequently because of the risk of inducing life-threatening arrhythmias.

Anomalous aortic origins of the coronary arteries are usually minor defects, but a potentially dangerous abnormality exists when the left main coronary artery arises from the right coronary sinus and passes between the pulmonary artery and aorta. This defect has been associated with cardiac symptoms and sudden death, as has the origin of the right coronary artery from the left coronary sinus (usually when the right coronary is dominant). The etiology of ischemia in both defects is thought to be related to the acute angle of origin and slitlike orifice of the anomalous vessel and the extrinsic compression created by the apposing walls of the aorta and pulmonary artery. These defects usually present in older patients. Symptomatic patients are treated surgically by coronary artery bypass.

Myocardial bridging occurs when a segment of an epicardial coronary artery (usually the left anterior descending) takes an intramyocardial course over a short segment. Although this is a common incidental finding at cardiac catheterization, this defect has been associated in some cases with myocardial ischemia. Treatment involves dividing the muscle bridge to free the coronary, coronary bypass beyond the bridge, or transcatheter stenting.

Coronary aneurysms occur rarely, usually in conjunction with an inflammatory condition such as Kawasaki syndrome, polyarteritis nodosa, Takayasu arteritis, or syphilis. Coronary aneurysms may thrombose or lead to distal coronary stenosis or embolization. Rupture occurs uncommonly. Treatment ranges from antiplatelet therapy to coronary artery bypass grafting, and possible transplantation.

B. Treatment

All symptomatic fistulas should be occluded, either surgically or by transcatheter techniques. In some cases, coronary bypass grafting may be necessary when distal flow is compromised by fistula occlusion. Treatment of asymptomatic fistulas is controversial, but occlusion should probably be undertaken when significant left-to-right shunting is present.

Surgical repair is indicated for all patients with ALCAPA. Historically, the initial surgical approach involved ligation of the proximal left coronary artery. This served to eliminate coronary steal and allow perfusion of the left coronary system by collaterals from the right. Despite the ease of simple ligation, most centers have abandoned this approach in favor of establishment of a 2-coronary system, which offers better long-term freedom from ischemia. In older patients, this may be achieved by proximal ligation of the left coronary artery in conjunction with coronary artery bypass, ideally with a left internal mammary graft. Coronary bypass is technically difficult in neonates, and a number of alternative operations have been devised to create a direct connection between the aorta and the anomalous coronary artery. Most commonly, this can be achieved by removing the origin of the left coronary artery (along with a button of adjacent pulmonary artery) and reimplanting the vessel directly into the side of the aorta. Another approach involves creation of a side-to-side connection between the aorta and pulmonary artery with placement of an intrapulmonary baffle to direct flow from this connection to the anomalous left coronary ostium.

C. Prognosis

Survival following surgical repair of ALCAPA has improved over the years. Recent reports have suggested an operative mortality of 6% or less. Ventricular function tends to normalize after surgery. In most patients, mitral valve function also improves, but for patients with severe mitral regurgitation, concurrent mitral valve repair may be indicated.

De Wolf D et al: Major coronary anomalies in childhood. Eur J Pediatr 2002;161:637.

Friedman AH et al: Identification, imaging, functional assessment and management of congenital coronary arterial abnormalities in children. Cardiol Young 2007;17:56.

Lange R et al: Long-term results of repair of anomalous origin of the left coronary artery from the pulmonary artery. Ann Thorac Surg 2007;83:1463.

Satou GM, Giamelli J, Gewitz MH: Kawasaki disease: diagnosis, management, and long-term implications. Cardiol Rev 2007; 15:163.

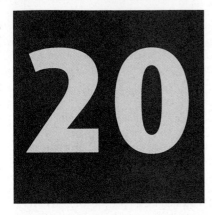

20

Esophagus & Diaphragm

Marco G. Patti, MD

Piero M. Fisichella, MD

▼ I. THE ESOPHAGUS

ANATOMY

The esophagus (Figure 20–1) is a muscular tube that serves as a conduit for the passage of food and fluids from the pharynx to the stomach. It originates at the level of the sixth cervical vertebra, posterior to the cricoid cartilage. In the thorax, the esophagus passes behind the aortic arch and the left main stem bronchus, enters the abdomen through the esophageal hiatus of the diaphragm, and terminates in the fundus of the stomach. Its muscle fibers originate from the cricoid cartilage and pharynx above and interdigitate with those of the stomach below. About 2–4 cm of esophagus are normally below the diaphragm. The junction between the esophagus and stomach is maintained in its normal intra-abdominal position by the reflection of the peritoneum onto the stomach and of the phrenoesophageal ligament onto the esophagus. The latter is a fibroelastic membrane that lies beneath the peritoneum, on the inferior surface of the diaphragm. When it reaches the esophageal hiatus, the ligament is reflected in an orad direction onto the lower esophagus, where it inserts into the circular muscle layer above the gastroesophageal sphincter, 2–4 cm above the diaphragm.

Three anatomic areas of narrowing occur in the esophagus: (1) at the level of the cricoid cartilage (pharyngoesophageal or upper esophageal sphincter); (2) in the mid thorax, from compression by the aortic arch and the left main stem bronchus; and (3) at the level of the esophageal hiatus of the diaphragm (gastroesophageal or lower esophageal sphincter).

In the adult, the distance as measured from the upper incisor teeth to the cricopharyngeus muscle is 15–20 cm; to the aortic arch, 20–25 cm; to the inferior pulmonary vein, 30–35 cm; and to the gastroesophageal junction, approximately 40–45 cm.

The musculature of the pharynx and upper third of the esophagus is skeletal in type (striated muscle); the remainder is smooth muscle. Physiologically, the entire organ behaves as a single functioning unit, so that no distinction can be made between the upper and lower esophagus from the standpoint of propulsive activity. As in the intestinal tract, the muscle fibers are arranged into inner circular and outer longitudinal layers. The arterial supply to the esophagus is quite consistent. The upper end is supplied by branches from the inferior thyroid arteries. The thoracic portion receives blood from the bronchial arteries and from esophageal branches originating directly from the aorta. The intercostal arteries may also contribute. The diaphragmatic and abdominal segments are nourished by the left inferior phrenic artery and by the esophageal branches of the left gastric artery.

The venous drainage is more complex and variable. The most important veins are those that drain the lower esophagus. Blood from this region passes into the esophageal branches of the coronary vein, a tributary of the portal vein. This connection constitutes a direct communication between the portal circulation and the venous drainage of the lower esophagus and upper stomach. When the portal system is obstructed, as in cirrhosis of the liver, blood is shunted upward through the coronary vein and the esophageal venous plexus to eventually pass by way of the azygos vein into the superior vena cava. The esophageal veins may eventually form varices as they become distended when portal hypertension is present.

The mucosal lining of the esophagus consists of stratified squamous epithelium that contains scattered mucous glands throughout. The esophagus has no serosal layer and, for this reason, does not heal as readily after injury or surgical anastomosis as other portions of the gastrointestinal tract.

PHYSIOLOGY

The coordinated activity of the upper esophageal sphincter (UES), the esophageal body and the lower esophageal sphincter (LES) is responsible for the motor function of the esophagus.

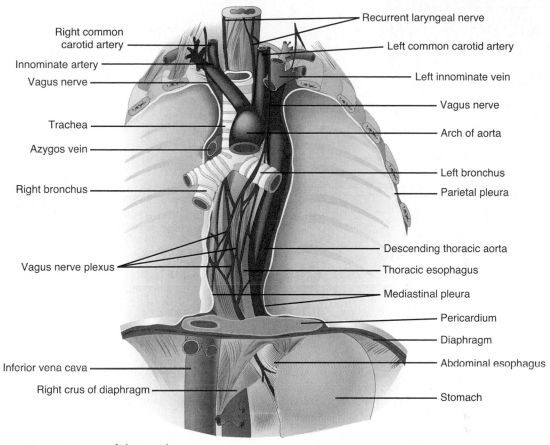

Right common carotid artery

Innominate artery

Vagus nerve

Trachea

Azygos vein

Right bronchus

Vagus nerve plexus

Inferior vena cava

Right crus of diaphragm

Recurrent laryngeal nerve

Left common carotid artery

Left innominate vein

Vagus nerve

Arch of aorta

Left bronchus

Parietal pleura

Descending thoracic aorta

Thoracic esophagus

Mediastinal pleura

Pericardium

Diaphragm

Abdominal esophagus

Stomach

▲ **Figure 20–1.** Anatomy of the esophagus.

1. Upper Esophageal Sphincter

The UES receives motor innervation directly from the brain (nucleus ambiguous). The sphincter is continuously in a state of tonic contraction, with a resting pressure of about 100 mm Hg (anteroposterior axis). The sphincter prevents passage of air from the pharynx into the esophagus and reflux of esophageal contents into the pharynx. During swallowing, a food bolus is moved by the tongue into the pharynx, which contracts while the UES relaxes. After the food bolus has reached the esophagus, the UES regains its resting tone (Figure 20–2).

2. Esophageal Body

When food passes through the UES, a contraction is initiated in the upper esophagus, which progresses distally toward the stomach. The wave initiated by swallowing is referred as primary peristalsis (Figure 20–2). It travels at a speed of 3 to 4 cm/s and reaches amplitudes of 60–140 mm Hg in the distal esophagus. Local stimulation by distention at any point in the body of the esophagus will elicit a peristaltic wave from the point of stimulus. This is called secondary

peristalsis and aids esophageal emptying when the primary wave has failed to clear the lumen of ingested food, or when gastric contents reflux from the stomach. Tertiary waves are considered abnormal, but they are frequently seen in elderly subjects who have no symptoms of esophageal disease.

3. Lower Esophageal Sphincter

The LES measures 3–4 cm in length and its resting pressure ranges between 15 and 24 mm Hg. At the time of swallowing, the LES relaxes for 5–10 seconds to allow the food bolus to enter the stomach and then regains its resting tone (Figure 20–2). The LES relaxation is mediated by vasoactive intestinal polypeptide and nitric oxide, both nonadrenergic, noncholinergic neurotransmitters. The resting tone depends mainly on intrinsic myogenic activity. The LES has a tendency to relax periodically at times independent from swallowing. These periodic relaxations are called **transient lower esophageal sphincter relaxations** to distinguish them from relaxations triggered by swallows. The cause of these transient relaxations is not known, but gastric distention

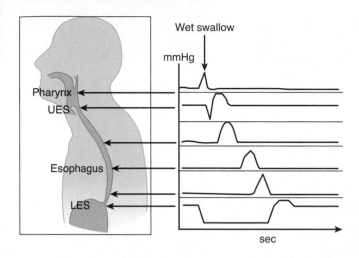

▲ **Figure 20–2.** Swallowing process. Upper esophageal sphincter, esophageal peristalsis, and lower esophageal sphincter in response to swallowing.

probably plays a role. Transient LES relaxations account for the small amount of physiologic gastroesophageal reflux present in any individual, and are also the most common cause of reflux in patients with gastroesophageal reflux disease (GERD). Decrease in length or pressure of the LES (or both) is responsible for abnormal reflux in the remaining patients. Overall, it is thought that while transient LES relaxation is the most common mechanism of reflux in volunteers and patients with either absent or mild esophagitis, the prevalence of a mechanically defective sphincter

(hypotensive and short) increases in patients with severe esophagitis, particularly when Barrett metaplasia is present. The crus of the esophageal hiatus of the diaphragm contributes to the resting pressure of the LES. This *pinchcock* action of the diaphragm is particularly important because it protects against reflux caused by sudden increases of intraabdominal pressure, such as with coughing or bending. This synergistic action of the diaphragm is lost when a sliding hiatal hernia is present, as the gastroesophageal junction is displaced above the diaphragm (Figure 20–3).

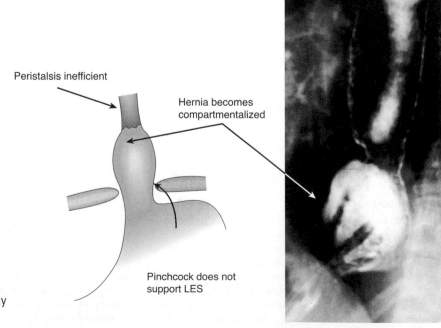

▲ **Figure 20–3.** Pathophysiology of hiatal hernia.

DIAGNOSTIC APPROACH TO ESOPHAGEAL DISEASES

▶ Symptomatic Evaluation

Dysphagia is a unique symptom as it points to an esophageal disorder, either functional (secondary to abnormalities of esophageal peristalsis or lack of coordination between different parts of the esophagus) or mechanical (secondary to a peptic or malignant stricture or an intraluminal mass). Heartburn and regurgitation are considered *typical* of GERD, but they can also be caused by nonesophageal disorders such as biliary disease, irritable bowel syndrome, coronary artery disease, and psychiatric diseases. GERD can also be responsible for *atypical* symptoms such as cough, hoarseness, and chest pain (Table 20–1).

▶ Upper Gastrointestinal Series

The test is performed by giving the patient barium to swallow. Subsequently, multiple images are taken, including the esophagus, the gastroesophageal junction, the stomach, and the duodenum (a barium swallow focuses just on the esophagus and the gastroesophageal junction). This test characterizes a hiatal hernia, an esophageal stricture, an esophageal diverticulum, or an intraluminal mass. A cine-esophagram is instead a dynamic evaluation of the swallowing process, and it is particularly useful in patients with functional dysphagia (secondary to a motility disorder, in the absence of a mechanical cause).

▶ Upper Endoscopy

This test allows visualization of the mucosal surface of the esophagus (plus stomach and duodenum). The endoscopist can determine the presence and degree of esophagitis and the presence of an intraluminal mass, and take biopsies.

▶ Endoscopic Ultrasound

An ultrasonographic evaluation can be performed during endoscopy. This test is used in patients with esophageal cancer to define the depth of penetration of the tumor through the esophageal wall (T) and the presence of enlarged periesophageal lymph nodes (N). Fine-needle aspiration of these nodes can be done, and cytologic analysis of the aspirate performed.

▶ Esophageal Manometry

Esophageal manometry allows determination of (1) LES location, length, pressure, and relaxation in response to swallowing; (2) pressure, duration, and velocity of propagation of the peristaltic waves; and (3) location, pressure, relaxation of the UES, and coordination with the pharyngeal contraction. The test lasts about 20 minutes, and it is performed by inserting a water-perfused or solid-state cath-

Table 20–1. Clinical Presentation of GERD.

Esophageal	Heartburn
	Regurgitation
	Dysphagia
Gastric	Bloating
	Early satiety
	Belching
	Nausea
Pulmonary	Aspiration
	Asthma
	Wheezing
	Cough
	Dyspnea
	Fibrosis
Ears, nose, throat	Globus
	Water brash
	Hoarseness
Cardiac	Chest pain

eter through the nostrils (using topical anesthesia) down the esophagus into the stomach, and then withdrawing it gradually while giving the patient sips of water.

▶ Ambulatory 24-hour pH Monitoring

This test measures reflux of acid from the stomach into the esophagus, and it is considered the gold standard for the diagnosis of GERD. By convention, the catheter is placed 5 cm above the upper border of the manometrically determined LES and is kept in place for 24 hours, during which the patient does not alter the daily activities and diet. In patients in whom cough or hoarseness are thought to be secondary to the upward extent of the gastric refluxate, acid can be measured at different levels in the esophagus. In addition to defining whether a pathologic amount of gastroesophageal reflux is present, the test establishes if there is a temporal correlation between episodes of reflux and symptoms such as heartburn, cough, and chest pain (Figure 20–4). Esophageal impedance is a technique that measures flow of liquids and gas across the gastroesophageal junction, independently of the pH of the gastric refluxate. In association with pH monitoring, impedance is indicated in patients with proton pump inhibitors–resistant typical reflux symptoms and chronic unexplained cough.

▶ Computerized Axial Tomography

A CT scan is used to assess the presence of metastases (lung, liver, adrenals) in patients with esophageal cancer (M).

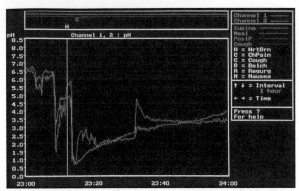

▲ **Figure 20–4.** Ambulatory pH monitoring. Temporal correlation between episodes of reflux (pH less than 4.0) and cough (C). (Reproduced, with permission, from Patti MG, Debas HT, Pellegrini CA. Clinical and functional characterization of high gastroesophageal reflux. Am J Surg 1993;165:163.)

▶ Positron Emission Tomography

A PET scan is used to assess the metastatic spread of esophageal cancer (M). In addition, it might help predict the response of esophageal cancer to neoadjuvant therapy.

▶ Laparoscopy/Thoracoscopy

Laparoscopy or thoracoscopy can be used to stage esophageal cancer, particularly when liver metastases or extensive lymphadenopathy are suspected.

Bredenoord AJ et al: Technology review: Esophageal impedance monitoring. Am J Gastroenterol 2007;102:187.
Cerfolio RJ et al: The accuracy of endoscopic ultrasonography with fine needle aspiration, integrated positron emission tomography with computed tomography in restaging patients with esophageal cancer after neoadjuvant therapy. J Thorac Cardiovasc Surg 2005;129:1232.
Hirano I et al: New technologies for the evaluation of esophageal motility disorders. Impedance, high resolution manometry and intraluminal ultrasound. Gastroenterol Clin North Am 2007; 36:531.
Patti MG et al: Role of esophageal function tests in the diagnosis of gastroesophageal reflux disease. Dig Dis Sci 2001;46:597.
Pech O et al: The impact of endoscopic ultrasound and computed tomography on the TNM staging of early cancer in Barrett's esophagus. Am J Gastroenterol 2006;101:2223.
Westerterp M et al: Esophageal cancer: CT, endoscopic us, and FDG PET for assessment of response to neoadjuvant therapy. Radiology 2005;236:841-851.

ESOPHAGEAL MOTILITY DISORDERS

The named primary esophageal motility disorders are achalasia, diffuse esophageal spasm, nutcracker esophagus, and the hypertensive LES. They occur in the absence of any other esophageal disorder such as reflux, and their cause is unknown. These disorders present with a combination of dysphagia, regurgitation, chest pain, and heartburn. Esophageal manometry is the key test that differentiates these disorders.

ACHALASIA

 ESSENTIALS OF DIAGNOSIS

▶ Dysphagia.
▶ Regurgitation.
▶ Radiologic evidence of distal esophageal narrowing.
▶ Absence of esophageal peristalsis on esophageal manometry.

▶ General Considerations

Esophageal achalasia is a primary esophageal motility disorder characterized by the absence of esophageal peristalsis. In addition, in most patients, the LES is hypertensive and fails to relax appropriately in response to swallowing. These abnormalities lead to impaired propulsion of food with consequent stasis in the esophagus. The incidence of achalasia is about 1 in 100,000 persons. It affects men more than women, and it can occur at any age.

▶ Pathogenesis

The etiology of esophageal achalasia is still unknown, but two theories exist: (1) a degenerative disease of the neurons and (2) infections of the neurons by a virus (eg, herpes zoster) or another infectious agent. The latter is supported by the fact that similar findings occur in patients with **Chagas disease** (American trypanosomiasis), a condition in which the infective organism destroys parasympathetic ganglion cells throughout the body, including the heart and the gastrointestinal, urinary, and respiratory tracts. The degeneration of the myenteric plexus of Auerbach determines loss of the postganglionic inhibitory neurons (which contain nitric oxide and vasoactive intestinal polypeptide), which mediate LES relaxation. Because the postganglionic cholinergic neurons are spared, there is unopposed cholinergic stimulation, which increases LES resting pressure and decreases LES relaxation. There is no propagation of peristaltic waves in response to swallowing, but rather the presence of simultaneous contractions, which are often a mirror image of each other.

▶ Clinical Findings

A. Symptoms and Signs

Dysphagia is the most common symptom, experienced by virtually every patient. It is often for both solids and liquids.

Most patients adapt with changes in their diet and are able to maintain a stable weight, while other eventually experience some weight loss. Regurgitation of undigested food is the second-most common symptom and is present in about 60% of patients. It occurs more often in the supine position and may lead to aspiration. Heartburn is present in about 40% of patients. It is not due to gastroesophageal reflux, but rather to stasis and fermentation of undigested food in the distal esophagus. Chest pain also occurs in about 40% of patients, due to esophageal distension, and it is usually experienced at the time of a meal.

B. Imaging Studies

A barium swallow should be the first test performed in the evaluation of a patient with dysphagia. It usually shows narrowing at the level of the gastroesophageal junction (Figure 20–5). A dilated, sigmoid esophagus may be present in patients with longstanding achalasia. Endoscopy is performed to rule out a tumor of the gastroesophageal junction.

C. Special Tests

Esophageal manometry is the key test for establishing the diagnosis of esophageal achalasia. The classic manometric findings are (1) absence of esophageal peristalsis and (2) hypertensive LES (in about 50% of patients) that relaxes only partially in response to swallowing. When the esophagus is dilated and sigmoid in shape, it may be difficult to pass the catheter through the gastroesophageal junction into the stomach: In these cases, the catheter may be placed under fluoroscopic or endoscopic guidance.

▶ Differential Diagnosis

Benign strictures due to gastroesophageal reflux and esophageal carcinoma may mimic the clinical presentation of achalasia. Sometimes an infiltrating tumor of the gastroesophageal junction can mimic not only the clinical and radiological presentation of achalasia but also the manometric profile. This condition is called **secondary or pseudo-achalasia** and should be suspected in patients older than 60 years with recent onset of dysphagia (less than 6 months) and excessive weight loss. An endoscopic ultrasound or a CT scan can help establishing the diagnosis.

▶ Complications

Aspiration of retained and undigested food can cause repeated episodes of pneumonia. Achalasia is also a risk factor for esophageal cancer. Squamous cell carcinoma is probably due to the continuous irritation of the mucosa by the retained and fermenting food. Adenocarcinoma can occur in patients who develop gastroesophageal reflux after either pneumatic dilatation or myotomy.

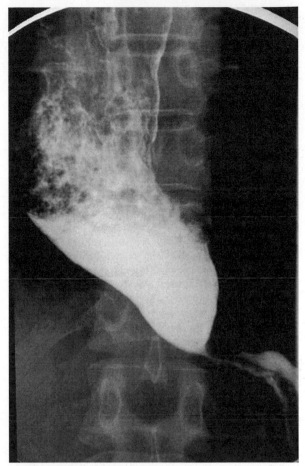

▲ **Figure 20–5.** Esophageal achalasia. Note dilation of the esophageal body, retained barium, and distal esophageal narrowing (bird's beak).

▶ Treatment

Therapy is palliative, and it is directed toward relief of symptoms by decreasing the outflow resistance caused by the dysfunctional LES. Because peristalsis is absent and does not return after any form of treatment, gravity becomes the key factor that allows emptying of food from the esophagus into the stomach. The following treatment modalities are available to achieve this goal.

▶ Medical Therapy

Calcium-channel blockers are used to decrease LES pressure. However, because only 10% of patients benefit from this treatment, it should be used primarily in elderly patients who have contraindications to either pneumatic dilatation or to surgery.

A. Endoscopic Treatment

Intrasphincteric injection of botulinum toxin is used to block the release of acetylcholine at the level of the LES, thereby restoring the balance between excitatory and inhibitory neurotransmitters. This treatment, however, is of limited value: Only 60% of treated patients still have relief of dysphagia 6 months after treatment, and this number further decreases to 30% (even after multiple injections) 2.5 years later. In addition, it often causes an inflammatory reaction at the level of the gastroesophageal junction, which makes a subsequent myotomy more difficult. It should be used primarily in elderly patients who are poor candidates for dilatation or surgery.

Pneumatic dilatation has been the main modality of treatment for many years. A balloon is inflated at the level of the gastroesophageal junction to rupture the muscle fibers while trying to leave the mucosa intact. The initial success rate is between 70% and 80%, but it decreases to 50% at 10 years, even after multiple dilatations. The perforation rate is 2–5%. If a perforation occurs, patients are taken emergently to the operating room, where closure of the perforation and a myotomy are performed through a left thoracotomy. The incidence of postdilatation gastroesophageal reflux is about 25–35%. Patients who fail pneumatic dilatation are usually treated by a Heller myotomy.

B. Surgical Treatment

A laparoscopic Heller myotomy and partial fundoplication is the procedure of choice for esophageal achalasia. The operation consists of a controlled division of the muscle fibers (myotomy) of the lower esophagus (6 cm) and proximal stomach (2 cm), followed by an anterior or a posterior partial fundoplication to prevent reflux. Patients remain in the hospital for 24–48 hours and return to regular activities in about 2 weeks. The operation effectively relieves symptoms in about 90% of patients and is effective even in patients who have a low LES pressure after previous dilatation or whose esophagus is dilated. The incidence of postoperative reflux is around 15%. Because of the excellent results, the short hospital stay, and the fast recovery time, a laparoscopic Heller myotomy and partial fundoplication is considered today the primary treatment modality for esophageal achalasia. Persistent or recurrent dysphagia after myotomy can be treated with pneumatic dilatation or a second myotomy. Esophagectomy is reserved for patients with severe dysphagia who have failed both dilatation and myotomy.

▶ Prognosis

A laparoscopic Heller myotomy allows excellent relief of symptoms in the majority of patients and should be preferred to pneumatic dilatation whenever surgical expertise is available. Botulinum toxin and medications should be used only in patients who are not candidates for pneumatic dilatation or laparoscopic Heller myotomy. Periodic follow-up by endoscopy is recommended to rule out the development of esophageal cancer.

DIFFUSE ESOPHAGEAL SPASM

 ESSENTIALS OF DIAGNOSIS

▶ Dysphagia.

▶ Chest pain.

▶ Intermittent symptoms.

▶ Radiologic evidence of tertiary contractions (corkscrew esophagus).

▶ Intermittent normal and absent peristaltic waves on manometry (> 10%, < 100%).

▶ Normal 24-hour ambulatory pH monitoring.

▶ General Considerations

The cause of this disorder is not known. Stress might play a role. Progression of diffuse esophageal spasm to achalasia has been documented (complete loss of esophageal peristalsis).

▶ Clinical Findings

A. Symptoms and Signs

The most common symptom is intermittent chest pain, which varies from slight discomfort to severe spasmodic pain that simulates the pain of coronary artery disease. Most patients complain of dysphagia, but weight loss is uncommon.

B. Imaging Studies

The barium swallow is abnormal in about 70% of patients. Fluoroscopic studies show segmental spasms, areas of narrowing, and irregular uncoordinated peristalsis (*corkscrew esophagus*) in about 30% of patients. An epiphrenic diverticulum is sometimes present.

C. Manometry

Esophageal manometry is the key test for establishing the diagnosis of diffuse esophageal spasm. The classic manometric findings are (1) alternation of esophageal peristalsis and simultaneous contractions (> 10% and < 100%)—contrary to old beliefs, the contractions are not hypertensive but of normal or even low amplitude—and (2) normal LES function or abnormalities similar to those seen in achalasia (elevated resting pressure and decreased relaxation in response to swallowing).

D. Ambulatory 24-hour pH Monitoring

This test is essential as the symptoms and the manometric picture of diffuse esophageal spasm can be caused by GERD. In such cases, treatment should be directed toward reflux because the dysmotility is secondary. Therefore, it is crucial to be certain about the diagnosis, as treatment of GERD (acid-reducing medications or a fundoplication) is completely different from that of a primary esophageal motility disorder (pneumatic dilatation or myotomy).

Differential Diagnosis

When chest pain is the predominant symptom, a complete cardiac workup is necessary to exclude a cardiac reason for the pain. Once the heart disease has been excluded, ambulatory pH monitoring must be performed to rule out abnormal gastroesophageal reflux, which is the most common cause of noncardiac chest pain. Esophageal manometry is the only test that distinguishes diffuse esophageal spasm from other primary esophageal motor disorders. An endoscopy should be performed to confirm the absence of intraluminal lesions.

Complications

Regurgitation and aspiration may occur, possibly leading to repeated pneumonic infections. An epiphrenic diverticulum may be present, secondary to the motor disorder.

Treatment

The therapeutic approach to diffuse esophageal spasm is similar to that of achalasia. Both disorders can be conceptualized as different points in a spectrum of esophageal motility, where peristalsis is progressively lost and progression from diffuse spasm to achalasia has been documented. In patients with diffuse esophageal spasm, dysphagia is secondary to abnormalities of the peristalsis and the LES, while the chest pain probably results from esophageal distension from poor emptying. Medical therapy (long-acting nitrates, calcium-channel blocking agents) is relatively ineffective. Pneumatic dilatation improves the dysphagia in about 25% of patients. Intrasphincteric injection of botulinum toxin has also given poor results. In contrast, a laparoscopic Heller myotomy and partial fundoplication (as for patients with achalasia) improves both dysphagia and chest pain in about 80% of patients.

The **hypertensive lower esophageal sphincter** is a rare disorder that manifests with dysphagia and is characterized manometrically by a hypertensive LES (resting pressure > 45 mm Hg), which relaxes in response to swallowing, and normal esophageal peristalsis. Treatment is similar to that of esophageal achalasia.

NUTCRACKER ESOPHAGUS

ESSENTIALS OF DIAGNOSIS

▶ Chest pain.

▶ Dysphagia.

▶ Intermittent symptoms.

▶ Peristaltic waves propagate normally but have very high amplitude and long duration.

▶ Normal 24-hour ambulatory pH monitoring.

General Considerations

The cause of this disorder is not known.

Clinical Findings

A. Symptoms and Signs

Chest pain is the most common symptom. Patients often come to the attention of gastroenterologists only after a thorough cardiac workup has been performed. About half of the patients complain of dysphagia in addition to chest pain.

B. Imaging Studies

The barium swallow is usually normal. An epiphrenic diverticulum is sometimes present.

C. Manometry

Esophageal manometry is the key test for establishing the diagnosis of nutcracker esophagus. The classic manometric findings are as follows: (1) normal propagation of the peristalsis waves (there are no simultaneous contractions)—the peristaltic waves in the distal esophagus, however, have very high amplitude (> 180 mm Hg) and duration (> 6 seconds)—and (2) normal LES function or abnormalities similar to those seen in achalasia and diffuse esophageal spasm.

D. Ambulatory 24-hour pH Monitoring

This test is essential because the symptoms and the manometric picture of nutcracker esophagus can be caused by GERD. In such cases, treatment should be directed toward reflux because the dysmotility is secondary.

Differential Diagnosis

When chest pain is the predominant symptom, a complete cardiac work up is necessary to exclude a cardiac reason for the pain. Once the heart has been excluded as a cause of the symptom, ambulatory pH monitoring must be performed to rule out abnormal gastroesophageal reflux, which is the most common cause of noncardiac chest pain. Esophageal manometry is the only test that distinguishes nutcracker esophagus from other primary esophageal motility disorders.

Complications

Regurgitation and aspiration may occur, possibly leading to repeated pneumonic infections. An epiphrenic diverticulum may be present, secondary to the motor disorder.

Treatment

The nutcracker esophagus is not as well defined as the other primary esophageal motility disorders for both pathophysiology and treatment. Initially, it was thought that the high pressure of the peristaltic contractions were the cause of the chest pain, so treatment was aimed at decreasing the high amplitude of the peristaltic waves. However, calcium-channel blockers are unable to improve the chest pain even though they decrease the strength of the contractions. Similarly, the results of surgery have been disappointing, as chest pain persists after myotomy in about 50% of patients. Dysphagia is improved in 80% of patients.

Eckardt VF et al: Pneumatic dilatation for achalasia: late results of a prospective follow-up investigation. Gut 2004;53:629.

Gockel I et al: Persistent and recurrent achalasia after Heller myotomy. Analysis of different patterns and long term results of reoperation. Arch Surg 2007;142:1093.

Patti MG et al: Spectrum of esophageal motility disorders. Implications for diagnosis and treatment. Arch Surg 2005;140:442.

Patti MG et al: Impact of minimally invasive surgery on the treatment of esophageal achalasia. A decade of change. J Am Coll Surg 2003;196:698.

Richards WO et al: Heller myotomy versus Heller myotomy with Dor fundoplication for achalasia. A prospective double-blind clinical trial. Ann Surg 2004;240:405.

Rosemurgy A et al: Laparoscopic Heller myotomy provides durable relief from achalasia and salvages failures after botox or dilation. Ann Surg 2005;241:725.

West RL et al: Long-term results of pneumatic dilatation in achalasia followed for more than 5 years. Am J Gastroenterol 2002;97:1346.

Zaninotto G et al: Randomized controlled trial of botulinum toxin versus laparoscopic Heller myotomy for esophageal achalasia. Ann Surg 2004;239:364.

ESOPHAGEAL DIVERTICULA

Diverticula of the esophagus are located above the UES (pharyngoesophageal or Zenker diverticulum) or the LES (epiphrenic diverticulum). They are considered pulsion diverticula and are secondary to abnormalities of the sphincters in terms of resting pressure, relaxation in response to swallowing, and coordination with the segment above the sphincter. As a consequence, mucosa and submucosa protrude through the muscular layers, forming the outpouching.

1. Pharyngoesophageal Diverticulum (Zenker Diverticulum)

ESSENTIALS OF DIAGNOSIS

▶ Dysphagia.
▶ Regurgitation of undigested food (with risk of aspiration).
▶ Gurgling sounds in the neck.
▶ Halitosis.

▶ General Considerations

This is the most common of the esophageal diverticula and is three times more frequent in men than in women. Most patients are over age 60. The condition originates from the posterior wall of the esophagus, in a triangular area of weakness (Killian triangle), limited inferiorly by the cricopharyngeus muscle and superiorly by the inferior constrictor muscles of the pharynx. As the diverticulum enlarges, it tends to deviate from the midline, mostly to the left.

▶ Pathogenesis

A Zenker diverticulum is due either to lack of coordination between the pharyngeal contraction and the opening time of the UES or to a hypertensive UES. Because of the increased intraluminal pressure, there is progressive herniation of mucosa and submucosa through the Killian triangle. Occasionally, UES dysfunction can occur in the absence of a diverticulum (cricopharyngeal achalasia). A hereditary syndrome called oculopharyngeal muscular dystrophy, consisting of ptosis and dysphagia, has been described in patients of French-Canadian ancestry. The dysphagia is the result of weak pharyngeal musculature in the face of normal UES function; it is considerably improved by UES myotomy. This syndrome also manifests with cervical dysphagia. A chronic cough may develop in some patients from aspiration of saliva and ingested food.

▶ Clinical Findings

A. Symptoms

Dysphagia is the most common symptom. Regurgitation of undigested food from the diverticulum often occurs and can lead to aspiration into the tracheobronchial tree and pneumonia. Patients frequently have halitosis and can hear gurgling sounds in the neck. About 30% of patients have associated GERD.

B. Imaging Studies

A barium swallow clearly shows the position and size of the diverticulum or a prominent cricopharyngeal bar without diverticulum (Figure 20–6). In some patients, a hiatal hernia is present.

C. Special Tests

Esophageal manometry shows lack of coordination between the pharynx and the cricopharyngeus muscle and often a hypertensive UES. In addition, it can show a hypotensive LES and abnormal esophageal peristalsis. Ambulatory pH monitoring determines if abnormal esophageal acid exposure is present.

Endoscopy may be dangerous because the instrument can enter the diverticulum rather than the esophageal lumen and cause a perforation.

▶ Differential Diagnosis

Differential diagnosis includes esophageal stricture, achalasia, and esophageal cancer. Pulmonary infection is the most

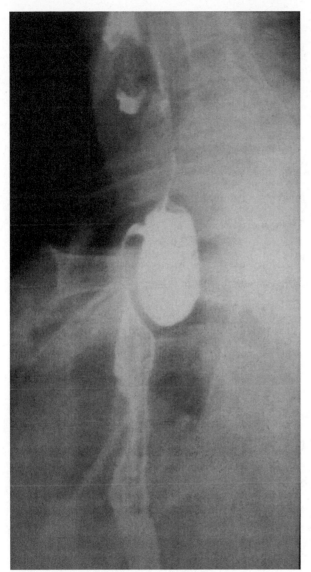

▲ **Figure 20–6.** Pharyngoesophageal diverticulum (Zenker diverticulum).

frequent serious complication, and many patients are first seen after experiencing repeated episodes of pneumonia.

Treatment

The standard treatment consists of excision of the diverticulum and myotomy of the cricopharyngeus muscle and the upper 3 cm of the posterior esophageal wall. For small diverticula (< 2 cm), the myotomy alone is sufficient. As an alternative to the conventional treatment, a transoral endoscopic approach (using an endoscopic stapling device that

ablates the septum between the diverticulum and the cervical esophagus) can be used for diverticula between 3 and 6 cm in size. If gastroesophageal reflux is present, it should be corrected before dividing the UES in order to avoid aspiration.

Prognosis

The prognosis is excellent in about 90% of cases. Complications are rare and the patients are usually able to eat the day after the procedure.

Bonavina L et al: Long term results of endosurgical and open surgical approach for Zenker diverticulum. World J Gastroenterol 2007;13:2586.
Chang CY et al: Endoscopic staple diverticulostomy for Zenker's diverticulum. Review of the literature and experience in 159 consecutive cases. Laryngoscope 2003;113:957.
Constantini M et al: Oesophageal diverticula. Best Practice & Research Clinical Gastroenterology 2004;18:3.
Morse CR et al: Preliminary experience by a thoracic service with endoscopic transoral stapling of cervical (Zenker's) diverticulum. J Gastrointest Surg 2007;11:1091.

2. Epiphrenic Diverticulum

 ESSENTIALS OF DIAGNOSIS

▶ Dysphagia.

▶ Regurgitation.

▶ Diverticulum evident on barium swallow.

▶ Esophageal motility disorder shown by esophageal manometry.

General Considerations

Epiphrenic diverticula are located just above the diaphragm. The diverticulum is not a primary anatomic abnormality but rather the consequence of an underlying motility disorder of the esophagus (achalasia is the most common, followed by diffuse esophageal spasm and nutcracker esophagus). The disorder causes an outflow obstruction at the level of the gastroesophageal junction, with consequent increase in intraluminal pressure and progressive herniation of mucosa and submucosa through the esophageal muscle layers.

Clinical Findings

A. Symptoms

The symptoms experienced by the patient are in part due to the underlying motility disorder (dysphagia, chest pain) and in part due to the diverticulum per se (regurgitation with the risk of aspiration). Some diverticula, however, can be asymptomatic.

B. Imaging Studies

A chest radiograph can show an air-fluid level in the posterior mediastinum. A barium swallow clearly shows the position and size of the diverticulum (Figure 20–7).

C. Special Tests

In the majority of cases, esophageal manometry shows the underlying motility disorder. Sometimes it is difficult to position the manometry catheter, and endoscopic or fluoroscopic guidance might be necessary.

▶ Differential Diagnosis

A paraesophageal hernia can be confused with an epiphrenic diverticulum. The barium swallow and the endoscopy help in establishing the diagnosis.

▶ Treatment

The treatment is surgical, and the laparoscopic approach is preferred. It consists of the following:

1. Resection of the diverticulum.
2. Long myotomy. This is performed in the side of the esophagus opposite to where the diverticulum is located. It extends proximally to the upper border of the neck of the diverticulum and distally for about 2 cm onto the gastric wall.
3. A partial fundoplication to prevent gastroesophageal reflux.

▶ Prognosis

A laparoscopic diverticulectomy, with myotomy and fundoplication, is successful in 80–90% of cases.

Fasano NC et al: Epiphrenic diverticulum: clinical and radiographic findings in 27 patients. Dysphagia 2003;18:9.

Nehra D et al: Physiologic basis for the treatment of epiphrenic diverticulum. Ann Surg 2002;235:346.

Tedesco P et al: Cause and treatment of epiphrenic diverticula. Am J Surg 2005;190:891.

Varghese TK et al: Surgical treatment of epiphrenic diverticula: a 30 year experience. Ann Thorac Surg 2007;84:1801.

ESOPHAGEAL MANIFESTATIONS IN SCLERODERMA & OTHER SYSTEMIC DISEASES

Scleroderma and several other systemic diseases may involve the esophagus.

In scleroderma or progressive systemic sclerosis, there is involvement of the gastrointestinal tract in up to 90% of patients. The most common site of gastrointestinal involvement is the smooth muscle portion of the esophagus, where atrophy and fibrosis occur. The upper esophagus (striated muscle) and the UES are not involved. As a consequence, the LES has a low pressure and the peristalsis is weak (low ampli-

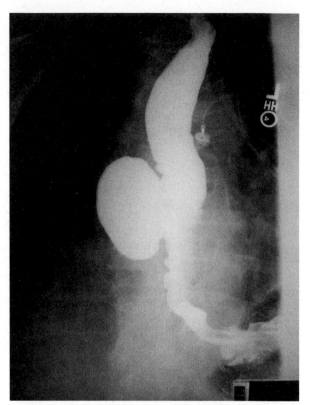

▲ **Figure 20–7.** Epiphrenic diverticulum.

tude or abnormal propagation of the peristaltic waves). These changes can be followed by an increased amount of gastroesophageal reflux with delayed clearance of the refluxed gastric contents. Esophageal symptoms usually appear in patients with the characteristic skin changes and Raynaud syndrome. In addition to heartburn and regurgitation, patients may have respiratory symptoms due to the upward extent of the gastric refluxate and aspiration. Dysphagia may be due to the abnormal peristalsis or to the presence of a peptic stricture. The diagnostic approach is similar to that of patients with GERD:

- A barium swallow may show a hiatal hernia or a stricture.
- Endoscopy shows esophagitis in 50–60% of patients. Barrett esophagus is present in about 10% of patients.
- Esophageal manometry usually shows a hypotensive LES. Dysmotility is frequent and can progress to complete loss of peristalsis.
- Ambulatory pH monitoring is essential to establish the diagnosis. It can also measure the presence of acid in the proximal esophagus and pharynx in patients with cough or vocal cord problems.
- Gastric scintigraphy is indicated in patients who experience postprandial bloating and fullness to measure the gastric emptying of solids and liquids.

Similar esophageal changes may also occur in rheumatoid arthritis, Sjögren syndrome, Raynaud disease, and systemic lupus erythematosus. Similar motor abnormalities are occasionally seen in alcoholism, diabetes mellitus, myxedema, multiple sclerosis, and amyloidosis.

Medical management should always be tried first. A proton pump inhibitor is the drug of choice. If gastroparesis is present, a prokinetic medication such as metoclopramide should be added. A fundoplication should be considered particularly in patients with regurgitation, cough, or vocal cord problems.

Ebert EC: Esophageal disease in scleroderma. J Clin Gastroenterol 2006;40:769.

Mandel T et al: Dysphagia and dysmotility of the pharynx and oesophagus in patients with primary Sjogren's syndrome. Scand J Rheumatol 2007;36:394.

Ntoumazios SK et al: Esophageal involvement in scleroderma: gastroesophageal reflux, the common problem. Semin Arthritis Rheum 2006;36:173.

GASTROESOPHAGEAL REFLUX DISEASE

ESSENTIALS OF DIAGNOSIS

- ▶ Heartburn.
- ▶ Regurgitation.
- ▶ Sliding hiatal hernia on barium swallow.
- ▶ Esophagitis on endoscopy.
- ▶ Abnormal esophageal motility on manometry.
- ▶ Abnormal esophageal exposure on ambulatory pH monitoring.

▶ General Considerations

GERD is the most common upper gastrointestinal disorder of the Western world and accounts for about 75% of esophageal diseases. Heartburn, usually considered synonymous with the presence of abnormal gastroesophageal reflux, is experienced by 20–40% of the adult population of Western countries. However, because many symptomatic patients treat themselves with over-the-counter medications without consulting a physician, the prevalence of the disease is probably higher than reported. The incidence of reflux symptoms increases with age, and both sexes seem to be equally affected. Symptoms are more common during pregnancy, probably due to hormonal effects on the LES and the increased intra-abdominal pressure due to the enlarging uterus. Recent studies have demonstrated a link between obesity and GERD whereby the body mass index is an independent factor and has a direct effect on the severity of reflux.

▶ Pathogenesis

GERD is caused by the abnormal retrograde flow of gastric contents into the esophagus, resulting in symptoms and mucosal damage. A defective LES is the most common cause of GERD. Transient LES relaxations account for the majority of reflux episodes in patients without mucosal damage or with mild esophagitis, while a short and hypotensive LES is more frequently found in patients with more severe esophagitis. In 40–60% of patients with GERD, abnormalities of esophageal peristalsis are also present. Because esophageal peristalsis is the main determinant of esophageal clearance (the ability of the esophagus to clear gastric contents refluxed through the LES), patients with abnormal esophageal peristalsis have more severe reflux and slower clearance. Therefore, these patients often have more severe mucosal injury and more frequent atypical symptoms such as cough or hoarseness. A hiatal hernia also contributes to the incompetence of the gastroesophageal junction by altering the anatomic relationship between the esophageal crus and the LES. As the gastroesophageal junction is displaced above the diaphragm, the *pinchcock* action of the esophageal crus is lost. In patients with large hiatal hernias, the LES is usually shorter and weaker, and the amount of reflux is greater.

▶ Clinical Findings

A. Symptoms

Heartburn, regurgitation, and dysphagia are considered *typical* symptoms of GERD. However, a clinical diagnosis of GERD based on these symptoms is correct in only 70% of patients (when compared with the results of pH monitoring). A good response to therapy with proton pump inhibitors is a good predictor of the presence of abnormal reflux. GERD can also cause *atypical* symptoms such as cough, wheezing, chest pain, hoarseness, and dental erosions. Two mechanisms have been postulated for GERD-induced respiratory symptoms: (1) a vagal reflex arc resulting in bronchoconstriction and (2) microaspiration into the tracheobronchial tree. Ear, nose, and throat symptoms such as hoarseness or dental erosions are instead secondary to the upward extent of the acid with direct damage of the vocal cords or teeth.

B. Barium Swallow

A barium swallow provides information about the presence and size of a hiatal hernia, the presence and length of a stricture, and the length of the esophagus. This test, however, is not diagnostic of GERD, as a hiatal hernia or reflux of barium can be present in the absence of abnormal reflux.

C. Endoscopy

Fifty percent of patients with abnormal reflux do not have esophagitis on endoscopy. Therefore, endoscopy is useful for diagnosing complications of GERD such as esophagitis,

Barrett esophagus, or a stricture. In addition, there is major interobserver variation among endoscopists for the low grades of esophagitis (Table 20–2).

D. Esophageal Manometry

This test provides information about the LES (resting pressure, length, and relaxation) and the quality of esophageal peristalsis. In addition, manometry is essential for proper placement of the pH probe for ambulatory pH monitoring (5 cm above the upper border of the LES).

E. Ambulatory pH Monitoring

This test has a sensitivity and specificity of about 92% and is considered the gold standard for diagnosing GERD (Table 20–3). Medications that affect the production of acid by the parietal cells must be stopped 3 days (H_2-blocking agents) to 14 days (proton pump inhibitors) prior to the study. Diet and exercise are unrestricted during the test in order to mimic a typical day of the patient's life. This test should be performed (1) in patients who do not respond to medical therapy, (2) in patients who relapse after discontinuation of medical therapy, (3) before antireflux surgery, or (4) when evaluating atypical symptoms such as cough, hoarseness, and chest pain. Because fewer than 50% of these patients experience heartburn or have esophagitis on endoscopy, a pH monitoring study becomes the only way to establish a link between reflux and symptoms. A pH probe with 2 sensors, located 5 cm and 20 cm above the LES, allows determination of the upward extent of the reflux. Tracings are analyzed for a temporal correlation between symptoms and episodes of reflux.

▶ Differential Diagnosis

Heartburn can be the presenting symptom of irritable bowel syndrome, achalasia, cholelithiasis, coronary artery disease, or psychiatric disorders. Esophageal manometry and pH monitoring are essential to determine with certainty if GERD is present and if reflux is the cause of the symptoms.

▶ Complications

Esophagitis is the most common complication. Peptic strictures are uncommon, particularly in the era of proton pump

Table 20–2. Endoscopic Grading System for Esophagitis.

Grade 1	Reddening of the mucosa without ulceration
Grade 2	Linear ulcerations lined with granulation tissue that bleeds easily when touched
Grade 3	Ulcerations have coalesced to leave islands of epithelium
Grade 4	Stricture

Table 20–3. Normal Values for Ambulatory 24-hour pH Monitoring.

Percentage of total time pH < 4.0	4.5%
Percentage of upright time pH < 4.0	8.4%
Percentage of supine time pH < 4.0	3.5%
Number of episodes of reflux < 4.0	47
Number of episodes > 5 minutes	3.5
Longest episode (minutes)	20
Composite score[1]	14.7

[1]The composite score indicates the extent to which the patient's values deviate from the normal means of the six variables. It allows one to express in a single figure the degree of the patient's abnormality.

inhibitors. Barrett esophagus (metaplasia of the esophageal mucosa from squamous to columnar epithelium) is found in about 10–15% of patients with reflux documented by pH monitoring. Some patients may eventually progress to high-grade dysplasia and adenocarcinoma. Respiratory complications vary from chronic cough to asthma, aspiration pneumonia, and even pulmonary fibrosis. Vocal cord and dental damage can also occur.

▶ Treatment

A. Lifestyle Modifications

Patients should eat frequent small meals during the day (to avoid gastric distention), avoiding fatty foods, spicy foods, and chocolate, as they lower LES pressure. The last meal should be no less than 2 hours before going to bed. In order to increase the effect of gravity, the head of the bed should be elevated over 4-inch to 6-inch blocks.

B. Medical Therapy

Antacids are useful for patients with mild intermittent heartburn. Acid-suppressing medications are the mainstay of medical therapy. H_2-blocking agents are usually prescribed for patients with mild symptoms or mild esophagitis. Proton pump inhibitors are superior to H_2-blocking agents because they determine a more profound control of the acid secretion, with healing of esophagitis in 80–90% of patients. However, symptoms and esophagitis tend to recur in the majority of patients after discontinuation of therapy, so most patients need chronic maintenance therapy. In addition, about 50% of patients on maintenance proton pump inhibitors require increasing doses to maintain healing of esophagitis. Medical therapy is largely ineffective for the treatment of the extraesophageal manifestations of GERD due to the upward extension of the refluxate. In these patients, acid-suppressing medications only alter the pH of the gastric refluxate, but reflux and aspiration can still occur because of an incompetent LES and ineffective esophageal peristalsis. Proton pump inhibitors can interfere with calcium absorption causing fractures. In addition, they have been shown to cause delay in gastric emptying and abnormal cardiac contractility.

C. Surgical Therapy

In the past, antireflux operation was considered only for patients who did not respond to medical treatment with antacids or H_2-blocking agents. Today the ideal patient is the one whose heartburn is well controlled by proton pump inhibitors and in whom ambulatory pH monitoring shows abnormal reflux. The operation is indicated in (1) young patients who require chronic therapy with proton pump inhibitors for control of symptoms, (2) patients in whom regurgitation persists during therapy, (3) patients with respiratory symptoms (cough, asthma, aspiration pneumonia, pulmonary fibrosis), (4) patients with vocal cord damage, and (5) patients with Barrett esophagus. Recent evidence suggests that an effective antireflux operation may promote regression of the columnar epithelium in up to 50% of patients who have a short segment of Barrett esophagus (< 3 cm). In addition, it may arrest the progression from metaplasia to dysplasia. However, since the response to therapy is unpredictable, endoscopic surveillance after laparoscopic fundoplication in patients with Barrett esophagus is recommended.

The goal of surgical therapy is to restore the competence of the LES. A laparoscopic Nissen fundoplication (360°) is considered today the procedure of choice (Figure 20–8) because it increases the resting pressure and length of the LES and decreases the number of transient LES relaxations. The success of the operation is based on the following technical elements:

1. Dissection of the esophagus in the posterior mediastinum to allow 3–4 cm of esophagus to lie without tension below the diaphragm. By bringing the entire stomach and gastroesophageal junction below the diaphragm, a sliding hiatal hernia is reduced.

2. Division of the short gastric vessels in order to create a "floppy" fundoplication.

3. Approximation of the esophageal crus to decrease the size of the esophageal hiatus, thereby avoiding herniation of the wrap.

4. Construction of a 360° fundoplication over a 56–60 French bougie.

The hospital stay is usually 1 day only, and the postoperative discomfort is minimal. Most patients return to work within 2–3 weeks.

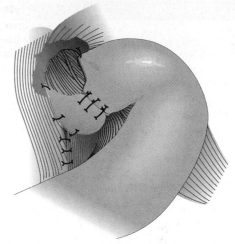

▲ **Figure 20–8.** Nissen fundoplication (360 degrees).

▶ Prognosis

Control of *typical* symptoms is obtained in about 90% of patients after a fundoplication. Failures are treated with either medications or a second operation. The success rate is in the 70–90% range for patients with *atypical* symptoms, because it is often more difficult to establish preoperatively a strong correlation between gastroesophageal reflux and symptoms.

Diener U et al: Esophageal dysmotility and gastroesophageal reflux disease. J Gastrointest Surg 2001;5:260.

Halum SL et al: Patients with isolated laryngopharyngeal reflux are not obese. Laryngoscope 2005;115:1042.

Herbella FA et al: Gastroesophageal reflux disease and obesity. Pathophysiology and implications for treatment. J Gastrointest Surg 2007;11:286.

Patti MG et al: Total fundoplication is superior to partial fundoplication even when esophageal peristalsis is weak. J Am Coll Surg 2004;198:863.

Patti MG et al: Role of esophageal function tests in the diagnosis of gastroesophageal reflux disease. Dig Dis Sci 2001;46:597.

Shillinger W et al: Negative inotropy of the gastric proton pump inhibitor. Pantoprazole in myocardium from human and rabbits. Circulation 2007;116:57.

Smith CD et al: When fundoplication fails: redo? Ann Surg 2005;241:861.

Sweet MP et al: The prevalence of distal and proximal gastroesophageal reflux in patients awaiting lung transplantation. Ann Surg 2006;244:491.

Takahashi Y et al: Influence of acid suppressants on gastric emptying: cross-analysis in healthy volunteers. J Gastroenterol and Hepatol 2006;21:1664.

Tamhankar AP et al: Omeprazole does not reduce gastroesophageal reflux: new insights using multichannel intraluminal impedance technology. J Gastrointest Surg 2004;8:888.

Young YX et al: Long-term proton pump inhibitors therapy and risk of hip fracture. JAMA 2006;296:2947-2953.

BARRETT ESOPHAGUS

ESSENTIALS OF DIAGNOSIS

▶ GERD symptoms (typical and atypical).

▶ Endoscopic evidence of "salmon pink" epithelium above gastroesophageal junction.

▶ Specialized columnar epithelium on esophageal biopsy.

▶ General Considerations

Barrett esophagus is caused by a change in the esophageal mucosa with replacement of the squamous epithelium by columnar epithelium. About 10–12% of patients undergoing endoscopy for symptoms of GERD are found to have Barrett epithelium, usually classified in short segment (less than 3 cm in length) or long segment (3 cm or longer). It occurs more frequently in white men older than 50 years. This metaplasia may progress to high-grade dysplasia and eventually adenocarcinoma. Thus, adenocarcinoma represents the final step of a sequence of events in which a benign disease (GERD) evolves into a preneoplastic disease and eventually into cancer.

▶ Pathogenesis

Barrett esophagus is due to reflux of gastric contents (acid and duodenal juice) into the esophagus. Barrett metaplasia is considered an advanced stage of GERD, characterized by a panesophageal motor disorder. When compared with patients with GERD with no mucosal injury or less severe esophagitis, patients with Barrett esophagus have a shorter and weaker LES and decreased amplitude of esophageal peristalsis. As a consequence, the amount of reflux is greater and esophageal clearance is slower. In addition, hiatal hernia is more common in patients with Barrett metaplasia.

▶ Clinical Findings

A. Symptoms

Patients with Barrett esophagus typically have a long history of GERD. While most patients experience both typical and atypical symptoms of GERD, others may become asymptomatic over time due to the decreased sensitivity of the metaplastic epithelium.

B. Imaging Studies

Barium swallow may show ulcerations, a hiatal hernia, or a stricture. Endoscopy shows presence of "salmon pink" epithelium above the gastroesophageal junction, replacing the whitish squamous epithelium. The diagnosis is confirmed by pathologic examination of the esophageal mucosa and requires the identification of intestinal type epithelium, characterized by the presence of goblet cells.

C. Special Tests

Esophageal manometry often shows a short and hypotensive LES and abnormal esophageal peristalsis (decreased amplitude of peristaltic waves, simultaneous waves). Ambulatory pH monitoring usually shows a severe amount of acid reflux. Esophageal exposure to duodenal juice can be quantified by a fiberoptic probe that measures intraluminal bilirubin as a marker for duodenal reflux. In GERD patients, the prevalence of esophageal bilirubin exposure parallels the degree of mucosal injury, being higher in patients with Barrett esophagus.

▶ Treatment

A. Barrett Esophagus: Metaplasia

The treatment options are similar to those of patients with GERD without metaplasia and consist of either proton pump inhibitors or a fundoplication. A surgical approach might offer an advantage over medical therapy for the following reasons:

1. Successful elimination of reflux symptoms with proton pump inhibitors does not guarantee control of acid reflux. When pH monitoring is performed in asymptomatic Barrett patients treated with these medications, up to 80% of them still have abnormal acid reflux.

2. Proton pump inhibitors do not eliminate the reflux of bile, a major contributor to the pathogenesis of Barrett esophagus. In contrast, an antireflux operation prevents any form of reflux by restoring the competence of the gastroesophageal junction

3. A fundoplication may promote regression of the columnar epithelium. Many studies have shown that regression occurs in 15–50% of patients when the length of the Barrett segment is less than 3 cm. Regardless of the effect of the fundoplication on symptoms, surveillance endoscopy should be performed every 12–24 months.

B. Barrett Esophagus: Low-Grade Dysplasia

Patients with low-grade dysplasia should be treated for 1–2 months with high doses of proton pump inhibitors (3–4 pills per day), and subsequently the endoscopy should be repeated with multiple biopsies. The rationale for this approach is to decrease the mucosal inflammation by blocking acid secretion, allowing the pathologist a more accurate reading. If the repeated biopsies show metaplasia or high-grade dysplasia, the patient will be treated accordingly. If low-grade dysplasia is confirmed, the patient can continue taking acid-reducing medications or have a laparoscopic fundoplication. There is evidence that regression to metaplasia or even disappearance of the columnar epithelium can occur after a successful fundoplication. Surveillance endoscopy should be performed every 6–12 months.

C. Barrett Esophagus: High-Grade Dysplasia

When high-grade dysplasia is found (the diagnosis must be confirmed by two experienced pathologists), two treatment options are available:

(1) Patients can enroll in a program of strict endoscopic surveillance, with endoscopy performed every 3 months and 4-quadrant biopsies obtained for every centimeter of Barrett epithelium. The goal is to detect cancer as soon as it develops but before it becomes invasive and spreads to lymph nodes. Progression from high-grade dysplasia to cancer occurs in about 50% of patients 5 years after the initial diagnosis is established. This approach is reasonable if the patient is willing to undergo endoscopy every 3 months but unwilling to have an esophagectomy or if severe comorbid conditions (cardiac or respiratory disease) are present.

(2) For young and medically fit patients who are unwilling to undergo endoscopy every 3 months, an esophagectomy should be considered. The rationale for an operation is based on the following considerations: (a) cancer is already found in about 30% of patients thought to have high-grade dysplasia; (b) cancer develops in about 50% of patients during follow-up; (c) recent studies have shown that in specialized centers the operation can be performed with minimal morbidity, no mortality, and postoperative quality of life similar to that of the general population; and (d) because the prognosis depends on the pathologic staging, waiting exposes patients to the risk of development of invasive cancer with lymph node metastases.

D. Endoscopic Treatment Modalities

Because either acid-reducing medications or a fundoplication determine regression in some patients with a short segment only, and because there is no evidence that they block progression to cancer, different modalities have been developed for the endoscopic ablation of the Barrett epithelium. Photodynamic therapy is based on the administration of a photosensitizing drug, which is retained in the Barrett epithelium. Light of proper wavelength is then delivered endoscopically, producing an oxidative reaction with destruction of the abnormal mucosa. Complete destruction of the columnar epithelium can be achieved in about 50% of patients. This technique, however, is associated with the development of esophageal strictures in about 30% of patients. In addition, islands of columnar epithelium can still be present under the regenerated squamous epithelium. A new technique based on radio frequency ablation seems to avoid these problems and is effective in about 70% of patients. In selected patients with short islands of Barrett epithelium, the mucosa can be resected endoscopically.

Chang LC et al: Long-term outcome of esophagectomy for high grade dysplasia or cancer found during surveillance for Barrett's esophagus. J Gastrointest Surg 2006;10:341.

Corley DA et al: Surveillance and survival in Barrett's adenocarcinomas: a population-based study. Gastroenterology 2002; 122:633.

Ganapathy AP et al: Long-term survival following endoscopic and surgical treatment of high-grade dysplasia in Barrett's esophagus. Gastroenterology 2007;132:1226.

Gerson LB et al: Prevalence of Barrett's esophagus in asymptomatic individuals. Gastroenterology 2002;123:461.

Moraca RJ et al: Outcomes and health-related quality of life after esophagectomy for high-grade dysplasia and intramucosal cancer. Arch Surg 2006;141:545.

Oelschlager BK et al: Clinical and pathologic response of Barrett's esophagus to laparoscopic antireflux surgery. Ann Surg 2003;238:458.

Shaheen NJ: Advances in Barrett's esophagus and esophageal adenocarcinoma. Gastroenterology 2005;128:1554.

Sharma VK et al: Balloon-based circumferential, endoscopic radiofrequency ablation of Barrett's esophagus: one year follow-up of 100 patients. Gastrointest Endosc 2007;65:185.

Smith CD et al: Endoscopic ablation of intestinal metaplasia containing high-grade dysplasia in esophagectomy patients using a balloon-based ablation system. Surg Endosc 2007; 21:560.

HIATAL HERNIA

PARAESOPHAGEAL HIATAL HERNIA

 ESSENTIALS OF DIAGNOSIS

▶ May be asymptomatic.

▶ Symptoms secondary to mechanical obstruction: dysphagia, epigastric discomfort, bleeding.

▶ Symptoms secondary to gastroesophageal reflux: heartburn, regurgitation.

▶ General Considerations

There are two types of esophageal hiatal hernia: paraesophageal and sliding (the sliding type was discussed in the section on Gastroesophageal Reflux Disease); see Figures 20–9 and 20–10. Obesity, aging, and general weakening of the musculofascial structures set the stage for enlargement of the esophageal hiatus and herniation of the stomach into the posterior mediastinum.

There are two types of paraesophageal hernia. In one type, the less common, part of the stomach herniates into the thorax immediately adjacent to an undisplaced gastroesophageal junction (Figures 20–11 and 20–12). Since the gastroesophageal sphincteric mechanism functions normally in most of these cases, reflux of gastric contents is uncommon. More commonly, however, the paraesophageal herniation occurs in association with the sliding type, and symptoms due to gastroesophageal reflux may occur along with symptoms secondary to the mechanical obstruction.

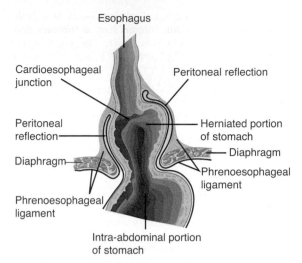

▲ **Figure 20–9.** Sliding esophageal hiatal hernia.

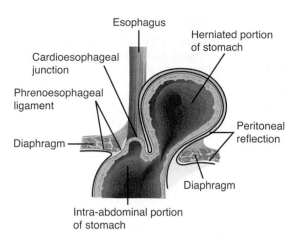

▲ **Figure 20–11.** Paraesophageal hernia.

▶ Clinical Findings

Symptoms usually develop late in adult life. Patients can experience epigastric discomfort, postprandial bloating, or dysphagia or have anemia secondary to gastric erosions. In addition, they may experience symptoms due to gastroesophageal reflux.

▶ Diagnosis

A barium swallow will delineate the anatomy and the type of hiatal hernia. Endoscopy is important to determine if gastric or esophageal inflammation is present and to rule out cancer. If reflux symptoms are present, manometry and pH monitoring should be performed.

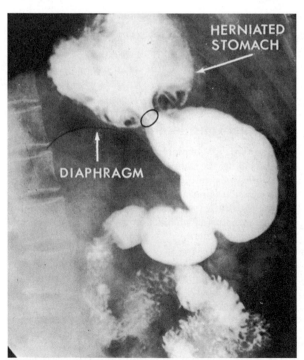

▲ **Figure 20–10.** Large sliding hiatal hernia. Diaphragmatic hiatus is circled.

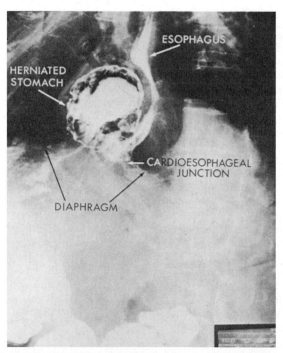

▲ **Figure 20–12.** Paraesophageal hernia. Note that the cardioesophageal junction remains in its normal anatomic position below the diaphragm.

Complications

The most frequent complications of paraesophageal hernia are hemorrhage, incarceration, obstruction, and strangulation. The herniated portion of the stomach often becomes congested, and bleeding occurs from erosions of the mucosa. Obstruction may occur, most often at the esophagogastric junction as a result of torsion and angulation at this point—especially if a large portion (or all) of the stomach herniates into the chest. In paraesophageal hiatal hernia—in contrast to the sliding type—other viscera such as the small and large intestines and spleen may also enter the mediastinum along with the stomach.

Treatment

Operative repair is indicated in symptomatic patients. The usual method is to return the herniated stomach below the diaphragm into the abdomen, repair the enlarged esophageal hiatus, and then add a fundoplication. In most cases, the operation can be performed laparoscopically.

Prognosis

The results of surgical management are excellent in about 90% of patients.

Aly A et al: Laparoscopic repair of larger hiatal hernias. Br J Surg 2005;92:648.
Oelschlager BK et al: Biologic prosthesis reduces recurrence after laparoscopic paraesophageal hernia repair. A multicenter, prospective, randomized trial. Ann Surg 2006;244:481.
Zaninotto G et al: Objective follow-up after laparoscopic repair of large type III hiatal hernia. Assessment of safety and durability. World J Surg 2007;31:2177.

TUMORS OF THE ESOPHAGUS

1. Benign Tumors of the Esophagus

ESSENTIALS OF DIAGNOSIS

► Dysphagia, epigastric discomfort.
► Radiographic demonstration of a smooth filling defect within the esophageal lumen.

General Considerations

Esophageal leiomyomas are the most common benign tumors of the esophagus. They represent 10% of all gastrointestinal leiomyomas. They originate in the smooth muscle layers, mostly in the lower two thirds of the esophagus, and they narrow the esophageal lumen. These tumors consist of smooth muscle cells surrounded by a capsule of fibrous tissue. The mucosa overlying the tumor is generally intact, but occasionally it may become ulcerated as a result of pressure necrosis by an enlarging lesion. Leiomyomas are not associated with the development of cancer. Other tumors such as fibromas, lipomas, fibromyomas, and myxomas are rare. Congenital cysts or duplications of the esophagus (the second-most common benign lesion after leiomyomas) may occur at any level, although they are most common in the lower esophagus.

Clinical Findings

Many benign lesions are asymptomatic and are discovered incidentally during upper gastrointestinal fluoroscopic examination. Benign tumors or cysts grow slowly and become symptomatic only after reaching a size of 5 cm or more. On barium swallow, leiomyomas appear as a smooth filling defect within the esophageal lumen (Figure 20–13). An intraluminal mass covered by normal mucosa can be easily recognized during endoscopy, but biopsies should not be taken because they may make subsequent enucleation of the tumor more difficult. Endoscopic ultrasound and chest CT help in the characterization of the tumor and in the differential diagnosis.

Differential Diagnosis

Leiomyomas, cysts, and duplications can be distinguished from cancer by their classic radiographic appearance. Intraluminal papillomas, polyps, or granulomas may be indistinguishable radiographically from early carcinoma, so their exact nature must be confirmed histologically.

Treatment

Small polypoid intraluminal lesions may be removed endoscopically. The treatment of choice for symptomatic leiomyomas

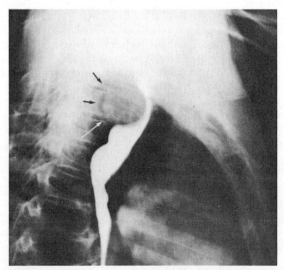

▲ **Figure 20–13.** Leiomyoma of esophagus. Note smooth, rounded density causing extrinsic compression of esophageal lumen.

is enucleation. While in the past a thoracotomy or a laparotomy was used to expose the esophagus and remove the tumor, today enucleation can be accomplished by either a thoracoscopic or a laparoscopic approach.

Herbella FA et al: Thoracoscopic resection of esophageal duplication cysts. Dis Esophagus 2006;19:132.

Kent M et al: Minimally invasive resection of benign esophageal tumors. J Thorac Cardiovasc Surg 2007;134:177.

Mutrie CJ et al: Esophageal leiomyomas: A 40-year experience. Ann Thorac Surg 2005;79:1122.

2. Carcinoma of the Esophagus

 ESSENTIALS OF DIAGNOSIS

▶ Progressive dysphagia, initially for solids and later for liquids.

▶ Progressive weight loss.

▶ Diagnosis established by endoscopy and biopsies.

▶ Staging established by endoscopic ultrasound, computed tomography of chest and abdomen, and positron emission tomography. Bronchoscopy indicated for cancer of the mid thoracic esophagus.

General Considerations

In the United States, esophageal carcinoma accounts for 10,000–11,000 deaths per year. The epidemiology of esophageal cancer in the United States has changed considerably during the last 30 years. In the 1970s, squamous cell carcinoma was the most common type of esophageal cancer, accounting for about 90% of the total cases. It was located in the thoracic esophagus and affected mostly black men. Over the past three decades, there has been a progressive increase in the incidence of adenocarcinoma of the distal esophagus and gastroesophageal junction, so that today it accounts for more than 70% of all new cases of esophageal cancer. Adenocarcinoma is more frequent in white men with GERD. Squamous cell cancer is still the most common type worldwide. Esophageal cancer occurs mostly during the fifth to seventh decades of life and is more common in men than in women.

Pathogenesis

The most common contributing factors for squamous cell carcinoma are cigarette smoking and chronic alcohol exposure. Chronic ingestion of hot liquids or foods, poor oral hygiene, and nutritional deficiencies may play a role. Certain medical conditions such as achalasia, caustic injuries of the esophagus, and Plummer-Vinson syndrome are associated with an increased incidence of squamous cell cancer. GERD is the most common predisposing factor for adenocarcinoma of the esophagus, where adenocarcinoma represents

the last event of a sequence that starts with GERD and progresses to metaplasia, high-grade dysplasia, and cancer. Esophageal cancer arises in the mucosa and subsequently invades the submucosa and the muscle layers. Ultimately, structures located next to the esophagus may be infiltrated (tracheobronchial tree, aorta, recurrent laryngeal nerve). At the same time, the tumor tends to metastasize to the lymph nodes (celiac, mediastinal, cervical) and to the liver, lungs, adrenals, and bones.

Clinical Findings

A. Symptoms

Dysphagia is the most common presenting symptom. Dysphagia is initially for solids but eventually it progresses to liquids. Weight loss occurs in more than 50% of patients. Patients can have pain when swallowing. Pain over bony structures may be due to metastases. Hoarseness is usually due to invasion of the right or left recurrent laryngeal nerves with paralysis of the ipsilateral vocal cord. Respiratory symptoms may be due to regurgitation and aspiration of undigested food or to invasion of the tracheobronchial tree, with development of a tracheoesophageal fistula.

B. Imaging Studies

Barium swallow shows the location and the extent of the tumor. Esophageal cancer usually presents as an irregular intraluminal mass or a stricture (Figure 20–14). Endoscopy allows direct visualization and biopsies of the tumor. For tumors of the upper and midesophagus, bronchoscopy is indicated to rule out invasion of the tracheobronchial tree.

C. Special Tests

After the diagnosis is established, it is important to determine the staging of the cancer (Table 20–4). Abdominal and chest CT scans are useful to detect distant organ metastases (M, metastases) and invasion of structures next to the esophagus. Alternatively, PET can be used. Endoscopic ultrasound is the most sensitive test to determine the penetration of the tumor (T, tumor), the presence of enlarged periesophageal lymph nodes (N, nodes), and invasion of structures next to the esophagus. Fine-needle aspiration of enlarged periesophageal lymph nodes can be done under ultrasound guidance. A bone scan is indicated in patients with new onset of bone pain.

Differential Diagnosis

The differential diagnosis includes peptic strictures due to reflux, achalasia, and benign esophageal tumors.

Treatment

Patients with esophageal cancer are considered candidates for esophageal resection if the following criteria are met:

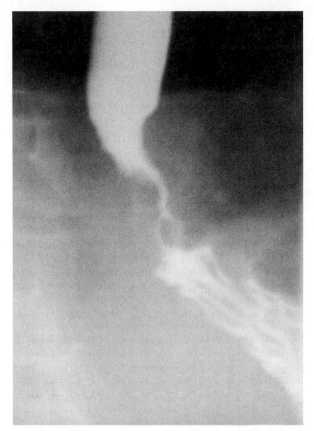

▲ **Figure 20–14.** Barium swallow demonstrating a distal esophageal carcinoma.

Table 20–4. American Joint Committee on Cancer (AJCC) Staging System (pTNM) of Esophageal Cancer.

Primary tumor (T)	
Tx	Primary tumor cannot be assessed
T0	No evidence of primary tumor
T1	Tumor invades lamina propria or submucosa
T2	Tumor invades muscularis propria
T3	Tumor invades adventitia
T4	Tumor invades adjacent structures
Regional lymph nodes (N)	
Nx	Regional nodes cannot be assessed
N0	No regional node metastasis
N1	Regional node metastasis
Distant metastasis (M)	
Mx	Presence of distant metastasis cannot be assessed
M0	No distant metastasis
M1a	Celiac node metastasis (lower esophagus)/supraclavicular node metastasis (upper esophagus)
M1b	Nonregional nodal metastasis or distant metastasis

Reproduced, with permission, from *AJCC Cancer Staging Manual,* 6th ed. Springer, 2002.

(1) there is no evidence of spread of the tumor to structures next to the esophagus such as the tracheobronchial tree, the aorta, or the recurrent laryngeal nerve; (2) there is no evidence of distant metastases; (3) the patient is fit from a cardiac and respiratory point of view. An esophagectomy can be performed by using an abdominal and a cervical incision (with blunt dissection of the thoracic esophagus through the esophageal hiatus; transhiatal esophagectomy) or by using an abdominal and a right chest incision (transthoracic esophagectomy). After removal of the esophagus, continuity of the gastrointestinal tract is reestablished by using either the stomach or the colon. The transhiatal esophagectomy offers the advantage of avoiding the chest incision, with decreased compromise of lung function and decreased postoperative discomfort. The validity of the transhiatal esophagectomy as a cancer operation was initially questioned because part of the operation is not done under direct vision and because of the small number of resected lymph nodes. However, many retrospective studies and prospective randomized trials have shown no difference in survival between the two operations, suggesting that it is not the type of operation that influences survival but rather the stage of the disease at the time the operation is performed. The morbidity rate of the operation is around 30%, and it is mostly due to cardiac (arrhythmias), respiratory (atelectasis, pleural effusion), and septic complications (anastomotic leak, pneumonia). The mortality rate in specialized centers is less than 5%. As with other complex operations (cardiac operation, liver and pancreatic resections), a lower mortality rate is obtained in "high-volume centers" and is due to the presence of an experienced team composed of surgeons, anesthesiologists, intensivists, cardiologists, radiologists, and nurses.

Because most patients already have lymph node metastases at the time of surgery, the 5-year survival for this disease remains poor. Neoadjuvant therapy based on a combination of radiotherapy and chemotherapy is used in order to improve local (radiotherapy) and distant control of the disease (chemotherapy). Overall, it seems that the combination of neoadjuvant therapy followed by surgery offers the best survival benefit. This is particularly true in the subgroup of patients (about 20%) who have a "complete pathologic response" (no tumor found in the specimen).

Nonoperative therapy is reserved for patients who are not candidates for surgery because of local invasion of the tumor, metastases, or a poor functional status. The goal of therapy in these patients is palliation of the dysphagia, allowing them to eat. The following treatment modalities are available to achieve this goal:

1. Expandable, coated, metallic stents can be deployed by endoscopy under fluoroscopic guidance in order to keep the esophageal lumen open. They are particularly useful when a tracheoesophageal fistula is present.

2. Laser therapy (Nd:YAG laser) relieves dysphagia in up to 70% of patients. However, multiple sessions are usually required to keep the esophageal lumen open.

3. Radiation therapy is successful in relieving dysphagia in about 50% of patients.

▶ Prognosis

The stage of the disease is the most important prognostic factor. Overall 5-year survival for esophageal cancer remains around 25%.

American Joint Committee on Cancer. *AJCC Cancer Staging Manual,* 6th ed. Springer Verlag, 2002:91.

Gebski V et al: Survival benefits from neoadjuvant chemoradiotherapy or chemotherapy in oesophageal carcinoma: a meta-analysis. Lancet Oncol 2007;8:226.

Hofstetter W et al: Proposed modification of nodal status in AJCC esophageal cancer staging system. Ann Thorac Surg 2007;84:365.

Kwon RS et al: Gastrointestinal cancer imaging: deeper than the eye can see. Gastroenterology 2005;128:1538.

Luketich JD et al: Minimally invasive esophagectomy. Outcomes in 222 patients. Ann Surg 2003;238:486.

Mariette C et al: Therapeutic strategies in oesophageal carcinoma: role of surgery and other modalities. Lancet Oncol 2007;8:545.

Orringer MB et al: Two thousand transhiatal esophagectomies. Changing trends, lessons learned. Ann Surg 2007;246:363.

Rasanen JV et al: Prospective analysis of accuracy of positron emission tomography, computed tomography, and endoscopic ultrasonography in staging of adenocarcinoma of the esophagus and esophagogastric junction. Ann Surg Oncol 2003;10:954.

Wang KK et al: American Gastroenterological Association technical review on the role of the gastroenterologists in the management of esophageal carcinoma. Gastroenterology 2005;128:1471.

OTHER SURGICAL DISORDERS OF THE ESOPHAGUS

PERFORATION OF THE ESOPHAGUS

ESSENTIALS OF DIAGNOSIS

▶ History of recent instrumentation of the esophagus or severe vomiting.

▶ Pain in the neck, chest, or upper abdomen.

▶ Signs of mediastinal or thoracic sepsis within 24 hours.

▶ Radiographic evidence of an esophageal leak.

▶ General Considerations

Esophageal perforations can result from iatrogenic instrumentation (eg, endoscopy, balloon dilation), severe vomiting, external trauma, and other rare causes. The subsequent clinical manifestations are influenced by the site of the perforation (ie, cervical or thoracic) and, in the case of thoracic perforations, whether or not the mediastinal pleura has been ruptured. Morbidity resulting from esophageal perforation is principally due to infection. Immediately after injury, the tissues are contaminated by esophageal contents, but infection has not become established; surgical closure of the defect will usually prevent the development of serious infection. If more than 24 hours have elapsed since the time of injury, severe contamination has occurred. At this time, the esophageal defect usually breaks down if it is surgically closed, and measures to treat mediastinitis and empyema may not be adequate to avoid a fatal outcome. Although serious infection usually occurs if surgical repair is delayed, a few cases of minor instrumental perforations can be managed by antibiotics without operation.

A. Instrumental Perforations

Medical instrumentation is the most common cause of esophageal perforation (diagnostic or therapeutic endoscopy). Instrumental perforations are most likely to occur in the cervical esophagus. The endoscope may press the posterior wall of the esophagus against osteoarthritic spurs of the cervical vertebrae, causing contusion or laceration. The cricopharyngeal area is the most common site of injury. Perforations of the thoracic esophagus may occur at any level but are most common at the natural sites of narrowing, at the level of the left main stem bronchus and at the diaphragmatic hiatus. Perforations during pneumatic dilatation for achalasia (2–6%) occur proximal to the gastroesophageal junction.

B. Spontaneous (Postemetic) Perforation (Boerhaave Syndrome)

Spontaneous perforation usually occurs in the absence of preexisting esophageal disease, but 10% of patients have reflux esophagitis, esophageal diverticulum, or carcinoma. Most cases follow a bout of heavy eating and drinking. The rupture usually involves all layers of the esophageal wall and most frequently occurs in the left posterolateral aspect, 3–5 cm above the gastroesophageal junction. The tear results from excessive intraluminal pressure, usually caused by violent retching and vomiting. Some cases have also been associated with childbirth, defecation, convulsions, heavy lifting, and forceful swallowing. The overlying pleura are also torn, so both the mediastinum and the pleural cavity are contaminated with esophageal contents. The second-most common site of perforation is at the midthoracic esophagus, on the right side at the level of the azygos vein.

Clinical Findings

A. Signs and Symptoms

The principal early manifestation is pain, which is felt in the neck with cervical perforations and in the chest or upper abdomen with perforations of the thoracic esophagus. The pain may radiate to the back. With cervical perforations, pain is followed by crepitus in the neck, dysphagia, and signs of infection. Perforations of the thoracic esophagus, which communicate with the pleural cavity in about 75% of cases, are usually accompanied by tachycardia, tachypnea, dyspnea, and the early development of hypotension. With perforation into the chest, pneumothorax is produced, followed by hydrothorax and, if not promptly treated, empyema. The left chest is involved in 70% and the right chest in 20%; involvement is bilateral in 10%. Escape of air into the mediastinum may result in a "mediastinal crunch," which is produced by the heart beating against air-filled tissues (Hamman sign). If the pleura remain intact, mediastinal emphysema appears more rapidly, and pleural effusion is slow to develop.

B. Imaging Studies

X-ray studies are important to demonstrate that perforation has occurred and to locate the site of the injury. In perforations of the cervical esophagus, x-rays show air in the soft tissues, especially along the cervical spine. The trachea may be displaced anteriorly by air and fluid. Later, widening of the superior mediastinum may be seen. With thoracic perforations, mediastinal widening and pleural effusion with or without pneumothorax are the usual findings. An esophagogram using water-soluble contrast medium should be performed promptly in every patient suspected of having an esophageal perforation (Figure 20–15). If a leak is not seen, the examination should be repeated using barium. A CT scan of the chest is also useful to localize the perforation and eventually to drain mediastinal fluid collections.

C. Special Studies

Thoracentesis will reveal cloudy or purulent fluid, depending on how much time has passed since the time of perforation. The amylase content of the fluid is elevated, and serum amylase levels may also be high as a result of absorption of amylase from the pleural cavity.

Treatment

Antibiotics should be given immediately. The infection is usually polymicrobial with *Staphylococcus, Streptococcus, Pseudomonas,* and *Bacteroides.* Early operation is appropriate for all but a few cases, and every effort should be made to operate before the perforation is 24 hours old. For lesions treated within this time limit, the operation should consist of closure of the perforation and external drainage. External drainage alone may suffice for small cervical perforations, which may be difficult to find. Patients with achalasia in

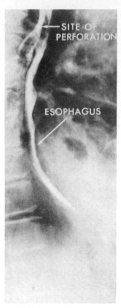

▲ **Figure 20–15.** Extravasation of contrast material through instrumental perforation of upper thoracic esophagus. Note loculi of air and fluid anterior to esophagus, indicating that mediastinitis has already developed.

whom perforation has resulted from balloon dilation should have the tear in the esophagus repaired and a Heller myotomy performed on the opposite side of the esophagus. Definitive therapy (eg, resection) should also be performed in patients with other surgical conditions, such as esophageal carcinoma.

Primary repair has a high failure rate if the perforation is older than 24 hours. The classic recommendation in this situation has been to isolate the perforation (ie, to minimize further contamination) by performing a temporary cervical esophagostomy, ligating the esophagus just proximal to the gastroesophageal junction, and placing a feeding jejunostomy for enteral nutrition. Alternatively, the segment of esophagus where the perforation is located can be resected, bringing the proximal end of esophagus out through the neck and closing the distal end. The mediastinum is drained, and a feeding jejunostomy is created. Later, the esophagostomy is taken down, and stomach or colon are interposed to bridge the gap. Blunt esophagectomy may be feasible as emergency treatment of instrumental perforation in a patient with lye stricture.

Nonoperative management consisting of antibiotics alone may be all that is necessary in a few selected cases of instrumental perforation. This approach should be confined to patients without thoracic involvement (eg, pneumothorax or hydrothorax) whose esophagogram demonstrates just a short extraluminal sinus tract without wide mediastinal spread (ie, the contamination is limited) and who have no systemic signs of sepsis (eg, hypotension and tachypnea). Recently, esophageal stents have been placed for the treatment of iatrogenic, intrathoracic esophageal perforations.

► Prognosis

The survival rate is 90% when surgical treatment is accomplished within 24 hours. The rate drops to about 50% when treatment is delayed.

Freeman RK et al: Esophageal stent placement for the treatment of iatrogenic, intrathoracic esophageal perforation. Ann Thorac Surg 2007;83:2003.

Kiev J et al: A management algorithm for esophageal perforation. Am J Surg 2007;194:103.

Vogel SB et al: Esophageal perforation in adults: aggressive, conservative treatment lowers morbidity and mortality. Ann Surg 2005;241:1016.

INGESTED FOREIGN OBJECTS

Most cases of ingested foreign objects occur in children who swallow coins or other small objects. In adults, the problem most often consists of esophageal meat impaction or, less commonly, lodged bones or toothpicks. Dentures and esophageal disease, such as a benign stricture, are the principal predisposing factors in adults. Prisoners and mentally ill persons occasionally swallow foreign objects intentionally.

About 90% of swallowed foreign objects pass into the stomach and from there into the intestine and are eventually passed without problems. Ten percent hang up in the esophagus. If they traverse the esophagus, objects whose dimensions exceed 2–5 cm tend to remain in the stomach. Ten percent of ingested foreign objects require endoscopic removal, and 1% requires surgery. About 10% of ingested foreign objects enter the tracheobronchial tree.

The patient's history usually defines the problem adequately. The patient with a foreign object in the esophagus may or may not experience dysphagia or chest pain.

► Specific Kinds of Ingested Foreign Objects

A. Coins

Pennies and dimes usually pass into the stomach, but larger coins will lodge in the esophagus at or just beyond the cricopharyngeus. It is important to know if a swallowed coin has remained in the esophagus, and whether or not the patient has symptoms is an unreliable basis for making the determination. Therefore, anteroposterior and lateral chest x-rays should be obtained to determine whether the coin is in the esophagus or trachea. Small children should be x-rayed from the base of the skull to the anus in order to find any additional coins in the gut.

Coins in the esophagus should be removed promptly, since complications may occur if treatment delay exceeds 24 hours. The procedure is best accomplished with a grasping forceps passed through a flexible endoscope. Sedation is adequate for older children or adults, but general endotracheal anesthesia is required in order to protect the airway of infants and young children. A smooth foreign body too large to grasp with a forceps can be removed by passing a dilating balloon beyond it and then withdrawing the endoscope and balloon as a unit. If the object is small enough (< 20 mm), it may be pushed into the stomach.

Once a coin has passed into the stomach, it can be observed by periodic x-rays for as long as a month before the conclusion is reached that spontaneous elimination is unlikely and endoscopic removal is indicated.

B. Meat Impaction

Meat is the most common foreign object that lodges in the esophagus of adults, and many affected patients have underlying esophageal disease. The site of meat impaction is usually at the cricopharyngeus muscle or in the distal esophagus in patients with achalasia, diffuse esophageal spasm, or a stricture.

No x-rays (especially barium studies) are indicated, for they make the endoscopist's task more difficult. If obstruction is complete and the patient cannot handle saliva, endoscopy should be performed as an emergency to prevent aspiration. If the clinical findings are minor, however, endoscopy can be postponed for up to 12 hours (but no longer) to see whether the food will pass spontaneously.

Meat can usually be removed as a single piece using a polypectomy snare passed through a flexible endoscope. In some cases, a meat bolus can be pushed into the stomach, which is safe so long as it passes with minimal pressure. After the esophagus has been cleared, it should be checked endoscopically for underlying disease. An esophageal stricture should be dilated if the esophageal wall is not acutely inflamed as a result of the meat impaction.

C. Sharp and Pointed Objects

Bones, safety pins, hat pins, razor blades, toothpicks, nails, and many others constitute this group of foreign objects. The general principles of management are (1) to remove these objects endoscopically by grasping and pulling a blunt side (eg, the hinge of an open safety pin) with forceps, (2) to remove a piece of glass or a razor blade by pulling it into the lumen of a rigid esophagoscope, or (3) to operate if neither of these methods appears to be safe. Sharp or pointed objects in the stomach should be removed surgically, since 25% of them will perforate the intestine, usually near the ileocecal valve, if they exit the pylorus.

D. Button Batteries

These small batteries are swallowed by children, just like coins, but unlike coins, they are highly corrosive and should be removed urgently before a serious complication such as an esophagotracheal or esophagoaortic fistula develops.

E. Cocaine Packets

Cocaine smugglers may swallow small packets of cocaine in balloons or condoms. Rupture of just one of these packets can be fatal, so attempts at endoscopic removal are unsafe. If it appears that the packets will pass spontaneously, the patient may be watched; otherwise, surgical removal is indicated.

Louie JP et al: Witnessed and unwitnessed esophageal foreign bodies in children. Pediatr Emerg Care 2005;21:582.

Tokar B et al: Ingested gastrointestinal foreign bodies: predisposing factors for complications in children having surgical or endoscopic removal. Pediatr Surg Int 2007;23:135.

CAUSTIC INJURIES OF THE ESOPHAGUS

ESSENTIALS OF DIAGNOSIS

▶ History of ingestion of caustic liquids or solids.

▶ Burns of the lips, mouth, tongue, and oropharynx.

▶ Chest pain and dysphagia.

▶ General Considerations

Ingestion of strong solutions of acid or alkali or of solid substances of similar nature produces extensive chemical burns. The injury usually represents a suicide attempt in adults and accidental ingestion in children. Strong alkali produces "liquefaction necrosis," which involves dissolution of protein and collagen, saponification of fats, dehydration of tissues, thrombosis of blood vessels, and deep penetrating injuries. Acids produce a "coagulation necrosis" involving eschar formation, which tends to shield the deeper tissues from injury. Depending upon the concentration and the length of time the irritant remains in contact with the mucosa, sloughing of the mucous membrane, edema and inflammation of the submucosa, infection, perforation, and mediastinitis may develop.

Ingested lye in solid form tends to adhere to the mucosa of the pharynx and proximal esophagus. Severe acute esophageal necrosis is rare, and the main clinical problems are early edema and late stricture formation, principally of the proximal esophagus. Liquid caustics commonly produce much more extensive esophageal necrosis, and occasionally even tracheoesophageal and esophagoaortic fistulas. If the patient survives the acute phase, a lengthy nondilatable stricture often develops.

Ingestion of strong acid characteristically produces greatest injury to the stomach, with the esophagus remaining intact in over 80% of cases. The result may be immediate gastric necrosis or late antral stenosis.

Nearly all severe injuries are caused by strong alkali. Weak alkali and acid are associated with less extensive lesions.

▶ Clinical Findings

A. Symptoms and Signs

Systemic symptoms roughly parallel the severity of the caustic burn. The most common finding is inflammatory edema of the lips, mouth, tongue, and oropharynx; in the absence of visible injury in this area, severe esophageal damage is rare. Patients with serious esophageal burns often experience chest pain and dysphagia and drooling of large amounts of saliva. Pain on swallowing may be intense. If the damage is severe, the patient often appears toxic, with high fever, prostration, and shock. The absence of toxicity does not rule out severe injury. Tracheobronchitis accompanied by coughing and increased bronchial secretions is frequently noted. Stridor may be present, and in a few patients respiratory obstruction progresses rapidly and requires tracheostomy for relief. Complete esophageal obstruction due to edema, inflammation, and mucosal sloughing may develop within the first few days.

B. Esophagoscopy

Endoscopy is the key test in the evaluation of caustic trauma to the esophagus. Determination of the extent of injury by esophagoscopy contributes substantially to therapeutic decisions. Endoscopy should be performed after the initial resuscitation, usually within 24 hours of admission. The scope is inserted far enough to gauge the most serious degree of burn, which is classified as first-, second-, or third-degree, as defined in Table 20–5.

Table 20–5. Endoscopic Grading of Corrosive Burns of Esophagus and Stomach.

Grade	Definition	Endoscopic Findings
First-degree	Superficial mucosal injury	Mucosal hyperemia and edema; superficial mucosal desquamation.
Second-degree	Full-thickness mucosal involvement. No or partial-thickness muscular injury.	Sloughing of mucosa. Hemorrhage, exudate, ulceration, pseudomembrane formation, and granulation tissue when examined late.
Third-degree	Full-thickness esophageal or gastric injury with extension into adjacent tissues.	Sloughing of tissues with deep ulceration. Complete obliteration of esophageal lumen by edema; charring and eschar formation; full-thickness necrosis; perforation.

Reproduced, with permission, from Estrera A et al: Corrosive burns of the esophagus and stomach: a recommendation for an aggressive surgical approach. Ann Thorac Surg 1986;41:276.

C. Radiology

A chest x-ray should be taken in all patients. It may show signs of esophageal perforation (subcutaneous emphysema, pneumomediastinum, pneumothorax) or aspiration (pulmonary infiltrates).

An esophagogram is indicated in the initial evaluation if perforation is suspected and in later stages to detect the presence of a stricture.

▶ Treatment

Patients should be hospitalized and intravenous fluids started. Intravenous antibiotics should be administered. The use of steroids is still controversial. A nasogastric tube placed under fluoroscopic or endoscopic guidance allows stenting of the esophagus, preventing complete obstruction of the lumen.

Patients with first-degree burns do not require aggressive therapy and may be discharged from the hospital after a short period of observation. Second-degree and minor spotty third-degree injuries are treated by inserting a nasogastric tube. Nutrition can be given through the nasogastric tube or parenterally. Periodic esophagograms are obtained in follow-up to look for stricture formation, which is treated early in its development by dilations and eventually resection.

Third-degree burns involving extensive esophagogastric necrosis require emergency esophagogastrectomy, esophagostomy, and feeding jejunostomy. Esophagectomy is best performed by the blunt technique using a laparotomy and cervical incision. It is sometimes necessary to resect adjacent organs (eg, transverse colon) that have also been damaged. Reconstruction by substernal colon interposition is performed 8–12 weeks later.

▶ Prognosis

Early and proper management of caustic burns provides satisfactory results in most cases. The ingestion of strong acid or alkaline solutions with extensive immediate destruction of the mucosa produces profound pathologic changes that may result in fibrous strictures that require dilations and, in some cases, esophagectomy and colon interposition.

Ertekin C et al: The results of caustic ingestions. Hepatogastroenterology 2004;51:1397.
Keh SM et al: Corrosive injury to upper gastrointestinal tract: still a major surgical dilemma. World J Gastroenterol 2006;12:5223.

ESOPHAGEAL BANDS, WEBS, OR RINGS

A narrow mucosal ring (**Schatzki ring**) may develop at the lower end of the esophagus. Most patients are relatively free from symptoms. Dysphagia occurs when the ring is less than 12 mm in diameter. In most cases, the ring is located at the squamocolumnar junction and occurs in a patient with GERD. Being confined to the mucosa, it differs from an inflammatory (peptic) stricture, which involves all layers of the esophagus. A barium swallow clearly identifies the problem. Treatment consists of endoscopic dilatation of the ring and treatment of the associated reflux (acid-reducing medications or fundoplication).

Jalil S, Castell DO: Schatzki's ring: a benign cause of dysphagia in adults. J Clin Gastroenterol 2002;35:295.
Sgouros SN et al: Single-session, graded esophageal dilation without fluoroscopy in outpatients with lower esophageal (Schatzki) rings: a prospective, long-term follow-up study. J Gastroenterol Hepatol 2007;22:653.

▌ II. THE DIAPHRAGM

The diaphragm (Figure 20–16) is a musculotendinous, dome-shaped structure attached posteriorly to the first, second, and third lumbar vertebrae, anteriorly to the lower sternum and laterally to the costal arches. It separates the abdominal and the thoracic cavities. The diaphragm allows the passage of various normal structures through anatomic foramina. The aortic hiatus lies posteriorly at the level of the 12th thoracic vertebra, and through it pass the aorta, the thoracic duct, and the azygos venous system. The esophageal hiatus lies immediately anteriorly and slightly to the left at the level of the tenth thoracic vertebra and is separated from the aortic hiatus by the decussation of the right crus of the diaphragm. Through this hiatus pass the esophagus and the vagus nerves. At the level of the ninth thoracic vertebra and slightly to the right of the esophageal hiatus is the vena caval foramen, which allows passage of the inferior vena cava and small branches of the phrenic nerve. The phrenic arteries arising directly from the aorta supply the diaphragm along with the lower intercostal arteries and the terminal branches of the internal mammary arteries.

PARASTERNAL OR RETROSTERNAL (FORAMEN OF MORGAGNI) HERNIA & PLEUROPERITONEAL (FORAMEN OF BOCHDALEK) HERNIA

Failure of fusion of the sternal and costal portions of the diaphragm anteriorly in the midline creates a defect (foramen of Morgagni) through which hernias can occur. Normally, the diaphragm becomes fused, allowing only the internal mammary arteries and their superior epigastric branches, along with lymphatics, to pass through this area. Posterolaterally, failure of fusion of the pleuroperitoneal canal creates a defect through which viscera may herniate to produce a foramen of Bochdalek hernia (Figure 20–17).

Although both types of hernia are congenital, symptoms in the Morgagni hernia usually do not develop until middle life or later. This type of hernia is more frequent in women. These hernias are mostly right-sided and have a hernia sac. The most common contents are the omentum, the colon, and the stomach. On the other hand, the Bochdalek hernia

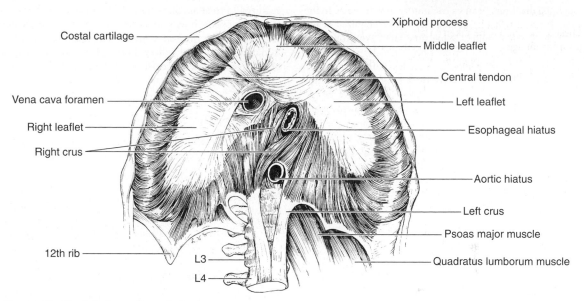

▲ **Figure 20–16.** Inferior surface of diaphragm.

occurs more frequently on the left side and may cause severe respiratory distress at birth, requiring an emergent operation. Routine chest films show a retrosternal solid mass, a retrosternal air-filled viscus, or similar findings in the posterolateral thorax if a Bochdalek hernia is present. Chest CT confirms the diagnosis and identifies the contents of the hernia.

Elective surgical repair is indicated in most instances to prevent complications. An emergent operation may become necessary in the newborn infant who develops progressive cardiorespiratory insufficiency. Repair of the defect by a transabdominal approach is preferable, and the results are excellent. A minimally invasive approach (laparoscopic or thoracoscopic) has been recently used.

Dutta S et al: Use of a prosthetic patch for laparoscopic repair of Morgagni diaphragmatic hernia in children. J Laparoendoscop Adv Surg Tech 2007;17:391.
Minneci PC et al: Foramen of Morgagni hernia: changes in diagnosis and treatment. Ann Thorac Surg 2004;77:1956.

TRAUMATIC DIAPHRAGMATIC HERNIA

Traumatic rupture of the diaphragm may occur as a result of penetrating wounds or severe blunt external trauma. Lacerations usually occur in the tendinous portion of the diaphragm, most often on the left side. The liver provides protection to diaphragmatic injury on the right side except from penetrating wounds. Abdominal viscera may immediately herniate through the defect in the diaphragm into the pleural cavity or may gradually insinuate themselves into the thorax over a period of months or years.

▶ Clinical Findings

Diaphragmatic ruptures present in two ways. In the acute form, the patient has recently experienced blunt trauma or a penetrating wound to the chest, abdomen, or back. The clinical manifestations are essentially those of the associated injuries, but occasionally, massive herniation of abdominal viscera

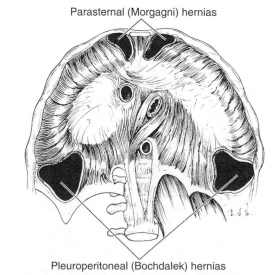

▲ **Figure 20–17.** Sites of congenital diaphragmatic herniation.

through the diaphragm causes respiratory insufficiency. In the chronic form, the diaphragmatic tear is unrecognized at the time of the original injury. Some time later, symptoms (eg, pain, bowel obstruction) appear from herniation of viscera. Respiratory symptoms in such cases are less common.

Plain films of the chest may show a radiopaque area and occasionally an air-fluid level if hollow viscera have herniated. If the stomach has entered the chest, the abnormal path of a nasogastric tube may be diagnostic. Ultrasonography, CT scan, and MRI may demonstrate the diaphragmatic rent. Barium study of the colon may show irregular patches of barium in the colon above the diaphragm or a smooth colonic outline if the colon does not contain feces.

Differential Diagnosis

Traumatic rupture of the diaphragm must be differentiated from atelectasis, space-consuming tumors of the lower pleural space, pleural effusion, and intestinal obstruction due to other causes.

Complications

Hemorrhage and obstruction may occur. If herniation is massive, progressive cardiorespiratory insufficiency may threaten life. The most severe complication is strangulating obstruction of the herniated viscera.

Treatment

For acute ruptures, a transabdominal (most commonly) or transthoracic route is used depending on the procedure required to treat ancillary injuries. When the diaphragmatic tear is the only injury, it is usually fixed by laparotomy. Chronic injuries can be repaired by either approach. Asymptomatic tears of the diaphragm with herniated viscera should be repaired, because the risk of strangulating obstruction is high. Laparoscopy is very useful for both diagnosis and treatment.

Prognosis

Surgical repair of the rent in the diaphragm is curative, and the prognosis is excellent. The diaphragm supports sutures well, so recurrence is practically unknown.

Baldassarre E et al: The role of laparoscopy in the diagnosis and treatment of missed diaphragmatic hernia after penetrating trauma. J Laparoendoscop Adv Surg Tech 2007;17:302.
Matthews BD et al: Laparoscopic repair of traumatic diaphragmatic injuries. Surg Endosc 2003;17:254.

TUMORS OF THE DIAPHRAGM

Primary tumors of the diaphragm are not common. The majority are benign lipomas. Pericardial cysts develop in the space between the heart and the diaphragm and are usually unilocular and on the right side. Fibrosarcoma, the most common primary malignant diaphragmatic tumor, is extremely rare.

Benign tumors are usually asymptomatic. Since their benign nature cannot be established except by histology, all lesions of this type should be excised through an appropriate thoracotomy or thoracoabdominal approach.

The Acute Abdomen

Gerard M. Doherty, MD

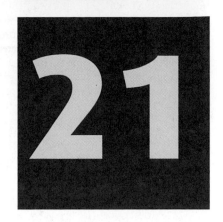

"An acute abdomen" denotes any sudden, spontaneous, nontraumatic disorder whose chief manifestation is in the abdominal area and for which urgent operation may be necessary. Because there is frequently a progressive underlying intra-abdominal disorder, undue delay in diagnosis and treatment adversely affects outcome.

The approach to a patient with an acute abdomen must be orderly and thorough. An acute abdomen must be suspected even if the patient has only mild or atypical complaints. The history and physical examination should suggest the probable causes and guide the choice of initial diagnostic studies. The clinician must then decide if in-hospital observation is warranted, if additional tests are needed, if early operation is indicated, or if nonoperative treatment would be more suitable.

All clinicians should be thoroughly familiar with the presenting pattern of the most common causes of an acute abdomen (Table 21–1). Moreover, they should be familiar with the disease patterns specific to the region and locality where they practice. Other chapters in this book provide detailed descriptions of specific diseases and their management.

HISTORY

▶ Abdominal Pain

History taking by an experienced physician is an active process whereby a cluster of diagnostic possibilities is considered in order to systematically eliminate less likely conditions. Pain is the most common and predominant presenting feature of an acute abdomen. Careful consideration of the location, the mode of onset and progression, and the character of the pain will suggest a preliminary list of differential diagnoses.

A. Location of Pain

Because of the complex dual visceral and parietal sensory network innervating the abdominal area, pain is not as pre-cisely localized as in the extremities. Fortunately, some general patterns do emerge that provide clues to diagnosis. Visceral sensation is mediated primarily by afferent C fibers located in the walls of hollow viscera and in the capsules of solid organs. Unlike cutaneous pain, **visceral pain** is elicited by distention, by inflammation or ischemia stimulating the receptor neurons, or by direct involvement (eg, malignant infiltration) of sensory nerves. The centrally perceived sensation is generally slow in onset, dull, poorly localized, and protracted. Different visceral structures are associated with different sensory levels in the spine (Table 21–2). Because of this, increased wall tension due to luminal distention or forceful smooth muscle contraction (colic) produces diffuse, deep-seated pain felt in the midepigastrium, periumbilical area, lower abdomen, or flank areas (Figure 21–1). Visceral pain is most often felt in the midline because of the bilateral sensory supply to the spinal cord.

By contrast, **parietal pain** is mediated by both C and A delta nerve fibers, the latter being responsible for the transmission of more acute, sharper, better-localized pain sensation. Direct irritation of the somatically innervated parietal peritoneum (especially the anterior and upper parts) by pus, bile, urine, or gastrointestinal secretions leads to more precisely localized pain. The cutaneous distribution of parietal pain corresponds to the T6–L1 areas. Parietal pain is more easily localized than visceral pain because the somatic afferent fibers are directed to only one side of the nervous system. Abdominal parietal pain is conventionally described as occurring in one of the four abdominal quadrants or in the epigastric or central abdominal area.

Abdominal pain may be referred or may shift to sites far removed from the primarily affected organs (Figure 21–2). **Referred pain** denotes noxious (usually cutaneous) sensations perceived at a site distant from that of a strong primary stimulus. Distorted central perception of the site of pain is due to the confluence of afferent nerve fibers from widely disparate areas within the posterior horn of the spinal cord. For example, pain due to subdiaphragmatic irritation by air,

Table 21–1. Common Causes of the Acute Abdomen.[1]

Gastrointestinal tract disorders
  Nonspecific abdominal pain
  Appendicitis
  Small and large bowel obstruction
  Perforated peptic ulcer
  Incarcerated hernia
  Bowel perforation
  Meckel's diverticulitis
  Boerhaave's syndrome
  Diverticulitis
  Inflammatory bowel disorders
  Mallory-Weiss syndrome
  Gastroenteritis
  Acute gastritis
  Mesenteric adenitis
  Parasitic infections
Liver, spleen, and biliary tract disorders
  Acute cholecystitis
  Acute cholangitis
  Hepatic abscess
  Ruptured hepatic tumor
  Spontaneous rupture of the spleen
  Splenic infarct
  Biliary colic
  Acute hepatitis
Pancreatic disorders
  Acute pancreatitis
Urinary tract disorders
  Ureteral or renal colic
  Acute pyelonephritis
  Acute cystitis
  Renal infarct
Gynecologic disorders
  Ruptured ectopic pregnancy
  Twisted ovarian tumor
  Ruptured ovarian follicle cyst
  Acute salpingitis
  Dysmenorrhea
  Endometriosis
Vascular disorders
  Ruptured aortic and visceral aneurysms
  Acute ischemic colitis
  Mesenteric thrombosis
Peritoneal disorders
  Intra-abdominal abscesses
  Primary peritonitis
  Tuberculous peritonitis
Retroperitoneal disorders
  Retroperitoneal hemorrhage

[1]The most common causes are marked with an asterisk. Conditions in italic type often require urgent operation.

Table 21–2. Sensory Levels Associated with Visceral Structures.

Structures	Nervous System Pathways	Sensory Level
Liver, spleen, and central part of diaphragm	Phrenic nerve	C3–5
Peripheral diaphragm, stomach, pancreas, gallbladder, and small bowel	Celiac plexus and greater splanchnic nerve	T6–9
Appendix, colon, and pelvic viscera	Mesenteric plexus and lesser splanchnic nerve	T10–11
Sigmoid colon, rectum, kidney, ureters, and testes	Lowest splanchnic nerve	T11–L1
Bladder and rectosigmoid	Hypogastric plexus	S2–4

peritoneal fluid, blood, or a mass lesion is referred to the shoulder via the C4-mediated (phrenic) nerve. Pain may also be referred to the shoulder from supradiaphragmatic lesions such as pleurisy or lower lobe pneumonia, especially in young patients. Although more often perceived in the right scapular region, referred biliary pain may mimic angina pectoris if it is perceived in the anterior chest or left shoulder areas. Posterolateral right flank pain may be seen in retrocecal appendicitis.

Spreading or shifting pain parallels the course of the underlying condition. The site of pain at onset should be distinguished from the site at presentation. Beginning classically in the epigastric or periumbilical region, the incipient visceral pain of acute appendicitis (due to distention of the appendix) later shifts to become sharper parietal pain localized in the right lower quadrant when the overlying peritoneum becomes directly inflamed (Figure 21–2). In perforated peptic ulcer, pain almost always begins in the epigastrium, but as the leaked gastric contents track down the right paracolic gutter, pain may descend to the right lower quadrant with even diminution of the epigastric pain.

The location of pain serves only as a rough guide to the diagnosis—"typical" descriptions are reported in only two thirds of cases. This great variability is due to atypical pain patterns, a shift of maximum intensity away from the primary site, or advanced or severe disease. In cases presenting late with diffuse peritonitis, generalized pain may completely obscure the precipitating event. Pain confined to either upper quadrant may be evaluated by anatomic consideration of acute conditions that affect the underlying organs.

B. Mode of Onset and Progression of Pain

The mode of onset of pain reflects the nature and severity of the inciting process. Onset may be explosive (within seconds), rapidly progressive (within 1–2 hours), or gradual (over several hours). Unheralded, excruciating generalized pain suggests an intra-abdominal catastrophe such as a perforated viscus or rupture of an aneurysm, ectopic pregnancy, or abscess. Accompanying systemic signs (tachycardia, sweating, tachypnea, shock) soon supersede the abdom-

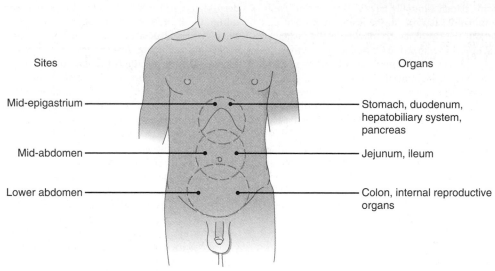

Sites

Mid-epigastrium

Mid-abdomen

Lower abdomen

Organs

Stomach, duodenum, hepatobiliary system, pancreas

Jejunum, ileum

Colon, internal reproductive organs

▲ **Figure 21–1.** Visceral pain sites.

inal disturbances and underscore the need for prompt resuscitation and laparotomy.

A less dramatic clinical picture is steady, mild pain becoming intensely centered in a well-defined area within 1–2 hours.

Any of the above conditions may present in this manner, but this mode of onset is more typical of acute cholecystitis, acute pancreatitis, strangulated bowel, mesenteric infarction, renal or ureteral colic, and high (proximal) small bowel obstruction.

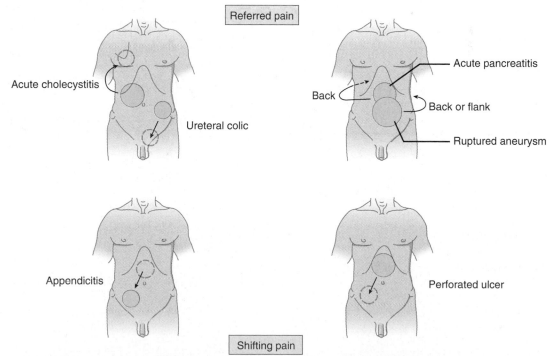

Referred pain

Acute cholecystitis

Ureteral colic

Acute pancreatitis

Back

Back or flank

Ruptured aneurysm

Appendicitis

Perforated ulcer

Shifting pain

▲ **Figure 21–2.** Referred pain and shifting pain in the acute abdomen. Solid circles indicate the site of maximum pain; dashed circles indicate sites of lesser pain.

Finally, some patients initially have slight—at times only vague—abdominal discomfort that is fleetingly present diffusely throughout the abdomen. It may be unclear whether these patients even have an acute abdomen or whether the illness is likely to be a matter for medical rather than surgical attention. Associated gastrointestinal symptoms are infrequent at first, and systemic symptoms are absent. Eventually, the pain and abdominal findings become more pronounced and steady and are localized to a smaller area. This pattern may reflect a slowly developing condition or the body's defensive efforts to cordon off an acute process. This broad category includes acute appendicitis (especially retrocecal or retroileal), incarcerated hernias, low (distal) small bowel and large bowel obstructions, uncomplicated peptic ulcer disease, walled-off (often malignant) visceral perforations, some genitourinary and gynecologic conditions, and milder forms of the rapid-onset group mentioned in the first paragraph.

C. Character of Pain

The nature, severity, and periodicity of pain provide useful clues to the underlying cause (Figure 21–3). Steady pain is most common. Sharp superficial constant pain due to severe peritoneal irritation is typical of perforated ulcer or a ruptured appendix, ovarian cyst, or ectopic pregnancy. The gripping, mounting pain of small bowel obstruction (and occasionally early pancreatitis) is usually intermittent, vague, deep-seated, and crescendo at first but soon becomes sharper, unremitting, and better localized. Unlike the disquieting but bearable pain associated with bowel obstruction, pain caused by lesions occluding smaller conduits (bile ducts, uterine tubes, and ureters) rapidly becomes unbearably intense. Pain is appropriately referred to as **colic** if there are pain-free intervals that reflect intermittent smooth muscle contractions, as in ureteral colic. In the strict sense, the term "biliary colic" is a misnomer because biliary pain does not remit. The reason is that the gallbladder and bile duct, in contrast to the ureters and intestine, do not have peristaltic movements. The "aching discomfort" of ulcer pain, the "stabbing, breathtaking" pain of acute pancreatitis and mesenteric infarction, and the "searing" pain of ruptured aortic aneurysm remain apt descriptions. Despite the use of such descriptive terms, the quality of visceral pain is not a reliable clue to its cause.

Agonizing pain denotes serious or advanced disease. Colicky pain is usually promptly alleviated by analgesics. Ischemic pain due to strangulated bowel or mesenteric thrombosis is only slightly assuaged even by narcotics. Nonspecific abdominal pain is usually mild, but mild pain may also be found with perforated ulcers that have become localized and in mild acute pancreatitis. An occasional patient will deny pain but complain of a vague feeling of abdominal fullness that feels as though it might be relieved by a bowel movement. This visceral sensation (**gas stoppage sign**) is due to reflex ileus induced by an inflammatory lesion

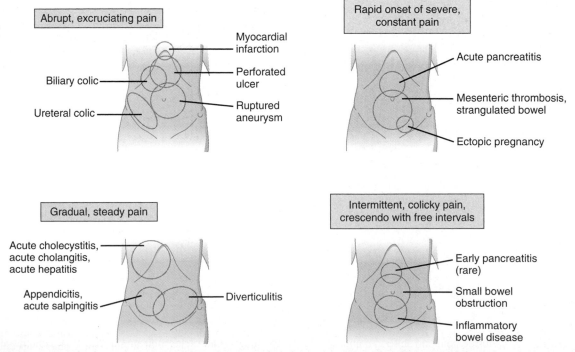

▲ **Figure 21–3.** The location and character of pain are helpful in the differential diagnosis of the acute abdomen.

walled off from the free peritoneal cavity, as in retrocecal or retroileal appendicitis.

Past episodes of pain and factors that aggravate or relieve pain should be noted. Pain caused by localized peritonitis, especially when it affects upper abdominal organs, tends to be exacerbated by movement or deep breathing.

The clinician should be familiar with the pathophysiology and salient features of the common causes of acute abdomen. The location, character, and severity of the pain in relation to its duration of onset along with the presence or absence of systemic symptoms help to differentiate rapidly progressive (and usually more serious) surgical conditions (eg, intestinal ischemia) from more indolent or medical causes (eg, ruptured ovarian cysts).

▶ Other Symptoms Associated with Abdominal Pain

Anorexia, nausea and vomiting, constipation, or diarrhea often accompanies abdominal pain, but since these are nonspecific symptoms, they do not have much diagnostic value.

A. Vomiting

When sufficiently stimulated by secondary visceral afferent fibers, the medullary vomiting centers activate efferent fibers to induce reflex vomiting. Hence, pain in the acute surgical abdomen usually precedes vomiting, whereas the reverse holds true in medical conditions. Vomiting is a prominent symptom in upper gastrointestinal diseases such as Boerhaave syndrome, Mallory-Weiss syndrome, acute gastritis, and acute pancreatitis. Severe, uncontrollable retching provides temporary pain relief in moderate attacks of pancreatitis. The absence of bile in the vomitus is a feature of pyloric stenosis. Where associated findings suggest bowel obstruction, the onset and character of vomiting may indicate the level of the lesion. Recurrent vomiting of bile-stained fluid is a typical early sign of proximal small bowel obstruction. In distal small or large bowel obstruction, prolonged nausea precedes vomiting, which may become feculent in late cases. Disorders that induce vomiting in younger patients may give rise only to anorexia or nausea in older patients. Although vomiting may present in either acute appendicitis or nonspecific abdominal pain, coexisting nausea and anorexia are more suggestive of the former condition.

B. Constipation

Reflex ileus is often induced by visceral afferent fibers stimulating efferent fibers of the sympathetic autonomic nervous system (splanchnic nerves) to reduce intestinal peristalsis. Hence, paralytic ileus undermines the value of constipation in the differential diagnosis of an acute abdomen. Constipation itself is hardly an absolute indicator of intestinal obstruction. However, **obstipation** (the absence of passage of both stool and flatus) strongly suggests mechanical bowel

obstruction if there is progressive painful abdominal distention or repeated vomiting.

C. Diarrhea

Copious watery diarrhea is characteristic of gastroenteritis and other medical causes of an acute abdomen. Blood-stained diarrhea suggests ulcerative colitis, Crohn disease, or bacillary or amebic dysentery. It is also common with ischemic colitis but often absent in intestinal infarction due to superior mesenteric artery occlusion.

D. Other Specific Symptoms

These are extremely helpful if present. **Jaundice** suggests hepatobiliary disorders; **hematochezia** or **hematemesis,** a gastroduodenal lesion or Mallory-Weiss syndrome; or **hematuria,** ureteral colic or cystitis. The passage of blood clots or necrotic mucosal debris may be the sole evidence of advanced intestinal ischemia.

▶ Other Relevant Aspects of the History

A. Gynecologic History

The menstrual history is crucial to the diagnosis of ectopic pregnancy, mittelschmerz (due to a ruptured ovarian follicle), and endometriosis. A history of vaginal discharge or dysmenorrhea may denote pelvic inflammatory disease.

B. Drug History

Anticoagulants have been implicated in retroperitoneal and intramural duodenal and jejunal hematomas; oral contraceptives have been implicated in the formation of benign hepatic adenomas and in mesenteric venous infarction. Corticosteroids, in particular, may mask the clinical signs of even advanced peritonitis. Pyloric perforation has been caused by "crack" smoking.

C. Family History

Family history often provides the best information about medical causes of an acute abdomen.

D. Travel History

Travel history may raise the possibility of amebic liver abscess or hydatid cyst, malarial spleen, tuberculosis, *Salmonella typhi* infection of the ileocecal area, or dysentery.

E. Operation History

Any history of a previous abdominal, groin, vascular, or thoracic operation may be relevant to the current illness. Particular attention to the mode of operation (laparoscopic, open, endovascular) and any anatomic reconstructions may clarify aspects of the current complaint. If possible within the time constraints imposed by the urgency of the current problem, operative notes and pathology reports should be obtained and reviewed.

PHYSICAL EXAMINATION

The tendency to concentrate on the abdomen should be resisted in favor of a methodical and complete general physical examination. A systematic approach to the abdominal examination is outlined in Table 21–3. One should search for specific signs that confirm or rule out differential diagnostic possibilities (Table 21–4).

(1) General observation: General observation affords a fairly reliable indication of the severity of the clinical situation. Most patients, although uncomfortable, remain calm. The writhing of patients with visceral pain (eg, intestinal or ureteral colic) contrasts with the rigidly motionless bearing of those with parietal pain (eg, acute appendicitis, generalized peritonitis). Diminished responsiveness or an altered sensorium often precedes imminent cardiopulmonary collapse.

(2) Systemic signs: Systemic signs usually accompany rapidly progressive or advanced disorders associated with an acute abdomen. Extreme pallor, hypothermia, tachycardia, tachypnea, and sweating suggest major intra-abdominal hemorrhage (eg, ruptured aortic aneurysm or tubal pregnancy). Given such findings, one must proceed rapidly with the subsequent examination and tests in order to exclude extra-abdominal causes and to institute treatment.

(3) Fever: Constant low-grade fever is common in inflammatory conditions such as diverticulitis, acute cholecystitis, and appendicitis. High fever with lower abdominal tenderness in a young woman without signs of systemic illness suggests acute salpingitis. Disorientation or extreme lethargy combined with a very high fever (> 39 °C) or swinging fever or with chills and rigors signifies impending septic shock. This is most often due to advanced peritonitis, acute cholangitis, or pyelonephritis. However, fever is often mild or absent in elderly, chronically ill, or immunosuppressed patients with a serious acute abdomen.

(4) Examination of the acute abdomen

(a) Inspection: The abdomen should be thoughtfully inspected before palpation. A tensely distended abdomen with an old surgical scar suggests both the presence and the cause (adhesions) of small bowel obstruction. A scaphoid contracted abdomen is seen with perforated ulcer; visible peristalsis occurs in thin patients with advanced bowel

Table 21–3. Steps in Physical Examination of the Acute Abdomen.

1. Inspection	7. Bump tenderness
2. Auscultation	Costal area
3. Cough tenderness	Costovertebral area
4. Percussion	8. Special signs
5. Guarding or rigidity	9. External hernias and
6. Palpation	male genitalia
One-finger	10. Rectal and pelvic
Rebound tenderness	examination
Deep	

Table 21–4. Physical Findings in Various Causes of Acute Abdomen.

Condition	Helpful Signs
Perforated viscus	Scaphoid, tense abdomen; diminished bowel sounds (late); loss of liver dullness; guarding or rigidity.
Peritonitis	Motionless; absent bowel sounds (late); cough and rebound tenderness; guarding or rigidity.
Inflamed mass or abscess	Tender mass (abdominal, rectal, or pelvic); bump tenderness; special signs (Murphy, psoas, or obturator).
Intestinal obstruction	Distention; visible peristalsis (late); hyperperistalsis (early) or quiet abdomen (late); diffuse pain without rebound tenderness; hernia or rectal mass (some).
Paralytic ileus	Distention; minimal bowel sounds; no localized tenderness.
Ischemic or strangulated bowel	Not distended (until late); bowel sounds variable; severe pain but little tenderness; rectal bleeding (some).
Bleeding	Pallor, shock; distention; pulsatile (aneurysm) or tender (eg, ectopic pregnancy) mass; rectal bleeding (some).

obstruction; and soft doughy fullness is seen in early paralytic ileus or mesenteric thrombosis.

(b) Auscultation: Auscultation of the abdomen should also precede palpation. Peristaltic rushes synchronous with colic are heard in mid small bowel obstruction and in early acute pancreatitis. These tend to last longer but occur less frequently than in normal patients or in those with acute cholecystitis. They differ from the high-pitched hyperperistaltic sounds unrelated to the crampy pain of gastroenteritis, dysentery, and fulminant ulcerative colitis. An abdomen that is silent except for infrequent tinkly or squeaky sounds characterizes late bowel obstruction or diffuse peritonitis. Except for these more extreme patterns, the many auscultatory variants heard in paralytic ileus and other conditions render them largely useless for specific diagnosis.

(c) Coughing to elicit pain: The patient should be asked to cough and point to the area of maximal pain. Peritoneal irritation so demonstrated may be confirmed afterward without causing unnecessary pain by rigorous testing for rebound tenderness. Unlike the parietal pain of peritonitis, colic is visceral pain and is seldom aggravated by deep inspiration or coughing.

(d) Percussion: Percussion serves several purposes. Tenderness on percussion is akin to eliciting rebound tenderness; both reflect peritoneal irritation and parietal pain. With a perforated viscus, free air accumulating under the diaphragm may efface normal liver dullness. Tympany near the midline in a distended abdomen denotes air trapped within distended bowel loops. Free peritoneal fluid may be detected by demonstrating shifting dullness.

(e) Palpation: Palpation is performed with the patient resting in a comfortable supine position. Incisional and periumbilical hernias are noted. **Guarding** is assessed by placing both hands over the abdominal muscles and depressing the fingers gently. Properly performed, this maneuver is comforting to the patient. If there is voluntary spasm, the muscle will be felt to relax when the patient inhales deeply through the mouth. With true involuntary spasm, however, the muscle will remain taut and rigid ("boardlike") throughout respiration. Except for rare neurologic disorders—and, for unknown reasons, renal colic—only peritoneal inflammation (by reflex afferent stimulation of efferent motor fibers) produces rectus muscle rigidity. Unlike peritonitis, renal colic induces spasm confined to the ipsilateral rectus muscle.

Tenderness that connotes localized peritoneal inflammation is the most important finding in patients with an acute abdomen. Its extent and severity are determined first by one- or two-finger palpation, beginning away from the area of cough tenderness and gradually advancing toward it. Tenderness is usually well demarcated in acute cholecystitis, appendicitis, diverticulitis, and acute salpingitis. If there is poorly localized tenderness unaccompanied by guarding, one should suspect gastroenteritis or some other inflammatory intestinal process without peritonitis. Compared with the degree of pain, unexpectedly little and only vague tenderness is elicited in uncomplicated hollow viscus obstruction, walled-off or deep-seated perforations (eg, retrocecal or retroileal appendicitis or diverticular phlegmons), and in very obese patients.

When the patient raises his or her head from the bed or examination table, the abdominal muscles will be tensed. Tenderness persists in abdominal wall conditions (eg, rectus hematoma), whereas deeper peritoneal pain due to intraperitoneal disease is lessened (Carnett test). Hyperesthesia may be demonstrable in abdominal wall disorders or localized peritonitis, but it is more prominent in herpes zoster, spinal root compression, and other neuromuscular problems. Trigger point sensitivity, lateral costal rib tip tenderness, and pain exacerbated by spinal motion reflect parietal abdominal wall conditions that subside dramatically after infiltration with local anesthetic agents.

Abdominal masses are usually detected by deep palpation. Superficial lesions such as a distended gallbladder or appendiceal abscess are often tender and have discrete borders. If one suspects that abdominal guarding is masking an acutely inflamed gallbladder, the right subcostal area should be palpated while the patient inhales deeply. Inspiration will be arrested abruptly by pain (**Murphy sign**), or the gallbladder fundus may be felt as it strikes the examining fingers during descent of the diaphragm.

Deeper masses may be adherent to the posterior or lateral abdominal wall and are often partially walled off by overlying omentum and small bowel. As a result, their borders are ill-defined, and only dull pain may be elicited by palpation. Examples include pancreatic phlegmon and ruptured aortic aneurysm.

Even if a mass cannot be directly felt, its presence may be inferred by other maneuvers. A large psoas abscess arising from a perinephric abscess or perforated Crohn enteritis may cause pain when the hip is passively extended or actively flexed against resistance (**iliopsoas sign**). Similarly, internal and external rotation of the flexed thigh may exert painful pressure (**obturator sign**) on a loop of the small bowel entrapped within the obturator canal (obturator hernia). **Bump tenderness** over the lower costal ribs indicates an inflammatory condition affecting the diaphragm, liver, or spleen or its adjacent structures. While this may suggest a hepatic, splenic, or subphrenic abscess, it is also common in acute cholecystitis, acute hepatitis, or splenic infarct. **Costovertebral angle tenderness** is common in acute pyelonephritis. Since they are not invariably present, these special signs are helpful only in conjunction with a compatible history and related physical findings.

(f) Inguinal and femoral rings; male genitalia: The inguinal and femoral rings in both sexes and the genitalia in male patients should be examined next.

(g) Rectal examination: A rectal examination should be performed in most patients with an acute abdomen. Diffuse tenderness is nonspecific, but right-sided rectal tenderness accompanied by lower abdominal rebound tenderness is indicative of peritoneal irritation due to pelvic appendicitis or abscess. Other useful findings include a rectal tumor, blood-stained stool, or occult blood (detected by guaiac testing). Rectal examination may be dispensed with in children diagnosed as having appendicitis because of marked right lower quadrant tenderness, guarding, or rigidity.

(h) Pelvic examination: An acute abdomen is incorrectly diagnosed more often in women than in men, particularly in younger age groups. A pelvic examination is vital in women with a vaginal discharge, dysmenorrhea, menorrhagia, or left lower quadrant pain. A properly performed pelvic examination is invaluable in differentiating among acute pelvic inflammatory diseases that do not require operation and acute appendicitis, twisted ovarian cyst, or tubo-ovarian abscess.

INVESTIGATIVE STUDIES

The history and physical examination by themselves provide the diagnosis in two thirds of cases of an acute abdomen. Supplementary laboratory and radiologic examinations are indispensable for diagnosis of many surgical conditions, for exclusion of medical causes ordinarily not treated by operation, and for assistance in preoperative preparation. Even in the absence of a specific diagnosis, there may already be enough information on which to base a rational decision about management. Additional studies are worthwhile only if they are likely to significantly alter or improve therapeutic decisions. A more liberal use of diagnostic studies is justified in elderly or seriously ill patients, in whom the history and physical findings may be less reliable and an early diagnosis vital to ensure a successful outcome.

The availability and reliability of certain studies vary in different hospitals. The invasiveness, risks, and cost-effectiveness of a test should be weighed when the physician selects diagnostic studies. Test results must always be interpreted within the clinical context of each case. Basic studies should be obtained in all but the most desperately ill patients. Other less vital tests may be requested later as indicated (Table 21–5).

▶ Laboratory Investigations

A. Blood Studies

Hemoglobin, hematocrit, and white blood cell and differential counts taken on admission are highly informative. Only a rising or marked leukocytosis (> 13,000/μL), especially in the presence of a shift to the left on the blood smear, is indicative of serious infection. Moderate leukocytosis, commonly encountered in medical as well as surgical inflammatory conditions, is nonspecific and may be even absent in elderly or debilitated patients with infections. A low white blood cell count (< 8000/μL) is a feature of viral infections such as mesenteric adenitis or gastroenteritis and nonspecific abdominal pain.

A specimen of clotted blood for crossmatching should be sent whenever urgent surgery is anticipated. An additional tube of clotted blood may be reserved in case of such need.

Serum electrolytes, urea nitrogen, and creatinine are important, especially if hypovolemia is expected (ie, due to shock, copious vomiting or diarrhea, tense abdominal distention, or delay of several days after onset of symptoms). Arterial blood gas determinations should be obtained in patients with hypotension, generalized peritonitis, pancreatitis, possible ischemic bowel, and septicemia. Unsuspected metabolic acidosis may be the first clue to serious disease.

A raised serum amylase level corroborates a clinical diagnosis of acute pancreatitis. Moderately elevated values must be interpreted with caution, since abnormal levels frequently accompany strangulated or ischemic bowel, twisted ovarian cyst, or perforated ulcer. Moreover, a normal or even low amylase value may be seen in hemorrhagic pancreatitis or pseudocyst. Cloudy (lactescent) serum in a patient with abdominal pain suggests pancreatitis even though the serum amylase is normal.

In patients with suspected hepatobiliary disease, liver function tests (serum bilirubin, alkaline phosphatase, aspartate aminotransferase, alanine aminotransferase, albumin, and globulin) are useful to differentiate medical from surgical hepatic disorders and to gauge the severity of underlying parenchymal disease.

Clotting studies (platelet counts, prothrombin time, and partial thromboplastin time) and a peripheral blood smear should be requested if the history hints at a possible hematologic abnormality (cirrhosis, petechiae, etc). The erythrocyte sedimentation rate, often nonspecifically raised in the acute abdomen, is of dubious diagnostic value; a normal value does not exclude serious surgical illness.

Antibody titers for amebic, typhoid, or viral disease and other special blood tests may pinpoint a specific disease, but therapeutic decisions often cannot await their results.

B. Urine Tests

Urinalysis is easily performed and may reveal useful information. Dark urine or a raised specific gravity reflects mild dehydration in patients with normal renal function. Hyperbilirubinemia may give rise to tea-colored urine that froths

---

Table 21–5. General Principles of Timing of Diagnostic Studies in an Acute Abdomen.

	Immediate	Same Day[1]	Next Day[1]
Blood	Hematocrit, white blood cell count, urea, creatinine, crossmatching,[1] arterial gases.[1]	Clotting studies, amylase, liver function tests.	Specific tests.
Urine	Microscopy, dipstick testing, culture.[1]		Specific tests.
Stool	Occult blood.	Warm smear, culture.	
Radiography and ultrasound	Chest, abdomen.	Ultrasonography or CT scan, angiography, water-soluble upper gastrointestinal series, HIDA scan.	Repeat abdominal films; barium enema or small bowel follow-through, intravenous urogram, and percutaneous transhepatic cholangiography; liver-spleen, gallium, and technetium scans.
Endoscopy		Proctosigmoidoscopy, upper endoscopy.	ERCP, colonoscopy, laparoscopy.
Other		Paracentesis, culdocentesis.	

[1]When indicated.

when shaken. Microscopic hematuria or pyuria can confirm ureteral colic or urinary tract infection and obviate a needless operation. Initial antibiotic treatment should be adjusted after culture and sensitivity reports are available. Dipstick testing (for albumin, bilirubin, glucose, and ketones) may reveal a medical cause of an acute abdomen. Pregnancy tests should be ordered if there is a history of a missed period.

C. Stool Tests

Gastrointestinal bleeding is not a common feature of the acute abdomen. Nonetheless, testing for occult fecal blood should be routinely performed. A positive test points to a mucosal lesion that may be responsible for large bowel obstruction or chronic anemia, or it may reflect an unsuspected carcinoma.

Warm stool smears for bacteria, ova, and animal parasites may demonstrate amebic trophozoites in patients with bloody or mucous diarrhea. Stool samples for culture should be taken in patients with suspected gastroenteritis, dysentery, or cholera.

▶ Imaging Studies

A. Plain Chest X-Ray Studies

An erect chest x-ray is essential in all cases of an acute abdomen. Not only is it vital for preoperative assessment, but it may also demonstrate supradiaphragmatic conditions that simulate an acute abdomen (eg, lower lobe pneumonia or ruptured esophagus). An elevated hemidiaphragm or pleural effusion may direct attention to subphrenic inflammatory lesions.

B. Plain Abdominal X-Ray Studies

Plain supine films of the abdomen should be obtained only selectively. In general, erect (or lateral decubitus) views contribute little additional information except in suspected intestinal obstruction. Even though radiologic abnormalities are present in up to 40% of patients, these are diagnostic only half the time. Plain films are indicated in patients who have appreciable abdominal tenderness or distention, abnormal bowel sounds, a history of abdominal surgery, suspected foreign body ingestion, or who have a depressed sensorium or are in a high-risk category. They are helpful in patients with possible intestinal obstruction or ischemia, perforated viscus, renal or ureteral calculi, or acute cholecystitis. They are seldom of value in patients suspected to have appendicitis or urinary tract infection. They are inappropriate in pregnant patients, unstable individuals in whom clear-cut physical signs mandating laparotomy already exist, or patients with only mild, resolving nonspecific pain. Maximal information is obtained by an experienced radiologist apprised of the clinical situation. However, the surgeon who is familiar with the clinical details should review all x-rays.

One should observe the gas pattern of the hollow viscera; free or abnormal air patterns under the diaphragm, within the biliary radicles, or outside the bowel wall; the outline of solid organs and the peritoneal fat lines; and radiopaque densities.

An abnormal bowel gas pattern suggests paralytic ileus, mechanical bowel obstruction, or pseudo-obstruction. A diffuse gas pattern with air outlining the rectal ampulla suggests paralytic ileus, especially if bowel sounds are absent. Gaseous distention is the rule in bowel obstruction. Air-fluid levels are usually seen in distal small bowel obstruction and a distended cecum with small bowel dilation in large bowel obstruction. Along with the clinical findings, the distinctive radiologic appearances of colonic dilation in toxic megacolon or volvulus establish the diagnosis (see Figure 30–15). Adynamic ileus associated with longstanding acute appendicitis or with an atypical appendix location often produces a pattern that suggests localized right lower quadrant ileus. This radiologic picture in a patient without previous abdominal surgery should influence the diagnostic decision toward appendicitis or other ileocecal disease (tumor, inflammatory disorders). "Thumbprint" impressions on the colonic wall are noted in about half of patients with ischemic colitis. A displaced gastric or colonic air shadow may be the only sign of subcapsular splenic hematoma.

Free gas under the hemidiaphragm must be looked for specifically. Its presence in approximately 80% of perforated ulcers corroborates the clinical diagnosis. Massive pneumoperitoneum is observed in free colonic perforations.

Biliary tree air designates a biliary-enteric communication, such as a spontaneous or surgically created choledochoduodenal fistula or gallstone ileus. Air delineating the portal venous system characterizes pylephlebitis. Air between loops of small bowel may arise from a small localized perforation.

Obliteration of the psoas muscle margins or enlargement of the kidney shadows indicates retroperitoneal disease.

Radiopaque densities of characteristic appearance and location may confirm a clinical suspicion of biliary, renal staghorn, or ureteral calculi; appendicitis; or aortic aneurysm. Whereas pelvic phleboliths are readily distinguishable, a migrant gallstone may be mistaken for a calcified mesenteric lymph node if the accompanying small bowel distention or biliary tree air is overlooked in gallstone ileus.

C. Angiography

Percutaneous invasive angiographic studies, or magnetic resonance angiography (MRA), are indicated if intraabdominal intestinal ischemia or ongoing hemorrhage is suspected. They should precede any gastrointestinal contrast study that might obscure film interpretation. Selective visceral angiography is a reliable method of diagnosing mesenteric infarction. Emergency angiography may confirm a ruptured liver adenoma or carcinoma or an aneurysm of the splenic artery or other visceral artery. In patients with massive lower gastrointestinal bleeding, angiography may identify the bleeding site, may suggest the likely diagnosis (eg, vascular ectasia, polyarteritis nodosa) and may even be therapeutic if embolization can be performed. Angiography is of little value in ruptured aortic aneurysm or if frank peritoneal findings (peritonitis) are present. It is contraindicated in unstable patients with severe shock or sepsis and seldom warranted if other findings or tests already dictate the need for laparotomy or laparoscopy. Magnetic resonance angiography is most useful to evaluate the aortic, celiac, and mesenteric vasculature in the setting of possible subacute or chronic mesenteric ischemia.

D. Gastrointestinal Contrast X-Ray Studies

Gastrointestinal contrast studies should not be requested routinely or be regarded as screening studies. They are helpful only if a specific condition being considered can be verified or treated by a contrast x-ray examination. For suspected perforations of the esophagus or gastroduodenal area without pneumoperitoneum, a water-soluble contrast medium (eg, meglumine diatrizoate [Gastrografin]) is preferred. If there is no clinical evidence of bowel perforation, a barium enema may identify the level of a large bowel obstruction or even reduce a sigmoid volvulus or intussusception. Only if there is no likelihood of large bowel obstruction should a barium small bowel follow-through study be used to study a partial small bowel obstruction or to look for an intramural duodenal (or jejunal) hematoma that is best managed conservatively.

An emergency intravenous urogram is seldom necessary to evaluate nontraumatic causes of hematuria. It should be performed electively after microscopic examination of a stained and centrifuged urine specimen and cystoscopic examination. Ultrasonography and dimethyl iminodiacetic acid (HIDA) scans have replaced intravenous cholangiography in the evaluation of jaundiced patients and those suspected of having acute cholecystitis.

E. Ultrasonography

Ultrasonography is useful in evaluating upper abdominal pain that does not resemble ulcer pain or bowel obstruction and in investigating abdominal masses. Ultrasonography has a diagnostic sensitivity of about 80% for acute appendicitis and is most useful in pregnant patients and those presenting with features suggestive of atypical appendicitis or in young women with midabdominal or lower abdominal pain. Color Doppler studies can distinguish avascular cysts and twisted masses from inflammatory and infectious processes. CT scanning may be more useful if excessive bowel gas, so common in elderly and ill patients, precludes satisfactory ultrasound examination. It is particularly helpful in pancreatic and retroperitoneal lesions and any severe localized infections (eg, acute diverticulitis).

F. CT Scan

Urgent or emergent CT scan of the abdomen is now generally routinely and rapidly available. This has proved extremely useful in the evaluation of abdominal complaints for patients who do not already have clear indications for laparotomy or laparoscopy. CT is helpful in identifying small amounts of free intraperitoneal gas and sites of inflammatory diseases that may prompt (appendicitis, tubo-ovarian abscess) or postpone (diverticulitis, pancreatitis, hepatic abscess) operation. It should not replace or delay operation in a patient for whom the scan will not change the decision to operate.

G. Radionuclide Scans

The utility of radionuclide scans has been greatly decreased by the routine availability of urgent CT scans. Liver-spleen scans, HIDA scans, and gallium scans may be useful for localizing intra-abdominal abscesses in rare cases. Radionuclide blood pool or Tc-sulfur colloid scans may identify sources of slow or intermittent intestinal bleeding. Technetium pertechnetate scans may reveal ectopic gastric mucosa in Meckel diverticulum.

► Endoscopy

Proctosigmoidoscopy is indicated in any patient with suspected large bowel obstruction, grossly bloody stools, or a rectal mass. Minimal air should be used for bowel insufflation. Besides reducing a sigmoid volvulus, colonoscopy may also locate the source of bleeding in cases of lower gastrointestinal hemorrhage that has subsided. Gastroduodenoscopy and endoscopic retrograde cholangiopancreatography (ERCP) are usually done electively to evaluate less urgent inflammatory conditions (eg, gastritis, peptic disease) in patients without alarming abdominal signs.

► Paracentesis

In patients with free peritoneal fluid, aspiration of blood, bile, or bowel contents is a strong indication for urgent laparotomy. On the other hand, infected ascitic fluid may establish a diagnosis in spontaneous bacterial peritonitis, tuberculous peritonitis, or chylous ascites, which rarely require surgery. Culdocentesis may be useful for suspected ruptured corpus luteum cyst.

Peritoneal cytology (obtained by direct aspiration through a fine catheter) or diagnostic peritoneal lavage may disclose tumor or an acute intra-abdominal inflammatory problem. These investigations should be used selectively after imaging studies in patients with equivocal findings and in those who would poorly tolerate a negative laparotomy.

► Laparoscopy

Laparoscopy is now a therapeutic as well as a diagnostic modality. In young women, it may distinguish a nonsurgical problem (ruptured graafian follicle, pelvic inflammatory disease, tubo-ovarian disease) from appendicitis. In obtunded, elderly, or critically ill patients, who often have deceptive manifestations of an acute abdomen, it may facilitate earlier treatment in those with positive findings while eliminating the added morbidity of a laparotomy in negative cases. Where appendicitis is confirmed, laparoscopic appendectomy may be performed. Increasingly, surgeons must acquire new laparoscopic skills in order to deal with other acute intra-abdominal conditions (eg, adhesive bowel obstruction) that previously demanded a formal laparotomy.

DIFFERENTIAL DIAGNOSIS

The age and gender of the patient help in the differential diagnosis: Mesenteric adenitis mimics acute appendicitis in the young, gynecologic disorders complicate the evaluation of lower abdominal pain in women of childbearing age, and malignant and vascular diseases are more common in the elderly. Causes of an acute abdomen reflect the disease patterns of the indigenous population, and an awareness of common causes within the physician's locale will improve diagnostic accuracy. The clinical picture in early cases is often unclear. The following observations should be borne in mind:

(1) Any patient with acute abdominal pain persisting for over 6 hours should be regarded as having a surgical problem requiring in-hospital evaluation. Well-localized pain and tenderness usually indicate a surgical condition. Systemic hypoperfusion in conjunction with generalized abdominal pain is seldom due to a nonsurgical problem.

(2) Acute cholecystitis, appendicitis, bowel obstruction, cancer, and acute vascular conditions are the most common causes of the surgical acute abdomen in older patients. In children, appendicitis accounts for one third of all cases and nonspecific abdominal pain for nearly all of the remainder.

(3) Acute appendicitis and intestinal obstruction are the most frequent final diagnoses in cases erroneously believed at first to be nonsurgical. Appendicitis should always remain a foremost concern if sepsis or an inflammatory lesion is suspected. It is the commonest cause of bizarre peritoneal findings that produce ileus or intestinal obstruction. Half of children with appendicitis present with a marked facial flush (due to high serotonin levels). The presence of the gas stoppage sign or x-ray findings of right lower quadrant ileus should raise the possibility of retrocecal or retroileal appendicitis. Appendicitis is less likely in previously healthy individuals if the history exceeds 3 days' duration and the patient has no fever, appreciable tenderness, ileus, or leukocytosis.

Pelvic appendicitis, with mild abdominal pain, vomiting, and frequent loose stools, simulates gastroenteritis. The initial abdominal signs may be mild and the rectal and pelvic examinations unremarkable. A low white blood cell count or lymphocytosis favors gastroenteritis.

Atypical presentations of appendicitis are encountered during pregnancy. Maternal illness and fetal death in such cases are caused mainly by complications following delayed diagnosis. Appendectomy is well tolerated during pregnancy, and removal of a normal appendix is more frequently tolerated than observation of a perforation.

(4) Salpingitis, dysmenorrhea, ovarian lesions, and urinary tract infections complicate the evaluation of the acute abdomen in young women. Many diagnostic errors can be avoided by taking a careful menstrual history and performing a pelvic examination and urinalysis. Ultrasound study and pregnancy tests are helpful in appropriate cases. Compared with patients with appendicitis, patients with acute salpingitis tend to present with a longer history of pain, often related to the menstrual cycle, and to have higher fever, bilateral pelvic signs, and a markedly elevated white blood cell count.

(5) Unusual types or atypical manifestations of intestinal obstruction, especially early cases, are easily missed. Emesis, abdominal distention, and air-fluid levels on x-ray may be negligible in Richter hernia, proximal or closed-loop small bowel obstructions, and early cecal volvulus.

Intestinal obstruction in an elderly woman who has not had a previous operation suggests an incarcerated femoral hernia or, rarely, an obturator hernia or gallstone ileus. There may be no pain or tenderness in the area of the hernia. Carefully examine the inguinofemoral region; repeat the rectal and pelvic examinations; and check for an obturator sign. Transient mild upper abdominal pain followed several days later by signs of intestinal obstruction is typical of gallstone ileus. Look for a radiopaque stone and air outlining the biliary tree on the plain abdominal x-ray.

(6) Elderly or cardiac patients with severe unrelenting diffuse abdominal pain but without commensurate peritoneal signs or abnormalities on plain abdominal films may have intestinal ischemia. Arterial blood pH should be measured and visceral angiography performed expediently.

(7) Medical causes of the acute abdomen should be considered and excluded if possible before exploratory laparotomy is planned (Table 21–6). Upper abdominal pain may be encountered in myocardial infarction, acute pulmonary conditions (pneumothorax, lower lobe pneumonia, pleurisy, empyema, infarction), and acute hepatitis. Generalized or migratory abdominal discomfort may be felt in acute rheumatic fever, polyarteritis nodosa and other types of diffuse vasculitis, acute intermittent porphyria, and acute pleurodynia. Sharp flank pain, often accompanied by rectus spasm and cutaneous hyperesthesia, may be caused by osteoarthritis with thoracic or spinal nerve compression. Likewise, acute bursitis and hip joint disorders may produce pain radiating into the lower quadrants. Exquisite tingling or pinpricking sensations along a flank dermatome are characteristic of preeruptive herpes zoster.

Medical conditions usually can be distinguished from surgical ones by a careful assessment of the history and

Table 21–6. Medical Causes of an Acute Abdomen for which Surgery Is Not Indicated.

Endocrine and metabolic disorders	Infections and inflammatory disorders
Uremia	Tabes dorsalis
Diabetic crisis	Herpes zoster
Addisonian crisis	Acute rheumatic fever
Acute intermittent porphyria	Henoch-Schönlein purpura
Acute hyperlipoproteinemia	Systemic lupus erythematosus
Hereditary Mediterranean fever	Polyarteritis nodosa
Hematologic disorders	**Referred pain**
Sickle cell crisis	Thoracic region
Acute leukemia	Myocardial infarction
Other dyscrasias	Acute pericarditis
Toxins and drugs	Pneumonia
Lead and other heavy metal poisoning	Pleurisy
Narcotic withdrawal	Pulmonary embolus
Black widow spider poisoning	Pneumothorax
	Empyema
	Hip and back

physical examination. The family history may furnish the first clue. The history is usually atypical in some aspects, and thoughtful scrutiny will disclose details such as unusual or exaggerated symptoms—or concomitant extra-abdominal complaints—that point to the true cause. Despite the apparent severity of pain, localized abdominal tenderness with involuntary guarding is seldom present. Fever and associated systemic signs may be disproportionate to the degree of pain. Laboratory and x-ray studies will verify the diagnosis and avoid an operation.

(8) Beware of acute cholecystitis, acute appendicitis, and perforated peptic ulcer in patients already hospitalized for an illness affecting another organ system. The presentation of these conditions is often atypical, leading to delayed diagnosis and complications.

(9) Exploration is most often undertaken without benefit for salpingitis, mesenteric adenitis, gastroenteritis, pyelonephritis, and acute viral hepatitis.

(10) Nonspecific abdominal pain, comprising one third of all cases, is the most common cause of the acute abdomen, especially in children. Generally mild, short-lived, and seldom associated with other serious symptoms, it resolves without specific treatment. Most cases represent undiagnosed viral and mild bacterial infections, irritable bowel syndrome, gynecologic problems, abdominal wall pain, psychosomatic pain, or worm infection.

INDICATIONS FOR SURGICAL EXPLORATION

The need for operation is apparent when the diagnosis is certain, but surgery sometimes must be undertaken before a precise diagnosis is reached. Table 21–7 lists some indications for urgent laparotomy or laparoscopy. Among patients with acute abdominal pain, those over age 65 more often require operation (33%) than do younger patients (15%).

A liberal policy of exploration is advisable in patients with inconclusive but persistent right lower quadrant tenderness. Pain in the left upper quadrant infrequently requires urgent laparotomy, and its cause can usually await elective confirmatory studies.

PREOPERATIVE MANAGEMENT

After initial assessment, parenteral analgesics for pain relief should not be withheld. In moderate doses, analgesics neither obscure useful physical findings nor mask their subsequent development. Indeed, abdominal masses may become obvious once rectus spasm is relieved. Pain that persists in spite of adequate doses of narcotics suggests a serious condition often requiring operative correction.

Resuscitation of acutely ill patients should proceed based on their intravascular fluid deficits and systemic diseases. Medications should be restricted to only essential requirements. Particular care should be given to use of cardiac drugs and corticosteroids and to control of diabetes. Antibiotics are indicated for some infectious conditions or as prophylaxis during the perioperative period.

Table 21–7. Indications for Urgent Operation in Patients with an Acute Abdomen.

Physical findings
  Involuntary guarding or rigidity, especially if spreading
  Increasing or severe localized tenderness
  Tense or progressive distention
  Tender abdominal or rectal mass with high fever or hypotension
  Rectal bleeding with shock or acidosis
  Equivocal abdominal findings along with septicemia (high fever, marked or rising leukocytosis, mental changes, or increasing glucose intolerance in a diabetic patient)
      Bleeding (unexplained shock or acidosis, falling hematocrit)
      Suspected ischemia (acidosis, fever, tachycardia)
      Deterioration on conservative treatment
Radiologic findings
  Pneumoperitoneum
  Gross or progressive bowel distention
  Free extravasation of contrast material
  Space-occupying lesion on scan, with fever
  Mesenteric occlusion on angiography
Endoscopic findings
  Perforated or uncontrollably bleeding lesion
Paracentesis findings
  Blood, bile, pus, bowel contents, or urine

A nasogastric tube should be inserted in patients likely to undergo surgery and for those with hematemesis or copious vomiting, suspected bowel obstruction, or severe paralytic ileus. This precaution may prevent aspiration in patients suffering from drug overdose or alcohol intoxication, patients who are comatose or debilitated, or elderly patients with impaired cough reflexes. However, since the tube interferes with coughing and is uncomfortable, it should be removed once it is safe to do so.

A urinary catheter should be placed in patients with systemic hypoperfusion. In some elderly patients, it eliminates the cause of pain (acute bladder distention) or unmasks relevant abdominal signs.

Informed consent for surgery may be difficult to obtain when the diagnosis is uncertain. It is prudent to discuss with the patient and family the possibility of multiple-staged operations, temporary or permanent stomal openings, impotence or sterility, and postoperative intubation for mechanical ventilation. Whenever the exact diagnosis is uncertain—especially in young or frail or severely ill patients—a frank preoperative discussion of the diagnostic dilemma and reasons for laparotomy or laparoscopy will reduce postoperative anxieties and misunderstanding.

Kilpatrick CC, Monga M: Approach to the acute abdomen in pregnancy. Obstet Gynecol Clin North Am 2007;34:389.

Langell JT, Mulvihill SJ: Gastrointestinal perforation and the acute abdomen. Med Clin North Am 2008;92:599.

Lyon C, Clark DC: Diagnosis of acute abdominal pain in older patients. Am Fam Physician 2006;74:1537.

Nicolaou S et al: Imaging of acute small-bowel obstruction. Am J Roentgenol 2005;185:1036.

Rabah R: Pathology of the appendix in children: an institutional experience and review of the literature. Pediatr Radiol 2007;37:15.

Yu J et al: Helical CT evaluation of acute right lower quadrant pain: part I, common mimics of appendicitis. Am J Roentgenol 2005;184:1136.

Yu J et al: Helical CT evaluation of acute right lower quadrant pain: part II, uncommon mimics of appendicitis. Am J Roentgenol 2005;184:1143.

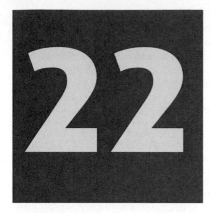

Peritoneal Cavity

Gerard M. Doherty, MD

The peritoneal cavity is lined by the **parietal peritoneum,** a mesothelial lining. This lining is called the **visceral peritoneum** where it is reflected onto the enclosed abdominal organs. Its relationship to intraperitoneal structures defines discrete compartments within which abscesses may form (see Intra-abdominal Abscesses). The peritoneal surface area is a semipermeable membrane with an area comparable to that of the cutaneous body surface. Nearly 1 m^2 of the total 1.7 m^2 area participates in fluid exchange with the extracellular fluid space at rates of 500 mL or more per hour. Normally, there is less than 50 mL of free peritoneal fluid, a transudate with the following characteristics: specific gravity below 1.016, protein concentration less than 3 g/dL, white blood cell count less than 3000/μL, complement-mediated antibacterial activity, and lack of fibrinogen-related clot formation. The circulation of peritoneal fluid is directed toward lymphatics in the undersurface of the diaphragm. There, particulate matter—including bacteria up to 20 μm in size—is cleared via stomas in the diaphragmatic mesothelium and lymphatics and discharged mainly into the right thoracic duct.

The peritoneal cavity is normally sterile. Small numbers of bacteria can be efficiently disposed of, but peritonitis ensues if the defense mechanisms are overwhelmed by massive or continued contamination. In response to tissue damage, mast cells in the delicate mesothelial lining discharge histamine and other vasoactive substances that enhance vascular permeability. The resulting fibrinogen-rich plasma exudate supplies complement and opsonic proteins that promote bacterial destruction. Tissue thromboplastin released by injured mesothelial cells converts fibrinogen into fibrin, which may in turn lead to collagen deposition and formation of fibrous adhesions. In health, this reaction is limited by a plasminogen activator in the cell lining, but the plasminogen activator is inactivated by injury or infection. Bacterial lipopolysaccharide (endotoxin) and cytokines can stimulate production of tumor necrosis factor (TNF). TNF, in turn, mediates the release of

plasminogen activator inhibitor produced by inflamed peritoneal mesothelial cells, which can lead to persistence of fibrin. Fibrin clots segregate bacterial deposits, a source of endotoxins that contribute to sepsis, but segregation may also inadvertently shield bacteria from bacteria-clearing mechanisms.

The **omentum** is a well-vascularized, pliable, mobile double fold of peritoneum and fat that participates actively in the control of peritoneal inflammation and infection. Its composition is well suited to sealing off a leaking viscus (eg, perforated ulcer) or area of infection (eg, resulting from a ruptured appendix) and for carrying a collateral blood supply to ischemic viscera. Its bacteria scavenger functions include absorption of small particles and delivery of phagocytes that destroy unopsonized bacteria.

ACUTE SECONDARY BACTERIAL PERITONITIS

▶ Pathophysiology

Peritonitis is an inflammatory or suppurative response of the peritoneal lining to direct irritation. Peritonitis can occur after perforating, inflammatory, infectious, or ischemic injuries of the gastrointestinal or genitourinary system. Common examples are listed in Table 22–1. **Secondary peritonitis** results from bacterial contamination originating from within viscera or from external sources (eg, penetrating injury). It most often follows disruption of a hollow viscus. Extravasated bile and urine, although only mildly irritating when sterile, are markedly toxic if infected and provoke a vigorous peritoneal reaction. Gastric juice from a perforated duodenal ulcer remains mostly sterile for several hours, during which time it produces a chemical peritonitis with large fluid losses; but if left untreated, it evolves within 6–12 hours into bacterial peritonitis. Intraperitoneal fluid dilutes opsonic proteins and impairs phagocytosis. Furthermore,

Table 22–1. Common Causes of Peritonitis.

Severity	Cause	Mortality Rate
Mild	Appendicitis	< 10%
	Perforated gastroduodenal ulcers	
	Acute salpingitis	
Moderate	Diverticulitis (localized perforations)	< 20%
	Nonvascular small bowel perforation	
	Gangrenous cholecystitis	
	Multiple trauma	
Severe	Large bowel perforations	20–80%
	Ischemic small bowel injuries	
	Acute necrotizing pancreatitis	
	Postoperative complications	

when hemoglobin is present in the peritoneal cavity, *Escherichia coli* growing within the cavity can elaborate leukotoxins that reduce bactericidal activity. Limited, localized infection can be eradicated by host defenses, but continued contamination invariably leads to generalized peritonitis and eventually to septicemia with multiple organ failure.

Factors that influence the severity of peritonitis include the type of bacterial or fungal contamination, the nature and duration of the injury, and the host's nutritional and immune status. The grade of peritonitis varies with the cause. Clean (eg, proximal gut perforations) or well-localized (eg, ruptured appendix) contaminations progress to fulminant peritonitis relatively slowly (eg, 12–24 hours). In contrast, bacteria associated with distal gut or infected biliary tract perforations quickly overwhelm host peritoneal defenses. This degree of toxicity is also characteristic of postoperative peritonitis due to anastomotic leakage or contamination. Conditions that ordinarily cause mild peritonitis may produce life-threatening sepsis in an immunocompromised host.

▶ Causative Organisms

Systemic sepsis due to peritonitis occurs in varying degrees depending on the virulence of the pathogens, the bacterial load, and the duration of bacterial proliferation and synergistic interaction. Except for spontaneous bacterial peritonitis, peritonitis is almost invariably polymicrobial; cultures usually contain more than one aerobic and more than two anaerobic species. The microbial picture reflects the bacterial flora of the involved organ. As long as gastric acid secretion and gastric emptying are normal, perforations of the proximal bowel (stomach or duodenum) are generally sterile or associated with relatively small numbers of gram-positive organisms. Perforations or ischemic injuries of the distal small bowel (eg, strangulated hernia) lead to infection with

aerobic bacteria in about 30% of cases and anaerobic organisms in about 10% of cases. Fecal spillage, with a bacterial load of 10^{12} or more organisms per gram, is extremely toxic. Positive cultures with gram-negative and anaerobic bacteria are characteristic of infections originating from the appendix, colon, and rectum. The predominant aerobic pathogens include the gram-negative bacteria *E coli,* streptococci, proteus, and the Enterobacter-klebsiella groups. Besides *Bacteroides fragilis,* anaerobic cocci and clostridia are the prevalent anaerobic organisms. Synergism between fecal anaerobic and aerobic bacteria increases the severity of infections.

▶ Clinical Findings

By estimating the severity of peritonitis from clinical and laboratory findings, the need for specific organ-supportive care and surgery can be determined.

See Chapter 21 for details of radiologic and other investigations.

A. Symptoms and Signs

The clinical manifestations of peritonitis reflect the severity and duration of infection and the age and general health of the patient. Physical findings can be divided into (1) abdominal signs arising from the initial injury and (2) manifestations of systemic infection. Acute peritonitis frequently presents as an acute abdomen. **Local findings** include abdominal pain, tenderness, guarding or rigidity, distention, free peritoneal air, and diminished bowel sounds—signs that reflect parietal peritoneal irritation and resulting ileus. **Systemic findings** include fever, chills or rigors, tachycardia, sweating, tachypnea, restlessness, dehydration, oliguria, disorientation, and, ultimately, refractory shock. Shock is due to the combined effects of hypovolemia and septicemia with multiple organ dysfunction. *Recurrent unexplained shock is highly predictive of serious intraperitoneal sepsis.*

The findings in abdominal sepsis are modified by the patient's age and general health. Physical signs of peritonitis are subtle or difficult to interpret in both very young and very old patients as well as in those who are chronically debilitated, immunosuppressed, or receiving corticosteroids and in postoperative patients. Paracentesis or diagnostic peritoneal lavage may be occasionally useful in equivocal cases and in senile or confused patients. A white blood cell count of greater than 200 cells/μL is indicative of peritonitis, with virtually no false-positive and minimal false-negative errors. Delayed recognition is a major cause of the high mortality rate of peritonitis.

B. Laboratory Findings

Laboratory studies gauge the severity of peritonitis and guide therapy. Blood studies should include a complete blood cell count, crossmatching, arterial blood gases, electrolytes, a blood clotting profile, and liver and renal function tests. Samples for culture of blood, urine, sputum, and peritoneal fluid should be taken before antibiotics are started. A positive blood culture is usually present in toxic patients.

Differential Diagnosis

Specific kinds of infective (eg, gonococcal, amebic, candidal) and noninfective peritonitis may be seen. In the elderly, systemic diseases (eg, pneumonia, uremia) may produce intestinal ileus so striking that it resembles bowel obstruction or peritonitis.

Familial Mediterranean fever (periodic peritonitis, familial paroxysmal polyserositis) is a rare genetic condition that affects individuals of Mediterranean genetic background. Its exact cause is unknown. Patients present with recurrent bouts of abdominal pain and tenderness along with pleuritic or joint pain. Fever and leukocytosis are common. Colchicine prevents but does not treat acute attacks. Provocative testing by infusion of metaraminol (10 mg) induces abdominal pain within 2 days.

Laparoscopy has superseded laparotomy in suspect individuals. Free fluid and inflamed peritoneal surfaces are found, but smears and cultures are negative. The appendix should be removed to simplify diagnosis in subsequent episodes. Amyloidosis with renal failure is a late complication that is preventable by long-term colchicine therapy.

Treatment

Fluid and electrolyte replacement, operative control of sepsis, and systemic antibiotics are the mainstays of treatment of peritonitis.

A. Preoperative Care

1. Intravenous fluids—The massive transfer of fluid into the peritoneal cavity must be replaced by an appropriate amount of intravenous fluid. If systemic toxicity is evident or if the patient is old or in fragile health, a central venous pressure (or pulmonary artery wedge pressure) line and bladder catheter should be inserted, a fluid balance chart should be kept, and serial body weight measurements should be taken to monitor fluid requirements. Sufficient balanced or lactated Ringer solution must be infused rapidly enough to correct intravascular hypovolemia promptly and to restore blood pressure and urine output to satisfactory levels. Potassium supplements are withheld until tissue and renal perfusion are adequate and urine is produced. Blood is reserved for anemic patients or those with concomitant bleeding.

2. Care for advanced septicemia—Cardiovascular agents and mechanical ventilation in an intensive care unit are essential in patients with advanced septicemia. An arterial line for continuous blood pressure recording and blood sampling is helpful. Cardiac monitoring with a Swan-Ganz catheter is essential if inotropic drugs are used. (See Chapters 9, 10, and 13 for details of fluid resuscitation and the management of septic shock.)

3. Antibiotics—Loading doses of intravenous antibiotics directed against the anticipated bacterial pathogens should be given after fluid samples have been obtained for culture. Initial antibiotics employed include third-generation cephalosporins, ampicillin-sulbactam, ticarcillin-clavulanic acid, aztreonam or imipenem-cilastatin for gram-negative coliforms, and metronidazole or clindamycin for anaerobic organisms. The choice of single-, double-, or triple-drug therapy is of less importance than adequate coverage of both anticipated aerobic and anaerobic organisms. Inadequate initial drug dosing and scheduling contribute to treatment failures. Aminoglycosides should be used judiciously because renal impairment is often a feature of peritonitis and because lowered intraperitoneal pH may impair their in vivo activity.

Empirically chosen antibiotics should be modified postoperatively by culture and sensitivity results if there is persistent or subsequent infection (seen in 15–20% of patients). Antibiotics are continued until the patient has remained afebrile with a normal white count and a differential count of less than 3% bands.

B. Operative Management

1. Control of sepsis—The objectives of surgery for peritonitis are to remove all infected material, correct the underlying cause, and prevent late complications. Except in early, localized peritonitis, a midline incision offers the best surgical exposure. Materials for aerobic and anaerobic cultures of fluid and infected tissue are obtained immediately after the peritoneal cavity is entered. Occult pockets of infection are located by thorough exploration, and contaminated or necrotic material is removed. Routine radical debridement of all peritoneal and serosal surfaces does not increase survival rates. The primary disease is then treated. This may require resection (eg, ruptured appendix or gallbladder), repair (eg, perforated ulcer), or drainage (eg, acute pancreatitis). Attempts to reanastomose resected bowel in the presence of extensive sepsis or intestinal ischemia often lead to leakage. Temporary stomas are safer, and these can be taken down several weeks later after the patient has recovered from the acute illness. Surgical wounds should seldom be closed primarily. They should be left open in grossly soiled cases or delayed primary closure employed in those with less contamination.

2. Peritoneal lavage—In diffuse peritonitis, lavage with copious amounts (> 3 L) of warm isotonic crystalloid solution removes gross particulate matter as well as blood and fibrin clots and dilutes residual bacteria. The addition of antiseptics or antibiotics to the irrigating solution is generally useless or even harmful because of induced adhesions (eg, tetracycline, povidone-iodine). Antibiotics given parenterally will reach bactericidal levels in peritoneal fluid and may afford no additional benefit when given by lavage. Furthermore, lavage with aminoglycosides can produce respiratory depression and complicate anesthesia because of the neuromuscular blocking action of this group of drugs. After lavage is completed, all fluid in the peritoneal cavity must be aspirated because it may hamper local defense mechanisms by diluting opsonins and removing surfaces upon which phagocytes destroy bacteria.

3. Peritoneal drainage—Drainage of the free peritoneal cavity is ineffective and often undesirable. Not only are drains quickly isolated from the rest of the peritoneal cavity, but they still act as a channel for exogenous contamination. Prophylactic drainage in diffuse peritonitis does not prevent abscess formation and may even predispose to abscesses or fistulas. Drainage is useful for residual focal infection or when continued contamination is present or likely to occur (eg, fistula). It is indicated for localized inflammatory masses that cannot be resected or for cavities that cannot be obliterated. Soft sump drains with continuous suction through multiple side perforations are effective for large volumes of fluid. Smaller volumes of fluid are best handled with closed drainage systems (eg, Jackson-Pratt drains). Large cavities with thick walls may be drained by several large Penrose drains placed in a dependent position.

To achieve more effective peritoneal drainage in severe peritonitis, some surgeons have previously left the entire abdominal wound open to widely expose the peritoneal cavity. Besides requiring intensive nursing and medical support to cope with massive protein and fluid losses (averaging 9 L the first day), there are serious complications such as spontaneous fistulization, wound sepsis, segmental colonic necrosis, and large incisional hernias. Consequently, this method is seldom employed now.

An alternative method is to re-explore the abdomen every 1–3 days until all loculations have been adequately drained. The wound may be closed temporarily with a sheet of polypropylene (Marlex) mesh that contains a nylon zipper or Velcro to avoid a tight abdominal closure and to facilitate repeated opening and closing. Other options include the use of a plastic sheet (Bogota bag) or a wound vacuum device bridging over the open fascia. Exploration may even be performed in the intensive care unit with heavy sedation. Available data suggest that this method should be restricted to selected patients with long-standing (more than 48 hours) extensive intraperitoneal sepsis associated with multiple organ failure (high sepsis scores). One prospective study failed to demonstrate a significant difference in mortality rates between the conventional closed (31%) and open (44%) techniques.

4. Management of abdominal distention—Abdominal distention caused by ileus frequently accompanies peritonitis, and decompression of the intestine is often ineffective in reliably decreasing the distention. An alternative approach is to close the abdomen temporarily with a sheet of plastic (Bogota bag) to avoid further distention, increased intra-abdominal pressure, and respiratory or renal problems (abdominal compartment syndrome). A **gastrostomy** may

be advantageous if prolonged nasogastric decompression is expected, especially in elderly patients or those with chronic respiratory disease. A central total parenteral nutrition (TPN) line or needle jejunostomy catheter (for proximal gut lesions) is placed when prolonged nutritional support is anticipated.

C. Postoperative Care

Intensive care monitoring, often with ventilatory support, is mandatory in unstable and frail patients. Achieving hemodynamic stability to perfuse major organs is the immediate objective, and this may entail the use of cardiac inotropic agents besides fluid and blood product supportive measures. Antibiotics are given for 10–14 days, depending on the severity of peritonitis. A favorable clinical response is evidenced by well-sustained perfusion with good urine output, reduction in fever and leukocytosis, resolution of ileus, and a returning sense of well-being. The rate of recovery varies with the duration and degree of peritonitis.

The early removal of all nonessential catheters (arterial, central venous, urinary, and nasogastric) reduces the risk of secondary infected foci. Drains should be removed or advanced once drainage diminishes and becomes more serous in nature. Excessive or prolonged suction may produce fistulas or bleeding even within a few days.

Growing awareness of the association between proximal gut colonization with candida, *Streptococcus faecalis*, pseudomonas, and coagulase-negative staphylococci and secondary nosocomial infections and subsequent multiple organ failure has encouraged early gut feeding and discontinuation of unnecessary antibiotics whenever feasible.

▶ Complications

Postoperative complications are frequent and may be divided into local and systemic problems. Deep wound infections, residual abscesses and intraperitoneal sepsis, anastomotic breakdown, and fistula formation usually become manifest toward the end of the first postoperative week. Persistent high or swinging fever, inability to wean off cardiac inotropes, generalized edema with unexplained continued high fluid requirements, increased abdominal distention, prolonged mental apathy and weakness, or general failure to improve despite intensive treatment may be the sole indicators of residual intra-abdominal infection. This should prompt a thorough examination of the patient for infected catheters and an abdominal CT scan. Percutaneous catheter drainage of localized abscesses or open reexploration is undertaken as needed (see next section).

Uncontrolled sepsis leads inexorably to sequential multiple organ failure affecting the respiratory, renal, hepatic, clotting, and immune systems. Supportive measures, including mechanical ventilation, transfusions, total parenteral nutrition, and hemodialysis, are ineffectual unless primary septic foci are eliminated by combined surgical and antibiotic therapy.

Prognosis

The overall mortality rate of generalized peritonitis is about 40% (Table 22–1). Factors contributing to a high mortality rate include the type of primary disease and its duration, associated multiple organ failure before treatment, and the age and general health of the patient. Mortality rates are consistently below 10% in patients with perforated ulcers or appendicitis; in young patients; in those having less extensive bacterial contamination; and in those diagnosed and operated upon early. Patients with distal small bowel or colonic perforations or postoperative sepsis tend to be older, to have concurrent medical illnesses and greater bacterial contamination, and to have a greater propensity to renal and respiratory failure; their mortality rates are about 50%. Markedly poor physiologic indices (eg, APACHE II or Mannheim Peritonitis Index), reduced cardiac status, and low preoperative albumin levels identify high-risk patients who require intensive treatment to reduce a daunting mortality rate.

INTRA-ABDOMINAL ABSCESSES

1. Intraperitoneal Abscesses

Pathophysiology

An intra-abdominal abscess is a collection of infected fluid within the abdominal cavity. Gastrointestinal perforations, postoperative complications, penetrating trauma, and geni-tourinary infections are the most common causes. An abscess forms by one of two modes: It may develop (1) adjacent to a diseased viscus (eg, with perforated appendix, Crohn entero-colitis, or diverticulitis) or (2) as a result of external contamination (eg, postoperative subphrenic abscesses). In one third of cases, the abscess occurs as a sequela of generalized peritonitis. Interloop and pelvic abscesses form if extravasated fluid gravitating into a dependent or localized area becomes secondarily infected (Figure 22–1).

Bacteria-laden fibrin and blood clots and neutrophils contribute to the formation of an abscess. The pathogenic organisms are similar to those responsible for peritonitis, but anaerobic organisms occupy an important role. Experimentally, mixed aerobic (*E coli*) and anaerobic (*B fragilis*) infections, especially in conjunction with adjuvants (eg, feces or barium), reduce intraperitoneal O_2 and pH, thereby fostering anaerobic proliferation and abscess formation.

Sites of Abscesses

The areas in which abscesses commonly occur are defined by the configuration of the peritoneal cavity with its dependent lateral and pelvic basins (Figure 22–1), together with the natural divisions created by the transverse mesocolon and the small bowel mesentery. The supracolic compartment, located above the transverse mesocolon, broadly defines the subphrenic spaces (Figure 22–2A). Within this area, the subdiaphragmatic (suprahepatic) and subhepatic areas of the sub-

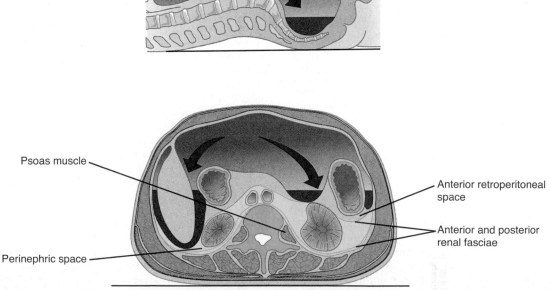

▲ **Figure 22–1.** Lateral (*top*) and cross-sectional (*bottom*) views of the abdomen, showing fluid gravitating to the dependent areas of the peritoneal cavity. The retroperitoneal compartments are also outlined.

phrenic space may be distinguished. The **subdiaphragmatic space** on each side occupies the concavity between the hemidiaphragms and the domes of the hepatic lobes. The inferior limits of its posterior recess are the attachments of the coronary and triangular ligaments on the dorsal—not superior—aspect of the diaphragm. Anteriorly, the lower limits are defined on the right by the transverse colon and on the left by the anterior stomach surface, omentum, transverse colon, spleen, and phrenicocolic ligament. Although each subdiaphragmatic space is continuous over the convex liver surface, inflammatory adhesions may delimit an abscess in an anterior or posterior position (Figure 22–2B). The falciform ligament separates the right and left subdiaphragmatic divisions.

The **right subhepatic division** (Figure 22–2B) of the subphrenic space is located between the undersurfaces of the liver and gallbladder superiorly and the right kidney and mesocolon inferiorly. The anterior bulge of the kidney partitions this space into an anterior (gallbladder fossa) and posterior (Morison pouch) section.

The **left subhepatic space** also has an anterior and posterior part (Figure 22–2C). The smaller anterior subhepatic space lies between the undersurface of the left lobe and the anterior surface of the stomach. Left subdiaphragmatic collections often extend into this anterior subhepatic area. The posterior subhepatic space is the lesser sac, which is situated behind the lesser omentum and stomach and lies anterior to the pancreas,

duodenum, transverse mesocolon, and left kidney. It extends posteriorly to the attachment of the left triangular ligament superiorly on to the hemidiaphragm. The lesser sac communicates with both the right subhepatic and right paracolic spaces through the narrow foramen of Winslow.

The **infracolic compartment,** below the transverse mesocolon, includes the pericolic and pelvic areas (Figure 22–3). The diagonally aligned root of the small bowel mesentery divides the midabdominal area between the fixed right and left colons into right and left infracolic spaces. Each lateral paracolic gutter and lower quadrant area communicates freely with the pelvic cavity. However, while right paracolic collections may track upward into the subhepatic and subdiaphragmatic spaces, the phrenicocolic ligament hinders fluid migration along the left paracolic gutter into the left subdiaphragmatic area.

The most common abscess sites are in the lower quadrants, followed by the pelvic, subhepatic, and subdiaphragmatic spaces (Table 22–2).

▶ Clinical Findings
A. Symptoms and Signs

An intraperitoneal abscess should be suspected in any patient with a predisposing condition. Fever, tachycardia, and pain may be mild or absent, especially in patients receiving antibiotics. A deep-seated or posteriorly situated abscess may exist

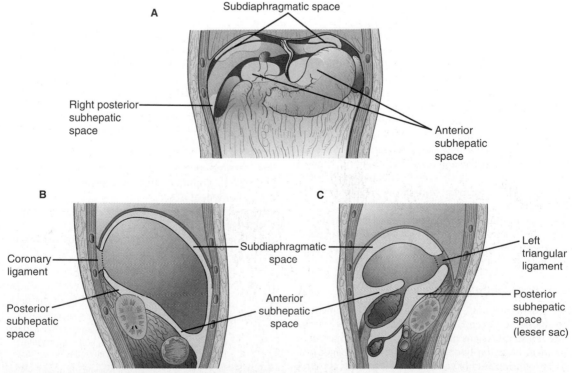

▲ **Figure 22–2.** Subphrenic spaces. **A:** Anterior view. **B:** Right lateral view. **C:** Left lateral view.

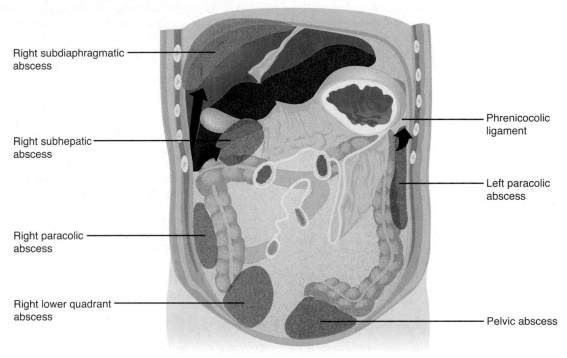

▲ **Figure 22–3.** The infracolic peritoneal compartment and common abscess sites. Note how paracolic fluid on the right side can migrate up into the subphrenic spaces, whereas collections on the left side are prevented from doing so by the phrenicocolic ligament.

in seemingly well individuals whose only symptom is persistent fever. Not infrequently, prolonged ileus or a sluggish recovery in a patient who has had recent abdominal surgery or peritoneal sepsis, rising leukocytosis, or nonspecific radiologic abnormality provides the initial clue. A mass is seldom felt except late in patients with lower quadrant or pelvic lesions. Irritation of contiguous structures may produce lower chest pain, dyspnea, referred shoulder pain or hiccup, or basilar atelectasis or effusion in subphrenic abscesses; or diarrhea or urinary frequency in pelvic abscesses. The diagnosis is more difficult in postoperative, chronically ill, confused, or diabetic patients and in those receiving immunosuppressive drugs, a group particularly susceptible to septic complications.

Sequential multiple organ failure—principally respiratory, renal, or hepatic failure—or stress-induced gastrointestinal bleeding with disseminated intravascular coagulopathy is highly suggestive of intra-abdominal infection.

B. Laboratory Findings

A raised leukocyte count, abnormal liver or renal function test results, hyperglycemia, and abnormal arterial blood gases are nonspecific signs of infection. Serial postoperative measurement of serum lysozyme (derived from phagocytic cells) is a promising but not widely available test that appears to be highly specific for intra-abdominal pus. Persistently positive blood cultures point strongly to an intra-abdominal focus. A cervical smear demonstrating gonococcal infection is of specific value in diagnosing tubo-ovarian abscess.

C. Imaging Studies

1. X-ray studies—Plain x-rays may suggest an abscess in up to one half of cases. In subphrenic abscesses, the chest x-ray

Table 22–2. Common Sites and Causes of Intraperitoneal Abscesses.

Site	Cause
Right lower quadrant	Appendicitis, perforated ulcer, regional enteritis
Left lower quadrant	Colorectal perforation (diverticulitis, carcinoma, inflammatory bowel diseases)
Pelvis	Appendicitis, colorectal perforation, gynecologic sepsis, postoperative complications
Subphrenic region	Postoperative complications following gastric or hepatobiliary surgery or splenectomy, perforated ulcer, acute cholecystitis, appendicitis, pancreatitis (lesser sac)
Interloop	Postoperative bowel perforation

may show pleural effusion, a raised hemidiaphragm, basilar infiltrates, or atelectasis. Abnormalities on plain abdominal films include an ileus pattern, soft tissue mass, air-fluid levels, free or mottled gas pockets, effacement of properitoneal or psoas outlines, and displacement of viscera. Many of these findings are vague or nonspecific, but they may suggest the need for a CT scan. Barium contrast studies interfere with and have been largely superseded by other imaging techniques. A water-soluble upper gastrointestinal series may reveal an unsuspected perforated viscus or outline perigastric and lesser sac abscesses.

2. Ultrasonography—Real-time ultrasonography is sensitive (about 80% of cases) in diagnosing intra-abdominal abscesses. The findings consist of a sonolucent area with well-defined walls containing fluid or debris of variable density. Bowel gas, intervening viscera, skin incisions, and stomas interfere with ultrasound examinations, limiting their efficacy in postoperative patients. Nevertheless, the procedure is readily available, portable, and inexpensive, and the findings are specific when correlated with the clinical picture. Ultrasonography is most useful when an abscess is clinically suspected, especially for lesions in the right upper quadrant and the paracolic and pelvic areas.

3. CT scan—CT scan of the abdomen, the best diagnostic study, is highly sensitive (over 95% of cases) and specific. Neither gas shadows nor exposed wounds interfere with CT scanning in postoperative patients, and the procedure is reliable even in areas poorly seen on ultrasonography. Abscesses appear as cystic collections with density measurements of between 0 and 15 attenuation units. Resolution is increased by contrast media (eg, sodium diatrizoate) injected intravenously or instilled into hollow viscera adjacent to the abscess. One drawback of CT scan is that diagnosis may be difficult in areas with multiple thick-walled bowel loops or if a pleural effusion overlies a subphrenic abscess, so occasionally a very large abscess is missed. CT-guided or ultrasonography-guided needle aspiration can distinguish between sterile and infected collections in uncertain cases.

4. Radionuclide scan—Gallium-67 citrate and indium 111-labeled autologous leukocyte scans are rarely indicated because, compared to other modalities, they do not provide a timely answer, have high false-positive and false-negative rates, and provide less anatomic localization.

5. Magnetic resonance imaging—The scanning time, patient inaccessibility during scan acquisition, and upper respiratory motion have limited the usefulness of MRI in the investigation of upper abdominal abscesses. CT scan is generally preferable.

▶ Treatment

Treatment consists of prompt and complete drainage of the abscess, control of the primary cause, and adjunctive use of effective antibiotics. Depending upon the abscess site and the condition of the patient, drainage may be achieved by operative or nonoperative methods. **Percutaneous drainage** is the preferred method for single, well-localized, superficial bacterial abscesses that do not have fistulous communications or contain solid debris. Following CT scan or ultrasonographic delineation, a needle is guided into the abscess cavity, infected material is aspirated for culture, and a suitably large drainage catheter is inserted.

Postoperative irrigation is vital to remove debris and ensure catheter patency. This technique is not appropriate for multiple or deep (especially pancreatic) abscesses or for patients with ongoing contamination, fungal infections, or thick purulent or necrotic material. Percutaneous drainage can be performed in about 75% of cases. The success rate exceeds 80% in simple abscesses but is often less than 50% in more complex ones. It is heavily influenced by the availability of appropriate equipment and the experience of the radiologist performing the drainage. Complications include septicemia, fistula formation, bleeding, and peritoneal contamination.

Open drainage is reserved for abscesses for which percutaneous drainage is inappropriate or unsuccessful. These include many cases where there is a persistent focus of infection (eg, diverticulitis or anastomotic dehiscence) that needs to be controlled. In cases without evidence of continued soiling, the direct extraserous route has the advantage of establishing dependent drainage without contaminating the rest of the peritoneal cavity. Only light general anesthesia or even local anesthesia is necessary, and surgical trauma is minimized. Right anterior subphrenic abscesses can be drained by a subcostal incision (Figure 22–4). Posterior subdiaphragmatic and subhepatic lesions can be decompressed

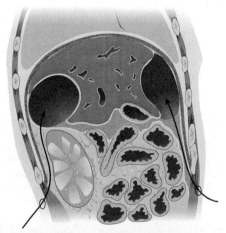

▲ **Figure 22–4.** Extraperitoneal approaches to the right subphrenic spaces. An abscess in the anterior subhepatic space usually requires transperitoneal drainage. Posterior abscesses may also be drained laterally.

posteriorly through the bed of the resected twelfth rib (Figure 22–4) or by a lateral extraserous method. Most lower quadrant and flank abscesses can be drained through a lateral extraperitoneal approach. Pelvic abscesses can often be detected on pelvic or rectal examination as a fluctuant mass distorting the contour of the vagina or rectum. If needle aspiration directly through the vaginal or rectal wall returns pus, the abscess is best drained by making an incision in that area. In all cases, digital or direct exploration must ensure that all loculations are broken down. Penrose and sump drains are used to allow continued drainage postoperatively until the infection has resolved. Serial sonograms or imaging studies help document obliteration of the abscess cavity.

Transperitoneal exploration is indicated if the abscess cannot be localized preoperatively, if there are several or deep-lying lesions, if an enterocutaneous fistula or bowel obstruction exists, or if previous drainage attempts have been unsuccessful. This is especially likely in postoperative patients with multiple abscesses and persistent peritoneal soiling. The need to achieve complete drainage fully justifies the greater stress of laparotomy and the small possibility that infection might be spread to other uninvolved areas. Laparoscopy alone is often inadequate, especially in critically toxic patients without a localized focus.

Satisfactory drainage is usually evidenced by improving clinical findings within 3 days after starting treatment. Failure to improve indicates inadequate drainage, another source of (or ongoing) sepsis, or organ dysfunction. Additional localizing studies and repeated percutaneous or operative drainage should be undertaken urgently (ie, within 24–48 hours, depending on the seriousness of the case). Failure to acknowledge adequate progress delays essential studies and incurs higher mortality.

▶ Prognosis

The mortality rate of serious intra-abdominal abscesses is about 30%. Deaths are related to the severity of the underlying cause, delay in diagnosis, multiple organ failure, and incomplete drainage. Right lower quadrant and pelvic abscesses are usually caused by perforated ulcers and appendicitis in younger individuals. They are readily diagnosed and treated, and the mortality rate is less than 5%. Diagnosis is often delayed in older patients; this increases the likelihood of multiple organ failure. Decompensation of two major organ systems is associated with a mortality rate of over 50%. Shock is an especially ominous sign. Subphrenic, deep, and multiple abscesses frequently require operative drainage and are associated with a mortality rate of over 40%. An untreated residual abscess is nearly always fatal.

Kim S et al: The perihepatic space: comprehensive anatomy and CT features of pathologic conditions. Radiographics 2007;27:129.
Kaplan M: Negative pressure wound therapy in the management of abdominal compartment syndrome. Ostomy Wound Manage 2004;50:20S.

Lubner M et al: Blood in the belly: CT findings of hemoperitoneum. Radiographics 2007;27:109.
Schimp VL et al: Vacuum-assisted closure in the treatment of gynecologic oncology wound failures. Gynecol Oncol 2004;92:586.

2. Retroperitoneal & Retrofascial Abscesses
▶ Pathophysiology

The large retroperitoneal space, extending from the diaphragm to the pelvis, is divided into anterior and posterior compartments (Figure 22–1). The **anterior portion** includes structures between the posterior peritoneum and the perinephric fascia (pancreas; parts of the duodenum and the ascending and descending colon). The **posterior portion** contains the adrenals, kidneys, and perinephric spaces. The compartment posterior to the transversalis fascia is involved in retrofascial abscesses.

Abscesses occur less commonly in the retroperitoneum than in the peritoneal cavity. Retroperitoneal abscesses arise chiefly from injuries or infections in adjacent structures: gastrointestinal tract abscesses due to appendicitis, pancreatitis, penetrating posterior ulcers, regional enteritis, diverticulitis, or trauma; genitourinary tract abscesses due to pyelonephritis; and spinal column abscesses due to osteomyelitis or disk space infections.

Psoas abscesses may be primary or secondary. Primary psoas abscesses, which occur without associated disease of other organs, are caused by hematogenous spread of *Staphylococcus aureus* from an occult source and are predominantly seen in children and young adults. They are more common in underdeveloped countries. Secondary psoas abscesses result from spread of infection from adjacent organs, principally from the intestine, and are therefore most often polymicrobial. The most common cause is Crohn disease.

The pyogenic bacteria (*E coli*, bacteroides, proteus, klebsiella) have replaced *Mycobacterium tuberculosis* as the major causative organism. Surprisingly, only a single causative organism is involved in over one half of cases. A positive blood culture—especially with *Bacteroides*—is an ominous finding.

▶ Clinical Findings

Although they may be symptomless, retroperitoneal abscesses tend to develop in patients with obvious acute illnesses. Fever and abdominal or flank pain are prominent features, sometimes accompanied by anorexia, weight loss, and nausea and vomiting. The clinical findings in patients with psoas abscess consist of hip pain, flexion of the hip with pain on extension, and a positive iliopsoas sign. Abdominal, thigh, and back pain may also occur. The diagnosis is apt to be overlooked when pain in the hip aggravated by walking is the major complaint. The differential diagnosis includes retroperitoneal tumors and hematomas. Radionuclide scanning, bowel contrast studies, and urograms are the common preliminary investigations, but CT scanning most accurately delineates these lesions. Gas bubbles are diagnostic of an abscess. Awareness of the overall clinical picture is essential for CT scanning to differentiate retroperitoneal abscesses from neoplasms or hematomas. Abscesses are confined to specific compartments, whereas malignant lesions, by contrast, frequently violate peritoneal and fascial barriers and can invade bone.

▶ Treatment

Failure to institute prompt and adequate drainage in addition to systemic antibiotics leads to a fatal outcome. Apart from multiloculated pancreatic abscesses, many retroperitoneal abscesses are amenable to percutaneous CT scan–guided needle aspiration and catheter drainage. Drainage by catheter, however, has a lower success rate for retroperitoneal than intraperitoneal abscesses for the following reasons: (1) Retroperitoneal abscesses often dissect along planes, giving a stellate instead of globular shape; (2) they often contain necrotic debris that will not pass through catheters; and (3) they often invade adjacent muscle (eg, psoas abscess). Operation is indicated if there is no clinical improvement after 2 days of percutaneous drainage. An extraperitoneal approach via the flank is preferred for upper retroperitoneal and perirenal abscesses—and one via the perineum presacrally between the anus and the coccyx for pelvic lesions. Transperitoneal exploration may be unavoidable for deep anterior retroperitoneal abscesses. Resection of necrotic or diseased organs, debridement of the affected compartment, and thorough drainage should be accomplished. In general, retroperitoneal abscesses are difficult to drain completely, and residual or recurrent abscesses are common (especially with regional enteritis). Psoas abscesses may invade the spine or ipsilateral hip to cause osteomyelitis or may track across the midline to cause a contralateral psoas abscess.

The surgical mortality rate is about 25%. Failure of the fever to subside within 3 days indicates inadequate drainage and persistent sepsis that will prove fatal if not corrected promptly.

PRIMARY PERITONITIS

Primary ("spontaneous") peritonitis occurring in the absence of gastrointestinal perforation is caused mainly by hematogenous spread but occasionally by transluminal or direct bacterial invasion of the peritoneal cavity. Impairment of the hepatic reticuloendothelial system and compromised peripheral destruction of bacteria by neutrophils promotes bacteremia, which readily infects ascitic fluid that has reduced bacterium-killing capacity. Primary peritonitis is most closely associated with cirrhosis and advanced liver disease with a low ascitic fluid protein concentration. It is also seen in patients with the nephrotic syndrome or systemic lupus erythematosus, or after splenectomy during childhood. Recurrence is common in cirrhosis and often proves fatal.

▶ Clinical Findings

The clinical presentation simulates secondary bacterial peritonitis, with abrupt onset of fever, abdominal pain, distention, and rebound tenderness. However, one fourth of patients have minimal or no peritoneal symptoms. Most have clinical and biochemical manifestations of advanced cirrhosis or nephrosis. Leukocytosis, hypoalbuminemia, and a prolonged prothrombin time are characteristic findings. The diagnosis hinges upon examination of the ascitic fluid, which reveals a white blood cell count greater than 500/μL and more than 25% polymorphonuclear leukocytes. A blood-ascitic fluid albumin gradient greater than 1.1 g/dL, a raised serum lactic acid level (> 33 mg/dL), or a reduced ascitic fluid pH (< 7.31) supports the diagnosis. Bacteria are seen on Gram-stained smears in only 25% of cases. Culture of ascitic fluid inoculated immediately into blood culture media at the bedside usually reveals a single enteric organism, most commonly E coli, klebsiella, or streptococci, but Listeria monocytogenes has been reported in immunocompromised hosts.

▶ Treatment

Antibiotic prophylaxis is of no proven value. Systemic antibiotics with third-generation cephalosporins (eg, cefotaxime) or a beta-lactam-clavulanic acid combination along with supportive treatment are begun once the diagnosis has been established. The 50% average mortality rate is due to peritonitis in only about a third of cases. Multiple organ failure as indicated by gastrointestinal bleeding, hepatic encephalopathy, and renal failure are ominous signs.

Troidle L et al: Differing outcomes of gram positive and gram-negative peritonitis. Am J Kidney Dis 1998;32:623.

TUBERCULOUS PERITONITIS

▶ Pathophysiology

Tuberculosis peritonitis is encountered in 0.5% of new cases of tuberculosis. It presents as a primary infection without active pulmonary, intestinal, renal, or uterine tube involvement. Its cause is reactivation of a dormant peritoneal focus derived from hematogenous dissemination from a distant nidus or breakdown of mesenteric lymph nodes. Some cases occur as a systemic manifestation of extra-abdominal infection. Multiple small, hard, raised, whitish tubercles studding the peritoneum, omentum, and mesentery are the distinctive finding. A cecal tuberculoma, matted lymph nodes, or omental involvement may form a palpable mass.

The disease affects young persons, particularly women, and is more prevalent in countries where tuberculosis is still endemic. AIDS patients are especially susceptible to development of extrapulmonary tuberculosis.

▶ Clinical Findings

Chronic symptoms (lasting more than a week) include abdominal pain and distention, fever, night sweats, weight loss, and altered bowel habits. Ascites is present in about half of cases, especially if the disease is of long standing, and may be the primary manifestation. A mass may be felt in a third of cases. The differential diagnosis includes Crohn disease, carcinoma, hepatic cirrhosis, and intestinal lymphoma. One fourth of patients have acute symptoms suggestive of acute bowel obstruction or peritonitis that mimics appendicitis, cholecystitis, or a perforated ulcer.

Detection of an extra-abdominal site of tuberculosis, evident in half of cases, is the single most useful diagnostic clue. Pleural effusion is present in up to 50% of patients. Paracentesis, laparoscopy, or peritoneal biopsy is applicable only in patients with ascites. The peritoneal fluid is characterized by a protein concentration above 3 g/dL with less than 1.1 g/dL serum-ascitic fluid albumin difference and lymphocyte predominance among white blood cells. Definitive diagnosis is possible in 80% of cases by culture (often taking several weeks) and direct smear. A purified protein derivative (PPD) skin test is useful only when positive (about 80% of cases). Hematologic and biochemical studies are seldom helpful, and leukocytosis is uncommon. The sedimentation rate is elevated in many cases. The presence of high-density ascites or soft tissue masses on ultrasonography or CT scan supports the diagnosis. Young patients from endemic areas who present with classic symptoms or who have suggestive imaging findings should undergo diagnostic laparoscopy, which may obviate laparotomy.

▶ Treatment

In chronic cases, nonoperative therapy is preferable if the diagnosis can be established. Most patients presenting with acute symptoms are diagnosed only by laparotomy. In the absence of intestinal obstruction or perforation, only a biopsy of a peritoneal or omental nodule should be taken. Obstruction due to constriction by a tuberculous lesion usually develops in the distal ileum and cecum, although multiple skip areas along the small bowel may exist. Localized short segments of diseased bowel are best treated by resection with primary anastomosis. Multiple strictured areas may be managed either by side-to-side bypass or a stricturoplasty of partially narrowed segments.

Combination antituberculosis chemotherapy should be started once the diagnosis is confirmed or considered likely. A favorable response is the rule, but isoniazid and rifampin must be continued for 18 months postoperatively.

GRANULOMATOUS PERITONITIS

▶ Pathophysiology

Talc (magnesium silicate), cornstarch glove lubricants, gauze fluffs, and cellulose fibers from disposable surgical fabrics may elicit a vigorous granulomatous (probably a delayed hypersensitivity) response in some patients 2–6 weeks after laparotomy. The condition is uncommon now that surgeons wipe clean their gloves before handling abdominal viscera. Less rarely, granulomatous peritonitis may develop as a hypersensitivity reaction to other foreign material (eg, intestinal ascariasis or food particles from a perforated ulcer). This process should be distinguished from congenital peritoneal encapsulation or abdominal cocoon.

▶ Clinical Findings

Besides abdominal pain, which is often out of proportion to the low-grade fever, there may be nausea and vomiting, ileus, and other systemic complaints. Abdominal tenderness is usually diffuse but mild. Free abdominal fluid, if detectable, should be tapped and inspected for the diagnostic Maltese cross pattern of starch particles.

▶ Treatment

Reoperation achieves little and should be avoided if the diagnosis can be made. Most patients undergo reexploration because they present an erroneous impression of postoperative bowel obstruction or peritoneal sepsis. The diffuse hard, white granulomatous masses studding the peritoneum and omentum are easily mistaken for cancer or tuberculosis unless a biopsy specimen is taken to demonstrate foreign body granulomas.

If granulomatous peritonitis is suspected, the response to treatment with corticosteroids or other anti-inflammatory agents is often so dramatic as to be diagnostic in itself. After clinical improvement, intravenous methylprednisolone can be replaced by oral prednisone for 2–3 weeks. The disease is self-limited and does not predispose to late intestinal obstruction.

ASCITES

1. Chylous Ascites

The accumulation of free chyle in the peritoneal cavity is a rare form of ascites. Most patients are adults—many of them elderly women—with occult cancer, often a lymphoma or adenocarcinoma (of the pancreas or stomach), causing lymphatic obstruction. Chylous ascites resulting from external trauma or operative mishap (portosystemic decompression, abdominal aneurysmectomy and retroperitoneal lymphadenectomy procedures) has a more favorable prognosis. About 15% of cases occur in young children (usually < 1 year old) with congenital lymphatic anomalies.

▶ Clinical Findings

The typical presentation is of abdominal distention and pain along with vague constitutional symptoms. Physical findings—besides ascites—include concomitant pleural effusion and peripheral edema. The combination of fever, night sweats, and lymphadenopathy should arouse suspicion of a lymphoma. The discovery of milky ascitic fluid on paracentesis suggests the correct diagnosis. Only a rough correlation exists between the gross appearance of the fluid and its triglyceride content (> 200 mg/dL, with a mean level of 1500 mg/dL). The fluid leukocyte count (mostly lymphocytes) averages 1000/μL. Hypoalbuminemia, lymphocytopenia, and anemia are frequently present.

Conventional radiologic investigations, particularly CT scan of the abdomen, may be helpful. Lymph node biopsy, where applicable, and laparotomy have the highest diagnostic value.

▶ Treatment

Treatment of spontaneous chylous ascites is largely supportive rather than operative. Symptomatic relief can be obtained by intermittent abdominal and pleural tapping. Repeated punctures seldom arrest the chylous leakage and are not without hazard. Dietary measures should begin with a low-fat diet supplemented by medium-chain triglycerides, the latter being transported via the portal rather than the lymphatic circulation. Two thirds of pediatric cases resolve spontaneously on expectant management within a month or so as collaterals develop. If dietary measures fail, oral findings should be halted and total parenteral nutrition instituted. In adults, the most hopeful situation is if an underlying cancer (which is rarely amenable to curative resection) producing the chylous ascites regresses with chemotherapy or irradiation. Spontaneous improvement is the rule in posttraumatic cases.

Except for resectable congenital chylous cysts, surgery has little to offer. In refractory traumatic cases, intraoperative lymphangiography or perioperative injection of lipophilic dyes at times identifies a leaking site that can be plicated. At operation, the root of the small bowel mesentery around the superior mesenteric vessels should be carefully examined, as a discrete tear is more common at this site. Peritoneovenous shunting has been successful in some postoperative cases. Other surgical endeavors such as bowel resection and retroperitoneal dissection are uniformly futile.

2. Malignant Ascites

Ascites due to advanced cancer is a distressing complication that often necessitates in-hospital care. Peritoneal implants stimulate production of ascitic fluid while impeding its resorption by diaphragmatic lymphatics. Malignant ascites also occurs in the absence of free peritoneal tumor cells if there is advanced venous or lymphatic obstruction. A positive cytologic diagnosis is obtained in 60–90% of cases and supported by a high lactate dehydrogenase (> 500 IU/L) or carcinoembryonic antigen (CEA) content. DNA aneuploidy on flow cytometry analysis is confirmatory in cytology-negative cases.

Since this is often a preterminal condition, conservative management is preferred, with diuretics (especially spirono-

lactone), paracentesis if warranted by the symptoms, and chemotherapy.

Peritoneovenous shunting (preferably with the Denver shunt) should be considered in symptomatic patients who have ascites refractory to conservative methods and an expected survival time of at least 2 months. Shunting is not effective for viscous or loculated ascites, heavily bloodstained ascites, or ascites with an unusually high cell count. The procedure is most suitable in patients with breast, gastric, or ovarian adenocarcinoma or cytology-negative ascites. Complications include shunt obstruction, disseminated intravascular coagulation, fluid overload, and sepsis. Surprisingly, dissemination of the tumor is rare. About half of the patients derive substantial benefits but few survive beyond 6 months.

Arroyo V et al: Complications of cirrhosis. II. Renal and circulatory dysfunction. Lights and shadows in an important clinical problem. J Hepatol 2000;32(1 Suppl):157.
Dugernier T et al: Ascites fluid in severe acute pancreatitis: from pathophysiology to therapy. Acta Gastroenterol Belg 2000; 63:264.
Heneghan MA et al: Pathogenesis of ascites in cirrhosis and portal hypertension. Med Sci Monit 2000;6:807.
Uriz J et al: Pathophysiology, diagnosis and treatment of ascites in cirrhosis. Baillieres Best Pract Res Clin Gastroenterol 2000; 14:927.

PERITONEAL ADHESIONS

Tissue ischemia, mechanical or thermal trauma, infection, radiation injury, and foreign body reaction predispose to adhesion formation. The peritoneal injury underlying these noxious stimuli evokes a serosanguineous inflammatory reaction that leads to fibrin deposition. Ordinarily, local plasminogen activators initiate lysis of the fibrin strands within 3 days of their formation. Metamorphosis of mesodermal cells regenerates a single layer of new mesothelium as early as 5 days after injury. Inadequate fibrinolysis due to reduced mesothelial plasminogen activator activity allows fibroblastic proliferation to produce fibrous adhesions. Adhesions are now the most prevalent cause of acute and recurrent small bowel obstruction (see Chapter 29) and a persistent bane of abdominal and especially pelvic surgery. However, adhesions may also provide useful vascular bridges that promote tissue healing, such as in ischemic areas of a bowel anastomosis.

Adhesions develop in two thirds of patients after laparotomy, especially after extensive procedures, pelvic operations, or multiple abdominal operations. Spontaneous adhesions, presumably related to subclinical inflammation, are also found in one quarter of patients on postmortem examination. Postoperative adhesions are most heavily distributed near the operative site. The omentum, small bowel, colon, and rectum (in descending order of frequency) are involved most often. Short, obese female patients seem to have a greater tendency to form adhesions.

► Prevention & Treatment

Precise operative technique with avoidance of serosal trauma will reduce but not eliminate adhesion formation. Ischemic tissue trauma caused by crushing, cautery, and mass ligation should be minimized. Reperitonealization of the pelvic floor under tension has been shown to promote rather than hinder adhesion formation. Indeed, well-vascularized peritoneal edges will resurface adjacent denuded areas with epithelium within 2 weeks. The use of an omental flap or synthetic absorbable or nonabsorbable material (eg, GORE-TEX) appears useful after extensive pelvic dissections. Abdominal packs, moist or dry, should be used sparingly, because they produce abrasive serosal tears. Blood and foreign bodies alone induce only a slight peritoneal reaction, but this becomes extensive when there are accompanying serosal injuries. Precise hemostasis is vital, because unclotted blood in the peritoneal cavity acts as an additional source of fibrin, and platelets themselves stimulate serosal inflammation. Starch glove powder, lint gauze fluffs, and cellulose fibers from disposable drapes provoke a rigorous foreign body reaction, and care should be taken to prevent such contamination. The differences between similar types of nonreactive suture material are less critical than the manner in which they are employed: A large number of coarse sutures creates more adhesions than well-placed finer sutures. Laparoscopic procedures tend to produce fewer adhesions than laparotomy.

Hyaluronic acid-carboxymethylcellulose film (Sepra film) placed during laparotomy decreases the formation of intraperitoneal adhesions. It is particularly useful in patients likely to need early reoperation, such as those with a temporary bowel diversion.

Beck DE et al: A prospective, randomized, multicenter, controlled study of the safety of Seprafilm adhesion barrier in abdomino-pelvic surgery of the intestine. Dis Col Rectum 2003;46:1310.

TUMORS OF THE PERITONEUM & RETROPERITONEUM

Most tumors affecting the peritoneum are secondary implants from primary intraperitoneal cancers. Some unusual peritoneal and retroperitoneal lesions present with abdominal masses or ascites that may be confused with carcinomatosis or chronic inflammatory peritonitis.

► Peritoneal Mesothelioma

These rare primary neoplasms are derived from the meso-dermal lining of the peritoneum. The malignant variety develops most commonly in men, with a long latent period (averaging 40 years) after prolonged asbestos exposure. Pleural malignant mesotheliomas outnumber peritoneal ones by a ratio of 3:1. Patients present typically with weight loss, crampy abdominal pain, a large mass or distention due to ascites, and a history of asbestos contact. Fewer than half of these patients have asbestosis demonstrated on plain chest films. In contrast to peritoneal carcinomatosis, mesotheliomas are associated with less ascites than the degree of abdominal distention would suggest, and cytologic studies of ascitic fluid are rarely positive. CT scan of the lower thorax and abdomen will demonstrate ascites, peritoneal and mesenteric thickening, pleural plaques, and soft tissue masses involving the omentum and peritoneum. Multiple fine-needle aspiration biopsies guided by ultrasonography, CT scan, or laparoscopy can establish the diagnosis. Electron microscopy is confirmatory in equivocal cases.

Patients usually undergo laparotomy either for diagnosis or because of bowel obstruction. Localized masses should be resected to avoid subsequent obstruction. Metastases to the liver and lung occur late. Encouraging results have been reported with long-term survival following cytoreductive operation and intraperitoneal cisplatin-based combination chemotherapy. Long-term survivors (beyond 1 year) have been reported with combined treatment by surgical debulking, intraperitoneal cisplatin-doxorubicin, and whole-abdomen irradiation. One should differentiate malignant mesotheliomas from cystic mesotheliomas and well-differentiated papillary mesotheliomas in women, which are less malignant and carry a better prognosis even though they tend to recur locally.

► Pseudomyxoma Peritonei

This unusual disease is caused by a low-grade mucinous cystadenocarcinoma of the appendix or ovary that secretes large amounts of mucus-containing epithelial cells. It should be distinguished from benign appendiceal mucocele, which may also have local mucinous deposits but carries a favorable outlook. Patients seldom complain until advanced stages of disease, at which time they have abdominal distention and pain and, in many instances, intermittent or chronic partial small bowel obstruction. Weight loss and other features of cancer are uncommon. The shed neoplastic cells spread freely to two main areas: the upper abdominal sites of peritoneal fluid resorption (undersurface of diaphragm and omentum) and the dependent peritoneal areas (pelvis and lateral abdominal gutters). Distant metastases and visceral involvement are rare. Ultrasonography and CT scans show a distinctive peritoneal scalloping of the liver margin, calcified plaques, ascites, and low-density masses.

At laparotomy, the surgeon should remove as much of the primary lesion and gelatinous material as possible. The omentum also should be resected and existing or impending bowel obstruction relieved. This often necessitates right hemicolectomy. If there is no apparent primary tumor, the appendix, and, in women, both ovaries should be removed. Some surgeons advocate radical peritonectomy (including splenectomy, cholecystectomy, appendectomy, sigmoid colectomy, and hysterectomy) to eliminate potential areas of microscopic spread. Whether the higher morbidity incurred is justified remains debated.

Current therapy favors very early intraperitoneal fluoro-uracil-based adjuvant chemotherapy. Systemic chemotherapy is generally useless. Adjuvant intracavitary radiotherapy has also been advocated, especially for patients with residual disease. Reexploration should be undertaken either as a planned second-look laparotomy or to debulk residual tumor responsible for recurrent obstruction or debilitating mucous ascites. Two thirds of patients eventually succumb to local or regional disease. The survival rate is about 50% at 5 years and 30% at 10 years.

Bijelic L, Jonson A, Sugarbaker PH: Systematic review of cytoreductive surgery and heated intraoperative intraperitoneal chemotherapy for treatment of peritoneal carcinomatosis in primary and recurrent ovarian cancer. Ann Oncol 2007;18:1943.

Esquivel J. et al: Cytoreductive surgery and hyperthermic intraperitoneal chemotherapy in the management of peritoneal surface malignancies of colonic origin: a consensus statement. Society of Surgical Oncology. Ann Surg Oncol 2007;14:128.

Yan TD et al: Perioperative outcomes of cytoreductive surgery and perioperative intraperitoneal chemotherapy for non-appendiceal peritoneal carcinomatosis from a prospective database. J Surg Oncol 2007;96:102.

▶ Cysts of the Mesentery & Retroperitoneum

These rare developmental lesions are usually ectopic pockets of lymphatic tissue or, more rarely, mucinous ovarian cystadenomas. Patients—one third of whom are children—present with an asymptomatic abdominal mass, chronic pain, or an acute abdomen. The mass is often large, smooth, round, compressible, and more mobile transversely than longitudinally. CT or ultrasonographic scans along with contrast studies of the gastrointestinal and urinary tracts reveal the cystic nature and location of the mass. The differential diagnosis includes pancreatic pseudocysts, enteric duplication (in children), inflammatory cysts, and retroperitoneal tumors. Laparotomy or laparoscopy reveals the cyst, which contains serous fluid if it is in the mesocolon; chylous fluid if it is in the small bowel mesentery; or blood-stained fluid. Most lesions are benign, and enucleation suffices. Segmental resection may be necessary for cysts that impinge upon the bowel wall or its blood supply. Recurrences are more frequent with retroperitoneal cysts, because they may not be amenable to complete excision, and marsupialization may be required instead.

▶ Mesenteric Lipodystrophy (Mesenteric Panniculitis)

There are fewer than 200 reported cases of mesenteric lipodystrophy, in which chronic fat degeneration and fibrosis affecting the root of the mesentery produce diffuse mesenteric thickening or masses. Its cause is unknown, but it may be a localized form of Weber-Christian disease.

The patient, often an elderly man, has recurrent abdominal pain, weight loss, or symptoms of partial intestinal obstruction. A hard irregular abdominal mass, usually in the left upper quadrant, is felt in over half of patients. CT or ultrasound examination and barium follow-up studies can outline the lesion. CT scanning shows the characteristic features of nonhomogeneous masses of fat and soft tissue density. MRI may suggest the fibrous nature of the lesion and delineates vascular involvement. The diagnosis is usually made only by biopsy at laparotomy, but resection is neither feasible nor indicated. An occasional patient will require a side-to-side intestinal bypass to relieve obstruction.

The process subsides spontaneously in most cases. A more serious variant (**retractile mesenteritis**) associated with obstruction of the mesenteric lymphatics and veins often proves fatal. Corticosteroids, cyclophosphamide, and azathioprine should be reserved for such cases and for patients with clinical deterioration. Lymphoma occurs in 15% of cases on follow-up.

RETROPERITONEAL FIBROSIS

This uncommon entity is characterized by extensive fibrotic encasement of retroperitoneal tissues. Over two thirds of cases are idiopathic and the rest secondary to drugs (eg, methysergide, beta-adrenergic blocking agents), retroperitoneal hemorrhage, perianeurysmal inflammation, irradiation, urinary extravasation, or cancer. The fibrosis represents an allergic reaction to insoluble lipid (ceroid) that has leaked from atheromatous plaques, especially those within the aorta. The urinary tract may be involved with a diagnostic triad of hydronephrosis and hydroureter (usually bilateral), medial deviation of the ureters, and extrinsic ureteric compression near the L4–5 level. Desmoplastic involvement of the small and large bowel may give rise to obstructive symptoms. Most patients are men over age 50 who present with renal failure or obstructive uropathy. Pain in the low back or flank is common. Pyuria is present in most patients. The diagnosis is suggested by a CT scan that shows the fibrotic process and any coexisting aneurysmal changes in the aorta. MRI may distinguish fibrosis from lymphoma or metastatic carcinoma. Withdrawal of suspect drugs is usually followed by gradual improvement.

Severe urinary obstruction should be decompressed by ureteric stents or nephrostomy. Prednisone (30–60 mg daily) and immunosuppression have been tried but with inconclusive benefits. These agents should be started early postoperatively before marked fibrosis develops. Tamoxifen has produced regression of desmoid tumors. If surgery becomes necessary, a thick rubbery or fibrotic plaque containing chronic inflammatory cells is found at exploration. Multiple biopsy specimens should be taken to exclude cancer. Ureterolysis should be attempted, and there may be some advantage to wrapping omentum around the freed ureters to reduce the risk of subsequent entrapment. Laparoscopic ureterolysis may occasionally be feasible. The outlook is good as long as there is no underlying cancer.

Marcolongo R et al: Immunosuppressive therapy for idiopathic retroperitoneal fibrosis: a retrospective analysis of 26 cases. Am J Med 2004;116:194.

Marzano A et al: Treatment of idiopathic retroperitoneal fibrosis using cyclosporin. Ann Rheum Dis 2001;60:427.

Vaglio A, Salvarani C, Buzio C: Retroperitoneal fibrosis. Lancet 2006;367:241.

DISORDERS INVOLVING THE OMENTUM

▶ Infection

The omentum plays an important role in protecting against spreading peritonitis. In chronic infections such as tuberculosis, it may become infected and appear as a rolled-up thickened, inflamed mass. Nonspecific inflammation of the omentum, often a sequela of previous torsion, causes vague abdominal pain.

▶ Torsion & Infarction

Primary (spontaneous) torsion of the omentum may develop if a free portion is fixed by an adhesion or trapped within a hernia. Rotation around the pedicle occludes the blood supply and leads to ischemic necrosis. Infarction may also be secondary to abdominal trauma or vascular conditions such as polyarteritis nodosa. Paraesophageal omental herniation may predispose to a hiatal hernia and may mimic a mediastinal lipoma.

Clinically, torsion presents as acute abdominal pain with nausea and vomiting. Tenderness is confined to the involved area, usually on the right side but away from McBurney point. A mobile, tender mass is noted in one third of cases. These features may suggest acute appendicitis or cholecystitis but are not typical of those diseases. The clinical findings usually mandate surgical exploration, which reveals serosanguineous fluid, a normal appendix, and the hemorrhagic necrotic segment of omentum. Resection of the affected portion is curative.

▶ Tumors & Cysts of the Omentum

The omentum is frequently involved secondarily by intra-abdominal malignant tumors, especially gastrointestinal and ovarian adenocarcinomas. Primary cysts or vascular anomalies, usually incidentally discovered at laparotomy, are readily resected.

Stomach & Duodenum

Gerard M. Doherty, MD
Lawrence W. Way, MD

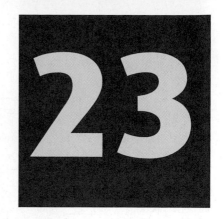

I. STOMACH

The stomach receives food from the esophagus and has four functions: (1) It acts as a reservoir that permits eating reasonably large quantities of food at intervals of several hours. (2) Food contained in the stomach is mixed, triturated, and delivered into the duodenum in amounts regulated by its chemical nature and texture. (3) The first stages of protein and carbohydrate digestion are carried out in the stomach. (4) A few substances are absorbed across the gastric mucosa.

ANATOMY

The anatomy of the stomach may be seen in Figures 23–1, 23–2, and 23–3.

The **cardia** is located at the gastroesophageal junction. The **fundus** is the portion of the stomach that lies cephalad to the gastroesophageal junction. The **corpus** is the capacious central part; division of the corpus from the pyloric antrum is marked approximately by the angular incisure, a crease on the lesser curvature just proximal to the "crow's-foot" terminations of the nerves of Latarjet (Figure 23–3). The **pylorus** is the boundary between the stomach and the duodenum.

The **cardiac gland area** is the small segment located at the gastroesophageal junction. Histologically, it contains principally mucus-secreting cells, though a few parietal cells are sometimes present. The **oxyntic gland area** is the portion containing parietal (oxyntic) cells and chief cells (Figure 23–2). The boundary between this region and the adjacent pyloric gland area is reasonably sharp, since the zone of transition spans a segment of only 1–1.5 cm. The **pyloric gland** area constitutes the distal 30% of the stomach and contains the G cells that manufacture gastrin. Mucous cells are common in the oxyntic and pyloric gland areas.

As in the rest of the gastrointestinal tract, the muscular wall of the stomach is composed of an outer longitudinal and an inner circular layer. An additional incomplete inner layer of obliquely situated fibers is most prominent near the lesser curvature but is of less substance than the other two layers.

▶ Blood Supply

The blood supply of the stomach and duodenum is illustrated in Figure 23–3. The left gastric artery supplies the lesser curvature and connects with the right gastric artery, a branch of the common hepatic artery. In 60% of persons, a posterior gastric artery arises off the middle third of the splenic artery and terminates in branches on the posterior surface of the body and the fundus. The greater curvature is supplied by the right gastroepiploic artery (a branch of the gastroduodenal artery) and the left gastroepiploic artery (a branch of the splenic artery). The mid portion of the greater curvature corresponds to a point at which the gastric branches of this vascular arcade change direction. The fundus of the stomach along the greater curvature is supplied by the vasa brevia, branches of the splenic and left gastroepiploic arteries.

The blood supply to the duodenum is from the superior and inferior pancreaticoduodenal arteries, which are branches of the gastroduodenal artery and the superior mesenteric artery, respectively. The stomach contains a rich submucosal vascular plexus. Venous blood from the stomach drains into the coronary, gastroepiploic, and splenic veins before entering the portal vein. The lymphatic drainage of the stomach, which largely parallels the arteries, partially determines the direction of spread of gastric neoplasms.

▶ Nerve Supply

The parasympathetic nerves to the stomach are shown in Figure 23–3. As a rule, two major vagal trunks pass through the esophageal hiatus in close approximation to the esophageal muscle. The nerves are originally located to the right and left of the esophagus and stomach during embryonic development. When the foregut rotates, the lesser curvature turns to the right and the greater curvature to the left, and corresponding shifts in location of the vagal trunks follow.

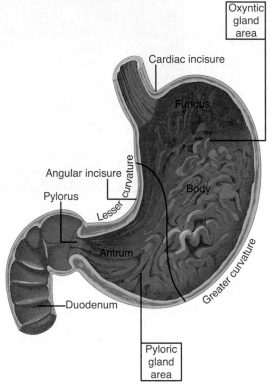

▲ Figure 23–1. Names of the parts of the stomach. The line drawn from the lesser to the greater curvature depicts the approximate boundary between the oxyntic gland area and the pyloric gland area. No prominent landmark exists to distinguish between antrum and body (corpus). The fundus is the portion craniad to the esophagogastric junction.

Hence, the right vagus supplies the posterior and the left the anterior gastric surface. About 90% of the vagal fibers are sensory afferent; the remaining 10% are efferent.

In the region of the gastroesophageal junction, each trunk bifurcates. The anterior trunk sends to the liver a division that travels in the lesser omentum. The bifurcation of the posterior trunk gives rise to fibers that enter the celiac plexus and supply the parasympathetic innervation to the remainder of the gastrointestinal tract as far as the mid transverse colon. Both trunks, after giving rise to their extragastric divisions, send some fibers directly onto the surface of the stomach and others along the lesser curvature (anterior and posterior nerves of Latarjet) to supply the distal part of the organ. As shown in Figure 23–3, a variable number of vagal fibers ascend with the left gastric artery after having passed through the celiac plexus.

The preganglionic motor fibers of the vagal trunks synapse with ganglion cells in the Auerbach plexus (plexus myentericus) between the longitudinal and circular muscle layers. Postganglionic cholinergic fibers are distributed to the cells of the smooth muscle layers and the mucosa.

The adrenergic innervation to the stomach consists of postganglionic fibers that pass along the arterial vessels from the celiac plexus.

PHYSIOLOGY

▶ Motility

Storage, mixing, trituration, and regulated emptying are accomplished by the muscular apparatus of the stomach. Peristaltic waves originate in the body and pass toward the pylorus. The thickness of the smooth muscle increases in the antrum and corresponds to the stronger contractions that can be measured in the distal stomach. The pylorus behaves as a sphincter, though it normally allows a little to-and-fro movement of chyme across the junction.

An electrical pacemaker situated in the fundal musculature near the greater curvature gives rise to regular (3/min) electrical impulses (pacesetter potential, basic electrical rhythm) that pass toward the pylorus in the outer longitudinal layer. Every impulse is not always followed by a peristaltic muscular contraction, but the impulses determine the maximal peristaltic rate. The frequency of peristalsis is governed by a variety of stimuli mentioned below. Each contraction follows sequential depolarization of the underlying circular muscle resulting from arrival of the pacesetter potential.

Peristaltic contractions are more forceful in the antrum than the body and travel faster as they progress distally. Gastric chyme is forced into the funnel-shaped antral chamber by peristalsis; the volume of contents delivered into the duodenum by each peristaltic wave depends on the strength of the advancing wave and the extent to which the pylorus closes. Most of the gastric contents that are pushed into the antral funnel are propelled backward as the pylorus closes and pressure within the antral lumen rises. Five to 15 mL enter the duodenum with each gastric peristaltic wave.

The volume of the empty gastric lumen is only 50 mL. By a process called receptive relaxation, the stomach can accommodate about 1000 mL before intraluminal pressure begins to rise. Receptive relaxation is an active process mediated by vagal reflexes and abolished by vagotomy. Peristalsis is initiated by the stimulus of distention after eating. Various other factors have positive or negative influences on the rate and strength of contractions and the rate of gastric emptying. Vagal reflexes from the stomach have a facilitating influence on peristalsis. The texture and volume of the meal both play a role in the regulation of emptying; small particles are emptied more rapidly than large ones, which the organ attempts to reduce in size (trituration). The osmolality of gastric chyme and its chemical makeup are monitored by duodenal receptors. If osmolality is greater than 200 mosm/L, a long vagal reflex (the enterogastric reflex) is activated, delaying emptying. Gastrin causes delay in emptying. Gastrin is the only circulating gastrointestinal hormone to have a physiologic effect on emptying.

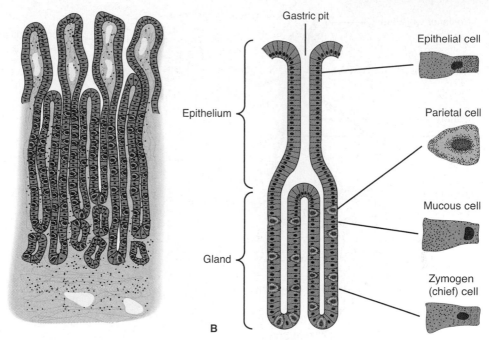

▲ **Figure 23–2.** Histologic features of the mucosa in the oxyntic gland area. Each gastric pit drains three to seven tubular gastric glands. **A:** The neck of the gland contains many mucous cells. Oxyntic (parietal) cells are most numerous in the mid portion of the glands; peptic (chief) cells predominate in the basal portion. **B:** Drawing from photomicrograph of the gastric mucosa.

▶ Gastric Juice

The output of gastric juice in a fasting subject varies between 500 and 1500 mL/d. After each meal, about 1000 mL are secreted by the stomach.

The components of gastric juice are as follows:

A. Mucus

Mucus is a heterogeneous mixture of glycoproteins manufactured in the mucous cells of the oxyntic and pyloric gland areas. Mucus provides a weak barrier to the diffusion of H^+ and probably protects the mucosa. It also acts as a lubricant and impedes diffusion of pepsin.

B. Pepsinogen

Pepsinogens are synthesized in the chief cells of the oxyntic gland area (and to a lesser extent in the pyloric area) and are stored as visible granules. Cholinergic stimuli, either vagal or intramural, are the most potent pepsigogues, though gastrin and secretin are also effective. The precursor zymogen is activated when pH falls below 5.00, a process that entails severance of a polypeptide fragment from the larger molecule. Pepsin cleaves peptide bonds, especially those containing phenylalanine, tyrosine, or leucine. Its optimal pH is

about 2.00. Pepsin activity is abolished at pH greater than 5.00, and the molecule is irreversibly denatured at pH greater than 8.00.

C. Intrinsic Factor

Intrinsic factor, a mucoprotein secreted by the parietal cells, binds with vitamin B_{12} of dietary origin and greatly enhances absorption of the vitamin. Absorption occurs by an active process in the terminal ileum.

Intrinsic factor secretion is enhanced by stimuli that evoke H^+ output from parietal cells. Pernicious anemia is characterized by atrophy of the parietal cell mucosa, deficiency in intrinsic factor, and anemia. Subclinical deficiencies in vitamin B_{12} have been described after operations that reduce gastric acid secretion, and abnormal Schilling tests in these patients can be corrected by the administration of intrinsic factor. Total gastrectomy creates a dependence on parenteral administration of vitamin B_{12}.

D. Blood Group Substances

Seventy-five percent of people secrete blood group antigens into gastric juice. The trait is genetically determined and is associated with a lower incidence of duodenal ulcer than in nonsecretors.

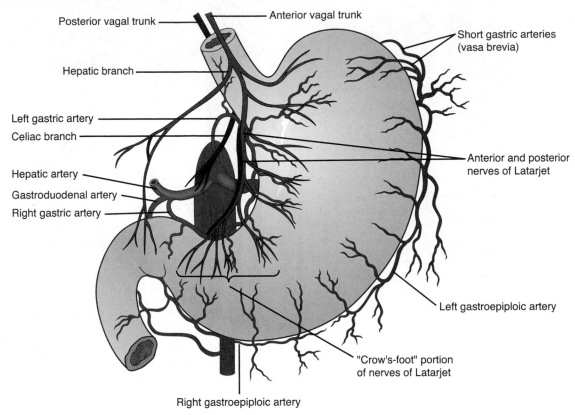

Posterior vagal trunk ————
Anterior vagal trunk

Short gastric arteries
(vasa brevia)

Hepatic branch ————

Left gastric artery ————
Celiac branch ————

Anterior and posterior
nerves of Latarjet

Hepatic artery ————
Gastroduodenal artery ————
Right gastric artery ————

Left gastroepiploic artery

"Crow's-foot" portion
of nerves of Latarjet

Right gastroepiploic artery

▲ **Figure 23–3.** Blood supply and parasympathetic innervation of the stomach and duodenum.

E. Electrolytes

The unique characteristic of gastric secretion is its high concentration of hydrochloric acid, a product of the parietal cells. As the concentration of H$^+$ rises during secretion, that of Na$^+$ drops in a reciprocal fashion. K$^+$ remains relatively constant at 5–10 meq/L. Chloride concentration remains near 150 meq/L, and gastric juice maintains its isotonicity at varying secretory rates.

▶ The Parietal Cell & Acid Secretion

Many of the key events in acid secretion by gastric parietal cells are illustrated in Figure 23–4. The onset of secretion is accompanied by striking morphologic changes in the apical membranes. Resting parietal cells are characterized by an infolding of the apical membrane, called the secretory canaliculus, which is lined by short microvilli. Multiple membrane-bound tubulovesicles and mitochondria are present in the cytoplasm. With stimulation, the secretory canaliculus expands, the microvilli become long and narrow and filled with microfilaments, and the cytoplasmic tubulovesicles disappear. The proton pump mechanism for acid secretion is

located in the tubulovesicles in the resting state and in the secretory canaliculus in the stimulated state.

The basal lateral membrane contains the receptors for secretory stimulants and transfers HCO$_3^-$ out of the cell to balance the H$^+$ output at the apical membrane. Active uptake of Cl$^-$ and K$^+$ conduction also occur at the basal lateral membrane. Separate membrane-bound receptors exist for histamine (H$_2$ receptor), gastrin, and acetylcholine. The intracellular second messengers are thought to be cAMP for histamine and Ca^{2+} for gastrin and acetylcholine.

Acid secretion at the apical membrane is accomplished by a membrane-bound H$^+$/K$^+$-ATPase (the proton pump); H$^+$ is secreted into the lumen in exchange for K$^+$.

▶ Mucosal Resistance in the Stomach & Duodenum

The healthy mucosa of the stomach and duodenum is provided with mechanisms that allow it to withstand the potentially injurious effects of high concentrations of luminal acid. Disruption of these mechanisms may contribute to acute or chronic ulceration.

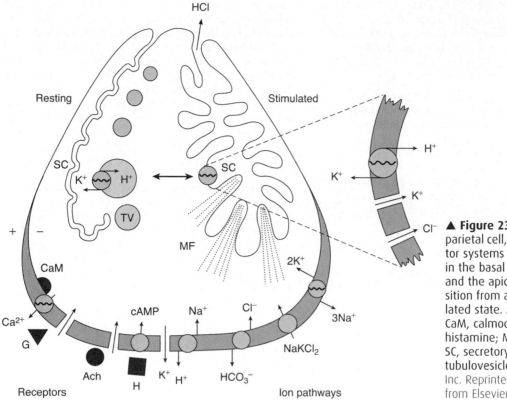

▲ **Figure 23–4.** Diagram of a parietal cell, showing the receptor systems and ion pathways in the basal lateral membrane and the apical membrane transition from a resting to a stimulated state. Ach, acetylcholine; CaM, calmodulin; G, gastrin; H, histamine; MF, microfilaments; SC, secretory canaliculus; TV, tubulovesicles. (© 1984 Elsevier Inc. Reprinted with permission from Elsevier.)

The surface of the gastric mucosa is coated with mucus and secretes HCO_3^- in addition to H^+. Protected by the blanket of mucus, the surface pH is much higher than the luminal pH. HCO_3^- secretion is stimulated by cyclic adenosine monophosphate (cAMP), prostaglandins, cholinomimetics, glucagon, cholecystokinin (CCK), and by as yet unidentified paracrine hormones. Inhibitors of HCO_3^- secretion include nonsteroidal anti-inflammatory agents, alpha-adrenergic agonists, bile acids, ethanol, and acetazolamide. Increases in luminal H^+ result in increased HCO_3^- secretion, probably mediated by tissue prostaglandins.

Gastric mucus is a gel composed of high-molecular-weight glycoproteins and 95% water. Since it forms an unstirred layer, it helps the underlying mucosa to maintain a higher pH than that of gastric juice, and it also acts as a barrier to the diffusion of pepsin. At the surface of the layer of mucus, peptic digestion continuously degrades mucus, while below it is continuously being replenished by mucous cells. Gastric acid is thought to enter the lumen through thin spots in the mucus overlying the gastric glands. Secretion of mucus is stimulated by luminal acid and perhaps by cholinergic stimuli. The layer of mucus is damaged by exposure to nonsteroidal anti-inflammatory agents and is enhanced by topical prostaglandin E_2.

Mucosal defects produced by mechanical or chemical trauma are rapidly repaired by adjacent normal cells that spread to cover the defect, a process that can be enhanced experimentally by adding HCO_3^- to the nutrient side of the mucosa. This important phenomenon has not yet been thoroughly studied.

The duodenal mucosa possesses defenses similar to those in the stomach: the ability to secrete HCO_3^- and mucus and rapid repair of mucosal injuries.

▶ Regulation of Acid Secretion

The regulation of acid secretion can best be described by considering separately those factors that enhance gastric acid production and those that depress it. The interaction of these forces is what determines the levels of secretion observed during fasting and after meals.

A. Stimulation of Acid Secretion

Acid production is usually described as the result of three phases that are excited simultaneously after a meal. The separation into phases is of value principally for descriptive purposes.

1. Cephalic phase—Stimuli that act upon the brain lead to increased vagal efferent activity and acid secretion. The sight, smell, taste, or even thought of appetizing food may elicit this response. The effect is entirely vagally mediated and is abolished by vagotomy. The vagal stimuli have a direct effect on the parietal cells to increase acid output.

2. Gastric phase—Food in the stomach (principally protein hydrolysates and hydrophobic amino acids) stimulates gastrin release from the antrum. Gastric distention has a similar but less intense effect.

The presence of food in the stomach excites long vagal reflexes, impulses that pass to the central nervous system via vagal afferents and return to stimulate the parietal cells.

A third aspect of the gastric phase involves the sensitizing effect of distention of the parietal cell area to gastrin that is probably mediated through local intramural cholinergic reflexes.

3. Intestinal phase—The role of the intestinal phase in the stimulation of gastric secretion has been incompletely investigated. Various experiments have shown that the presence of food in the small bowel releases a humoral factor, named entero-oxyntin, that evokes acid secretion from the stomach.

B. Inhibition of Acid Secretion

Without systems to limit secretion, unchecked acid production could become a serious clinical problem. Examples can be found (eg, Billroth II gastrectomy with retained antrum) where acid production rose after surgical procedures that interfered with these inhibitory mechanisms.

1. Antral inhibition—pH below 2.50 in the antrum inhibits the release of gastrin regardless of the stimulus. When the pH reaches 1.20, gastrin release is almost completely blocked. If the normal relationship of parietal cell mucosa to antral mucosa is changed so that acid does not flow past the site of gastrin production, serum gastrin may increase to high levels, with marked acid stimulation. Somatostatin in gastric antral cells serves a physiologic role as an inhibitor of gastrin release (a paracrine function).

2. Intestinal inhibition—The intestine participates in controlling acid secretion by liberating hormones that inhibit both the release of gastrin and its effects on the parietal cells. Secretin blocks acid secretion under experimental conditions but not as a physiologic action. Fat in the intestine is the most potent method of inhibition, affecting gastrin release and acid secretion. Neither somatostatin nor gastric inhibitory polypeptide (GIP), both released by food in the intestine, seems able to account for the inhibition, and the term enterogastrone is used to denote the still unidentified hormone presumably responsible.

▶ Integration of Gastric Physiologic Function

Ingested food is mixed with salivary amylase before it reaches the stomach. The mechanisms stimulating gastric secretion are activated. Serum gastrin levels increase from a mean fasting concentration of about 50 pg/mL to 200 pg/mL, the peak occurring about 30 minutes after the meal. Food in the lumen of the stomach is exposed to high concentrations of acid and pepsin at the mucosal surface. Food settles in layers determined by sequence of arrival, but fat tends to float to the top. The greatest mixing occurs in the antrum. Antral contents therefore become more uniformly acidic than those in the body of the organ, where the central portion of the meal tends to remain alkaline for a considerable time, allowing continued activity of the amylase.

Peptic digestion of protein in the stomach is only about 5–10% complete. Carbohydrate digestion may reach 30–40%. A lipase originating from the tongue initiates the first stages of lipolysis in the stomach.

The gastric contents are delivered to the duodenum at a rate determined by the volume and texture of the meal, its osmolality and acidity, and its content of fat. A meal of lean meat, potatoes, and vegetables leaves the stomach within 3 hours. A meal with a very high fat content may remain in the stomach for 6–12 hours.

Calam J, Baron JH: ABC of the upper gastrointestinal tract: pathophysiology of duodenal and gastric ulcer and gastric cancer. BMJ 2001;323:980.

PEPTIC ULCER

Peptic ulcers result from the corrosive action of acid gastric juice on a vulnerable epithelium. Depending on circumstances, they may occur in the esophagus, the duodenum, the stomach itself, the jejunum after surgical construction of a gastrojejunostomy, or the ileum in relation to ectopic gastric mucosa in Meckel diverticulum. When the term peptic ulcer was first used, it was thought that the most important factor was the peptic activity in gastric juice. Since then, evidence has implicated acid as the chief injurious agent; in fact, it is axiomatic that if gastric juice contains no acid, a (benign) peptic ulcer cannot be present. Appreciation of the role of acid has led to the emphasis on therapy with antacids and H_2 blocking agents for the medical therapy of ulcers and to operations that reduce acid secretion as the major surgical approach. In the case of duodenal and gastric ulcers, *Helicobacter pylori* must colonize and weaken the mucosa before acid is able to do the damage, and therapy directed against this organism has a more definitive effect on the disease.

It has been estimated that about 2% of the adult population in the United States suffers from active peptic ulcer disease, and about 10% of the population will have the disease during their lifetime. Men are affected three times as often as women. Duodenal ulcers are ten times more common than gastric ulcers in young patients, but in the older age groups the frequency is about equal. Probably as a result of a declining prevalence of *H pylori* infection, the incidence has declined to less than half what it was 25 years ago.

In general terms, the ulcerative process can lead to four types of disability: (1) **Pain** is the most common. (2) **Bleeding** may occur as a result of erosion of submucosal or extraintestinal vessels as the ulcer becomes deeper. (3) Penetration of the ulcer through all layers of the affected gut results in **perforation** if other viscera do not seal the ulcer. (4) **Obstruction** may result from inflammatory swelling and scarring and is most likely to occur with ulcers located at the pylorus or gastroesophageal junction, where the lumen is narrowest.

The clinical features and prognosis of duodenal ulcer and gastric ulcer are sufficiently different to be dealt with separately here.

DUODENAL ULCER

ESSENTIALS OF DIAGNOSIS

▶ Epigastric pain relieved by food or antacids.

▶ Epigastric tenderness.

▶ Normal or increased gastric acid secretion.

▶ Signs of ulcer disease on upper gastrointestinal x-rays or endoscopy.

▶ Evidence of *Helicobacter pylori* infection.

▶ General Considerations

Duodenal ulcers may occur in any age group but are most common in the young and middle-aged (20–45 years). They appear in men more often than women. About 95% of duodenal ulcers are situated within 2 cm of the pylorus, in the duodenal bulb.

Considerable evidence implicates *H pylori* as the principal cause of duodenal ulcer disease. This microaerophilic gram-negative curved bacillus can be found colonizing patches of gastric metaplasia within the duodenum in 90% of patients with this disease. The bacilli remain on the surface of the mucosa rather than invading it. They are thought to render the duodenum more vulnerable to the injurious effects of acid and pepsin by releasing urease or other toxins.

The epidemiology of peptic ulcer disease reflects the prevalence of *H pylori* infection in different populations. In areas of the world where peptic ulcer is uncommon (eg, rural Africa), human infection is rare. Duodenal ulcer disease has emerged as a major clinical entity in Western society only since the latter part of the 19th century. The incidence reached a peak about 30 years ago and then declined to reach a lower plateau a few years ago. These changes are thought to be explained by variations in *H pylori* infection resulting from public health factors. Within countries like the United States, the distribution of *H pylori* is explainable by a fecal-oral theory of transmission. The prevalence of infection is higher among lower socioeconomic groups. Interestingly, only a minority of infected persons develop ulcers. *H pylori* also has an important role in the etiology of gastric ulcer, gastric cancer, and gastritis. The 10% of duodenal ulcers that are not associated with helicobacter infection are caused by nonsteroidal anti-inflammatory drugs and other agents.

Gastric acid secretion is characteristically higher than normal in patients with duodenal ulcer compared with normal subjects, but only one sixth of the duodenal ulcer population have secretory levels that exceed the normal range (ie, acid secretion in normal subjects and those with duodenal ulcer overlap considerably), so the disease cannot be explained simply as a manifestation of increased acid production. Whether acid secretion increases in response to helicobacter infection is doubted. One possibility is that the patches of metaplastic gastric epithelium in the duodenum on which helicobacter take up residence result from the action of acid. Then the colonized patches undergo ulceration.

Chronic liver disease, chronic lung disease, and chronic pancreatitis have all been implicated as increasing the possibility of duodenal ulceration.

▶ Clinical Findings

A. Symptoms and Signs

Pain, the presenting symptom in most patients, is usually located in the epigastrium and is variably described as aching, burning, or gnawing. Radiologic survey studies indicate, however, that some patients with active duodenal ulcer have no gastrointestinal complaints.

The daily cycle of the pain is often characteristic. The patient usually has no pain in the morning until an hour or more after breakfast. The pain is relieved by the noon meal, only to recur in the later afternoon. Pain may appear again in the evening, and in about half of cases it arouses the patient during the night. Food, milk, or antacid preparations give temporary relief.

When the ulcer penetrates the head of the pancreas posteriorly, back pain is noted; concomitantly, the cyclic pattern of pain may change to a more steady discomfort, with less relief from food and antacids.

Varying degrees of nausea and vomiting are common. Vomiting may be a major feature even in the absence of obstruction.

The abdominal examination may reveal localized epigastric tenderness to the right of the midline, but in many instances no tenderness can be elicited.

B. Endoscopy

Gastroduodenoscopy is useful in evaluating patients with an uncertain diagnosis, those with bleeding from the upper intestine, and those who have obstruction of the gastroduodenal segment and for assessing response to therapy.

C. Diagnostic Tests

1. Gastric analysis—A gastric analysis may be indicated in certain cases. The standard gastric analysis consists of the following: (1) Measurement of acid production by the unstimulated stomach under basal fasting conditions; the result is expressed as H^+ secretion in meq/h and is termed the **basal acid output (BAO)**. (2) Measurement of acid production during stimulation by histamine or pentagastrin given in a dose maximal for this effect. The result is expressed as H^+ secretion in meq/h and is termed the **maximal acid output (MAO)**.

Interpretation of the results is outlined in Table 23–1.

2. Serum gastrin—Depending on the laboratory, normal basal gastrin levels average 50–100 pg/mL, and levels over 200 pg/mL can almost always be considered high.

Gastrin concentrations may rise in hyposecretory and hypersecretory states. In the former conditions (eg, atrophic gastritis, pernicious anemia, acid-suppressant medications), the cause is higher antral pH with loss of antral inhibition for gastrin release. More important clinically is elevated gastrin levels with concomitant hypersecretion, where the high gastrin level is responsible for the increased acid and resulting peptic ulceration. The best-defined clinical condition in this category is Zollinger-Ellison syndrome (gastrinoma). Antrum attached to the duodenum, but out of continuity with the gastric alimentary flow after gastrectomy ("retained antrum"), is another cause of elevated gastrin driving excess gastric acid secretion.

A fasting serum gastrin determination should be obtained in patients with peptic ulcer disease that is unusually severe or refractory to therapy.

D. Radiographic Studies

On an upper gastrointestinal series, the changes induced by duodenal ulcer consist of duodenal deformities and an ulcer niche. Inflammatory swelling and scarring may lead to distortion of the duodenal bulb, eccentricity of the pyloric channel, or pseudodiverticulum formation. The ulcer itself may be seen either in profile or, more commonly, en face.

▶ Differential Diagnosis

The most common diseases simulating peptic ulcer are (1) chronic cholecystitis, in which cholecystograms show either nonfunctioning of the gallbladder or stones in a functioning gallbladder; (2) acute pancreatitis, in which the serum amylase is elevated; (3) chronic pancreatitis, in which endoscopic retrograde cholangiopancreatography (ERCP) shows an abnormal pancreatic duct; (4) functional indigestion, in which x-rays are normal; and (5) reflux esophagitis.

▶ Complications

The common complications of duodenal ulcer are hemorrhage, perforation, and duodenal obstruction. Each of these

Table 23–1. Mean Values for Acid Output during Gastric Analysis for Normals and Patients with Duodenal Ulcer. The Upper Limits of Normal are Basal, 5 meq/h; Maximal, 30 meq/h.

	Sex	Mean Acid Output (meq/h)	
		Normal	**Duodenal Ulcer**
Basal	Male	2.5	5.5
	Female	1.5	3
Maximal (pentagastrin)	Male	30	40
	Female	20	30

is discussed in a separate section. Less common complications are pancreatitis and biliary obstruction.

▶ Prevention

Prevention of ulcer disease entails avoidance of *H pylori* infection.

▶ Treatment

Acute duodenal ulcer can be controlled by suppressing acid secretion in most patients, but the long-term course of the disease (ie, frequency of relapses and of complications) is unaffected unless *H pylori* infection is eradicated. Surgical therapy is recommended principally for the treatment of complications: bleeding, perforation, or obstruction.

A. Medical Treatment

The goals of medical therapy are (1) to heal the ulcer and (2) to cure the disease. Treatment in the first category is aimed at decreasing acid secretion or neutralizing acid. The principal drugs consist of H_2 receptor antagonists (eg, cimetidine, ranitidine) and proton pump blockers (eg, omeprazole). One of the H_2 receptor antagonists is usually the first choice, and when given in therapeutic doses, it will bring about healing of the ulcer in 80% of patients within 6 weeks. Omeprazole is reserved for patients whose ulcers are refractory to H_2 antagonists or for those with Zollinger-Ellison syndrome. Antacids may be used alternatively as primary therapy or on an as-needed basis to treat ulcer pain. Antacids are just as effective as H_2 receptor antagonists but slightly more difficult to administer.

After the ulcer has healed, discontinuation of therapy results in an 80% recurrence rate within 1 year, which may be avoided by chronic nighttime administration of a single dose of H_2 receptor antagonists. A better approach is to treat the *H pylori* infection along with the ulcer, since eradication of *H pylori* eliminates recurrent ulceration unless the infection recurs—an uncommon event. At present, the optimal daily regimen consists of the following combination of drugs:

lansoprazole, 30 mg twice daily for 14 days; amoxicillin, 1 g twice daily for 14 days; and clarithromycin, 500 mg twice daily for 14 days.

B. Surgical Treatment

If medical treatment has been optimal, a persistent ulcer may be judged intractable, and surgical treatment is indicated. This is now uncommon.

The surgical procedures that can cure peptic ulcer are aimed at reduction of gastric acid secretion. Excision of the ulcer itself is not sufficient for either duodenal or gastric ulcer; recurrence is nearly inevitable with such procedures.

The surgical methods of treating duodenal ulcer are vagotomy (several varieties) and antrectomy plus vagotomy. All of these procedures can be performed laparoscopically.

With rare exceptions, one of the vagotomy operations is sufficient (Figure 23–5).

1. Vagotomy—Truncal vagotomy consists of resection of a 1- or 2-cm segment of each vagal trunk as it enters the abdomen on the distal esophagus. The resulting vagal denervation of the gastric musculature produces delayed emptying of the stomach in many patients unless a drainage procedure is performed. The method of drainage most often selected is **pyloroplasty (Heineke-Mikulicz procedure;** Figure 23–6); **gastrojejunostomy** is used less often. Neither procedure gives a superior functional result, and pyloroplasty is less time consuming.

Vagal denervation of just the parietal cell area of the stomach is called **parietal cell vagotomy** or **proximal gastric vagotomy.** The technique spares the main nerves of Latarjet

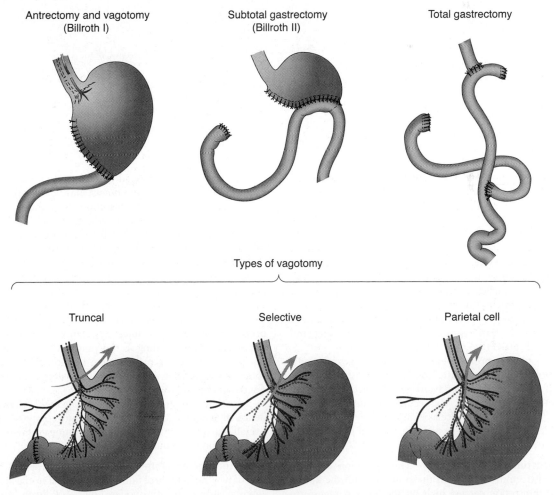

▲ **Figure 23–5.** Various types of operations currently popular for treating duodenal ulcer disease. Total gastrectomy is reserved for Zollinger-Ellison syndrome. The choice among the other procedures should be individualized according to principles discussed in the text.

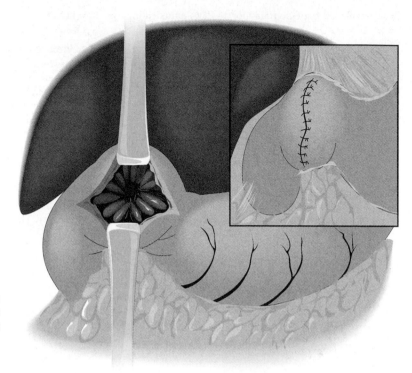

▲ **Figure 23–6.** Heineke-Mikulicz pyloroplasty. A longitudinal incision has been made across the pylorus, revealing an active ulcer in the duodenal bulb. The insert shows the transverse closure of the incision that widens the gastric outlet. The accompanying vagotomy is not shown.

(Figures 23–3 and 23–5) but divides all vagal branches that terminate on the proximal two thirds of the stomach. Since antral innervation is preserved, gastric emptying is relatively normal, and a drainage procedure is unnecessary. Nevertheless, parietal cell vagotomy plus pyloroplasty gives better results (ie, fewer recurrent ulcers) than parietal cell vagotomy alone. Parietal cell vagotomy appears to have about the same effectiveness as truncal or selective vagotomy for curing the ulcer disease, but dumping and diarrhea are much less frequent. It is probably the procedure of choice for intractable and perforated duodenal ulcers and is relatively less useful for obstructing and bleeding ulcers.

The vagotomy procedures have the advantages of technical simplicity and preservation of the entire gastric reservoir capacity. The principal disadvantage is recurrent ulceration in about 10% of patients. The recurrence rate after parietal cell vagotomy is about twice as high in patients with prepyloric ulcer, and most surgeons use a different operation for an ulcer in this location.

2. Antrectomy and vagotomy—This operation entails a distal gastrectomy of 50% of the stomach, with the line of gastric transection carried high on the lesser curvature to conform with the boundary of the gastrin-producing mucosa.

The terms antrectomy and hemigastrectomy are loosely synonymous. The proximal remnant may be reanastomosed to the duodenum (**Billroth I resection**) or to the side of the proximal jejunum (**Billroth II resection**). The Billroth I technique is most popular, but there is no conclusive evidence that the results are superior. When creating a Billroth II (gastrojejunostomy) reconstruction, the surgeon may bring the jejunal loop up to the gastric remnant either anterior to the transverse colon or posteriorly through a hole in the transverse mesocolon. Since either method is satisfactory, an antecolic anastomosis is elected in most cases because it is simpler. Truncal vagotomy is performed as described in the preceding section; antrectomy by itself will not prevent a high recurrence rate. In most instances, the surgeon will be able to remove the ulcerated portion of duodenum in the course of resection.

Vagotomy and antrectomy is associated with a low incidence of marginal ulceration (2%) and a generally good overall outcome, but the risk of complications is higher than after vagotomy without resection.

3. Subtotal gastrectomy—This operation consists of resection of two thirds to three fourths of the distal stomach. After subtotal gastrectomy for duodenal ulcer, a Billroth II reconstruction is preferable. Subtotal gastrectomy is largely of historical interest.

▶ Complications of Surgery for Peptic Ulcer

A. Early Complications

Duodenal stump leakage, gastric retention, and hemorrhage may develop in the immediate postoperative period.

B. Late Complications

1. Recurrent ulcer (marginal ulcer, stomal ulcer, anastomotic ulcer)—Recurrent ulcers form in about 10% of duodenal ulcer patients treated by vagotomy and pyloroplasty or parietal cell vagotomy; and in 2–3% after vagotomy and antrectomy or subtotal gastrectomy. These figures were accumulated before the emergence of effective treatment against *H pylori*, however, and are likely to be lower with current management. Recurrent ulcers nearly always develop immediately adjacent to the anastomosis on the intestinal side.

The usual complaint is upper abdominal pain, which is often aggravated by eating and improved by antacids. In some patients, the pain is felt more to the left in the epigastrium, and left axillary or shoulder pain is occasionally reported. About a third of patients with stomal ulcer will experience major gastrointestinal hemorrhage. Free perforation is less common (5%).

Diagnosis and treatment are essentially the same as for the original ulcer.

2. Gastrojejunocolic and gastrocolic fistula—A deeply eroding ulcer may occasionally produce a fistula between the stomach and colon. Most examples have resulted from recurrent peptic ulcer after an operation that included a gastrojejunal anastomosis.

Severe diarrhea and weight loss are the presenting symptoms in over 90% of cases. Abdominal pain typical of recurrent peptic ulcer often precedes the onset of the diarrhea. Bowel movements number 8–12 or more a day; they are watery and often contain particles of undigested food.

The degree of malnutrition ranges from mild to very severe. Laboratory studies reveal low serum proteins and manifestations of fluid and electrolyte depletion. Appropriate tests may reflect deficiencies in both water-soluble and fat-soluble vitamins.

An upper gastrointestinal series reveals the marginal ulcer in only 50% of patients and the fistula in only 15%. Barium enema unfailingly demonstrates the fistulous tract.

Initial treatment should replenish fluid and electrolyte deficits. The involved colon and ulcerated gastrojejunal segment should be excised and colonic continuity reestablished. Vagotomy, partial gastrectomy, or both are required to treat the ulcer diathesis and prevent another recurrent ulcer. Results are excellent in benign disease. In general, the outlook for patients with a malignant fistula is poor.

3. Dumping syndrome—Symptoms of the dumping syndrome are noted to some extent by most patients who have an operation that impairs the ability of the stomach to regulate its rate of emptying. Within several months, however, dumping is a clinical problem in only 1–2% of patients. Symptoms fall into two categories: cardiovascular and gastrointestinal. Shortly after eating, the patient may experience palpitations, sweating, weakness, dyspnea, flushing, nausea, abdominal cramps, belching, vomiting, diarrhea, and, rarely, syncope. The degree of severity varies widely, and not all symptoms are reported by all patients. In severe cases, the patient must lie down for 30–40 minutes until the discomfort passes.

Diet therapy to reduce jejunal osmolality is successful in all but a few cases. The diet should be low in carbohydrate and high in fat and protein content. Sugars and carbohydrates are least well tolerated; some patients are especially sensitive to milk. Meals should be taken dry, with fluids restricted to between meals. This dietary regimen ordinarily suffices, but anticholinergic drugs may be of help in some patients; others have reported improvement with supplemental pectin in the diet, and the use of somatostatin analogues offers some promise.

4. Alkaline gastritis—Reflux of duodenal juices into the stomach is an invariable and usually innocuous situation after operations that interfere with pyloric function, but in some patients, it may cause marked gastritis. The principal symptom is postprandial pain, and the diagnosis rests on endoscopic and biopsy demonstration of an edematous inflamed gastric mucosa. Since a minor degree of gastritis is found in most patients after Billroth II gastrectomy, the endoscopic findings are to some degree nonspecific. Persistent severe pain is an indication for surgical reconstruction. Roux-en-Y gastrojejunostomy with a 40-cm efferent jejunal limb is the treatment of choice.

5. Anemia—Iron deficiency anemia develops in about 30% of patients within 5 years after partial gastrectomy. It is caused by failure to absorb food iron bound in an organic molecule. Before this diagnosis is accepted, the patient should be checked for blood loss, marginal ulcer, or an unsuspected tumor. Inorganic iron—ferrous sulfate or ferrous gluconate—is indicated for treatment and is absorbed normally after gastrectomy.

Vitamin B_{12} deficiency and megaloblastic anemia appear in a few cases after gastrectomy.

6. Postvagotomy diarrhea—About 5–10% of patients who have had truncal vagotomy require treatment with antidiarrheal agents at some time, and perhaps 1% are seriously troubled by this complication. The diarrhea may be episodic, in which case the onset is unpredictable after symptom-free intervals of weeks to months. An attack may consist of only one or two watery movements or, in severe cases, may last for a few days. Other patients may continually produce 3–5 loose stools per day.

Most cases of postvagotomy diarrhea can be treated satisfactorily with constipating agents.

7. Chronic gastroparesis—Chronic delayed gastric emptying is seen occasionally after gastric surgery. Prokinetic agents (eg, metoclopramide) are often helpful, but some cases are refractory to any therapy except a completion gastrectomy and Roux-en-Y esophagojejunostomy (ie, total gastrectomy).

Donahue PE: Parietal cell vagotomy versus vagotomy-antrectomy: ulcer surgery in the modern era. World J Surg 2000;24:264.

Jamieson GG: Current status of indications for surgery in peptic ulcer disease. World J Surg 2000;24:256.

Logan RP, Walker MM: ABC of the upper gastrointestinal tract: epidemiology and diagnosis of *Helicobacter pylori* infection. BMJ 2001;323:920.

Leontiadis GI et al: Systematic reviews of the clinical effectiveness and cost-effectiveness of proton pump inhibitors in acute upper gastrointestinal bleeding. Health Technol Assess 2007;11:iii, 1.

Schubert ML. Peura DA. Control of gastric acid secretion in health and disease. Gastroenterology 2008;134:1842.

Zittel TT, Jehle EC, Becker HD: Surgical management of peptic ulcer disease today—indication, technique and outcome. Langenbecks Arch Surg 2000;385:84.

ZOLLINGER-ELLISON SYNDROME (GASTRINOMA)

 ESSENTIALS OF DIAGNOSIS

▶ Peptic ulcer disease (often severe) in 95%.

▶ Gastric hypersecretion.

▶ Elevated serum gastrin.

▶ Non-B islet cell tumor of the pancreas or duodenum.

General Considerations

Zollinger-Ellison syndrome is manifested by gastric acid hypersecretion caused by a gastrin-producing tumor (gastrinoma). Although the normal pancreas does not contain appreciable amounts of gastrin, most gastrinomas occur in the pancreas; others are found submucosally in the duodenum and rarely in the antrum or ovary. The gastrin-producing lesions (called **apudomas** from the theory of their histogenesis) in the pancreas are non-B islet cell carcinomas (60%), solitary adenomas (25%), and hyperplasia or microadenomas (10%); the remaining cases (5%) are due to solitary submucosal gastrinomas in the first or second portion of the duodenum. About one third of patients have the multiple endocrine neoplasia type I syndrome (MEN 1), which is characterized by a family history of endocrinopathy and the presence of tumors in other glands, especially the parathyroids and pituitary. Patients with MEN 1 usually have multiple benign gastrinomas. Those without MEN 1 usually have solitary gastrinomas that are often malignant. The tumors may be as small as 2–3 mm and are often difficult to find. In about one third of cases, the tumor cannot be located at laparotomy.

The diagnosis of cancer can be made only with findings of metastases or blood vessel invasion, because the histologic pattern is similar for benign and malignant tumors. In most patients with malignant gastrinomas, the illness caused by hypergastrinemia (ie, severe peptic ulcer disease) is a greater threat to health than the illness caused by malignant growth and spread.

▶ Clinical Findings

A. Symptoms and Signs

Symptoms associated with gastrinoma are principally a result of acid hypersecretion—usually from peptic ulcer disease. Some patients with gastrinoma have severe diarrhea from the large amounts of acid entering the duodenum, which can destroy pancreatic lipase and produce steatorrhea, damage the small bowel mucosa, and overload the intestine with gastric and pancreatic secretions. About 5% of patients present with diarrhea only.

Ulcer symptoms are often refractory to large doses of antacids or standard doses of H_2 blocking agents. Hemorrhage, perforation, and obstruction are common complications. Marginal ulcers appear after surgical procedures that would cure the ordinary ulcer diathesis.

B. Laboratory Findings

Hypergastrinemia in the presence of acid hypersecretion is almost diagnostic of gastrinoma. Gastrin levels are normally inversely proportionate to gastric acid output; therefore, diseases that result in increased gastric pH may cause a rise in serum gastrin concentration (eg, pernicious anemia, atrophic gastritis, gastric ulcer, postvagotomy state, acid-suppressing medications). Serum gastrin levels should be measured in any patient with suspected gastrinoma or ulcer disease severe enough to warrant consideration of surgical treatment. H_2 receptor blocking agents, omeprazole, or antacids frequently increase serum gastrin concentrations and should be avoided for several days before gastrin measurements are made. It is often helpful to measure gastric acid secretion to rule out H^+ hyposecretion as a cause of hypergastrinemia.

The normal gastrin value is less than 200 pg/mL. Patients with gastrinoma usually have levels exceeding 500 pg/mL and sometimes 10,000 pg/mL or higher. Very high gastrin levels (eg, > 5000 pg/mL) or the presence of alpha chains of hCG in the serum usually indicate cancer. Patients with borderline gastrin values (eg, 200–500 pg/mL) and acid secretion in the range associated with ordinary duodenal ulcer disease should have a secretin provocative test. Following intravenous administration of secretin (2 units/kg as a bolus), a rise in the gastrin level of > 150 pg/mL within 15 minutes is diagnostic.

Marked basal acid hypersecretion (> 15 meq H^+ per hour) occurs in most Zollinger-Ellison patients who have an intact stomach. In a patient who has previously undergone gastrectomy, a basal acid output of 5 meq/h or more is highly suggestive. Since the parietal cells are already under near maximal stimulation from hypergastrinemia, there is little increase in acid secretion following an injection of pentagastrin, and the ratio of basal to maximal acid output (BAO/MAO) characteristically exceeds 0.6.

Hypergastrinemia and gastric acid hypersecretion may be seen in gastric outlet obstruction, retained antrum after a Billroth II gastrojejunostomy, and antral gastrin cell hyperactivity (hyperplasia). These conditions may be differentiated from gastrinoma by use of the secretin test. Because associated hyperparathyroidism is so common, serum calcium concentrations should be measured in all patients with gastrinoma.

Serum levels of neuron-specific enolase, β-hCG, and chromogranin-A are often elevated in patients with functioning apudomas. Although they are probably of no physiologic importance, the high levels of these peptides may be useful in diagnosing apudomas and following the results of therapy.

C. Imaging Studies

A CT or MR scan will often demonstrate the pancreatic tumors. Somatostatin-receptor scintigraphy is extremely sensitive for detection of gastrinoma primary and metastatic sites. Transhepatic portal vein blood sampling to find gradients of gastrin production has been supplanted by the intra-arterial secretin test. Infusion of secretin into the artery supplying a functional gastrinoma causes an increase in hepatic vein gastrin levels. This invasive test is usually reserved for difficult situations.

Although used less frequently now with the availability of endoscopy, an upper gastrointestinal series can show ulceration in the duodenal bulb, though ulcers sometimes appear in the distal duodenum or proximal jejunum. The presence of ulcers in these distal ("ectopic") locations is nearly diagnostic of gastrinoma. The stomach contains prominent rugal folds, and secretions are present in the lumen despite overnight fasting. The duodenum may be dilated and exhibit hyperactive peristalsis. Edema may be detected in the small bowel mucosa. The barium flocculates in the intestine, and transit time is accelerated.

▶ Treatment

A. Medical Treatment

Initial treatment should consist of H_2 blocking agents (eg, cimetidine, 300–600 mg, four times daily; ranitidine, 300–450 mg, four times daily) or proton pump inhibitor (eg, omeprazole 20–40 mg, once or twice daily). The dose should be adjusted to keep gastric H^+ output below 5 meq in the hour preceding the next dose. Although the response to H_2 blocking agents is usually excellent at first, with time, the dose must be increased in order to maintain the same level

of control. A proton pump inhibitor is indicated sooner or later in nearly all patients.

B. Surgical Treatment

Resection is the ideal treatment for gastrinoma and is appropriate in all patients with apparently localized disease and no other significant limitations to their survival. Surgical cure may be possible when there are resectable metastases in peripancreatic lymph nodes or the liver. Overall, about 70% of patients have immediate biochemical cure, and about 30% of patients remain disease-free after 5 years.

Every patient with sporadic Zollinger-Ellison syndrome should be considered a candidate for tumor resection. The preoperative workup should include a CT or MR scan of the pancreas and somatostatin-receptor scintigraphy. Regardless of other findings, exploratory laparotomy is then recommended in the absence of evidence of unresectable metastatic disease. If the tumor is found in the pancreas, it is enucleated if possible. Operative ultrasound may help in the examination of the pancreas. Most lesions will be found either in the head of the pancreas or in the duodenum. All patients should have longitudinal duodenotomy and palpation of the duodenal mucosa to identify the frequent primary tumors in this site.

▶ Prognosis

Since H_2 blocking agents become less effective with time, omeprazole is eventually required in medically treated patients. Because it is usually multifocal, the disease can rarely be cured surgically in patients with MEN 1. Malignant gastrinomas can cause death from growth of metastases.

Gibril F, Jensen RT: Advances in evaluation and management of gastrinoma in patients with Zollinger-Ellison syndrome. Curr Gastroenterol Rep 2005;7:114.

Norton JA: Surgical treatment and prognosis of gastrinoma. Best Pract Res Clin Gastroenterol 2005;19:799.

Pisegna JR: The effect of Zollinger-Ellison syndrome and neuropeptide-secreting tumors on the stomach. Curr Gastroenterol Rep 1999;1:511.

GASTRIC ULCER

 ESSENTIALS OF DIAGNOSIS

- ▶ Epigastric pain.
- ▶ Ulcer demonstrated by x-ray.
- ▶ Acid present on gastric analysis.

▶ General Considerations

The peak incidence of gastric ulcer is in patients aged 40–60 years, or about 10 years older than the average for those with duodenal ulcer. Ninety-five percent of gastric ulcers are located on the lesser curvature, and 60% of these are within 6 cm of the pylorus. The symptoms and complications of gastric ulcer closely resemble those of duodenal ulcer.

Gastric ulcers may be separated into three types with different causes and different treatments. **Type I ulcers,** the most common variety, are found in patients who on the average are 10 years older than patients with duodenal ulcers and who have no clinical or radiographic evidence of previous duodenal ulcer disease; gastric acid output is normal or low. The ulcers are usually located within 2 cm of the boundary between parietal cell and pyloric mucosa, but always in the latter. As noted above, 95% are on the lesser curvature, usually near the incisura angularis.

Antral gastritis is universally present, being most severe near the pylorus and gradually diminishing. This is associated in most cases with the presence of *H pylori* beneath the mucus layer, on the luminal surface of epithelial cells, and gastric ulcer disease is probably the result of infection with this organism.

Type II ulcers are located close to the pylorus (prepyloric ulcers) and occur in association with (most often following) duodenal ulcers. The risk of cancer is very low in these gastric ulcers. Acid secretion measured by gastric analysis is in the range associated with duodenal ulcer.

Type III ulcers occur in the antrum as a result of chronic use of nonsteroidal anti-inflammatory agents.

Ulcer identified on x-ray or by endoscopy could be an ulcerated malignant tumor rather than a simple benign ulcer. Efforts must be expended during the *initial* stage of the workup to establish this distinction. Despite the generally discouraging results of surgery for gastric adenocarcinoma, those whose tumors are difficult to distinguish from benign ulcer have a 50–75% chance of cure after gastrectomy.

▶ Clinical Findings

A. Symptoms and Signs

The principal symptom is epigastric pain relieved by food or antacids, as in duodenal ulcer. Epigastric tenderness is a variable finding. Compared with duodenal ulcer, the pain in gastric ulcer tends to appear earlier after eating, often within 30 minutes. Vomiting, anorexia, and aggravation of pain by eating are also more common with gastric ulcer.

Achlorhydria is defined as no acid (pH > 6.00) after pentagastrin stimulation. Achlorhydria is incompatible with the diagnosis of benign peptic ulcer and suggests a malignant gastric ulcer. About 5% of malignant gastric ulcers will be associated with this finding.

B. Gastroscopy and Biopsy

Gastroscopy should be performed as part of the initial workup to attempt to find malignant lesions. The rolled-up margins of the ulcer that produce the meniscus sign on x-ray can often be distinguished from the flat edges characteristic of a benign ulcer. Multiple (preferably six) biopsy specimens and brush biopsy should be obtained from the edge of the lesion. False positives are rare; false negatives occur in 5–10% of malignant ulcers.

C. Imaging Studies

Upper gastrointestinal x-rays can show an ulcer, usually on the lesser curvature in the pyloric area. In the absence of a tumor mass, the following suggest that the ulcer is malignant: (1) the deepest penetration of the ulcer is not beyond the expected border of the gastric wall; (2) the meniscus sign is present (ie, a prominent rim of radiolucency surrounding the ulcer), caused by heaped-up edges of tumor; and (3) cancer is more common (10%) in ulcers greater than 2 cm in diameter. Coexistence of duodenal deformity or ulcer favors a diagnosis of benign ulcer in the stomach.

▶ Differential Diagnosis

The characteristic symptoms of gastric ulcer are often clouded by numerous nonspecific complaints. Uncomplicated hiatal hernia, atrophic gastritis, chronic cholecystitis, irritable colon syndrome, and undifferentiated functional problems are distinguishable from peptic ulcer only after appropriate radiologic studies and sometimes not even then.

Gastroscopy and biopsy of the ulcer should be performed to rule out malignant gastric ulcer.

▶ Complications

Bleeding, obstruction, and perforation are the principal complications of gastric ulcer. They are discussed separately elsewhere in this chapter.

▶ Treatment

A. Medical Treatment

Medical management of gastric ulcer is the same as for duodenal ulcer. The patient should be questioned regarding the use of ulcerogenic agents, which should be eliminated as far as possible.

Repeat endoscopy should be obtained to document the rate of healing. After 4–16 weeks (depending on the initial size of the lesion and other factors), healing usually has reached a plateau. In order to cure the disease and avoid recurrent ulcers, *H pylori* must be eradicated. The success of therapy in this regard can be checked by serologic testing for *H pylori* antibodies.

B. Surgical Treatment

Before the significance of *H pylori* in the etiology of gastric ulcer was appreciated, the most effective surgical treatment was distal hemigastrectomy (including the ulcer); somewhat less effective but still useful in high-risk patients was vagotomy and pyloroplasty. Parietal cell vagotomy for prepyloric ulcers was followed by a high (eg, 30%) recurrence rate, but parietal cell vagotomy plus pyloroplasty worked well.

Intractability to medical therapy has now become a rare indication for surgery in gastric ulcer disease, since H_2 receptor antagonists or omeprazole can bring the condition under control, and treatment of *H pylori* infection can almost eliminate the problem of recurrence. Consequently, surgery is needed principally for complications of the disease: bleeding, perforation, or obstruction.

Atherton JC. The pathogenesis of *Helicobacter pylori*-induced gastro-duodenal diseases. Annu Rev Patholog 2006;1:63.

Calam J, Baron JH: ABC of the upper gastrointestinal tract: pathophysiology of duodenal and gastric ulcer and gastric cancer. BMJ 2001;323:980.

Lai LH, Sung JJ: Helicobacter pylori and benign upper digestive disease. Best Pract Res Clin Gastroenterol 2007;21:261.

Pai R, Tarnawski A: Signal transduction cascades triggered by EGF receptor activation: relevance to gastric injury repair and ulcer healing. Dig Dis Sci 1998;43(9 Suppl):14S.

Peskar BM, Maricic N: Role of prostaglandins in gastroprotection. Dig Dis Sci 1998;43(9 Suppl):23S.

UPPER GASTROINTESTINAL HEMORRHAGE

Upper gastrointestinal hemorrhage may be mild or severe but should always be considered an ominous manifestation that deserves thorough evaluation. Bleeding is the most common serious complication of peptic ulcer, portal hypertension, and gastritis, and these conditions taken together account for most episodes of upper gastrointestinal bleeding in the average hospital population.

The major factors that determine the diagnostic and therapeutic approach are the amount and rate of bleeding. Estimates of both should be made promptly and monitored and revised continuously until the episode has been resolved. It is important to know at the outset that bleeding stops spontaneously in 75% of cases; the remainder includes those who will require surgery, experience complications, or die.

Hematemesis or melena is present except when the rate of blood loss is minimal. **Hematemesis** of either bright-red or dark blood indicates that the source is proximal to the ligament of Treitz. It is more common from bleeding that originates in the stomach or esophagus. In general, hematemesis denotes a more rapidly bleeding lesion, and a high percentage of patients who vomit blood require surgery. Coffee-ground vomitus is due to vomiting of blood that has been in the stomach long enough for gastric acid to convert hemoglobin to methemoglobin.

Most patients with **melena** (passage of black or tarry stools) are bleeding from the upper gastrointestinal tract, but melena can be produced by blood entering the bowel at any point from mouth to cecum. The conversion of red blood to dark depends more on the time it resides in the intestine than on the site of origin. The black color of melenic stools is probably caused by hematin, the product of oxidation of heme by intestinal and bacterial enzymes. Melena can be produced by as little as 50–100 mL of blood in the stomach. When 1 L of blood was instilled into the upper intestine of experimental subjects, melena persisted for 3–5 days, which shows that the rate of change in character of the stool is a poor guide to the time bleeding stops after an episode of hemorrhage.

Hematochezia is defined as the passage of bright-red blood from the rectum. Bright-red rectal blood can be produced by bleeding from the colon, rectum, or anus. However, if intestinal transit is rapid during brisk bleeding in the upper intestine, bright-red blood may be passed unchanged in the stool.

▶ Tests for Occult Blood

Normal subjects lose about 2.5 mL of blood per day in their stools, presumably from minor mechanical abrasions of the intestinal epithelium. Between 50 and 100 mL of blood per day will produce melena. Tests for occult blood in the stool should be able to detect amounts between 10 and 50 mL/d. False-positive results may be due to dietary hemoglobin, myoglobin, or peroxidases of plant origin. Iron ingestion does not give positive reactions. The various tests using guaiac, benzidine, phenolphthalein, or orthotoluidine have similar specificities. The sensitivity of the guaiac slide test (Hemoccult) is in the desired range, and this is the best test available at present.

▶ Initial Management

In an apparently healthy patient, melena of a week or more suggests that the bleeding is slow. In this type of patient, admission to the hospital should be followed by a deliberate but nonemergency workup. However, patients who present with hematemesis or melena of less than 12 hours' duration should be handled as if exsanguination were imminent. The approach entails a simultaneous series of diagnostic and therapeutic steps with the following initial goals: (1) Assess the status of the circulatory system and replace blood loss as necessary. (2) Determine the amount and rate of bleeding. (3) Slow or stop the bleeding by ice-water lavage. (4) Discover the lesion responsible for the episode. The last step may lead to more specific treatment appropriate to the underlying condition.

The patient should be admitted to the hospital and a history and physical examination performed. Experienced clinicians are able to make a correct diagnosis of the cause of bleeding from clinical findings in only 60% of patients. Peptic ulcer, acute gastritis, esophageal varices, esophagitis, and Mallory-Weiss tear account for over 90% of cases (see Table 23–2). Questions concerning the symptoms and predisposing factors should be asked. The patient should be questioned about salicylate intake and any history of a bleeding tendency.

Table 23–2. Causes of Massive Upper Gastrointestinal Hemorrhage. Note That Cancer Is Rarely the Cause.

		Relative Incidence
Common causes		
Peptic ulcer		45%
Duodenal ulcer	25%	
Gastric ulcer	20%	
Esophageal varices		20%
Gastritis		20%
Mallory-Weiss syndrome		10%
Uncommon causes		5%
Gastric carcinoma		
Esophagitis		
Pancreatitis		
Hemobilia		
Duodenal diverticulum		

Of the diseases commonly responsible for acute upper gastrointestinal bleeding, only portal hypertension is associated with diagnostic clues on physical examination. However, gastrointestinal bleeding should not be automatically attributed to esophageal varices in a patient with jaundice, ascites, splenomegaly, spider angiomas, or hepatomegaly; over half of cirrhotic patients who present with acute hemorrhage are bleeding from gastritis or peptic ulcer.

Blood should be drawn for crossmatching, hematocrit, hemoglobin, creatinine, and tests of liver function. An intravenous infusion should be started and, in the massive bleeder, a large-bore nasogastric tube inserted. In cases of melena, the gastric aspirate should be examined to verify the gastroduodenal source of the hemorrhage, but about 25% of patients with bleeding duodenal ulcers have gastric aspirates that test negatively for blood. The tube must be larger than the standard nasogastric tube (16F) so the stomach can be lavaged free of liquid blood and clots. After its contents have been removed, the stomach should be irrigated with copious amounts of ice water or saline solution until blood no longer returns. If the patient was bleeding at the time the nasogastric tube was inserted, iced saline irrigation usually stops it. The large tube can then be exchanged for a standard nasogastric tube attached to continuous suction so further blood loss can be measured.

It is common to give H_2 receptor antagonists or omeprazole, though controlled trials have shown no benefit. If bleeding continues or if tachycardia or hypotension is present, the patient should be monitored and treated as for hemorrhagic shock.

In acute rapid hemorrhage, the hematocrit may be normal or only slightly low. A very low hematocrit without obvious signs of shock indicates more gradual blood loss.

All of the above tests and procedures can be performed within 1 or 2 hours after admission. By this time, in most instances, bleeding is under control, blood volume has been restored to normal, and the patient is being adequately monitored so that recurrent bleeding can be detected promptly. When this stage is reached, additional diagnostic tests should be performed.

▶ Diagnosis of Cause of Bleeding

Once the patient is stabilized, endoscopy should be the first study. In general, endoscopy should be performed within 24 hours after admission, and under these circumstances the source of bleeding can be demonstrated in about 80% of cases. Longer delays have a lower diagnostic yield. Two lesions are seen in about 15% of patients. An upper gastrointestinal series should be performed if endoscopy is equivocal or unavailable. Although the diagnostic information provided by endoscopy does not appear to have resulted in decreased blood loss or improved outcome, endoscopic therapy, in the form of sclerosis of varices or injection of a bleeding ulcer, may do so. Having the diagnosis will also help in planning subsequent treatment, including the surgical approach if operation becomes necessary.

Rarely, selective angiography will have diagnostic or therapeutic usefulness. For diagnosis, it is most helpful when other studies fail to demonstrate the cause of bleeding. Infusion through the angiographic catheter of vasoconstrictors (eg, vasopressin) and embolization of the bleeding vessel with Gelfoam may be able to halt the bleeding in special cases.

▶ Later Management

Although a precise diagnosis of the cause of the bleeding may be valuable in later management, the patient must not be allowed to slip out of clinical control during the search for definitive diagnostic information. *The decision for emergency surgery depends more on the rate and duration of bleeding than on its specific cause.*

The need for transfusion should be determined on a continuing basis, and blood volume must be maintained. Blood pressure, pulse, central venous pressure, hematocrit, hourly urinary volume, and amount of blood obtained from the gastric tube or from the rectum all enter into this assessment. Many studies have shown the tendency to underestimate blood loss and inadequately transfuse massively bleeding patients who truly need aggressive therapy. Continued slow bleeding is best monitored by serial determinations of the hematocrit.

The following criteria define patients with a very low risk of serious bleeding: age less than 75 years, no unstable comorbid illness, no ascites evident on physical examination, normal prothrombin time, and, within 1 hour after admission, a systolic blood pressure above 100 mm Hg, and nasogastric aspirate free of fresh blood. Patients with all six of these findings may be spared emergency endoscopy and discharged from the hospital early to undergo outpatient workup.

Several factors are associated with a worse prognosis with continued medical management of the bleeding episode. These are not absolute indications for laparotomy, but they should alert the clinician that emergency surgery may be required.

High rates of bleeding or amounts of blood loss predict high failure rates with medical treatment. Hematemesis is usually associated with more rapid bleeding and a greater blood volume deficit than melena. The presence of hypotension on admission to the hospital or the need for more than four units of blood to achieve circulatory stability implies a worse prognosis; if bleeding continues and subsequent transfusion requirements exceed 1 unit every 8 hours, continued medical management is usually unwise. The level of serum fibrin degradation products, indicating endogenous fibrinolysis, correlates with the severity of hemorrhage and the death rate. This may be a useful prognostic test, and the results could be used as a guide for the administration of fibrinolytic inhibitors in therapy. Evidence for or against this view is not yet available.

Total transfusion requirements also correlate with death rates. Death is uncommon when fewer than 7 units of blood have been used, and the death rate rises progressively thereafter.

In general, bleeding from a gastric ulcer is more dangerous than bleeding from gastritis or duodenal ulcer, and patients with gastric ulcer should always be considered for early surgery. Regardless of the cause, if bleeding recurs after it has once stopped, the chances of success without operation are low. Most patients who rebleed in the hospital should have surgery.

Patients over age 60 tolerate continued blood loss less well than younger patients, and their bleeding should be stopped before secondary cardiovascular, pulmonary, or renal complications arise.

In 85% of patients, bleeding stops within a few hours of admission. About 25% of patients rebleed once bleeding has stopped. Rebleeding episodes are concentrated within the first 2 days of hospitalization, and if the patient has had no further bleeding for a period of 5 days, the chance of rebleeding is only 2%. Rebleeding is most common in patients with varices, peptic ulcer, anemia, or shock. About 10% of patients require surgery to control bleeding, and most of these patients have bleeding ulcers or, less commonly, esophageal varices. The death rate is 30% among patients who rebleed and 3% among those who do not. The mortality rate is also high in the elderly and in patients who are already hospitalized at the onset of bleeding. Analyses of large series of patients suggest that a number of those who died would not have done so if operations had been performed earlier and more often.

Dallal HJ, Palmer KR: ABC of the upper gastrointestinal tract: upper gastrointestinal haemorrhage. BMJ 2001;323:1115.

Leontiadis GI et al: Systematic reviews of the clinical effectiveness and cost-effectiveness of proton pump inhibitors in acute upper gastrointestinal bleeding. Health Technol Assess 2007;11:iii, 1.
Spiegel BM, Vakil NB, Ofman JJ: Endoscopy for acute nonvariceal upper gastrointestinal tract hemorrhage: is sooner better? A systematic review. Arch Intern Med 2001;161:1393.
Van Dam J, Brugge KR: Endoscopy of the upper gastrointestinal tract. N Engl J Med 1999;341:1738.

HEMORRHAGE FROM PEPTIC ULCER

Approximately 20% of patients with peptic ulcer will experience a bleeding episode, and this complication is responsible for about 40% of the deaths from peptic ulcer. Peptic ulcer is the most common cause of massive upper gastrointestinal hemorrhage, accounting for over half of all cases. Chronic gastric and duodenal ulcers have about the same tendency to bleed, but the former produce more severe episodes. Bleeding ulcers are more common in persons with blood group O, though the reason for this association is not known.

Bleeding ulcers in the duodenum are usually located on the posterior surface of the duodenal bulb. As the ulcer penetrates, the gastroduodenal artery is exposed and may become eroded. Since no major blood vessels lie on the anterior surface of the duodenal bulb, ulcerations at this point are not as prone to bleed. Patients with concomitant bleeding and perforation usually have two ulcers, a bleeding posterior ulcer and a perforated anterior one. Postbulbar ulcers (those in the second portion of the duodenum) bleed frequently, though ulcers are much less common in this site than near the pylorus.

In some patients, the bleeding is sudden and massive, manifested by hematemesis and shock. In others, chronic anemia and weakness due to slow blood loss are the only findings. The diagnosis is unreliable when based on clinical findings, so endoscopy should be performed early (ie, within 24 hours) in most cases.

In the preceding section, the management of acute upper gastrointestinal hemorrhage, the selection of diagnostic tests, and the factors suggesting the need for operation were discussed. Most patients (75%) with bleeding peptic ulcer can be successfully managed by medical means alone. Initial therapeutic efforts usually halt the bleeding. H_2 blockers and proton pump inhibitors decrease the risk of bleeding but have no effect on active bleeding.

After 12–24 hours have passed and the bleeding has clearly stopped, a patient who feels hungry should be fed. Twice-daily hematocrit readings should be ordered as a check on slow continued blood loss. Stools should be tested daily for the presence of blood; they will usually remain guaiac-positive for several days after bleeding stops.

Rebleeding in the hospital has been attended by a death rate of about 30%. A policy of early surgery for those who rebleed would improve this figure. Patients who are over age 60, present with hematemesis, are actively bleeding at the time of endoscopy, or whose admission hemoglobin is below

8 g/dL have a higher risk of rebleeding. About three times as many patients with gastric ulcer (30%) rebleed compared with those with duodenal ulcer. Most instances of rebleeding occur within 2 days from the time the first episode has stopped. In one study, only 3% of patients who stopped bleeding for this long bled again.

Endoscopic Therapy

Treatments administered through the endoscope may stop active bleeding or prevent rebleeding. Effective methods include injection into the ulcer of epinephrine, epinephrine plus 1% polidocanol (a sclerosing agent), or ethanol; or cautery using the heater probe, monopolar electrocautery, or the Nd:YAG laser. At least two modalities should be available to the endoscopist in the event one is unsuitable for a specific case or fails to work. Except for the laser, all are inexpensive. The indications for treatment are (1) active bleeding at the time of endoscopy and (2) the presence of a visible vessel in the base of the ulcer. Endoscopic therapy decreases transfusion requirements (by about half) and the rate of rebleeding (by about three quarters) compared with sham-treated controls. When treatment fails the first time, it may often be repeated with a good chance of success. It is important, however, not to allow the patient to deteriorate during nonoperative attempts at halting the bleeding.

Emergency Surgery

Less than 10% of patients bleeding from a peptic ulcer require emergency surgery. Selection of those most likely to survive with surgical compared with medical treatment rests on the rate of blood loss and the other factors associated with a poor prognosis.

The overall death rate is significantly less after vagotomy and pyloroplasty than after gastrectomy for bleeding ulcer, and rebleeding occurs with about equal frequency after either procedure.

During laparotomy, the first step is to make a pyloroplasty incision if the endoscopic diagnosis is a bleeding duodenal ulcer. If a duodenal ulcer is found, the bleeding vessel should be suture-ligated and the duodenum and antrum inspected for additional ulcers. The pyloroplasty incision should then be closed and a truncal vagotomy performed. If the posterior wall of the duodenal bulb has been destroyed by a giant duodenal ulcer, a gastrectomy and Billroth II gastrojejunostomy may be preferable, since this somewhat uncommon ulcer is especially prone to bleed again if left in continuity with the stomach. Gastric ulcers can be handled by either gastrectomy or vagotomy and pyloroplasty. A thorough search should always be made for second ulcers or other causes of bleeding.

Prognosis

The death rate for an acute massive hemorrhage is about 15%. Careful study of the causes of death suggests that this figure could be improved by (1) more precise blood replacement, since undertransfusion is the cause of some complications and deaths; and (2) earlier surgery in selected patients who fall into serious-risk categories, since the tendency has been to perform surgery on too few patients too late in the illness. Patients who stop bleeding should be treated as outlined in the section on duodenal ulcer.

Cappell MS, Friedel D: Initial management of acute upper gastrointestinal bleeding: from initial evaluation up to gastrointestinal endoscopy. Med Clin North Am 2008;92:491.

MALLORY-WEISS SYNDROME

Mallory-Weiss syndrome is responsible for about 10% of cases of acute upper gastrointestinal hemorrhage. The lesion consists of a 1- to 4-cm longitudinal tear in the gastric mucosa near the esophagogastric junction; it usually follows a bout of forceful retching. The disruption extends through the mucosa and submucosa but not usually into the muscularis mucosae. About 75% of these lesions are confined to the stomach, 20% straddle the esophagogastric junction, and 5% are entirely within the distal esophagus. Two thirds of patients have a hiatal hernia.

The majority of patients are alcoholics, but the tear may appear after severe retching for any reason. Several cases have been reported following closed-chest cardiac compression.

Clinical Findings

Typically, the patient first vomits food and gastric contents. This is followed by forceful retching and then bloody vomitus. Rapid increases in gastric pressure, sometimes aggravated by hiatal hernia, cause the tear. Actual rupture of the distal esophagus can also be produced by vomiting (Boerhaave syndrome), but the difference seems to depend on vomiting of food in rupture and nonproductive retching in gastric mucosal tear.

Esophagogastroscopy is the most practical means of making the diagnosis.

Treatment & Prognosis

Initially, the patient is handled according to the general measures prescribed for upper gastrointestinal hemorrhage. In about 90% of patients, the bleeding stops spontaneously after ice-water lavage of the stomach. Patients who are still bleeding vigorously by the time endoscopy is performed are likely to require surgery. The bleeding can sometimes be controlled by endoscopic therapy (eg, electrocautery). If bleeding persists, surgical repair of the tear will be required.

If the diagnosis has been made before laparotomy, the surgeon should make a long, high gastrotomy after the abdomen is opened. The tear may be difficult to expose adequately. The search must be thorough, since in about 25% of patients there are two tears. A running polyglycolic acid (not catgut) suture should be used to oversew the lesion. Postoperative recurrence is rare.

Kortas DY: Mallory-Weiss tear: predisposing factors and predictors of a complicated course. Am J Gastroenterol 2001;96:2863.
Younes Z, Johnson DA: The spectrum of spontaneous and iatrogenic esophageal injury: perforations, Mallory-Weiss tears, and hematomas. J Clin Gastroenterol 1999;29:306.

PYLORIC OBSTRUCTION DUE TO PEPTIC ULCER

The cycles of inflammation and repair in peptic ulcer disease may cause obstruction of the gastroduodenal junction as a result of edema, muscular spasm, and scarring. To the extent that the first two factors are involved, the obstruction may be reversible with medical treatment. Obstruction is usually due to duodenal ulcer and is less common than either bleeding or perforation. The few gastric ulcers that obstruct are close to the pylorus. Obstruction due to peptic ulcer must be differentiated from that caused by a malignant tumor of the antrum or of the pancreas. Malignancy is becoming the more common cause, and it may be difficult to identify.

▶ Clinical Findings

A. Symptoms and Signs

Most patients with obstruction have a long history of symptomatic peptic ulcer, and as many as 30% have been treated for perforation or obstruction in the past. The patient often notes gradually increasing ulcer pains over weeks or months, with the eventual development of anorexia, vomiting, and failure to gain relief from antacids. The vomitus often contains food ingested several hours previously, and absence of bile staining reflects the site of blockage. Weight loss may be marked if the patient has delayed seeking medical care.

Dehydration and malnutrition may be obvious on physical examination but are not always present. A succussion splash can often be elicited from the retained gastric contents. Peristalsis of the distended stomach may be visible on gross inspection of the abdomen, but this sign is relatively rare. Most patients have upper abdominal tenderness. Tetany may appear with advanced alkalosis.

B. Laboratory Findings

Anemia is found in about 25% of patients. Prolonged vomiting leads to a unique form of metabolic alkalosis with dehydration. Measurement of serum electrolytes shows hypochloremia, hypokalemia, hyponatremia, and increased bicarbonate. Vomiting depletes the patient of Na^+, K^+, and Cl^-; the latter is lost in excess of Na^+ and K^+ as HCl. Gastric HCl loss causes extracellular HCO_3^- to rise, and renal excretion of HCO_3^- increases in an attempt to maintain pH. Large amounts of Na^+ are excreted in the urine with the HCO_3^-. Increasing Na^+ deficit evokes aldosterone secretion, which in turn brings about renal Na^+ conservation at the expense of

more renal loss of K^+ and H^+. Glomerular filtration rate (GFR) may drop and produce a prerenal azotemia. The eventual result of the process is a marked deficit of Na^+, Cl^-, K^+, and H_2O. Treatment involves replacement of water and NaCl until a satisfactory urine flow has been established. KCl replacement should then be started. Details of management are found in Chapter 9.

C. Saline Load Test

This is a simple means of assessing the degree of pyloric obstruction and is useful in following the patient's progress during the first few days of nasogastric suction.

Through the nasogastric tube, 700 mL of normal saline (at room temperature) is infused over 3–5 minutes, and the tube is clamped. Thirty minutes later, the stomach is aspirated and the residual volume of saline recorded. Recovery of more than 350 mL indicates obstruction. It must be recognized that the results of a saline load test do not predict how well the stomach will handle solid food. Solid emptying can be measured with technetium-99m-labeled chicken liver.

D. Imaging Studies

Plain abdominal x-rays may show a large gastric fluid level. An upper gastrointestinal series should not be performed until the stomach has been emptied, because dilution of the barium in the retained secretions makes a worthwhile study impossible.

E. Endoscopy

Gastroscopy is usually indicated to rule out the presence of an obstructing neoplasm.

▶ Treatment

A. Medical Treatment

A large (32F) Ewald tube should be passed and the stomach emptied of its contents and lavaged until clean. After the stomach has been completely decompressed, a smaller tube should be inserted and placed on suction for several days to allow pyloric edema and spasm to subside and to permit the gastric musculature to regain its tone. A saline load test may be performed at this point to provide a baseline for later comparison. If chronic obstruction has produced severe malnutrition, total parenteral nutrition should be instituted.

After decompression of the stomach for 48–72 hours, the saline load test should be repeated. If this indicates sufficient improvement, the tube should be withdrawn and a liquid diet may be started. Gradual resumption of solid foods is permitted as tolerated.

B. Surgical Treatment

If 5–7 days of gastric aspiration do not result in relief of the obstruction, the patient should be treated surgically.

Persistence of nonoperative effort beyond this point in the absence of progress rarely achieves the result hoped for. Failure of the obstruction to resolve completely (eg, if the patient can take only liquids) and recurrent obstruction of any degree are indications for surgery.

Surgical treatment may consist of a truncal or parietal cell vagotomy and drainage procedure (Figure 23–5). Truncal vagotomy and gastrojejunostomy is the easiest to perform laparoscopically.

▶ Prognosis

About two thirds of patients with acute obstruction fail to improve sufficiently on medical therapy and require operation to relieve the blockage. Patients who respond to medical treatment should be treated as outlined in the section on duodenal ulcer.

Jamieson GG: Current status of indications for surgery in peptic ulcer disease. World J Surg 2000;24:256.

PERFORATED PEPTIC ULCER

Perforation complicates peptic ulcer about half as often as hemorrhage. Most perforated ulcers are located anteriorly, though occasionally gastric ulcers perforate into the lesser sac. The 15% death rate correlates with increased age, female sex, and gastric perforations. The diagnosis is overlooked in about 5% of patients, most of whom do not survive.

Anterior ulcers tend to perforate instead of bleed because of the absence of protective viscera and major blood vessels on this surface. In less than 10% of cases, acute bleeding from a posterior "kissing" ulcer complicates the anterior perforation, an association that carries a high death rate. Immediately after perforation, the peritoneal cavity is flooded with gastroduodenal secretions that elicit a chemical peritonitis. Early cultures show either no growth or a light growth of streptococci or enteric bacilli. Gradually, over 12–24 hours, the process evolves into bacterial peritonitis. Severity of illness and occurrence of death are directly related to the interval between perforation and surgical closure.

In an unknown percentage of cases, the perforation becomes sealed by adherence to the undersurface of the liver. In such patients, the process may be self-limited, but a subphrenic abscess will develop in many.

▶ Clinical Findings
A. Symptoms and Signs

The perforation usually elicits a sudden, severe upper abdominal pain whose onset can be recalled precisely. The patient may or may not have had preceding chronic symptoms of peptic ulcer disease. Perforation rarely is heralded by nausea or vomiting, and it typically occurs several hours after the last meal. Shoulder pain, if present, reflects diaphragmatic irritation. Back pain is uncommon.

The initial reaction consists of a chemical peritonitis caused by gastric acid or bile and pancreatic enzymes. The peritoneal reaction dilutes these irritants with a thin exudate, and as a result the patient's symptoms may temporarily improve before bacterial peritonitis occurs. The physician who sees the patient for the first time during this symptomatic lull must not be misled into interpreting it as representing bona fide improvement.

The patient appears severely distressed, lying quietly with the knees drawn up and breathing shallowly to minimize abdominal motion. Fever is absent at the start. The abdominal muscles are rigid owing to severe involuntary spasm. Epigastric tenderness may not be as marked as expected because the boardlike rigidity protects the abdominal viscera from the palpating hand. Escaped air from the stomach may enter the space between the liver and abdominal wall, and upon percussion the normal dullness over the liver will be tympanitic. Peristaltic sounds are reduced or absent. If delay in treatment allows continued escape of air into the peritoneal cavity, abdominal distention and diffuse tympany may result.

The above description applies to the typical case of perforation with classic findings. In as many as one third of patients, the presentation is not as dramatic, diagnosis is less obvious, and serious delays in treatment may result from failure to consider this condition and to obtain the appropriate abdominal x-rays. Many of these atypical perforations occur in patients already hospitalized for some unrelated illness, and the significance of the new symptom of abdominal pain is not appreciated. The only way to improve this record is to routinely obtain abdominal films on patients with abdominal pain of recent onset.

Lesser degrees of shock with minimal abdominal findings occur if the leak is small or rapidly sealed. A small duodenal perforation may slowly leak fluid that runs down the lateral peritoneal gutter, producing pain and muscular rigidity in the right lower quadrant and thus raising a problem of confusion with acute appendicitis.

Perforations may be sealed by omentum or by the liver, with the later development of a subhepatic or subdiaphragmatic abscess.

B. Laboratory Findings

A mild leukocytosis in the range of 12,000/μL is common in the early stages. After 12–24 hours, this may rise to 20,000/μL or more if treatment has been inadequate. The mild rise in the serum amylase value that occurs in many patients is probably caused by absorption of the enzyme from duodenal secretions within the peritoneal cavity. Direct measurement of fluid obtained by paracentesis may show very high levels of amylase.

C. Imaging Studies

Plain x-rays of the abdomen reveal free subdiaphragmatic air in 85% of patients. Films should be taken with the patient both supine and upright. A film in the left lateral decubitus position may be a more practical way to demonstrate free air in the uncomfortable patient. If the findings are questionable, 400 mL of air can be insufflated into the stomach through a nasogastric tube and the films repeated. Free air in the abdomen in a patient with sudden upper abdominal pain should clinch the diagnosis.

If no free air is demonstrated and the clinical picture suggests perforated ulcer, an emergency upper gastrointestinal series should be performed. If the perforation has not sealed, the diagnosis is established by noting escape of the contrast material from the lumen. Barium is more reliable than water-soluble contrast media, and, contrary to previous views, does not appear to aggravate infection or to be difficult to remove.

▶ Differential Diagnosis

The differential diagnosis includes acute pancreatitis and acute cholecystitis. The former does not have as explosive an onset as perforated ulcer and is usually accompanied by a high serum amylase level. Acute cholecystitis with perforated gallbladder could mimic perforated ulcer closely but free air would not be present with ruptured gallbladder. Intestinal obstruction has a more gradual onset and is characterized by less severe pain that is crampy and accompanied by vomiting.

The simultaneous onset of pain and free air in the abdomen in the absence of trauma usually means perforated peptic ulcer. Free perforation of colonic diverticulitis and acute appendicitis are other rare causes.

▶ Treatment

The diagnosis is often suspected before the patient is sent for confirmatory x-rays. Whenever a perforated ulcer is considered, the first step should be to pass a nasogastric tube and empty the stomach to reduce further contamination of the peritoneal cavity. Blood should be drawn for laboratory studies, and intravenous antibiotics (eg, cefazolin, cefoxitin) should be started. If the patient's overall condition is precarious owing to delay in treatment, fluid resuscitation should precede diagnostic measures. X-rays should be obtained as soon as the clinical status will permit.

The simplest surgical treatment, laparoscopy (or laparotomy) and suture closure of the perforation solves the immediate problem. The closure most often consists of securely plugging the hole with omentum (Graham-Steele closure) sutured into place rather than bringing together the two edges with sutures. All fluid should be aspirated from the peritoneal cavity, but drainage is not indicated. Reperforation is rare in the immediate postoperative period.

About three fourths of patients whose perforation is the culmination of a history of chronic symptoms continue to have clinically severe ulcer disease after simple closure. This has gradually led to a more aggressive treatment policy involving a definitive ulcer operation for most patients with acute

perforation (eg, parietal cell vagotomy plus closure of the perforation or truncal vagotomy and pyloroplasty). Now that ulcer disease can be cured by eradicating *H pylori*, the value of anything more than simple closure will have to be reexamined.

Concomitant hemorrhage and perforation are most often due to two ulcers, an anterior perforated one and a posterior one that is bleeding. Perforated ulcers that also obstruct obviously cannot be treated by suture closure of the perforation alone. Vagotomy plus gastroenterostomy or pyloroplasty should be performed. Perforated anastomotic ulcers require a vagotomy or gastrectomy, since in the long run, closure alone is nearly always inadequate.

Nonoperative treatment of perforated ulcer consists of continuous gastric suction and the administration of antibiotics in high doses. Although this has been shown to be effective therapy, with a low death rate, it is occasionally accompanied by a peritoneal and subphrenic abscess, and side effects are greater than with laparoscopic closure.

▶ Prognosis

About 15% of patients with perforated ulcer die, and about a third of these are undiagnosed before surgery. The death rate of perforated ulcer seen early is low. Delay in treatment, advanced age, and associated systemic diseases account for most deaths.

Donovan AJ, Berne TV, Donovan JA: Perforated duodenal ulcer: an alternative therapeutic plan. Arch Surg 1998;133:1166.

Hernandez-Diaz S, Rodriguez LA: Association between nonsteroidal anti-inflammatory drugs and upper gastrointestinal tract bleeding/perforation: an overview of epidemiologic studies published in the 1990s. Arch Intern Med 2000;160:2093.

Memon MA, Fitzgibbons RJ Jr: The role of minimal access surgery in the acute abdomen. Surg Clin North Am 1997;77:1333.

Millat B, Fingerhut A, Borie F: Surgical treatment of complicated duodenal ulcers: controlled trials. World J Surg 2000;24:299.

Svanes C: Trends in perforated peptic ulcer: incidence, etiology, treatment, and prognosis. World J Surg 2000;24:277.

STRESS GASTRODUODENITIS, STRESS ULCER & ACUTE HEMORRHAGIC GASTRITIS

The term stress ulcer has been used to refer to a heterogeneous group of acute gastric or duodenal ulcers that develop following physiologically stressful illnesses. There are four major etiologic factors associated with such lesions: (1) shock, (2) sepsis, (3) burns, and (4) central nervous system tumors or trauma.

▶ Etiology

A. Stress Ulcer

Acute ulcers following major surgery, mechanical ventilation, shock, sepsis, and burns (Curling ulcers) have enough common features to suggest they evolve by a similar pathogenetic mechanism.

Hemorrhage is the major clinical problem, though perforation occurs in about 10% of cases. Despite the predilection of stress ulcers to develop in the parietal cell mucosa, in about 30% of patients the duodenum is affected, and sometimes both stomach and duodenum are involved. Morphologically, the ulcers are shallow, discrete lesions with congestion and edema but little inflammatory reaction at their margins. Gastroduodenal endoscopy performed early in traumatized or burned patients has shown acute gastric erosions in the majority of patients within 72 hours after the injury (Figures 23–7 and 23–8). Such studies illustrate how frequently the disease process remains subclinical; clinically apparent ulcers develop in about 20% of susceptible patients. Clinically evident bleeding is usually seen 3–5 days after the injury, and massive bleeding generally does not appear until 4–5 days later.

Decreased mucosal resistance is the first step, which may involve the effects of ischemia (with production of toxic superoxide and hydroxyl radicals) and circulating toxins, followed by decreased mucosal renewal, decreased production of endogenous prostanoids, and thinning of the surface mucus layer. Decreased gastric mucosal blood flow also plays a role by decreasing the supply of blood buffers available to neutralize hydrogen ions that are diffusing into the weakened mucosa. Experimental evidence has implicated platelet-activating factor, released by endotoxin, as a possible mediator of gut ulceration in sepsis. The mucosa is thus rendered more vulnerable to acid-pepsin ulceration and lysosomal enzymes. Acid hypersecretion may be involved to some extent, since burn patients who manifest serious bleeding have higher gastric acid output than patients with a more benign course. Disruption of the gastric mucosal barrier to back diffusion of acid has been found in less than half of patients and is now thought to be a manifestation of the disease rather than a cause.

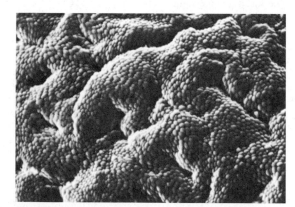

▲ **Figure 23–7.** Scanning electron photomicrograph of the surface epithelium of a normal subject showing individual cells and numerous gastric pits. (Reduced from × 350.) (Courtesy of Jeanne M. Riddle.)

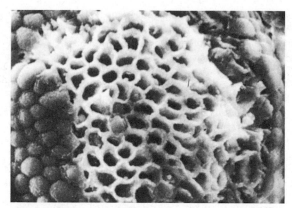

▲ **Figure 23–8.** Scanning electron photomicrograph of the surface epithelium of a patient with acute gastric mucosal erosions, showing a patch of cellular defoliation. Lesions such as this may account for back diffusion of H^+. (Reduced from × 1145.) (Courtesy of Jeanne M. Riddle.)

B. Cushing Ulcers

Acute ulcers associated with central nervous system tumors or injuries differ from stress ulcers because they are associated with elevated levels of serum gastrin and increased gastric acid secretion. Morphologically, they are similar to ordinary gastroduodenal peptic ulcers. Cushing ulcers are more prone to perforate than other kinds of stress ulcers.

C. Acute Hemorrhagic Gastritis

This disorder may share some causative factors with the above conditions, but the natural history is different and the response to treatment considerably better. Most of these patients can be controlled medically. When surgery is required for alcoholic gastritis, a high proportion of patients are cured by pyloroplasty and vagotomy.

▶ Clinical Findings

Hemorrhage is nearly always the first manifestation. Pain rarely occurs. Physical examination is not contributory except to reveal gross or occult fecal blood or signs of shock.

▶ Prevention

H_2 receptor antagonists given prophylactically to critically ill patients decrease the incidence of stress erosions and overt bleeding. The drug may be given orally (eg, ranitidine, 150 mg through a nasogastric tube every 12 hours) or intravenously (eg, cimetidine, 50–100 mg/h). Sucralfate is also effective. Patients receiving total parenteral nutrition appear to be protected by this therapy and experience no increased benefit from H_2 antagonists. A concern that decreasing gastric acidity with H_2 blocking agents would increase the rate and severity of nosocomial pneumonia (from gastric bacterial overgrowth) has not been justified by experience.

▶ Treatment

Initial management should consist of gastric lavage with chilled solutions and measures to combat sepsis if present. H_2 receptor blockers are of no value in the actively bleeding patient, but they probably decrease the rate of rebleeding once bleeding has stopped.

Some success has been reported with the selective infusion of vasoconstricting agents (eg, vasopressin) into the left gastric artery through a percutaneously placed catheter. In the sickest patients, if facilities and trained personnel are available, this technique should probably be attempted before operation is considered.

Perform laparotomy if the nonoperative regimen fails to halt the bleeding. Surgical treatment should consist of vagotomy and pyloroplasty, with suture of the bleeding points, or vagotomy and subtotal gastrectomy. There is a trend toward the first of these options, particularly in the sickest patients. When it occurs, rebleeding is nearly always from an ulcer left behind at the initial procedure. Rarely, total gastrectomy has had to be used because of the extent of ulceration and severity of bleeding or because of rebleeding after a lesser operation.

Felig DM, Carafa CJ: Stress ulcers of the stomach. Gastrointest Endosc 2000;51:596.

Phillips JO et al: A randomized, pharmacokinetic and pharmacodynamic, cross-over study of duodenal or jejunal administration compared to nasogastric administration of omeprazole suspension in patients at risk for stress ulcers. Am J Gastroenterol 2001;96:367.

GASTRIC CARCINOMA

There are about 20,000 new cases of carcinoma of the stomach in the United States annually. The incidence has dropped to one third of what it was 35 years ago. This may reflect changes in the prevalence of *H pylori* infection, which has a role in the etiology of this disease. *H pylori* is known to be a cause of chronic atrophic gastritis, which in turn is a recognized precursor of gastric adenocarcinoma. Epidemiologic studies have linked gastric *H pylori* infection with a 3.6-fold to 18-fold (all patients versus women) increase in the risk of developing carcinoma of the body or antrum (not the cardia), and the risk is proportionate to serum levels of *H pylori* antibodies.

The present incidence in American males is 10 new cases per 100,000 population per year. The highest rate, 63 per 100,000 males, is seen in Costa Rica; in eastern and central European countries, it is about 35 per 100,000 per year. Epidemiologic studies suggest that the incidence of gastric carcinoma is related to low dietary intake of vegetables and fruits and high intake of starches. Carcinoma of the stomach is rare under age 40, from which point the risk gradually climbs. The mean age at discovery is 63. It is about twice as common in men as in women.

Gastric epithelial cancers are nearly always adenocarcinomas. Squamous cell tumors of the proximal stomach involve the stomach secondarily from the esophagus. Five morphologic subdivisions correlate loosely with the natural history and outcome.

1. Ulcerating carcinoma (25%)—This consists of a deep, penetrating ulcer-tumor that extends through all layers of the stomach. It may involve adjacent organs in the process. The edges are shallow by contrast with overhanging edges noted in benign ulcers.

2. Polypoid carcinomas (25%)—These are large, bulky intraluminal growths that tend to metastasize late.

3. Superficial spreading carcinoma (15%)—Also known as early gastric cancer, superficial spreading carcinoma is confined to the mucosa and submucosa. Metastases are present in only 30% of cases. Even when metastases are present, the prognosis after gastrectomy is much better than for the more deeply invading lesions of advanced gastric cancer. In Japan, screening programs have been so successful that early gastric cancer now constitutes 30% of surgical cases, and survival rates have improved accordingly.

4. Linitis plastica (10%)—This variety of spreading tumor involves all layers with a marked desmoplastic reaction in which it may be difficult to identify the malignant cells. The stomach loses its pliability. Cure is rare because of early spread.

5. Advanced carcinoma (35%)—This largest category contains the big tumors that are found partly within and partly outside the stomach. They may originally have qualified for inclusion in the preceding groups but have outgrown that early stage.

Gastric adenocarcinomas can also be classified by degree of differentiation of their cells. In general, rate and extent of spread correlate with lack of differentiation. Some tumors are found histologically to excite an inflammatory cell reaction at their borders, and this feature indicates a relatively good prognosis. Tumors whose cells form glandular structures (intestinal type) have a somewhat better prognosis than tumors whose cells do not (diffuse type); the diffuse type is often associated with a substantial stromal component. The intestinal type of tumor accounts for a much larger proportion of cases in countries such as Japan and Finland where gastric cancer is especially common. The gradual decline in incidence in these areas is due principally to decreased occurrence of the intestinal type of tumor. Signet ring carcinomas, which contain more than 50% signet ring cells, have become increasingly more common and now constitute one third of all cases. They behave as the diffuse type of cancer and occur more frequently in women, in younger patients, and in the distal part of the stomach. Previous *H pylori* infection is not associated with the development of any specific histologic type of gastric cancer.

Extension occurs by intramural spread, direct extraluminal growth, and lymphatic metastases. Pathologic staging, which correlates closely with survival, is illustrated in Figure 23–9. Three fourths of patients have metastases when first seen. Within the stomach, proximal spread exceeds distal spread. The pylorus acts as a partial barrier, but tumor is found in 25% of cases in the first few centimeters of the bulb.

Early gastric cancer, defined as a primary lesion confined to the mucosa and submucosa with or without lymph node metastases, is associated with an excellent prognosis (5-year survival rate of 90%) after resection. In Japan, mass screening programs detect about 30% of patients with this lesion, whereas in the United States, only 10% of patients have early gastric cancer.

Forty percent of tumors are in the antrum, predominantly on the lesser curvature; 30% arise in the body and fundus, 25% at the cardia, and 5% involve the entire organ. Frequency of location has gradually changed, so that proximal lesions are more common now than 10–20 years ago. Benign ulcers develop at the greater curvature and cardia less commonly than malignant ones. Ulcers at these points are particularly suspect for neoplasm.

▶ Clinical Findings

A. Symptoms and Signs

The earliest symptom is usually vague postprandial abdominal heaviness that the patient does not identify as a pain. Sometimes the discomfort is no different from other vague dyspeptic symptoms that have been intermittently present for years, but the frequency and persistence are new.

Anorexia develops early and may be most pronounced for meat. Weight loss, the most common symptom, averages about 6 kg. True postprandial pain suggesting a benign gastric ulcer is relatively uncommon, but if it is present, one may be misled if subsequent x-rays show an ulcer. Vomiting may be present and becomes a major feature if pyloric obstruction occurs. It may have a coffee-ground appearance owing to bleeding by the tumor. Dysphagia may be the presenting symptom of lesions at the cardia.

An epigastric mass can be felt on examination in about one fourth of cases. Hepatomegaly is present in 10% of cases. The stool will be positive for occult blood in half of patients, and melena is seen in a few. Otherwise, abnormal physical findings are confined to signs of distant spread of the tumor. Metastases to the neck along the thoracic duct may produce a Virchow node. Rectal examination may reveal a Blumer shelf, a solid peritoneal deposit anterior to the rectum. Enlarged ovaries (Krukenberg tumors) may be caused by intraperitoneal metastases. Further dissemination may involve the liver, lungs, brain, or bone.

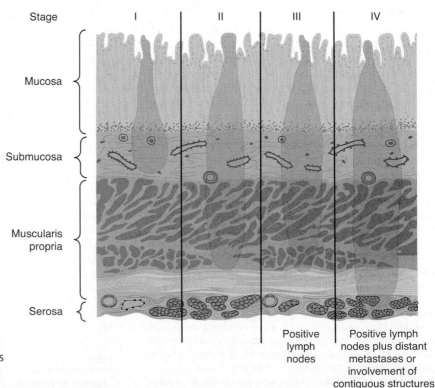

▲ **Figure 23–9.** Staging system for gastric carcinoma. The darkly shadowed areas represent cancers with different depths of mucosal penetration.

B. Laboratory Findings

Anemia is present in 40% of patients. Carcinoembryonic antigen (CEA) levels are elevated in 65%, usually indicating extensive spread of the tumor.

C. Imaging Studies

An upper gastrointestinal series is diagnostic for many tumors, but the overall false-negative rate is about 20%. Major diagnostic problems are posed by ulcerating tumors, a few of which may not be distinguishable radiologically from benign peptic ulcers. The differential features are listed in the section on gastric ulcer, but x-rays alone will not establish a diagnosis of benign ulcer. All patients with a newly discovered gastric ulcer should undergo gastroscopy and gastric biopsy.

D. Gastroscopy and Biopsy

Large gastric carcinomas can usually be identified as such by their gross appearance at endoscopy. All gastric lesions, whether polypoid or ulcerating, should be examined by taking multiple biopsy and brush cytology specimens during endoscopy. False results are seen occasionally as a result of sampling error, and a minimum of six biopsies is necessary for greatest accuracy.

▶ Treatment

Surgical resection is the only curative treatment. About 85% of patients are operable, and in 50% the lesions are amenable to resection; of the resectable lesions, half are potentially curable (ie, no signs of spread beyond the limits of resection).

The surgical objective should be to remove the tumor, an adjacent uninvolved margin of stomach and duodenum, the regional lymph nodes, and, if necessary, portions of involved adjacent organs. The proximal margin should be a minimum of 6 cm from the gross tumor. If the tumor is located in the antrum, a curative resection would entail distal gastrectomy with en bloc removal of the omentum, a 3- to 4-cm cuff of duodenum and the subpyloric lymph nodes, and, in some instances, excision of the left gastric artery and nearby lymph nodes. Reconstruction after gastrectomy may be by either a Billroth I or II procedure, but the latter is preferable because postoperative growth of residual tumor near the pylorus may obstruct a gastroduodenal anastomosis early.

Total gastrectomy with splenectomy is required for tumors of the proximal half of the stomach and for extensive tumors (eg, linitis plastica). Whether or not the spleen should be removed in such cases is a subject of debate. Alimentary continuity is most often reestablished by a Roux-en-Y esophagojejunostomy. Construction of an intestinal pouch as a substitute food reservoir (eg, Hunt-Lawrence pouch) is of no nutritional value, and it increases the risks of immediate complications.

Esophagogastrectomy plus splenectomy with intrathoracic esophagogastrostomy is the operation usually performed for tumors of the cardia. The procedure is usually done through two separate incisions: first, a laparotomy for the gastric part, and then a right posterolateral thoracotomy for the anastomosis.

Japanese surgeons have devised a more detailed staging system than the one used in most other countries and have also recommended more aggressive lymphadenectomy as a matter of routine in the resection of gastric cancers. The results of resections as reported from Japan are better than those obtained by the standard operations described above, so attempts are being made to determine whether the difference is due to the more radical operations. Most Western surgeons are skeptical, and radical lymphadenectomy (eg, clearing all nodal levels up to and including the para-aortic nodes) is not recommended at present.

The propensity for proximal submucosal spread must be appreciated at surgery. It is often advisable to perform a frozen section at the proximal margin before constructing the anastomosis. If tumor is found, the gastrectomy should be extended.

Palliative resection is usually indicated if the stomach is still movable and life expectancy is estimated to be more than 1–2 months. Palliative gastrectomy is usually performed to remove an antral lesion and prevent obstruction, but in selected cases, total gastrectomy is appropriate palliative treatment if the operation can be done safely and the amount of extragastric tumor is minimal. Whenever technically feasible, palliative gastrectomy is preferable to palliative gastrojejunostomy.

Adjuvant chemotherapy after curative surgery has not been of value with the regimens tested to date. For advanced disease, doxorubicin or fluorouracil alone, each of which results in a 20% response rate, is as good as a combination of chemotherapeutic agents.

▶ Prognosis

In the United States, the overall 5-year survival rate is about 12%. The 5-year survival rate for patients with early gastric cancer is about 90%. The 5-year survival rates in relation to the extent of spread are stage I, 70%; stage II, 30%; stage III, 10%; and stage IV, 0%.

Death from tumor may follow dissemination to other organs or may be the result of progressive gastric obstruction and malnutrition.

Gastric cancer and *Helicobacter pylori*: a combined analysis of 12 case control studies nested within prospective cohorts. Gut 2001;49:347.

Hulscher JB et al: Prospective analysis of the diagnostic yield of extended en bloc resection for adenocarcinoma of the oesophagus or gastric cardia. Br J Surg 2001;88:715.

Huntsman DG et al: Early gastric cancer in young, asymptomatic carriers of germ-line E-cadherin mutations. N Engl J Med 2001;344:1904.

Kalmar K et al: Comparison of quality of life and nutritional parameters after total gastrectomy and a new type of pouch construction with simple Roux-en-Y reconstruction: preliminary results of a prospective, randomized, controlled study. Dig Dis Sci 2001;46:1791.

Kelly S et al: A systematic review of the staging performance of endoscopic ultrasound in gastro-oesophageal carcinoma. Gut 2001;49:534.

Lee HK et al: Influence of the number of lymph nodes examined on staging of gastric cancer. Br J Surg 2001;88:1408.

Macdonald JS et al: Chemoradiotherapy after surgery compared with surgery alone for adenocarcinoma of the stomach or gastroesophageal junction. N Engl J Med 2001;345:725.

Wu AW et al: Neoadjuvant chemotherapy versus none for resectable gastric cancer. Cochrane Database Syst Rev 2007;2:CD005047.

Yasuda K et al: Risk factors for complications following resection of large gastric cancer. Br J Surg 2001;88:873.

GASTRIC POLYPS

Gastric polyps are single or multiple benign tumors that occur predominantly in the elderly. Those located in the distal stomach are more apt to cause symptoms. Whenever gastric polyps are discovered, gastric cancer must be ruled out.

Gastric polyps can be classified histologically as hyperplastic, adenomatous, or inflammatory. Other polypoid lesions, such as leiomyomas and carcinoid tumors, are discussed elsewhere. Hyperplastic polyps, which constitute 80% of cases, consist of an overgrowth of normal epithelium; they are not true neoplasms and have no relationship to gastric cancer. About 30% of adenomatous polyps contain a focus of adenocarcinoma, and adenocarcinoma can be found elsewhere in the stomach in 20% of patients with a benign adenomatous polyp. The incidence of cancer in an adenomatous polyp rises with increasing size. Lesions with a stalk and those less than 2 cm in diameter are usually not malignant. About 10% of benign adenomatous polyps undergo malignant change during prolonged follow-up.

Anemia may develop from chronic blood loss or deficient iron absorption. Over 90% of patients are achlorhydric after maximal stimulation. Vitamin B_{12} absorption is deficient in 25%, although megaloblastic anemia is present in only a few. Exfoliative cytologic examination of specimens obtained by endoscopy and brush biopsy should be performed in all patients.

Excision with a snare through the endoscope can be performed safely for most polyps. Otherwise, laparotomy is indicated for polyps greater than 1 cm in diameter or when cancer is suspected. Single polyps may be excised through a gastrotomy and a frozen section performed. If the polyp is found to be carcinoma, an appropriate type of gastrectomy is indicated. Partial gastrectomy should be performed for multiple polyps in the distal stomach. If 10–20 polyps are distributed throughout the stomach, the antrum should be removed and the fundic polyps excised. Total gastrectomy may be required for symptomatic diffuse multiple polyposis.

These patients should be followed because they have an increased risk of late development of pernicious anemia or gastric cancer. Recurrent polyps are uncommon.

Abraham SC et al: Hyperplastic polyps of the stomach: associations with histologic patterns of gastritis and gastric atrophy. Am J Surg Pathol 2001;25:500.

Ohkusa T et al: Disappearance of hyperplastic polyps in the stomach after eradication of *Helicobacter pylori*. A randomized, clinical trial. Ann Intern Med 1998;129:712.

GASTRIC LYMPHOMA & PSEUDOLYMPHOMA

Lymphoma is the second-most common primary cancer of the stomach but constitutes only 2% of the total number, 95% being adenocarcinomas. Almost all are non-Hodgkin lymphomas and are generally classified as B cell mucosa-associated lymphoid tissue (MALT) lymphomas. They are further subclassified as low-grade or high-grade based on nuclear pattern. About 20% of patients manifest a second primary cancer in another organ.

The principal symptoms are epigastric pain and weight loss, similar to those of carcinoma. Characteristically, the tumor has attained bulky proportions by the time it is discovered; by comparison with adenocarcinoma of the stomach, the symptoms from a gastric lymphoma are usually mild in relation to the size of the lesion. A palpable epigastric mass is present in 50% of patients. Barium x-ray studies will demonstrate the lesion, although it usually is mistaken for adenocarcinoma or, in 10% of cases, for benign gastric ulcer. Gastroscopy with biopsy and brush cytology provides the correct diagnosis preoperatively in about 75% of cases. If a pathologic diagnosis has not been made, the surgeon may incorrectly judge the lesion to be inoperable carcinoma because of its large size. Preoperative staging should include a CT scan and bone marrow biopsy.

Treatment of low-grade gastric lymphoma consists of long-term chemotherapy with cyclophosphamide. Surgical resection followed by total abdominal radiotherapy may be the treatment of choice for high-grade lymphomas, but the subject is debated. Intraoperative staging should consist of needle biopsies of both lobes of the liver and biopsies of celiac and para-aortic lymph nodes. Splenectomy should be performed only if the spleen is directly invaded. Extension into the duodenum or esophagus should not lead to resection of these organs but to postoperative adjunctive therapy. The 5-year disease-free survival rate is 50%. Survival correlates with stage of disease, extent of penetration of the gastric wall, and histologic grade of the tumor. Most recurrences appear within 2 years of surgery. Because two thirds of recurrences are outside the abdomen, patients at high risk of recurrence should receive postoperative chemotherapy also.

Gastric pseudolymphoma consists of a mass of lymphoid tissue in the gastric wall, often associated with an overlying mucosal ulcer. It is thought to represent a response to chronic inflammation. The lesion is not malignant, though the presentation, which includes pain, weight loss, and a mass on barium studies, cannot be distinguished from that of a malignant lesion.

Treatment of gastric pseudolymphoma consists of resection. The distinction from lymphoma is made on histologic examination of the specimen, which shows mature germinal centers in pseudolymphoma. No additional therapy is indicated postoperatively.

Crump M, Gospodarowicz M, Shepherd FA: Lymphoma of the gastrointestinal tract. Semin Oncol 1999;26:324.

Kolve ME, Fischbach W, Wilhelm M: Primary gastric non-Hodgkin's lymphoma: requirements for diagnosis and staging. Recent Results Cancer Res 2000;156:63.

Steinbach G et al: Antibiotic treatment of gastric lymphoma of mucosa-associated lymphoid tissue. An uncontrolled trial. Ann Intern Med 1999;131:88.

Yamashita H et al: When can complete regression of low-grade gastric lymphoma of mucosa-associated lymphoid tissue be predicted after *Helicobacter pylori* eradication? Histopathology 2000;37:131.

GASTRIC LEIOMYOMAS & GASTROINTESTINAL STROMAL TUMOR (GIST)

Leiomyomas are common submucosal growths that are usually asymptomatic but may cause intestinal bleeding. GIST (previously called leiomyosarcomas) may grow to a large size and most often present with bleeding. Radiologically, the tumor usually contains a central ulceration caused by necrosis from outgrowth of its blood supply. In most cases the tumor arises from the proximal stomach. It may grow into the gastric lumen, remain entirely on the serosal surface, or even become pedunculated within the abdominal cavity. Spread is by direct invasion or blood-borne metastases. CT scans provide useful information on the amount of extragastric extension. Leiomyomas should be removed by enucleation or wedge resection. After the more radical resections required for leiomyosarcomas, the 5-year survival rate is 20%. If technically possible, complete resection of metastases (eg, peritoneal, hepatic) in addition to the primary tumor may improve the outcome. The results are affected by tumor size, DNA ploidy pattern, and tumor grade. Lesions that exhibit ten or more mitoses in a high-powered field rarely can be cured. The tumor is resistant to radiotherapy. Imatinib mesylate (Gleevec) is an effective systemic agent. It is used for disseminated disease and is in trials for adjuvant use.

MÉNÉTRIER DISEASE

Ménétrier disease, a form of hypertrophic gastritis, consists of giant hypertrophy of the gastric rugae; high, normal, or low acid secretion; and excessive loss of protein from the thickened mucosa into the gut, with resulting hypoproteinemia. The etiology may involve altered expression of TGF-α. Clinical manifestations include edema, diarrhea, anorexia, weight loss, and skin rash. Chronic blood loss may also be a

problem. Indigestion may respond to antacids, but this treatment does not improve the gastric pathologic process or secondary hypoproteinemia. The hypertrophic rugae present as enormous filling defects on upper gastrointestinal series and are frequently misinterpreted as carcinoma. The protein leak from the gastric mucosa may respond to atropine (and other anticholinergic drugs), hexamethonium bromide, eradication of *H pylori*, or H_2 blocking agents or omeprazole. Rarely, total gastrectomy is indicated for severe intractable hypoproteinemia, anemia, or inability to exclude cancer. Medical management is best for most patients, though the gastric abnormalities and hypoproteinemia may persist. Some cases gradually evolve into atrophic gastritis. In children the disease characteristically is self-limited and benign. There is an increased risk of adenocarcinoma of the stomach in adults with Ménétrier disease.

Badov D et al: *Helicobacter pylori* as a pathogenic factor in Ménétrier's disease. Am J Gastroenterol 1998;93:1976.

Burdick JS et al: Treatment of Ménétrier's disease with a monoclonal antibody against the epidermal growth factor receptor. N Engl J Med 2000;343:1697.

Madsen LG et al: Ménétrier's disease and *Helicobacter pylori*: normalization of gastrointestinal protein loss after eradication therapy. Dig Dis Sci 1999;44:2307.

PROLAPSE OF THE GASTRIC MUCOSA

This uncommon lesion occasionally accompanies small prepyloric gastric ulcers. Episodes of vomiting and abdominal pain simulate peptic ulcer disease. X-ray shows prolapse of antral folds into the duodenum. One must be alert to the presence of gastric or duodenal ulcer as the underlying cause.

Antrectomy with a Billroth I anastomosis is occasionally required. Generally, conservative treatment suffices.

GASTRIC VOLVULUS

The stomach may rotate about its longitudinal axis (organoaxial volvulus) or a line drawn from the mid lesser to the mid greater curvature (mesenteroaxial volvulus). The former is more common and is often associated with a paraesophageal hiatal hernia. In other patients, eventration of the left diaphragm allows the colon to rise and twist the stomach by pulling on the gastrocolic ligament.

Acute gastric volvulus produces severe abdominal pain accompanied by a diagnostic triad (Borchardt triad): (1) vomiting followed by retching and then inability to vomit, (2) epigastric distention, and (3) inability to pass a nasogastric tube. The situation calls for immediate laparotomy to prevent death from acute gastric necrosis and shock. An emergency upper gastrointestinal series will show a block at the point of the volvulus. The death rate is high.

Chronic volvulus is more common than acute. It may be asymptomatic or may cause crampy intermittent pain. Cases associated with paraesophageal hiatal hernia should be treated by repair of the hernia and anterior gastropexy.

When cases are due to eventration of the diaphragm, the gastrocolic ligament should be divided the entire length of the greater curvature. The colon rises to fill the space caused by the eventration, and the stomach will resume its normal position, to be fastened by a gastropexy.

GASTRIC DIVERTICULA

Gastric diverticula are uncommon and usually asymptomatic. Most are pulsion diverticula consisting of mucosa and submucosa only, located on the lesser curvature within a few centimeters of the esophagogastric junction. Those in the prepyloric region generally possess all layers and are more likely to be symptomatic. A few patients have symptoms from hemorrhage of inflammation within a gastric diverticulum, but for the most part these lesions are incidental findings on upper gastrointestinal series. Radiologically, they can be confused with a gastric ulcer.

BEZOAR

Bezoars are concretions formed in the stomach. Trichobezoars are composed of hair and are usually found in young girls who pick at their hair and swallow it. Phytobezoars consist of agglomerated vegetable fibers. Pressure by the mass can create a gastric ulcer that is prone to bleed or perforate.

The postgastrectomy state predisposes to bezoar formation because pepsin and acid secretion are reduced and the triturating function of the antrum is gone. Orange segments or other fruits that contain a large amount of cellulose have been implicated in most cases. Improper mastication of food is a contributing factor that can sometimes be obviated by providing the patient with properly fitted dentures. The fruit may remain in the stomach or pass into the small intestine and cause obstruction. Some surgeons routinely warn postgastrectomy patients to avoid citrus fruits.

Large semisolid bezoars of *Candida albicans* have also been found in postgastrectomy patients. Some can be fragmented with the gastroscope. The patient should also be treated with oral nystatin.

Patients with symptomatic gastric bezoars may complain of abdominal pain. Ulceration and bleeding are associated with a death rate of 20%.

Nearly all gastric bezoars can be broken up and dispersed by endoscopy. Neglected lesions with complications (ie, bleeding or perforation) require gastrectomy.

II. DUODENUM

DUODENAL DIVERTICULA

Diverticula of the duodenum are found in 20% of autopsies and 5–10% of upper gastrointestinal series. Symptoms are uncommon, and only 1% of those found by x-ray warrant surgery.

Duodenal pulsion diverticula are acquired outpouchings of the mucosa and submucosa, 90% of which are on the medial aspect of the duodenum. They are rare before age 40. Most are solitary and within 2.5 cm of the ampulla of Vater. There is a high incidence of gallstone disease of the gallbladder in patients with juxtapapillary diverticula. Diverticula are not seen in the first portion of the duodenum, where diverticular configurations are due to scarring by peptic ulceration or cholecystitis.

A few patients have chronic postprandial abdominal pain or dyspepsia caused by a duodenal diverticulum. Treatment is with antacids and anticholinergics.

Serious complications are hemorrhage or perforation from inflammation, pancreatitis, and biliary obstruction. Bile acid-bilirubinate enteroliths are occasionally formed by bile stasis in a diverticulum. Enteroliths can precipitate diverticular inflammation or biliary obstruction and, rarely, have caused bowel obstruction after entering the intestinal lumen.

Surgical treatment is required for complications and, rarely, for persistent symptoms. Excision and a two-layer closure are usually possible after mobilization of the duodenum and dissection of the diverticulum from the pancreas. Removal of the diverticulum and closure of the defect are superior to simple drainage in the case of perforation. If biliary obstruction appears in a patient whose bile duct empties into a diverticulum, excision might be more hazardous than a side-to-side choledochoduodenostomy.

The rare wind sock type of intraluminal diverticulum usually presents with vague epigastric pain and postprandial fullness, though intestinal bleeding or pancreatitis is occasionally seen. The diagnosis can be made by barium x-ray studies. The diverticulum can be excised through a nearby duodenotomy. In some cases, the narrow diverticular outlet can be enlarged endoscopically.

Lobo DN et al: Periampullary diverticula and pancreaticobiliary disease. Br J Surg 1999;86:588.

DUODENAL TUMORS

Tumors of the duodenum are rare. Carcinoma of the ampulla of Vater is discussed in Chapter 26.

1. Malignant Duodenal Tumors

Most malignant duodenal tumors are adenocarcinomas, leiomyosarcomas, or lymphomas. They appear in the descending duodenum more often than elsewhere. Pain, obstruction, bleeding, obstructive jaundice, and an abdominal mass are the modes of presentation. Duodenal carcinomas, particularly those in the third and fourth portions of the duodenum, are often missed on barium x-ray studies. Endoscopy and biopsy will usually be diagnostic if the examiner is suspicious enough and can reach the lesion.

If possible, adenocarcinomas and leiomyosarcomas should be resected. Pancreaticoduodenectomy is usually necessary if the tumor is localized. Unresectable lesions should be treated by radiotherapy. Biopsy and radiotherapy are recommended for lymphoma.

After curative resections, the 5-year survival rate is 30%. The overall 5-year survival rate is 18%.

2. Benign Duodenal Tumors

Brunner gland adenomas are small submucosal nodules that have a predilection for the posterior duodenal wall at the junction of the first and second portions. Sessile and pedunculated variants are seen. Symptoms are due to bleeding or obstruction. Leiomyomas may also be found in the duodenum and ordinarily are asymptomatic.

Carcinoid tumors of the duodenum are often endocrinologically active, producing gastrin, somatostatin, or serotonin. Simple excision is the treatment of choice.

Heterotopic gastric mucosa, presenting as multiple small mucosal nodules, is an occasional endoscopic finding of no clinical significance.

Villous adenomas of the duodenum may give rise to intestinal bleeding or may obstruct the papilla of Vater and cause jaundice. As in the colon, the risk of malignant change is high—about 50%. Small pedunculated villous adenomas may be snared during endoscopy, but sessile tumors must be locally excised via laparotomy. Tumors that contain malignant tissue should be treated by a Whipple procedure.

Alarcon FJ et al: Familial adenomatous polyposis: efficacy of endoscopic and surgical treatment for advanced duodenal adenomas. Dis Colon Rectum 1999;42:1533.

Bakaeen FG et al: What prognostic factors are important in duodenal adenocarcinoma? Arch Surg 2000;135:635.

Bouvet M et al: Factors influencing survival after resection for periampullary neoplasms. Am J Surg 2000;180:13.

Kaklamanos IG et al: Extent of resection in the management of duodenal adenocarcinoma. Am J Surg 2000;179:37.

Ryder NM et al: Primary duodenal adenocarcinoma: a 40-year experience. Arch Surg 2000;135:1070.

Wallace MH et al: Randomized, placebo-controlled trial of gastric acid-lowering therapy on duodenal polyposis and relative adduct labeling in familial adenomatous polyposis. Dis Colon Rectum 2001;44:1585.

SUPERIOR MESENTERIC ARTERY OBSTRUCTION OF THE DUODENUM

Rarely, obstruction of the third portion of the duodenum is produced by compression between the superior mesenteric vessels and the aorta. It most commonly appears after rapid weight loss following injury, including burns. Patients in body casts are particularly susceptible.

The superior mesenteric artery normally leaves the aorta at an angle of 50–60 degrees, and the distance between the two vessels where the duodenum passes between them is 10–20 mm. These measurements in patients with superior mesenteric artery syndrome average 18 degrees and 2.5 mm. Acute loss of mesenteric fat is thought to permit the artery to drop posteriorly, trapping the bowel like a scissors.

Skepticism exists regarding the frequency of this condition in adults who have not experienced acute loss of weight. Most often the patient in question is a thin, nervous woman whose complaints of dyspepsia and occasional emesis are more properly explained on a functional basis. When a clear-cut example is encountered, it may actually represent a form of intestinal malrotation with duodenal bands.

The patient complains of epigastric bloating and crampy pain relieved by vomiting. The symptoms may remit in the prone position. Anorexia and postprandial pain lead to additional malnutrition and weight loss.

Upper gastrointestinal x-rays demonstrate a widened duodenum proximal to a sharp obstruction at the point where the artery crosses the third portion of the duodenum. When the patient moves to the knee-chest position, the passage of barium is suddenly unimpeded. Further verification can be provided if angiography shows an angle of 25 degrees or less between the superior mesenteric artery and the aorta. However, this procedure is not recommended for routine evaluation of obvious cases.

Many patients whose superior mesenteric artery makes a prominent impression on the duodenum are asymptomatic, and in ambulatory patients one should hesitate to attribute vague chronic complaints to this finding.

Involvement of the duodenum by scleroderma leads to duodenal dilatation and hypomotility and an x-ray and clinical picture highly suggestive of superior mesenteric artery syndrome. In the latter, increased duodenal peristalsis should be demonstrable proximal to the arterial blockage, whereas diminished peristalsis characterizes scleroderma. Patients with duodenal scleroderma usually have dysphagia from concomitant esophageal involvement.

Malrotation with duodenal obstruction by congenital bands can mimic this syndrome.

Postural therapy may suffice. The patient should be placed prone when symptomatic or in anticipation of postprandial difficulties. Ambulatory patients should be instructed to assume the knee-chest position, which allows the viscera and the artery to rotate forward off the duodenum.

Chronic obstruction may require section of the suspensory ligament and mobilization of the duodenum, or a duodenojejunostomy to bypass the obstruction. Patients with various forms of malrotation should be treated by mobilizing the duodenojejunal flexure, which releases the duodenum from entrapment by congenital bands.

Diwakaran HH, Stolar CG, Prather CM: Superior mesenteric artery syndrome. Gastroenterology 2001;121:516, 746.

Richardson WS, Surowiec WJ: Laparoscopic repair of superior mesenteric artery syndrome. Am J Surg 2001;181:377.

REGIONAL ENTERITIS OF THE STOMACH & DUODENUM

The proximal intestine and stomach are rarely involved in regional enteritis, though this disease has now been reported in every part of the gastrointestinal tract from the lips to the anus. Most patients with Crohn disease in the stomach or duodenum have ileal involvement as well.

Pain can in many instances be relieved by antacids. Intermittent vomiting from duodenal stenosis or pyloric obstruction is frequent. The x-ray finding of a cobblestone mucosa or stenosis would be suggestive when associated with typical changes in the ileum. The endoscopic appearance is fairly characteristic, and biopsy with the peroral suction device usually gives an adequate specimen for histologic confirmation of the diagnosis.

Medical treatment is nonspecific and consists principally of corticosteroids during exacerbations. Surgery may be indicated for disabling pain or obstruction. If the disease is localized to the stomach, a partial gastrectomy can be performed. Duodenal involvement most often requires a gastrojejunostomy to bypass the obstruction. Vagotomy should also be performed to prevent development of a marginal ulcer. Recurrent Crohn disease involving the anastomosis is an occasional late complication, but it can usually be managed successfully by reoperation.

Internal fistulas involving the stomach or duodenum usually represent extensions from primary disease in the ileum or colon. Surgical treatment consists of resection of the diseased ileum or colon and closure of the fistulous opening in the upper gut.

Mansari OE et al: Adenocarcinoma complicating Crohn's disease of the duodenum. Eur J Gastroenterol Hepatol 2001;13:1259.

Reynolds HL Jr, Stellato TA: Crohn's disease of the foregut. Surg Clin North Am 2001;81:117.

Worsey MJ et al: Strictureplasty is an effective option in the operative management of duodenal Crohn's disease. Dis Colon Rectum 1999;42:596.

Liver & Portal Venous System

William R. Jarnagin, MD

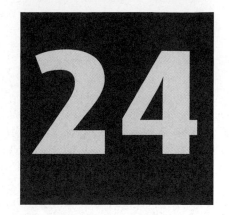

SURGICAL ANATOMY

▶ Segments

The liver develops as an embryologic outpouching from the duodenum by a process described in Chapter 25. The liver is one of the largest organs in the body, representing 2% of the total body weight. In classic descriptions, the liver was characterized as having four lobes: right, left, caudate, and quadrate; however, this is an overly simplistic view that fails to consider the much more complex segmental anatomy, which is depicted in Figure 24–1.

The liver is divided into eight segments based on the branching of the portal triads and hepatic veins. The structures of the portal triad (hepatic artery, portal vein, and biliary duct) are separate extrahepatically but enter the hepatic hilus ensheathed within a thickened layer of the Glisson capsule. The three main hepatic veins divide the liver into four sectors, each of which is supplied by a **portal pedicle.** The caudate lobe is an exception because its venous drainage is directly into the vena cava and therefore independent of the major hepatic veins. The four sectors delimited by the hepatic veins are called the **portal sectors,** and these portions of the parenchyma are supplied by independent portal pedicles arising from the right or left main pedicles. The divisions separating the sectors are called **portal scissurae,** within each of which runs a hepatic vein. Further branching of the pedicles subdivides the sectors into segments. The liver is thus subdivided into eight segments, with the caudate lobe designated as segment I. Segments I–IV comprise the left liver, and segments V–VIII, the right. Each segment is supplied by an independent portal pedicle, which forms the basis of sublobar segmental resections.

The anatomical right and left hemilivers are separated by an imaginary line running from the medial aspect of the gallbladder fossa to the inferior vena cava, running parallel with the fissure of the round ligament. This division is known as the Cantlie line or the principal plane and marks the course of the middle hepatic vein. The right hepatic vein further subdivides the right liver into anterior (segments V and VIII) and posterior (segments VI and VII) sectors, while the umbilical fissure subdivides the left liver into the medial sector (segment IV) and left lateral segment (segments II and III). The relationship of the liver to the other abdominal organs is shown in Figure 24–2.

▶ Portal Circulation

The portal vein is formed by the confluence of the splenic and superior mesenteric veins at the level of the second lumbar vertebra behind the head of the pancreas (Figure 24–3). It runs for approximately 6–9 cm to the hilum of the liver, where it divides into the main right and left branches. The left gastric vein usually enters the portal vein on its anteromedial aspect just cephalad to the margin of the pancreas, in which case it must be ligated during the surgical construction of a portacaval shunt; in 25% of cases, the left gastric vein joins the splenic vein. Other small venous tributaries from the pancreas and duodenum are less constant but must be anticipated during surgical mobilization of the portal vein.

The inferior mesenteric vein often drains into the splenic vein to the left of its junction with the superior mesenteric vein; alternatively, it may empty directly into the superior mesenteric vein.

In the hepatoduodenal ligament, the portal vein lies dorsal and slightly medial to the common bile duct. Portocaval lymph nodes are encountered along the right lateral aspect of the portal vein, running from the level of the duodenum to the liver and extending posteriorly. These lymph nodes are routinely removed during resections for certain malignancies and must be dissected before a portocaval shunt can be created.

▶ Venous Blood Supply

The anatomy of venous blood supply is shown in Figure 24–4. Both the portal and hepatic venous systems lack valves. The main portal vein terminates in the porta hepatis by dividing

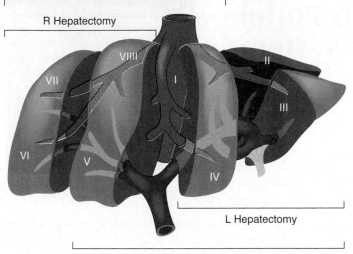

R Extended hepatectomy

R Hepatectomy

VIII
VII
I
II
VI
V
III
IV

L Hepatectomy

L Extended hepatectomy

▲ **Figure 24–1.** Segmental anatomy of the liver is shown, with each of the individual segments numbered. Segment I (caudate) is indicated at the back of the liver, posterior to the middle hepatic vein. The most common major hepatic resections performed and the segments removed with each are indicated.

into right and left branches. The right branch typically has a short extrahepatic course before subsequently dividing into anterior and posterior sectoral divisions, often high within the

porta hepatic or intrahepatically. The left branch has a longer extrahepatic course, running first along the base of segment IV and then entering the umbilical fissure, where it gives rise to branches to segments II, III, and IV; a large branch to the caudate lobe generally arises from the left portal vein prior to its entry into the umbilical fissure. Variations in the normal portal venous anatomy occur but are less common than aberrancies in the arterial supply or biliary drainage. The most common anomaly of the portal venous system is separate origins of the right anterior and posterior sectoral branches.

The hepatic veins represent the final common pathway for the central veins of the lobules of the liver. There are three major hepatic veins: left, right, and middle. The right

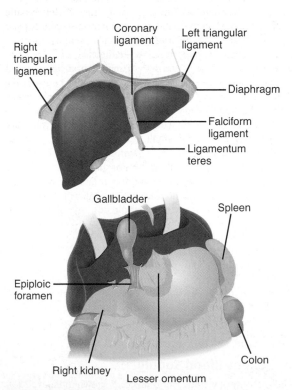

Right triangular ligament

Coronary ligament

Left triangular ligament

Diaphragm

Falciform ligament

Ligamentum teres

Gallbladder

Spleen

Epiploic foramen

Right kidney   Lesser omentum

Colon

▲ **Figure 24–2.** Relationships of the liver to adjacent abdominal organs.

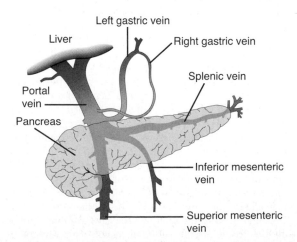

Left gastric vein

Liver

Right gastric vein

Portal vein

Splenic vein

Pancreas

Inferior mesenteric vein

Superior mesenteric vein

▲ **Figure 24–3.** Anatomic relationships of portal vein and branches.

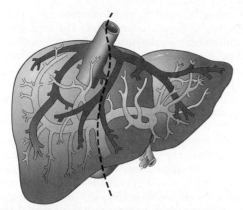

▲ **Figure 24–4.** Anatomy of the veins of the liver. The major lobar fissure is represented by the dashed line. Branches of the hepatic artery and biliary ducts follow those of the portal vein. The darker vessels represent the hepatic veins and vena cava; the lighter system represents the portal vein and its branches.

hepatic vein drains into the vena cava independently, while the middle and left hepatic veins typically join just outside of the liver, forming a common trunk. The middle hepatic vein runs in the principal plane (Cantlie line) and provides drainage for segment IV and the anterior sector of the right liver (segments V and VIII). The left hepatic vein drains segments II and III, while the right hepatic vein drains the posterior sector (segments VI and VII) and provides additional drainage to the anterior sector. A small umbilical vein runs within the umbilical fissure, providing accessory drainage of segments III and IV and emptying into the left hepatic vein. Several small accessory veins enter the inferior vena cava directly from the posterior aspect of the right lobe and must be carefully ligated during mobilization and resection of the right liver.

Arterial Blood Supply

The common hepatic artery arises from the celiac axis, ascends in the hepatoduodenal ligament, and gives rise to the right gastric, gastroduodenal, and proper hepatic arteries; the proper hepatic artery then divides into the right and left hepatic arterial branches in the liver hilum. The hepatic artery supplies approximately 25% of the 1500 mL of blood that enters the liver each minute; the remaining 75% is supplied by the portal vein.

Variations of the standard arterial anatomy of the liver are relatively common, seen in up to 40% of patients. The most common variants involve different origins of the right or left hepatic artery. A replaced right hepatic artery arises entirely from the superior mesenteric artery and courses to the right of the common bile duct within the porta hepatis, which is in contrast to its normal position to the left of the

duct. Recognition of this anatomical variant is critical during operations on the extrahepatic biliary tree. An accessory right hepatic artery also arises from the superior mesenteric artery and is found in the same location within the porta hepatis but supplies only a portion of the right liver; in this situation, a separate right branch arising from its normal position off the proper hepatic artery is typically present. An accessory or replaced left hepatic artery arises from the left gastric artery and enters the liver through the gastrohepatic ligament. Up to 25% of patients have a replaced or accessory right hepatic artery, and a similar proportion have a replaced or accessory left hepatic artery. Within the liver, the hepatic arterial branches travel with segmental bile ducts and portal vein branches.

Biliary Drainage

The biliary tree arises within the liver from bile canaliculi, formed from specialized segments of the hepatocyte membrane. Bile canaliculi join to form progressively larger channels, resulting in segmental bile ducts that drain each segment. The right anterior and right posterior sectoral ducts unite to form the main right hepatic duct, while the union of ducts draining segments II, III, and IV forms the left hepatic duct. The left hepatic duct typically is longer and has a longer extrahepatic course than the right hepatic duct. Drainage of segment I (caudate lobe) is principally into the left hepatic duct, but additional smaller ducts enter the right hepatic duct or drain directly into the hepatic duct confluence, which is formed by the union of the major lobar ducts to form the common hepatic duct. The common hepatic duct descends within the hepatoduodenal ligament for a variable distance to the point of insertion of the cystic duct of the gallbladder to give rise to the common bile duct.

Anatomic variations in the biliary ductal anatomy are seen in approximately 30% of patients and most often involve the right hepatic duct. In approximately 25% of patients, the duct from the right posterior sector joins the common hepatic duct or the left hepatic duct independently. Variations are far less common on the left side.

Lymphatics

Lymphatics draining superficial lobules of the liver follow a subcapsular course to the diaphragm, to the suspensory ligaments of the liver, or to the posterior mediastinum, while others enter the porta hepatis. Lymphatics arising from lobules deep within the liver travel either with the hepatic veins along the vena cava or with the portal veins into the porta hepatis. Most of the lymphatic drainage of the liver is to the hepatoduodenal ligament.

NERVES

The liver and biliary tree are innervated by sympathetic fibers arising from T7 to T10 and by parasympathetic fibers from the right and left vagus nerves. The postganglionic sympathetic nerves arise from the celiac ganglia. Fibers derived from the celiac ganglia and vagus nerves form a plexus of nerves that run along the anterior and posterior aspects of the hepatic artery.

PHYSIOLOGY

Total hepatic blood flow (about 1500 mL/min; 30 mL/min per kg body weight) constitutes 25% of the cardiac output, though the liver accounts for only 2.5% of body weight. About 30% of the hepatic volume is blood (12% of total blood volume). Two thirds of the flow enters through the portal vein and one-third through the hepatic artery. Pressure in the portal vein is normally low (10–15 cm H_2O [7–11 mm Hg]). The liver derives half of its oxygen from hepatic arterial blood and half from portal venous blood.

Blood flow within the liver is uniform, as demonstrated by an even distribution of microspheres injected into the hepatic artery or portal vein. Hepatic blood flow to the liver is regulated by a number of factors. Muscular sphincters at the inlet and outlet of sinusoids represent a major control point and respond to a number of different stimuli, including the autonomic nervous system, circulating hormones, bile salts, and metabolites. The cells lining the hepatic sinusoids (endothelial cells, Kupffer cells, and stellate cells) can also regulate flow to some extent.

Portal venous and hepatic arterial blood becomes pooled after entering the periphery of the hepatic sinusoid (Figure 24–5). Hepatic arterial flow increases or decreases reciprocally with changes in portal flow; however, portal venous flow does not increase with reductions in arterial flow. This arterial compensatory response is controlled largely by adenosine, which is released into the space of Mall surrounding the hepatic arterial resistance vessels. High concentrations of adenosine dilate the vessels, which increases flow and washes out the adenosine.

Sudden occlusion of the portal vein results in an immediate 60% rise in hepatic arterial flow. The total flow then gradually returns toward normal. On the other hand, sudden reductions in hepatic arterial supply are not immediately met by significant increases in portal vein flow. In both normal subjects and cirrhotics, total hepatic flow and portal pressure drop following hepatic arterial occlusion. Arterial collaterals develop, and arterial perfusion is ultimately restored.

It is for this reason that interruption of hepatic arterial flow to the right or left liver generally has little impact on hepatic function. The one notable exception is in the setting of biliary obstruction. Decreased hepatic arterial flow to portions of the liver with impaired biliary drainage carries a high risk of hepatic necrosis. Clinically, this is an important consideration in patients undergoing hepatic arterial embolization of liver tumors and in patients undergoing resection of periampullary tumors, where jaundice is common and dissection within the porta hepatic could potentially put the hepatic artery at risk for injury. On the other hand, portal venous flow plays a critical role in maintaining normal hepatic architecture and function. This point is underscored by the observation that occlusion of the right or left portal venous branches results in profound ipsilateral hepatic atrophy and contralateral hypertrophy. Portal vein occlusion is clinically relevant in a number of disease processes, particularly carcinoma of the hepatic duct confluence (hilar cholangiocarcinoma), in which portal venous involvement is common and has important therapeutic implications. Additionally, intentional occlusion of a major portal vein branch (usually the right side) is a procedure being used with greater frequency prior to major hepatic resection, primarily when the regenerative capacity of the future liver remnant (that portion of the liver that will remain behind after the resection) is questionable because of either size concerns (too small) or underlying parenchymal disease (steatohepatitis, cirrhosis). By causing atrophy of the liver to be resected, and therefore hypertrophy of the future liver remnant, the risk of postoperative hepatic failure may be reduced.

HEPATIC RESECTION

Liver resection is most commonly indicated for primary and secondary malignant tumors and symptomatic benign tumors; less common indications include traumatic injury, infection/abscesses, and living donor transplantation. Removal of as much as 80–85% of the normal liver can be performed with the expectation that the liver remnant will regenerate sufficiently for the patient to survive. It must be emphasized, however, that such extensive resections should be considered only in patients with normal hepatic function; those with cirrhosis or significant fibrosis or steatosis (fatty infiltration of the liver) are less likely to tolerate a major hepatic resection. Liver function may be impaired for several weeks after an extensive resection, but the extraordinary regenerative capacity of the liver rapidly provides new func-

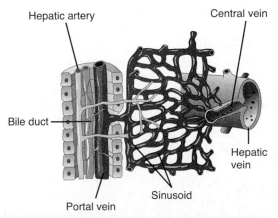

▲ **Figure 24–5.** Vascular anatomy of the liver lobule.

tioning hepatocytes. Within 24 hours after partial hepatectomy, cell replication becomes active and continues until the original volume of hepatic tissue is restored. Considerable regeneration occurs within 10 days, and the process is essentially complete by 4–5 weeks. Excised portions of liver are not re-formed; rather, the growth consists of formation of new lobules and expansion of residual lobules. The stimuli for hepatic regeneration are thought to include the following: hepatocyte growth factor, tumor growth factor (TGF)-α, heparin-binding growth factor, hepatopoietin B, and disinhibition by TGF-β_1 (ie, decreased levels of this inhibitor of hepatic growth).

▶ Preoperative Evaluation

Several different disease-related and patient-related factors must be assessed before deciding to proceed with hepatic resection. Among the most important of these is the preoperative functional status of the liver. Cirrhosis is a relative contraindication for partial hepatectomy because the limited reserve of the residual cirrhotic liver may be insufficient to meet essential metabolic demands, and the cirrhotic liver has a reduced capacity for regeneration. Cirrhosis is a particular concern in patients with hepatocellular carcinoma, which frequently arises in the setting of chronic hepatic parenchymal disease. An increasingly important concern in patients with hepatic colorectal metastases is chemotherapy-induced liver damage, which may also impair regeneration of the liver remnant.

Several tests are available to assess hepatic function prior to operation, none of which is perfect. The Child-Pugh classification is the oldest and most widely employed and remains the most useful assessment. The Child-Pugh system classifies hepatic function on the basis of several measures (Table 24–1). Originally used to assess mortality related to portosystemic shunts, the Child-Pugh score also predicts mortality in patients with cirrhosis after hepatic resection. In general, only Child-Pugh A and highly selected Child-Pugh B cirrhotics would be candidates for resection. The indocyanine green clearance (IGC) test is commonly used in centers outside of North America but has not been proven superior to the Child-Pugh scoring system.

▶ Extent of Hepatic Resection

Hepatic resections are classified as anatomical (based on the segmental liver anatomy) or nonanatomical. Wedge resections, enucleations, and resectional debridement of devitalized tissue are examples of the latter. In general, anatomical resections are preferred because they are associated with lower blood loss and, when performed for malignancy, a lower incidence of positive resection margins.

Major resections must be performed in accordance with the segmental anatomy. Major resections (right or left hepatectomy or extended hepatectomy) are commonly performed; however, the segmental anatomy of the liver allows smaller resections or bilateral resections to be performed when necessary and appropriate. For example, in selected situations, a resection of the anterior (segments V and VIII) or posterior (segments VI and VII) sectors may be performed rather than sacrificing the entire right liver. Such parenchymal-sparing resections on one side would then allow a resection of part of the contralateral lobe, if necessary.

The terminology and extent of the common types of major resections are in Figure 24–1. The operation entails removal of a lobe or segment with its afferent and efferent vessels while avoiding injury to vessels and bile ducts supplying the residual tissue.

Most elective hepatic resections can be performed through an abdominal incision, although selected situations (very large right lobe tumors) are probably best performed with a thoracoabdominal approach. Laparoscopic resections are being performed with greater frequency, although the open approach is most common and remains the standard. The best perioperative results are obtained by minimizing blood, which is accomplished by (1) achieving vascular inflow and outflow control prior to parenchymal transaction, (2) performing careful division of the liver with precise control of intrahepatic vascular structures, and (3) using low central venous pressure anesthesia, which reduces hepatic venous blood loss. Clamping of the portal inflow pedicle (Pringle maneuver) for periods of 10–15 minutes is commonly used to minimize blood loss via intrahepatic arterial and portal venous branches, although hepatic venous bleeding is unaffected.

Table 24–1. Child-Pugh Classification of Functional Status in Liver Diseases.

	Class: A Risk: Low	B Moderate	C High
Ascites	Absent	Slight to moderate	Tense
Encephalopathy	None	Grades I–II	Grades III–IV
Serum albumin (g/dL)	> 3.5	3.0–3.5	< 3.0
Serum bilirubin (mg/dL)	< 2.0	2.0–3.0	> 3.0
Prothrombin time (seconds above control)	< 4.0	4.0–6.0	> 6.0

Preoperative Portal Vein Embolization

As discussed previously, preoperative portal vein embolization is a technique that can be used to potentially improve the safety of major hepatic resections. By inducing hypertrophy of the future liver remnant prior to operation, the risk of postoperative liver failure is potentially reduced. The risk of such complications increases significantly with resections that leave behind a liver remnant of less than 25% in patients with normal liver or less than 40% in patients with liver disease.

Postoperative Course

Patients submitted to major resections require close monitoring for the first several postoperative days; however, a prolonged stay in the intensive care unit is unnecessary in most cases. The major concern in the immediate postoperative period is hemorrhage, although in practice, reoperation for bleeding is rarely necessary. Patients without cirrhosis usually exhibit some metabolic changes consistent with mild liver insufficiency, but these quickly normalize, and they are often ready for discharge on the seventh or eighth postoperative day. In the presence of significant hepatic parenchymal disease (ie, cirrhosis, fibrosis, steatosis) or septic complications, postoperative liver function may be significantly impaired.

Many of the postoperative abnormalities can be predicted on the basis of the liver's normal function. The serum bilirubin often increases after major resections but returns to normal as regeneration progresses. A persistent or rising serum bilirubin level should raise concern for a perihepatic fluid collection (biloma) or hepatic failure (especially if other measures of hepatic function are also deteriorating). The serum albumin level usually falls, and the prothrombin time often increases; treatment of the latter with fresh frozen plasma is generally needed only when the international normalized ratio (INR) is markedly elevated (> 2). Some patients may develop ascites, which can be treated with diuresis. Although the liver's glycogen stores are necessarily reduced after a major partial hepatectomy, hypoglycemia is almost never a problem postoperatively; normoglycemia can be easily maintained with 5% dextrose solutions, and profound hypoglycemia should raise concern for pending liver failure. Serum levels of phosphate, magnesium, and potassium often decrease during the first several postoperative days and require replacement. The liver enzymes (aspartate aminotransferase [AST], alanine aminotransferase [ALT]) are usually increased in the first few days after operation and then normalize. By contrast, the alkaline phosphatase is often initially normal and then increases and can remain elevated for several days to weeks after surgery.

Complications

Complications occur in up to 40% of patients after major liver resection (≥ 3 segments), but many are relatively minor, and the overwhelming majority are readily managed and resolve without sequelae. Liver-related complications are the most frequent; perihepatic fluid collections requiring drainage occur in approximately 10–15% of patients. Relative hepatic insufficiency (hyperbilirubinemia, ascites, coagulopathy) is common but resolves in most patients as the liver regenerates; however, hepatic failure is distinctly uncommon in high-volume centers. Pulmonary complications are also seen with some frequency, underscoring the need for aggressive pulmonary toilet postoperatively. The most common pulmonary problems are symptomatic pleural effusions or atelectasis; pneumonia is infrequent. Despite the potential complications associated with major liver resection, mortality rates are low, typically on the order of 1–3% in high-volume centers. Less extensive liver resections (< 3 segments) are associated with even lower morbidity and mortality rates.

Ardito F et al: Laparoscopic liver resection for benign disease. Arch Surg 2007;142:1188.

Belghiti et al: Seven hundred forty-seven hepatectomies in the 1990s: an update to evaluate the actual risk of liver resection. J Am Coll Surg 2000;191:38.

Ettorre GM et al: Postoperative liver function after elective right hepatectomy in elderly patients. Br J Surg 2001;88:73.

Giraudo G et al: Preoperative contralateral protal vein embolization before major hepatic resection is a safe and efficient procedure: a large single institution experience. Surgery 2009;143:476.

Jackson PG et al: Predictors of outcome in 100 consecutive laparoscopic antireflux procedures. Am J Surg 2001;181:231.

Jarnagin et al: Improvement in perioperative outcome after hepatic resection: analysis of 1803 cases over the past decade. Ann Surg 2002;236:397.

Kinoshita H et al: Preoperative portal vein embolization for hepatocellular carcinoma. World J Surg 1986;10:803

Nagino M et al: Liver regeneration after major hepatectomy for biliary cancer. Br J Surg 2001;88:1084.

Nuzzo G et al: Liver resections with or without pedicle clamping. Am J Surg 2001;181:238.

Papadimitriou JD et al: The impact of new technology on hepatic resection for malignancy. Arch Surg 2001;136:1307.

Strasberg SM: Terminology of liver anatomy and liver resections: coming to grips with hepatic Babel. J Am Coll Surg 1997;184:413.

Takayama T et al: Randomized comparison of ultrasonic vs clamp transection of the liver. Arch Surg 2001;136:922.

Yamashita Y et al: Bile leakage after hepatic resection. Ann Surg 2001;233:45.

DISEASES & DISORDERS OF THE LIVER

HEPATIC TRAUMA

Based on the mechanism of injury, liver trauma is classified as penetrating or blunt. Penetrating wounds, constituting more than half of cases, are typically due to projectiles (such as bullets or shrapnel) or knives. In civilian practice, most of these tend to be clean wounds that are dangerous because of intra-abdominal bleeding but do not result in much devitalization of liver tissue. In contrast, high-velocity projectiles are associated with greater energy that is transferred to the abdominal viscera and can shatter the parenchyma, even if the projectile does not enter the liver directly.

Blunt trauma can be inflicted by a direct blow to the upper abdomen or lower right rib cage or can follow sudden deceleration, as occurs with a fall from a great height. Most often a consequence of automobile accidents, direct blunt trauma tends to produce explosive bursting wounds or linear lacerations of the hepatic surface, often with considerable parenchymal destruction. The stellate, bursting type of injury tends to affect the posterior and superior aspect of the right liver (segments VI, VII, and VIII) because of its relatively vulnerable location, convex surface, fixed position, and concentration of hepatic mass. Damage to the left lobe is much less common than damage to the right. Injuries that involve shearing forces can tear the hepatic veins where they enter the liver substance, producing an exsanguinating retrohepatic injury in an area difficult to surgically expose and repair. The staging system described in Table 24–2 is used to categorize liver injuries and provide a common language in order to allow comparisons of results of treatment between institutions.

The principal surgical goals are to stop bleeding and debride devitalized liver. Because some degree of liver failure is common postoperatively, efforts should be made during each step to maintain adequate oxygenation and perfusion of the liver. Also, when one is debriding liver tissue, care should be taken to avoid injury to the vascular supply of adjacent viable parenchyma.

▶ Clinical Findings

A. Symptoms and Signs

The clinical manifestations of liver injury are those of hypovolemic shock: hypotension, decreased urinary output, low central venous pressure, and, in some cases, abdominal distention.

B. Laboratory Findings

With major injuries, particularly those associated with disruption of hepatic veins, the rate of blood loss is usually so rapid that anemia does not develop. Leukocytosis greater than 15,000/μL is common following rupture of the liver from blunt trauma.

C. Imaging Techniques

CT scans should be obtained in most stable patients suspected of having a hepatic injury. The scans demonstrate the extent of the injury and provide a rough estimate of the amount of blood loss. The findings are useful for triaging, since minor injuries rarely require surgical treatment, whereas extensive injuries usually do. One must exercise caution, however, in using CT estimates of injury grade,

Table 24–2. Liver Injury Scale.[1]

Grade	Type	Description
I	Hematoma	Subcapsular, nonexpanding, < 10% surface area.
	Laceration	Capsular tear, nonbleeding; < 1 cm deep in parenchyma.
II	Hematoma	Subcapsular, nonexpanding, 10–50% surface area; intraparenchymal, nonexpanding, < 2 cm in diameter.
	Laceration	Capsular tear, active bleeding; 1–3 cm deep into the parenchyma, < 10 cm long.
III	Hematoma	Subcapsular, > 50% surface area or expanding; ruptured subcapsular hematoma with active bleeding; intraparenchymal hematoma > 2 cm or expanding.
	Laceration	> 3 cm deep into the parenchyma.
IV	Hematoma	Ruptured intraparenchymal hematoma with active bleeding.
	Laceration	Parenchymal disruption involving > 50% of hepatic lobe.
V	Laceration	Parenchymal disruption involving > 50% of hepatic lobe.
	Vascular	Juxtahepatic venous injuries; ie, retrohepatic vena cava or major hepatic veins.
VI	Vascular	Hepatic avulsion.

[1]Increase by one grade when there are two or more injuries to the liver. Grading applied based on best available evidence, whether from x-rays, operative findings, or autopsy findings.

because they correlate poorly (ie, they both understage and overstage) with what is found at surgery. CT scanning is also useful for identifying injuries to other organs, which are not uncommon, particularly in the setting of blunt trauma.

Sonography has not been helpful other than as the rapid abdominal sonogram to identify fluid in the abdomen. It does not help to define the injury. Angiography is generally not helpful in the acute setting but may be used to diagnose and treat specific postinjury problems, such as hemobilia.

▶ Treatment

Patients with stable minor liver injuries (and no associated injuries requiring exploration) may be managed expectantly unless symptoms or signs of bleeding appear. The CT findings in patients who may be considered for nonoperative management include contained subcapsular or intrahepatic hematoma, unilobar fracture, absence of devitalized liver, minimal intraperitoneal blood, and absence of injuries to other intra-abdominal organs. Serial CT scans should be obtained to verify that the lesion is stable rather than expanding.

Most patients have CT or clinical evidence of active bleeding or a major injury, however, and require prompt exploration. Most lacerations have stopped bleeding by the time operation is performed. In the absence of active hemorrhage, these wounds need not be sutured. Active bleeding should be managed by clipping or direct suture of identifiable vessels, if possible, rather than by mass ligatures. Subcapsular hematomas often overlie an active bleeding site or parenchyma in need of debridement and should be explored even though the injury appears to be tamponaded and of limited severity. Blunt injuries associated with substantial amounts of parenchymal destruction may be particularly difficult to manage. Rarely, a very severe pulverizing injury requires formal lobectomy.

Temporary occlusion of the hepatic artery and portal vein can be done quickly by placing a vascular clamp around the entire hepatoduodenal ligament (Pringle maneuver). This can be done for periods of 15–20 minutes and reduce the hemorrhage sufficiently to permit more accurate ligation of bleeding vessels. With major hepatic venous injuries, however, a Pringle maneuver has little effect, and precise repair of the injury may not be possible. Absorbable gauze mesh (eg, polyglycolic acid) can sometimes be wrapped around an injured lobe and sutured in a way that maintains pressure and tamponades the bleeding; this is difficult to accomplish without rendering the involved liver ischemic, however, and such an approach is rarely applicable. In some cases, control of arterial hemorrhage requires ligation of the hepatic artery or one of the accessible lobar branches in the hilum.

The most difficult problems involve lacerations of the major hepatic veins behind the liver. With such injuries, temporary clamping of the inflow vessels will not slow the bleeding to allow inspection and repair of the injured vessels. For persistent bleeding, the abdominal incision can be extended into a median sternotomy to improve exposure. An ancillary technique, which is used only rarely, is to place a tube through the atrial appendage into the inferior vena cava past the origin of the hepatic veins. Appropriately placed ligatures around the vena cava permit total isolation of the liver circulation without interrupting venous return from the lower extremities to the heart. Resection of the right liver improves exposure of the retrohepatic vena cava but is a difficult to perform in the face of overwhelming hemorrhage.

In many cases, when bleeding is difficult to control and especially when other injuries must be addressed, the best strategy is to pack the liver to achieve hemostasis. The packs are generally left in place for 48–72 hours, during which time the patient remains sedated and intubated in the intensive care unit where adequate resuscitative measures are undertaken. The packs are removed in the operating room; if persistent bleeding is noted, definitive repair of the injury can then be performed.

The majority of patients who come to operation require little in the way of surgical intervention to control bleeding; drainage of substantial liver lacerations and other injuries is reasonable, since bile leakage can occur. Suture ligation of bleeding hepatic vessels and debridement of devitalized tissue are indicated in about 30% and 10% of cases, respectively. More extensive procedures are indicated even less often.

Penetrating injuries that also involve the small bowel or colon may result in contamination of perihepatic fluid or devitalized liver tissue, leading to a subhepatic abscess. Placement of drains may help prevent this problem, but a high index of suspicion should be maintained.

► Postoperative Complications

With present techniques, hemorrhage at laparotomy is rarely uncontrollable except with retrohepatic venous injuries. Patients who rebled from the liver wound after initial suture ligation should be treated by reexploration or packing; rarely is a major resection required. Angiography and CT scanning may provide useful diagnostic information preoperatively in such patients. Subhepatic sepsis develops in about 20% of cases; it is more frequent if lobectomy has been done.

Hemobilia may be responsible for gastrointestinal bleeding in the postoperative period and can be diagnosed by selective angiography. Treatment consists of embolization through the arteriography catheter.

► Prognosis

The death rate of 10–15% following hepatic trauma depends largely on the type of injury and the extent of associated injury to other organs. About one third of patients admitted to the emergency department in shock cannot be saved. Only 1% of penetrating civilian wounds are lethal, whereas a 20% death rate attends blunt trauma. The death rate in blunt hepatic injury is 10% when only the liver is injured. If three major organs are damaged, the death rate is close to 70%. Bleeding causes more than half of deaths associated with liver trauma.

Carrillo EH et al: Non-operative management of blunt hepatic trauma. Br J Surg 1998;85:461.

Chen RJ et al: Factors determining operative mortality of grade V blunt hepatic trauma. J Trauma 2000;49:886.

David Richardson J et al: Evolution in the management of hepatic trauma: a 25-year perspective. Ann Surg 2000;232:324.

Leone RJ Jr, Hammond JS: Nonoperative management of pediatric blunt hepatic trauma. Am Surg 2001;67:138.

Oniscu GC, Parks RW, Garden OJ: Classification of liver and pancreatic trauma. HPB 2006;8:4.

Pryor JP, Stafford PW, Nance ML: Severe blunt hepatic trauma in children. J Pediatr Surg 2001;36:974.

Yanar H et al: Nonoperative treatment of multiple intra-abdominal solid organ injury after blunt abdominal trauma. J Trauma 2008;64:943.

SPONTANEOUS HEPATIC RUPTURE

Spontaneous rupture of the liver is not common. Many cases of ruptured normal liver occur during or after pregnancy and are related to preeclampsia-eclampsia and/or HELLP syndrome (hemolysis, elevated liver enzymes, low platelet count). Most cases of ruptured diseased liver are due to hepatic tumors (hepatocellular carcinoma or hepatic adenoma). Hepatic rupture should be suspected in any pregnant or postpartum patient (especially if hypertensive) who complains of acute discomfort in the upper abdomen. Spontaneous rupture has also been reported in association with a number of other conditions, including hepatic hemangioma, typhoid fever, malaria, tuberculosis, syphilis, polyarteritis nodosa, and diabetes mellitus. The diagnosis is best made by CT scanning. Rupture of the liver in the newborn is related to birth trauma in larger infants after difficult deliveries. The typical progression is intrahepatic hemorrhage expanding to subcapsular hematoma and eventually capsular rupture and free intra-abdominal hemorrhage.

Angiography and hepatic artery embolization can be quite effective for controlling hemorrhage in the setting of spontaneous rupture. Emergency laparotomy and intraoperative management (as one would for a traumatic liver injury) are reserved for those who fail hepatic artery embolization or are unsuitable for the procedure. Patients who experience hemoperitoneum from spontaneous rupture of hepatocellular carcinoma appear to be at increased risk for peritoneal dissemination of tumor.

Lai EC, Lau WY: Spontaneous rupture of hepatocellular carcinoma: a systematic review. Arch Surg 2006;141:191.

Risseeuw JJ et al: Liver rupture postpartum associated with preeclampsia and HELLP syndrome. J Matern Fetal Med 1999;8:32.

Stoot JH et al: Life-saving therapy for haemorrhaging liver adenomas using selective arterial embolization. Br J Surg 2007;94:1249.

Sutton BC et al: Fatal postpartum spontaneous liver rupture: case report and literature review. J Forensic Sci 2008;53:472.

PRIMARY LIVER CANCER

Liver malignancy may arise from hepatocytes (hepatocellular carcinoma, the most common) or biliary epithelial cells (intrahepatic cholangiocarcinoma). Tumors arising from both cell types (mixed hepatocellular carcinoma/cholangiocarcinoma) have also been described. Neonates may also develop a variant of hepatocellular carcinoma called hepatoblastoma because it is morphologically similar to fetal liver and the occasional presence of hematopoiesis. Primary malignancy arising from other liver cell types (endothelial cells, stellate cells, neuroendocrine cells, or lymphocytes) is exceedingly rare.

Primary hepatic cancer is relatively uncommon in the United States, but its incidence is increasing. In Asia and Africa, however, primary liver cancer is extremely common and in some areas represents the single-most frequent abdominal tumor and the most common cause of cancer-related death. The etiologic factors in these high-risk areas are environmental or cultural, since persons of similar racial background in the United States are at only slightly greater risk than Caucasians. About 9000 cases—distributed equally between men and women—occur in the United States each

year. Most arise in persons over age 50, but a few are found in children, mainly under 2 years of age.

Chronic hepatitis B and C virus (HBV and HCV) infection is the principal etiologic factor worldwide for hepatocellular carcinoma. Patients chronically seropositive for HBsAg constitute a high-risk group for development of hepatocellular carcinoma, which in some cases may be detected early by screening for serum α-fetoprotein (AFP) levels. Hepatitis B virus DNA has been detected integrated into the genome of host hepatocytes and hepatoma cells and has a direct oncogenic effect. Patients with chronic hepatitis B infection may therefore develop hepatocellular carcinoma in the absence of cirrhosis; by contrast, hepatocellular carcinoma arising in the setting of chronic hepatitis C infection is typically associated with cirrhotic change. Cirrhosis from almost any cause (eg, alcoholism, hemochromatosis, α_1-antitrypsin deficiency, or primary biliary cirrhosis) is associated with an increased risk of hepatocellular carcinoma, and the great majority of these tumors arise in the setting of chronic underlying liver disease. Certain fungal metabolites called aflatoxins have been shown experimentally to be capable of producing liver tumors. These substances are present in staple foods (eg, ground nuts and grain) in some parts of Africa where hepatomas are common.

Unlike hepatocellular carcinoma, intrahepatic cholangiocarcinoma is infrequently associated with cirrhosis. Primary sclerosing cholangitis is a predisposing condition in a small minority of patients. Widespread infection with liver flukes (*Clonorchis sinensis*) is at least partly responsible for the higher incidence of these tumors in some parts of Asia. Emerging evidence has implicated chronic hepatitis C infection, obesity, diabetes mellitus, chronic liver disease, and cigarette smoking as risk factors for intrahepatic cholangiocarcinoma. In Western centers, the vast majority of intrahepatic cholangiocarcinomas are sporadic. Intrahepatic cholangiocarcinoma generally presents as a large mass within the liver and is therefore clinically distinct from cholangiocarcinoma arising from the extrahepatic biliary tree.

Hepatomas constitute about 85–95% of primary hepatic cancers. Previously, differences in morphology were used to separate tumors into three types: **mass-forming** type, characterized by a single predominant mass clearly demarcated from the surrounding liver, occasionally with small satellite nodules; **nodular** type, composed of multiple nodules, often distributed throughout the liver; and a **diffuse** type, characterized by infiltration of tumor throughout the remaining parenchyma. A number of staging systems for hepatocellular carcinoma are in current use: American Joint Commission on Cancer tumor node-metastasis (TNM) staging system, Okuda, and Cancer of the Liver Italian Program (CLIP); none fully accounts for extent of disease and underlying hepatic parenchymal function, which is an important predictor of outcome.

About 50% of resectable tumors are surrounded by a fibrous capsule, which develops as a result of compression of adjacent liver stroma. Encapsulated tumors exhibit a lower incidence of tumor microsatellites and venous permeation compared with nonencapsulated tumors, and the finding is a favorable sign. An uncommon variant, **fibrolamellar hepatocellular carcinoma,** contains numerous fibrous septa and may resemble focal nodular hyperplasia. Fibrolamellar hepatoma occurs in a younger age group (average 25 years) and is not associated with cirrhosis or hepatitis B virus infection.

A large proportion of patients will have intrahepatic or extrahepatic metastases at presentation. Multiple intrahepatic tumors can arise as a result of infiltration of the portal venous system with subsequent dissemination of tumor cells. Vascular invasion is more common with larger tumors (> 5 cm). The extrahepatic sites most commonly involved with metastatic disease include the hilar and celiac lymph nodes and the lungs; metastases to bone and brain are less common, and peritoneal disease (ie, carcinomatosis) is distinctly unusual. Major portal or hepatic veins are often invaded by tumor, and venous occlusion may occur as a result.

Microscopically, there is usually little stroma between the malignant cells, and the tumor has a soft consistency. The tumor may be highly vascularized, a feature that rarely can result in massive intraperitoneal hemorrhage following spontaneous rupture.

Cholangiocarcinoma makes up a small fraction of primary liver cancers, although several reports have documented a marked increase in incidence worldwide. Histologically, these tumors are most often invasive adenocarcinomas, although rare variants have been reported. Intrahepatic or extrahepatic spread of disease is not uncommon by the time the tumor is detected. These tumors infrequently cause symptoms at early stages and therefore often grow to a large size before they become apparent, frequently because of pain. Infrequently, these tumors may contain cells of both cholangiocellular and hepatocellular origin. These mixed tumors are similar to intrahepatic cholangiocarcinoma in that they are infrequently associated with chronic liver disease.

Angiosarcoma of the liver, a rare fatal tumor, has been seen in workers intensively exposed to vinyl chloride for prolonged periods in polymerization plants.

▶ Clinical Findings

A. Symptoms and Signs

The diagnosis at early and more treatable stages is often difficult, since symptoms are often absent. Screening and surveillance of high-risk patients (with cirrhosis, chronic hepatitis, etc) is helpful in this regard. Patients with more advanced tumors may have epigastric or right upper quadrant pain, which may be associated with referred pain in the right shoulder. Weight loss may be present. Jaundice is rare in patients with small tumors and good liver function; the presence of jaundice suggests either very advanced cancer or deteriorating liver function or both.

Hepatomegaly or a mass is palpable in many patients. An arterial bruit or a friction rub may be audible over the liver. Intermittent fever may be a presenting feature. Ascites or gastrointestinal bleeding from varices indicates advanced disease, and ascites fluid with blood should always suggest hepatoma. An acute deterioration in a previously well-compensated cirrhotic patient should also raise the suspicion of hepatocellular carcinoma.

The patterns of presentation can thus be extremely variable and may include (1) pain with or without hepatomegaly; (2) sudden deterioration of the condition of a cirrhotic patient with the onset of hepatic failure, bleeding varices, or ascites; (3) sudden, massive intraperitoneal hemorrhage; (4) acute illness with fever and abdominal pain; (5) symptoms related to distant metastases; and (6) no clinical findings or symptoms.

B. Laboratory Findings

Depending on the disease extent and underlying hepatic function, laboratory values may range from entirely normal to suggestive of impending liver failure. Serum transaminase levels (AST and ALT) and alkaline phosphatase may be increased but are nonspecific and often seen in patients with chronic liver disease without hepatocellular carcinoma. The presence of a moderate to large liver tumor may bring about an increase in the serum alkaline phosphatase in the absence of underlying liver disease. An elevated serum bilirubin is a more ominous finding and reflects some degree of liver dysfunction, either from the underlying chronic liver disease or from a large volume of cancer within the liver. Tumor extension within the portal venous system is not uncommon, and involvement of the right and left portal trunks or the main portal vein may result in jaundice due to compromised portal venous inflow. Less often, jaundice is the result of tumor involvement of the biliary confluence by direct compression or by intrabiliary tumor extension. Other signs of compromised hepatic function include hypoalbuminemia, coagulopathy, and thrombocytopenia. A large number of patients will be positive for HBsAg or HCV antibody; the proportions of each will vary somewhat by geography.

C. Liver Scan

CT scans, ultrasound scans, and MRI scans demonstrate the principal lesion in nearly all patients. MRI scans with MR angiography or CT angiography may provide more detail regarding vascular involvement. A triple-phase, contrast-enhanced helical CT scan generally provides the best images of disease extent within the liver and will also assess for extrahepatic spread.

D. Angiography

Diagnostic angiography was previously used often to assess liver tumors but is now rarely needed for this purpose; it is reserved primarily for treatment (ie, chemoembolization). Hepatomas are supplied primarily by the hepatic artery, and the vast majority are more vascular than adjacent paren-chyma (hypervascular). In some cases, the center of the tumor has become necrotic, and only the peripheral areas are hypervascular. Arterial branches supplying the tumor have an irregular appearance compared to the native hepatic artery, and arterial-venous shunting may be seen. By con-trast, cholangiocarcinomas usually appear less vascular than adjacent tissue. Hemangiomas have a distinctive pattern of peripheral nodular enhancement and patchy vascular pool-ing. Other benign tumors, particularly adenomas and focal nodular hyperplasia, are more difficult to diagnose based on angiographic features alone.

The venous phase of a superior mesenteric arterial injection may show invasion or occlusion of the portal vein by tumor.

Angiography may be equivocal in small tumors, which may be demonstrated with greater certainty by a selective injection of iodized oil (Lipiodol) followed 1–2 weeks later by CT scanning. In a normal liver, the contrast medium is cleared quickly but hepatomas retain it and remain opacified.

E. Liver Biopsy

The diagnosis can be established by percutaneous core biopsy or aspiration biopsy. Fine-needle aspiration biopsy is associated with an approximately 30% false-negative rate. A negative result therefore does not rule out malignant disease, and a core biopsy should be pursued if the index of suspicion is high. Percutaneous biopsy carries some risk of bleeding, although this is rare in experienced hands; tumor dissemina-tion resulting from a biopsy has been reported but is uncom-mon. In patients with cirrhosis, the presence of a hypervas cular mass larger than 2 cm on two different imaging studies (ultrasound, CT, MRI, or angiography) or a hypervascular mass larger than 2 cm on one imaging study combined with a serum AFP level higher than 400 ng/mL is diagnostic of hepatocellular carcinoma, and a biopsy is generally not required.

F. Surveillance

In high-risk patients, surveillance with periodic imaging studies is recommended in order to detect early hepatocellu-lar carcinoma, which is more amenable to treatment. The optimal type and timing of imaging studies is the subject of debate, but such programs have proved useful in areas with a high incidence of chronic hepatitis, such as Asia, where a large proportion of patients are now identified with a mass 2 cm in diameter or smaller; other studies in high-risk patients have also proved valuable.

G. Tumor Markers

AFP, a glycoprotein normally present only in the fetal circu-lation, is present in high concentrations in the serum of many patients with primary hepatomas and testicular tumors. Increased levels are rarely seen as a product of other tumor types, such as the lung, stomach, pancreas, and biliary tree.

The upper limit of normal in the serum is 20 ng/mL; values above 200 ng/mL are suggestive of hepatoma, while levels above 400 ng/mL in a cirrhotic patients with a hyper-vascular liver mass larger than 2 cm in diameter are diagnos-tic. Levels in the intermediate range are nonspecific and may occur with benign liver diseases, such as cirrhosis and chronic hepatitis, where they represent a manifestation of liver cell proliferation. As imaging methods have improved, the diagnosis of liver cancer is being made earlier, when AFP levels may be normal or only minimally elevated. Addition-ally, some patients may have normal AFP levels despite the presence of advanced disease. In general, AFP levels correlate with tumor size and vascular invasion, and a number of studies have shown a correlation between high AFP levels and recurrent cancer after resection. AFP levels can also provide a measure of tumor response in patients treated nonoperatively.

Differential Diagnosis

The clinical picture is often nonspecific, and the presenting symptoms may provide little in the way of diagnostic clues. Primary liver cancer may initially be confused with meta-static cancer arising from other abdominal sites. The pres-ence of cirrhosis and findings consistent with chronic liver disease make hepatocellular carcinoma the leading diagnosis, and this is often confirmed with further testing. In patients without cirrhosis or normal AFP levels (or both), a hypervas-cular mass in the liver should raise other diagnostic consid-erations, such as hepatic adenoma, which can be difficult to distinguish from hepatocellular carcinoma on the basis of imaging alone. In addition, certain types of cancer may give rise to hypervascular liver metastases, including melanoma, neuroendocrine carcinoma, and renal cell carcinoma.

When complications develop suddenly in a cirrhotic patient, the possibility of hepatoma must always be consid-ered. In rare instances, primary hepatocellular cancer is associated with metabolic or endocrine abnormalities such as erythrocytosis, hypercalcemia, hypoglycemic attacks, Cushing syndrome, or virilization.

Complications

Sudden intra-abdominal hemorrhage may occur from spon-taneous bleeding. Obstruction of the portal vein may pro-duce portal hypertension, and obstruction of the hepatic veins may produce the Budd-Chiari syndrome. Liver failure is a common cause of death in these situations.

Treatment
A. Partial Hepatectomy

Resection is the most effective therapy and is the treatment of choice in selected patients without cirrhosis or in cirrhotics with well-preserved hepatic function. Initial diagnostic lap-aroscopy, immediately prior to planned laparotomy, may identify previously undetected spread of tumor within the liver or abdominal cavity that would preclude resection; however, with better imaging, the yield of laparoscopy has decreased. The minimal criteria of resectability that must be met are (1) disease confined to the liver and (2) disease amenable to a complete resection. Multiple tumors in the liver and tumor invasion into major portal or hepatic veins are bad prognostic findings, even if resection is technically feasible; such patients generally are not good candidates for resection. For small and peripherally placed lesions, particularly in cirrhotics, sublobar, segmental resections are preferred if technically feasible. Anatomical segmentectomies are preferred to nonanatomical resections. Larger or more central tumors will require more extensive resections. In Western centers, about 25–30% of patients with hepatocellular carcinoma prove to be candidates for resection; this proportion is over 60% in Japan due largely to widespread surveillance programs.

If gross tumor is left behind or if the margins of resection are involved microscopically, progressive disease is the rule. After a complete resection, the prognosis is best for patients with a solitary, small, and asymptomatic tumor and well-preserved hepatic function. Several adverse predictors of outcome have been identified, which vary somewhat among studies. However, the presence of vascular invasion (even if microscopic) has been identified in nearly all studies to predict recurrent cancer and poor outcome. Large tumor size (> 5 cm), the presence of satellite tumors, and markedly elevated AFP (> 2000 ng/mL) are also associated with a worse outcome, in part because of their correlation with vascular invasion. Additionally, patients with coexistent hepatocellular disease (ie, cirrhosis) tend to do worse, and this is especially true in the face of significant hepatocellular dysfunction or portal hypertension.

In general, cirrhosis constitutes the major obstacle to resection in patients with hepatocellular carcinoma. Careful patient selection (Child-Pugh A, no portal hypertension) is critical in order to avoid acute liver failure. In addition to this immediate perioperative concern, cirrhotic patients have a late risk of death from progression of the underlying liver disease (bleeding esophageal varices or liver failure) and a high rate (> 75%) of new tumors developing in the residual liver. For these reasons, highly selected patients may be better treated with liver transplantation rather than resection.

Overall, the rate of tumor recurrence is approximately 70% at 5 years (although it is higher, as mentioned above, in patients with cirrhosis). Some patients may be candidates for repeat resection or ablative procedures. The 5-year survival rate is approximately 40% but is lower for patients with cirrhosis.

After surgery, patients should be followed by periodic physical examinations and blood work to assess liver function. Imaging studies and AFP measurements (if elevated before resection) at regular intervals may help identify early, localized recurrences that may be amenable to repeat resection or palliative therapy.

B. Liver Transplantation

Hepatocellular carcinoma is the only solid neoplasm for which transplantation plays a significant role. Liver transplantation has the advantage of treating not only the malignant disease but also the underlying cirrhosis. Previously, the selection criteria for transplanting hepatoma patients were broad and included patients with very advanced disease. Consequently, 5-year survival rates were less than 40%, too low to justify use of a scarce resource. The lessons learned from this early experience have allowed identification of patients most likely to benefit, specifically those with a single tumor no larger than 5 cm in diameter or up to three tumors with none exceeding 3 cm in diameter and no major vascular invasion. Using these strict criteria (the Milan criteria), 5-year survival rates of 70% can be achieved. It should be emphasized that the benefit of transplantation is realized only when the waiting time for a new graft is under 6 months. Since waiting times can exceed 12 months in many centers, up to 50% of patients will develop cancer progression or otherwise become ineligible. This problem has led a number of centers to adopt living donor transplantation as a means of increasing the donor pool, an approach that remains controversial because of donor-related morbidity and mortality.

A major concern of transplantation in cancer patients has been that the immunosuppressive therapy required to support the graft would remove an important defense mechanism against progression of residual microscopic disease. Indeed, calculated tumor doubling times for lesions in transplanted patients have been shown to be greater compared to patients not on immunosuppressive agents. Despite this possibility and although the logistical problems and expense are enormous, transplantation is a reasonable option in patients with cirrhosis who are not candidates for resection and have limited malignant disease, as specified in the selection criteria.

At present, transplantation has no role in patients with intrahepatic cholangiocarcinoma outside of controlled clinical trials, since the results to date have been poor.

C. Ethanol Injection

Percutaneous ablative techniques are a reasonable option in patients with small, unresectable hepatocellular carcinoma, of which ethanol injection is the cheapest, easiest, and least morbid. Using ultrasound or CT guidance, 95% ethanol (5–20 mL) is injected through a 22-gauge needle directly into the tumor. This approach can achieve complete necrosis in 90–100% of tumors small than 2 cm, but its efficacy declines rapidly as the tumor size increases. The patient is followed up and retreatment given for residual or new primary tumors. In one multi-institutional series from Italy, survival 1, 2, and 3 years after treatment for patients with solitary, small tumors was 90%, 80%, and 63%, respectively.

D. Radiofrequency Ablation

Radiofrequency ablation (RFA) is another percutaneous ablative approach, useful for treating selected patients with unresectable, small tumors. RFA has generally supplanted ethanol injection as the percutaneous treatment of choice. Under ultrasound or CT guidance, a needle is used to access the lesion; the needle is attached to a radiofrequency generator that generates thermal energy to bring about tumor destruction. RFA can be used percutaneously, laparoscopically, or at laparotomy.

The goal of RFA is the same at that of ethanol injection: to achieve complete tumor necrosis. The efficacy of RFA is limited by tumor size but may be somewhat greater than ethanol injection in this regard; RFA is less effective for tumors adjacent to major vascular structures. A randomized study comparing the two techniques found no differences in survival, although RFA may offer better local tumor control rates. In carefully selected patients, 5-year survival rates of 30–40% have been reported.

E. Arterial Embolization

Hepatic artery embolization is another ablative technique that is more broadly applicable than RFA or ethanol injection. This approach takes advantage of the fact that primary liver cancers derive disproportionately greater blood supply from the hepatic arterial circulation compared to the surrounding liver. The strategy is to combine selective hepatic arterial injection of cancer chemotherapeutic agents with arterial embolization, the latter to produce tumor necrosis and slow the washout of the drugs. Embolization can be used in patients with much larger tumors than can be effectively treated with percutaneous procedures, and the procedure can be staged to treat bilobar disease. Patients must have adequate liver function; those with Child-Pugh C cirrhosis or thrombosis of the portal vein are not suitable candidates.

A variety of techniques have been used. Embolization is often performed with Gelfoam, which dissolves after a few weeks, but other inert agents are also used. Doxorubicin, mitomycin, and cisplatin in various combinations are the drugs most often given. Lipiodol, which lodges in the tumor, has occasionally been used as a carrier for the drugs. It remains unclear if the addition of chemotherapeutic agents provides much benefit beyond the necrosis produced by occlusion of the hepatic arterial supply. Many patients require multiple treatments, although the optimal schedule is ill defined. Embolization achieves partial responses in up to 55% of patients. The best 3-year survival rates are approximately 50%. Histologic studies of tumors resected shortly after treatment reveal viable neoplastic cells in the tumor capsule, which receives blood from the portal vein as well as the hepatic artery.

A recent randomized prospective trial showed that the combination of RFA and chemoembolization provides superior disease control rates than either technique alone.

Bergsland EK, Venook AP: Hepatocellular carcinoma. Curr Opin Oncol 2000;12:357.

Cheng BQ et al: Chemoembolization combined with radiofrequency ablation for patients with hepatocellular carcinoma larger than 3 cm: a randomized controlled trial. JAMA 2008;299:1669.

Endo I et al: Intrahepatic cholangiocarcinoma: rising frequency, improved survival, and determinants of survival after resection. Ann Surg 2008;247:994

Fong Y et al: Hepatocellular Carcinoma: An analysis of 412 HCC at a Western center. Ann Surg 1999;229:790.

Grasso A et al: Radiofrequency ablation in the treatment of hepatocellular carcinoma—a clinical viewpoint. J Hepatol 2000;33:667.

Krinsky GA, Lee VS, Theise ND: Focal lesions in the cirrhotic liver: high resolution ex vivo MRI with pathologic correlation. J Comput Assist Tomogr 2000;24:189.

Llovet JM et al: Hepatocellular carcinoma. Lancet 2003;362:1907.

Mazzaferro V et al: Liver transplantation for the treatment of small hepatocellular carcinomas in patients with cirrhosis. N Engl J Med 1996;334:693.

Mor E et al: Treatment of hepatocellular carcinoma associated with cirrhosis in the era of liver transplantation. Ann Intern Med 1998;129:643.

Patel T: Increasing incidence and mortality of primary intrahepatic cholangiocarcinoma in the United States. Hepatology. 2001;33:1353.

Trevisani F et al: Randomized control trials on chemoembolization for hepatocellular carcinoma: is there room for new studies? J Clin Gastroenterol 2001;32:383.

Tung-Ping Poon R, Fan ST, Wong J: Risk factors, prevention, and management of postoperative recurrence after resection of hepatocellular carcinoma. Ann Surg 2000;232:10.

Weber SM et al: Intrahepatic cholangiocarcinoma: resectability, recurrence pattern and outcome. J Am Coll Surg 2001:193;384.

Welzel TM et al: Risk factors for intrahepatic and extrahepatic cholangiocarcinoma in the United States: a population-based case-control study. Clin Gastroenterol Hepatol 2007;5:1221.

METASTATIC NEOPLASMS OF THE LIVER

In Western countries, metastatic cancer is much more common than primary tumors in the liver. Nearly all solid tumors can potentially give rise to liver metastases; primary cancers of the gastrointestinal tract (colon, pancreas, esophagus, stomach, neuroendocrine), breast, lung, genitourinary system (kidney, adrenal), ovary and uterus, melanoma, and sarcomas account for the overwhelming majority of cases. Spread to the liver may be via the systemic or portal venous circulation. The cirrhotic liver, which often gives rise to primary hepatic tumors, seems to be less susceptible than normal liver to implantation of metastases.

Individual tumor types have characteristic patterns of spread. For example, colorectal cancer spreads to the liver as the first site of metastatic disease in a very high proportion of patients; the lung is the next most common site, but bone, brain, or adrenal metastases are distinctly unusual. By contrast, metastatic lung cancer to the liver typically occurs concomitantly with spread to other sites, with brain, bone, and adrenal among the most common. In general, the vast majority of patients with metastases to the liver also have disease at other sites. A notable exception is colorectal cancer, which in many cases involves the liver only for a prolonged period. In the past, approximately 20% of patients with hepatic metastases had additional tumor deposits in the liver not seen on preoperative imaging studies. As imaging technology has improved, however, this proportion has become increasingly smaller.

Clinical Findings

A. Symptoms and Signs

The signs and symptoms will vary with the clinical scenario, the disease extent within the liver, and the presence or absence of metastatic disease to other sites. Patients with an undiagnosed primary tumor may come to attention because of symptoms caused by the metastatic disease. Weight loss, fatigue, pain, and anorexia are the presenting general complaints in many such patients. Signs of liver failure, such as ascites and jaundice, are uncommon and suggestive of very advanced cancer. Fever without demonstrable infection is present in 15% of cases. By contrast, patients with a known history of cancer undergoing routine surveillance often develop liver metastases that cause no symptoms; in a small proportion of cases, liver metastases are found on studies done for unrelated reasons.

Physical examination is frequently unrevealing. Hepatomegaly or a palpable tumor in the upper abdomen may be present, and either may be tender. Portal hypertension may be manifested by abdominal venous collaterals or splenomegaly. A friction rub is sometimes heard over the liver.

B. Laboratory Findings

Laboratory values may be entirely normal or at most reflect only minor nonspecific changes. Patients with advanced cancer will have anemia and hypoalbuminemia. The alkaline phosphatase is increased in most patients. More significant derangements in liver function will occur in patients with a large volume of liver disease, although this is uncommon at initial presentation. Tumor marker levels (carcinoembryonic antigen [CEA], cancer antigen [CA] 19-9, CA-125) are often elevated, depending on the tumor type, and may be helpful for monitoring treatment.

The diagnosis can be established in most cases by CT-guided or ultrasound-guided percutaneous liver biopsy or fine-needle aspiration for malignant cells.

C. Imaging Studies

The detection of liver metastases relies on CT and/or MRI scans; ultrasonography will identify tumors in the liver and will distinguish solid from cystic lesions but cannot provide the same degree of anatomical detail. MRI provides useful additional information and may help distinguish benign from malignant disease. However, a high-quality triple phase CT scan with intravenous and oral contrast medium provides excellent assessment of disease extent in the liver and elsewhere in the abdomen. In the past, CT portography was superior to ordinary contrast-enhanced CT and was obtained routinely in patients being considered for hepatic resection, but this is no longer the case. Positron emission tomography using 14-fluorodeoxyglucose (FDG-PET) is a commonly used staging study and may help identify extrahepatic disease, a finding that could change the treatment recommendations. During surgery, intraoperative ultrasound is used to assess the liver for disease not appreciated on imaging studies.

Treatment

For most patients with metastatic liver disease, chemotherapy is the only treatment option, particularly with coexisting metastases outside the liver. Such therapy is usually not curative but rather palliative in most cases. A notable exception is metastatic colorectal cancer, for which resection or other treatments aimed at the liver disease are effective and potentially curative; the recent advent of several active chemotherapeutic agents has further improved the results of treatment. Carefully selected patients with metastases from other primary tumors (sarcoma, breast, ovary, lung, neuroendocrine) may also benefit from resection but represent a small minority of cases.

A. Hepatic Resection

Hepatic resection is most commonly indicated in patients with metastatic colorectal cancer. Of the approximately 130,000 patients diagnosed with colorectal cancer annually in the United States, approximately 50% either have liver metastases at diagnosis or develop liver metastases at some point. In 40% of the latter group, the liver is the only demonstrable site of disease. Hepatic metastases from colorectal cancer thus affect approximately 20,000 patients per year, which is comparable to the annual incidence of pancreatic or esophageal carcinoma.

After a complete resection, the 5-year survival rate has historically been 25–40%; systemic or regional chemotherapy or both are frequently given after resection and appear to enhance the results of surgery, with more recent series reporting 5-year survival figures of approximately 50%. The presence of extrahepatic metastases and inability to achieve a complete resection are contraindications to resection in most cases. However, as more effective chemotherapeutic options have emerged, the indications for resection have expanded to include selected patients with multiple bilobar tumors and even some with extrahepatic metastatic disease. Extensive use of chemotherapy prior to surgery can cause changes in the liver, particularly steatosis and steatohepatitis, which can impair the liver's normal regenerative response. Caution is therefore needed when considering such patients for major hepatic resections, since operative morbidity and mortality may be increased; preoperative portal vein embolization may reduce the incidence of serious postoperative complications.

The following variables are associated with a worse prognosis after resection: (1) original tumor with involved lymph nodes (stage III or Dukes C), (2) multiple liver lesions, (3) less than 1 year since resection of the colon primary (disease-free interval), and (4) CEA level higher than 20 ng/mL. Variables that do not influence the outcome include (1) histologic grade of the tumor, (2) bilateral rather than unilateral disease, (3) site of the primary tumor within the large intestine, and (4) the gender of the patient. The mortality rate for resection of hepatic metastases is 1–2% in hospitals where this operation is performed frequently.

The liver is the most common site of cancer recurrence after a complete resection. A small proportion of patients with hepatic recurrence may be amenable to a second resection. The use of adjuvant hepatic arterial chemotherapy appears to reduce the risk of intrahepatic recurrence.

The efficacy of liver resection for colorectal cancer has been clearly established and is the most common indication for this procedure. By contrast, for most other tumor types, particularly those arising from the gastrointestinal tract other than the colon or rectum, the benefit of liver resection is much more limited. Rare patients with metastases from renal cell carcinoma, ovarian cancer, adrenocortical carcinoma, or sarcomas appear to derive the most benefit; by contrast, liver resection for metastatic esophageal, gastric or pancreatic cancer is almost never warranted. In selecting patients with noncolorectal liver metastases for resection, the most important factors are (1) long disease-free interval, (2) solitary resectable liver tumor, and (3) absence of extrahepatic metastases.

Neuroendocrine carcinomas (pancreatic islet cell tumors, carcinoids) represent a unique class of tumors that often give rise to liver metastases. Unlike patients with other metastatic tumor types, those with neuroendocrine tumors often survive for many years. Multiple liver metastases are the rule with this disease, so complete resection is usually not possible. However, debulking liver resections are sometimes indicated to palliate tumor-related pain or hormonal symptoms. Partial hepatectomy is also sometimes worthwhile to extirpate a tumor invading directly from a contiguous organ.

B. Radiofrequency Ablation

RFA has been used to treat metastases to the liver from a variety of tumor types. The indications for this procedure remain ill defined. The best candidates are those with a limited number of small liver lesions with no evidence of extrahepatic cancer.

C. Chemotherapy

In a large proportion of patients with metastatic colorectal cancer, the liver is the only evident site of disease. If the lesions cannot be resected, regional intrahepatic chemotherapy can be given by placing a catheter in the gastroduodenal artery (at its origin with the common hepatic artery) connected to an implantable, subcutaneous infusion pump, which allows the delivery of much higher concentrations of drug to the tumor than is possible with systemic administration. This regimen is generally not used for metastases from other kinds of tumors. The pump is primed with floxuridine, which is delivered by continuous infusion (0.1–0.2 mg/kg/d) for 14-day periods alternating with 14-day rests. Systemic chemotherapy is usually given concomitantly. The discovery of extrahepatic lesions at laparotomy for pump placement is a relative contraindication to proceeding with this approach. Treatment is continued until disease progression or excessive toxicity is seen or, rarely, until the response is complete. Toxicity consists mainly of gastroduodenal erosions (caused by unintentional perfusion of these areas), chemical hepatitis, or chemical sclerosing cholangitis. Survival is related principally to the initial amount of liver involvement by tumor, objective response to treatment (which is seen in about 60% of patients), and extent of prior chemotherapy. The median survival of patients with less than 30% of liver replaced by tumor is 24 months, compared with 10 months if the extent of replacement exceeds 30%. There is a general perception that hepatic artery infusion therapy improves survival, but the objective evidence is inconclusive. Cure is not a realistic objective.

Hepatic artery infusion chemotherapy may be a useful adjunctive therapy after complete tumor resection or RFA. Studies of this option are under way.

Systemic chemotherapy (eg, with fluorouracil, irinotecan, or oxaliplatin) after liver resection has not been proved to improve survival, although it is often prescribed.

D. Miscellaneous

Hepatic artery ligation or angiographic embolization of the tumor has been of benefit in a few patients with hepatic metastases from specific tumor types, particularly neuroendocrine tumors.

▶ Prognosis

Survival varies with the site of origin of the primary tumor and the extent of metastatic disease. Patients with extensive hepatic replacement by multiple lesions have a dismal outlook, with a survival measured in months, compared to perhaps 2–3 years for patients with small solitary lesions. The range of treatment options and effective chemotherapeutic agents is greatest for metastatic colorectal cancer compared to most other tumor types, and survival is generally better in this group.

Adam et al: Two-stage hepatectomy: a planned strategy to treat irresectable liver tumors. Ann Surg 2000;232:777.

Andres A et al: Improved long-term outcome of surgery for advanced colorectal liver metastases: reasons and implications for management on the basis of a severity score. Ann Surg Onc 2007;15:134.

Cho CS et al: Histologic grade is correlated with outcome after resection of hepatic neuroendocrine neoplasms. Cancer 2008; 113:126.

DeMatteo RP et al: Results of hepatic resection for sarcoma metastatic to liver. Ann Surg 2001;234:540.

Fong et al: Clinical score for predicting recurrence after hepatic resection for metastatic colorectal cancer: analysis of 1001 consecutive cases. Ann Surg 1999;230:309.

Heslin MJ et al: Colorectal hepatic metastases: resection, local ablation, and hepatic artery infusion pump are associated with prolonged survival. Arch Surg 2001;136:318.

Kokudo N et al: Anatomical major resection versus nonanatomical limited resection for liver metastases from colorectal carcinoma. Am J Surg 2001;181:153.

Lambert LA, Colacchio TA, Barth RJ Jr: Interval hepatic resection of colorectal metastases improves patient selection. Arch Surg 2000;135:473.

Nagakura S, Shirai Y, Hatakeyama K: Computed tomographic features of colorectal carcinoma liver metastases predict posthepatectomy patient survival. Dis Colon Rectum 2001; 44:1148.

Nordlinger B et al: Perioperative chemotherapy with FOLFOX4 and surgery versus surgery alone for resectable liver metastases from colon cancer (EORTC Intergroup trial 40983): a randomized controlled trial. Lancet 2008;371:1007.

Primrose JN: Treatment of colorectal metastases: surgery, cryotherapy, or radiofrequency ablation. Gut 2002;50:1.

Strasberg SM et al: Survival of patients evaluated by FDG-PET before hepatic resection for metastatic colorectal carcinoma: a prospective database study. Ann Surg 2001;233:293.

Tomlinson JS et al: Actual 10-year survival after resection of colorectal liver metastases defines cure. J Clin Oncol 2007; 25:4575.

Vauthey JN et al: Chemotherapy regimen predicts steatohepatitis and an increase in 90-day mortality after surgery for hepatic colorectal metastases. J Clin Oncol 2006;24:2065.

Weitz J et al: Partial hepatectomy for metastases from non-colorectal, non-neuroendocrine carcinoma. Ann of Surg 2005;241:269.

BENIGN TUMORS & CYSTS OF THE LIVER*

► Hemangiomas

Hemangioma is the most common benign hepatic tumor, and except for the skin and mucous membranes, the liver is the most common site of origin. Women are affected more often than men—in some series, up to 75% of patients are female. Histologically, hepatic hemangiomata are of the cavernous type rather than the capillary type. Most are small, solitary subcapsular growths that are found incidentally during laparotomy or autopsy or on imaging studies. Rarely, hemangiomata grow to very large dimensions (giant hemangiomata) and cause abdominal pain or a palpable mass. Most are small to moderate-sized lesions, however; pain is uncommon in tumors smaller than 8–10 cm in diameter.

Rare complications of liver hemangiomata include hemorrhagic shock resulting from spontaneous rupture and the Kasabach-Merritt syndrome, which is usually seen in children and is associated with thrombocytopenia and a consumptive coagulopathy; both of these complications are exceedingly uncommon. Large congenital hemangiomas of the liver may be associated with others in the skin. Large hemangiomata may also give rise to large-volume arteriovenous shunting, resulting in cardiac hypertrophy and congestive heart failure.

Large-bore needle biopsy is hazardous due to bleeding risks; aspiration biopsy with a fine needle is safe but rarely helpful. Fortunately, biopsy is very rarely indicated, since the diagnosis can be made with certainty in most cases by contrast-enhanced CT or MRI scans. The hallmark features of hemangiomata are nodular peripheral enhancement with progressive central enhancement on the more delayed images. MRI is a particularly good study for hemangiomata, which appear very bright on the T2-weighted images. Angiography is unnecessary, and nuclear scans lack sufficient sensitivity and specificity.

The only reasons to resect hemangiomata are for symptoms, most commonly pain, or diagnostic uncertainty. Symptomatic hemangiomas should be excised by lobectomy or enucleation. Even large lesions can be safely removed. Radiotherapy or embolization via a catheter in the hepatic artery may be tried in patients who are poor candidates for surgery, but the efficacy of these approaches is limited. The natural history of asymptomatic hemangiomas, whether large or small, is benign. The vast majority of incidentally discovered hemangiomata remain stable in follow-up, do not give rise to symptoms, and therefore do not require resection. Progressive growth of asymptomatic hemangiomata over a relatively short time interval, particularly in young patients, is considered a relative indication for resection.

Bykov S et al: The role of hepatobiliary scintigraphy in the follow-up of benign liver tumors secondary to oral contraceptive use. Clin Nucl Med 2001;26:946.

Charny CK et al: The management of 155 patients with benign liver tumours. Br J Surg 2001;88:1.

Cherqui D et al: Laparoscopic liver resections: a feasibility study in 30 patients. Ann Surg 2000;232:753.

Clarke D et al: Hepatic resection for benign non-cystic liver lesions. HPB 2004;6:115.

Popescu I et al: Liver hemangioma revisited: current surgical indications, technical aspects, results. Hepatogastroenterology 2001;48:770.

Terkivatan T et al: Indications and long-term outcome of treatment for benign hepatic tumors: a critical appraisal. Arch Surg 2001;136:1033.

Van den Bos IC et al: Magnetic resonance imaging of liver lesions: exceptions and atypical lesions. Curr Probl Diagn Radiol 2008;37:95.

► Cysts

A number of different cystic lesions may affect the liver. Simple hepatic cysts, the most common, are unilocular fluid-filled lesions that generally produce no symptoms. The occasional large cyst may present as an upper abdominal

---

*Echinococcal cysts are discussed in Chapter 8.

mass or discomfort. Small, simple cysts may be difficult to diagnose on CT and may be confused for metastatic disease; ultrasound and MRI are better modalities to assess the character of cystic lesions. Many patients have multiple simple cysts, which should not be confused with polycystic liver disease, a progressive condition characterized by cystic replacement of virtually the entire liver. Polycystic liver disease is associated in about half of cases with polycystic renal disease. The possibility of echinococcosis (see Chapter 8) should be considered in patients with cystic liver lesions and the appropriate exposure history, although their radiographic appearance is usually quite distinctive.

Most simple cysts have a serous lining and a smooth, thin wall. Intracystic hemorrhage can occur, which can confuse the radiographic appearance. Solitary cysts lined with cuboidal epithelium are classified as cystadenomas and should be resected, since they are premalignant. Cystadenomas are characterized radiographically as complex, with internal septae, an irregular lining, and papillary projections. Complex, multilocular (septated) cysts (if not echinococcal) are often neoplastic and should be resected. However, cystadenomas and cystadenocarcinomas are rare, while internal hemorrhage into a simple cyst is a more common entity and may have a similar appearance. Nevertheless, complex cysts of the liver must be approached with some caution in order to avoid inappropriate interventions. There are few indications for aspirating hepatic cysts— simple cysts reaccumulate fluid quickly, neoplastic cysts must be excised, and parasitic cysts might rupture and the parasite thus be allowed to spread. It is possible to eliminate small cysts by aspiration of the contents followed by an injection into the lumen of 20–100 mL of absolute alcohol; however, small cysts almost never cause symptoms and generally require no treatment.

Large symptomatic cysts are difficult to eradicate with alcohol injections, and serious superinfection of the cyst cavity may occur. The simplest method of treatment consists of laparoscopic cyst fenestration (wide excision of the cyst wall). A tongue of omentum is fixed so it lies in the residual cyst cavity as an ancillary measure to prevent the edges from coapting. The operation is curative in nearly all patients.

Multiple, small, simple cysts do not usually require treatment, but large polycystic livers that cause discomfort or are associated with obstructive jaundice can be managed by partial resection or surgically unroofing the cysts on the surface of the liver and creating windows between superficial cysts and adjacent deep cysts. The opened cysts are allowed to drain into the abdominal cavity. The results of surgery for polycystic liver disease are often disappointing, with quick return of symptoms in many patients.

Cowles RA, Mulholland MW: Solitary hepatic cysts. J Am Coll Surg 2000;191:311.
Del Poggio P, Buonacore M: Cystic tumors of the liver: a practical approach. World J Gastroenterol 2008;14:3616.

Hansen P, Ludemann R, Swanstrom LL: Minimally invasive approaches to hepatic surgery. Hepatogastroenterology 2001; 48:37.
Inaba Y et al: Focal attenuation differences in pericystic liver tissue as seen on CT hepatic arteriography and CT arterial portography: observation using a unified helical CT and angiography system. Abdom Imaging 1999;24:360.

▶ Hepatic Adenoma

Hepatic adenomas occur predominantly in women and appear to be related to the use of oral contraceptives. Mestranol-containing compounds have been associated with a disproportionate number of cases, but mestranol has been in use longer than the other agents.

The tumors are soft, yellow-tan, well-circumscribed masses that are usually of moderate size (range of 2–15 cm in diameter). Most of those that cause symptoms are in the 8–15-cm range. Two thirds of hepatic adenomas are solitary; other benign tumors (such as focal nodular hyperplasia, see next section) are present in some cases. Transition from benign hepatic adenoma to hepatocellular carcinoma may occur, with liver cell dysplasia as an intermediate step. Histologically, hepatic adenomas consist of an encapsulated homogeneous mass of normal-appearing hepatocytes without bile ducts or central veins. Intratumoral hemorrhage or central necrosis may be present.

About half of patients are asymptomatic. Most of those with symptoms present with right upper quadrant pain. Spontaneous hemorrhage into the substance of the tumor with subsequent rupture and intraperitoneal bleeding is a well-known potential complication of adenomas; patients with this life-threatening problem present with acute pain or even hemorrhagic shock. There is a strong association of acute bleeding episodes with pregnancy.

Liver function tests and AFP levels are usually normal or minimally deranged. Adenomas typically appear hypervascular compared to the surrounding liver parenchyma, a feature that is apparent on contrast-enhanced CT or MRI scans or angiography. Adenomas can be difficult to distinguish from focal nodular hyperplasia, another benign tumor often found in young women. Differences in tumor vascularity may be demonstrated on angiography; however, MRI is probably the best study for differentiating these lesions. Adenomas often cannot be distinguished from well-differentiated hepatocellular carcinoma on imaging studies and even on biopsy specimens. Needle biopsy is generally safe but often inconclusive and is associated with a small risk of bleeding.

The general recommendation is that adenomas should be resected because of the risks of malignant change and spontaneous hemorrhage. Unfortunately, the true likelihood of these events is difficult to estimate, since most series include only treated patients. Symptomatic and large asymptomatic adenomas clearly should be resected. Emergent resection or hepatic artery embolization should be undertaken in patients with evidence of hemorrhage. Small peripheral lesions may be removed with wedge excisions, but larger tumors require more extensive resections. Small adenomas may regress when oral contraceptive agents are discontinued, and close follow-up with imaging studies is not unreasonable in such cases; however, any change in symptoms or imaging characteristics (growth, hemorrhage) should prompt resection. The possibility that a presumed adenoma is actually a well-differentiated hepatocellular carcinoma or contains a focus of malignancy must always be kept in mind; there is no completely reliable means of making the differentiation other than pathologic analysis of the resected specimen.

Most patients recover without sequelae after surgical removal; recurrence is rare. Oral contraceptives should be proscribed permanently in all cases. Radiotherapy and chemotherapy are of no value, but elective hepatic artery embolization may be helpful in patients who are not surgical candidates. Embolization may be particularly helpful in the very rare patient with multiple hepatic adenomas (hepatic adenomatosis), since resection is usually not possible.

▶ Focal Nodular Hyperplasia

Focal nodular hyperplasia is a benign lesion with no malignant potential. Like hepatic adenoma, focal nodular hyperplasia is much more common in young women. The average age is about 40 years, but the tumor can occur at any age. Unlike hepatic adenoma, however, the use of oral contraceptive agents does not appear to predispose to the development of focal nodular hyperplasia, although it has been suggested that these agents may stimulate growth.

Grossly, the tumor is a well-circumscribed, firm, tan, usually subcapsular mass measuring 2–3 cm in diameter. In patients with symptoms, the lesions are much larger, usually around 10 cm. Multiple tumors can occur; 80% are solitary. The gross appearance on cut section is quite characteristic, consisting of a central stellate scar (which is actually an aggregation of blood vessels) with radiating fibrous septa that compartmentalize the lesion into lobules. Histologically, there are nodular aggregations of normal-appearing hepatocytes without central veins or portal triads. Bile duct proliferation is present in the nodules.

Most patients with focal nodular hyperplasia are asymptomatic. The few with symptoms present with a right upper quadrant discomfort. Unlike hepatic adenomas, these lesions rarely, if ever, bleed, and the natural history of asymptomatic lesions is benign. Very rare patients with diffuse focal nodular hyperplasia develop portal hypertension.

Hepatic function tests and AFP levels are usually normal. Hepatic scintiscans usually do not show a filling defect but are of little practical value. CT scans demonstrate the tumor and may also show the central stellate scar. The arteriographic pattern is one of hypervascularity. In most cases, the diagnosis of focal nodular hyperplasia can be made with noninvasive studies, although distinguishing focal nodular hyperplasia from hepatic adenomas can be difficult, even for experienced radiologists. MRI scanning is the best modality, but the imaging features of both tumors overlap somewhat, and they occur in similar patient populations. Fine-needle aspiration biopsies are generally not helpful.

Symptomatic lesions should be removed, while asymptomatic tumors (the majority) should be left undisturbed, provided that the diagnosis has been made confidently. In the latter circumstance, a period of observation with imaging studies is recommended to ensure stability. Inability to distinguish focal nodular hyperplasia from adenoma or malignant disease is an indication for resection in some patients. Discontinuation of oral contraceptives probably has no impact. Focal nodular hyperplasia can be reliably identified on examination of frozen sections.

Bioulac-Sage P, Balabaud C, Wanless IR: Diagnosis of focal nodular hyperplasia: not so easy. Am J Surg Pathol 2001;25:1322.

Bonney GK et al: Indication for treatment and long-term outcome of focal nodular hyperplasia. HPB 2007;9:368.

Cho SW et al: Surgical management of hepatocellular adenoma: take it or leave it. Ann Surg Oncol 2008; in press.

Kim YI, Chung JW, Park JH: Feasibility of transcatheter arterial chemoembolization for hepatic adenoma. J Vasc Interv Radiol 2007;18:862.

Leconte I et al: Focal nodular hyperplasia: natural course observed with CT and MRI. J Comput Assist Tomogr 2000;24:61.

Terkivatan T et al: Indications and long-term outcome of treatment for benign hepatic tumors: a critical appraisal. Arch Surg 2001;136:1033.

Terkivatan T et al: Treatment of ruptured hepatocellular adenoma. Br J Surg 2001;88:207.

PORTAL HYPERTENSION

▶ Etiology

The major causes of portal hypertension are listed in Table 24–3. In all but a few instances, the basic lesion is increased resistance to portal flow. Those associated with increased resistance can be subclassified according to the site of the block as prehepatic, hepatic, and posthepatic; hepatic causes of portal hypertension are further subclassified as presinusoidal, sinusoidal, and postsinusoidal. Cirrhosis accounts for about 85% of cases of portal hypertension in the United States, most commonly from heavy alcohol use. Postnecrotic cirrhosis is next in frequency, followed by biliary cirrhosis. The other intrahepatic causes of portal hypertension are relatively rare in Western countries, although in some parts of the world, hepatic schistosomiasis constitutes the largest single group. Idiopathic portal hypertension occurs with greater frequency in southern Asia.

After cirrhosis, extrahepatic portal venous thrombosis or occlusion is the most common cause of portal hypertension in the United States. Patients with this condition are generally younger than cirrhotics, and many are children. Posthepatic obstruction due to Budd-Chiari syndrome or constrictive pericarditis is rare.

Pathophysiology

Portal hypertension is defined as a portal pressure gradient greater than 5 mm Hg. Since pressure in the portal venous system is determined by the relationship Pressure = Flow × Resistance, portal hypertension could result either from increased volume of portal blood flow or increased resistance to flow. In practice, however, the liver has tremendous reserve capacity to accommodate increased blood flow, and portal hypertension due to this mechanism is extremely uncommon. Nearly all clinically relevant cases result from increased resistance, although the site of the resistance varies in different diseases. A pathophysiologic classification of the causes of portal hypertension is given in Table 24–3.

Portal venous pressure normally ranges from 7 to 10 mm Hg. In portal hypertension, portal pressure exceeds 10 mm Hg, averaging around 20 mm Hg and occasionally rising as high as 50–60 mm Hg.

In alcoholic liver disease, the abnormal resistance is predominantly postsinusoidal, as indicated by the results of wedged hepatic vein pressure studies.*

The causes of increased resistance in this disease are thought to be (1) distortion of the hepatic veins by regenerative nodules and (2) fibrosis of perivascular tissue around the hepatic veins and the sinusoids.

Even in the absence of cirrhosis, acute alcoholic hepatitis can raise portal pressure by producing centrilobular swelling and fibrosis. Sinusoidal resistance to flow is also increased by engorgement of adjacent hepatocytes with fat and resultant distortion and narrowing of vascular channels. Documented cases of normalization or reduction in portal pressure have occurred with resolution of the pathologic changes.

Schistosomiasis can produce a unique form of presinusoidal obstruction to blood flow from deposition of parasite ova in small portal venules. The subsequent chronic inflammatory reaction leads to fibrosis and cirrhosis. Many patients with schistosomiasis are also at risk for chronic hepatitis, which can exacerbate the liver damage.

Fluctuations in the level of portal hypertension may occur in conjunction with changes in blood volume. This is almost never a problem in patients with a normal liver. However, administration of colloid solutions to a patient with underlying liver disease and a normal or expanded blood volume could theoretically aggravate the clinical manifestations of portal hypertension.

Budd-Chiari syndrome (hepatic vein thrombosis) results from obstruction of flow through the hepatic veins. The resulting sinusoidal hypertension produces prominent ascites and hepatomegaly. Conditions (veno-occlusive dis-

---

*A catheter wedged in a tributary of the hepatic vein permits estimation of the pressure in the afferent veins to the sinusoid. The gradient between the wedged pressure and that in the hepatic vein reflects resistance at any point between the wedged position and the periphery of the sinusoid. The current view holds that the site of principal resistance in normal persons is in reasonably large hepatic veins. In cirrhosis, it is probably in the sinusoids as well as the hepatic veins.

Table 24–3. Causes of Portal Hypertension.

I. Increased resistance to flow
  A. Prehepatic (portal vein obstruction)
   1. Congenital atresia or stenosis
   2. Thrombosis of portal vein
   3. Thrombosis of splenic vein
   4. Extrinsic compression (eg, tumors)
  B. Hepatic
   1. Cirrhosis
     a. Portal cirrhosis (nutritional, alcoholic, Laënnec)
     b. Postnecrotic cirrhosis
     c. Biliary cirrhosis
     d. Others (Wilson disease, hemochromatosis)
   2. Acute alcoholic liver disease
   3. Chronic active hepatitis
   4. Congenital hepatic fibrosis
   5. Idiopathic portal hypertension (hepatoportal sclerosis)
   6. Schistosomiasis
   7. Sarcoidosis
  C. Posthepatic
   1. Budd-Chiari syndrome (hepatic vein thrombosis)
   2. Veno-occlusive disease
   3. Cardiac disease
     a. Constrictive pericarditis
     b. Valvular heart disease
     c. Right heart failure
II. Increased portal blood flow
  A. Arterial-portal venous fistula
  B. Increased splenic flow
   1. Banti syndrome
   2. Splenomegaly (eg, tropical splenomegaly, myeloid metaplasia)

ease, inferior vena cava obstruction by tumor or congenital webs, right-sided heart failure) that reduce flow through the hepatic veins will result in a similar clinical picture.

Banti syndrome was defined as liver disease secondary to primary splenic disease and was incorrectly considered as the cause of portal hypertension now known to result from cirrhosis and other hepatic disorders rather than a consequence of such conditions. Portal hypertension from splenomegaly and increased splenic vein flow has been described in patients with hematologic diseases or tropical splenomegaly and apparently normal liver function. This is extremely uncommon, however, and given the great reserve of the liver to handle increases in portal flow, many such patients probably have some component of liver disease. In cirrhosis, the increased splenic blood flow accompanying "congestive" splenomegaly may occasionally be great enough to warrant splenic artery ligation or splenectomy to decrease portal pressure and improve symptoms, but this situation is rare.

Increased flow may contribute to portal hypertension in patients with arterial-portal venous fistulae (traumatic, congenital). When an arteriovenous fistula occurs, portal hypertension and its clinical manifestations usually do not appear for several months, because sinusoidal capacity is so great that the immediate rise in portal pressure is only moderate. With time, however, sinusoidal sclerosis develops, resistance increases, and portal pressure gradually reaches high levels, leading to the formation of varices.

The average portal flow in cirrhotic patients with complications of portal hypertension is about 30% of normal, ranging from 0 to 700 mL/min. Hepatic arterial flow is usually reduced by a similar proportion. The range of portal flow rates in different patients may vary greatly; in some, blood in the portal vein moves sluggishly or the direction of flow may even be reversed (hepatofugal) so that the portal vein functions as an outflow tract from the liver. These states of low flow predispose to spontaneous thrombosis of the portal vein, a complication of cirrhosis that usually is associated with acute clinical deterioration and renders the portal vein unsuitable for a shunt to decompress the portal venous system. Along with these changes, blood flow through the splanchnic vascular bed increases as a result of decreased resistence, the consequence of increased production of local vasodilators (eg, nitric oxide) and mesenteric angiogenesis.

The obstacle to flow through the liver promotes expansion of collateral channels between the portal and systemic venous systems. As the pathologic process develops, portal pressure increases until a level of about 40 cm H_2O (30 mm Hg) is reached. At this point, increasing hepatic resistance, even to the point of occlusion of the portal vein, diverts a greater fraction of portal flow through collaterals without significant increments in portal pressure.

The type of collateral that develops depends partly on the cause of the portal hypertension. In extrahepatic portal vein thrombosis (without liver disease), collaterals in the diaphragm and in the hepatocolic, hepatoduodenal, and gastrohepatic ligaments transport blood into the liver around the occluded vein (hepatopetal). In cirrhosis, collateral vessels circumvent the liver and deliver portal blood directly into the systemic circulation (hepatofugal); these collaterals give rise to esophageal and gastric varices. Other common spontaneous collaterals are through a recanalized umbilical vein to the abdominal wall, from the superior hemorrhoidal vein into the middle and inferior hemorrhoidal veins, and through numerous small veins (of Retzius) connecting the retroperitoneal viscera with the posterior abdominal wall.

Isolated thrombosis of the splenic vein causes localized splenic venous hypertension and gives rise to large collaterals from spleen to gastric fundus. From there, the blood returns to the main portal system through the coronary vein. In this condition, gastric varices are often present without esophageal varices.

Of the many large collaterals that form as a result of portal hypertension, spontaneous bleeding is relatively uncommon except from those at the gastroesophageal junction; spontaneous bleeding from gastric varices can sometimes occur. Compared with adjacent areas of the esophagus and stomach, the gastroesophageal junction is especially rich in submucosal veins, which expand disproportionately in patients with portal hypertension. The cause of variceal bleeding is most probably rupture due to sudden increases in hydrostatic pressure. Esophagitis is usually mild or absent.

Debernardi-Venon W et al: CO_2 wedged hepatic venography in the evaluation of portal hypertension. Gut 2000;46:856.

Krige JE, Beckingham IJ: ABC of diseases of liver, pancreas, and biliary system. Portal hypertension—1: varices. BMJ 2001; 322:348.

Krige JE, Beckingham IJ: ABC of diseases of liver, pancreas, and biliary system: portal hypertension—2. Ascites, encephalopathy, and other conditions. BMJ 2001;322:416.

Sanyal AJ et al: Portal hypertension and its complications. Gastroenterology 2008;134:1715

CIRRHOSIS

Hepatic cirrhosis remains a major public health problem worldwide, with and annual mortality of approximately 23,000 per year in the United States alone. The incidence of cirrhosis is increasing, due in large measure to hepatitis C, and at present is the third-most common cause of death in men in the fifth decade of life.

Alcohol abuse remains the leading cause of cirrhosis in most Western countries. Alcohol exerts direct toxic effects on the liver that are magnified in the presence of protein and other dietary deficiencies that are often present. Even still, cirrhosis develops in a small minority of patients who abuse alcohol. Alcohol induces a specific cytochrome P450 in the liver (ie, P450 2E1) that participates in its metabolism to acetaldehyde, which has a number of deleterious effects, including antibody formation, decreased DNA repair, enzyme inactivation, and alterations in microtubules, mitochondria, and plasma membranes. Acetaldehyde also promotes glutathione depletion, free radical–mediated toxicity, lipid peroxidation, and hepatic collagen synthesis. Hepatic steatosis and alcoholic hepatitis are stages of alcoholic liver injury that may precede cirrhosis. Alcoholic hyalin, a glycoprotein, accumulates in centrilobular hepatocytes of patients with alcoholic hepatitis. There is some evidence that immunologic responses to alcoholic hyalin may be important in the pathogenesis of cirrhosis.

Collagen deposition in cirrhosis results from increased fibroblastic activity as well as from repair following hepatocellular injury and necrosis. The ultimate result is a liver containing regenerative nodules and connective tissue septa linking portal fields with central canals.

The natural history of cirrhosis is difficult to predict. Once the diagnosis has been established, up to 30% of patients die within a year from hepatic failure or complications of portal hypertension, of which bleeding esophageal varices is the most feared. In newly diagnosed cirrhotics, the chances of dying within the subsequent 2–3 years are influenced by the status of liver function (as reflected by the Child-Pugh classification), the presence of varices, and the portal pressure. A group of cirrhotics with varices followed by the Boston Interhospital Liver Group experienced a 1-year death rate of 66%. Cirrhotics without varices may benefit substantially by abstaining from alcohol. Bleeding episodes occur in up to 40% of all patients with cirrhosis, and the initial episode of variceal hemorrhage is fatal in 50% or more. At least two thirds of those who survive their initial hemorrhage will bleed again, and the risk of dying from the second is similarly high. It is principally for such patients that portal decompressive procedures are recommended.

Reuben A: Alcohol and the liver. Curr Opin Gastroenterol 2008; 24:328.

Schuppan D, Afdhal NH: Liver cirrhosis. Lancet 2008;371:838.

ACUTELY BLEEDING VARICES

Varices will develop in 5–15% of cirrhotic patients per year. Most patients with cirrhosis will develop varices, but only about one third will experience variceal hemorrhage. Each bleeding episode is associated with a mortality rate of up to 25%, and 70% of untreated patients will die within a year of the first episode. This high death rate reflects not only the massive hemorrhage but also the frequent presence of severely compromised liver function and other systemic disease that may or may not be related to alcohol abuse. Malnutrition, pulmonary aspiration, infections, and coronary artery disease are frequent coexisting conditions. Additional complicating factors in this patient population include lack of cooperation with treatment and acute alcohol withdrawal, which in its worst manifestation (delirium tremens) adds greatly to the already high mortality rate.

▶ Clinical Findings

A. Symptoms and Signs

The initial management of the patient with massive gastrointestinal hemorrhage is discussed in Chapter 23. Critical initial steps include airway protection, particularly in patients with altered mental status or those with hemodynamic instability, and resuscitation with fluid and blood products; correction of coagulopathy and thrombocytopenia should also be initiated early. Patients admitted with variceal hemorrhage are often bacteremic as a result of a concomitant infectious process (spontaneous bacterial peritonitis, urinary tract infection, or pneumonia). Clinical trials have shown better outcomes when empiric antibiotic therapy is initiated, usually a third-generation cephalosporin such as ceftriaxone.

It must be emphasized that bleeding from varices cannot be accurately diagnosed on clinical grounds alone even though the history or the appearance of the patient may strongly suggest the presence of cirrhosis or portal hypertension. Most patients with bleeding varices have alcoholic cirrhosis, and the diagnosis may seem obvious in a patient with hepatomegaly, jaundice, and vascular spiders who admits to recent binge drinking. Splenomegaly, the most constant physical finding, is present in 80% of patients with portal hypertension regardless of the cause. Ascites is frequently present. Massive ascites and hepatosplenomegaly in a nonalcoholic would suggest the much less common Budd-Chiari syndrome. If cirrhosis or varices have been documented on previous examinations, hematemesis would strongly suggest bleeding varices as the cause.

B. Laboratory Findings

Most patients with alcoholic liver disease and acute upper gastrointestinal bleeding have compromised liver function. The bilirubin is usually elevated, and the serum albumin is often below 3 g/dL. The leukocyte count may be elevated. Anemia may be a reflection of chronic alcoholic liver disease or hypersplenism as well as acute hemorrhage. The development of a hepatoma by a cirrhotic may first manifest by hemorrhage from varices; CT scan and marked elevation of the serum α-fetoprotein will make the diagnosis. Thrombocytopenia and coagulopathy are common.

C. Special Examinations

1. Esophagogastroscopy—Emergency esophagogastroscopy is the most useful procedure for diagnosing bleeding varices and should be performed as soon as the patient's general condition is stabilized by blood transfusion and other supportive measures. Endotracheal intubation is usually necessary for airway control. Varices appear as three or four large, tortuous submucosal bluish vessels running longitudinally in the distal esophagus. The bleeding site may be identified, but in some cases the lumen fills with blood so rapidly that the lesion is obscured.

2. Upper gastrointestinal series—A barium swallow outlines the varices in about 90% of affected patients, but barium studies are neither as sensitive nor as specific as endoscopy, and they are difficult and dangerous studies to perform in the bleeding patient.

▶ Treatment of Acute Bleeding

The general goal of treatment is to control the bleeding as quickly and reliably as possible using methods with the fewest possible side effects. The methods currently in use for acute variceal bleeding are listed in Table 24–4.

The patient's condition is stabilized to the extent possible by following the general guidelines for treating major upper gastrointestinal bleeding described in Chapter 23. Other therapy should include measures to treat or prevent encephalopathy, parenteral vitamin K to correct a prolonged prothrombin time, intravenous antibiotics, and electrolyte replacement (especially potassium) as required to restore electrolyte balance.

Vasoactive drugs aimed at reducing portal pressure (vasopressin and terlipressin, somatostatin and its analogues) and endoscopic variceal ablation (sclerotherapy and banding) are the most commonly used initial therapies. In general, vasoac-

Table 24–4. Measures to Control Acute Bleeding from Esophageal Varices.

Medical
    1. Vasopressin, terlipressin
    2. Somatostatin analogues
Mechanical
    3. Balloon tamponade
Interventional, nonsurgical
    4. Endoscopic sclerotherapy
    5. Transhepatic embolization and sclerotherapy
Surgical
    6. Emergency portasystemic shunts
    7. Esophageal transection and reanastomosis
    8. Esophagogastric devascularization
    9. Suture ligation of varices

tive compounds should be used immediately in all patients, since control of bleeding can be achieved in 80–85% of episodes. Endoscopic intervention in the very acute setting can be equally effective but requires a skilled endoscopist; banding has been shown to be more effective and is considered the treatment of choice, although very profuse bleeding makes ligation a challenge, and sclerotherapy is useful in this setting. A meta-analysis showed that combined endoscopic and pharmacologic treatment is more effective in controlling acute bleeding than after endoscopic treatment alone. Balloon tamponade is no longer used routinely but is rather reserved for special situations when other methods fail.

These measures are successful in approximately 90% of cases, but the early rebleeding rate is about 30%. When bleeding continues after initial treatment and if the patient is a good operative risk, an emergency shunt procedure should be considered.

Death rates rise rapidly in patients requiring more than 10 units of blood, and in general, patients still bleeding after 6 units—or those whose bleeding is still unchecked 24 hours after admission—should be considered for portal decompression procedures. Even when the bleeding is brought under control by the initial intervention, the mortality rate remains high (about 35%) as a result of liver failure and other complications.

Specific Measures

1. Acute endoscopic sclerotherapy or ligation—Via fiberoptic endoscopy, 1–3 mL of sclerosant solution is injected into the lumen of each varix, causing it to become thrombosed. Variations in the type of endoscope or sclerosant solution or whether or not the varices are physically compressed appear to have little influence on the outcome. Endoscopy is usually repeated within 48 hours and then once or twice again at weekly intervals, at which time any residual varices are injected.

Sclerotherapy controls acute bleeding in 80–85% of patients, and rebleeding during the same hospitalization is

about half (25% versus 50%) the rebleeding rate of patients treated with a combination of vasopressin and balloon tamponade. Even though controlled trials show improvement in the control of bleeding with sclerotherapy, the evidence for increased patient survival is conflicting.

A similar effect is achieved by endoscopic ligation of the varices. The varix is lifted with a suction tip, and a small rubber band is slipped around the base. The varix necroses to leave a superficial ulcer. Several controlled trials have reported rubber band ligation to be more effective in controlling long-term bleeding episodes compared to sclerotherapy, although comparisons in the acute setting are limited. Band ligation is associated with fewer complications and fewer procedures are needed for complete eradication and has thus emerged as the initial endoscopic treatment of choice.

2. Vasopressin and terlipressin (triglycyl lysine vasopressin)—Vasopressin and terlipressin lower portal blood flow and portal pressure by directly constricting splanchnic arterioles, thereby reducing inflow. Vasopressin or terlipressin alone controls acute bleeding in about 80–85% of patients, and this rate is increased when combined with endoscopic therapy or balloon tamponade. Cardiac output, oxygen delivery to the tissues, hepatic blood flow, and renal blood flow are also decreased—effects that occasionally produce complications such as myocardial infarction, cardiac arrhythmias, and intestinal necrosis. These unwanted side effects may sometimes be prevented without interfering with the decrease in portal pressure by simultaneous administration of nitroglycerin or isoproterenol. Terlipressin, a long-acting synthetic vasopressin analogue, has fewer untoward cardiovascular side effects than vasopressin.

Although the results are somewhat contradictory, controlled trials generally indicate that vasopressin plus nitroglycerin is superior to vasopressin alone and that vasopressin alone is superior to placebo in controlling active variceal bleeding. Survival is not increased, however. In fact, while several vasoactive agents effectively stop acute hemorrhage, only terlipressin has been shown to improve survival after an acute event. Vasopressin is given as a peripheral intravenous infusion (at about 0.4 units/min), which is safer than bolus injections. Nitroglycerin can be given intravenously or sublingually. Terlipressin undergoes gradual conversion to vasopressin in the body and is safe to give by intravenous bolus injection (2 mg intravenously every 6 hours).

3. Somatostatin—Somatostatin infusion reduces portal pressure without any impact on systemic hemodynamics. By contrast, octreotide (a longer lasting somatostatin analogue) appears to have less of an impact on portal pressure. Somatostatin has been shown, in a prospective randomized trial, to effectively control acute bleeding, although other studies have had equivocal results. A meta-analysis of all studies using somatostatin or its analogues did show a significant risk reduction in control of hemorrhage. The efficacy of octreotide remains uncertain, but it appears to reduce the rebleeding rate when used in conjunction with endoscopic therapy. It should be emphasized that no study of somatostatin or octreotide has shown improved survival after an acute bleeding episode. Somatostatin is typically administered as a bolus of 250 micrograms followed by an infusion of 250 µg/hour for 24 hours. Octreotide is given as an initial bolus of 50–100 µg followed by a continuous infusion of 25–50 µg/h for 24 hours.

4. Balloon tamponade—See Figure 24–6. Tubes designed for tamponade have two balloons that can be inflated in the lumen of the gut to compress bleeding varices. There are three or four lumens in the tube, depending on the type: two are for filling balloons within the stomach and the esophagus, and the third permits aspiration of gastric contents. A fourth lumen in the Minnesota tube is used to aspirate the esophagus orad to the esophageal balloon. The main effect results from traction applied to the tube, which forces the gastric balloon to compress the collateral veins at the cardia of the stomach. Inflating the esophageal balloon probably contributes little, since barium x-rays suggest that it does not actually compress the varices.

The most common serious complication is aspiration of pharyngeal secretions and pneumonitis. Another serious hazard is the occasional instance of esophageal rupture caused by inflation of the esophageal balloon. The esophageal balloon is therefore infrequently used.

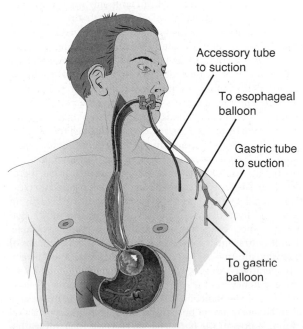

▲ Figure 24–6. Sengstaken-Blakemore tube with both gastric and esophageal balloons inflated.

Accessory tube to suction

To esophageal balloon

Gastric tube to suction

To gastric balloon

About 75% of actively bleeding patients can be controlled by balloon tamponade. When bleeding has stopped, the balloons are left inflated for another 24 hours. They are then decompressed, leaving the tube in place. If bleeding does not recur, the tube should be withdrawn. The efficacy of other therapies combined with potential complications associated with balloon catheters have led to a marked reduction in the use of the latter approach, which is now reserved as a salvage treatment in patients who fail initial measures.

5. Transjugular intrahepatic portasystemic shunt (TIPS)—TIPS is a minimally invasive means of creating a portasystemic shunt by creating a direct communication between the portal and hepatic venous systems within the liver parenchyma. A catheter is introduced through the jugular vein and, under radiologic control, positioned in the hepatic vein. From this point, the portal vein is accessed through the liver, the tract is dilated, and the channel is kept open by inserting an expandable metal stent, which is left in place. This technique is of great value in controlling portal hypertension and variceal bleeding and can be used to stop acute bleeding or to prevent rebleeding in a patient who has recovered from an acute episode. The shunts remain open in most patients for up to a year, at which point intimal overgrowth lead to thrombosis and occlusion in many cases. The use of polytetrafluoroethylene (PTFE)-covered stents may improve the patency rate.

TIPS is used most commonly as a salvage procedure in patients who continue to bleed after treatment with pharmacologic agents and endoscopic banding or sclerotherapy. TIPS has proved most useful as a bridge to transplantation. It should not be regarded as definitive therapy, however, even though the shunt will usually remain patent for many months. Thus, patients with advanced liver disease are the principal candidates for TIPS, whereas those with less severe cirrhosis should be considered for beta-blocker therapy or surgery (shunt or devascularization procedure).

6. Surgery—The operative procedures to control active bleeding are emergency portasystemic shunt and variceal ligation or esophageal transection.

A. EMERGENCY PORTACAVAL SHUNT—An emergency portasystemic shunt has a 95% rate of success in stopping variceal bleeding. Like TIPS, surgical intervention in the acute setting is generally used to salvage patients with persistent hemorrhage. The death rate of the operation is not insignificant, generally related to the status of the patient's liver function (eg, Child-Pugh classification; Table 24–1) as well as the rate and amount of bleeding and its effects on cardiac, renal, and pulmonary function. Some patients with advanced liver disease, especially those with severe encephalopathy and ascites, have an extraordinarily poor survival regardless of the treatment. In such patients, surgery is usually not warranted, even in the face of continued bleeding. On the other hand, patients with good liver function usually recover after an emergency shunt. A controlled trial showed that the death rate in acutely bleeding Child-Pugh C patients was insignificantly lower after endoscopic sclerotherapy (44%) than after emergency portacaval shunt (50%).

For active bleeding, an end-to-side portacaval shunt or H-mesocaval shunt is most commonly performed.

The distal splenorenal (Warren) shunt is usually too time-consuming for use in emergency operations. The central splenorenal shunt is more complicated than an end-to-side portacaval shunt and has no specific advantages. A side-to-side portacaval shunt might be preferable in an acutely bleeding patient with severe ascites, and this approach (or a variant such as an H-mesocaval shunt) would be required for someone with Budd-Chiari syndrome.

Hepatic failure is the cause of death in about two thirds of those who die after an emergency portacaval shunt. Renal failure, which is often accompanied by ascites, is another potentially lethal problem. Metabolic alkalosis and delirium tremens are not uncommon postoperatively in alcoholics.

B. ESOPHAGEAL TRANSECTION—Varices may be obliterated by firing the end-to-end stapler in the distal esophagus after tucking a full-thickness ring of tissue into the cartridge with a circumferential tie. This procedure has gained popularity in the past decade, and in many surgical units it is the first choice for therapy when nonsurgical methods fail. If transection is performed, it must be done as soon as it is recognized that a second attempt at sclerotherapy or band ligation has failed. As a last-ditch effort—after many units of blood have been transfused—death from liver failure is all but certain. The results (eg, survival) are better in patients with nonalcoholic cirrhosis. Stapled transection has replaced the older technique of direct suture ligation of the varices. Transection must be viewed as an emergency measure to stop persistent bleeding—not as definitive treatment—since the underlying portal hypertension is not corrected and varices recur months later in many patients.

Bambha K et al: Predictors of early re-bleeding and mortality after acute variceal hemorrhage in patients with cirrhosis. Gut 2008; 57:814.

Bendtsen F, Krag A, Moller S: Treatment of acute variceal bleeding. Dig Liver Dis 2008;40:328.

Cales P et al: Early administration of vapreotide for variceal bleeding in patients with cirrhosis. French Club for the Study of Portal Hypertension. N Engl J Med 2001;344:23.

Gerbes AL et al: Transjugular intrahepatic portosystemic shunt (TIPS) for variceal bleeding in portal hypertension: comparison of emergency and elective interventions. Dig Dis Sci 1998; 43:2463.

Mercado MA et al: Comparative study of 2 variants of a modified esophageal transection in the Sugiura-Futagawa operation. Arch Surg 1998;133:1046.

Orozco H et al: A comparative study of the elective treatment of variceal hemorrhage with beta-blockers, transendoscopic sclerotherapy, and surgery: a prospective, controlled, and randomized trial during 10 years. Ann Surg 2000;232:216.

Shibata D et al: Transjugular intrahepatic portosystemic shunt for treatment of bleeding ectopic varices with portal hypertension. Dis Colon Rectum 1999;42:1581.

Toubia N, Sanyal AJ: Portal hypertension and variceal hemorrhage. Med Clin N Am 2008;92:551.

Woods JE, Kiely JM: Short-term international medical service. Mayo Clin Proc 2000;75:311.

NONBLEEDING VARICES

Patients with varices that have never bled have a 30% chance of bleeding at some point; of those who bleed, 50% die. For patients who do not bleed during the first year after diagnosis of varices, the risk of bleeding subsequently decreases by half and continues to drop thereafter. Patients who have bled once from esophageal varices have a 60–70% chance of bleeding again, and about two thirds of repeat bleeding episodes are fatal.

▶ Evaluation

A. Portal Flow and Pressure Measurements

Measurements of pressure and flow in the splanchnic vasculature have been used for diagnosis and as a guide to therapy and prognosis in portal hypertension. Portal pressure can be measured directly at surgery or preoperatively by any of the following techniques: (1) Wedged hepatic venous pressure (WHVP) accurately reflects free portal pressure when portal hypertension is caused by a postsinusoidal (or sinusoidal) resistance, as in cirrhosis. The portal pressure can be determined with the catheter in the wedged position, corrected by subtracting the free hepatic venous pressure (FHVP); the hepatic venous pressure gradient (HVPG, the pressure gradient from the portal to the hepatic venous systems) can also be determined. This is the most commonly used technique. (2) Direct measurement of splenic pulp pressure is obtained by a percutaneously placed needle. (3) Percutaneous transhepatic catheterization of the intrahepatic branches of the portal vein is the method of choice in patients thought to have presinusoidal block or Budd-Chiari syndrome. (4) Catheterization of the umbilical vein is accomplished through a small incision, and the catheter is threaded into the portal system. With each of these methods, one may also obtain anatomic information by performing angiography through the catheter.

HVPG predicts decompensation and death. Reduction in the HVPG, either spontaneously or after therapy, may help predict the risk of rebleeding in some patients. It has therefore been suggested that HVPG can be used to guide therapy. However, its value currently has been shown primarily in alcoholic liver disease. Also, it is an invasive study that requires special expertise and is not always readily available. Duplex ultrasonography is an accurate noninvasive means of assessing the amount and direction of flow in the portal vein. Preoperatively, duplex ultrasonography is useful to determine patency of the portal vein and direction of flow. Because of spontaneous thrombosis, about 10% of patients with cirrhosis have a portal vein unsuitable for a portacaval shunt. If flow in the portal vein is reversed (hepatofugal), a selective shunt is not recommended, because it compromises the ability of portal tributaries to serve as an outflow tract for liver blood. Duplex ultrasonography can also be used to follow changes in portal perfusion after shunt operations.

B. Portal Angiography

The portal venous anatomy is often studied preoperatively by angiographic techniques. The objectives are to determine the patency, location, and size of the veins tentatively chosen for a shunt, to demonstrate the presence of varices, and to estimate the degree of prograde portal flow. Some of this information can now be obtained less invasively by duplex ultrasonography. When a splenorenal shunt is contemplated, the left renal vein should be opacified, either by injection of the renal artery or renal vein.

▶ Treatment

The treatment options consist of expectant management, endoscopic sclerotherapy, nonselective beta-blocker (eg, propranolol, nadolol), portasystemic shunts, devascularization of the esophagogastric junction, and miscellaneous rarely used operations. The treatment of patients with varices that have never bled is usually referred to as prophylactic therapy (eg, prophylactic sclerotherapy or prophylactic propranolol). By convention, procedures performed on patients who have bled previously are referred to as therapeutic (eg, therapeutic shunts).

A. Prophylactic Therapy

Prophylactic therapy is of value, since the mortality rate of variceal bleeding is high (25%), the risk of bleeding in patients with varices is relatively high (30%), and varices can often be diagnosed before the initial episode of bleeding. In patients who have never had a bleeding episode, the following have been shown to be related to the risk of hemorrhage: Child-Pugh classification, the size of the varices, and the presence of red wale markings (longitudinal dilated venules resembling whip marks) on the varices. This information can be used to identify high-risk patients (up to 65% risk of bleeding within a year) who are most likely to benefit from prophylactic treatment.

In patients who have never bled but have a high risk (medium to large varices or small varices with red wale markings and/or decompensated cirrhosis), treatment in the form of nonselective beta-blocker or endoscopic band ligation is recommended. Both of these therapies are effective in this setting. It has been suggested that beta-blocker therapy should be the first-line treatment, with endoscopic variceal ligation (EVL) used in patients who cannot tolerate or have contraindications to beta-blockade. Endoscopic sclerotherapy is no longer routinely used as primary prophylaxis.

B. Therapy of Patients Who Have Bled Previously

As noted earlier, patients who recover from an episode of variceal bleeding an approximately 60–70% chance of bleed-

ing again. Much effort has been expended to ascertain the best treatment for these patients. The methods of greatest interest include beta-blocker therapy, endoscopic band ligation, and portasystemic shunts.

1. Nonselective beta-blocker therapy—As with patients who have never bled, nonselective beta-adrenergic blocking agents (propranolol, nadolol) effectively reduce the risk of recurrent bleeding episodes. These agents work by decreasing cardiac output and splanchnic blood flow and consequently portal blood pressure. Chronic propranolol therapy, 20–160 mg twice daily (a dose that reduces resting pulse rate by 25%), decreases by about 40% the frequency of rebleeding from esophageal or gastric varices, deaths from rebleeding, and overall mortality. The benefits are greater in Child-Pugh A and B than in Child-Pugh C cirrhotics. Beta-blocker therapy has been compared to endoscopic sclerotherapy, with no difference in rebleeding or mortality seen but with higher complications in the sclerotherapy group. The addition of isosorbide mononitrate to beta-blocker therapy appears to result in a greater reduction of portal pressure compared to beta-blockade alone. Abstinence from alcohol should always be emphasized and may help prevent further bleeding but may not necessarily decrease the mortality related specifically to variceal hemorrhage, as was previously thought.

2. Endoscopic band ligation—Endoscopic band ligation, as described earlier, is an effective means of preventing recurrent bleeding episodes and has been shown to be superior to sclerotherapy in this regard. Both band ligation and beta-blocker therapy appear to be similarly effective in preventing rebleeding. However, the combination of both therapies has been shown to significantly reduce not only the risk of rebleeding but also the recurrence of varices. Thus, combination therapy appears to be the most effective treatment after an initial bleeding episode.

3. Endoscopic sclerotherapy—The technique of endoscopic sclerotherapy was described earlier in this chapter. Sclerotherapy was previously used routinely to reduce the risk of rebleeding but has been replaced by band ligation.

4. Transjugular intrahepatic portasystemic shunt—The TIPS technique is described in the preceding section. TIPS is effective in preventing rebleeding episodes, more so than either endoscopic or pharmacologic therapy alone. However, this advantage is offset by its higher morbidity and mortality rate from the development of hepatic encephalopathy and liver failure. For this reason, as well as the lack of a clear survival or cost-benefit advantage, TIPS is used mainly to salvage patients who fail endoscopic and/or pharmacologic treatment.

TIPS has generally superseded shunt surgery in most patients who fail first-line therapy. A recent large multicenter randomized trial showed that TIPS and surgical shunts had similar rates of rebleeding, encephalopathy, and mortality in

Child-Pugh A and B cirrhotic patients. There was a higher incidence of shunt dysfunction in the TIPS patients, perhaps because of the type of stent used. Given the similar outcomes but more durable patency compared to TIPS, surgical shunts still have a role in the management of these patients.

C. Surgical Approaches

The objective of surgical procedures used to treat portal hypertension is either to obliterate the varices or to reduce blood flow and pressure within the varices (Table 24–5). A third option, particularly in patients with advanced cirrhosis, is liver transplantation.

1. Liver transplantation—Any relatively young patient with cirrhosis who has survived an episode of variceal hemorrhage should be considered a candidate for liver transplantation, since any other form of therapy carries a much higher (about 80%) mortality rate within the subsequent 1–2 years as a result of repeat bleeding or complications of hepatic failure. Obviously, continued alcohol use is a contraindication to transplantation in most patients. The good transplantation candidates, however, should not be subjected to portasystemic shunts or other procedures if it appears that they will come to transplantation in the near future. In general, Child-Pugh A patients are candidates for portal decompression; Child-Pugh C patients are candidates for a transplant. A transjugular intrahepatic shunt (see previous section) is an excellent way to control bleeding while the patient is being prepared for a transplant.

2. Portasystemic shunts—The advent of TIPS has resulted in a marked decline in the number of shunt operations performed. However, surgical shunts are much more durable than TIPS, and good risk patients appear to benefit from theses procedures.

Portasystemic shunts can be grouped into those that shunt the entire portal system (total shunts) and those that selectively shunt blood from the gastrosplenic region while preserving the pressure-flow relationships in the rest of the portal bed (selective shunts). All of the shunt operations commonly used today reduce the incidence of rebleeding to less than 10%, compared with about 75% in unshunted patients. Unfortunately, the price of this achievement is an operative mortality rate of 5–20% (depending on the Child-Pugh classification [Table 24–1]), further impairment of liver function, and an increase in encephalopathy (greater with total shunts). Therefore, since shunts have these potential drawbacks, clinical trials are needed to pinpoint their place within an overall treatment strategy.

In one well-designed trial, patients who had bled previously were randomized to chronic sclerotherapy or a distal splenorenal shunt (Warren shunt). Patients randomized to chronic sclerotherapy who had recurrent episodes of bleeding during treatment (ie, treatment failures, which amounted to 30% of the sclerotherapy group) were then treated surgically (ie, shunted). The results showed that 2-year survival

Table 24–5. Surgical Procedures for Esophageal Varices.

A. Direct variceal obliteration
 1. Variceal suture ligation
  a. Transthoracic
  b. Transabdominal
 2. Esophageal transection and reanastomosis
  a. Suture technique
  b. Staple technique
 3. Variceal sclerosis
  a. Esophagoscopic
  b. Transhepatic
 4. Variceal resection
  a. Esophagogastrectomy
  b. Subtotal esophagectomy
B. Reduction of variceal blood flow and pressure
 1. Portasystemic shunts
  a. End-to-side
  b. Side-to-side
   1. Side-to-side portacaval
   2. Mesocaval
   3. Central splenorenal
   4. Renosplenic
 2. Selective shunts
  a. Distal splenorenal (Warren)
  b. Left gastric vena caval (Inokuchi)
 3. Reduction of portal blood flow
  a. Splenectomy
  b. Splenic artery ligation
 4. Reduction of proximal gastric blood flow
  a. Esophagogastric devascularization
  b. Gastric transection and reanastomosis (Tanner)
 5. Stimulation of additional portasystemic venous collaterals
  a. Omentopexy
  b. Splenic transposition
C. Measures to preserve hepatic blood flow after portacaval shunt
 1. Arterialization of portal vein stump

was better among those originally randomized to sclerotherapy (90%) than among those originally assigned to the shunt group (60%). This trial supports a general treatment plan consisting initially of endoscopic therapy and reserving portasystemic shunts for the patients in whom the former fails to control bleeding adequately.

The choice of shunt has been the subject of much debate and several randomized trials. The principal question in recent years has been whether encephalopathy and survival are better with a selective shunt (eg, a distal splenorenal shunt) than with a total shunt (eg, a mesocaval or an end-to-side portacaval shunt). The results are conflicting, but in general they support the contention that there is about half as much severe encephalopathy following selective shunts. None of the trials have shown any particular shunt to be associated with longer survival.

3. Severity of hepatic disease and operative risk—The immediate death rate of an elective shunt procedure can be predicted from the patient's hepatic function as reflected by the Child-Pugh classification (Table 24–1). In addition to operative death rate, the figures also correlate with the death rate in the first postshunt year. Thereafter, survival curves of the different risk classes become reasonably parallel.

The severity of histopathologic changes in liver biopsies correlates with the immediate surgical death rate, the most ominous findings being hepatocellular necrosis, polymorphonuclear leukocyte infiltration, and the presence of Mallory bodies. The extent of histologic change also correlates with the more easily obtained data in the Child-Pugh classification (ie, severe changes occur in class C patients), so results of biopsies have no independent predictive value.

A. TYPES OF PORTASYSTEMIC SHUNTS—Figure 24–7 depicts the various shunts in use currently. Although they differ technically, physiologically there are only three different types: end-to-side, side-to-side, and selective.

(1) Total shunts—The end-to-side shunt completely disconnects the liver from the portal system. The portal vein is transected near its bifurcation in the liver hilum and anastomosed to the side of the inferior vena cava. The hepatic stump of the vein is oversewn. Postoperatively, the WHVP (sinusoidal pressure) drops slightly, reflecting the inability of the hepatic artery to compensate fully for the loss of portal inflow. The side-to-side portacaval, mesocaval, mesorenal, and central splenorenal shunts are all physiologically similar, since the shunt preserves continuity between the hepatic limb of the portal vein, the portal system, and the anastomosis. Flow through the hepatic limb of the standard side-to-side shunt is nearly always away from the liver and toward the anastomosis. The extent to which hepatofugal flow is produced by the other types of side-to-side shunts listed previously is not known.

The end-to-side portacaval shunt gives immediate and permanent protection from variceal bleeding and is somewhat easier to perform than a side-to-side portacaval or central splenorenal shunt. Encephalopathy may be slightly more common after side-to-side than end-to-side portacaval shunts. Side-to-side shunts are required in patients with Budd-Chiari syndrome or refractory ascites (when the latter is treated by a portasystemic shunt).

The mesocaval shunt interposes a segment of prosthetic graft or internal jugular vein between the inferior vena cava and the superior mesenteric vein where the latter passes in front of the uncinate process of the pancreas. The mesocaval shunt is particularly useful in the presence of severe scarring in the right upper quadrant or portal vein thrombosis, and in some cases it may be technically easier than a conventional side-to-side portacaval shunt if a side-to-side type of shunt is necessary. In most cases, portal flow to the liver is lost after this shunt. Evidence has been presented, however, that by limiting the diameter of the prosthetic graft to 8 mm (compared with 12- to 20-mm grafts), prograde flow is preserved in the portal vein, which decreases the incidence of postoperative encephalopathy while still preventing variceal hemorrhage.

(2) Selective shunts—Selective shunts lower pressure in the gastroesophageal venous plexus while preserving blood flow through the liver via the portal vein.

The distal splenorenal (Warren) shunt involves anastomosing the distal (splenic) end of the transected splenic vein to the side of the left renal vein, plus ligation of the major collaterals between the remaining portal and isolated gastrosplenic venous system. The latter step involves division of the gastric vein, the right gastroepiploic vein, and the vessels in the splenocolic ligament. The operation is more difficult and time consuming than conventional shunts and except for the experienced operator is probably too complex for emergency portal decompression. If mobilization of the splenic vein is hazardous, the renal vein may be transected and its caval end joined to the side of the undisturbed splenic vein. The segment of splenic vein between the anastomosis and the portal vein is then ligated. Surprisingly, this seems to have

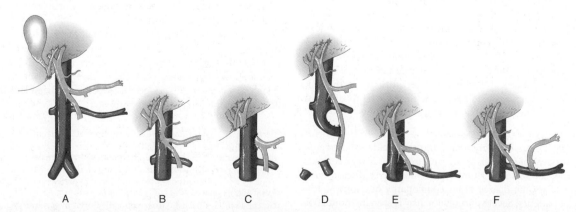

▲ **Figure 24–7.** Types of portacaval anastomoses: **A:** Normal. **B:** Side-to-side. **C:** End-to-side. **D:** Mesocaval. **E:** Central splenorenal. **F:** Distal splenorenal (Warren). The H-mesocaval shunt is not illustrated.

little permanent effect on renal function as long as the remaining tributaries are preserved on the oversewn renal vein stump.

In contrast to total shunts, the Warren shunt does not improve ascites and should not be performed in patients whose ascites has been difficult to control. Preoperative angiography should be performed to determine if the splenic vein and left renal vein are large enough and close enough together for performance of this shunt. Recent pancreatitis may preclude safe dissection of the splenic vein from the undersurface of the pancreas.

Another type of selective shunt (Inokuchi shunt) consists of joining the left gastric vein to the inferior vena cava by a short segment of autogenous saphenous vein. The procedure has not become popular, perhaps because of its technical complexity.

Selective shunts tend to become less selective over several years as new collaterals develop between the high-pressure and low-pressure regions of the portal system. This is accompanied by a gradual decrease in portal pressure (measured by WHVP) and evolution of the procedure into a version of side-to-side total shunt. The enlargement postoperatively of small venous tributaries entering the distal splenic vein from the pancreas suggests that this is the path by which nonselectivity develops. It is possible that this can be avoided by mobilizing the splenic vein all the way to the hilum (dividing these small vessels) before performing the splenorenal anastomosis.

B. CHOICE OF SHUNT—A reasonable approach to shunt selection is as follows: The distal splenorenal shunt is the first choice for elective portal decompression. If ascites is present or the anatomy is unfavorable, an end-to-side portacaval shunt is preferred. Side-to-side shunts would be done for patients with severe ascites or Budd-Chiari syndrome. The H-mesocaval and central splenorenal shunts are reserved for special anatomic situations in which the above operations are unsuitable. An end-to-side shunt or H-mesocaval shunt is performed for emergency decompression.

Portacaval and distal splenorenal shunts are often followed by a rise in platelet count in patients with secondary hypersplenism. The response is unpredictable, however, and hypersplenism need not necessarily dictate the type of shunt since it rarely produces clinical manifestations. A central splenorenal shunt, in which splenectomy is performed, should not be considered preferable to other kinds of shunt just because the patient has a low platelet count.

C. RESULTS OF PORTASYSTEMIC SHUNTS—Over 90% of portasystemic shunts remain patent, and the incidence of recurrent variceal bleeding is less than 10%. The 5-year survival rate after a portacaval shunt for alcoholic liver disease averages 45%. Some degree of encephalopathy develops in 15–25% of patients. Severe encephalopathy is seen in about 20% of alcoholics following a total shunt; its occurrence is not related to the severity of preshunt encephalopathy.

D. Devascularization Operations

The objective of devascularization is to destroy the venous collaterals that transport blood from the high-pressure portal system into the veins in the submucosa of the esophagus.

The Sugiura-Futugawa procedure is done in two stages. In the first stage, performed through a thoracotomy, the dilated venous collaterals between esophagus and adjacent structures are divided, and the esophagus at the level of the diaphragm is transected and reanastomosed. The second stage, a laparotomy, is performed immediately after the thoracotomy if the patient is actively bleeding but is deferred 4–6 weeks in elective cases. In the second stage of the operation, the upper two thirds of the stomach is devascularized, and selective vagotomy, pyloroplasty, and splenectomy are performed. It is possible in some cases to perform the entire operation through the left chest. An analogous operation has been described that consists of splenectomy, gastroesophageal devascularization, and resection of a 5-cm segment of the gastroesophageal junction. Continuity of the gut is restored by esophagogastrostomy with pyloroplasty.

In studies from Japan, where these operations originated, operative mortality is around 5%, variceal rebleeding is 2–4%, and 5-year survival is approximately 80%. Operations of this type performed in patients with alcoholic cirrhosis in North America have had poor results, owing to a high rate (40%) of late rebleeding.

E. Miscellaneous Operations

Attempts have also been made to decrease portal pressure by decreasing splanchnic inflow through splenectomy or splenic artery ligation. Diseases characterized by marked splenomegaly may rarely be associated with portal hypertension as a consequence of increased splenic blood flow, which has been known to reach levels as high as 1000 mL/min. Splenic blood flow may occasionally be increased enough in patients with cirrhosis to contribute significantly to the portal hypertension. However, splenectomy or splenic artery ligation in cirrhosis most often gives only a transient decrease in portal pressure, and over half of patients having these operations bleed again. Some workers have suggested that the absolute size of the splenic artery (a crude index of splenic flow) correlates with the clinical effectiveness of splenic artery ligation, a good result being predictable if the diameter of the artery is 1 cm or greater.

Berzigotti A, Garcia-Pagan JC: Prevention of recurrent variceal bleeding. Dig Liv Dis 2008;40:337.

de Franchis R: Updating consensus in portal hypertension: report of the Baveno III Consensus Workshop on definitions, methodology and therapeutic strategies in portal hypertension. J Hepatol 2000;33:846.

Garcia-Tsao G, Bosch J, Groszmann RJ: Portal hypertension and variceal bleeding: unresolved issues. Summary of an AASLD and EASLD single topic conference. Hepatology 2008;47:1764.

Gentilini P et al: Ascites and hepatorenal syndrome during cirrhosis: two entities or the continuation of the same complication? J Hepatol 1999;31:1088.

Gonzalez R et al: Combination endoscopic and drug therapy to prevent variceal rebleeding in cirrhosis. Ann Intern Med 2008;149:109.

Henderson JM et al: Distal splenorenal shunt versus TIPS for refractory variceal bleeding: a prospective randomized controlled trial. Gastroenterology 2006;130:1643.

Krige JE, Beckingham IJ: ABC of diseases of liver, pancreas, and biliary system. Portal hypertension—1: varices. BMJ 2001; 322:348.

Lebrec D: Drug therapy for portal hypertension. Gut 2001;49:441.

Masson S et al: Hepatic encephalopathy after transjugular intrahepatic portosystemic shunt insertion: a decade of experience. QJM 2008;101:493.

Sarin SK et al: Comparison of endoscopic ligation and propranolol for the primary prevention of variceal bleeding. N Engl J Med 1999;340:988.

Suzuki H, Stanley AJ: Current management and novel therapeutic strategies for refractory ascites and hepatorenal syndrome. QJM 2001;94:293.

Vlachogiannakos J et al: Angiotensin converting enzyme inhibitors and angiotensin II antagonists as therapy in chronic liver disease. Gut 2001;49:303.

EXTRAHEPATIC PORTAL VENOUS OCCLUSION

Extrahepatic portal vein obstruction is one of many causes of noncirrhotic portal hypertension, the other common cause being noncirrhotic portal fibrosis. These disorders are distinct but appear to share several similar etiological and pathogenetic features, the most notable of which is the clinical manifestation of portal hypertension in the absence of significant hepatic parenchymal dysfunction.

Idiopathic portal vein thrombosis (in the absence of liver disease) is a relatively common cause of portal hypertension in developing countries but is less prevalent in the West. This diagnosis accounts for most cases of portal hypertension in childhood (80–90%) and for a smaller proportion of cases in adults. Neonatal septicemia, omphalitis, umbilical vein catheterization for exchange transfusion, and dehydration have all been incriminated as possible causes, but collectively they can be implicated in less than half of cases. The causes of portal vein thrombosis in adults include hepatic tumors, cirrhosis, trauma, pancreatitis, pancreatic pseudocyst, myelofibrosis, thrombotic states (eg, protein C deficiency), and sepsis; in particular, cirrhosis and/or hepatocellular carcinoma need to be considered in adult patients.

Although clinical manifestations may be delayed until adulthood, 80% of patients present between 1 and 6 years of age with variceal bleeding, although hemorrhage from ectopic varices at other locations in the gastrointestinal tract is not uncommon. About 70% of hemorrhages are preceded by a recent upper respiratory tract infection. Some of these children first come to medical attention because of splenomegaly and pancytopenia. Failure to recognize the underlying problem has occasionally led to splenectomy, with the result that portal decompression using the splenic vein is precluded.

Ascites is uncommon except transiently after bleeding. Liver function is either normal or only slightly impaired, which probably accounts for the low incidence of overt encephalopathy. There is an increased frequency of neuropsychiatric problems, which may be a subtle form of encephalopathy.

Portal biliopathy refers to abnormalities of the extrahepatic bile ducts, usually the result of bile duct compression from large, dilated venous collaterals within the porta hepatis. These changes result in marked irregularities of the biliary wall that can progress to strictures and even obstructive jaundice and cholangitis in some cases; secondary biliary cirrhosis has been reported. Biliopathy is commonly seen on imaging studies, but most patients remain free of related symptoms.

Because the patient's general condition and liver function are good, the death rate for sudden massive bleeding is below that for other types of portal hypertension. The diagnosis can be confirmed with cross-sectional imaging or direct mesenteric angiography. WHVP is normal to slightly elevated; liver biopsies are normal or may show mild to moderate periportal fibrosis.

Bleeding episodes in children under age 8 are usually self-limited and often do not require endoscopic sclerotherapy, administration of vasopressin, or balloon tamponade. Even if such interventions are necessary, however, the bleeding episodes are self-limited and uncommonly fatal, so emergency operations are rarely necessary.

Thrombosed portal veins are unsuitable for shunt procedures. Cavomesenteric shunts are best for young children, whose vessels are small. In older individuals, treatment should be started with sclerotherapy; if that fails to control the bleeding, a distal splenorenal shunt is preferred. Splenectomy alone has no permanent effect and sacrifices the splenic vein, which might be needed later for a shunt operation. Shunts in small children have a high rate of spontaneous thrombosis and should be avoided, if possible, until approximately 8–10 years of age, when the vessels are of larger caliber. Even still, using precise technique, some surgeons have obtained a high rate of anastomotic patency in the very young. Encephalopathy and hepatic dysfunction many years after a total shunt may be improved if converted to a selective shunt.

Splenectomy alone is never indicated in this disease, either for hypersplenism or in an attempt to reduce portal pressure, because the rebleeding rate is 90% and fatal postsplenectomy sepsis is not uncommon. If it is not possible to construct an adequate shunt, expectant management is the best strategy. Repeated severe bleeding episodes should be treated by transendoscopic sclerosis. Esophagogastrectomy with colonic interposition may be effective but should be considered a last resort.

Janssen HL et al: Extrahepatic portal vein thrombosis: aetiology and determinants of survival. Gut 2001;49:720.

Sarin SK, Kumar A: Noncirrhotic portal hypertension. Clin Liver Dis 2006;10:627.

Sheen CL et al: Clinical features, diagnosis and outcome of acute portal vein thrombosis. QJM 2000;93:531.

Valla DC, Condat B: Portal vein thrombosis in adults: pathophysiology, pathogenesis and management. J Hepatol 2000;32:865.

van't Riet M et al: Diagnosis and treatment of portal vein thrombosis following splenectomy. Br J Surg 2000;87:1229.

SPLENIC VEIN THROMBOSIS

Isolated thrombosis of the splenic vein is a rare cause of variceal bleeding that can be cured by splenectomy. The splenic venous blood, blocked from its normal route, flows through the short gastric vessels to the gastric fundus and then into the left gastric vein, continuing toward the liver. As the blood traverses the stomach, large gastric varices are produced that may rupture and bleed. Characteristically, the collateral pattern does not involve the esophagus, so esophageal varices are uncommon.

The principal causes of this syndrome are pancreatitis, pancreatic pseudocyst, neoplasm, and trauma. Splenomegaly is present in two thirds of patients. Diagnosis can be made by selective splenic arteriography that opacifies the venous phase. Splenectomy is curative. Many cases of splenic vein thrombosis are unaccompanied by bleeding varices, and in such cases, no therapy is required. Treatment of acute bleeding from gastric varices is generally endoscopic, and endoscopic variceal obturation with tissue glue appears to be superior to band ligation or sclerotherapy.

de Franchis R: Updating consensus in portal hypertension: report of the Baveno III Consensus Workshop on definitions, methodology and therapeutic strategies in portal hypertension. J Hepatol 2000;33:846.

Gentilini P et al: Ascites and hepatorenal syndrome during cirrhosis: two entities or the continuation of the same complication? J Hepatol 1999;31:1088.

Krige JE, Beckingham IJ: ABC of diseases of liver, pancreas, and biliary system. Portal hypertension—1: varices. BMJ 2001; 322:348.

Lebrec D: Drug therapy for portal hypertension. Gut 2001;49:441.

Mercado MA et al: Results of surgical treatment (modified Sugiura-Futagawa operation) of portal hypertension associated to complete splenomesoportal thrombosis and cirrhosis. HPB Surg 1999;11:157.

Sarin SK et al: Comparison of endoscopic ligation and propranolol for the primary prevention of variceal bleeding. N Engl J Med 1999;340:988.

Sakorafas GH, Tsiotou AG: Splenic-vein thrombosis complicating chronic pancreatitis. Scand J Gastroenterol 1999;34:1171.

Sakorafas GH et al: The significance of sinistral portal hypertension complicating chronic pancreatitis. Am J Surg 2000;179:129.

Stein M, Link DP: Symptomatic spleno-mesenteric-portal venous thrombosis: recanalization and reconstruction with endovascular stents. J Vasc Interv Radiol 1999;10:363.

Suzuki H, Stanley AJ: Current management and novel therapeutic strategies for refractory ascites and hepatorenal syndrome. QJM 2001;94:293.

Vlachogiannakos J et al: Angiotensin converting enzyme inhibitors and angiotensin II antagonists as therapy in chronic liver disease. Gut 2001;49:303.

BUDD-CHIARI SYNDROME

Budd-Chiari syndrome is a rare disorder resulting from obstruction of hepatic venous outflow, which can arise at several different levels, from the small hepatic venous tributaries within the liver parenchyma to the major hepatic venous trunks to the inferior vena cava up to the level of the right atrium. Most cases are caused by spontaneous thrombosis of the hepatic veins, often associated with myeloproliferative disorders (polycythemia vera, essential thrombocytosis) or the use of birth control pills. Other common associated conditions include factor V Leiden and factor II gene mutations. Other predisposing factors include protein C and S deficiencies, antiphospholipid syndrome, antithrombin III deficiency, paroxysmal nocturnal hemoglobinuria, Behçet syndrome, and trauma. Some patients present with idiopathic membranous stenosis of the inferior vena cava located between the hepatic veins and right atrium, which is usually associated with secondary thrombosis of the hepatic veins; this condition appears to be more common in Asia than in Western countries. Many patients with Budd-Chiari syndrome are HBsAg-positive, and others have malignancies (eg, hepatocellular carcinoma). Vena caval webs were once thought to be congenital, but more recent evidence suggests that they are the consequence of thrombus formation. Primary Budd-Chiari syndrome originates from within the lumen of the hepatic veins or venules, and occlusion results from thrombosis, webs, or endophlebitis. By contrast, secondary Budd-Chiari syndrome results from extrinsic compression of the venous outflow tract, usually related to a neoplasm or abscess.

Veno-occlusive disease and congestive hepatopathy are two conditions that can cause hepatic venous outflow obstruction, and although the clinical picture of both may be indistinguishable from that of Budd-Chiari syndrome, they differ in the level of obstruction and in predisposing conditions. Veno-occlusive disease is primarily a problem affecting the sinusoids and terminal venules, while congestive hepatopathy reflects a problem at the level of the heart.

Posthepatic (postsinusoidal) obstruction raises sinusoidal pressure, which is transmitted proximally to cause portal hypertension. Because the parenchyma is relatively free of fibrosis, filtration across the sinusoids and hepatic lymph formation increase greatly, producing marked ascites.

Symptoms usually begin with a mild prodrome consisting of vague right upper quadrant abdominal pain, postprandial bloating, and anorexia. After weeks or months, a more florid picture develops consisting of gross ascites, hepatomegaly, and hepatic failure. At this stage, the AST is usually markedly increased, the serum bilirubin is slightly elevated, and the alkaline phosphatase is inconsistently abnormal.

Except in patients with membranous obstruction of the vena cava, liver scans (CT or MRI) usually demonstrate a marked perfusion abnormality throughout most of the liver except for a small central area representing the caudate lobe, whose venous outflow is spared (it goes directly to the vena cava through multiple small tributaries). CT scans show pooling of intravenous contrast media in the periphery of the liver; patent hepatic veins cannot be seen on ultrasound scans. An enlarged azygos vein may be seen on chest x-rays of patients with caval obstruction. Liver biopsy reveals grossly dilated central veins and sinusoids, pericentral necrosis, and replacement of hepatocytes by red blood cells. Centrilobular fibrosis develops late. The clinical diagnosis should be confirmed by venography, which shows the hepatic veins to be obstructed, usually with a beaklike deformity at their orifice. The inferior vena cava should be opacified to verify its patency, which is a requirement for a successful portacaval shunt. Previously, direct venography was used, but the required information may now be obtained using noninvasive methods, such as CT or MR angiography. The x-rays may show compression of the intrahepatic cava by the congested liver.

In patients without cancer and in whom the obstruction is confined to the hepatic veins, a side-to-side portacaval or mesocaval shunt can be considered; TIPS is not an option in this situation because the hepatic veins are not patent. Focal membranous obstruction of the suprahepatic cava may be treated by excision of the lesion with or without the addition of a patch angioplasty. Some cases may be managed nonsurgically by percutaneous transluminal balloon dilation of the stenosis.

Occlusion of the inferior vena cava by thrombosis or compression from the liver requires a mesoatrial shunt using a prosthetic vascular graft. Because the incidence of graft thrombosis is relatively high, it may be advisable to perform a second-stage side-to-side portacaval shunt a few months after mesoatrial shunt decompression of the liver in patients with hepatic vein thrombosis whose vena cava was originally blocked by a congested liver. Development of hepatocellular carcinoma is common in patients with membranous obstruction of the vena cava. The postoperative results are excellent in patients without malignant neoplasms.

Liver transplantation is indicated in patients with advanced hepatic decompensation either from cirrhosis or as part of the acute syndrome. The results are excellent, and the risk of later hepatocellular carcinoma is eliminated.

Bayraktar UD, Seren S, Bayraktar Y: Hepatic venous outflow obstruction: three similar syndromes. World J Gastroenterol 2007;13:1912.

Garcia-Pagan JC et al: TIPS for Budd-Chiari syndrome: long-term results and prognostic factors in 124 patients. Gastroenterology 2008;135:808.

Horton JD, San Miguel FL, Ortiz JA: Budd Chiari syndrome: illustrated review of current management. Liver Int 2008; 28:455.

Olzinski AT, Sanyal AJ: Treating Budd-Chiari syndrome: making rational choices from a myriad of options. J Clin Gastroenterol 2000;30:155.

Orloff MJ et al: A 27-year experience with surgical treatment of Budd-Chiari syndrome. Ann Surg 2000;232:340.

ASCITES

Ascites is a common manifestation of chronic liver disease, resulting from sinusoidal hypertension as the specific pathophysiologic abnormality. Ascites in hepatic disease results from (1) increased formation of hepatic lymph (from sinusoidal hypertension), (2) increased formation of splanchnic lymph (from splanchnic vasodilatation), (3) hypoalbuminemia, and (4) salt and water retention by the kidneys. Before therapy is started, paracentesis should be performed and the following examinations made on a sample of ascitic fluid: (1) Culture and leukocyte count: Spontaneous bacterial peritonitis is common and may be clinically silent. A white count above 250/μL is highly suggestive of infection. (2) LDH levels: A ratio of LDH in ascites to serum that exceeds 0.6 suggests the presence of cancer or infection. (3) Serum amylase: A high level suggests pancreatic disease. (4) Albumin: The ratio of serum to ascites albumin concentrations is above 1.1 in liver disease and below 1.1 in malignant ascites. (5) Cytology: This is pertinent only in patients with a cancer diagnosis or a suspicion of cancer.

▶ Medical Treatment

In general, the intensity of medical therapy required to control ascites can be predicted from the pretreatment 24-hour urine Na^+ output as follows: A Na^+ output below 5 meq/24 h will require strong diuretics; 5–25 meq/24 h, mild diuretics; and above 25 meq/24 h, no diuretics. Initial treatment is usually with spironolactone, 200 mg/d. The objective is to stimulate a weight loss of 0.5–0.75 kg/d except in patients with peripheral edema who can mobilize fluid faster. If spironolactone alone is insufficient, another drug such as furosemide should be added. A loop diuretic (eg, furosemide, ethacrynic acid) should be given only in combination with a distally acting diuretic (eg, spironolactone, triamterene). Alternatively, massive ascites may be treated by one or more large volume (eg, 5-L) paracenteses; this is often accompanied by an intravenous infusion of albumin, although the benefits of albumin remain controversial. Close monitoring of serum electrolytes should be done. Salt or water restriction is recommended in refractory cases. Caution is required in patients with evidence of renal dysfunction, since aggressive fluid removal can result in renal failure.

▶ Surgical Treatment

A. Portacaval Shunt

A history of ascites that has been easy to control need not influence the choice of shunt operation intended to treat variceal bleeding. When ascites has been severe, however, a side-to-side shunt (eg, side-to-side portacaval, H-mesocaval, central splenorenal) may be considered, because it reduces sinusoidal as well as splanchnic venous pressure. A side-to-side portacaval shunt is rarely indicated just to treat ascites (eg, in patients in whom several LeVeen shunts have thrombosed), although the incidence of severe postoperative encephalopathy is high under these circumstances. TIPS is another effective intervention for refractory ascites, probably a better option than repeated paracentesis in good-risk patients, although there is an associated risk of hepatic encephalopathy.

B. Peritoneal-Jugular Shunt (LeVeen Shunt, Denver Shunt)

Refractory ascites can be treated with a LeVeen shunt—a subcutaneous Silastic catheter that transports ascitic fluid from the peritoneal cavity to the jugular vein. A small unidirectional valve sensitive to a pressure gradient of 3–5 cm H_2O prevents backflow of blood. A modification called the Denver shunt contains a small chamber that can be used as a pump to clear the line by external pressure. In practice, Denver shunts become blocked more often than LeVeen shunts.

In patients with ascites due to cirrhosis, use of a LeVeen shunt should be confined to those who fail to respond to high doses of diuretics (eg, 400 mg of spironolactone and 400 mg of furosemide daily) or who repeatedly develop encephalopathy or azotemia during diuretic therapy.

Peritoneovenous shunts may also be used for ascites associated with cancer. The best results occur in patients whose ascitic fluid contains no malignant cells. A LeVeen shunt is of benefit in Budd-Chiari syndrome but is ineffective for chylous ascites. Because the incidence of complications and early shunt thrombosis is high, a LeVeen shunt is relatively contraindicated if the ascitic fluid is grossly bloody, contains many malignant cells, or has a high protein concentration (> 4.5 g/dL). The incidence of tumor embolization is low (5%).

The ascitic fluid should be cultured a few days before the shunt is inserted. Antibiotic coverage should be given for the procedure. The operation can be done with local anesthesia.

Postoperatively, the patient is outfitted with an abdominal binder and instructed to perform respiratory exercises against mild pressure to increase abdominal pressure and flow through the shunt. Dietary salt should not be restricted. A functioning LeVeen shunt alone is unable to fully eliminate the ascites, but it improves symptoms related to distention and renders the patient much more responsive to diuretics. Therefore, furosemide should be administered postoperatively.

An average of 10 kg of weight is lost during the first 10 days after the operation, and eventually the abdomen assumes a normal configuration. Nutrition and serum albumin levels often improve postoperatively. Urinary sodium excretion increases promptly, and renal function may improve in patients with the hepatorenal syndrome. Serious complications and deaths are most common in patients with advanced hepatorenal syndrome or a serum bilirubin level greater than 4 mg/dL. Although some patients eventually bleed from varices following insertion of a LeVeen shunt, the shunt itself does not increase the risk of bleeding and actually decreases portal pressure. Thus, a previous episode of variceal bleeding is not a contraindication for this procedure.

Disseminated intravascular coagulation (manifested by increased fibrin split products, decreased platelet count, etc) occurs in more than half of cases but is clinically relevant in only a few. The frequency and severity of disseminated intravascular coagulation may be minimized by emptying most of the ascitic fluid from the abdomen during operation and partially replacing it with Ringer lactate solution. Lethal septicemia may occur if the ascitic fluid is infected at the time the shunt is inserted. In about 10% of cases, the valve becomes thrombosed and must be replaced.

Hydrothorax, usually on the right side, may develop in patients with cirrhosis and ascites. The fluid reaches the chest through a pinhole opening in the membranous portion of the diaphragm, a pathway that can be demonstrated by aspirating the thoracic fluid, injecting technetium ^{99m}Tc colloid into the ascites fluid, and observing rapid accumulation of the label in the chest. Treatment consists of a peritoneovenous shunt and injection of a sclerosing agent into the pleural cavity after it has been tapped dry. If a leak persists, it may be closed surgically by thoracotomy.

Helton WS et al: Transjugular intrahepatic portasystemic shunt vs surgical shunt in good-risk cirrhotic patients: a case-control comparison. Arch Surg 2001;136:17.

Krige JE, Beckingham IJ: ABC of diseases of liver, pancreas, and biliary system: portal hypertension-2. Ascites, encephalopathy, and other conditions. BMJ 2001;322:416.

Kuiper JJ, van Buuren HR, de Man RA: Ascites in cirrhosis: a review of management and complications. Neth J Med 2007;65:283.

Laffi G et al: Is the use of albumin of value in the treatment of ascites in cirrhosis? The case in favour. Dig Liv Dis 2003;35:660.

Rossle M et al: A comparison of paracentesis and transjugular intrahepatic portosystemic shunting in patients with ascites. N Engl J Med 2000;342:1701.

Suzuki H, Stanley AJ: Current management and novel therapeutic strategies for refractory ascites and hepatorenal syndrome. QJM 2001;94:293.

Zervos EE, Rosemurgy AS: Management of medically refractory ascites. Am J Surg 2001;181:256.

HEPATIC ENCEPHALOPATHY

Central nervous system abnormalities may be seen in patients with chronic liver disease and are especially likely after portocaval shunts. Portosystemic encephalopathy, ammonia intoxication, hepatic coma, and meat intoxication are older terms used to refer to this condition. The manifestations range from lethargy to coma—from minor personality changes to psychosis—from asterixis to paraplegia. Hypothermia and hyperventilation may precede coma. The changes may be quite subtle and detectable only with the use of neuropsychological or neurophysiological testing.

▶ Pathogenesis

Hepatic encephalopathy is a reversible metabolic neuropathy that results from the action of chemicals absorbed from the gut on the brain. Increased exposure of the brain to these agents is the result of impaired hepatic metabolism due to cirrhosis or spontaneous or surgically created shunts of portal venous blood around the liver and increased permeability of the blood-brain barrier. The chemical agents responsible for encephalopathy form from the action of colonic bacteria on protein within the gut. Potential aggravating factors include gastrointestinal hemorrhage, constipation, azotemia, hypokalemic alkalosis, infection, excessive dietary protein, and sedatives (Table 24–6). Four main chemical mediators of this syndrome currently attract the most attention. Low-grade cerebral edema appears to be a major component of the pathophysiologic process.

A. Amino Acid Neurotransmitters

Gamma-aminobutyric acid (GABA), the principal inhibitory neurotransmitter in the brain, produces a state similar to hepatic encephalopathy when given experimentally. It is normally synthesized in the brain and by bacteria within the colon; GABA in the gastrointestinal tract is normally degraded by the liver and is found in increased levels in the serum of patients with hepatic encephalopathy. The passage of GABA across the blood-brain barrier is increased in hepatic encephalopathy. Experiments also indicate the presence of increased numbers of GABA receptors in encephalopathy and increased GABA-ergic tone, perhaps due to a benzodiazepine receptor agonist ligand on the receptor complex (GABA/benzodiazepine receptor). This has raised the possibility of treating encephalopathy with benzodiazepine antagonists, and the drug flumazenil has shown promise in preliminary trials.

B. Ammonia

Ammonia is produced in the colon by bacteria and is absorbed and transported in portal venous blood to the liver, where it is extracted and converted to glutamine. Ammonia concentrations are elevated in the arterial blood and cerebrospinal fluid of patients with encephalopathy, and experimental administration of ammonia produces central nervous system symptoms.

C. False Neurotransmitters

According to this theory, cerebral neurons become depleted of normal neurotransmitters (norepinephrine and dopamine), which are partially replaced by false neurotransmitters (octopamine and phenylethanolamine). The result is inhibition of neural function. Serum levels of branched-chain amino acids (leucine, isoleucine, valine) are decreased, and levels of aromatic amino acids (tryptophan, phenylalanine, tyrosine) are elevated in patients with encephalopathy. Because these two classes of amino acids compete for transport across the blood-brain barrier, the aromatic amino acids have increased access to the central nervous system, where they serve as precursors for false neurotransmitters. Trials of therapy with supplements of branched-chain amino acids have given conflicting results.

Table 24–6. Factors Contributing to Encephalopathy.

A. Increased systemic toxin levels
1. Extent of portal-systemic venous shunt
2. Depressed liver function
3. Intestinal protein load
4. Intestinal flora
5. Azotemia
6. Constipation

B. Increased sensitivity of central nervous system
1. Age of patient
2. Hypokalemia
3. Alkalosis
4. Diuretics
5. Sedatives, narcotics, tranquilizers
6. Infection
7. Hypoxia, hypoglycemia, myxedema

D. Synergistic Neurotoxins

This theory postulates that ammonia, mercaptans, and fatty acids, none of which accumulate in the brain in amounts capable of producing encephalopathy, have synergistic effects that produce the full-blown syndrome in patients with liver disease.

▶ Prevention

Encephalopathy is a major side effect of portacaval shunt and is to some extent predictable. Elderly patients are considerably more susceptible. Patients with alcoholic liver disease fare better than those with postnecrotic or cryptogenic cirrhosis, apparently owing to the invariable progression of liver dysfunction in the latter. Good liver function partially protects against encephalopathy. If the liver has adapted to complete or nearly complete diversion of portal blood before operation, a surgical shunt is less apt to depress liver function further. For example, patients with thrombosis of the portal vein (complete diversion and normal liver function) rarely experience encephalopathy after portasystemic shunt. Encephalopathy is less common after a distal splenorenal (Warren) shunt than after other kinds of shunts.

Increased intestinal protein, whether of dietary origin or from intestinal bleeding, aggravates encephalopathy by providing more substrate for intestinal bacteria. Constipation allows more time for bacterial action on colonic contents. Azotemia results in higher concentration of blood urea, which diffuses into the intestine, is converted to ammonia, and is then reabsorbed. Hypokalemia and metabolic alkalosis aggravate encephalopathy by shifting ammonia from extracellular to intracellular sites where the toxic action occurs.

▶ Laboratory Findings

Arterial ammonia levels are usually high, although encephalopathy can certainly be present with a normal ammonia level. The presence of high levels of glutamine in the cerebrospinal fluid may help distinguish hepatic encephalopathy from other causes of coma. Electroencephalography is more sensitive than clinical evaluation in detecting minor involvement. The changes are nonspecific and consist of slower mean frequencies. Studies performed at different times can be compared to assess the effects of therapy.

▶ Treatment

Acute encephalopathy is treated by controlling precipitating factors, halting all dietary protein intake, cleansing the bowel with purgatives and enemas, and administering antibiotics (neomycin or ampicillin) or lactulose. Neomycin may be given orally or by gastric tube (two to four times daily) or rectally as an enema (1% solution one or two times daily). At least 1600 kcal of carbohydrate should be provided daily, along with therapeutic amounts of vitamins. Blood volume must be maintained to avoid prerenal azotemia. After the patient responds to initial therapy, dietary protein may be started at 20 g/d and increased by increments of 10–20 g every 2–5 days as tolerated.

Chronic encephalopathy is treated by restriction of dietary protein, avoidance of constipation, and elimination of sedatives, diuretics, and tranquilizers. To avoid protein depletion, protein intake must not be chronically reduced below 50 g/d. Vegetable protein in the diet is tolerated better than animal protein. Lactulose, a disaccharide unaffected by intestinal enzymes, is the drug of choice for long-term control. When given orally (20–30 g three or four times daily), it reaches the colon, where it stimulates bacterial anabolism (which increases ammonia uptake) and inhibits bacterial enzymes (which decreases the generation of nitrogenous toxins). Its effect is independent of colonic pH. A related compound outside the United States, lactitol (β-galactoside sorbitol), is also effective and appears to work faster. As a powder, it is easier to use than liquid lactulose. Intermittent courses of oral neomycin or metronidazole may be given if lactulose therapy and preventive measures are inadequate.

Butterworth RF: Hepatic encephalopathy: a neuropsychiatric disorder involving multiple neurotransmitter systems. Curr Opin Neurol 2000;13:727.
Haussinger D, Schliess F: Pathogenetic mechanisms of hepatic encephalopathy. Gut 2008;57:1156.
Lockwood AH: Early detection and treatment of hepatic encephalopathy. Curr Opin Neurol 1998;11:663.

HEPATIC ABSCESS

Hepatic abscesses may be bacterial, parasitic, or fungal in origin. In the United States, pyogenic abscesses are the most common, followed by amebic abscesses (see Chapter 8). Unless otherwise indicated, the remarks in this section refer to bacterial abscesses.

Cases are about evenly divided between those with a single abscess and those with multiple abscesses. About 90% of right lobe abscesses are solitary, while only 10% of left lobe abscesses are solitary.

In most cases, the development of a hepatic abscess follows a suppurative process elsewhere in the body. Many abscesses are due to direct spread from biliary infections such as empyema of the gallbladder or protracted cholangitis. Abdominal infections such as appendicitis or diverticulitis may spread through the portal vein to involve the liver with abscess formation. About 40% of patients have an underlying malignancy. Other cases develop after generalized sepsis from bacterial endocarditis, renal infection, or pneumonitis. In 25% of cases, no antecedent infection can be documented ("cryptogenic" abscesses). Rare causes include secondary bacterial infection of an amebic abscess, hydatid cyst, or congenital hepatic cyst.

In most cases, the organism is of enteric origin. *Escherichia coli, Klebsiella pneumoniae,* bacteroides, enterococci (eg, *Streptococcus faecalis*), anaerobic streptococci (eg, Peptostreptococcus), and microaerophilic streptococci are most common. Staphylococci, hemolytic streptococci, or other gram-positive organisms are usually found if the primary infection is bacterial endocarditis or pneumonitis.

▶ Clinical Findings

A. Symptoms and Signs

When liver abscess develops in the course of another intra-abdominal infection such as diverticulitis, it is accompanied by increasing toxicity, higher fever, jaundice, and a generally deteriorating clinical picture. Right upper quadrant pain and chills may appear.

In other cases, the diagnosis is much less obvious, since the illness develops insidiously in a previously healthy person. In these, the first symptoms are usually malaise and fatigue, followed after several weeks by fever. Epigastric or right upper quadrant pain is present in about half of cases. The pain may be aggravated by motion or may be referred to the right shoulder.

The course of fever is often erratic, and spikes to 40–41 °C are common. Chills are present in about 25% of cases. The liver is usually enlarged and may be tender to palpation. If tenderness is severe, the condition may be confused with cholecystitis.

Jaundice is unusual in solitary abscesses unless the patient's condition is worsening. Jaundice is often present in patients with multiple abscesses and primary disease in the biliary tree and in general is a bad prognostic sign.

B. Laboratory Findings

Leukocytosis is present in most cases and is usually over 15,000/µL. A small group of patients, usually the most seriously ill, may fail to develop leukocytosis. Anemia is present in most. The average hematocrit is 33%.

Serum bilirubin is usually normal except in patients with multiple abscesses or biliary obstruction or when hepatic failure has supervened. Alkaline phosphatase is often elevated even in the presence of a normal bilirubin.

C. Imaging Studies

X-ray changes present in the right lung in about one third of cases consist of basilar atelectasis or pleural effusion. The right diaphragm may be elevated and less mobile than the left.

Plain films of the abdomen are usually normal or show only hepatomegaly. In a few patients, an air-fluid level in the region of the liver reveals the presence and location of the abscess. Distortion of the contour of the stomach on upper gastrointestinal series may be seen with large abscesses involving the left lobe.

Ultrasound and CT scans are the most useful diagnostic tests, providing accurate information regarding the presence, size, number, and location of abscesses within the liver. CT scans have the added advantage of being able to demonstrate abscesses or neoplasms elsewhere in the abdomen. The radioisotope liver scintiscan is able to demonstrate most liver abscesses but is nonspecific, gives little other useful information, and is therefore not helpful.

Differential Diagnosis

In many cases, early findings may be so vague that hepatic abscess is not even considered. The multiple other causes of malaise, weight loss, and anemia would enter into the differential diagnosis. With spiking fevers, one must consider all the causes of fever of unknown origin. Failure to entertain the idea of hepatic abscess and to obtain the necessary scans leads to most errors in diagnosis.

Once imaging tests have demonstrated the abscess, the responsible organisms must be identified. Amebiasis should be considered in cases of a solitary abscess. Compared with amebic abscesses, pyogenic liver abscesses are seen more often in patients older than 50 years and are associated with jaundice, pruritus, sepsis, a palpable mass, and elevated bilirubin and alkaline phosphatase levels. Patients with amebic abscesses more often have been to an endemic area and have abdominal pain and tenderness, diarrhea, hepatomegaly, and positive serologic tests for amebiasis.

Complications

Intrahepatic spread of infection may create multiple additional abscesses and is responsible for some failures after treatment of an apparently solitary abscess. As the untreated abscess expands, rupture may occur into the pleural or peritoneal cavity, usually with catastrophic results. Septicemia and septic shock are common terminal complications of diffuse hepatic infection. Hepatic failure may develop in addition to uncontrolled sepsis, or it may predominate over signs of infection.

Hemobilia may follow bleeding from the vascular wall into the abscess cavity. In this case, hepatic artery embolization or ligation may be required to control bleeding.

Treatment

Antibiotics should be started promptly. Initial coverage, before culture results are available, should be adequate for *E coli, K pneumoniae,* bacteroides, enterococci, and yanaerobic streptococci and consequently would usually include an aminoglycoside, clindamycin or metronidazole, and ampicillin. The regimen may be modified later according to the results of cultures.

About 80% or more of patients with liver abscesses are adequately treated by drainage catheters inserted percutaneously under ultrasound or CT guidance. Whether the patient has a single abscess or multiple abscesses, this is usually the most appropriate initial therapy. The catheters can be removed in 1–2 weeks after output becomes nonpurulent and scant.

In about 40% of patients, the catheters do not drain well following initial placement and must be repositioned. The principal advantage of percutaneous drainage is lower morbidity compared to open drainage, although not necessarily lower mortality. It is easier to provide thorough drainage surgically, so when difficulties are encountered with percutaneous drainage, laparotomy should be performed promptly. Surgical intervention is more often necessary in cases of multiple, loculated collections or when the abscess cavity contains a large amount of necrotic debris. In such cases, open debridement should be considered early. Likewise, early surgical intervention is indicated for patients who are seriously ill (APACHE II score $\geq$ 15). Rarely, multiple abscesses are confined to a single lobe and can be cured by lobectomy. Biliary obstruction or other causes of sepsis must also be corrected.

Prognosis

The overall mortality rate of 15% is more closely related to the underlying disease than to any other factor. The mortality rate is about 40% in patients with malignant disease. Pleural effusion, leukocytosis over 20,000/μL, hypoalbuminemia, and polymicrobial infection correlate with a poor outcome. In the United States, whether the abscess is solitary or multiple no longer has a major influence on survival, but where benign biliary disease remains a major cause of this disease, multiple hepatic abscesses are associated with a worse prognosis. Death is rare in patients with a cryptogenic liver abscess.

Chen SC et al: Predictors of mortality in patients with pyogenic liver abscess. Neth J Med 2008;66:183.

Hsieh HF et al: Aggressive hepatic resection for patients with pyogenic liver abscess and APACHE II score $\geq$ 15. Am J Surg 2008;196:346.

Johannsen EC, Sifri CD, Madoff LC: Pyogenic liver abscesses. Infect Dis Clin North Am 2000;14:547.

Molle I et al: Increased risk and case fatality rate of pyogenic liver abscess in patients with liver cirrhosis: a nationwide study in Denmark. Gut 2001;48:260.

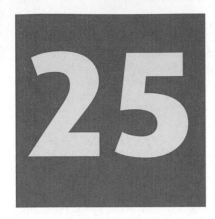

25

Biliary Tract

Gerard M. Doherty, MD

EMBRYOLOGY & ANATOMY

The anlage of the biliary ducts and liver consists of a diverticulum that appears on the ventral aspect of the foregut in 3 mm embryos. The cranial portion becomes the liver, a caudal bud forms the ventral pancreas, and an intermediate bud develops into the gallbladder. Originally hollow, the hepatic diverticulum becomes a solid mass of cells that later recanalizes to form the ducts. The smallest ducts—the bile canaliculi—are first seen as a basal network between the primitive hepatocytes that eventually expands throughout the liver (Figure 25–1). Numerous microvilli increase the canalicular surface area. Bile secreted here passes through the interlobular ductules (canals of Hering) and the lobar ducts and then into the hepatic duct in the hilum. In most cases, the common hepatic duct is formed by the union of a single right and left duct, but in 25% of individuals, the anterior and posterior divisions of the right duct join the left duct separately. The origin of the common hepatic duct is close to the liver but always outside its substance. It runs about 4 cm before joining the cystic duct to form the common bile duct. The common duct begins in the hepatoduodenal ligament, passes behind the first portion of the duodenum, and runs in a groove on the posterior surface of the pancreas before entering the duodenum. Its terminal 1 cm is intimately adherent to the duodenal wall. The total length of the common duct is about 9 cm.

In 80–90% of individuals, the main pancreatic duct joins the common duct to form a common channel about 1 cm long. The intraduodenal segment of the duct is called the hepatopancreatic ampulla, or ampulla of Vater.

The gallbladder is a pear-shaped organ adherent to the undersurface of the liver in a groove separating the right and left lobes. The fundus projects 1–2 cm below the hepatic edge and can often be felt when the cystic or common duct is obstructed. It rarely has a complete peritoneal covering, but when this variation does occur, it predisposes to infarction by torsion. The gallbladder holds about 50 mL of bile when fully distended. The neck of the gallbladder tapers into the narrow cystic duct, which connects with the common duct. The lumen of the cystic duct contains a thin mucosal septum, the spiral valve of Heister, which offers mild resistance to bile flow. In 75% of persons, the cystic duct enters the common duct at an angle. In the remainder, it runs parallel to the hepatic duct or winds around it before joining the common duct (Figure 25–2).

In the hepatoduodenal ligament, the hepatic artery is to the left of the common duct and the portal vein is posterior and medial. The right hepatic artery usually passes behind the hepatic duct and then gives off the cystic artery before entering the right lobe of the liver, but variations are common.

The mucosal epithelium of the bile ducts varies from cuboidal in the ductules to columnar in the main ducts. The gallbladder mucosa is thrown into prominent ridges when the organ is collapsed, and these flatten during distention. The tall columnar cells of the gallbladder mucosa are covered by microvilli on their luminal surface. Wide channels, which play an important role in water and electrolyte absorption, separate the individual cells.

The walls of the bile ducts contain only small amounts of smooth muscle, but the termination of the common duct is enveloped by a complex sphincteric muscle. The gallbladder musculature is composed of interdigitated bundles of longitudinal and spirally arranged fibers.

The biliary tree receives parasympathetic and sympathetic innervation. The former contains motor fibers to the gallbladder and secretory fibers to the ductal epithelium. The afferent fibers in the sympathetic nerves mediate the pain of biliary colic.

PHYSIOLOGY

▶ Bile Flow

Bile is produced at a rate of 500–1500 mL/d by the hepatocytes and the cells of the ducts. Active secretion of bile salts into the biliary canaliculus is responsible for most of the

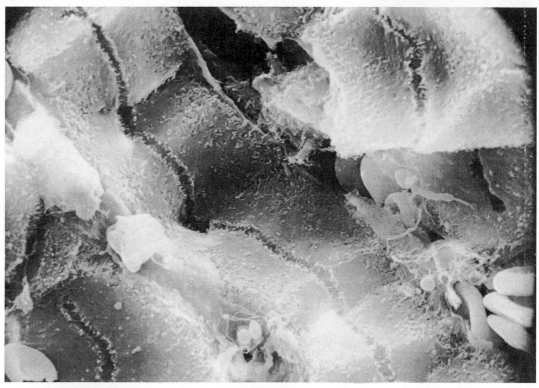

▲ **Figure 25–1.** Scanning electron photomicrograph of a hepatic plate with adjacent sinusoids and sinusoidal microvilli and a bile canaliculus running in the center of the liver cells. Although their boundaries are indistinct, about four hepatocytes constitute the section of the plate in the middle of the photograph. Occasional red cells are present within the sinusoids. (Reduced from × 2000.) (Courtesy of Dr James Boyer.)

volume of bile and its fluctuations. Na^+ and water follow passively to establish isosmolality and electrical neutrality. Lecithin and cholesterol enter the canaliculus at rates that correlate with variations in bile salt output. Bilirubin and a number of other organic anions (estrogens, sulfobromophthalein, etc) are actively secreted by the hepatocyte by a different transport system from that which handles bile salts.

The columnar cells of the ducts add a fluid rich in HCO_3^- to that produced in the canaliculus. This involves active secretion of Na^+ and HCO_3^- by a cellular pump stimulated by secretin, vasoactive intestinal polypeptide (VIP), and cholecystokinin. K^+ and water are distributed passively across the ducts (Figure 25–3).

Between meals, bile is stored in the gallbladder, where it is concentrated at rates of up to 20% per hour. Na^+ and either HCO_3^- or Cl^- are actively transported from its lumen during absorption. The changes in composition brought about by concentration are shown in Figure 25–4.

Three factors regulate bile flow: hepatic secretion, gallbladder contraction, and choledochal sphincteric resistance. In the fasting state, pressure in the common bile duct is 5–10 cm H_2O, and bile produced in the liver is diverted into the gallbladder. After a meal, the gallbladder contracts, the sphincter relaxes, and bile is forced into the duodenum in squirts as ductal pressure intermittently exceeds sphincteric resistance. During contraction, pressure within the gallbladder reaches 25 cm H_2O, and that in the common bile duct reaches 15–20 cm H_2O.

Cholecystokinin (CCK) is the major physiologic stimulus for postprandial gallbladder contraction and relaxation of the sphincter, but vagal impulses facilitate its action. CCK is released into the bloodstream from the mucosa of the small bowel by fat or lipolytic products in the lumen. Amino acids and small polypeptides are weaker stimuli, and carbohydrates are ineffective. Bile flow during a meal is augmented by turnover of bile salts in the enterohepatic circulation and stimulation of ductal secretion by secretin, VIP, and CCK. Motilin stimulates episodic partial gallbladder emptying in the interdigestive phase.

► Bile Salts & the Enterohepatic Circulation

Bile salts, lecithin, and cholesterol comprise about 90% of the solids in bile, the remainder consisting of bilirubin, fatty

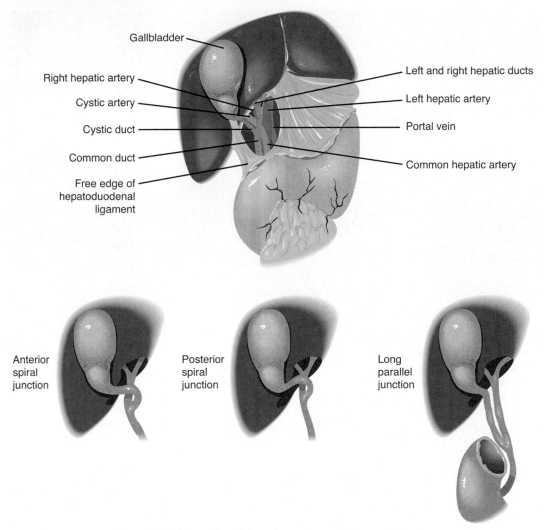

▲ Figure 25–2. Anatomy of the gallbladder and variations in anatomy of the cystic duct.

acids, and inorganic salts. Gallbladder bile contains about 10% solids and has a bile salt concentration between 200 and 300 mmol/L (Figure 25–4).

Bile salts are steroid molecules formed from cholesterol by hepatocytes. The rate of synthesis is under feedback control and can be increased a maximum of about 20-fold. Two **primary** bile salts—cholate and chenodeoxycholate—are produced by the liver. Before excretion into bile, they are conjugated with either glycine or taurine, which enhances water solubility. Intestinal bacteria alter these compounds to produce the **secondary** bile salts, deoxycholate and lithocholate. The former is reabsorbed and enters bile, but lithocholate is insoluble and is excreted in the stool. Bile is composed of 40% cholate, 40% chenodeoxy-

cholate, and 20% deoxycholate, conjugated with glycine or taurine in a ratio of 3:1.

The functions of bile salts are (1) to induce the flow of bile, (2) to transport lipids, and (3) to bind calcium ions in bile. The importance of the last of these is unknown. Bile acid molecules are amphipathic (ie, they have hydrophilic and hydrophobic poles). In bile, they form multimolecular aggregates called micelles in which the hydrophilic poles become aligned to face the aqueous medium. Water-insoluble lipids, such as cholesterol, can be dissolved within the hydrophobic centers of bile salt micelles. Molecules of lecithin, a water-insoluble but polar lipid, aggregate into hydrated bilayers that form vesicles in bile, and they also become incorporated into bile acid micelles to form mixed micelles. Mixed micelles

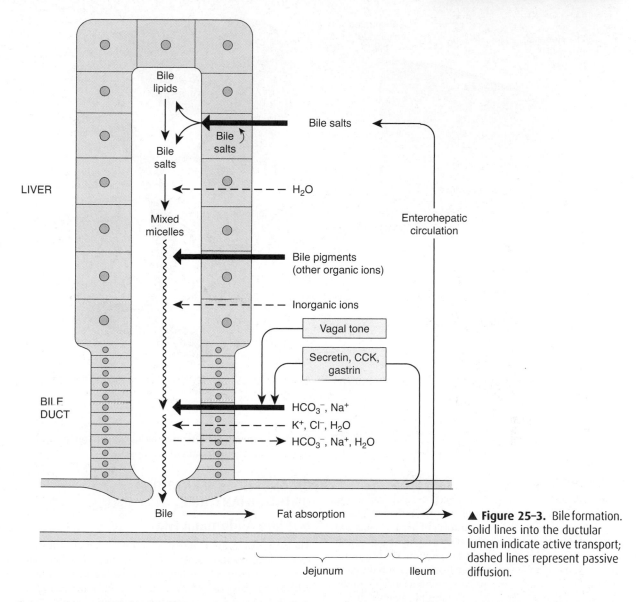

▲ Figure 25–3. Bile formation. Solid lines into the ductular lumen indicate active transport; dashed lines represent passive diffusion.

have an increased lipid-carrying capacity compared with pure bile acid micelles. Cholesterol in bile is transported within the phospholipid vesicles and the bile salt micelles.

Bile salts remain in the intestinal lumen throughout the jejunum, where they participate in fat digestion and absorption (Figure 25–5). Upon reaching the distal small bowel, they are reabsorbed by an active transport system located in the terminal 200 cm of ileum. Over 95% of bile salts arriving from the jejunum are transferred by this process into portal vein blood; the remainder enter the colon, where they are converted to secondary bile salts. The entire bile salt pool of 2.5–4 g circulates twice through the enterohepatic circulation during each meal, and six to eight

cycles are made each day. The normal daily loss of bile salts in the stool amounts to 10–20% of the pool and is restored by hepatic synthesis.

Arias IM et al: The biology of the bile canaliculus. Hepatology 1993;17:318.

Gustafsson U, Sahlin S, Finarsson C: Biliary lipid composition in patients with cholesterol and pigment gallstones and gallstone-free subjects: deoxycholic acid does not contribute to formation of cholesterol gallstones. Eur J Clin Invest 2000;30:1099.

Hofmann AF: The continuing importance of bile acids in liver and intestinal disease. Arch Intern Med 1999;159:2647.

Kullak-Ublick GA: Regulation of organic anion and drug transporters of the sinusoidal membrane. J Hepatol 1999;31:563.

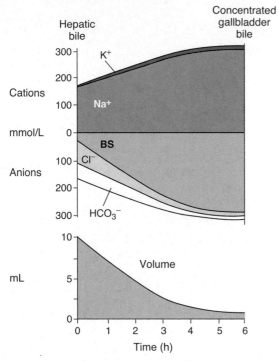

▲ Figure 25–4. Changes in gallbladder bile composition with time. (Courtesy of J Dietschy.)

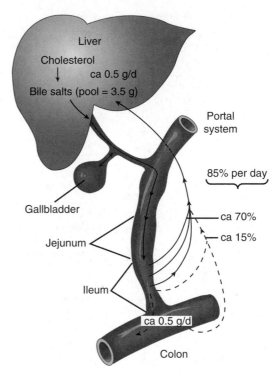

▲ Figure 25–5. Enterohepatic circulation of bile salts. (Courtesy of M Tyor.)

Sahin M et al: Effect of octreotide (Sandostatin 201-995) on bile flow and bile components. Dig Dis Sci 1999;44:181.

▶ Bilirubin

About 250–300 mg of bilirubin is excreted each day in the bile, 75% of it from breakdown of red cells in the reticuloendothelial system and 25% from turnover of hepatic heme and hemoproteins. First, heme is liberated from hemoglobin, and the iron and globin are removed for reuse by the organism. Biliverdin, the first pigment formed from heme, is reduced to unconjugated bilirubin, the indirect-reacting bilirubin of the van den Bergh test. Unconjugated bilirubin is insoluble in water and is transported in plasma bound to albumin.

Unconjugated bilirubin is extracted from blood by hepatocytes, where it is conjugated with glucuronic acid to form bilirubin diglucuronide, the water-soluble direct bilirubin. Conjugation is catalyzed by glucuronyl transferase, an enzyme on the endoplasmic reticulum. Bilirubin is transported within the hepatocyte by cytosolic binding proteins, which rapidly deliver the molecule to the canalicular membrane for active secretion into bile. Within bile, conjugated bilirubin is largely transported in association with mixed lipid micelles.

After entering the intestine, bilirubin is reduced by intestinal bacteria to several compounds known as urobilinogens, which are subsequently oxidized and converted to pigmented urobilins. The term urobilinogen is often used to refer to both urobilins and urobilinogens.

DIAGNOSTIC EXAMINATION OF THE BILIARY TREE

▶ Plain Abdominal Film

The posteroanterior supine view of the abdomen will show gallstones in the 10–15% of cases where they are radiopaque. The bile itself sometimes contains sufficient calcium (milk of calcium bile) to be seen. An enlarged gallbladder can occasionally be identified as a soft tissue mass in the right upper quadrant indenting an air-filled hepatic flexure.

In several types of biliary disease, the diagnosis may be suggested by air seen in the bile ducts on a plain film. This usually signifies the presence of a biliary-intestinal fistula (from disease or surgery) but also occurs rarely in severe cholangitis, emphysematous cholecystitis, and biliary ascariasis.

▶ Oral Cholecystography

Tyropanoate sodium or iopanoic acid is taken orally the night before the examination, along with a light meal. The drug is absorbed, bound to albumin in portal blood, extracted by hepatocytes, and secreted in bile. Opacification occurs only with concentration in the gallbladder and on the average is optimal 10 hours after tyropanoate ingestion. Posteroanterior and oblique supine views and an upright or lateral decubitus film are obtained.

Oral cholecystograms are unsatisfactory if the contrast agent is inefficiently absorbed from the intestine or poorly excreted by the liver. Absorption is often impaired in acute abdominal illnesses with ileus, vomiting, or diarrhea. If the bilirubin level is over 3 mg/dL, hepatic excretion will probably be inadequate. False-negative results are obtained in 5% of tests. A normal gallbladder may not opacify for several weeks after severe trauma or a major illness.

Nonopacification occurs in 20% of patients after the usual single-dose regimen. When a second dose is given and x-rays repeated the following day, opacification is obtained in 25% of these patients. Persistent nonopacification is a highly reliable (> 95% true positive) indication of gallbladder disease. Instead of performing a double-dose oral cholecystogram as the next step when a single dose fails to opacify, it is simpler to obtain an ultrasound scan.

▶ Percutaneous Transhepatic Cholangiography (THC, PTC)

Percutaneous transhepatic cholangiography is performed by passing a fine needle through the right lower rib cage and the hepatic parenchyma and into the lumen of a bile duct. Water-soluble contrast material is injected, and x-ray films are taken.

The technical success is related to the degree of dilatation of the intrahepatic bile ducts. THC is especially valuable in demonstrating the biliary anatomy in patients with benign biliary strictures, malignant lesions of the proximal bile duct, or when endoscopic retrograde cholangiopancreatography (ERCP; see next section) has been unsuccessful. Failure of the contrast medium to enter a duct does not prove that obstruction is absent. THC should not be done in patients with cholangitis until the infection has been controlled with antibiotics. Virtually all patients should be premedicated with antibiotics regardless of whether they have cholangitis—septic shock has been produced by sudden inoculation of organisms from bile into the systemic circulation. Otherwise, the contraindications are the same as for percutaneous liver biopsy.

▶ Endoscopic Retrograde Cholangiopancreatography (ERCP)

ERCP involves cannulating the sphincter of Oddi under direct vision through a side-viewing duodenoscope. It requires special training involving more than familiarity with the use of fiberoptic endoscopes. Usually, it is possible to opacify the pancreatic as well as the bile ducts. It is usually the preferred method of examining the biliary tree in patients with presumed choledocholithiasis or obstructing lesions in the periampullary region.

▶ Ultrasound

Ultrasonography is both sensitive and specific in detecting gallbladder stones and dilatation of bile ducts. In the investigation of gallbladder disease, false-positive diagnoses for stones are rare, and false-negative reports owing to small stones or a contracted gallbladder occur in only 5% of patients examined by real-time ultrasound. Ultrasound usually misses stones in the common duct.

Dilatation of bile ducts in a jaundiced patient indicates bile duct obstruction, but it is fairly common for the ducts to be normal in the presence of obstruction. When ultrasound shows dilated ducts, THC will nearly always be technically successful.

The ultrasonographer occasionally reports that the gallbladder contains "sludge." This material is sonographically opaque, does not cast an acoustic shadow, and forms a dependent layer in the gallbladder. On clinical analysis, it is a fine precipitate of calcium bilirubinate. Sludge may accompany gallstone disease or may be a solitary finding. It is seen in a variety of clinical settings, many of which are characterized by gallbladder stasis (eg, prolonged fasting). By itself, sludge is not an indication for cholecystectomy.

▶ Radionuclide Scan (HIDA Scan)

Technetium 99m-labeled derivatives of iminodiacetic acid (IDA) are excreted in high concentration in bile and produce excellent gamma camera images. Following intravenous injection of the radionuclide, imaging of the bile ducts and gallbladder normally appears within 15–30 minutes and of the intestine within 60 minutes. In patients with acute right upper quadrant pain and tenderness, a good image of the bile duct accompanied by no image of the gallbladder indicates cystic duct obstruction and strongly supports a diagnosis of acute cholecystitis. The test is easy to perform and is occasionally a useful method of confirming this diagnosis.

JAUNDICE

Jaundice is categorized as prehepatic, hepatic, or posthepatic, depending upon the site of the underlying disease. Hemolysis, the most common cause of prehepatic jaundice, involves increased production of bilirubin. Less common causes of prehepatic jaundice are Gilbert disease and the Crigler-Najjar syndrome.

Hepatic parenchymal jaundice is subdivided into hepatocellular and cholestatic types. The former includes acute viral hepatitis and chronic alcoholic cirrhosis. Some cases of intrahepatic cholestasis may be indistinguishable clinically and biochemically from cholestasis due to bile duct obstruction. Primary biliary cirrhosis, toxic drug jaundice, cholestatic jaundice of pregnancy, and postoperative cholestatic jaundice are the most common forms.

Extrahepatic jaundice most often results from biliary obstruction by a malignant tumor, choledocholithiasis, or biliary stricture. Pancreatic pseudocyst, chronic pancreatitis, sclerosing cholangitis, metastatic cancer, and duodenal diverticulitis are less common causes.

The cause of jaundice can be ascertained in the majority of patients from clinical and laboratory findings alone. In the remainder, THC or ERCP and ultrasound or CT scans will be necessary. The indications for these tests are discussed in later sections.

History

The age, sex, and parity of the patient and possible deleterious habits should be noted. Most cases of infectious hepatitis occur in patients under age 30. A history of drug addiction may suggest serum hepatitis transmitted by shared hypodermic equipment. Chronic alcoholism can usually be documented in patients with cirrhosis, and acute jaundice in alcoholics usually follows a recent binge. Obstructing gallstones or tumors are more common in older people.

Patients with jaundice due to choledocholithiasis may have associated biliary colic, fever, and chills and may report previous similar attacks. The pain in malignant obstruction is deepseated and dull and may be affected by changes in position. Pain in the region of the liver is frequently experienced in the early stages of viral hepatitis and acute alcoholic liver injury. The patient with extrahepatic obstruction may report that stools have become lighter in color and the urine dark.

Cholestatic diseases are often accompanied by pruritus—a source of severe discomfort in some cases. Pruritus may precede jaundice, but usually it appears at about the same time. The itching is most severe on the extremities and is aggravated by warm, humid weather. The cause remains obscure; itching does not correlate with bile salt levels in the skin, as was once believed. Cholestyramine, an anion exchange resin, usually provides relief by binding bile salts in the intestinal lumen and preventing their reabsorption.

Physical Examination

Hepatomegaly is common in both hepatic and posthepatic jaundice. In some cases, palpation of the liver may suggest cirrhosis or metastatic cancer, but impressions of this kind are unreliable. Secondary stigmas of cirrhosis usually accompany acute alcoholic jaundice; liver palms, spider angiomas, ascites, collateral veins on the abdominal walls, and splenomegaly suggest cirrhosis. A nontender, palpable gallbladder in a jaundiced patient suggests malignant obstruction of the common duct (Courvoisier law), but absence of a palpable gallbladder is of little significance in ruling out cancer.

Laboratory Tests

In hemolytic disease, the increased bilirubin is principally in the unconjugated indirect fraction. Since unconjugated bilirubin is insoluble in water, the jaundice in hemolysis is acholuric. The total bilirubin in hemolysis rarely exceeds 4–5 mg/dL, because the rate of excretion increases as the bilirubin

concentration rises, and a plateau is quickly reached. Greater values suggest concomitant hepatic parenchymal disease.

Jaundice due to hepatic parenchymal disease is characterized by elevations of both conjugated and unconjugated serum bilirubin. An increase in the conjugated fraction always signifies disease within the hepatobiliary system. The direct bilirubin predominates in about half of cases of hepatic parenchymal disease.

Both intrahepatic cholestasis and extrahepatic obstruction raise the direct bilirubin fraction, though the indirect fraction also increases somewhat. Since direct bilirubin is water-soluble, bilirubinuria develops. With complete extrahepatic obstruction, the total bilirubin rises to a plateau of 25–30 mg/dL, at which point loss in the urine equals the additional daily production. Higher values suggest concomitant hemolysis or decreased renal function. Obstruction of a single hepatic duct does not usually cause jaundice.

In extrahepatic obstruction caused by neoplasms, the serum bilirubin usually exceeds 10 mg/dL, and the average concentration is about 18 mg/dL. Obstructive jaundice due to common duct stones often produces transient bilirubin increases in the range of 2–4 mg/dL, and the level rarely exceeds 15 mg/dL. Serum bilirubin values in patients with alcoholic cirrhosis and acute viral hepatitis vary widely in relation to the severity of the parenchymal damage.

In extrahepatic obstruction, modest rises of aspartate aminotransferase (AST) levels are common, but levels as high as 1000 units/L are seen (though rarely) in patients with common duct stones and cholangitis. In the latter patients, the high values last for only a few days and are associated with increases in lactate dehydrogenase (LDH) concentrations. In general, AST levels above 1000 units/L suggest viral hepatitis.

Serum alkaline phosphatase comes from three sites: liver, bone, and intestine. In normal subjects, liver and bone contribute about equally, and the intestinal contribution is small. Hepatic alkaline phosphatase is a product of the epithelial cells of the cholangioles, and increased alkaline phosphatase levels associated with liver disease are the result of increased enzyme production. Alkaline phosphatase levels go up with intrahepatic cholestasis, cholangitis, or extrahepatic obstruction. Since the elevation is from overproduction, it may occur with focal hepatic lesions in the absence of jaundice. For example, a solitary hepatic metastasis or pyogenic abscess in one lobe or a tumor obstructing only one hepatic duct may fail to obstruct enough hepatic parenchyma to cause jaundice but usually is associated with increased alkaline phosphatase. In cholangitis with incomplete extrahepatic obstruction, serum bilirubin levels may be normal or mildly elevated, but serum alkaline phosphatase may be very high.

Bone disease may complicate the interpretation of abnormal alkaline phosphatase levels (Figure 25–6). If one suspects that the increased serum enzyme may be from bone, serum calcium, phosphorus, and 5'-nucleotidase or leucine aminopeptidase levels should be determined. These last two

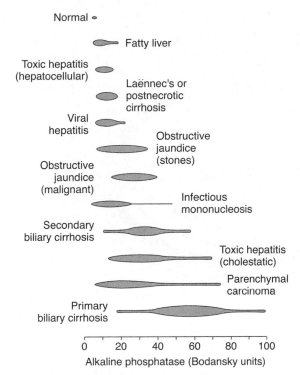

▲ Figure 25–6. Range of alkaline phosphatase values in various hepatobiliary disorders.

enzymes are also produced by cholangioles and are elevated in cholestasis, but their serum concentrations remain unchanged with bone disease.

Changes in serum protein levels may reflect hepatic parenchymal dysfunction. In cirrhosis, the serum albumin falls and the globulins increase. Serum globulins reach high values in some patients with primary biliary cirrhosis. Biliary obstruction generally produces no changes unless secondary biliary cirrhosis has developed.

▶ Diagnosis

The principal diagnostic objective is to distinguish surgical (obstructive) from nonsurgical jaundice. The history, physical examination, and basic laboratory data allow an accurate diagnosis to be made in most cases without invasive tests (eg, liver biopsy, cholangiograms).

Since most jaundiced patients are not critically ill when first seen, diagnosis and therapy may be conducted in a stepwise fashion, with each test selected according to the information available at that point. Only severe or worsening cholangitis requires urgent intervention. If the jaundice is mild and recent, it often passes within 24–48 hours, at which time an oral cholecystogram or ultrasound scan can be ordered to verify gallstone disease.

In patients with persistent jaundice, the first test is usually an ultrasound scan, which may show dilated intrahepatic bile ducts (indicating ductal obstruction) or gallbladder stones. The lesion may be further delineated by ERCP or THC. ERCP is preferable when the lower end of the duct is thought to be obstructed (eg, suspected carcinoma of the pancreas or other periampullary tumors). THC is usually preferred for proximal lesions (eg, biliary stricture, neoplasm of the bifurcation of the hepatic ducts), because it gives better opacification of the ducts proximal to the obstruction and therefore provides more information that can be used in planning surgery. If the clinical presentation suggests neoplastic obstruction, a CT scan could be selected in preference to an ultrasound scan, because CT gives better definition of mass lesions while also demonstrating the presence and general location of bile duct obstruction.

If ultrasound or CT scans suggest biliary obstruction, a decision must be made about whether cholangiograms are indicated. In general, patients with gallstone disease do not require preoperative cholangiograms, whereas cholangiograms would be routine in patients with neoplastic obstruction, benign biliary stricture, or rare or unknown causes of obstructive jaundice.

PATHOGENESIS OF GALLSTONES

More than 20 million people in the United States have gallstones in their gallbladders; about 300,000 operations are performed annually for this disease, and at least 6000 deaths result from its complications or treatment. The incidence of gallstones rises with age, so that between 50 and 65 years of age, about 20% of women and 5% of men are affected (Figure 25–7).

The gallstones in 75% of patients are composed predominantly (70–95%) of cholesterol and are called cholesterol stones. The remaining 25% are pigment stones. Regardless of composition, all gallstones give rise to similar clinical sequelae.

▶ Cholesterol Gallstones

Cholesterol gallstones result from secretion by the liver of bile supersaturated with cholesterol. Influenced by various factors present in bile, the cholesterol precipitates from solution and the newly formed crystals grow to macroscopic stones. Except when the common bile duct is dilated or partially obstructed, the stones in this disease form almost exclusively within the gallbladder. Those found in the ducts usually reach that location after passing through the cystic duct.

The incidence of cholesterol gallstone disease is highest in Native Americans, lower in Caucasians, and lowest in blacks, with a twofold gradient from one group to the next. More than 75% of Native American women over age 40 are affected. Before puberty, the disease is rare but of equal frequency in both sexes. Thereafter, women are more commonly affected than men until after menopause, when the

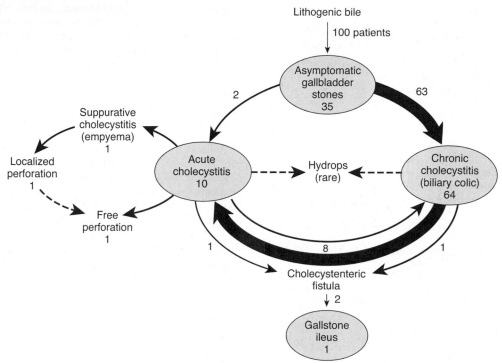

▲ **Figure 25–7.** The natural history of gallbladder stones. The numbers approximate the percentage of patients in each category. Note that most patients with acute cholecystitis have previously had biliary colic.

discrepancy lessens. Hormonal effects are also reflected in the increased incidence of gallstones with multiparity and the increased cholesterol saturation of bile and greater incidence of gallstones following ingestion of oral contraceptives. Obesity is the other major risk factor. The relative risk rises proportionately to the extent of overweight due to a progressively increasing output of cholesterol in bile.

As noted previously, cholesterol is insoluble and in bile must be transported within bile salt micelles and phospholipid (lecithin) vesicles. When the amount of cholesterol in bile exceeds the cholesterol holding capacity, cholesterol crystals begin to precipitate from the phospholipid vesicles.

The secretion of bile salt and cholesterol into bile is linked. Bile salt elutes cholesterol from the hepatocyte membrane during passage into the bile canaliculus. At higher bile salt output levels, the amount of cholesterol relative to bile salt entering bile decreases. This means that during low bile flow (eg, during fasting), bile holding capacity for cholesterol is more saturated than during high bile flow. In fact, almost half of persons in Western cultures have bile supersaturated with cholesterol in the morning after an overnight fast. The bile salt pool in patients with cholesterol gallstone disease is about half the size of that of normal subjects, but this is a result of the gallstone disease (eg, gallstones displace bile in the gallbladder) and not a cause.

The occurrence of cholesterol gallstone disease requires cholesterol supersaturation of bile, but that in itself is not sufficient. Cholesterol in supersaturated bile from individuals without gallstone disease precipitates spontaneously at a much slower rate than does the cholesterol in similar bile from patients with gallstones. Furthermore, among individuals with supersaturated bile, only those with gallstone disease demonstrate cholesterol crystal formation in vivo. These observations are the result of specific bile proteins that either stabilize or destabilize cholesterol-laden phospholipid vesicles. For gallstone formation, the pronucleating factors (eg, immunoglobulin, mucus glycoprotein, fibronectin, orosomucoid) appear to be more important than the antinucleating factors (eg, glycoprotein, apolipoprotein, cytokeratin). Variations in these proteins may be the critical factor determining which of the many individuals with saturated bile develop gallstones.

The fact that gallstones form almost exclusively in the gallbladder even though the composition of hepatic bile is abnormal underscores the important role of the gallbladder in gallstone pathogenesis. This includes concentrating the bile, providing nidi (eg, small grains of pigment) for crystallization of cholesterol, supplying mucoprotein to paste the stones together, and serving as an area of stasis to allow stone formation and growth.

▶ Pigment Stones

Pigment stones account for 25% of gallstones in the United States and 60% of those in Japan. Pigment stones are black to dark brown, 2–5 mm in diameter, and amorphous. They are composed of a mixture of calcium bilirubinate, complex bilirubin polymers, bile acids, and other unidentified substances. About 50% are radiopaque, and in the United States they constitute two thirds of all radiopaque gallstones. The incidence is similar in men and women and in blacks and whites. Pigment stones are rare in Native Americans.

Predisposing factors are cirrhosis, bile stasis (eg, a strictured or markedly dilated common duct), and chronic hemolysis. Some patients with pigment stones have increased concentrations of unconjugated bilirubin in their bile. Scanning electron microscopy demonstrates that about 90% of pigment stones are composed of dense mixtures of bacteria and bacterial glycocalix along with pigment solids. This suggests that bacteria have a primary role in pigment gallstone formation, and it also helps to explain why patients with pigment gallstone disease have sepsis more often than do those with cholesterol gallstone disease. It seems likely that bacterial β-glucuronidase is responsible for deconjugating the soluble bilirubin-diglucuronide to insoluble unconjugated bilirubin, which subsequently becomes agglomerated by glycocalix into macroscopic stones.

Beckingham IJ: ABC of diseases of liver, pancreas, and biliary system. Gallstone disease. BMJ 2001;322:91.

Caroli-Bosc FX et al: Cholelithiasis and dietary risk factors: an epidemiologic investigation in Vidauban, Southeast France. General Practitioner's Group of Vidauban. Dig Dis Sci 1998;43:2131.

Cicala M et al: Increased sphincter of Oddi basal pressure in patients affected by gall stone disease: a role for biliary stasis and colicky pain? Gut 2001;48:414.

Glasgow RE et al: The spectrum and cost of complicated gallstone disease in California. Arch Surg 2000;135:1021.

Han T et al: Apolipoprotein B-100 gene Xba I polymorphism and cholesterol gallstone disease. Clin Genet 2000;57:304.

Ko CW, Sekijima JH, Lee SP: Biliary sludge. Ann Intern Med 1999;130(4 Part 1):301.

Wells JE et al: Isolation and characterization of cholic acid 7alpha-dehydroxylating fecal bacteria from cholesterol gallstone patients. J Hepatol 2000;32:4.

Zapata R et al: Gallbladder motility and lithogenesis in obese patients during diet-induced weight loss. Dig Dis Sci 2000; 45:421.

▼ DISEASES OF THE GALLBLADDER & BILE DUCTS

ASYMPTOMATIC GALLSTONES

Data on the prevalence of gallstones in the United States indicate that only about 30% of people with cholelithiasis come to surgery. Symptoms of gallstone disease generally do not change in severity. Each year, about 2% of patients with asymptomatic gallstones develop symptoms, usually biliary colic rather than one of the complications of gallstone disease. Patients with chronic colic tend to have symptoms of the same level of severity and frequency. The present practice of operating only on symptomatic patients, leaving the millions without symptoms alone, seems appropriate. A question is often raised about what to advise the asymptomatic patient found to have gallstones during the course of unrelated studies. The presence of either of the following portends a more serious course and should probably serve as a reason for prophylactic cholecystectomy: (1) large stones (> 2 cm in diameter), because they produce acute cholecystitis more often than small stones; and (2) a calcified gallbladder, because it so often is associated with carcinoma. However, most asymptomatic patients have no special features. If coexistent cardiopulmonary or other problems increase the risk of surgery, operation should not be considered. For the average asymptomatic patient, it is not reasonable to make a strong recommendation for cholecystectomy. The tendency, however, is to operate on younger patients and temporize in the elderly.

Beckingham IJ: ABC of diseases of liver, pancreas, and biliary system. Gallstone disease. BMJ 2001;322:91.

GALLSTONES & CHRONIC CHOLECYSTITIS (BILIARY COLIC)

 ESSENTIALS OF DIAGNOSIS

- ▶ Episodic abdominal pain.
- ▶ Dyspepsia.
- ▶ Gallstones on cholecystography or ultrasound scan.

▶ General Considerations

Chronic cholecystitis is the most common form of symptomatic gallbladder disease and is associated with gallstones in nearly every case. In general, the term cholecystitis is applied whenever gallstones are present regardless of the histologic appearance of the gallbladder. Repeated minor episodes of obstruction of the cystic duct cause intermittent biliary colic and contribute to inflammation and subsequent scar formation. Gallbladders from symptomatic patients with gallstones who have never had an attack of acute cholecystitis are of two types: (1) In some, the mucosa may be slightly flattened, but the wall is thin and unscarred and, except for the stones, appears normal. (2) Others exhibit obvious signs of chronic inflammation, with thickening, cellular infiltration, loss of elasticity, and fibrosis. The clinical history in these two groups cannot always be distinguished, and inflammatory changes may also be found in patients with asymptomatic gallstones.

▶ Clinical Findings

A. Symptoms and Signs

Biliary colic, the most characteristic symptom, is caused by transient gallstone obstruction of the cystic duct. The pain usually begins abruptly and subsides gradually, lasting for a few minutes to several hours. The pain of biliary colic is usually steady—not intermittent, like that of intestinal colic. In some patients, attacks occur postprandially; in others, there is no relationship to meals. The frequency of attacks is quite variable, ranging from nearly continuous trouble to episodes many years apart. Nausea and vomiting may accompany the pain.

Biliary colic is usually felt in the right upper quadrant, but epigastric and left abdominal pain are common, and some patients experience precordial pain. The pain may radiate around the costal margin into the back or may be referred to the region of the scapula. Pain on top of the shoulder is unusual and suggests direct diaphragmatic irritation. In a severe attack, the patient usually curls up in bed, changing position frequently in order to be more comfortable.

During an attack, there may be tenderness in the right upper quadrant, and, rarely, the gallbladder is palpable.

Fatty food intolerance, dyspepsia, indigestion, heartburn, flatulence, nausea, and eructations are other symptoms associated with gallstone disease. Because they are also frequent in the general population, their presence in any given patient may only be incidental to the gallstones.

B. Laboratory Findings

An ultrasound scan of the gallbladder should usually be the first test. Gallstones can be demonstrated in about 95% of cases, and a positive reading for gallstones is almost never in error. An oral cholecystogram should be obtained if the ultrasound study is equivocal, if the patient is a candidate for lithotripsy or ursodiol therapy, or if symptoms are highly suggestive and an ultrasound study has been read as normal.

About 2% of patients with gallstone disease have normal ultrasound studies and oral cholecystograms. Therefore, if the clinical suspicion of gallbladder disease is high and these two tests are negative, the patient should be studied by ERCP (to opacify the gallbladder in the search for stones) or duodenal intubation and examination of duodenal bile for cholesterol crystals or bilirubinate granules.

▶ Differential Diagnosis

Gallbladder colic may be strongly suggested by the history, but the clinical impression should always be verified by an ultrasound study. Biliary colic may simulate the pain of duodenal ulcer, hiatal hernia, pancreatitis, and myocardial infarction.

An electrocardiogram and a chest x-ray should be obtained to investigate cardiopulmonary disease. It has been suggested that biliary colic may sometimes aggravate cardiac

disease, but angina pectoris or an abnormal electrocardiogram should rarely be indications for cholecystectomy.

Right-sided radicular pain in the T6–T10 dermatomes may be confused with biliary colic. Osteoarthritic spurs, vertebral lesions, or tumors may be shown on x-rays of the spine or may be suggested by hyperesthesia of the abdominal skin.

An upper gastrointestinal series may be indicated to search for esophageal spasm, hiatal hernia, peptic ulcer, or gastric tumors. In some patients, the irritable colon syndrome may be mistaken for gallbladder discomfort. Carcinoma of the cecum or ascending colon may be overlooked on the assumption that postprandial pain in these conditions is due to gallstones.

▶ Complications

Chronic cholecystitis predisposes to acute cholecystitis, common duct stones, and adenocarcinoma of the gallbladder. The longer the stones have been present, the higher the incidence of all of these complications. Complications are infrequent, however, and the presence of gallstones is not reason enough for prophylactic cholecystectomy in a person with asymptomatic or mildly symptomatic disease.

▶ Treatment

A. Medical Treatment

Avoidance of offending foods may be helpful.

1. Dissolution—Cholesterol gallstones in the gallbladder can be dissolved in some cases by chronic treatment with ursodiol, which reduces the cholesterol saturation of bile by inhibiting cholesterol secretion. The resulting undersaturated bile slowly dissolves the solid cholesterol in the gallstones.

Unfortunately, bile salt therapy has marginal efficacy. The gallstones must be small (eg, < 5 mm) and devoid of calcium (ie, nonopaque on CT scans), and the gallbladder must opacify on oral cholecystography (an indication of unobstructed flow of bile between bile duct and gallbladder). About 15% of patients with gallstones are candidates for treatment. Dissolution is achieved within 2 years in about 50% of highly selected patients. Stones recur, however, in 50% of cases within 5 years. In general, dissolution therapy—alone or in conjunction with lithotripsy—is used very rarely.

2. Lithotripsy and dissolution—Extracorporeal shock wave lithotripsy (ESWL) involves focusing shock waves, which pass through tissue and fluids, upon the gallstones. The stones are fragmented by explosion of small air bubbles within interstices of the solid material.

Lithotripsy is of little therapeutic value because the fragments remain in the gallbladder unless they can be dissolved. Consequently, candidates for lithotripsy must also use ursodiol therapy. Complete elimination of gallbladder stones is attained within 9 months in about 25% of appropriately selected patients. Because of the many drawbacks of this form of treatment, it has not been approved by the US Food and Drug Administration.

B. Surgical Treatment

Cholecystectomy is indicated in most patients with symptoms. The procedure can be scheduled at the patient's convenience, within weeks or months after diagnosis. Active concurrent disease that increases the risk of surgery should be treated before operation. In some chronically ill patients, surgery should be deferred indefinitely.

Cholecystectomy is most often performed laparoscopically, but when the laparoscopic approach is contraindicated (eg, too many adhesions) or unsuccessful, it may be performed through a laparotomy. The difference consists of 4 fewer days in the hospital and fewer weeks off work when done laparoscopically. Regardless of how it is done, operative cholangiography is often included to look for common duct stones. If stones are found, common duct exploration may be performed (see section on Choledocholithiasis).

▶ Prognosis

Serious complications and deaths related to the operation itself are rare. The operative death rate is about 0.1% in patients under age 50 and about 0.5% in patients over age 50. Most deaths occur in patients recognized preoperatively to have increased risks. The operation relieves symptoms in 95% of cases.

Beyer AJ 3rd, Delcore R, Cheung LY: Nonoperative treatment of biliary tract disease. Arch Surg 1998;133:1172.

Binmoeller KF, Schafer TW: Endoscopic management of bile duct stones. J Clin Gastroenterol 2001;32:106.

Calland JF et al: Outpatient laparoscopic cholecystectomy: patient outcomes after implementation of a clinical pathway. Ann Surg 2001;233:704.

Fletcher DR et al: Complications of cholecystectomy: risks of the laparoscopic approach and protective effects of operative cholangiography: a population-based study. Ann Surg 1999;229:449.

Gadacz TR: Update on laparoscopic cholecystectomy, including a clinical pathway. Surg Clin North Am 2000;80:1127.

Maxwell JG et al: Cholecystectomy in patients aged 80 and older. Am J Surg 1998;176:627.

Montori A et al: Endoscopic and surgical integration in the approach to biliary tract disease. J Clin Gastroenterol 1999;28:198.

Moonka R et al: The presentation of gallstones and results of biliary surgery in a spinal cord injured population. Am J Surg 1999;178:246.

Sakuramoto S et al: Preoperative evaluation to predict technical difficulties of laparoscopic cholecystectomy on the basis of histological inflammation findings on resected gallbladder. Am J Surg 2000;179:114.

Stuart SA et al: Routine intraoperative laparoscopic cholangiography. Am J Surg 1998;176:632.

Tocchi A et al: The need for antibiotic prophylaxis in elective laparoscopic cholecystectomy: a prospective randomized study. Arch Surg 2000;135:67.

Traverso LW: Risk factors for intraoperative injury during cholecystectomy: an ounce of prevention is worth a pound of cure. Ann Surg 1999;229:458.

Yerdel MA et al: Direct trocar insertion versus Veress needle insertion in laparoscopic cholecystectomy. Am J Surg 1999;177:247.

ACUTE CHOLECYSTITIS

ESSENTIALS OF DIAGNOSIS

▶ Acute right upper quadrant pain and tenderness.

▶ Fever and leukocytosis.

▶ Palpable gallbladder in one third of cases.

▶ Nonopacified gallbladder on radionuclide excretion scan.

▶ Sonographic Murphy sign.

▶ General Considerations

In 80% of cases, acute cholecystitis results from obstruction of the cystic duct by a gallstone impacted in the Hartmann pouch. The gallbladder becomes inflamed and distended, creating abdominal pain and tenderness. The natural history of acute cholecystitis varies, depending on whether the obstruction becomes relieved, the extent of secondary bacterial invasion, the age of the patient, and the presence of other aggravating factors such as diabetes mellitus. Most attacks resolve spontaneously without surgery or other specific therapy, but some progress to abscess formation or free perforation with generalized peritonitis.

The pathologic changes in the gallbladder evolve in a typical pattern. Subserosal edema and hemorrhage and patchy mucosal necrosis are the first changes. Later, polymorphonuclear (PMN) leukocytes appear. The final stage involves development of fibrosis. Gangrene and perforation may occur as early as 3 days after onset, but most perforations occur during the second week. In cases that resolve spontaneously, acute inflammation has largely cleared by 4 weeks, but some residual evidence of inflammation may last for several months. About 90% of gallbladders removed during an acute attack show chronic scarring, although many of these patients deny having had any previous symptoms.

The cause of acute cholecystitis is still partially conjectural. Obstruction of the cystic duct is present in most cases, but in experimental animals, cystic duct obstruction does not result in acute cholecystitis unless the gallbladder is filled with concentrated bile or bile saturated with cholesterol. There is also evidence that trauma from gallstones releases phospholipase from the mucosal cells of the gallbladder. This is followed by conversion of lecithin in bile to lysolecithin, which is a toxic compound that may cause more inflammation.

Bacteria appear to have a minor role in the early stages of acute cholecystitis, even though most complications of the disease involve suppuration.

About 20% of cases of acute cholecystitis occur in the absence of cholelithiasis (acalculous cholecystitis). Some of these are due to cystic duct obstruction by another process such as a malignant tumor. Rarely, acute acalculous cholecystitis results from cystic artery occlusion or primary bacterial infection by *Escherichia coli,* clostridia, or, occasionally, *Salmonella typhi.* Most cases occur in patients hospitalized with some other illness; acute acalculous cholecystitis is particularly common in trauma victims (civilian or military) and in patients receiving total parenteral nutrition. Small-vessel occlusion occurs early, and unless treatment is given promptly, the disease progresses rapidly to gangrenous cholecystitis and septic complications, at which point the death rate is high.

▶ Clinical Findings

A. Symptoms and Signs

The first symptom is abdominal pain in the right upper quadrant, sometimes associated with referred pain in the region of the right scapula. In 75% of cases, the patient will have had previous attacks of biliary colic, at first indistinguishable from the present illness. However, in acute cholecystitis, the pain persists and becomes associated with abdominal tenderness. Nausea and vomiting are present in about half of patients, but the vomiting is rarely severe. Mild icterus occurs in 10% of cases. The temperature usually ranges from 38 to 38.5 °C. High fever and chills are uncommon and should suggest the possibility of complications or an incorrect diagnosis.

Right upper quadrant tenderness is present, and in about a third of patients the gallbladder is palpable (often in a position lateral to its normal one). Voluntary guarding during examination may prevent detection of an enlarged gallbladder. In others, the gallbladder is not enlarged because scarring of the wall restricts distention. If instructed to breathe deeply during palpation in the right subcostal region, the patient experiences accentuated tenderness and sudden inspiratory arrest (Murphy sign).

B. Laboratory Findings

The leukocyte count is usually elevated to 12,000–15,000/µL. Normal counts are common, but if the count goes much above 15,000, one should suspect complications. A mild elevation of the serum bilirubin (in the range of 2–4 mg/dL) is common, presumably owing to secondary inflammation of the common duct by the contiguous gallbladder. Bilirubin values above this range would most likely indicate the associated presence of common duct stones. A mild increase in alkaline phosphatase may accompany the attack. Occasionally, the serum amylase concentration transiently reaches 1000 units/dL or more.

C. Imaging Studies

A plain x-ray of the abdomen may occasionally show an enlarged gallbladder shadow. In 15% of patients, the gallstones contain enough calcium to be seen on the plain film.

Ultrasound scans show gallstones, sludge, and thickening of the gallbladder wall, and the ultrasonographer can determine even better than the clinician whether the point of maximum tenderness is over the gallbladder (ultrasonographic Murphy sign). This last finding is often absent, however, when the gallbladder is gangrenous. Usually, ultrasound is the only test needed to make the diagnosis of acute cholecystitis.

If additional diagnostic information is desirable (eg, if ultrasound is equivocal or negative), a radionuclide excretion scan (eg, HIDA scan) should be performed. This test cannot demonstrate gallstones, but if the gallbladder is imaged, acute cholecystitis is ruled out except in rare cases of acalculous cholecystitis (the test is positive in most cases of acute acalculous cholecystitis). Imaging of the duct but not the gallbladder supports the diagnosis of acute cholecystitis. A few false positives are seen in advanced gallstone disease without acute inflammation and in acute biliary pancreatitis.

▶ Differential Diagnosis

The differential diagnosis includes other common causes of acute upper abdominal pain and tenderness. An acute peptic ulcer with or without perforation might be suggested by a history of epigastric pain relieved by food or antacids. Most cases of perforated ulcer demonstrate free air under the diaphragm on x-ray. An emergency upper gastrointestinal series may help.

Acute pancreatitis can be confused with acute cholecystitis, especially if cholecystitis is accompanied by an elevated amylase level. Furthermore, HIDA scans fail to outline the gallbladder in most cases of acute biliary pancreatitis. Sometimes the two diseases coexist, but pancreatitis should not be accepted as a second diagnosis without specific findings.

Acute appendicitis in patients with a high cecum may closely simulate acute cholecystitis.

Severe right upper quadrant pain with high fever and local tenderness may develop in acute gonococcal perihepatitis (Fitz-Hugh-Curtis syndrome). Clues to the proper diagnosis may be found in tenderness in the adnexa, vaginal discharge that shows gonococci on a Gram-stained smear, and a disparity between the patient's high fever and her general lack of toxicity.

▶ Complications

The major complications of acute cholecystitis are empyema, gangrene, and perforation.

A. Empyema

In empyema (suppurative cholecystitis), the gallbladder contains frank pus, and the patient becomes more toxic, with high spiking fever (39–40 °C), chills, and leukocytosis greater than 15,000/μL. Parenteral antibiotics should be given, and percutaneous cholecystostomy or cholecystectomy should be performed.

B. Perforation

Perforation may take any of three forms: (1) localized perforation with pericholecystic abscess, (2) free perforation with generalized peritonitis, and (3) perforation into an adjacent hollow viscus, with the formation of a fistula. Perforation may occur as early as 3 days after the onset of acute cholecystitis or not until late in the second week. The total incidence of perforation is about 10%.

1. Pericholecystic abscess—Pericholecystic abscess, the most common form of perforation, should be suspected when the signs and symptoms progress, especially when accompanied by the appearance of a palpable mass. The patient often becomes toxic, with fever to 39 °C and a leukocyte count above 15,000/μL, but sometimes there is no correlation between the clinical signs and the development of local abscess. Cholecystectomy and drainage of the abscess can be performed safely in many of these patients, but if the patient's condition is unstable, percutaneous cholecystostomy is preferable.

2. Free perforation—Free perforation occurs in only 1–2% of patients, most often early in the disease when gangrene develops before adhesions wall off the gallbladder. The diagnosis is made preoperatively in less than half of cases. In some patients with localized pain, sudden spread of pain and tenderness to other parts of the abdomen suggests the diagnosis. Whenever it is suspected, free perforation must be treated by emergency laparotomy. Abdominal paracentesis may be misleading and has proved to be of little diagnostic usefulness. Cholecystectomy should be performed if the patient's condition will permit; otherwise, cholecystostomy is done. The death rate depends partly on whether the cystic duct remains obstructed or the stone becomes dislodged after perforation. The former leads to a purulent peritonitis that is lethal in 20% of cases. In the latter, a true bile peritonitis ensues and over 50% of patients die. The earlier operation is performed, the better the prognosis.

3. Cholecystenteric fistula—If the acutely inflamed gallbladder becomes adherent to adjacent stomach, duodenum, or colon and necrosis develops at the site of one of these adhesions, perforation may occur into the lumen of the gut. The resulting decompression often allows the acute disease to resolve. If the gallbladder stones discharge through the fistula and if they are large enough, they may obstruct the small intestine (gallstone ileus; see later in chapter). Rarely, patients vomit gallstones that have entered the stomach through a cholecystogastric fistula. In most patients, the acute attack subsides and the cholecystenteric fistula is clinically unsuspected.

Cholecystenteric fistulas do not usually cause symptoms unless the gallbladder is still partially obstructed by stones or scarring. Neither oral nor intravenous cholangiograms will opacify the gallbladder or the fistula, but the latter may be shown on upper gastrointestinal series, where it must be differentiated from a fistula due to perforated peptic ulcer. Malabsorption and steatorrhea have been reported in isolated cases of cholecystocolonic fistulas. Steatorrhea in this situation could be due either to absence of bile in the proximal bowel following diversion into the colon or, more rarely, to excess bacteria in the upper intestine.

Symptomatic cholecystenteric fistulas should be treated by cholecystectomy and closure of the fistula. The majority are discovered incidentally during cholecystectomy for symptomatic gallbladder disease.

▶ Treatment

Intravenous fluids should be given to correct dehydration and electrolyte imbalance, and a nasogastric tube should be inserted. For acute cholecystitis of average severity, parenteral cefazolin (2–4 g daily) should be given. Parenteral penicillin (20 million units daily), clindamycin, and an aminoglycoside should be given for severe disease. Single-drug therapy using imipenem is a good alternative.

There are two schools of thought about the treatment of acute cholecystitis. Since the disease resolves with antibiotics and supportive care in about 60% of cases, one approach is to manage the patient expectantly, with a plan to perform elective cholecystectomy after recovery, reserving surgery during the acute attack for those with severe or worsening disease. (This approach is untenable in acute acalculous cholecystitis.)

The preferred plan is to perform cholecystectomy in all patients unless there are specific contraindications to operation (eg, serious concomitant disease). Four controlled trials have supported this approach with the following data: (1) the incidence of technical complications is no greater with early surgery; (2) early surgery reduces the total duration of illness by approximately 30 days, length of hospitalization by 5–7 days, and direct medical costs by several thousand dollars; and (3) the death rate is slightly lower with early surgery because of earlier treatment for some patients whose condition would have worsened during expectant management. Since these trials were completed, the average case appears to have become more severe, and the arguments against expectant management are now even more compelling.

The following are the major factors that affect the decision (Figure 25–8): (1) whether the diagnosis is established; (2) the general health of the patient as modified by coexistent disease or the present illness; and (3) signs of local complications of acute cholecystitis. The diagnosis should be clear-cut and the patient optimally prepared; if perforation or empyema is suspected, emergency surgery is indicated.

In about 30% of cases, the diagnosis of acute cholecystitis is established but the general condition of the patient is

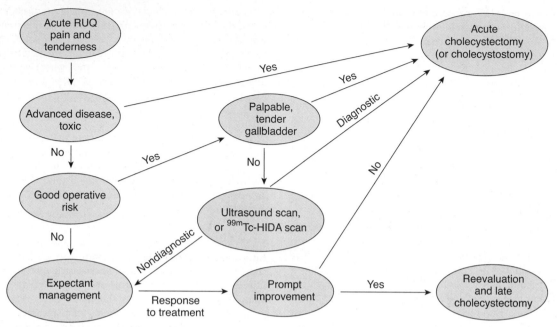

▲ **Figure 25–8.** Scheme for the management of acute cholecystitis.

unsatisfactory. If possible, surgery should be postponed in these cases until the ancillary disease is controlled. Expectant management cannot be rigidly adhered to, however, if the manifestations of cholecystitis worsen.

About 10% of patients require emergency treatment. These are generally clinical situations in which the disease appears to have become complicated or is about to. High fever (39 °C), marked leukocytosis (> 15,000/μL), or chills suggest suppurative progression. Acalculous acute cholecystitis should automatically be placed in this category. When the patient's general condition is poor, percutaneous catheter cholecystostomy is the preferable treatment. Patients in better overall health should be treated by cholecystectomy.

The sudden appearance of generalized abdominal pain may indicate free perforation. Appearance of a mass while the patient is under observation may be a sign of local perforation and abscess formation. Changes of this sort are indications for emergency surgery.

Cholecystectomy is the preferable operation in acute cholecystitis, and it can be performed laparoscopically in about 50% of patients. Operative cholangiography should be performed in most cases, and the common bile duct explored if appropriate indications are present (see section on Choledocholithiasis). Patients with severe acute cholecystitis who are in poor condition for emergency cholecystectomy should be treated by percutaneous cholecystostomy. Percutaneous cholecystostomy may also be the preferred therapy for acute acalculous cholecystitis. A catheter inserted under ultrasound or CT guidance is allowed to drain the gallbladder of its bile or pus. The resulting decompression

controls the acute disease, including any local infection, but the gallstones cannot be removed. Therefore, cholecystectomy should be performed after the patient recovers in order to avoid recurrent attacks. Cholecystectomy is definitive therapy in the patient with acalculous cholecystitis. At one time, cholecystostomy was performed surgically, but most hospitals now have radiologists skilled in the simpler percutaneous method.

▶ **Prognosis**

The overall death rate of acute cholecystitis is about 5%. Nearly all of the deaths are in patients over age 60 or those with diabetes mellitus. In the older age group, secondary cardiovascular or pulmonary complications contribute substantially to the death rate. Uncontrolled sepsis with peritonitis and intrahepatic abscesses are the most important local conditions responsible for death.

Common duct stones are present in about 15% of patients with acute cholecystitis, and some of the more seriously ill patients have simultaneous cholangitis from biliary obstruction. Acute pancreatitis may also complicate acute cholecystitis, and the combination carries a greater risk.

Patients who develop the suppurative forms of gallbladder disease such as empyema or perforation are less likely to recover. Earlier admission to the hospital and early cholecystectomy reduce the chances of these complications.

Berber E et al: Selective use of tube cholecystostomy with interval laparoscopic cholecystectomy in acute cholecystitis. Arch Surg 2000;135:341.

Borzellino G et al: Emergency cholecystostomy and subsequent cholecystectomy for acute gallstone cholecystitis in the elderly. Br J Surg 1999;86:1521.

Davis CA et al: Effective use of percutaneous cholecystostomy in high-risk surgical patients: techniques, tube management, and results. Arch Surg 1999;134:727.

Eldar S et al: The impact of patient delay and physician delay on the outcome of laparoscopic cholecystectomy for acute cholecystitis. Am J Surg 1999;178:303.

Geoghegan JG, Keane FB: Laparoscopic management of complicated gallstone disease. Br J Surg 1999;86:145.

Greenwald JA et al: Standardization of surgeon-controlled variables: impact on outcome in patients with acute cholecystitis. Ann Surg 2000;231:339.

Kim KH et al: Percutaneous gallbladder drainage for delayed laparoscopic cholecystectomy in patients with acute cholecystitis. Am J Surg 2000;179:111.

Laycock WS et al: Variation in the use of laparoscopic cholecystectomy for elderly patients with acute cholecystitis. Arch Surg 2000;135:457.

Lillemoe KD: Surgical treatment of biliary tract infections. Am Surg 2000;66:138.

Lobe TE: Cholelithiasis and cholecystitis in children. Semin Pediatr Surg 2000;9:170.

Svanvik J: Laparoscopic cholecystectomy for acute cholecystitis. Eur J Surg 2000;(Suppl 585):16.

EMPHYSEMATOUS CHOLECYSTITIS

Emphysematous cholecystitis is a rare condition in which bubbles of gas from anaerobic infection appear in the lumen of the gallbladder, its wall, the pericholecystic space, and, on occasion, the bile ducts. Clostridia species are the most commonly implicated organisms, but other gas-forming anaerobes such as *E coli* or anaerobic streptococci may be found. Three times as many men as women are affected, and 20% of patients have diabetes mellitus. In contrast to the usual form of acute cholecystitis, the disease probably is a bacterial infection from the earliest moment. In many cases, the gallbladder contains no stones.

The disease begins with sudden and rapidly progressive right upper quadrant pain. Fever and leukocytosis reach high levels quickly, and the patient is considerably more toxic than is usually the case in acute cholecystitis. On examination, a mass can usually be found in the right upper quadrant.

Plain films of the abdomen show tissue emphysema outlining the gallbladder and, in some cases, an air-fluid level in the lumen. The clinical and x-ray pictures are characteristic enough so that the diagnosis is usually obvious. If the changes on plain films are equivocal, a CT scan may bring them out.

The patient should be treated with high doses of antibiotics effective against clostridia and the other species mentioned above. Emergency surgical treatment should follow the initial resuscitative measures. Cholecystectomy can be safely performed in most cases, but the most critically ill might fare better with cholecystostomy. The types of complications are the same as in other forms of acute cholecystitis, but illness is more severe and death rates are higher.

Danse EM, Laterre PF: Images in clinical medicine. Emphysematous cholecystitis. N Engl J Med 1999;341:1126.

Garcia-Sancho Tellez L et al: Acute emphysematous cholecystitis. Report of twenty cases. Hepatogastroenterology 1999;46:2144.

Zeebregts CJ et al: Percutaneous drainage of emphysematous cholecystitis associated with pneumoperitoneum. Hepatogastroenterology 1999;46:771.

GALLSTONE ILEUS

Gallstone ileus is mechanical intestinal obstruction caused by a large gallstone lodged in the lumen. It is seen most often in women, and the average age is about 70.

▶ Clinical Findings

A. Symptoms

The patient usually presents with obvious small bowel obstruction, either partial or complete. The obstructing gallstone enters the intestine through a cholecystenteric fistula located in the duodenum, colon, or, rarely, the stomach or jejunum. The gallbladder may contain one or several stones, but stones that cause gallstone ileus are almost always 2.5 cm or more in diameter. The lumen in the proximal bowel will allow most of these large calculi to pass caudally until the ileum is reached. Obstruction of the large intestine may follow passage of a gallstone through a fistula at the hepatic flexure or may occur even after the stone has traversed the entire small bowel.

B. Signs

In most patients, the findings on physical examination are typical of distal small bowel obstruction. Obstruction of the duodenum or jejunum may give a perplexing clinical picture because of the lack of distention. Right upper quadrant tenderness and a mass may be present in some cases, but the distended abdomen may be difficult to examine accurately.

C. Imaging Studies

In addition to dilated small intestine, plain films of the abdomen may show a radiopaque gallstone, and unless one is alert to the possibility of gallstone ileus, the ectopic stone can be a puzzling finding. In about 40% of cases, careful examination of the film will reveal gas in the biliary tree, a manifestation of the cholecystenteric fistula. When the clinical picture is unclear, an upper gastrointestinal series should be obtained, which will demonstrate the cholecystoduodenal fistula and verify intestinal obstruction.

▶ Treatment

The proper treatment is emergency laparotomy and removal of the obstructing stone through a small enterotomy. The proximal intestine must be carefully inspected for the presence of a second calculus that might cause a postoperative recurrence. The gallbladder should be left undisturbed at the original operation.

Once the patient has recovered, an elective cholecystectomy should be scheduled if the patient complains of chronic gallbladder symptoms. On this basis, interval cholecystectomy will be required in about 30% of patients. The fistula itself is rarely the source of trouble and closes spontaneously in most patients.

▶ Prognosis

The death rate of gallstone ileus remains about 20%, largely because of the poor general condition of elderly patients at the time of laparotomy. In many cases, the patient has developed cardiac or pulmonary complications during a preoperative delay when the diagnosis was unclear.

Lobo DN, Jobling JC, Balfour TW: Gallstone ileus: diagnostic pitfalls and therapeutic successes. J Clin Gastroenterol 2000;30:72.
Scarpa F et al: Gallstone ileus: diagnostic pitfalls and therapeutic successes. J Clin Gastroenterol 2000;30:72.

CHOLANGITIS (BACTERIAL CHOLANGITIS)

Bacterial infection of the biliary ducts always signifies biliary obstruction, since in the absence of obstruction even heavy bacterial contamination of the ducts fails to produce symptoms or pathologic changes. The block to flow may be partial or, less commonly, complete. The principal causes are choledocholithiasis, biliary stricture, and neoplasm. Less common causes are chronic pancreatitis, ampullary stenosis, pancreatic pseudocyst, duodenal diverticulum, congenital cyst, and parasitic invasion. Iatrogenic cholangitis may complicate transhepatic or T tube cholangiography. Not all obstructing lesions are followed by cholangitis, however. For example, biliary infection develops in only 15% of patients with neoplastic obstruction. The likelihood of cholangitis is greatest when the obstruction occurs after the duct has acquired a resident bacterial population.

With obstruction, ductal pressure rises, and bacteria proliferate and escape into the systemic circulation via the hepatic sinusoids. Experimentally, the incidence of positive blood cultures with ductal infection is directly proportionate to the absolute height of the pressure in the duct.

The symptoms of cholangitis (sometimes called the Charcot triad) are biliary colic, jaundice, and chills and fever, though a complete triad is present in only 70% of cases. Laboratory findings include leukocytosis and elevated serum bilirubin and alkaline phosphatase levels. The predominant organisms in bile (in approximately decreasing frequency) are *E coli*, klebsiella, pseudomonas, enterococci, and proteus. *Bacteroides fragilis* and other anaerobes (eg, *Clostridium perfringens*) can be detected in about 25% of cases, and their presence correlates with multiple previous biliary operations (often including a biliary enteric anastomosis), severe symptoms, and a high incidence of postoperative suppurative complications. Anaerobes are nearly always seen in the company of aerobes. Two species of bacteria can be cultured in about 50% of cases. Bacteremia probably occurs in most cases, and blood cultures obtained at the appropriate time contain the same organisms as the bile. Early

in an attack, an ultrasound scan will often give useful diagnostic information. Further workup (THC, ERCP, etc) can proceed later after the acute manifestations are brought under control. Cholangiography is dangerous during active cholangitis.

The term **suppurative cholangitis** has been used for the most severe form of this disease, when manifestations of sepsis overshadow those of hepatobiliary disease. The diagnostic pentad of suppurative cholangitis consists of abdominal pain, jaundice, fever and chills, mental confusion or lethargy, and shock. The diagnosis is often missed because the signs of biliary disease are overlooked.

Most cases of cholangitis can be controlled with intravenous antibiotics. A cephalosporin antibiotic (eg, cefazolin, cefoxitin) is the drug of choice in the average mild to moderately severe case. If disease is severe or progressively worsens, an aminoglycoside plus clindamycin or metronidazole should be added to the regimen.

For patients with severe cholangitis or unremitting cholangitis despite antibiotic therapy, the bile duct must be promptly decompressed. Most cases of severe acute cholangitis are associated with choledocholithiasis, where the best treatment consists of emergency endoscopic sphincterotomy. In the uncommon case where this is unsuccessful, laparotomy is indicated in order to decompress the bile duct. Cholangitis accompanying neoplastic obstruction may be managed by insertion of a transhepatic drainage catheter into the bile duct. A cholangiogram should not be obtained because the procedure could worsen sepsis.

Urgent intervention (eg, endoscopic sphincterotomy, percutaneous transhepatic drainage, or operative decompression) is required in about 10% of patients with acute cholangitis. The remaining 90% are eventually treated by elective surgery or endoscopic sphincterotomy following antibiotic therapy and a thorough diagnostic evaluation.

Elsakr R et al: Antimicrobial treatment of intra-abdominal infections. Dig Dis 1998;16:47.
Hanau LH, Steigbigel NH: Acute (ascending) cholangitis. Infect Dis Clin North Am 2000;14:521.
Poon RT et al: Management of gallstone cholangitis in the era of laparoscopic cholecystectomy. Arch Surg 2001;136:11.
Raraty MG, Finch M, Neoptolemos JP: Acute cholangitis and pancreatitis secondary to common duct stones: management update. World J Surg 1998;22:1155.

CHOLEDOCHOLITHIASIS

ESSENTIALS OF DIAGNOSIS

- ▶ Biliary pain.
- ▶ Jaundice.
- ▶ Episodic cholangitis.
- ▶ Gallstones in gallbladder or previous cholecystectomy.

General Considerations

Approximately 15% of patients with stones in the gallbladder are found to harbor calculi within the bile ducts. Common duct stones are usually accompanied by others in the gallbladder, but in 5% of cases, the gallbladder is empty. The number of duct stones may vary from one to more than 100.

There are two possible origins for common duct stones. The evidence suggests that most cholesterol stones develop within the gallbladder and reach the duct after traversing the cystic duct. These are called secondary stones. Pigment stones may have a similar pedigree or, more often, develop de novo within the common duct. These are called primary common duct stones. About 60% of common duct stones are cholesterol stones and 40% are pigment stones. The latter are generally associated with more severe clinical manifestations.

Patients may have one or more of the following principal clinical findings, all of which are caused by obstruction to the flow of bile or pancreatic juice: biliary colic, cholangitis, jaundice, and pancreatitis (Figure 25–9). It seems likely, however, that as many as 50% of patients with choledocholithiasis remain asymptomatic.

The common duct may dilate to 2–3 cm proximal to an obstructing lesion, and truly huge ducts develop in patients with biliary tumors. In choledocholithiasis or biliary stricture, the inflammatory reaction restricts dilation, so the dilatation is less marked. Dilation of the ductal system within the liver can also be limited by cirrhosis.

Biliary colic is the result of rapid rises in biliary pressure whether the block is in the common duct or neck of the gallbladder. Gradual occlusion of the duct—as in cancer—rarely produces the same kind of pain as gallstone disease.

Clinical Findings

A. Symptoms

Choledocholithiasis may be asymptomatic or may produce sudden toxic cholangitis, leading to a rapid demise. The seriousness of the disease parallels the degree of obstruction, the length of time it has been present, and the extent of secondary bacterial infection (see earlier section on Cholangitis). Biliary colic, jaundice, or pancreatitis may be isolated findings or may occur in any combination along with signs of infection (cholangitis).

Biliary colic from common duct obstruction cannot be distinguished from that caused by stones in the gallbladder. The pain is felt in the right subcostal region, epigastrium, or even the substernal area. Referred pain to the region of the right scapula is common.

Choledocholithiasis should be strongly suspected if intermittent chills, fever, or jaundice accompanies biliary colic. Some patients notice transient darkening of their urine during an attack even though jaundice is not evident.

Pruritus is usually the result of persistent, longstanding obstruction. The itching is more intense in warm weather when the patient perspires and is usually worse on the

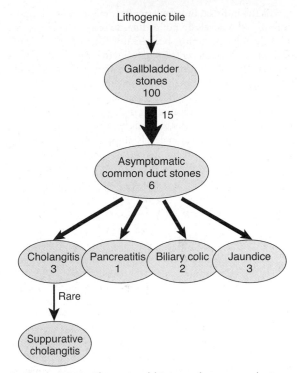

▲ **Figure 25–9.** The natural history of common duct stones. Of every 100 patients with gallbladder stones, 15 will have common duct stones, which will produce the spectrum of syndromes illustrated. Note that the individual syndromes overlap, indicating that they may appear together in various combinations.

extremities than on the trunk. It is much more common with neoplastic obstruction than with gallstone obstruction.

B. Signs

The patient may be icteric and toxic, with high fever and chills, or may appear to be perfectly healthy. A palpable gallbladder is unusual in patients with obstructive jaundice from common duct stone because the obstruction is transient and partial, and scarring of the gallbladder renders it inelastic and nondistensible. Tenderness may be present in the right upper quadrant but is not often as marked as in acute cholecystitis, perforated peptic ulcer, or acute pancreatitis. Tender hepatic enlargement may occur.

C. Laboratory Findings

In cholangitis, leukocytosis of 15,000/μL is usual, and values above 20,000/μL are common. A rise in serum bilirubin often appears within 24 hours after the onset of symptoms. The absolute level usually remains under 10 mg/dL, and most are in the range of 2–4 mg/dL. The direct fraction exceeds the indirect, but the latter becomes elevated in most cases. Bilirubin levels do not ordinarily reach the high values seen in malignant tumors because the obstruction is usually incomplete and transient. In fact, fluctuating jaundice is so characteristic of choledocholithiasis that it fairly reliably differentiates between benign and malignant obstruction.

The serum alkaline phosphatase level usually rises and may be the only chemical abnormality in patients without jaundice. When the obstruction is relieved, the alkaline phosphatase and bilirubin levels should return to normal within 1–2 weeks, with the exception that the former may remain elevated longer if the obstruction was prolonged.

Mild increases in AST and ALT are often seen with extrahepatic obstruction of the ducts; rarely, AST levels transiently reach 1000 units.

D. Imaging Studies

Radiopaque gallstones may be seen on plain abdominal films or CT scans. Ultrasound scans will usually show gallbladder stones and, depending on the degree of obstruction, dilatation of the bile duct. Ultrasound and CT scans are insensitive in the search for stones in the common duct. ERCP is indicated if the patient has had a previous cholecystectomy. If cholecystectomy has not been performed, cholangiography should be part of operative management. Some clinicians choose preoperative ERCP for patients scheduled for cholecystectomy in order to clear the common bile duct. If ERCP is not technically successful, the surgeon will be forced to convert to open common bile duct exploration to clear the duct of stones.

Bilirubin values above 10 mg/dL are so uncommon in choledocholithiasis that when this finding is present, cholangiography should be performed to rule out the possibility of neoplastic obstruction.

▶ Differential Diagnosis

The workup should consider the same possibilities in differential diagnosis as for cholecystitis.

Serum amylase levels above 500 units/dL can result from acute pancreatitis, acute cholecystitis, or choledocholithiasis. Other manifestations of pancreatic disease should be documented before an unqualified diagnosis of pancreatitis is accepted.

Alcoholic cirrhosis or acute alcoholic hepatitis may present with jaundice, right upper quadrant tenderness, and leukocytosis. The differentiation from cholangitis may be impossible from clinical data. A history of a recent binge suggests acute liver disease. A percutaneous liver biopsy may be specific.

Intrahepatic cholestasis from drugs, pregnancy, chronic active hepatitis, or primary biliary cirrhosis may be difficult to distinguish from extrahepatic obstruction. ERCP would be appropriate to make the distinction, particularly if other studies (eg, ultrasound scan) failed to provide evidence of

gallstone disease. If jaundice has persisted for 4–6 weeks, a mechanical cause is probable. Since most patients improve during this interval, persistent jaundice should never be assumed to be the result of parenchymal disease unless a normal cholangiogram rules out obstruction of the major ducts.

Intermittent jaundice and cholangitis after cholecystectomy are compatible with biliary stricture, and the distinction requires ERCP.

Biliary tumors usually produce intense jaundice without biliary colic or fever, and once it begins, the jaundice rarely remits.

▶ Complications

Longstanding ductal infection can produce intrahepatic abscesses. Hepatic failure or secondary biliary cirrhosis may develop in unrelieved obstruction of long duration. Since the obstruction is usually incomplete and intermittent, cirrhosis develops only after several years in untreated disease. Acute pancreatitis, a fairly common complication of calculous biliary disease, is discussed in Chapter 26. Rarely, a stone in the common duct may erode through the ampulla, resulting in gallstone ileus. Hemorrhage (hemobilia) is also a rare complication.

▶ Treatment

Patients with acute cholangitis should be treated with systemic antibiotics and other measures as described in the preceding section; this usually controls the attack within 24–48 hours. If the patient's condition worsens or if marked improvement is not observed within 2–4 days, endoscopic sphincterotomy or surgery and common bile duct exploration should be performed.

The typical patient presents with mild cholangitis and evidence on ultrasound scans of gallbladder stones. Laparoscopic cholecystectomy is indicated, and depending on the experience of the surgeon, laparoscopic exploration of the common duct should be done if an operative cholangiogram or laparoscopic ultrasound demonstrates the expected common duct stones. Laparoscopic common duct exploration is usually accomplished through the cystic duct (which may have to be dilated), but when the common duct is enlarged (> 1.5 cm), it may be accomplished through a choledochotomy incision, just as in open surgery. Eventually, nearly all cases of common duct stones should be manageable by laparoscopic techniques, but at this stage the requisite laparoscopic skills are not available in most hospitals. If the surgeon thinks the common duct stones cannot be removed laparoscopically, it is probably best to remove the gallbladder laparoscopically and the common duct stones by endoscopic sphincterotomy. If the stones cannot be removed by sphincterotomy, a second (open) operation may be necessary.

There is also a lack of consensus regarding the importance of operative cholangiography or ultrasound during cholecystectomy when there are no clues suggesting stones in the duct. In such cases, the chances of finding a stone are only 3–5%, and some consider the effort unwarranted. On the other hand, operative cholangiograms also provide confirmation of the biliary anatomy, which contributes to avoidance of bile duct injuries, and the natural history of the few overlooked stones is worrisome. Therefore, we side with those who perform operative cholangiography liberally in such cases.

When the common duct is explored through the cystic duct and gallstones are removed, the cystic duct must be ligated, but a drainage catheter is not usually left within the common duct. When the common duct is explored through a choledochotomy (either during a laparoscopic or open operation), a T tube is usually left in the duct, and cholangiograms are taken a week or so postoperatively. Any residual stones discovered on these postoperative x-rays can be extracted 4–6 weeks later through the T tube tract.

Patients with common duct stones who have had a previous cholecystectomy are best treated by **endoscopic sphincterotomy.** Using a side-viewing duodenoscope, the ampulla is cannulated, and a 1-cm incision is made in the sphincter with an electrocautery wire. The opening created in the sphincter permits stones to pass from the duct into the duodenum. Endoscopic sphincterotomy is unlikely to be successful in patients with large stones (eg, > 2 cm), and it is contraindicated in the presence of stenosis of the bile duct proximal to the sphincter. Laparotomy and common duct exploration are required in a few cases.

Stones in the intrahepatic branches of the bile duct can usually be removed without difficulty during common duct exploration. In some cases, however, one or more of the intrahepatic ducts have become packed with stones, and the associated chronic inflammation has produced stenosis of the duct near its junction with the common hepatic duct. It is often impossible in these cases to clear the duct of stones, and if the disease involves only one lobe (usually the left lobe), hepatic lobectomy is indicated.

Binmoeller KF, Schafer TW: Endoscopic management of bile duct stones. J Clin Gastroenterol 2001;32:106.

Lauter DM, Froines EJ: Laparoscopic common duct exploration in the management of choledocholithiasis. Am J Surg 2000; 179:372.

Prat F et al: Prediction of common bile duct stones by noninvasive tests. Ann Surg 1999;229:362.

Rosenthal RJ, Rossi RL, Martin RF: Options and strategies for the management of choledocholithiasis. World J Surg 1998;22:1125.

Soetikno RM, Montes H, Carr-Locke DL: Endoscopic management of choledocholithiasis. J Clin Gastroenterol 1998;27:296.

Soper NJ: Intraoperative detection: intraoperative cholangiography vs. intraoperative ultrasonography. J Gastrointest Surg 2000; 4:334.

Suc B et al: Surgery vs endoscopy as primary treatment in symptomatic patients with suspected common bile duct stones: a multicenter randomized trial. French Associations for Surgical Research. Arch Surg 1998;133:702.

Tranter SE, Thompson MH: Potential of laparoscopic ultrasonography as an alternative to operative cholangiography in the detection of bile duct stones. Br J Surg 2001;88:65.

Wu JS, Dunnegan DL, Soper NJ: The utility of intracorporeal ultrasonography for screening of the bile duct during laparoscopic cholecystectomy. J Gastrointest Surg 1998;2:50.

POSTCHOLECYSTECTOMY SYNDROME

Postcholecystectomy syndrome has been used to signify the heterogeneous group of disorders affecting patients who continue to complain of symptoms after cholecystectomy. It is not really a syndrome, and the term is confusing.

The usual reason for incomplete relief after cholecystectomy is that the preoperative diagnosis of chronic cholecystitis was incorrect. The only symptom entirely characteristic of chronic cholecystitis is biliary colic. When a calculous gallbladder is removed in the hope that the patient will gain relief from dyspepsia, fatty food intolerance, belching, and other symptoms, the operation may leave the symptoms unchanged.

The presenting symptom may be dyspepsia or pain. An organic cause for the symptoms is more likely to be discovered in patients with severe episodic pain than in those with other complaints. Abnormal liver function studies, jaundice, and cholangitis are other manifestations that indicate residual biliary disease. Patients with suspicious findings should be studied by ERCP or THC. Choledocholithiasis, biliary stricture, and chronic pancreatitis are the most common causes of symptoms. Evidence is accumulating to implicate sphincter of Oddi dysmotility as a cause of pain in some patients. The diagnosis may be possible by biliary manometry, but experience is still too meager to justify acceptance of this entity without question. Relief of pain may follow endoscopic sphincterotomy. Stenosis of the hepatobiliary ampulla, a long cystic duct remnant, and neuromas have been blamed for continued symptoms, but well-verified cases are uncommon.

CARCINOMA OF THE GALLBLADDER

Carcinoma of the gallbladder is an uncommon neoplasm that occurs in elderly patients. It is associated with gallstones in 70% of cases, and the risk of malignant degeneration correlates with the length of time gallstones have been present. The tumor is twice as common in women as in men, as one would expect from the association with gallstones.

Most primary tumors of the gallbladder are adenocarcinomas that appear histologically to be scirrhous (60%), papillary (25%), or mucoid (15%). Dissemination of the tumor occurs early by direct invasion of the liver and hilar structures and by metastases to the common duct lymph nodes, liver, and lungs. In an occasional case, where carcinoma is an incidental finding after cholecystectomy for gallstone disease, the tumor is confined to the gallbladder as a carcinoma in situ or an early invasive lesion. Most invasive carcinomas, however, have spread by the time of surgery, and spread is virtually certain if the tumor has progressed to the point where it causes symptoms.

Clinical Findings

A. Symptoms and Signs

The most common presenting complaint is of right upper quadrant pain similar to previous episodes of biliary colic but more persistent. Obstruction of the cystic duct by tumor sometimes initiates an attack of acute cholecystitis. Other cases present with obstructive jaundice and, occasionally, cholangitis due to secondary involvement of the common duct.

Examination usually reveals a mass in the region of the gallbladder, which may not be recognized as a neoplasm if the patient has acute cholecystitis. If cholangitis is the principal symptom, a palpable gallbladder would be an unusual finding with choledocholithiasis alone and should suggest gallbladder carcinoma.

B. Imaging Studies

Oral cholecystograms almost never opacify except in patients with small incidental cancers. CT and ultrasound scans may demonstrate the extent of disease, but more often they show only gallstones.

The correct diagnosis is made preoperatively in only 10% of cases.

Complications

Obstruction of the common duct may produce multiple intrahepatic abscesses. Abscesses in or next to the tumor-laden gallbladder are frequent.

Prevention

The incidence of gallbladder cancer has decreased in recent years as the frequency of cholecystectomy has increased. It has been estimated that one case of gallbladder cancer is prevented for every 100 cholecystectomies performed for gallstone disease.

Treatment

If a localized carcinoma of the gallbladder is recognized at laparotomy, cholecystectomy should be performed along with en bloc wedge resection of an adjacent 3–5 cm of normal liver and dissection of the lymph nodes in the hepatoduodenal ligament. If a small invasive carcinoma overlooked during cholecystectomy for gallstone disease is later discovered by the pathologist, reoperation is indicated to perform a wedge resection of the liver bed plus regional lymphadenectomy. Some surgeons also recommend that the common duct be included routinely (ie, even in the absence of gross invasion) in the lymph node dissection for any

lesion that involves the full thickness of the gallbladder wall. In the few cases where cancer has not penetrated the muscularis mucosae, cholecystectomy alone should suffice. More extensive hepatectomies (eg, right lobectomy) are not worthwhile. Lesions that invade the bile duct and produce jaundice should be resected if possible. When not, a stent should be inserted endoscopically or percutaneously. There is little that surgery can offer in cases with hepatic metastases or more distant spread.

Prognosis

Radiotherapy and chemotherapy are not effective palliative measures. About 85% of patients are dead within a year after diagnosis.

The 10% of patients who presently survive more than 5 years consist of those whose carcinoma was an incidental finding during cholecystectomy for symptomatic gallstone disease and those in whom an aggressive resection has removed all gross tumor.

Baillie J: Tumors of the gallbladder and bile ducts. J Clin Gastroenterol 1999;29:14.

Bismuth H, Majno PE: Hepatobiliary surgery. J Hepatol 2000; 32(1 Suppl):208.

Kondo S et al: Regional and para-aortic lymphadenectomy in radical surgery for advanced gallbladder carcinoma. Br J Surg 2000;87:418.

Mainprize KS, Gould SW, Gilbert JM: Surgical management of polypoid lesions of the gallbladder. Br J Surg 2000;87:414.

Scott TE et al: A case-control assessment of risk factors for gallbladder carcinoma. Dig Dis Sci 1999;44:1619.

Sugiyama M, Atomi Y, Yamato T: Endoscopic ultrasonography for differential diagnosis of polypoid gall bladder lesions: analysis in surgical and follow up series. Gut 2000;46:250.

MALIGNANT TUMORS OF THE BILE DUCT

 ESSENTIALS OF DIAGNOSIS

- ▶ Intense cholestatic jaundice and pruritus.
- ▶ Anorexia and dull right upper quadrant pain.
- ▶ Dilated intrahepatic bile ducts on ultrasound or CT scan.
- ▶ Focal stricture on transhepatic or retrograde endoscopic cholangiogram.

General Considerations

Primary bile duct tumors are not more common in patients with cholelithiasis, and men and women are affected with equal frequency. Tumors appear at an average age of 60 years but may appear at any time between 20 and 80 years of age. More young people have been seen with this disease in recent years. Ulcerative colitis is a common associated condition, and in occasional cases, bile duct cancer develops in a patient with ulcerative colitis who has been known to have sclerosing cholangitis for several years. Chronic parasitic infestation of the bile ducts in the Orient may be responsible for the greater incidence of bile duct tumors in that area.

Most malignant biliary tumors are adenocarcinomas located in the hepatic or common bile duct. The histologic pattern varies from typical adenocarcinoma to tumors composed principally of fibrous stroma and few cells. The acellular tumors may be mistaken for benign strictures or sclerosing cholangitis if adequate biopsies are not obtained. About 10% are bulky papillary tumors, which tend to be less invasive and less apt to metastasize.

At presentation, metastases are uncommon, but the tumor has often grown into the portal vein or hepatic artery.

▶ Clinical Findings

A. Symptoms and Signs

The illness presents with gradual onset of jaundice or pruritus. Chills, fever, and biliary colic are usually absent, and except for a deep discomfort in the right upper quadrant, the patient feels well. Bilirubinuria is present from the start, and light-colored stools are usual. Anorexia and weight loss develop insidiously with time.

Icterus is the most obvious physical finding. If the tumor is located in the common duct, the gallbladder may distend and become palpable in the right upper quadrant. The tumor itself is never palpable. Patients with tumors of the hepatic duct do not develop palpable gallbladders. Hepatomegaly is common. If obstruction is unrelieved, the liver may eventually become cirrhotic, and splenomegaly, ascites, or bleeding varices become secondary manifestations.

B. Laboratory Findings

Since the duct is often completely obstructed, the serum bilirubin is usually over 15 mg/dL. Serum alkaline phosphatase is also increased. Fever and leukocytosis are not common, since the bile is sterile in most cases. The stool may contain occult blood, but this is more common with tumors of the pancreas or hepatopancreatic ampulla than those of the bile ducts.

C. Imaging Studies

Ultrasound or CT scans usually detect dilated intrahepatic bile ducts. THC or ERCP clearly depicts the lesion, and both are indicated in most cases. THC is of greater value, since it better demonstrates the ductal anatomy on the hepatic side of the lesion. With tumors involving the bifurcation of the common hepatic duct (Klatskin tumors), it is important to determine the proximal extent of the lesion (ie, whether the first branches of the lobar ducts are also involved). ERCP is of value with proximal tumors because if it shows concomitant obstruction of the cystic

duct, the diagnosis will most often prove to be gallbladder cancer invading the common duct (not a primary common duct neoplasm). The typical pattern with distal bile duct cancers consists of stenosis of the bile duct with sparing of the pancreatic duct. Adjacent stenoses of both ducts (the double-duct sign) indicate primary cancer of the pancreas. MR cholangiopancreatography may be useful if high-quality studies are available.

Occasionally, bile samples obtained at the time of THC will show malignant cells on cytologic study, but this is not a particularly useful test, since the diagnosis of cancer must be presumed from the cholangiographic findings and a negative cytologic study is unreliable. Angiography may suggest invasion of the portal vein or encasement of the hepatic artery. False positives may occur, however.

▶ Differential Diagnosis

The differential diagnosis must consider other causes of extrahepatic and intrahepatic cholestatic jaundice. Choledocholithiasis is characterized by episodes of partial obstruction, pain, and cholangitis, which contrast with the unremitting jaundice of malignant obstruction. Bilirubin concentrations rarely surpass 15 mg/dL and are usually below 10 mg/dL in gallstone obstruction, whereas bilirubin levels almost always exceed 10 mg/dL and are usually above 15 mg/dL in neoplastic obstruction. A rapid rise of the bilirubin level to above 15 mg/dL in a patient with sclerosing cholangitis should suggest superimposed neoplasm. Dilatation of the gallbladder may occur with tumors of the distal common duct but is rare with calculous obstruction.

The combination of an enlarged gallbladder with obstructive jaundice is usually recognized as being due to tumor. If the gallbladder cannot be felt, primary biliary cirrhosis, drug-induced jaundice, chronic active hepatitis, metastatic hepatic cancer, and common duct stone must be ruled out. In general, any patient with cholestatic jaundice of more than 2 weeks' duration whose diagnosis is uncertain should be studied by THC or ERCP. The finding of focal bile duct stenosis in the absence of previous biliary surgery is almost pathognomonic of neoplasm.

▶ Treatment

Patients without evidence of metastases or other signs of advanced cancer (eg, ascites) are candidates for laparotomy. The 30% of patients who do not qualify may be treated by insertion of a tube stent into the bile duct transhepatically under radiologic control or from the duodenum under endoscopic control. The tube is positioned so that holes above and below the tumor reestablish flow of bile into the duodenum. If both lobar ducts are blocked by a tumor at the bifurcation of the common hepatic duct, it is usually necessary to place a transhepatic tube into only one lobar duct. If the lesion blocks the takeoff of the segmental ducts, stents are rarely beneficial.

Laparotomy is indicated in most cases, however, with the objective of removing the tumor. Preoperative decompression of the bile duct with a percutaneous catheter to relieve jaundice does not lower the incidence of postoperative complications. At operation, which may be immediately preceded by diagnostic laparoscopy, the extent of the tumor should be determined by external examination of the bile duct and the adjacent portal vein and hepatic artery.

Tumors of the distal common duct should be treated by radical pancreaticoduodenectomy (Whipple procedure) if it appears that all tumor would be removed. Secondary involvement of the portal vein is the usual reason for unresectability of tumors in this location. Mid common duct or low hepatic duct tumors should also be removed if possible. If the tumor cannot be excised, bile flow should be reestablished into the intestine by a cholecystojejunostomy or Roux-en-Y choledochojejunostomy. The choice is based on technical considerations.

Tumors at the hilum of the liver should be resected if possible and a Roux-en-Y hepaticojejunostomy performed. The anastomosis is usually between hilum and bowel rather than between individual bile ducts and bowel. A curative operation nearly always requires resection of either the right or the left lobe of the liver and, in all cases, the caudate lobe. Extension into the lobar and segmental ducts and secondary involvement of the hepatic artery and portal vein are the most common reasons for inability to resect the tumor. Subtotal resections offer little in the way of palliation.

Postoperative radiotherapy is commonly recommended.

► Prognosis

The average patient with adenocarcinoma of the bile duct survives less than a year. The overall 5-year survival rate is 15%. Following a thorough radical operation, 5-year survival is about 40%. Biliary cirrhosis, intrahepatic infection, and general debility with terminal pneumonitis are the usual causes of death. Palliative resections and stents may improve the length and quality of survival in this disease even though surgical cure is uncommon. Limited experience with liver transplantation for this disease has been discouraging: tumor has recurred postoperatively in most patients.

Ahrendt SA, Nakeeb A, Pitt HA: Cholangiocarcinoma. Clin Liver Dis 2001;5:191.

Burke EC et al: Hilar cholangiocarcinoma: patterns of spread, the importance of hepatic resection for curative operation, and a presurgical clinical staging system. Ann Surg 1998;228:385.

Chamberlain RS, Blumgart LH: Hilar cholangiocarcinoma: a review and commentary. Ann Surg Oncol 2000;7:55.

Jarnagin WR: Cholangiocarcinoma of the extrahepatic bile ducts. Semin Surg Oncol 2000;19:156.

Kosuge T et al: Improved surgical results for hilar cholangiocarcinoma with procedures including major hepatic resection. Ann Surg 1999;230:663.

Lillemoe KD, Cameron JL: Surgery for hilar cholangiocarcinoma: the Johns Hopkins approach. J Hepatobiliary Pancreat Surg 2000;7:115.

Molmenti EP et al: Hepatobiliary malignancies. Primary hepatic malignant neoplasms. Surg Clin North Am 1999;79:43.

BENIGN TUMORS & PSEUDOTUMORS OF THE GALLBLADDER

Various unrelated lesions appear on the cholecystogram as projections from the gallbladder wall. The differentiation from gallstones is based upon observing whether a shift in position of the projections follows changes in posture of the patient, since stones are not fixed. Cancer should be suspected in any polypoid lesion that exceeds 1 cm in diameter.

► Polyps

Most of these are not true neoplasms but cholesterol polyps, a local form of cholesterosis. Histologically, they consist of a cluster of lipid-filled macrophages in the submucosa. They easily become detached from the wall when the gallbladder is handled at surgery. It is not known whether cholesterol polyps are important in the genesis of gallstones. Some patients experience gallbladder pain, but whether this is related to the presence of the polyps per se or is a manifestation of functional gallbladder disease has not been established.

Inflammatory polyps have also been reported, but they are quite rare.

► Adenomyomatosis

On cholecystography, this entity presents as a slight intraluminal convexity that is often marked by central umbilication. It is usually found in the fundus but may occur elsewhere. It is unclear whether adenomyomatosis is an acquired degenerative lesion or a developmental abnormality (ie, hamartoma). The following synonyms for this lesion appear in the literature: adenomatous hyperplasia, cholecystitis glandularis proliferans, and diverticulosis of the gallbladder. Although the condition is probably asymptomatic in many cases, adenomyomatosis can cause abdominal pain. Cholecystectomy should be performed in such patients.

► Adenomas

These appear as pedunculated adenomatous polyps, true neoplasms that may be papillary or nonpapillary histologically. In a few cases, they have been found in association with carcinoma in situ of the gallbladder.

BENIGN TUMORS OF THE BILE DUCTS

Benign papillomas and adenomas may arise from the ductal epithelium. Only 90 cases have been reported to date. The neoplastic propensity of the ductal epithelium is widespread, so the tumors are often multiple, and recurrence is common after excision. The affected duct must be radically excised for permanent cure to result.

BILE DUCT INJURIES & STRICTURES

ESSENTIALS OF DIAGNOSIS

▶ Episodic cholangitis.
▶ Previous biliary surgery.
▶ Transhepatic cholangiogram often diagnostic.

▶ General Considerations

Benign biliary injuries and strictures are caused by surgical trauma in about 95% of cases. The remainder result from external abdominal trauma or, rarely, from erosion of the duct by a gallstone. Prevention of injury to the duct depends on a combination of technical skill, experience, and a thorough knowledge of the normal anatomy and its variations in the hilum of the liver. The number of bile duct injuries has risen sharply in the past few years along with the shift from open to laparoscopic cholecystectomy.

The most common lesion consists of excision of a segment of the common duct as a result of mistaking it for the cystic duct. Partial transection, occlusion with metal clips, injury to the right hepatic duct, and leakage from the cystic duct are other examples. A full discussion of how these injuries occur and how they can be prevented is beyond the scope of this text.

A clean incision of the duct without additional damage is best managed by opening the abdomen and suturing the incision with fine absorbable suture material.

▶ Clinical Findings

A. Symptoms

Manifestations of injury to the duct may or may not be evident in the postoperative period. Following laparoscopic surgery, bile ascites, manifested by abdominal distention, bloating, and pain plus mild jaundice, is the usual presentation, since the duct is usually open to the abdomen. The symptoms are relatively mild and may for a time be thought to represent only ileus until a worsening picture requires further investigation.

Injuries following open cholecystectomy more often present with intermittent cholangitis or jaundice as a consequence of a biliary stricture. The first clear-cut symptoms may not be evident for weeks or months after surgery.

B. Signs

Findings are not distinctive. Bile ascites produces abdominal distention and ileus and, rarely, true bile peritonitis with toxicity. The right upper quadrant may be tender but usually is not. Jaundice is usually present during an attack of cholangitis.

C. Laboratory Findings

The serum alkaline phosphatase concentration is elevated in cases of stricture. The serum bilirubin fluctuates in relation to symptoms but usually remains well below 10 mg/dL.

Blood cultures are usually positive during acute cholangitis.

D. Imaging Studies

Bile ascites can be suspected on ultrasound or CT scan. Fluid should be aspirated, and if it is bile, the diagnosis is clear. THC and ERCP are necessary to depict the anatomy. After laparoscopic cholecystectomy, the most common pattern is a blocked (by a metal clip) lower duct and an upper duct draining freely into the abdomen. With a stricture, the findings most often consist of focal narrowing of the common hepatic duct within 2 cm of the bifurcation and mild to moderate dilatation of the intrahepatic ducts.

▶ Differential Diagnosis

Choledocholithiasis is the condition that most often must be differentiated from biliary stricture because the clinical and laboratory findings can be identical. A history of trauma to the duct would point toward stricture as the more likely diagnosis. The final distinction must often await radiologic or surgical findings. THC or ERCP should be definitive.

Other causes of cholestatic jaundice may have to be ruled out in some cases.

▶ Complications

Complications develop quickly if the leak is not controlled. Bile peritonitis and abscesses may form. With stricture, persistent cholangitis may progress to multiple intrahepatic abscesses and a septic death.

▶ Treatment

Bile duct injuries should be surgically repaired in all but a few patients who are likely to improve with a nonoperative approach. Excision of the damaged duct and Roux-en-Y hepaticojejunostomy is indicated for most acute and chronic injuries. The entire biliary tree must be outlined by cholangiograms preoperatively. The key to success is the thoroughness of the dissection and the ability ultimately to suture healthy duct to healthy bowel. This, in turn, depends on the experience of the surgeon with this particular operation.

When a definitive repair is technically impossible, the stricture may be dilated with a transhepatic balloon-tipped catheter. This is particularly applicable to patients with portal hypertension, whose hepatic hilum contains numerous venous collaterals that make operation hazardous.

▶ Prognosis

The death rate from biliary injuries is about 5%, and severe illness is frequent. If the stricture is not repaired, episodic cholangitis and secondary liver disease are inevitable.

Surgical correction of the stricture should be successful in about 90% of cases. Experience at centers with a special interest in this problem indicates that good results can be obtained even if several previous attempts did not relieve the obstruction. There is essentially no place for liver transplantation in this disease.

Nealon WH, Urrutia F: Long-term follow-up after bilioenteric anastomosis for benign bile duct stricture. Ann Surg 1996;223:639.

Savader SJ et al: Laparoscopic cholecystectomy-related bile duct injuries: a health and financial disaster. Ann Surg 1997;225:268.

Strasberg SM, Eagon CJ, Drebin JA: The "hidden cystic duct" syndrome and the infundibular technique of laparoscopic cholecystectomy: the danger of the false infundibulum. J Am Coll Surg 2000;191:661.

Strasberg SM, Hertl M, Soper NJ: An analysis of the problem of biliary injury during laparoscopic cholecystectomy. J Am Coll Surg 1995;180:101.

Strasberg SM, Picus DD, Drebin JA: Results of a new strategy for reconstruction of biliary injuries having an isolated right-sided component. J Gastrointest Surg 2001;5:266.

Yeh TS et al: Value of magnetic resonance cholangiopancreatography in demonstrating major bile duct injuries following laparoscopic cholecystectomy. Br J Surg 1999;86:181.

UNCOMMON CAUSES OF BILE DUCT OBSTRUCTION

▶ Congenital Choledochal Cysts

About 30% of congenital choledochal cysts produce their first symptoms in adults, usually presenting with jaundice, cholangitis, and a right upper quadrant mass. Diagnosis can be made by THC or ERCP. The optimal surgical procedure is excision of the cyst and construction of a Roux-en-Y hepaticojejunostomy. If this is not technically possible or if the patient's condition will not permit a prolonged operation, the cyst should be emptied of precipitated biliary sludge and a cystenteric anastomosis constructed. Congenital cysts of the biliary tree have a high incidence of malignant degeneration, which is another argument for excision rather than drainage.

Vercruysse R, Van den Bossche MR: Choledochal cyst in adults. Acta Chir Belg 1998;98:220.

Watanatittan S, Niramis R: Choledochal cyst: review of 74 pediatric cases. J Med Assoc Thai 1998;81:586.

▶ Caroli Disease

Caroli disease, another form of congenital cystic disease, consists of saccular intrahepatic dilatation of the ducts. In some cases, the biliary abnormality is an isolated finding, but more often it is associated with congenital hepatic fibrosis and medullary sponge kidney. The latter patients often present in childhood or as young adults with complications of portal hypertension. Others have cholangitis and obstructive jaundice as initial manifestations. There is no definitive

surgical solution to the problem except in rare cases with isolated involvement of one hepatic lobe, where lobectomy is curative. Intermittent antibiotic therapy for cholangitis is the usual regimen.

Hara H et al: Surgical treatment for congenital biliary dilatation, with or without intrahepatic bile duct dilatation. Hepatogastroenterology 2001;48:638.

Parada LA et al: Clonal chromosomal abnormalities in congenital bile duct dilatation (Caroli's disease). Gut 1999;45:780.

Waechter FL et al: The role of liver transplantation in patients with Caroli's disease. Hepatogastroenterology 2001;48:672.

▶ Hemobilia

Hemobilia presents with the triad of biliary colic, obstructive jaundice, and occult or gross intestinal bleeding. Most cases in Western cultures follow several weeks after hepatic trauma with bleeding from an intrahepatic branch of the hepatic artery into a duct. It is seen with less frequency now, because the general principles of management of hepatic trauma are better understood. In the Orient, hemobilia usually follows ductal parasitism (*Ascaris lumbricoides*) or Oriental cholangiohepatitis. Other causes are hepatic neoplasms, rupture of a hepatic artery aneurysm, hepatic abscess, and choledocholithiasis. The diagnosis may be suspected from a technetium-99m-labeled red blood cell scan, but an arteriogram is usually required for diagnosis and planning of therapy. Sometimes the bleeding can be stopped by embolizing the lesion with stainless steel coils, Gelfoam, or autologous blood clot infused through a catheter selectively positioned in the hepatic artery. If this is unsuccessful, either direct ligation of the bleeding point in the liver or proximal ligation of an upstream branch of the hepatic artery in the hilum is required.

Green MH et al: Haemobilia. Br J Surg 2001;88:773.

▶ Pancreatitis

Pancreatitis can cause obstruction of the intrapancreatic portion of the bile duct by inflammatory swelling, encasement with scar, or compression by a pseudocyst. The patient may present with painless jaundice or cholangitis. Occasionally, a distended gallbladder can be felt on abdominal examination. Differentiation from choledocholithiasis and secondary acute pancreatitis depends on biliary x-rays or surgical exploration if the jaundice persists. Jaundice due to inflammation alone rarely lasts more than 2 weeks; persistent jaundice following an attack of acute pancreatitis suggests the development of a pseudocyst, underlying chronic pancreatitis with obstruction by fibrosis, or even an obstructing neoplasm.

Biliary obstruction from chronic pancreatitis may have few or no clinical manifestations. Jaundice is usually present, but the average peak bilirubin level is only 4–5 mg/dL. Some patients with functionally significant stenosis have persistently elevated alkaline phosphatase levels as the only abnormality; when surgical decompression of the bile duct is not performed, these patients often develop secondary biliary cirrhosis within a year or so. Diagnosis of stricture is made by ERCP, which shows a long stenosis of the intrapancreatic portion of the duct, proximal dilatation, and either a gradual or abrupt tapering of the lumen at the pancreatic border, occasionally accompanied by ductal angulation. If cholangiograms show stenosis and if alkaline phosphatase or bilirubin levels remain more than twice normal for longer than 2 months, the stenosis is functionally significant and unlikely to resolve and requires surgical correction. Choledochoduodenostomy is done in most cases. Cholecystoduodenostomy is unreliable because the cystic duct is often too narrow to provide continued biliary decompression.

Patients with obstructive jaundice and pseudocyst usually respond to surgical drainage of the pseudocyst. However, occasionally they do not respond, because chronic scarring—not the cyst—is the cause of obstruction. Procedures to drain both the bile duct and the pseudocyst are indicated if operative cholangiograms demonstrate persistent bile duct obstruction after the cyst has been decompressed.

▶ Ampullary Dysfunction & Stenosis

Stenosis of the hepatopancreatic ampulla (ampullary stenosis) has been implicated as a cause of pain and other manifestations of ampullary obstruction and is often considered as a cause of postcholecystectomy complaints. Some cases are idiopathic, whereas others may be the result of trauma from gallstones. If the patient has secondary manifestations of biliary obstruction (eg, jaundice, increased alkaline phosphatase concentration, cholangitis) in the absence of gallstones or some other obstructing lesion, and cholangiography shows dilatation of the common duct, ampullary stenosis is a plausible explanation. However, the diagnosis is more often proposed as a reason for upper abdominal pain without these more objective findings. Ampullary dysfunction is postulated in these cases.

Sphincter of Oddi dysfunction may be the cause of biliary-like pain and is often considered in patients who remain uncomfortable after cholecystectomy. The pathogenesis of the symptoms is thought to be similar to that of esophageal dysmotility and the irritable bowel syndrome. The patients typically experience severe, intermittent upper abdominal pain that lasts for 1–3 hours, sometimes following a meal.

Residual gallstone and pancreatic disease must first be ruled out. Ampullary dysfunction can then be diagnosed by sphincter of Oddi manometry. Patients are placed in one of three groups depending on the presence of three objective manifestations of biliary obstruction: abnormal liver function tests, prolonged (> 45 minutes) common bile duct emptying of contrast media after ERCP; and a common duct greater than 12 mm in diameter. Patients in group I have all

three findings; patients in group II have one or two findings; and patients in group III have none of the findings. Group I patients are thought to have enough evidence of disease that sphincterotomy should be performed without manometry. Group I patients have abnormal motility so rarely that they should not be considered further for sphincterotomy. Thus, motility studies are most often of value in determining which of the group II patients will improve after sphincterotomy.

The abnormalities sought on the motility studies include an elevated (> 40 mm Hg) basal sphincter pressure and a paradoxic rise in sphincter pressure in response to CCK. The former is most reliable. About 50% of group II patients have elevated sphincter pressures, and these are the ones who benefit from sphincterotomy.

A scintigraphic test may be just as accurate. The patient is given a bolus of CCK followed by technetium-99m diisopropyl iminodiacetic acid (^{99m}Tc-DISIDA). Gamma camera images of the liver and bile duct are obtained for 60 minutes. A scoring system (score: 0–12) is based on the rate of passage of the imaging agent past various relevant points (eg, appearance and clearance through the liver, bile duct, and bowel). The normal range is 0–5; abnormal is 6–12.

Sphincter of Oddi dysfunction is an uncommon explanation for abdominal pain, and it is appropriate to remain skeptical unless the objective findings of biliary obstruction are clear-cut. In well-selected cases, however, endoscopic sphincterotomy is truly beneficial.

Chen JW, Saccone GT, Toouli J: Sphincter of Oddi dysfunction and acute pancreatitis. Gut 1998;43:305.

Rosenblatt ML et al: Comparison of sphincter of Oddi manometry, fatty meal sonography, and hepatobiliary scintigraphy in the diagnosis of sphincter of Oddi dysfunction. Gastrointest Endosc 2001;54:697.

Silverman WB et al: Hybrid classification of sphincter of Oddi dysfunction based on simplified Milwaukee criteria: effect of marginal serum liver and pancreas test elevations. Dig Dis Sci 2001;46:278.

Thomas PD et al: Use of (99m)Tc-DISIDA biliary scanning with morphine provocation for the detection of elevated sphincter of Oddi basal pressure. Gut 2000;46:838.

Toouli J et al: Manometry based randomized trial of endoscopic sphincterotomy for sphincter of Oddi dysfunction. Gut 2000;46:98.

▶ Duodenal Diverticula

Duodenal diverticula usually arise on the medial aspect of the duodenum within 2 cm of the orifice of the bile duct, and in some individuals the duct empties directly into a diverticulum. Even in the latter circumstance, duodenal diverticula are usually innocuous. Occasionally, distortion of the duct entrance or obstruction by enterolith formation in the diverticulum produces symptoms. Either choledochoduodenostomy or Roux-en-Y choledochojejunostomy is usually a safer method of reestablishing biliary drainage than attempts to excise the diverticulum and reimplant the duct.

Ascariasis

When the worms invade the duct from the duodenum, ascariasis can produce symptoms of ductal obstruction. Air may sometimes be seen within the ducts on plain films. Antibiotics should be used until cholangitis is controlled, and anthelmintic therapy (mebendazole, albendazole, or pyrantel pamoate) should then be given. The acute symptoms usually subside with antibiotics, but if they do not, endoscopic sphincterotomy should be performed and attempts made to extricate the worms. If this is unsuccessful and the patient remains acutely ill, the duct should be emptied surgically.

Recurrent Pyogenic Cholangitis (Oriental Cholangiohepatitis)

Oriental cholangiohepatitis is a type of chronic recurrent cholangitis prevalent in coastal areas from Japan to Southeast Asia. In Hong Kong, it is the third-most common indication for emergency laparotomy and the most frequent type of biliary disease. The disease is currently thought to result from chronic portal bacteremia, with portal phlebitis antedating the biliary disease. *E coli* causes secondary infection of the bile ducts, which initiates pigment stone formation within the ducts.

Biliary obstruction from the stones gives rise to recurrent cholangitis, which, unlike gallstone disease in Western countries, may be unaccompanied by gallbladder stones. The gallbladder is usually distended during an attack and may contain pus.

Chronic recurrent infection often leads to biliary strictures and hepatic abscess formation. The strictures are usually located in the intrahepatic bile ducts, and for some unknown reason, the left lobe of the liver is more severely involved. Intrahepatic gallstones are common, and their surgical removal may be difficult or impossible. Acute abdominal pain, chills, and high fever are usually present, and jaundice develops in about half of cases. Right upper quadrant tenderness is usually marked, and in about 80% of cases the gallbladder is palpable. ERCP or THC is the best way to study the biliary tree and can help in determining the need for surgery and the type of procedure.

Systemic antibiotics should be given for acute cholangitis. Surgical treatment consists of cholecystectomy, common duct exploration, and removal of stones. Sphincteroplasty should also be performed to allow any residual or recurrent stones to escape from the duct. A Roux-en-Y choledochojejunostomy is indicated for patients with strictures, markedly dilated ducts (eg, > 3 cm), or recurrent disease after a previous sphincteroplasty. The results of surgery are good in 80% of patients. Chronic intrahepatic stones and infection, which often involve only one lobe, may require hepatic lobectomy.

Although many patients are cured, prolonged illness from repeated infection is almost unavoidable once strictures have appeared or the intrahepatic ducts have become packed with stones.

Cosenza CA et al: Current management of recurrent pyogenic cholangitis. Am Surg 1999;65:939.
Harris HW et al: Recurrent pyogenic cholangitis. Am J Surg 1998;176:34.
Kim M et al: MR imaging findings in recurrent pyogenic cholangitis. AJR Am J Roentgenol 1999;173:1545.
Park MS et al: Recurrent pyogenic cholangitis: comparison between MR cholangiography and direct cholangiography. Radiology 2001;220:677.

Sclerosing Cholangitis

Sclerosing cholangitis is a rare chronic disease of unknown cause characterized by nonbacterial inflammatory narrowing of the bile ducts. About 60% of cases occur in patients with ulcerative colitis, and sclerosing cholangitis develops in about 5% of patients with that disorder. Other less commonly associated conditions are thyroiditis, retroperitoneal fibrosis, and mediastinal fibrosis. The disease chiefly affects men 20–50 years of age. In most cases, the entire biliary tree is affected by the inflammatory process, which causes irregular partial obliteration of the lumen of the ducts. The narrowing may be confined, however, to the intrahepatic or extrahepatic ducts, though it is almost never so short as to resemble a posttraumatic or focal malignant stricture. The woody-hard duct walls contain increased collagen and lymphoid elements and are thickened at the expense of the lumen.

The clinical onset usually consists of the gradual appearance of mild jaundice and pruritus. Symptoms of bacterial cholangitis (eg, fever and chills) are uncommon in the absence of previous biliary surgery. Laboratory findings are typical of cholestasis. The total serum bilirubin averages about 4 mg/dL and rarely exceeds 10 mg/dL. ERCP is usually diagnostic, demonstrating ductal stenoses and irregularity, which often gives a beaded appearance. Liver biopsy may show pericholangitis and bile stasis, but the changes are nonspecific.

The complications of sclerosing cholangitis include gallstone disease and adenocarcinoma of the bile duct. The latter is most common in patients with ulcerative colitis. Furthermore, patients with ulcerative colitis and sclerosing cholangitis appear to be at greater risk for colonic mucosal dysplasia and colon cancer than those with ulcerative colitis not associated with sclerosing cholangitis.

Ursodiol (ursodeoxycholic acid), 10 mg/kg/d, improves liver function tests and symptoms. Cholestyramine will give relief from pruritus. Percutaneous transhepatic balloon dilatation can be of value to treat dominant strictures. In cases where the disease is largely confined to the distal extrahepatic duct and the proximal ducts are dilated, a Roux-en-Y hepaticojejunostomy may be indicated. For patients with severe intrahepatic involvement, hepatic transplantation should be considered.

The natural history of sclerosing cholangitis is one of chronicity and unpredictable severity. Some patients seem to obtain nearly complete remission after treatment, but this is not common. Bacterial cholangitis may develop after operation if adequate drainage has not been established. In these cases, antibiotics will be required at intervals. Most patients experience the gradual evolution of secondary biliary cirrhosis after many years of mild to moderate jaundice and pruritus. Liver transplantation is indicated when the disease becomes advanced. The results are good.

Ghosh S, Shand A, Ferguson A: Ulcerative colitis. BMJ 2000;320:1119.

Kim WR et al: A revised natural history model for primary sclerosing cholangitis. Mayo Clin Proc 2000;75:688.

Kubicka S et al: K-ras mutations in the bile of patients with primary sclerosing cholangitis. Gut 2001;48:403.

Ryder SD, Beckingham IJ: ABC of diseases of liver, pancreas, and biliary system. Other causes of parenchymal liver disease. BMJ 2001;322:290.

van Hoogstraten HJ et al: Ursodeoxycholic acid therapy for primary sclerosing cholangitis: results of a 2-year randomized controlled trial to evaluate single versus multiple daily doses. J Hepatol 1998;29:417.

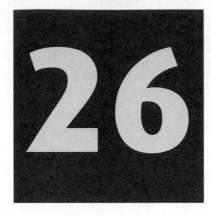

26

Pancreas

Gerard M. Doherty, MD
Lawrence W. Way, MD

EMBRYOLOGY

The pancreas arises in the fourth week of fetal life from the caudal part of the foregut as dorsal and ventral pancreatic buds. Both anlagen rotate to the right and fuse near the point of origin of the ventral pancreas. Later, as the duodenum rotates, the pancreas shifts to the left. In the adult, only the caudal portion of the head and the uncinate process are derived from the ventral pancreas. The cranial part of the head and all of the body and tail are derived from the dorsal pancreas. Most of the dorsal pancreatic duct joins with the duct of the ventral pancreas to form the main pancreatic duct (**duct of Wirsung**); a small part persists as the accessory duct (**duct of Santorini**). In 5–10% of people, the ventral and dorsal pancreatic ducts do not fuse, and most regions of the pancreas drain through the duct of Santorini and the orifice of the minor papilla. In this case, only the small ventral pancreas drains with the common bile duct through the papilla of Vater.

ANATOMY

The pancreas is a thin elliptic organ that lies within the retroperitoneum in the upper abdomen (Figures 26–1 and 26–2). In the adult, it is 12–15 cm long and weighs 70–100 g. The gland can be divided into three portions: head, body, and tail. The head of the pancreas is intimately adherent to the medial portion of the duodenum and lies in front of the inferior vena cava and superior mesenteric vessels. A small tongue of tissue called the uncinate process lies behind the superior mesenteric vessels as they emerge from the retroperitoneum. Anteriorly, the stomach and the first portion of the duodenum lie partly in front of the pancreas. The common bile duct passes through a posterior groove in the head of the pancreas adjacent to the duodenum. The body of the pancreas is in contact posteriorly with the aorta, the left crus of the diaphragm, the left adrenal gland, and the left kidney. The tail of the pancreas lies in the hilum of the spleen. The main pancreatic duct (the duct of Wirsung) courses along the gland from the tail to the head and joins the common bile duct just before entering the duodenum at the ampulla of Vater. The accessory pancreatic duct (the duct of Santorini) enters the duodenum 2–2.5 cm proximal to the ampulla of Vater (Figure 26–1).

The blood supply of the pancreas is derived from branches of the celiac and superior mesenteric arteries (Figure 26–2). The superior pancreaticoduodenal artery arises from the gastroduodenal artery, runs parallel to the duodenum, and eventually meets the inferior pancreaticoduodenal artery, a branch of the superior mesenteric artery, to form an arcade. The splenic artery provides tributaries that supply the body and tail of the pancreas. The main branches are termed the dorsal pancreatic, pancreatica magna, and caudal pancreatic arteries. The venous supply of the gland parallels the arterial supply. Lymphatic drainage is into the peripancreatic nodes located along the veins.

The innervation of the pancreas is derived from the vagal and splanchnic nerves. The efferent fibers pass through the celiac plexus from the celiac branch of the right vagal nerve to terminate in ganglia located in the interlobular septa of the pancreas. Postganglionic fibers from these synapses innervate the acini, the islets, and the ducts. The visceral afferent fibers from the pancreas also travel in the vagal and splanchnic nerves, but those that mediate pain are confined to the latter. Sympathetic fibers to the pancreas pass from the splanchnic nerves through the celiac plexus and innervate the pancreatic vasculature.

PHYSIOLOGY

▶ Exocrine Function

The external secretion of the pancreas consists of a clear, alkaline (pH 7.0–8.3) solution of 1–2 L/d containing digestive enzymes. Secretion is stimulated by the hormones secretin and cholecystokinin (CCK) and by parasympathetic vagal discharge. Secretin and cholecystokinin are synthesized, stored, and released from duodenal mucosal cells in response to specific stimuli. Acid in the lumen of the duodenum

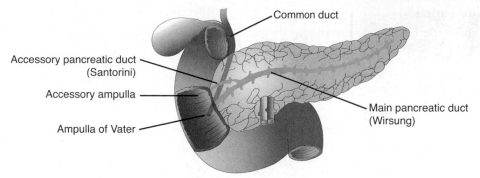

▲ **Figure 26–1.** Anatomic configuration of pancreatic ductal system. (Courtesy of W Silen.)

causes the release of secretin, and luminal digestion products of fat and protein cause the release of cholecystokinin.

The water and electrolyte secretion is formed by the centroacinar and intercalated duct cells principally in response to secretin stimulation. The secretion is modified by exchange processes and active secretion in the ductal collecting system. The cations sodium and potassium are present in the same concentrations as in plasma. The anions bicarbonate and chloride vary in concentration according to the rate of secretion: With increasing rate of secretion, the bicarbonate concentration increases and chloride concentration falls, so that the sum of the two is the same throughout the secretory range. Pancreatic juice helps neutralize gastric acid in the duodenum and adjusts luminal pH to the level that gives optimal activity of pancreatic enzymes.

Pancreatic enzymes are synthesized, stored (as zymogen granules), and released by the acinar cells of the gland, principally in response to cholecystokinin and vagal stimula-tion. Pancreatic enzymes are proteolytic, lipolytic, and amy-lolytic. Lipase and amylase are stored and secreted in active forms. The proteolytic enzymes are secreted as inactive pre-cursors and are activated by the duodenal enzyme enteroki-nase. Other enzymes secreted by the pancreas include ribonu-cleases and phospholipase A. Phospholipase A is secreted as an inactive proenzyme activated in the duodenum by trypsin. It catalyzes the conversion of biliary lecithin to lysolecithin.

Turnover of protein in the pancreas exceeds that of any other organ in the body. Intravenously injected amino acids are incorporated into enzyme protein and may appear in the pancreatic juice within 1 hour. Three mechanisms prevent autodigestion of the pancreas by its proteolytic enzymes: (1) The enzymes are stored in acinar cells as zy-mogen granules, where they are separated from other cell proteins. (2) The enzymes are secreted in an inactive form. (3) Inhibitors of proteolytic enzymes are present in pancre-atic juice and pancreatic tissue.

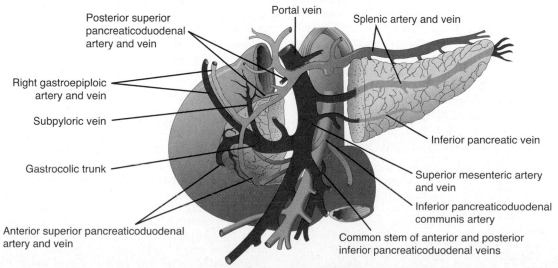

▲ **Figure 26–2.** Arterial supply and venous drainage of the pancreas. (Courtesy of W Silen.)

Endocrine Function

The function of the endocrine pancreas is to facilitate storage of foodstuffs by release of insulin after a meal and to provide a mechanism for their mobilization by release of glucagon during periods of fasting. Insulin and glucagon, as well as pancreatic polypeptide and somatostatin, are produced by the islets of Langerhans.

Insulin, a polypeptide (MW 5734) consisting of 51 amino acid residues, is formed in the β cells of the pancreas via the precursor proinsulin. Insulin secretion is stimulated by rising or high serum concentrations of metabolic substrates such as glucose, amino acids, and perhaps short-chain fatty acids. The major normal stimulus for insulin release appears to be glucose. The release and synthesis of insulin are stimulated by activation of specific glucoreceptors located on the surface membrane of the beta cell. Insulin release is also stimulated by calcium, glucagon, secretin, cholecystokinin, vasoactive intestinal polypeptide (VIP), and gastrin, all of which sensitize the receptors on the beta cell to glucose. Epinephrine, tolbutamide, and chlorpropamide release insulin by acting on the adenylyl cyclase system.

Glucagon, a polypeptide (MW 3485) consisting of 29 amino acid residues, is formed in the α cells of the pancreas. The release of glucagon is stimulated by a low blood glucose concentration, amino acids, catecholamines, sympathetic nervous discharge, and cholecystokinin. It is suppressed by hyperglycemia and insulin.

The principal functions of insulin are to stimulate anabolic reactions involving carbohydrates, fats, proteins, and nucleic acids. Insulin decreases glycogenolysis, lipolysis, proteolysis, gluconeogenesis, ureagenesis, and ketogenesis. Glucagon stimulates glycogenolysis from the liver and proteolysis and lipolysis in adipose tissue as well as in the liver. With the increase in lipolysis, there is an increase in ketogenesis and gluconeogenesis. Glucagon increases cAMP in the liver, heart, skeletal muscle, and adipose tissue. The short-term regulation of gluconeogenesis depends on the balance between insulin and glucagon. Studies on insulin and glucagon suggest that the hormones exert their effects via receptors on the cell membrane. Before entering the systemic circulation, blood draining from the islets of Langerhans perfuses the pancreatic acini, and this exposure to high levels of hormones is thought to influence acinar function.

ANNULAR PANCREAS

Annular pancreas is a rare congenital condition in which a ring of pancreatic tissue from the head of the pancreas surrounds the descending duodenum. The abnormality usually presents in infancy as duodenal obstruction with postprandial vomiting. There is bile in the vomitus if the constriction is distal to the entrance of the common bile duct. X-rays show a dilated stomach and proximal duodenum (double-bubble sign) and little or no air in the rest of the small bowel.

After correction of fluid and electrolyte imbalance, the obstructed segment should be bypassed by a duodenojejunostomy or other similar procedure. No attempt should be made to resect the obstructing pancreas, because a pancreatic fistula or acute pancreatitis often develops postoperatively.

Occasionally, annular pancreas will present in adult life with similar symptoms.

PANCREATITIS

Pancreatitis is a common nonbacterial inflammatory disease caused by activation, interstitial liberation, and autodigestion of the pancreas by its own enzymes. The process may or may not be accompanied by permanent morphologic and functional changes in the gland. Much is known about the causes of pancreatitis, but despite the accumulation of much experimental data, understanding of the pathogenesis of this disorder is still incomplete.

In **acute pancreatitis,** there is sudden upper abdominal pain, nausea and vomiting, and elevated serum amylase. **Chronic pancreatitis** is characterized by chronic pain, pancreatic calcification on x-ray, and exocrine (steatorrhea) or endocrine (diabetes mellitus) insufficiency. Attacks of acute pancreatitis often occur in patients with chronic pancreatitis. **Acute relapsing pancreatitis** is defined as multiple attacks of pancreatitis without permanent pancreatic scarring, a picture most often associated with biliary pancreatitis. The unsatisfactory term **chronic relapsing pancreatitis,** denoting recurrent acute attacks superimposed on chronic pancreatitis, is not used in this chapter. Alcoholic pancreatitis often behaves in this way. The term **subacute pancreatitis** has also been used by some to denote the minor acute attacks that typically appear late in alcoholic pancreatitis.

Etiology

Most cases of pancreatitis are caused by gallstone disease or alcoholism; a few result from hypercalcemia, trauma, hyperlipidemia, and genetic predisposition; and the remainder are idiopathic. Important differences exist in the manifestations and natural history of the disease as produced by these various factors.

A. Biliary Pancreatitis

About 40% of cases of pancreatitis are associated with gallstone disease, which, if untreated, usually gives rise to additional acute attacks. For unknown reasons, even repeated attacks of acute biliary pancreatitis seldom produce chronic pancreatitis. Eradication of the biliary disease nearly always prevents recurrent pancreatitis. The etiologic mechanism most likely consists of transient obstruction of the ampulla of Vater and pancreatic duct by a gallstone. Choledocholithiasis is found in only 25% of cases, but because over 90% of patients excrete a gallstone in feces passed within 10 days after an acute attack, it is assumed that most attacks are caused by a gallstone or biliary sludge traversing the common duct and ampulla of Vater. Other possible steps in pathogenesis initiated by passage of the gallstone are discussed below.

B. Alcoholic Pancreatitis

In the United States, alcoholism accounts for about 40% of cases of pancreatitis. Characteristically, the patients have been heavy users of hard liquor or wine; the condition is relatively infrequent in countries where beer is the most popular alcoholic beverage. Most commonly, 6 years or more of alcoholic excess precede the initial attack of pancreatitis, and even with the first clinical manifestations, signs of chronic pancreatitis can be detected if the gland is examined microscopically. Thus, alcoholic pancreatitis is often considered to be synonymous with chronic pancreatitis no matter what the clinical findings.

Acetaldehyde, an ethanol metabolite, has been implicated as a mediator, since it can generate toxic oxygen metabolites under the influence of xanthine oxidase. In experimental studies, alcohol decreases incorporation of phosphate into parenchymal phospholipids, decreases zymogen synthesis, and produces ultrastructural changes in acinar cells. Acute administration of alcohol stimulates pancreatic secretion and induces spasm in the sphincter of Oddi. This has been compared to experiments that produce acute pancreatitis by combining partial ductal obstruction and secretory stimulation. If the patient can be persuaded to stop drinking, acute attacks may be prevented, but parenchymal damage continues to occur owing to persistent ductal obstruction and fibrosis.

C. Hypercalcemia

Hyperparathyroidism and other disorders accompanied by hypercalcemia are occasionally complicated by acute pancreatitis. With time, chronic pancreatitis and ductal calculi appear. It is thought that the increased calcium concentrations in pancreatic juice that result from hypercalcemia may prematurely activate proteases. They may also facilitate precipitation of calculi in the ducts.

D. Hyperlipidemia

In some patients—especially alcoholics—hyperlipidemia appears transiently during an acute attack of pancreatitis; in others with primary hyperlipidemia (especially those associated with elevated chylomicrons and very low-density lipoproteins), pancreatitis seems to be a direct consequence of the metabolic abnormality. Hyperlipidemia during an acute attack of pancreatitis is usually associated with normal serum amylase levels, because the lipid interferes with the chemical determination for amylase; urinary output of amylase may still be high. One should inspect the serum of every patient with acute abdominal pain, because if it is lactescent, pancreatitis will almost always be the correct diagnosis. If a primary lipid abnormality is present, dietary control reduces the chances of additional attacks of pancreatitis as well as other complications.

E. Familial Pancreatitis

In this condition, attacks of abdominal pain usually begin in childhood. The genetic defect appears to be transmitted as a non-X-linked dominant with variable penetrance. Some affected families also have aminoaciduria, but this is not a universal finding. Diabetes mellitus and steatorrhea are uncommon. Chronic calcific pancreatitis develops eventually in most patients, and many patients become candidates for operation for chronic pain. Pancreatic carcinoma is more frequent in patients with familial pancreatitis.

F. Protein Deficiency

In certain populations where dietary protein intake is markedly deficient, the incidence of chronic pancreatitis is high. The reason for this association is obscure, especially in view of the observation that pancreatitis afflicts alcoholics with higher dietary protein and fat intake than those who consume less protein and fat.

G. Postoperative (Iatrogenic) Pancreatitis

Most cases of postoperative pancreatitis follow common bile duct exploration, especially if sphincterotomy was performed. Two practices, now largely abandoned, were often responsible: (1) use of a common duct T tube with a long arm passing through the sphincter of Oddi and (2) dilation of the sphincter to 5–7 mm during common duct exploration. Operations on the pancreas, including pancreatic biopsy, are another cause. A few cases follow gastric surgery or even operations remote from the pancreas. Pancreatitis is particularly common after cardiac surgery with cardiopulmonary bypass, where the risk factors are preoperative renal failure, valve surgery, postoperative hypotension, and (particularly) the perioperative administration of calcium chloride (> 800 mg calcium chloride per square meter of body surface area). Pancreatitis may also complicate endoscopic retrograde pancreatography or endoscopic sphincterotomy.

Rarely, pancreatitis follows Billroth II gastrectomy, owing to acute obstruction of the afferent loop and reflux of duodenal secretions under high pressure into the pancreatic ducts. The condition has been recreated experimentally in dogs (Pfeffer loop preparation).

H. Drug-Induced Pancreatitis

Drugs are probably responsible for more cases of acute pancreatitis than is generally suspected. The most commonly incriminated drugs are corticosteroids, estrogen-containing contraceptives, azathioprine, thiazide diuretics, and tetracyclines. Pancreatitis associated with use of estrogens is usually the result of drug-induced hypertriglyceridemia. The mechanisms involved in the case of other drugs are unknown.

I. Obstructive Pancreatitis

Chronic partial obstruction of the pancreatic duct may be congenital or may follow healing after injury or inflammation.

Over time, the parenchyma drained by the obstructed duct is replaced by fibrous tissue, and chronic pancreatitis develops. Sometimes there are episodes of acute pancreatitis as well.

Pancreas divisum may predispose to a kind of obstructive pancreatitis. If this anomaly is present and further narrowing of the opening of the minor papilla occurs (eg, by an inflammatory process), the orifice may be inadequate to handle the flow of pancreatic juice. The diagnosis of pancreas divisum may be made by endoscopic retrograde cholangiopancreatography (ERCP). If a patient with the anomaly is found to have documented episodes of acute pancreatitis and no other cause is found, it is reasonable to assume that the anomaly is the cause.

Surgical sphincteroplasty of the minor papilla or the insertion of a stent has been proposed as treatment, but results have been suboptimal. This may be due to the presence of irreversible parenchymal changes and the persistence of chronic inflammation. In patients with obvious changes of chronic pancreatitis, surgical treatment should consist of pancreatic resection or drainage (see p 584).

J. Idiopathic Pancreatitis and Miscellaneous Causes

In about 15% of patients, representing the third-largest group after biliary and alcoholic pancreatitis, there is no identifiable cause of the condition. If investigated in greater than usual detail (eg, duodenal drainage examination for cholesterol crystals), many of these patients will be found to have gallstones or biliary sludge undetectable by ultrasound scans. Recent data have linked mutations of the cystic fibrosis gene to idiopathic pancreatitis.

Viral infections and scorpion stings may cause pancreatitis.

▶ Pathogenesis

The concept that pancreatitis is due to enzymatic digestion of the gland is supported by the finding of proteolytic enzymes in ascitic fluid and increased amounts of phospholipase A and lysolecithins in pancreatic tissue from patients with acute pancreatitis. Experimentally, pancreatitis can be created readily if activated enzymes are injected into the pancreatic ducts under pressure. Trypsin has not been found in excessive amounts in pancreatic tissue from affected humans, possibly because of inactivation by trypsin inhibitors. Nevertheless, although the available evidence is inconclusive, the autodigestion theory is almost universally accepted. Other proposed factors are vascular insufficiency, lymphatic congestion, and activation of the kallikrein-kinin system.

For many years, trypsin and other proteases were held to be the principal injurious agents, but recent evidence has emphasized phospholipase A, lipase, and elastase as perhaps of greater importance. Trypsin ordinarily does not attack living cells, and even when trypsin is forced into the interstitial spaces, the resulting pancreatitis does not include coagulation necrosis, which is so prominent in human pancreatitis.

Phospholipase A, in the presence of small amounts of bile salts, attacks free phospholipids (eg, lecithin) and those bound in cellular membranes to produce extremely potent lysocompounds. Lysolecithin, which would result from the action of phospholipase A on biliary lecithin, or phospholipase A itself, plus bile salts, is capable of producing severe necrotizing pancreatitis. Trypsin is important in this scheme, because small amounts are needed to activate phospholipase A from its inactive precursor.

Elastase, which is both elastolytic and proteolytic, is secreted in an inactive form. Because it can digest the walls of blood vessels, elastase has been thought to be important in the pathogenesis of hemorrhagic pancreatitis.

If autodigestion is the final common pathway in pancreatitis, earlier steps must account for the presence of active enzymes and their reaction products in the ducts and their escape into the interstitium. The following are the most popular theories that attempt to link the known etiologic factors with autodigestion.

A. Obstruction-Secretion

In animals, ligation of the pancreatic duct generally produces mild edema of the pancreas that resolves within a week. Thereafter, atrophy of the secretory apparatus occurs. On the other hand, partial or intermittent ductal obstruction, which more closely mimics what seems to happen in humans, can produce frank pancreatitis if the gland is simultaneously stimulated to secrete. The major shortcoming of these experiments has been the difficulty encountered in attempting to cause severe pancreatitis in this way. However, since the human pancreas manufactures 10 times as much phospholipase A as does the dog or rat pancreas, the consequences of obstruction in humans conceivably could be more serious.

B. Common Channel Theory

Opie, having observed pancreatitis in a patient with a gallstone impacted in the ampulla of Vater, speculated that reflux of bile into the pancreatic ducts might have initiated the process. Flow between the biliary and pancreatic ducts requires a common channel connecting these two systems with the duodenum. Although these ducts converge in 90% of humans, only 10% have a common channel long enough to permit biliary-pancreatic reflux if the ampulla contained a gallstone. Experimentally, pancreatitis produced by pancreatic duct obstruction alone is similar in severity to pancreatitis following obstruction of a common channel, so biliary reflux is discounted as an etiologic factor in this disease.

C. Duodenal Reflux

The above theories do not explain activation of pancreatic enzymes, a process that normally takes place through the action of enterokinase in the duodenum. In experimental animals, if the segment of duodenum into which the pancreatic duct empties is surgically converted to a closed loop, reflux of duodenal juice initiates severe pancreatitis (Pfeffer loop). Pancreatitis associated with acute afferent loop obstruction after Billroth II gastrectomy is probably the result of similar factors. Other than in this specific example, there is no direct evidence for duodenal reflux in the pathogenesis of pancreatitis in humans.

D. Back Diffusion Across the Pancreatic Duct

Just as the gastric mucosa must serve as a barrier to maintain high concentrations of acid, so must the epithelium of the pancreatic duct prevent diffusion of luminal enzymes into the pancreatic parenchyma. Experiments in cats have shown that the barrier function of the pancreatic duct is vulnerable to several injurious agents, including alcohol and bile acids. Furthermore, the effects of alcohol can occur even after oral ingestion, because alcohol is secreted in the pancreatic juice. Injury to the barrier renders the duct permeable to molecules as large as MW 20,000, and enzymes from the lumen may be able to enter the gland and produce pancreatitis.

The studies by Steer and his coworkers have shown that a very early event in several forms of experimental pancreatitis, including that due to pancreatic duct obstruction, consists of zymogen activation within acinar cells by lysosomal hydrolases (eg, cathepsin B). This may represent the long-sought unifying explanation. Other factors must be postulated, however, to account for the variations in severity of the disease. In biliary pancreatitis, transient obstruction of the ampulla of Vater by a gallstone is most likely the first event. Alcoholic pancreatitis probably has several causes, including partial ductal obstruction, secretory stimulation, acute effects on the ductal barrier, and toxic actions of alcohol on parenchymal cells.

E. Systemic Manifestations

Severe acute pancreatitis may be complicated by multiple organ failure, principally respiratory insufficiency (acute respiratory distress syndrome [ARDS]), myocardial depression, renal insufficiency, and gastric stress ulceration. The pathogenesis of these complications is similar in many respects to that of multiple organ failure in sepsis, and in fact, sepsis due to pancreatic abscess formation is a contributing factor in some of the most severe cases of acute pancreatitis. During acute pancreatitis, pancreatic proteases, bacterial endotoxins, and other active agents are liberated into the systemic circulation. The concentrations of serum factors able to complex with the proteases (eg, α_2-macroglobulin) decrease in proportion to the severity of the illness, and complexed α_2-macroglobulin, which normally is cleared rapidly by macrophages, accumulates. These circulating complexes, which retain proteolytic activity, are thought to contribute to systemic toxicity. The endotoxin probably originates from bacteria that translocate through an abnormally permeable intestinal mucosa. Within the circulation, the proteases and the endotoxin activate the complement system (especially C5) and kinins. Complement activation leads to granulocyte aggregation and accumulation of aggregates in the pulmonary capillaries. The granulocytes release neutrophil elastase, superoxide anion, hydrogen peroxide, and hydroxide radicals, which in concert with bradykinin exert local toxic effects on the pulmonary epithelium that result in increased permeability. Arachidonate metabolites (eg, PGE_2, PGI_2, leukotriene B_4) may also be involved in some way. Analogous events are thought to occur in other organs.

Chen JW, Saccone GT, Toouli J: Sphincter of Oddi dysfunction and acute pancreatitis. Gut 1998;43:305.

Cohn JA et al: Relation between mutations of the cystic fibrosis gene and idiopathic pancreatitis. N Engl J Med 1998;339:653.

Eckerwall G, Andersson R: Early enteral nutrition in severe acute pancreatitis: a way of providing nutrients, gut barrier protection, immunomodulation, or all of them? Scand J Gastroenterol 2001;36:449.

Etemad B, Whitcomb DC: Chronic pancreatitis: diagnosis, classification, and new genetic developments. Gastroenterology 2001;120:682.

Granger J, Remick D: Acute pancreatitis: models, markers, and mediators. Shock 2005;24(Suppl 1):45.

Halangk W et al: Role of cathepsin B in intracellular trypsinogen activation and the onset of acute pancreatitis. J Clin Invest 2000;106:773.

Layer P, Keller J: Pancreatic enzymes: secretion and luminal nutrient digestion in health and disease. J Clin Gastroenterol 1999;28:3.

Miskovitz P: Role of selectins in acute pancreatitis. Crit Care Med 2001;29:686.

Opie EL: The theory of retrojection of bile into the pancreas. Rev Surg 1970;27:1.

Sharer N et al: Mutations of the cystic fibrosis gene in patients with chronic pancreatitis. N Engl J Med 1998;339:645.

Spanier BW, Dijkgraaf MG, Bruno MJ: Epidemiology, aetiology and outcome of acute and chronic pancreatitis: An update. Best Pract Res Clin Gastroenterol 2008;22:45.

Steer ML: How and where does acute pancreatitis begin? Arch Surg 1992;127:1350.

1. Acute Pancreatitis

 ESSENTIALS OF DIAGNOSIS

▶ Abrupt onset of epigastric pain, frequently with back pain.

▶ Nausea and vomiting.

▶ Elevated serum or urinary amylase.

▶ Cholelithiasis or alcoholism (many patients).

▶ General Considerations

While edematous and hemorrhagic pancreatitis are manifestations of the same pathologic processes and the general principles of treatment are the same, hemorrhagic pancreatitis has more complications and a higher death rate. In edematous pancreatitis, the glandular tissue and surrounding retroperitoneal structures are engorged with interstitial fluid, and the pancreas is infiltrated with inflammatory cells that surround small foci of parenchymal necrosis. Hemorrhagic pancreatitis is characterized by bleeding into the parenchyma and surrounding retroperitoneal structures and extensive pancreatic necrosis. In both forms, the peritoneal surfaces may be studded with small calcifications representing areas of fat necrosis.

▶ Clinical Findings

A. Symptoms and Signs

The acute attack frequently begins following a large meal and consists of severe epigastric pain that radiates through to the back. The pain is unrelenting and usually associated with vomiting and retching. In severe cases, the patient may collapse from shock.

Depending on the severity of the disease, there may be profound dehydration, tachycardia, and postural hypotension. Myocardial function is depressed in severe pancreatitis, presumably because of circulating factors that affect cardiac performance. Examination of the abdomen reveals decreased or absent bowel sounds and tenderness that may be generalized but more often is localized to the epigastrium. Temperature is usually normal or slightly elevated in uncomplicated pancreatitis. Clinical evidence of pleural effusion may be present, especially on the left. If an abdominal mass is found, it probably represents a swollen pancreas (phlegmon) or, later in the illness, a pseudocyst or abscess. In 1–2% of patients, bluish discoloration is present in the flank (**Grey Turner sign**) or periumbilical area (**Cullen sign**), indicating hemorrhagic pancreatitis with dissection of blood retroperitoneally into these areas.

B. Laboratory Findings

The hematocrit may be elevated as a consequence of dehydration or low as a result of abdominal blood loss in hemorrhagic pancreatitis. There is usually a moderate leukocytosis, but total white blood cell counts over 12,000/μL are unusual in the absence of suppurative complications. Liver function studies are usually normal, but there may be a mild elevation of the serum bilirubin concentration (usually < 2 mg/dL).

The serum amylase concentration rises to more than $2\frac{1}{2}$ times normal within 6 hours after the onset of an acute episode and generally remains elevated for several days. Values in excess of 1000 IU/dL occur early in the attack in 95% of patients with biliary pancreatitis and 85% of patients with acute alcoholic pancreatitis. Those with the most severe disease are more apt to have amylase levels below 1000 IU/dL.

Elevated serum lipase is detectable early and for several days after the acute attack. Since the lipase level tends to be higher in alcoholic pancreatitis and the amylase level higher in gallstone pancreatitis, the lipase/amylase ratio has been suggested as a means to help distinguish the two.

Elevated amylase levels may occur in other acute abdominal conditions, such as gangrenous cholecystitis, small bowel obstruction, mesenteric infarction, and perforated ulcer, though levels rarely exceed 500 IU/dL. Episodes of acute pancreatitis may occur without rises in serum amylase; this is the rule if hyperlipidemia is present. Furthermore, high levels may return to normal before blood is drawn.

The methods most commonly used for measuring amylase in the serum detect pancreatic amylase, salivary amylase, and macroamylase. However, hyperamylasemia is sometimes present in patients with abdominal pain when the elevated amylase levels consist entirely of salivary amylase or macroamylase and the pancreas is not inflamed.

Urine amylase excretion is also increased and is of diagnostic value. Excretion of more than 5000 units/24 h is abnormal. The urinary clearance of amylase increases during acute pancreatitis owing to a decrease in tubular reabsorption of amylase (normally 75% of filtered amylase). This was once thought to be specific, and the amylase-to-creatinine clearance ratio was used as a diagnostic test for acute pancreatitis. However, the increased amylase clearance results from overload of the tubular reabsorptive pathway with various urine proteins and is a nonspecific effect of tissue damage seen in many acute illnesses or following trauma.

In severe pancreatitis, the serum calcium concentration may fall as a result of calcium being complexed with fatty acids (liberated from retroperitoneal fat by lipase) and impaired reabsorption from bone owing to the action of calcitonin (liberated by high levels of glucagon). Relative hypoparathyroidism and hypoalbuminemia have also been implicated.

C. Imaging Studies

In about two thirds of cases, a plain abdominal film is abnormal. The most frequent finding is isolated dilation of a segment of gut (**sentinel loop**) consisting of jejunum, transverse colon, or duodenum adjacent to the pancreas. Gas distending the right colon that abruptly stops in the mid or left transverse colon (**colon cutoff sign**) is due to colonic spasm adjacent to the pancreatic inflammation. Both of these findings are relatively nonspecific. Glandular calcification may be evident, signifying chronic pancreatitis. An upper gastrointestinal series may show a widened duodenal loop, swollen ampulla of Vater, and, occasionally, evidence of gastric irritability. Chest films may reveal pleural effusion on the left side.

A CT scan of the pancreas using intravenous contrast media should be obtained in any patient with acute pancreatitis whose illness is not resolving after 48–72 hours. The radiologic findings may be consistent with any of the following: relatively normal appearing pancreas, pancreatic **phlegmon**, pancreatic phlegmon with extension of the inflammatory process to adjacent extrapancreatic spaces, pancreatic **necrosis**, or pancreatic pseudocyst or **abscess** formation.

Occasionally, radiopaque gallstones will be apparent on plain x-rays. Ultrasound study may demonstrate gallstones early in the attack and may be used as a baseline for sequential examinations of the pancreas.

Several weeks after the pancreatitis has subsided, ERCP may be of value in patients with a tentative diagnosis of idiopathic pancreatitis (ie, those who have no history of alcoholism and no evidence of gallstones on ultrasound and oral cholecystogram). This examination demonstrates gallstones or changes of chronic pancreatitis in about 40% of such patients.

▶ Differential Diagnosis

To some extent, acute pancreatitis is a diagnosis of exclusion, for other acute upper abdominal conditions (eg, acute cholecystitis, penetrating or perforated duodenal ulcer, high small bowel obstruction, acute appendicitis, and mesenteric infarction) must always be seriously considered. In most cases, the distinction is possible on the basis of the clinical picture, laboratory findings, and CT scans. The critical point is that the diseases with which acute pancreatitis is most likely to be confused are often lethal if not treated surgically. Therefore, diagnostic laparotomy is indicated if they cannot be ruled out on clinical grounds.

Chronic hyperamylasemia occurs rarely without any relation to pancreatic disease. Some cases are associated with renal failure, chronic sialadenitis, salivary tumors, ovarian tumors, or liver disease, but often there is no explanation. Analysis of serum amylase isoenzymes is the only way to determine whether the amylase originates from salivary glands or pancreas. **Macroamylasemia** is a chronic hyperamylasemia in which normal amylase (usually salivary) is bound to a large serum glycoprotein or immunoglobulin molecule and is therefore not excreted into urine. The diagnosis rests on the combination of hyperamylasemia and low urinary amylase. Macroamylasemia has been found in patients with other diseases such as malabsorption, alcoholism, and cancer. Many patients have abdominal pain, but the relationship of the pain and the macroamylasemia is uncertain.

▶ Complications

The principal complications of acute pancreatitis are abscess and pseudocyst formation. These are discussed in separate sections. Gastrointestinal bleeding may occur from adjacent inflamed stomach or duodenum, ruptured pseudocyst, or peptic ulcer. Intraperitoneal bleeding may occur spontaneously from the celiac or splenic artery or from the spleen following acute splenic vein thrombosis. Involvement of the transverse colon or duodenum by the inflammatory process may result in partial obstruction, hemorrhage, necrosis, or fistula formation.

Early identification of patients at greatest risk of complications allows them to be managed more aggressively, which appears to decrease the mortality rate. The criteria of severity that have been found to be reliable are based either on the systemic manifestations of the disease as reflected in the clinical and laboratory findings or on the local changes in the pancreas as reflected by the findings on CT scan. Ranson used the former approach to develop the staging criteria listed in Table 26–1. Just the single finding of fluid sequestration (ie, fluid administered minus urine output) exceeding 2 L/d for more than 2 days is a reasonably accurate dividing line between severe (life-threatening) and mild-to-moderate disease. The local changes in the pancreas as shown on CT scans may be even more revealing. The presence of any of the following indicates a high risk of local infection in the pancreatic bed: involvement of extrapancreatic spaces in the inflammatory process, pancreatic necrosis (areas in the pancreas that do not enhance with intravenous contrast media), and early signs of abscess formation (eg, gas bubbles in the tissue).

▶ Treatment

A. Medical Treatment

The goals of medical therapy are reduction of pancreatic secretory stimuli and correction of fluid and electrolyte derangements.

1. Gastric suction—Oral intake is withheld, and a nasogastric tube is inserted to aspirate gastric secretions, although the latter has no specific therapeutic effect. Oral feeding should be resumed only after the patient appears much improved, appetite has returned, and serum amylase levels have dropped to normal. Premature resumption of eating may result in exacerbation of disease.

2. Fluid replacement—Patients with acute pancreatitis sequester fluid in the retroperitoneum, and large volumes of intravenous fluids are necessary to maintain circulating blood volume and renal function. Patients with severe pancreatitis should receive albumin to combat the capillary leak that contributes to the pathophysiology. In severe hemorrhagic

Table 26–1. Ranson Criteria of Severity of Acute Pancreatitis.[1]

Criteria present initially
Age > 55 years
White blood cell count > 16,000/μL
Blood glucose > 200 mg/dL
Serum LDH > 350 IU/L
AST (SGOT) > 250 IU/dL
Criteria developing during first 24 hours
Hematocrit fall > 10%
BUN rise > 8 mg/dL
Serum Ca^{2+} < 8 mg/dL
Arterial Po_2 < 60 mm Hg
Base deficit > 4 meq/L
Estimated fluid sequestration > 600 mL

[1]Morbidity and mortality rates correlate with the number of criteria present. Mortality rates correlate as follows: 0–2 criteria present = 2%; 3 or 4 = 15%; 5 or 6 = 40%; 7 or 8 = 100%.

pancreatitis, blood transfusions may also be required. The adequacy of fluid replacement is the single most important aspect of medical therapy. In fact, undertreatment with fluids may actually contribute to the progression of pancreatitis. Fluid replacement may be judged most accurately by monitoring the volume and specific gravity of urine.

3. Antibiotics—Antibiotics are not useful in mild cases of acute pancreatitis. However, recent studies have shown benefit of antibiotics that penetrate pancreatic tissue for patients with severe pancreatitis. Imipenem is the most commonly used antibiotic. Antibiotics should also be used for treatment of specific operative complications.

4. Calcium and magnesium—In severe attacks of acute pancreatitis, hypocalcemia may require parenteral calcium replacement in amounts determined by serial calcium measurements. Recognition of hypocalcemia is important because it may produce cardiac dysrhythmias. Hypomagnesemia is also common, especially in alcoholics, and magnesium should also be replaced as indicated by serum levels.

5. Oxygen—Hypoxemia severe enough to require therapy develops in about 30% of patients with acute pancreatitis. It is often insidious, without clinical or x-ray signs, and out of proportion to the severity of the pancreatitis. The most pronounced examples accompany severe pancreatitis, often in association with hypocalcemia. The basic lesion, a form of adult respiratory distress syndrome, is poorly understood. Pulmonary changes include decreased vital capacity and an oxygen diffusion defect.

Hypoxemia must be suspected in every patient, and arterial blood gases should be measured every 12 hours for the first few hospital days. Supplemental oxygen therapy is indicated for PaO_2 levels below 70 mm Hg. An occasional patient requires endotracheal intubation and mechanical ventilation. Diuretics may be useful in decreasing lung water and improving arterial oxygen saturation.

6. Peritoneal lavage—Peritoneal lavage has been employed in severe refractory cases to remove toxins in the peritoneal fluid that would otherwise have been absorbed into the systemic circulation. Some patients appear to improve in response to this therapy although controlled trials have not substantiated its efficacy. Severe pancreatitis that fails to show clinical improvement after 24–48 hours of standard inpatient treatment is the usual indication for peritoneal lavage. The technique involves infusing and withdrawing 1–2 L of lactated Ringer solution through a peritoneal dialysis catheter every hour for 1–3 days. Meta-analysis of the existing data shows no benefit; this treatment is not recommended outside of a clinical trial.

7. Nutrition—Total parenteral nutrition avoids pancreatic stimulation and should be used for nutritional support in any severely ill patient who will be unable to eat for more than 1 week. Elemental diets ingested orally or given by tube into the small intestine do not avoid secretory stimulation.

Neither form of nutrition directly affects recovery of the pancreas.

8. Other drugs—Octreotide, H_2 receptor blockers, anticholinergic drugs, glucagon, and aprotinin have shown no beneficial effects in controlled trials.

B. Endoscopic Sphincterotomy

Biliary pancreatitis is caused by a gallstone becoming lodged in the ampulla of Vater. In most cases, the stone passes into the intestine, but occasionally it becomes impacted in the ampulla, which results in more severe disease. Less than 10% of cases of biliary pancreatitis are severe (ie, three or more three Ranson criteria), but in severe cases, endoscopic sphincterotomy performed within 72 hours of the onset of the disease has been shown to decrease the incidence of concomitant biliary sepsis and lower the mortality rate from the pancreatitis.

C. Surgical Treatment

Surgery is generally contraindicated in uncomplicated acute pancreatitis. However, when the diagnosis is uncertain in a patient with severe abdominal pain, diagnostic laparotomy is not thought to aggravate pancreatitis.

When laparotomy has been performed for diagnosis and mild to moderate pancreatitis is found, cholecystectomy and operative cholangiography should be performed if gallstones are present, but the pancreas should be left undisturbed. For *severe* edematous pancreatitis, the gastrocolic omentum should be divided and the pancreas inspected. Although some surgeons place drains and irrigating catheters in the region of the pancreas, we prefer to keep foreign bodies out of this area.

The diagnosis of biliary pancreatitis can usually be suspected on the basis of ultrasound studies of the gallbladder early in the acute attack. Cholecystectomy should be performed on these patients during hospitalization for the acute attack soon after the attack resolves. A longer delay (even a few weeks) is associated with a high incidence (80%) of recurrent pancreatitis. Since life-threatening attacks are uncommon in gallstone pancreatitis, operation (common duct exploration; sphincteroplasty) or endoscopic therapy (sphincterotomy) early in an attack is rarely justified. However, when the attack is especially severe, elective cholecystectomy should be deferred up to several months to allow complete recovery from pancreatitis.

It is currently thought that debridement of dead peripancreatic tissue, which is often (40% of cases) colonized by bacteria, reduces the mortality rate of acute severe necrotizing pancreatitis. Historical controls place the mortality rate at 50–80% in the absence of operative treatment and 10–40% among patients subjected to necrosectomy. The diagnosis of necrotizing pancreatitis is suspected from the clinical findings; patients treated surgically have three or more Ranson criteria and average about $4^1/_2$ criteria. Contrast-enhanced

CT scans obtained early in the course of the disease are studied for the presence of nonenhancing areas, which indicate lack of vascular perfusion and reflect the presence of necrotic peripancreatic fat or pancreatic parenchyma. Percutaneous needle aspiration of these areas is used to detect the presence of bacterial colonization. A distinction is made between these cases of "infected necrotizing pancreatitis" and "pancreatic abscess," which may appear later in the course of the disease. Patients with infected necrotizing pancreatitis and severe clinical findings benefit most from surgical therapy, but laparotomy may be undertaken just because of a deteriorating condition in patients with necrotizing pancreatitis in the absence of bacterial colonization. At surgery, all peripancreatic spaces are opened and any necrotic tissue is removed by gentle blunt dissection. A T tube is inserted if there is bile duct obstruction, and cholecystectomy is performed for gallstone disease. Two large drains are placed within the debrided spaces and are used postoperatively for sterile lavage. About 8 L of fluid are infused through this system daily for an average of 2 weeks. Other than CT evidence of necrotic tissue with or without infection, there are presently no other criteria in general use that call for pancreatic surgery in patients with severe pancreatitis.

Surgery for complications of acute pancreatitis, such as abscess, pseudocyst, and pancreatic ascites, is discussed later in this chapter.

▶ Prognosis

The death rate associated with acute pancreatitis is about 10%, and nearly all deaths occur in a first attack and among patients with three or more Ranson criteria of severity. Respiratory insufficiency and hypocalcemia indicate a poor prognosis. The death rate associated with severe necrotizing pancreatitis is 50% or more, but surgical therapy lowers the figure to about 20%. Persistent fever or hyperamylasemia 3 weeks or longer after an attack of pancreatitis usually indicates the presence of a pancreatic abscess or pseudocyst.

Abu-Zidan FM, Bonham MJ, Windsor JA: Severity of acute pancreatitis: a multivariate analysis of oxidative stress markers and modified Glasgow criteria. Br J Surg 2000;87:1019.

Beckingham IJ, Bornman PC: ABC of diseases of liver, pancreas, and biliary system. Acute pancreatitis. BMJ 2001;322:595.

Bornman PC, Beckingham IJ: ABC of diseases of liver, pancreas, and biliary system. Chronic pancreatitis. BMJ 2001;322:660.

Brivet FG, Emilie D, Galanaud P: Pro- and anti-inflammatory cytokines during acute severe pancreatitis: an early and sustained response, although unpredictable of death. Parisian Study Group on Acute Pancreatitis. Crit Care Med 1999;27:749.

Chang L et al: Preoperative versus postoperative endoscopic retrograde cholangiopancreatography in mild to moderate gallstone pancreatitis: a prospective randomized trial. Ann Surg 2000; 231:82.

Dervenis C, Bassi C: Evidence-based assessment of severity and management of acute pancreatitis. Br J Surg 2000;87:257.

Frakes JT: Biliary pancreatitis: a review. Emphasizing appropriate endoscopic intervention. J Clin Gastroenterol 1999;28:97.

Gumaste V: Prophylactic antibiotic therapy in the management of acute pancreatitis. J Clin Gastroenterol 2000;31:6.

Hamano H et al: High serum IgG4 concentrations in patients with sclerosing pancreatitis. N Engl J Med 2001;344:732.

Nealon WH, Matin S: Analysis of surgical success in preventing recurrent acute exacerbations in chronic pancreatitis. Ann Surg 2001;233:793.

Platell C, Cooper D, Hall JC: A meta-analysis of peritoneal lavage for acute pancreatitis. J Gastroenterol Hepatol 2001;16:689.

Schmid SW et al: The role of infection in acute pancreatitis. Gut 1999;45:311.

Toh SK, Phillips S, Johnson CD: A prospective audit against national standards of the presentation and management of acute pancreatitis in the South of England. Gut 2000;46:239.

Uhl W et al: Acute gallstone pancreatitis: timing of laparoscopic cholecystectomy in mild and severe disease. Surg Endosc 1999;13:1070.

Williams M, Simms HH: Prognostic usefulness of scoring systems in critically ill patients with severe acute pancreatitis. Crit Care Med 1999;27:901.

Windsor JA, Hammodat H: Metabolic management of severe acute pancreatitis. World J Surg 2000;24:664.

2. Pancreatic Pseudocyst

 ESSENTIALS OF DIAGNOSIS

▶ Epigastric mass and pain.

▶ Mild fever and leukocytosis.

▶ Persistent serum amylase elevation.

▶ Pancreatic cyst demonstrated by ultrasound or CT scan.

▶ General Considerations

Pancreatic pseudocysts are encapsulated collections of fluid with high enzyme concentrations that arise from the pancreas. They are usually located either within or adjacent to the pancreas in the lesser sac, but pancreatic pseudocysts have also been found in the neck, mediastinum, and pelvis. The walls of a pseudocyst are formed by inflammatory fibrosis of the peritoneal, mesenteric, and serosal membranes, which limits spread of the pancreatic juice as the lesion develops. The term pseudocyst denotes absence of an epithelial lining, whereas true cysts are lined by epithelium.

Two different processes are involved in the pathogenesis of pancreatic pseudocysts. Many occur as complications of severe acute pancreatitis, where extravasation of pancreatic juice and glandular necrosis form a sterile pocket of fluid that is not reabsorbed as inflammation subsides. Superinfection of such collections leads to pancreatic abscess instead of pseudocyst. In other patients, usually alcoholics or trauma victims, pseudocysts appear without preceding acute pancreatitis. The mechanism in these cases consists of ductal obstruction and formation of a retention cyst that loses its epithelial lining as it grows beyond the confines of the gland. In posttraumatic pseudocyst, symptoms usually do not appear until several weeks after the injury. Some are iatrogenic, eg, occurring during splenectomy; others follow an external blow to the abdomen.

Pseudocysts develop in about 2% of cases of acute pancreatitis. The cysts are single in 85% of cases and multiple in the remainder.

► Clinical Findings

A. Symptoms and Signs

A pseudocyst should be suspected when a patient with acute pancreatitis fails to recover after a week of treatment or when, after improving for a time, symptoms return. Since it is now fairly routine to obtain a CT scan early in an attack of severe acute pancreatitis, the early stages of pseudocyst formation are often demonstrated radiographically before specific clinical findings appear. The first clinical manifestation is usually a palpable tender mass in the epigastrium, consisting of a swollen pancreas and contiguous viscera (a phlegmon). With time, the mass may subside, but if it persists it most likely represents a pseudocyst.

In other cases, the pseudocyst develops insidiously without an obvious attack of acute pancreatitis.

Regardless of the type of prodromal phase, pain is the most common finding. Fever, weight loss, tenderness, and a palpable mass are present in about half of patients. A few have jaundice, a manifestation of obstruction of the intrapancreatic segment of the bile duct.

B. Laboratory Findings

An elevated serum amylase and leukocytosis are present in about half of patients. When present, elevated bilirubin levels reflect biliary obstruction. Of those patients with acute pancreatitis whose serum amylase remains elevated for as long as 3 weeks, about half will have a pseudocyst.

C. Imaging Studies

CT scan (Figure 26–3) is the diagnostic study of choice. The size and shape of the cyst and its relationship to other viscera can be seen. Acute pseudocysts are often irregular in shape; chronic pseudocysts are most often circular or nearly so. An enlarged pancreatic duct may be demonstrated in patients with chronic pancreatitis. A dilated common bile duct would suggest biliary obstruction, either from the cyst or from underlying chronic pancreatitis.

The gallbladder should be studied by ultrasound to look for gallstones, especially in patients with acute pancreatitis. Although ultrasound can also demonstrate pseudocysts, the amount of important detail obtained is less than that from CT scans, and consequently the role of ultrasound is mainly to follow changes in size of an acute pseudocyst already imaged by CT scans so the amount of x-ray exposure can be kept to a minimum.

ERCP should be performed if there are thought to be significant abnormalities of the bile or pancreatic duct as suggested by CT scans or the results of liver function tests. Either duct may be dilated and in need of surgical drainage in conjunction with drainage of the pseudocyst. ERCP usually opacifies the pseudocyst as well, but the information is not usually of major value in planning treatment, so ERCP is not obtained routinely.

An upper gastrointestinal series will often reveal a mass in the lesser sac that distorts the stomach or duodenum, but this is not particularly useful information. The principal indication

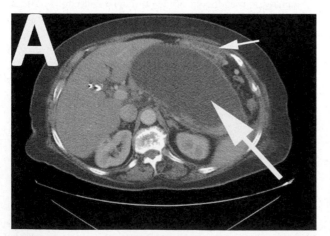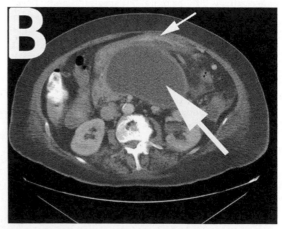

▲ **Figure 26–3.** CT scan of a large pancreatic pseudocyst impinging on the posterior wall of the stomach. The large arrow indicates the pseudocyst; the smaller arrow indicates the stomach. **A:** More cephalad in the abdomen, the pseudocyst abuts the stomach and liver. **B:** More caudad in the abdomen, the pseudocyst is immediately posterior to the gastric antrum. The stomach is compressed against the anterior wall of the abdomen, and the duodenum is stretched over the pseudocyst, causing early satiety. A cyst in this location is usually best drained into the stomach.

for an upper gastrointestinal series is to search for a site of gastric or duodenal obstruction in patients who are vomiting.

With wide use of sensitive imaging studies in the diagnosis of pancreatic disease, small asymptomatic pseudocysts are often demonstrated. The natural history of these subclinical lesions is benign, and there is no indication for prophylactic surgical treatment.

▶ Differential Diagnosis

Pancreatic pseudocysts must be distinguished from pancreatic abscess and acute pancreatic phlegmon. Patients with an abscess exhibit signs of infection.

Rarely, patients with pseudocyst present with weight loss, jaundice, and a nontender palpable gallbladder and are first thought to have pancreatic carcinoma. CT scans show that the lesion is fluid-filled, which suggests the correct diagnosis.

Neoplastic cysts—either cystadenoma or cystadenocarcinoma—account for about 5% of all cases of cystic pancreatic masses and may be indistinguishable preoperatively from pseudocyst. The correct diagnosis can be made from the gross appearance supplemented by a biopsy obtained at operation.

▶ Complications

A. Infection

Infection is a rare complication resulting in high fever, chills, and leukocytosis. Drainage is required as soon as the diagnosis is suspected. Some lesions can be drained externally via a catheter placed percutaneously using ultrasound guidance. Internal drainage of infected pseudocysts adherent to the stomach can be achieved surgically by cystogastrostomy; otherwise, drainage should be external, because the suture line of a Roux-en-Y cystojejunostomy may not heal.

B. Rupture

Sudden perforation into the free peritoneal cavity produces severe chemical peritonitis, with boardlike abdominal rigidity and severe pain. Rapid enlargement of the pseudocyst is sometimes noted before it ruptures. The treatment is emergency surgery with irrigation of the peritoneal cavity and a drainage procedure for the pseudocyst. The wall of a ruptured pseudocyst is usually too flimsy to hold sutures securely, so most ruptured cysts must be drained externally. Rupture of a pseudocyst occurs in less than 5% of cases, but even with prompt treatment it may be fatal.

C. Hemorrhage

Bleeding may occur into the cyst cavity or an adjacent viscus into which the cyst has eroded. Intracystic bleeding may present as an enlarging abdominal mass with anemia resulting from blood loss. If the cyst has eroded into the stomach, there may be hematemesis, melena, and blood in the nasogastric aspirate. The rapidity of the blood loss often produces hemorrhagic shock, which may preclude arteriography. If time permits, however, emergency arteriography should be performed to delineate the site of bleeding, which is usually a false aneurysm of an artery in the cyst wall, and to embolize it if possible. If embolization successfully occludes the bleeding vessel, several weeks should elapse to ensure that bleeding will not recur, and at that point the pseudocyst should be drained surgically in the same fashion as a nonbleeding pseudocyst. If the bleeding cannot be stopped by embolization, emergency surgery should be performed. Usually, all that can be done is to open the cyst and suture ligate the bleeding vessel in the cyst wall, followed by external or internal drainage of the cyst. Sometimes it is possible to excise the cyst, which is desirable because doing so more certainly avoids the risk of recurrent hemorrhage.

▶ Treatment

The principal indications for treating pancreatic pseudocysts are to improve symptoms and to prevent complications. Recent data indicate that the natural history of these lesions is more benign than previously thought—that in the absence of symptoms or radiographic evidence of enlargement (and irrespective of cyst size), expectant management is not unreasonable and that a few untreated cysts resolve spontaneously even after being stable for months. Expectant management is especially important in the first 6–12 weeks of existence of cysts that have arisen during an attack of acute pancreatitis. The chances of spontaneous resolution are about 40%; catheter drainage at this stage is meddlesome; and internal drainage of the cyst by surgery may be difficult or even impossible. Thereafter, for cysts greater than 5 cm, treatment is usually recommended over expectant management (in the absence of contraindications, such as serious concomitant disease), because most cysts can be promptly eliminated by percutaneous catheter drainage or surgical drainage into the stomach or intestine. This obviates the need for prolonged follow-up with repeated ultrasound or CT scans and avoids the risks, albeit low, of complications. Patients who present with a symptomatic pseudocyst and no history of recent acute pancreatitis may be treated without the 6–12-week delay, because their cyst wall is tough (mature) enough to hold sutures and allow an anastomosis with the gut. Jaundice in a patient with a pseudocyst is usually caused by pressure from the cyst on the bile duct. Draining the pseudocyst usually relieves the obstruction, but an operative cholangiogram should be obtained to make sure.

A. Excision

Excision is the most definitive treatment but is usually confined to chronic pseudocysts in the tail of the gland. This approach is recommended especially for cysts that follow trauma, where the head and body of the gland are normal. Most cysts should be drained either externally or internally into the gut.

B. External Drainage

External drainage is best for critically ill patients or when the cyst wall has not matured sufficiently for anastomosis to other organs. A large tube is sewn into the cyst lumen, and its end is brought out through the abdominal wall. External drainage is complicated in a third of patients by a pancreatic fistula that sometimes requires surgical drainage but on the average closes spontaneously in several months. The incidence of recurrent pseudocyst is about four times greater after external drainage than after drainage into the gut.

C. Internal Drainage

The preferred method of treatment is internal drainage, where the cyst is anastomosed to a Roux-en-Y limb of jejunum (cystojejunostomy), to the posterior wall of the stomach (cystogastrostomy), or to the duodenum (cystoduodenostomy). The interior of the cyst should be inspected for evidence of a tumor and biopsy performed as appropriate. Cystogastrostomy is preferable for cysts behind and densely adherent to the stomach. This may well be done laparoscopically in the future. To accomplish free, dependent drainage, Roux-en-Y cystojejunostomy provides better drainage of cysts in various other locations. Cystoduodenostomy is indicated for cysts deep within the head of the gland and adjacent to the medial wall of the duodenum—lesions that would be difficult to drain by any other technique. The procedure consists of making a lateral duodenotomy, opening into the cyst through the medial wall of the duodenum, and then closing the lateral duodenotomy. Following internal drainage, the cyst cavity becomes obliterated within a few weeks. Even after cystogastrostomy, an unrestricted diet can be allowed within a week after surgery, and x-rays taken at this time usually show only a small residual cyst cavity.

D. Nonsurgical Drainage

External drainage can be established by a percutaneous catheter placed into the cyst under radiographic or ultrasound control. This is the preferred method for infected pseudocysts. In some centers, it is also used for the majority of uncomplicated pseudocysts as the primary mode of therapy. About two thirds of cysts so treated are permanently eradicated. It may also be useful to shrink a truly huge pseudocyst (eg, one that occupies half of the abdominal cavity), because it is technically difficult to obtain adequate internal drainage of these lesions into the gut. Occasionally, a sterile cyst may become infected when a narrow catheter is inserted into it. This is more likely when the cyst lumen contains debris that is not drained effectively by this technique. Chronic external pancreatic fistula is a potential complication of this method.

Two other drainage techniques have been tried: (1) Passing a catheter percutaneously through the anterior abdominal wall, the anterior wall of the stomach, and through the posterior stomach into the cyst. After several weeks, the catheter is removed, and a chronic tract remains from cyst to gastric lumen. (2) Using a fiberoptic gastroscope to make a small incision through the back wall of the stomach into the cyst. Because of questions about efficacy and safety, neither method is widely used.

▶ Prognosis

The recurrence rate for pancreatic pseudocyst is about 10%, and recurrence is more frequent after treatment by external drainage. Serious postoperative hemorrhage from the cyst occurs rarely—most often after cystogastrostomy. In most cases, however, surgical treatment of pseudocysts is uncomplicated and definitively solves the immediate problem. Many patients later experience chronic pain as a manifestation of underlying chronic pancreatitis.

Cooperman AM: Surgical treatment of pancreatic pseudocysts. Surg Clin North Am 2001;81:411.

Heider R et al: Percutaneous drainage of pancreatic pseudocysts is associated with a higher failure rate than surgical treatment in unselected patients. Ann Surg 1999;229:781.

Heider R, Behrns KE: Pancreatic pseudocysts complicated by splenic parenchymal involvement: results of operative and percutaneous management. Pancreas 2001;23:20.

Mori T et al: Laparoscopic pancreatic cystgastrostomy. J Hepatobiliary Pancreat Surg 2000;7:28.

Neff R: Pancreatic pseudocysts and fluid collections: percutaneous approaches. Surg Clin North Am 2001;81:399.

Vidyarthi G, Steinberg SE: Endoscopic management of pancreatic pseudocysts. Surg Clin North Am 2001;81:405.

3. Pancreatic Abscess

Pancreatic abscess, which complicates about 5% of cases of acute pancreatitis, is invariably fatal if it is not treated surgically. It tends to develop in severe cases accompanied by hypovolemic shock and pancreatic necrosis and is an especially frequent complication of postoperative pancreatitis. Abscess formation follows secondary bacterial contamination of necrotic pancreatic debris and hemorrhagic exudate. The organisms may spread to the pancreas hematogenously as well as directly through the wall of the transverse colon. It is unknown whether prophylactic antibiotics given early in the course of severe acute pancreatitis decrease the incidence of abscess.

▶ Clinical Findings

An abscess should be suspected when a patient with severe acute pancreatitis fails to improve and develops rising fever or when symptoms return after a period of recovery. In most cases, there is improvement for a while before signs of infection appear 2–4 weeks after the attack began. Epigastric pain and tenderness and a palpable tender mass are clues to diagnosis. In many cases, the findings are not especially striking (ie, the temperature is only modestly elevated and the patient does not appear septic). Vomiting or jaundice may be present, but in some cases fever and leukocytosis are the only findings. The serum amylase may be elevated but usually is normal. Characteristically, the serum albumin is below 2.5 g/dL and the alkaline phosphatase is elevated. Pleural fluid and diaphragmatic paralysis may be evident on chest x-rays. An upper gastrointestinal series may show deformity of the stomach or duodenum by a mass, but it usually does not, and the changes are nonspecific in any case. Diagnostic CT scans will usually indicate the presence of a fluid collection in the area of the pancreas. Gas in the collection on plain films or CT scans is virtually diagnostic. Percutaneous CT scan–guided aspiration may be used to aid in diagnosis and obtain a specimen for Gram stain and culture.

In general, the diagnosis is difficult, treatment is often instituted late, illness is severe, and death rates are high.

▶ Treatment

The collection of pus must be drained. Percutaneous catheter drainage may be helpful as a first step in order to decrease toxicity or to obtain a specimen for culture. In some cases, catheter drainage will prove to be definitive, but most often the infected retroperitoneal space is honeycombed and contains necrotic debris that cannot pass through the catheter, so surgical debridement is necessary. It is best to consider catheter drainage as a preparatory step for surgery rather than a curative treatment, for that is the usual relationship. Otherwise, there may be a tendency to delay surgery for too long as futile efforts are repeatedly made to manipulate the catheters into better positions. In fact, the two measures—surgical debridement and catheter drainage—are complementary.

Preoperatively, the patient should be given broad-spectrum antibiotics, since the organisms are usually a mixed flora (most often *Escherichia coli, Bacteroides, Staphylococcus, Klebsiella, Proteus, Candida albicans,* etc). Necrotic debris should be removed and external drainage instituted.

Postoperative hemorrhage (immediate or delayed) from the abscess cavity occurs occasionally.

▶ Prognosis

The death rate is about 20%, a consequence of the severity of the condition, incomplete surgical drainage, and the inability in some cases to make the diagnosis.

Baril NB et al: Does an infected peripancreatic fluid collection or abscess mandate operation? Ann Surg 2000;231:361.

Beger HG, Rau B, Isenmann R: Prevention of severe change in acute pancreatitis: prediction and prevention. J Hepatobiliary Pancreat Surg 2001;8:140.

Kang CY et al: Development of HIV/AIDS vaccine using chimeric gag-env virus-like particles. Biol Chem 1999;380:353.

Tsiotos GG, Sarr MG: Management of fluid collections and necrosis in acute pancreatitis. Curr Gastroenterol Rep 1999;1:139.

Venu RP et al: Endoscopic transpapillary drainage of pancreatic abscess: technique and results. Gastrointest Endosc 2000;51(4 Part 1):391.

4. Pancreatic Ascites & Pancreatic Pleural Effusion

Pancreatic ascites consists of accumulated pancreatic fluid in the abdomen without peritonitis or severe pain. Since many of these patients are alcoholic, they are often thought at first to have cirrhotic ascites. The syndrome is most often due to chronic leakage of a pseudocyst, but a few cases are due to disruption of a pancreatic duct. The principal causative factors are alcoholic pancreatitis in adults and traumatic pancreatitis in children. Marked recent weight loss is a major clinical manifestation, and unresponsiveness of the ascites to diuretics is an additional diagnostic clue. The ascitic fluid, which ranges in appearance from straw-colored to blood-tinged, contains elevated protein (> 2.9 g/dL) and amylase levels. Once this condition is suspected, definitive diagnosis is based on chemical analysis of the ascitic fluid and endoscopic retrograde pancreatography. The latter procedure frequently demonstrates the point of fluid leak and allows a rational surgical approach if operation is required.

Initial therapy should consist of a period of intravenous hyperalimentation and somatostatin. This often cures the problem. If considerable improvement has not occurred within 2–3 weeks, surgery should be performed. A preoperative ERCP is essential to demonstrate the site of the leak. If it is not entirely obvious from the films taken during ERCP, a CT scan should be performed immediately afterward, while contrast media is still in the pancreatic duct. The greater sensitivity of the CT scan will be enough to reveal the tiny trickle from the pancreatic duct into the abdomen. The operation involves suturing a Roux-en-Y limb of jejunum to the site of the leak on the surface of the pancreas or a pancreatic pseudocyst. With appropriate therapy, the outlook is excellent. The death rate is low in patients treated before debilitation becomes severe.

Chronic pleural effusions of pancreatic origin represent a variant in which the pancreatic fistula drains into the chest. The diagnosis is made by measuring high concentrations of amylase (usually > 3000 IU/dL) in the fluid. A CT scan of the pancreas and retrograde pancreatogram should be obtained. Medical therapy consists of draining the fluid with a chest tube, somatostatin, and total parenteral nutrition. If after several weeks the fistula persists or if it recurs after the tube has been removed, the source of the leak on the pancreas should either be drained into a Roux-en-Y limb of jejunum or excised as part of a distal pancreatectomy.

Dugernier T, Laterre PF, Reynaert MS: Ascites fluid in severe acute pancreatitis: from pathophysiology to therapy. Acta Gastroenterol Belg 2000;63:264.

Kaman L et al: Internal pancreatic fistulas with pancreatic ascites and pancreatic pleural effusions: recognition and management. Aust N Z J Surg 2001;71:221.

Takeo C, Myojo S: Marked effect of octreotide acetate in a case of pancreatic pleural effusion. Curr Med Res Opin 2000;16:171.

5. Chronic Pancreatitis

ESSENTIALS OF DIAGNOSIS

▶ Persistent or recurrent abdominal pain.

▶ Pancreatic calcification on x-ray in 50%.

▶ Pancreatic insufficiency in 30%; malabsorption and diabetes mellitus.

▶ Most often due to alcoholism.

▶ General Considerations

Chronic alcoholism causes most cases of chronic pancreatitis, but a few are due to gallstones, hypercalcemia, hyperlipidemia, duct obstruction from any cause, or inherited predisposition (familial pancreatitis). Direct trauma to the gland, either from an external blow or from surgical injury, can produce chronic pancreatitis if a ductal stricture develops during the healing process. In such cases, disease is often localized to the segment of gland drained by the obstructed duct. Although gallstone disease may cause repeated attacks of acute pancreatitis, this uncommonly leads to chronic pancreatitis.

There is evidence that pancreatic juice normally contains a specific protein responsible for maintaining calcium carbonate in solution. Levels of this protein are decreased in patients with chronic pancreatitis, a situation that allows calcium carbonate to precipitate and form calculi. Pressure within the duct is increased in patients with chronic pancreatitis (about 40 cm H_2O) compared with normal subjects (about 15 cm H_2O). This is a result of increased viscosity of pancreatic juice, partial obstruction by calculi, and impaired distensibility of the gland because of diffuse fibrosis (eg, a compartment syndrome). Sphincteric pressure remains in the normal range. The increased pressure causes dilation of the duct in the patient whose pancreas has not yet become fixed by scarring. It may also impair nutrient blood flow, causing further functional damage. Pathologic changes in the gland include destruction of parenchyma, fibrosis, dedifferentiation of acini, calculi, and ductal dilation.

▶ Clinical Findings

A. Symptoms and Signs

Chronic pancreatitis may be asymptomatic, or it may produce abdominal pain, malabsorption, diabetes mellitus, or (usually) all three manifestations. The pain is typically felt deep in the upper abdomen and radiating through to the back, and it waxes and wanes from day to day. Early in the course of the disease, the pain may be episodic, lasting for days to weeks and then vanishing for several months before returning again. Attacks of acute pancreatitis may occur, superimposed on the pattern of chronic pain. Many patients become addicted to the narcotics prescribed for pain.

B. Laboratory Findings

Abnormal laboratory findings may result from (1) pancreatic inflammation, (2) pancreatic exocrine insufficiency, (3) diabetes mellitus, (4) bile duct obstruction, or (5) other complications such as pseudocyst formation or splenic vein thrombosis.

1. Amylase—In acute exacerbations, serum and urinary amylase levels may be elevated, but most often they are not, perhaps because pancreatic fibrosis has destroyed so much of the enzyme-forming capacity of the parenchyma.

2. Tests of exocrine pancreatic function—The secretin and cholecystokinin stimulation tests are the most sensitive tests to detect exocrine malfunction but are difficult to perform.

3. Diabetes mellitus—About 75% of patients with calcific pancreatitis and 30% of those with noncalcific pancreatitis have insulin-dependent diabetes. Most of the rest have either abnormal glucose tolerance curves or abnormally low serum insulin levels after a test meal. The margin of reserve is such that partial pancreatectomy is quite likely to convert a patient who does not require insulin into one who does require it postoperatively.

4. Biliary obstruction—Elevated bilirubin or alkaline phosphatase levels may result from fibrotic entrapment of the lower end of the bile duct. The differential diagnosis of biliary obstruction in these patients must consider acute pancreatic inflammation, pseudocyst, or pancreatic neoplasm.

5. Miscellaneous—Splenic vein thrombosis may produce secondary hypersplenism or gastric varices.

C. Imaging Studies

Endoscopic retrograde pancreatography is helpful in establishing the diagnosis of chronic pancreatitis, in ruling out pancreatic pseudocyst and neoplasm, and in preoperative planning for patients thought to be candidates for surgery. The typical findings are ductal stones and irregularity, with dilation and stenoses and, occasionally, ductal occlusion. The discovery of small unsuspected pseudocysts is common. Retrograde cholangiography should be performed simultaneously to determine whether the common bile duct is narrowed by the pancreatitis, to determine whether biliary calculi are present, and to aid the surgeon in avoiding injury to the bile duct during operation.

▶ Complications

The principal complications of chronic pancreatitis are pancreatic pseudocyst, biliary obstruction, duodenal obstruction, malnutrition, and diabetes mellitus. Adenocarcinoma of the pancreas occurs with greater frequency in patients with familial chronic pancreatitis than in the general population.

▶ Treatment

A. Medical Treatment

Malabsorption and steatorrhea are managed with support and measures. Controlled trials have shown that administering pancreatic enzymes has little effect on the pain.

Patients with chronic pancreatitis should be urged to discontinue the use of alcohol. Abstention from alcohol will reduce chronic or episodic pain in more than half of cases even though damage to the pancreas is irreversible. Psychiatric treatment may be beneficial. Diabetes in these patients usually requires insulin.

B. Surgical Treatment

Surgical therapy is principally of value to relieve chronic intractable pain. It is essential that every effort be made to eliminate alcohol abuse. The best surgical candidates are those whose pain persists after alcohol has been abandoned.

Surgical treatment in most cases involves a procedure that facilitates drainage of the pancreatic duct or resects diseased pancreas—or that serves both purposes. The choice of operation can usually be made preoperatively based on the findings of a retrograde pancreatogram and CT scans. Coincidental bile duct obstruction is common and should be treated by simultaneous choledochoduodenostomy.

1. Drainage procedures—A dilated ductal system reflects obstruction, and when dilation is present, procedures to improve ductal drainage usually relieve pain. Calcific alcoholic pancreatitis most often falls into this category.

The usual finding is an irregular, widely dilated duct (1–2 cm in diameter) with points of stenosis ("chain of lakes" appearance) and ductal calculi. For such patients, a longitudinal pancreaticojejunostomy (**Puestow procedure**) is appropriate (Figure 26–4). The duct is opened anteriorly from the tail into the head of the gland and anastomosed side to side to a Roux-en-Y segment of proximal jejunum. Pain improves postoperatively in about 80% of patients, but improvement of pancreatic insufficiency is uncommon. This procedure, however, has a low rate of success when the pancreatic duct is narrow (ie, < 8 mm).

Sphincteroplasty and distal (caudal) pancreaticojejunostomy (**Du Val procedure**) are other drainage techniques that were used more often in the past. The latter is only of historical interest, but surgical sphincteroplasty plus extraction of pancreatic ductal calculi continuous in use. Attempts are currently being made to accomplish something similar by subjecting pancreatic calculi to external shock wave lithotripsy, followed by endoscopic sphincterotomy and stone extraction. Another experimental method involves decompression of the duct by an endoscopically placed stent. Questions of safety and efficacy have tempered the early enthusiasm for these procedures.

2. Pancreatectomy—In the absence of a dilated duct, pancreatectomy is the best procedure, and the extent of resection can often be determined from a CT scan and pancreatogram.

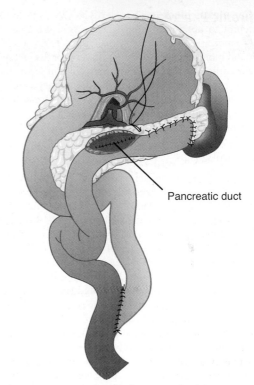

▲ **Figure 26–4.** Longitudinal pancreaticojejunostomy (Puestow) for chronic pancreatitis.

In patients with small ducts, the most severe disease is usually located in the head of the gland, and **pancreaticoduodenectomy** (Whipple procedure) is the operation of choice. A variant of this procedure involves resection of the head of the gland while preserving the duodenum. A Roux-en-Y limb of jejunum is anastomosed to both cut surfaces of the pancreas. If the duct is also dilated in the body and tail, resection of the head can also be combined with longitudinal pancreaticojejunostomy in that part of the gland. Pain relief is satisfactory in about 80% of patients treated by these operations. **Total pancreatectomy** is indicated when a previous pancreaticoduodenectomy or distal pancreatectomy has failed to give satisfactory pain relief. The reported results are contradictory; pain relief has been excellent in reports from the United Kingdom but less than excellent in reports from the United States. Difficulties in controlling diabetes mellitus occur in 30–40% of patients who have had total pancreatectomy and are responsible for occasional deaths. For this reason, total pancreatectomy is contraindicated in unreformed alcoholics. For chronic alcoholic pancreatitis, resections from the left of the gland (eg, **distal subtotal pancreatectomy**) are much less successful than resections of the head and are rarely performed nowadays. The most common indication is chronic focal posttraumatic pancreatitis, in which the head may be normal.

3. Celiac plexus block—Celiac plexus block may be used in an attempt to obtain pain relief before proceeding with a major pancreatic resection in small duct pancreatitis. A newer and more effective variant of this approach consists of **thoracoscopic splanchnicectomy**—resection of segments of the greater and lesser splanchnic nerves as they enter the thorax from the abdomen. When performed thoracoscopically, the procedure is relatively minor, and it interrupts the pain afferents with greater certainty.

▶ Prognosis

Longitudinal pancreaticojejunostomy relieves pain in about 80% of patients with a dilated duct. Weight gain is common but less predictable. The results of pancreaticoduodenectomy are good in 80% of patients, but removal of the distal pancreas is less successful. Total pancreatectomy, which is principally reserved for failures of other operations, gives satisfying relief in 30–90% of patients depending on the series. The reasons for these widely differing results are not known. Celiac plexus block is of lasting benefit to no more than 30% of patients. In some patients, pain subsides with advancing pancreatic insufficiency.

Except in advanced cases with continuous pain, alcoholics who can be persuaded to stop drinking often experience relief from pain and recurrent attacks of pancreatitis. In familial pancreatitis, the progress of the disease is inexorable, and many of these patients require surgery. The results of longitudinal pancreaticojejunostomy are excellent in familial pancreatitis. Narcotic addiction, diabetes, and malnutrition are serious problems in many patients.

Adamek HE et al: Long term follow up of patients with chronic pancreatitis and pancreatic stones treated with extracorporeal shock wave lithotripsy. Gut 1999;45:402.

Apte MV, Keogh GW, Wilson JS: Chronic pancreatitis: complications and management. J Clin Gastroenterol 1999;29:225.

Berney T et al: Long-term metabolic results after pancreatic resection for severe chronic pancreatitis. Arch Surg 2000;135:1106.

Bornman PC, Beckingham IJ: ABC of diseases of liver, pancreas, and biliary system. Chronic pancreatitis. BMJ 2001;322:660.

Izbicki JR et al: Extended drainage versus resection in surgery for chronic pancreatitis: a prospective randomized trial comparing the longitudinal pancreaticojejunostomy combined with local pancreatic head excision with the pylorus-preserving pancreatoduodenectomy. Ann Surg 1998;228:771.

Jimenez RE et al: Outcome of pancreaticoduodenectomy with pylorus preservation or with antrectomy in the treatment of chronic pancreatitis. Ann Surg 2000;231:293.

McCutcheon AD: Neurological damage and duodenopancreatic reflux in the pathogenesis of alcoholic pancreatitis. Arch Surg 2000;135:278.

Pitchumoni CS: Chronic pancreatitis: pathogenesis and management of pain. J Clin Gastroenterol 1998;27:101.

Sakorafas GH et al: Pancreatoduodenectomy for chronic pancreatitis: long-term results in 105 patients. Arch Surg 2000;135:517.

Whitcomb DC: Hereditary pancreatitis: new insights into acute and chronic pancreatitis. Gut 1999;45:317.

PANCREATIC INSUFFICIENCY (STEATORRHEA; MALABSORPTION)

Pancreatic exocrine insufficiency may follow pancreatectomy or pancreatic disease, especially chronic pancreatitis. Many patients with varying degrees of pancreatic insufficiency have no symptoms and require no treatment, whereas others may benefit greatly from a rational medical regimen.

Malabsorption and steatorrhea do not appear until more than 90% of pancreatic exocrine function is lost; with 2–10% of normal function, steatorrhea is mild to moderate; with less than 2% of normal function, steatorrhea is severe. On a diet containing 100 g of fat per day, normal subjects excrete 5–7 g/d, and the efficiency of assimilation is similar over a wide range of fat intake. Total pancreatectomy causes about 70% fat malabsorption. If the pancreatic remnant is normal, subtotal resections may have little effect on absorption.

Pancreatic insufficiency affects fat absorption more than that of protein or carbohydrate, because protein digestion is aided by gastric pepsin and carbohydrate digestion by salivary and intestinal amylase. Malabsorption of vitamins is rarely a significant problem. Water-soluble B vitamins are absorbed throughout the small intestine, and fat-soluble vitamins, although dependent on micellar solubilization by bile salts, do not require pancreatic enzymes for absorption. Vitamin B_{12} malabsorption has been detected in some patients with pancreatic insufficiency, but it is rarely a clinical problem, and vitamin B_{12} replacement is unnecessary.

Thus, the principal problem in otherwise uncomplicated pancreatic insufficiency is fat malabsorption and accompanying caloric malnutrition.

▶ Tests of Pancreatic Exocrine Function

A. Secretin or Cholecystokinin Test

Pancreatic juice is obtained by peroral duodenal intubation, and the response to an intravenous injection of secretin or cholecystokinin is measured. The results vary, depending on the dose and preparation of hormone used. Both tests (using purified hormones or the synthetic octapeptide of cholecystokinin) seem to be reliable. Pancreatic fluid should normally have a bicarbonate concentration greater than 80 meq/L and bicarbonate output above 15 meq/30 min.

B. Pancreolauryl Test

Fluorescein dilaurate is given orally with breakfast, and urinary fluorescein excretion is measured. Release and absorption of fluorescein depend on the action of pancreatic esterase. The test is relatively specific, but considerable exocrine insufficiency is required for a positive result. It is currently the most widely used test of exocrine function because it is inexpensive and easy to do.

C. PABA Excretion (Bentiromide) Test

The patient ingests 1 g of the synthetic peptide bentiromide (Bz-Ty-PABA), and urinary excretion of aromatic amines (PABA) is measured. Cleavage of the peptide to liberate PABA depends on intraluminal chymotrypsin activity. Patients with chronic pancreatitis excrete about 50% of the normal amount of PABA.

D. Fecal Fat Balance Test

The patient ingests a diet containing 75–100 g fat each day for 5 days. The amounts of dietary fat should be measured and should be the same each day. Excretion of less than 7% of ingested fat is normal. Clinically significant steatorrhea is present when fat malabsorption exceeds about 25%. Total pancreatectomy results in about 70% fat malabsorption.

Examination of a stool specimen for fat globules (obviously much simpler than the fat balance test) is specific and relatively sensitive for fat malabsorption.

▶ Treatment

The diet should aim for 3000–6000 kcal/d, emphasizing carbohydrate (400 g or more) and protein (100–150 g). Patients with steatorrhea may or may not have diarrhea, and dietary restriction of fat is important mainly to control diarrhea. Patients with diarrhea may be restricted to 50 g of fat and the amount increased until diarrhea appears. Permissible fat intake averages 100 g/d distributed equally among four meals.

Pancrelipase replacement may be accomplished with pancreatic extracts containing 30,000–50,000 units of lipase distributed throughout each of four daily meals. Lesser amounts are much less effective; an hourly dosage regimen probably has no advantages.

If enzymes alone do not improve the malabsorption enough, the problem is probably due to destruction of lipase by gastric acid. This can be largely alleviated by adding an H_2 receptor blocking agent to the enzyme regimen. A preparation of enzymes as enteric-coated microspheres (Pancrease) is less vulnerable to low pH and may be more effective in refractory cases.

Medium-chain triglycerides (MCT), which can be obtained as a powder or an oil, may be used as a caloric supplement. This product is more rapidly hydrolyzed and the fatty acids more readily absorbed than are long-chain triglycerides, which make up 98% of the fat in a normal diet. Unfortunately, MCT oil is relatively unpalatable and is frequently associated with nausea and vomiting, bloating, and diarrhea, which limit patient acceptance.

DiMagno EP: Gastric acid suppression and treatment of severe exocrine pancreatic insufficiency. Best Pract Res Clin Gastroenterol 2001;15:477.

Durie PR: Pancreatic aspects of cystic fibrosis and other inherited causes of pancreatic dysfunction. Med Clin North Am 2000; 84:609.

Layer P, Keller J: Pancreatic enzymes: secretion and luminal nutrient digestion in health and disease. J Clin Gastroenterol 1999; 28:3.

Tsiotos GG et al: Long-term outcome of necrotizing pancreatitis treated by necrosectomy. Br J Surg 1998;85:1650.

ADENOCARCINOMA OF THE PANCREAS

An estimated 37,680 patients will develop pancreatic cancer in the United States in 2008, and 34,290 will die of the disease. These nearly equal numbers illustrate the dismal prognosis generally associated with pancreatic carcinoma. The death rate per 100,000 people has been basically unchanged since the mid-1960s at about 13/100,000 for men and 10/100,000 for women. After tumors of the lung, colon, breast for women, and prostate for men, pancreatic carcinoma is the fourth leading cause of death due to cancer accounting for 6% of all cancer deaths. Factors associated with an increased risk of pancreatic cancer are cigarette smoking, obesity, chronic pancreatitis, diabetes, cirrhosis, and use of smokeless tobacco.

The peak incidence is in the fifth and sixth decades. In two thirds of cases, the tumor is located in the head of the gland; the remainder occur in the body or tail. Ductal adenocarcinoma, mainly of a poorly differentiated cell pattern, accounts for 80% of the cancers; the remainder are islet cell tumors and cystadenocarcinomas, tumors that are discussed later in this chapter. Pancreatic adenocarcinoma is characterized by early local extension to contiguous structures and metastases to regional lymph nodes and the liver. Pulmonary, peritoneal, and distant nodal metastases occur later.

▶ Clinical Findings

A. Symptoms and Signs

1. Carcinoma of the head of the pancreas—About 75% of patients with carcinoma of the head of the pancreas present with weight loss, obstructive jaundice, and deep-seated abdominal pain. Back pain occurs in 25% of patients and is associated with a worse prognosis. In general, smaller tumors confined to the pancreas are associated with less pain. Weight loss averages about 20 lb (44 kg). Hepatomegaly is present in half of patients but does not necessarily indicate spread to the liver. A palpable mass, which is found in 20%, nearly always signifies surgical incurability. Jaundice is unrelenting in most patients but fluctuates in about 10%. Cholangitis occurs in only 10% of patients with bile duct obstruction. A palpable nontender gallbladder in a jaundiced patient suggests neoplastic obstruction of the common duct (**Courvoisier sign**), most often due to pancreatic cancer; this finding is present in about half of cases. Jaundice is often accompanied by pruritus, especially of the hands and feet.

2. Carcinoma of the body and tail of the pancreas—Since carcinomas of the body and tail of the pancreas are remote from the bile duct, less than 10% of patients are jaundiced. The presenting complaints are weight loss and pain, which sometimes occurs in excruciating paroxysms. In the few patients with jaundice or hepatomegaly, metastatic involvement has usually occurred. Migratory thrombophlebitis develops in 10% of cases. Once considered relatively specific as a clue to pancreatic cancer, this complication is now known to affect patients with other types of malignant disease.

The diagnosis of pancreatic carcinoma may be extremely difficult. The typical patient who presents with abdominal pain, weight loss, and obstructive jaundice rarely presents a problem, but those with just weight loss, vague abdominal pain, and nondiagnostic x-rays are occasionally labeled psychoneurotics until the existence of cancer becomes obvious. If back pain predominates, orthopedic or neurosurgical causes may be sought at first. One characteristic feature is the tendency for the patient to seek relief of pain by assuming a sitting position with the spine flexed. Recumbency, on the other hand, aggravates the discomfort and sometimes makes sleeping in bed impossible. Sudden onset of diabetes mellitus is an early manifestation in 25% of patients.

B. Laboratory Findings

Elevated alkaline phosphatase and bilirubin levels reflect either common duct obstruction or hepatic metastases. The bilirubin level with neoplastic obstruction averages 18 mg/dL, much higher than that generally seen with benign disease of the bile ducts. Only rarely are serum aminotransferase levels markedly elevated. Repeated examination of stool specimens for occult blood gives a positive reaction in many cases.

Serum levels of the tumor marker CA 19-9 are elevated in most patients with pancreatic cancer, but the sensitivity in resectable (< 4 cm) lesions is probably too low (50%) for this to serve as a screening tool. Elevated levels also occur with other gastrointestinal cancers. The greatest usefulness of CA 19-9 measurements may be in following the results of treatments. After complete resection of a tumor, elevated levels drop to normal, but they rise again with recurrence.

C. Imaging Studies

Nearly all patients should have a CT scan.

1. CT scan—CT scans show a pancreatic mass in 95% of cases, usually with a central zone of diminished attenuation, and in over 90% of patients with a mass there are signs of extension beyond the boundaries of the pancreas. The upstream pancreatic duct is noted to be dilated in 70% of patients, and the bile duct is dilated in 60% (principally in those with jaundice). The presence of both bile duct and pancreatic duct dilation is strong evidence for pancreatic cancer even in the absence of a mass. Findings suggesting unresectability include local tumor extension (eg, behind the pancreas; into the liver hilum), contiguous organ invasion (eg, duodenum, stomach), distant metastases, involvement of the superior mesenteric or portal vessels, or ascites. In general, size of the mass is only loosely related to resectability. CT scans using modern dynamic scanning techniques are as accurate as angiography in assessing vascular involvement.

2. ERCP—In patients with a typical clinical history and a pancreatic mass on CT, ERCP is unnecessary. In the absence of a mass, an ERCP is indicated. It is the most sensitive test (95%) for detecting pancreatic cancer, though specificity in differentiating between cancer and pancreatitis is low. Consequently, a pancreatogram should be obtained early in cases where the existence of a pancreatic lesion is suspected but unproved. The findings consist of stenosis or obstruction of the pancreatic duct. Adjacent lesions of the bile duct and pancreatic duct (double-duct sign) are highly suggestive of neoplastic disease, especially if the biliary involvement is focal. Although ERCP is useful to distinguish between the various kinds of periampullary tumors, that information rarely alters management.

3. Upper gastrointestinal series—An upper gastrointestinal series is not sensitive in detecting pancreatic cancer, but it provides information about patency of the duodenum that may be useful in deciding whether a gastrojejunostomy will have to be performed. The classic findings consist of widening of the duodenal sweep, narrowing of the lumen, and the "reversed-3 sign," named for the duodenal configuration.

4. Other studies—Angiography has not proved reliable in detecting or staging pancreatic neoplasms, and ultrasound is a poor second to CT scans for imaging.

D. Aspiration Biopsy

Percutaneous aspiration biopsy of pancreatic mass lesions is positive in 85% of malignant tumors. The procedure is relatively safe, but there is a risk of spreading a localized (resectable) tumor, so it is contraindicated in patients who are candidates for surgery. Aspiration biopsy in them should be performed, if desired, during laparotomy. Percutaneous aspiration biopsy is principally of value to verify a presumptive diagnosis of adenocarcinoma of the pancreas in patients with radiographic evidence of unresectability. In these cases, cytologic proof is important, for treatment decisions should not be made solely on the basis of the indirect evidence provided by CT scans and other imaging tests. There is too great a risk of misdiagnosing something unusual, such as a retroperitoneal lymphoma or sarcoma, and administering inappropriate treatment.

▶ Differential Diagnosis

The other periampullary neoplasms—carcinoma of the ampulla of Vater, distal common bile duct, or duodenum—may also present with pain, weight loss, obstructive jaundice, and a palpable gallbladder. Preoperative cholangiography and gastrointestinal x-rays may suggest the correct diagnosis, but laparotomy is sometimes required.

▶ Complications

Obstruction of the splenic vein by tumor may cause splenomegaly and segmental portal hypertension with bleeding gastric or esophageal varices.

▶ Treatment

Pancreatic resection for pancreatic cancer is appropriate only if all gross tumor can be removed with a standard resection. The lesion is considered resectable if the following areas are free of tumor: (1) the hepatic artery near the origin of the gastroduodenal artery; (2) the superior mesenteric artery where it courses under the body of the pancreas; and (3) the liver and regional lymph nodes. Since the pancreas is so close to the portal vein and the superior mesenteric vessels, these structures may be involved early. About 20% of cancers of the head of the pancreas can be resected, but because of local and distant spread, this is rarely possible for lesions of the body and tail.

A histologic diagnosis can usually be made at operation by aspiration biopsy. With small lesions of the head of the gland, it may be difficult to obtain a specimen for histologic diagnosis because much of the palpable mass may consist of inflamed pancreatic tissue. Occasionally, histologic diagnosis is impossible, and clinical decisions must rest on indirect evidence.

For curable lesions of the head, pancreaticoduodenectomy (**Whipple procedure**) is required (Figure 26–5). This involves resection of the common bile duct, the gallbladder, the duodenum, and the pancreas to the midbody. There is an increasing tendency to preserve the antrum and pylorus. Involvement of a short (< 1.5 cm) segment of the portal vein is not a contraindication to a curative resection. This is managed by a partial or circumferential resection of the affected area.

When the procedure is performed by surgeons who do it frequently, the operative mortality rate is less than 5%. When it is performed by less experienced surgeons, the mortality rate is 20–30%. Postoperative deaths are due to complications such as pancreatic and biliary fistulas, hemorrhage, and infection.

In an attempt to increase the cure rate, total pancreatectomy has been given a trial on the theory that many pancreatic cancers are multicentric. However, total pancreatectomy produces a brittle type of diabetes mellitus that compromises the quality of life, and cure rates were not higher.

For unresectable lesions, cholecystojejunostomy or choledochojejunostomy provides relief of jaundice and pruritus. A cholangiogram should be obtained to verify patency between the cystic and common bile ducts unless it is grossly obvious. Percutaneous or endoscopically placed biliary stents may also provide effective palliation and are preferable to surgical biliary decompression if the lesion is known to be unresectable. Gastrojejunostomy is required if the tumor blocks the duodenum. If laparotomy has been performed, gastrojejunostomy should be considered regardless of the presence of duodenal obstruction, because with time this often develops before other life-threatening complications.

Laparoscopy is a useful first step in patients scheduled for a possible Whipple procedure. If metastases are seen that militate against a curative resection, laparoscopic gastrojejunostomy or cholecystojejunostomy (or both) can be performed. If not, one should proceed with the laparotomy. About 15% of patients thought to have localized disease from preoperative studies are found to be unresectable at laparoscopy.

Gemcitabine-based chemotherapy has clear benefits in patients with metastatic disease. Its utility in combination with radiation therapy and as adjuvant therapy is being defined.

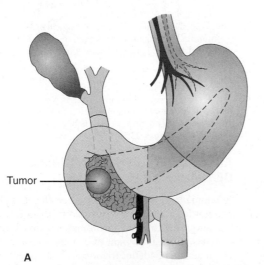 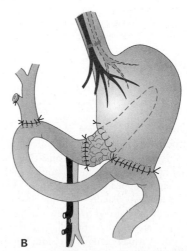

Tumor

A   B

▲ **Figure 26–5.** Pancreaticoduodenectomy (Whipple procedure). **A:** Preoperative anatomic relationships showing a tumor in the head of the pancreas. **B:** Postoperative reconstruction showing pancreatic, biliary, and gastric anastomoses. A cholecystectomy and bilateral truncal vagotomy are also part of the procedure. In many cases, the distal stomach and pylorus can be preserved, and vagotomy is then unnecessary.

▶ Prognosis

The mean survival following palliative therapy is 7 months. Following a Whipple procedure, survival averages about 18 months. Factors associated with tumor recurrence and shorter survival include lymph node involvement, tumor size over 2.5 cm, blood vessel invasion, and amount of blood transfused. If tumor cells extend to the margins of the resected specimen, long-term survival is rare. If the margins are clear, about 20% of patients live more than 5 years. Overall 5-year survival is about 10%, but only 60% of these patients are actually free of tumor.

Balci NC, Semelka RC: Radiologic diagnosis and staging of pancreatic ductal adenocarcinoma. Eur J Radiol 2001;38:105.

Bodner WR, Hilaris BS, Mastoras DA: Radiation therapy in pancreatic cancer: current practice and future trends. J Clin Gastroenterol 2000;30:230.

Bornman PC, Beckingham IJ: ABC of diseases of liver, pancreas, and biliary system. Pancreatic tumours. BMJ 2001;322:721.

Crane CH et al: Combining gemcitabine with radiation in pancreatic cancer: understanding important variables influencing the therapeutic index. Semin Oncol 2001;28(3 Suppl 10):25.

Farnell MB, Nagorney DM, Sarr MG: The Mayo clinic approach to the surgical treatment of adenocarcinoma of the pancreas. Surg Clin North Am 2001;81:611.

Kozuch P et al: Treatment of metastatic pancreatic adenocarcinoma: a comprehensive review. Surg Clin North Am 2001;81:683.

Madura JA et al: Adenosquamous carcinoma of the pancreas. Arch Surg 1999;134:599.

Mangray S, King TC: Molecular pathobiology of pancreatic adenocarcinoma. Front Biosci 1998;3:D1148.

Molinari M, Helton WS, Espat NJ: Palliative strategies for locally advanced unresectable and metastatic pancreatic cancer. Surg Clin North Am 2001;81:651.

Rose DM et al: [18]Fluorodeoxyglucose-positron emission tomography in the management of patients with suspected pancreatic cancer. Ann Surg 1999;229:729.

Sohn TA, Yeo CJ: The molecular genetics of pancreatic ductal carcinoma: a review. Surg Oncol 2000;9:95.

CYSTIC NEOPLASMS

Cystic neoplasms of the pancreas usually present with abdominal pain, a mass, or jaundice and are diagnosed from the findings on CT scans.

Cystadenomas can be classified as serous or mucinous. Serous cystadenomas, which are usually microcystic adenomas, are well-circumscribed lesions consisting of multiple small cysts ranging in size from microscopic to about 2 cm. The cut surface has the appearance of a sponge. The multicystic nature of the lesion is usually—but not always—evident on CT scans, which may also show a few calcifications. The epithelium, which is flat to cuboidal, has no malignant potential. Treatment usually entails excision, but in the rare case where this is too hazardous, the lesion may be left in place with the knowledge that complications are rare. An occasional serous cystadenoma will consist of one or more large cysts (ie, macrocystic).

Mucinous cystadenomas (macrocystic adenomas), which are much more common in women than in men, are unilocular or, more often, multilocular lesions that have a smooth lining with papillary projections. The septate appearance on CT scans is characteristic. The cystic spaces measure 2–20 cm in diameter and contain mucus. The lining consists of tall columnar and goblet cells, which are often arranged in a papillary pattern. In time, most mucinous cystadenomas will evolve into cystadenocarcinomas, so total excision is the required treatment.

Cystadenocarcinomas invariably present as a focus of malignancy within an existing mucinous cystadenoma. The tumors are often quite large (eg, 10–20 cm) at the time of diagnosis. Metastases occur in about 25% of cases. Complete excision results in a 5-year survival rate of 70%.

An uncommon lesion, referred to as solid-and-papillary or papillary-cystic neoplasm of the pancreas, occurs almost exclusively in young women (under age 25 years). The tumor is usually large. It may be locally invasive, but metastases are uncommon, and cure is to be expected after resection.

Balci NC, Semelka RC: Radiologic features of cystic, endocrine and other pancreatic neoplasms. Eur J Radiol 2001;38:113.

Balcom JH 4th et al: Cystic lesions in the pancreas: when to watch, when to resect. Curr Gastroenterol Rep 2000;2:152.

Le Borgne J, de Calan L, Partensky C: Cystadenomas and cystadenocarcinomas of the pancreas: a multiinstitutional retrospective study of 398 cases. French Surgical Association. Ann Surg 1999;230:152.

Sarr MG et al: Cystic neoplasms of the pancreas: benign to malignant epithelial neoplasms. Surg Clin North Am 2001;81:497.

Sarr MG et al: Clinical and pathologic correlation of 84 mucinous cystic neoplasms of the pancreas: can one reliably differentiate benign from malignant (or premalignant) neoplasms? Ann Surg 2000;231:205.

Shima Y et al: Diagnosis and management of cystic pancreatic tumours with mucin production. Br J Surg 2000;87:1041.

Verdolini K et al: Laryngeal adduction in resonant voice. J Voice 1998;12:315.

Vihtelic TS, Doro CJ, Hyde DR: Cloning and characterization of six zebrafish photoreceptor opsin cDNAs and immunolocalization of their corresponding proteins. Vis Neurosci 1999;16:571.

Wilentz RE et al: Pathologic examination accurately predicts prognosis in mucinous cystic neoplasms of the pancreas. Am J Surg Pathol 1999;23:1320.

ADENOMA & ADENOCARCINOMA OF THE AMPULLA OF VATER

Adenoma and adenocarcinoma of the ampulla of Vater account for about 10% of neoplasms that obstruct the distal bile duct. One third are adenomas and two thirds adenocarcinomas. Since a remnant of benign adenoma can be found in a majority of adenocarcinomas, it is suspected that malignant change in an adenoma gives rise to most carcinomas. The presenting symptom is most often jaundice or occasionally gastrointestinal bleeding. Weight loss and pain are more common with carcinoma than with adenoma, but the differences are not great enough to allow a distinction to be made on this basis alone.

CT and ultrasound scans reveal dilation of the biliary tree and pancreatic duct. Gallstones are an incidental finding in 20% of patients, and when common duct stones are present, they may incorrectly be held responsible for the biliary obstruction. The most important diagnostic study is ERCP. In 75% of cases, tumor is visible on duodenoscopy as an exophytic papillary lesion, an ulcerated tumor, or an infiltrating mass. An adequate biopsy usually can be obtained of these lesions. In 25% of cases, there is no intraduodenal growth, and endoscopic sphincterotomy is necessary to display the tumor. It is best to wait 10–14 days to biopsy these tumors because of transient artifacts that result from the sphincterotomy. ERCP also demonstrates dilation of the biliary and pancreatic ducts. It has become common to perform a sphincterotomy whenever possible, not only to facilitate performance of a biopsy but also to decompress the biliary tree and allow jaundice to subside in anticipation of subsequent surgical therapy. The value of this step has not been established.

Although some adenomas have been successfully treated by snare excision or, preferably, by neodymium:YAG laser destruction, local resection or pancreaticoduodenectomy is preferable because of the significant chance that an invasive carcinoma will be undertreated at a time that it is curable. These nonsurgical methods should be reserved for patients who are poor candidates for resection.

Treatment of adenocarcinoma consists of pancreaticoduodenectomy as for pancreatic carcinoma. The operative mortality rate is less than 5%, and the 5-year survival rate is about 50%. The presence of metastases in resectable peripancreatic lymph nodes is not a contraindication to pancreaticoduodenectomy, for the 5-year survival rate under these circumstances is still a respectable 25%. Local excision is an alternative for noninfiltrating papillary adenocarcinomas in patients who are too poor a risk for pancreaticoduodenectomy, but this operation is not as successful as pancreaticoduodenectomy. Endoscopic sphincterotomy alone or with retrograde stent placement (the combination is usually required) is indicated when there is definite evidence (eg, hepatic metastases) that the tumor is incurable. Survival averages less than a year with this approach, however.

Bakaeen FG et al: What prognostic factors are important in duodenal adenocarcinoma? Arch Surg 2000;135:635.

Crucitti A et al: Ampullary carcinoma: prognostic significance of ploidy, cell-cycle analysis and proliferating cell nuclear antigen (PCNA). Hepatogastroenterology 1999;46:1187.

Howe JR et al: Factors predictive of survival in ampullary carcinoma. Ann Surg 1998;228:87.

Lee JH et al: Outcome of pancreaticoduodenectomy and impact of adjuvant therapy for ampullary carcinomas. Int J Radiat Oncol Biol Phys 2000;47:945.

Roberts RH et al: Pancreaticoduodenectomy of ampullary carcinoma. Am Surg 1999;65:1043.

PANCREATIC ISLET CELL TUMORS

Islet cell tumors may be functioning (ie, hormone-producing) or nonfunctioning, malignant or nonmalignant. More than half are functioning; less than half are malignant. Insulinoma, the most common functioning islet cell neoplasm, arises from beta cells and produces insulin and symptoms of hypoglycemia. Tumors of the δ or α_1 cells produce gastrin and the Zollinger-Ellison syndrome. α_2 Cell neoplasms may produce excess glucagon and hyperglycemia. Non-β islet cell tumors may secrete serotonin, adrenocorticotropic hormone (ACTH), melanocyte-stimulating hormone (MSH), and kinins (and evoke the carcinoid syndrome). Some produce pancreatic cholera, a severe diarrheal illness.

1. Nonfunctioning Islet Cell Tumors

Most of these lesions are malignant tumors of the head of the gland, which present with abdominal and back pain, weight loss, and, in many cases, a palpable abdominal mass. Jaundice is seen occasionally. CT scans reveal a pancreatic mass, and angiography typically shows it to be hypervascular. The histologic pattern on biopsy specimens is diagnostic of islet cell tumor, but whether or not the lesion is malignant rests on evidence of invasiveness or metastases, not the appearance of the cells. Immunohistochemical staining of the tissue is positive for chromogranin and neuron-specific enolase (markers of amine precursor uptake and decarboxylation [APUD] tumors). Metastases are present at the time of diagnosis in 80% of patients. Resection of all gross tumor (eg, by a Whipple procedure), the preferred treatment, is possible in less than half of patients because of local extension or distant metastases. A combination of streptozocin and doxorubicin is the most effective chemotherapeutic regimen. The 5-year disease-free survival rate is about 15%.

Bartsch DK et al: Management of nonfunctioning islet cell carcinomas. World J Surg 2000;24:1418.

Jensen RT: Carcinoid and pancreatic endocrine tumors: recent advances in molecular pathogenesis, localization, and treatment. Curr Opin Oncol 2000;12:368.

Somogyi L, Mishra G: Diagnosis and staging of islet cell tumors of the pancreas. Curr Gastroenterol Rep 2000;2:159.

2. Insulinoma

Insulinomas have been reported in all age groups. About 75% are solitary and benign. About 10% are malignant, and metastases are usually evident at the time of diagnosis. The remaining 15% are manifestations of multifocal pancreatic disease—either adenomatosis, nesidioblastosis, or islet cell hyperplasia.

The symptoms (related to cerebral glucose deprivation) are bizarre behavior, memory lapse, or unconsciousness. Patients may be mistakenly treated for psychiatric illness. There may be profuse sympathetic discharge, with palpitations, sweating, and tremulousness. Hypoglycemic episodes are usually precipitated by fasting and are relieved by food, so weight gain is common. The classic diagnostic criteria (**Whipple triad**) are present in most cases: (1) hypoglycemic symptoms produced by fasting, (2) blood glucose below 50 mg/dL during symptomatic episodes, and (3) relief of symptoms by intravenous administration of glucose.

The most useful diagnostic test and the only one indicated in all but a few patients is demonstration of fasting hypoglycemia in the presence of inappropriately high levels of insulin. The patient is fasted, and blood samples are obtained every 6 hours for glucose and insulin measurements. The fast is continued until hypoglycemia or symptoms appear or for a maximum of 72 hours. If hypoglycemia has not developed after 70 hours, the patient should be exercised for the final 2 hours. Although insulin levels are not always elevated in patients with insulinoma, they will be high relative to the blood glucose concentration. A ratio of plasma insulin to glucose greater than 0.3 is diagnostic. Ratios should be calculated before and during the fast. Proinsulin, which constitutes more than 25% of total insulin (the upper limit of normal) in about 85% of patients with insulinomas, should also be measured. Proinsulin levels greater than 40% suggest a malignant islet cell tumor.

Drugs that release insulin (tolbutamide, glucagon, leucine, arginine, calcium) were used in the past as provocative tests. No provocative tests are currently used.

Localization of the tumor is important but may be difficult. In about 10% of cases, the tumor is so small or located so deeply that it is difficult or impossible to find at laparotomy. High-resolution CT and MR scans are successful in demonstrating about 40% of tumors. Endoscopic (gastroscopic) ultrasound examination of the pancreas may be able to show a much higher percentage. The most important examination is intraoperative ultrasound, which can identify a pancreatic tumor in nearly all cases. It is more sensitive than any preoperative test.

In patients who have had previous resection or significant upper abdominal surgery, exploration with intraoperative ultrasound may be difficult. Invasive preoperative testing may then be useful. Angiography gives a yield of about 50%. Transhepatic portal venous sampling has proved an accurate preoperative localizing method, demonstrating the position in the pancreas in about 95% of lesions. However, this test is time-consuming and somewhat invasive, involving entering the portal vein with a catheter passed percutaneously through the liver and testing blood at various sites within the portal, superior mesenteric, and splenic veins for insulin levels. The point where insulin concentrations rise sharply indicates the site of the tumor. An alternative invasive localizing test uses arteriography with selective calcium infusion into arteries supplying the pancreas. Blood samples from the hepatic veins reveal an increase in insulin level when calcium is infused into an artery supplying the tumor.

Differential Diagnosis

Fasting hypoglycemia may be a manifestation of some nonpancreatic, non–islet cell tumors. Clinically, the condition is identical to that resulting from insulinoma, but the cause is rarely secretion of insulin by the tumors, as serum insulin levels are normal. Most non–islet cell tumors associated with hypoglycemia are large and readily detected on physical examination. The majority are of mesenchymal origin (eg, hemangiopericytoma, fibrosarcoma, leiomyosarcoma) and are located in the abdomen or thorax, but hepatoma, adrenocortical carcinoma, and a variety of other lesions may also produce hypoglycemia. The principal means by which these tumors produce hypoglycemia are the following: (1) secretion by the tumor of insulinlike growth factor II (IGF-II), an insulinlike peptide that normally mediates the effects of growth hormone; and (2) inhibition of glycogenolysis or gluconeogenesis. Rapid utilization of glucose by the tumor, replacement of liver tissue by metastases, and secretion of insulin are other postulated mechanisms that are probably uncommon.

Surreptitious self-administration of insulin is seen occasionally, most often in an individual with access to insulin on the job. If insulin injections have been given for as long as 2 months, insulin antibodies will be detectable in the patient's serum. Circulating C peptide levels are normal in these patients but elevated in most patients with insulinoma. Sulfonylurea ingestion can be detected by measuring the drug in plasma.

Treatment

Surgery should be done promptly, because with repeated hypoglycemic attacks, permanent cerebral damage occurs and the patient becomes progressively more obese. Moreover, the tumor may be malignant. Medical treatment is reserved for surgically incurable lesions.

A. Medical Treatment

Diazoxide is administered to suppress insulin release. For incurable islet cell carcinomas, streptozocin is the best chemotherapeutic agent. Sixty percent of patients live up to 2 additional years. Toxicity is considerable; streptozocin is not recommended as a routine adjunct to surgical therapy.

B. Surgical Treatment

At surgery, the entire pancreas must be palpated carefully because the tumors are usually small and difficult to find. The gland should also be examined intraoperatively with ultrasound, which may be able to locate a tumor that cannot be felt or to demonstrate signs of invasion (ie, irregular borders) that indicate malignancy—something that cannot be detected by palpation. When the tumor is found, it may be enucleated if it is superficial or resected as part of a partial pancreatectomy if it is deep-seated or invasive. Insulinomas in the head of the gland can nearly always be enucleated.

Tumors that can be localized preoperatively, and that are placed in favorable anatomic locations, can sometimes be resected using a laparoscopic approach. The same principles of local, complete resection should be followed. Laparoscopic ultrasound is often useful to guide this exploration.

In the past, the tumor could not be detected in about 5% of cases by these methods. The traditional recommendation was to resect the distal half of the pancreas and have the pathologist slice the specimen into thin sections and look for the tumor. If the tumor was found, the operation was concluded; if it was not found, additional pancreas would be resected until an 80% distal pancreatectomy had been performed. Since the tumors are evenly distributed, this strategy is 80% successful in removing the tumor. Intraoperative monitoring of blood glucose is often done as a means of determining if the tumor has been excised, but it is unreliable. With the use of operative ultrasound scanning, however, no more than 1–2% of insulinomas remain occult, and blind distal pancreatectomy is rarely even considered.

Patients with insulinoma associated with multiple endocrine neoplasia (MEN)-1 usually have multiple (average of three) lesions. Because persistence of the disease is much more likely in this condition following the standard surgical approach, the operation recommended here is distal pancreatectomy plus enucleation of any lesions found in the head of the gland.

For islet cell hyperplasia, nesidioblastosis, or multiple benign adenomas, distal subtotal pancreatectomy usually decreases insulin levels enough that medical management is simplified. For islet cell carcinomas, resection of both primary and metastatic lesions is warranted if technically feasible.

Patients with sporadic insulinomas lead a normal life after the tumor has been removed. The outcome is less predictable in patients with MEN-1, who may have several insulin-producing tumors.

Dolan JP, Norton JA: Occult insulinoma. Br J Surg 2000;87:385.
Grant CS: Surgical aspects of hyperinsulinemic hypoglycemia. Endocrinol Metab Clin North Am 1999;28:533.
Grant CS: Insulinoma. Surg Oncol Clin N Am 1998;7:819.
Service FJ: Classification of hypoglycemic disorders. Endocrinol Metab Clin North Am 1999;28:501.

3. Pancreatic Cholera (WDHA Syndrome: Watery Diarrhea, Hypokalemia, & Achlorhydria)

Most cases of pancreatic cholera are caused by a non-β islet cell tumor of the pancreas that secretes VIP (vasoactive intestinal polypeptide) and peptide histidine isoleucine. The syndrome is characterized by profuse watery diarrhea, massive fecal loss of potassium, low serum potassium, and extreme weakness. Gastric acid secretion is usually low or absent even after stimulation with betazole or pentagastrin. Stool volume averages about 5 L/d during acute episodes and contains over 300 meq of potassium (20 times normal). Severe metabolic acidosis frequently results from loss of bicarbonate in the stool. Many patients are hypercalcemic, possibly from secretion by the tumor of a parathyroid hormonelike substance. Abnormal glucose tolerance may result from hypokalemia and altered sensitivity to insulin. Patients who complain of severe diarrhea must be studied carefully for other causes before the diagnosis of WDHA syndrome is entertained seriously. Chronic laxative abuse is a frequent explanation.

CT scan is the best initial imaging test; somatostatin receptor scintigraphy is also very useful for localization. Approximately 80% of the tumors are solitary, located in the body or tail, and can be removed easily. About half of the lesions are malignant, and three fourths of those have metastasized by the time of exploration. Even if all of the tumor cannot be removed, resection of most of it alleviates symptoms in about 40% of patients even though the average survival is only 1 year. Streptozocin has produced remissions in several cases, but nephrotoxicity may limit its effectiveness. Treatment with long-acting somatostatin analogues decreases VIP levels, controls diarrhea, and may even reduce tumor size. The effect persists indefinitely in most patients, but in a few it is transient.

Jensen RT: Overview of chronic diarrhea caused by functional neuroendocrine neoplasms. Semin Gastrointest Dis 1999; 10:156.
Soga J, Yakuwa Y: Vipoma/diarrheogenic syndrome: a statistical evaluation of 241 reported cases. J Exp Clin Cancer Res 1998;17:389.

4. Glucagonoma

Glucagonoma syndrome is characterized by migratory necrolytic dermatitis (usually involving the legs and perineum), weight loss, stomatitis, hypoaminoacidemia, anemia, and mild to moderate diabetes mellitus. Scotomas and changes in visual acuity have been reported in some cases. The age range is 20–70 years, and the condition is more common in women. The diagnosis may be suspected from the distinctive skin lesion; in fact, the presence of a prominent rash in a patient with diabetes mellitus should be enough to raise suspicions. Glucagonoma should also be suspected in any patient with new onset of diabetes after age 60. Confirmation of the diagnosis depends on measuring elevated serum glucagon levels. CT scans demonstrate the tumor and sites of spread. Angiography is not essential but reveals a hypervascular lesion.

Glucagonomas arise from α_2 cells in the pancreatic islets. Most are large at the time of diagnosis. About 25% are benign and confined to the pancreas. The remainder have metastasized by the time of diagnosis, most often to the liver, lymph nodes, adrenal gland, or vertebrae. A few cases have been the result of islet cell hyperplasia.

Severe malnutrition should be corrected preoperatively with a period of total parenteral nutrition and treatment with somatostatin analogues. Surgical removal of the primary lesion and resectable secondaries is indicated if technically feasible. If the tumor is confined to the pancreas, cure is possible. Even if it is not possible to remove all the tumor deposits, considerable palliation may result from subtotal removal, so surgery is indicated in almost every case. Low-dose heparin therapy should be administered preoperatively and postoperatively because of a high risk of deep venous thrombosis and pulmonary embolism. Streptozocin and dacarbazine are the most effective chemotherapeutic agents for unresectable lesions. Somatostatin therapy normalizes serum glucagon and amino acid levels, clears the rash, and promotes weight gain. The clinical course generally parallels changes in serum levels of glucagon in response to therapy.

Bernstein M et al: Amino acid, glucose, and lipid kinetics after palliative resection in a patient with glucagonoma syndrome. Metabolism 2001;50:720.

Chastain MA: The glucagonoma syndrome: a review of its features and discussion of new perspectives. Am J Med Sci 2001;321:306.

El Rassi Z et al: Necrolytic migratory erythema, first symptom of a malignant glucagonoma: treatment by long-acting somatostatin and surgical resection. Report of three cases. Eur J Surg Oncol 1998;24:562.

Metz DC: Diagnosis of non-Zollinger-Ellison syndrome, non-carcinoid syndrome, enteropancreatic neuroendocrine tumours. Ital J Gastroenterol Hepatol 1999;31(Suppl 2):S153.

5. Somatostatinoma

Somatostatinomas are characterized by diabetes mellitus (usually mild), diarrhea and malabsorption, and dilation of the gallbladder (usually with cholelithiasis). Serum calcitonin and IgM concentrations may be elevated. The syndrome results from secretion of somatostatin by an islet cell tumor of the pancreas, half of which are malignant and accompanied by hepatic metastases. The lesion is usually large and readily demonstrated by CT scan. The diagnosis may be made by recognizing the clinical syndrome and measuring increased concentrations of somatostatin in the serum. Often, however, the somatostatin syndrome is unsuspected until histologic evidence of metastatic islet cell carcinoma has been obtained. When the disease is localized, resection is able to cure about 50% of cases. Enucleation is inappropriate for these tumors. Chemotherapy with streptozocin, dacarbazine, or doxorubicin is the best treatment for unresectable tumors. Small somatostatin-rich tumors of the duodenum or ampulla of Vater have also been reported, but none of these lesions have been associated with high serum levels of somatostatin or the clinical syndrome.

Metz DC: Diagnosis of non-Zollinger-Ellison syndrome, non-carcinoid syndrome, enteropancreatic neuroendocrine tumours. Ital J Gastroenterol Hepatol 1999;31(Suppl 2):S153.

Soga J, Yakuwa Y: Somatostatinoma/inhibitory syndrome: a statistical evaluation of 173 reported cases as compared to other pancreatic endocrinomas. J Exp Clin Cancer Res 1999;18:13.

Tanaka S et al: Duodenal somatostatinoma: a case report and review of 31 cases with special reference to the relationship between tumor size and metastasis. Pathol Int 2000;50:146.

Spleen

Douglas L. Fraker, MD

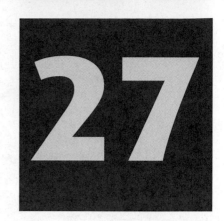

27

ANATOMY

The spleen is a dark purplish, highly vascular, coffee bean–shaped organ of mesodermal origin situated in the left upper quadrant of the abdomen at the level of the 8th to 11th ribs between the fundus of the stomach, the diaphragm, the splenic flexure of the colon, and the left kidney (Figure 27–1). The adult spleen weighs 100–150 g, measures about $12 \times 7 \times 4$ cm, and usually cannot be palpated. It is attached to adjacent viscera, the abdominal wall, and the diaphragm by peritoneal folds or "ligaments." The gastrosplenic ligament carries the short gastric vessels. The other ligaments are avascular except in patients with portal hypertension or myelofibrosis.

The splenic capsule consists of peritoneum overlying a 1- to 2-mm fibroelastic layer that contains a few smooth muscle cells. The fibroelastic layer sends into the pulp numerous fibrous bands (trabeculae) that form the framework of the spleen. Corrosion cast studies demonstrate that the spleen consists of specific segments based on arterial supply numbering between two and six separated by an avascular plane.

The splenic artery enters the hilum of the spleen, branches into the trabecular arteries, and then branches into the central arteries that course through the surrounding white pulp and send radial branches to the peripheral marginal zone and the more distant red pulp. The white pulp consists of lymphatic tissue including T cells adjacent to the central artery (periarteriolar lymphoid sheets [PALS]), with a surrounding area containing lymphoid follicles rich in B cells interspersed with dendritic and reticular cells important in antigen presentation. The vascular spaces of the marginal zone between the red and white pulp channel blood into the splenic Billroth cords and out to the associated sinuses. The red pulp vascular structures have a noncontiguous basement membrane that filters cells such as senescent erythrocytes into the macrophage-lined sinuses.

Accessory spleens (splenunculi) are seen in 10–15% of the normal population and are located primarily in the gastrosplenic, gastrocolic, and lienorenal ligaments, but they can also be found throughout the peritoneal cavity in the omentum, bowel mesentery, and pelvis. Accessory spleens probably result from a failure of infusion of splenic embryologic tissues. Ordinarily of no significance, they may play a role in recurrence of certain hematologic disorders for which splenectomy is performed. Removal of accessory spleens may lead to remission of disease in these patients. Accessory spleens are more difficult to identify with laparoscopic procedures, but the use of a hand port has allowed identification and resection of accessory spleens with a minimally invasive approach. Patients who fail to respond to initial splenectomy should undergo scanning with technetium 99m-labeled red cells or indium 111-labeled platelets to identify potential sites of missed accessory spleens and can be identified intraoperatively with a handheld gamma counter.

Ectopic spleen (wandering spleen) is an unusual condition in which a long splenic pedicle allows the spleen to move within the peritoneum. It often resides in the lower abdomen or pelvis, where even a normal-sized spleen can be felt as a mass. The condition is 13 times more common in women than in men. Diagnostic radionuclide scan can diagnose the mass as a spleen. Acute torsion of the pedicle occurs occasionally, necessitating emergency splenectomy, and elective removal of wandering spleens in the pelvis is recommended.

PHYSIOLOGY

The spleen has a dual function as a secondary lymphoid organ important in host immunity and as a large filter for blood removing senescent erythrocytes and recycling iron. The anatomy of the spleen provides an ideal environment for these two functions with the immune activity in the white pulp and the hematologic function in the red pulp.

The spleen receives 5% of the total cardiac output, or approximately 150–300 mL/min, such that each red cell averages 1000 passes through the spleen each day. Normal blood cells pass rapidly through the spleen, while abnormal and senescent cells are slowed and entrapped. As they travel

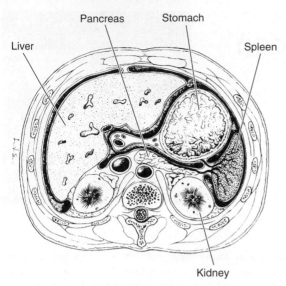

Liver   Pancreas   Stomach   Spleen   Kidney

▲ **Figure 27–1.** Normal anatomic relations of the spleen.

through the hypoxic, acidic, glucose-deprived splenic cords and sinuses of the red pulp, senescent erythrocytes pass into the vascular spaces and are phagocytosed by macrophages in a process called culling. Part of the membrane of erythrocytes can be removed through the gaps between endothelial cells lining the vascular spaces in a similar process called pitting. In the presence of splenomegaly and other disease states, the flow patterns of the spleen become more circuitous as the red pulp volume expands, so that even normal cells may be trapped.

The spleen is considered to be a secondary organ of the immune system and represents the largest single collection of lymphoid tissue in the body. The white pulp of the spleen contains the various cellular components needed to generate an immune response, with structural and functional relationships similar to those of lymph nodes. Lymphocytes and circulating antigen-presenting cells enter the white pulp via the marginal zone capillaries and traverse the T cell–rich PALS before passing through bridging channels into the red pulp. Primary follicles or germinal centers with secondary follicles at the periphery of the white pulp are sites of B cell expansion and immunoglobulin production. Blood passing through the spleen is exposed to all the key cellular components necessary for both humoral and cellular immune responses. Tissue macrophage in the spleen are key components of generating an immune response, particularly in encapsulated organs. Moreover, the concentration of macrophages in the red pulp vascular spaces facilitates opsonization of particles coated with IgG and plays an important role in the filtration and removal of senescent erythrocytes, the autoimmune hematologic diseases, as well as explaining the increased risk of sepsis that follows splenectomy in children

under 2 years of age. Even in adults, splenectomy leads to a slight but definite reduction in immune function.

Normally, about 30% of the total platelet pool is sequestered in the spleen. Splenomegaly typically involves expansion of the red pulp, which increases this sequestration to between 80% and 95% of the platelet cell mass. Storage of erythrocytes and granulocytes in the spleen is limited in humans, but newly formed reticulocytes released from the bone marrow concentrate in the spleen to undergo a maturational process.

Brendolan et al: Development and function of the mammalian spleen. Bioessays 2007;29:166.

Hilmes MA et al: The pediatric spleen. Semin Ultrasound CT MR 2007;28:3.

Mebius RE, Kraal C: Structure and function of the spleen. Nat Rev Immunol 2005;5:606.

Scandella JT et al: Form follows function: lymphoid tissue microarchitecture in antimicrobial immune defence. Nature Reviews. Immunology 2008;8:764.

▼ OPERATIVE INDICATIONS FOR SPLENECTOMY

To better describe and understand operative indications in surgery of the spleen, one could categorize the indications for splenectomy or procedures of the spleen into eight general areas:

(1) Hypersplenism is characterized by diffuse enlargement of the spleen by neoplastic disorders, hematopoietic disorders of the bone marrow, and metabolic or storage disorders. These various disease processes result in diffuse enlargement of the spleen and amplify the normal function of elimination of circulating blood cells resulting in general pancytopenia. Erythrocytes and platelets are most commonly affected. Hypersplenism also may cause symptoms of early satiety due to the splenic size.

(2) Autoimmune/erythrocyte disorders. Specific cytopenias are related either to antibodies targeting platelets, erythrocytes, or neutrophils. A second category of diseases relates to intrinsic structural changes within the erythrocyte that lead to a shortened red blood cell half-life with accelerated splenic clearance. There is nothing intrinsically wrong with the spleen, and splenic size is typically normal.

(3) Trauma or injury to the spleen.

(4) Vascular diseases. Splenic vein thrombosis and splenic artery aneurysm may require splenectomy for treatment.

(5) Cysts, abscesses, and primary splenic tumors are mass lesions of the spleen. This category includes treatment of simple cysts, echinococcal cysts, splenic abscess, and various benign neoplasms, including hamartomas, hemangiomas, lymphangiomas, and rare malignant lesions.

(6) Diagnostic procedures. This category of splenectomy occurs when the spleen is removed primarily to make a clinical diagnosis when none is available. A subcategory is

staging laparotomy for Hodgkin disease, which has all but been eliminated based on alternative imaging techniques and current treatment regimens.

(7) Iatrogenic splenectomy. Splenectomy that is performed due to an incidental injury to the spleen during surgery within the general abdominal cavity or, specifically, the left upper quadrant, can be categorized as iatrogenic splenectomy. This category is likely underreported and may be considered a subcategory of trauma.

(8) Incidental splenectomy. The spleen may be removed as part of a standard operation to remove the distal pancreas most commonly, and also for gastric cancers, left-sided renal cell carcinomas, adrenal cancers, and retroperitoneal sarcomas in the left upper quadrant. The spleen is removed in these instances because of direct tumor extension, vascular involvement, or the need for excision of splenic hilum lymph nodes.

With the increase in splenic preservation for trauma, many institutional series list medical conditions as the most frequent indications for splenectomy. Most recent series report 40–50% for hematologic conditions, 35–40% for trauma, and 20–30% for neoplastic disease. Within the category, idiopathic thrombocytopenia purpura has the highest incidence for splenectomy. Each category of disease, including the etiology and pathophysiology of the disorder, specific indications for splenectomy, alternative treatments, and the results of splenectomy, is discussed in this chapter.

Harbrecht BG et al: Is splenectomy after trauma an endangered species? Am Surg 2008;74:410.

Katz SC et al: Indications for splenectomy. Am Surg 2006;72:565.

Morgenstern L et al: Love in the time of spleen: a personal memoir. J Am Coll Surg 2006;202:335.

Wood L et al: Splenectomy in haematology—a 5-year single centre experience 2005;10:505.

HYPERSPLENISM

In the past, the term hypersplenism or increased splenic function has been used to denote the syndrome characterized by splenic enlargement, deficiency of one or more blood cell lines, normal or hyperplastic cellularity of deficient cell lines in the marrow, and increased turnover of affected cells. Increased understanding of the pathophysiology of specific disorders has shown that hypersplenism is not synonymous with splenomegaly. Some disorders in which there is spleen-dependent destruction of blood elements do not manifest all features of hypersplenism. For example, splenomegaly is rarely a feature of immune thrombocytopenic purpura, and splenectomy is not always curative. Conversely, other conditions that enlarge the spleen may not result in destruction or sequestration of blood elements with resultant cytopenias. In disorders with known pathogenesis, the recent trend has been to classify them as separate disease entities rather than as hypersplenic conditions.

The defects in hypersplenism are exaggerations of normal splenic functions primarily associated with the red pulp. The principal cause of cytopenias in hypersplenism is increased sequestration and destruction of blood cells in the spleen, which is hypertrophied or increased in volume in a variety of diseases. Etiologic factors include (1) neoplastic infiltration, (2) disease of the bone marrow in which the spleen becomes a site of extramedullary hematopoiesis, and (3) metabolic/genetic disorders such as Gaucher disease. The hyperplastic spleen is not selective in its hyperfunction in most of these disorders. The splenomegaly can lead to an increased turnover in erythrocytes and platelets, with a lesser effect on leukocytes. For example, about 60% of patients with cirrhosis develop splenomegaly and 15% develop hypersplenism. The hypersplenism of cirrhosis is seldom of clinical significance; the anemia and thrombocytopenia are usually mild and rarely are indications for splenectomy.

▶ **Clinical Findings**

A. Symptoms and Signs

The clinical findings depend largely on the underlying disorder or are secondary to the depletion of circulating blood elements caused by the hypersplenism (Table 27–1). Manifestations of hypersplenism usually develop gradually, and the diagnosis often follows a routine physical or laboratory examination. Some patients experience left upper quadrant fullness, discomfort (can be severe), or early satiety. Others have hematemesis due to gastroesophageal varices.

Purpura, bruising, and diffuse mucous membrane bleeding are unusual symptoms despite the presence of thrombocytopenia. Anemia may produce significant fatigue that may be the chief complaint in this patient population. Recurrent infections may be seen in patients with severe leukopenia.

B. Laboratory Findings

Patients with primary hypersplenism usually exhibit pancytopenia of moderate degree and generalized marrow hyperplasia. Anemia is most prominent, reflecting the destruction of erythrocytes in the hypertrophied red pulp of the spleen. Thrombocytopenia occurs because of sequestration of platelets but also possibly because of increased turnover. In most

Table 27–1. Disorders Associated with Secondary Hypersplenism.

Congestive splenomegaly (cirrhosis, portal or splenic vein obstruction)
Neoplasm (leukemia, metastatic carcinoma)
Inflammatory disease (sarcoid, lupus erythematosus, Felty syndrome)
Acute infections with splenomegaly
Chronic infection (tuberculosis, brucellosis, malaria)
Storage diseases (Gaucher disease, Letterer-Siwe disease, amyloidosis)
Chronic hemolytic diseases (spherocytosis, thalassemia, glucose-6-phosphate dehydrogenase deficiency, elliptocytosis)
Myeloproliferative disorders (myelofibrosis with myeloid metaplasia)

cases, more immature cell types such as reticulocytes are present, reflecting the overactivity of the bone marrow to compensate for the pancytopenias. One exception is myeloid metaplasia, in which dysfunction of the bone marrow is the primary defect.

C. Evaluation of Splenic Size

Before it becomes palpable, an enlarged spleen may cause dullness to percussion above the left costal margin. Splenomegaly is manifested on supine x-rays of the abdomen by medial displacement of the stomach and downward displacement of the transverse colon and splenic flexure. CT scan is useful for differentiating the spleen from other abdominal masses and for demonstrating splenic enlargement or intrasplenic lesions. Some of the largest massive spleens (spleen weight > 1500 g) occur in these types of disease. Finding the edge of the spleen below the iliac crest and across the abdominal midline is frequent.

▶ Differential Diagnosis

Leukemia and lymphoma are diagnosed by marrow aspiration, lymph node biopsy, and examination of the peripheral blood (white count and differential). In hereditary spherocytosis, there are spherocytes, osmotic fragility is increased, and platelets and white cells are normal. The hemoglobinopathies with splenomegaly are differentiated on the basis of hemoglobin electrophoresis or the demonstration of an unstable hemoglobin level. Thalassemia major becomes apparent in early childhood, and the blood smear morphology is characteristic. In myelofibrosis, the bone marrow shows proliferation of fibroblasts and replacement of normal elements. In idiopathic thrombocytopenic purpura, the spleen is normal or only slightly enlarged. In aplastic anemia, the spleen is not enlarged and the marrow is fatty.

▶ Treatment & Prognosis

The course, response to treatment, and prognosis of the hypersplenic syndromes differ widely depending on the underlying disease and its response to treatment; these are discussed for each particular disorder. The indications for splenectomy are given in Table 27–2.

Splenectomy may decrease transfusion requirements, decrease the incidence and number of infections, prevent hemorrhage, and reduce pain. The course of congestive splenomegaly due to portal hypertension depends on the degree of venous obstruction and liver damage. The hypersplenism is rarely a major problem and is almost always overshadowed by variceal bleeding or liver dysfunction.

NEOPLASTIC DISEASES

Neoplastic diseases in which splenectomy may play a role in management of hypersplenism include chronic lymphocytic leukemia (CLL), hairy cell leukemia, and non-Hodgkin lym-

Table 27–2. Indications for Splenectomy.

Splenectomy always indicated
    Primary splenic tumor (rare)
    Hereditary spherocytosis (congenital hemolytic anemia)
Splenectomy usually indicated
    Primary hypersplenism
    Chronic immune thrombocytopenic purpura
    Splenic vein thrombosis causing gastric varices
    Splenic abscess (rare)
Splenectomy sometimes indicated
    Splenic injury
    Autoimmune hemolytic disease
    Elliptocytosis with hemolysis
    Nonspherocytic congenital hemolytic anemias
    Hodgkin disease (for staging)
    Thrombotic thrombocytopenic purpura
    Idiopathic myelofibrosis
    Splenic artery aneurysm
    Wiscott-Aldrich syndrome
    Gaucher disease
    Mastocytosis-aggressive disease
Splenectomy rarely indicated
    Chronic leukemia
    Splenic lymphoma
    Macroglobulinemia
    Thalassemia major
    Sickle cell anemia
    Congestive splenomegaly and hypersplenism due to portal
      hypertension
    Felty syndrome
    Hairy cell leukemia
    Chédiak-Higashi syndrome
    Sarcoidosis
Splenectomy not indicated
    Asymptomatic hypersplenism
    Splenomegaly with infection
    Splenomegaly associated with elevated IgM
    Hereditary hemolytic anemia of moderate degree
    Acute leukemia
    Agranulocytosis

phoma. Lymphoma is discussed in detail in Chapter 44. Related neoplastic disorders of idiopathic myelofibrosis and mastocytosis are also discussed as precursors or variants of neoplastic diseases in which splenectomy are occasionally indicated.

1. Chronic Lymphocytic Leukemia

CLL is a low-grade neoplasm of B cell lineage characterized by accumulations of populations of lymphocytes that are mature morphologically but functionally incompetent. In the United States, CLL occurs as 25–30% of all leukemias with mean age at diagnosis of 72. The clinical manifestations and natural history are variable, but initially the disease tends to be indolent. In more advanced stages, splenomegaly, which is frequently massive, is a common characteristic of CLL. Most symptoms related to the spleen are from thrombocytopenia and anemia due to secondary hypersplenism

(80–90% of splenic symptoms). Ten to 20 percent of patients may have symptoms primarily related to pressure from the size of the enlarged spleen.

Other causes of cytopenia in CLL relate to decreased cellular production from the bone marrow. Bone marrow failure can be due to replacement with leukemic cells or to depletion of the bone marrow as a toxic effect of prior antitumor chemotherapy.

Splenectomy in patients with CLL corrects thrombocytopenia in 70–85% of cases, neutropenia in 60–70%, and anemia in 50–60% of cases. The median duration of benefit for both platelets and red cell populations is well over 1 year. Patients with smaller spleens preoperatively, lower preoperative platelet counts, and extensive prior chemotherapy are less likely to respond to splenectomy. However, a positive bone marrow aspirate for leukemic cells is not a contraindication to splenectomy in CLL. Patients who do not have a good performance status should not undergo splenectomy, since patients in terminal stages have unacceptable operative morbidity.

Hill J et al: Laparoscopic splenectomy for autoimmune hemolytic anemia in patients with chronic lymphocytic leukemia: a case series and review of the literature. Am J Hematol 2004;75:134.
Petroianu A et al: Subtotal splenectomy for the treatment of chronic lymphocytic leukemia. Ann Hematol 2003;82:708.
Ruchlemer R et al: Splenectomy in mantle cell lymphoma with leukemia: a comparison with chronic lymphocytic leukemia. Br J Haematol 2002;118:952.
Subbiah V et al: Outcomes of splenectomy in T-cell large granular lymphocyte leukemia with splenomegaly and cytopenia. Exp Hematol 2008;36:1078.

2. Hairy Cell Leukemia

Hairy cell leukemia is a low-grade lymphoproliferative disorder with characteristic "hairy cells" (ie, B lymphocytes with irregular cytoplasmic protrusions positive for tartrate reaction acid phosphatase), which infiltrate the bone marrow and spleen. Patients are typically male, and onset of the disease is in the fifth or sixth decade of life. Symptoms relate to pancytopenia, with anemia requiring transfusions; and to neutropenia, characterized by increased susceptibility to infections and increased bleeding tendencies. Some patients may have symptoms from splenomegaly, which is present in 80% of patients at the time of diagnosis of hairy cell leukemia. The cytopenias are due to a combination of bone marrow replacement and secondary hypersplenism.

The standard therapy for hairy cell leukemia between 1960 and 1995 was splenectomy, but recent advances in pharmacotherapy have superseded this surgical approach. First-line therapy is now treatment with purine nucleoside analogs, primarily cladribine, with a complete response rate of 80–90%. It has never been shown that splenectomy offers survival benefit in this indolent disease, and the operation should be reserved for palliation of splenomegaly in patients who have failed treatment with cladribine and second-line agent rituximab and α-interferon.

Gidron A et al: Hairy cell leukemia: towards a curative strategy. Hematol Oncol Clin North Am 2006;20:1152.
Haberman TM, et al: Splenectomy, interferon, and treatments of historical interest in hairy cell leukemia. Hematol Oncol Clin North Am 2006;20:1075.
Riccioni R et al: Hairy cell leukemia. Curr Treat Options Oncol 2007;8:129.

3. Myelodysplastic Syndrome

Myelodysplastic syndromes are a heterogeneous group of clinical hematopoietic stem cell disorders manifested by pancytopenias and dysplasia of the bone marrow.

Pathologic changes include extensive bone marrow fibrosis, extramedullary hematopoiesis in the spleen and liver, and a leukoerythroblastic blood reaction that may evolve into acute myeloid leukemia over time.

The bone marrow is usually almost completely replaced by fibrous tissue, although in some cases it is hyperplastic and fibrosis is minimal. Extramedullary hematopoiesis develops mainly in the spleen, liver, and long bones. Symptoms are attributable to anemia (weakness, fatigue, dyspnea) and to splenomegaly (abdominal fullness and pain, which may be severe). Pain over the spleen from splenic infarcts is common. Spontaneous bleeding, fatigue, secondary infection, bone pain, and a hypermetabolic state are frequent. Portal hypertension develops in some cases as a result of fibrosis of the liver, greatly increased splenic blood flow, or both.

Hepatomegaly is present in 75% of cases and splenomegaly with a firm and irregular spleen in all cases. Striking changes in the peripheral blood are referable to the combination of extramedullary hematopoiesis and hypersplenism. Patients are uniformly anemic, and red cells vary greatly in size and shape, many of them distorted and fragmented. The white count is usually high (20,000–50,000/µL). The platelet count may be elevated, but values less than 100,000/µL are seen in 30% of cases due to secondary hypersplenism. Bone marrow aspirates frequently result in a dry tap because marrow is replaced with fibrosis. It was once incorrectly thought that the spleen performed a crucial function of extramedullary hematopoiesis in this disease and that splenectomy could be lethal. In fact, many patients with myeloid metaplasia feel better if the massive spleen is removed, and their hypersplenism is often corrected.

About 30% of patients are asymptomatic at the time of initial diagnosis and require no therapy. When cytopenias and splenomegaly produce symptoms, treatment is primarily supportive using transfusions, androgenic steroids, antimetabolites, and hematopoietic growth factors as indicated. Newer therapies include treatment with immunomodulatory drugs such as thalidomide or antibodies to vascular endothelial growth factor and tumor necrosis factor. A subset of patients with myeloid metaplasia has a component of autoimmune hemolytic anemia, and in this group of patients, immunosuppressive therapy may be beneficial. Splenectomy is indicated in the following situations: (1) major hemolysis unresponsive to medical management, (2) severe symptoms of massive splenomegaly with mass effect of the spleen, (3) life-threatening thrombocytopenia, and (4) portal hypertension with variceal hemorrhage. This is one of the rare occasions when portal hypertension may be cured by splenectomy.

Splenectomy in myeloid metaplasia is associated with a 7–10% death rate and frequent complications often related to postsplenectomy hepatic morbidity. Splenectomy best relieves symptoms of splenomegaly and portal hypertension, but only about 75% of patients get relief from anemia and thrombocytopenia. Younger patients with normal platelet counts and symptoms are the best candidates for splenectomy in idiopathic myelofibrosis.

Mesa R et al: Myeloproliferative disorder-associated massive splenomegaly. Clin Adv Hematol Oncol 2008;6:278.

Mesa RA et al: Palliative goals, patient selection, and perioperative platelet management: outcomes and lessons from 3 decades of splenectomy for myelofibrosis with myeloid metaplasia at the Mayo Clinic. Cancer 2006;107:361.

Reilly JT et al: Idiopathic myelofibrosis: pathogenesis to treatment. Hematol Oncol 2006;24:56.

4. Systemic Mast Cell Disease

Systemic mast cell disease, or mastocytosis, is a rare condition characterized by mast cell infiltration of a number of tissues, including the spleen. There are two types: indolent and aggressive. In indolent systemic mass cell disease, there is no need for consideration of splenectomy. The aggressive type is associated with hematologic diseases with characteristics of lymphoma. Splenomegaly may occur, with the predominant symptoms resulting from thrombocytopenia due to hypersplenism. In this subgroup of patients with aggressive disease, splenectomy improves platelet counts and is associated with longer median survival time than for patients with aggressive disease who do not undergo splenectomy, although systemic therapy including α-interferon has been shown to be effective.

Hennessy B et al: Management of patients with systemic mastocytosis: review of the M.D. Anderson Cancer Center experience. Am J Hematol 2004;77:209.

Maalouf M et al: Portal vein thrombosis after laparoscopic splenectomy for systemic mastocytosis: a case report and review of the literature. Surgical Laparosc Endosc Percutan Tech 2008;18:219.

METABOLIC DISORDERS

Metabolic disorders amenable to splenectomy are rare inherited diseases that include as a component splenic enlargement due to the pathologic deposition of material within the spleen. In Gaucher disease, excess sphingolipid is deposited in the spleen. In sarcoidosis, the spleen becomes involved with noncaseating granulomas, as can be seen in lymph nodes. Inherited disorders also include disease in which there is a specific immunologic target with associated destruction in the spleen.

1. Gaucher Disease

Gaucher disease is an autosomal recessive disorder characterized by a deficiency in β-glucosidase, a lysosomal enzyme that degrades the sphingolipid glucocerebroside. There is an increased incidence of this disorder in Ashkenazi Jews. Three types of this disease exist, and the one amenable to splenectomy is type I, or the adult type. Pathologically, Gaucher disease results in lipid accumulation within the white pulp of the spleen, the liver, or the bone marrow. Predominant symptoms relate to massive splenomegaly either from the direct effects of the size of the spleen or secondary to cytopenias from hypersplenism.

▶ Treatment & Prognosis

Treatment by total splenectomy alleviates the symptoms but results in accelerated hepatic and bone disease as well as a significant increased risk of postsplenectomy infections. Treatment with partial or subtotal splenectomy has been studied over the past 10 years for both adults and children with Gaucher disease. Removing most of the spleen corrects the symptoms of splenomegaly, but leaving a splenic remnant provides a site for further deposition of lipid that protects the liver and bone. The major problem with partial splenectomy is the eventual recurrence and enlargement of the splenic remnant accompanied by recurrent symptoms. As with hereditary spherocytosis, there is an increased incidence of pigmented gallstones occurring in up to two thirds of female patients and one third of male patients. The goal of subtotal splenectomy in Gaucher disease is to leave a small fragment approximately the size of the fist of the patient. Replacement therapy with recombinant glucocerebrosidase enzyme has recently become available, but the cost of chronic treatment is prohibitive.

Cox TM et al: Management of non-neuronopathic Gaucher disease with special reference to pregnancy, splenectomy, bisphosphonate therapy, use of biomarkers and bone disease monitoring. J Inherit Metab Dis 2008;31:319.

Jmoudiak M et al: Gaucher disease: pathological mechanisms and modern management. Br J Haematol 2005;129:178.

2. Wiskott-Aldrich Syndrome

Wiskott-Aldrich syndrome is an X-linked disease characterized by thrombocytopenia, combined B and T cell immunodeficiency, eczema, and a propensity to develop malignancies. Thrombocytopenia is the major feature of this rare disorder, with most patients presenting with bloody diarrhea, epistaxis, and petechiae at a young age. Platelet counts typically range between 20,000/μL and 40,000/μL, and the platelets that are present are between one fourth and one half of normal size. The spleen sequesters and destroys platelets in this disease, releasing "microplatelets" back into the circulation. The genetic defect in this disorder may be related to an abnormal adhesion molecule affecting immune as well as platelet cell-to-cell interaction.

Treatment & Prognosis

Splenectomy in Wiskott-Aldrich syndrome was at one time withheld, since the postoperative course was characterized by severe and fatal infections due to the underlying immune defect of this disorder combined with loss of the immune function of the spleen. However, splenectomy does normalize platelet shape, size, and numbers, and the use of prophylactic antibiotics after splenectomy has significantly increased survival rates. The optimal treatment of Wiskott-Aldrich syndrome is a human leukocyte antigen (HLA)-matched sibling bone marrow transplantation. However, splenectomy with antibiotics results in better survival than an unmatched bone marrow transplantation. Patients who do not undergo bone marrow transplantation or splenectomy typically do not survive past the age of 5 years.

Conley ME et al: An international study examining therapeutic options used in the treatment of Wiskott-Aldrich syndrome. Clin Immunol 2003;109:272.

Verni W et al: The spleen in the Wiskott-Aldrich syndrome: histopathologic abnormalities of the white pulp correlate with the clinical phenotype of the disease. Am J Surg Pathol 1999;23:192.

3. Chédiak-Higashi Syndrome

Chédiak-Higashi syndrome is a rare autosomal recessive disease characterized by immunodeficiency that increases the susceptibility to bacterial and viral infections and is manifested by recurrent fever, nystagmus, and photophobia. Most patients experience widespread infiltration of tissues with histiocytes similar to a lymphoma. Secondary hepatosplenomegaly with lymphadenopathy, leukopenia, and bleeding complications occur in the accelerated phase of Chédiak-Higashi syndrome. Standard treatment includes chemotherapy, steroids, and ascorbic acid, but these patients have a poor prognosis. Splenectomy has been used in the accelerated phase with beneficial results.

Dinauer MC et al: Disorders of neutrophil function. Methods Mol Biol 2007;412:489.

Harfi HA et al: Chédiak-Higashi syndrome: clinical, hematologic, and immunologic improvement after splenectomy. Ann Allergy 1992;69:147.

4. Sarcoidosis

Sarcoidosis is a granulomatous disease of unknown origin that can involve virtually any organ or area of the body. Pulmonary disease is most common, but autopsy studies have shown that the spleen is the second-most common site, with enlargement by noncaseating granulomas in 50–60% of patients. However, most patients do not have massive splenomegaly. When this does occur, patients can have significant cytopenias related to hypersplenism as well as the constitutional symptoms and hypercalcemia of sarcoidosis. In this subgroup of patients, splenectomy is indicated as a potential curative procedure for each of these symptoms.

Rodriguez-Garcia JL: Systemic sarcoidosis with spleen involvement. Postgrad Med J 2001;77:265.

Xiao GQ et al: Asymptomatic sarcoidosis presenting as massive splenomegaly. Am J Med 2002:113:698.

ERYTHROCYTE DISORDERS

In this category of diseases, there is generally no intrinsic abnormality of the spleen, as opposed to hypersplenism, in which the spleen is primarily infiltrated by neoplasia or storage products and causes cytopenias due to increased volume of splenic tissue. In the autoimmune disorders, there is a humoral antibody response against proteins on circulating blood cells, resulting in depletion primarily within the spleen. Disorders involving platelets, erythrocytes, and neutrophils are listed in decreasing order of incidence. Erythrocyte disorders are genetic defects in structural components or hemoglobin that increase the clearance of red cells in the spleen, causing a significant decrease in erythrocyte half-life.

1. Hereditary Spherocytosis

 ESSENTIALS OF DIAGNOSIS

▶ Malaise, abdominal discomfort.

▶ Jaundice, anemia, splenomegaly.

▶ Spherocytosis, increased osmotic fragility of red cells, negative Coombs test.

General Considerations

Hereditary spherocytosis (congenital hemolytic jaundice, familial hemolytic anemia), the most common congenital hemolytic anemia (affecting 1:5000 individuals), is transmitted as an autosomal dominant trait. It is caused by a variety of genetic defects related to abnormal cellular structural proteins, primarily ankyrin band 3, alpha and beta spectrum, and protein 4-2, which alter binding of the cytoskeleton to the cellular membrane, causing a decreased cellular plasticity with membrane loss. The normal shape of the erythrocyte is changed from a biconcave disk into a sphere, and the decreased membrane-to-cell volume ratio causes a lack of deformability that delays passage through the channels of the splenic red pulp. Significant cell destruction occurs only in the presence of the spleen. Hemolysis is largely relieved by splenectomy.

The condition is seen in all races but is more frequent in whites than in blacks. When discovered early in infancy, it may resemble hemolytic disease of the newborn due to ABO incompatibility. In occasional instances, the diagnosis is not made until later in adult life, but it is usually discovered in the first 3 decades.

▶ Clinical Findings

A. Symptoms and Signs

The principal manifestations are splenomegaly, mild to moderate anemia, and jaundice. The patient may complain of easy fatigability. The spleen is almost always enlarged and may cause fullness and discomfort in the left upper quadrant. However, most patients are diagnosed during a family survey at a time when they are asymptomatic.

Periodic exacerbations of hemolysis can occur. The rare hypoplastic crises, which often follow acute viral illnesses, may be associated with profound anemia, headache, nausea, abdominal pain, pancytopenia, and hypoactive marrow.

B. Laboratory Findings

The red cell count and hemoglobin are moderately reduced. Some of the asymptomatic patients detected by family surveys have normal red cell counts when first seen. The red cells are usually normocytic, but microcytosis may occur. Macrocytosis may present during periods of marked reticulocytosis. Spherocytes in varying numbers, sizes, and shapes are seen on a Wright-stained smear. The reticulocyte count is increased to 5–20%.

The indirect serum bilirubin and stool urobilinogen are usually elevated, and serum haptoglobin is usually decreased to absent. The Coombs test is negative. Osmotic fragility is increased; hemolysis of 5–10% of cells may be observed at saline concentrations of 0.6%. A more accurate reflector of fragility is the cryohemolysis test, which has a sensitivity and specificity of almost 95% for spherocytosis. Occasionally, the osmotic fragility is normal but the incubated fragility test (defibrinated blood incubated at 37 °C for 24 hours) will show increased hemolysis. Autohemolysis of defibrinated blood incubated under sterile conditions for 48 hours is usually greatly increased (10–20%, compared to a normal value of < 5%). The addition of 10% glucose before incubation will decrease the abnormal osmotic fragility and autohemolysis. Infusion of the patient's own blood labeled with ^{51}Cr shows a greatly shortened red cell life span and sequestration in the spleen. Normal red cells labeled with ^{51}Cr have a normal life span when transfused into a spherocytotic patient, indicating that splenic function is normal.

▶ Differential Diagnosis

At present, there is no pathognomonic test for hereditary spherocytosis, although the cryohemolysis test is very promising. Spherocytes in large numbers may occur in autoimmune hemolytic anemias, in which osmotic fragility and autohemolysis may be increased but are usually not improved by incubation with glucose. The positive Coombs test, negative family history, and sharply reduced survival of normal donor red cells are diagnostic of autoimmune hemolysis. Spherocytes are also seen in hemoglobin C disease, in some alcoholics, and in some severe burns.

▶ Complications

Pigment gallstones occur in about 85% of adults with spherocytosis but are uncommon under age 10. On the other hand, gallstones in a child should suggest congenital spherocytosis.

Chronic leg ulcers unrelated to varicosities are a rare complication but, when present, will heal only after the spleen is removed.

▶ Treatment

Splenectomy is the sole treatment for hereditary spherocytosis and is indicated even when the anemia is fully compensated and the patient is asymptomatic. The longer the hemolytic process persists, the greater the potential risk of complications such as hypoplastic crises and cholelithiasis. At operation, the gallbladder should be inspected for stones and accessory spleens should be sought. When there is associated cholelithiasis, cholecystectomy should be performed along with the splenectomy. Unless the clinical manifestations are severe, splenectomy should be delayed in children until age 6 to avoid the risk of increased infection due to loss of reticuloendothelial function. For children under age 5 with severe disease and high transfusion requirements, a partial (80%) splenectomy may correct symptoms while maintaining the normal immune functions of the spleen.

▶ Prognosis

Splenectomy cures the anemia and jaundice in all patients. The membrane abnormality, spherocytosis, and increased osmotic fragility persist, but red cell life span becomes almost normal. An overlooked accessory spleen is an occasional cause of failure of splenectomy. The presence of Howell-Jolly bodies in red cells makes the presence of accessory spleens unlikely.

Diesen DL et al: Partial splenectomy for children with congenital hemolytic anemia and massive splenomegaly. J Pediatr Surg 2008;43:466.

Perrotta S: Hereditary spherocytosis. Lancet 2008;372:1411.

Tracy ET et al: Partial splenectomy for hereditary spherocytosis. Pediatr Clin North Am 2008;55:503.

2. Hereditary Elliptocytosis

This autosomal dominant genetic disorder, also known as ovalocytosis, is usually of little clinical significance. Normally, up to 15% oval or elliptic red blood cells can be seen on a peripheral blood smear. In elliptocytosis, at least 25% and up to 90% of circulating erythrocytes are elliptic. As with hereditary spherocytosis, this disease is due to a variety of genetic defects in cytoskeletal proteins such as spectrin. The predominant abnormality is that this structural protein exists as a dimer instead of a tetramer, leading to change in the erythrocyte's shape, decreased plasticity, and a shortened life span of the cell.

Most affected individuals are asymptomatic; about 10% have clinical manifestations consisting of moderate anemia, slight jaundice, and a palpable spleen.

Symptomatic patients should have splenectomy and, if gallstones are present, cholecystectomy. The red cell defect persists after splenectomy, but the hemolysis and anemia are cured.

Gallagher PG: Update on the clinical spectrum and genetics of red blood cell membrane disorders. Curr Hematol Rep 2004;3:85.
Silveira P et al: Red blood cell abnormalities in hereditary elliptocytosis and their relevance to variable clinical expression. Am J Clin Pathol 1997;108:391.

3. Hereditary Nonspherocytic Hemolytic Anemia

This is a heterogeneous group of rare hemolytic anemias caused by inherited intrinsic red cell defects that lead to oxidative hemolysis. Included in the group are pyruvate kinase deficiency and glucose 6-phosphate dehydrogenase (G6PD) deficiency. They are usually manifested in early childhood with anemia, jaundice, reticulocytosis, erythroid hyperplasia of the marrow, and normal osmotic fragility. As with other hemolytic anemias, there may be associated cholelithiasis.

Multiple blood transfusions are often required. Splenectomy, while not curative, may ameliorate some of these conditions, especially pyruvate kinase deficiency. In G6PD deficiency, splenectomy is not beneficial, and treatment consists of avoidance of dietary oxidants.

Baronciani L et al: Hematologically important mutations: red cell pyruvate kinase. Blood Cells Mol Dis 1998;24:273.

4. Thalassemia Major (Mediterranean Anemia; Cooley Anemia)

In the most common form of this autosomal dominant disorder, a structural defect in the β-globin chain causes excess α chains to precipitate on the inner surface of the membrane of the erythrocyte and produces abnormal red cells (eg, target cells). Heterozygotes usually have mild anemia (thalassemia minor); however, starting early in infancy, homozygotes have severe chronic anemia accompanied by jaundice, hepatosplenomegaly (often massive), retarded body growth, and enlargement of the head. The peripheral blood smear reveals target cells, nucleated red cells, and a hypochromic microcytic anemia. Gallstones are present in about 25% of patients. A characteristic feature is the persistence of fetal hemoglobin (Hb F).

Since the anemia of thalassemia is due to both increased destruction of red cells and decreased hemoglobin production, splenectomy does not cure the anemia, as in spherocytosis, but it may reduce transfusion requirements by removing an enlarged, uncomfortable spleen. Treatment is by iron chelation and transfusion.

Aessopos A et al: Cardiovascular effects of splenomegaly and splenectomy in beta-thalassemia. Ann Hematol 2005;84:353.
Konstadoulakis MM et al: Laparoscopic versus open splenectomy in patients with beta thalassemia major. J Laparoendosc Adv Surg Tech A 2006;16:5.

AUTOIMMUNE DISORDERS

The production of IgG autoantibodies specific for cell membrane proteins on erythrocytes causes autoimmune hemolytic anemia; on platelets, it causes idiopathic thrombocytopenic purpura (ITP) and may cause neutropenia in Felty syndrome. Macrophages express Fc receptors for IgG, and antibody-coated cells that pass through the splenic sinuses of the red pulp come into contact with these phagocytic cells. Furthermore, the microenvironment of the red pulp with slow flow of blood with a high cellular content through circuitous spaces facilitates opsonization of cells in the spleen. Production of autoantibodies in the white pulp germinal centers may also enhance cellular destruction, particularly in ITP. Understanding this pathophysiologic mechanism is important, since autoimmune hemolytic anemia caused by IgM autoantibodies (ie, cold agglutinin hemolytic anemia) does not respond to splenectomy because macrophages do not have Fc receptors for IgM. This mechanism also explains why treatment with high-dose intravenous immune globulin is beneficial in these diseases because it blocks the macrophage Fc receptor.

1. Acquired Hemolytic Anemia

 ESSENTIALS OF DIAGNOSIS

► Fatigue, pallor, jaundice.
► Splenomegaly.
► Persistent anemia and reticulocytosis.

General Considerations

The **autoimmune hemolytic anemias** have also been classified according to the optimal temperature at which autoantibodies react with the red cell surface (warm or cold antibodies). This classification is particularly useful, since patients with cold antibodies will not benefit from splenectomy but those with warm antibodies may.

Although hemolysis without demonstrable antibody (negative Coombs test) may occur in uremia, cirrhosis of the liver, cancer, and certain infections, in most cases the red cell membranes are coated with either immunoglobulin or complement (positive Coombs test). The antibody in IgG autoimmune hemolytic anemia is specifically directed against the Rh locus on the erythrocyte. Initiation of this disease is either idiopathic (40–50%) or secondary to drug exposure, connective tissue disorders, or lymphoproliferative disorders.

Hemolytic anemia due to cold antibodies is less common and always a secondary immune response. Cold agglutinin hemolytic anemia is due typically to an IgM directed against the I red cell antigen, and hemolysis occurs intravascularly by complement fixation and not within the spleen making splenectomy not beneficial in the setting of cold antibodies.

About 20% of cases of secondary immune hemolytic anemia are due to drug use, and hemolysis is usually mediated by warm antibodies. Penicillin, quinidine, hydralazine, and methyldopa have been most commonly implicated in this syndrome (Table 27–3).

▶ Clinical Findings

A. Symptoms and Signs

Autoimmune hemolytic anemia may be encountered at any age but is most common after age 50; it occurs twice as often in women. The onset is usually acute, consisting of anemia, mild jaundice, and sometimes fever. The spleen is palpably enlarged in over 50% of patients, and pigment gallstones are present in about 25%. Rarely, a sudden severe onset produces hemoglobinuria, renal tubular necrosis, and a 40–50% death rate.

B. Laboratory Findings

Hemolytic anemia is diagnosed by demonstrating a normocytic normochromic anemia, reticulocytosis (over 10%), erythroid hyperplasia of the marrow, and elevation of serum indirect bilirubin. Stool urobilinogen may be greatly increased, but there is no bile in the urine. Serum haptoglobin is usually low or absent. The direct Coombs test is positive because the red cells are coated with immunoglobulins or complement (or both).

▶ Treatment

Associated diseases must be carefully sought and appropriately treated. For drug-induced secondary hemolytic anemia, further exposure to the offending agent must be terminated. Corticosteroids produce a remission in about 75% of patients, but only 25% of remissions are permanent. Transfusion should be avoided if possible, since crossmatching may be extremely difficult, requiring washed red cells and saline-active antisera. Rituximab is an effective second-line therapy now producing durable responses 40% of steroid resistant cases.

Splenectomy is indicated for patients with warm-antibody hemolysis who fail to respond to 4–6 weeks of high-dose corticosteroid therapy, for patients who relapse after an initial response when steroids are withdrawn, and for patients in whom steroid therapy is contraindicated (eg, those with active pulmonary tuberculosis). Patients who require chronic high-dose steroid therapy should also be considered for splenectomy, since the risks of long-term steroid administration are substantial.

Table 27–3. Disorders Associated with Immune Hemolysis.

Immune drug reaction (penicillin, quinidine, hydralazine, methyldopa, cimetidine)
Collagen vascular disease (lupus erythematosus, rheumatoid arthritis)
Tumors (lymphoma, myeloma, leukemia, dermoid cysts, ovarian teratoma)
Infection (*Mycoplasma,* malaria, syphilis, viremia)

Splenectomy is effective because it removes the principal site of red cell destruction. Occasionally, splenectomy identifies the presence of an underlying disorder such as lymphoma. About half of patients who fail to respond to splenectomy will respond to azathioprine or cyclophosphamide. Plasmapheresis has been employed as salvage therapy in patients with refractory hemolytic anemia.

▶ Prognosis

Relapses may occur after splenectomy but are less frequent if the initial response was good. The ultimate prognosis in the secondary cases depends on the underlying disorder.

Packman CH et al: Hemolytic anemia due to warm autoantibodies. Blood Rev 2008;22:17.
Valent P et al: Diagnosis and treatment of autoimmune haemolytic aneaemias in adults: a clinical review. Wien Klin Wochenschr 2008;120:136.

2. Immune Thrombocytopenic Purpura (Idiopathic Thrombocytopenic Purpura, ITP)

 ESSENTIALS OF DIAGNOSIS

- ▶ Petechiae, ecchymoses, epistaxis, easy bruising.
- ▶ No splenomegaly.
- ▶ Decreased platelet count, prolonged bleeding time, poor clot retraction, normal coagulation time.

▶ General Considerations

Immune thrombocytopenic purpura is a hemorrhagic syndrome with diverse causes that can occur in an acute or chronic form and is characterized by marked reduction in the number of circulating platelets, abundant megakaryocytes in the bone marrow, and a shortened platelet life span. It may be idiopathic or secondary to a lymphoproliferative disorder, drugs or toxins, bacterial or viral infection (especially in children), systemic lupus erythematosus, or other conditions. Although responses to corticosteroids and to splenectomy in these patients are comparable to the responses observed in other patients with immune thrombocytopenic purpura, splenectomy should be reserved for those with signs of blood loss, since surgical complications are high and survival may be short. However, due to the incidence of ITP, this disease is typically the most common indication for splenectomy in most institutional series.

The pathogenesis of both primary and secondary disorders involves a circulating antiplatelet IgG autoantibody usually directed against a membrane protein, which is the fibrinogen receptor (glycoprotein IIb/IIIa). In this disorder, the spleen is primarily the site of platelet destruction and may also be a significant source of autoantibody production. Splenomegaly, present in only 2% of cases, is usually a manifestation of another underlying disease such as lymphoma or lupus erythematosus. Of HIV-positive patients, 5–15% have thrombocytopenia independent of the immunologic state of their disease that is clinically indistinguishable from typical chronic ITP. The precise pathophysiologic mechanism in relation to HIV infection is not known.

▶ Clinical Findings

A. Symptoms and Signs

The onset may be acute, with ecchymoses or showers of petechiae, and may be accompanied by bleeding gums, vaginal bleeding, gastrointestinal bleeding, and hematuria. Central nervous system bleeding occurs in 3% of patients. The acute form is most common in children, usually occurring before 8 years of age, and often begins 1–3 weeks after a viral upper respiratory illness.

The chronic form, which may start at any age, is more common in women. It characteristically has an insidious onset, often with a long history of easy bruisability and menorrhagia. Showers of petechiae may occur, especially over pressure areas. Cyclic remissions and exacerbations may continue for several years.

B. Laboratory Findings

The platelet count is moderately to severely decreased (always below 100,000/µL), and platelets may be absent from the peripheral blood smear. Although white and red cell counts are usually normal, iron deficiency anemia may be present as a result of bleeding. The bone marrow shows increased numbers of large megakaryocytes without platelet budding.

The bleeding time is prolonged, capillary fragility (Rumpel-Leede test) greatly increased, and clot retraction poor. Partial thromboplastin time, prothrombin time, and coagulation time are normal. Specific determinations of antiplatelet antibody titers can now be routinely assessed to aid in diagnosis. Reduced red cell or platelet survival can be measured by labeling the patient's cells with ^{51}Cr or the platelets with indium-111 and measuring the rate of disappearance of radioactivity from the blood. The spleen's role in producing the anemia or thrombocytopenia can be determined by measuring the ratio of radioactivity that accumulates in the liver and spleen during destruction of the tagged cells; a spleen–liver ratio greater than 2:1 indicates significant splenic pooling and suggests that splenectomy would be beneficial.

▶ Differential Diagnosis

Other causes of nonimmunologic thrombocytopenia must be ruled out, such as leukemia, aplastic anemia, and macroglobulinemia. Thrombocytopenia and purpura may be caused by ineffective thrombocytopoiesis (eg, pernicious anemia, preleukemic states) or by nonimmune platelet destruction (eg, septicemia, disseminated intravascular coagulation, or other causes of hypersplenism).

▶ Treatment

Treatment of immune thrombocytopenic purpura depends on the age of the patient, the severity of the disease, the duration of the thrombocytopenia, and the clinical variant. Secondary immune thrombocytopenias are best managed by treating the underlying primary disorder (eg, if it is drug-induced, the drug should be stopped).

Patients with mild or no symptoms need no specific therapy but should avoid contact sports, elective surgery, and all unessential medications. Corticosteroids are indicated in patients with moderate to severe purpura of short duration. Usually, 60 mg of prednisone (or equivalent) is required daily; this is continued until the platelet count returns to normal and then is gradually tapered after 4–6 weeks. Corticosteroids produce a response in 70–80%, but sustained remissions in only 20% of adults. Second-line therapy with rituximab improves platelet counts in 30–40% of patients and sustained complete response in 10–20%. New agents to stimulate platelet production such as thrombopoietin (TPO) against AMG531 and eltrombopag are being studied as third-line medical therapies.

Splenectomy is the most effective form of therapy and is indicated for patients who do not respond to corticosteroids, for those who relapse after an initial remission on steroids, and for steroid-dependent patients. Corticosteroid therapy is not necessary in the immediate preoperative period unless bleeding is severe or the patient was receiving steroids before the operation. If indicated, platelet transfusions are given intraoperatively only after ligation of the splenic artery or removal of the spleen, since platelets from earlier transfusion would be rapidly sequestered in the spleen. For temporary treatment of the thrombocytopenia, intravenous immunoglobulin (IGIV) is effective.

Splenectomy produces a sustained remission in about 68% of patients. As with corticosteroids, success rates are better with acute than chronic immune thrombocytopenic purpura. Two factors associated with better outcomes are shorter duration of disease and younger age. The platelet count usually rises promptly following splenectomy (eg, it may double in 24 hours) and reaches a peak after 1–2 weeks.

If the platelet count remains elevated after 2 months, the patient can be considered cured. When corticosteroids and splenectomy have failed, immunosuppressive drugs (azathioprine, vincristine) will achieve a remission in 25% of cases.

The benefit of splenectomy for HIV-associated ITP has been less clear. The risk of infection and the overall shortened survival in this population argue against splenectomy. However, in HIV patients without AIDS, clinically significant thrombocytopenia responds completely in 70%, and there is partial improvement in 20% following splenectomy. Splenectomy does not appear to alter the overall natural history of HIV infection.

► Prognosis

Acute immune thrombocytopenic purpura in children under age 16 has an excellent prognosis; approximately 80% of patients have a complete and permanent spontaneous remission. This occurs rarely in adults. Splenectomy is successful in about 80% of patients, but more often in idiopathic cases than in those secondary to another disorder. The proportion of patients undergoing splenectomy for ITP has decreased due to medical treatment other than steroids that have efficacy, although the incidence of chronic ITP has increased. Agents to stimulate thrombopoietin may have significant benefit for patients who have no improvement in platelet count after splenectomy.

Arnold DM et al: Current options for the treatment of idiopathic thrombocytopenic purpura. Semin Hematol 2007;44:512.

Cooper N et al: Should rituximab be used before or after splenectomy in patients with immune thrombocytopenic purpura? Curr Opin Hematol 2007;14:642.

Dolan JP et al: Splenectomy for immune thrombocytopenic purpura. Am J Hematol 2008;83:93.

Godeau B et al: Rituximab efficacy and safety in adult splenectomy candidates with chronic immune thrombocytopenic purpura: results of a prospective multicenter phase 2 study. Blood 2008; 112:999.

Kuter DJ et al: Efficacy of romiplostim in patients with chronic immune thrombocytopenic purpura: a double-blind randomized controlled trial. Lancet 2008;371:395.

Neunert CE et al: Severe chronic refractory immune thrombocytopenic purpura during childhood: a survey of physician management. Pediatr Blood Cancer 2008;51:513.

Newland W et al: Emerging strategies to treat chronic immune thrombocytopenic purpura. Eur J Haematol 2008;69:27.

Rodeghiero F et al: First-line therapies for immune thrombocytopenic purpura: re-evaluating the need to treat. Eur J Haematol 2008;69:19.

Shojaiefard A et al: Prediction of response to splenectomy in patients with idiopathic thrombocytopenic purpura. World J Surg 2008;32:488.

Stasi R et al: Idiopathic thrombocytopenic purpura: current concepts in pathophysiology and management. Thromb Haemost 2008;99:4.

Tarantino MD et al: Update on the management of immune thrombocytopenic purpura in children. Curr Opin Hematol 2007;14:526.

3. Felty Syndrome

Approximately 1% of patients with rheumatoid arthritis have splenomegaly and neutropenia—a triad known as Felty syndrome. High levels of IgG have been identified on the surface of neutrophils with evidence of increased of granulopoiesis in the bone marrow. Pathologic analysis of the spleen in Felty syndrome patients shows a larger proportionate increase in the white pulp as opposed to most conditions of splenomegaly. There is evidence of excess accumulation of neutrophils in both the T cell zone of the white pulp as well as the cord and sinuses of the red pulp.

Patients with severe neutropenia have clinical symptoms of recurring infections in Felty syndrome. Symptomatic patients who have evidence of IgG on the surface of neutrophils should be considered for splenectomy. Neutropenia will improve in 60–70% of these patients, but relapse of neutropenia as well as recurrent infections in the presence of normal neutrophil counts may occur, and these untoward events have dampened enthusiasm for splenectomy in this disease.

Balint GP, Balint PV: Felty's syndrome. Best Pract Res Clin Rheumatol 2004;18:631.

Burks EJ, Loughran TP: Pathogenesis of neutropenia in large granular cells leukemia and Felty's syndrome. Blood Rev 2006;20:265.

4. Thrombotic Thrombocytopenic Purpura

Thrombotic thrombocytopenic purpura (TTP) is a rare disease with a pentad of clinical features: (1) fever, (2) thrombocytopenic purpura, (3) hemolytic anemia, (4) neurologic manifestations, and (5) renal failure. The cause is unknown, but autoimmunity to endothelial cells or a primary platelet defect has been implicated, and its occurrence in patients with AIDS has been reported. It is most common between ages 10 and 40 years.

The thrombocytopenia is probably due to a shortened platelet life span. The microangiopathic hemolytic anemia is produced by passage of red cells over damaged small blood vessels containing fibrin strands. Rigid red cells are trapped and fragmented in the spleen, whereas those that escape the spleen may be more vulnerable to damage and destruction in the abnormal microvasculature. The anemia is often severe, and it may be aggravated by hemorrhage secondary to thrombocytopenia. Hepatomegaly and splenomegaly occur in 35% of cases.

► Treatment & Prognosis

Until recently, there was no effective therapy for this disorder, and mortality rates as high as 95% were reported. Most patients died of renal failure or cerebral bleeding. Plasmapheresis with plasma exchange has recently emerged as an effective form of treatment that is superior to simple plasma infusion with complete response rate of 55–65%. Plasma exchange failure can be salvaged with splenectomy with 60% having a substantial response and a 20–30% relapse rate.

Kappers-Klunne MC et al: Splenectomy for the treatment of thrombotic thrombocytopenic purpura. Br J Haematol 2005; 130:768.

Outschoorn UM et al: Outcomes in the treatment of thrombotic thrombocytopenic purpura with splenectomy: a retrospective cohort study. Am J Hematol 2006;81:895.

VASCULAR DISORDERS OF THE SPLEEN

Vascular disease of the spleen treated by splenectomy can occur both with the arterial inflow and the venous outflow. The most common disease is splenic vein thrombosis; this can be treated in a straightforward manner by splenectomy. Splenic artery aneurysms are one of the most common sites of visceral aneurysms and may require splenectomy.

1. Splenic Vein Thrombosis

▶ Etiology

Thrombosis of the splenic vein can occur as an isolated event not due to any pathologic findings in the spleen but due to diseases that impact the splenic vein as it travels along the superior border of the pancreas. The most common cause is acute or chronic pancreatitis or a pseudocyst of the body/tail of the pancreas, with the general inflammatory reaction in the pancreas resulting in thrombosis of the splenic vein in 20% of patients. Inflammation from a posterior gastric ulcer is another cause. Direct extension of carcinoma of the pancreas or stomach into the lesser sac may cause splenic vein thrombosis, but the diagnosis is generally not subtle because of other manifestations of these malignancies. Idiopathic retroperitoneal fibrosis may be an alternative cause of splenic vein thrombosis.

Splenic vein thrombosis presents as upper gastrointestinal hemorrhage due to isolated gastric varices. With occlusion of the splenic vein, outflow of blood from the spleen is diverted into the short gastric veins as the remaining collateral vessels. These veins dilate and become varices primarily in the fundus of the stomach, resulting in bleeding in 15–20% of patients.

▶ Diagnosis

Splenic vein thrombosis is suspected when there are isolated varices of the stomach particularly in the proximal greater curvature without any esophageal varices. Since there is no portal hypertension, there are no associated signs or symptoms of cirrhosis. Definitive diagnosis is made by confirming that there is no blood flow in the main splenic vein. Invasive venography is no longer needed because this diagnosis can be confirmed by CT scan or MRI scans with contrast material or by high-resolution ultrasound. CT or MRI is preferred because the splenic vein may be hidden from ultrasound by bowel gas, and CT or MRI allows characterization of the surrounding structures (pancreas, stomach) to assess for causative pathology.

▶ Treatment & Prognosis

Splenectomy is curative in patients with splenic vein thrombosis. All of the symptoms relate to increased splenic blood flow through collateral vessels; eliminating that blood flow is curative. If a splenic vein thrombosis is diagnosed—even if the patients have not had an episode of upper gastrointestinal hemorrhage—an elective or prophylactic splenectomy is indicated if the patients are otherwise healthy. In patients with portal vein thrombosis, the magnitude of the disease and associated problems is greatly amplified, and splenectomy is almost never indicated because it is not curative.

Agarwal AK et al: Significance of splenic vein thrombosis in chronic pancreatitis. Am J Surg 2008;196:149.

2. Cysts & Tumors of the Spleen

Parasitic cysts are almost always echinococcal. They may be asymptomatic, but usually the patient notices splenomegaly. Calcification of the cyst wall may be seen on x-ray. Eosinophilia may be found, and serologic tests may confirm the diagnosis. The treatment of choice is splenectomy.

Other cysts are dermoid, epidermoid, endothelial, and pseudocysts. The latter are thought to be late results of infarction or trauma. Splenectomy may be indicated to exclude tumor; however, partial splenectomy or observation has been advocated.

The rare primary tumors of the spleen include lymphoma, sarcoma, hemangioma, and hamartoma. Hamartomas may be confused grossly with splenic lymphoma at laparotomy. These lesions are usually asymptomatic until splenomegaly causes abdominal discomfort or a palpable mass. The benign vascular tumors of the spleen (angiomas) can produce hypersplenism. Spontaneous rupture with massive hemorrhage can occur. Splenectomy is indicated if the tumor appears to be limited to the spleen. Inflammatory pseudotumors are benign lesions composed of a mixture of inflammatory cells and a granulomatous reaction that can occur in a variety of organs, including the spleen. Constitutional symptoms of lethargy, weight loss, and fatigue occur and can be alleviated by splenectomy.

The spleen is a common site for metastases in advanced cancers, especially of the lung and breast and melanoma. Splenic metastases are common autopsy findings but are rarely clinically significant.

Atmatzidis K et al: Splenectomy versus spleen-preserving surgery for splenic echinococcosis. Dig Surg 2003;20:527.

Kraus MD, Fleming MD, Vonderheide RH: The spleen as a diagnostic specimen: a review of 10 years' experience at two tertiary care institutions. Cancer 2001;91:2001.

Mackenzie RK, Youngson GG, Mahomed AA: Laparoscopic decapsulation of congenital splenic cysts: a step forward in splenic preservation. J Ped Surg 2004;39:88.

Wu HM et al: Management of splenic pseudocysts following trauma: a retrospective case series. Am J Surg 2006;191:631.

Yu RS, Zhang SZ, Hua JM: Imaging findings of splenic hamartoma. World J Gastroent 2004;10:13.

INFECTIONS OF THE SPLEEN (SPLENIC ABSCESS)

Splenic abscesses are uncommon but are important because the death rate ranges between 40% and 100%. They may be caused by hematogenous seeding of the spleen with bacteria from remote sepsis such as endocarditis, by direct spread of infection from adjacent structures, or by splenic trauma resulting in a secondarily infected splenic hematoma. Splenic abscess is a complication of intravenous drug abuse. In 80% of cases, one or more abscesses exist in organs other than the spleen, and the splenic abscess develops as a terminal manifestation of uncontrolled sepsis in other organs. Enteric organisms are found in over two thirds of splenic abscesses, with staphylococci and nonenteric streptococci comprising the majority of the remainder. In some patients, unexplained sepsis, progressive splenic enlargement, and abdominal pain are the presenting manifestations. The spleen may not be palpable, because of left upper quadrant tenderness and guarding. A left pleural effusion combined with unexplained leukocytosis in a septic patient suggests a splenic abscess. The finding of gas in the spleen on plain abdominal x-ray is pathognomonic of splenic abscess, but CT scan is the optimal way to define and diagnose a splenic abscess.

Most splenic abscesses remain localized, periodically seeding the bloodstream with bacteria, but spontaneous rupture and peritonitis may occur. Splenectomy is essential for cure if sepsis is localized to the spleen. Percutaneous drainage of large, solitary juxtacapsular abscesses may occasionally be feasible but is associated with an extremely high mortality rate and should be reserved for patients unable to withstand an operation.

Tung CC et al: Splenic abscess: an easily overlooked disease? Am Surg 2006;72:322.

DIAGNOSTIC SPLENECTOMY

One indication for splenectomy is for diagnosis in an otherwise asymptomatic patient. Splenectomy may be needed to make a diagnosis when an asymptomatic mass lesion is seen within the spleen on CT scan, ultrasound, or MRI scan for which a definitive diagnosis cannot be made radiographically. Another example is when a patient has either a palpable spleen on physical examination or an enlarged spleen by scan, and otherwise has no clear diagnostic disorder.

▶ Splenic Mass Lesions

For the patients who have an isolated splenic mass, 60% turned out to be malignant lesions and 40% turned out to be benign lesions. Most malignant lesions are lymphoma; the next most common is metastatic carcinomas, including some in which the primary diagnosis had not been made previously. In patients with benign lesions, more than half were cysts, and there were also splenic hamartomas and splenic hemangiomas.

In diagnosing an isolated splenic mass, most of these lesions can be diagnosed by doing a fine-needle aspiration biopsy. Certain lesions—such as the cystic lesions or hemangioma—have classic appearance on gadolinium-enhanced MRI scan, and these scans are another imaging modality that could be utilized to sort out mass lesions without tissue biopsy. PET scans will reliably identify high-grade lymphoma and metastatic tumors but may miss low-grade or mantle zone lymphoma. The risk of bleeding is significant in patients with hemangiomas. These benign tumors of endothelial cells can be definitively diagnosed with gadolinium-enhanced MRI, and this imaging test is optimal for characterizing an isolated splenic mass.

▶ Splenomegaly without a Diagnosis

The second diagnostic indication for splenectomy is unexplained splenomegaly. Most of these enlarged spleens will be shown to have lymphoma. The minority will have benign diagnoses including benign lymphoid proliferation, benign vascular lesions, and granulomatous disease, as well as splenic infarction and hemorrhage. The role of the fine-needle aspiration and other percutaneous biopsies for non-diagnosed splenomegaly is quite limited with no distinct mass to biopsy; there would be very low yield in terms of being able to make that diagnosis by that form of biopsy.

▶ Staging Laparotomy for Hodgkin Disease

Another type of diagnostic procedure is a staging laparotomy for Hodgkin disease. Discussion of this procedure is more of a historical note because it has limited use in today's current practice in treating this form of lymphoma.

A standard practice for pathologic staging between 1960 and 1990 was performance of a staging laparotomy in most patients with Hodgkin disease. The reason for performing this invasive procedure was based on reports that laparotomy altered the clinical stage of disease in approximately 35% of patients. There are several reasons why the incidence of performing staging laparotomy has decreased over the past 10–15 years. The primary reason is that it does not alter treatment of Hodgkin disease, according to results of recent clinical series. Since systemic chemotherapy treats the whole patient, accurate pathologic staging makes no impact on the treatment outcome or treatment decisions.

Kraus MD, Fleming MD, Vonderheide RH: The spleen as a diagnostic specimen: a review of 10 years' experience at two tertiary care institutions. Cancer 2001;91:2001.

Rose AT et al: The incidence of splenectomy is decreasing: lessons learned from trauma experience. Am Surg 2000;66:481.

Rutherford SC et al: FDG-PET in prediction of splenectomy findings in patients with known or suspected lymphoma. Leuk Lymphoma 2008;49:719.

Procedures in which mobilization of the left upper quadrant is done (such as reflection of the spleen and pancreas medially to expose retroperitoneal tissue, left adrenalectomy, and left nephrectomy) put the spleen at risk for injury during the dissection. Simple mobilization of the splenic flexure of the colon can lead to bleeding from the inferior pole of the spleen that may be difficult to control. The ligaments that go directly from the omentum to the capsule of the spleen may be the most common cause of iatrogenic splenic trauma, as it is a common practice to aggressively retract the omentum as needed for exposure. If there are direct branches that sometimes may be sizable from the omentum to the splenic capsule, this could lead to capsular disruption and troublesome bleeding. A national database on antireflux procedures of 86,411 patients reported an incidence of iatrogenic splenectomy of 2.3%, which translates into 1987 iatrogenic splenectomies for that indication alone over a 6-year period. An outcome study for colon cancer of 42,000 reported iatrogenic splenectomy in less than 1% of all patients but 6% of colon cancers at the splenic flexure. Splenectomy had a significant increase in length of stay and a 40% increase in morbidity.

A recent series listed 73 iatrogenic splenectomies over a 10-year period, or an average of 7 per year. This comprised 8.1% of all splenectomies performed during that time interval. There are probably several times that number of minor or moderate injuries to the spleen during unrelated operations in which the spleen was not removed but was repaired or salvaged. Just as in trauma to the spleen, the techniques of splenorrhaphy can be employed to preserve the spleen. A recent report indicates that use of a mesh wrap splenorrhaphy, even in the setting of bowel surgery, does not lead to an increased incidence of infection. For minor capsular disruption, the use of the argon beam coagulator for surface cautery is a helpful technique.

The primary teaching point regarding iatrogenic injuries is that the best way to preserve the spleen is to not damage it in the first place. This requires caution in mobilizing tissue in and around the spleen as well as visual inspection of the attachments of the spleen prior to blunt mobilization. Whenever possible, attempts should be made to preserve the spleen to decrease the risk of postsplenectomy sepsis.

Berry MF, Rosato EF, Williams NN: Dexon mesh splenorrhaphy for intraoperative splenic injuries. Am Surg 2003;69:176.

Cassar K, Munro A: Iatrogenic splenic injury. J Roy Coll Surg Edinburgh 2002;47:731.

Flum DR et al: The nationwide frequency of major adverse outcomes in antireflux surgery and the role of surgeon experience. J Am Coll Surg 2002;195:611.

McGory ML et al: The significance of inadvertent splenectomy during colorectal cancer resection. Arch Surgery 2007;142:668.

2. Incidental Splenectomy

In a recent large series evaluating reasons for splenectomy from tertiary institutions, the single-most common indication for splenectomy was as an incidental procedure on operations on an adjacent organ. In these situations, the spleen needs to be removed either for completeness of resection or because of division of the splenic vasculature The actual primary treatments of those various disease entities in adjacent organs are subjects of multiple other chapters within this textbook, but a few comments need to be made regarding the reasons for splenectomy and whether splenic preservation procedures are possible.

One common indication for an incidental splenectomy is to remove tumors located in the distal pancreas. For decades, it was standard practice to remove the spleen when removing the body and tail of the pancreas because the splenic vein is intimately associated with the distal pancreas. Because of the interest in splenic preservation due to the incidence of postsplenectomy infection, operations have been developed to remove the distal pancreas without removing the spleen. The more technically challenging operation is a distal pancreatectomy with preservation of the splenic artery and vein. A second spleen-preserving distal pancreatectomy involves ligation of the splenic artery and vein but preservation of short gastric vessels and utilizing those vessels as collateral inflow and outflow to maintain splenic viability. Removal of the distal pancreas with splenic preservation has also been recently reported as a laparoscopic procedure. For patients with tumors that mandate removal of the lymph nodes of the splenic hilum or with direct association of the tumor with splenic parenchyma, certainly it is more appropriate to do an operation based on neoplastic principles and perform a distal pancreatectomy/splenectomy. In other indications, if the anatomy is appropriate and the completeness of tumor resection is not compromised, splenic preservation is certainly possible.

Additional procedures in which it is common to perform a splenectomy include proximal gastric cancers. The importance of complete nodal dissection in long-term results in gastric resections has been debated for several decades. Level X lymph nodes are located in the splenic hilum, and for 20–25% of proximal gastric cancers, these nodes will have metastatic cancer mandating removal. A randomized trial showed increased morbidity with a splenectomy and a marginal improvement in survival. Other tumors of the left upper quadrant and retroperitoneum may require splenectomy, including large renal cell carcinomas, left adrenal tumors, and retroperitoneal sarcomas that may infiltrate upward into the spleen. Although the asplenic state does make patients susceptible to infections (see earlier section on Hyposplenism), the spleen should be viewed as an expendable organ if necessary to accomplish complete resection of malignancies, and there should be no hesitation to remove the spleen in these situations to do an appropriate cancer operation.

Carrere N et al: Spleen-preserving distal pancreatectomy with excision of splenic artery and vein: a case matched comparison with conventional distal pancreatectomy with splenectomy. World J Surg 2007;31:375.

Hartgrink HH et al: Extended lymph node dissection for gastric cancer: who may benefit? Final results of the randomized Dutch gastric cancer group trial. J Clin Oncol 2004;22:2069.

Pryor A et al: Laparoscopic distal pancreatectomy with splenic preservation. Surg Endosc 2007;21:2326.

Yu W et al: Randomized clinical trial of splenectomy versus splenic preservation in patients with proximal gastric cancer. Br J Surg 2006;93:559.

SPLENOSIS (SPLENIC AUTOTRANSPLANTATION)

In splenosis, multiple small implants of splenic tissue grow in scattered areas on the peritoneal surfaces throughout the abdomen. They arise from dissemination and autotransplantation of splenic fragments following traumatic rupture of the spleen. Splenic implants or intentional autotransplants are capable of cell culling, and some immunologic function appears to be exhibited in cases of intentional autotransplantation. Aggressive attempts at surgical excision are not warranted. Splenosis is usually an incidental finding discovered much later during laparotomy for an unrelated problem. However, the implants stimulate formation of adhesions and may be a cause of intestinal obstruction. They must be distinguished from peritoneal nodules of metastatic carcinoma and from accessory spleens. Histologically, they differ from accessory spleens by the absence of elastic or smooth muscle fibers in the delicate capsule.

Cothren CC et al: Radiographic characteristics of postinjury splenic autotransplantation: avoiding a diagnostic dilemma. J Trauma-Injury Infection & Crit Care 2004;57:537.

Young JT et al: Splenosis: a remote consequence of traumatic splenectomy. J Am Coll Surg 2004;199:500.

SPLENECTOMY

Preoperative preparation of patients undergoing elective splenectomy should correct coagulation abnormalities and deficits in red cell mass, treat infections, and control immune reactions. Because platelets are removed so rapidly from the circulation, they usually are not given for thrombocytopenia until after the splenic artery has been ligated. Antibodies in the patient's serum may complicate crossmatching of blood. Many patients with autoimmune disorders require corticosteroid coverage in the perioperative period. For emergency splenectomy, hypovolemia should be corrected by whole blood transfusions. For elective cases, prophylactic vaccination with a polyvalent pneumococcal vaccine that protects against a common encapsulated offending organism in postsplenectomy infection is recommended. Elective splenectomy is now most commonly performed as a laparoscopic procedure. This reduces the recovery period and is significantly better tolerated by most patients.

Details of surgical technique are not within the scope of this text, but it should be noted that there are two approaches to open splenectomy (Figure 27–2). In one, which is of value chiefly in traumatic rupture of the spleen, the organ is immediately mobilized and the splenic artery is secured from behind as it enters the hilum. In the other, which is of vital importance in the removal of massively enlarged spleens, the organ is left in situ. The gastrocolic ligament is opened, and the splenic artery is ligated as it courses along the upper edge of the pancreas. This permits blood to leave the spleen through the splenic vein while all other attachments (ie, the short gastric vessels and colic attachments) are divided before the spleen is delivered. This

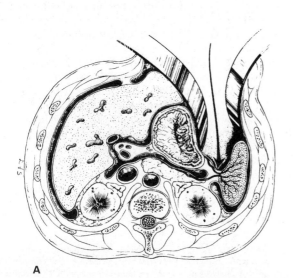
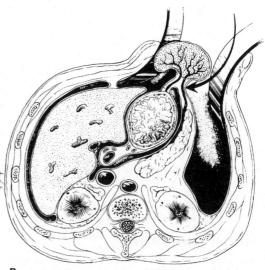

A

B

▲ **Figure 27–2. A:** Anterior approach to splenic artery. **B:** Mobilization of spleen with posterior exposure of splenic artery.

method permits the removal of massively enlarged vascular spleens with practically no loss of blood.

Splenorrhaphy is operative repair of the spleen following trauma. The principles of splenorrhaphy are to debride the devitalized tissue and to attempt to approximate the normal contour of the spleen with capsular sutures or external wraps of material. Partial splenic resections may be performed for trauma or for disease states in which splenic debulking is indicated but may be unsuccessful with a higher immediate complication rate. Partial splenectomy for Gaucher disease, large cysts, or benign tumors has been reported using automatic stapling devices as well as microwave coagulators. On the other hand, for autoimmune disorders, it is absolutely essential for cure to remove the spleen completely, including excision of accessory spleens. There may be some benefit to obtain a preoperative nuclear scan and intraoperative identification with a handheld gamma counter.

Massive splenomegaly is defined as a spleen weight of greater than 1500 g, or 8–10 times the normal size. Disease processes leading to massive splenomegaly include lymphoma, leukemia, and metabolic storage diseases. The morbidity and mortality rates of splenectomy for massive splenomegaly are increased primarily as a result of the risk of severe and rapid intraoperative blood loss. The operative approach in these cases is initial ligation of the splenic artery through the lesser sac at the superior border of the pancreas. Next, ligation of the short gastric vessels along the greater curvature all the way to the gastroesophageal junction is performed, allowing the stomach and left lobe of the liver to be retracted away from the spleen. Only after decreasing the splenic arterial inflow by the above maneuvers should mobilization of the lateral and superior attachments be performed, leading to removal of the massive spleen.

Laparoscopic splenectomy is now the standard of care in most major centers with high volumes of splenic surgery. Virtually any indication for elective splenectomy qualifies for a laparoscopic approach, including patients with severe thrombocytopenia, patients with massive splenomegaly, patients needing partial splenectomy, and for the removal of accessory spleens and the wandering spleen. Contraindications to laparoscopic splenectomy include portal hypertension and severe comorbid disease. With improved techniques, laparoscopic partial splenectomy has now been reported for focal mass lesions and hereditary hematologic diseases.

Laparoscopic splenectomy is performed typically using four ports. Midline ports for the cannula as well as for retraction of the stomach away from the splenic hilum are placed. Left subcostal ports are used as operating sites for dissection of the splenic hilum. An angled laparoscope is required for visualization of the superior and lateral attachments of the spleen. Vessels are divided with clips, sutures, or stapling devices. Precise exposure of the hilum with gentle upward traction on the spleen to stretch and expose the vessels is preferred to blind stapling of the hilum. Clinical conditions such as idiopathic thrombocytopenic purpura

and hereditary spherocytosis are the most common indications for laparoscopic splenectomy as the spleen is of normal size. Search via the laparoscope for accessory spleens is important in these procedures for a successful outcome, and this may be facilitated by the use of a hand port for palpation.

Bergeron E et al: The use of a handheld gamma probe for identifying two accessory spleens in difficult locations in the same patient. Ann Nucl Med 2007;22:331.

Becmeur HG et al: Laparoscopic partial splenectomy: indications and results of a multicenter retrospective study. Surg Endosc 2008;22:45.

Feldman LS et al: Refining the selection criteria for laparoscopic versus open splenectomy for splenomegaly. J Lapraroendosc Adv Surg Tech A 2008;18:13.

Grahn SW et al: Trends in laparoscopic splenectomy for massive splenomegaly. Arch Surg 2006;141:755.

Habermalz B et al: Laparoscopic splenectomy: the clinical practice e guidelines of the European Association for Endoscopic Surgery. Surg Endosc 2008;22:821.

Kasaje N et al: Short-term outcomes of splenectomy avoidance in trauma patients. Am J Surg 2008;196:213.

Rescoria FJ et al: Laparoscopic splenic procedures in children: experience in 231 children. Ann Surg 2007;246:683.

Stamou KM et al: Prospective study of the incidence and risk factors of postsplenectomy thrombosis of the portal, mesenteric, and splenic veins. Arch Surg 2006;141:663.

HEMATOLOGIC EFFECTS OF SPLENECTOMY

Absence of the spleen in a normal adult usually has few clinical consequences. Red cell count and indices do not change, but red cells with cytoplasmic inclusions may appear (eg, Heinz bodies, Howell-Jolly bodies, and siderocytes). Granulocytosis occurs immediately after splenectomy but is replaced in several weeks by lymphocytosis and monocytosis. Platelets are usually increased, occasionally markedly so, and may stay at levels of 400,000–500,000/μL for over a year. Even more striking thrombocytosis (eg, 2–3 million/μL) may develop after splenectomy for hemolytic anemia. A platelet count of over a million is not an indication for anticoagulants, but antiplatelet agents such as aspirin may help prevent thrombosis.

William BM et al: Hyposplenism: a comprehensive review. Part I: basic concepts and causes. Hematology 2007;12:1.

William BM et al: Hyposplenism: a comprehensive review. Part II: clinical manifestations, diagnosis, and management. Hematology 2007;12:89.

POSTSPLENECTOMY SEPSIS & OTHER POSTSPLENECTOMY PROBLEMS

Complications related to splenectomy per se are relatively few, with atelectasis, pancreatitis, and postoperative hemorrhage being the most common. If splenectomy is done for thrombocytopenia, secondary bleeding may occur even though the platelet count usually rises promptly. Platelet transfusions should be given if primary hemostasis is abnormal (ie, oozing occurs) and the platelet count remains low. Thromboembolic complications may be more common following splenectomy, but this complication does not correlate with the degree of thrombocytosis. The risk of portal vein thrombosis is 3% and occurs most commonly after splenectomy for massive spleens hemolytic anemia and not after trauma or splenectomy for thrombocytopenia. Symptoms include fever, abdominal pain, diarrhea, and abnormal liver function tests. Treatment consists of anticoagulation plus antibiotics.

Individuals are more susceptible to fulminant bacteremia after splenectomy, and cases have been reported between 1 week and greater than 20 years after splenectomy. This is a result of the following changes that occur after splenectomy: (1) decreased clearance of bacteria from the blood, (2) decreased levels of IgM, and (3) decreased opsonic activity. The risk is greatest in young children, especially in the first 2 years after surgery (80% of cases) and when the disorder for which splenectomy was required was a disease of the reticuloendothelial system. In general, the younger the patient undergoing splenectomy and the more severe the underlying condition, the greater the risk for developing overwhelming postsplenectomy infection. There is a low but significant risk of infection even in otherwise normal adults following splenectomy. Most of these infections occur after the first year, and nearly half occur more than 5 years after splenectomy. Lethal sepsis is very rare in adults. There is a distinct clinical syndrome: mild, nonspecific symptoms are followed by high fever and shock from sepsis, which may rapidly lead to death. *Streptococcus pneumoniae, Haemophilus influenzae,* and meningococci are the most common pathogens. Disseminated intravascular coagulation is a common complication. Awareness of this fatal complication has led to efforts to avoid splenectomy or to perform partial splenectomy or splenic repair for ruptured spleens (analogous to surgical management of liver trauma) to maintain adequate splenic function. Splenic autotransplantation may also achieve partial restoration of splenic function after splenectomy.

The risk of fatal sepsis is less after splenectomy for trauma than for hematologic disorders, probably due to splenic autotransplantation. Prophylactic vaccination against pneumococcal sepsis should be used in all surgically or functionally asplenic patients. Since splenic function may be important in the immune response to vaccine, early administration of polyvalent pneumococcal vaccine (Pneumovax) is advisable. The vaccine provides protection in adults and older children for 4–5 years, after which revaccination is advisable. Since the vaccine is effective against only about 80% of organisms, some authorities have recommended a 2-year course, treatment until age 16, or lifelong prophylaxis with penicillin following splenectomy. Others have advocated use of ampicillin to provide coverage for *H influenzae* as well as pneumococci. Antibiotic prophylaxis is essential in children under 2 years of age and should be continued until at least age 6. In general, splenectomy should be deferred until age 6 unless the hematologic problem is especially severe.

Cadili A et al: Complications of splenectomy. Am J Med 2008; 121:371.

Krauth MT et al: The postoperative splenic/portal vein thrombosis after splenectomy and its prevention—an unresolved issue. Haematologica 2008;93:1227.

Okabayashi T et al: Overwhelming postsplenectomy infection syndrome in adults: a clinically preventable disease. World J Gastroenterol 2008;14:176.

Price VE et al: The prevention and management of infections in children with asplenia or hyposplenia. Infect Dis Clin North Am 2007;21:697.

Shatz DV et al: Vaccination practices among North American trauma surgeons in splenectomy for trauma. J Trauma-Injury Inf & Crit Care 2002;53:950.

Shatz DV et al: Antibody responses in postsplenectomy trauma patients receiving the 23-valent pneumococcal polysaccharide vaccine at 14 versus 28 days postoperatively. J Trauma-Injury Inf & Crit Care 2002;53:1037.

Spelman D et al: Guidelines for the prevention of sepsis in asplenic and hyposplenic patients. Intern Med J 2008;38:349.

Appendix

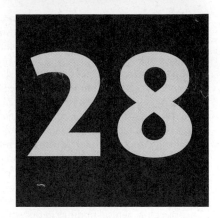

Gerard M. Doherty, MD

ANATOMY & PHYSIOLOGY

In infants, the appendix is a conical diverticulum at the apex of the cecum, but with differential growth and distention of the cecum, the appendix ultimately arises on the left and dorsally approximately 2.5 cm below the ileocecal valve. The taeniae of the colon converge at the base of the appendix, an arrangement that helps in locating this structure at operation. The appendix is fixed retrocecally in 16% of adults and is freely mobile in the remainder.

The appendix in youth is characterized by a large concentration of lymphoid follicles that appear 2 weeks after birth and number about 200 or more at age 15. Thereafter, progressive atrophy of lymphoid tissue proceeds concomitantly with fibrosis of the wall and partial or total obliteration of the lumen.

If the appendix has a physiologic function, it is probably related to the presence of lymphoid follicles. Reports of a statistical relationship between appendectomy and subsequent carcinoma of the colon and other neoplasms in humans are not supported by controlled studies.

Schumpelick V et al: Appendix and cecum. Embryology, anatomy, and surgical applications. Surg Clin North Am 2000;80:295.

ACUTE APPENDICITIS

 ESSENTIALS OF DIAGNOSIS

► Abdominal pain.
► Anorexia, nausea and vomiting.
► Localized right lower quadrant abdominal tenderness.
► Low-grade fever.
► Leukocytosis.

► General Considerations

Approximately 7% of people in Western countries have appendicitis at some time during their lives, and about 200,000 appendectomies for acute appendicitis are performed annually in the United States. The incidence has been steadily dropping over the past 25 years, however, while the incidence in developing countries—which in the past has been quite low—has been rising in proportion to economic gains and changes in lifestyle.

Obstruction of the proximal lumen by fibrous bands, lymphoid hyperplasia, fecaliths, calculi, or parasites has long been considered to be the major cause of acute appendicitis, though that theory is doubted by many experts. Evidence of temporal and geographic clustering of cases has suggested a primary infectious etiology. A fecalith or calculus is found in only 10% of acutely inflamed appendices.

As appendicitis progresses, the blood supply is impaired by bacterial infection in the wall and distention of the lumen by pus; gangrene and perforation occur at about 24 hours, though the timing is highly variable. Gangrene implies microscopic perforation and bacterial peritonitis (which may be localized by adhesions from nearby viscera).

► Clinical Findings

Acute appendicitis has protean manifestations. It may simulate almost any other acute abdominal illness and in turn may be mimicked by a variety of conditions. Progression of symptoms and signs is the rule—in contrast to the fluctuating course of some other diseases.

A. Symptoms and Signs

Typically, the illness begins with vague midabdominal discomfort followed by nausea, anorexia, and indigestion. The pain is persistent and continuous but not severe, with occasional mild cramps. There may be an episode of vomiting, and within several hours the pain shifts to the right lower quadrant, becoming localized and causing discomfort on moving, walking, or coughing. The patient may feel constipated.

Examination at this point shows localized tenderness to one-finger palpation and perhaps slight muscular guarding. Rebound or percussion tenderness (the latter provides the same information more humanely) may be elicited in the same area. Peristalsis is normal or slightly reduced. Rectal and pelvic examinations are likely to be negative. The temperature is only slightly elevated (eg, 37.8 °C) in the absence of perforation.

Contrary to traditional teaching, tenderness on rectal examination is not a sign of acute appendicitis. If present, it more often points to another cause of the symptoms. Another common misconception is that inflammation in a retrocecal appendix produces an atypical syndrome. This too is incorrect; the clinical findings in this situation are the same as for ordinary (antececal) appendicitis.

Rarely, the cecum may lie on the left side of the abdomen, and appendicitis may be mistaken for sigmoid diverticulitis. An inflamed appendix in the right upper quadrant may mimic acute cholecystitis or perforated ulcer. Even when the cecum is normally situated, a long appendix may reach to other parts of the abdomen, and acute appendicitis in these circumstances may be very confusing indeed.

A couple of general points are worth remembering: (1) People with early (nonperforated) appendicitis often do not appear ill and may even apologize for taking your time. Finding localized tenderness over the McBurney point is the cornerstone of diagnosis. (2) A rule that will help considerably with atypical cases is never to place appendicitis lower than second in the differential diagnosis of acute abdominal pain in a previously healthy person.

B. Laboratory Findings

The average leukocyte count is 15,000/μL, and 90% of patients have counts over 10,000/μL. In three fourths of patients, the differential white count shows more than 75% neutrophils. It must be emphasized, however, that 1 patient in 10 with acute appendicitis has a leukocyte count indistinguishable from normal, and many have normal differential cell counts. Appendicitis in patients infected with HIV produces the same syndrome as in other people, but the white blood cell count is usually normal.

The urine is usually normal, but a few leukocytes and erythrocytes and occasionally even gross hematuria may be noted, particularly in retrocecal or pelvic appendicitis.

C. Imaging Studies

Localized air-fluid levels, localized ileus, or increased soft tissue density in the right lower quadrant is present in 50% of patients with early acute appendicitis. Less common findings are a calculus, an altered right psoas shadow, or an abnormal right flank stripe. The finding on plain films of a calculus in the right lower quadrant coupled with pain in this area strongly supports a diagnosis of appendicitis. Although perforated peptic ulcer is by far the most common cause of free intraperitoneal air, free air is also a rare manifestation of perforated appendicitis. In general, however, the findings on plain films are nonspecific and rarely of help in diagnosis. A suggestion that barium enema may contribute to the diagnosis has not been supported by experience.

A spiral CT examination of the appendix may be of help in diagnosis. An enlarged appendix with wall thickening or enhancement or periappendiceal fat stranding are the most useful CT findings of acute appendicitis. Other findings may be present, including focal cecal thickening, appendicoliths, extraluminal air, intramural air, and pericecal phlegmon, but are less reliable. CT scans are of greatest value in patients with less than typical clinical and laboratory findings, where a positive study would be an indication for appendectomy. In the face of typical time course of disease, right lower quadrant pain and tenderness plus signs of inflammation (eg, fever, leukocytosis), a CT scan would be superfluous and, if negative, even misleading. Ultrasound imaging is much less reliable than CT. When appendicitis is accompanied by a right lower quadrant mass, an ultrasound or CT scan should be obtained to differentiate between a periappendiceal phlegmon and an abscess.

D. Appendicitis during Pregnancy

Appendicitis is the most common nonobstetric surgical disease of the abdomen during pregnancy. Pregnant women develop appendicitis with the same frequency as do nonpregnant women of the same age, and the cases are equally distributed through the three trimesters of pregnancy. By far the most common presentation is right lower quadrant pain and tenderness—the classic syndrome—but the enlarged uterus occasionally will have pushed the appendix into the right upper quadrant, which gives rise to pain in this location. Fever is less common than with appendicitis in the absence of pregnancy. Leukocytosis is typical, but it too may be absent. The main problem is to recognize the possibility of appendicitis and perform appendectomy promptly. Delay in operation runs a higher than usual risk of perforation and diffuse peritonitis, because omentum is less available to wall off the infection. The mother is in greater jeopardy of serious abdominal infection, and the fetus is more vulnerable to premature labor with complications. Laparoscopic appendectomy (specifically the pneumoperitoneum) is well tolerated by the mother and fetus, but the frequency of technical complications is higher than with the open approach. Appendectomy during pregnancy is often followed by preterm labor but rarely by preterm delivery. Early appendectomy has decreased the maternal death rate to under 0.5% and the fetal death rate to under 10%.

▶ Diagnosis & Differential Diagnosis

The clinical diagnosis of appendicitis rests on a combination of localized pain and tenderness accompanied by signs of inflammation, such as fever, leukocytosis, and elevated C-reactive protein levels. Migration of pain from the periumbilical area to the right lower quadrant is also diagnostically significant. In the absence of signs of inflammation, the diagnosis is less certain (ie, falsely positive), and in this situation a CT scan might be of value. The best strategy in equivocal cases is to observe the patient for a period of 6 hours or more. During this time, patients with appendicitis experience increasing pain and signs of inflammation and those without appendicitis generally improve. False-positive diagnoses often involve cases where the surgeon has accorded more significance to the patient's pain than to the presence or absence of inflammatory signs. Anorexia, nausea, and rectal tenderness are not indicative of appendicitis. During the past 15 years, the overall false-positive rate for the diagnosis of appendicitis has dropped from 15% to 10% without an accompanying rise in the number of perforations. Thus, diagnostic accuracy appears to be improving.

The diagnosis of acute appendicitis is particularly difficult in the very young and in the elderly. These are the groups in which diagnosis is most often delayed and perforation most common. Infants manifest only lethargy, irritability, and anorexia in the early stages, but vomiting, fever, and pain are apparent as the disease progresses. Classic symptoms may not be elicited in aged patients, and the diagnosis is often not considered by the examining physician. The course of appendicitis is more virulent in the elderly, and suppurative complications occur earlier.

The highest incidence of false-positive diagnosis (20%) is in women between ages 20 and 40 and is attributable to pelvic inflammatory disease and other gynecologic conditions. Compared with appendicitis, pelvic inflammatory disease is more often associated with bilateral lower quadrant tenderness, left adnexal tenderness, onset of illness within 5 days of the last menstrual period, and a history that does not include nausea and vomiting. Cervical motion tenderness is common in both diseases.

▶ Complications

The complications of acute appendicitis include perforation, peritonitis, abscess, and pylephlebitis.

A. Perforation

Delay in seeking medical care appears to be the principal reason for perforations; the disease has just been allowed to progress according to its natural history. Perforation is accompanied by more severe pain and higher fever (average, 38.3 °C) than in appendicitis. It is unusual for the acutely inflamed appendix to perforate within the first 12 hours. The appendicitis has progressed to perforation by the time of appendectomy in about 50% of patients under age 10 or over age 50. Nearly all deaths occur in the latter group.

The acute consequences of perforation vary from generalized peritonitis to formation of a tiny abscess that may not appreciably alter the symptoms and signs of appendicitis.

Perforation in young women increases the subsequent risk of tubal infertility about fourfold.

B. Peritonitis

Localized peritonitis results from microscopic perforation of a gangrenous appendix, while spreading or generalized peritonitis usually implies gross perforation into the free peritoneal cavity. Increasing tenderness and rigidity, abdominal distention, and adynamic ileus are obvious in patients with peritonitis. High fever and severe toxicity mark progression of this catastrophic illness in untreated patients.

C. Appendiceal Abscess (Appendiceal Mass)

Localized perforation occurs when the periappendiceal infection becomes walled off by omentum and adjacent viscera. The clinical presentation consists of the usual findings in appendicitis plus a right lower quadrant mass. An ultrasound or CT scan should be performed; if an abscess is found, it is best treated by percutaneous ultrasound-guided aspiration. Opinion differs about how small abscesses and phlegmons should be handled. Some surgeons prefer a regimen consisting of antibiotics and expectant management followed by elective appendectomy 6 weeks later. The purpose is to avoid spreading the localized infection, which usually resolves in response to the antibiotics. Other surgeons recommend immediate appendectomy, which some believe shortens the duration of the illness. However, the immediate surgery approach has significant complications in a higher percentage of patients. There is not currently a consensus.

When the surgeon encounters an unsuspected abscess during appendectomy, it is usually best to proceed and remove the appendix. If the abscess is large and further dissection would be hazardous, drainage alone is appropriate.

Appendicitis recurs in only 10% of patients whose initial treatment consisted of antibiotics or antibiotics plus drainage of an abscess. Therefore, when the presence of ancillary conditions increases the risks of surgery, interval appendectomy may be postponed unless symptoms recur.

D. Pylephlebitis

Pylephlebitis is suppurative thrombophlebitis of the portal venous system. Chills, high fever, low-grade jaundice, and, later, hepatic abscesses are the hallmarks of this grave condition. The appearance of shaking chills in a patient with acute appendicitis demands vigorous antibiotic therapy to prevent the development of pylephlebitis.

CT scanning is the best means of detecting thrombosis and gas in the portal vein. In addition to antibiotics, prompt surgery is indicated to treat appendicitis or other primary sources of infection (eg, diverticulitis).

▶ Prevention

In the past it was common to perform an incidental appendectomy in people under age 50 during the course of an abdominal operation for another illness—as long as the exposure was adequate and there were no specific contraindications. The declining lifetime risk of appendicitis now calls this practice into question. A related question concerns the appropriate course when a laparoscopy is performed for presumptive appendicitis and the appendix looks normal. The trend in this case is to leave the appendix intact—not to remove it prophylactically or on the assumption that the visual assessment may be inaccurate.

▶ Treatment

With few exceptions, the treatment of appendicitis is surgical (ie, appendectomy). The operation can be done open (see Figure 28–1) or laparoscopically. The results of clinical trials comparing the two methods show no clear-cut advantage of one method over the other, though patients treated laparoscopically return to work a few days earlier. A laparoscopic approach is desirable when the preoperative diagnosis is uncertain because the morbidity is less if the appendix is found to be uninflamed and an appendectomy is not done.

Prophylactic antibiotics are indicated preoperatively. A single-drug regimen, usually a cephalosporin, is as effective as more aggressive multiple-drug combinations. Routinely culturing abdominal fluid is of no practical value even when the appendix has perforated. The organisms obtained are the usual fecal flora.

Abdominal drains are called for only to treat established abscesses, not for diffuse inflammation or abdominal fluid.

If a patient with appendicitis cannot be taken to a modern surgical facility for care, treatment should consist of antibiotics alone. The complication-free success rate of this approach is high.

▶ Prognosis

Although a death rate of zero is theoretically attainable in acute appendicitis, deaths still occur, some of which are avoidable. The death rate in simple acute appendicitis is approximately 0.1% and has not changed significantly since 1930. Progress in preoperative and postoperative care—particularly the emphasis on fluid replacement before operation—has reduced the death rate from perforation to about 5%. Nonetheless, postoperative infections still occur in 30% of cases of gangrenous or perforated appendix. Although most of these patients survive, many near fatalities require prolonged hospitalization. The substantial increase in tubal infertility that follows perforation in young women is also avoidable by early appendectomy.

Andersen BR, Kallehave FL, Andersen HK: Antibiotics versus placebo for prevention of postoperative infection after appendicectomy. Cochrane Database Syst Rev 2005;3:CD001439.

Andersson RE et al: Repeated clinical and laboratory examinations in patients with an equivocal diagnosis of appendicitis. World J Surg 2000;24:479.

Andersson RE et al: Why does the clinical diagnosis fail in suspected appendicitis? Eur J Surg 2000;166:796.

Asfar S et al: Would measurement of C-reactive protein reduce the rate of negative exploration for acute appendicitis? J R Coll Edinb 2000;45:21.

Blomqvist PG et al: Mortality after appendectomy in Sweden, 1987–1996. Ann Surg 2001;233:455.

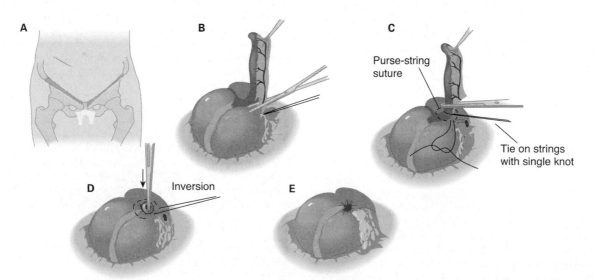

▲ **Figure 28–1.** Technique of appendectomy. **A:** Incision. **B:** After delivery of the tip of the cecum, the mesoappendix is divided. **C:** The base is clamped and ligated with a simple throw of the knot. The next step—inversion of the stump—is optional. **D:** A clamp is placed to hold the knot during inversion with a purse-string suture of fine silk. **E:** The loosely tied inner knot on the stump assures that there is no closed space for the development of a stump abscess.

Brown CV et al: Appendiceal abscess: immediate operation or percutaneous drainage? Am Surg 2003;69:829.

Carr NJ: The pathology of acute appendicitis. Ann Diagn Pathol 2000;4:46.

Choi D et al: The most useful findings for diagnosing acute appendicitis on contrast-enhanced helical CT. Acta Radiologica 2003;44:574.

Lee SL et al: Computed tomography and ultrasonography do not improve and may delay the diagnosis and treatment of acute appendicitis. Arch Surg 2001;136:556.

Long KH et al: A prospective randomized comparison of laparoscopic appendectomy with open appendectomy: clinical and economic analyses. Surgery 2001;129:390.

Mourad J et al: Appendicitis in pregnancy: new information that contradicts long-held clinical beliefs. Am J Obstet Gynecol 2000;182:1027.

Pinto Leite N et al: CT evaluation of appendicitis and its complications: imaging techniques and key diagnostic findings. Am J Roentgenol 2005;185:406.

Rucinski J et al: Gangrenous and perforated appendicitis: a meta-analytic study of 2532 patients indicates that the incision should be closed primarily. Surgery 2000;127:136.

Sauerland S, Lefering R, Neugebauer EA: Laparoscopic versus open surgery for suspected appendicitis. Cochrane Database Syst Rev 2004;4:CD001546.

Weyant MJ et al: Interpretation of computed tomography does not correlate with laboratory or pathologic findings in surgically confirmed acute appendicitis. Surgery 2000;128:145.

CHRONIC APPENDICITIS

Chronic abdominal pain is a common problem, and when the complaints are confined to the right lower quadrant, the question of chronic appendicitis is usually raised. Patients with genuine chronic appendicitis experience pain that lasts for 3 weeks or more. The history usually includes an acute illness at some time in the past, compatible with acute appendicitis, which was managed nonoperatively. On examination, the appendix is chronically inflamed or fibrotic. The symptoms resolve with appendectomy.

Chronic intermittent pain in the right lower quadrant is most often caused by something other than appendicitis, such as Crohn disease or renal disease. Barium x-rays are sometimes helpful, particularly in children. In many patients, the diagnosis is not obvious. Appendectomy relieves symptoms occasionally, but laparotomy for chronic abdominal pain is generally unproductive in the absence of objective findings (eg, localized tenderness, palpable mass, leukocytosis).

Roumen RM et al: Randomized clinical trial evaluating elective laparoscopic appendicectomy for chronic right lower-quadrant pain. Br J Surg 2008;95:169.

TUMORS OF THE APPENDIX

Benign tumors, including carcinoids, were found in 4.6% of 71,000 human appendix specimens examined microscopically. Benign neoplasms may arise from any cellular element and are usually incidental findings. Occasionally, a neoplasm obstructs the appendiceal lumen and produces acute appendicitis. No treatment other than appendectomy is indicated.

▶ Malignant Tumors

Primary malignant tumors were found in 1.4% of appendices in the same large series. Carcinoid and argentaffin tumors comprise the majority of appendiceal cancers, and the appendix is the commonest location of carcinoid tumors of the gastrointestinal tract. Carcinoid tumors of the appendix are usually benign, but the uncommon tumor that is over 2 cm in diameter may exhibit malignant behavior. Most appendiceal carcinoids are found in the tip of the organ, while a few are at the base. About half of these tumors are discovered during an appendectomy for acute appendicitis, and the remainder are identified incidentally. Lesions less than 2 cm in diameter invade the appendiceal wall in 25% of cases, but only 3% metastasize to lymph nodes, and hepatic metastases and the carcinoid syndrome are truly rare. Appendectomy alone is adequate treatment unless the lymph nodes are visibly involved, the tumor is more than 2 cm in diameter, mucinous elements are present in the tumor (adenocarcinoid), or the mesoappendix or base of the cecum is invaded. Right hemicolectomy is recommended for these more aggressive lesions.

Adenocarcinoma of the colonic type can arise in the appendix and spread rapidly to regional lymph nodes or implant on ovaries or other peritoneal surfaces. Ten percent of patients have widespread metastases when first seen. Adenocarcinoma is virtually never diagnosed preoperatively; about half of cases present as acute appendicitis, and 15% have formed appendiceal abscesses. Right hemicolectomy should be performed if disease is localized to the appendix and regional lymph nodes. The 5-year survival rate is 60% after right hemicolectomy and only 20% after appendectomy alone, but the latter group includes patients with distant metastases at the time of diagnosis.

▶ Mucocele

Mucocele of the appendix is a cystic, dilated appendix filled with mucin. Simple mucocele is not a neoplasm and results from chronic obstruction of the proximal lumen, usually by fibrous tissue. If the appendiceal contents distally are sterile, mucous cells continue to secrete until distention of the lumen thins the wall and interferes with nutrition of the lining cells; histologically, simple mucocele is lined by flattened cuboidal epithelium or no epithelium at all. Simple mucocele is cured by appendectomy.

Less commonly, mucocele is caused by a neoplasm—cystadenoma, or adenocarcinoma grade 1 in the older terminology. This lesion may arise de novo or (perhaps) in a preceding simple mucocele. In cystadenoma, the lumen is filled with mucin but the wall is lined by columnar epithelium with papillary projections. Tumor does not infiltrate the appendiceal wall and does not metastasize, although it may recur locally after appendectomy. Cystadenoma is believed to undergo malignant change in some instances. Appendectomy is adequate treatment.

Chiou YY et al: Rare benign and malignant appendiceal lesions: spectrum of computed tomography findings with pathologic correlation. J Comput Assist Tomogr 2003;27:297.

Murphy EM, Farquharson SM, Moran BJ: Management of an unexpected appendiceal neoplasm. Br J Surg 2006;93:783.

Sippel RS, Chen H: Carcinoid tumors. Surg Oncol Clin North Am 2006;15:463.

Sugarbaker PH: Peritoneal surface oncology: review of a personal experience with colorectal and appendiceal malignancy. Tech Coloproctol 2005;9:95.

Tchana-Sato V et al: Carcinoid tumor of the appendix: a consecutive series from 1237 appendectomies. World J Gastroentero 2006; 12:6699.

Small Intestine

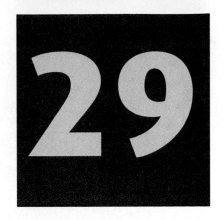

Andrew A. Shelton, MD

George J. Chang, MD, MS

Mark L. Welton, MD

The small intestine is the portion of the alimentary tract extending from the pylorus to the cecum. The structure, function, and diseases of the duodenum are discussed in Chapter 23; the jejunum and ileum are described in this chapter.

ANATOMY

Gross Anatomy

The small intestine in an adult is 5–6 m long from the ligament of Treitz to the ileocecal valve. The upper two fifths of the small intestine distal to the duodenum is termed the **jejunum,** and the lower three fifths is the **ileum.** There is no sharp demarcation between the jejunum and the ileum; however, as the intestine proceeds distally, the lumen narrows, the mesenteric vascular arcades become more complex, and the circular mucosal folds become shorter and fewer (Figure 29–1). In general, the jejunum resides in the left side of the peritoneal cavity, and the ileum occupies the pelvis and right lower quadrant.

The small bowel is attached to the posterior abdominal wall by the mesentery, a reflection from the posterior parietal peritoneum. This peritoneal fold arises along a line originating just to the left of the midline and passing obliquely to the right lower quadrant. Although the mesentery joins the intestine along one side, the peritoneal layer of the mesentery envelops the bowel and is called the visceral peritoneum, or serosa.

The mesentery contains fat, blood vessels, lymphatics, lymph nodes, and nerves. The arterial blood supply to the jejunum and ileum derives from the superior mesenteric artery. Branches within the mesentery anastomose to form arcades (Figure 29–1), and small straight arteries travel from these arcades to enter the mesenteric border of the gut. The antimesenteric border of the intestinal wall is less richly supplied with arterial blood than the mesenteric side, so when blood flow is impaired, the antimesenteric border becomes ischemic first. Venous blood from the small intestine drains into the superior mesenteric vein and then enters the liver through the portal vein.

Submucosal lymphoid aggregates (Peyer patches) are much more numerous in the ileum than in the jejunum. Lymphatic channels within the mesentery drain through regional lymph nodes and terminate in the cisterna chyli.

Parasympathetic nerves from the right vagus and sympathetic fibers from the greater and lesser splanchnic nerves reach the small intestine through the mesentery. Both types of autonomic nerves contain efferent and afferent fibers, but intestinal pain appears to be mediated by the sympathetic afferents only.

Microscopic Anatomy

The wall of the small intestine consists of four layers: mucosa, submucosa, muscularis, and serosa.

A. Mucosa

The absorptive surface of the mucosa is multiplied by circular mucosal folds termed plicae circulares (valvulae conniventes) that project into the lumen; they are taller and more numerous in the proximal jejunum than in the distal ileum (Figure 29–1). On the surface of the plicae circulares are delicate villi less than 1 mm in height, each containing a central lacteal, a small artery and vein, and fibers from the muscularis mucosae that lend contractility to the villus. Villi are in turn covered by columnar epithelial cells that have a brush border consisting of microvilli 1 μm in height. The presence of villi multiplies the absorptive surface about 8 times, and microvilli increase it another 14–24 times; the total absorptive area of the small intestine is 200–500 m².

The major cell types in the epithelium of the small intestine are absorptive enterocytes, mucous cells, Paneth cells, endocrine cells, and M cells. Absorptive enterocytes are responsible for absorption; they arise from continually proliferating undifferentiated cells in the crypts of Lieberkühn (Figure 29–2) and migrate to the tips of villi over a 3–7-day period. Peptide growth factors regulate this process. The life span of enterocytes in humans is 5–6 days.

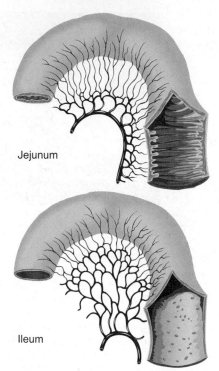

▲ Figure 29–1. Blood supply and luminal surface of the small bowel. The arterial arcades of the small intestine increase in number from one or two in the proximal jejunum to four or five in the distal ileum, a finding that helps to distinguish proximal from distal bowel at operation. Plicae circulares are more prominent in the jejunum.

Mucous cells originate in crypts and migrate to the tips of villi also; mature mucous cells are termed goblet cells. Paneth cells are found only in the crypts; their function is unknown but may be secretory. Endocrine cells have abundant cytoplasmic granules that contain 5-hydroxtryptamine and various peptides. Enterochromaffin cells are the most numerous; N cells (containing neurotensin), L cells (glucagon), and other cells containing motilin and cholecystokinin are also present. M cells are thin membranous cells that cover Peyer patches. They have the ability to sample luminal antigens such as proteins and microorganisms. Mucosal T lymphocytes of several phenotypes play an important role in mucosal cell–mediated immunity. Mast cells in the lamina propria are closely applied to nerve fibers, thus providing an anatomic basis for communication between these two structures in disease processes such as inflammation.

B. Other Layers

The submucosa is a fibroelastic layer containing blood vessels and nerves. Submucosa is the strongest component of bowel wall and must be included in intestinal sutures. The

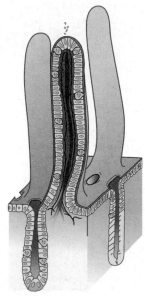

▲ Figure 29–2. Schematic representation of villi and crypts of Lieberkühn.

muscularis consists of an inner circular layer and an outer longitudinal coat of smooth muscle. The serosa is the outermost covering of the intestine.

Jones MP. Bratten JR: Small intestinal motility. Curr Opin Gastroenterol 2008;24:164.
Walters JR: Recent findings in the cell and molecular biology of the small intestine. Curr Opin Gastroenterol 2005;21:135.

PHYSIOLOGY

The principal function of the small intestine is absorption.

▶ Motility

Smooth muscles of the small intestine undergo spontaneous oscillations of membrane potential; these cyclic changes are termed pacesetter potentials or electrical control activity. Each segment of intestine has a characteristic frequency of pacesetter potentials; it is highest proximally, and it decreases progressively from duodenum to ileum. In intact intestine, higher-frequency pacesetter potentials can drive adjacent distal intestine so that both segments have the same frequency (said to be phase-locked). In humans, the duodenum determines the frequency of pacesetter potentials for the entire small intestine.

As pacesetter potentials spread distally, they bring the onset of action potentials and muscular contractions into phase. One type of muscular contraction (nonpropagating, or stationary) causes segmentation, which mixes chyme with digestive juices, repeatedly exposes the mixture to the absorptive surface, and moves chyme slowly in an aboral direction. Another type of muscular contraction (propagating) is peristaltic. Normal peristalsis is a short, weak propulsive movement that travels at about 1 cm/s for a distance of 10–15 cm before subsiding. Mean transit time for a solid meal is 4 hours from mouth to colon.

The enteric nervous system is a dominant regulator of all aspects of motility of the small intestine. The two major types of nerve plexuses in the enteric nervous system are the myenteric plexus, mainly responsible for control of peristaltic activity, and the submucosal plexus, which regulates secretion and absorption. The enteric nervous system contains four types of neurons: motor, secretory, sensory, and interneurons (which provide communication between neurons in the intestinal wall). Neurotransmitters found in the enteric nervous system include cholinergic, adrenergic, serotonergic, and peptidergic substances. Among the numerous peptides secreted by neurons in the enteric nervous system are cholecystokinin, vasoactive intestinal peptide (VIP), somatostatin, neurotensin, enkephalin, galanin, and substance P. In general, intestinal action potentials and muscular contractions are stimulated by substance P and galanin, and motility is inhibited by VIP, somatostatin, neurotensin, and enkephalin. Nitric oxide mediates neural inhibition in circular muscle of human small intestine.

Peristalsis is initiated by stretch of the intestinal wall by a food bolus, and a dual reflex is set in motion. The circular smooth muscle orad to the bolus contracts; this reflex is mediated by enteric neurons with acetylcholine and substance P as neurotransmitters. Simultaneous relaxation of the intestinal circular muscle below is mediated by enteric neurons using VIP as the neurotransmitter.

The interdigestive migrating myoelectric complex (MMC) originates every 1.5–2 hours in the stomach and duodenum of fasting mammals. It is an aborally progressive front of action potentials and muscular contractions consisting of three successive phases: a quiescent phase 1 with slow waves only, phase 2 with increasing action potential activity, and phase 3 with action potentials on every slow wave. The MMC progresses aborally until it reaches the colon, and then another burst of potentials and contractions begins proximally. The MMC has been called the "intestinal housekeeper" because it cleans up remnants of the preceding meal and gets rid of microorganisms that escaped destruction by gastric acid. The MMC is controlled by the enteric nervous system; motilin and 5-hydroxytryptamine may play regulatory roles. The MMC is abolished by ingestion of food, and some features are altered by major abdominal operations or peritonitis.

Numerous peptides have been found to act in the brain to alter gastrointestinal motility. Hypothalamic hormones (eg, corticotropin-releasing factor and thyrotropin-releasing hormone), calcitonin, and nearly all of the enteric nervous system neurotransmitters have central nervous system actions that affect motility, at least in animals. Exogenous opioids, including codeine and loperamide, exert antidiarrheal action by inhibition or disruption of the pattern of circular muscle contraction; some of these effects are mediated by the μ-opioid receptor on the smooth muscle of the bowel wall. The vagus plays an important role in many of these phenomena.

Paralytic (adynamic) ileus is routine after abdominal operations, and it also accompanies inflammatory conditions in the abdomen, intestinal ischemia, ureteral colic, pelvic fractures, and back injuries. Abdominal surgery abolishes gastrointestinal motility for a period of time that varies with the type of operation; the MMC returns within 3 hours after cholecystectomy, the small intestine recovers in 12–24 hours, and the colon may not regain normal motility until the sixth postoperative day. The clinical manifestations of postoperative ileus do not correlate well with the myoelectric parameters, however, and the pathophysiology of ileus remains incompletely understood. Corticotropin-releasing factor may be an important mediator of postoperative ileus.

Orocecal transit time is an important indicator of small bowel function. Transit may be accelerated in patients with diarrhea and delayed in constipation; a variety of disease states are responsible. Orocecal transit time can be measured by the lactulose breath hydrogen test. An ingested solution of lactulose reaches the cecum in about 90 minutes; colonic fermentation of lactulose produces hydrogen, which is detected in the breath. Several techniques of gamma scintigraphy, including the use of isotopically labeled pellets, are alternative methods of estimating small bowel transit time.

▶ Digestion, Secretion, & Absorption

With a few exceptions (eg, iron, calcium), the normal small intestine absorbs indiscriminately without regard to body composition. Absorption of fat, carbohydrate, and protein is just as complete in the obese patient as in the slender individual. The enteric nervous system regulates secretion and absorption in the small intestine; VIP is one mediator, and neuropeptide Y may be another.

A. Water and Electrolytes

Ingested fluid and salivary, gastric, biliary, pancreatic, and intestinal secretions present a total of 5–9 L of water to the absorptive surface of the small intestine each day, and 1–2 L are discharged from the ileum into the colon. Water is absorbed throughout the intestine, but the major site of absorption after a meal is in the upper tract.

The net flow of water and electrolytes across the intestinal mucosa is equal to the difference between absorption and secretion. The villi are mainly absorbing structures, and secretion of water and electrolytes is localized to the crypts. Much of the transfer of water and small solutes occurs via paracellular "shunt" pathways. The intercellular tight junctions between cells are actually rather loose, and it is through these "pores" that water moves passively in response to osmotic and hydrostatic pressures in the lumen and in the interstitial fluid. The pores are larger in the jejunum (0.7–0.9 nm) than in the ileum (0.3–0.4 nm). Hypertonic solutions in the duodenum and upper jejunum are rapidly brought into osmotic equilibrium with blood, and as the osmotic pressure of luminal contents is increased further by breakdown of large molecules into smaller ones, still more water enters the lumen. Net absorption of water accompanies active transport of ions and small molecules such as glucose and amino acids. If the lumen contains nonabsorbable solute, water is retained to maintain isotonicity.

Three mechanisms are responsible for sodium and chloride absorption in the small intestine: (1) active electrogenic transport of sodium, which establishes an electrical gradient for passive absorption of chloride, mostly through the paracellular pathway; (2) sodium absorption directly coupled to the absorption of water-soluble organic solutes such as hexoses, amino acids, and triglycerides, with passive absorption of chloride; and (3) neutral sodium chloride cotransport, in which a carrier at the mucosal membrane mediates the one-for-one entry of both ions into the cell. The ileum has low permeability to chloride, so that active absorption processes are needed for chloride in that part of the gut.

Potassium diffuses passively along electrical and concentration gradients. Calcium diffuses passively and also is actively transported, a process stimulated by vitamin D. Calcium absorption is most efficient in the duodenum, but because intestinal contents are in the jejunum and ileum longer, most calcium is absorbed in these areas. Magnesium is absorbed by all segments of the intestine, but relatively poorly. Iron is absorbed in the duodenum and jejunum, primarily as the ferrous ion.

Bicarbonate is absorbed by secretion of hydrogen ions in exchange for sodium ions; one bicarbonate ion is released into the interstitial fluid for every hydrogen ion secreted, and CO_2 is generated in the intestinal lumen. Phosphate is absorbed in all portions of the small bowel.

Epithelial transport of water and electrolytes is under partial control of the enteric nervous system. Ingestion of a meal increases the magnitude of jejunal water and electrolyte absorption by neuroendocrine mechanisms that have not been clarified. Intramural nervous reflexes elicited by luminal stimuli increase fluid secretion from the crypts. The afferent part of these reflexes is not well understood, but acetylcholine and perhaps substance P and VIP are secretory neurotransmitters on the efferent side. Absorption and secretion are influenced by other polypeptides such as somatostatin, corticosteroids, prostaglandins, neuropeptide YY, cyclic adenosine monophosphate (cAMP), various drugs, and bacterial toxins.

B. Carbohydrate

The polysaccharides starch and glycogen and the disaccharides sucrose and lactose comprise about half the calories ingested by humans. Digestion of starch is begun by salivary amylase and is completed by pancreatic amylase in the duodenum and upper jejunum. The products of hydrolysis are further hydrolyzed by contact with enzymes contained in the brush border of intestinal epithelial cells. The monosac-

charides glucose, galactose, and fructose are actively transported against a concentration gradient by a carrier-mediated mechanism that is dependent on and coupled to the absorption of sodium. Monosaccharides are delivered directly into portal blood from the intestinal mucosa.

Although the entire small intestine has the capacity for carbohydrate digestion and absorption, under normal circumstances most absorption of monosaccharides occurs in the duodenum and proximal jejunum. About 10% of dietary starch passes unabsorbed into the colon.

Fiber is an insoluble matrix substance of plant cells and is mostly indigestible by human enzymes. It is composed of the carbohydrates cellulose and hemicellulose and the noncarbohydrate lignin. Dietary fiber increases the osmotic load to the distal small intestine and colon and therefore increases stool mass.

C. Protein

Protein is denatured and partially digested in the stomach, but these steps are not essential. Pancreatic enzymes digest protein to form free amino acids and oligopeptides; oligopeptides are attacked by carboxypeptidases and aminopeptidases in the brush border, liberating amino acids, dipeptides, and tripeptides. Amino acids are absorbed by means of an active, carrier-mediated transport mechanism. Dipeptides and tripeptides are actively absorbed into columnar cells, where they are hydrolyzed completely to constituent amino acids. More than 80% of protein absorption occurs in the proximal 100 cm of jejunum. Absorption of ingested protein is virtually complete, and the protein excreted in feces is derived from bacteria, desquamated cells, and mucoproteins.

Important changes occur in the intestine during critical illness (eg, following trauma or abdominal surgery). The intestinal epithelial barrier to absorption of bacteria and endotoxins may be compromised, permitting translocation of bacteria into the circulation. Furthermore, glutamine extraction from the circulation by the small intestine is impaired in septic patients. Glutamine is the preferred fuel for oxidative metabolism by the enterocyte, and diminished uptake of this mucosal nutrient may be significant. In stressed states, glutamine deficiency is associated with mucosal atrophy.

D. Fat

Dietary fat is largely in the form of triglycerides, which are water-insoluble oil droplets until attacked by pancreatic lipase. Colipase, a protein in pancreatic juice, helps lipase adhere to the surface of these oil droplets as the triglycerides are partially hydrolyzed to fatty acids and 2-monoglycerides. These products of digestion are also water-insoluble, and their efficient absorption depends on the presence of bile acids. When the concentration of bile acids exceeds a certain level (the critical micellar concentration), they spontaneously aggregate to form micelles. Bile acids in micelles are arranged with the fat-soluble portion of the molecule toward the center of the aggregate and the water-soluble portion at the periphery; hydrophobic molecules such as fatty acids, monoglycerides, cholesterol, and fat-soluble vitamins are carried in the centers of the micelles.

Micelles release monoglycerides and fatty acids to enter the mucosal cells, where triglycerides are resynthesized, aggregated with phospholipid and cholesterol, and delivered to the lymph as chylomicrons. Medium-chain triglyceride is a synthetic substance that is hydrolyzed to water-soluble fatty acids that do not require bile acids for absorption. Also, these fatty acids are not reesterified to triglycerides in the mucosal cells; they pass directly into portal blood.

Normally, most of the ingested fat is digested and absorbed in the duodenum and proximal jejunum. Conjugated bile acids are actively absorbed in the distal ileum and returned via portal blood to the liver, where they again are secreted into the bile. Disease or resection of the terminal ileum disrupts this enterohepatic circulation, and increased amounts of bile acids enter the colon, where they induce net secretion of water and electrolytes and cause diarrhea (cholerrheic diarrhea). Malabsorbed fatty acids contribute to diarrhea by an effect similar to that of castor oil.

E. Vitamins

Vitamin B_{12} (cyanocobalamin) is a water-soluble cobalt compound that requires a special mechanism for absorption, because of its large molecular weight. Dietary vitamin B_{12} complexes with intrinsic factor, a mucoprotein secreted by the gastric parietal cells. The complex dissociates at the surface of cells in the distal ileum, and vitamin B_{12} enters the cells, perhaps by receptor-mediated endocytosis. Folic acid, thiamin, and ascorbic acid are also absorbed by active transport. Other water-soluble vitamins diffuse passively across the mucosa.

Fat-soluble vitamins—notably vitamins A, D, E, and K—are dissolved in mixed micelles and absorbed like other lipids. Since they are totally nonpolar lipids, the absence of bile seriously impairs their absorption.

Crenn P, Messing B, Cynober L: Citrulline as a biomarker of intestinal failure due to enterocyte mass reduction. Clin Nutr 2008;27:328.

De Block CE et al: Current concepts in gastric motility in diabetes mellitus. Curr Diabetes Rev 2006;2:113.

Jones MP, Bratten JR: Small intestinal motility. Curr Opin Gastroenterol 2008;24:164.

BLIND LOOP SYNDROME

The normal concentration of bacteria in the small intestine is about 10^5/mL. Mechanisms that limit bacterial populations include the continual flow of luminal contents, resulting from peristalsis, the interdigestive migrating myoelectric complex, gastric acidity, local effects of immunoglobulins, and the prevention of reflux of colonic contents by the ileocecal valve. Disturbance of any of these mechanisms can lead to bacterial overgrowth and blind loop (contaminated small bowel, intestinal bacterial overgrowth) syndrome. Strictures, diverticula, fistulas, or blind (poorly emptying) segments of intestine are anatomic lesions that cause stagnation and permit bacterial proliferation. In many patients, stasis of intestinal contents is the result of a functional abnormality of motility (eg, scleroderma). Bacterial overgrowth is observed in patients with immunodeficiency syndromes.

Steatorrhea, diarrhea, megaloblastic anemia, and malnutrition are the hallmarks of blind loop syndrome. Steatorrhea is the consequence of bacterial deconjugation and dehydroxylation of bile salts in the proximal small bowel. Deconjugated bile salts have a higher critical micellar concentration, and micelle formation is inadequate to solubilize ingested fat in preparation for absorption. The presence of partially digested triglycerides in the distal ileum inhibits jejunal motility; nevertheless, the unabsorbed fatty acids enter the colon, where they increase net secretion of water and electrolytes, and diarrhea results. Hypocalcemia occurs because calcium is bound to unabsorbed fatty acids in the intestinal lumen. Macrocytic anemia is due to malabsorption of vitamin B_{12}, largely because of binding of the vitamin by anaerobic bacteria. Malabsorption of carbohydrate and protein is due partly to bacterial catabolism and partly to impaired absorption of these nutrients because of direct damage to the small intestinal mucosa. All of these mechanisms contribute to malnutrition in blind loop syndrome.

Quantitative culture of upper intestinal aspirates is valuable if properly performed; bacterial counts of more than 10^5 per mL are generally abnormal. Endoscopic biopsies of duodenum can be helpful in patients with suspected small intestinal malabsorption. Laboratory studies reveal impaired absorption of orally administered vitamin B_{12} (Schilling test), D-xylose, and ^{14}C triolein. Fecal fat measurement is an obsolete procedure. A large variety of breath tests have been studied, but most have proved to be unreliable. The ^{14}C-D-xylose breath test is the best of these methods available at present. Anaerobic bacteria in the small bowel metabolize xylose, releasing $^{14}CO_2$, which is detected in the breath.

Surgical treatment of the underlying neoplasm, fistula, blind loop, diverticula, or other lesion is carried out whenever possible. A majority of patients do not have a problem that is amenable to surgical correction, however, and treatment consists of broad-spectrum antibiotics and drugs to control diarrhea. It may be necessary to use different antibiotics in sequence, guided by culture results and response to therapy. Damage to enterocytes appears to be reversible with treatment. Octreotide (somatostatin analog) may reduce bacterial overgrowth and improve abdominal symptoms in patients with scleroderma, according to a recent report.

Goulet O, Ruemmele F: Causes and management of intestinal failure in children. Gastroenterology 2006;130(2 suppl 1):S16.

Rana SV, Bhardwaj SB: Small intestinal bacterial overgrowth. Scand J Gastroenterol 2008;43:1030.

SHORT BOWEL SYNDROME

ESSENTIALS OF DIAGNOSIS

▶ Extensive small bowel resection.

▶ Diarrhea.

▶ Steatorrhea.

▶ Malnutrition.

▶ General Considerations

The absorptive capacity of the small intestine is normally far in excess of need. Short bowel syndrome may develop after extensive resection of the small intestine for trauma, mesenteric thrombosis, regional enteritis, radiation enteropathy, strangulated small bowel obstruction, or neoplasm. Necrotizing enterocolitis and congenital atresia are the most common pediatric causes.

The ability of a patient to maintain nutrition after massive small bowel resection depends on the extent and site of resection, the presence or absence of the colon, the absorptive function of the intestinal remnant, adaptation of remaining bowel, and the nature of the underlying disease process and its complications. When 3 m or less of the small intestine remain, serious nutritional abnormalities can develop. With 2 m or less remaining, function is clinically impaired in most patients, and many patients with 1 m or less of normal bowel require parenteral nutrition at home indefinitely. Some patients with a very short small bowel are net absorbers, and others are net secretors (ie, they put out more intestinal fluid than they take orally).

If the jejunum is resected, the ileum is able to take over most of its absorptive function. Because transport of bile salts, vitamin B_{12}, and cholesterol is localized to the ileum, resection of this region is poorly tolerated (Figure 29–3). Bile salt malabsorption causes diarrhea, and steatorrhea occurs if 100 cm or more of distal ileum is resected. Abdominal gamma counting after oral administration of 23-selena-25-homocholyltaurine (^{75}SeHCAT) is a test of bile acid absorption in the distal ileum. Blind loop syndrome due to bacterial overgrowth in the shortened small bowel (see previous section) compounds the problems. Patients who undergo colectomy in addition to extensive small bowel resection are among the most difficult to manage.

Calcium oxalate urinary tract calculi form in 7–10% of patients who have extensive ileal resection (or disease) and an intact colon. This condition, called **enteric hyperoxaluria,** results from excessive absorption of oxalate from the colon. Two synergistic mechanisms are responsible: (1) Unabsorbed fatty acids combine with calcium, preventing the formation of insoluble calcium oxalate and allowing oxalate to remain available for absorption. (2) Unabsorbed fatty acids and bile acids increase the permeability of the colon to oxalate.

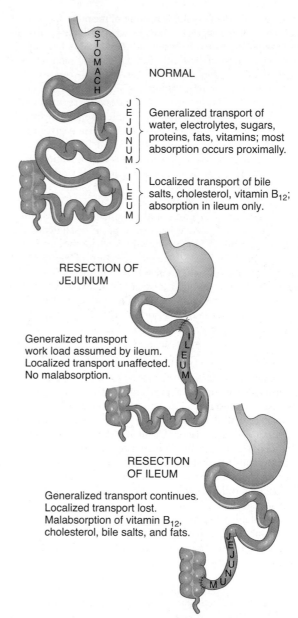

NORMAL

Generalized transport of water, electrolytes, sugars, proteins, fats, vitamins; most absorption occurs proximally.

Localized transport of bile salts, cholesterol, vitamin B_{12}; absorption in ileum only.

RESECTION OF JEJUNUM

Generalized transport work load assumed by ileum. Localized transport unaffected. No malabsorption.

RESECTION OF ILEUM

Generalized transport continues. Localized transport lost. Malabsorption of vitamin B_{12}, cholesterol, bile salts, and fats.

▲ **Figure 29–3.** The consequences of complete resection of jejunum or ileum are predictable in part from the loss of regionally localized transport processes.

D-Lactic acidosis may result from colonic fermentation of unabsorbed carbohydrate; symptoms of confusion, loss of memory, slurred speech, unsteady gait, and inappropriate behavior resemble those associated with alcoholic intoxication. Treatment includes correction of the acidosis with bicarbonate infusion, thiamine replacement, and antibiotics to reduce colonic flora.

Some patients develop gastric hypersecretion after extensive small bowel resection. It is more marked after proximal resection, and it improves with time. The outpouring of gastric juice may damage the mucosa of the upper intestine, inactivate lipase and trypsin by lowering intraluminal pH, and present an excessive solute load to the intestinal remnant. The increased acid production results from loss of inhibitory hormones normally secreted by the small intestine. Elevated basal and postprandial serum gastrin levels have been detected in some cases.

► Clinical Course

During the immediate postoperative period, more than 2 L of daily fluid and electrolyte losses from diarrhea are characteristic. The diarrhea is less severe after a few weeks, and eventually a reasonably normal existence is possible in most cases. The progression of a patient from strict dependence on intravenous feeding to nutritional maintenance by oral intake is possible because of intestinal **adaptation,** a compensatory increase of absorptive capacity in the intestinal remnant. The mucosa becomes hyperplastic, the villi lengthen and the crypts become deeper, the wall thickens, and the intestine elongates and dilates. The intensity of these responses is proportionate to the amount of intestine removed, the segment remaining (greater after proximal than after distal small bowel resection), and the presence of a luminal stream. Nutritional support is essential, and although nutrition must be provided intravenously at first, food in the lumen of the intestine is required for full adaptation. Short-chain fatty acids and long-chain triglycerides, sugars, and proteins are all important trophic nutrients. Glutamine is the principal fuel utilized by the small intestine, and gut glutamine extraction is increased in the first week after massive small bowel resection in animals, but it is not clear whether glutamine needs to be provided to patients to aid in adaptation. Circulating peptide factors no doubt are important. Enteroglucagon, epidermal growth factor (urogastrone), neurotensin, and insulinlike growth factors are implicated as trophic agents, and somatostatin and transforming growth factor-β (TGF-β) may play inhibitory roles.

► Treatment

A. General Measures

Treatment of severe short bowel syndrome may be divided into three stages:

1. Stage 1 (intravenous feeding)—During this stage, which lasts 1–3 months, diarrhea is massive and patients should receive nothing by mouth. Careful intravenous fluid and electrolyte therapy and parenteral nutrition must be given. Catheter sepsis is a common complication in this setting. Other important measures include reduction of gastric secretion with intravenous H_2 blockers or proton pump inhibitors, control of diarrhea (eg, with loperamide, diphenoxylate, or deodorized tincture of opium), and protection of perianal skin from irritation. Somatostatin has limited value in reduction of fecal output.

2. Stage 2 (intravenous and oral feeding)—Oral feedings should not be initiated until diarrhea subsides to less than 2.5 L/d. Intravenous nutrition should continue while oral intake begins. Oral rehydration solutions that are used for diarrheal diseases in developing countries are applicable to short bowel syndrome as well. An oral solution of sodium and potassium salts and glucose takes advantage of the phenomenon of cotransport whereby sodium ions are absorbed with the hexose molecules across the intestinal epithelium. Other liquid diets are best tolerated if they are isotonic. Liquid polymeric diets are the next step, and then a more liberal selection of food is allowed. A diet with normal fat content is more palatable and just as effective as a low-fat diet.

Milk may aggravate diarrhea, because total intestinal lactase activity is severely reduced after extensive resection; cheese is tolerated because lactose has been digested in this product. There may be some advantage in making breakfast the largest meal of the day, because as a result of gallbladder filling during the overnight fast, morning may be the time when the greatest amount of bile salts are present in the proximal intestine.

3. Stage 3 (complete oral feeding)—After a few months, complete dependence on oral intake may be expected in patients with 1–2 m of remaining small bowel, but full adaptation may require up to 2 years. Maintenance of body weight at levels 20% or more below normal, acceptable bowel habits, and return to productive life are reasonable expectations in many patients. Chronic parenteral nutrition at home is required if oral intake is not tolerated.

Patients with extensive ileal resection require parenteral vitamin B_{12} (1000 μg intramuscularly every 2–3 months) for life. Hyperoxaluria often can be prevented by a diet low in fat and oxalate; supplementary oral calcium or citrate may be helpful. Oral cholestyramine to minimize diarrhea is usually rejected by patients due to texture and taste; loperamide (Imodium) and Lomotil are well tolerated. Pancreatic enzyme supplements may reduce diarrhea also. Deficiencies in magnesium, vitamins D, A, and K, and water-soluble vitamins should be prevented. Osteomalacia is common. Blind loop syndrome may require treatment. H_2 receptor antagonists or proton pump inhibitors reduce acid secretion and improve absorption in the early stages but probably are not needed long term. The incidence of cholelithiasis is increased in patients with short bowel syndrome, and symptoms should be investigated. Interestingly, the stones may be composed of pigment rather than cholesterol.

B. Adjunctive Surgical Procedures

Surgical procedures to slow intestinal transit, reduce gastric acidity, or increase the absorptive surface are not recommended routinely and are rarely used. Reversed segments, recirculating loops, and construction of valve mechanisms have been tried in the hope of slowing transit and improving absorption. None of these methods have a clearly established role. By enhancing bacterial growth, damaging additional bowel, and obstructing the intestine, they are likely to make matters worse. Gastric hyperacidity is controlled by H_2 receptor antagonists, and operation is rarely necessary for this problem. A method of lengthening the small intestine by longitudinal division of the bowel and its mesentery has been described for certain pediatric situations.

C. Small Bowel Transplantation

Small bowel transplantation has become the treatment of choice for patients with life-threatening complications of intestinal failure. It is estimated that 15–20% of patients on chronic total parenteral nutrition for short bowel syndrome or intestinal failure will eventually require small bowel transplantation. Long-term parenteral nutrition frequently leads to liver failure, so a combined liver and small bowel transplantation is often necessary. Early attempts at intestinal transplantation were unsuccessful due to both technical and immunologic failure. However, the introduction of newer immunosuppressive drugs, such as tacrolimus, as well as improvement in surgical technique make intestinal transplantation a viable option for select patients with short bowel syndrome who are dependent on total parenteral nutrition.

Buchman AL, Scolapio J, Fryer J: AGA technical review on short bowel syndrome and intestinal transplantation. Gastroenterology 2003;124:1111.

Jeppesen PB: Glucagon-like peptide 2 improves nutrient absorption and nutritional status in short-bowel patients with no colon. Gastroenterology 2001;120:806.

Langnas AN: Advances in small-intestine transplantation. Transplantation 2004;77:S75.

OBSTRUCTION OF THE SMALL INTESTINE

 ESSENTIALS OF DIAGNOSIS

Complete proximal obstruction:

▶ Vomiting.
▶ Abdominal discomfort.
▶ Abnormal oral contrast x-rays or CT scan.

Complete mid or distal obstruction:

▶ Colicky abdominal pain.
▶ Vomiting.
▶ Abdominal distention.
▶ Constipation-obstipation.
▶ Peristaltic rushes.
▶ Dilated small bowel on x-ray.
▶ Transition point on CT scan.

▶ General Considerations

Obstruction is the most common surgical disorder of the small intestine.

Mechanical obstruction implies a physical barrier that impedes aboral progress of intestinal contents; it may be complete or partial. **Simple obstruction** occludes the lumen only; **strangulation obstruction** impairs the blood supply also and leads to necrosis of the intestinal wall. Most simple obstructions occur at only one point. Closed loop obstruction, in which the lumen is occluded in at least two places (eg, in a volvulus), is commonly associated with strangulation. Ileus is a term whose definition includes mechanical obstruction, but in the United States, it usually refers to **paralytic ileus** (adynamic ileus), a disorder in which there is neurogenic failure of peristalsis to propel intestinal contents but no mechanical obstruction.

A. Etiology

1. Adhesions—Adhesions are by far the most common cause of mechanical small bowel obstruction (Table 29–1). Congenital bands are seen in children, but adhesions acquired from abdominal operations or inflammation are much more frequent in adults.

2. Neoplasms—Intrinsic small bowel neoplasms can progressively occlude the lumen or serve as a leading point in intussusception. Symptoms may be intermittent, onset of obstruction is slow, and signs of chronic anemia are present. Neoplasms extrinsic to small bowel may entrap loops, and strategically situated lesions of the colon—particularly those near the ileocecal valve—may present as small bowel obstruction.

3. Hernia—Incarceration of an external hernia is uncommon since prophylactic repair of hernias became routine. Inguinal, femoral, or umbilical hernias may have been present for years, or the patient may be unaware of the defect before the onset of obstructive symptoms. An incarcerated hernia may be overlooked by the examining surgeon, particularly if the patient is obese or if the hernia is of the femoral type, and a careful search for external hernias must be made

Table 29–1. Causes of Obstruction of the Small Intestine in Adults.

Causes	Relative Incidence (%)
Adhesions	60
External hernia	10
Neoplasms	20
Intrinsic	3
Extrinsic	17
Miscellaneous	10

during evaluation of every patient with acute abdominal illness. Internal hernias into the obturator foramen, foramen epiploicum (Winslow), or other anatomic defects are rare, but internal herniation is one of several mechanisms by which acquired adhesions produce obstruction. Surgical defects—lateral to an ileostomy, for example—also provide sites for internal herniation of small bowel loops.

4. Intussusception—Invagination of one loop of intestine into another is rarely encountered in adults and is usually caused by a polyp or other intraluminal lesion. Intussusception is more often seen in children; an organic lesion is not required, and the syndrome of colicky pain, passage of blood per rectum, and a palpable mass (the intussuscepted segment) is characteristic.

5. Volvulus—Volvulus results from rotation of bowel loops about a fixed point, often the consequence of congenital anomalies or acquired adhesions. Onset of obstruction is abrupt, and strangulation develops rapidly. Malrotation of the intestine is a cause of volvulus in infants and rarely in adults.

6. Foreign bodies—Bezoars and ingested foreign bodies may pass into the intestine and block the lumen.

7. Gallstone ileus—Passage of a large gallstone into the intestine through a cholecystenteric fistula may produce obstruction of the small bowel. Gallstone ileus is discussed in Chapter 25.

8. Inflammatory bowel disease—Inflammatory bowel disease (Regional enteritis) often causes obstruction when the lumen is narrowed by inflammation or fibrosis of the wall.

9. Stricture—Stricture due to ischemia or radiation injury or surgical trauma can result in mechanical obstruction.

10. Cystic fibrosis—Cystic fibrosis causes chronic partial obstruction of the distal ileum and right colon in adolescents and adults. It is equivalent to meconium ileus in newborns.

11. Hematoma—Hematoma may develop spontaneously in the intestinal wall in a patient taking anticoagulants.

B. Pathophysiology

The small bowel proximal to a point of obstruction distends with gas and fluid. Swallowed air is the major source of gaseous distention, at least in the early stages, because nitrogen is not well absorbed by mucosa. When bacterial fermentation occurs later on, other gases are produced; the partial pressure of nitrogen within the lumen is lowered, and a gradient for diffusion of nitrogen from blood to lumen is established.

Enormous quantities of fluid from the extracellular space are lost into the gut and from the serosa into the peritoneal cavity. Fluid fills the lumen proximal to the obstruction, because the bidirectional flux of salt and water is disrupted and net secretion is enhanced. Mediator substances (eg,

endotoxin, prostaglandins) released from proliferating bacteria in the static luminal contents are responsible. Somatostatin effectively inhibits secretion in animal models of intestinal obstruction, but it has no defined role in humans. Reflexly induced vomiting accentuates the fluid and electrolyte deficit. Hypovolemia leads to multiorgan system failure and is the cause of death in patients with nonstrangulating obstruction.

Audible peristaltic rushes are manifestations of attempts by the small bowel to propel its contents past the obstruction. The vomitus becomes feculent—particularly with distal obstruction—as the illness progresses. Bacterial translocation from lumen to mesenteric nodes and the bloodstream occurs even in simple obstruction. Abdominal distention elevates the diaphragm and impairs respiration, so that pulmonary complications are frequent.

Strangulation is a threat early in the course of closed loop obstruction but must be feared in any complete mechanical obstruction. Incarcerated inguinal hernia and volvulus are examples of obstructing mechanisms that occlude the vascular supply as well as the intestinal lumen. Strangulation rarely if ever results just from progressive distention. Venous drainage is more apt to be interrupted than arterial inflow when the mesentery is trapped. Gangrenous intestine bleeds into the lumen and into the peritoneal cavity, and eventually it perforates. The luminal contents of strangulated intestine are a toxic mixture of bacteria, bacterial products, necrotic tissue, and blood. Some of this fluid may enter the circulation by way of intestinal lymphatics or by absorption from the peritoneal cavity; septic shock is the result.

▶ Clinical Findings

A. Simple Obstruction

1. Symptoms and signs—(Figure 29–4). Proximal (high) small bowel obstruction usually presents as profuse vomiting that seldom becomes feculent even in prolonged obstruction. Abdominal pain is variable and often is described as upper abdominal discomfort rather than cramping pain.

Obstruction of the mid or distal small intestine causes cramping periumbilical or poorly localized abdominal pain. Each episode of cramps has a crescendo-decrescendo pattern, lasts for a few seconds to a few minutes, and recurs every few minutes. Between cramps, the patient may be entirely free of pain. Vomiting follows the onset of pain after an interval that varies with the level of obstruction; it may not occur until several hours later. The more distal the obstruction, the more likely it is that vomitus will become feculent. Gas and feces present in the colon may be expelled after the onset of pain, but obstipation always occurs eventually in complete obstruction.

Vital signs may be normal in the early stages, but dehydration is noted with continued loss of fluid and electrolytes. Temperature is normal or mildly elevated. Abdominal distention is minimal to absent in proximal obstruction but is pronounced in more distal obstruction. Peristalsis in dilated

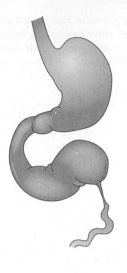
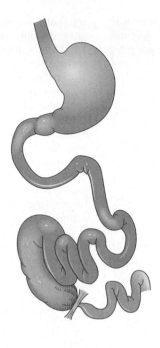
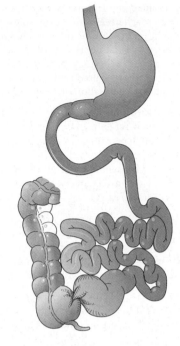

High	**Middle**	**Low**
Frequent vomiting. No distention. Intermittent pain but not classic crescendo type.	Moderate vomiting. Moderate distention. Intermittent pain (crescendo, colicky) with free intervals.	Vomiting late, feculent. Marked distention. Variable pain; may not be classic crescendo type.

▲ **Figure 29–4.** Small bowel obstruction. Variable manifestations of obstruction depend on the level of blockage of the small bowel.

loops of small bowel may be visible beneath the abdominal wall in thin patients. Mild tenderness may be elicited. Peristaltic rushes, gurgles, and high-pitched tinkles are audible in coordination with attacks of cramping pain in distal obstruction. Incarcerated hernias should be sought. Rectal examination is usually normal.

2. Laboratory findings—In the early stages, laboratory findings may be normal; with progression of disease, there are hemoconcentration, leukocytosis, and electrolyte abnormalities that depend on the level of obstruction and the severity of dehydration. Serum amylase is often elevated.

3. Imaging studies—Supine and upright plain abdominal films reveal a ladderlike pattern of dilated small bowel loops with air-fluid levels (Figure 29–5). These features may be minimal or absent in early obstruction, proximal obstruction, or closed loop obstruction or in some cases when fluid-filled loops contain little gas. The colon is often devoid of gas unless the patient has been given an enema, has undergone sigmoidoscopy, or has only a partial obstruction. Opaque gallstones and air in the biliary tree should be looked for.

Administration of contrast media orally confirms the presence of mechanical obstruction and its completeness. CT scan is highly accurate in making the diagnosis of and determining the level of a small bowel obstruction.

B. Strangulation Obstruction

Although certain clinical features should make the surgeon suspicious of strangulation, no historical, physical, or laboratory findings entirely exclude the possibility of strangulation in complete small bowel obstruction. At least one third of strangulation obstructions are unsuspected before operation, which underscores the need for early operation whenever obstruction is complete.

1. Symptoms and signs—Shock that appears early in the course of obstruction suggests a strangulated closed loop. When strangulation supervenes in simple obstruction, high fever may develop, previously cramping abdominal pain may become a severe continuous ache, vomitus may contain gross or occult blood, and abdominal tenderness and rigidity may appear.

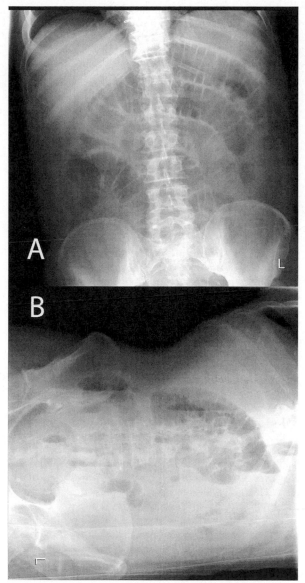

▲ **Figure 29–5.** Small bowel obstruction. **A:** Supine film showing dilated loops of small bowel and no gas in the colon. **B:** Decubitus film showing air-fluid levels consistent with obstruction.

2. Laboratory findings—Marked leukocytosis not accounted for by hemoconcentration alone should suggest strangulation, as does lactic acidosis that does not resolve with volume resuscitation.

3. Imaging studies—Intraperitoneal fluid is seen as widened spaces between adjacent loops of dilated bowel on plain films and is often found in simple obstruction as well as in strangulation. Thumbprinting, loss of mucosal pattern, and gas within the bowel wall or within intrahepatic branches of the portal vein may be seen in strangulation. Air-fluid levels outside the bowel indicate perforation. CT scanning is reported to have a sensitivity of 90% or higher in detecting complete or high-grade small bowel obstruction. It also provides information as to the cause of the obstruction and the severity of bowel injury. The CT scan may reveal a whirling pattern in the mesentery of patients with a volvulus and closed loop obstruction as well as raise the suspicion of intestinal ischemia by documenting thickening and edema of the bowel wall or, in late cases, intramural air.

► **Differential Diagnosis**

Pain from paralytic ileus is usually not severe but is constant and diffuse, and the abdomen is distended and mildly tender. If ileus has resulted from an acute intraperitoneal inflammatory process (eg, acute appendicitis), there should be symptoms and signs of the primary problem as well as the ileus. Plain films show gas mainly in the colon in uncomplicated postoperative ileus; gas in the small bowel suggests peritonitis. CT may be required in order to distinguish ileus from mechanical obstruction in postoperative patients.

Obstruction of the large intestine is characterized by obstipation and abdominal distention; pain is less often colicky, and vomiting is an inconstant symptom. X-rays usually make the diagnosis by demonstrating colonic dilation proximal to the obstructing lesion. If the ileocecal valve is incompetent, the distal small bowel will be dilated, and a barium enema may be needed to determine the level of obstruction. This subject is covered in detail in Chapter 30.

Acute gastroenteritis, acute appendicitis, and acute pancreatitis can mimic simple intestinal obstruction. Strangulation obstruction may be confused with acute hemorrhagic pancreatitis or mesenteric vascular occlusion.

Intestinal pseudoobstruction is a diverse group of disorders in which there are symptoms and signs of intestinal obstruction without evidence for an obstructing lesion. Acute pseudoobstruction of the colon carries the risk of cecal perforation and is discussed in Chapter 30. Chronic or recurrent pseudoobstruction affecting the small bowel with or without colonic involvement is often idiopathic. In other cases, pseudoobstruction is associated with scleroderma, myxedema, lupus erythematosus, amyloidosis, drug abuse (eg, phenothiazine ingestion), radiation injury, or progressive systemic sclerosis. Several variations of familial visceral *myopathy* have been identified with seemingly distinct patterns of intestinal pseudoobstruction. Patients with familial visceral *neuropathy* have degeneration of axons and neurons of the myenteric plexus of the gastrointestinal tract, and pseudoobstruction results.

Patients with chronic pseudoobstruction have recurrent attacks of vomiting, cramping abdominal pain, and abdominal distention. In some patients the esophagus, stomach, small bowel, colon, and urinary bladder all have abnormal motility, but in others one or more of these organs may be spared. Treatment is directed at the underlying disease if there is one. Management of idiopathic pseudoobstruction is largely supportive.

▶ Treatment

Partial small bowel obstruction can be treated expectantly as long as there is continued passage of stool and flatus. Plain abdominal x-rays show gas in the colon, and small bowel contrast x-rays prove the diagnosis. Decompression with a nasogastric tube is successful in 90% of such patients. Operation may be required if obstruction persists for several days even though it is incomplete. The decision of when—if ever—to operate for repeatedly recurring partial small bowel obstructions that resolve with nonoperative treatment can be a difficult one.

Complete obstruction of the small intestine is treated by operation after a period of careful preparation. The compelling reason for operation is that strangulation cannot be excluded with certainty, and strangulation is associated with high rates of complications and death. The surgeon must avoid being lulled into a false sense of security by the improvement in symptoms and signs that almost invariably occurs after resuscitation.

There are exceptions to the general rule that operation must be performed promptly: Incomplete obstruction, postoperative obstruction, a history of numerous previous operations for obstruction, radiation therapy, inflammatory bowel disease, and abdominal carcinomatosis are situations demanding mature judgment, and judicious nonoperative management may be in the patient's best interests. A long intestinal tube (eg, Miller-Abbott tube) may be passed in these cases to decompress the intestine.

A. Preparation

Proper timing of the operation is determined by the requirements of individual patients. The risk of strangulation must be weighed against the severity of fluid and electrolyte abnormalities and the need for evaluation and treatment of associated systemic diseases.

1. Nasogastric suction—A nasogastric tube should be inserted immediately upon admission to the emergency ward in order to relieve vomiting, avoid aspiration, and reduce the contribution of further swallowed air to the abdominal distention.

2. Fluid and electrolyte resuscitation—Depending upon the level and duration of obstruction, fluid and electrolyte deficits are mild to severe. Hemoconcentration induced by longstanding obstruction cannot be corrected by dextrose solutions alone. Fluid losses are isotonic, and resuscitation should begin with infusion of isotonic saline solution. Losses of gastrointestinal fluid also entail acid-base deficits, and since there is no neuroendocrine mechanism for correcting these deficits, the surgeon must do so. Serum electrolyte concentrations and arterial blood gas determinations are

guides to electrolyte therapy; potassium is best withheld until urine output is satisfactory, but patients should not undergo operation until hypokalemia has been treated. The volume of fluid required and its exact electrolyte composition must be calculated for each patient, and careful monitoring of clinical signs and associated systemic diseases is imperative. Some patients—notably those with strangulation obstruction—require plasma or blood. Antibiotics should be given if strangulation is even remotely suspected.

B. Operation

Operation may commence when the patient has been rehydrated and vital organs are functioning satisfactorily. Occasionally, the toxic effects of strangulation may force operation at an earlier time.

A standard groin incision is used for patients with incarcerated inguinal or femoral hernias. Laparoscopic adhesiolysis may be performed in carefully selected patients by surgeons skilled in this procedure. Generally, however, an open procedure is performed through an incision that is partly dictated by the location of scars from previous operations.

Details of the operative procedure vary according to the cause of obstruction. Adhesive bands causing obstruction should be lysed; an obstructing tumor should be resected; and an obstructing foreign body should be removed through an enterotomy. Gangrenous intestine must be resected, but it may be difficult to determine whether obstructed bowel is viable or not. The loop should be wrapped in a warm saline-soaked pack and inspected for color, mesenteric pulsation, and peristalsis several minutes later. Intraoperative use of Doppler ultrasound is a method of determining viability of obstructed intestine. The qualitative fluorescein test may be helpful; 1000 mg of fluorescein is injected into a peripheral vein over 30–60 s, and the bowel is then inspected under ultraviolet (Wood) light. If the loop appears nonviable, resection with end-to-end anastomosis is the safest course.

Extirpation of the obstructing lesion is not possible in some patients with carcinoma or radiation injury. Anastomosis of proximal small bowel to small or large intestine distal to the obstruction (bypass) may be the best procedure in these patients. Rarely, adhesions are so dense that the intestine cannot be freed and bypass cannot be accomplished. Prolonged decompression through a gastrostomy or jejunostomy tube and provision of nutrition via the parenteral route may allow spontaneous resolution over a period of a few weeks.

Decompression of massively dilated small bowel loops facilitates closure of the abdomen and may shorten the time for recovery of bowel function postoperatively. Decompression is accomplished by threading down a long tube passed orally or by needle aspiration through the bowel wall.

Attempts to prevent uncontrolled adhesion formation by suturing loops of bowel so that they are fixed in a suitable relation to one another (Nobel plication procedures) are unsuccessful. However, another procedure in which a long tube is inserted through a gastrostomy or jejunostomy for 10 days to provide intraluminal stenting has some proponents. Adhesion prevention with a hyaluronic acid methylcellulose bioabsorbable barrier has proved effective in decreasing adhesion formation and decreasing reoperative times. Studies proving efficacy in reducing the incidence of small bowel obstructions have shown a small benefit.

▶ Prognosis

Nonstrangulating obstruction has a death rate of about 2%; most of these deaths occur in the elderly. Strangulation obstruction has a mortality rate of approximately 8% if operation is performed within 36 hours of the onset of symptoms and 25% if operation is delayed beyond 36 hours. Recurrent obstruction after lysis of adhesions is uncommon.

Beck DE et al: A prospective, randomized, multicenter, controlled study of the safety of Sepra film adhesion barrier in abdomino-pelvic surgery of the intestine. Dis Colon Rectum 2003;46:1310.

Fevang BT et al: Long-term prognosis after operation for adhesive small bowel obstruction. Ann Surg 2004;240:193.

Jenkins JT: Secondary causes of intestinal obstruction: rigorous preoperative evaluation is required. Am Surg 2000;66:662.

Lazarus DE et al: Frequency and relevance of the "small-bowel feces" sign on CT in patients with small-bowel obstruction. Am J Roentgenol 2004;183:1361.

Miller G et al: Natural history of patients with adhesive small bowel obstruction. Br J Surg 2000;87:1240.

Ryan MD et al: Adhesional small bowel obstruction after colorectal surgery. ANZ J Surg 2004;74:1010.

Scaglione M et al: Helical CT diagnosis of small bowel obstruction in the acute clinical setting. Eur J Radiol 2004;50:15.

Zalcman M et al: Helical CT signs in the diagnosis of intestinal ischemia in small-bowel obstruction. Am J Roentgenol 2000; 175:1601.

ACQUIRED INTESTINAL DIVERTICULA*

Congenital diverticula of the jejunum are rare, but acquired diverticula are found in the jejunum (or ileum) in 1.3% of radiographic studies or autopsy series when specifically sought. Jejunal diverticula are wide-mouthed sacs measuring 1–25 cm in diameter. Most contain all layers of the intestinal wall (true diverticula), but some consist of mucosa and submucosa herniated through thickened muscularis (false diverticula). Diverticula in the small bowel are often multiple; they diminish in frequency from the ligament of Treitz to the ileocecal valve and are associated with diverticulosis of the duodenum or colon in 30% of cases. Most symptomatic patients are over age 60.

Jejunal diverticulosis is a heterogeneous disorder associated with abnormalities of smooth muscle or the myenteric plexus. Intestinal pseudoobstruction is a common associated problem, also reflecting the presence of an underlying motility disorder such as familial visceral myopathy or progressive systemic sclerosis.

Symptoms may be due to pseudoobstruction or to inflammation of the diverticula. Acute intestinal bleeding and diverticulitis leading to perforation may occur. Blind loop syndrome is caused by bacterial overgrowth in the stagnant bowel with pseudoobstruction or in large diverticula.

Barium x-rays may outline the diverticula and reveal the underlying motility disorder. The primary cause should be sought.

Operation is required for perforation or bleeding. Symptoms of the underlying motility disorder are not improved by resection of the segment containing diverticula.

Woods K et al: Acquired jejunoileal diverticulosis and its complications: a review of the literature. Am Surg 2008;74:849.

REGIONAL ENTERITIS†

ESSENTIALS OF DIAGNOSIS

- ▶ Diarrhea.
- ▶ Abdominal pain and palpable mass.
- ▶ Low-grade fever, lassitude, weight loss.
- ▶ Anemia.
- ▶ Radiographic findings of thickened, stenotic bowel with ulceration and internal fistulas.

▶ General Considerations

Regional enteritis (Crohn disease) is a chronic progressive granulomatous inflammatory disorder of the gastrointestinal tract. In the United States and Europe, 2–9 cases per 100,000 population are detected annually. The prevalence ranges broadly from 20 to 90 per 100,000 population. There is geographic variation (more common in urban dwellers and Northern U.S. residents), and there is a relatively high incidence among Ashkenazi Jews. The peak incidence occurs between the second and fourth decades. Cigarette smoking and a high intake of sugar are independent risk factors for regional enteritis.

A. Etiology

Considerable progress has been made recently elucidating the underlying etiology of regional enteritis. A complex interaction between genetic factors, environmental factors, host immune response, and inflammatory pathways is thought to result in inappropriate and ongoing activation of the mucosal immune system. A genetic influence is supported by several studies showing that first-degree relatives of patients with regional enteritis have an incidence of

---

*Meckel diverticulum and other congenital diverticula of the small intestine are discussed in Chapter 43.

†Crohn disease of the colon is discussed in Chapter 30.

regional enteritis that is 4–20 times that of the general population. The cause of regional enteritis is unknown; a number of candidate genes have been identified and are the subject of intense study. However, despite the role that genetics certainly plays in the development of regional enteritis, environmental factors contribute as well, including the host immune response to luminal flora.

B. Pathology

Regional enteritis may affect any part of the gastrointestinal tract from the lips to the anus and may even spill over into the larynx or extend beyond the gut to the skin. "Metastatic" skin lesions have been described. The distal ileum is the most frequent site of involvement, eventually becoming diseased in about three fourths of patients. The small bowel alone is involved in 15–30%, both the distal ileum and the colon in 40–60%, and the large bowel alone in 25–30%. Duodenal regional enteritis is found in 0.5–7% of patients. Discontinuous areas of disease with segments of normal bowel between them ("skip lesions") occur in 15% of patients. Subtle histologic changes can be seen in "normal," grossly uninvolved intestine of patients with regional enteritis, suggesting that the mucosa of the entire bowel may be abnormal in this disorder.

The earliest lesion is a focal accumulation of inflammatory cells adjacent to an epithelial crypt. Candidate mediators of inflammation include plasma activating factor, leukotrienes, complement, cytokines, enterotoxin, interleukins, tumor necrosis factor, phospholipase A_2, and neurotransmitters of the enteric nervous system. In a process similar to that seen in ischemia, reactive molecules such as oxygen radicals are generated; they propagate the inflammatory response and contribute to tissue damage. Erosions, crypt abscesses, and granulomas result.

Granulomas are seen in the bowel wall in 50–70% and in mesenteric lymph nodes in 25% of patients. The number of granulomas is related to the duration of disease and the site of involvement. It has been speculated that granuloma formation reflects efforts to localize or eliminate the causative agent of regional enteritis. Mucosal lesions appear grossly as tiny (pinpoint) hemorrhagic spots or shallow ulcers with white bases and elevated margins (aphthous ulcers). Punched-out ulcers are seen with progression of the disease. The next stage is development of fissures—knifelike clefts beginning in mucosa and extending deeply into the wall. These fissures and the serpiginous or linear ulcers surrounding islands of intact mucosa overlying edematous submucosa give a cobblestone appearance to the luminal surface. Regional enteritis ultimately becomes a transmural inflammatory process with thickening of the bowel wall, and it often progresses to stricture formation. The bowel and its mesentery are foreshortened in advanced cases, and on gross inspection, mesenteric fat seems to have advanced over the surface of the bowel toward the antimesenteric border.

▶ Clinical Findings

A. Symptoms and Signs

Regional enteritis has many modes of presentation:

1. Diarrhea—Continuous or episodic diarrhea is noted in about 90% of patients. Stools are liquid or semisolid and characteristically contain no blood if small bowel alone is diseased. One third of patients with colonic involvement pass blood, and a few present with bloody diarrhea resembling that seen in ulcerative colitis.

2. Recurrent abdominal pain—Mild colic initiated by meals, centered in the lower abdomen, and relieved by defecation is common. These symptoms are due to chronic partial obstruction of the small bowel, colon, or both. Some patients progress to complete obstruction, and they have severe cramping, vomiting, and abdominal distention.

3. Abdominal symptoms and constitutional effects—Episodic attacks of abdominal pain and diarrhea accompanied by lassitude, malaise, weight loss, fever, and anemia are a common syndrome. A mass is often palpable in the right lower quadrant in these patients. Occasionally, fever of unknown origin is the only clinical finding.

4. Anorectal lesions—Chronic anal fissures, large ulcers, edematous skin tags, complex anal fistulas, or pararectal abscesses are seen in 15–25% of patients with regional enteritis otherwise confined to small bowel and in 50–75% of those with colonic involvement. These problems may appear many years before the intestinal disease. Histologic features of regional enteritis, including granulomas, are often found in biopsies of anorectal lesions even when the only other identifiable disease is located much higher in the gastrointestinal tract.

5. Anemia—Iron deficiency anemia or macrocytic anemia resulting from vitamin B_{12} or folate deficiency due to poor absorption from terminal ileal disease may occur in the absence of abdominal symptoms.

6. Malnutrition—Protein-losing enteropathy, steatorrhea, chronic obstruction, and diminished dietary intake from chronic illness contribute to malnutrition and weight loss. Mineral and vitamin deficiencies (especially vitamin D deficiency) are common. Deficiencies of water-soluble and fat-soluble vitamins are common in patients with regional enteritis of the small intestine, but clinical symptoms of vitamin deficiency are rare. Zinc deficiency has been recognized. Children afflicted with extensive regional enteritis fail to grow and may have severely retarded sexual maturation. Reversal of growth arrest by parenteral feeding emphasizes the importance of malnutrition as a cause of growth failure in regional enteritis.

7. Acute onset—Acute abdominal pain and right lower quadrant tenderness mimicking acute appendicitis may be found at operation to be due to acute inflammation of the distal ileum. Only 15% of such cases evolve into chronic regional enteritis, suggesting that most patients with acute ileitis have an infectious process unrelated to regional enteritis. This condition is discussed further in the section on Acute Enteritis & Mesenteric Lymphadenitis.

8. Systemic complications—Any of the systemic complications described below may prompt the patient to seek medical advice.

B. Laboratory Findings

Test results are nonspecific and vary greatly according to the site of intestinal involvement, the severity of disease, and the presence of complications such as abscess or fistula. The sedimentation rate may not be elevated in patients with disease of the small intestine. Hypoalbuminemia, anemia, and steatorrhea are common. Abnormal D-xylose absorption suggests extensive disease or fistula formation, since carbohydrate is normally absorbed in the jejunum. Breath tests, as described in the section on Blind Loop Syndrome, are abnormal if the ileum is diseased or if bacterial overgrowth has occurred, but are rarely used clinically.

C. Imaging Studies

Radiographic studies contribute substantially to the diagnosis of regional enteritis. The appearance of small bowel during a barium small bowel follow-through is a composite of proliferative and destructive changes. The principal findings include thickened bowel wall with stricture ("string sign"), longitudinal ulceration that is shallow at first but becomes deep and undermining, deep transverse fissures resembling spicules, and cobblestone formation (Figure 29–6). Deformity of the cecum, fistulas, abscesses, and skip lesions are additional findings of importance. Enteroclysis provides excellent detail. CT scan is useful for identifying thickened, abnormal loops of small bowel, strictured areas leading to obstruction, and abscesses due to contained perforation of the intestine.

D. Endoscopy

Upper gastrointestinal endoscopy diagnoses esophageal, gastric, and duodenal lesions. Colonoscopy reveals typical changes of regional enteritis in the colon if it is involved or in the ileum if it can be examined. Ileoscopy after colectomy is accurate for the diagnosis of regional enteritis in the ileum.

E. Capsule Endoscopy

The capsule endoscope is a disposable plastic capsule that weighs 3.7 g and measures 11 mm in diameter and 26 mm in length. The contents include a silicon chip camera, a short focal-length lens, four white light-emitting diode (LED) illumination sources, two silver oxide batteries, and a UHF band radio telemetry transmitter. Peristalsis propels the capsule through the intestine and pictures are received at a rate of 2 frames per second. Although the diagnostic yield of

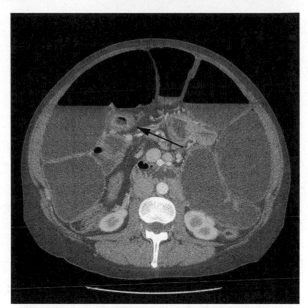

▲ **Figure 29–6.** CT scan showing a markedly thickened loop of distal ileum (*arrow*) causing obstruction of the more proximal small bowel in regional enteritis.

capsule endoscopy in regional enteritis is high, its use has a positive impact on clinical outcome in only a small number of patients. Capsule endoscopy should not be used in the setting of a known stricture, as its use may lead to complete obstruction or perforation requiring surgery that may have otherwise not been needed.

▶ Differential Diagnosis

A. Ulcerative Colitis

Regional enteritis of the colon may be difficult to distinguish from ulcerative colitis. This topic is covered in detail in Chapter 30.

B. Appendicitis

Acute ileitis may be the presenting manifestation, and differentiation from appendicitis may be impossible without operation.

B. Tuberculosis

Tuberculosis may affect any part of the gastrointestinal tract but is uncommon distal to the cecum. Small bowel tuberculosis is discussed elsewhere in this chapter.

D. Lymphoma

Radiographic findings help differentiate lymphoma from regional enteritis, but histologic examination of the tissue is occasionally required before the diagnosis is certain. Rectal or colonic biopsies that show granulomas or colitis may support the diagnosis of regional enteritis.

E. Other Diseases

Carcinoma, amebiasis, ischemia, eosinophilic gastroenteritis, nonsteroidal anti-inflammatory enteropathy, and other inflammatory conditions may simulate regional enteritis.

▶ Complications

A. Intestinal

Some intestinal complications, such as obstruction, abscess, fistula, and anorectal lesions, are so common that they are regarded as part of the characteristic clinical picture. Free perforation and massive hemorrhage are uncommon. The risk of cholelithiasis is increased. Oral manifestations of regional enteritis may cause disabling pain. Carcinoma may occur in segments of small or large bowel that are involved with regional enteritis, especially in segments excluded from the fecal stream by surgical bypass procedures.

B. Systemic

Systemic complications such as hepatobiliary disease, uveitis, arthritis, ankylosing spondylitis, aphthous ulcers, erythema nodosum, amyloidosis, thromboembolism, and vascular disorders are found both in regional enteritis and in ulcerative colitis. These manifestations are described more fully in Chapter 30. "Metastatic" (distant cutaneous) regional enteritis is a cutaneous ulcer with a granulomatous reaction at a site separated from gut by normal skin. Urinary complications include cystitis, calculi, and ureteral obstruction.

▶ Treatment

A. Medical

The initial treatment of regional enteritis is nonoperative. Physical rest, relief of emotional stress, and a confiding patient-doctor relationship have favorable effects. A low-residue, milk-free, high-protein diet may provide adequate nutrition. Malnourished patients benefit from elemental or polymeric diets if standard food is not tolerated, and total or supplementary parenteral nutrition is an important adjunct. As nutrition improves, infection is more successfully treated, and complications such as fistulas may be reversed. Chronic intermittent elemental diet improves growth failure in prepubertal children. Most clinicians prefer enteral feeding over the parenteral route when conditions permit, though comparative studies are inconclusive on this issue. Preoperative total parenteral nutrition prolongs the hospital stay and does not reduce the incidence or severity of postoperative complications. Chronic parenteral nutrition at home allows some patients with extensive disease to postpone operation, but it does not reduce the necessity of operation over the long term.

Enteral nutrition alone is insufficient therapy for active regional enteritis compared with pharmacologic treatment. The standard drugs for regional enteritis are aminosalicylates, immunosuppressive and immunoregulatory agents, antibiotics, steroids, and antitumor necrosis factor alpha (anti-TNF-α). Prednisone, prednisolone, and methylprednisolone are the most common corticosteroids for this purpose. Studies suggest that steroids are most effective for regional enteritis of the small intestine, but they are applied to regional enteritis involving the colon as well. Prednisone (0.25–0.75 mg/d) is superior to placebo in the control of acute disease over the short term but should not be used for long-term maintenance therapy. Relief of symptoms is seen in up to 70% of patients after 4 weeks of treatment. Steroids are then tapered once improvement is seen. The utility of prednisone is limited by side effects, including bone loss and osteopenia, cataract formation, weight gain, immunosuppression, and delayed wound healing. Sulfasalazine, an aminosalicylate, has been a cornerstone of therapy of regional enteritis for many years. It is superior to placebo in control of acute disease, but its use is complicated by adverse reactions. The active principle of sulfasalazine is 5-aminosalicylic acid (5-ASA). Other aminosalicylates, including mesalamine, olsalazine, and balsalazide, are now used widely and are considered to be therapeutically equivalent to sulfasalazine. Not only are they beneficial for patients with active regional enteritis involving the colon and ileocolitis, but oral aminosalicylates also may succeed in maintaining remission of regional enteritis, a goal that has not been achieved by any other agents to date.

Azathioprine and mercaptopurine are the immunosuppressive drugs with the longest records. They are effective in regional enteritis affecting the colon and regional enteritis of the small bowel; they spare steroids (allow reduction of steroid doses), help close fistulas, maintain remissions, and heal perianal disease. The disadvantage of azathioprine and mercaptopurine is their slow action. Bone marrow suppression may be seen in patients on these drugs, and monitoring of blood counts during therapy is necessary. Acute pancreatitis can also be a complication of therapy with 6-MP. 6-MP is also used to delay recurrence after surgical therapy of regional enteritis. Various broad-spectrum antibiotics have been tried, most commonly metronidazole and ciprofloxacin for perianal disease. Infliximab (anti-TNF-α monoclonal chimeric antibody) is now FDA approved for use in patients with active regional enteritis. Infliximab is given as an intravenous infusion. Studies have shown prompt response to treatment with infliximab both for intestinal and perianal disease, although maintenance infusions are required. Despite medical advances in management, there is still no cure for regional enteritis.

B. Surgical Therapy

Surgery is not curative for regional enteritis, but its judicious use is often warranted to manage complications of the disease. The indication for operation in regional enteritis of the small bowel is obstruction in about half of cases; perforation, internal fistula, external fistula, abscess, perianal disease, and growth failure in children are other reasons for operation. Over the long term, about 70% of patients with regional enteritis undergo definitive surgery. Conservative resection of diseased bowel with a large side-to-side anastomosis is the preferred surgical procedure. The guiding principle in the surgical treatment of regional enteritis is preservation of intestinal length. Increasingly, surgical resection of ileocolic regional enteritis is being performed laparoscopically. Resection is usually limited to the area responsible for the complications that prompted operation. If multiple symptomatic strictures are encountered, they can be treated by "strictureplasty," a procedure in which the bowel is incised through the stricture and the wall is sutured or stapled in such a way that the lumen is widened. Strictureplasty is indicated for (1) diffuse involvement of the small bowel with multiple strictures, (2) stricture(s) in a patient who has previously undergone major resection of the small bowel, (3) rapid recurrence of regional enteritis manifested as obstruction, and (4) a nonphlegmonous fibrotic stricture.

▶ Prognosis

Regional enteritis is a chronic condition. It may progress to involve additional portions of bowel or may seem to spread no farther. Surgical procedures are palliative, not curative, but operations contribute greatly to rehabilitation of patients with refractory disease. The recurrence rate after resection of ileal or ileocolic disease increases with time. Symptomatic recurrence rates are 25–50% at 5 years, 35–80% at 10 years, and 45–85% at 15 years. The marked variability is due to differences in patient populations, type of surgical procedures, and criteria for recurrence. Extensive confluent ulcers seen endoscopically in the ileum at the anastomosis within 1 year after ileocolectomy strongly predict symptomatic recurrence. Strictureplasty is effective for obstructive lesions, and there are few postoperative complications. Reoperation is needed in about 10% of patients within a year after strictureplasty and in one third of patients by 10 years; surprisingly, however, the strictureplasty sites are usually not the source of symptoms.

Surgery should be used to manage complications in coordination with medical therapy. This team approach enables 80–85% of patients who require surgery to lead normal lives. Community-based studies have shown that long-term survival of people with regional enteritis is similar to that of the general population irrespective of the age at diagnosis. There is little evidence that pregnancy affects the course of regional enteritis or that inactive regional enteritis alters the course of pregnancy.

Behm BW, Bickston SJ: Tumor necrosis factor-alpha antibody for maintenance of remission in Crohn's disease. Cochrane Database Syst Rev 2008;1:CD006893.

Benchimol EI et al: Traditional corticosteroids for induction of remission in Crohn's disease. Cochrane Database Syst Rev 2008; 2:CD006792.

Dietz DW et al: Safety and long-term efficacy of strictureplasty in 314 consecutive patients with obstructing small bowel Crohn's Disease. J Am Coll Surg 2001;192:330.

McDonald JW et al: Cyclosporine for induction of remission in Crohn's disease. Cochrane Database Syst Rev 2005;2:CD000297.

Milsom JW et al: Prospective, randomized trial comparing laparoscopic vs. conventional surgery for refractory ileocolic Crohn's Disease. Dis Colon Rectum 2001;44:1.

Podolsky DK: Inflammatory bowel disease. N Engl J Med 2002;347:417.

Rastogi A, Schoen RE, Slivka A: Diagnostic yield and clinical outcomes of capsule endoscopy. Gastrointest Endosc 2004; 60:959.

Ricart E et al: Infliximab for Crohn's disease in clinical practice at the Mayo Clinic: the first 100 patients. Am J Gastroenterol 2001;96:722.

Sutherland LR et al: Prevention of relapse of Crohn's disease. Inflamm Bowel Dis 2000;6:321.

OTHER INFLAMMATORY & ULCERATIVE DISEASES OF THE SMALL INTESTINE

▶ Acute Enteritis & Mesenteric Lymphadenitis

Acute inflammation of the small intestine (enteritis) often also affects the stomach (**gastroenteritis**) or the colon (**enterocolitis**). Involvement of regional lymph nodes is termed **mesenteric adenitis.** These usually self-limiting illnesses may be caused by viruses, bacteria, parasites, toxins, or unknown agents. These conditions are of importance to the surgeon when they mimic acute appendicitis or other problems that require operative treatment.

▶ HIV-Associated Enteropathy

Gastrointestinal infections are frequent in AIDS patients. Enteric pathogens recoverable from these patients include *Cryptosporidium,* cytomegalovirus, *Entamoeba histolytica, Giardia lamblia, Mycobacterium avium-intracellulare, Salmonella typhimurium, Shigella,* and *Campylobacter jejuni.*

Many symptomatic patients have no identifiable intestinal pathogen, and there is evidence to support the existence of an enteropathy caused by the human immunodeficiency virus itself. Intestinal perforation is a rare but devastating complication in these patients.

Giovanni B et al: HIV enteropathy: undescribed ultrastructural changes of duodenal mucosa and their regression after triple antiviral therapy. A case report. Dig Dis Sci 2005;50:617.

Kotler DP: HIV infection and the gastrointestinal tract. AIDS 2005;19:107.

▶ Yersinia Enteritis

Much attention has focused on *Yersinia enterocolitica;* this pathogen may cause acute gastroenteritis, terminal ileitis, enterocolitis, colitis, mesenteric lymphadenitis, hepatic and splenic abscesses, and autoimmune processes such as erythema nodosum and polyarthritis. *Y enterocolitica* has also been implicated in other disease (especially in women), including carditis, glomerulonephritis, Graves disease, and Hashimoto thyroiditis.

Acute gastroenteritis with fever, diarrhea, and sometimes vomiting is the most common clinical syndrome, especially in children. Acute mesenteric lymphadenitis and acute terminal ileitis are more frequent in adolescents and adults. These infections may cause enough abdominal pain and tenderness that appendicitis seems a likely diagnosis. If operation is performed, large inflamed lymph nodes are found in the mesentery of the distal ileum, and the bowel itself may be grossly inflamed. In these circumstances, appendectomy is usually performed. Organisms can be cultured from stool, and antibody titers may rise and then fall in some patients. *Y enterocolitica* may respond to trimethoprim-sulfamethoxazole or doxycycline, and complicated *Y enterocolitica* infections should be treated. Fatal septicemia has been reported. No patient with *Y enterocolitica* enteritis has progressed to classic regional enteritis.

▶ Campylobacter Enteritis

Campylobacter jejuni is a gram-negative rod that is now recognized as an important cause of human illness in all parts of the world. *C jejuni* infection is more common than infection by either salmonella or shigella. Raw milk, untreated drinking water, and undercooked poultry are recognized vehicles of transmission. Clinical features vary from mild abdominal pain, fever, emesis, and diarrhea indistinguishable from viral gastroenteritis to severe chronic or relapsing bloody diarrhea that resembles ulcerative or granulomatous colitis. *C jejuni* produces an enterotoxin that may play a role in causing diarrhea.

Darkfield or phase-contrast microscopy of stool samples may reveal the characteristic darting motility of *C jejuni* and allow for a presumptive diagnosis. Stool and occasionally blood cultures are positive. Colonoscopy may reveal colonic lesions, and x-rays show inflammation of the small bowel or colon.

Although *C jejuni* infection is self-limited in most patients and symptoms subside within a week, relapses occur in 20% of untreated patients. The appropriate antibiotic is erythromycin, ciprofloxacin, or doxycycline, depending on the results of in vitro sensitivity studies. Disease can be spread by symptomatic patients; once diarrhea subsides, transmission is unlikely.

▶ Tuberculosis

Primary tuberculous infection of the intestine, caused by ingestion of the bovine strain of *Mycobacterium tuberculosis,* is rare in the United States. Secondary infection is due to swallowing the human tubercle bacillus. About 1% of patients with pulmonary tuberculosis have intestinal involvement. Recent immigration from endemic areas has increased the incidence. Tuberculosis is prevalent in individuals infected with HIV.

The distal ileum is the most common site of disease. The bacillus localizes in the mucosal glands and spreads to Peyer patches, where inflammation, sloughing of tissue, and local attempts at walling off give rise to symptoms. The pathologic reaction is hypertrophic or ulcerative. Hypertrophic tuberculous enteritis results in stenosis, and the symptoms and signs are those of obstruction. The ulcerative form causes abdominal pain, alternating constipation and diarrhea, and, occasionally, progressive inanition. Free perforation, fistula formation, or hemorrhage may occur in severe untreated disease.

The diagnosis of intestinal tuberculosis can be difficult, but medical treatment should not be based on clinical suspicion alone, since carcinoma and regional enteritis cause similar symptoms and signs. Less than half of patients in a recent study had an abnormality on chest x-ray, and none had a positive sputum result. Biopsy by colonoscopy, laparoscopy, or even laparotomy is needed to demonstrate the presence of the organism.

Antituberculosis chemotherapy is the mainstay of management. Surgery is required if the diagnosis is uncertain, if disease is resistant to chemotherapy, or if complications develop. Some surgeons recommend early operation because medical treatment results in healing by fibrosis with resultant obstruction. Resection is the preferred surgical procedure, and bypass is done only if abscesses or fistulas are present. The prognosis is good if the patient is operated on in the early stages of the illness.

Engin G, Balk E: Imaging findings of intestinal tuberculosis. J Comput Assist Tomogr 2005;29:37.

Misra SP et al: Endoscopic biopsies from normal-appearing terminal ileum and cecum in patients with suspected colonic tuberculosis. Endoscopy 2004;36:612.

▶ Typhoid

Salmonella typhi may cause ulcers in the distal ileum or cecum. Bleeding or perforation presents a formidable surgical challenge. Early operation offers the best hope for survival.

▶ Enteropathy from Nonsteroidal Anti-inflammatory Drugs

Nonsteroidal anti-inflammatory drugs increase intestinal permeability within hours after ingestion, exposing the mucosa to macromolecules and toxins in the lumen. Bacterial invasion may contribute to inflammation. Perhaps 70% of patients of any age and either sex who have taken these agents for 6 months or longer develop enteropathy, with subclinical intestinal inflammation and occult blood loss. Fewer than 1% of patients develop mucosal ulceration or transmural inflammation with submucosal fibrosis and circumferential diaphragmlike strictures. These patients may have obstruction, perforation, or anemia. The differential diagnosis includes regional enteritis, ischemia, tuberculosis, and lymphoma.

The drug should be withdrawn. Strictures require resection.

Graham DY et al: Visible small-intestinal mucosal injury in chronic NSAID users. Clin Gastroenterol Hepatol 2005;3:55.

Radiation Enteropathy

Aggressive radiation therapy for abdominal or pelvic cancer is almost always associated with some gastrointestinal injury, because proliferating intestinal epithelial cells are extremely radiosensitive. Degeneration of cells and edema of bowel wall may produce abdominal pain, nausea and vomiting, and sometimes bloody diarrhea during therapy or a few months later. Symptoms are usually minor and transient for most patients with modern irradiation techniques.

Injury to blood vessels in the bowel wall is far more serious than the early mucosal lesion. Endothelial proliferation and fibrosis in the media may gradually obliterate the vessel lumen over months or years, producing chronic intestinal ischemia. Carcinoma arising in irradiated small intestine is a rare late complication.

The incidence of significant bowel injury is dose-related and varies from 5% after 4500 cGy to 30% after 6000 cGy. Fixation of small bowel loops in the radiation field by adhesions from previous operations greatly increases the risk of intestinal complications. Absorbable polyglycolic acid mesh can be used to keep the small bowel out of the pelvis when radiation therapy is planned following pelvic surgery. Oral glutamine protects the small bowel mucosa from some of the morbidity of irradiation in preliminary animal studies.

Symptoms necessitating operation appear as early as 1 month or as late as 30 years after completion of therapy. Operation is required for obstruction due to stricture or entrapment in pelvic fibrosis, perforation with abscess or fistula formation, or hemorrhage from ulcerated mucosa. Symptoms should not be attributed to cancer until residual cancer is proved to be present.

The objective of operation is relief of symptoms. If resection of the involved segment is not possible, bypass is performed. It is imperative that normal bowel be used for anastomoses, because suture lines in irradiated bowel are likely to disrupt. The bowel is friable despite its thickness, and care must be taken in freeing adhesions. If the distal colon and rectum are involved, diverting colostomy is the safest course. Radiation proctitis is discussed in Chapter 31.

The operative death rate is 10–15%, and the prognosis thereafter depends on the extent of involvement and the presence of untreatable fistulas, short bowel syndrome, and cancer. Only 30–45% of patients with significant intestinal complications of radiation therapy are alive 5 years after operation.

Jain G et al: Chronic radiation enteritis: a ten-year follow-up. J Clin Gastroenterol 2002;35:214.

Zimmerer T et al: Medical prevention and treatment of acute and chronic radiation induced enteritis—is there any proven therapy? A short review. Z Gastroenterol 2008;46:441.

SMALL INTESTINE FISTULAS

 ESSENTIALS OF DIAGNOSIS

▶ Fever and sepsis.

▶ Abdominal pain.

▶ Localized abdominal tenderness.

▶ External drainage of small bowel contents.

▶ Dehydration and malnutrition.

General Considerations

External fistulas of the small bowel may form spontaneously as a result of disease, but about 95% are complications of surgical procedures (anastomotic dehiscence or injury to bowel during dissection). Fistulas are particularly prone to develop when the surgeon encounters extensive adhesions, inflamed intestine, or radiation enteropathy.

Fistulas can be classified according to anatomic site, characteristics of the tract (simple or complex), and volume of output (high or low). A high-output fistula produces more than 500 mL/24 h. Other descriptive terms are also used, such as end fistula, which encompasses the entire diameter of the bowel, and lateral fistula, which arises from one side only.

Clinical Findings

A. Symptoms and Signs

Postoperative fistula formation is heralded by fever and abdominal pain until bowel contents discharge through the abdominal incision. Spontaneous fistulas from neoplasms or inflammatory disease usually develop in a more indolent manner. Most fistulas are associated with one or more abscesses, which often drain incompletely with fistulization, so that persistent sepsis is a common feature. Intestinal fluid escaping through the fistula may severely excoriate the skin and abdominal wall tissues. Fluid and electrolyte losses may be severe, especially if the fistula is large, if it is located in the upper tract, or if there is partial or complete intestinal obstruction distal to the fistula. Persistent sepsis and difficulty in nourishing the patient contribute to rapid weight loss.

B. Laboratory Findings

Routine laboratory tests reflect the severity of deficits in red cell mass, plasma volume, and electrolytes. Leukocytosis due to sepsis and hemoconcentration is common. Disease of other organs such as liver and kidneys may be detected.

C. Imaging Studies

Abscesses and intestinal obstruction may be evident on plain abdominal films. Contrast medium administered orally, per rectum, or through the fistula (fistulogram) delineates the abnormal anatomy, including intrinsic bowel disease, and demonstrates the location and number of fistulas, the length and course of fistula tracts, associated abscess cavities, and the presence of distal obstruction. Radiologists can manipulate catheters into tracts and provide detailed diagnostic information; this procedure may also be therapeutic (see below). Chest films, CT scans, ultrasound, endoscopy, and other special studies may be indicated in certain individuals.

► Complications

Fluid and electrolyte losses, malnutrition, and sepsis contribute to multiple-organ failure and death unless effective therapy is instituted promptly.

► Treatment

A systematic approach combining diagnostic, supportive, and operative procedures is essential in the management of patients with fistulas (Table 29–2). In few other conditions is the proper timing of operative intervention more critical.

A. Fluid and Electrolyte Resuscitation

Many fistula patients are profoundly depleted of intravascular and interstitial volume, and replacement of this fluid with isotonic saline solution takes first priority. Central venous pressure, urine output, and skin turgor are guides to the progress of volume resuscitation. Blood is sent to the laboratory for measurement of serum electrolyte concentrations and arterial blood gases. Results of these studies assist in correcting electrolyte deficits and deranged acid-base balance.

Table 29–2. Treatment of Fistulas.

First:
　Restore blood volume and begin correction of fluids and electrolyte imbalance.
　Drain accessible abscesses.
　Control fistula and measure losses.
　Begin nutritional support.
Second:
　Delineate anatomy of fistulas by radiographic studies.
Third:
　Maintain caloric intake of 2000–3000 kcal or more per day, depending on status of nutrition and energy expenditure.
　Drain abscesses as they appear.
Fourth:
　Operate if fistula fails to close.

Body weight is recorded daily. Fluid and electrolyte resuscitation can usually be accomplished within the first day or two. Subsequent maintenance of homeostasis depends on accurately measuring losses and replacing them.

B. Control of Fistula

Fistula drainage fluid must be collected to avoid excoriation of skin and abdominal wall tissues and to record volume losses. An ostomy appliance may fit around the fistula, or a catheter inserted by a radiologist under x-ray guidance may work best. Skilled and experienced nursing care is indispensable.

C. Control of Sepsis

Abscesses should be drained as soon as they are diagnosed. The source of sepsis is often obscure, and a continuous diligent search for abscesses must be made by repeated physical examination and imaging studies until the infection is located and treated. Blind therapy with broad-spectrum antibiotics is not a substitute for drainage of abscesses. In many cases, an incompletely drained abscess can be managed by an interventional radiologist, who passes a catheter through a fistula tract into the associated abscess cavity. Drainage is accomplished, and the fistula may close.

D. Delineation of Fistula

Radiographic contrast studies (see above) should be obtained as soon as feasible.

E. Nutrition

Adequate nutrition and control of sepsis make the difference between survival and death for these patients. A useful general rule is to avoid all oral intake at the outset. Nasogastric suction may be necessary temporarily. As soon as intravascular fluid and electrolytes are restored, parenteral nutrition should be instituted via a central intravenous catheter.

For many patients, total parenteral nutrition is the principal exogenous source of calories and nitrogen until the fistula heals or is closed surgically. For patients with low-output or distal fistulas, the enteral route for nutrition is preferred, and elemental or polymeric diets can be delivered into the distal gut in some patients with proximal fistulas.

F. Other Measures

H_2 receptor antagonists and proton pump inhibitors are useful adjuncts in patients with proximal fistulas. By reducing gastric acid secretion, fistula output is decreased and fluid and electrolyte management is simplified. Somatostatin analogs decrease fistula output and may accelerate fistula closure.

G. Operation

About 30% of fistulas close spontaneously; regional enteritis, irradiated bowel, cancer, foreign body, distal obstruction, extensive disruption of intestinal continuity, and a short (< 2 cm) fistula tract are associated with failure of fistulas to heal. Fibrin glue has been effective in some small bowel fistulas; in particular, it may be considered in complicated patients with a history of a hostile abdomen. Treatment may be successful if the fistula is long and the output is low. If they are going to heal spontaneously, fistulas usually close within a month after eradication of infection and institution of adequate nutritional support, and persistence much beyond a month indicates the need for surgical closure in most cases. Serum levels of short-turnover proteins, particularly transferrin, might be useful in predicting which patients are unlikely to close their fistulas. The operation should be postponed, however, until one can predict that intra-abdominal inflammation has resolved—typically 2–3 months or more after the last operation. The fistulous segment should be resected, associated obstruction relieved, and continuity reestablished by a functional end-to-end anastomosis.

▶ Prognosis

The plan of management outlined above results in survival rates of 80–95% in patients with external fistulas. Uncontrolled sepsis is the chief cause of death.

Becker HP, Willms A, Schwab R: Small bowel fistulas and the open abdomen. Scand J Surg 2007;96:263.

Evenson AR, Fischer JE: Current management of enterocutaneous fistula. J Gastrointest Surg 2006;10:455.

Hollington P et al: An 11-year experience of enterocutaneous fistula. Br J Surg 2004;91:1646.

Lynch AC et al: Clinical outcome and factors predictive of recurrence after enterocutaneous fistula surgery. Ann Surg 2004; 240:825.

ACUTE VASCULAR LESIONS OF THE SMALL INTESTINE & MESENTERY

Lesions producing acute or chronic ischemia or hemorrhage may result from intrinsic vascular disease, systemic illness, pharmacologic agents, and surgical procedures. Chronic occlusion may be amenable to vascular reconstruction and is discussed in Chapter 34. Acute mesenteric ischemia is discussed here.

1. Acute Mesenteric Vascular Occlusion

ESSENTIALS OF DIAGNOSIS

▶ Severe, diffuse abdominal pain.

▶ Gross or occult intestinal bleeding.

▶ Minimal physical findings.

▶ Radiographic findings (sometimes).

▶ Operative findings.

▶ General Considerations

Sudden occlusion of major small bowel arteries or veins is catastrophic. It is predominantly a disease of the elderly and is highly lethal. Mesenteric **arterial emboli** account for 50% of cases of acute mesenteric ischemia; they most commonly originate from mural thrombus in an infarcted left ventricle or clot in a fibrillating left atrium in patients with mitral stenosis. **Thrombosis of a mesenteric artery** (25% of cases) is the end result of atherosclerotic stenosis, and these patients often give a history of intestinal angina before the acute thrombosis occurs. Other causes of acute arterial occlusions, such as dissecting aortic aneurysm or fusiform aortic aneurysm, are rare. Occlusions of smaller mesenteric arteries often are associated with connective tissue or other systemic disorders. Cocaine ingestion is another cause. Nonocclusive disease is responsible for about 20% of patients with acute mesenteric ischemia.

Thrombosis of mesenteric veins (5% of cases) is associated with portal hypertension, abdominal sepsis, hypercoagulable states, or trauma, or there may be no apparent underlying disease. Mesenteric venous or arterial thrombosis can occur in women taking oral contraceptives. Some venous occlusions develop peripherally and progress insidiously, causing segmental infarction that resembles strangulation obstruction. Others have acute, severe, rapidly progressive ischemia.

The consequences of major vascular occlusion depend on the vessel involved, the level of occlusion, the status of other visceral vessels, the development of collaterals, the establishment of reperfusion, and other factors. Tissue injury is caused by events related to the ischemia itself (ischemic injury) and by return of blood flow, either spontaneous or as a result of treatment (reperfusion injury). Complete interruption of oxygen supply to the intestine produces necrosis first at the tips of villi. Mucosal slough begins within 3 hours after onset of ischemia, and ulceration and bleeding soon become extensive. Full-thickness infarction of bowel wall occurs as early as 6 hours after onset in total ischemia; in partial ischemia, it may take several days for this stage to be reached. Hemorrhage into the lumen, accumulation of bloody abdominal fluid, perforation, and death from sepsis are the end results of infarction. Sepsis and multiorgan system failure may develop even in the absence of full-thickness necrosis or perforation; bacteria proliferate in the necrotic segment; the mucosal barrier is disrupted; and bacteria and their toxic products translocate into the circulation. A variety of plasma substances, including tumor necrosis factor and platelet-activating factor, arise at the site of intestinal injury, enter the circulation and damage target organs such as the lung and kidneys.

There is increasing recognition of the importance of reperfusion injury in the outcome of intestinal ischemia. Return of arterial blood flow from spontaneous events, lysis of clot by anticoagulants, or arterial reconstruction converts the enzyme xanthine dehydrogenase to xanthine oxidase, resulting in the release of superoxide and hydrogen peroxide. These oxygen radicals destabilize cell membranes, disrupt the mucosal barrier, and flood the systemic circulation with mediators of damage to other organs. Most of the data come from experimental animals, but there is little doubt that reperfusion injury is an important and potentially lethal phenomenon in patients.

▶ Clinical Findings

A. Symptoms and Signs

The most constant symptom is severe, poorly localized abdominal pain that is often unresponsive to narcotics. Nausea and vomiting, diarrhea, and constipation are variable in occurrence.

In the early stages, there is a striking paucity of abdominal findings; in fact, pain out of proportion to the objective findings is a hallmark of mesenteric vascular occlusion. Ischemia can also occur with much less severe pain, and serious illness may be recognized only when secondary toxicity develops. Later in the course, abdominal distention and tenderness occur. Shock and generalized peritonitis eventually develop, but by that time the opportunity for salvage has been lost. In some instances—particularly with a high venous occlusion—shock is an early finding. Stool or gastric contents contain blood in 75–95% of patients later in the course. Paracentesis does not help to establish the diagnosis in the reversible stages.

B. Laboratory Findings

There is no laboratory test to definitively rule in or out a diagnosis of mesenteric ischemia. Striking leukocytosis is present. Serum amylase is elevated in about half of patients, and creatine kinase (BB isoenzyme) correlates with intestinal infarction. Significant base deficits may be observed. Increased inorganic phosphate levels in serum and peritoneal fluid are a sign of irreversible ischemia. Hemoconcentration and the effects of hemorrhage into the lumen or mesentery are reflected in laboratory tests in the late stages. Antithrombin III deficiency and other abnormalities of coagulation should be sought.

C. Imaging Studies

Plain abdominal films allow a presumptive diagnosis of vascular occlusion to be made in about 20% of patients. Absence of intestinal gas, diffuse distention with air-fluid levels, and distention of small bowel and colon up to the splenic flexure are nonspecific but suggestive. Blunt plicae, thickened bowel wall, and small bowel loops that remain unchanged over several hours are seen occasionally. Specific findings of intestinal necrosis, including intramural gas and gas in the portal venous system, which may be seen on either a CT scan or plain abdominal films, occur late. Barium studies may reveal thumbprinting and disordered motility

(either slow or rapid). CT gives useful information in 50% of patients, though a specific diagnosis is possible in only 25% of cases. MRI may be useful. Mesenteric arteriography may be helpful but is logistically cumbersome in acutely ill patients and is not sensitive enough to rule out the diagnosis. It is important to recognize that short of mesenteric arteriography, imaging studies such as plain films, CT, and barium studies cannot be relied on to definitively rule out a diagnosis of acute mesenteric ischemia.

▶ Differential Diagnosis

Acute pancreatitis and strangulation obstruction of the intestine may be difficult to distinguish from mesenteric vascular occlusion. A very high serum amylase early in the disease or an edematous pancreas on CT scan suggests pancreatitis. Differentiation from strangulation obstruction is less important, since both conditions require operation. Angiography may be definitive. Even surgeons with a special interest in this condition are unable to make an early diagnosis in more than half of cases.

▶ Treatment

Survival depends upon diagnosis and operative treatment within 12 hours after onset of symptoms. Although acute occlusion of major arteries or veins requires operation, preoperative and postoperative intra-arterial infusion of papaverine (30–60 mg/h) has been recommended if the angiogram demonstrates embolic occlusion of the superior mesenteric artery.

Acute venous thrombosis is diagnosed by the edematous mesentery and extrusion of clots when mesenteric veins are cut. Resection of all of the involved gut and its mesentery is the treatment of choice; direct mesenteric venous surgery (thrombectomy) is seldom successful. Administration of heparin postoperatively is recommended. Antithrombin III deficiency and other causes of hypercoagulability should be treated.

In arterial occlusion, there is segmental or diffuse ischemia or infarction of small bowel and colon in the distribution of the occluded vessel. Arterial pulsations are absent or reduced, and mesenteric edema is not so striking as in venous occlusion. Many methods of helping the surgeon judge viability have been suggested, but most have not proved their worth. The Doppler ultrasonic flowmeter is of some help, and the laser Doppler system is promising. The qualitative fluorescein test is not as sensitive as once believed. Quantitative fluorescence, as measured by a perfusion fluorometer, is under investigation.

Necrotic bowel should be resected unless the extent of damage is so great that satisfactory life could not be expected. With the availability of home parenteral nutrition, more patients are salvageable now than before. It is not clear how to integrate the new information about reperfusion injury into management of patients with reversibly ischemic bowel. Perhaps it is better to just resect the affected intestine, particularly in the elderly, even though vascular reconstruction may be technically possible by embolectomy, thrombo-endarterectomy, or arterial bypass. Vascular reconstruction was attempted in 10% or less of patients before reperfusion injury became recognized, and it is likely that even fewer patients will be treated by a direct approach to the vessels in the future.

Massive volume support and antibiotics are mandatory, and anticoagulants or drugs that inhibit platelet aggregation are given by some surgeons. A second-look operation is performed 24–48 hours later if marginally viable bowel was left in.

Percutaneous transluminal angioplasty and stent placement has been used to treat acute mesenteric ischemia, but its role is yet to be defined, and abdominal operation remains the standard treatment.

▶ Prognosis

Acute mesenteric vascular occlusion is often lethal, because diagnosis and treatment are delayed, infarction is extensive, and arterial reconstruction is difficult. The overall mortality rate of arterial occlusion is about 45%, although a recent report of deaths occurring in only 24% is encouraging. If infarction is so extensive that over half of the small bowel must be resected, the death rate is 45–85%. Reconstruction of acutely thrombosed visceral arteries is often not feasible, and patency rates are poor. In a few patients, the acute ischemic episode goes unrecognized, and the process resolves spontaneously with stricture formation. The prognosis is excellent in this situation. Acute venous thrombosis has a death rate of 30%, and if long-term anticoagulants are not used, approximately 25% of patients have another episode of thrombosis. Administration of coumarin anticoagulants for at least 3 months is recommended to minimize the possibility of recurrence.

2. Nonocclusive Intestinal Ischemia

In about one fourth of patients with intestinal ischemia, vascular occlusion does not involve a major artery or vein (although arterial stenosis is usually present). In the presence of some other acute disease, such as a cardiac dysrhythmia or sepsis, splanchnic vasoconstriction occurs, and the intestine becomes ischemic because of low perfusion pressure and flow. Arterial blood is shunted away from the villi in these circumstances, and the ischemic villi are destroyed if the condition persists.

The diagnosis is suspected when a potentially susceptible patient develops acute abdominal pain. The clinical picture is similar to that of arterial thrombosis, but the onset is less often sudden. Arteriography documents the absence of major vascular occlusion but is not otherwise diagnostic in most cases.

Direct infusion of vasodilator agents into the superior mesenteric artery may reverse splanchnic vasoconstriction in selected cases. Papaverine is the drug of choice, but other drugs are under investigation. Operation is usually required to exclude other diseases that simulate intestinal ischemia and to resect infarcted bowel.

Patchy or diffuse ischemia varies in extent and severity. Ischemia is most pronounced on the antimesenteric border, and the mucosa may be extensively involved before abnormalities are visible on the serosal surface. There are often ischemic areas in other organs such as the liver and spleen. Vascular reconstruction is ineffective, and surgical procedures are limited to resection of infarcted bowel. Decisions about when to perform a primary anastomosis or second-look operation are individualized. The death rate was about 90% until recently, mainly because the underlying disease often could not be corrected. Intra-arterial vasodilator therapy has lowered this figure.

Angelelli G et al: Acute bowel ischemia: CT findings. Eur J Radiol 2004;50:37.

Cleveland TJ, Nawaz S, Gaines PA: Mesenteric arterial ischaemia: diagnosis and therapeutic options. Vasc Med 2002;7:311.

Sarkar R: Evolution of the management of mesenteric occlusive disease. Cardiovasc Surg 2002;10:395.

Schoots IG et al: Systematic review of survival after acute mesenteric ischaemia according to disease aetiology. Br J Surg 2004;91:17.

3. Other Vascular Lesions

▶ Vasculitis

Vascular lesions associated with systemic disorders such as polyarteritis nodosa and systemic lupus erythematosus may cause patchy infarction of the small intestine. Similar lesions have been seen in patients with a history of amphetamine abuse. The presenting manifestation is usually perforation with peritonitis or intraluminal bleeding, but strictures occur as well. The prognosis depends on the underlying pathologic process and the severity of peritoneal contamination. These patients are often on corticosteroid therapy and do not tolerate infection well. Survival is rare.

▶ Mesenteric Apoplexy

Mesenteric apoplexy is a rare disorder caused by spontaneous rupture of mesenteric arteries. The more general category of **abdominal apoplexy** includes spontaneous hemorrhage into the peritoneal cavity from tumors (particularly hepatomas), the spleen, or other organs. Arteriosclerotic lesions are the cause of arterial rupture in older individuals; the superior mesenteric, right colic, and branches of the celiac artery are the usual sites. Sudden hemorrhage from congenital aneurysms occurs in younger patients; the splenic artery is most commonly involved and is particularly prone to rupture during pregnancy. The typical picture is sudden onset of diffuse abdominal pain followed by hypotension. Operation is imperative.

▶ Bleeding Lesions

Arteriovenous malformations and other bleeding lesions in the small intestine are discussed under Acute Lower Gastrointestinal Hemorrhage in Chapter 30.

GAS CYSTS (PNEUMATOSIS CYSTOIDES INTESTINALIS)

Pneumatosis cystoides intestinalis is a rare condition characterized by gas-filled cysts in the wall of the gut and sometimes in the mesentery. When the process is limited to the large intestine, the term **pneumatosis coli** is used. Cysts vary in size from microscopic to several centimeters in diameter.

Pneumatosis may be primary or secondary. About 15% of cases are primary and idiopathic; the cysts are submucosal and usually are limited to the left colon. Secondary pneumatosis comprises 85% of cases. Cysts are subserosal and may be located anywhere in the gastrointestinal tract or its mesentery. Conditions that underlie secondary pneumatosis intestinalis or pneumatosis coli include inflammatory bowel disease, infectious gastroenteritis or colitis, steroid therapy, connective tissue disorders, intestinal obstruction, diverticulitis, chronic obstructive pulmonary disease, acute leukemia, lymphoma, AIDS, and organ transplantation.

The mechanism of cyst formation may not be the same in all patients. In some, anaerobic bacterial fermentation of carbohydrates leads to excess production of hydrogen gas, which enters the intestinal wall by diffusion. Some patients have greatly diminished activity of methanogenic and sulfate-reducing bacteria, which normally consume or metabolize hydrogen. Patients with impaired pulmonary function are less able to excrete excessive hydrogen gas through the lungs, and they are more prone to develop pneumatosis. Cysts are maintained because additional hydrogen is generated with each meal, thus replacing gas that may have diffused into the bloodstream since the previous meal. High breath hydrogen levels have been reported in pneumatosis patients even during fasting.

Symptoms are absent or nonspecific. In secondary pneumatosis, symptoms are due to the underlying disease. In the primary form, patients may complain of abdominal discomfort, distention, diarrhea with mucus, or passing of excessive amounts of gas. Rarely, perforation of a cyst, hemorrhage, obstruction, or malabsorption may bring benign pneumatosis to medical attention. **Fulminant pneumatosis** is associated with acute bacterial infection and necrosis of the bowel wall. Such patients are toxic and may have underlying impaired immunologic defenses. Gas may also be seen within the intestinal wall late in intestinal infarction. Pneumoperitoneum is sometimes present.

Treatment of secondary pneumatosis intestinalis is directed toward the underlying disease. Resolution of cysts can be accomplished in either primary or secondary pneumatosis by having patients breathe oxygen by mask for several days interrupted only at mealtime. Response to hyperbaric oxygen is more rapid. Recurrence of cysts after oxygen treatment reflects continued production of hydrogen, and in these patients it is necessary to reduce the amount of gas being generated. The amount of substrate can be controlled by dietary manipulation, and the fecal flora can be suppressed by antibacterial agents such as ampicillin or metronidazole. Surgical resection of bowel involved with benign primary pneumatosis is rarely required, but underlying disease may need operative treatment in the secondary form of this condition. Fulminant pneumatosis is treated surgically, but the mortality rate is high.

Deniz K et al: Intestinal involvement in Wegener's granulomatosis. J Gastrointestin Liver Dis 2007;16:329.
Ebert EC: Gastric and enteric involvement in progressive systemic sclerosis. J Clin Gastroenterol 2008;42:5.

TUMORS OF THE SMALL INTESTINE

Neoplasms of the jejunum and ileum comprise 1–5% of all tumors of the gastrointestinal tract. The terminal ileum is the favored site, followed by proximal jejunum. Approximately 85% of patients are over age 40. There is a high correlation of small bowel tumors with primary neoplasms elsewhere.

Only 10% of small bowel tumors are symptomatic. Benign lesions are 10 times as common as malignant ones. Lymphoma is now the most common primary malignant tumor of the small intestine. At least 75% of symptomatic neoplasms are malignant. Bleeding and obstruction, sometimes due to intussusception, are the most frequent symptoms.

1. Benign Tumors

▶ Polyps

Adenomatous or villous polyps of the type seen in the colon are rare in the small bowel; they are usually solitary and cause symptoms by intussusception or bleeding.

Polypoid **hamartomas** may be solitary in patients who are free of associated anomalies. Hamartomas are multiple in 50% of cases, and 10% of these have **Peutz-Jeghers syndrome,** a familial disorder characterized by diffuse gastrointestinal polyposis and mucocutaneous pigmentation. The malignant potential of these polyps is very small. Operation is indicated only for symptoms (eg, obstruction, bleeding), at which time all polyps greater than about 1 cm should be removed. A combined surgical and endoscopic approach is the best strategy.

Familial adenomatous polyposis (familial polyposis coli, Gardner syndrome; see Chapter 30) is characterized by multiple intestinal and colonic polyps, osteomas, and subcutaneous cysts or fibromas. The polyps are true neoplasms, and malignant degeneration of colonic polyps is common; there is a predilection for periampullary duodenal cancer as well.

Juvenile (retention) polyps may bleed or obstruct. They are more common in the colon than in the small bowel and usually autoamputate before adolescence. Some pathologists regard these lesions as hamartomas.

Other Tumors

Leiomyomas, lipomas, neurofibromas, and fibromas may cause symptoms that require operation. Endometriosis can implant on the small bowel. Hemangiomas are discussed in the section on Acute Lower Gastrointestinal Hemorrhage in Chapter 30.

Gore RM et al: Diagnosis and staging of small bowel tumours. Cancer Imaging 2006;6:209.

Hyland R, Chalmers A: CT features of jejunal pathology. Clin Radiol 2007;62:1154.

Miettinen M, Lasota J: Gastrointestinal stromal tumors: review on morphology, molecular pathology, prognosis, and differential diagnosis. Arch Pathol Lab Med 2006;130:1466.

Rondonotti E et al: Small bowel capsule endoscopy in 2007: indications, risks and limitations. World J Gastroenterol 2007;13:6140.

Schwartz GD, Barkin JS: Small bowel tumors. Gastrointest Endosc Clin N Am 2006;16:267.

2. Malignant Tumors

Primary

Adenocarcinoma is often asymptomatic or causes only minimal symptoms for prolonged periods. It usually arises in the proximal jejunum, except in regional enteritis, in which bypassed distal ileum is at greatest risk. Metastases are present in 80% of cases at the time of operation. Segmental resection of bowel and adjacent mesentery is done when possible, but metastases near the superior mesenteric artery may make the procedure difficult. Five-year survival is 25% in patients undergoing intestinal resection.

Primary small intestinal lymphomas of the Western type arise focally. These lymphomas develop in the proximal jejunum in patients with celiac disease, and in another group of patients, the lymphomas arise de novo in the distal ileum. Most primary lymphomas of the small intestine involve B-cell proliferation, but a few cases of primary T-cell lymphoma have been reported. In the Middle East, primary small bowel lymphoma is the most common form of extranodal lymphomatous disease. **Immunoproliferative small intestinal disease** is a geographic variant in that part of the world; it is characterized by diffuse infiltration of the small intestine by abnormal lymphoid cells. The infiltrate is probably benign in the initial phase of alpha-chain disease, but the other cases are malignant. AIDS-associated non-Hodgkin lymphomas of B-cell origin can involve the small intestine; the prognosis in these patients is very poor.

Western-type lymphomas develop as a nodular, polypoid, or ulcerating mass. Lesions are multiple in 20% of patients. Obstruction, bleeding, and perforation bring the lesion to attention. Abdominal operation is often required to establish a histologic diagnosis by conservative resection of the intestinal lesion. Operation is followed by whole abdominal radiation, with or without chemotherapy, in some patients. The overall 5-year survival rate is about 40%.

Small bowel gastrointestinal stromal tumors (GIST) tend to ulcerate centrally and bleed. Other types of primary malignant neoplasm are rare.

Metastatic

Small bowel metastases are found in 50% of patients dying of malignant melanoma. Carcinomas of the cervix, kidney, breast, lung, etc, may also spread to bowel. Obstruction or hemorrhage may require operation if life expectancy is reasonably good. Significant palliation may be achieved, particularly in patients with solitary metastatic lesions.

Delaunoit T et al: Pathogenesis and risk factors of small bowel adenocarcinoma: a colorectal cancer sibling? Am J Gastroenterol 2005;100:703.

Kummar S, Ciesielski TE, Fogarasi MC: Management of small bowel adenocarcinoma. Oncology (Huntington) 2002;16:1364.

Schwartz GD, Barkin JS: Small bowel tumors. Gastrointest Endosc Clin N Am 2006;16:267.

3. Carcinoid Tumors & Carcinoid Syndrome

Carcinoid tumors are apudomas that arise from enterochromaffin cells throughout the gut. Carcinoids may be associated with multiple endocrine neoplasia (MEN) type 1 and type 2. Rare familial clustering not associated with MEN has been reported. Neoplasms of other organs—most commonly the colon, lung, stomach, or breast—are present in 15% of patients. Carcinoids occur in patients 25–45 years of age.

The origin of carcinoid tumors of the gastrointestinal tract is foregut, 5%; midgut, 88%; and hindgut, 6%. Most carcinoids associated with MEN are of foregut origin. Midgut carcinoids produce serotonin and substance P; neurotensin, gastrin, somatostatin, motilin, secretin, and pancreatic polypeptide are also common. Foregut and hindgut carcinoids do not produce serotonin, but they often contain gastrin, somatostatin, pancreatic polypeptide, and glucagon.

The appendix is the most common site of carcinoid tumors, and the small intestine is the second-most common location; about 10 times as many originate in the ileum as in the jejunum. Multiple tumors are present in 40% of cases. Grossly, carcinoids are firm, yellowish submucosal nodules. Special stains may demonstrate argentaffin or argyrophil reactions in microscopic sections.

Carcinoid of the small bowel should be regarded as "a malignant neoplasm in slow motion." At the time of surgical diagnosis, 40% of tumors have invaded the muscularis and 45% have metastasized to lymph nodes or liver. Of primary tumors less than 1 cm in diameter, fewer than 2% metastasize, but 80% of those larger than 2 cm have spread at the time of operation. Huge metastatic deposits emanating from a minute primary are sometimes encountered.

Clinical Findings

A. Symptoms and Signs

Small tumors are usually asymptomatic. Overall, 30% of small bowel carcinoids cause symptoms of obstruction, pain, bleeding, or the carcinoid syndrome. Obstruction due to sclerosis and kinking of the bowel may be related to elaboration of vasoactive materials by metastases in the mesentery. Intestinal ischemia has been reported.

About 10% of patients with small bowel carcinoids present with **carcinoid syndrome,** and others develop it later. The syndrome consists of cutaneous flushing, diarrhea, bronchoconstriction, and right-sided cardiac valvular disease due to collagen deposition. Biologically active substances secreted by carcinoids are usually inactivated in the liver, but hepatic metastases or primary ovarian or bronchial carcinoids release these compounds directly into the systemic circulation, where they produce symptoms. Serotonin production in large quantities occurs in almost all cases of carcinoid syndrome; it is responsible for much of the diarrhea. A host of other vasoactive substances may participate, including amines (histamine, dopamine, 5-hydroxytryptophan, and 5-HIAA), tachykinins (kallikrein, substance P, and neuropeptide K), peptides (pancreatic polypeptide, chromogranins, neurotensin, and motilin), and prostaglandins.

B. Laboratory Findings

Some carcinoid tumors are detected by radiographic methods. Elevated urinary levels of 5-HIAA or of serum chromogranin A are the diagnostic hallmark of carcinoid syndrome. An injection of pentagastrin can be used as a provocative test: Symptoms appear, and serum levels of serotonin and substance P increase.

▶ Treatment

All accessible carcinoid tumor in small bowel, mesentery, and the peritoneal cavity should be removed. If intestinal obstruction is the principal serious manifestation of incur-able abdominal disease, it should be treated aggressively because tumor growth is so slow. Extensive enterectomy followed by chronic total parenteral nutrition may even be justified in some cases. Patients are followed up postoperatively with CT and octreotide scans.

Localized hepatic metastases should be resected. Unresectable hepatic metastases can sometimes be palliated by hepatic artery embolization or hepatic artery infusion chemotherapy. In some instances, longstanding metastatic disease isolated to the liver has been successfully treated with liver transplantation. Octreotide can be used to suppress tumor growth and control the symptoms of carcinoid syndrome. Octreotide inhibits release of gastrointestinal hormones; in carcinoid syndrome, it relieves flushing, wheezing, and severe diarrhea refractory to other measures.

▶ Prognosis

Carcinoid tumors grow slowly over months and years. The overall 5-year survival rate after resection of small bowel carcinoid is 70%; 40% of patients with inoperable metastases and 20% of those with hepatic metastases survive 5 years or longer. Median survival from the time of histologic diagnosis is 14 years, and from onset of the carcinoid syndrome, it is 8 years.

Horton KM, Fishman EK: Multidetector-row computed tomography and 3-dimensional computed tomography imaging of small bowel neoplasms: current concept in diagnosis. J Comput Assist Tomogr 2004;28:106.

Horton KM et al: Carcinoid tumors of the small bowel: a multitechnique imaging approach. AJR 2004;182:559.

Karatzas G et al: Gastrointestinal carcinoid tumors: 10-year experience of a general surgical department. Int Surg 2004;89:21.

Large Intestine

George J. Chang, MD, MS
Andrew A. Shelton, MD
Mark L. Welton, MD

30

ANATOMY

The colon extends from the end of the ileum to the rectum. The cecum, ascending colon, hepatic flexure, and proximal transverse colon comprise the **right colon.** The distal transverse colon, splenic flexure, descending colon, sigmoid colon, and rectosigmoid comprise the **left colon** (Figure 30–1). The ascending and descending portions are fixed to the retroperitoneum, and the transverse colon and sigmoid colon are suspended in the peritoneal cavity by their mesocolons. The caliber of the lumen is greatest at the cecum and diminishes distally. The wall of the colon has four layers: mucosa, submucosa, muscularis, and serosa (Figure 30–2). The muscularis propria consists of an inner circular layer and an outer longitudinal layer. The longitudinal muscle completely encircles the colon in a very thin layer, and at three points around the circumference it is gathered into thick bands called taeniae coli. Sacculations (haustra) are the result of shortening of the colon by the taeniae and contractions of the circular muscle. The haustra are not fixed anatomic structures and may be observed to move longitudinally. There are fatty appendages (the appendices epiploicae) on the serosal surface. The wall of the colon is so thin that it becomes markedly distended when obstructed.

The length of the **rectum** varies from 12 to 16 cm, and it is dependent on an individual's body habitus. The taeniae coli spread out at the rectosigmoid junction and are not apparent distal to that area. The upper rectum is invested by peritoneum anteriorly and laterally, but posteriorly it is retroperitoneal up to the junction with the sigmoid colon. The anterior peritoneal reflection dips low into the pelvis and may be as low as 5–8 cm above the anal verge. The anterior peritoneal reflection lies behind the bladder in males and behind the uterus (the rectouterine pouch of Douglas) in females. Tumor masses or abscesses in this location are readily palpated on digital rectal or pelvic examination. The rectum is normally distensible and serves a function as a capacitance organ. When its capacity to distend is lost or impaired by surgery or disease, fecal urgency and frequency are noted.

The rectal valves of Houston are prominent spirally arranged mucosal folds within the rectum. Less than half of people have the so-called normal three valves, two on the left and one on the right. The valves are at variable distances from the anal verge in different individuals. Normally, the valves appear thin, with sharp edges, but they become thickened and blunted when inflamed.

In men, the prostate gland, the seminal vesicles, and the seminal ducts lie anterior to the rectum. The prostate usually is easily felt, but the seminal vesicles are not palpable unless distended, because the firm, unyielding rectovesical fascia of Denonvilliers intervenes. The neurovascular bundle including the nervi-erigentes run along the posterolateral aspects of the prostate gland with Denonvilliers fascia and are subject to injury or trauma during proctectomy. In women, the rectovaginal septum and uterus lie anterior and the uterine adnexa anterolateral to the rectum. The structures are easily palpated with one finger in the vagina and one in the rectum.

▶ Blood Supply & Lymphatic Drainage

The arterial supply of the right colon, from the ileocecal junction to approximately the midtransverse colon, is from the superior mesenteric artery through its ileocolic, right colic, and middle colic branches. The anatomy of the right colic artery is variable but usually arises from the ileocolic trunk and may arise separately from the superior mesenteric artery. The venous anatomy is even more variable. The right colic vein is only present in 50% of people.

The inferior mesenteric artery arises from the abdominal aorta and gives off the left colic and before it becomes the superior hemorrhoidal artery. The vasa recta are the terminal arterial branches to the colon and run directly to the mesocolic wall or through the bowel wall to the antimesocolic border.

The colic arteries bifurcate and form arcades about 2.5 cm from the mesocolic border of the bowel, forming a pathway of communicating vessels called the **marginal artery of Drummond.** The marginal artery thus forms an anastomosis between the superior mesenteric and inferior mesenteric

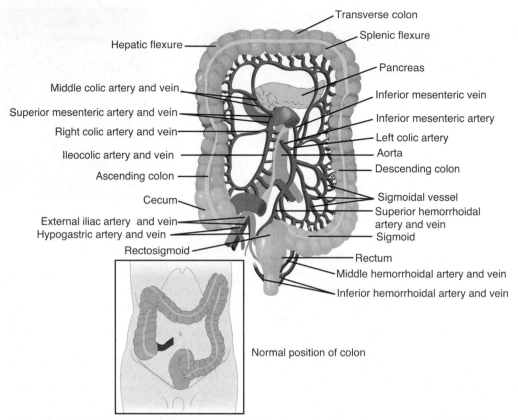

▲ **Figure 30–1.** The large intestine: anatomic divisions and blood supply. The veins are shown in black. The insert shows the usual configuration of the colon.

arteries. The configuration of the blood supply, however, varies greatly; the typical pattern is present in only 15% of individuals. The arc of Riolan comprises another collateral circuit between the superior mesenteric and inferior mesenteric arteries.

The middle hemorrhoidal artery arises on each side from the anterior division of the internal iliac artery or from the internal pudendal artery and runs inward at the level of the pelvic floor. The inferior hemorrhoidal arteries derive from the internal pudendal arteries and pass through Alcock canal. The anastomoses between the superior hemorrhoidal vessels and branches of the internal iliac arteries provide collateral circulation; this is important after surgical interruption or atherosclerotic occlusion of the vascular supply of the left colon.

The veins accompany the corresponding arteries and drain into the liver through the portal vein or into the systemic circulation by way of the hypogastric veins. Continuous lymphatic plexuses in the submucosal and subserosal layers of the bowel wall drain into the lymphatic channels and lymph nodes that accompany the blood vessels.

▶ **Nerve Supply**

The sympathetic nerves originating in T10–12 travel in the thoracic splanchnic nerves to the celiac plexus and then to the preaortic and superior mesenteric plexuses, from which postganglionic fibers are distributed along the superior mesenteric artery and its branches to the right colon. The left colon is supplied by sympathetic fibers that arise in L1–3, synapse in the paravertebral ganglia, and accompany the inferior mesenteric artery to the colon. The parasympathetic nerves to the right colon come from the right vagus and travel with the sympathetic nerves. The parasympathetic supply to the left colon derives from S2–4. These fibers emerge from the spinal cord as the nervi erigentes, which form the pelvic plexus and send branches to rectum.

Al-Fallouji MA, Tagart RE: The surgical anatomy of the colonic intramural blood supply and its influence on colorectal anastomosis. J R Coll Surg Edinb 1985;30:380.

Irving MH, Catchpole B: ABC of colorectal diseases: Anatomy and physiology of the colon, rectum, and anus. Br Med J 1992;304:1106.

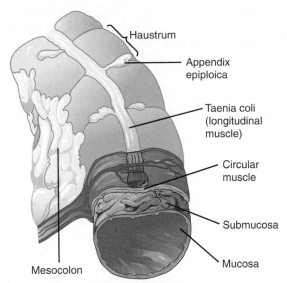

Haustrum

Appendix
epiploica

Taenia coli
(longitudinal
muscle)

Circular
muscle

Submucosa

Mucosa

Mesocolon

▲ **Figure 30–2.** Cross section of colon. The longitudinal muscle encircles the colon but is thickened in the region of the taeniae coli.

Pace JL: The anatomy of the haustra of the human colon. Proc R Soc Med 1968;61:934.
Ward SM: Interstitial cells of Cajal in enteric neurotransmission. Gut 2000;47(Suppl 4):40.

PHYSIOLOGY

The primary functions of the colon are absorption, secretion, motility, and intraluminal digestion. These interrelated phenomena process ileal effluent and convert it into semisolid feces that are stored until defecation is convenient. Regional variations in function are significant. The proximal colon absorbs electrolytes and water more efficiently than do the descending colon and rectum, and motility and intraluminal digestion differ by region also. Loss of colonic function through disease or surgery results in a continuous discharge of food wastes and increases daily intestinal losses of water and electrolytes, chiefly sodium and chloride.

The small intestine digests and absorbs most nutrients from ingested foods. The role of the colon in human nutrition is not well defined. Metabolism of carbohydrate to absorbable volatile fatty acids is probably important. Ureolysis—conversion of circulating urea to ammonia, which is reabsorbed and reused—may be significant. The colon also absorbs amino acids, bile acids, and vitamin K, but the contribution of the colon to homeostasis by these mechanisms has not been quantified.

▶ Intestinal Gas

The volume and composition of intestinal gas vary greatly among normal individuals. The small intestine contains approximately 100 mL of gas and the colon somewhat more. Some gas is absorbed through the mucosa and excreted through the lungs, and the remaining 400–1200 mL/d are discharged as flatus.

Nitrogen (N_2) comprises 30–90% of intestinal gas. Swallowed air is the principal source of intestinal N_2, but N_2 also can diffuse across the mucosa from blood to lumen when other gases are produced in sufficient volume to lower the partial pressure of N_2 and establish a gradient for diffusion. Other intestinal gases include oxygen (O_2), carbon dioxide (CO_2), hydrogen (H_2), methane (CH_4), and odoriferous trace substances such as methyl sulfide, hydrogen sulfide, indole, and skatole. H_2 and CO_2 are generated by fermentation of ingested nonabsorbed carbohydrate, especially carbohydrate present in polysaccharides (eg, fiber) and some starches. Lactose in milk provides the substrate in lactase-deficient persons. Mucus is the main endogenous source of carbohydrate in the colon; intestinal glycoproteins are 80% carbohydrate. Only about one third of the population produces CH_4, which is a product of colonic bacteria that use hydrogen to reduce CO_2. Stools of CH_4 producers nearly always float, even in the absence of fecal fat. CH_4, like H_2, can be measured in the breath. H_2 and CH_4 are explosive gases, and caution must be exercised when using electrocautery in the bowel lumen.

Patients with excessive gas may complain of abdominal pain and distention, increased flatus, and watery stools. Some of these patients have irritable bowel syndrome. Increased flatus may reflect extreme sensitivity of the rectum to small volumes, resulting in frequent passage of gas. Alternatively, gas may be produced in excessive quantities in symptomatic patients. Almost invariably, hydrogen is the culprit. Measurement of breath hydrogen is a potentially useful test for malabsorption states. Treatment of overproduction of gas at present is directed toward elimination of lactose, legumes, and wheat from the diet.

▶ Motility

Motor activity of the colon occurs in three patterns, and there is marked regional variation between the right and left colon. A pacemaker in the transverse colon has been postulated, perhaps pacing the proximal colon retrograde to facilitate storage and absorption while pacing the distal colon in the aboral direction to favor propulsion. **Retrograde peristalsis (antiperistalsis)**—annular contractions moving orad—dominates in the right colon. This kind of activity churns the contents and tends to confine them to the cecum and ascending colon. As ileal effluent continually enters the cecum, some of the column of liquid stool in the right colon is displaced and flows into the transverse colon. **Segmentation** is the most common type of motor activity in the transverse and descending colon. Annular contractions divide the lumen into uniform segments, propelling feces over short distances in both directions. Segmental contractions form, relax, and re-form in different locations, seemingly at random. **Mass movement** is a strong ring contraction moving aborad over long distances in the transverse and descending colon. It occurs infrequently—perhaps only a few times daily—most commonly after meals.

The enteric nervous system coordinates and programs motility (see Chapter 29). Eating produces a group of alterations in colonic myoelectrical and motor activity collectively termed the gastrocolic response. As a result, more fluid is emptied from the ileum into the colon; mass movements are increased; and the urge to defecate is perceived. The magnitude of the gastrocolic response depends on the caloric content of the meal. Dietary fat is the principal stimulus.

Physical activities such as changes in posture, walking, and lifting are physiologically important stimuli of movement of colonic contents. Colonic motility is also affected by emotional states. Transit through the colon is speeded by a diet containing large amounts of fiber from vegetables or bran. Fiber is defined as insoluble plant cell matrix and consists of cellulose, hemicellulose, and lignin. Dietary fiber slows transit through the jejunum.

Normal colonic movements are slow, complex, and extremely variable, making it difficult to define altered motility in disease states. The fecal stream itself does not move along in anything resembling orderly laminar flow. Some of the material entering the cecum flows past feces remaining from earlier periods. Portions of the stream enter the periphery of haustra, where they may fail to progress for 24 hours or more. In most persons with normal bowel function, residue from a meal reaches the cecum after 4 hours and the rectosigmoid by 24 hours. The transverse colon is the primary site for fecal storage. Mixing of bowel content in the colon results in passage of residue from a single meal in movements for up to 3–4 days afterward.

The urge to defecate is perceived when small amounts of feces enter the rectum and stimulate stretch receptors in the rectal wall or the levator muscles. Rectal distention elicits the rectoanal inhibitory reflex, the reflex relaxation of the internal anal sphincter, which allows the rectal contents to be "sampled" by the specialized mucosa at the anorectal transition zone. Almost immediately after the internal sphincter relaxes, the external sphincter contracts, forcing the contents proximally into the rectum. This complex reflex mechanism is thought to allow the rectal contents to descend distally into the rectum, contacting the sensory fibers in the surgical anal canal. If it is a socially acceptable time and flatus is present, it may be expelled. If stool is present and defecation must be deferred, the rectum accommodates and the sense of rectal fullness abates. Defecation cannot be deferred indefinitely, and with continued rectal filling the urge to defecate is impossible to deny.

Defecation is facilitated by assuming the sitting position, performing a Valsalva maneuver, and relaxing the anal sphincters. The pelvic floor relaxes and the rectum loses its curves as the feces are discharged from the anus. Afterward, the sphincters resume their tone.

▶ Absorption

The colon participates in maintaining the body economy by absorption of water and electrolytes, but the absorptive function of the colon is not essential to life. Although amino acids, fatty acids, and some vitamins can be absorbed slowly from the large bowel, only a small amount of these nutrients reaches the colon normally. Perhaps 10–20% of ingested starch, however, passes unabsorbed into the colon, where bacterial fermentation converts starch to short-chain volatile fatty acids (eg, acetate). Absorption of fatty acids contributes importantly to assimilation of calories. Dietary celluloses and hemicelluloses are degraded by colonic bacteria.

Approximately 1000–2000 mL of ileal effluent consisting of 90% water enters the cecum each day. This material is desiccated during transit through the colon, so that only 100–200 mL of water is excreted in the feces. Table 30–1 gives average values for the electrolyte and water composition of ileal effluent and feces; the differences provide a rough estimate of colonic absorption and secretion. Data are listed also for the estimated maximal absorptive capacity, which is greater in the right colon than in the left. This capacity depends on the rate at which fluid enters the cecum. Normally, formed feces are composed of 70% water and 30% solids. Almost half of these solids are bacteria; the remainder is food waste and desquamated epithelium.

Table 30–1. Mean Values for Electrolyte and Water Balance in the Normal Colon. A Plus (+) Sign Indicates Absorption from the Colonic Lumen; A Minus (–) Sign Indicates Secretion into the Lumen.

	Ileal Effluent		Fecal Fluid		Net Colonic Absorption (per 24 h)	
	Concentration (meq/L)	Quantity (per 24 h)	Concentration (meq/L)	Quantity (per 24 h)	Normal	Maximal Capacity
Na^+	120	180 meq	30	2 meq	+178 meq	+400 meq
K^+	6	10 meq	67	5 meq	+5 meq	–45 meq
Cl^-	67	100 meq	20	1.5 meq	+98 meq	+500 meq
HCO_3	40	60 meq	50	4 meq	+56 meq	
H_2O		1500 mL		100 mL	+1400 mL	+5000 mL

Sodium is absorbed by an active transport mechanism that is enhanced by mineralocorticoids, glucocorticoids, and volatile fatty acids produced by bacteria. Volatile fatty acids may be essential mucosal nutrients for normal colonic absorption of electrolytes and water. There are segmental differences in the mode of absorption of sodium and water. Normally, sodium absorption is so efficient that a person can remain in balance on as little as 5 meq in the daily diet, but colectomy increases the minimum daily requirements to 80–100 meq to offset losses from the ileostomy. Potassium enters feces by passive diffusion and by secretion in mucus. Excessive mucus production may occur in colitis or with certain tumors such as villous adenomas and may lead to substantial potassium losses in the stool. Chloride is absorbed in exchange for bicarbonate.

▶ Bowel Habits

The frequency of defecation is influenced by social and dietary customs. The average interval between bowel movements among the population of Western countries is a little over 24 hours but may vary in normal subjects from 8–12 hours to 2–3 days. Dietary fiber content and physical activity influence stool frequency to a great extent. Many bedridden patients have infrequent, hard stools. Self-reported constipation in the general population of the United States has a prevalence of about 10% in men and 20% in women; gender differences in colonic function (slower transit and smaller fecal mass in women under controlled conditions) may be responsible for the difference in frequency of constipation. Diarrhea is reported by 5% of men and women. These complaints are more frequent with aging.

A change in bowel habits demands investigation for organic disease. Diarrhea may be debilitating and even fatal, because it is associated with loss of large amounts of water and electrolytes. Diarrhea is usually said to be present if stools contain more than 300 mL of fluid daily. Osmotic diarrhea results when excess water-soluble molecules remain in the bowel lumen, causing osmotic retention of water; this is one mechanism by which saline laxatives act. Colonic diseases that produce diarrhea usually cause excessive fluid secretion more so than impaired absorption. Bile salts, hydroxy fatty acids, and castor oil (ricinoleic acid) are a few of the many substances that stimulate secretion of fluid by the colon by increasing mucosal cyclic adenosine monophosphate (cAMP). Increased secretion by the small bowel may also cause diarrhea. Loss of absorptive surface (eg, after intestinal resection) and exudative diseases are other reasons for feces to contain excess fluid. Disordered intestinal motility is not primarily responsible for increased fecal excretion of water. The physician should be alert to surreptitious laxative abuse among patients who complain of diarrhea.

Constipation means infrequent stools (fewer than two per week), excessive straining, or incomplete evacuation. Recent onset of this complaint in an adult should prompt a search for obstructing lesions. Constipation affects up to

25% or more of the population in Western countries, with females more likely to be affected than males.

Severe idiopathic constipation refractory to usual remedies is more common in women; it often begins in adolescence and worsens during the 20s or 30s, or it may be precipitated by childbirth or hysterectomy. A heterogeneous group of disorders is responsible. Slow colonic transit (colonic inertia) is one mechanism of constipation. A decrease in the number of interstitial cells of Cajal has been implicated in this disorder. Failure of the pelvic floor to relax during defecation (obstructed defecation) is a separate category. A classification of disorders in which constipation and obstructed defecation are symptoms is given in Table 30–2. Conditions giving rise to obstructed defecation are part of a larger group of abnormalities termed disorders of the pelvic floor.

A thorough history and physical examination may elucidate the origin of the symptoms, eg, depression, psychotropic or other drugs, or anatomic abnormalities. Further investigation of chronic idiopathic constipation requires assessment of colonic transit and study of pelvic floor function. Colonic transit is evaluated by obtaining serial plain abdominal x-rays after ingestion of tiny radiopaque markers or by scintigraphy after ingestion of radiolabeled solid pellets. Tests of pelvic floor function include defecography, anorectal manometry, electromyography, nerve conduction studies and dynamic magnetic resonance imaging.

Severe slow-transit constipation does not respond to dietary fiber; lactulose or an irritant laxative (eg, Senokot, Dulcolax) or retrograde enemas may be effective. A number of pharmacologic agents have been evaluated and recently a selective chloride channel (CIC-2) activator (lubiprostone) in the apical membrane of the intestinal epithelium increases the intestinal chloride secretion and therefore fluid in the gut, facilitating the transit of stool. Tegaserod, a partial 5-hydroxytryptamin-4 (5-HT4) receptor agonist, was approved for chronic idiopathic constipation in both men and women in

Table 30–2. Classification of Constipation and Obstructed Defecation.[1]

Constipation
Normal colon
Normal transit
Slow transit
Megacolon/megarectum
Congenital
Acquired
Obstructed defecation
Solitary rectal ulcer syndrome
Descending perineum syndrome
Rectal intussusception
Complete rectal prolapse
Anismus (inappropriate sphincter contraction)

[1]Modified from Bartolo DCG: Pelvic floor disorders: incontinence, constipation, and obstructed defecation. Perspect Colon Rectal Surg 1988;1:1.

2004; however, it was subsequently withdrawn in 2007 after a meta-analysis demonstrated an increased number of cardiovascular events in patients treated with the agent.

Selected patients qualify for a surgical procedure (colectomy and ileorectal anastomosis). Although associated with a significant improvement in quality of life, postoperative persistence of abdominal pain and the development of incontinence or diarrhea are limitations. Obstructed defecation related to rectal prolapse responds to operative repair of the prolapse. Rectal intussusception is treated with fiber, water, and stimulating bowel movements with suppositories for mild to moderate situations. Patients are instructed to stimulate a bowel movement in the morning with a suppository and to ignore the urge to defecate during the day. The sense of rectal fullness that the patient experiences is a result of the proximal bowel prolapsing into the distal rectum. With this behavioral modification, the symptoms usually resolve. Biofeedback therapy may be a helpful adjunct. Surgical repair is reserved for severe cases of rectal intussusception.

Agarwal R, Afzalpurkar R, Fordtran JS: Pathophysiology of potassium absorption and secretion by the human intestine. Gastroenterology 1994;107:548.

Bassotti G et al: Colonic motility in man: features in normal subjects and in patients with chronic idiopathic constipation. Am J Gastroenterol 1999;94:1760.

Brown SR et al: Biofeedback avoids surgery in patients with slow-transit constipation: report of four cases. Dis Colon Rectum 2001;44:737.

FitzHarris GP et al: Quality of life after subtotal colectomy for slow-transit constipation: both quality and quantity count. Dis Colon Rectum 2003;46:433.

He CL et al: Decreased interstitial cell of Cajal volume in patients with slow-transit constipation. Gastroenterology 2000;118:14.

Johanson JF et al: Multicenter, 4-week, double-blind, randomized, placebo-controlled trial of lubiprostone, a locally-acting type-2 chloride channel activator, in patients with chronic constipation. Am J Gastroenterol 2008;103:170.

Knowles CH, Scott SM, Lunniss PJ: Slow transit constipation: a disorder of pelvic autonomic nerves? Dig Dis Sci 2001;46:389.

Locke GR 3rd, Pemberton JH, Phillips SF: AGA technical review on constipation. American Gastroenterological Association. Gastroenterology 2000;119:1766.

Mollen RM, Kuijpers HC, Claassen AT: Colectomy for slow-transit constipation: preoperative functional evaluation is important but not a guarantee for a successful outcome. Dis Colon Rectum 2001;44:577.

Monahan DW, Peluso FE, Goldner F: Combustible colonic gas levels during flexible sigmoidoscopy and colonoscopy. Gastrointest Endosc 1992;38:40.

Moran BJ, Jackson AA: Function of the human colon. Br J Surg 1992;79:1132.

Pikarsky AJ et al: Long-term follow-up of patients undergoing colectomy for colonic inertia. Dis Colon Rectum 2001;44:179.

Robertson G et al: Effects of exercise on total and segmental colon transit. J Clin Gastroenterol 1993;16:300.

Scheppach W, Luehrs H, Menzel T: Beneficial health effects of low-digestible carbohydrate consumption. Br J Nutr 2001; 85(Suppl 1):S23.

Tack J, Vanden Berghe P: Neuropeptides and colonic motility: it's all in the little brain. Gastroenterology 2000;119:257.

Thakur A et al: Surgical treatment of severe colonic inertia with restorative proctocolectomy. Am Surg 2001;67:36.

MICROBIOLOGY

The colon of the fetus is sterile, and the bacterial flora is established soon after birth. The type of organisms present in the colon depends in part on dietary and environmental factors. It is estimated that stool contains up to 400 different species of autochthonous (native) bacteria.

Over 99% of the normal fecal flora is anaerobic. *Bacteroides fragilis* is most prevalent, and counts average 10^{10}/g of wet feces. *Lactobacillus bifidus,* clostridia, and cocci of various types are other common anaerobes. Aerobic fecal bacteria are mainly coliforms and enterococci. *Escherichia coli* is the predominant coliform and is present in counts of 10^7/g of feces; other aerobic coliforms include klebsiella, proteus, and *Enterobacter. Streptococcus faecalis* is the principal enterococcus. *Methanobrevibacter smithii* is the predominant methane-producing organism in humans.

The fecal flora participates in numerous physiologic processes. Bacteria degrade bile pigments to give the stool its brown color, and the characteristic fecal odor is due to the amines indole and skatole produced by bacterial action. Fecal organisms deconjugate bile salts (only free bile salts are found in feces) and alter the steroid nucleus. Bacteria influence colonic motility and absorption, consume and generate intestinal gases, supply vitamin K to the host, and may be important in the defense against infection. Nutrition of colonic mucosal cells may be partially derived from fuels (eg, fatty acids) produced by bacteria. Intestinal bacteria participate in the pathophysiology of a variety of disease processes. Bacterial translocation from the small and large bowel in critically ill or traumatized patients is believed to contribute to multiple organ system failure. There is evidence that bacteria play a role in the pathogenesis of carcinoma of the large bowel.

Bourquin LD et al: Fermentation of dietary fibre by human colonic bacteria: disappearance of, short-chain fatty acid production from, and potential water-holding capacity of, various substrates. Scand J Gastroenterol 1993;28:249.

Chapman MA: The role of the colonic flora in maintaining a healthy large bowel mucosa. Ann R Coll Surg Engl 2001;83:75.

Gibson GR, MacFarlane GT, Cummings JH: Sulphate reducing bacteria and hydrogen metabolism in the human large intestine. Gut 1993;34:437.

Strocchi A et al: Methanogens outcompete sulphate reducing bacteria for H_2 in the human colon. Gut 1994;35:1098.

X-RAY EXAMINATION

Plain films of the abdomen depict the distribution of gas in the intestines, calcifications, tumor masses, and the size and position of the liver, spleen, and kidneys. In the presence of acute intra-abdominal disease, upright, lateral, and oblique projections and lateral decubitus views are helpful.

Although plain radiographs of the abdomen are generally nonspecific, they often give clues to the underlying problems. Free air in the abdominal cavity is best seen on upright views. An obstructing colon cancer may demonstrate dilation of the proximal colon with a paucity of gas distal to the mass. Air-fluid levels in the bowel in the absence of air within the rectum suggest a complete bowel obstruction. Volvulus of the sigmoid colon or cecum may demonstrate their characteristic radiographic findings.

The lumen of the colon can be seen radiographically by instilling a suspension of barium sulfate through the anus (barium enema) (Figure 30–3). Adequate preparation of the bowel is imperative before barium enema examination so that the colon will be as free as possible of fecal material and gas. Although many rectal lesions can be demonstrated by barium enema, x-rays are not as accurate here as with lesions above the rectosigmoid. Proctosigmoidoscopy is the best method for inspecting the rectum. Postevacuation films reveal the mucosal pattern and small lesions.

Barium enemas are performed as single-column or double-column studies. In the double-column (air contrast) barium enema, a higher-density, more viscous barium is used. After the mucosa is first coated with barium, carbon dioxide or air is insufflated to distend the colon and provide a second contrast medium. The double-column barium enema is more sensitive for detection of small lesions, but it is more strenuous and for that reason less well tolerated by frail or elderly patients.

Water-soluble contrast agents such as diatrizoate meglumine (Gastrografin) or diatrizoate sodium (Hypaque) may be used as alternatives to barium. Fine resolution with these agents is not as good as with barium; however, they can be used when barium is contraindicated, such as when there is a concern for perforation.

CT scan is very useful in the diagnosis of masses (neoplasms and abscesses) and is also the most sensitive for detecting intra-abdominal free air and acute inflammatory processes such as appendicitis or diverticulitis. CT colography, or *virtual colonoscopy*, is a technique that utilizes 3D reconstruction of the air-distended colon. In a series of 1223 average-risk adults who subsequently underwent conventional (optical) colonoscopy, virtual colonoscopy was as good as or better at detecting relevant lesions. A subsequent study demonstrated similar detection rates for advanced neoplasia with CT colonography and optical colonoscopy with a reduced rate of polypectomies and complications. Therefore, studies are ongoing to evaluate the efficacy of virtual colonoscopy in both screening and surveillance. Thus far, the major limitations include the need for full bowel preparation and follow-up colonoscopy for tissue diagnosis of radiographic abnormalities. Because virtual colonoscopy is considerably time and labor intensive from the standpoint of the radiologists, active investigations into methods of automating the evaluation process are ongoing.

MRI is proving reliable for staging of cancer. Sonography (external, endorectal, and endovaginal) is useful in the diagnosis of masses as well in the evaluation of anatomy, such as

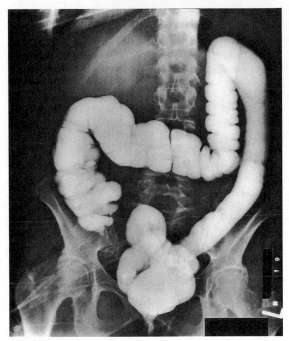

▲ **Figure 30–3.** X-ray of normal colon. The colon has been rendered radiopaque by a barium enema (single-column technique).

depth of penetration of rectal cancers or presence of pelvic nodal metastases. Positron emission tomography with fused computed tomography (PET/CT) has emerged as an increasingly valuable tool in the management of patients with colon and rectal cancer. PET has been shown to be 95% sensitive, 98% specific, and 96% accurate in the detection of cancer recurrence and is an important modality in the evaluation of suspected disease. The technique utilizes the glucose analogue fluorodeoxyglucose, which accumulates in metabolically active tissues. Semiquantitative analysis uses a standardized uptake value to help discriminate benign from malignant disease. When used appropriately, it can help to distinguish patients who would benefit from surgery for recurrent cancer from those who have unresectable disease, particularly when the other imaging modalities fail to localize the disease.

Arteriography is used to detect bleeding sites and is discussed in the section on acute lower gastrointestinal hemorrhage.

Extramural depth of tumor invasion at thin-section MR in patients with rectal cancer: results of the MERCURY study. Radiology 2007;243:132.

Fenlon HM et al: A comparison of virtual and conventional colonoscopy for the detection of colorectal polyps. N Engl J Med 1999;341:1496.

Freeman AH: CT and bowel disease. Br J Radiol 2001;74:4.

Garcia-Aguilar J et al: Accuracy of endorectal ultrasonography in preoperative staging of rectal tumors. Dis Colon Rectum 2002;45:10.

Hageman MJHH, Goei R: Cleansing enema prior to double-contrast barium enema examination: is it necessary? Radiology 1993;187:109.

Jensen DM: What to choose for diagnosis of bleeding colonic angiomas: colonoscopy, angiography, or helical computed tomography angiography? Gastroenterology 2000;119:581.

Kim DH et al: CT colonography versus colonoscopy for the detection of advanced neoplasia. N Engl J Med 2007;357:1403.

Libutti SK et al: A prospective study of 2-[18F]fluoro-2-deoxy-D-glucose/positron emission tomography scan, 99m Tc-labeled arcitumomab (CEA-scan), and blind second-look laparotomy for detecting colon cancer recurrence in patients with increasing carcinoembryonic antigen levels. Ann Surg Oncol 2001; 8:779.

Pickhart PJ et al: Computed tomographic virtual colonoscopy to screen for colorectal neoplasia in asymptomatic adults. N Engl J Med 2003;349:2191.

Suri S et al: Comparative evaluation of plain films, ultrasound and CT in the diagnosis of intestinal obstruction. Acta Radiol 1999;40:422.

Veit-Haibach P et al: Diagnostic accuracy of colorectal cancer staging with whole-body PET/CT colonography. JAMA 2006; 296:2590.

Vernava AM 3rd et al: Lower gastrointestinal bleeding. Dis Colon Rectum 1997;40:846.

FIBEROPTIC COLONOSCOPY & SIGMOIDOSCOPY

The flexible colonoscope permits examination of the entire colon in most individuals, and permits diagnostic and therapeutic intervention under direct vision.

Diagnostic colonoscopy is indicated in adults age 50 and over and repeated every 5–10 years if normal (Table 30–3). It is indicated also in those with a personal or family history of colorectal cancer, polyps, or specific familial cancer syndromes; after an abnormal or equivocal radiographic screening test or episode of unexplained rectal bleeding; after

Table 30–3. Indications for Colonoscopy.

Diagnostic indications
Age ≥ 50
Personal or family history of colorectal cancer, polyps, or specific familial cancer syndromes
Unexplained rectal bleeding or change in bowel habits
Unexplained anemia
Abnormal or equivocal barium enema
Abnormal sigmoidoscopy (eg, polyps)
Inflammatory bowel disease
Therapeutic indications
Excision of polyps
Control of bleeding
Removal of a foreign body
Detorsion of volvulus
Decompression of pseudoobstruction
Dilation of strictures
Destruction of neoplasms

abnormal sigmoidoscopy (eg, polyps); and for any patient with a diagnosis of inflammatory bowel disease. Therapeutic uses of colonoscopy include excision of polyps, control of bleeding, removal of a foreign body, detorsion of volvulus, decompression of pseudoobstruction, dilation of strictures, placement of endoluminal stents, and destruction of neoplasms when formal surgical resection is contraindicated. Relative contraindications to colonoscopy are fulminant colitis and suspected colonic perforation. The main complications of diagnostic colonoscopy procedures include perforation (0.1–0.2%) and bleeding (0.2%). Success may be limited by such technical difficulties as diverticular disease, strictures, angulation, redundant colon, or previous pelvic surgery.

Flexible sigmoidoscopy uses an instrument 70 cm long. The complications of flexible sigmoidoscopy are similar to colonoscopy, although a higher rate of perforation (0.8%) has been reported. Flexible sigmoidoscopes have replaced the rigid variety for most but not all purposes.

Botoman VA, Pietro M, Thirlby RC: Localization of colonic lesions with endoscopic tattoo. Dis Colon Rectum 1994;37:775.

Lieberman DA et al: Use of colonoscopy to screen asymptomatic adults for colorectal cancer. Veterans Affairs Cooperative Study Group 380. N Engl J Med 2000;343:162.

Sieg A, et al: Prospective evaluation of complications in outpatient GI endoscopy: a survey among German gastroenterologists. Gastrointest Endosc 2001;53:620.

Winawer SJ et al: A comparison of colonoscopy and double-contrast barium enema for surveillance after polypectomy. National Polyp Study Work Group. N Engl J Med 2000; 342:1766.

▼ DISEASES OF THE COLON & RECTUM

OBSTRUCTION OF THE LARGE INTESTINE

 ESSENTIALS OF DIAGNOSIS

► Constipation or obstipation.

► Abdominal distention and sometimes tenderness.

► Abdominal pain.

► Nausea and vomiting (late).

► Characteristic x-ray findings.

► General Considerations

Approximately 15% of intestinal obstructions in adults occur in the large bowel. The obstruction may be in any portion of the colon but most commonly is in the sigmoid. Complete colonic obstruction is most often due to carcinoma; volvulus, diverticular disease, inflammatory disorders, benign tumors, fecal impaction, and miscellaneous rare problems account for the remainder (Table 30–4). Adhesive bands seldom obstruct the colon, and intussusception is uncommon in adults.

Obstruction by a lesion at the ileocecal valve produces the symptoms and signs of small bowel obstruction. The pathophysiology of more distal colonic obstruction depends on the competence of the ileocecal valve (Figure 30–4). In 10–20% of individuals, the ileocecal valve is incompetent, and colonic pressure is relieved by reflux into the ileum. If the colon is not decompressed through the ileocecal valve, a closed loop is formed between the valve and the obstructing point. The colon distends progressively because the ileum continues to empty gas and fluid into the obstructed segment. If luminal pressure becomes very high, circulation is impaired and gangrene and perforation can result. The wall of the right colon is thinner than that of the left colon and its luminal caliber is larger, so the cecum is at greatest risk of perforation in these circumstances (law of Laplace). In general, if the cecum acutely reaches a diameter of 10–12 cm, the risk of perforation is great.

► Clinical Findings

A. Symptoms and Signs

Simple mechanical obstruction of the colon may develop insidiously. Deep, visceral, cramping pain from obstruction of the colon is usually referred to the hypogastrium. Lesions of the fixed portions of the colon (cecum, hepatic flexure, splenic flexure) may cause pain that is felt immediately anteriorly. Pain originating from the sigmoid is often located to the left in the lower abdomen. Severe, continuous abdominal pain suggests intestinal ischemia or peritonitis. Borborygmus may be loud and coincident with cramps. Constipation or obstipation is a universal feature of complete obstruction, though the colon distal to the obstruction may empty after the initial symptoms begin. Vomiting is a late finding and may not occur at all if the ileocecal valve prevents reflux. If reflux decompresses the cecal contents into the small intestine, the symptoms of small bowel as well as large bowel obstruction appear. Feculent vomiting is a late manifestation.

Physical examination discloses abdominal distention and tympany, and peristaltic waves may be seen if the abdominal

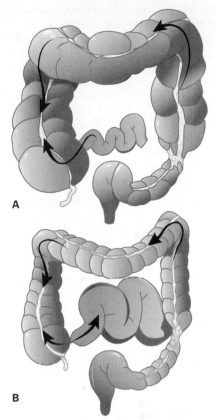

▲ **Figure 30–4.** The role of the ileocecal valve in obstruction of the colon. The obstruction is in the upper sigmoid. **A:** The ileocecal valve is competent, creating a closed loop between the obstruction and the valve. Tension in the closed loop is increased further by emptying of gas and fluid from the ileum into the colon. **B:** The ileocecal valve is incompetent. Reflux into the ileum is permitted. The colon is relieved of some of its distention, and the small bowel has become distended.

wall is thin. High-pitched, metallic tinkles associated with rushes and gurgles may be heard on auscultation. Localized tenderness or a tender, palpable mass may indicate a strangulated closed loop. Signs of localized or generalized peritonitis suggest gangrene or rupture of the bowel wall. Fresh blood may be found in the rectum in intussusception and in carcinoma of the rectum or colon. Sigmoidoscopy may disclose a neoplasm. Colonoscopy may be diagnostic and perhaps therapeutic in some patients with strictures or neoplasms.

B. Imaging Studies

The distended colon frequently creates a "picture frame" outline of the abdominal cavity. The colon can be distin-

Table 30–4. Causes of Colonic Obstruction in Adults.

Cause	Relative Incidence (%)*
Carcinoma of colon	65
Diverticulitis	20
Volvulus	5
Miscellaneous	10

*Obstruction due to diverticulitis is usually incomplete; volvulus is second to carcinoma as a cause of complete obstruction.

guished from the small intestine by its haustral markings, which do not cross the entire lumen of the distended colon. A contrast enema or CT scan with rectal contrast will confirm the diagnosis of colonic obstruction and identify its exact location. Water-soluble contrast medium should be used if strangulation or perforation is suspected. Barium should not be given orally in the presence of suspected colonic obstruction. A CT scan with rectal contrast is the most useful single test for large bowel obstruction because it can yield information regarding the location and etiology of the bowel obstruction.

▶ Differential Diagnosis

A. Small Versus Large Bowel Obstruction

Large bowel obstruction is frequently slow in onset, causes less pain, and may not cause vomiting in spite of considerable distention. Elderly patients with no history of abdominal surgery or prior attacks of obstruction frequently have carcinoma of the large bowel. Plain abdominal x-rays and contrast studies are helpful in establishing the diagnosis.

B. Paralytic Ileus

Paralytic ileus may be a result of peritonitis or trauma to the back or pelvis. The abdomen is silent, and abdominal cramping is not present. There may be tenderness. Plain films show a dilated colon. Contrast enema may be required to exclude an obstruction.

C. Pseudo-obstruction

Acute pseudo-obstruction of the colon (**Ogilvie syndrome**) is massive colonic distention in the absence of a mechanically obstructing lesion (Figure 30–5). It is a severe form of ileus and arises in bedridden patients who have serious extraintestinal illness (renal, cardiac, respiratory) or trauma (eg, vertebral fracture). Aerophagia and impairment of colonic motility by drugs are contributing factors. Abdominal distention without pain or tenderness is the earliest manifestation, but later symptoms mimic those of true obstruction. Plain x-rays of the abdomen show marked gaseous distention of the colon. Although the entire colon may contain gas, the distention is typically localized to the right colon, with a cutoff at the hepatic or splenic flexure. Contrast enema proves the absence of obstruction, but instillation of radiopaque material should cease as soon as the dilated colon is reached.

Conservative treatment with nasogastric suction and enemas may succeed in resolving colonic pseudoobstruction. Neostigmine is highly effective in treating colonic pseudoobstruction. It should be avoided in patients with a mechanical colonic obstruction, bradycardia, bronchospasm, or renal insufficiency. If the cecum is markedly dilated, the risk of perforation is high, and direct intervention must be prompt. Colonoscopic decompression is the method of choice if an expert is available. Initial success is claimed in 90% of

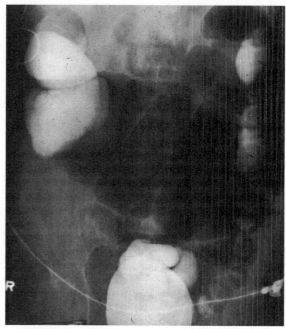

▲ **Figure 30–5.** Plain radiograph demonstrating the dilated colon with pseudoobstruction (Ogilvie syndrome). (Courtesy of Dr. Santhat Nivatvongs.)

patients, but recurrence is common (25% or more). Often, it is possible to place a tube into the proximal colon during colonoscopy to maintain decompression. Placement of a decompressive tube per rectum under fluoroscopic guidance has been described recently. Another alternative is cecostomy, performed either in the standard open fashion or by an endoscopic percutaneous method, similar to the technique for gastrostomy, using laparoscopic assistance.

▶ Complications

Cecal perforation, described earlier, is a potentially lethal complication. Partially obstructive lesions of the colon may be complicated by acute colitis in the bowel proximal to the obstruction; it is probably a form of ischemic colitis secondary to impaired mucosal blood flow in the distended segment.

▶ Treatment

An operation is almost always required. The primary goals of treatment are resection of all necrotic bowel and decompression of the obstructed segment. Removal of the obstructing lesion is a secondary goal, but a single operation to accomplish both objectives is preferred whenever possible.

Colonoscopic balloon dilation with endoluminal stent placement across obstructing benign strictures or neoplasms may be performed in selected circumstances. Stent placement may allow for decompression of the obstruction as a bridge to elective resection. Stents may be considered also for palliation in patients whose life expectancy is less than 6 months, which is the expected patency of a colonic stent placed for malignancy. Laser photocoagulation of an obstructing cancer, especially in the rectum, may enlarge the lumen to permit an elective operation later under better circumstances, and occasionally a patient with advanced cancer may avoid operation entirely. Permanent diverting colostomy may be the only possible choice in a debilitated patient with unresectable obstructing rectal cancer.

Obstructing lesions of the right colon are resected in one stage, with ileotransverse colostomy if the patient's condition is good. If the patient's condition is precarious or if the colon has perforated, the bowel is resected but no anastomosis is done; an ileostomy is established, and anastomosis is performed at a second operation. Unresectable lesions may be bypassed.

Obstructing lesions of the left colon are best treated by resection in patients who seem likely to tolerate this procedure. After resection has been achieved, anastomosis may be postponed and a temporary end colostomy created (two-stage procedure; Figure 30–6). Alternatively, intraoperative colonic lavage has previously been advocated to cleanse the colon well enough so that primary anastomosis can be performed safely. In this setting, subtotal colectomy results in similar morbidity and mortality as on-table lavage and still permits a one-stage procedure using healthy bowel. If the proximal bowel is healthy, a primary anastomosis with a proximal defunctioning (diverting) loop ileostomy may be possible. Two other options may be entertained. A colonic stent may be deployed preoperatively to decompress the obstructed bowel, allowing for an elective resection under better circumstances. Alternatively, in unfavorable circumstances, a diverting transverse colostomy may utilized. However, a serious disadvantage is the need for three operations if this approach is elected: (1) colostomy, (2) resection of the obstructing lesion with anastomosis, and (3) closure of the colostomy.

▶ Prognosis

The prognosis depends upon the age and general condition of the patient, the extent of vascular impairment of the bowel, the presence or absence of perforation, the cause of obstruction, and the promptness of surgical management. The overall mortality rate is about 20%. Cecal perforation carries a 40% mortality rate. Obstructing cancer of the colon has a worse prognosis than nonobstructing cancer because it is more likely to be locally extensive or metastatic to nodes or distant sites.

Baron TH: Expandable metal stents for the treatment of cancerous obstruction of the gastrointestinal tract. N Engl J Med 2001; 344:1681.

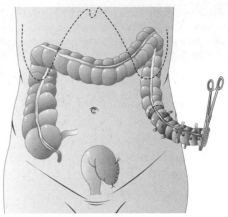

▲ **Figure 30–6.** Primary resection for diverticulitis of the colon. The affected segment (shaded) has been divided at its distal end. If primary anastomosis is to be done, the proximal margin (dotted line) is transected, and the bowel is anastomosed end to end. If a two-stage procedure will be used, a colostomy is formed at the proximal margin, and the distal stump is oversewn (Hartmann procedure, as shown) or exteriorized as a mucous fistula. The second stage consists of colostomy takedown and anastomosis.

Bharucha AE et al: Acute, toxic, and chronic. Curr Treat Options Gastroenterol 1999;2:517.

Boorman P et al: Endoluminal stenting of obstructed colorectal tumours. Ann R Coll Surg Engl 1999;81:251.

Breitenstein S et al: Systematic evaluation of surgical strategies for acute malignant left-sided colonic obstruction. Br J Surg 2007;94:1451.

Chapman AH, McNamara M, Porter G: The acute contrast enema in suspected large bowel obstruction: value and technique. Clin Radiol 1992;46:273.

Gooszen AW et al: Operative treatment of acute complications of diverticular disease: primary or secondary anastomosis after sigmoid resection. Eur J Surg 2001;167:35.

Gooszen AW et al: Prospective study of primary anastomosis following sigmoid resection for suspected acute complicated diverticular disease. Br J Surg 2001;88:693.

Ponec RJ, Saunders MD, Kimmey MB: Neostigmine for the treatment of acute colonic pseudo-obstruction. N Engl J Med 1999;341:137.

SCOTIA Study Group. Single-stage treatment for malignant left-sided colonic obstruction: a prospective randomized clinical trial comparing subtotal colectomy with segmental resection following intraoperative irrigation. Br J Surg 1995; 82(12):1622.

Stewart J, Diament RH, Brennan TG: Management of obstructing lesions of the left colon by resection, on-table lavage, and primary anastomosis. Surgery 1993;114:502.

Suri S et al: Comparative evaluation of plain films, ultrasound and CT in the diagnosis of intestinal obstruction. Acta Radiol 1999;40:422.

Tilney HS et al: Comparison of colonic stenting and open surgery for malignant large bowel obstruction. Surg Endosc 2007; 21:225.

CANCER OF THE LARGE INTESTINE

ESSENTIALS OF DIAGNOSIS

Right colon:

▶ Unexplained weakness or anemia.

▶ Occult blood in feces.

▶ Dyspeptic symptoms.

▶ Persistent right abdominal discomfort.

▶ Palpable abdominal mass.

▶ Characteristic x-ray findings.

▶ Characteristic colonoscopic findings.

Left colon:

▶ Change in bowel habits.

▶ Gross blood in stool.

▶ Obstructive symptoms.

▶ Characteristic x-ray findings.

▶ Characteristic colonoscopic or sigmoidoscopic findings.

Rectum:

▶ Rectal bleeding.

▶ Change in bowel habits.

▶ Sensation of incomplete evacuation.

▶ Intrarectal palpable tumor.

▶ Sigmoidoscopic findings.

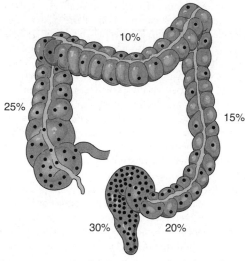

▲ **Figure 30–7.** Distribution of cancer of the colon and rectum.

▶ General Considerations

In Western countries, cancer of the colon and rectum ranks second after cancer of the lung in incidence and death rates. An estimated 150,000 new cases of colorectal cancer are diagnosed and over 50,000 people die of this disease in the United States each year. The overall death rates from colorectal cancer in the United States has been declining since the mid-1980s, perhaps related to earlier detection. The incidence increases with age, from 0.39/1000 persons per year at age 50 to 4.5/1000 persons per year at age 80. Carcinoma of the colon, particularly the right colon, is more common in women, and carcinoma of the rectum is more common in men. The distribution of cancers of the colon and rectum is shown in Figure 30–7. An apparent "proximal shift" of cancer (increased incidence in the right colon and decreased incidence in the rectum) in recent decades is at least partially explainable by improved diagnostic accuracy for proximal lesions as a result of total colonoscopy. Multiple synchronous colonic cancers (ie, two or more carcinomas occurring simultaneously) are found in 5% of patients. Metachronous cancer is a new primary lesion in a patient who has had a

previous resection for cancer. The cumulative risk of metachronous colorectal cancer was 6.3% at 18 years in one study and as high as 10% at a mean follow-up of 39 months in another series. Ninety-five percent of malignant tumors of the colon and rectum are adenocarcinomas.

Genetic predisposition to cancer of the large bowel is well recognized in persons with familial adenomatous polyposis (FAP; discussed in the Treatment section under Polyps of the Colon & Rectum). The most common form of hereditary colorectal cancer is **hereditary nonpolyposis colorectal cancer (HNPCC)**, also called Lynch syndrome. There are four cardinal features of HNPCC: (1) earlier average age (45 years) at onset of cancer than in the general population, (2) the presence of HNPCC-associated cancers within the pedigree, (3) improved survival when compared stage for stage to sporadic cases, (4) the presence of a germline mutation in affected family members. The gene responsible for this syndrome has been localized to chromosome 2p, and the genetic defect is in DNA mismatch repair genes (*MLH1, MSH2, MSH6, PMS1,* and *PMS2*). The defects occur in the setting of microsatellite instability. There may be other genes not as of yet identified. The Amsterdam I and II criteria and Revised Bethesda criteria (Tables 30–5a and 30–5b) were developed to identify patients with HNPCC. The presence of the Amsterdam criteria defines HNPCC by history alone and the presence of any one of the Revised Bethesda criteria warrants further investigation for HNPCC. However, all patients with early-onset colorectal cancer should be offered screening for a familial colorectal cancer syndrome. First-degree relatives of patients with sporadic colorectal cancer have a twofold to threefold increased risk of large bowel cancer, and it is estimated that approximately 10% of cancers of the large

Table 30–5a. Amsterdam I and II criteria.

Amsterdam I criteria:	
At least three relatives must have histologically verified colorectal cancer.	(1) One must be a first-degree relative of the other two. (2) At least two successive generations must be affected. (3) At least one of the relatives with colorectal cancer must have received the diagnosis before age 50.
Amsterdam II criteria:	
At least three relatives must have a cancer associated with hereditary nonpolyposis colorectal cancer (HNPCC) (colorectal, endometrial, stomach, ovary, ureter or renal-pelvis, brain, small bowel, hepatobiliary tract, skin (sebaceous tumors)	(1) One must be a first-degree relative of the other two. (2) At least two successive generations must be affected. (3) At least one of the relatives with HNPCC-associated cancer must have received the diagnosis before age 50.

bowel are due primarily to an inherited genetic defect. (Polyposis-associated familial colorectal cancer syndromes are discussed later in chapter.)

Ulcerative colitis, Crohn colitis, schistosomal colitis, exposure to radiation, and the presence of an ureterocolostomy are conditions that predispose to cancer of the large bowel. It was previously thought that a prior history of cholecystectomy predisposed to the development of colorectal cancer, but this has largely been disproved.

The main behavioral risk factors for the development of advanced colorectal neoplasia include cigarette smoking and excessive alcohol consumption. Additional contributing factors may include obesity, lack of dietary fiber, and excessive red meat consumption. Mitigating factors include nonsteroidal anti-inflammatory drug (NSAID) use, vitamin D consumption, and physical activity.

Table 30–5b. Revised Bethesda Criteria.

1. Colorectal cancer (CRC) diagnosed in individual under age 50 years.
2. Presence of synchronous, metachronous colorectal or other HNPCC-associated tumors, regardless of age.
3. CRC with the microsatellite instability-high (MSI-H) histology (presence of tumor-infiltrating lymphocytes, Crohn-like lymphocytic reaction, mucinous/signet-ring differentiation, or medullary growth pattern) in patient 60 years of age.
4. CRC in one or more first-degree relatives with an HNPCC-related tumor, with one of the cancers being diagnosed under age 50 years.
5. CRC diagnosed in two or more first- or second-degree relatives with HNPCC-related tumors, regardless of age.

A high incidence of colorectal cancer occurs in populations that are economically prosperous. This observation has focused attention on environmental factors, particularly diet, in the etiology of this tumor. Increased intake of saturated fat, increased caloric intake, decreased dietary calcium, and decreased intake of fiber are among the possible dietary influences. Dietary fat enhances cholesterol and bile acid synthesis by the liver, and the amounts of these sterols in the colon increase. Anaerobic colonic bacteria convert these compounds to secondary bile acids, which are promoters of carcinogenesis. Other possible mechanisms by which saturated fat promotes colorectal cancer include changes in immunity, effects on lipid peroxidation, and modulation of prostaglandin synthesis through arachidonic acid metabolism. Experimental studies have suggested that dietary fish oil, rich in unsaturated fatty acids of the omega-3 type, is protective against colorectal cancer, and the mechanism may be inhibition of prostaglandin synthesis from arachidonic acid.

The mechanism by which dietary fiber is protective remains elusive. Effects of fiber on fecal bulk, water content, transit time, and pH are less important than once thought. Plant lignans in fiber are fermented to a group of human lignans by colonic bacteria, and these substances may be important in some way. Metabolic activity of gut microflora is altered by dietary fiber, perhaps with important inhibitory effects on tumor promoters such as bile acids. Another possible mechanism is chelation of dietary iron by the phytate content of high-fiber foods. Iron catalyzes oxidation of lipid to substances that are genotoxic, and iron has been associated with the initiating and promoting phases of carcinogenesis in experimental systems. Ingested calcium affects colonic epithelial cell proliferation topically and by absorption into the bloodstream. If these concepts are correct, reducing dietary saturated fat and calories and increasing the intake of calcium and fermentable fiber can minimize the risk of colorectal cancer. Populations with a high incidence of colon cancer tend to have low serum cholesterol levels, and average serum cholesterol levels are higher in groups with less cancer of the colon.

Carcinogenesis in the large bowel and elsewhere is a long, multistep process. Colorectal cancer involves multiple genetic alterations, ie, oncogene activation, including K-ras point mutation, c-myc amplification and overexpression, and c-src kinase activation. Tumor-suppressor gene inactivation is also important; these events may include point mutations in the APC gene (adenomatous polyposis coli, at chromosome 5q21), the DCC gene (deleted in colorectal carcinoma, on chromosome 18q), and TP53 (on chromosome 17). Genetic damage is initiated by carcinogenic agents. In addition, DNA microsatellite instability has been demonstrated to be another pathway for colorectal carcinogenesis. Promoters, such as bile acids, may stimulate growth of a benign neoplasm, and it may be that still other promoters cause malignant change to occur. There is evidence that estrogen may have a protective effect for the development of colon cancer. Aspirin and other

NSAIDs, particularly the cyclooxygenase-2 inhibitors, may also reduce the incidence of and mortality rate from colorectal cancer by inhibition of the prostaglandins implicated in immune suppression and the promotion of metastasis. The use of such agents is the subject of several clinical trials for the chemoprevention of colon cancer.

Cancer of the colon and rectum spreads in the following ways:

A. Direct Extension

Carcinoma grows circumferentially and may completely encircle the bowel before it is diagnosed; this is especially true in the left colon, which has a smaller caliber than the right. It takes about 1 year for a tumor to encircle three fourths of the circumference of the bowel. Longitudinal submucosal extension occurs with invasion of the intramural lymphatic network, but it rarely goes beyond 2 cm from the edge of the tumor unless there is concomitant spread to lymph nodes. As the lesion extends radially, it penetrates the outer layers of the bowel wall, and it may extend by contiguity into neighboring structures: the liver, the greater curvature of the stomach, the duodenum, the small bowel, the pancreas, the spleen, the bladder, the vagina, the kidneys and ureters, and the abdominal wall. Cancer of the rectum may invade the vaginal wall, bladder, prostate, or sacrum, and it may extend along the levators. Subacute perforation with inflammatory attachment of bowel to an adjacent viscus may be indistinguishable from actual invasion on gross examination.

B. Hematogenous Metastasis

Lymphovascular invasion may allow tumor cells be carried via the portal venous system to establish hepatic metastases. Tumor embolization also occurs through lumbar and vertebral veins to the lungs and elsewhere. Rectal cancer spreads through tributaries of the hypogastric veins. Metastases to ovaries are mostly hematogenous; they are found in 1–10.3% of women with colorectal cancer. Venous invasion occurs in 15–50% of cases even though it does not always cause distant metastases. An attempt is made to avoid producing hematogenous metastases during operation by minimizing manipulation of the tumor prior to ligation of the blood supply.

C. Regional Lymph Node Metastasis

This is the most common form of tumor spread (Figure 30–8). Longitudinal spread via extramural lymphatics is an important mechanism. Rectal cancer metastasizes proximally to the mesorectal, iliac, and inferior mesenteric lymph nodes, and radially along lymphatics to the pelvic side walls, where obturator nodes can become involved. The lymphatic drainage of the tumor must be removed in curative operations, and some nodal involvement will be found in over half of the specimens. Over the past several years, sentinel lymph node mapping for colorectal cancer has been under investigation in an effort to improve identification of candidates for adjuvant chemother-

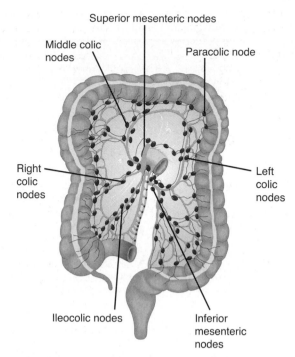

▲ **Figure 30–8.** Lymphatic drainage of the colon. The lymph nodes (black) are distributed along the blood vessels to the bowel.

apy. However, results have been inconsistent with several large single and multi-institutional studies demonstrating an unacceptably high false-negative rate with the technique. The completeness of lymph node evaluation as reflected in the total number of lymph nodes examined at the time of colectomy for cancer is associated with survival. The size of the lesion bears little relationship to the degree of nodal involvement. The more anaplastic the lesion, the more likely that lymph node metastasis will occur. Up to 10–25% of T1 rectal cancers may harbor occult lymph node metastases.

D. Transperitoneal Metastasis

"Seeding" may occur when the tumor has extended through the serosa and tumor cells enter the peritoneal cavity, producing local implants or generalized abdominal carcinomatosis. Large metastatic deposits in the pelvic cul-de-sac are palpable as a hard shelf (Blumer shelf).

E. Intraluminal Metastasis

Malignant cells shed from the surface of the tumor can be swept along in the fecal current. Implantation more distally on intact mucosa occurs rarely, if ever, but viable exfoliated cells presumably can be trapped in an anastomotic suture or staple line during operation.

▶ Clinical Findings

A. Symptoms and Signs

Adenocarcinoma of the colon and rectum has a median doubling time (the time required for the tumor to double in volume) of 130 days, suggesting that at least 5 years—and often 10–15 years—of silent growth are required before a cancer reaches symptom-producing size. During this asymptomatic phase, diagnosis depends on routine examination.

The value of **routine screening** of asymptomatic populations who lack high-risk factors for development of large bowel cancer has been established. Screening should be initiated at age 50. The goals of screening are detection of early cancers and prevention of cancer by finding and removing adenomas. The screening recommendations of the American Society of Colon and Rectal Surgery are listed in (Table 30–6). Screening for occult blood detects has been shown to have a survival benefit in a US prospective trial of occult blood testing followed by colonoscopy in those with positive tests. Improved survival in the screened group was related to a lower percentage of advanced cancers—the lesions that more commonly prove fatal. It is not clear whether the survival benefit in this study should be attributed mainly to the tests for occult blood or the colonoscopy, because the latter test alone might have achieved the same outcome. Four case-control studies have demonstrated that sigmoidoscopy is associated with a reduced mortality for colorectal cancer. However, its utility as a screening test for colorectal neoplasia is limited by the amount of colon visualized with a 70 cm sigmoidoscope. Cancer mortality is reduced for lesions within the reach of the sigmoidoscope but not in the area beyond the reach of the sigmoidoscope. Therefore, flexible sigmoidoscopy should be used in conjunction with radiographic evaluation of the more proximal colon or annual fecal occult blood testing. Dissatisfaction with the poor specificity of guaiac slide tests has led to

Table 30–6. American Society of Colon and Rectal Surgeons Guidelines for Colorectal Cancer Screening.[1]

Risk	Procedure	Onset (Age, yr)	Frequency
I. Low Risk			
A. Asymptomatic—no risk factors	Fecal occult blood testing and flex-sig	50	FOBT yearly. Flex-sig every 5 years
B. Colorectal cancer in none of first-degree relatives	Total colon examination (colonoscopy or double-contrast barium enema and proctosigmoidoscopy)	50	Every 5–10 years
II. Moderate Risk (20–30% of people)			
A. Colorectal cancer in first-degree relative, age 55 or younger, or two or more first-degree relatives of any ages	Colonoscopy	40, or 10 yrs. before the youngest case in the family, whichever is earlier	Every 5 years
B. Colorectal cancer in a first-degree relative over the age of 55	Colonoscopy	50, or 10 yrs. before the age of the case, whichever is earlier	Every 5–10 years
C. Personal history of large (> 1 cm) or multiple colorectal polyps of any size	Colonoscopy	One year after polypectomy	If recurrent polyps—1 year If normal—5 years
D. Personal history of colorectal malignancy—surveillance after resection for curative intent	Colonoscopy	1 year after resection	If normal—3 years If still normal—5 years If abnormal—as above
III. High Risk (6–8 percent of people)			
A. Family history of hereditary adenomatous polyposis	Flex-sig; consider genetic counseling and genetic testing	12–14 (Puberty)	Every 1–2 years
B. Family history of hereditary nonpolyposis colon cancer	Colonoscopy; consider genetic counseling and genetic testing	21–40 40	Every 2 years Every year
C. Inflammatory bowel disease			
1. Left-side colitis	Colonoscopy	15th	Every 1–2 years
2. Pancolitis	Colonoscopy	8th	Every 1–2 years

[1]FOBT, fecal occult blood testing; Flex-sig, flexible sigmoidoscopy.

development of alternative methods, including immunochemical fecal occult blood tests and fecal tests for DNA mutations. If fecal occult blood testing is positive, total colonoscopy should be performed. As a screening test, flexible sigmoidoscopy, when normal, should be repeated every 5 years. Alternatively, total colonoscopy can be performed as the initial examination, since all roads eventually lead to colonoscopy for diagnosis or therapy (as in the case of a lesion on barium enema).

Screening colonoscopy has been widely recognized to save lives by preventing the development of colorectal cancer. However, as a screening test, it is operator dependent. The incidence of missed polyps may be as high as 10% and related to the duration of time the operator spends during the examination. In addition, the yield particularly for small lesions may be augmented by new technologies such as high-definition video and chromoendography. Yet there is still controversy regarding the cost effectiveness of routine colonoscopic screening when compared to other modalities.

More recently, fecal immunohistochemical testing and fecal DNA testing has been studied with great interest, as they may potentially have improved rates of sensitivity and specificity when compared to fecal occult blood tests. The principle advantage of these tests is the potential for improved population participation rates when compared to invasive modalities such as flexible sigmoidoscopy with air-contrast barium enema or colonoscopy.

The need for colonoscopic screening of patients in high-risk groups has been established, but the timing of initial evaluations must be individualized. Children with possible FAP should have annual or biannual sigmoidoscopy (then colonoscopy as indicated) starting at puberty. Biannual colonoscopy beginning at age 21 is the recommendation for members of families with HNPCC. Colonoscopy every year is probably the best advice for patients with ulcerative colitis for longer than 10 years. People with a history of colorectal cancer in one first-degree relative should undergo colonoscopy starting by age 50 years or at an age 10 years younger than the age at which the index relative was diagnosed.

Symptoms in patients with large bowel cancer depend upon the anatomic location of the lesion, its type and extent, and upon complications, including perforation, obstruction, and hemorrhage. Marked systemic manifestations such as cachexia are indications of advanced disease. The average delay between the onset of symptoms and definitive therapy is 7–9 months; both patients and physicians are responsible.

The **right colon** has a large caliber and a thin and distensible wall, and the fecal content is fluid. Because of these anatomic features, carcinoma of the right colon may attain large size before it is diagnosed. Patients often see a physician for complaints of fatigue and weakness due to severe anemia. Unexplained microcytic hypochromic anemia should always raise the question of carcinoma of the colon. Gross blood may not be visible in the stool, but occult blood may be detected. Patients may complain of vague right abdominal discomfort, which is often postprandial and may be mistakenly attributed to gallbladder or gastroduodenal disease. Alterations in bowel habits are not characteristic of carcinoma of the right colon, and obstruction is uncommon. In about 10% of cases, the first evidence of the disease is discovery of a mass by the patient or the physician.

The **left colon** has a smaller lumen than the right, and the feces are semisolid. Tumors of the left colon can gradually occlude the lumen, causing changes in bowel habits with alternating constipation and increased frequency of defecation (not true watery diarrhea). Partial or complete obstruction may be the initial picture. Bleeding is common but is rarely massive. The stool may be streaked or mixed with bright red or dark blood, and mucus is often passed together with small blood clots.

In **cancer of the rectum,** the most common symptom is the passage of bright red blood with bowel movements (hematochezia). Bleeding is usually persistent; it may be slight or (rarely) copious. Blood may or may not be mixed with stool or mucus. Predictions of an anal source of bleeding based on color and pattern are unreliable. *Whenever persistent rectal bleeding occurs, even in the presence of hemorrhoids, cancer must be ruled out.* There may be tenesmus (an ineffectual urge to evacuate the rectum).

Physical examination is important to determine the extent of local disease, to identify distant metastases, and to detect diseases of other organ systems that may influence treatment. The supraclavicular areas should be carefully palpated for metastatic nodes. Examination of the abdomen may disclose a mass, enlargement of the liver, ascites, or engorgement of the abdominal wall veins if there is portal obstruction. If a mass is palpated, its location and extent of fixation are important.

Distal rectal cancers can be felt as a flat, hard, oval or encircling tumor with rolled edges and a central depression. Its extent, the size of the lumen at the site of the tumor, and the degree of fixation should be noted. Blood may be found on the examining finger. Vaginal and rectovaginal examination will yield additional information on the extent of the tumor. Retrorectal nodes may be palpable. Rigid proctoscopic examination is essential to accurately determine the location of the tumor within the rectum in order to inform subsequent treatment decisions.

B. Laboratory Findings

Urinalysis, leukocyte count, and hemoglobin determination should be done. Serum proteins, calcium, bilirubin, alkaline phosphatase, and creatinine should be measured if clinically indicated.

The most familiar chemical marker for cancer of the large bowel is **carcinoembryonic antigen (CEA)**, a glycoprotein found in the cell membranes of many tissues, including colorectal cancer. Some of the antigen enters the circulation and is detected by radioimmunoassay of serum; CEA is also detectable in various other body fluids, urine, and feces. Elevated serum CEA is not specifically associated with colorectal cancer; abnormally high levels are also found in sera of patients with other gastrointestinal cancers, nonalimentary cancers, and various benign diseases. CEA levels are high in 70% of patients with cancer of the large intestine, but less than half of patients with localized disease are CEA-positive. CEA does not, therefore, serve as a useful screening procedure, nor is it an accurate diagnostic test for colorectal cancer in a curable stage. CEA is helpful in detecting recurrence after curative surgical resection; if high CEA levels return to normal after operation and then rise progressively during the follow-up period, recurrence of cancer is likely.

C. Imaging Studies

Chest films should be obtained routinely. Barium enema examination is a radiographic means of diagnosing cancer of the colon and is mainly of historical importance, but unnecessary in patients who have undergone complete colonoscopy. Carcinoma of the left colon appears as a fixed filling defect, with an annular ("apple core") configuration. Lesions of the right colon may appear as a constriction or an intraluminal mass. These are the typical findings of locally advanced carcinoma and earlier stages of the disease may produce less characteristic filling defects that should be investigated with colonoscopy. Artifacts (stool, spasm) can resemble carcinoma. Barium should not be administered by mouth if there is evidence of carcinoma of the colon, especially on the left side, since it may precipitate acute large bowel obstruction.

CT scans of the chest, abdomen, and pelvis with oral, intravenous, rectum contrast are essential in patients with cancer of the colon. They are informative for identifying the primary tumor location, assessing extramural extension in patients with colon or rectal cancer and for detecting metastatic disease in distant organs or regional lymph node basin (Figure 30–9). In many situations a combined resection of the primary lesion with the metastatic lesion (eg, hepatic) can be performed. MRI may be useful for this purpose as well. PET/CT scans are useful for detecting recurrences and metastatic disease but are probably not necessary as part of the routine initial evaluation. Detection of liver metastases by CT scan and other methods is discussed further in Chapter 24.

D. Special Examinations

1. Proctosigmoidoscopy—Fifty to sixty-five percent of colorectal cancers are within the reach of a 70 cm flexible sigmoidoscope. Only 20% can be seen with a rigid sigmoidoscope. The typical cancer is raised, red, centrally ulcerated, and may bleed. Mobility of the lesion can be determined by manipulation with the tip of the instrument. The size of the lumen should be noted, and the sigmoidoscope should be passed beyond the lesion to inspect the proximal bowel if possible. The tumor should be biopsied.

2. Colonoscopy—Endoscopic examination of the entire colon should be performed in every patient with suspected or known cancer of the colon or rectum if the intention is curative treatment. Colonoscopy allows for tissue diagnosis, evaluation for synchronous lesions, and opportunity for ink-spot tattoo marking of the colon for tumor localization.

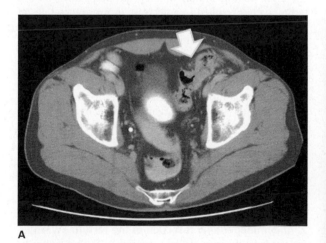

A

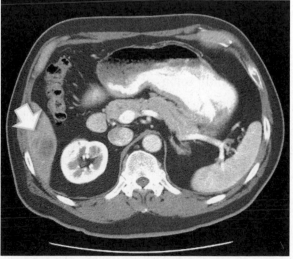

B

▲ **Figure 30–9.** CT scan images. **A:** Primary, circumferential carcinoma of the sigmoid colon (arrow). **B:** Hepatic metastasis (arrow).

When complete colonoscopy cannot be performed, the evaluation of the colon may be completed by CT colonography or air-contrast barium enema.

3. Endorectal ultrasound—Endorectal ultrasound for the evaluation of a newly diagnosed rectal cancer is performed using either a rigid or flexible probe. In the United States, endorectal ultrasound is one of the principal diagnostic tests for the clinical evaluation of rectal cancer. However, recently there has been increasing interest in high-resolution pelvic MRI for the determination of surgical resection margin status and lymph node involvement.

▶ Differential Diagnosis

An initial erroneous diagnosis is made in as many as 25% of patients with cancer of the colon and rectum after gastrointestinal symptoms appear. Symptoms may be attributed mistakenly to disease of the upper gastrointestinal tract, particularly gallstones or peptic ulcer. Chronic anemia may be attributed to a primary hematologic disorder if fecal occult blood testing is not done. Acute pain in the right side of the abdomen owing to carcinoma can simulate appendicitis.

Most errors are made when the clinical findings are ascribed to benign disease, and patients may even be operated upon for benign anorectal conditions in the presence of undetected cancer. Cancer must be sought out in every patient with recent onset of significant rectal bleeding even if there are obvious hemorrhoids.

Carcinoma may be difficult to distinguish from diverticular disease; colonoscopy is useful in these cases. Other colonic diseases—including ulcerative colitis, Crohn colitis, ischemic colitis, and amebiasis—usually can be diagnosed by colonoscopy, sigmoidoscopy, or barium enema. Symptoms should be attributed to irritable bowel syndrome only after neoplasm has been ruled out.

▶ Treatment

A. Cancer of the Colon

Treatment consists of wide surgical resection of the lesion and its regional lymphatic drainage. Resection of the primary tumor may be indicated, even if unresectable distant metastases have occurred, in order to prevent obstruction or bleeding and allow for maximization of systemic therapy.

The abdomen is explored to determine resectability of the tumor and to search for distant metastases, and associated abdominal disease. Care is taken not to contribute to spread of the tumor by unnecessary palpation. The cancer-bearing portion of colon is mobilized and removed according to anatomic criteria based on the vascular distribution of the segment of colon containing the tumor. The extent of resection of the colon and mesocolon for cancers in various locations and the methods for restoration of continuity are shown in Figure 30–10.

B. Cancer of the Rectum

For cancer of the rectum, the choice of operation depends on the location of the lesion within the rectum, the extent of tumor invasion into the rectal wall, histopathologic features such as the degree of differentiation or presence of lymphatic or venous invasion, and the patient's size, habitus, and general condition. Preoperative evaluation and staging by digital rectal examination, proctoscopy, endorectal ultrasound, CT and or MRI, is essential in order to tailor the treatment to the patient. Preservation of the anal sphincter and avoidance of colostomy are desirable if possible.

The principal procedures for rectal tumors are as follows:

1. Low anterior resection of the rectum—This operation, performed through an abdominal incision, is the curative procedure of choice provided a margin of 1–2 cm or more of normal bowel can be resected below the lesion but above the dentate line. The proximal extent of resection should include the sigmoid colon as it makes for a poor replacement for the rectum due to hypertrophy of the muscle and common presence of diverticula. For more proximal lesions within the rectum, it is important to excise at least 5 cm of mesorectum distal to the tumor to minimize the chance of local recurrence from cancer in lymph nodes. The technique of **total mesorectal excision (TME)** described by Heald in 1982 entails an en bloc resection of the rectum as an intact unit with its lymphovascular drainage contained within the fascia propria (Figure 30–11). The mesorectum tapers and diminishes at the level of the Waldeyer fascia. TME allows for preservation of the radial resection margins. Surgeons now recommend a "tumor-specific" sharp mesorectal excision preserving the mesorectal fascia integrity for at least 5 cm distal to the tumor. Widespread acceptance of this technique has resulted in a decrease in recurrence rates of rectal cancer from 20–30% to 5–10%. The descending or sigmoid colon is anastomosed to the rectum. The end-to-end stapling device facilitates very low anastomosis, sometimes even as low as the anal canal (coloanal anastomosis). Unfortunately, such low reconstruction can be associated with functional difficulties including seepage, urgency, and frequent bowel movements. This improves over time (1–2 years); however, the specific treatment should be tailored to the patient. It may be preferable to construct a colonic J-pouch when technically feasible to diminish the severity of these symptoms in the first year. However, J-pouch reconstruction may be associated with evacuation difficulties, and the relative benefits of such a reconstruction should be considered.

2. Abdominoperineal resection of the rectum—When adequate distal margins for low anterior resection cannot be obtained, or the patient's functional status obviates a sphincter-sparing approach, an abdominoperineal resection is performed. The distal sigmoid colon, rectum, and anus are removed through combined abdominal and perineal approaches. A permanent end colostomy is required.

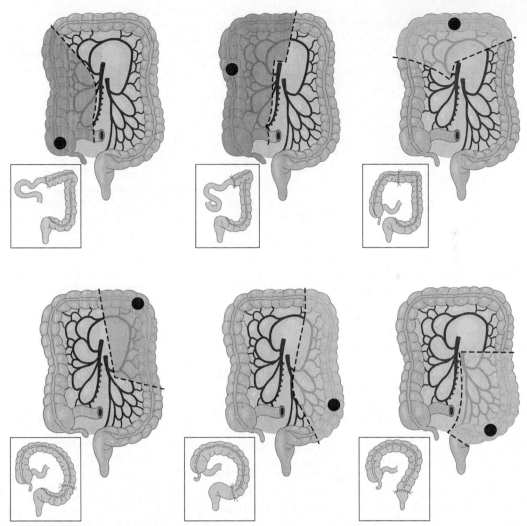

▲ **Figure 30–10.** Extent of surgical resection for cancer of the colon at various sites. The cancer is represented by a black disk. Anastomosis of the bowel remaining after resection is shown in the small insets. The extent of resection is determined by the distribution of the regional lymph nodes along the blood supply. The lymph nodes may contain metastatic cancer.

3. Laparoscopic-assisted resection of the colon or rectum—Curative resections for cancer of the colon or rectum can be carried out by laparoscopic-assisted techniques. Laparoscopic resection has been shown to improve postoperative recovery with less pain, faster return of bowel function, and shorter duration of hospitalization. Initial concerns of port-site metastases from early reports have been dispelled. A number of phase III randomized controlled clinical trials have demonstrated that oncologic outcomes with laparoscopic surgery are equivalent to open surgery for colon cancer. The laparoscopic approach differs from open surgery only in the approach, but the same oncologic resection is performed as with open surgery.

4. Local excision—In carefully selected patients with small, well-differentiated, superficial, mobile polypoid lesions, a full-thickness excision, with margins greater than 1 cm, of the rectal wall containing the tumor can be performed as definitive therapy. This technique of resection should be limited to selected T1 lesions because patient survival with salvage radical surgery for recurrence after local excision of T2 and deeper lesions may be much poorer when compared to initial radical surgery. Lymph nodes are not sampled or treated by local excision, and success is based on adherence to strict criteria that predict a low likelihood of nodal spread. Even T1 tumors have been reported to be associated with a 7–14% chance of nodal metastasis. A strategy of chemoradiation and local

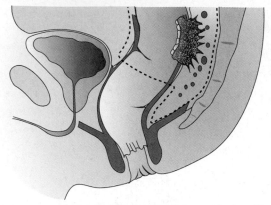

▲ **Figure 30–11.** Total mesorectal excision as depicted in Heald's original publication.

excision has been reported in small case series for lesions more advanced than T1; however, the long-term results are not well documented, and this approach should subject to clinical trials such as one currently ongoing sponsored by the American College of Surgeons Oncology Group (ACoSOG). **Transanal endoscopic microsurgery (TEM)** is a minimally invasive technique for the local resection of rectal tumors, best suited for more proximal rectal lesions. The same criteria are applied to patients for conventional local excision or TEM.

5. Palliative procedures—Unresectable rectal cancers can be palliated by fulguration (electrocoagulation) or laser photocoagulation. Unfortunately, symptom relief—of bleeding, tenesmus, and mucus discharge—in patients with these advanced lesions is often less than anticipated. A diverting colostomy can be performed for obstructing rectal cancer that cannot be resected. However, in such cases, colonoscopically deployed endoluminal stents can provide relief of obstruction even when the lumen is too small to accommodate a pediatric colonoscope. Tumor ingrowth will cause stent occlusion within 6–9 months, but this can be prolonged with laser photocoagulation.

6. Radiation therapy—Adjuvant external beam radiation therapy, given with chemotherapy as a radiation sensitizer has been demonstrated to reduce local failure risk following curative surgical resection. The strategy of preoperative treatment (**neoadjuvant therapy**) is more effective than postoperative treatment for improving local control, sphincter preservation, and reducing treatment related toxicity. Complete clinical response has been reported to be as high as 30% after neoadjuvant treatment; however, many of these patients will still have pathologically detectable disease and therefore complete clinical response does not eliminate the need for surgical resection. Although the benefit of radiation on decreasing local recurrence rates has been well demonstrated in several randomized trials, only one major randomized trial has demonstrated a benefit in survival. It should be noted, however, that the boundaries of resection for curative intent should be based on the pretreat-

ment evaluation of tumor extent and not on the visible tumor after treatment. Irradiation is not used for cancer of the colon. Intraoperative radiation therapy at the time of curative resection is a promising method of reducing local recurrence risk among patients with locally advance or recurrent rectal cancer.

C. Adjuvant Therapy

Chemotherapy and radiation therapy have been studied extensively as adjuvants to curative resection of cancer of the large intestine. Strategies are different for cancer of the colon and cancer of the rectum. Patients with stage I lesions in either site do not benefit from adjuvant therapy. Some stage II and stage III rectal cancer patients have improved local control and survival with combined neoadjuvant chemoradiation therapy followed by postoperative adjuvant chemotherapy. Stage III colon cancer patients benefit from adjuvant chemotherapy. Current regimens include either intravenous 5-fluorouracil or oral capecitabine in combination with oxaliplatin as first-line therapy (Table 30–7). Other agents effective in the metastatic setting are currently under investigation in the adjuvant setting. Some patients with stage II colon cancer may benefit from adjuvant therapy, and these patients should be enrolled into clinical trials, many of which currently use molecular markers to help select patients for adjuvant therapy.

▶ Treatment of Complications

A. Obstruction

Obstructing cancer of the left or right colon is treated by immediate resection in good-risk patients. (See earlier section on Obstruction of the Large Intestine.)

B. Perforation

An aggressive approach to perforated cancer of the colon is advisable, but anastomosis is often delayed based on the degree of contamination and the health of the bowel. If contamination is severe or if bowel health is compromised, the proximal end is exteriorized as a colostomy (or ileostomy), and the distal end is exteriorized or closed. Secondary anastomosis is performed after inflammation subsides. Alternatively, the anastomosis may be performed and "covered" with a defunctioning loop ileostomy. Closure of a loop ileostomy is a simpler and less morbid procedure than reexploration and closure of an end stoma.

C. Direct Extension

When carcinoma of the colon has spread by contiguity to adjacent viscera such as the small intestine, spleen, kidney, uterus, prostate, or urinary bladder, the involved viscus—or a portion of it—should be resected en bloc with the colon.

▶ Prognosis

The **clinicopathologic stage** of disease is the most important determinant of survival. In general the results of surgical

Table 30–7. Currently Used Chemotherapeutic Agents Effective in the Treatment of Colon Cancer.

Agent	Route	Class	Indication
5-fluorouracil	Intravenous	Antimetabolite	Adjuvant Metastatic
Capecitabine	Oral	Antimetabolite	Adjuvant Metastatic
Uracil and tegafur	Oral	Antimetabolite	Adjuvant Metastatic
Oxaliplatin	Intravenous	DNA alkylation and cross-linking	Adjuvant Metastatic
Irinotecan	Intravenous	Inhibit DNA repair by topoisomerase I	Metastatic
Bevacizumab	Intravenous	MAb to VEGF	Metastatic
Cetuximab	Intravenous	MAb to EGFR	Metastatic (k-ras wild type)
Panitumumab	Intravenous	MAb to EGFR	Metastatic

treatment are better for cancer of the colon than for cancer of the rectum, and low rectal cancer has a worse prognosis than cancer higher in the rectum. The Dukes classification was introduced decades ago but has been replaced by the TNM system developed by the American Joint Committee for Cancer. Table 30–8 lists the definitions of TNM and the stage grouping along with the corresponding historical Dukes classification. Clinical data are used for determination of M, and both clinical and pathologic information is included in assessment of T and N. Survival rates differ considerably in various series; actuarial rates are higher than crude survival rates. Adjuvant therapy, particularly with some of the newer agents, in addition to improved surgical techniques, has led to 5-year survival rates of 40–80% for stage III disease.

Up to 20% of patients have liver or other distant metastases at presentation. However, in selected patients with metastases in whom all metastatic disease can be completely resected, operation for cure should be performed. The operative mortality rate is 1–4%.

The prognosis is adversely affected by complications such as obstruction or perforation. The histologic features—including the degree of differentiation of the tumor, intravascular tumor cells, or malignant cells in the perineural space—also have a bearing on prognosis and may influence the decision to recommend adjuvant chemotherapy in node-negative patients.

One limitation of AJCC/TNM staging is that patients with TNM stage may have widely different potentials for local recurrence, distant metastasis, and survival. Ultrastaging techniques include immunohistochemistry for markers such as cytokeratins and reverse transcription polymerase chain reaction for CEA to look for evidence of micrometastasis within regional lymph nodes or genotypic subset analysis. Loss of heterozygosity at chromosome 18q (affecting expression of DCC, Smad4, and Smad2) is predictive of a poor outcome. Other markers of poor prognosis include loss of heterozygosity at chromosome 17p (affecting

p53) and 8q, and a mutation in the *BAX* gene. Favorable prognostic factors include the presence of microsatellite instability in the genes of the mismatch repair family and increased expression of the cyclin-dependent kinase inhibitor p21$^{WAF1/CIP1}$ protein. Further study is required before clinicians can base therapeutic decisions on assays of these and other molecular markers.

Studies from several countries show that low-income people have more advanced disease when diagnosed and that their stage-for-stage survival rates are worse; these observations have not been explained satisfactorily. An association of perioperative blood transfusions with poorer prognosis from colorectal cancer has been found by some, but not all, investigators; if it is genuine, the association may reflect other effects—larger tumors requiring more extensive surgery and transfusions, for example—rather than some consequence of transfusion itself.

Follow-up after curative resection of cancer of the large bowel is controversial. There are good data to support the view that periodic colonoscopy to detect and remove adenomas after colonoscopic polypectomy prevents subsequent cancer, and colonoscopy at 3 years is just as beneficial as colonoscopy at 1 and 3 years after complete removal of the index adenoma. It is not known whether these observations can be extrapolated to follow-up after curative resection of cancer, but in the absence of data, many clinicians perform surveillance colonoscopy periodically for the purpose of detecting adenomas and metachronous carcinomas. In addition, presence of a distracting lesion may result in an increased risk for missed lesions during colonoscopy. Other goals of follow-up are the diagnosis of recurrent cancer or metastatic cancer. The physician should tailor the follow-up strategy to the patient's ability and interest in pursuing an aggressive approach should recurrent disease be discovered. Follow-up programs include a complete blood count, liver function tests, serum CEA levels, chest x-rays, and CT scans in addition to colonoscopy.

Table 30–8. TNM Classification of Cancer of the Colon and Rectum.[1]

	Primary Tumor (T)
TX	Primary tumor cannot be assessed
T0	No evidence of primary tumor
Tis	Carcinoma in situ
T1	Tumor invades submucosa
T2	Tumor invades muscularis propria
T3	Tumor invades through the muscularis propria into the subserosa or into nonperitonealized pericolic or perirectal tissues
T4	Tumor perforates the visceral peritoneum, or directly invades other organs or structures

	Regional Lymph Nodes (N)
NX	Regional lymph nodes cannot be assessed
N0	No regional lymph node metastasis
N1	Metastasis in 1 to 3 pericolic or perirectal lymph nodes
N2	Metastasis in 4 or more pericolic or perirectal lymph nodes
N3	Metastasis in any lymph node along the course of a named vascular trunk

	Distant Metastasis (M)
MX	Presence of distant metastasis cannot be assessed
M0	No distant metastasis
M1	Distant metastasis

Stage Grouping				Dukes	Modified Astler-Coller
Stage 0	Tis	N0	M0		
Stage I	T1	N0	M0	A	A
	T2	N0	M0	A	B1
Stage IIA	T3	N0	M0	B	B2
Stage IIB	T4	N0	M0	B	B3
IIIA	T1-2	N1	M0	C	C1
IIIB	T3-4	N1	M0	C2/C3	
IIIC	Any T	N2	M0	C1/C2/C3	
Stage IV	Any T	Any N	M1		

[1]Used with the permission of the American Joint Committee on Cancer (AJCC), Chicago, IL. The original source for this material is *AJCC Cancer Staging Manual*, 6th ed. Lippincott-Raven, 2002.

If recurrent cancer or metastatic cancer is discovered, the patient is evaluated for potential surgical resection of the lesions. This is particularly true for hepatic or pulmonary metastases where a survival benefit has been demonstrated. Local recurrences can be resected, sometimes in combination with intraoperative radiation therapy. Five-year survival rates of 25–35% after multimodality therapy, including preoperative chemoradiation and surgical resection with intraoperative radiation therapy, have been reported for recurrent rectal cancer. Unfortunately, the prognosis of patients with local recurrence is generally poor. If recurrent cancer is suggested on the basis of rising serum CEA levels, it can usually be located by CT, MRI, or PET scan. A second-look laparotomy is now rarely required because of improvements in the quality of cross-sectional imaging.

Allen E, Nicolaidis C, Helfand M: The evaluation of rectal bleeding in adults. A cost-effectiveness analysis comparing four diagnostic strategies. J Gen Intern Med 2005;20:81.

Allison JE et al: A comparison of fecal occult-blood tests for colorectal-cancer screening. N Engl J Med 1996;334:155.

Barclay RL et al: Colonoscopic withdrawal times and adenoma detection during screening colonoscopy. N Engl J Med 2006;355:2533.

Bruinvels DJ et al: Follow-up of patients with colorectal cancer. A meta-analysis. Ann Surg 1994;219:174.

Busch ORC et al: Blood transfusions and prognosis in colorectal cancer. N Engl J Med 1993;328:1372.

Chang GJ et al: Lymph node evaluation and survival after curative resection of colon cancer: systematic review. J Natl Cancer Inst 2007;99:433.

Clinical Outcomes of Surgical Therapy Study Group (COST): A comparison of laparoscopically assisted and open colectomy for colon cancer. N Engl J Med 2004;350:2050.

Chu KC et al: Temporal patterns in colorectal cancer incidence, survival, and mortality from 1950 through 1990. J Natl Cancer Inst 1994;86:997.

Gann PH et al: Low-dose aspirin and incidence of colorectal tumors in a randomized trial. J Natl Cancer Inst 1993;85:1220.

Giardiello FM et al: The use and interpretation of commercial *APC* gene testing for familial adenomatous polyposis. N Engl J Med 1997;336:823.

Gryfe R et al: Tumor microsatellite instability and clinical outcome in young patients with colorectal cancer. N Engl J Med 2000; 342:69.

Howe GR et al: Dietary intake of fiber and decreased risk of cancers of the colon and rectum: evidence from the combined analysis of 13 case-control studies. J Natl Cancer Inst 1992; 84:1887.

Jessup JM et al: The National Cancer Data Base. Report on colon cancer. Cancer 1996;78:918.

Kapiteijn E et al: Preoperative radiotherapy combined with total mesorectal excision for resectable rectal cancer. Dutch ColoRectal Cancer Group. N Engl J Med 2001;345:638.

Lichtenstein P et al: Environmental and heritable factors in the causation of cancer: analyses of cohorts of twins from Sweden, Denmark, and Finland. N Engl J Med 2000;343:78.

Lieberman DA et al: Use of colonoscopy to screen asymptomatic adults for colorectal cancer. Veterans Affairs Cooperative Study Group 380. N Engl J Med 2000;343:162.

Lieberman DA et al for the VA Cooperative Study Group: Risk factors for advanced colonic neoplasia and hyperplastic polyps in asymptomatic individuals. JAMA 2003;290:2959.

Lim SJ et al: Sentinel lymph node evaluation does not improve staging accuracy in colon cancer. Ann Surg Oncol 2008;15:46.

Lin KM et al: Colorectal and extracolonic cancer variations in MLH1/MSH2 hereditary nonpolyposis colorectal cancer kindreds and the general population. Dis Colon Rectum 1998; 41:428.

Lynch HT, de la Chapelle A: Hereditary colorectal cancer. N Engl J Med 2003;348:919.

Macdonald JS, Astrow AB: Adjuvant therapy of colon cancer. Semin Oncol 2001;28:30.

Pignone M et al: Cost-effectiveness analyses of colorectal cancer screening: a systematic review for the U.S. Preventive Services Task Force. Ann Intern Med 2002;137:96.

Steinbach G et al: The effect of celecoxib, a cyclooxygenase-2 inhibitor, in familial adenomatous polyposis. N Engl J Med 2000;342:1946.

Rex DK et al: Quality in the technical performance of colonoscopy and the continuous quality improvement process for colonoscopy: recommendations of the U.S. Multi-Society Task Force on Colorectal Cancer. Am J Gastroenterol 2002;97:1296.

Ribic CM et al: Tumor microsatellite-instability status as a predictor of benefit from fluorouracil-based adjuvant chemotherapy for colon cancer. N Engl J Med 2003;349:247.

Saha S et al: Sentinel lymph node mapping in colorectal cancer—a review. Surg Clinics North Am 2000;80:1811.

Sanchez W, Harewood GC, Petersen BT: Evaluation of polyp detection in relation to procedure time of screening or surveillance colonoscopy. Am J Gastroenterol 2004;99:1941.

Sauer R et al: Preoperative versus postoperative chemoradiotherapy for rectal cancer. N Engl J Med 2004;351:1731.

Scholefield JH: ABC of colorectal cancer: screening. BMJ 2000;321:1004.

Swedish Rectal Cancer Trial: Improved survival with preoperative radiotherapy in resectable rectal cancer. N Engl J Med 1997;336:980.

Watanabe T et al: Molecular predictors of survival after adjuvant chemotherapy for colon cancer. N Engl J Med 2001;344:1196.

Weeks JC et al: Short-term quality-of-life outcomes following laparoscopic-assisted colectomy vs open colectomy for colon cancer. A randomized trial. JAMA 2002;287:321.

Winawer SJ, Zauber AG: Colonoscopic polypectomy and the incidence of colorectal cancer. Gut 2001;48:753.

POLYPS OF THE COLON & RECTUM

ESSENTIALS OF DIAGNOSIS

► Family history.

► Sigmoidoscopic, colonoscopic, or radiologic discovery of polyps.

► General Considerations

Colorectal polyps are masses of tissue that project into the lumen. They comprise a heterogeneous group of sessile or pedunculated, benign or malignant, mucosal, submucosal, or muscular lesions. "Polyp" is a morphologic term, and no histologic diagnosis is implied. The most common epithelial polyps of the colon and rectum are listed in Table 30–9. Most adenomas are tubular, tubulovillous, or villous. Hyperplastic

Table 30–9. Polyps of the Large Intestine.

Type	Histologic Diagnosis
Neoplastic	Adenoma
	Tubular adenoma (adenomatous polyp)
	Tubulovillous adenoma (villoglandular adenoma)
	Villous adenoma (villous papilloma)
	Carcinoma
Hamartomas	Juvenile polyp
	Peutz-Jeghers polyp
Inflammatory	Inflammatory polyp (pseudopolyp)
	Benign lymphoid polyp
Unclassified	Hyperplastic polyp
Miscellaneous	Lipoma, leiomyoma, carcinoid

polyps are diminutive lesions most often found in the left colon. Hamartomas are uncommon. Polyposis, discussed later in this section, is a term reserved for the presence of many polyps in the large bowel.

Estimates of the incidence of colonic and rectal polyps in the general population range from 9% to 60%—the higher figure includes small polyps found at autopsy. Polypoid adenomas are found in about 25% of asymptomatic adults who undergo screening colonoscopy. The prevalence of adenomas is 30% at age 50 years, 40% at age 60, 50% at age 70, and 55% at age 80. The mean age is 55 years, about 5–10 years younger than the mean age of patients with colorectal cancer. Approximately 50% of polyps occur in the sigmoid or rectum. About 50% of patients with adenoma have more than one lesion, and 15% have more than two lesions.

Inflammatory polyps have no malignant potential. Cancer developing in association with hamartomas is rare but has been reported. Patients with the Peutz-Jeghers hamartomatous polyposis syndrome, however, do have an increased lifetime risk for a variety of cancers, including colorectal cancer. Hyperplastic polyps are not neoplastic and therefore do not become malignant. However, they may be difficult to distinguish from serrated adenomas, which do have malignant potential.

Adenomas are a premalignant lesion. The vast majority of adenocarcinomas of the large bowel develop through an orderly progression from normal mucosa to adenomas to carcinomas, the polyp–cancer sequence. In 1990, Fearon and Vogelstein described a model for colorectal cancer and provided a framework to elucidate the mutations in the genetic regulatory elements that lead to uncontrolled cell growth. Further studies have elaborated this multistep pathway, commonly referred as loss of heterozygosity (LOH), which can be observed in inherited and sporadic colorectal cancer. In Western populations, both adenomas and cancer increase in incidence with age, and the distribution of adenomas and cancer in the bowel is similar. Patients who have more adenomatous polyps at the time of examination are more likely to have a synchronous colon cancer. About one third of colonic and rectal specimens resected for cancer also harbor adenomas; if a surgical specimen contains two or more synchronous carcinomas, the incidence of associated adenomas is 75%. All gradations of malignancy—from total absence to dysplasia to invasive cancer to a gross cancer with remnants of benign tumor at one margin—may be seen in colonic neoplasms; on the other hand, cancers that are smaller than 0.5 cm in diameter and contain no benign adenoma are extremely rare.

The malignant potential of an adenoma depends on size, growth pattern, and the degree of epithelial atypia. Cancer is found in 1% of adenomas under 1 cm in diameter, 10% of adenomas 1–2 cm in size, and up to 45% of adenomas larger than 2 cm. So-called flat adenomas, more commonly reported in Asian populations, are small, flat or depressed tubular adenomas that tend to occur in the right colon and

may arise through a different pathway of carcinogenesis. They may also become malignant when still only a few millimeters in diameter. The three histologic patterns of adenoma are variations of one neoplastic process; about 5% of tubular adenomas, 22% of tubulovillous adenomas, and 40% of villous adenomas become malignant. The potential for cancerous transformation rises with increasing degrees of epithelial dysplasia. Sessile lesions are more apt than pedunculated ones to be malignant. It probably takes at least 5 years, and more often 10 years, for an adenoma to become malignant.

▶ Clinical Findings

A. Symptoms and Signs

Most polyps are asymptomatic, but the larger the lesion, the more likely it is to cause symptoms. Rectal bleeding is by far the most frequent complaint. Blood is bright red or dark red depending on the location of the polyp, and bleeding is usually intermittent. Profuse hemorrhage from polyps is rare.

Changes in bowel habits are more common in the presence of frank carcinoma particularly in the left side of the colon or in the rectum, but large benign tumors may produce tenesmus, constipation, or increased frequency of bowel movements. Some polyps, notably large villous adenomas, may secrete copious amounts of mucus that are evacuated per rectum. Polypoid tumors may induce peristaltic cramps or varying degrees of intussusception, but most often obstructive symptoms are due to associated diverticular disease or irritable bowel syndrome and persist after polypectomy. Occasionally, a polyp on a very long pedicle will prolapse through the anus; this is most apt to occur with juvenile polyps.

General physical examination yields little information about the colonic polyps themselves, although other manifestations of diseases such as Peutz-Jeghers syndrome may be found. A polyp may be palpable by digital rectal examination, and proctosigmoidoscopy may disclose polyps in the rectum or sigmoid. Blood-tinged mucus strongly suggests the presence of a neoplasm situated farther proximally. Since polyps are often multiple and may occur synchronously with cancer, further investigation of the colon is mandatory even if a lesion is found by sigmoidoscopy.

B. Imaging Studies (Barium Enema)

No longer used as the primary diagnostic modality for colorectal cancer, a polyp or mass appears as a rounded filling defect with smooth, sharply defined margins on air-contrast barium enema. Thorough cleansing of the colon and careful examination are essential if small polyps are to be demonstrated.

C. Colonoscopy

This is the most reliable way to diagnose colonic polyps. Polypectomy can be done at the same time. However, small polyps may still be missed at a rate of 5–10%. The sensitivity of colonoscopy is in part dependent on the operator and associated with the duration of time to perform endoscope withdrawal. The entire colon should be carefully examined by colonoscopy in every patient with known polyps or symptoms suggestive of their presence.

D. CT Colonography

CT colonography continues to evolve as a potentially important technique for colonic polyp diagnosis and screening. The principal advantage is the potential for a more complete evaluation of the mucosal and extraluminal surfaces. The main disadvantage is the continued need for a bowel prep and the need for a subsequent colonoscopy should an abnormality be identified.

▶ Differential Diagnosis

Abnormal findings seen on barium enema and CT colonography should be further evaluated by colonoscopy for histologic confirmation.

▶ Treatment

Polyps of the colon and rectum are treated because they produce symptoms, because they may be malignant when first discovered, or because they may become malignant later. The cumulative risk of eventual cancer in untreated polyps is approximately 2.5% at 5 years, 8% at 10 years, and 24% at 20 years.

Polyps should be completely removed endoscopically when possible. Polyps located within the rectum may be removed with a transanal mucosal resection. Histologic examination of the complete specimen should be performed. Whenever possible, the entire polyp should be removed in one piece in order to allow for adequate histologic examination of the margins and proper classification of a polyp-associated carcinoma. The finding of invasive carcinoma within a polyp removed piecemeal requires completion of therapy with formal surgical resection, whereas complete en bloc endoscopic resection may have been sufficient in some cases.

Endoscopic mucosal resection (EMR), with saline injection elevation of the submucosa, is preferred because it allows for a more complete polypectomy, including the submucosa, with improved evaluation of the deep margin of resection. If a polyp is suspected to harbor early invasive carcinoma and cannot endoscopically be completely removed intact, polypectomy should not be performed and the patient should be referred for formal oncologic surgical resection. Patients with HNPCC and others with multiple polyps may require total abdominal colectomy with ileorectal or ileal J-pouch anal anastomosis (IPAA).

From 2% to 4% of colonoscopically excised polyps contain invasive adenocarcinoma, and a decision must be made whether to resect the segment of colon or simply follow the patient. In 1985, Haggitt and coworkers proposed a morpho-

logic classification for pedunculated malignant polyps (Table 30–10). The risk of lymph node metastasis in Haggitt levels 1–3 lesions is < 1%. Haggitt level 4 and sessile lesions are associated with a 10% or greater risk for lymph node metastasis. In the case of malignant polyps, resection of the colon is not required if the following criteria are met: (1) Gross margin is clear at endoscopy; (2) microscopic margin is clear; (3) cancer is well-differentiated; (4) there is no lymphatic or venous invasion; and (5) cancer does not invade the stalk (Haggitt level 0–2). Other malignant polyps of the colon (eg, sessile) should be managed by resection of involved bowel. In the context of EMR of sessile malignant polyps, the depth of invasion into the submucosa, classified as sm1–sm3, is predictive of metastatic potential. Sm1 and some sm2 lesions may be treated with endoscopic polypectomy because their risk for nodal metastasis is low. However, reliable determination of sm classification requires both an excellent en bloc EMR polypectomy and expert histopathologic examination. Molecular markers may help make the determination for surgical resection in the future. Since early rectal cancers are sometimes treated definitively by local excision, it may not be necessary to do a radical resection if the malignant polyp arose in the distal rectum.

Familial adenomatous polyposis (adenomatous polyposis coli) is a rare but important disease because colorectal cancer develops before age 40 in nearly all untreated patients. The trait is autosomal dominant. Genetic advances have been explosive. The *APC* gene (*FAP* had already been used in the genetics nomenclature) was localized to chromosome 5q21 in 1991, and since then more than 100 different mutations have been identified. Genetic testing of at-risk individuals is currently available. Patients present with hundreds to thousands of polyps of varying size and configuration in the colon and rectum. A subset of patients have attenuated FAP (previously known as hereditary flat adenoma syndrome) characterized by the presence of fewer polyps (usually < 100), later onset of

Table 30–10. Haggitt Classification.[1]

Level	Depth
0	Carcinoma in situ or intramucosal carcinoma
1	Carcinoma invading through muscularis mucosa into the submucosa but limited to the head of the polyp
2	Carcinoma invading the neck of the polyp
3	Carcinoma invading any part of the stalk
4	Carcinoma invading into the submucosa of the bowel wall below the stalk of the polyp but above the muscularis propria (T1)
Sessile	By definition, equivalent to level 4

[1]From Haggitt RC et al: Prognostic factors in colorectal carcinomas arising in adenomas: implications for lesions removed by endoscopic polypectomy. Gastroenterology 1985;89:328.

colon cancer, and characteristic different mutations of the *APC* gene. A long list of benign and malignant extracolonic manifestations are associated with FAP (Table 30–11). **Gardner syndrome** (polyposis, desmoid tumors, osteomas of mandible or skull, and sebaceous cysts) and **Turcot syndrome** (polyposis and childhood cerebellar medulloblastoma) are examples of FAP with variations in expression of the extracolonic manifestations; both syndromes are associated with mutations in the *APC* gene, although Turcot syndrome may also be associated with HNPCC and defects in mismatch repair genes (colon cancer with childhood or adult gliomas). Congenital hypertrophy of retinal pigment epithelium is present as early as at 3 months of age in affected members of two thirds of families with FAP; this abnormality (always bilateral, more than four lesions on each side) predicts FAP with 97% sensitivity. Polyps begin to appear at puberty, at which time colonoscopy should be performed. Once the *APC* gene mutation or polyposis is diagnosed, colectomy should be done. Upper gastrointestinal endoscopy is performed to look for gastroduodenal lesions.

Although total proctocolectomy eliminates the risk of cancer, it leaves the patient with a permanent ileostomy. Abdominal colectomy ("subtotal colectomy") with ileorectal anastomosis may be favored when the number of rectal polyps is few, the patient is compliant with regular follow-up, and the patient is otherwise not a candidate for a total colectomy with ileal J-pouch anal anastomosis. Following ileorectal anastomosis, it is hoped that cancer can be prevented by sigmoidoscopic destruction of the remaining rectal polyps every 6–12 months. With rigorous surveillance, the incidence of cancer in the remaining rectum is low. Sulindac and celecoxib have both been reported to induce regression of polyps and may be considered for chemoprevention in the remaining rectum. If the rectal mucosa is excised completely, the risk of subsequent rectal neoplasia is essentially nil. Case reports of cancer arising in the anal canal after this operation may reflect incomplete excision of susceptible mucosa at the time of ileoanal anastomosis. Prophylactic colectomy does not alter the extracolonic manifestations.

Duodenal and periampullary adenomatous polyps are found in 30–70% of individuals affected by FAP, and the lifetime risk approaches 100%. These lesions lag in time of presentation from colorectal adenomas by approximately 10–20 years with median age of presentation at 38 years. Patients with FAP have a 100-fold to 330-fold higher risk of developing duodenal cancer than the general population with an estimated cumulative risk of up to 10% by age 60. Development of duodenal cancer is the second-most common cause of disease-related mortality in patients with FAP, surpassed only by advanced and metastatic colorectal cancer.

MYH (mutY homolog)-associated polyposis syndrome has recently been identified in subgroups of patients in FAP registries who have tested negative for *APC* gene mutations. The pattern or inheritance is autosomal recessive, and the phenotype demonstrates multiple colorectal polyps (> 10)

Table 30–11. Extracolonic Manifestations of Familial Adenomatous Polyposis.[1]

Benign	Malignant
Endocrine adenoma	Duodenal carcinoma
Osteoma	Bile duct carcinoma
Epidermoid cyst	Pancreatic carcinoma
Hypertrophic retinal pigmentation	Desmoid tumor
	Carcinoma of the stomach
Gastric fundic gland polyp	Adrenal carcinoma
Duodenal adenoma	Medulloblastoma
Small bowel adenoma	Glioblastoma
	Thyroid carcinoma
	Small bowel carcinoma
	Carcinoid tumor of the ileum
	Osteogenic sarcoma
	Hepatoblastoma

[1]Reproduced, with permission, from Jagelman DG: The expanding spectrum of familial adenomatous polyposis. Perspect Colon Rectal Surg 1998;1:30.

but typically fewer than in individuals with classic FAP. The age at onset of colorectal cancer in patients with biallelic *MYH* mutations has been reported to be less than 50 years. Colorectal cancers in *MYH* polyposis syndrome are associated with G:C to T:A transversions resulting from defects in base excision repair. This colorectal cancer–associated polyposis syndrome continues to be defined.

Four syndromes of juvenile polyposis have been defined: (1) **juvenile polyposis syndrome** (1/100,000 population), (2) **Cronkhite-Canada syndrome** (juvenile polyposis and ectodermal lesions), (3) **Bannayan-Riley-Ruvalcaba syndrome** (juvenile polyposis and macrocephaly and genital hyperpigmentation), and (4) **Cowden disease** (juvenile polyposis and facial trichilemmomas, thyroid goiter and cancer, and breast cancer). Although juvenile polyps are hamartomas with a low malignant potential, the risk of gastrointestinal cancer is increased in familial juvenile polyposis patients and their relatives. The lifetime risk of colorectal cancer with juvenile polyposis syndrome is 30–60%. Furthermore, hamartomas can coexist with adenomas, and one must not assume that a polyp is a hamartoma without proof. Colonoscopic excision is performed for large or symptomatic (bleeding, intussusception) lesions. Some juvenile polyps autoamputate. Colectomy is required in some patients with familial forms of juvenile polyposis.

Peutz-Jeghers syndrome is an uncommon autosomal dominant disease (1/200,000 population) in which multiple hamartomatous polyps appear in the stomach, small bowel, and colon. Affected individuals have melanotic pigmentation of the skin and mucous membranes, especially about the lips and gums. Until recently the Peutz-Jeghers hamartomas were thought to be without malignant potential, but adenomatous changes and the development of malignancy have been described. The lifetime risk of colorectal cancer has been reported to be 39%. Prophylactic colectomy has not been studied in the Peutz-Jeghers syndrome population, and polyps are generally removed only if symptomatic, but patients should undergo continued surveillance. Carcinoma also develops at an increased rate in other tissues (eg, stomach, duodenum, pancreas, small intestine, and breast).

▶ Prognosis

Villous adenomas recur at the excision site in about 15% of cases after local removal. Tubular adenomas seldom recur, but new ones may develop, and a patient who has had any type of adenoma is at greater risk of developing adenocarcinoma than the general population. The risk of metachronous neoplasms following excision of a colorectal adenoma is greatest if there were multiple index lesions or if an adenoma was sessile, villous, or over 2 cm in diameter. The risk is somewhat higher in men than in women. In one study, the cumulative risk of developing further adenomas was linear over time, reaching about 50% by 15 years after removal of one or more colorectal adenomas; the cumulative incidence of cancer in the same population rose to 7% at 15 years. If the colon is cleared by total colonoscopy at the time of excision of the index polyp, follow-up colonoscopy at 3 years is just as effective as colonoscopy at 1 and 3 years in preventing development of ominous neoplasms.

Al-Tassan N et al: Inherited variants of MYH associated with somatic G:C–>T:A mutations in colorectal tumors. Nat Genet 2002;30:227.

Boardman LA: Heritable colorectal cancer syndromes: recognition and preventive management. Gastroenterol Clin North Am 2002;31:1107.

Church J et al: Staging intra-abdominal desmoid tumors in familial adenomatous polyposis: a search for a uniform approach to a troubling disease. Dis Colon Rectum 2005;48:1528.

Frazier ML et al: Current applications of genetic technology in predisposition testing and microsatellite instability assays. J Clin Oncol 2000;18(21 Suppl):70S.

Gelfand DW: Decreased risk of subsequent colonic cancer in patients undergoing polypectomy after barium enema: analysis based on data from the preendoscopic era. AJR Am J Roentgenol 1997;169:1243.

Levin B et al: Screening and surveillance for the early detection of colorectal cancer and adenomatous polyps, 2008: a joint guideline from the American Cancer Society, the US Multi-Society Task Force on Colorectal Cancer, and the American College of Radiology. Gastroenterology 2008;134:1570.

Lynch HT, Lynch JF, Lynch PM: Toward a consensus in molecular diagnosis of hereditary nonpolyposis colorectal cancer (Lynch syndrome). J Natl Cancer Inst 2007;99:261.

Lynch PM: Prevention of colorectal cancer in high-risk populations: the increasing role for endoscopy and chemoprevention in FAP and HNPCC. Digestion 2007;76:68.

Marshall JR: Prevention of colorectal cancer: diet, chemoprevention, and lifestyle. Gastroenterol Clin North Am 2008;37:73.

Soravia C et al: Desmoid disease in patients with familial adenomatous polyposis. Dis Colon Rectum 2000;43:363.

Winawer SJ, Zauber AG: Colonoscopic polypectomy and the incidence of colorectal cancer. Gut 2001;48:753.

OTHER TUMORS OF THE COLON & RECTUM

Carcinoids of the large bowel are uncommon, and most of them occur in the rectum. Lesions less than 2 cm in diameter usually are asymptomatic, behave benignly, and can be managed by local excision. Larger tumors arising in the colon (mainly the right side) or rectum cause local symptoms, metastasize, and require standard cancer operations. In contrast to carcinoid tumors of the small intestine, carcinoid syndrome appears in less than 5% of patients with metastatic carcinoid of the large bowel.

Lymphomas are the most common noncarcinomatous malignant tumors of the large bowel. Diffuse lymphomatous polyposis is a rare gastrointestinal manifestation. Non-Hodgkin B cell lymphoma and Kaposi sarcoma are two AIDS-related cancers that affect the colon and rectum. Lymphoma is often aggressive, but Kaposi sarcoma may cause few colonic or systemic symptoms.

Lipomas may be difficult to distinguish with barium enema from mucosal neoplasms, but CT examination may demonstrate a mass with fat density, and colonoscopy may demonstrate a soft "pillow" lesion, often permitting accurate diagnosis. Lipomas are usually asymptomatic but can cause obstruction. Removal is recommended if they cause symptoms.

Leiomyomas are much less common in the colon than in the stomach or small intestine. Colonic tumors are less apt to cause significant hemorrhage than those of the upper bowel. Some leiomyomas become malignant. Fifteen percent of **gastrointestinal stromal tumors** (GIST), previously known as leiomyosarcoma, may occur in the colon or rectum.

Endometriomas are masses of endometrial tissue that implant on the surface of the rectum, sigmoid colon, appendix, cecum, or distal ileum and may invade locally into the muscularis, submucosa, and even mucosa. Endoscopically, they may even have the appearance of a primary colon cancer. The ectopic tissue responds to cyclic hormonal stimulation, causing inflammation and fibrosis. Intestinal symptoms of endometriosis include altered bowel habits, rectal pain, and rectal bleeding during menstruation. Tender nodularities are palpable in the pelvis in 90% of cases. Sigmoidoscopy, fiberoptic colonoscopy, and barium enema x-rays may make the diagnosis, but diagnostic laparoscopy may be necessary to be certain of the problem. Therapeutic laparoscopy is performed if symptoms are not controlled by endocrine therapy or if cancer cannot be excluded. Endometrial lesions on peritoneal surfaces in the pelvis may be excised or destroyed by laser or cautery; colonic or rectal lesions may be managed by partial or full-thickness resection of the bowel. Relief of intestinal symptoms is reported in 90–100% of patients who undergo surgical treatment.

Other benign colorectal tumors include neurofibromas associated with Recklinghausen disease, teratomas, enterocystomas (duplication of rectum), lymphangiomas, and cavernous hemangiomas. Adenosquamous carcinoma, primary squamous cell carcinoma, and primary melanoma of the colon or rectum are extremely rare malignant tumors.

Henkel A, Christensen B, Schindler AE: Endometriosis: a clinically malignant disease. Eur J Obstet Gynecol Reprod Biol 1999;82:209.

Jerby BL et al: Laparoscopic management of colorectal endometriosis. Surg Endosc 1999;13:1125.

Kawamoto K et al: Colonic submucosal tumors: a new classification based on radiologic characteristics. AJR Am J Roentgenol 1993;160:315.

Londono-Schimmer EE, Ritchie JK, Hawley PR: Coloanal sleeve anastomosis in the treatment of diffuse cavernous haemangioma of the rectum: long-term results. Br J Surg 1994;81:1235.

Saclarides TJ, Szeluga D, Staren ED: Neuroendocrine cancers of the colon and rectum: results of a ten-year experience. Dis Colon Rectum 1994;37:635.

Soga J: Carcinoids of the colon and ileocecal region: a statistical evaluation of 363 cases collected from the literature. J Exp Clin Cancer Res 1998;17:139.

Spread C et al: Colon carcinoid tumors. A population-based study. Dis Colon Rectum 1994;37:482.

DIVERTICULAR DISEASE OF THE COLON

Diverticula are more common in the colon than in any other portion of the gastrointestinal tract. Colonic diverticula are acquired and are classified as false because they consist of mucosa and submucosa that have herniated through the muscular coats. True diverticula containing all layers of the bowel wall are rare in the colon. Colonic diverticula are pulsion (rather than traction) diverticula, because they are pushed out by intraluminal pressure. They vary from a few millimeters to several centimeters in diameter; the necks may be narrow or wide; and some contain inspissated fecal matter. Approximately 95% of patients with diverticula have involvement of the sigmoid colon. The descending, transverse, and ascending portions of the colon are involved in decreasing order of frequency. The presence of a solitary diverticulum of the cecum and the occurrence of multiple diverticula limited to the right colon are distinct entities most often seen in Asian people but seldom encountered in other populations. Giant colonic diverticulum is a very rare lesion of huge dimensions, usually arising from the sigmoid colon.

In Western countries, perhaps 50% of individuals develop diverticula—10% by age 40 years and 65% by age 80 years. Diverticular disease is more common in Western nations than in Asia or in developing countries of the tropics. The prevalence of diverticulosis is 20%; in Singapore, 70% of the cases are right-sided. Cultural factors, especially diet, play an important etiologic role. Chief among the dietary influences is the fiber content of foods.

The pathogenesis of diverticula requires defects in the colonic wall and increased pressure in the lumen relative to the serosal surface. Small openings in the circular muscle layer for penetration of nutrient blood vessels are the sites of diverticula formation (Figure 30–12). Diverticulosis of the colon comprises a spectrum with two extremes: (1) diverticulosis associated with hypermotility and (2) simple massed diverticulosis. In the first type, colonic musculature is shortened and thickened (myochosis coli); colonic pressures are high in response to meals or pharmacologic stimuli; patients may have pain and altered bowel habits; and diverticula are limited to the sigmoid, at least initially. It is hypothesized that myochosis reflects work hypertrophy from a lifetime of fiber-deficient diet and the consequent scybalous stools. High intraluminal pressures are possible because the colon forms closed compartments when opposite walls of the thickened bowel actually touch and occlude the lumen. The propensity for diverticula to develop in the sigmoid is explained by the law of Laplace, which states that pressure within a tube is inversely proportionate to the radius. It had been speculated that irritable bowel syndrome was a prediverticular state, but patterns of colonic motility are different in diverticular disease and irritable bowel syndrome. Moreover, it is clear that irritable bowel syndrome can affect the esophagus and small bowel in addition to the colon, so an etiologic link to colonic diverticula now seems unlikely. The two conditions can coexist, however, and irritable bowel syndrome may be the reason for symptoms.

Patients with simple massed diverticulosis have grossly normal colonic musculature, normal pressures, often no symptoms, and diverticula throughout the colon. Presumably, the primary abnormality is weakness of the colonic wall from aging or illness. It is of interest that Ehlers-Danlos syndrome and Marfan syndrome, both of which involve

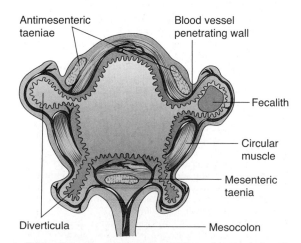

▲ **Figure 30–12.** Cross section of the colon depicting the sites where diverticula form. Note that the antimesocolic portion is spared. The longitudinal layer of muscle completely encircles the bowel and is not limited to the taeniae as depicted here.

abnormal connective tissue, are associated with colonic diverticulosis.

1. Diverticulosis

Diverticulosis is the presence of multiple false diverticula.

▶ Clinical Findings

A. Symptoms and Signs

Diverticulosis probably remains asymptomatic in about 80% of people and is detected incidentally on barium enema x-rays, CT scans, or endoscopy if it is discovered at all. Symptoms attributable to the diverticula themselves are actually complications—bleeding and diverticulitis—each described in separate sections. Symptoms (episodic pain, constipation, diarrhea) in patients with uncomplicated diverticulosis are due to the associated motility disorder, and the diverticula are coincidental. Physical examination may disclose mild tenderness in the left lower quadrant, and the left colon is sometimes palpable as a firm tubular structure. Fever and leukocytosis are absent in patients with pain but no inflammation.

B. Imaging Studies

In addition to diverticula, barium enema films may show segmental spasm and muscular thickening that narrow the lumen and give it a sawtoothed appearance.

C. Colonoscopy

There is little role for colonoscopy in the evaluation of diverticulosis. Its role in diverticulitis is discussed in the section on Diverticulitis.

▶ Differential Diagnosis

Pain from the colonic muscular abnormality in the absence of inflammation can be difficult to differentiate from diverticulitis. The presence or absence of systemic signs of inflammation is the chief differential point, but the natural history of the acute episode may be the only way to make the distinction. Diverticulosis must be differentiated from other causes of rectal bleeding, especially carcinoma. Colonoscopy is essential in patients with bleeding.

▶ Complications

Diverticulitis and massive hemorrhage are discussed in the section on Diverticulitis.

▶ Treatment

A. Medical Treatment

Asymptomatic persons with diverticulosis may be given a high-fiber diet, though it is not certain that complications of diverticulosis can be avoided by dietary changes once the diverticula have formed. Symptomatic patients also can be treated with a high-fiber diet; constipation is improved, but abdominal pain is not. Wheat bran is the least expensive source of fiber; patients should take 10–25 g daily with cereal, soup, salad, or other food. Palatable bran products are now available. Other sources of wheat fiber include whole-grain bread and breakfast cereals. Commercial bulk agents (eg, psyllium seed or hemicellulose products) are also available at greater cost. One problem in prescribing bulk agents is that different types of fiber may have dissimilar effects on the colon. Anticholinergic agents, sedatives, tranquilizers, antidepressants, and antibiotics have no value. Analgesics should be avoided, but if pain relief is necessary, nonopioid medications are preferred. Education, reassurance, and a warm personal relationship between physician and patient are important to successful management.

B. Surgical Treatment

Operation is necessary for massive hemorrhage or to rule out carcinoma in some patients, but colonoscopy usually resolves the question of cancer. Colon resection for uncomplicated diverticular disease or irritable bowel syndrome is rarely necessary or advisable.

▶ Prognosis

The natural history of diverticulosis has not been defined. Ten to 20 percent of patients with diverticulosis develop diverticulitis or hemorrhage when followed for many years. These patients are selected, however, and the incidence of complications in the population at large may be much lower. About 75% of complications of diverticular disease develop in patients with no prior colonic symptoms. Some evidence suggests that diverticulitis is more common with the hyper-motility type of diverticulosis, and bleeding is the more frequent complication in simple massed diverticulosis. Irritable bowel syndrome is a chronic relapsing disorder distinct from diverticulosis that affects patients over long periods of their lives. There is hope that better understanding of the pathophysiologic mechanisms will soon lead to more rational therapy.*

2. Diverticulitis

ESSENTIALS OF DIAGNOSIS

- ▶ Acute abdominal pain.
- ▶ Left lower quadrant tenderness and mass.
- ▶ Fever and leukocytosis.
- ▶ Characteristic radiologic signs.

*See references at end of next section.

General Considerations

Acute colonic diverticulitis is the result of perforation of a diverticulum and may be due to intraluminal pressure. Only one diverticulum is involved at a time, usually in the sigmoid colon. Disease severity is a continuum from mild inflammation localized to a segment of the bowel wall to feculent peritonitis.

Contained perforation of a diverticulum leads to localized inflammation in the colonic wall or paracolic tissues and may progress to more serious complications including formation of a phlegmon, abscess, or fistula. Generally, the original perforation seals quickly and the paracolic infection is isolated from the colonic lumen. An abscess may be confined by adjacent structures or may enlarge and spread; small abscesses may resorb with antibiotic treatment; others may drain spontaneously into the lumen of the bowel or into an adjacent viscus to form a fistula or require surgical drainage either percutaneously or by laparotomy. Free perforation results in purulent or feculent peritonitis. Chronic colonic obstruction can result from fibrosis in response to repeated episodes of microperforation (stricture). Also, small bowel may adhere acutely to an inflamed area and cause small bowel obstruction. Cecal diverticulitis resembles appendicitis clinically.

Clinical Findings

A. Symptoms and Signs

The acute attack consists of localized abdominal pain that is mild to severe, aching, and either steady or cramping; it resembles acute appendicitis except that it is situated in the left lower quadrant. Occasionally, pain is suprapubic, in the right lower quadrant, or throughout the lower abdomen. Constipation or increased frequency of defecation (or both in the same patient) is common, and passage of flatus may give some relief of pain. Inflammation adjacent to the bladder may produce dysuria. Nausea and vomiting depend on the location and severity of the inflammation. Physical findings characteristically include low-grade fever, mild abdominal distention, left lower quadrant tenderness, and a left lower quadrant or pelvic mass. Neither occult nor gross blood in the stools is common, and presence of blood may suggest malignancy. Leukocytosis is variably present.

The clinical picture described above is typical, but acute diverticulitis has other modes of presentation. Free perforation of a diverticulum produces generalized peritonitis rather than localized inflammation. An acute attack of diverticulitis may go unnoticed until a complication such as stricture or fistula develops, and the complication may be the reason for the patient to seek help. The course of diverticulitis may be so insidious, particularly in old people, that vague abdominal pain associated with an abscess in the groin or a colovesical fistula is the initial presentation. In some cases, pain and inflammatory signs are not marked, but a palpable mass and signs of large bowel obstruction are present, so that carcinoma of the left colon seems the more likely diagnosis. In one series of women with proved diverticulitis, 38% were initially misdiagnosed as having a gynecologic pelvic mass because gastrointestinal symptoms and signs were mild or absent.

B. Imaging Studies

Plain abdominal films may show free abdominal air if a diverticulum has perforated into the general peritoneal cavity. If inflammation is localized, there is a picture of ileus, partial colonic obstruction, small bowel obstruction, or left lower quadrant mass.

CT scan of the abdomen and pelvis is the preferred initial imaging study and should be obtained early in the patient's course, with intravenous, oral, and rectal contrast to enhance the image. Stranding of pericolic fat is seen in diverticulitis, and complications such as abscess or fistula may be evident. (See Figure 30–13.) Findings on CT scan may also be predictive of the need for surgical intervention or successful non-operative expectant management. In an effort to provide standardization for the discussion of perforated diverticulitis, Hinchey and coworkers described four stages of the disease: (1) pericolic abscess confined to the mesentery of the colon, (2) pelvic abscess resulting from an extension of a pericolic abscess, (3) purulent peritonitis, and (4) feculent peritonitis. Repeat CT or operative intervention is indicated when patients fail to improve or when they deteriorate over the initial 48 hours of medical therapy.

Barium enema is contraindicated during the initial stages of an acute attack of diverticulitis lest barium leak into the peritoneal cavity, but water-soluble contrast media used under low pressure is safe. Barium enema can be performed a week or more after the attack began if the patient has recovered promptly but is rarely necessary with modern CT scan imaging.

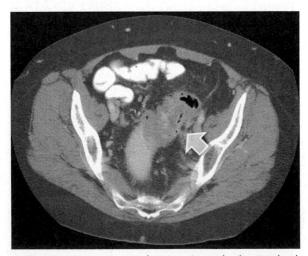

▲ **Figure 30–13.** CT scan showing sigmoid colon involved with diverticulitis. Note the pericolonic stranding, bowel wall thickening, and intramural abscess.

C. Special Examinations

The rigid sigmoidoscope usually cannot be passed beyond the rectosigmoid junction because of acute angulation and fixation at that level with a decrease in size of the lumen. Erythema, edema, and spasm may be noted. A purulent discharge can sometimes be seen coming from above. Flexible sigmoidoscopy or colonoscopy should be avoided during an acute attack but is helpful in ruling out cancer and evaluating strictures and other persistent abnormalities later. Small-bore upper tract instruments may be needed to examine narrow segments. Cystoscopy may reveal bullous edema of the bladder wall.

▶ Differential Diagnosis

Free perforation of a diverticulum with generalized peritonitis often cannot be differentiated from the other causes of perforation, including foreign bodies and stercoraceous perforation. Acute diverticulitis with localized perforation may simulate appendicitis, perforated colonic carcinoma, obstruction with strangulation, mesenteric vascular insufficiency, Crohn disease, and many other conditions. Differentiation from appendicitis is especially difficult when a redundant sigmoid colon lies in the right lower quadrant. A history of colonic symptoms on prior occasions, palpation of a mass, ultrasonography, CT, or water-soluble contrast enema may be helpful in differentiating these conditions. Colonoscopy may detect carcinoma, vascular insufficiency, or inflammatory disease of the colon. A difficult differential diagnosis lies between diverticulitis and carcinoma of the colon, particularly in the more silent forms of diverticulitis that present with a mass or fistula. Although barium enema and colonoscopy may clarify the issue, the diagnosis may not be known until the surgical specimen is examined by the pathologist.

▶ Complications

The clinical spectrum of diverticulitis includes such complications as free perforation, abscess formation, fistulization, and partial obstruction. Colonic obstruction is usually slow in onset and incomplete. If acute, it generally resolves with nasogastric decompression and intravenous antibiotics, allowing for elective resection when necessary. Small bowel obstruction may result from the attachment of a loop of small intestine to the inflamed sigmoid.

Fistulas in males usually involve the bladder (see Colovesical Fistula, later). Fistulas may also occur to the ureter, urethra, vagina, uterus, cecum, small bowel, ovaries, fallopian tubes, perineum, and abdominal wall.

▶ Treatment

A. Expectant Treatment

Patients with acute diverticulitis may need to be hospitalized. Details of management vary with the severity of the attack. Generally, nothing is given by mouth, nasogastric suction may be necessary, intravenous fluids are given, and systemic broad-spectrum antibiotics are administered. Oral nonabsorbable antibacterial drugs are of little value. Opioid pain medications should be given prudently so as to allow for serial abdominal examination. As acute manifestations subside, oral feeding is resumed gradually, and bulk-forming agents are prescribed if there is no stricture. It is estimated that such treatment is successful in more than 70% of patients. Recurrence following nonoperative management is expected in approximately 30% of patients following their first episode.

Colonoscopy is performed 6–8 weeks after the resolution of symptoms. Colonoscopy is mandatory in the presence of rectal bleeding or if x-rays show a possible neoplasm (stricture, mass, equivocal findings). The entire colon should always be evaluated for polyps or malignancy whenever elective resection for diverticular disease is planned. It is recommended—even if barium x-rays reveal only diverticula—in patients with abdominal pain or change in bowel habits attributed to diverticular disease. Colonoscopy will disclose a colonic neoplasm in about 30% of such patients.

B. Surgical Treatment

Indications for colectomy include perforation with generalized peritonitis or failure to improve with medical therapy. Elective resection was traditionally recommended for recurrent disease, a history of complicated disease (ie, phlegmon or abscess resolved with medical therapy or percutaneous drainage, stricture, or fistula), or the inability to rule out carcinoma. Age under 50 years was also an indication for resection. However, such traditional indications for colectomy are currently being reconsidered, and many experts now advocate close observation of such patients with surgery reserved for recurrent, chronic, or complicated disease. Obstruction and fistula are seldom indications for urgent operation during acute diverticulitis; both of these clinical problems are discussed separately in this chapter.

Percutaneous catheter drainage of well-localized paracolic abscesses can be performed by the interventional radiologist. This technique is especially useful because it converts a potential emergency operation to an elective one that can be performed when the acute inflammation has resolved. Colonic resection is indicated after an episode of complicated diverticulitis.

At laparotomy for severe acute diverticulitis, peritoneal fluid varies from turbid to purulent to grossly fecal. The sigmoid colon is involved in an inflammatory mass composed of large bowel, mesocolon, omentum, and sometimes small bowel. Except in cases of free perforation with generalized fecal peritonitis, the diseased diverticulum may not be visible. An abscess cavity may be hidden beneath colon or omentum and discovered when the bowel is mobilized; abscesses are commonly found lateral or medial to the colon, in the mesocolon, or in the pelvis. Microperforation of a diverticulum is not associated with a grossly apparent abscess. The extent of colonic inflammation, the amount of peritonitis, the patient's general condition, and the surgeon's experience and preferences determine the type of operation to be performed.

1. Primary resection with anastomosis—Resection of the diseased colon and primary colonic anastomosis has the advantage of solving the entire problem in one operation. It is not possible to anastomose the colon safely if there is gross infection in the surgical field after the diseased bowel has been removed, because the risk of anastomotic leakage is great. Intraoperative lavage of the colon may make it possible to perform primary anastomosis if other conditions permit.

2. Primary resection without anastomosis (two-stage procedure)—The diseased bowel is removed, the proximal end of the colon is brought out as a temporary colostomy, and the distal colonic stump is closed (Hartmann procedure; Figure 30–6) or exteriorized as a mucous fistula. Intestinal continuity is restored in a second operation after the inflammation subsides. Increasingly, percutaneous drainage of abscesses avoids the need for staged procedures and allows for primary resection with anastomosis once the inflammation has resolved with drainage. However, if percutaneous drainage is unsuccessful, percutaneous drainage is indicated.

3. Three-stage procedure—The three-stage procedure consists of a first operation during which a transverse colostomy is created and the paracolic abscess is drained, a second operation during which the left colon is resected, and a third operation during which the colostomy is taken down. The three-stage approach is uncommonly used in the United States today because it is associated with a higher mortality than the two-stage approach.

Definitive resection for sigmoid diverticulitis should include the sigmoid colon distally to the point where the taeniae become confluent so that anastomosis is performed to the uninvolved rectum. The proximal extent of resection should be the point at which the bowel is soft and appears healthy—this generally includes the entire sigmoid colon. It is unnecessary to resect additional bowel proximally; even if it is involved with diverticula, they are unlikely to become symptomatic in the absence of the sigmoid high-pressure zone. The laparoscopic approach may have advantages when compared to the open approach but may be difficult or technically not possible due to the persistence of inflammation.

▶ **Prognosis**

Approximately 25% of patients hospitalized with acute diverticulitis require surgical treatment. The operative mortality rate is about 5% in recent reports, compared with 25% historically. Some of this improvement is attributable to the greater use of primary resection following percutaneous drainage of abscess.

Diverticulitis recurs in about one third of medically treated cases. Most of these recurrences develop within the

first 5 years. It is unknown whether recurrent attacks of diverticulitis can be prevented by increasing dietary fiber, although this measure is generally recommended. Recurrent diverticulitis after resection is unusual (about 3–7%) if the distal extent of the resection is at the rectum.

Abbas S: Resection and primary anastomosis in acute complicated diverticulitis, a systematic review of the literature. Int J Colorectal Dis 2007;22:351.

Aldoori WH et al: A prospective study of dietary fiber types and symptomatic diverticular disease in men. J Nutr 1998;128:714.

Ambrosetti P: Acute diverticulitis of the left colon: value of the initial CT and timing of elective colectomy. J Gastrointest Surg 2008;12:1318.

Baker ME: Imaging and interventional techniques in acute left-sided diverticulitis. J Gastrointest Surg 2008;12:1314.

Chapman JR et al: Diverticulitis: a progressive disease? Do multiple recurrences predict less favorable outcomes? Ann Surg 2006;243:876.

Desai DC et al: The utility of the Hartmann procedure. Am J Surg 1998;175:152.

Jacobs DO: Clinical practice. Diverticulitis. N Engl J Med 2007; 357:2057.

Lee EC et al: Intraoperative colonic lavage in nonelective surgery for diverticular disease. Dis Colon Rectum 1997;40:669.

Miura S et al: Recent trends in diverticulosis of the right colon in Japan: retrospective review in a regional hospital. Dis Colon Rectum 2000;43:1383.

Nagorney DM, Adson MA, Pemberton JH: Sigmoid diverticulitis with perforation and generalized peritonitis. Dis Colon Rectum 1985;28:71.

Rafferty et al: Practice parameters for sigmoid diverticulitis. The Standards Committee of The American Society of Colon and Rectal Surgeons. Dis Colon Rectum 2006;49:939.

Salem L, Flum DR: Primary anastomosis or Hartmann's procedure for patients with diverticular peritonitis? A systematic review. Dis Colon Rectum 2004;47:1953.

Schwandener O et al: Laparoscopic colectomy for recurrent and complicated diverticulitis: a prospective study of 396 patients. Langenbecks Arch Surg 2004;389:97.

COLOVESICAL FISTULA

Colovesical fistula is the most common type of fistulous communication between the urinary bladder and the gastrointestinal tract. There is a 3:1 ratio of men to women with this condition, presumably because in women the uterus and adnexa are situated between the colon and the bladder.

Diverticulitis is the most common cause of colovesical fistula. This complication occurs in 2–4% of cases of diverticulitis, though an even higher incidence is reported from specialized referral centers. Carcinoma of the colon, cancer of other organs such as the bladder, Crohn disease, radiation injury, external trauma, foreign bodies, and iatrogenic injuries are other causes or underlying conditions.

A colovesical fistula may cause surprisingly little disturbance to the patient, and some patients remain completely asymptomatic. The appearance of a fistula from diverticulitis or colon cancer is seldom accompanied by dramatic or sudden abdominal symptoms; more typically, refractory urinary tract infection is the presenting complaint. Fecaluria and pneumaturia may have been obvious to the patient, or it may be recollected only in response to direct questioning. The episode of diverticulitis may have gone entirely unnoticed.

Physical examination may disclose a pelvic mass or no abnormalities. Leukocytosis is absent in most cases, and routine blood chemistries are normal. Urinalysis may reveal fecaluria or infected urine. Rigid sigmoidoscopy is usually unrevealing; flexible sigmoidoscopy or colonoscopy may disclose colon cancer or inflammation at the fistula site. Cystoscopy shows bullous edema, but the fistula is usually not visible. CT detects small amounts of air in the bladder in 90% of patients. Barium enema, sonography, and cystography may demonstrate the fistula, but small communications escape detection. In some cases, the fistula is not demonstrable because it has closed, at least temporarily.

Colovesical fistulas require surgical treatment if they persist, but there is no need for emergency or urgent operation. Patients may recover well from spontaneous drainage of a paracolic abscess through a fistula into the bladder, and operation can be delayed to be sure it is necessary and by then the conditions will be more favorable. Inability to rule out cancer may prompt earlier operation. If a fistula closes spontaneously, as it may do in up to 50% of patients with diverticulitis, requirements for resection depend on the nature of the underlying colonic disease. Some patients tolerate a colovesical fistula so well that operation is deferred indefinitely.

At operation, patients with diverticulitis or colonic carcinoma have mild to moderate inflammatory reaction around the sigmoid colon, which has dropped into the pelvis and adhered to the bladder; severe active diverticulitis with abscess or peritonitis is exceptional. If the fistula was caused by cancer of the colon, the adherent bladder should not be separated from the colon lest tumor cells be spilled into the pelvis; a disk of bladder wall should be excised in continuity with the colon, the bladder closed primarily, and catheter drainage of the bladder provided for 7–10 days. Fortunately, most colovesical fistulas enter the bladder away from the trigone. Diverticulitis is managed by bluntly dissecting the colon from the bladder, resecting the colon, and performing a primary anastomosis. The bladder side of the fistula is sutured, and the bladder is decompressed with a Foley catheter. It is rarely necessary to delay performance of the colonic anastomosis.

Lavery IC: Colonic fistulas. Surg Clin North Am 1996;76:1183.
Vasilevsky CA et al: Fistulas complicating diverticulitis. Int J Colorectal Dis 1998;13:57.

ACUTE LOWER GASTROINTESTINAL HEMORRHAGE

Acute hemorrhage per rectum can originate from lesions in the gastroduodenum, small bowel, colon, or anorectum. A source in the lower gastrointestinal tract is suggested by the passage of dark to bright red blood, but the color of evacuated blood is a function of the length of time it remained in the intestinal tract, and bright red blood may come from a duodenal ulcer or hemorrhoids as well as any point in between. If a patient passing bright red blood is not in shock, the bleeding site is probably in the distal small bowel or colon.

Exsanguinating hemorrhage from the colon in adults is caused by diverticular disease, angiodysplasia, solitary ulcer, ulcerative colitis, ischemic colitis, or a variety of uncommon lesions such as coagulation disorders, radiation injury, chemotherapeutic toxicity, and others. Bleeding occurs in the right colon about as often as in the left colon, probably because angiodysplasias are more prominent on the right side, but right-sided diverticula can also bleed. Bleeding lesions in the small intestine are rare and include hereditary hemorrhagic telangiectasia (Rendu-Osler-Weber syndrome).

Chronic rectal bleeding, typically seen in patients with cancer, polyps, hemorrhoids, fissures, and other conditions, does not require emergent evaluation. Anorectal examination, colonoscopy, and x-rays if indicated can be performed electively. Acute severe hemorrhage, however, is a potentially life-threatening problem, and prompt evaluation and treatment are critical. Some patients bleed rapidly, but the bleeding stops spontaneously after only a small amount of blood is lost, and these patients are never in danger. Usually, however, one cannot be sure that bleeding will not recur, so this type of bleeding must be taken seriously too, which means that aggressive evaluation is needed.

A plan of management of acute lower gastrointestinal hemorrhage is outlined in Figure 30–14. Many decisions depend on the rate of bleeding, which is difficult to include in an algorithm. Bleeding stops spontaneously in 90% of patients before transfusion requirements exceed two units.

The patient with severe rectal bleeding is resuscitated with intravenous fluids and transfusions while the diagnostic procedures are begun. Clotting parameters should be measured and deficits corrected, and associated medical conditions should be identified and treated as soon as possible. Digital rectal examination, anoscopy, and sigmoidoscopy should be performed with no attempt to prepare the bowel. If a bleeding lesion is found in the anorectum, it should be treated. Examples include hemorrhoids, polypoid neoplasm, and ulcerative proctitis.

A nasogastric tube should be inserted and the aspirate inspected for bile, gross blood, and occult blood. Blood in the stomach is an indication of bleeding from a site proximal to the ligament of Treitz (ie, upper gastrointestinal bleeding), and esophagogastroduodenoscopy is performed. Occasionally, a patient bleeds from the duodenum but blood does not reflux back into the stomach; bile in the nasogastric aspirate would seem to eliminate this possibility, but in the absence of blood or bile, esophagogastroduodenoscopy should be done.

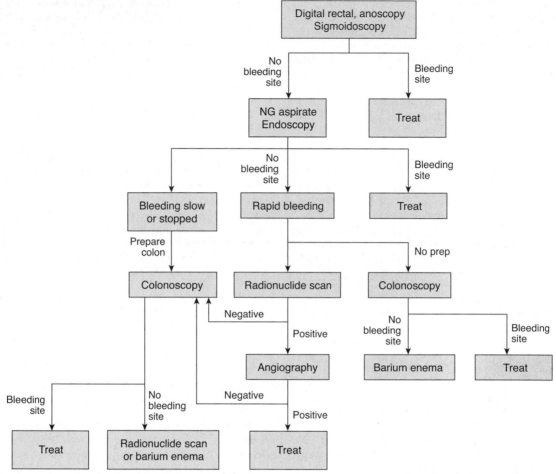

▲ **Figure 30–14.** Plan for diagnosis and treatment of acute lower gastrointestinal hemorrhage. (NG = nasogastric.)

If esophagogastroduodenoscopy is negative and bleeding has presumably stopped or continues at a slow rate, the colon can be prepared and colonoscopy performed within a few hours. The bleeding site is identified in 25–94% of cases, depending in part on skill, experience, and, very importantly, the criteria for inclusion of a patient in this category of bleeding. Some bleeding lesions can be treated colonoscopically with a bipolar probe, heater probe, or laser. Colonoscopy with negative results probably means that bleeding has stopped. Barium enema discloses abnormalities such as diverticula but does not reveal which lesions have been bleeding. If the esophagogastroduodenoscopy and colonoscopy are both negative, a capsule videoendoscopy may be performed to evaluate for a small bowel source.

The optimal method for evaluating patients who are bleeding rapidly is controversial, and the decision may hinge on available resources. A radionuclide "bleeding" scan after injection of ^{99m}Tc-labeled red blood cells may show whether bleeding persists and can detect a 0.1 mL/min rate of bleeding. Localization of bleeding is not reliable, but valuable information may be obtained. Angiography is seldom successful in demonstrating an active bleeding site if the bleeding scan is negative, so colonoscopy should be undertaken. Active bleeding shown on radionuclide scan should be followed by angiography.

Selective mesenteric angiography identifies the bleeding site in 14–70% of patients (threshold 0.5 mL/min); here, too, experience of the angiographer is important. If the bleeding site is seen, intra-arterial infusion of vasopressin controls bleeding, at least transiently, in 35–90% of patients. Definitive treatment with highly selective arterial embolization may be performed with success in 75% of patients.

The other option for rapid bleeding is emergency colonoscopy without preliminary bowel cleansing. Blood is a cathartic, and the colon may be free of stool. Even so, colonoscopy in this situation is difficult. Experts can see the bleeding point in up to 50% of patients, and in 70% of cases, bleeding can be localized to one region. Endoscopic therapeutic measures can be applied in up to 40% of patients, with success in half of them.

Operation is indicated for bleeding that persists or recurs despite angiographic and endoscopic therapeutic maneuvers. Operation is advisable also in good-risk patients who have stopped bleeding if the bleeding source is known and cannot be managed in some other way (eg, colonoscopic coagulation). Operation is limited to segmental colonic resection if the bleeding site has been localized conclusively. More extensive resection is usually warranted in patients who are bleeding from the right colon and have multiple diverticula in the left colon. If the surgeon has no preoperative localizing data and intraoperative examination is unrevealing, the stomach, small bowel, and colon can be endoscoped during the procedure to search for the source of blood. If all localizing efforts fail and the colon is the likely bleeding site, total abdominal colectomy (usually with primary anastomosis) may be the only recourse. Fortunately, extensive "blind" colectomy is seldom required today.

The mortality rate from lower gastrointestinal hemorrhage is about 10–15%.

American Society for Gastrointestinal Endoscopy: The role of endoscopy in the patient with lower gastrointestinal bleeding. Gastrointest Endosc 1998;48:685.

Eisen GM et al: An annotated algorithmic approach to acute lower gastrointestinal bleeding. Gastrointest Endosc 2001;53:859.

Farrell JJ, Friedman LS: Gastrointestinal bleeding in the elderly. Gastroenterol Clin North Am 2001;30:377.

Gordon RL et al: Selective arterial embolization for the control of lower gastrointestinal bleeding. Am J Surg 1997;174:24.

Jensen DM: What to choose for diagnosis of bleeding colonic angiomas: colonoscopy, angiography, or helical computed tomography angiography? Gastroenterology 2000;119:581.

Luchtefeld MA et al: Evaluation of transarterial embolization for lower gastrointestinal bleeding. Dis Colon Rectum 2000;43:532.

Suzman MS et al: Accurate localization and surgical management of active lower gastrointestinal hemorrhage with technetium-labeled erythrocyte scintigraphy. Ann Surg 1996;224:29.

ANGIODYSPLASIA

Angiodysplasia is an acquired condition most often affecting people over age 60. It is a focal submucosal vascular ectasia that has a propensity to bleed spontaneously. Most lesions are located in the cecum and proximal ascending colon, but in younger persons they are occasionally found in the small bowel, principally the jejunum. Multiple lesions occur in 25% of cases. Aortic stenosis is found in patients with angiodysplasias, but whether they are truly related is still being argued. Von Willebrand disease is present in some patients, and it has been suggested that the two conditions may be reflections of a generalized tissue disorder. Bleeding is typically intermittent and is rarely massive; a typical episode requires transfusion of 2–4 units of blood and is not associated with hypotension. Angiodysplasia may also present clinically as melena or as iron deficiency anemia and guaiac-positive stools.

The diagnosis is made in some cases by colonoscopy, and colonoscopic therapy is often successful. Incidental angiomas should be ignored. The lesions are characterized angiographically by (1) an early-filling vein (ie, within 4–5 seconds after injection), (2) a vascular tuft, and (3) a delayed-emptying vein. It is generally thought that two of the three features should be seen for the diagnosis to be secure. Active bleeding (ie, extravasation) is rarely demonstrated by angiography. As many as 25% of persons over age 60 with no history of gastrointestinal bleeding have angiodysplasias of the cecum, so the finding of a lesion is not proof that it has caused bleeding.

The natural history of angiodysplasia is not well delineated, and in elderly, poor-risk patients who have bled only once, expectant management may be preferable to surgery if colonoscopic therapeutic methods are unsuccessful. Operation should be directed to the affected segment of colon. In one series, 23% of patients who underwent operation for presumably bleeding colonic angiodysplasias were eventually found to have a small bowel lesion also.

Foutch PG: Colonic angiodysplasia. Gastroenterologist 1997; 5:148.

Orsi P, Guatti-Zuliani C, Okolicsanyi L: Long-acting octreotide is effective in controlling rebleeding angiodysplasia of the gastrointestinal tract. Dig Liver Dis 2001;33:330.

Rockey DC: Occult gastrointestinal bleeding. N Engl J Med 1999;341:38.

Sharma R, Gorbien MJ: Angiodysplasia and lower gastrointestinal tract bleeding in elderly patients. Arch Intern Med 1995; 155:807.

Veyradier A et al: Abnormal von Willebrand factor in bleeding angiodysplasias of the digestive tract. Gastroenterology 2001; 120:346.

VOLVULUS

 ESSENTIALS OF DIAGNOSIS

► Colicky abdominal pain, usually with persistence of pain between spasms.

► Abdominal distention.

► Vomiting sometimes.

► Usually older age groups.

► Characteristic x-ray findings.

► General Considerations

Rotation of a segment of the intestine on an axis formed by its mesentery may result in partial or complete obstruction of the lumen and may be followed by circulatory impairment of the bowel (Figure 30–15). Volvulus of the colon involves the cecum (30%), sigmoid (65%), transverse colon (3%), or splenic flexure (2%). Volvulus of the colon accounts for 5–10% of cases of large bowel obstruction in the United States and is the second-most common cause of complete colonic obstruction. In certain countries where the population consumes a high-residue diet, volvulus is the most frequent cause of large bowel obstruction. Volvulus—sigmoid more often than cecal—accounts for 25% of intestinal obstructions during pregnancy; it occurs most often in the last trimester, probably because the enlarging uterus displaces the colon.

Elongation of the sigmoid and rectosigmoid is a predisposing factor in sigmoid volvulus; 50% of patients are over age 70, and many patients are mentally ill or bedridden persons who do not evacuate stool with regularity. Chagas disease of the colon is an important cause of sigmoid volvulus in South America. Formation of cecal volvulus requires a cecum that is hypermobile owing to incomplete embryologic fixation of the ascending colon. The bowel twists about the mesentery, forming a closed-loop obstruction as the entry and exit points of the twist engage; obstruction of the lumen usually occurs when the rotation is 180 degrees. When the twist is 360 degrees, the veins are occluded, and the circulatory impairment leads to gangrene and perforation if treatment is not instituted promptly. A related condition called **cecal bascule** involves folding of the ascending colon so that the cecum moves anteriorly and superiorly, causing obstruction at the site of the transverse fold. Patients may describe intermittent bloating, pain, and obstructive symptoms improved by lying down and massaging the abdomen. Since no axial twist of the mesentery is involved in this situation, early strangulation from occlusion of the main vessels is not a factor.

▶ Clinical Findings

A. Cecal Volvulus

Not only the cecum but also the terminal ileum are involved in the rotation, so the symptoms generally include those of distal small bowel obstruction. Severe intermittent colicky pain begins in the right abdomen. Pain eventually becomes continuous, vomiting ensues, and passage of gas and feces per rectum decreases to the point of obstipation. Abdominal distention is variable; occasionally, a bulging tympanitic mass may be detected. There may be a history of similar but milder attacks, and valid examples of chronic intermittent cecal volvulus exist; they can be detected and operated on electively.

The diagnosis is seldom made without x-ray examination. Plain films show a hugely dilated ovoid cecum that may change position but favors the epigastrium or left upper quadrant. The distended loop may assume a "coffee bean" shape. In cecal volvulus, the concavity of the coffee bean points toward the right lower abdominal quadrant, and in sigmoid volvulus, it points toward the left lower quadrant. In

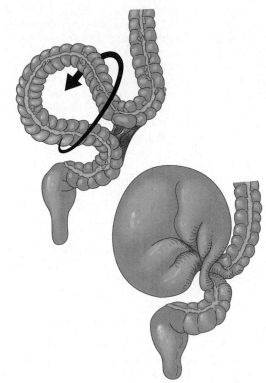

▲ **Figure 30–15.** Volvulus of the sigmoid colon. The twist is counterclockwise in most cases of sigmoid volvulus.

the early stages, there is a single fluid level that may be mistaken for gastric dilation, but large amounts of gas or fluid cannot be aspirated from the stomach, and the x-ray picture is not changed by this maneuver. Later, the radiologic findings of small bowel obstruction are superimposed on the cecal volvulus. The success rate of diagnosis based on plain abdominal films is extremely variable, ranging from 5% to 90%. Radiographic contrast enema may be diagnostic.

B. Sigmoid Volvulus

In volvulus of the sigmoid, there are intermittent cramplike pains, increasing in severity as obstipation becomes complete. Abdominal distention may be marked. There may be a history of transient attacks in which spontaneous reduction of the volvulus has occurred. On a plain film of the abdomen, a single greatly distended loop of bowel that has lost its haustral markings is usually seen rising up out of the pelvis, frequently as high as the diaphragm. On barium enema, a "bird's beak" or "ace of spades" deformity with spiral narrowing of the upper end of the lower segment is pathognomonic (Figure 30–16). Between attacks, barium enema may reveal sigmoid megacolon. The entire colon may be termed a megacolon in some cases.

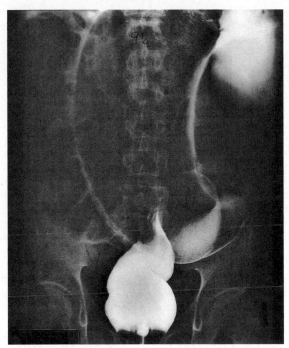

▲ **Figure 30–16.** Volvulus of the sigmoid colon. Barium enema taken with the patient in the supine position. Note the massively dilated sigmoid colon. The distinct vertical crease, which represents juxtaposition of adjacent walls of the dilated loop, points toward the site of torsion. The barium column resembles a "bird's beak" or "ace of spades" because of the way in which the lumen tapers toward the volvulus.

Differential Diagnosis

Cecal volvulus must be differentiated from colonic pseudoobstruction and from other causes of small bowel and colonic obstruction. Sigmoid volvulus mimics other types of large bowel obstruction. Alertness to the possibility and correct interpretation of x-rays are the essentials of diagnosis.

Complications

Early diagnosis and treatment are imperative because perforation may occur if circulation to the bowel is impaired. Delay may be due to incorrect diagnosis or to futile attempts at proximal decompression by gastric intubation.

Treatment

In cecal volvulus decompression is advisable as soon as the patient can be prepared by replacing fluid and electrolyte deficits. Colonoscopic detorsion and decompression may be attempted if an expert is available, especially in patients who have serious associated disease that would make operation

hazardous. Resection and anastomosis is the preferred operation, even if the bowel is viable, due to better long-term results than with lesser procedures. A laparoscopic or open approach may be utilized. Cecopexy (suture fixation of the bowel to the parietal peritoneum) has been reported and gives good immediate results, but the long-term success rate is controversial; recurrent volvulus developed in 29% of patients after cecopexy in one review. Tube cecostomy both decompresses the cecum and fixes it, but problems with tube management and a high risk for recurrence make this a less favorable option. Gangrenous colon or small bowel is found in about 20% of cases.

In many patients with sigmoid volvulus, the distended sigmoid can be decompressed by gentle insertion of a flexible colonoscope or sigmoidoscope. Decompression by passage of a tube through a rigid sigmoidoscope is also possible when flexible endoscopy is unavailable. Endoscopic decompression is contraindicated if there is evidence of strangulation or perforation. Percutaneous decompression of sigmoid volvulus has been reported, but it cannot be recommended for general use. If decompression is successful, good-risk young patients should be scheduled for elective resection of the affected bowel as soon as the colon can be prepared, because the recurrence rate after decompression alone is 50%. However, in patients with severe disease of other organ systems, one may need to tailor this approach. Emergency operation is performed if strangulation or perforation is suspected or if attempts to decompress the bowel per rectum are unsuccessful. Gangrenous bowel is found in about one third of such patients and is treated by resection. If the sigmoid is viable, most surgeons proceed with resection, deferring anastomosis to a later time if the bowel is unprepared. If the entire colon is a megacolon, total abdominal colectomy should be considered. Recurrent volvulus in nonoperated patients is managed by transrectal decompression followed by a definitive surgical procedure in all patients but those with very severe associated disease.

Prognosis

The mortality rate after emergency operation in patients with cecal volvulus is 12%; if the bowel is gangrenous, 35% of patients die after resection. Recurrence after cecopexy or resection is very unusual.

Sigmoid volvulus is fatal in about 50% of patients with perforation; mortality rates are much lower with gangrene alone, and only 5% of patients die after operation if the bowel is viable. Elective resection after endoscopic decompression has a low mortality rate, and recurrent volvulus is rare. Nonresection therapies are ineffective at preventing recurrence.

Feldman D: The coffee bean sign. Radiology 2000;216:178.
Grossmann EM et al: Sigmoid volvulus in Department of Veterans Affairs Medical Centers. Dis Colon Rectum 2000;43:414.
Madiba TE, Thomson SR: The management of sigmoid volvulus. J R Coll Surg Edinb 2000;45:74.

COLITIS

Colitis is a nonspecific term. Patients have diarrhea, abdominal pain, systemic symptoms, and abnormal endoscopic, radiographic, and laboratory tests. The task of the clinician is to differentiate among the various causes of colitis discussed below.

1. Idiopathic Mucosal Ulcerative Colitis

ESSENTIALS OF DIAGNOSIS

- ▶ Diarrhea, usually bloody.
- ▶ Abdominal cramps.
- ▶ Fever, weight loss, anemia.
- ▶ Absence of specific fecal pathogens.
- ▶ Endoscopic and radiographic abnormalities.

▶ General Considerations

The age at onset of ulcerative colitis has a bimodal distribution, with the first peak between ages 15 and 30 years and a second, lower peak in the sixth to eighth decades. Females are affected slightly more often than males. The annual incidence varies from 5 to 12 per 100,000 population, and the prevalence is 50–150 per 100,000 population. The disease is found worldwide but is more common in Western countries. It is uncommon in Asia. In the United States, Jews are more commonly affected than non-Jews, but in Israel, the prevalence among new immigrants is low.

The cause of ulcerative colitis is not known. A combination of genetic, environmental, and host immune response factors appear to be important in the pathogenesis of inflammatory bowel disease. It is also possible that ulcerative colitis and Crohn disease are different manifestations of a mechanistic continuum. Genetic factors contribute to the susceptibility to inflammatory bowel disease but cannot be explained by simple Mendelian inheritance. In 15–40% of patients, there is a family history of ulcerative colitis or Crohn disease. Based on genomewide association studies, the nucleotide-binding oligomerization domain 2 (NOD2) within the IBD1 locus on chromosome 16q, as well as the IB5 locus on chromosome 5q, appears to be important for Crohn disease but not for ulcerative colitis. Patients with two mutations of NOD2 have a 20-fold to 40-fold increased risk of developing Crohn disease. Chromosomes 3, 5, 7, and 12 have been linked to ulcerative colitis but not Crohn disease.

Environmental factors are also important; only 45% of identical twins are concordant for Crohn disease. Luminal flora is a requisite and perhaps central factor in the development of inflammatory bowel disease. This may explain the therapeutic benefits seen with broad-spectrum antibiotics

and probiotics in specific subgroups of patients. Perhaps the best environmental association is seen with Crohn disease and the use of NSAIDs, which can induce disease flares. Appendectomy has been associated with a decreased risk for later development of ulcerative colitis. Cigarette smoking appears to be protective against ulcerative colitis, but it increases the risk of Crohn disease.

The host immune response to mucosal antigens and environmental factors is also important. Differences may be on the basis of altered immune activation or a failure of counterregulation. The mucosa immune-cell population in Crohn disease is dominated by CD4+ T lymphocytes with a type 1 helper T cell (Th1), characterized by the production of interferon-γ and interleukin-2 (IL-2). In contrast, patients with ulcerative colitis exhibit a predominance of the type 2 helper T-cell (Th2) phenotype, characterized by the production of transforming growth factor β (TGF-β) and IL-5, but not IL-4. Ultimately, the activation of immune-cell populations results in the production of a variety of nonspecific inflammatory mediators that include cytokines, chemokines, and growth factors, as well as metabolites of arachidonic acid (eg, prostaglandins and leukotrienes). These mediators eventually play a critical role in the manifestation of inflammatory bowel disease.

Ulcerative colitis is a diffuse but contiguous inflammatory disease confined to the mucosa initially. Abscesses form in the crypts of Lieberkühn and penetrate the superficial submucosa, and by spreading horizontally, they cause the overlying mucosa to slough. Vascular congestion and hemorrhage are prominent. The margins of the ulcers are raised as mucosal tags that project into the lumen (pseudopolyps or inflammatory polyps). Except in the most severe forms, the muscular layers are spared; the serosal surface usually shows only dilated congested blood vessels. In fulminant disease, when the full thickness is involved, the colon may dilate or perforate. The colon is shortened, but the mesocolon remains thin—in contrast to Crohn disease.

Ulcerative colitis can manifest as ulcerative proctitis (involvement limited to the rectum), ulcerative proctosigmoiditis (involvement limited to the rectum and sigmoid colon), left-sided ulcerative colitis (inflammation is distal to the splenic flexure), and pancolitis (inflammation extends proximal to the splenic flexure or involves the entire colon). A few centimeters of distal ileum are ulcerated in 10% of patients with pancolitis (backwash ileitis). The diseased areas are contiguous and extend proximally from the rectum. The presence of segmental involvement or skip lesions should prompt the evaluation for Crohn disease.

▶ Clinical Findings
A. Symptoms and Signs

The cardinal symptoms are rectal bleeding and diarrhea: frequent discharges of watery stool mixed with blood, pus, and mucus accompanied by tenesmus, rectal urgency, and even anal incontinence. Nearly two thirds of patients have cramping abdominal pain and variable degrees of fever, vomiting, weight loss, and dehydration. The onset may be insidious or acute and fulminating, and the clinical findings differ accordingly. Mild disease may be manifested only by loose or frequent stools, and, paradoxically, a few patients complain of constipation. In isolated instances, the only symptoms may be from systemic complications such as arthropathy or pyoderma. Dairy products may aggravate diarrhea.

If the disease is mild, physical examination may be normal, but in severe disease the abdomen is tender, especially in the left lower quadrant, and the colon may be distended. As a rule, in contrast to Crohn disease, the anus is spared in ulcerative colitis. However, severe rectal inflammation may result in considerable tenderness and spasticity during digital rectal examination. The examining finger may be covered with blood, mucus, or pus.

A simple classification of the severity of an attack was devised by Truelove and Witts. The assessment of disease severity is based on six simple clinical signs (Table 30–12).

Proctosigmoidoscopy is essential. The characteristic mucosal changes of loss of vascular pattern, granularity, friability, hyperemia, and ulceration may be identified. These findings begin in the distal rectum and proceed proximally in a continuous fashion. Gross ulcers are not visible in the rectum in ulcerative colitis because of the superficial nature of these lesions. In more advanced disease, the mucosa is purplish-red, velvety, and extremely friable. Blood mixed with mucous is evident in the lumen. The disease is uniform in the affected bowel, and patches of normal mucosa are not seen. If the mucosa is not grossly diseased, biopsy may be helpful to confirm the diagnosis. In the recovery phase, mucosal hyperemia and edema subside and inflammatory polyps may be seen. The healing mucosa is typically dull and granular and has a neovascular pattern of telangiectatic vessels that differs from the normal pink mucosa.

B. Laboratory Findings

Anemia, leukocytosis, and an elevated sedimentation rate are usually present. Severe disease leads to hypoalbuminemia; depletion of water, electrolytes, and vitamins; and laboratory evidence of steatorrhea. Reduced plasma antithrombin III

levels may contribute to thromboembolic complications. Smears of the stool should be examined for parasites, bacteria, and leukocytes, and stool should be sent for cultures.

C. Imaging Studies

Barium enema examination should not be preceded by catharsis in acute cases and should not be performed at all in severely ill patients, because it may precipitate acute colonic dilation. Plain films may reveal severe colonic dilation (megacolon) with fulminant disease.

Barium x-rays in acute ulcerative colitis show mucosal irregularity that varies from fine serrations to rough, ragged, undermined ulcers. As the disease progresses, haustrations are gradually effaced, and the colon narrows and shortens because of muscular rigidity (Figure 30–17). Pseudopolyposis signifies severe ulceration. Widening of the space between the sacrum and rectum is due either to periproctitis or to shortening of the bowel. The presence of a stricture should always arouse suspicion of cancer. An upper gastrointestinal contrast examination with small bowel follow through should be performed to rule out Crohn disease.

CT scanning with oral, rectal, and intravenous contrast has largely replaced barium enema examination for assessing patients with severe disease. CT scanning also permits enterographic evaluation of the small bowel.

D. Colonoscopic Findings

Proctosigmoidoscopy or colonoscopy should be performed in most situations. Usually, the instrument need be inserted only into the sigmoid in order to make the initial diagnosis. Because of the danger of perforation, colonoscopy should be performed with great care if the disease is active, and it should not be done in the presence of colonic dilation. In chronic disease, colonoscopy with biopsies is valuable in surveillance for cancer. Strictures and other x-ray abnormalities can be investigated by colonoscopy also.

▶ Differential Diagnosis

Malignant neoplasms of the colon (including lymphomas) and diverticular disease must be considered in the differential

Table 30–12. Ulcerative Colitis Disease Severity (Based on the Truelove and Witt Classification).

Symptoms	Mild	Severe	Fulminant
Stools (per day)	< 4	> 6	> 10
Hematochezia	Intermittent	Frequent	Continuous
Temperature	Normal	> 37.5 °C	
Pulse (beats/min)	Normal	> 90	
Hemoglobin	Normal	< 75% of normal	Requires transfusion
ESR	< 30 mm/h	> 30 mm/h	

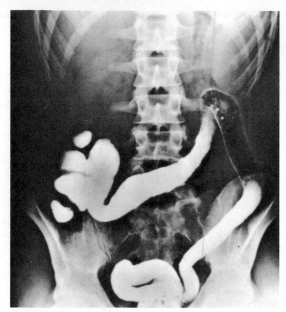

▲ **Figure 30–17.** Ulcerative colitis. Barium enema x-ray of colon. Note shortening of colon, loss of haustral markings ("lead pipe" appearance), and fine serrations at the edges of the bowel wall that represent multiple small ulcers.

diagnosis. Salmonellosis and other bacillary dysenteries are diagnosed by repeated stool cultures. Shigellosis may be suspected on the basis of a positive methylene blue stain for fecal leukocytes. *Campylobacter jejuni* is a common cause of bloody diarrhea; the organisms can be cultured from the stool, and serum antibody titers rise during the illness. Hemorrhagic colitis—a syndrome of bloody diarrhea and abdominal cramps but no fever—is associated with infection by *Escherichia coli* O157:H7. Legionella infections can mimic ulcerative colitis. Gonococcal proctitis is detected by culture of rectal swabs. Herpes simplex virus is the most common cause of nongonococcal proctitis in homosexual men. *Chlamydia trachomatis* infections are also common in this group; the mucosa is markedly inflamed and resembles Crohn disease; the organism can be cultured. It is most important in every case to rule out amebiasis (see Chapter 8) by microscopic examination of stool, rectal swabs, or rectal biopsies; serologic tests confirm that clinical infection has occurred. Corticosteroids must never be given to a patient with presumed idiopathic ulcerative colitis until amebiasis has been excluded.

Rare cases of histoplasmosis, tuberculosis, cytomegalovirus disease, schistosomiasis, amyloidosis, or Behçet disease may be very difficult to diagnose. AIDS-related gastrointestinal infections are increasingly common. Colitis caused by antibiotics is discussed separately below; the history is important in this type of disease. NSAIDs can cause mucosal inflammation and even strictures in the large intestine. Collagenous colitis may or may not be related to NSAID usage. Watery diarrhea is the main symptom of this syndrome, endoscopy is grossly normal, and biopsies show a thickened band of collagen just beneath the surface. Treatment to date has been difficult, but most patients are not seriously troubled by this condition. Ischemic colitis has a segmental pattern of involvement quite unlike the contiguous distribution of ulcerative colitis. Functional diarrhea can mimic colitis, but organic disease must be excluded before it can be concluded that the diarrhea is functional. Malacoplakia is a rare chronic granulomatous disease that can cause colonic strictures and may resemble colitis.

Diversion colitis is inflammation of a previously normal segment of colon or rectum following construction of a temporary colostomy (eg, in a two-stage approach to diverticulitis). Deficiency of mucosal nutrients may be responsible, and inflammation may resolve with topical application of short-chain fatty acids. Restoration of intestinal continuity also solves the problem.

The most difficult differential diagnosis is between mucosal ulcerative colitis and Crohn colitis (Table 30–13). None of the features are specific for one or the other disease, and often the differentiation can be made only after all the data have been assembled. Serum perinuclear antineutrophil cytoplasmic antibodies (pANCA) are found in 60–70% of patients with ulcerative colitis but also are found in up to 40% of patients with Crohn disease. The combination of a positive pANCA and a negative anti-saccharomyces cerevisiae antibody (ASCA) has a positive predictive value for ulcerative colitis of 75%, whereas a negative pANCA and positive ASCA has a positive predictive value of 86% for Crohn disease. Thus serologic testing in patients with inflammatory bowel disease may be helpful when considered in the context of other clinical factors. About 10% of cases cannot be classified (indeterminate colitis).

► Complications

The following **extracolonic manifestations** may occur in association with ulcerative colitis. There is an inexact relationship between the severity of the colitis and these complications: (1) lesions of the skin and mucous membranes (eg, erythema nodosum, erythema multiforme, pyoderma gangrenosum, pustular dermatitis, and aphthous stomatitis); (2) uveitis; (3) bone and joint lesions (eg, arthralgia, arthritis, and ankylosing spondylitis); (4) hepatobiliary and possibly pancreatic lesions (eg, fatty infiltration, pericholangitis, cirrhosis, sclerosing cholangitis, bile duct carcinoma, gallstones, and pancreatic insufficiency); (5) anemia, usually due to iron deficiency; (6) malnutrition and growth retardation; and (7) pericarditis. Sclerosing cholangitis may require liver transplantation.

Perianal diseases may affect patients with ulcerative colitis just as they do the general population. The presence of perianal findings in a patient with ulcerative colitis, however, should prompt a thorough reassessment of the patient's presentation to exclude Crohn disease.

Table 30–13. Comparison of Various Features of Ulcerative Colitis with Those of Granulomatous Colitis.

	Ulcerative (Mucosal) Colitis	Crohn (Granulomatous) Colitis
Signs and symptoms		
Diarrhea	Marked.	Present; less severe.
Gross bleeding	Characteristic.	Infrequent.
Perianal lesions	Infrequent, mild.	Frequent, complex; may precede diagnosis of intestinal disease.
Toxic dilatation	Yes (3–10%).	Yes (2–5%).
Perforation	Free.	Localized.
Systemic manifestations (arthritis, uveitis, pyoderma, hepatitis)	Common.	Common.
X-ray studies	Confluent, diffuse. Tiny serrations, coarse mucosa, mucosal tags. Concentric involvement. Internal fistulas very rare. Colon only except in backwash ileitis; may be limited to left side.	Skip areas. Longitudinal ulcers, transverse ridges, "cobblestone" appearance. Eccentric involvement. Internal fistula common. Any portion of intestinal tract may be involved; may be limited to ileum and right colon.
Morphology		
Gross	Confluent involvement. Rectum usually involved. Mesocolon not involved; nodes enlarged. Widespread, ragged, superficial ulceration. Inflammatory polyps (pseudopolyps) common. No thickening of bowel wall.	Segmental involvement with or without skip areas. Rectum often not involved. Thickened mesocolon; pronounced lymph node enlargement. Large longitudinal ulcers or transverse fissures. Inflammatory polyps not prominent. Thickened bowel wall.
Microscopic	Inflammatory reaction usually limited to mucosa and submucosa; only in severe disease are muscle coats involved; no fibrosis. Granulomas rare.	Chronic inflammation of all layers of bowel wall; damage to muscle layers usual; submucosal fibrosis. Granulomas frequent.
Natural history	Exacerbations, remissions; may be explosive, lethal.	Indolent, recurrent.
Treatment		
Response to medical treatment	Good response in 85% of cases.	Difficult to evaluate; less well controlled over long term.
Type of surgical treatment and response	Colectomy with ileoanal anastomosis; proctocolectomy with ileostomy. No recurrence.	Segmental colectomy; total colectomy with ileorectal anastomosis; proctocolectomy if rectum severely diseased. Recurrence common.

Perforation of the colon, which occurs in about 3% of hospitalized patients, is responsible for more deaths than any other complication of ulcerative colitis. The risk of perforation is highest in the initial attack of the disease and correlates well with its extent and severity. It occurs most commonly in the sigmoid or splenic flexure and may result in a localized abscess or generalized fecal peritonitis. Any severely diseased colon may perforate, but patients with toxic dilation (megacolon) are especially vulnerable. Systemic therapy (corticosteroids and antibiotics) may mask the development of this complication.

Acute colonic dilation (toxic megacolon) occurs in approximately 3–10% of patients and in about 9% of patients coming to emergency operation. The patients are severely ill (toxic) and usually have one or more of the following contributing factors: inflammation involving the muscular coats, hypokalemia, opioid use, anticholinergic use, or barium enema examination. Toxic megacolon is diagnosed by plain abdominal x-rays or barium enemas, which show a thickened bowel wall and dilated lumen (> 6 cm in the transverse colon); often, the luminal air outlines irregular nodular pseudopolyps (Figure 30–18). Placing the patient in the knee-elbow position and use of a rectal tube are recommended medical measures to help the colon decompress. Toxic dilation also occurs in Crohn disease and in other types of colitis such as amebiasis and salmonellosis.

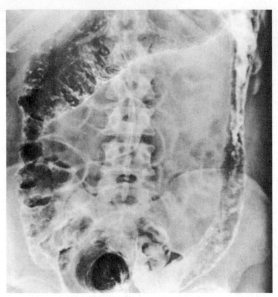

▲ **Figure 30–18.** Barium enema showing acute colonic dilation in ulcerative colitis. Note dilation of the transverse colon, the multiple irregular densities in the lumen that represent pseudopolyps, and the loss of haustral markings.

Massive hemorrhage is an uncommon but life-threatening complication.

Carcinoma of the colon or rectum begins to appear 8–10 years after onset of ulcerative colitis. The cumulative incidence increases by about 1% per year after 10 years. Factors thought to identify patients at greatest risk for cancer are the extent of colitis, the severity of disease, the duration of active disease, and the presence of primary sclerosing cholangitis. Cancers in ulcerative colitis tend to be multicentric and may be difficult to recognize grossly by endoscopy or x-ray because they are small and flat. Periodic surveillance colonoscopy with multiple random biopsies is recommended to search for epithelial dysplasia. The finding of high-grade dysplasia, a dysplasia associated lesion or mass, multifocal low-grade dysplasia, or low-grade dysplasia with a mass are indications for colectomy. In previous studies of prospective surveillance programs, the presence of dysplasia associated lesion or mass was associated with a synchronous cancer at colectomy in 43% of patients. With high-grade dysplasia, the chances of finding cancer in the colon are 30–50%, and some of the cancers are advanced. There is an intensive search for a more sensitive marker, and one or more of the molecular markers may fill the need eventually. Meanwhile, the risks and benefits of colectomy should be weighed against those of repeated colonoscopy in patients with a long history of ulcerative colitis; with the availability of ileoanal anastomosis, colectomy is more appealing to physicians and their patients than in the past.

▶ **Treatment**

A. Medical Therapy

The goals of conservative therapy are to terminate the acute attack as rapidly as possible and to maintain remission of symptoms. Management depends on the severity of the attack (classified as mild, moderate, severe, or fulminant) and the age group; children and the elderly present special problems.

1. Mild to moderate attack—Mild or insidious disease usually can be checked with outpatient management. Diet should be free of bovine milk products and any other food that exacerbates diarrhea in the individual patient. In controlled trials, sulfasalazine, 2–6 g/d orally, is effective for inducing and maintaining remission in mild to moderately active ulcerative colitis. Patients who are allergic to sulfonamide drugs can obtain similar benefit with oral mesalamine, 2–5 g/d. Other related drugs include olsalazine (1–3 g/d) and balsalazide (6.75 g/d). Drug-associated toxicity limits utility in up to 30% of patients treated with these regimens. Ulcerative proctitis and some cases of proctosigmoiditis can be treated with topical mesalamine or steroids. These agents can be delivered by suppository or foam if disease involves only 15–20 cm of distal bowel, and enemas can be used if colitis extends proximally for up to 60 cm; there are several choices of preparations. Topical mesalamine agents are superior to oral steroids or oral aminosalicylates, and the combination of oral and topical aminosalicylates improve efficacy.

Controlled trials have shown that high-dose oral corticosteroids, 100 mg/d cortisone or 40–60 mg/d prednisone, are effective for inducing remission in mild and severe ulcerative colitis. However, low-dose steroids are not effective at maintaining remission. Similar results have been obtained with rectally administered steroids for distal disease.

2. Severe attack—Severe or fulminant ulcerative colitis requires hospitalization. Nasogastric suction is required in patients with colonic dilation or those at risk of developing this complication. Otherwise, "bowel rest" has no special benefit, and when the danger of dilation has passed, polymeric total enteral nutrition is just as safe and effective as total parenteral nutrition in patients with acute, severe ulcerative colitis. Failure to improve within 7–10 days of maximal medical therapy is an indication for either colectomy or treatment with cyclosporine. Failure of medical therapy will occur in approximately 40% of patients with acute severe ulcerative colitis.

Corticosteroids are given intravenously initially as hydrocortisone (100–300 mg/d) or methylprednisolone (20–80 mg/d). Broad-spectrum antibiotics are often given to severely ill patients in an effort to prevent systemic sepsis from colonic bacterial translocation. Cyclosporine (4 mg/kg/d intravenously) is effective for severe colitis refractory to steroid therapy. Toxicity can be significant, however, and the long-term benefit of cyclosporine treatment is unknown. Hypokalemia is common and should be corrected. Caution should be exercised in administering anticholinergics and opioids because they may precipitate acute dilation of the colon.

Infliximab is a chimeric monoclonal antibody to the human tumor necrosis factor α and available in clinical practice since 1998. A highly effective agent for Crohn disease, infliximab has been used to induce (5 mg/kg, weeks 0, 2, 6) and maintain remission (q 8 week infusion) among patients with acute severe ulcerative colitis.

3. Maintenance—The maintenance regimen following induction of remission from the acute attack may include sulfasalazine, olsalazine, mesalamine, or balsalazide. Nightly mesalamine suppositories or oral mesalamine serves as maintenance therapy for patients with distal colitis. Oral mesalamine or 5-aminosalicylic acid reduces relapse rates of patients with more extensive colitis. Chronic steroid use should be avoided whenever possible because of the systemic side effects even if the drug is administered topically. Azathioprine at doses of 1.5–2.5 mg/kg/day has been shown to be effective for steroid sparing in patients with steroid-dependent ulcerative colitis. In addition, maintenance 6-mercaptopurine may enhance long-term remission. Transdermal nicotine reportedly has a therapeutic effect on ulcerative colitis, but clinicians are understandably reluctant to use this agent until more is learned about long-term safety and efficacy. There is no role for antibiotic therapy as primary treatment for ulcerative colitis.

B. Surgical Treatment

1. Indications

A. ACUTE DISEASE—Emergency operation is indicated for proved or suspected perforation of the colon. Operation on an urgent basis is required for an acute problem (toxic megacolon, hemorrhage, or refractory fulminant colitis) treated medically at first and then surgically if the response is inadequate. There are no firm guidelines for when to switch from medical to surgical therapy in these cases. If toxic megacolon does not respond to treatment, prompt operation is necessary to avoid perforation. Fulminant disease without megacolon should improve in 7–10 days or less; otherwise, operation may be advisable. Prolonged medical treatment may result in the need for a staged surgical approach, whereas earlier intervention may require only one operation.

B. CHRONIC DISEASE—Intractable disease is difficult to define. Frequent exacerbations, chronic continuous symptoms, malnutrition, weakness, inability to work, incapacity to enjoy a full social and sexual life—all are elements of intractable disease. Exacerbation of disease when corticosteroids are tapered—and thus inability to discontinue these drugs over months or even years—is a compelling indication for colectomy. Children with chronic colitis may have impaired growth and development and risk for cancer development. Prevention or treatment of carcinoma is an important indica-

tion for operation. Severe extracolonic manifestations, such as arthritis or pyoderma gangrenosum, may respond to colectomy, but other problems (eg, ankylosing spondylitis or sclerosing cholangitis) do not improve after the diseased colon is removed.

C. RISK FOR MALIGNANCY—Colectomy is also indicated for patients in whom carcinoma is suspected.

2. Surgical procedures—Total colectomy with ileoanal anastomosis (restorative proctocolectomy, ileal pouch–anal anastomosis) is the elective operation of choice in most patients. Obesity and advanced age are limiting factors. In this procedure, the entire colon and rectum are excised, and the ileum (made into a reservoir or pouch) is brought into the pelvis and anastomosed to the anal canal just above the dentate line (Figure 30–19). Rectal mucosectomy was once routine, but many surgeons now do not

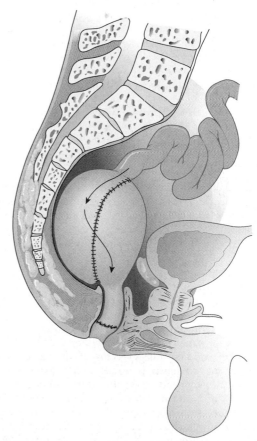

▲ **Figure 30–19.** View of the pelvis after colectomy and ileoanal anastomosis in a male. The J-pouch, shown here, is one of several types of reservoirs and is most commonly utilized. The pouch is anastomosed to the anal canal just above the dentate line.

strip the mucosa at all in patients with colitis; instead, the full thickness of rectum is excised to eliminate disease while preserving good rectal function. A temporary ileostomy to protect the ileoanal anastomosis for 2–3 months is not mandatory, but it is used if there is concern about the quality of the anastomosis or the patient's healing properties. Success is expected in 95% of patients. In a series of 1310 patients undergoing ileal pouch–anal anastomosis at the Mayo Clinic before 1994, overall operative mortality was 0.2%, and the postoperative pelvic sepsis rate was 3% in the most recent 4 years. Pouch survival was 98% at 1 year and 91% at 10 years. Pouchitis (inflammation of the reservoir) occurs in up to 40% of patients and the risk increases with time; it usually responds to antibiotics such as metronidazole or ciprofloxacin.

Proctocolectomy with permanent conventional ileostomy is chosen in patients who may not be candidates for the ileoanal procedure. In an emergency operation, the rectum is preserved to minimize operative complications in an ill patient and to make it possible to do an ileoanal procedure later. This staged operation therefore consists of total abdominal colectomy (subtotal colectomy) and ileostomy with a distal mucous fistula or Hartmann procedure. Ileorectal anastomosis (ileoproctostomy, ileorectostomy) and continent ileostomies are seldom used for ulcerative colitis today.

The procedures for ulcerative colitis are now increasingly performed laparoscopically with equivalent functional results and improved short-term outcomes.

▶ Prognosis

The mortality rate of ulcerative colitis has dropped sharply in the past 2 decades. First attacks are seldom fatal when treated by specialists. In one large series, emergency colectomy was required in 25% of patients with severe first attacks; 60% responded rapidly to medical therapy; and 15% improved slowly on medications alone. Overall, the colitis-related mortality rate during the year after onset is about 1%. Emergency colectomy has a mortality rate of 6%; most of these deaths are due to perforation, a complication that has a fatal outcome in 40% of cases.

The long-term prognosis of ulcerative proctitis is good; about 10% of patients will develop colonic disease by 10 years, and the mortality rate is very low. If colitis involves the left colon, the prognosis is worse, and in patients with pancolitis, the likelihood of operation during the first year is about 25% and the mortality rate is 5% over 10 years. Colorectal cancer in ulcerative colitis is more often diagnosed at an advanced stage than is sporadic cancer, but the stage-for-stage prognosis is the same. Screening with colonoscopy and biopsies seems to have reduced the cancer mortality rate, but there are still too many patients who escape detection until the malignancy has progressed to incurability. The problem is lack of a sensitive marker that predicts cancer before it develops.

The operative mortality rate is less than 1% for elective colectomy. Quality of life after restorative proctocolectomy with an ileal pouch is excellent. Most patients who undergo the procedure are pleased with the outcome compared with their preoperative symptoms and treatment. In an estimated 90% of survivors, colectomy with ileostomy is consistent with normal life, but a few patients experience problems such as small bowel obstruction and ileostomy dysfunction. Altered sexual function after proctectomy occurs in about 12% of men overall, limited mostly to those over age 50. True impotence is found in 3% of men. Sexual dysfunction is common in the first few months in women.

American Gastroenterological Association Institute Medical position statement on corticosteroids, immunomodulators, and infliximab in inflammatory bowel disease. Gastroenterology 2006;130:935.

Andersson RE et al: Appendectomy and protection against ulcerative colitis. N Engl J Med 2001;344:808.

Bernstein CN et al: Cancer risk in patients with inflammatory bowel disease: a population-based study. Cancer 2001;91:854.

Bernstein CN et al: The prevalence of extraintestinal diseases in inflammatory bowel disease: a population-based study. Am J Gastroenterol 2001;96:1116.

Cohen JL et al: Practice parameters for the surgical treatment of ulcerative colitis. Standards Committee of the American Society of Colon and Rectal Surgeons. Dis Colon Rectum 2005;48:1997

D'Haens G et al: Intravenous cyclosporine versus intravenous corticosteroids as single therapy for severe attacks of ulcerative colitis. Gastroenterology 2001;120:1323.

Eaden JA, Abrams KR, Mayberry JF: The risk of colorectal cancer in ulcerative colitis: a meta-analysis. Gut 2001;48:526.

Farmer M et al: Association of susceptibility locus for inflammatory bowel disease on chromosome 16 with both ulcerative colitis and Crohn's disease. Dig Dis Sci 2001;46:632.

Goudet P et al: Characteristics and evolution of extraintestinal manifestations associated with ulcerative colitis after proctocolectomy. Dig Surg 2001;18:51.

Hahnloser D et al: Results at up to 20 years after ileal pouch-anal anastomosis for chronic ulcerative colitis. Br J Surg 2007; 94:333.

Kornbluth A, Sachar DB: Ulcerative colitis practice guidelines in adults (update). American College of Gastroenterology, Practice Parameters Committee. Am J Gastroenterol 2004;99:1371

Lawrance IC, Fiocchi C, Chakravarti S: Ulcerative colitis and Crohn's disease: distinctive gene expression profiles and novel susceptibility candidate genes. Hum Mol Genet 2001;10:445.

Sandborn WJ et al: Evaluation of serologic disease markers in a population-based cohort of patients with inflammatory bowel disease. Inflamm Bowel Dis 2001;7:192.

Shelton AA et al: Retrospective review of colorectal cancer in ulcerative colitis at a tertiary center. Arch Surg 1996;131:806.

Thoeni RF, Cello JP. CT imaging of colitis. Radiology 2006; 240:623.

Thomas GA et al: Transdermal nicotine as maintenance therapy for ulcerative colitis. N Engl J Med 1995;332:988.

The Wellcome Trust Case Control Consortium. Genome-wide association study of 14,000 cases of seven common diseases and 3,000 shared controls. Nature 2007;447:661.

Winawer S et al: Colorectal cancer screening and surveillance: clinical guidelines and rational: update based on new evidence. Gastroenterology 2003;124:544.

2. Crohn Colitis (Granulomatous Colitis)

The general features of Crohn disease (regional enteritis, granulomatous colitis, transmural colitis) are described in Chapter 29. Approximately 40% of patients with Crohn disease have both small and large bowel involvement; 30% have disease limited to the small bowel, 25% have colonic disease alone; and another 8% have anorectal involvement only. Diarrhea, cramping abdominal pain, constitutional effects, and extraintestinal manifestations are approximately the same in colonic and enteric disease. Internal fistulas and abscesses and intestinal obstruction are usually complications of small bowel disease. Anorectal complications (anal fistula, fissure, abscess, and rectal stricture) and hemorrhage are more common when the large bowel is affected, and toxic dilation is limited to patients with inflammation of the colon.

Typical anal lesions of Crohn disease are large, undermined, indolent ulcers. The perianal skin has a violaceous hue, and if fistulas are present, they tend to be multiple and complex. Proctosigmoidoscopy discloses a normal rectum in 50% of patients with Crohn colitis. Diseased mucosa is patchily involved, with irregular ulcerations separated by edematous or even normal-appearing mucosa. Biopsy may confirm the diagnosis. Radiographic features include sparing of the rectum, right colonic and ileal involvement, skip areas, transverse fissures, longitudinal ulcers, strictures, and fistulas. Features differentiating Crohn disease from ulcerative colitis are summarized in Table 30–13. Ischemic colitis is another disease that may be confused with Crohn colitis, and the differential diagnosis is discussed below. *Chlamydia trachomatis* infection is diagnosed by culture of the organism. Malacoplakia is a rare chronic granulomatous disease that can cause colonic strictures, and Behçet disease is another rare condition that can mimic inflammatory bowel disease. Tuberculosis and amebiasis must be considered also.

Frank blood in the stools is observed in about one third of patients with granulomatous colitis, but massive hemorrhage is unusual. Acute colonic dilation (toxic megacolon) occurs in 5%; it responds to nonoperative treatment more often than it does in ulcerative colitis.

Actuarial methods suggest that the risk of colonic cancer in granulomatous colitis patients is 4 to 20 times that of the general population, and it appears that segments of intestine excluded from the fecal stream (eg, an isolated rectal stump or bypassed ileum) are especially vulnerable. Carcinoma can also arise in anorectal or rectovaginal fistulas. The small bowel is at risk for development of cancer in patients with regional enteritis with or without colitis. Epithelial dysplasia is associated with cancer in Crohn disease as well as in ulcerative colitis, but this indicator is not helpful for the areas at greatest risk (eg, bypassed segments of small bowel or colon) because they may not be able to be examined endoscopically. Surveillance colonoscopy should be routinely performed in patients with longstanding Crohn disease and resection performed for high-grade dysplasia or dysplasia associated lesion or mass lesions. Cancer should always be ruled out in colonic strictures.

Medical management of Crohn disease of the small bowel is described in Chapter 29. Steroids are effective for acute attacks, but they are not advisable for maintenance therapy because of limited benefit and frequent complications. Oral 5-aminosalicylates (sulfasalazine, 4 g/d; or mesalamine, 2–5 g/d) are effective treatment for Crohn colitis. Topical 5-aminosalicylates are beneficial for disease of the rectum and sigmoid. These agents are steroid sparing (ie, they allow the dosage of steroids to be reduced). Metronidazole, 10–20 mg/kg/d orally in three to five doses, is used for treatment of anal complications of Crohn disease. Abscesses and fistulas improve with less pain and drainage, but full permanent healing is unusual, and the disease worsens when the drug is discontinued. Immunosuppressants (azathioprine, mercaptopurine) are steroid-sparing drugs that seem to control Crohn colitis well enough that surgery is delayed or avoided. There are mixed reports of effectiveness of cyclosporine in refractory Crohn disease. Infliximab (5–10 mg/kg) is effective for inflammatory Crohn disease and is also specifically indicated for fistulizing disease. Patients who respond to infliximab induction should receive maintenance therapy.

Indications for surgical treatment of Crohn disease include failure of medical therapy, perforation, obstruction, severe inflammation with impending perforation, refractory hemorrhage, neoplasia, or growth retardation. Segmental colectomy with primary anastomosis is useful for limited colonic disease. Total colectomy with ileorectal anastomosis may be performed for pancolitis with rectal sparing. Proctocolectomy with ileostomy is needed if rectal disease is severe and the colon needs resection also. Diverting ileostomy or colostomy is only temporarily helpful. Perianal complications can be treated directly (eg, by fistulotomy) in carefully selected patients.

There is a high rate of recurrence at intestinal anastomoses (50–75% at 15 years). Recurrence is less common following proctocolectomy and ileostomy (about 15% at 15 years, but there is a wide disparity (3–46%) among different reports on this controversial topic). Cigarette smoking is an independent risk factor for recurrence of Crohn disease after resection.

Surgical procedures—like medical therapy—should be regarded as palliative, not curative, in patients with Crohn disease. Although recurrence rates are high and chronic disease is common, a productive life is usually possible with the aid of combined medical and surgical management. The mortality rate is about 15% over 30 years. Urolithiasis is a common sequela of resection for Crohn disease.

Hanauer SB, Sandborn W: Management of Crohn's disease in adults. Am J Gastroenterol 2001;96:635.

Lichtenstein GR et al: American Gastroenterological Association Institute medical position statement on corticosteroids, immunomodulators, and infliximab in inflammatory bowel disease. Gastroenterology 2006;130:935.

Nwokolo CU et al: Surgical resections in parous patients with distal ileal and colonic Crohn's disease. Gut 1994;35:220.

Sandborn WJ et al: AGA technical review on perianal Crohn's disease. Gastroenterology 2003;125:1508.

Strong SA et al: Practice parameters for the surgical management of Crohn's disease. Dis Colon Rectum 2007;50:1735.

Thirlby RC, Sobrino MA, Randall JB: The long-term benefit of surgery on health-related quality of life in patients with inflammatory bowel disease. Arch Surg 2001;136:521.

3. Antibiotic-Associated Colitis

A spectrum of adverse colonic responses may develop in hospitalized patients during or after antibiotic therapy. There may be diarrhea without gross mucosal abnormality (antibiotic-associated diarrhea), gross inflammation of the mucosa, or whitish-green or yellow plaques on the inflamed mucosa (pseudomembranous colitis). Patients may progress from mild to more severe disease. The differential diagnosis among these variations is based on endoscopic findings and the clinical picture.

Clostridium difficile is a resident of the gut in 3% of people in the general population and in up to 25% of patients admitted to hospital. It is the major known cause of nosocomial antibiotic-associated diarrhea and colitis. Certain antibiotics allow the organism to proliferate, and it is then transmitted among patients and hospital personnel. Epidemics of *C difficile* infection have been noted on surgical wards, and increasingly virulent and resistant strains have been recently isolated. The organism can be transmitted by people caring for the patient, and gloving or hand-washing is essential. Infection with *C difficile* can be very severe in patients with AIDS.

C difficile may colonize the upper gastrointestinal tract as well as the colon, but the symptomatic infection appears at present to be colonic alone. The organism elaborates at least four toxins, including toxin A (an enterotoxin) and toxin B (a cytotoxin). Together these substances—and perhaps others—produce the symptoms and signs. Clindamycin causes watery diarrhea in 15–30% of patients and true pseudomembranous colitis in 1–10%, but all antibiotics that alter the gut flora, including metronidazole, may incite pathologic infections with *C difficile*. Approximately 15–25% of antibiotic-associated diarrhea result from *C difficile* infection. Colitis may develop as early as 2 days after beginning antibiotics or as late as many weeks after they are discontinued.

Symptoms and signs include diarrhea, which is usually watery, occasionally bloody, and has a characteristic foul odor; abdominal cramps; vomiting; fever; and leukocytosis. Sigmoidoscopy in pseudomembranous colitis shows elevated plaques or a confluent pseudomembrane, and the mucosa is erythematous and edematous. Biopsies reveal acute inflammation; the pseudomembrane is made up of leukocytes, necrotic epithelial cells, and fibrin. The rectum is spared in about one fourth of cases, and colonoscopy may be necessary to detect the presence of pseudomembranous colitis. Demonstration of *C difficile* cytotoxin in the stool is sensitive and specific. The cell cytotoxicity test is the best available test and has been reported to have a sensitivity and specificity of up to 98% and 99%, respectively. However, it is a technically demanding test and requires 24–48 hours to perform. The enzyme-linked immunoassay for toxins A and B are popular because of their ease of performance but limited because of their lack of sensitivity: only 40–75% compared with the cell cytotoxicity assay. Stool culture is less efficient, since some strains of *C difficile* are nontoxicogenic, but it has the advantage of identifying the specific strains for epidemiologic purposes, especially during an outbreak. In the appropriate clinical setting, the demonstration of leukocytes in the stool is sufficient evidence for initiating treatment for *C difficile*. Radiographic studies may reveal colonic wall thickening due to submucosal edema (so called "accordion sign" or "target sign").

C difficile infection may also cause a paralytic ileus and therefore present without diarrhea. Other associated symptoms and signs, such as pain and leukocytosis, may be present and, in the appropriate setting following recent antibiotic exposure, should raise concern for *C difficile* infection.

Management consists first of discontinuing the inciting antibiotic agent. In most patients, the colitis resolves in 1–2 weeks after the offending agent is withdrawn, but severe symptoms or persistent diarrhea calls for additional treatment. Vancomycin (125–500 mg orally four times daily for 7–10 days) is expensive but effective—though the relapse rate is 15–20% after vancomycin is discontinued. Vancomycin may also be effective as a retention enema. Metronidazole, 1.5–2 g/d orally for 7–14 days, is also effective and much less expensive. Other agents which have been tested and appear to be also equally effective at achieving symptomatic cure include bacitracin, rifaximin, nitazoxanide, and fusidic acid. Teicoplanin is the most effective agent for both symptomatic and bacteriocidal cure. Paradoxically, however, the antibiotics used for treatment can also cause antibiotic-associated colitis. Antidiarrheal drugs may prolong symptoms and should be avoided. Oral administration of *Saccharomyces boulardii*, a nonpathogenic yeast, has been successful in treatment of recurrent *C difficile* colitis in an experimental setting. In such refractory cases, cholestyramine may be an effective adjunct by binding the toxin produced by *C difficile* bacteria.

The outcome of pseudomembranous colitis and the other forms of antibiotic-associated colonic disease is usually excellent if the disease is recognized and treated. Untreated pseudomembranous colitis, however, may lead to severe dehydration and electrolyte imbalance, toxic megacolon, or colonic perforation with a high risk for mortality. Operation is required for perforation or toxic dilation.

Bartlett JG, Gerding DN: Clinical recognition and diagnosis of *Clostridium difficile* infection. Clin Infect Dis 2008;46(Suppl 1):S12.

Dallal RM et al: Fulminant *Clostridium difficile*: an underappreciated and increasing cause of death and complications. Ann Surg 2002;235:363.

Hall JF, Berger D: Outcome of colectomy for *Clostridium difficile* colitis: a plea for early surgical management. Am J Surg 2008; 196:384.

Kelly CP, Pothoulakis C, LaMont JT: *Clostridium difficile* colitis. N Engl J Med 1994;330:257.

Medich DS et al: Laparotomy for fulminant pseudomembranous colitis. Arch Surg 1992;127:847.

Nelson R: Antibiotic treatment for *Clostridium difficile*–associated diarrhea in adults. Cochrane Database Syst Rev 2007;3:CD004610.

Synnott K et al: Timing of surgery for fulminating pseudomembranous colitis. Br J Surg 1998;85:229.

Zerey M et al: The burden of *Clostridium difficile* in surgical patients in the United States. Surg Infect (Larchmt) 2007;8:557.

4. Ischemic Colitis

Ischemic colitis is caused by mesenteric vascular occlusion or nonocclusive mechanisms. A common precipitating event is abdominal aortic reconstruction with interruption of a vital blood supply such as the inferior mesenteric artery. An entity that resembles ischemic colitis sometimes develops proximal to obstructing colonic carcinoma. Isolated ischemia of the right colon is seen in patients with chronic heart disease, especially aortic stenosis. Ischemic colitis most often afflicts the elderly (average age, 60 years), but it also occurs in younger adults in association with diabetes mellitus, systemic lupus erythematosus, or sickle cell crisis. Pancreatitis can occlude mesocolic vessels.

The most common location is the sigmoid colon (40%) followed by the transverse colon (17%), splenic flexure (11%), ascending colon (12%), and the rectum (6%). Ischemic colitis is categorized as reversible or irreversible. Reversible ischemia heals with nonoperative treatment, sometimes with stricture formation. Over half of the patients have a reversible injury. The severe form is fulminant from onset or may pursue an indolent course without resolution for weeks. Both of the severe forms require operation.

Patients with ischemic colitis have an abrupt onset of abdominal pain, diarrhea (commonly bloody), and systemic symptoms. The abdomen may be tender diffusely, in a localized area (eg, left lower quadrant), or not at all. Blood is seen coming from above at endoscopy which, when performed carefully, is the diagnostic modality of choice; the mucosa of the involved segment is edematous, hemorrhagic, friable, and sometimes ulcerated. A grayish membrane may be present, resembling pseudomembranous colitis, but the presence of hyalinized, hemorrhagic lamina on biopsy will differentiate colonic ischemia from *C difficile* colitis. Serum amylase or alkaline phosphatase is elevated in some cases. Serum acidosis may be present. Plain abdominal x-rays are nonspecific. Barium enema x-rays show "thumbprints" or pseudotumors but is primarily of historical importance. CT scan shows a thickened colonic wall or pneumatosis and helps to exclude other conditions. Mesenteric arteriography may show major arterial occlusion if associated with an acute vascular event but more typically shows no abnormalities.

Differentiating ischemic colitis from carcinoma, ulcerative colitis, and diverticulitis should not be difficult, but Crohn disease presents a greater diagnostic problem. Rectal bleeding—especially gross hemorrhage—is less common in Crohn disease, and the rapid onset of ischemic colitis is also different from Crohn disease. Radiographic findings and, in some cases, the colonoscopic appearance may be helpful, but the natural history of the acute attack is often the only way to make the distinction. Acute mesenteric ischemia may be difficult to exclude (see Chapter 29), but the more benign presentations of reversible ischemic colonic injury are not seen with ischemia of the small intestine. *C difficile* toxin is present in stool in pseudomembranous colitis.

Therapy for reversible ischemic colitis consists of intravenous fluids, antibiotics, and observation to be certain the problem is in fact reversible. The most common cause is hypotension from underlying sepsis or cardiogenic causes. Strenuous physical activity has also been implicated with endurance activities such as running or cycling. Irreversible disease, whether fulminant from the beginning, becoming more severe over several days, or just failing to resolve after treatment, should be treated by operation. The diseased colon is resected; anastomosis is usually deferred because of the risk for leak, and a second-look laparotomy is commonly performed 12–24 hours later. Because patients with severe ischemia often have multiple other medical problems, the overall mortality rate is 50%.

Balthazar EJ, Yen BC, Gordon RB: Ischemic colitis: CT evaluation of 54 cases. Radiology 1999;211:381.

Houe T et al: Can colonoscopy diagnose transmural ischaemic colitis after abdominal aortic surgery? An evidence-based approach. Eur J Vasc Endovasc Surg 2000;19:304.

Hwang RF, Schwartz RW: Ischemic colitis: a brief review. Curr Surg 2001;58:192.

Hyun H, Pai E, Blend MJ: Ischemic colitis: Tc-99m HMPAO leukocyte scintigraphy and correlative imaging. Clin Nucl Med 1998;23:165.

Valentine RJ et al: Gastrointestinal complications after aortic surgery. J Vasc Surg 1998;28:404.

5. Neutropenic Colitis

Neutropenic colitis (neutropenic enterocolitis, neutropenic typhlitis, ileocecal syndrome, necrotizing enteropathy, agranulocytic colitis) occurs as colonic necrosis in neutropenic patients. Although the cecum and right colon are most often affected, all parts of the small or large bowel can be involved. Acute leukemia, aplastic anemia, and cyclic neutropenia are the most common underlying diseases in which this lesion occurs. However it may occur in any patient with severe neutropenia from causes such as chemotherapy for malignancies other than leukemia. Colonic perforation during treatment with IL-2 is probably related. The pathogenesis is not well understood, but responsible factors probably include mucosal ischemia, necrosis of intramural leukemic infiltrates, shock, hemorrhage into the bowel wall, chemotherapy, and corticosteroid therapy. *Clostridium septicum* has been implicated in some cases. The mucosa ulcerates, permitting bacterial invasion into the bowel wall, thrombosis of intramural vessels, necrosis, and perforation.

Approximately 25% of neutropenic cancer patients with abdominal pain requiring surgical consultation will have neutropenic colitis. Fever, watery or bloody diarrhea, abdominal discomfort and distention, and nausea are noted first. Pain and tenderness may then become localized to the right lower quadrant, and systemic toxicity increases. Careful examination and x-ray studies are required. Nasogastric suction, parenteral nutrition, and antibiotic therapy are instituted. Operation (resection of the involved segment of colon) is performed for persistent unresponsive sepsis, perforation, obstruction, severe bleeding, or abscess formation but is associated with a high mortality. Neutropenic colitis can recur after medical therapy.

Badgwell BD et al: Challenges in surgical management of abdominal pain in the neutropenic cancer patient. Ann Surg 2008;248:104.

Gorbach SL: Neutropenic enterocolitis. Clin Infect Dis 1998; 27:700.

Sayfan J et al: Acute abdomen caused by neutropenic enterocolitis: surgeon's dilemma. Eur J Surg 1999;165:502.

Song HK et al: Changing presentation and management of neutropenic enterocolitis. Arch Surg 1998;133:979.

INTESTINAL STOMAS (ILEOSTOMY & COLOSTOMY)

An intestinal stoma is an opening of the bowel onto the surface of the abdomen. It may be temporary or permanent. Esophagostomy, gastrostomy, jejunostomy, and cecostomy are usually temporary, but ileostomy, colostomy, and some urinary tract stomas are often permanent. Although "stoma" is the preferred medical term, "ostomy" is used by lay organizations devoted to the rehabilitation of these patients.

Few surgical alterations of anatomy are surrounded by as much misunderstanding as intestinal stomas, and few pronouncements by surgeons are as horrifying to patients as the indication that a stoma will be necessary. For these and other reasons, a paramedical profession, **enterostomy therapy,** has emerged. The enterostomal therapist (ET) is usually a registered nurse who has taken specialized training and is certified in the field. The enterostomal therapist provides the following services: (1) preoperative education and counseling of patient and family; (2) immediate postoperative care of the stoma; (3) training in the use of equipment and supervision of self-care; (4) fitting of a permanent appliance; (5) advice on day-to-day living with a stoma; (6) management of skin problems and odor control; (7) recognition of surgical stoma problems; (8) long-term emotional, moral, and physical support; and (9) information about the United Ostomy Association, an organization with chapters in many localities.

ILEOSTOMY

Permanent ileostomy is sometimes performed after proctocolectomy for ulcerative colitis; patients with Crohn disease, familial polyposis, and other conditions may also require ileostomy. A temporary (loop) ileostomy often is used to divert the fecal stream for 3 months when ileoanal or coloanal anastomosis is performed. An ileostomy discharges small quantities of liquid material continuously; it does not require irrigation; and an appliance must be worn at all times.

The optimal position of the ileostomy is in the right lower quadrant (Figure 30–20). The ileum is brought through the rectus abdominis muscle and everted upon itself, and the mucosa is sutured to the skin (surgically matured). An appliance is placed immediately; it consists of a plastic bag attached to a square sheet of protective material containing a central opening for the stoma. A reusable appliance can be fitted after a few weeks, but modern disposable appliances are so satisfactory that most patients never do change to the other type. Appliances lie flat against the abdomen, adhere firmly to the skin, are inconspicuous and odor-proof, and in most cases need to be changed only every 3–5 days. They are drained at intervals during the day through an opening in the bottom of the pouch.

A **continent ileostomy** (reservoir ileostomy; Kock pouch) is designed to avoid the continual discharge of ileal effluent that necessitates construction of a protruding stoma and the wearing of an appliance at all times. A reservoir is constructed out of the distal ileum, and the outlet from the reservoir is arranged as a valve so that fluid cannot escape onto the abdominal wall. The reservoir is emptied several times a day by inserting a catheter into the stoma. However, virtually all patients will experience nipple failure, and the ileal pouch anal anastomosis has replaced this procedure for most indications.

Physiologic changes after ileostomy are due to the loss of the water-absorbing and salt-absorbing capacity of the colon. If the small bowel is free of disease and extensive resection has not been done, an ileostomy puts out 1–2 L of fluid per day initially (Table 30–1). The volume of effluent diminishes to between 500 and 800 mL/d after a month or two. This loss of fluid is obligatory and is not reduced by manipulations of diet. Obligatory sodium losses are about 50 meq/d greater than in patients with an intact colon, and potassium losses are also increased. Healthy ileostomates (patients with ileostomies) have low total exchangeable sodium and potassium but normal serum electrolyte concentrations. The depletion, therefore, is primarily intracellular. The ileostomy patient is susceptible to acute or subacute salt and water depletion manifested by fatigue, anorexia, irritability, headache, drowsiness, muscle cramps, and thirst. Gastroenteritis or diarrhea from any cause and exposure to hot weather or vigorous exercise are situations that require caution; salt and water intake must be increased in these circumstances. Ileostomy patients must never be in a position where salt and water are unavailable (eg, on long hikes in the desert). Low-salt diets and diuretics may also induce salt depletion or dehydration. Patients should be counseled

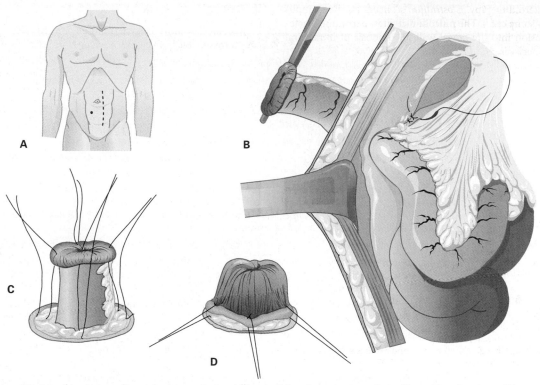

▲ **Figure 30–20.** Ileostomy after colectomy. **A:** A midline incision for colectomy is indicated by the dotted line and the site of the ileostomy by the black dot. **B:** The ileum has been brought through the abdominal wall. **C and D:** The ileostomy stoma has been everted and its margins sutured to the edges of the wound.

to salt food liberally, but salt tablets will not be required in usual circumstances. Patients with unusually high ileostomy outputs may need supplemental potassium in the form of bananas or orange juice. Water intake in response to thirst may not be adequate to maintain hydration, and patients should consume enough water to keep the urine pale or to maintain a urine output of at least 1 L/d.

Patients must be informed about these physiologic alterations and measures to compensate for them. Otherwise, instructions are simple, and ileostomy patients should live normally. A constipating, bland diet should be advised initially (eg, breads, cereals, rice, diary, peanut butter, bananas). Certain foods (eg, fish, eggs, broccoli) may cause excessive odor or gas. Oral fiber supplementation and antimotility agents such as loperamide or diphenoxylate can be sequentially added to slow down ileostomy output and prevent dehydration. Ordinary physical activity, employment, and social activities are encouraged. Bathing, swimming, sexual intercourse, and pregnancy and delivery are unrestricted.

Complications (Table 30–14) are reported in about 40% of patients with conventional ileostomy; about 15% require operative correction, usually minor. In long-term follow-up of ileostomy patients, most return to their previous occupation and consider their health to be good to excellent.

Sexual consequences of proctocolectomy should be discussed before and after operation. Some degree of sexual impairment occurs in 10–20% of men after removal of the rectum for inflammatory bowel disease. Up to three fourths of women report dyspareunia or reduced orgasmic sensation in the first few months after proctectomy and ileostomy, but only 12% experience long-term sexual dysfunction. Infertility is more frequent among women after excision of the rectum, and cesarean delivery is necessary more often; both problems are related to pelvic fibrosis and not the ileostomy.

COLOSTOMY

Colostomies are made for the following purposes: (1) to decompress an obstructed colon; (2) to divert the fecal stream in preparation for resection of an inflammatory, obstructive, or perforated lesion or following traumatic injury; (3) to serve as the point of evacuation of stool when the distal colon or rectum is removed; and (4) to protect a distal anastomosis following resection. The colostomy may be temporary, in which event it is subsequently closed; or it may be permanent. Colostomies can be constructed by making an opening in a loop of colon (**loop colostomy**) or by dividing the colon and bringing out one end (**end [terminal] colostomy**).

Table 30–14. Ileostomy Complications.

Complication	Causes and Comment
Intestinal obstruction	May be due to adhesive bands, volvulus, or paraileostomy herniation of bowel.
Stenosis	Circumferential scar formation at the skin or subcutaneous level is usually at fault. Stenosis may cause profuse watery discharge from the ileostomy. Treatment requires a minor local procedure to release the scar.
Retraction	The stoma should protrude 2–3 cm above the skin level to avoid leakage beneath the ileostomy pouch. A flush or retracted stoma functions poorly and should be revised.
Prolapse	Uncommon if the mesentery has been sutured to the parietal peritoneum.
Paraileostomy abscess and fistula	Perforation of the ileum by sutures, pressure necrosis from an ill-fitted appliance, or recurrent disease may cause abscess and fistula.
Skin irritation	The single-most common complication of ileostomy, due to leakage of ileal effluent onto the peristomal skin. Usually minor but can be severe if neglected. Treatment is directed toward the cause of leakage, usually an ill-fitted pouch. Protection of the skin by a barrier material (eg, karaya [*Sterculia*] gum) or a variety of synthetic products will resolve the problem. Enterostomy therapists manage these problems expertly.
Offensive odors	Odor-proof appliances, commercial deodorants placed in the appliance, and attention to diet usually control the problem.
Diarrhea	Excessive output should be reported to the physician promptly, and supplemental water, salt, and potassium should be given. Codeine, diphenoxylate with atropine, or loperamide may slow the output. Recurrent intestinal disease, bowel obstruction, or ileostomy stenosis should be looked for.
Urinary tract calculi	Uric acid and calcium stones occur in about 5–10% of patients after ileostomy and are probably the result of chronic dehydration due to inadequate fluid intake. Ileostomy is associated with lower urine pH and volume and higher urine concentration of calcium, oxalate, and uric acid than in patients with intact gastrointestinal tracts.
Gallstones	Cholesterol gallstones are three times more common in ileostomy patients than in the general population. Altered bile acid absorption preoperatively may be responsible.
Ileitis	Patients who develop inflammation of the ileum just proximal to the ileostomy usually have recurrence of their original inflammatory bowel disease. Stenosis of the stoma is another cause.
Varices	Varices develop around the stoma in patients with portal hypertension. Bleeding can be troublesome.

The most common permanent colostomy is a **sigmoid colostomy** made at the time of abdominoperineal resection for cancer of the rectum (Figure 30–21). Such a colostomy is compatible with a normal life except for the route of fecal evacuation. A sigmoid colostomy expels stool approximately once a day, but the frequency varies among individuals just as bowel habits vary in the general population. An appliance is not required, though many patients find that wearing a light pouch is reassuring. Some patients achieve a regular pattern of evacuation on their own; others require irrigation daily or every other day. Irrigation is performed by inserting a catheter into the stoma and instilling water, 500 mL at a time, by gravity flow from a reservoir held at shoulder height. A plastic olive-shaped tip on the catheter fits snugly into the stoma and greatly reduces the risk of perforation. Diet is individualized; generally, patients are able to eat the same foods they enjoyed preoperatively. Fresh fruits, fruit juices, and other foods may cause diarrhea. A properly functioning colostomy need not be dilated.

Transverse colostomy should not be constructed as a permanent stoma if it can be avoided. Unlike sigmoid colostomy, transverse colostomy is "wet" (ie, it discharges semiliquid waste frequently) and usually requires an appliance. These stomas are bulky, foul-smelling, and extremely difficult to manage. They are prone to leak under the appliance, and prolapse is common. The needs of most patients who require a permanent stoma are better served by an ileostomy than by a transverse colostomy.

The overall complication rate of colostomies is higher than 20%, and 15% of complications require operative correction. Chronic paracolostomy hernia is a frequent complication; it develops because the abdominal wall aperture enlarges with time, allowing colon, omentum, or small bowel to herniate adjacent to the colostomy. Hernia—and prolapse—are more apt to occur in obese patients. Stenosis may require revision. Necrosis and retraction are due to technical errors in constructing the stoma. Paracolostomy abscess occurs occasionally regardless of precautions. Perforation is avoided by the plastic catheter tip and by keeping the irrigation reservoir at no greater than shoulder height. Less serious complications include diarrhea, fecal impaction, and skin irritation.

Leong APK, Londono-Schimmer EE, Phillips RKS: Life-table analysis of stomal complications following ileostomy. Br J Surg 1994;81:727.

Lyons AS: Ileostomy and colostomy support groups. Mt Sinai J Med 2001;68:110.

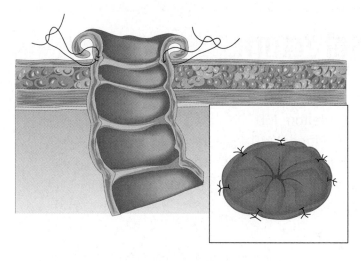

▲ **Figure 30–21.** End colostomy. The margins of the stoma are fixed to the skin with sutures.

Oliveira L et al: Laparoscopic creation of stomas. Surg Endosc 1997;11:19.

Rubin MS, Schoetz DJ Jr, Matthews JB: Parastomal hernia: is stoma relocation superior to fascial repair? Arch Surg 1994; 129:413.

Rullier E et al: Loop ileostomy versus loop colostomy for defunctioning low anastomoses during rectal cancer Surgery. World J Surg 2001;25:274.

Sakai Y et al: Temporary transverse colostomy vs loop ileostomy in diversion: a case- matched study. Arch Surg 2001;136:338.

▼ PREOPERATIVE PREPARATION OF THE COLON

Complications of colonic surgery, such as wound infection and anastomotic dehiscence, are partially related to the high bacterial content of the large bowel. It has been widely accepted that elimination of the fecal mass and reduction of the numbers of bacteria prior to operation is desirable, and measures taken to achieve this purpose are known as the "bowel prep." Patients in good health can have preparation as an outpatient on the day before surgery and undergo operation on the day of admission. However, more recent evidence suggests that the use of bowel preparation prior to colonic surgery results in an increased risk for infectious complications and potentially anastomotic leaks, calling into question the convention of routine preparation.

Mechanical cleansing is typically achieved with whole-gut lavage, which involves ingestion (or instillation through a nasogastric tube) of large quantities of unabsorbed fluid, such as a solution containing polyethylene glycol (PEG), to minimize the risk of fluid overload and excessive dehydration. Oral sodium phosphate compares favorably with PEG solutions. It requires only a small volume for ingestion but causes an osmotic diarrhea; therefore dehydration and electrolyte abnormalities are a concern, and patients need to be admonished to generously hydrate during the preparation.

Gut sterilization with oral antibiotics (neomycin and erythromycin base) remains controversial despite many years of study but has largely fallen out of favor. Oral antibiotics are associated with significant patient discomfort, poor compliance, and no appreciable reduction in infectious complications.

Only the use of parenteral antibiotic prophylaxis given just prior to incision has been clearly associated with improved wound infection rates and is currently mandated. Until a multicenter randomized trial of mechanical preparation can be performed, the debate is likely to continue.

Bleday R et al: Quantitative cultures of the mucosal-associated bacteria in the mechanically prepared colon and rectum. Dis Colon Rectum 1993;36:844.

Burke P et al: Requirement for bowel preparation in colorectal surgery. Br J Surg 1994;81:907.

Cohen SM et al: Prospective, randomized, endoscopic-blinded trial comparing precolonoscopy bowel cleansing methods. Dis Colon Rectum 1994;37:689.

Guenaga KF, Matos D, Castro AA, et al: Mechanical bowel preparation for elective colorectal surgery. Cochrane Database Syst Rev 2005;1:CD001544.

Henderson JM et al: Single-day, divided-dose oral sodium phosphate laxative versus intestinal lavage as preparation for colonoscopy: efficacy and patient tolerance. Gastrointest Endosc 1995;42:238.

Miettinen RP et al: Bowel preparation with oral polyethylene glycol electrolyte solution vs. no preparation in elective open colorectal surgery: prospective, randomized study. Dis Colon Rectum 2000;43:669.

Platell C, Hall J: What is the role of mechanical bowel preparation in patients undergoing colorectal surgery? Dis Colon Rectum 1998;41:875.

Santos JC Jr et al: Prospective randomized trial of mechanical bowel preparation in patients undergoing elective colorectal surgery. Br J Surg 1994;81:1673.

Wolters U et al: Prospective randomized study of preoperative bowel cleansing for patients undergoing colorectal surgery. Br J Surg 1994;81:598.

Zamora O, Pikarsky AJ, Wexner SD: Bowel preparation for colorectal surgery. Dis Colon Rectum 2001;44:1537.

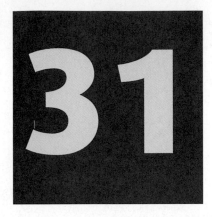

Anorectum

Mark L. Welton, MD
Carlos E. Pineda, MD
George J. Chang, MD, MS
Andrew A. Shelton, MD

GENERAL ANATOMIC CONSIDERATIONS

The rectum, endodermal in origin, is the dorsal component of the cloaca, which is partitioned by the anorectal septum. The anal canal is an invagination of ectodermal tissue. The anorectum develops from fusion of the rectum and the anal canal, which occurs at 8 weeks, when the anal membrane ruptures. The dentate line marks the point of fusion and the transition from endodermal to ectodermal tissue.

The rectum is 12–15 cm long. It extends from the rectosigmoid junction, marked by the fusion of the tenia, to the anal canal, marked by the passage into the pelvic floor musculature (Figure 31–1). The rectum lies in the sacrum and forms three distinct curves, creating folds known as the **valves of Houston.** The proximal and distal curves are convex to the left and the middle curve is convex to the right. The middle curve roughly marks the anterior peritoneal reflection, which is 6–8 cm above the anus. The rectum gradually undergoes transition from intraperitoneal to extraperitoneal beginning 12–15 cm from the anus and becoming completely extraperitoneal 6–8 cm from the anus. The rectum is fixed posteriorly, laterally, and anteriorly by the presacral (Waldeyer) fascia, the lateral ligaments, and Denonvilliers fascia, respectively.

The anatomic anal canal starts at the **dentate line,** the junction of colorectal mucosa and anal mucosa, and ends at the **anal verge,** the junction of the anal mucosa with the perianal skin. However, for practical purposes, the surgical anal canal extends from the muscular diaphragm of the pelvic floor to the anal verge. The **anal canal** is a collapsed anteroposterior slit 3–4 cm long. The anal canal is supported by the surrounding **anal sphincter mechanism,** composed of the internal and external sphincters. The **internal sphincter** is a specialized continuation of the circular muscle of the rectum. It is an involuntary muscle that is normally contracted at rest. The structure and function of the **external sphincter** is the subject of some controversy, but it acts as a spout on a funnel of one continuous circumferential func-

tional muscle mass that includes the external sphincter caudally and extends cranially to the conical puborectalis and levator ani muscles. The external sphincter is composed of voluntary striated muscle. The conjoined longitudinal muscle separates the internal and external sphincters. This intersphincteric plane is created by the continuation of the longitudinal muscle of the rectum joined by fibers from the levator ani and puborectalis, forming the conjoined muscle. Some fibers from this muscle become the corrugator cutis ani and insert on the perianal skin, creating rugal folds and a puckered appearance. Other fibers traverse the internal sphincter and support the internal hemorrhoids as the mucosal suspensory ligaments.

Familiarity with the histology of the rectum and anal canal is important in order to understand the disease processes of these areas. The rectum is composed of an innermost layer of mucosa that overlies the submucosa, two continuous sheaths of muscle—the circular and longitudinal muscles—and, in the proximal rectum, serosa. The mucosa is subdivided into three layers: (1) epithelial cells, (2) lamina propria, and (3) muscularis mucosae. The **muscularis mucosae** is a fine sheet of muscle containing a network of lymphatics. Lymphatics are essentially absent above this level, so the muscularis mucosae determines the metastatic potential of malignancies.

As the rectum enters the narrow musculature of the pelvic floor and becomes the anal canal, the tissue is thrown into folds known as the **columns of Morgagni.** At the lower end of the columns lie crypts, some of which communicate with anal glands lying in the intersphincteric plane. The epithelium of the anal canal is of three types: colorectal mucosa is present in the proximal 2–3 cm, transitional epithelium is at and just above the dentate line, and the anoderm is below the dentate line. The anoderm is squamous mucosa rich in nerve fibers. The anal verge marks the true mucocutaneous junction.

The pelvic floor is composed of the levator ani and puborectalis muscles. The levator ani, two broad, thin, sym-

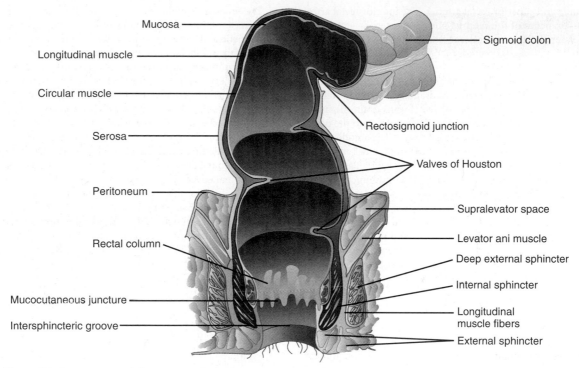

▲ **Figure 31-1.** Anatomy of the anorectal canal.

metric muscular sheets that originate from the pelvic side-wall and sacrospinous ligament, form the principal support of the pelvic viscera. The puborectalis muscle originates on the posterior aspect of the pubis, forms a sling around the rectum, and returns to the posterior aspect of the pubis. The fibers of the puborectalis are situated immediately adjacent to and below the innermost component of the levator ani muscle, where they are intimately associated with the upper posterolateral fibers of the deep external anal sphincter. Thus, the puborectalis serves as a bridge between the broad sheetlike component of the funnel created by the levators and the narrow spout of the funnel created by the external anal sphincter. The puborectalis in the contracted state is responsible for the normal acute anorectal angle between the levators and the external sphincters. It is also responsible for the shelf that is normally palpable on digital examination as one passes from the distal narrow lumen of the anus to the more proximal capacious lumen of the rectum.

The innervation of the rectum is via the sympathetic and parasympathetic nervous systems. The sympathetic nerves originate from the lumbar segments L1–3, form the inferior mesenteric plexus, travel through the superior hypogastric plexus, and descend as the hypogastric nerves to the pelvic plexus.

The parasympathetic nerves arise from the second, third, and fourth sacral roots and join the hypogastric nerves anterior and lateral to the rectum to form the pelvic plexus, from which fibers pass to form the periprostatic plexus. Sympathetic and parasympathetic fibers pass from the pelvic and periprostatic plexuses to the rectum and internal anal sphincter as well as the prostate, bladder, and penis. Injury to these nerves can lead to impotence, bladder dysfunction, and loss of normal defecatory mechanisms.

The internal anal sphincter is innervated with sympathetic and parasympathetic fibers. Both are inhibitory and keep the sphincter in a constant state of contraction. The external sphincters are skeletal muscles innervated by the pudendal nerve with fibers that originate from S2–4. Above the dentate line, noxious stimuli are experienced as ill-defined, dull sensations conducted through afferent fibers of the parasympathetic nerves. Below the dentate line, the epithelium is exquisitely sensitive. Cutaneous sensations of heat, cold, pain, and touch are conveyed through the inferior rectal and perineal branches of the pudendal nerve.

The arterial supply of the anorectum is via the superior, middle, and inferior rectal arteries. The superior rectal artery is the terminal branch of the inferior mesenteric artery and descends in the mesorectum. It supplies the upper and middle rectum. The middle rectal arteries arise from the internal iliac arteries and enter the rectum anterolaterally at the level of the pelvic floor musculature. They supply the lower two thirds of the rectum. Collaterals exist between the middle and superior rectal arteries. The inferior rectal arteries—branches of the internal pudendal arteries—enter posterolaterally, do not anastomose with the blood supply to the middle rectum, and provide blood to the anal sphincters and epithelium.

The venous drainage of the anorectum is via the superior, middle, and inferior rectal veins draining into the portal and systemic systems. The superior rectal veins drain the upper and middle thirds of the rectum. They empty into the portal system via the inferior mesenteric vein. The middle rectal veins drain the lower rectum and the upper anal canal into the systemic system via the internal iliac veins. The inferior rectal veins drain the lower anal canal, communicating with the pudendal veins and draining into the internal iliac veins. Communication between the venous systems allows low rectal cancers to spread via the portal and systemic systems.

Lymphatic drainage of the upper and middle rectum is into the inferior mesenteric nodes. Lymph from the lower rectum may also drain into the inferior mesenteric system or into the systems along the middle and inferior rectal arteries, posteriorly along the middle sacral artery, and anteriorly through channels in the retrovesical or rectovaginal septum. These drain to the iliac nodes and ultimately to the periaortic nodes. Lymphatics from the anal canal above the dentate line drain via the superior rectal lymphatics to the inferior mesenteric lymph nodes and laterally to the internal iliac nodes. Below the dentate line, drainage occurs primarily to the inguinal nodes but can occur to the inferior or superior rectal lymph nodes.

NORMAL FUNCTION OF THE ANORECTUM

The normal function of the anorectum is storage and release of intestinal waste products. The rectum functions mainly as a capacitance storage vessel. The normal volume of the rectum is 650–1200 mL. Resting rectal pressure is approximately 10 mm Hg. Changes in intrarectal pressure are primarily a reflection of intra-abdominal pressure changes since the rectum itself has little peristaltic function.

The function of the pelvic floor is complex and poorly understood. The complexity of the interactions of the pelvic floor structures and the nature of material passed per rectum compromises the ability to study function with intraluminal monitors, as is done in the upper intestinal tract.

The levators ani form a funnel that suspends the rectum in a muscular sling which ends where the puborectalis angulates the rectum forward at the anorectal junction. The levators may contain sensory fibers that report pelvic fullness and thus may be important in the sensation of the urge to defecate. The acuity of the anorectal angle (created by the puborectalis) is critical for maintaining continence. The puborectalis contracts, increasing the angle during Valsalva maneuvers, where continence is maintained (coughing, straining) but relaxes to open the angle during similar efforts performed as part of normal defecation.

The internal sphincter, composed of smooth muscle, accounts for 85% of the resting tone. It is innervated by sympathetic and parasympathetic fibers. Both are inhibitory and keep the sphincter in a constant state of contraction. The external sphincters are skeletal muscles innervated by the pudendal nerve with fibers from S2–4. The muscles provide 15% of the resting tone and 100% of the voluntary squeeze pressure. The external sphincter, pelvic floor, and cricopharyngeus muscles are unique skeletal muscles in being able to maintain a state of tonic contraction. The strength of contraction in the first two is increased by factors that increase intra-abdominal pressure such as erect posture, coughing, or Valsalva maneuver. Voluntary contraction of the external sphincter doubles the resting pressure but it cannot be sustained longer than 3 minutes.

The normal hemorrhoidal cushions are important participants in maintaining continence and minimizing trauma during defecation. They function as protective pillows that engorge with blood during the act of defecation, protecting the anoderm from direct trauma due to passage of stool. They also seal the anal canal and prevent leakage of gas and stool. The internal and external sphincters alone cannot close the anal canal, but when sphincter action is combined with interdigitating internal hemorrhoidal cushions, continence is achieved. Hemorrhoidal tissues become engorged when intra-abdominal pressure is increased (eg, obesity, pregnancy, lifting, and defecation).

Through complex mechanisms not clearly understood, the anal sphincters function as a unit in concert with the levator ani, the puborectalis, and the rectum, allowing defecation to be controlled. Continence is maintained when intrarectal pressures are lower than the pressures generated by the resting internal and external sphincters. In the resting state, the rectum is not completely empty, but the contents are not sensed. Sensory fibers in the levators that initially signal the presence of pelvic fullness adapt and the rectum accommodates (decreases muscle tone), allowing the contents to remain. Periodically, the internal sphincter relaxes, allowing the rectal contents to drop down into the anal canal where the contents can be sensed by the anoderm. In response, the external sphincter contracts and the contents are pushed back into the rectum. This "sampling reflex," or **rectoanal inhibitory reflex**, also results from rectal distention, allowing determination of rectal contents as the rectum fills. The sampling reflex occurs up to seven times a day. Progressive distention of the rectum causes continuous inhibition of the internal sphincter and relaxation of the external sphincter, resulting in the urge to defecate. If solid waste is noted and one wishes to evacuate, a sitting or squatting position is assumed (straightening the anorectal angle), intra-abdominal pressure is increased by a Valsalva maneuver, the puborectalis relaxes, and reflex relaxation of the internal sphincter occurs as the contents enter the anal canal. As the puborectalis relaxes, the anorectal angle straightens, further shortening the anal canal and increasing the funnel shape of the musculature. The Valsalva maneuver is the principal force behind evacuation. Thus, normal defecation is a complex event involving multiple steps.

▼ DYSFUNCTION OF THE ANORECTUM

INCONTINENCE

Continence is maintained through rectal compliance, anorectal sensation, anorectal reflexes, and anal sphincter function. The nature and quantity of stool and colonic transit are important as well. The incidence of fecal incontinence is difficult to determine because of underreporting and lack of a standard definition of the term. Obstetric trauma is the major cause of mechanical injury to the external sphincter and nerves. The incidence of incontinence is increased after third-degree perineal tears, multiple vaginal deliveries, and infection of an episiotomy repair. Prolonged labor may mechanically disrupt the sphincter and stretch of the pudendal nerve. Although incontinence is most common in parous women, the prevalence in men is also high.

Neurogenic causes of incontinence include pudendal nerve stretch from to prolonged labor or multiple births and a history of chronic straining to defecate. Vaginal deliveries are associated with reversible pudendal nerve injury in 80% of primigravida births. The injury may be unilateral or bilateral. If it is permanent or repeated multiple times, denervation and weakening of the external sphincter and pelvic floor result. The neuropathy and associated sphincter dysfunction progress with time. A weakened pelvic floor is less able to withstand increased intra-abdominal pressure, leading to further perineal descent and stretch injury.

Chronic straining at stool and a sense of incomplete evacuation are common features of the descending perineum syndrome. Straining leads to descent of the pelvic floor and straightening of the anorectal angle. This may result in folding in or prolapse of the anterior rectal wall and further obstruction of defecation. The resultant increased straining and perineal descent cause pudendal nerve injury as the nerve is stretched over the ischial spine, leading to idiopathic fecal incontinence sometimes associated with internal rectal prolapse (intussusception).

Incontinence may result from the treatment of cryptogenic abscess or fistula disease or of perianal Crohn disease, where the external sphincter may be divided during fistulotomy. In women, the external sphincter is a thin band of muscle anteriorly and thus especially susceptible to complete transection in this location, resulting in incontinence.

Other causes of incontinence include systemic diseases affecting either the muscular or neurologic systems (eg, scleroderma, multiple sclerosis, dermatomyositis, diabetes) and causes unrelated to the function of the sphincter itself (severe diarrhea, fecal impaction with overflow incontinence, radiation proctitis with fibrosis, and tumors of the distal colon and rectum).

▶ Clinical Findings

A. Symptoms and Signs

Complete incontinence is lack of control of gas, liquid, and solid stool. Inability to control liquid and gas or gas alone is **partial incontinence.** Urgency, seepage, and soiling may occur regularly or intermittently, depending on the nature of the stool presenting to the rectum. Elicitation of these symptoms is important in establishing the nature of the injury. Validated fecal incontinence scores quantify these symptoms and are useful in establishing the patients' perceived baseline function and response to therapy. Patients who complain of soiling with urgency may have a poorly distensible rectum and normal sphincters, whereas patients complaining of inability to sense stool until it has passed may have a neurologic injury. The physical signs of incontinence may include a patulous anus, focal loss of corrugation of the anal verge, flattening and maceration of the perineum, exaggerated descent of the perineum with straining, decreased sphincter tone, diminished voluntary squeeze pressures, and loss of anal sensation.

B. Laboratory and Imaging Studies

Anorectal manometry, transrectal ultrasound, pudendal nerve latency studies, electromyography, and defecography may all be part of the evaluation of the incontinent patient.

Anorectal manometry defines the limits of the injury by measuring the maximum resting pressure, the maximum squeeze pressure, the sphincter length and symmetry, the minimum sensory volume, the presence or absence of the rectoanal inhibitory reflex, and the ability to relax the puborectalis muscle. Maximal resting pressures normally range from 40 mm Hg to 80 mm Hg, while maximal squeeze pressures range from 80 mm Hg to 160 mm Hg. The internal sphincter gives rise to 85% of the resting maximal pressure, while the external sphincter provides 15% of the resting pressure and 100% of the maximal squeeze pressure. The sphincter is typically 3 cm long and asymmetric (longer in back), and the whole complex is shorter in women. The minimum sensory volume is about 10 mL. The rectoanal inhibitory reflex is manifested as a decrease in resting anal pressure when an air-filled balloon distends the rectum. Finally, pelvic floor function and the ability to relax the pelvic floor to achieve defecation are assessed with the balloon expulsion test. This requires the patient to expel a fully inflated 60 mL latex balloon.

Transrectal ultrasound provides useful anatomic images for evaluating internal and external anal sphincter defects. Electromyographic changes correlate closely with ultrasonographic evidence of sphincter injury, allowing transrectal ultrasound to largely replace the more painful electromyography.

Pudendal nerve latency studies further define the nature of the injury. If one or both nerves are injured, surgical or nonsurgical treatment of incontinence may be predictably unsuccessful. The study is performed by inserting a gloved finger with a stimulating electrode at the fingertip in the rectum and stimulating the pudendal nerve as it traverses the ischial spine. An electrode at the base of the examining finger records the delay between stimulation and contraction of the external sphincter. The normal delay is 2 ± 0.2 s. It may be prolonged with age, after childbirth, in individuals with a history of excessive straining to defecate and perineal descent, and in systemic diseases such as diabetes and multiple sclerosis.

Defecography is useful in patients with both constipation and incontinence, for in a few patients with incontinence, rectal intussusception occurs during the act of straining to defecate and the intussusception produces obstruction and an inability to evacuate, which is later followed by uncontrolled release of liquid stool after the straining is stopped.

Differential Diagnosis

Incontinence may result from obstructions to defecation caused by tumors or intussusception. Varying degrees of incontinence may also result from obstetric injury, either from excessive straining and pudendal nerve injury or disruption of the sphincter mechanism. Incontinence may occur immediately or after many years as the patient ages, sphincter tone decreases, and an occult injury is manifested. Chronic straining at defecation stretches the pudendal nerve over the ischial spine, leading to idiopathic fecal incontinence in the elderly. An extreme example of this is seen in rectal prolapse, where 30% of patients experience incontinence after repair because of stretch injury from chronic prolapse. Secondary effects of systemic diseases such as multiple sclerosis, dermatomyositis, and diabetes mellitus should be considered. Incontinence may also stem from disease that overwhelms a normally functioning sphincter. Examples are severe diarrhea, fecal impaction with overflow, inflammatory bowel disease of the rectum, radiation proctitis, and fibrosis.

Treatment

An algorithm for the diagnosis and treatment of incontinence is given in (Figure 31–2). Patients with mild disease can initially be treated with medical therapy by increasing dietary fiber, avoiding foods that exacerbate the problem, and using antidiarrheal medications (with care). These measures can also be used as adjuncts to the therapies described subsequently. Biofeedback should be first-line therapy and in most series is reported to be highly effective in over two thirds of patients. If a muscular defect is limited and there is no neurologic injury, surgical correction with an overlapping sphincter reconstruction restores continence by reestablishing a complete ring of muscle. Overlapping sphincteroplasty is associated with excellent results in about 75% of candidate patients, but this result decreases to 50% at 10 years. If there

is extensive loss of sphincter muscle or severe neurologic injury, simple overlapping repair is not as successful, and consideration must be given to muscle flap procedures. The sacral nerve stimulator was initially designed for urinary incontinence and subsequently adapted for fecal incontinence. Ideal candidates have an anatomically intact sphincter and good results with a trial of "temporary" stimulation. The stimulating electrodes are applied to sacral nerve roots 2, 3, and 4 with a remotely implanted pulse generator. Excellent results with some improvement in virtually all patients can be achieved with appropriate patient selection, though long-term outcome data are still unavailable. The main complications are lead dislodgement and the need for device explantation due to intractable pain.

The stimulated-gracilis, the gracilis, and the gluteal muscle flap procedures are reserved for patients with complete neurologic injury or extensive muscle loss who wish to avoid a colostomy. The stimulated-gracilis procedure (dynamic graciloplasty) is similar to the gracilis procedure with the exception that a pacemaker is used to retrain the gracilis. Success rates range from 35–85%. The main limitation is a relatively high morbidity primarily due to infectious complications. An international multicenter trial and smaller single-institution trials of the artificial bowel sphincter have been completed. The multicenter trial reported a success rate of 53% based on an intent-to-treat analysis. However, a very high incidence of device-related adverse events and the need for revision surgery has limited its application.

Anal encirclement procedures with foreign material have been reserved for the critically ill or for patients with a short life expectancy. The anal canal is encircled with either a synthetic mesh or a silver wire. Patients are given daily enemas to evacuate the rectum, providing a form of continence involving artificial obstruction and stimulated evacuation. The obstructing foreign body is prone to infection and erosion into the rectum, often necessitating its removal.

The anal plug is a device that self-expands when soaked in fecal content. Advantages of this approach include less soilage and fewer skin complications. It may be better suited for those patients with neurological disorders.

If the aforementioned measures fail, consideration may be given to performing an end-colostomy. This option is radical, yet it often offers patients a better quality of life.

Prognosis

The incontinence associated with prolapse usually resolves after repair of the prolapse if there has not been severe nerve injury. Prior to repair, the prolapsing segment stimulates the rectoanal inhibitory reflex, decreasing internal sphincter pressure, fatiguing the external sphincter, and resulting in incontinence. The incontinence resolves after surgical repair in 70% of cases.

Baeten CG et al: Anal dynamic graciloplasty in the treatment of intractable fecal incontinence. N Engl J Med 1995;332:1600.

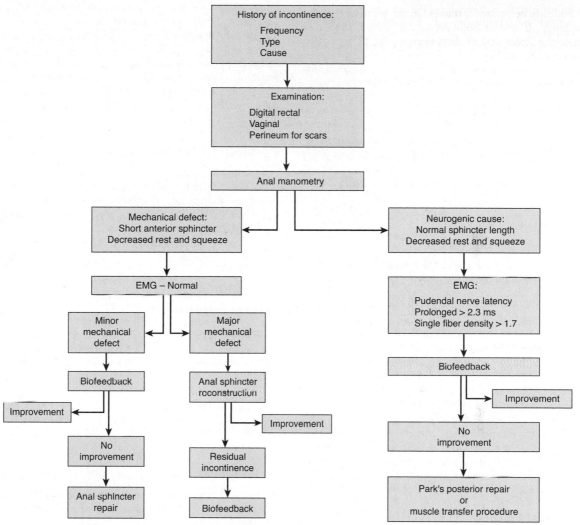

▲ **Figure 31–2.** Algorithm for workup and treatment of fecal incontinence. (Reproduced, with permission, from Grendel JH, McQuaid KR, Friedman SL: *Current Diagnosis & Treatment in Gastroenterology.* Originally published by Appleton & Lange. Copyright © 1996 by The McGraw-Hill Companies, Inc.)

Belyaev O et al: Neosphincter surgery for fecal incontinence: a critical and unbiased review of the relevant literature. Surg Today 2006;36:295

Cheong DM et al: Electrodiagnostic evaluation of fecal incontinence. Muscle Nerve 1995;18:612.

Falk PM et al: Transanal ultrasound and manometry in the evaluation of fecal incontinence. Dis Colon Rectum 1994;37:468.

Farouk R et al: Sustained internal sphincter hypertonia in patients with chronic anal fissure. Dis Colon Rectum 1994;37:424.

Hill JA et al: Pudendal neuropathy in patients with idiopathic fecal incontinence progresses with time. Br J Surg 1994;81:1492.

Johanson JF et al: Epidemiology of fecal incontinence: the silent affliction. Am J Gastroenterol 1996;91:33.

Ko CY et al: Biofeedback is effective therapy for fecal incontinence and constipation. Arch Surg 1997;132:829.

Lehur PA et al: Artificial anal sphincter: prospective clinical and manometric evaluation. Dis Colon Rectum 2000;43:1100.

Lestar B et al: The internal anal sphincter cannot close the anal canal completely. Int J Colorectal Dis 1992;7:159.

Madoff RD et al: Fecal incontinence. N Engl J Med 1992; 326:1002.

Nelson R et al: Community-based prevalence of anal incontinence. JAMA 1995;274:559.

Osterberg A et al: Results of neurophysiologic evaluation in fecal incontinence. Dis Colon Rectum 2000;43:1256.

Ryhammer AM et al: Long-term effect of vaginal deliveries on anorectal function in normal perimenopausal women. Dis Colon Rectum 1996;39:852.

Sangwan YP et al: Fecal incontinence. Surg Clin North Am J 1994;74:1377.

Sultan AH et al: Endosonography of the anal sphincters: normal anatomy and comparison with manometry. Clin Radiol 1994;49:368.

Tan JJ et al: Evolving therapies for fecal incontinence. Dis Colon Rectum 2007;50:1950

Wong WD et al: The safety and efficacy of the artificial bowel sphincter for fecal incontinence. Dis Colon Rectum 2002;45:1139.

PELVIC FLOOR DYSFUNCTION

ESSENTIALS OF DIAGNOSIS

▶ Inability to voluntarily evacuate rectal contents.

▶ Normal colonic transit time.

▶ General Considerations

Pelvic floor dysfunction, also called nonrelaxing puborectalis syndrome, anismus, or paradoxic pelvic floor contraction, is a functional disorder in that the muscle is normal but control is dysfunctional. In health, the puborectalis is contracted at rest, maintaining the anorectal angle. During defecation, the muscle relaxes and evacuation occurs. In nonrelaxing puborectalis syndrome, the muscle does not relax and maintains or increases (paradoxic contraction) the anorectal angle. The patient therefore performs a Valsalva maneuver against an obstructed outlet, and elimination does not occur or is significantly diminished.

Patients who chronically strain at stool, whether from colonic inertia or pelvic floor dysfunction, may develop lengthening of the attachments of the rectum to the sacrum or descending perineum syndrome. The increased mobility that results allows for internal prolapse (intussusception), solitary rectal ulcer, and rectal procidentia.

▶ Clinical Findings

A. Symptoms and Signs

Patients with pelvic floor dysfunction may complain of straining and anal or pelvic pain but also of constipation, incomplete evacuation, and a need to digitally evacuate rectal contents.

Digital examination of the patient with nonrelaxing puborectalis syndrome may reveal a tender pelvic muscular diaphragm. During the digital examination, if the patient is directed to squeeze to mimic holding in flatus, paradoxic relaxation and a Valsalva maneuver may occur. Similarly, if the patient is asked to bear down to simulate a bowel movement he may paradoxically contract the external sphincters and puborectalis muscles.

B. Laboratory and Imaging Studies

Patients with nonrelaxing puborectalis syndrome and internal intussusception should undergo defecography, colonic transit studies, anorectal manometry with the balloon expulsion test, and barium enema or colonoscopy.

The patient with isolated nonrelaxing puborectalis syndrome will have a normal colon on barium enema or colonoscopy and a normal colonic transit time to the rectosigmoid. Cinedefecography will demonstrate persistent anterior displacement of the rectum on the lateral view. The patient will be unable to expel the balloon during anorectal manometry evaluation.

▶ Differential Diagnosis

Complaints suggestive of obstructed defecation occur in patients with both functional and anatomic abnormalities. A functional abnormality is exemplified by the nonrelaxing puborectalis syndrome. Anatomic abnormalities include rectocele, internal intussusception, fecal impaction, and rectal or anal cancer. The workup of these complex patients is outlined in Figure 31–3.

▶ Treatment

A. Medical Treatment

Nonrelaxing puborectalis syndrome is best treated with biofeedback. The puborectalis is retrained to relax during the act of defecation, which allows the act to proceed without obstruction.

B. Surgical Treatment

Patients refractory to medical therapy may be offered a colostomy.

▶ Prognosis

Patients with nonrelaxing puborectalis syndrome have excellent results with biofeedback training but may require periodic retraining.

Glia A et al: Constipation assessed on the basis of colorectal physiology. Scand J Gastroenterol 1998;33:1273.

Mertz H et al: Symptoms and physiology in severe chronic constipation. Am J Gastroenterol 1999;94:131.

Nyam DC et al: Long-term results of surgery for chronic constipation. Dis Colon Rectum 1997;40:273. (Published erratum appears in Dis Colon Rectum 1997;40:529.)

ABNORMAL RECTAL FIXATION

ESSENTIALS OF DIAGNOSIS

▶ Increased mobility of the rectum.

▶ Altered defecation (constipation, incontinence, or both).

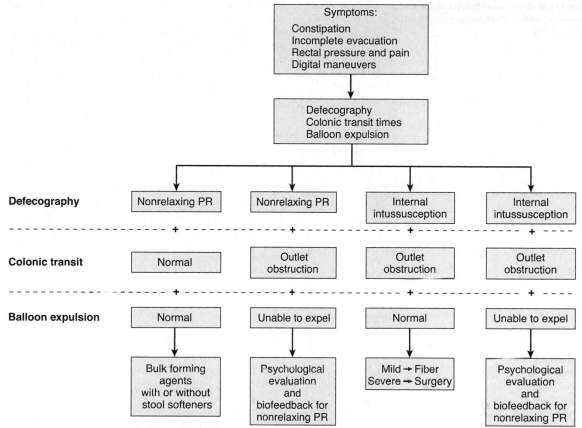

▲ **Figure 31–3.** Algorithm for workup and treatment of obstructed defecation. (Reproduced, with permission, from Grendel JH, McQuaid KR, Friedman SL: *Current Diagnosis & Treatment in Gastroenterology.* Originally published by Appleton & Lange. Copyright © 1996 by The McGraw-Hill Companies, Inc.)

▶ General Considerations

Abnormal rectal fixation is a group of diseases in which the attachment of the rectum to the sacrum has lengthened, allowing the rectum to block the act of defecation, to protrude into the vagina, or to prolapse through the anus. The reason for the increased mobility appears to be related to chronic straining. This may be secondary to colonic dysmotility or nonrelaxing puborectalis syndrome.

▶ Clinical Findings

A. Symptoms and Signs

Internal intussusception leads to complaints of rectal fullness, an urge to defecate, incomplete evacuation, incontinence, and, when associated with solitary rectal ulcers, rectal bleeding, mucus discharge, or tenesmus. Patients with rectal prolapse (rectal procidentia) complain of mucus discharge, progressive incontinence, pain, and bleeding, and upon direct questioning, they report that the rectum falls out.

Digital examination of the patient with internal intussusception may reveal a mass. This is the lead point of the intussusceptum and may be mistaken for a malignancy. The mass may be anterior and ulcerated (solitary rectal ulcer) or circumferential. The ulcer is 4–12 cm from the anal verge and is the ischemic traumatized lead point of the internal intussusceptum. Sigmoidoscopy may reveal the circumferential intussusceptum or an ulcerated mass that appears malignant. Pathologic examination reveals diffuse submucosal cysts with a characteristic fibrosis pattern and transverse smooth muscle cells within the lamina propria, distinguishing it from a malignancy. Physical examination of the patient with an acute rectal prolapse is not difficult. A large external mass of prolapsed tissue with concentric mucosal rings will be apparent. However, the diagnosis in a patient with a history of prolapse but without active prolapse may be more difficult. It may be necessary to give an enema, allow the patient to evacuate, and then examine the perineum. This often induces a prolapse, allowing for the diagnosis to be made in the office. An alternative is to demonstrate the prolapse on defecography. Digital examination may reveal decreased or absent sphincter tone. Anoscopy usually reveals a loss of normal hemorrhoidal tissue. The overlying distal rectal mucosa loses the dark plum color of the anal cushions and appears pink, resembling normal more proximal rectal mucosa right up to the dentate line.

B. Laboratory and Imaging Studies

Patients with internal intussusception and rectal prolapse may be evaluated with anorectal physiology testing, defecography or dynamic MRI, colonic transit studies, and barium enema or colonoscopy. Anorectal physiology testing may demonstrate obstructed defecation and exclude other causes of incontinence. Defecography or dynamic MRI will show the intussusceptum, making the diagnosis. Colonic transit time will be normal to the rectosigmoid, and barium enema or colonoscopy may document a normal colon. Rectal prolapse is usually diagnosed on physical examination without the need for further testing.

▶ Differential Diagnosis

Internal intussusception must be differentiated from adenocarcinoma. The symptoms, physical appearance, and histologic characteristics of the ulcer may be confused with malignancy.

Rectal prolapse should be distinguished from hemorrhoidal disease. Rectal prolapse is seen as uninterrupted circumferential rings of mucosa, while hemorrhoidal prolapse will be seen as prolapsing tissue with deep grooves between areas of prolapsing edematous tissue.

▶ Complications

The complications of intussusception and prolapse include progression of intussusception to prolapse, nerve injury from prolapse or chronic straining, descending perineum syndrome, bleeding, and incontinence. A severe rectal prolapse may become so edematous that it cannot be reduced, and it may progress to ischemia and gangrene.

▶ Treatment

A. Medical Treatment

Mild to moderate intussusception is treated with bulk agents, modification of bowel habits, and reassurance. The patient is instructed to stimulate a bowel movement in the morning and avoid the urge to defecate the remainder of the day because the fullness they sense is the proximal rectum intussuscepting into the distal rectum. With time, the urge to defecate resolves and so does the intussusception.

B. Surgical Treatment

There are two classes of operations for rectal prolapse: abdominal and perineal. The abdominal procedures have a lower recurrence rate and preserve the reservoir capacity of the rectum but carry more risk and have a higher incidence of postoperative constipation. The perineal procedures avoid an intra-abdominal anastomosis but remove the rectum, thereby eliminating the rectal reservoir, but have higher recurrence rates. The abdominal procedures are generally preferred in low-risk active patients under age 50 and in those who require other abdominal procedures simultaneously.

The abdominal procedures for patients with severe intussusception or rectal prolapse with normal sphincter function are sigmoid resection with or without rectopexy and rectopexy alone. Both operations—rectopexy or resection—require complete mobilization of the entire rectum to the pelvic floor in order to avoid distal intussusception.

Rectopexy aims to secure the rectum to the sacral hollow. It may be performed with sutures or prosthetic materials such as polypropylene mesh (Marlex), Gore-Tex, or polyglycolic acid or polyglactin mesh (Dexon or Vicryl). Many studies have suggested a higher complication rate with the prosthetics, a lower continence rate, and no difference in recurrence, suggesting that suture rectopexy is preferable. Suture rectopexy is performed with heavy nonabsorbable sutures, attaching the rectum to the sacral hollow. The suture may be placed through the lateral ligaments or through the muscularis propria of the rectum.

The addition of a sigmoid resection at the time of rectopexy lowers the recurrence rate and the incidence of postoperative constipation without increasing the morbidity. Rectopexy corrects the mobility of the rectum but does not correct the underlying disorder for patients with pelvic floor dysfunction or chronic constipation. Sigmoid resection removes the intussusceptum and the mobile portion of colon. Thus, in the constipated patient or the patient with a redundant sigmoid colon, resection is preferable to fixation alone.

Laparoscopic methods for repair of rectal prolapse involve fixation, with or without resection. Patients may experience less pain and faster return of bowel function and have a shorter duration of hospitalization than with the open abdominal approach.

Perineal operations for rectal prolapse consist of anal encirclement, the transanal Delorme procedure, and the Altemeier procedure. Anal encirclement has limited application and should be performed selectively only in patients with a very high operative risk or a limited life expectancy. The original Thiersch procedure involved placing a silver wire around the external sphincter within the ischiorectal fat. Now synthetic mesh or silicone tubes are used instead of wire. The foreign body creates an outlet obstruction, and laxatives or enemas are required for rectal evacuation. Erosion of the foreign material into the rectum and infection are significant complications that limit the utility of this technique.

The Delorme procedure is essentially a mucosal proctectomy with plication of the prolapsing rectal wall. The dissection is started 1–2 cm above the dentate line and carried to the apex of the prolapsing segment, where the mucosa is amputated. The muscle is reefed in with four to eight heavy absorbable sutures, and the mucosa is reapproximated with sutures or a circular stapler.

The Altemeier procedure is a complete proctectomy and often a partial sigmoidectomy. The apex of the prolapsing segment is delivered and placed on traction, and a full-thickness incision is made approximately 1 cm above the dentate line. The rectum is everted. The dissection is carried into the deep cul-de-sac anteriorly. Laterally and posteriorly, the vascular supply to the rectum is taken with electrocautery or clamps when necessary. The dissection is carried up onto the midline mesorectum and sigmoid mesentery until the redundant segment of bowel has been completely mobilized. If a levatoroplasty is planned, it is most easily carried out at this time with heavy absorbable suture. A levatoroplasty plicates the pelvic floor musculature and adds to improved continence by increasing the anorectal angle. The bowel is transected proximally, excising the redundant portion, and a hand-sewn (heavy absorbable suture) or stapled anastomosis is performed.

Sphincter function returns and incontinence resolves in 65% of patients who were incontinent preoperatively, but there is no way to predict who will respond. Those who do not have return of sphincter function will not tolerate a sigmoid resection. Therefore, perineal proctectomy and posterior sphincter enhancement are recommended in these patients. The posterior reconstruction may alter the angle of the rectum or obstruct the outlet sufficiently to bring about continence. Individuals with severe intussusception and those who have rectal prolapse without sphincter dysfunction should do well with either the abdominal or the perineal approach.

▶ Prognosis

The prognosis for patients with mild to moderate intussusception who are treated with bulking agents is excellent. Individuals with severe intussusception and those who have rectal prolapse without sphincter dysfunction should do well. Those with sphincter dysfunction have a 60–70% chance of regaining function. The abdominal approach is associated with approximately a 10% recurrence rate. The perineal approach is associated with a 20–30% recurrence rate. Reoperation for recurrence is possible after either approach but may be technically easier from the perineum if an abdominal resection has not been previously performed.

Athanasiadis S et al: The risk of infection of three synthetic materials used in rectopexy with or without colonic resection for rectal prolapse. Int J Colorectal Dis 1996;11:42.

Darzi A et al: Stapled laparoscopic rectopexy for rectal prolapse. Surg Endosc 1995;9:301.

Graf W et al: Laparoscopic suture rectopexy. Dis Colon Rectum 1995;38:211.

Huber FT et al: Functional results after treatment of rectal prolapse with rectopexy and sigmoid resection. World J Surg 1995;19:138;discussion 143.

Jacobs LK et al: The best operation for rectal prolapse. Surg Clin North Am 1997;77:49.

Mollen RM et al: Effects of rectal mobilization and lateral ligaments division on colonic and anorectal function. Dis Colon Rectum 2000;43:1283.

Novell JR et al: Prospective randomized trial of Ivalon sponge versus sutured rectopexy for full-thickness rectal prolapse. Br J Surg 1994;81:904.

Senagore AJ: Management of rectal prolapse: the role of laparoscopic approaches. Semin Laparosc Surg 2003;10:197.

Wexner SD et al: Laparoscopic colorectal surgery: analysis of 140 cases. Surg Endosc 1996;10:133.

HEMORRHOIDS

 ESSENTIALS OF DIAGNOSIS

Internal hemorrhoids:

▶ Painless bright red blood per rectum.

▶ Mucus discharge.

▶ Rectal fullness or discomfort.

External hemorrhoids:

▶ Sudden, severe perianal pain.

▶ Perianal mass.

▶ General Considerations

Hemorrhoidal tissues are part of the normal anatomy of the distal rectum and anal canal (Figure 31–1). **Internal hemorrhoids** are vascular and connective tissue cushions that originate above the dentate line and are lined with rectal or transitional mucosa. **External hemorrhoids** are vascular complexes underlying the richly innervated anoderm. Hemorrhoids function as protective pillows that become engorged with blood during the act of defecation, protecting the anal canal from direct trauma due to passage of stool. Hemorrhoidal tissues become engorged when intra-abdominal pressure is increased. This occurs with obesity, pregnancy, lifting, and straining for defecation.

Hemorrhoidal disease may involve the internal complex, the external complex, or both. Internal hemorrhoids become symptomatic when the internal complex becomes chronically engorged or the tissue prolapses into the anal canal due to laxity of the surrounding connective tissue and dilation of the veins. The external hemorrhoids become symptomatic with thrombosis, which leads to an acute onset of severe perianal pain. When the thrombosis resolves, the overlying skin becomes fibrotic, creating a skin tag.

Internal hemorrhoidal disease develops differently in older women and younger men. In older women, the principal cause appears to be chronic straining, which leads to vascular engorgement and dilatation, resulting in stretching and disruption of the supporting connective tissue surrounding the vascular channels. The most common cause of prolonged straining is the act of defecation. Contrary to popular belief, the stool may be liquid or solid. Hemorrhoid pathology has no correlation with constipation (infrequent passage of stool) or portal hypertension. Pathologic hemorrhoids are not dilated vascular channels, varices, or vascular hyperplasias. The principal mechanism in younger men is increased resting pressure within the anal canal, leading to decreased venous return, venous engorgement, and disruption of the supporting tissues. The cause of external hemorrhoidal disease is unknown but is associated with straining such as that which occurs with constipation or diarrhea.

Internal hemorrhoidal disease is classified based on *history* as follows: first-degree hemorrhoids bleed; second-degree hemorrhoids bleed and prolapse, but reduce spontaneously; third-degree hemorrhoids bleed, prolapse, and require manual reduction; and fourth-degree hemorrhoids bleed, cannot be reduced, and may strangulate.

► Clinical Findings

A. Symptoms and Signs

Pathologic internal hemorrhoids typically cause bright red bleeding per rectum, mucus discharge, and, when very large, a sense of rectal fullness or discomfort. Infrequently, internal hemorrhoids prolapse into the anal canal, where they may become incarcerated, thrombosed, and necrotic. In this instance, pain is common. Visual inspection may reveal a normal-appearing perineum, edema near the involved hemorrhoid, a prolapsed hemorrhoid, or an edematous, gangrenous, incarcerated hemorrhoid. The perineum may be macerated from chronic mucus discharge, the resulting moisture, and local irritation. Anoscopy may reveal tissue with evidence of chronic vascular dilatation, friability, mobility, and squamous metaplasia.

Acute intravascular thrombus may develop within external hemorrhoids associated with acute severe perianal pain. The pain usually peaks within 48–72 hours. An acutely thrombosed external hemorrhoid is a purple-black, edematous, tense subcutaneous perianal mass that is quite tender. The thrombus occasionally causes ischemia and necrosis of the overlying skin, resulting in bleeding.

B. Laboratory and Imaging Studies

Chronic bleeding from internal hemorrhoids may rarely cause anemia. However, until all other sources of blood loss have been ruled out, anemia must not be attributed to hemorrhoids regardless of the patient's age. Barium enema or colonoscopy is necessary to rule out malignancy and inflammatory bowel disease. Defecography is helpful in the patient in whom obstructed defecation and rectal prolapse is suspected.

► Differential Diagnosis

Patients with perianal diseases often come to the surgeon with an inaccurate preliminary diagnosis of "hemorrhoids." A thorough history often suggests the correct diagnosis. Painless bleeding attributed to hemorrhoids must be distinguished from rectal bleeding from colorectal malignancy, inflammatory bowel disease, diverticular disease, and adenomatous polyps. Painful bleeding associated with a bowel movement is caused by a rectal ulcer or anal fissure. Straining at stool may be caused by obstructed defecation. Similarly, rectal prolapse must be distinguished from hemorrhoids because it is safe to band a hemorrhoid but not a prolapsed rectum. Moisture or maceration may be secondary to hemorrhoids or condylomata acuminata.

► Complications

The complications of internal or external hemorrhoids are the indications for medical or surgical treatment: bleeding, pain, necrosis, mucus discharge, moisture, and, rarely, perianal sepsis.

► Treatment

A. Medical Treatment

Initial medical management is recommended for all but the most advanced cases. Dietary alterations, including elimination of constipating foods (eg, cheese, bananas) and the addition of bulking agents such as fiber, stool softeners, and increased intake of liquids, are advised. It is often beneficial to change daily routines by adding exercise and decreasing time spent on the commode.

B. Surgical Treatment

First-degree and second-degree hemorrhoids generally respond to medical management. Hemorrhoids that fail to respond to medical management may be treated with elastic band ligation, sclerosis, photocoagulation, cryosurgery, excisional hemorrhoidectomy, and many other local techniques that induce scarring and fixation of the hemorrhoids to the underlying tissues. The three classic techniques—elastic band ligation, sclerosis, and excisional hemorrhoidectomy—are discussed here along with the newer technique of stapled hemorrhoidopexy.

Elastic band ligation is a safe, office-based procedure that is effective in the treatment of first-degree, second-degree, third-degree, and selected fourth-degree hemorrhoids. Hemorrhoidal tissue 1–2 cm above the dentate line is grasped, pulled into the barrel of an elastic band applicator, and two bands are placed at the base of the hemorrhoidal complex. After 7–10 days, the hemorrhoid sloughs away, removing a portion of the offending redundant tissue and leaving a scar that inhibits further prolapse and bleeding of the remaining tissue. If the band is placed in the transitional zone or below, the patient may experience severe pain, as this mucosa and skin are highly innervated. If that happens, the band should be removed immediately. Immunocompromised patients or those with unrecognized rectal prolapse have occasionally developed severe sepsis after banding, a complication heralded by inordinate pain, fever, and urinary retention. Treatment requires intravenous antibiotics, band removal, debridement of necrotic tissue, and observation. Patients are advised to avoid nonsteroidal anti-inflammatory agents and aspirin for 10 days after ligation, since significant bleeding may otherwise occur when the hemorrhoid sloughs.

Injection sclerotherapy is often tried for first-degree and second-degree hemorrhoids that continue to bleed despite medical measures. One to two milliliters of sclerosant is injected into the loose submucosal connective tissue above the hemorrhoidal complex, which causes inflammation and scarring. This inhibits prolapse and bleeding of the remaining hemorrhoidal tissue. The depth of injection is critical, since mucosal sloughing, infection, and full-thickness injury have been reported.

Excisional hemorrhoidectomy is reserved for the larger third-degree and fourth-degree hemorrhoids, mixed internal and external hemorrhoids not amenable to banding of the internal component, and incarcerated internal hemorrhoids requiring urgent intervention. The base of the hemorrhoid is inspected through an anoscope. The vascular pedicle may be suture-ligated with absorbable suture. The hemorrhoidal tissue is excised, but care must be taken to avoid injuring the underlying internal sphincter while dissecting free the vascular cushion and overlying mucosa. The mucosal and skin defect may be left open, may be partially closed, or may be closed with the running the suture used to control the vascular pedicle.

Severe pain, urinary retention, bleeding, and fecal impaction are the most common complications of excisional hemorrhoidectomy. The incidence of these complications can be minimized with improved postoperative pain control, limited intraoperative intravenous fluid administration, attention to surgical technique, and stool bulking agents and stool softeners. Anal stenosis is a long-term complication that may be avoided by leaving enough anoderm between excised hemorrhoidal complexes.

Stapled hemorrhoidopexy is a technique that utilizes a circular stapling device to devascularize the hemorrhoidal tissue, reduce the mucosal prolapse, and perform an anopexy. The technique is safe, with improved postoperative pain control reported, but the cost of the device may limit its use. It is highly effective in the treatment of selected patients with circumferential advanced disease or mild rectal mucosal prolapse.

The acutely thrombosed external hemorrhoid may be treated with excision of the hemorrhoid or clot evacuation if the patient presents less than 48 hours after the onset of symptoms. Excision removes the clot and hemorrhoidal tissue, which decreases the chances of recurrence. However, many surgeons simply evacuate the thrombus, relieving the pressure and pain. If the patient presents over 48–72 hours after the symptoms begin, the thrombus will have started to organize and evacuation will be unsuccessful. Warm sitz baths, a high-fiber diet, stool softeners, and reassurance are appropriate at this point. Hemorrhoidal disease is not uncommon during pregnancy and can be treated in the immediate postpartum period should symptoms persist.

▶ Prognosis

The prognosis for recurrence of hemorrhoidal disease is mostly related to success in changing the patient's bowel habits. Increasing dietary fiber, decreasing constipating foods, introducing exercise, and decreasing time spent on the toilet all decrease the amount of time spent straining in the squatting position. These behavioral modifications are the most important steps in preventing recurrence.

Arbman G et al: Closed vs. open hemorrhoidectomy: is there any difference? Dis Colon Rectum 2000;43:31.

Corman ML et al: Stapled haemorrhoidopexy: a consensus position paper by an international working party: indications, contra-indications and technique. Colorectal Dis 2003;5:304.

Galizia G et al: Lateral internal sphincterotomy together with haemorrhoidectomy for treatment of haemorrhoids: a randomised prospective study. Eur J Surg 2000;166:223.

Hayssen TK et al: Limited hemorrhoidectomy: results and long-term follow-up. Dis Colon Rectum 1999;42:909; discussion 914.

Ho YH et al: Randomized controlled trial of open and closed haemorrhoidectomy. Br J Surg 1997;84:1729.

Hoff SD et al: Ambulatory surgical hemorrhoidectomy: a solution to postoperative urinary retention? Dis Colon Rectum 1994; 37:1242.

Komborozos VA et al: Rubber band ligation of symptomatic internal hemorrhoids: results of 500 cases. Dig Surg 2000;17:71.

Konsten J et al: Hemorrhoidectomy vs. Lord's method: 17-year follow-up of a prospective, randomized trial. Dis Colon Rectum 2000;43:503.

Lee HH et al: Multiple hemorrhoidal bandings in a single session. Dis Colon Rectum 1994;37:37.

Loder PB et al: Haemorrhoids: pathology, pathophysiology and aetiology. Br J Surg 1994;81:946.

MacRae HM et al: Comparison of hemorrhoidal treatment modalities. A meta-analysis. Dis Colon Rectum 1995;38:687.

O'Donovan S et al: Intraoperative use of Toradol facilitates outpatient hemorrhoidectomy. Dis Colon Rectum 1994;37:793.

Pescatori M: Urinary retention after anorectal operations. Dis Colon Rectum 1999;42:964.

Shalaby R, Desoky A: Randomized clinical trial of stapled versus Milligan-Morgan haemorrhoidectomy. Br J Surg 2001;88:1049.

ANAL STENOSIS

 ESSENTIALS OF DIAGNOSIS

▶ Obstructed defecation.

▶ Stenosis on rectal examination.

General Considerations

Anal stenosis is typically an iatrogenic complication of scarring after anal surgery. In particular, hemorrhoidectomies, single quadrant or circumferential (Whitehead), when inexpertly performed, may lead to stenosis. Other causes include anal tumors, Crohn disease, radiation injury, recurrent anal ulcers, infection, and trauma.

Clinical Findings

A. Symptoms and Signs

Anal stenosis causes increasing difficulty with—and straining at—defecation, thin and sometimes painful bowel movements, and bloating. Examination of the patient with anal stenosis may reveal postsurgical changes and a stenotic anal canal. Digital examination may be quite painful or impossible.

B. Laboratory and Imaging Studies

No additional studies of the patient with anal stenosis are required, although a contrast enema could help delineate the length of stenosis.

Differential Diagnosis

Patients with anal stenosis may complain of anal pain or obstructed defecation, and physical examination will assist with diagnosis. Other causes of anal pain include a fissure with or without concomitant stenosis, thrombosed external hemorrhoids, perirectal abscess, malignancy, foreign body, and proctalgia fugax. Proctalgia fugax (levator ani syndrome), a diagnosis of exclusion, is suggested when a patient complains of pain that awakens him or her from sleep. The pain is generally left-sided, short-lived, and relieved by heat, anal dilation, or muscle relaxants. The patient often has a history of migraine headaches and may report that the pain is triggered by stressful events.

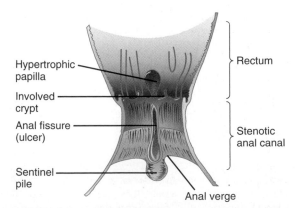

▲ **Figure 31–4.** Diagram of the anorectum showing the fissure or ulcer triad.

Hypertrophic papilla

Involved crypt

Anal fissure (ulcer)

Sentinel pile

Rectum

Stenotic anal canal

Anal verge

Treatment

Mild anal stenosis may be treated successfully with gentle dilation and bulk-forming agents. Severe anal stenosis is treated surgically if there is no evidence of active disease (eg, Crohn disease) and healthy tissue is available to perform the anoplasty. This can be achieved with a skin island or V-Y flap. Both procedures involve incision of the stenotic anus, mobilization of the surrounding skin, and advancement of the healthy tissue into the closure, relieving the stenosis. The prognosis for anal stenosis is excellent if there is no evidence of active disease of the anus.

ANAL FISSURE & ULCER

ESSENTIALS OF DIAGNOSIS

▶ Tearing pain upon defecation.
▶ Blood on tissue or stool.
▶ Persistent perianal pain or spasm following defecation.
▶ Sphincter spasm.
▶ Disruption of anoderm.

General Considerations

An anal fissure is a split in the anoderm. An anal ulcer is a chronic fissure. When mature, an ulcer is associated with a skin tag (**sentinel pile**) (Figure 31–4). Fissures typically occur in the midline just distal to the dentate line. Two studies have called into question the Goligher rule that 90% are posterior, 10% are anterior, and less than 1% occur simultaneously in the anterior and posterior positions. Both studies found anterior fissures to be more common than expected, but the fissures were still in the midline.

Fissures result from forceful dilation of the anal canal, most commonly during defecation. The anoderm is disrupted, exposing the underlying internal sphincter muscle. The muscle goes into spasm in response to exposure and fails to relax with the next dilation (bowel movement). This leads to further tearing, deepening of the fissure, and increased muscle irritation and spasm. The persistent muscle spasm leads to relative ischemia of the overlying anoderm and inhibits healing. Ultraslow waves—low-frequency, high-amplitude pressure changes—occur with increased frequency in patients with anal fissures and disappear with sphincterotomy and fissure healing, suggesting a relationship between spasm and persistent disease.

Classically, the initial insult is felt to be a firm bowel movement. The pain associated with the initial bowel movement is great, and the patient therefore ignores the urge to defecate for fear of experiencing the pain again. This allows the formation of harder stool that tears the anoderm more as it passes because of its size and the poor relaxation of the sphincter. A self-perpetuating cycle of pain, poor relaxation, and reinjury is the result.

Factors that may predispose to fissure formation are previous anorectal surgery (hemorrhoidectomy, fistulotomy, destruction of condylomas) resulting in scarring of the anoderm with loss of elasticity, which increases the probability that the anoderm will tear.

▶ Clinical Findings

A. Symptoms and Signs

Fissures cause pain and bleeding with defecation. The pain is often tearing or burning, worst during defecation, and subsides over a few hours. Blood is noted on the tissue and stool or dripping into the toilet water, but it is not mixed in the stool. Constipation may develop because of fear of recurrent pain. Although less common, fissures may present as painless nonhealing wounds that bleed intermittently.

Although anoscopy and sigmoidoscopy may not be tolerable in the initial evaluation of a patient with a fissure, they must be done later because associated anorectal malignancy or inflammatory bowel disease must be excluded. Any nonhealing midline fissure should be biopsied to exclude Crohn disease or malignancy.

Physical examination by simple, gentle traction on the buttocks will evert the anus enough to reveal a disruption of the anoderm in the midline at the mucocutaneous junction. This may be all there is in an acute fissure. In a chronic fissure, a sentinel pile may be seen at the inferior margin of the ulcer. Gentle, limited digital examination will confirm internal sphincter spasm. Anoscopy and proctosigmoidoscopy should be deferred until healing occurs, or alternatively the procedure can be performed under anesthesia. The classic triad of a proximal hypertrophied anal papilla above a fissure with the sentinel pile at the anal verge may be identified.

B. Laboratory and Imaging Studies

Anal manometry is unhelpful. Studies have shown increased anal pressures in patients with ulcers, but patients with high pressures have not been found to be at increased risk for fissure-ulcer disease.

▶ Differential Diagnosis

Fissure-ulcer disease occurs in the anterior or posterior midline and involves the epithelium immediately distal to the dentate line. Ulcers occurring off the midline or away from the dentate line are suspect. Crohn disease, anal tuberculosis, anal malignancy, abscess or fistula disease, cytomegalovirus, herpes, chlamydiosis, syphilis, AIDS, and some blood dyscrasias may all mimic fissure or ulcer disease. Initial manifestations of Crohn disease are limited to the anal canal in 10% of patients. Anal tuberculosis will be associated with a previous or concomitant history of pulmonary tuberculosis. Anal cancer may present as a painless ulcer. Nonhealing ulcers should be biopsied to rule out malignancy.

▶ Complications

The complications are related to persistence of the disease and its associated pain, bleeding, and alteration in bowel habits. The ulcers do not become malignant.

▶ Treatment

A. Medical Treatment

Stool softeners, bulking agents, and sitz baths will heal 90% of anal fissures. A second episode has a 70% chance of healing with this regimen. Sitz baths after painful bowel movements soothe the muscle spasm. Patients are instructed to soak in a hot bath and contract the sphincters to identify the muscle in spasm and to then concentrate on relaxing that muscle. The effect is twofold: it decreases the pain associated with the spasm and improves blood flow to the fissure, which benefits healing. Stool softeners and bulking agents make the stool more malleable, decreasing the trauma of each successive bowel movement. Chronic (> 1 month history) or chronic-recurrent ulcers should be considered for surgery.

Botulinum toxin infiltration into the internal sphincters aids healing of anal fissures. This agent inhibits the release of acetylcholine from presynaptic nerve fibers, creating a reversible paralysis that lasts several months. This allows for improved perfusion of the disrupted anoderm and healing at rates higher than can be achieved with standard medical therapy or topical nitroglycerin ointment therapy.

Nitroglycerin (0.2%) is also effective treatment. Nitroglycerin ointment is a nitric oxide source. Nitric oxide, an inhibitory neurotransmitter, relaxes the internal sphincter and improves blood flow to the anoderm. The major side effect, headache, persists at the lower therapeutic range (0.2% or 0.3%), causing some limitation of this therapy. An alternative approach is to use 0.3% nifedipine ointment. The calcium-channel blockade results in sphincter relaxation without the undesirable side effect of the headache associated with systemic absorption of nitroglycerin.

B. Surgical Treatment

Lateral internal anal sphincterotomy is the procedure of choice after conservative measures have failed. This may be performed open, where an incision is made in the skin and the hypertrophied distal one third of the internal sphincter is divided under direct vision. It may also be done closed, where a scalpel is passed in the intersphincteric plane and swept medially, dividing the internal sphincter blindly. Both techniques give similar results. It is possible to disrupt the internal sphincter with a four-finger stretch, but this is an uncontrolled disruption that is associated with a higher recurrence rate and incontinence.

Prognosis

Lateral internal anal sphincterotomy is over 90% successful in the treatment of chronic anal fissure-ulcer disease. Fewer than 10% of patients so treated are incontinent to mucus and gas. The recurrence rate is less than 10%.

Altomare DF et al: Glyceryl trinitrate for chronic anal fissure: healing or headache? Results of a multicenter, randomized, placebo-controlled, double-blind trial. Dis Colon Rectum 2000;43:174.

Argov S et al: Open lateral sphincterotomy is still the best treatment for chronic anal fissure. Am J Surg 2000;179:201.

Brisinda G et al: A comparison of injections of botulinum toxin and topical nitroglycerin ointment for the treatment of chronic anal fissure. N Engl J Med 1999;341:65.

Cook TA et al: Oral nifedipine reduces resting anal pressure and heals chronic anal fissure. Br J Surg 1999;86:1269.

Fernández López F et al: Botulinum toxin for the treatment of anal fissure. Dig Surg 1999;16:515.

Garcia-Aguilar J et al: Open vs. closed sphincterotomy for chronic anal fissure: long-term results. Dis Colon Rectum 1996;39:440.

Jost WH: One hundred cases of anal fissure treated with botulin toxin: early and long-term results. Dis Colon Rectum 1997;40:1029.

Keck JO et al: Computer-generated profiles of the anal canal in patients with anal fissure. Dis Colon Rectum 1995;38:72.

Lund JN et al: A randomised, prospective, double-blind, placebo-controlled trial of glyceryl trinitrate ointment in treatment of anal fissure. Lancet 1997;349:11.

Maria G et al: A comparison of botulinum toxin and saline for the treatment of chronic anal fissure. N Engl J Med 1998;338:217.

Maria G et al: Influence of botulinum toxin site of injections on healing rate in patients with chronic anal fissure. Am J Surg 2000;179:46.

Nelson RL: Meta-analysis of operative techniques for fissure-in-ano. Dis Colon Rectum 1999;42:1424; discussion 1428.

Nelson RL: Nonsurgical therapy for anal fissure. Cochrane Database Syst Rev 2003;4:CD003431.

Nyam DC et al: Long-term results of lateral internal sphincterotomy for chronic anal fissure with particular reference to incidence of fecal incontinence. Dis Colon Rectum 1999;42:1306.

Oettle GJ: Glyceryl trinitrate vs. sphincterotomy for treatment of chronic fissure-in-ano: a randomized, controlled trial. Dis Colon Rectum 1997;40:1318.

Richard CS et al: Internal sphincterotomy is superior to topical nitroglycerin in the treatment of chronic anal fissure: results of a randomized, controlled trial by the Canadian Colorectal Surgical Trials Group. Dis Colon Rectum 2000;43:1048.

Schouten WR et al: Ischaemic nature of anal fissure. Br J Surg 1996;83:63.

INFECTIONS OF THE ANORECTUM

ANORECTAL ABSCESS & FISTULA

 ESSENTIALS OF DIAGNOSIS

▸ Severe anal pain.

▸ Palpable mass usually present on perineal or digital rectal examination.

▸ Systemic sepsis.

General Considerations

Perirectal abscess and fistulous disease not associated with a specific systemic disease is most commonly cryptoglandular in origin. The anal canal has 6–14 glands that lie in or near the plane between the internal and external sphincters. Projections from the glands pass through the internal sphincters and drain into the crypts at the dentate line. Glands may become infected when a crypt is occluded, trapping stool and bacteria within the gland. Occlusion may follow impaction of vegetable matter or edema from trauma (firm stool or foreign body) or as a result of an adjacent inflammatory process. If the crypt does not decompress into the anal canal, an abscess may develop in the intersphincteric plane. The abscess may track within or across the intersphincteric plane. Abscesses are classified according to the space they invade (Figure 31–5). The most difficult to treat occurs when the abscess tracks proximally or circumferentially within the intersphincteric plane or within the ischiorectal fossa and deep postanal space. Regardless of location, the extent of an abscess may be difficult to determine without examination under anesthesia.

Antibiotics given while allowing the abscess to mature are not helpful. Early surgical operative drainage is the best way to avoid the potentially disastrous complications of undrained perineal sepsis. When the abscesses are drained,

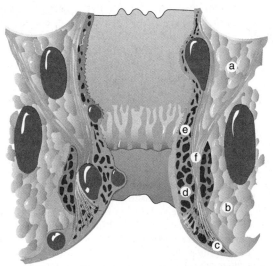

▲ **Figure 31–5.** Composite diagram of acute anorectal abscesses and spaces. (a) Pelvirectal (supralevator) space. (b) Ischiorectal space. (c) Perianal (subcutaneous) space. (d) Marginal (mucocutaneous) space. (e) Submucous space. (f) Intermuscular space.

either surgically or spontaneously, 50% have persistent communication with the crypt, creating a fistula from the anus to the perianal skin (fistula-in-ano). A fistula-in-ano is not a surgical emergency.

► Clinical Findings

A. Symptoms and Signs

An anorectal abscess typically causes severe and continuous throbbing pain that may worsen with ambulation and straining. Swelling and discharge are noted less frequently. Patients may present with fever, malaise, urinary retention, and life-threatening sepsis. People with diabetes mellitus or immune compromise are most vulnerable. A patient with fistula-in-ano may report a history of severe pain, bloody purulent drainage associated with resolution of the pain, and subsequent chronic mucopurulent discharge.

Physical examination reveals a tender perianal or rectal mass. The size is often difficult to assess until the patient is anesthetized. An apparently small abscess may extend high into the ischiorectal or supralevator space. A fistula is present when internal and external openings are identified. A firm connecting tract is often palpable.

B. Laboratory and Imaging Studies

No imaging studies are necessary in uncomplicated abscess fistulous disease. Sinograms, transrectal ultrasound, CT, and MRI may be useful in the evaluation of complex or recurrent disease. Transrectal ultrasound can identify branching of fistulous tracts, persistent undrained sepsis, and extent of sphincter involvement. Hydrogen peroxide injection of the tract may improve sensitivity of the ultrasound. CT scan may be helpful in finding an undiagnosed supralevator abscess. MRI and MRI with endorectal coil may be of use in identifying and classifying fistulas.

► Differential Diagnosis

Abscess and fistula disease of cryptoglandular origin must be differentiated from complications of Crohn disease, pilonidal disease, hidradenitis suppurativa, tuberculosis, actinomycosis, trauma, fissures, carcinoma, radiation injury, chlamydiosis, local dermal processes, retrorectal tumors, diverticulitis, and urethral injuries.

About 10% of patients with Crohn disease present with anorectal abscess fistulous disease with no antecedent history of inflammatory bowel disease. Tuberculosis may cause indolent, pale, granulomatous perianal disease, but there is usually a known history of tuberculosis. Hidradenitis suppurativa gives multiple chronic, draining fistulas, as might be seen with undiagnosed horseshoe abscess fistula disease. Pilonidal disease may extend toward the perineum; it is distinguished from cryptoglandular disease by the presence of inspissated hairs, the direction of the tract, and the presence of other openings in the sacrococcygeal area. A

colonic source may be suspected in a patient with known inflammatory bowel disease or diverticular disease. Other less common causes include tumors, radiation, infections, and urologic injuries.

► Complications

The complications of an undrained anorectal abscess may be severe. Unless drained, the infection may spread rapidly and result in extensive tissue loss, sphincter injury, and even death. In contrast, a fistula-in-ano, which develops when the abscess is drained, is not a surgical emergency. A chronic fistula may be associated with recurring perianal abscess formation and, rarely, with cancer of the fistulous tract.

► Treatment

Abscesses should be drained surgically. It is best done in the operating room, where anesthesia allows adequate evaluation of the extent of disease. Abscesses thought to be superficial in the office may be found to extend above the levators. Intersphincteric abscesses are treated by an internal sphincterotomy that drains the abscess and destroys the crypt. Perirectal and ischiorectal abscesses should be drained by a catheter or with adequate excision of skin to prevent premature closure and reaccumulation of the abscess. If the internal opening of the fistula is identified and external sphincter involvement is minimal, a fistulotomy may be performed when the abscess is drained. However, the internal opening is often hard to find because of the inflammation, and drainage is all that can be achieved. In this instance, catheter drainage is preferred to skin excision because the catheter (1) establishes drainage with minimal disruption of normal perianal skin, (2) facilitates identification of the internal opening at subsequent evaluation, and (3) facilitates patient compliance by eliminating the need for packing or leaving the wound open.

Patients with chronic or recurring abscesses after apparent adequate surgical drainage often have an undrained deep postanal space abscess that communicates with the ischiorectal fossa via a horseshoe fistula. Treatment involves opening the deep postanal space and counterdraining the tract through the ischiorectal external opening. The horseshoe fistula almost always arises from a posterior midline cryptoglandular origin. Once the postanal space heals, the counter drain may be removed.

Immunocompromised patients are a particular challenge. With moderate compromise (eg, diabetes mellitus), urgent drainage in the operating room is required, as these patients are prone to necrotizing anorectal infections. With severe compromise (eg, patients receiving chemotherapy), infection may occur without an abscess due to neutropenia. In these patients, it is important to attempt to localize the process, establish drainage, localize the internal opening, and obtain a biopsy for tissue examination and culture (to rule out leukemia and to select antibiotics).

The treatment of fistulas is dictated by the course of the fistula. The Salmon-Goodsall rule is of assistance in identifying the direction of the tract (Figure 31–6). If the tract passes superficially and does not involve sphincter muscle, a simple incision of the tract with ablation of the gland and saucerization of the skin at the external opening is all that is necessary. A fistula that involves a small amount of sphincter may be treated similarly. A tract that passes deep or that involves an undetermined amount of muscle may be initially treated with a collagen fistula plug, which has a success rate of 70.8% and 35% for simple and complex fistulas, respectively. Success rates for patients who have Crohn disease are lower than for those who do not have Crohn disease (26.6% versus 66.7%, respectively). If unsuccessful, the fistula is best treated with a mucosal advancement flap (described in the section on Rectovaginal Fistula) because immediate or delayed (as with a seton) muscle division is associated with a risk for incontinence.

▶ Prognosis

The prognosis for cryptoglandular abscess and fistula disease is excellent once the source of infection is identified. Fistulas persist when the source has not been identified or adequately drained, when the diagnosis is incorrect, or when postoperative care is insufficient.

Brook I et al: The aerobic and anaerobic bacteriology of perirectal abscesses. J Clin Microbiol 1997;35:2974.

Chapple KS et al: Prognostic value of magnetic resonance imaging in the management of fistula-in-ano. Dis Colon Rectum 2000;43:511.

Cho DY: Endosonographic criteria for an internal opening of fistula-in-ano. Dis Colon Rectum 1999;42:515.

Cintron JR et al: Repair of fistulas-in-ano using fibrin adhesive: long-term follow-up. Dis Colon Rectum 2000;43:944.

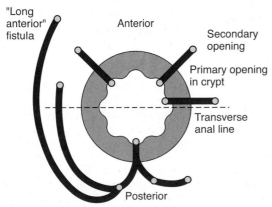

▲ **Figure 31–6.** Salmon-Goodsall rule. The usual relation of the primary and secondary openings of fistulas. When there is an anterior and also a posterior opening of the same fistula, the rule of the posterior opening applies; the long anterior fistula is an exception to the rule.

(Figure labels: "Long anterior" fistula; Anterior; Secondary opening; Primary opening in crypt; Transverse anal line; Posterior)

Garcia-Aguilar J et al: Anal fistula surgery. Factors associated with recurrence and incontinence. Dis Colon Rectum 1996;39:723.

Ho YH et al: Marsupialization of fistulotomy wounds improves healing: a randomized controlled trial. Br J Surg 1998;85:105.

Jun SH et al: Anocutaneous advancement flap closure of high anal fistulas. Br J Surg 1999;86:490.

Knoefel WT et al: The initial approach to anorectal abscesses: fistulotomy is safe and reduces the chance of recurrences. Dig Surg 2000;17:274.

Ky AJ et al: Collagen fistula plug for the treatment of anal fistulas. Dis Colon Rectum 2008;51:838

Miller GV et al: Flap advancement and core fistulectomy for complex rectal fistula. Br J Surg 1998;85:108.

Nelson RL et al: Dermal island-flap anoplasty for transsphincteric fistula-in-ano: assessment of treatment failures. Dis Colon Rectum 2000;43:681.

Park JJ et al: Repair of chronic anorectal fistulae using commercial fibrin sealant. Arch Surg 2000;135:166.

Practice parameters for treatment of fistula-in-ano—supporting documentation. The Standards Practice Task Force. The American Society of Colon and Rectal Surgeons. Dis Colon Rectum 1996;39:1363.

RECTOVAGINAL FISTULA

ESSENTIALS OF DIAGNOSIS

▶ Passing stool and flatus through the vagina.

▶ Altered continence.

▶ Tract generally visible or palpable.

▶ General Considerations

Rectovaginal fistulas occur as a result of obstetric injury, Crohn disease, diverticulitis, radiation, undrained cryptoglandular disease, foreign body trauma, surgical extirpation of anterior rectal tumors, and malignancies of the rectum, cervix, or vagina. The fistulas are classified as low, middle, or high. The location and cause of the fistula determine the operative approach.

▶ Clinical Findings

A. Symptoms and Signs

Passing stool and flatus through the vagina is characteristic of rectovaginal fistulas. There may be varying degrees of incontinence. An opening in the vagina or rectum may be seen or felt on physical examination.

B. Laboratory and Imaging Studies

A vaginogram or barium enema may identify the fistula. If the fistula is not demonstrated on radiographic or physical examination, a dilute methylene blue enema may be administered with a tampon in the vagina. If a fistula is present, it should be confirmed by methylene blue staining of the tampon.

▶ Differential Diagnosis

The signs and symptoms of a rectovaginal fistula are fairly unmistakable. The important differential is the cause of the fistula, as this affects management, as discussed shortly.

▶ Complications

The major complications of a rectovaginal fistula are impaired hygiene and incontinence.

▶ Treatment

The cause and location of the fistula determine the treatment. Involvement of surrounding tissue by the disease process that leads to the fistula may limit the surgical options. For example, in patients with active Crohn disease or radiation injury of the surrounding tissue, the fistula cannot be repaired with local procedures; Crohn disease must go into remission before a fistula can be repaired. Radiation injuries require that normal healthy tissue be brought from outside the irradiated field.

Low rectovaginal fistulas (rectal opening near the dentate line and vaginal opening just above the fourchette) commonly result from obstetric injuries, trauma from foreign bodies, cryptoglandular disease, or Crohn disease. Obstetric injuries often heal within the first 3 months. Waiting 3 months allows inflammation to resolve, which facilitates repair and allows for closure of those fistulas that will spontaneously heal. Similarly, traumatic fistulas may be repaired most easily after inflammation resolves. Fistulas secondary to cryptoglandular disease may close spontaneously once the primary process is drained.

Fistulas secondary to Crohn disease rarely heal spontaneously. Aggressive medical therapy and surgical control of perianal sepsis are necessary to conserve the sphincters. Once the disease is in remission, local advancement flap procedures may be performed. The principle is to bring fresh, uninvolved tissue down over the fistulous tract and excise the old rectal opening. This often delays proctectomy and preserves the anal sphincter and rectum. Patients with severe disease that does not respond to local measures may require a temporary diverting colostomy. After diversion, a single focus of disease is often found and an advancement procedure may be performed while the fecal stream is diverted. Extensive destruction of the rectum or sphincters may mandate immediate proctectomy without attempts at local preservation. Early surgical intervention and conservative drainage or diversion may postpone this situation.

Midrectal fistulas from cryptoglandular disease, Crohn disease, or obstetric injury should be treated as outlined previously. Those that occur secondary to radiation are not amenable to local procedures, as the surrounding tissue is similarly affected. Transabdominal resection and coloanal anastomosis is preferred. These are particularly challenging patients. Other surgical options are beyond the scope of this chapter.

High rectal fistulas result from Crohn disease, diverticular disease, operative injury, malignancy, and radiation. High rectovaginal fistulas are best treated via a transabdominal approach. This allows for resection of the diseased bowel that created the fistula.

▶ Prognosis

The prognosis is determined by the cause of the fistula.

Fry RD et al: Rectovaginal fistula. Surg Ann 1995;27:113.
Hull TL et al: Surgical approaches to low anovaginal fistula in Crohn's disease. Am J Surg 1997;173:95.
Hyman N: Endoanal advancement flap repair for complex anorectal fistula. Am J Surg 1999;178:337.
Khanduja KS et al: Reconstruction of rectovaginal fistula with sphincter disruption by combining rectal mucosal advancement flap and anal sphincteroplasty. Dis Colon Rectum 1999;42:1432.
Marchesa P et al: Advancement sleeve flaps for treatment of severe perianal Crohn's disease. Br J Surg 1998;85:1695.
Ozuner G et al: Long-term analysis of the use of transanal rectal advancement flaps for complicated anorectal/vaginal fistulas. Dis Colon Rectum 1996;39:10.
Simmang CL et al: Rectal sleeve advancement: repair of rectovaginal fistula associated with anorectal stricture in Crohn's disease. Dis Colon Rectum 1998;41:787.
Tsang CB et al: Anal sphincter integrity and function influences outcome in rectovaginal fistula repair. Dis Colon Rectum 1998;41:1141.
Tsang CB et al: Rectovaginal fistulas. Therapeutic options. Surg Clin North Am 1997;77:95.
Venkatesh KS et al: Fibrin glue application in the treatment of recurrent anorectal fistulas. Dis Colon Rectum 1999;42:1136.
Yee LF et al: Use of endoanal ultrasound in patients with rectovaginal fistulas. Dis Colon Rectum 1999;42:1057.

PILONIDAL DISEASE

 ESSENTIALS OF DIAGNOSIS

▶ Acute chronic recurring abscess or chronic draining sinus over the sacrococcygeal or perianal region.
▶ Pain, tenderness, purulent drainage, inspissated hair, induration.

▶ General Considerations

The incidence of pilonidal disease is highest in white males (3:1 male-to-female ratio) between ages 15 and 40, with a peak incidence between 16 and 20 years. It rarely occurs in patients more than 50 years old. It was once thought that pilonidal disease was a congenital condition that developed along an epithelialized tract of the natal cleft. It is now considered to be an acquired infection of natal cleft hair follicles, which become distended and obstructed and rupture into the subcutaneous tissues to form a pilonidal abscess. Hair from the surrounding skin is pulled into the abscess cavity by the friction generated by the gluteal muscles during walking.

Clinical Findings

Patients with pilonidal disease may present with small midline pits or abscesses on or off the midline near the coccyx or sacrum. The patients are generally heavy hirsute males who perspire profusely. The workup is limited to a physical examination unless one suspects Crohn disease, in which case a more extensive evaluation may be necessary. Physical examination may reveal a spectrum of disease from acute suppuration and an undrained abscess or chronic draining sinuses with multiple mature tracts with hairs protruding from the pitlike openings.

Differential Diagnosis

The differential diagnosis includes cryptoglandular abscess-fistulous disease of the anus, hidradenitis suppurativa, furuncle, and actinomycosis.

Complications

Untreated pilonidal disease may result in multiple draining sinuses with chronic recurrent abscess, drainage, soiling of clothing, and, rarely, necrotizing wound infections or malignant degeneration.

Treatment

Pilonidal abscesses may be drained under local anesthesia. A probe may be inserted into the primary opening and the abscess unroofed. Granulation tissue and inspissated hair are pulled out, but definitive therapy is not required at the first procedure. Cure rates of 60–80% have been reported after primary unroofing and extraction of hair. For those that fail to heal after 3 months or develop a chronic draining sinus, definitive therapy may be considered.

Nonoperative therapy with meticulous skin care (shaving of the natal cleft, perineal hygiene) and drainage of abscesses will substantially reduce the need for surgery.

Conservative excision of midline pits with removal of hair from lateral tracts and postoperative weekly shaving has a 90% success rate. Excision with open packing, marsupialization, or primary closure with or without flaps have all been advocated. Either open packing or marsupialization leaves the patient with painful wounds slow to heal, and marsupialization has a reported recurrence rate of 10%. Simple primary closure often results in dehiscence because the midline skin has a poor blood supply, the wounds are closed under tension, and there is often dead space at the base of the defect that is susceptible to infection. Closure over suction drainage or the use of lateral incisions with excision of the tracts decreases the rate of wound dehiscence. A recent Cochrane review showed no clear benefit supporting either primary closure or open healing by secondary intention. However, when primary closure was chosen, off-midline repairs were favored over midline repairs.

Prognosis

The prognosis after surgery is excellent. Recurrent or persistent disease has been reported to be 0–15% and is likely due to inadequate excision where external openings or occult tracts are missed. Inadequate postoperative hygiene with ingrowth of hair into the wound also leads to recurrence.

Abu Galala KH et al: Treatment of pilonidal sinus by primary closure with a transposed rhomboid flap compared with deep suturing: a prospective randomised clinical trial. Eur J Surg 1999;165:468.

Akinci OF et al: Simple and effective surgical treatment of pilonidal sinus: asymmetric excision and primary closure using suction drain and subcuticular skin closure. Dis Colon Rectum 2000;43:701.

Armstrong JH et al: Pilonidal sinus disease. The conservative approach. Arch Surg 1994;129:914.

Bozkurt MK et al: Management of pilonidal sinus with the Limberg flap. Dis Colon Rectum 1998;41:775.

McCallum I et al: Healing by primary versus secondary intention after surgical treatment for pilonidal sinus. Cochrane Database Syst Rev 2007;4:CD006213

Peterson S et al: Primary closure techniques in chronic pilonidal sinus: a survey of the results of different surgical approaches. Dis Colon Rectum 2002;45:1458.

Senapati A et al: Bascom's operation in the day-surgical management of symptomatic pilonidal sinus. Br J Surg 2000;87:1067.

Spivak H et al: Treatment of chronic pilonidal disease. Dis Colon Rectum 1996;39:1136.

PRURITUS ANI

 ESSENTIALS OF DIAGNOSIS

▶ Severe perianal itching, often at night.

▶ When chronic, skin becomes white, leathery, and thickened.

General Considerations

Pruritus ani is usually idiopathic. Most patients have tried many over-the-counter preparations without relief. These agents may exacerbate the problem by keeping the perineum moist, causing further irritation, or by creating a contact dermatitis (especially local anesthetics). Poor cleansing of the perineum may lead to irritation of the exquisitely sensitive anoderm and subsequent pruritus. In contrast, frequent washing with soaps and detergents dries the skin, also leading to pruritus. Pinworms (*Enterobius vermicularis*) are the most common cause of perianal itching in children.

Clinical Findings

A. Symptoms and Signs

The patient experiences severe perianal itching, often worse at night. The skin is thickened, white, and leathery in the chronic state but may be normal to weeping in the acute stage. In children with pinworms, perianal itching is most severe at night, when the pinworm deposits its eggs on the perianal skin.

B. Laboratory and Imaging Studies

The diagnosis of pinworms is made by applying cellophane tape to the perianal skin, which collects the eggs and allows them to be viewed under a microscope. Scrapings of the perianal skin viewed microscopically may reveal fungi or parasites. Biopsy and histologic evaluation may be necessary in refractory cases to rule out underlying malignancy.

Differential Diagnosis

Pruritus may be associated with other perianal lesions that distort normal anal anatomy, such as hemorrhoids, fistulas, fissures, tumors of the anorectum, previous surgery, and radiation therapy. As noted above, it may be secondary to excessive cleaning or application of ointments to the perianal region. Primary dermatologic diseases such as lichen planus, atopic eczema, psoriasis, and seborrheic dermatitis may all affect the perineum. Fungal (dermatophytosis, candidiasis), parasitic (*Enterobius vermicularis,* scabies, or pediculosis), and bacterial superinfection should be considered. Other causes include contact dermatitis from local anesthetic creams or soaps, recent antibiotic usage, systemic diseases (diabetes, liver disease), dietary factors, and perianal neoplasms (Bowen disease and extramammary Paget disease). Pruritus may result from tight clothing, obesity, and living in a hot climate. When a specific cause cannot be found, it is considered idiopathic.

Complications

Complications include severe excoriation, ulceration, and secondary infection of the perineum.

Treatment

Identifiable causes of pruritus ani, such as hemorrhoids, yeast infection, or parasites, should be treated. Patients should be educated about proper perineal care, and the use of soaps and topical ointments should be discouraged. The perineum should be kept dry. Use of a blow dryer on the perineum after bathing may be helpful. Alteration in dietary habits may be necessary. Coffee, tea, cola drinks, beer, chocolate, and tomatoes cause perianal itching and should be excluded from the diet for at least 2 weeks. Symptoms should resolve with alterations in dietary and cleaning habits. After symptoms resolve, each food group may be added

sequentially to identify the causative agent. Pruritus refractory to the above measures may be treated by intradermal injection of 1% methylene blue solution.

Prognosis

Relapse is common, and reeducation is often effective. In refractory cases, dermatologic and psychiatric consultation may be necessary.

PROCTITIS & ANUSITIS

Proctitis and anusitis are nonspecific terms for varying degrees of inflammation due to infectious or inflammatory diseases. The causative agent or event determines the symptoms, signs, and appropriate management. In considering these diseases, particular attention should be paid to sexual practices and sexually transmitted diseases.

1. Herpes Proctitis

Lesions appear as vesicles, which rupture to form ulcers that may become secondarily infected. Patients may present early with anal pain and vesicles or later with ulcerations, discharge, rectal bleeding, tenesmus, and even fear of defecation because of severe pain. Fever and generalized malaise are often noted. No history of anoreceptive intercourse is required, as the disease may spread by extension from the vagina. Viral culture of the vesicle or biopsy of the ulcer is diagnostic. Herpes simplex type 2 is most common.

Oral acyclovir is the treatment of choice but is not curative. It decreases the duration of outbreaks and viral shedding and increases the interval between attacks. The first episode is associated with the most pain and longest duration of ulceration. Subsequent episodes are generally shorter and not as painful.

2. Anorectal Syphilis

The chancre is an indurated, nontender perianal ulcer at the site of inoculation. Proctitis, pseudotumors, and condylomata lata may also be present. Condylomata lata are contiguous hypertrophic papules associated with secondary syphilis. Darkfield microscopy of exudate for *Treponema pallidum* and serologic testing are the preferred methods of diagnosis. Serologic tests may initially be negative and should be repeated several months later.

Penicillin is the treatment of choice. The prognosis is good. Contacts must be sought and treated.

3. Gonococcal Proctitis

Symptoms range from none to painful defecation. Rectal bleeding and discharge, perianal excoriation, and fistulas may develop. The mucosa may appear friable and edematous. Cultures of the anus, vagina, urethra, and pharynx should be obtained and plated on Thayer-Martin medium.

The gram-negative diplococcus *Neisseria gonorrhoeae* is the causative agent.

Intramuscular procaine penicillin G and oral probenecid is the treatment of choice. Resistant strains should be treated with spectinomycin. Follow-up examination and cultures should be performed to confirm adequate therapy. The prognosis is excellent.

4. Chlamydial Proctitis & Lymphogranuloma Venereum

As in gonococcal proctitis, the symptoms of chlamydial proctitis range from none to rectal pain, bleeding, and discharge. The small shallow ulcer of lymphogranuloma venereum (LGV) may go unnoticed, but the inguinal adenopathy may become quite marked. Late findings include hemorrhagic proctitis and rectal stricture. The causative agent is *Chlamydia trachomatis,* an intracellular parasite spread by anal intercourse or direct extension through the lymphatics of the rectovaginal septum. The diagnosis is made with the LGV complement fixation test. Tissue cultures are also used.

Treatment with 21 days of tetracycline is recommended, but erythromycin is an acceptable alternative. Early strictures may be dilated. Although uncommon, strictures may cause bowel obstruction and require colostomy.

5. Condylomata Acuminata

Human papilloma virus (HPV) is the cause of condylomata acuminata. Multiple types have been identified. Types HPV-6 and HPV-11 are associated with the common, benign genital wart, whereas HPV-16 and HPV-18 are associated with the development of high-grade anal dysplasia and anal cancer. In the United States, condyloma acuminatum is the most common sexually transmitted viral disease, with 1 million new cases reported per year. It is the most common anorectal infection of homosexual men and is particularly prevalent in HIV-positive patients. However, the disease is not limited to men or women who practice anoreceptive intercourse. In women, the virus may track down from the vagina, and in men it may pool and track from the base of the scrotum. Immunosuppression, either from drugs after transplantation or from HIV, increases susceptibility to condylomatous disease with prevalence rates of 5% and 85%, respectively.

▶ Clinical Findings

A. Symptoms and Signs

The most frequent complaint is that of a perianal growth. Pruritus, discharge, bleeding, odor, and anal pain are present to a lesser degree. Physical examination reveals the classic cauliflower-like lesion, which may be isolated, clustered, or coalescent. The warts tend to run in radial rows out from the anus. The lesions may be surprisingly large at the time of presentation.

B. Laboratory and Imaging Studies

Anoscopy or proctosigmoidoscopy are essential because the disease extends internally in more than three fourths of patients and because intra-anal disease is present in 95% of cases in homosexual men. Material for cultures and serologic tests for other venereal diseases may be taken from the penis, anus, mouth, and vagina.

▶ Differential Diagnosis

These lesions must be distinguished from condylomata lata, the lesions of secondary syphilis, and anal squamous cell carcinoma. Condylomata lata are flatter, paler, and smoother than condylomata acuminata. Anal squamous cell carcinoma is generally painful and may be tender and ulcerated, whereas condylomas are not tender or ulcerated.

▶ Complications

Squamous cell carcinoma of the anal canal is the major complication.

▶ Treatment & Prognosis

The extent of the disease and the risk of malignancy determine the treatment. Minimal disease is treated in the office with topical agents such as bichloracetic acid or 25% podophyllum resin in tincture of benzoin. The former is preferred, and there are fewer complications (scarring) because the latter must be washed off within 4–6 hours to limit pain. The warts respond promptly to therapy. Patients should be seen at regular intervals until resolution is complete. More extensive disease may require an initial treatment session under anesthesia so that random lesions can be excised for pathologic evaluation to rule out dysplasia and so that the remainder can be coagulated. Electrocautery coagulates the lesions. Care is taken to spare surrounding skin. Follow-up evaluation may reveal residual disease, but this is often easily treated with topical agents in the office.

Laser therapy is another method of condyloma destruction. Recurrence rates are low, but the equipment is expensive.

Recurrent disease may respond to repeat excision or destruction. Imiquimod is a topically applied immune modulator that induces interferon and cytokine release by the host tissues. It activates the host immune system to clear the HPV infection by both the innate and cell-mediated pathways. In select patients, external wart clearance has been achieved in 72–84%. Imiquimod may also be a useful adjunctive therapy following excision.

The first description of autologous vaccines was reported in 1944, but it is only recently that vaccines have shown more promise. The current vaccines target the late structural proteins of the viral capsid (E6, E7) to engender a cytotoxic T lymphocyte cell–mediated immune response. Recently, a quadrivalent vaccine that targets HPV-6, HPV-11, HPV-16, and HPV-18 has been developed for the prevention of cervical dysplasia and may have a role for the prevention of anal condylomas and anal dysplasia. Its impact on specifically preventing anal dysplasia is still being evaluated in a prospective trial.

HPV-16 and HPV-18 are causally associated with squamous cell carcinomas of the anal canal. This association has led to new screening techniques to evaluate high-risk patients for occult disease. These techniques are discussed in the section on Anal & Perianal Neoplasms. Representative biopsies of clinically apparent condylomas should be sent for pathologic study because unsuspected low-grade or high-grade dysplasia or squamous cell carcinoma of the anal canal may be found.

Buschke-Löwenstein tumors are giant condylomata acuminata that are locally aggressive and exhibit malignant behavior but benign histology. Radical excision is often the only therapeutic option for either palliation or cure. Wide local excision and even surgery with adjuvant chemotherapy and radiotherapy have been used with success.

6. Chancroid

Haemophilus ducreyi causes a soft perianal ulcer that is painful, often multiple, and bleeds easily. Autoinoculation is common. Inguinal lymph nodes become fluctuant, rupture, and drain. Cultures are diagnostic.

Treatment options include azithromycin, 1 g orally in a single dose; or ceftriaxone, 250 mg intramuscularly in a single dose; or ciprofloxacin, 500 mg orally twice daily for 3 days; or erythromycin base, 500 mg orally four times daily for 7 days. All are effective.

7. Inflammatory Proctitis

Inflammatory proctitis is a mild form of ulcerative colitis that is limited to the rectum. Rectal bleeding, discharge, diarrhea, and tenesmus are common. The rectal mucosa is inflamed and friable, but the remainder of the colon appears normal on examination. The disease course is often self-limited. Only about 10% of patients ever develop colonic manifestations of ulcerative colitis. Biopsies are taken at endoscopy to rule out infectious processes and Crohn disease.

An infectious process must be ruled out before initiating steroid therapy. Distinguishing between Crohn disease and inflammatory proctitis may be difficult. Lack of response to appropriate therapy calls for reassessment of the patient.

Steroid retention enemas are given for 2 weeks. If there is no response, a short course of oral steroids may be given. In addition, mesalamine (5-aminosalicylic acid) may be given orally or rectally in an enema or suppository. Patients should avoid milk and milk products, fruit, and dietary fiber. The disease usually responds to these measures and resolves rapidly.

8. Radiation Proctitis

Radiation proctitis in a patient with a history of radiation to the rectum is manifested early by diarrhea, rectal bleeding, discharge, tenesmus, pain, and incontinence. Late disease may develop months to years after the injury. Symptoms of late disease are secondary to strictures, fistulas, and telangiectasias, which may present as recurrent urinary tract infections, vaginal discharge, fecal incontinence, rectal bleeding, changes in stool caliber, and constipation. The symptoms include bleeding, change in bowel habits, urinary tract infections, and vaginal discharge. Endoscopy may reveal friable edematous mucosa, telangiectasias, or strictures and may show internal openings of fistulas.

Initial therapy includes bulk-forming agents, antidiarrheals, and antispasmodics. Topical steroids, mesalamine preparations, misoprostol suppositories, and short-chain fatty acids have all been used in acute and chronic disease. Refractory hemorrhagic proctitis may be treated with the application of formalin to the rectal mucosa. Dilatation of strictures and laser coagulation of telangiectasias are useful in late disease. The key to surgical success in treating fistulas to the bladder or vagina is interposition or transposition of healthy nonirradiated tissue into the field. Only infrequently is the rectum so badly irradiated that it must be removed. The prognosis, therefore, is good.

Babb RR: Radiation proctitis: a review. Am J Gastroenterol 1996;91:1309.

Berry JM, Palefsky JM: A review of human papillomavirus vaccines: from basic science to clinical trials. Frontiers Biosci 2003;8:s333.

Bjork M et al: Giant condyloma acuminatum (Buschke-Löwenstein tumor) of the anorectum with malignant transformation. Eur J Surg 1995;161:691.

Breese PL et al: Anal human papillomavirus infection among homosexual and bisexual men: prevalence of type-specific infection and association with human immunodeficiency virus. Sex Transm Dis 1995;22:7.

Chang GJ, Welton ML: Human papillomavirus, condylomata acuminata, and anal neoplasia. Clin Colon Rectal Surg 2004; 17:55.

Centers for Disease Control and Prevention: Sexually transmitted diseases treatment guidelines 2002. MMWR 2002;51.

Counter SF et al: Prospective evaluation of formalin therapy for radiation proctitis. Am J Surg 1999;177:396.

El-Attar SM et al: Anal warts, sexually transmitted diseases, and anorectal conditions associated with human immunodeficiency virus. Prim Care 1999;26:81.

Fantin AC et al: Argon beam coagulation for treatment of symptomatic radiation-induced proctitis. Gastrointest Endosc 1999; 49(4 Part 1):515.

Farouk R, Lee PW: Intradermal methylene blue injection for the treatment of intractable idiopathic pruritus ani. Br J Surg 1997;84:670.

Hakim AA et al: Indications and efficacy of the human papillomavirus vaccine. Curr Treat Options Oncol 2007;6:393.

Hemminki K et al: Cancer in husbands of cervical cancer patients. Epidemiology 2000;11:347.

Khan AM et al: A prospective randomized placebo-controlled double-blinded pilot study of misoprostol rectal suppositories in the prevention of acute and chronic radiation proctitis symptoms in prostate cancer patients. Am J Gastroenterol 2000;95:1961.

Kobal B: Herpes simplex genitalis type 2: our experiences. Clin Exp Obstet Gynec 1999;26:123.

Palefsky JM: Anal squamous intraepithelial lesions in human immunodeficiency virus-positive men and women. Semin Oncol 2000;27:471.

Palefsky JM: Anal squamous intraepithelial lesions: relation to HIV and human papillomavirus infection. J Acquir Immune Defic Syndr 1999;21(Suppl 1):S42.

Pinto A et al: Short-chain fatty acids are effective in short-term treatment of chronic radiation proctitis: randomized, double-blind, controlled trial. Dis Colon Rectum 1999;42:788.

Rompalo AM: Diagnosis and treatment of sexually acquired proctitis and proctocolitis: an update. Clin Infect Dis 1999;28(Suppl 1):S84.

Saclarides TJ et al: Formalin instillation for refractory radiation-induced hemorrhagic proctitis. Report of 16 patients. Dis Colon Rectum 1996;39:196.

Tabet SR et al: Incidence of HIV and sexually transmitted diseases (STD) in a cohort of HIV-negative men who have sex with men (MSM). AIDS 1998;12:2041.

Talley NA et al: Short-chain fatty acids in the treatment of radiation proctitis: a randomized, double-blind, placebo-controlled, cross-over pilot trial. Dis Colon Rectum 1997;40:1046.

Taylor JG et al: KTP laser therapy for bleeding from chronic radiation proctopathy. Gastrointest Endosc 2000;52:353.

FECAL IMPACTION

Fecal impaction may develop after excisional hemorrhoidectomy, in chronically debilitated patients, or from the use of constipating pain medications without stool softeners and fiber. In the hemorrhoidectomy population, preserving adequate anoderm between hemorrhoidal complexes minimizes the incidence of this complication. Postoperative pain control is essential because otherwise fear of defecation may develop. Limited use of constipating opioids, addition of nonsteroidal medications, stool bulking agents (fiber), and stool softeners will minimize the incidence of fecal impaction.

All hospitalized and postoperative patients are at risk for developing fecal impaction because of limitations on physical activity, disruption of dietary and bowel habits, and initiation of constipating medications (opioids, calcium-channel blockers, etc). Thus, patients at risk who do not suffer from diarrhea should be started on stool softeners and fiber-bulking agents to avoid this complication. Enemas and laxatives may be given as needed.

Patients with fecal impaction commonly present with diarrhea, as only liquid stool is able to pass the obstructing inspissated fecal bolus. Some may complain of pelvic pain with episodic severe spasms from the pressure of the mass on the pelvic floor. Digital rectal examination may reveal hard, dry stool that obstructs the rectum. Abdominal examination may reveal a pelvic or abdominal mass much like a gravid uterus.

Once detected, a fecal impaction may be digitally dislodged at the bedside, but treatment in the operating room with local or regional anesthesia may be necessary to provide pelvic floor relaxation and pain control. At completion of disimpaction, sigmoidoscopy is necessary to rule out an obstructing inflammatory or malignant mass or rectal injury incurred during the procedure.

Prather CM et al: Evaluation and treatment of constipation and fecal impaction in adults. Mayo Clin Proc 1998;73:881.

Tiongco FP et al: Use of oral GoLytely solution in relief of refractory fecal impaction. Dig Dis Sci 1997;42:1454.

ANAL & PERIANAL NEOPLASMS

Tumors of the anal canal account for 1.5% of malignancies of the gastrointestinal tract, with about 4650 new cases annually in the United States. The incidence has been increasing over the last 30 years. Chronic anal irritation has historically been related to the development of anal cancer, but there is an etiologic relationship between chronic infection with HPV and the development of anal cancer. Women are at increased risk for anal canal cancer, presumably because the virus may pool in the vagina and track down to the anus. Women also may practice anoreceptive intercourse in heterosexual relationships. Although in general women are at increased risk for anal cancer ($9:10^6$ versus $7:10^6$ women versus men, respectively), in HIV-negative and HIV-positive men who have sex with men, the incidence is $360:10^6$ and $700:10^6$, respectively. Other factors associated with an increased risk for anal cancer are anogenital warts; a history of sexually transmitted disease; more than 10 sexual partners (but if one has HPV, only one is necessary); a history of cervical, vulvar, or vaginal cancer; immunosuppression (HIV-positive or transplantation); long-term corticosteroids; and cigarette smoking.

High-grade squamous intraepithelial lesions (HSIL) are the putative precursor lesion to invasive squamous cell cancer of the anus. It is an increasingly prevalent condition associated with HPV infection. Treatment consists of targeted excision of involved tissues with the aid of the operating microscope and the use of acetic acid to aid in the identification of high-grade dysplasia. Such an approach is effective in controlling disease in both immunocompetent and immunocompromised patients. Recurrent disease is treated in the office with infrared coagulator ablation or trichloroacetic acid. In this way premalignant lesions can be controlled without radical surgery and with minimal morbidity.

Although women are at increased risk for anal canal cancer, this is not true of anal margin carcinoma, where men are at greater risk (4:1). This difference highlights the importance of classification based on anatomic landmarks such as the dentate line, the anal verge, and the anal sphincters. These landmarks distinguish tumors of the anal margin from tumors of the anal canal. Unfortunately, the literature is not clear with regard to these landmarks, and efforts have been made by the World Health Organization and the American Joint Committee on Cancer (AJCC) to establish anatomic landmarks to distinguish tumors of the anal canal from tumors of the anal margin. The definitions are as follows: The anal canal extends from the upper to the lower border of the internal anal sphincter (from the pelvic floor to the anal verge). Anal margin tumors occur outside the anal verge in the perianal skin but presumably within a 5–6 cm radius of the anus. Tumors of the anal canal tend to be aggressive, nonkeratinizing, and associated with HPV infection. Tumors of the anal margin are generally well-differentiated keratinizing tumors that behave similarly to other squamous cell carcinomas of the skin and are treated accordingly. The authors have proposed a new classification to aid clinicians across various specialties in the accurate description of anal neoplasms by dividing the region into three regions: intra-anal, perianal, and skin. Intra-anal lesions cannot be seen or are slightly visible upon gentle traction of the buttocks. Perianal lesions are completely visible and fall within a 5 cm radius of the anal opening upon gentle traction of the buttocks. Finally, skin lesions fall outside this 5 cm radius.

Staging of anal and perianal malignancies is clinical. Physical examination with digital rectal examination, paying attention to pararectal nodes, anoscopy, bilateral groin palpation, biopsy (examination under anesthesia, if necessary), endorectal ultrasound, CT, and MRI are used as needed to assess tumor size and establish nodal and distant disease. The AJCC staging classification for anal canal and anal margin tumors is presented in Table 31–1.

TUMORS OF THE ANAL MARGIN

1. Squamous Cell Carcinoma

Patients complain of a mass, bleeding, pain, discharge, itching, and pain or tenesmus (complaints common to most lesions of this region). Typically, the lesions are large and centrally ulcerated, with rolled, everted edges, and have been present for over 2 years before detection. All chronic or nonhealing ulcers of the perineum should be biopsied to rule out squamous cell carcinoma. Squamous cell carcinoma is more common in men.

Small, well-differentiated lesions (≤ 4 cm) are treated by wide local excision. Deep lesions that involve the sphincters require abdominoperineal resection. Chemoradiation is used for less favorable lesions. Spread is to the inguinal lymph nodes, which are generally included in the radiation fields. Excision of inguinal nodal disease is reserved for palpable and symptomatic disease. Disease recurring in the skin may be treated with reexcision or abdominoperineal resection. The T stage determines survival, with reports of 100% 5-year and 10-year survivals for T1 lesions, compared with 60% and 40% survival rates for T2 lesions at 5 and 10 years, respectively.

2. Basal Cell Carcinoma

Bleeding, itching, and pain are the presenting symptoms of basal cell carcinoma. The superficial, mobile lesions have raised, irregular edges and central ulceration. They are more frequent in men.

As with squamous cell carcinoma of the margin, treatment is by wide local excision when possible. Deeply invasive lesions may require abdominoperineal resection. Metastasis is rare, but the local recurrence rate is 30%. Local recurrence is treated with reexcision.

Table 31–1. Staging of Anal Cancer.

Anal Cancer			
Primary tumor (T stage)			
TX	Primary tumor cannot be assessed		
T0	No evidence of primary tumor		
Tis	Carcinoma in situ		
T1	≤ 2 cm		
T2	> 2–5 cm		
T3	> 5 cm		
T4	Invasion into adjacent organ(s)		
Nodal involvement (N stage)			
NX	Regional nodes cannot be assessed		
N0	No regional nodal involvement		
N1	Perirectal nodal involvement		
N2	Unilateral internal iliac/inguinal nodal involvement		
N3	Perirectal and/or bilateral internal iliac/inguinal nodal involvement		
Distant Metastasis (M stage)			
MX	Distant metastasis cannot be assessed		
M1	No distant metastasis		
M2	Distant metastasis present		
Stage Grouping			
Stage 0	Tis	N0	M0
Stage I	T1	N0	M0
Stage II	T2	N0	M0
	T3	N0	M0
Stage IIIA	T1	N1	M0
	T2	N1	M0
	T3	N1	M0
	T4	N0	M0
Stage IIIB	T4	N1	M0
	Any T	N2, N3	M0
Stage IV	Any T	Any N	M1

Adapted from *AJCC Cancer Staging Manual,* 6th ed. Springer, 2002.

3. Bowen Disease

Bowen disease (intraepithelial squamous cell carcinoma) is often associated with condylomas and can involve both the anal margin and the anal canal. Patients often complain of perianal burning, itching, or pain. Lesions are often found on routine histologic evaluation of specimens acquired during investigation of unrelated disorders. When grossly visible, the lesions appear scaly, discrete, erythematous, and sometimes pigmented. In immunocompromised patients

(HIV-positive, transplantation), a Pap smear is a useful screening technique to detect dysplasia. If the Pap smear is positive, high-resolution anoscopy with acetic acid painting may reveal otherwise occult condyloma with dysplasia.

Wide local excision with four-quadrant biopsies to establish that no residual disease persists has been the treatment of choice. Skin grafts may be necessary for larger lesions. However, there is no histologic difference between Bowen disease and HSIL, and radical skin excision ignores the intra-anal dysplastic lesions that may be even more aggressive than perianal disease. These intra-anal dysplastic lesions have been successfully managed with local excision or destruction, even in the immunocompromised host. Furthermore, fewer than 10% of patients with Bowen disease will develop invasive squamous cell carcinoma of the anus. Therefore, the need to perform radical excision and flap procedures has been questioned.

4. Paget Disease

Paget disease (intraepithelial adenocarcinoma) occurs predominantly in women. Patients are usually in the seventh or eighth decade of life. Severe, intractable anal pruritus is characteristic. On physical examination, an erythematous, eczematoid rash is apparent. Biopsy of any nonhealing lesion should be taken to rule out this diagnosis. If Paget disease is diagnosed, a thorough workup for an occult malignancy is indicated because up to 50% of patients have a coexistent gastrointestinal carcinoma.

Wide local excision is the treatment of choice. Abdominoperineal resection may be indicated for advanced disease. Lymph node dissection should be done only for palpable adenopathy. The role of chemoradiation is less clear. The prognosis is good unless there is metastatic disease or an underlying neoplasm.

Beck DE: Paget's disease and Bowen's disease of the anus. Semin Colon Rectal Surg 1995;6:143.

Chang GJ et al: Surgical treatment of high-grade anal squamous intraepithelial lesions: a prospective study. Dis Colon Rectum 2002;45:453.

Frisch M et al: Sexually transmitted infection as a cause of anal cancer. N Engl J Med 1997;337:1350.

Fuchshuber PR et al: Anal canal and perianal epidermoid cancers. J Am Coll Surg 1997;185:494.

Marchesa P et al: Perianal Bowen's disease: a clinicopathologic study of 47 patients. Dis Colon Rectum 1997;40:1286.

Marchesa P et al: Long-term outcome of patients with perianal Paget's disease. Ann Surg Oncol 1997;4:475.

Peiffert D et al: Conservative treatment by irradiation of epidermoid carcinomas of the anal margin. Int J Radiat Oncol Biol Phys 1997;39:57.

Pineda CE et al: High-resolution anoscopy targeted surgical destruction of anal high-grade squamous intraepithelial lesions: a ten-year experience. Dis Colon Rectum 2008;51:829.

Sarmiento JM et al: Paget's disease of the perianal region: an aggressive disease? Dis Colon Rectum 1997;40:1187.

Touboul E et al: Epidermoid carcinoma of the anal margin: 17 cases treated with curative-intent radiation therapy. Radiother Oncol 1995;34:195.

Welton ML et al: The etiology and epidemiology of anal cancer. Surg Oncol Clin North Am 2004;13:263.

TUMORS OF THE ANAL CANAL

1. Epidermoid (Squamous, Basaloid, Mucoepidermoid) Carcinoma

▶ Clinical Findings

In most cases, there is a long history of minor perianal complaints such as bleeding, itching, or discomfort. An indurated anal mass may be present. Disease may be extensive at presentation, with approximately half of the lesions extending beyond the bowel wall or perianal skin at presentation. Inguinal nodal metastases are found in 20% at diagnosis and another 15% over time. The workup is discussed in the section on Anal & Perianal Neoplasms.

Abdominal CT and chest radiographs may reveal liver or lung metastases. Endorectal ultrasound can determine the depth of invasion of the primary lesion and may identify pararectal nodes.

▶ Treatment

Early lesions that are small, mobile, confined to the submucosa, and well differentiated may be treated with local excision. Overall reported recurrence rates with local excision alone are high, with an average survival rate of 70% at 5 years. Local excision of the most favorable lesions results in less than 10% recurrence and 5-year survival of 100%. Larger lesions of the anal canal call for radiation therapy or multimodality treatment with chemotherapy and radiation.

Chemoradiation has now replaced surgery as first-line therapy for all but the earliest lesions, and surgery is advised only as a salvage procedure for persistent or recurrent disease. The Nigro regimen consisted of 30 Gy to the primary tumor and to the pelvic and inguinal nodes. Mitomycin (15 mg/m^2 as an intravenous bolus) was delivered on day 1 of radiation therapy. Two 4-day infusions of fluorouracil (5-FU) (1000 mg/m^2 per day) were given starting on days 1 and 28 of chemoradiation therapy. Excellent tumor responses with 80% disease-free survivals have been reported. Because of the morbidity associated with this regimen, the amount and type of chemotherapy and radiation have been modified. Radiation only, without chemotherapy, has resulted in higher local recurrence rates in multicenter randomized trials. Much of the chemotherapy toxicity is related to the mitomycin, which has increasingly been replaced by cisplatin, which is effective and is associated with fewer side effects. However, colostomy-free survival rates are higher with mitomycin C. External beam radiotherapy doses range from 35 Gy to 59 Gy; some centers use brachytherapy catheters as well.

Treatment failures occur most commonly in the pelvis at the primary site or in the locoregional lymph nodes, with disease occurring outside the pelvis in just 15% of patients. The most common site of extrapelvic failure is the liver. Salvage abdominoperineal resection for local failure with recurrent or persistent disease is associated with a 50% 5-year survival rate. Survival is related to the extent of disease at the time of failure and to nodal status before initiation of chemoradiation therapy.

Prophylactic groin dissection is not recommended, but some experts recommend that the groins be included in the radiation fields because the failure rate in the groins is 20% if they are not treated.

▶ Prognosis

Tumor size is the single-most important prognostic factor. Mobile lesions up to 2 cm in diameter have cure rates of 80%, but tumors 5 cm or more in diameter are associated with a 50% mortality. There are reports of excellent 10-year survival for T1–3 node-negative disease (88%) and T1–3 node-positive disease (50%). Metastatic disease is more likely to be present with increasing depth of invasion and size and worsening histologic grade. Distant disease is uncommon at the time of diagnosis but most commonly involves the liver when present. Subsequent metastasis out of the pelvis is not uncommon, and 40% of patients die with disease that has spread to distant sites. Lymph node involvement at the time of presentation is a bad prognostic sign.

2. Melanoma of the Anal Canal
▶ Clinical Findings

Melanoma of the anal canal accounts for less than 1% of all anal canal tumors, yet it is a common site of primary melanoma. As with other anal canal tumors, there is often a delay in diagnosis that results in advanced-stage disease at the time of presentation. Metastatic disease has been reported to be present in over one third of patients at the time of diagnosis. The lesions can be located in the anal canal, rectum, or both. The overall prognosis has been poor, with 5-year survival rates of less than 25% in several series. Most patients will die of disseminated disease.

▶ Treatment

Traditionally, treatment of primary melanoma of the anal canal has been radical surgery to include an abdomino-perineal resection (APR) with or without bilateral inguinal lymph node dissection, especially for localized small tumors. However, the uniformly poor prognosis of all patients has led many surgeons to question the appropriateness of this very morbid approach. The current approach favors wide local excision, reserving APR for those patients with bulky disease in whom a wide local excision is not possible. Very few patients present with isolated local recurrences; rather, most have disseminated disease at the time of recurrence.

▶ Prognosis

Unfortunately, the prognosis for anorectal melanoma remains poor. It remains a biologically aggressive disease that is often systemic at the time of diagnosis. It is poorly responsive to chemotherapy or radiation; however, some encouragement has been noted in a recent series of adjuvant chemoradiation after sphincter-sparing local excision, borrowing on the lessons learned from other disease sites, with an actuarial 5-year survival of 31% and actuarial local control rate of 74%. In addition to chemoradiation, some series have also used interferon-α with some improvement in survival. The development of novel therapies to treat malignant melanoma will hopefully improve the outlook for these patients.

Ajani JA et al: Fluorouracil, mitomycin, and radiotherapy vs fluorouracil, cisplatin and radiotherapy for carcinoma of the anal canal: a randomized controlled trial. JAMA 2008;299:1914.

Allal AS et al: Effectiveness of surgical salvage therapy for patients with locally uncontrolled anal carcinoma after sphincter-conserving treatment. Cancer 1999;86:405.

Ballo MT et al: Sphincter-sparing local excision and adjuvant radiation for anal-rectal melanoma. J Clin Oncol 2002;20:4555.

Brady MS et al: Anorectal melanoma. A 64-year experience at Memorial Sloan-Kettering Cancer Center. Dis Col Rectum 1995;38:146.

Doci R et al: Primary chemoradiation therapy with fluorouracil and cisplatin for cancer of the anus: results in 35 consecutive patients. J Clin Oncol 1996;14:3121.

Eng C et al: Chemotherapy and radiation of anal canal cancer: the first approach. Surg Onc Clinics N Am 2004;13:309.

Ellenhorn JD et al: Salvage abdominoperineal resection following combined chemotherapy and radiotherapy for epidermoid carcinoma of the anus. Ann Surg Oncol 1994;1:105.

Epidermoid anal cancer: results from the UKCCCR randomised trial of radiotherapy alone versus radiotherapy, 5-fluorouracil, and mitomycin. UKCCCR Anal Cancer Trial Working Party. UK Co-ordinating Committee on Cancer Research. Lancet 1996;348:1049.

Flam M et al: Role of mitomycin in combination with fluorouracil and radiotherapy, and of salvage chemoradiation in the definitive nonsurgical treatment of epidermoid carcinoma of the anal canal: results of a phase III randomized intergroup study. J Clin Oncol 1996;14:2527.

Homsi J et al: Melanoma of the anal canal: a case series. Dis Colon Rectum 2007;50:1004.

Klas JV et al: Malignant tumors of the anal canal: the spectrum of disease, treatment, and outcomes. Cancer 1999;85:1686.

Myerson RJ et al: Carcinoma of the anal canal. Am J Clin Oncol 1995;18:32.

Peiffert D et al: Preliminary results of a phase II study of high-dose radiation therapy and neoadjuvant plus concomitant 5-fluorouracil with CDDP chemotherapy for patients with anal canal cancer: a French cooperative study. Ann Oncol 1997;8:575.

Nilsson PJ et al: Salvage abdominoperineal resection in anal epidermoid cancer. Br J Surg 2002;89:1425.

Pocard M et al: Results of salvage abdominoperineal resection for anal cancer after radiotherapy. Dis Colon Rectum 1998;41:1488.

Ryan DP et al: Carcinoma of the anal canal. N Engl J Med 2000;342:792.

Smith DE et al: Cancer of the anal canal: treatment with chemotherapy and low-dose radiation therapy. Radiology 1994;191:569.

Thibault C et al: Anorectal melanoma: an incurable disease? Dis Col Rectum 1997;40:661.

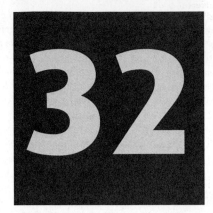

32

Hernias & Other Lesions of the Abdominal Wall*

Karen E. Deveney, MD

I. HERNIAS

An external hernia is an abnormal protrusion of intra-abdominal tissue through a fascial defect in the abdominal wall. Although the majority of hernias (75%) occurs in the groin, incisional hernias represent an increasing proportion (15–20%), with umbilical and other ventral hernias comprising the remainder. Generally, a hernial mass is composed of covering tissues (skin, subcutaneous tissues, etc), a peritoneal sac, and any contained viscera. Particularly if the neck of the sac is narrow where it emerges from the abdomen, bowel protruding into the hernia may become obstructed or strangulated. If the hernia is not repaired early, the defect may enlarge and operative repair may become more complicated. The definitive treatment of hernia is operative repair.

A **reducible hernia** is one in which the contents of the sac return to the abdomen spontaneously or with manual pressure when the patient is recumbent.

An **irreducible (incarcerated) hernia** is one whose contents cannot be returned to the abdomen, usually because they are trapped by a narrow neck. The term "incarceration" does not imply obstruction, inflammation, or ischemia of the herniated organs, though incarceration is necessary for obstruction or strangulation to occur.

Though the lumen of a segment of bowel within the hernia sac may become **obstructed,** there may initially be no interference with blood supply. Compromise to the blood supply of the contents of the sac (eg, omentum or intestine) results in a **strangulated hernia,** in which gangrene of the contents of the sac has occurred. The incidence of strangulation is higher in femoral than in inguinal hernias, but strangulation may occur in other hernias as well.

An uncommon and dangerous type of hernia, a **Richter hernia,** occurs when only part of the circumference of the bowel becomes incarcerated or strangulated in the fascial

defect. A strangulated Richter hernia may spontaneously reduce and the gangrenous piece of intestine be overlooked at operation. The bowel may subsequently perforate, with resultant peritonitis.

HERNIAS OF THE GROIN

Anatomy

All hernias of the abdominal wall consist of a peritoneal sac that protrudes through a weakness or defect in the muscular layers of the abdomen. The defect may be congenital or acquired.

Just outside the peritoneum is the **transversalis fascia,** an aponeurosis whose weakness or defect is the major source of groin hernias. Next are found the **transversus abdominis, internal oblique,** and **external oblique muscles,** which are fleshy laterally and aponeurotic medially. Their aponeuroses form investing layers of the strong **rectus abdominis muscles** above the semilunar line. Below this line, the aponeurosis lies entirely in front of the muscle. Between the two vertical rectus muscles, the aponeuroses meet again to form the **linea alba,** which is well defined only above the umbilicus. The subcutaneous fat contains the Scarpa fascia—a misnomer, since it is only a condensation of connective tissue with no substantial strength.

In the groin, an **indirect inguinal hernia** results when obliteration of the processus vaginalis, the peritoneal extension accompanying the testis in its descent into the scrotum, fails to occur. The resultant hernia sac passes through the **internal inguinal ring,** a defect in the transversalis fascia halfway between the anterior iliac spine and the pubic tubercle. The sac is located anteromedially within the spermatic cord and may extend partway along the **inguinal canal** or accompany the cord out through the subcutaneous (external) inguinal ring, a defect medially in the external oblique muscle just above the pubic tubercle. A hernia that passes fully into the scrotum is known as a **complete hernia.** The sac and the spermatic cord are invested by the **cremaster muscle,** an extension of fibers of the internal oblique muscle.

---

*See Chapter 43 for further discussion of hernias in the pediatric age group and Chapter 21 for a discussion of internal hernias.

Other anatomic structures of the groin that are important in understanding the formation of hernias and types of hernia repairs include the **conjoined tendon,** or falx inguinalis, a fusion of the medial aponeurotic transversus abdominis and internal oblique muscles that passes along the inferolateral edge of the rectus abdominis muscle and attaches to the pubic tubercle. Between the pubic tubercle and the anterior iliac spine passes the **inguinal (Poupart) ligament,** formed by the lowermost border of the external oblique aponeurosis as it rolls on itself and thickens into a cord.

Just deep and parallel to the inguinal ligament runs the **iliopubic tract,** a band of connective tissue that extends from the iliopsoas fascia, crosses below the deep inguinal ring, forms the superior border of the femoral sheath, and inserts into the superior pubic ramus to form the **lacunar (Gimbernat) ligament.** The lacunar ligament is about 1.25 cm long and triangular in shape. The sharp, crescentic lateral border of this ligament is the unyielding noose for the strangulation of a femoral hernia.

The **Cooper ligament** is a strong, fibrous band that extends laterally for about 2.5 cm along the iliopectineal line on the superior aspect of the superior pubic ramus, starting at the lateral base of the lacunar ligament.

The **Hesselbach triangle** is bounded by the inguinal ligament, the inferior epigastric vessels, and the lateral border of the rectus muscle. A weakness or defect in the transversalis fascia, which forms the floor of this triangle, results in a **direct inguinal hernia.** In most direct hernias, the transversalis fascia is diffusely attenuated, though a discrete defect in the fascia may occasionally occur. This **funicular** type of direct inguinal hernia is more likely to become incarcerated, since it has distinct borders.

A **femoral hernia** passes beneath the iliopubic tract and inguinal ligament into the upper thigh. The predisposing anatomic feature for femoral hernias is a small empty space between the lacunar ligament medially and the femoral vein laterally—the **femoral canal.** Because its borders are distinct and unyielding, a femoral hernia has the highest risk of incarceration and strangulation of groin hernias.

Surgeons must be familiar with the pathways of the nerves and blood vessels of the inguinal region to avoid injuring them when repairing groin hernias. The iliohypogastric nerve (T12, L1) emerges from the lateral edge of the psoas muscle and travels inside the external oblique muscle, emerging medial to the external inguinal ring to innervate the suprapubic skin. The ilioinguinal nerve (L1) parallels the iliohypogastric nerve and travels on the surface of the spermatic cord to innervate the base of the penis (or mons pubis), the scrotum (or labia majora), and the medial thigh. This nerve is the most frequently injured in anterior open inguinal hernia repairs. The genitofemoral (L1, L2) and lateral femoral cutaneous nerves (L2, L3) travel on and lateral to the psoas muscle and provide sensation to the scrotum and anteromedial thigh and to the lateral thigh, respectively. These nerves are subject to injury during lap-

aroscopic hernia repairs. The femoral nerve (L2–L4) travels from the lateral edge of the psoas and extends lateral to the femoral vessels. It can be injured during laparoscopic or femoral hernia repairs.

The external iliac artery travels along the medial aspect of the psoas muscle and beneath the inguinal ligament, giving off the inferior epigastric artery, which borders the medial aspect of the internal inguinal ring. The corresponding veins accompany the arteries. These vessels can be injured during hernia repairs of all types.

▶ Causes

Nearly all inguinal hernias in infants, children, and young adults are **indirect inguinal hernias.** Although these "congenital" hernias most often present during the first year of life, the first clinical evidence of hernia may not appear until middle or old age, when increased intra-abdominal pressure and dilation of the internal inguinal ring allow abdominal contents to enter the previously empty peritoneal diverticulum. An untreated indirect hernia will inevitably dilate the internal ring and displace or attenuate the inguinal floor. The peritoneum may protrude on either side of the inferior epigastric vessels to give a combined direct and indirect hernia, called a **pantaloon hernia.**

In contrast, **direct inguinal hernias** are acquired as the result of a developed weakness of the transversalis fascia in the Hesselbach area. There is some evidence that direct inguinal hernias may be related to hereditary or acquired defects in collagen synthesis or turnover. **Femoral hernias** involve an acquired protrusion of a peritoneal sac through the femoral ring. In women, the ring may become dilated by the physical and biochemical changes during pregnancy.

Any condition that chronically increases intra-abdominal pressure may contribute to the appearance and progression of a hernia. Marked obesity, abdominal strain from heavy exercise or lifting, cough, constipation with straining at stool, and prostatism with straining on micturition are often implicated. Cirrhosis with ascites, pregnancy, chronic ambulatory peritoneal dialysis, and chronically enlarged pelvic organs or pelvic tumors may also contribute. Loss of tissue turgor in the Hesselbach area, associated with a weakening of the transversalis fascia, occurs with advancing age and in chronic debilitating disease.

Skandalakis JE et al: Embryologic and anatomic basis of inguinal herniorrhaphy. Surg Clin North Am 1993;73:799.

INDIRECT & DIRECT INGUINAL HERNIAS

▶ Clinical Findings

A. Symptoms

Most hernias produce no symptoms until the patient notices a lump or swelling in the groin, though some patients may describe a sudden pain and bulge that occurred while lifting or straining. Frequently, hernias are detected in the course of routine physical examinations such as preemployment examinations. Some patients complain of a dragging sensation and, particularly with indirect inguinal hernias, radiation of pain into the scrotum. As a hernia enlarges, it is likely to produce a sense of discomfort or aching pain, and the patient must lie down to reduce the hernia.

In general, direct hernias produce fewer symptoms than indirect inguinal hernias and are less likely to become incarcerated or strangulated.

B. Signs

Examination of the groin reveals a mass that may or may not be reducible. The patient should be examined both supine and standing and also with coughing and straining, since small hernias may be difficult to demonstrate. The external ring can be identified by invaginating the scrotum and palpating with the index finger just above and lateral to the pubic tubercle (Figure 32–1). If the external ring is very small, the examiner's finger may not enter the inguinal canal, and it may be difficult to be sure that a pulsation felt on coughing is truly a hernia. At the other extreme, a widely patent external ring does not by itself constitute hernia. Tissue must be felt protruding into the inguinal canal during coughing in order for a hernia to be diagnosed.

Differentiating between direct and indirect inguinal hernia on examination is difficult and is of little importance, since most groin hernias should be repaired regardless of type. Nevertheless, each type of inguinal hernia has specific features more common to it. A hernia that descends into the scrotum is almost certainly indirect. On inspection with the patient erect and straining, a direct hernia more commonly appears as a symmetric, circular swelling at the external ring; the swelling disappears when the patient lies down. An indirect hernia appears as an elliptic swelling that may not reduce easily.

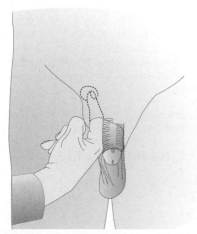

▲ **Figure 32–1.** Insertion of finger through upper scrotum into the external inguinal ring.

On palpation, the posterior wall of the inguinal canal is firm and resistant in an indirect hernia but relaxed or absent in a direct hernia. If the patient is asked to cough or strain while the examining finger is directed laterally and upward into the inguinal canal, a direct hernia protrudes against the side of the finger, whereas an indirect hernia is felt at the tip of the finger.

Compression over the internal ring when the patient strains may also help to differentiate between indirect and direct hernias. A direct hernia bulges forward through Hesselbach triangle, but the opposite hand can maintain reduction of an indirect hernia at the internal ring.

These distinctions are obscured as a hernia enlarges and distorts the anatomic relationships of the inguinal rings and canal. In most patients, the type of inguinal hernia cannot be established accurately before surgery.

▶ Differential Diagnosis

Groin pain of musculoskeletal or obscure origin may be difficult to distinguish from hernia. Herniography, in which x-rays are obtained after intraperitoneal injection of contrast medium, may aid in the diagnosis in cases of groin pain when no hernia can be felt even after multiple maneuvers to increase intra-abdominal pressure.

Herniation of preperitoneal fat through the inguinal ring into the spermatic cord ("lipoma of the cord") is commonly misinterpreted as a hernia sac. Its true nature may only be confirmed at operation. Occasionally, a femoral hernia that has extended above the inguinal ligament after passing through the fossa ovalis femoris may be confused with an inguinal hernia. If the examining finger is placed on the pubic tubercle, the neck of the sac of a femoral hernia lies lateral and below, while that of an inguinal hernia lies above.

Inguinal hernia must be differentiated from hydrocele of the spermatic cord, lymphadenopathy or abscesses of the groin, varicocele, and residual hematoma following trauma or spontaneous hemorrhage in patients taking anticoagulants. An undescended testis in the inguinal canal must also be considered when the testis cannot be felt in the scrotum.

The presence of an impulse in the mass with coughing, bowel sounds in the mass, and failure to transilluminate are features that indicate that an irreducible mass in the groin is a hernia.

▶ Treatment

Although inguinal hernias have traditionally been repaired electively to avoid the risks of incarceration, obstruction, and strangulation, asymptomatic or mildly symptomatic hernias may be safely observed in elderly, sedentary patients or those with high morbidity for operation. The annual risk of hernia incarceration is not precisely known but has been estimated at 2–3 per 1000 patients per year. All symptomatic groin hernias should be repaired if the patient can tolerate surgery.

Even elderly patients tolerate elective repair of a groin hernia very well when other medical problems are optimally controlled and local anesthetic is used. Emergency operation carries a much greater risk for the elderly than carefully planned elective operation.

If the patient has significant prostatic hyperplasia, it is prudent to solve this problem first, since the risks of urinary retention and urinary tract infection are high following hernia repair in patients with significant prostatic obstruction.

Although most direct hernias do not carry as high a risk of incarceration as indirect hernias, the difficulty in reliably differentiating them from indirect hernias makes the repair of all symptomatic inguinal hernias advisable. Direct hernias of the funicular type, which are particularly likely to incarcerate, should always be repaired.

Because of the possibility of strangulation, an incarcerated, painful, or tender hernia usually requires an emergency operation. Nonoperative reduction of an incarcerated hernia may first be attempted. The patient is placed with hips elevated and given analgesics and sedation sufficient to promote muscle relaxation. Repair of the hernia may be deferred if the hernia mass reduces with gentle manipulation and if there is no clinical evidence of strangulated bowel. Though strangulation is usually clinically evident, gangrenous tissue can occasionally be reduced into the abdomen by manual or spontaneous reduction. It is therefore safest to repair the reduced hernia at the earliest opportunity. At surgery, one must decide whether to explore the abdomen to make certain that the intestine is viable. If the patient has leukocytosis or clinical signs of peritonitis or if the hernia sac contains dark or bloody fluid, the abdomen should be explored.

A. Principles of Operative Treatment of Inguinal Hernia

(1) Successful repair requires that any correctable aggravating factors be identified and treated (chronic cough, prostatic obstruction, colonic tumor, ascites, etc) and that the defect be reconstructed with the best available tissues that can be approximated without tension.

(2) An indirect hernia sac should be anatomically isolated, dissected to its origin from the peritoneum, and ligated (Figure 32–2). In infants and young adults in whom the inguinal anatomy is normal, repair can usually be limited to high ligation, removal of the sac, and reduction of the internal ring to an appropriate size. For most adult hernias, the inguinal floor should also be reconstructed. The internal ring should be reduced to a size just adequate to allow egress of the cord structures. In women, the internal ring can be totally closed to prevent recurrence through that site.

(3) In direct inguinal hernia (Figure 32–3), the inguinal floor is usually so weak that a primary repair using the patient's own tissues would be under tension. Although a vertical relaxing incision in the anterior rectus abdominis sheath was traditionally used, most hernia repairs are now performed using mesh so that a tension-free repair can be accomplished.

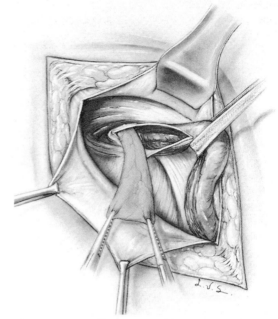

▲ **Figure 32–2.** Indirect inguinal hernia. Inguinal canal opened, showing spermatic cord retracted medially and indirect hernia peritoneal sac dissected free to above the level of the internal inguinal ring.

(4) Even though a direct hernia is found, the cord should always be carefully searched for a possible indirect hernia as well.

(5) In patients with large hernias, bilateral repair has traditionally been discouraged under the assumption that greater tension on the repair would result and therefore would increase the recurrence rate and surgical complications. If open mesh repair or laparoscopic methods are used, however, bilateral repairs can be done with low risk of recurrence. In children and adults with small hernias, bilateral hernia repair is usually recommended because it spares the patient a second anesthetic.

(6) Recurrent hernia within a few months or a year of operation usually indicates an inadequate repair, such as overlooking an indirect sac, missing a femoral hernia, or failing to repair the fascial defect securely. Any repair completed under tension is subject to early recurrence. Recurrences 2 or more years after repair are more likely to be caused by progressive weakening of the patient's fascia. Repeated recurrence after careful repair by an experienced surgeon suggests a defect in collagen synthesis. Because the fascial defect is often small, firm, and unyielding, recurrent hernias are much more likely than unoperated inguinal hernias to develop incarceration or strangulation, and they should nearly always be repaired again.

If recurrence is due to an overlooked indirect sac, the posterior wall is often solid and removal of the sac may be all

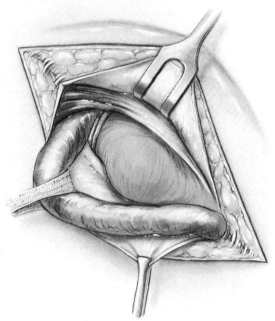

▲ **Figure 32–3.** Direct inguinal hernia. Inguinal canal opened and spermatic cord retracted inferiorly and laterally to reveal the hernia bulging through the floor of the Hesselbach triangle.

that is required. Occasionally, a recurrence is discovered to consist of a small, sharply circumscribed defect in the previous hernioplasty, in which case closure of the defect suffices.

B. Types of Operations for Inguinal Hernia

The goal of all hernia repairs is to reduce the contents of the hernia into the abdomen and to close the fascial defect in the inguinal floor. Traditional repairs approximated native tissues using permanent sutures. More recently, permanent mesh has supplanted tissue repairs because multiple prospective, randomized studies have shown lower recurrence with tension-free mesh repairs.

Over the past decade, increased experience has been gained with minimally invasive techniques for hernia repair. Although laparoscopic approaches offer less pain and more rapid return to work or normal activities, randomized trials comparing open-end laparoscopic hernia repairs do not demonstrate superiority of any specific approach with regard to overall complications or recurrence rates. The success of laparoscopic approaches is dependent on experience of the surgeon, as is also true for open repair.

Although repairs today overwhelmingly employ prosthetic material, the presence of infection or need to resect gangrenous bowel may make use of nonbiologic mesh unwise. In these situations, primary tissue repairs may still be

a preferable option. For this reason, surgeons need to know the traditional techniques even though they are rarely used today.

Among the traditional autologous tissue repairs, the **Bassini repair** is the most widely used method. In this repair, the conjoined tendon is approximated to the Poupart ligament, and the spermatic cord remains in its normal anatomic position under the external oblique aponeurosis. The **Halsted repair** places the external oblique beneath the cord but otherwise resembles the Bassini repair. **Cooper ligament (Lotheissen-McVay) repair** brings the conjoined tendon farther posteriorly and inferiorly to the Cooper ligament. Unlike the Bassini and Halsted methods, McVay repair is effective for femoral hernia but always requires a relaxing incision to relieve tension. Recurrence rates after these open nonmesh repairs vary widely according to skill and experience of the surgeon but range around 10%. Though the **Shouldice repair** has a low reported recurrence rate, it is not widely used, perhaps because of the more extensive dissection required and a belief that the skill of the surgeons may be as important as the method itself. In the Shouldice repair, the transversalis fascia is first divided and then imbricated to the Poupart ligament. Finally, the conjoined tendon and internal oblique muscle are also approximated in layers to the inguinal ligament.

The **open preperitoneal approach** exposes the groin from between the transversalis fascia and peritoneum via a lower abdominal incision to effect closure of the fascial defect. Because it requires more initial dissection and is associated with higher morbidity and recurrence rates in less experienced hands, it has not been widely used. For recurrent or large bilateral hernias, a preperitoneal approach using a large piece of mesh to span all areas of potential herniation has been described by Stoppa. Laparoscopic preperitoneal approaches have demonstrated excellent success, with low recurrence and complications in experienced hands.

A desire to decrease the recurrence rate of hernias has prompted the increased use of prosthetic materials in repair of both recurrent and first-time hernias. Methods include "plugs" of mesh inserted into the internal ring and sheets of mesh to create a tension-free repair. The most widely used technique is that of Lichtenstein, an open mesh repair that allows an early return to normal activities and a low complication and recurrence rate.

Virtually all laparoscopic approaches utilize mesh in the repair. Several methods have been explored, from a transabdominal intraperitoneal onlay of mesh (IPOM) to a transabdominal preperitoneal mesh technique (TAPP) to total extraperitoneal (preperitoneal) mesh placement (TEP). The high incidence of complications that occurred in early studies prompted revisions in the operative technique to avoid injury to lateral nerves. Several prospective randomized trials have subsequently been conducted comparing open with minimally invasive techniques and one type of minimally invasive technique with another. These studies generally have demonstrated decreased pain and faster return to work with the minimally invasive techniques but at increased time and cost of the procedure. Laparoscopic procedures also require general anesthesia and therefore are not appropriate for all patients. Because success of laparoscopic hernia repair is highly dependent on the skill and experience of the surgeon, few inguinal hernias are repaired laparoscopically. Specific situations in which minimally invasive procedures may be particularly advantageous include the repair of multiply recurrent hernias after anterior open repairs, repair of bilateral hernias simultaneously, and repair in patients who must return to work particularly quickly.

C. Nonsurgical Management (Use of a Truss)

The surgeon is occasionally called upon to prescribe a truss when a patient refuses operative repair or when there are absolute contraindications to operation. A truss should be fitted to provide adequate external compression over the defect in the abdominal wall. It should be taken off at night and put on in the morning before the patient arises. The use of a truss does not preclude later repair of a hernia, although it may cause fibrosis of the anatomic structures, so that subsequent repair may be more difficult.

► Preoperative & Postoperative Course

Although groin hernia repair is usually an outpatient procedure, a thorough preoperative evaluation should be completed before the day of surgery. The anesthetic may be general, spinal, or local. Local anesthetic is effective for most patients, and the incidence of urinary retention and pulmonary complications is lowest with local anesthesia. Recurrent hernias are more easily repaired with the patient under spinal or general anesthesia, since local anesthetic does not readily diffuse through scar tissue. A sedentary worker may return to work within a few days; heavy manual labor has traditionally not been performed for up to 4–6 weeks after hernia repair, though recent studies document no increase in recurrence when full activity is resumed as early as 2 weeks after surgery, particularly when open or laparoscopic mesh repairs have been used.

► Prognosis

In addition to chronic cough, prostatism, and constipation, poor tissue quality and poor operative technique may contribute to recurrence of inguinal hernia. Because tissue is often more attenuated in direct hernias, recurrence rates are higher than for indirect hernias. Placing the repair under tension leads to recurrence. Failure to find an indirect hernia, to dissect the sac high enough, or to adequately close the internal ring may lead to recurrence of indirect hernia. Postoperative wound infection is associated with increased recurrence. The recurrence rate is considerably increased in patients receiving chronic peritoneal dialysis—in one report, the rate was as high as 27%.

Recurrence rates after indirect hernia repair in adults are reported at best to be 0.6–3%, though the incidence is more probably 5–10%. Inadequate sac reduction or internal ring closure and failure to identify a femoral or direct hernia contribute to recurrence. A wide range of figures is quoted for recurrence after repair of direct hernias, from less than 1% to as high as 28%. The point of recurrence is most often just lateral to the pubic tubercle, implicating excessive tension on the repair and adding evidence to favor mesh repairs or the use of a relaxing incision in the rectus sheath if a traditional autologous tissue method is used in the repair of a direct hernia. The use of mesh in hernia repairs decreases the recurrence risk by 50–75%.

Another unappreciated sequela of groin hernia repair is chronic groin pain, which may occur in as high as 10% of patients and is usually attributed to nerve entrapment or neuroma.

Arvidsson D et al: Randomized clinical trial comparing 5-year recurrence rate after laparoscopic versus Shouldice repair of primary inguinal hernia. Br J Surg 2005;92:1085.

Cheek CM et al: Trusses in the management of hernia today. Br J Surg 1995;82:1611.

Eklund A et al: Recurrent inguinal hernia: randomized multicenter trial comparing laparoscopic and Lichtenstein repair. Surg Endosc 2007;21:634.

The EU Hernia Trialists Collaboration: Repair of groin hernia with synthetic mesh: Meta-analysis of randomized controlled trials. Ann Surg 2002;235:322.

Fitzgibbons R et al: Watchful waiting versus repair of inguinal hernia in minimally symptomatic men. JAMA 2006;295:285.

Grunwaldt L et al: Is laparoscopic inguinal hernia repair an operation of the past? JACS 2005;200:616.

Kark AE et al: 3175 primary inguinal hernia repairs: advantages of ambulatory open mesh repair using local anesthesia. J Am Coll Surg 1998;186:447.

Matthews R: Factors associated with postoperative complications and hernia recurrence for patients undergoing inguinal hernia repair: a report from the VA Cooperative Hernia Study Group. Am J Surg 2007;194:611.

McCormack K et al: Laparoscopic techniques versus open techniques for inguinal hernia repair. Cochrane Database Syst Rev 2004;4:CD001785.

Mellinger J et al: Primary inguinal hernia repair: open or laparoscopic, that is the question. Surg Endosc 2004;18:144.

Neumayer L et al: Open mesh versus laparoscopic mesh repair of inguinal hernia. New Engl J Med 2004;350:1819.

Scott NW et al: Open mesh versus non-mesh for groin hernia repair. Cochrane Database Syst Rev 2004;4:CD002197.

SLIDING INGUINAL HERNIA

A sliding inguinal hernia (Figures 32–4 and 32–5) is an indirect inguinal hernia in which the wall of a viscus forms a portion of the wall of the hernia sac. On the right side, the cecum is most commonly involved, and on the left side, the sigmoid colon. The development of a sliding hernia is related to the variable degree of posterior fixation of the large bowel or other sliding components (eg, bladder, ovary) and their proximity to the internal inguinal ring.

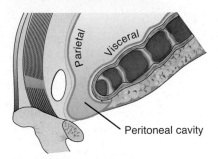

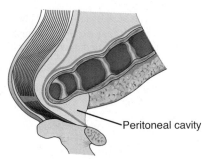

▲ Figure 32–4. Right-sided sliding hernia, sagittal view. *Top:* Note cecum and ascending colon sliding on fascia of posterior abdominal wall. *Bottom:* Hernia has entered internal inguinal ring. Note that one fourth of the hernia is not related to the peritoneal sac.

▶ Clinical Findings

Though sliding hernias have no special signs that distinguish them from other inguinal hernias, they should be suspected in any large hernia that cannot be completely reduced. Finding a segment of colon in the scrotum on contrast radiograph strongly suggests a sliding hernia. Recognition of this variation is of great importance at operation, since failure to recognize it may result in inadvertent entry into the lumen of the bowel or bladder.

▶ Treatment

It is essential to recognize the entity at an early stage of operation. As is true of all indirect inguinal hernias, the sac will lie anteriorly, but the posterior wall of the sac will be formed to a greater or lesser degree by colon or bladder.

After the cord has been dissected free from the hernia sac, most sliding hernias can be reduced by a series of inverting sutures (Bevan technique) and one of the standard types of inguinal repair performed. Very large sliding hernias may have to be reduced by entering the peritoneal cavity through a separate incision (La Roque technique), pulling the bowel back into the abdomen, and fixing it to the posterior abdominal wall. The hernia is then repaired in the usual fashion.

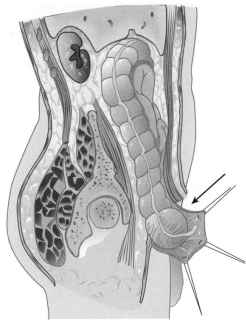

▲ Figure 32–5. Right-sided sliding hernia seen in sagittal section. At arrow, the wall of the cecum forms a portion of the hernia sac.

▶ Prognosis

Sliding hernias have a higher recurrence rate than uncomplicated indirect hernias.

The surgical complication most often encountered following sliding hernia repair is bowel or bladder injury. Injury can best be avoided by simply reducing the hernia and sac into the preperitoneal space and repairing the hernia defect.

Bendavid R: Sliding hernias. Hernia 2002;6:137.

FEMORAL HERNIA

A femoral hernia descends through the femoral canal beneath the inguinal ligament. Because of its narrow neck, it is prone to incarceration and strangulation. Femoral hernia is much more common in women than in men, but in both sexes femoral hernia is less common than inguinal hernia. Femoral hernias comprise about one third of groin hernias in women and about 2% of groin hernias in men.

▶ Clinical Findings

A. Symptoms

Femoral hernias are notoriously asymptomatic until incarceration or strangulation occurs. Even with obstruction or strangulation, the patient may feel discomfort more in the abdomen than in the femoral area. Thus, colicky abdominal pain and signs of intestinal obstruction frequently are the presenting manifestations of a strangulated femoral hernia, without discomfort, pain, or tenderness in the femoral region.

B. Signs

A femoral hernia may present in a variety of ways. If it is small and uncomplicated, it usually appears as a small bulge in the upper medial thigh just below the level of the inguinal ligament. Because it may be deflected anteriorly through the fossa ovalis femoris to present as a visible or palpable mass at or above the inguinal ligament, it can be confused with an inguinal hernia.

▶ Differential Diagnosis

Femoral hernia must be distinguished from inguinal hernia, a saphenous varix, and femoral adenopathy. A saphenous varix transmits a distinct thrill when a patient coughs, and it appears and disappears instantly when the patient stands or lies down—in contrast to femoral hernias, which are either irreducible or reduce gradually on pressure.

▶ Treatment

A. Principles

The principles of femoral hernia repair are as follows: (1) complete excision of the hernia sac, (2) the use of nonabsorbable sutures, (3) repair of the defect in the transversalis fascia that is responsible for the hernia, and (4) use of the Cooper ligament or iliopubic tract for the repair, since these structures give a firm support for sutures and form the natural line for closure of the defect.

B. Types of Repair for Femoral Hernia

A femoral hernia can be repaired through an inguinal, thigh, preperitoneal, or abdominal approach, though the inguinal approach is most commonly used. No matter what the approach, the hernia is often difficult to reduce. Reduction may be facilitated by carefully incising the iliopubic tract, Gimbernat ligament, or even the inguinal ligament. Occasionally, a counterincision in the thigh is required to free attachments below the inguinal ligament.

Irrespective of the approach used, successful femoral hernia repair must close the femoral canal. The Lotheissen-McVay repair, also used for inguinal hernia, is most commonly employed.

If the hernia sac and mass reduce when the patient is given opiates or anesthesia and if bloody fluid appears in the hernia sac when it is exposed and opened, one must strongly suspect the possibility of nonviable bowel in the peritoneal cavity. In such cases, it is mandatory to open and explore the abdomen, usually through a separate midline incision. The laparoscopic approach is well suited for repair of femoral hernias.

▶ Prognosis

Recurrence rates usually approximate the middle range for direct inguinal hernia: about 5–10%.

Glassow F: Femoral hernia: review of 2,105 repairs in a 17 year period. Am J Surg 1985;150:353.
Hernandez-Richter T: The femoral hernia: an ideal approach for the transabdominal preperitoneal technique (TAPP). Surg Endos 2000;14:736.

OTHER TYPES OF HERNIAS

UMBILICAL HERNIAS IN ADULTS

Umbilical hernia in adults occurs long after closure of the umbilical ring and is due to a gradual yielding of the cicatricial tissue closing the ring. It is more common in women than in men.

Predisposing factors include (1) multiple pregnancies with prolonged labor, (2) ascites, (3) obesity, and (4) large intra-abdominal tumors.

▶ Clinical Findings

In adults, umbilical hernia does not usually obliterate spontaneously, as in children, but instead increases steadily in size. The hernia sac may have multiple loculations. Umbilical hernias usually contain omentum, but small and large bowel may be present. Emergency repair is often necessary, because the neck of the hernia is usually quite narrow compared to the size of the herniated mass and incarceration and strangulation are common.

Umbilical hernias with tight rings are often associated with sharp pain on coughing or straining. Very large umbilical hernias more commonly produce a dragging or aching sensation.

▶ Treatment

Umbilical hernia in an adult should be repaired expeditiously to avoid incarceration and strangulation. Repairs utilizing mesh result in the lowest recurrence rate. The laparoscopic approach is associated with less postoperative pain and faster recovery than open techniques. Mesh should be used for all but the smallest umbilical hernias.

The presence of cirrhosis and ascites does not contraindicate repair of an umbilical hernia, since incarceration, strangulation, and rupture are particularly dangerous in patients with these disorders. If significant ascites exists, however, it should first be controlled medically or by TIPS (transjugular intrahepatic portosystemic shunt) if necessary, since mortality, morbidity, and recurrence are higher after hernia repair in patients with ascites. Preoperative correction of fluid and electrolyte imbalance and improvement of nutrition improves the outcome in these patients.

Prognosis

Factors that lead to a high rate of complication and recurrence after surgical repair include large size of the hernia, old age or debility of the patient, obesity, and the presence of related intra-abdominal disease. In healthy individuals, surgical repair of the umbilical defects gives good results with a low rate of recurrence.

Arroyo A et al: Randomized clinical trial comparing suture and mesh repair of umbilical hernia in adults. Br J Surg 2001;88:1321.

Hansen J et al: Danish nationwide cohort study of postoperative death in patients with liver cirrhosis undergoing hernia repair. Br J Surg 2002;89:805.

Lau H et al: Umbilical hernia in adults. Surg Endos 2003;17:2016.

EPIGASTRIC HERNIA

An epigastric hernia (Figure 32–6) protrudes through the linea alba above the level of the umbilicus. The hernia may develop through one of the foramina of egress of the small paramidline nerves and vessels or through an area of congenital weakness in the linea alba.

About 3–5% of the population have epigastric hernias. They are more common in men than in women and most common between the ages of 20 and 50. About 20% of epigastric hernias are multiple, and about 80% occur just off the midline.

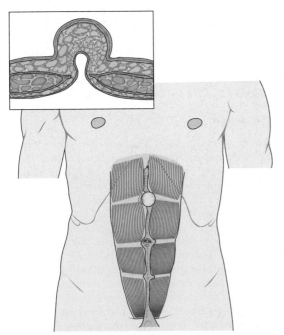

▲ **Figure 32–6.** Epigastric hernia. Note closeness to midline and presence in upper abdomen. The herniation is through the linea alba.

Clinical Findings

A. Symptoms

Most epigastric hernias are painless and are found on routine abdominal examination. If symptomatic, their presentation ranges from mild epigastric pain and tenderness to deep, burning epigastric pain with radiation to the back or the lower abdominal quadrants. The pain may be accompanied by abdominal bloating, nausea, or vomiting. The symptoms often occur after a large meal and on occasion may be relieved by reclining, probably because the supine position causes the herniated mass to drop away from the anterior abdominal wall. The smaller masses most frequently contain only preperitoneal fat and are especially prone to incarceration and strangulation. These smaller hernias are often tender. Larger hernias seldom strangulate and may contain, in addition to preperitoneal fat, a portion of the nearby omentum and, occasionally, a loop of small or large bowel.

B. Signs

If a mass is palpable, the diagnosis can often be confirmed by any maneuver that will increase intra-abdominal pressure and thereby cause the mass to bulge anteriorly. The diagnosis is difficult to make when the patient is obese, since a mass is hard to palpate; ultrasound, CT, or tangential radiographs may be needed in the very obese patient.

Differential Diagnosis

Differential diagnosis includes peptic ulcer, gallbladder disease, hiatal hernia, pancreatitis, and upper small bowel obstruction. On occasion, it may be impossible to distinguish the hernial mass from a subcutaneous lipoma, fibroma, or neurofibroma.

Another condition that must be distinguished from an epigastric hernia is **diastasis recti,** a diffuse widening and attenuation of the linea alba without a fascial defect. On examination, this condition appears as a fusiform, linear bulge between the two rectus abdominis muscles without a discrete fascial defect. Although this condition may be unsightly, repair should be avoided since there is no risk of incarceration, the fascial layer is weak, and the recurrence rate is high.

Treatment

Most epigastric hernias should be repaired, since small ones are likely to become incarcerated and large ones are often symptomatic and unsightly. Small defects can usually be closed primarily, although mesh should be used for large hernias. Herniated fat contents are usually dissected free and removed. Intraperitoneal herniating structures are reduced, but no attempt is made to close the peritoneal sac.

Prognosis

The recurrence rate is 10–20%, a higher incidence than with the routine inguinal or femoral hernia repair. This high recurrence rate may be partly due to failure to recognize and repair multiple small defects.

Muschaweck U: Umbilical and epigastric hernia repair. Surg Clin North Am 2003;83:1321.

INCISIONAL HERNIA (VENTRAL HERNIA)

About 10% of abdominal operations result in incisional hernias. The incidence of this iatrogenic type of hernia is not diminishing in spite of an awareness of the many causative factors.

▶ Etiology

The factors most often responsible for incisional hernia are listed below. When more than one factor coexists in the same patient, the likelihood of postoperative wound failure is greatly increased.

(1) Poor surgical technique. Inadequate fascial bites, tension on the fascial edges, or too tight a closure are most often responsible for incisional failure.

(2) Postoperative wound infection.

(3) Age. Wound healing is usually slower and less solid in older patients.

(4) General debility. Cirrhosis, carcinoma, and chronic wasting diseases are factors that affect wound healing adversely. Any condition that compromises nutrition increases the likelihood of incision breakdown.

(5) Obesity. Obese patients frequently have increased intra-abdominal pressure. The presence of fat in the abdominal wound masks tissue layers and increases the incidence of seromas and hematomas in wounds.

(6) Postoperative pulmonary complications that stress the repair as a result of vigorous coughing. Smokers and patients with chronic pulmonary disease are therefore at increased risk of fascial disruption.

(7) Placement of drains or stomas in the primary operative wound.

(8) Intraoperative blood loss greater than 1000 mL.

(9) Failure to close the fascia of laparoscopic trocar sites over 10 mm in size.

▶ Treatment

Small incisional hernias should be treated by early repair since they may cause bowel obstruction. If the patient is unwilling to undergo surgery or is a poor surgical risk, symptoms may be controlled by an elastic corset.

Defects too large to close easily may be left without surgical repair if they are asymptomatic, since they are unlikely to incarcerate.

A. Small Hernias

Small incisional hernias (< 2 cm in diameter) usually require only a direct fascia-to-fascia repair for satisfactory closure.

Interrupted or continuous closure may be used, but the sutures should be nonabsorbable. Sutures tied too tightly or tension on the repair will predispose to recurrence.

B. Large Hernias

Although no specific diameter distinguishes a small from a large hernia, a hernia can be considered large when the fascial edges cannot be approximated without tension.

In performing the repair, excess and scarred skin and subcutaneous tissues over the hernia are removed. The hernia sac is then carefully dissected free from the underlying muscles and fascial tissues. If there are no adherent intraperitoneal structures, the sac may be inverted and the repair done over the inverted sac. If there is incarceration or adhesion of intraperitoneal contents, the abdominal contents should be dissected free from the sac and dropped back into the abdomen. The edges of the fascial defect should be cleaned so that the closure will be to solid fascial tissue rather than to scar.

Primary closure of a large defect is not advisable, since tension on the closure increases the risk of hernia recurrence. Increasingly, repair of large or recurrent defects is performed using nonabsorbable mesh. Although a variety of techniques exist for placement of the mesh, a retrorectus underlay or a sandwich technique achieves a lower recurrence rate than an edge-to-edge or onlay placement. If a large dead space persists, a closed drainage system is usually employed in the space above the fascia. A primary fascial closure should be used only if the fascia can be brought together without tension and only for the smallest of defects.

Laparoscopic techniques are increasingly being used to repair incisional hernias and perform adhesiolysis electively. A sheet of synthetic material is secured to the abdominal wall as an underlay graft; the intraperitoneal placement of the graft enhances the durability of the repair, though it also increases the risk of bowel adhesions or fistula formation.

Alternative methods close the fascial defect using the patient's native tissues, such as a component separation technique, sliding myofascial flap, or lateral counterincisions in the anterior rectus sheath to allow primary closure in the midline. These techniques can be used to avoid the need for mesh and are especially indicated when the procedure is infected or contaminated, making synthetic mesh an unwise choice. Newer biologic mesh of human or animal origin may also be used, though recurrence rates with these materials are high.

▶ Prognosis

Results of randomized clinical trials show that mesh repair is superior to primary suture repair, even for small incisional hernias; in one study with a median follow up of 75 and 81 months for suture and mesh repairs, suture repairs showed 63% recurrence and mesh repair only 32%. Despite the increasing use of both open and laparoscopic mesh repairs, however, population-based studies show that incisional hernias continue to recur at a high rate after repair, and the 5-year reoperative rate increases with each subsequent reoperation for recurrence, reaching almost 40% on average after the third recurrence. It is yet to be known whether long-term results with laparoscopic mesh repairs will show improved results. Factors shown to increase risk of hernia recurrence include wound infection, presence of abdominal aneurysms, smoking, and poor nutrition. In all techniques employing mesh, the underlay technique with at least 3–4 cm of underlay of the mesh leads to the lowest recurrence rates. In addition to a high recurrence rate after operations, complications such as infected mesh, bleeding, seroma, and erosion of mesh into bowel causing a fistula occur in a small percentage of cases. Mesh infection is more likely after repair of a hernia occurring in a wound with a previous infection.

Burger JWA et al: Long-term follow-up of a randomized controlled trial of suture versus mesh repair of incisional hernia. Ann Surg 2004;240:578.

Cobb WS et al: Laparoscopic repair of incisional hernias. Surg Clin N Am 2005;85:91.

Flum DR et al: Have outcomes of incisional hernia repair improved with time? Ann Surg 2003;237:129.

Heniford BT et al: Laparoscopic repair of ventral hernias. Nine years' experience with 850 consecutive hernias. Ann Surg 2003;238:391.

Jezupors A et al: The analysis of infection after polypropylene mesh repair of abdominal wall hernia. World J Surg 2006;30:2270.

Klinge U et al: Incisional hernia: open techniques. World J Surg 2005;29:1066.

Leber GE et al: Long-term complications associated with prosthetic repair of incisional hernias. Arch Surg 1998;133:378.

McLanahan D et al: Retrorectus prosthetic mesh repair of midline abdominal hernia. Am J Surg 1997;173:445.

Sorensen LT et al: Smoking is a risk factor for incisional hernia. Arch Surg 2005;140:119.

VARIOUS RARE HERNIATIONS THROUGH THE ABDOMINAL WALL

▶ Littre Hernia

A Littre hernia is a hernia that contains a Meckel diverticulum in the hernia sac. Although Littre first described the condition in relation to a femoral hernia, the relative distribution of Littre hernias is as follows: inguinal, 50%; femoral, 20%; umbilical, 20%; and miscellaneous, 10%. Littre hernias of the groin are more common in men and on the right side. The clinical findings are similar to those of Richter hernia; when strangulation is present, pain, fever, and manifestations of small bowel obstruction occur late.

Treatment consists of repair of the hernia plus, if possible, excision of the diverticulum. If acute Meckel diverticulitis is present, the acute inflammatory mass may have to be treated through a separate abdominal incision.

▶ Spigelian Hernia

Spigelian hernia is an acquired ventral hernia through the linea semilunaris, the line where the sheaths of the lateral abdominal muscles fuse to form the lateral rectus sheath. Spigelian hernias are nearly always found above the level of the inferior epigastric vessels. They most commonly occur where the semicircular line (fold of Douglas) crosses the linea semilunaris.

The presenting symptom is pain that is usually localized to the hernia site and may be aggravated by any maneuver that increases intra-abdominal pressure. With time, the pain may become more dull, constant, and diffuse, making diagnosis more difficult.

If a mass can be demonstrated, the diagnosis presents little difficulty. The diagnosis is most easily made with the patient standing and straining; a bulge then presents in the lower abdominal area and disappears with a gurgling sound on pressure. Following reduction of the mass, the hernia orifice can usually be palpated.

Diagnosis is often made more difficult because the hernial defect may lie beneath an intact external oblique layer and therefore not be palpable. The hernia often dissects within the layers of the abdominal wall and may not present a distinct mass, or the mass may be located at a distance from the linea semilunaris. Patients with spigelian hernias should have a tender point over the hernia orifice, though tenderness alone is not sufficient to make the diagnosis. Both ultrasound and CT scan may help to confirm the diagnosis.

Spigelian hernias have a high incidence of incarceration and should be repaired. These hernias are quite easily cured by primary aponeurotic closure. Laparoscopic repair may decrease morbidity and hospital stay.

Moreno-Egea A et al: Open vs laparoscopic repair of spigelian hernia: a prospective randomized trial. Arch Surg 2002; 137:1266.

Skandalakis P et al: Spigelian hernia: Surgical anatomy, embryology, and technique of repair. Am Surg 2006;72:42.

▶ Lumbar or Dorsal Hernia

Lumbar or dorsal hernias (Figure 32–7) are hernias through the posterior abdominal wall at some level in the lumbar region. The most common sites (95%) are the superior (Grynfeltt) and inferior (Petit) lumbar triangles. A "lump in the flank" is the common complaint, associated with a dull, heavy, pulling feeling. With the patient erect, the presence of a reducible, often tympanitic mass in the flank usually makes the diagnosis. Incarceration and strangulation occur in about 10% of cases. Hernias in the inferior lumbar triangle are most often small and occur in young, athletic women. They present as tender masses producing backache and usually contain fat. Lumbar hernia must be differentiated from abscesses, hematomas, soft tissue tumors, renal tumors, and muscle strain.

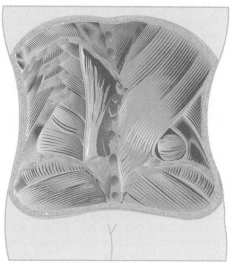

▲ **Figure 32–7.** Anatomic relationships of lumbar or dorsal hernia. On the left, lumbar or dorsal hernia into space of Grynfeltt. On the right, hernia into the Petit triangle (inferior lumbar space).

Acquired hernias may be traumatic or nontraumatic. Severe direct trauma, penetrating wounds, abscesses, and poor healing of flank incisions are the usual causes. Congenital hernias occur in infants and are usually isolated unilateral congenital defects.

Lumbar hernias increase in size and should be repaired when found. Repair is by mobilization of the nearby fascia and obliteration of the hernia defect by precise fascia-to-fascia closure. The recurrence rate is very low.

Heniford BT et al: Laparoscopic inferior and superior lumbar hernia repair. Arch Surg 1997;132:1141.
Killeen KL et al: Using CT to diagnose traumatic lumbar hernia. AJR Am J Roentgenol 2000;174:1413.

▶ Obturator Hernia

Herniation through the obturator canal is more frequent in elderly women and is difficult to diagnose preoperatively. The mortality rate (13–40%) of these hernias makes them the most lethal of all abdominal hernias. These hernias most commonly present as small bowel obstruction with cramping abdominal pain and vomiting. The hernia is rarely palpable in the groin, though a mass may be felt on pelvic or rectal examination. The most specific finding is a positive Howship-Romberg sign, in which pain extends down the medial aspect of the thigh with abduction, extension, or internal rotation of the knee. Since this sign is present in fewer than half of cases, diagnosis should be suspected in any elderly debilitated woman without previous abdominal operations who presents with a small bowel obstruction. Though diagnosis can be confirmed by CT scan, operation

should not be unduly delayed if complete bowel obstruction is present.

The abdominal approach gives the best exposure; these hernias should not be repaired from the thigh approach. The Cheatle-Henry approach (retropubic) may also be used. Simple repair is most often possible, though bladder wall, pectineal muscle, peritoneum, or mesh has been used when the defect cannot be approximated primarily.

Losanoff J et al: Obturator hernia. JACS 2002;194:657.

▶ Perineal Hernia

A perineal hernia protrudes through the muscles and fascia of the perineal floor. It may be primary but is usually acquired following perineal prostatectomy, abdominoperineal resection of the rectum, or pelvic exenteration.

These hernias present as easily reducible perineal bulges and usually are asymptomatic but may present with pain, dysuria, bowel obstruction, or perineal skin breakdown.

Repair is usually done by an abdominal approach, with an adequate fascial and muscular perineal repair. Occasionally, polypropylene (Marlex) mesh or flaps using the gracilis, rectus abdominis, or gluteus may be necessary, when the available tissues are too attenuated for adequate primary repair.

So JB et al: Post operative perineal hernia. Dis Colon Rectum 1997;40:954.

▶ Interparietal Hernia

Interparietal hernias, in which the sac insinuates itself between the layers of the abdominal wall, are usually of an indirect inguinal type but, rarely, may be direct or ventral hernias. Although interparietal hernias are rare, it is essential to recognize them, because strangulation is common and the mass is easily mistaken for a tumor or abscess. The lesion usually can be suspected on the basis of the physical examination provided it is kept in mind. In most cases, extensive studies for intra-abdominal tumors have preceded diagnosis. A lateral film of the abdomen will usually show bowel within the layers of the abdominal wall in cases with intestinal incarceration or strangulation, and an ultrasound or CT scan may be diagnostic.

As soon as the diagnosis is established, operation should be performed, usually through the standard inguinal approach.

▶ Sciatic Hernia

Sciatic hernia is the rarest of abdominal hernias and consists of an outpouching of intra-abdominal contents through the greater sciatic foramen. The diagnosis is made after incarceration or strangulation of the bowel occurs. The repair is usually made through the abdominal approach. The hernia sac and contents are reduced, and the weak area is closed by making a fascial flap from the superficial fascia of the piriformis muscle.

TRAUMATIC HERNIA

Abdominal wall hernias occur rarely as a direct consequence of direct blunt abdominal injury. The patient presents with abdominal pain. On examination, ecchymosis of the abdominal wall and a bulge are usually present. The existence of a hernia may not be obvious, however, and the patient may require CT scan to confirm it. Because of the high incidence of associated intra-abdominal injuries, laparotomy is usually required. The defect should be repaired primarily if possible.

Gill IS et al: Traumatic ventral abdominal hernia associated with small bowel gangrene: case report. J Trauma 1993;35:145.
Otero C et al: Injury to the abdominal wall musculature: the full spectrum of traumatic hernia. South Med J 1988;81:517.
Wood RJ et al: Traumatic abdominal hernia: a case report and review of the literature. Am Surg 1988;54:648.

II. OTHER LESIONS OF THE ABDOMINAL WALL

CONGENITAL DEFECTS

Congenital defects of the abdominal wall other than hernias or lesions of the urachus and umbilicus are rare. The important ones involving the urachus and umbilicus are discussed in Chapter 43.

TRAUMA TO THE ABDOMINAL WALL

▶ Rectus Sheath Hematoma

This is a rare but important entity that may follow mild trauma to the abdominal wall or may occur spontaneously in patients with disorders of coagulation, blood dyscrasia, or degenerative vascular diseases.

Abdominal pain localized to the rectus muscle is the presenting symptom. The pain may be sudden and severe in onset or slowly progressive. The key to diagnosis is the physical examination. Careful palpation will reveal a tender mass within the abdominal wall. When the patient tenses the rectus muscles by raising the head or body, the swelling becomes more tender and distinct on palpation, in contrast to an intra-abdominal mass or tenderness that disappears when the rectus muscles are contracted (Fothergill sign). In addition, there may be detectable discoloration or ecchymo-

sis. If the physical signs are not diagnostic, ultrasound or CT scan will demonstrate the hematoma in the abdominal wall.

The condition does not commonly require operation. The acute pain and discomfort usually disappear within 2 or 3 days, although a residual mass may persist for several weeks. If pain is severe, an acceptable alternative is evacuation of the clot and control of the bleeding.

Edlow JA et al: Rectus sheath hematoma. Ann Emerg Med 1999;34:671.

PAIN IN THE ABDOMINAL WALL

A number of conditions are characterized by pain in the abdominal wall without a demonstrable organic lesion. Pain from a diaphragmatic, supradiaphragmatic, or spinal cord lesion may be referred to the abdomen. Herpes zoster (shingles) may present as abdominal pain, in which case it will follow a dermatomal distribution.

Scars may be sensitive or painful, particularly in the first 6 months after surgery.

Entrapment of a nerve by a nonabsorbable suture may cause persistent incisional pain, sometimes quite severe. Hyperesthesia of the skin over the involved dermatome may provide a clue to the cause. If local anesthetic nerve block relieves the pain, nerve block with alcohol or nerve excision may be performed.

In all cases of localized pain in the abdominal wall, careful search should be made for a small hernia: MRI or CT scan may be helpful to rule out a hernia.

ABDOMINAL WALL TUMORS

Tumors of the abdominal wall are quite common, but most are benign, eg, lipomas, hemangiomas, and fibromas. Musculoaponeurotic fibromatoses (desmoid tumors), which often occur in abdominal wall scars or after parturition in women, are discussed in more detail in Chapter 44.

Endometriomas may also occur in the abdominal wall, particularly in the scars from gynecologic procedures and Caesarian sections. Most malignant tumors of the abdominal wall are metastatic. Metastases may appear by direct invasion from intra-abdominal lesions or by vascular dissemination. The sudden appearance of a sensitive nodule anywhere in the abdominal wall that is clearly not a hernia should arouse suspicion of an occult cancer, the lung and pancreas being the more likely primary sites.

Adrenals

Quan-Yang Duh, MD

Chienying Liu, MD

J. Blake Tyrrell, MD

Operations on the adrenal glands are performed for primary hyperaldosteronism, pheochromocytoma, hypercortisolism (Cushing disease or Cushing syndrome), and adrenocortical carcinoma. These conditions are usually characterized by hypersecretion of one or more of the adrenal hormones. Less commonly, surgery may also be performed for nonfunctioning tumors or metastases.

Anatomy & Surgical Principles

The normal combined weight of the adrenals is 7–12 g. The right gland lies posterior and lateral to the vena cava and superior to the kidney (Figure 33–1). The left gland lies medial to the superior pole of the kidney, just lateral to the aorta and immediately posterior to the superior border of the pancreas. An important surgical feature is the remarkable constancy of the adrenal veins. The right adrenal vein, 2–5 mm long and several millimeters wide, connects the anterior aspect of the adrenal gland with the posterolateral aspect of the vena cava. The left adrenal vein is several centimeters long and travels inferiorly from the lower pole of the gland, joining the left renal vein after receiving the inferior phrenic vein. The adrenal arteries are small, multiple, and inconstant. They usually come from the inferior phrenic artery, the aorta, and the renal artery.

With the exception of rare nonsecreting cancers, indications for adrenal surgery result from hypersecretory states. Diagnosis and treatment begin with confirmation of a hypersecretory state (ie, measurement of excess cortisol, aldosterone, or catecholamines in blood or urine). In order to determine whether the problem originates in the adrenal, levels of the trophic hormone in question (ie, adrenocorticotropic hormone [ACTH] or renin) must be measured. If levels of the trophic hormone are suppressed but hormone secretion is excessive, autonomous secretion is proved. The next step, except in pheochromocytoma, is to determine the degree of autonomy, a process that usually distinguishes hyperplasias (which respond to most but not all controlling mechanisms) from adenomas and adenomas from cancers.

In general, cancers are under little if any feedback control. If the primary problem is not in the adrenal, as in Cushing disease, treatment must be directed elsewhere when possible.

Adrenal masses are usually detected and localized by CT scan or MRI. Functioning tumors of the adrenal can be localized by adrenal scintigraphy, ^{131}I-6β-iodomethylnorcholesterol (NP-59) for cortical tumors and ^{131}I-metaiodobenzylguanidine (MIBG) for medullary tumors (pheochromocytomas). Functioning adrenal or pituitary tumors can also be localized by demonstrating a gradient of hormone levels between their venous drainage and a peripheral vein.

The major principles of adrenal surgery are as follows:

(1) Whenever possible, the surgeon must be certain of the diagnosis and the location of the lesion before undertaking the operation.

(2) The patient must be thoroughly prepared so he or she can withstand any metabolic problems caused by the disease or by the operation.

(3) The surgeon and consultants must be able to detect and treat any metabolic crisis that occurs during or after operation.

Surgical Approaches

Currently, almost all adrenal tumors are identified preoperatively by localization studies such as CT and MRI, so very few operations require general exploration of the abdomen. This permits the use of minimally invasive surgery. Almost all adrenal tumors can be removed laparoscopically. Traditional open adrenalectomy is necessary only when the tumor is especially large (eg, > 12 cm, depending on the surgeon's experience) or for locally invasive adrenocortical cancer where resection of lymph nodes or adjacent organs may be required.

Laparoscopic adrenalectomy can be performed using a transabdominal or retroperitoneal approach, but the former is preferable, especially for larger tumors. This involves medial rotation of the spleen and pancreas (on the left) or the liver (on the right), using gravity to drop the viscera away from the adrenal.

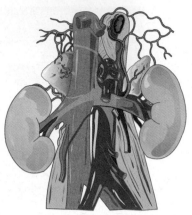

▲ **Figure 33–1.** Anatomy of the adrenals, showing venous return.

The traditional open surgical approach should be used only when laparoscopic expertise is not available or when required by the size and nature of the tumor. The advantages of the laparoscopic operation are so great that it is strongly preferred.

The open anterior (transperitoneal) approach through a long vertical midline incision or a bilateral subcostal incision allows wide exposure of the abdominal organs and the retroperitoneum. Unfortunately, this incision also causes more pain, ileus, and atelectasis and a much longer period of recovery. The risks of poor wound healing (Table 33–1) are greater, especially for patients with Cushing syndrome.

The open posterior approach, performed through incisions on each side of the spine and the bed of the 11th or 12th rib with the patient lying prone, is better tolerated postoperatively but provides a more limited exposure. It is adequate only for lesions smaller than 4–5 cm and has been superseded by the laparoscopic approach. An open lateral approach through the bed of the 11th rib to expose the adrenals retroperitoneally or a thoracoabdominal incision may be considered for large or invasive tumors.

▼ DISEASES OF THE ADRENALS

PRIMARY HYPERALDOSTERONISM

ESSENTIALS OF DIAGNOSIS

▶ Hypertension with or without hypokalemia.

▶ Elevated aldosterone secretion and suppressed plasma renin activity.

▶ Metabolic alkalosis, relative hypernatremia.

▶ Weakness, polyuria, paresthesias, tetany, cramps due to hypokalemia.

Table 33–1. Frequency of Manifestations of Hypercortisolism.

	Percentage
Obesity	95%
Hypertension	70%
Glucose tolerance	80%
Centripetal distribution of fat	80%
Weakness	20%
Muscle atrophy in upper and lower extremities	70%
Hirsutism	80%
Menstrual disturbance or impotence	75%
Purple striae	50%
Plethoric facies	85%
Easy bruisability	35%
Acne	40%
Psychological symptoms	40%
Edema	20%
Headache	15%
Back pain	60%

▶ General Considerations

Aldosterone, the most potent mineralocorticoid secreted by the adrenal cortex, regulates the body's electrolyte composition, fluid volume, and blood pressure. Excess aldosterone increases total body sodium, decreases potassium levels, increases extracellular fluid volume (without edema), and increases blood pressure. Under normal conditions, aldosterone secretion is regulated by the renin-angiotensin system in a feedback fashion and is also stimulated transiently by ACTH.

In primary hyperaldosteronism, aldosterone levels are elevated and renin levels are suppressed. In secondary hyperaldosteronism, increased aldosterone is due to increased renin secretion. Examples of secondary hyperaldosteronism include renal vascular disease, renin-secreting tumors, and cirrhosis with low intravascular volume or diuretic use. Among the subtypes of primary hyperaldosteronism, aldosterone-producing adenoma (aldosteronoma) and idiopathic hyperaldosteronism with adrenal hyperplasia are the most common types. Unilateral primary adrenal hyperplasia, aldosterone-producing adrenocortical carcinoma, and familial hyperaldosteronism (eg, glucocorticoid-remediable hyperaldosteronism) are rare. Surgery is beneficial only in patients with aldosterone-producing adenomas and in patients with unilateral primary adrenal hyperplasia.

Primary hyperaldosteronism in its classic form is characterized by hypertension, hypokalemia, increased aldosterone secretion, and suppressed plasma renin activity. However, hypokalemia is not required to make the diagnosis; recent studies have shown that many patients have a normal potassium level. Primary hyperaldosteronism was once thought to be present in about 1% of patients with hypertension, but its prevalence has increased to 5–13% based on various studies when plasma aldosterone concentration–to-plasma renin activity was used to screen for hyperaldosteronism in patients with hypertension who were not hypokalemic. Although rare, normotensive primary hyperaldosteronism has been described.

Aldosteronomas are usually solitary and small (0.5–2 cm). They have a characteristic chrome color when sectioned. Tumor cells typically have heterogeneous cytomorphology, resembling those of all three zones of the adrenal cortex, including hybrid cells having cytologic features of the zona glomerulosa and zona fasciculata. Hyperplasia is also often seen in glands harboring adenomas.

▶ Clinical Findings

Aldosterone facilitates the exchange of sodium for potassium and hydrogen ions in the distal nephron. Therefore, when aldosterone secretion is chronically increased, serum potassium and hydrogen ion concentrations fall (hypokalemia and alkalosis), total body sodium rises, and hypertension results.

A. Symptoms and Signs

Symptoms, if present, are usually those of hypokalemia and depend on the severity of potassium depletion. Patients complain of a sense of malaise, muscle weakness, polyuria, polydipsia, cramps, and paresthesias. Tetany and hypokalemic paralysis occur rarely. Headaches are common. Hypertension is usually moderate to severe and may be refractory to medical therapy, but advanced retinopathy is rare. Although extracellular fluid volume is increased, edema is not seen unless renal failure occurs.

B. Laboratory Findings

1. Screening test—Primary hyperaldosteronism should be suspected in patients with hypertension and hypokalemia—either spontaneous or following the administration of diuretics—and in patients with refractory hypertension. The diagnostic evaluation should start with screening tests. A simple ambulatory test determines the ratio of plasma aldosterone concentration (PAC), in nanograms per deciliter, to plasma renin activity (PRA), in nanograms per milliliter per hour, performed in the morning in a seated ambulant patient. A ratio greater than 20 with a plasma aldosterone concentration greater than 15 ng/dL suggests primary hyperaldosteronism and warrants confirmatory biochemical studies. Hypertensive individuals without primary hyperaldosteronism usually have ratios of less than 20. If the patient is taking an aldosterone receptor antagonist spironolactone or eplerenone, the data are uninterpretable, and estrogens increase plasma aldosterone concentrations by increasing

angiotensinogen. These agents should be discontinued for 6 weeks before the workup.

Angiotensin-converting enzyme inhibitors, angiotensin receptor blockers, diuretics, and calcium channel blockers raise PRA; therefore, a low PAC/PRA ratio in patients taking these medications does not exclude primary hyperaldosteronism. Beta-blockers decrease PRA and increase the PAC/PRA ratio. These medications may need to be discontinued for 2 weeks if needed.

Peripheral α-adrenergic blockers are the preferred antihypertensive agents during evaluation. In many patients, it is unwise to withdraw antihypertensive medications, and one must be content with imperfect data.

2. Confirmatory test—If the screening test is positive, failure to suppress aldosterone secretion with sodium loading will confirm the diagnosis of primary hyperaldosteronism in most patients. Aldosterone can be suppressed by oral salt loading or intravenous sodium chloride infusion. The patient should consume a high-sodium diet (5000 mg of sodium for 3 days) or be supplemented with NaCl tablets (2–3 g with each meal) if necessary. A 24-hour urine sample is collected for aldosterone and sodium on the third day. Serum potassium should be monitored because the high-salt diet increases kaliuresis, and potassium chloride should be supplemented to avoid hypokalemia, which interferes with the test results by decreasing aldosterone secretion and may cause cardiac arrhythmias. Urinary aldosterone excretion higher than 14 μg/24 h distinguishes most patients with primary hyperaldosteronism from those with essential hypertension on a high-salt diet, as confirmed by urinary sodium excretion exceeding 200 meq/24 h. Alternatively, a plasma aldosterone concentration higher than 10 ng/mL after an infusion of 2 L of normal saline over 4 hours is also consistent with primary hyperaldosteronism. However, the variability of aldosterone secretion throughout the day in patients with aldosteronomas makes this method less desirable than oral salt loading.

▶ Differential Diagnosis

Once the diagnosis is established, the surgically correctable forms—aldosterone-producing adenoma (aldosteronoma) and the rare unilateral primary adrenal hyperplasia—should be distinguished from idiopathic hyperaldosteronism due to bilateral adrenal hyperplasia, for which medical therapy is the best management. Aldosteronoma and idiopathic hyperaldosteronism are the most common subtypes. Compared with those with idiopathic hyperaldosteronism, patients with aldosteronoma have more severe hypertension, more severe hypokalemia, higher aldosterone secretion (> 20 ng/dL), higher 18-hydroxycorticosterone concentrations (> 100 ng/dL), and are younger.

The postural stimulation test may be helpful. The test is based on the observation that aldosteronomas are usually unaffected by the renin-angiotensin system but retain sensitivity to ACTH stimulation. Therefore, the plasma aldosterone concentration follows the diurnal variation of ACTH and cortisol. In contrast, idiopathic hyperaldosteronism is characterized by enhanced sensitivity to small changes in the renin-angiotensin axis but is unaffected by ACTH. Thus, if the patient remains upright for 4 hours, plasma aldosterone levels fall and renin remains suppressed in patients with aldosteronoma. In patients with idiopathic hyperaldosteronism, plasma aldosterone increases in response to a small increase in plasma renin.

Unfortunately, these features do not absolutely distinguish the two types. Combined biochemical studies and imaging studies are frequently necessary.

High-resolution thin-section CT identifies most adenomas and should be performed once the diagnosis of primary hyperaldosteronism is established. Adrenal vein sampling is indicated if the CT scan is equivocal or negative. Adrenal vein sampling is the most certain way to differentiate aldosteronoma from idiopathic hyperaldosteronism and to diagnose and localize an aldosteronoma. Routine use of selective adrenal venous sampling is advocated by some centers. Nevertheless, it is technically difficult, and failure to cannulate the adrenal veins, especially the right adrenal vein, is common.

Aldosterone-secreting adrenocortical carcinoma should be suspected if the tumor is larger than 4 cm. Glucocorticoid-remediable hyperaldosteronism (familial hyperaldosteronism type 1) is inherited in an autosomal dominant fashion. The genetic defect results in a chimeric gene. The mutated gene juxtaposes the promoter for expression of the 11-hydroxylase gene, which is ACTH-responsive, with the coding sequence of the aldosterone synthase gene. This leads to aldosterone production under ACTH stimulation in the zona fasciculata. Glucocorticoid therapy reverses this type of hyperaldosteronism. These patients have a family history of onset of hypertension at an early age. The diagnosis can be established by measuring elevated 24-hour urine 18-hydroxycortisol and 18-oxocortisol levels or by genetic testing.

▶ Tumor Localization

An aldosterone-producing adenoma can usually be demonstrated by high-resolution CT or MRI scanning. Some small aldosteronomas can be missed, and in such cases a patient with a small aldosteronoma not seen on CT may be misdiagnosed as having adrenal hyperplasia. Aldosteronomas that coexist with nonfunctional adenomas can be mislabeled as adrenal hyperplasia because of multinodularity or bilateral masses on CT. Small abnormalities on CT scans may represent hyperplasia rather than true aldosteronomas. Therefore, unless an unequivocal unilateral tumor, preferably larger than 1 cm, is present on the CT scan and the contralateral gland is normal, the diagnosis and localization of aldosteronoma cannot be considered certain. The clinical features and results of the postural stimulation test may offer clues but are not always predictive. When in doubt, adrenal vein sampling should be done; it is 95% accurate in identifying an aldosteronoma. Blood is sampled from the adrenal veins and the inferior vena cava for aldosterone and cortisol levels at baseline and after ACTH infusion. Proper catheter placement is confirmed by finding high cortisol levels in adrenal venous blood compared with the inferior vena cava. Corrected aldosterone levels are calculated from the ratio of aldosterone to cortisol in each venous sample. A lateralization ratio of the corrected aldosterone level higher than 4 indicates unilateral aldosterone secretion, thereby confirming a diagnosis of aldosteronoma in most patients. Adrenal vein sampling is invasive and requires considerable skill and experience. The success rate for cannulating both adrenal veins is about 90%. Unilateral catheterization of the left adrenal vein alone does not give useful information.

▶ Complications

Uncontrolled hypertension can lead to renal failure, stroke, and myocardial infarction. Severe hypokalemia can cause weakness, paralysis, and arrhythmia, especially in patients taking digitalis.

▶ Treatment

The goal of therapy is to prevent the complications of hypertension and hypokalemia. Unilateral adrenalectomy is recommended for patients with aldosteronoma and medical therapy for those with idiopathic hyperaldosteronism or those with aldosteronoma who are poor candidates for surgery.

A. Surgical Treatment

1. Preoperative preparation—Blood pressure and hypokalemia should be controlled before surgery. Spironolactone, a competitive aldosterone antagonist, has been the drug of choice. It blocks the mineralocorticoid receptor, promotes potassium retention, restores normal potassium concentrations, and reduces the extracellular fluid volume, thereby controlling blood pressure. Furthermore, it reactivates the suppressed renin-angiotensin-aldosterone system in the contralateral adrenal gland, reducing the risk of postoperative hypoaldosteronism. Initial dosages of 200–400 mg/d may be required to control hypokalemia and hypertension. Once blood pressure has normalized and hypokalemia is corrected, the dose can be tapered and maintained at about 100–150 mg/d. Spironolactone may have antiandrogenic side effects, such as impotence, gynecomastia, menstrual irregularity, and gastrointestinal disturbances.

Amiloride, 20–40 ng/d, a potassium-sparing diuretic, may be used alternatively or as a supplement to spironolactone. Other medications, such as calcium-channel blockers and diuretics, may be required to control hypertension. These agents can be continued to the day of operation. Hypokalemia and hypertension should be controlled preoperatively, and most patients require a minimum of 1–2 weeks of treatment with spironolactone. Glucocorticoids are unnecessary for patients undergoing unilateral adrenalectomy for aldosteronoma. Unlike spironolactone, which also blocks androgen and progesterone receptors, eplerenone is a selective mineralocorticoid receptor antagonist and has fewer endocrine side effects. It has been approved for treatment of hypertension and for heart failure after myocardial infarction. Eplerenone may become the treatment of choice for primary hyperaldosteronism because of its decreased side effects if it is proven as efficacious as spironolactone, in spite of its increased cost.

2. Surgery—Because aldosteronomas are almost always small and benign, laparoscopic adrenalectomy is the procedure of choice. It can be performed safely and with equally good results by several approaches. The lateral transabdominal approach uses gravity to help medially rotate the viscera (liver on the right and spleen and pancreas on the left) and exposes the adrenal gland. It is the most versatile approach and is preferred by most surgeons. The retroperitoneal approach, either laterally or posteriorly, is used occasionally. It may be best in patients with prior upper abdominal operations, but the working space is cramped. Although some surgeons perform a subtotal resection for aldosteronoma, most excise the adrenal gland with the tumor. The surrounding adrenal tissue frequently appears hyperplastic. A few small aldosteronomas may not be visible intraoperatively, so accurate preoperative localization is important. Bilateral adrenalectomy is not indicated, since patients with idiopathic hyperaldosteronism should be treated medically, and bilateral aldosteronomas are extremely rare.

3. Postoperative care—Occasional patients may develop transient aldosterone deficiency because of suppression of the contralateral adrenal gland by the hyperfunctioning adenoma. This is rare in patients treated with spironolactone preoperatively. Symptoms include postural hypotension and hyperkalemia. Adequate sodium intake is usually sufficient for treatment; rarely, short-term fludrocortisone replacement (0.1 mg/d orally) is required.

B. Medical Treatment

The goal is to control hypertension and hypokalemia. Spironolactone is the preferred agent, though amiloride may be better tolerated. Angiotensin-converting enzyme inhibitors and calcium-channel blockers have been used with some success. A combination of antihypertensive agents may be necessary.

▶ Prognosis

Hyperaldosteronism usually follows a prolonged and subtly changing course. Untreated hypertension may cause stroke, myocardial infarction, or renal failure.

Removal of an aldosteronoma normalizes potassium levels, but the hypertension is not always cured. About one third of patients have persistent mild hypertension that is usually easier to control than before the operation. Essential hypertension and atherosclerosis due to chronic hypertension are contributing factors. Although patients with idiopathic hyperaldosteronism should be treated medically, adrenalectomy is indicated for those with aldosteronoma because side effects of the medications and compliance make long-term medical treatment undesirable. The low morbidity, short hospitalization, and high success rate of laparoscopic adrenalectomy have made surgery preferable to long-term medical therapy.

Al Fehaily M, Duh QY: Clinical manifestation of aldosteronoma. Surg Clin North Am 2004;84:887.

Magill SB et al: Comparison of adrenal vein sampling and computed tomography in the differentiation of primary aldosteronism. J Clin Endocrinol Metab 2001;86;1066.

Mulatero P et al: Increased diagnosis of primary aldosteronism, including surgically correctable forms, in centers from five continents. J Clin Endocrin Metab 2004;89:1045.

Shen WT et al: Laparoscopic vs open adrenalectomy for the treatment of primary hyperaldosteronism. Arch Surg 1999; 134:628.

Walz MK et al: Retroperitoneoscopic adrenalectomy in Connís syndrome caused by adrenal adenomas or nodular hyperplasia. World J Surg 2008;32:847.

Weinberger MH, Fineberg NS: The diagnosis of primary aldosteronism and separation of two major subtypes. Arch Intern Med 1993;153:2125.

Young WF: Minireview: primary aldosteronism-changing concepts in diagnosis and treatment. Endocrinology 2003; 114:2208.

Young WF Jr et al: Role for adrenal venous sampling in primary aldosteronism. Surgery 2004;136:1227.

Zarnegar R et al: The aldosteronoma resolution score: predicting complete resolution of hypertension after adrenalectomy for aldosteronoma. Ann Surg 2008;247:511.

PHEOCHROMOCYTOMA

 ESSENTIALS OF DIAGNOSIS

▶ Hypertension, frequently sustained, with or without paroxysms.

▶ Episodic headache, excessive sweating, palpitation, and visual blurring.

▶ Postural tachycardia and hypotension.

▶ Elevated urinary catecholamines or their metabolites, hypermetabolism, hyperglycemia.

▶ General Considerations

Pheochromocytomas are tumors of the adrenal medulla and related chromaffin tissues elsewhere in the body (paragangliomas) that secrete epinephrine or norepinephrine, resulting in sustained or episodic hypertension and other symptoms of catecholamine excess.

Pheochromocytoma is found in less than 0.1% of patients with hypertension and accounts for about 5% of adrenal tumors incidentally discovered by CT scanning. Most pheochromocytomas occur sporadically without other diseases, but they may be associated with various familial syndromes such as multiple endocrine neoplasia (MEN) 2A (medullary thyroid carcinoma, pheochromocytoma, and hyperparathyroidism), MEN 2B (medullary thyroid carcinoma, pheochromocytoma, mucosal neuromas, marfanoid habitus, and ganglioneuromatosis), von Recklinghausen disease (café au lait spots, neurofibromatosis, pheochromocytoma), von Hippel-Lindau disease (retinal hemangioma, hemangioblastoma of the central nervous system, renal cysts and carcinoma, pheochromocytoma, pancreatic cysts, and epididymal cystadenoma), and familial paraganglioma syndromes caused by mutations of the succinate dehydrogenase genes *SDHB*, *SDHC*, and *SDHD* (malignant pheochromocytomas, extraadrenal paragangliomas, and chemodectomas). These syndromes should be considered especially in young patients and in patients with multifocal tumors. Family members of patients who have been diagnosed with these syndromes also need screening to determine whether they are gene carriers and are at risk for developing the various tumors, including pheochromocytoma.

On pathologic examination, pheochromocytoma appears reddish-gray and frequently has areas of necrosis, hemorrhage, and sometimes cysts. The usual size is about 100 g, or 5 cm in diameter, but they can be as small as 2–3 cm or as large as 12–16 cm. Cells are pleomorphic, showing prominent nucleoli and frequent mitoses. Cytologic findings cannot be used to determine whether a pheochromocytoma is malignant or benign. The veins and capsules may also be invaded even in clinically benign tumors. Malignancy can only be diagnosed in the presence of metastases or invasion into surrounding tissues.

▶ Clinical Findings

A. Symptoms and Signs

The clinical findings of pheochromocytoma are variable, and almost half of them come to attention because of an incidental finding of an adrenal tumor (incidentaloma) on CT or MRI scans performed to evaluate other diseases. Classically, the patient has episodic hypertension associated with the triad of palpitation, headache, and sweating. The patient may also complain of anxiety, tremors, weight loss, dizziness, nausea and vomiting, abdominal discomfort, constipation, and visual blurring. Some patients have diarrhea, which may be secondary to secretion of vasoactive intestinal peptide. The physical examination may be unremarkable except during an attack, when pallor and excess sweating may be observed. Tachycardia, postural hypotension, and hypertensive retinopathy are other signs.

Hypertension, the most common feature of pheochromocytoma, occurs in 90% of patients. More than half have sustained hypertension, which may be mild to moderate, with or without other signs and symptoms of catecholamine excess, and the diagnosis may be missed. In some cases, basal blood pressure may not be elevated, and severe hypertension occurs only while the patient is under stress, such as general anesthesia or trauma. Patients with diastolic hypertension and postural hypotension who are not receiving antihypertensive medications may have pheochromocytoma. Hyperglycemia may occur because epinephrine raises blood glucose and norepinephrine decreases insulin secretion.

Traditionally, catecholamine-secreting tumors have been said to be 10% malignant, 10% familial, 10% bilateral, 10% multiple, and 10% extra-adrenal. In children, hypertension is less prominent, and about 50% have multiple or extra-adrenal tumors. Malignancy may be more common in extra-adrenal pheochromocytomas and in patients with *SDHB* mutation. Pheochromocytomas occur in 40–50% of patients with MEN 2; they tend to be bilateral and multiple but are rarely extra-adrenal or malignant. Screening of MEN 2 patients and family members who are *ret* protooncogene mutation carriers by measuring urinary catecholamines and metanephrines or plasma-free metanephrines may diagnose pheochromocytomas before they produce clinical manifestations. Plasma-free metanephrines (metanephrine and normetanephrine) is the most sensitive test for pheochromocytoma in familial syndromes.

B. Laboratory Findings

The diagnosis of pheochromocytoma is best confirmed either by fractionated 24-hour urinary catecholamines and metanephrines measured in the same collection or by fractionated plasma-free metanephrines. Both tests have high diagnostic sensitivity and specificity. Plasma-free metanephrines is more sensitive than the urine test, but it has a higher false-positive rate, especially in elderly patients. Controversies exist as to which biochemical test is best (Figure 33–2). Urinary output of metanephrines and/or free catecholamines is elevated in more than 95% of patients with pheochromocytoma. In 80% of patients, the level exceeds twice normal. Measurement of urinary vanillylmandelic acid (VMA) is less sensitive, and this test should no longer be used. Assays using high-performance liquid chromatography (HPLC) reduce interference by drugs and diets, but not all HPLC assays are the same, and many drugs and diets can potentially interfere with certain HPLC assays or affect the secretion and metabolism of catecholamines. Examples include acetaminophen, labetalol, vasodilators (nitroglycerin and nitroprusside), nifedipine, theophylline, stimulants (amphetamine, caffeine, nicotine, methylphenidate), many antipsychotics, antidepressants (especially tricyclic antidepressants), buspirone, prochlorperazine, and methyldopa. Interpretation of the study may also be affected by coffee, ethanol, bananas, radiographic dyes, drugs that contain catecholamines, and withdrawal from clonidine. These agents should be discontinued for 2 weeks before measuring

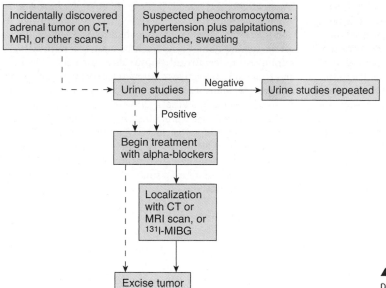

▲ Figure 33–2. Scheme for evaluation of a patient with suspected pheochromocytoma.

urinary catecholamines and metanephrines. The interfering substances vary depending on the specific assays used, so a list and protocol for preparing the patient should be obtained from the specific laboratory. Liquid chromatography-tandem mass spectrometry is a newer assay that has been shown to minimize drug interferences in the measurement of plasma and urinary metanephrines and may improve its diagnostic accuracy.

Overnight urinary collection and short collection periods following a paroxysm, indexed to creatinine, have also been used. Measuring plasma-free metanephrines is 96–100% sensitive and 85–89% specific. Depending on the particular assay, caffeic acid found in coffee, acetaminophen phenoxybenzamine, and tricyclic antidepressants may cause false-positive results. Provocative tests—using glucagon, histamine, or tyramine—are not accurate and are potentially dangerous; they are no longer used. Clonidine suppression tests are rarely used. Clonidine does not decrease plasma catecholamine levels in patients with pheochromocytoma as it may in normal, anxious individuals or in patients with essential hypertension.

C. Tumor Localization

Localization studies should be performed only after biochemical studies have confirmed the diagnosis of a catecholamine-secreting tumor. Ninety percent of pheochromocytomas are found in the adrenal glands and most are larger than 3 cm in diameter. Of the extra-adrenal pheochromocytomas (also called paragangliomas), 75% are in the abdomen, 10% in the bladder, 10% in the chest, 2% in the pelvis, and 3% in the head and neck. Both CT and MRI can localize most pheochromocytomas. CT scan is less expensive and gives

better anatomic details for the surgeons, but MRI avoids radiation exposure. Pheochromocytoma usually has a characteristic bright appearance on T2-weighted MRI. MIBG may be helpful for localizing extra-adrenal pheochromocytomas, and it should be considered when searching for extra-adrenal, multiple, malignant, or metastatic pheochromocytomas. MIBG is more specific but less sensitive compared with CT or MRI for localization. Arteriography and fine-needle aspiration biopsy can precipitate a hypertensive crisis. They do not contribute to the diagnosis and are not indicated. Venous sampling for catecholamines is no longer indicated.

▶ Differential Diagnosis

The differential diagnosis includes all causes of hypertension. Hyperthyroidism and pheochromocytoma have many features in common (weight loss, tremor, and tachycardia). The diagnosis of pheochromocytoma is easier if episodic hypertension is present. Acute anxiety attacks mimic the symptoms and may precipitate hypertensive episodes, but anxiety alone rarely produces severe hypertension. Carcinoid syndrome causing episodes of flushing may also be mistaken for pheochromocytoma. Urinary 5-HIAA level is usually markedly elevated, and CT scan may show liver metastases in patients with carcinoid syndrome. Labile essential hypertension is not associated with elevated catecholamine levels.

Pheochromocytoma in pregnancy, if not recognized, will kill half of the fetuses and nearly half of the mothers. Hypertension in pregnancy is usually ascribed to preeclampsia-eclampsia. The diagnosis of pheochromocytoma requires the same biochemical studies; MRI, instead of CT or MIBG, is indicated to localize the tumor when a biochemical diagnosis has been established to avoid radiation exposure. α-Adrenergic and β-adrenergic blockers appear to be well tolerated. Timing of the operation is individualized. If recognized early, the tumor is best removed early in the second trimester. Otherwise, α-adrenergic blockade is continued and then followed by a planned cesarean section at term. The pheochromocytoma can be resected either at the time of cesarean section—if easily accessible through the same incision—or electively a few weeks postpartum laparoscopically.

Pheochromocytoma crisis may develop in patients with pheochromocytoma, usually precipitated by trauma, certain medications, surgery, or other procedures. Trigger by glucocorticosteroids has been reported. Crisis usually occurs when α-adrenergic blockade has not been instituted. These patients may develop multisystem failure, mimicking severe sepsis. If the disease is not recognized, death is the usual result. Once pheochromocytoma is diagnosed, the patient should be stabilized and α-adrenergic blockade started. Emergent operation may rarely be necessary. Otherwise, resection during the same hospitalization after the patient is stabilized is preferred.

▶ Complications

Pheochromocytoma causes complications because of hypertension, cardiac arrhythmia, and hypovolemia. The sequelae of hypertension are stroke, renal failure, myocardial infarction, and congestive heart failure. Sudden death can result from ventricular tachycardia or fibrillation. α-Adrenergic stimulation by the catecholamines causes vasoconstriction and a low total blood volume. The patient is therefore unable to compensate for a sudden loss of blood volume (bleeding) or catecholamines (tumor removal) and is at risk of cardiovascular collapse. Preoperative α-adrenergic blockade and restoration of blood volume can prevent these complications.

▶ Treatment

A. Medical Treatment

Treatment with α-adrenergic blocking agents should be started as soon as the biochemical diagnosis is established. The aims of preoperative therapy are (1) to restore the blood volume, which has been depleted by excessive catecholamines; (2) to prevent a severe crisis, with its potential complications; and (3) to allow the patient to recover from cardiomyopathy. Close control of hypertension is necessary in order to keep blood volume normal.

Phenoxybenzamine, a nonselective α-adrenergic antagonist, has a long duration of action and is the preferred drug. It should be started at a dosage of 10 mg/12 h, and the dose should be increased by 10–20 mg every 2–3 days—as postural hypotension allows. Usual doses are 100–160 mg/d; however, dosages as high as 300 mg/d may be necessary. Most patients require 10–14 days of treatment, as judged by stabilization of blood pressure and reduction of symptoms.

Nasal stuffiness is usually present when alpha blockade is well established.

Metyrosine inhibits tyrosine hydroxylase and reduces catecholamine synthesis and can be added to phenoxybenzamine as preoperative therapy. Calcium-channel blockers and competitive selective α-adrenergic blocking agents such as doxazosin and prazosin may also be effective.

β-Adrenergic blocking agents are often used to treat arrhythmias and tachycardia but should only be given after alpha blockade has been achieved. Otherwise, a hypertensive crisis may be precipitated because of the unopposed α-adrenergic effect of the catecholamines. Opioids should be avoided because they may stimulate histamine release and precipitate a crisis.

B. Surgical Treatment

The definitive treatment of pheochromocytoma is excision. It was once recommended that both adrenal glands and other areas likely to harbor extra-adrenal tumors should be examined at the time of surgery, but that practice is now outmoded even for patients clinically at risk for bilateral or multiple tumors, because CT, MRI, and MIBG scans are so sensitive in finding all lesions.

Smaller (< 5–6 cm) adrenal pheochromocytomas can be safely resected by laparoscopic adrenalectomy. Very large (> 8–10 cm) and extra-adrenal tumors are technically more difficult and may require laparotomy.

During surgery, an arterial line is necessary for continuous blood pressure monitoring. Monitoring of pulmonary artery pressure is rarely necessary in patients who are well blocked.

Nitroprusside should be immediately available to treat sudden hypertension and beta-blockers to treat the cardiac dysrhythmias that may occur when the tumor is manipulated. Manipulation of the gland is less with laparoscopic than with open adrenalectomy, which minimizes fluctuations in plasma catecholamine levels.

Very large malignant tumors may require a thoracoabdominal incision. Malignant pheochromocytomas may invade the adrenal vein or vena cava. Extra-adrenal pheochromocytomas are usually found along the abdominal aorta and in the organ of Zuckerkandl near the aortic bifurcation. However, tumors have been found in widely scattered sites such as the bladder, the vagina, the mediastinum, the neck, and even the skull and pericardium. In general, extra-adrenal tumors should be localized with MIBG, CT, or MRI preoperatively to avoid a blind exploration.

In patients with MEN 2 and bilateral pheochromocytomas, cortical-sparing subtotal adrenalectomy on the side of the smaller tumor may avoid postoperative adrenal insufficiency, though it increases the risk for recurrence. In patients with MEN 2 and a unilateral pheochromocytoma, prophylactic resection of the contralateral normal-appearing adrenal gland is contraindicated, since bilateral adrenalectomy leads to lifelong hypoadrenalism requiring cortisol replacement. These patients should be followed with biochemical evaluations, and the contralateral adrenal gland should be resected only if pheochromocytoma develops.

Many patients undergoing resection of pheochromocytoma who are not adequately prepared preoperatively will have hypertensive crises, cardiac arrhythmia, myocardial infarction, or acute pulmonary edema. In addition, these patients may experience intractable hypotension and die in shock after tumor removal. If the patient has been properly prepared with alpha-blockers, the changes in blood pressure will not be severe. Otherwise, intravenous infusion of large amounts of saline and vasopressors may be necessary to maintain blood pressure after the tumor is removed. Although not common, hypoglycemia may develop after tumor removal.

▶ Prognosis

The outlook for patients with untreated pheochromocytoma is grim, whereas the operative mortality rate was decreased to 0–3% from 30% following the introduction of α-adrenergic blockade. Mild to moderate essential hypertension may persist after surgery. Second tumors in the remaining adrenal or metastatic tumors can occur years after excision of the primary pheochromocytoma; long-term follow-up is mandatory. Metastatic or recurrent malignant pheochromocytoma should be resected if possible to reduce the catecholamine load. Treatment with high-dose ^{131}I-MIBG may be helpful in these patients.

Bravo EL, Tagle R: Pheochromocytoma: state-of-the-art and future prospects. Endocr Rev 2003;24:539.

Duh Q-Y: Editorial: Evolving surgical management for patients with pheochromocytoma. J Clin Endocrinol Metab 2001;86:1477.

Jimenez C et al: Should patients with apparently sporadic pheochromocytomas or paragangliomas be screened for hereditary syndromes? J Clin Endocrinol Metab 2006;91:2851.

Kudva et al: The laboratory diagnosis of adrenal pheochromocytoma: the Mayo clinic experience. J Clin Endocrinol Metab 2003;88:4533.

Lenders JW et al: Biochemical diagnosis of pheochromocytoma. Which test is best? JAMA 2002;287:1427.

Mannelli M, Bemporad D: Diagnosis and management of pheochromocytoma during pregnancy. J Endocrinol Invest 2002; 25:567.

Rosas AL et al: Pheochromocytoma crisis induced by glucocorticoids: a report of four cases and review of the literature. Eur J Endocrinol. 2008;158:423.

Rose B et al: High dose ^{131}I-metaiodobenzylguanidine therapy for 12 patients with malignant pheochromocytoma. Cancer 2003; 98:239.

Scholz T et al: Clinical review: Current treatment of malignant pheochromocytoma. J Clin Endocrinol Metab 2007;92:1217.

Taylor RL, Singh RJ: Validation of liquid chromatography-tandem mass spectrometry method for analysis of urinary conjugated metanephrines and normetanephrines for screening of pheochromocytoma. Clin Chem. 2002;48:533.

Young WF Jr: Adrenal causes of hypertension: pheochromocytoma and primary aldosteronism. Rev Endocr Metab Disord 2007;8:309.

HYPERCORTISOLISM (CUSHING DISEASE & CUSHING SYNDROME)

 ESSENTIALS OF DIAGNOSIS

▶ Facial plethora, dorsocervical fat pad, supraclavicular fat pad, truncal obesity, easy bruisability, purple striae, acne, hirsutism, impotence or amenorrhea, muscle weakness, and psychosis.

▶ Hypertension, hyperglycemia, and osteopenia or osteoporosis.

▶ General Considerations

Cushing syndrome is due to chronic glucocorticoid excess. It may be caused by excess ACTH stimulation or by adrenocortical tumors that secrete glucocorticoids independently of ACTH stimulation. Excess ACTH may be produced by pituitary adenomas (Cushing disease) or extrapituitary ACTH-producing tumors (ectopic ACTH syndrome). Cushing syndrome not dependent on ACTH is usually caused by primary adrenal diseases such as adrenocortical adenoma and micronodular or macronodular hyperplasia or carcinoma.

The natural history of Cushing syndrome depends on the underlying disease and varies from a mild, indolent disease to rapid progression and death.

▶ Clinical Findings

A. Symptoms and Signs

See Table 33–1. The classic description of Cushing syndrome includes truncal obesity, hirsutism, moon facies, acne, buffalo hump, purple striae, hypertension, and diabetes, but other signs and symptoms are common. Weakness and depression are striking features. Weakness and other features are also seen after prolonged and excessive administration of adrenocortical steroids.

In children, Cushing syndrome is most commonly caused by adrenal cancers, but adenomas and nodular hyperplasia have been described. Cushing syndrome in children also causes growth retardation or arrest.

B. Pathologic Examination

The pathologic features of the adrenal gland depend on the underlying disease. Normal adrenal glands weigh 7–12 g combined. The hyperplastic adrenal glands in patients with Cushing disease weigh less than 25 g combined. In ectopic ACTH syndrome, the combined adrenal weight is greater—from 25 g to 100 g.

Adrenal adenomas in Cushing syndrome range in weight from a few grams to over 100 g, usually over 3 cm in diameter, and are larger than aldosterone-producing adenomas. The typical cells usually resemble those of the zona fasciculata. Variable degrees of anaplasia are seen, and differentiation of benign from malignant tumors is often difficult on the basis of cytology alone. These adrenal adenomas occur more frequently in women. Adrenal cancers are frequently very large—almost always over 5 cm in diameter. They are undifferentiated, invade the surrounding tissues, and metastasize via the blood stream.

Rare forms of ACTH-independent Cushing syndrome include macronodular hyperplasia, which in some cases is due to aberrant expression of receptors in the adrenals that respond to stimuli other than ACTH. In these cases, the adrenal glands can be massively enlarged. Pigmented micronodular hyperplasia is associated with the syndrome of Carney complex that also includes cardiac myxoma and lentigines.

Rarely, ectopic adrenal tissue can be the source of excessive cortisol secretion. It has been found in various locations, most commonly near the abdominal aorta.

Cushing disease is caused by pituitary adenomas.

Ectopic ACTH syndrome is usually caused by small-cell lung cancer and carcinoid tumors, but tumors of the pancreas, thymus, thyroid, prostate, esophagus, colon, and ovaries—as well as pheochromocytoma and malignant melanoma—may also secrete ACTH.

C. Laboratory Findings

Since no single test is specific, a combination of tests must be used.

Normal subjects have a circadian rhythm of ACTH secretion that is paralleled by cortisol secretion. Levels are highest in the early morning and decline during the day to their lowest levels in the late evening. In Cushing disease, the circadian rhythm is abolished, and total secretion of cortisol is increased. In mild cases, the plasma cortisol and ACTH levels may be within the normal range during much of the day but abnormally high in the evening.

When Cushing syndrome is suspected, the first objective is to establish the diagnosis; the second is to establish the cause. An algorithm for the diagnosis is presented in Figure 33–3. When hypercortisolism is suspected, an **overnight dexamethasone suppression test**—or measurement of 24-hour urinary free cortisol—is the first diagnostic step. Dexamethasone, 1 mg orally (equivalent to about 30 mg of cortisol), will suppress ACTH secretion and stop cortisol production. This low-dose dexamethasone, however, will not suppress excessive cortisol production from autonomous adrenocortical tumors or adrenals that are being stimulated by excess ACTH. Since dexamethasone does not cross-react in the assay for plasma cortisol, suppression of endogenous circulating cortisol is easily demonstrated. The test is done as follows: At 11 PM, the patient is given 1 mg of dexamethasone by mouth. A fasting plasma cortisol is measured the following morning between 8 and 9 AM. Suppression of plasma cortisol to 1.8 μg/dL (50 nmol/L) or less excludes Cushing

syndrome. Higher cutoff levels have been recommended, but some patients with mild ACTH-dependent Cushing syndrome may be suppressed easily; thus, the response is falsely negative and the diagnosis of Cushing syndrome is missed. On the other hand, this low cutoff level increases the likelihood of a false-positive result. False-positive results are more common in patients with depression, alcoholism, physiologic stress, marked obesity, or renal failure and in those taking estrogens or drugs that accelerate dexamethasone metabolism, such as phenytoin, rifampin, and phenobarbital. Estrogens increase cortisol-binding globulin and elevate total plasma cortisol concentrations. In these situations, measurement of 24-hour urinary free cortisol is preferred.

The results of the dexamethasone test should be confirmed with a measurement of 24-hour urinary excretion of free cortisol. It directly measures the physiologically active form of circulating cortisol, integrates the daily variations of cortisol production, and is very sensitive and specific for the diagnosis of Cushing syndrome.

The midnight plasma cortisol level also distinguishes Cushing syndrome from non-Cushing states, but because it requires hospitalization, it is impractical. In contrast, late-evening salivary cortisol sampling can be easily accomplished at home without stress. The procedure involves chewing a cotton tube for 2–3 minutes. Salivary cortisol levels correlate highly with plasma and serum-free cortisol levels. The test is underutilized, mainly because it is not widely available.

Once the diagnosis of Cushing syndrome is established, the next step is to determine the cause. Plasma ACTH measurement by immunoradiometric assay (IRMA) is the most direct method. A normal to elevated ACTH level is diagnostic of hypercortisolism due to pituitary adenoma or ectopic ACTH secretion. Suppressed ACTH levels are diagnostic of hypercortisolism due to a primary adrenal cause such as adenoma, carcinoma, or nodular hyperplasia.

The differential diagnosis of ACTH-dependent Cushing syndrome can be challenging. No test is perfect, and a combination of tests may be necessary. Since 90% of patients have Cushing disease, pituitary MRI is the first test to identify the source of ACTH secretion. However, 10% of normal adults have incidental pituitary lesions 3–6 mm in diameter on MRI, and many patients with Cushing disease have no detectable lesions. Lesions smaller than 3–4 mm are more likely to represent normal variation, artifacts, volume averaging, incidental nonfunctional adenomas, or cysts. An unequivocal pituitary lesion (ie, > 4–5 mm in diameter with decreased signal intensity on gadolinium) strongly suggests Cushing disease.

If the pituitary MRI does not show a definite lesion, the next step is inferior petrosal sinus sampling with corticotropin-releasing hormone (CRH) stimulation. Compared with other biochemical tests, such as high-dose dexamethasone suppression or CRH stimulation, petrosal sinus sampling is the most accurate way to identify an ACTH-secreting pituitary adenoma; the diagnostic accuracy is close to 100%. The

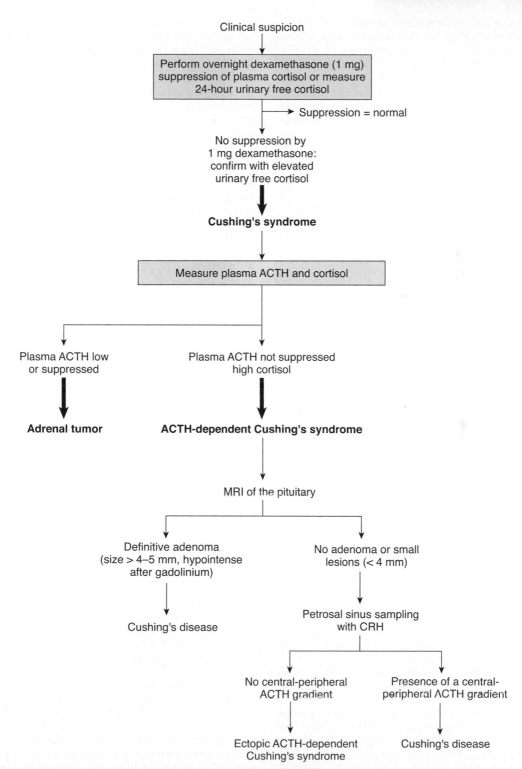

▲ **Figure 33–3.** Cushing syndrome: diagnosis and differential diagnosis.

test requires simultaneous bilateral venous sampling from the inferior petrosal sinuses. The inferior petrosal sinus connects the cavernous sinus and drains the pituitary. A central-to-peripheral ACTH ratio of 2 or greater without CRH stimulation is diagnostic of Cushing disease. CRH, 100 μg given intravenously as a bolus injection, can increase the diagnostic sensitivity to 100%; a peak central-to-peripheral ACTH ratio of 3 or greater is diagnostic of Cushing disease. The lack of a central-to-peripheral ACTH gradient is diagnostic of an ectopic ACTH-secreting tumor.

In Cushing syndrome caused by primary adrenal diseases, the plasma ACTH level is suppressed. Adenomas are usually 3–5 cm in diameter and secrete only cortisol. Adrenal carcinomas are typically larger than 5 cm in diameter, are usually rapidly progressive, and may cosecrete other hormones, such as adrenal androgens, deoxycorticosterone, aldosterone, and estrogens.

D. Imaging Studies

For Cushing syndrome caused by primary adrenal diseases, thin-section CT or MRI is able to detect virtually all of the adrenal tumors and hyperplasia. MRI of the sella is the imaging study of choice for pituitary adenomas. If a definitive adenoma is not seen, inferior petrosal sinus sampling with CRH stimulation can differentiate Cushing disease from ectopic Cushing syndrome. For ectopic Cushing syndrome, CT or MRI of the chest and abdomen may detect ACTH-secreting tumors. Bronchial carcinoids may be very small and difficult to find; high-resolution thin-cut CT of the chest is indicated. Occasionally, the source of an ectopic ACTH-secreting tumor cannot be determined (occult ectopic ACTH syndrome).

► Complications

Severe or lethal complications may result from sustained hypercortisolism, including hypertension, cardiovascular disease, stroke, thromboembolism, infection, severe debilitating muscle wasting, and weakness. Psychosis is common. Death may also be caused by the underlying tumors, such as adrenal carcinoma, small cell lung cancer, and others causing ectopic ACTH Cushing syndrome.

The truncal obesity and muscle weakness in patients with Cushing syndrome predispose them to postoperative pulmonary complications. Atrophic skin and easy bruisability also predict poor wound healing.

Nelson syndrome, the progression of an ACTH-secreting pituitary adenoma following bilateral adrenalectomy for Cushing disease, occurred in as many as 30% of patients in the era when bilateral adrenalectomy was used as primary therapy. However, since transsphenoidal resection has become the initial procedure of choice for Cushing disease, and because MRI now allows accurate diagnosis of pituitary adenomas larger than 5 mm, Nelson syndrome occurs in less than 5% of patients.

These tumors in patients with Nelson syndrome are among the most aggressive of pituitary tumors, causing sellar enlargement and extrasellar extension. Plasma ACTH levels are markedly elevated. Patients are frequently hyperpigmented and hypopituitary, with symptoms of mass effects including headaches, visual field deficits, and even blindness from optic nerve compression. Removal of feedback control from hypercortisolism at the pituitary level probably explains the aggressiveness of these tumors.

► Treatment

Resection is the best treatment for cortisol-producing adrenal tumors or ACTH-producing tumors. Other treatment options may be necessary to temporarily control hypercortisolism—or for patients not cured by resection or when complete resection is impossible.

A. Excision of Pituitary Adenoma

Patients with Cushing disease are usually treated by transsphenoidal microsurgical excision of the pituitary adenomas. Relief of symptoms is rapid, and the prognosis for adequate residual pituitary-adrenal function is good. Total or subtotal hypophysectomy may be performed in older patients if a discrete tumor is not found. Pituitary procedures fail in about 15–25% of patients because of failure to find the adenoma, pituitary hyperplasia, or recurrence of adenoma. When pituitary surgery fails, the disease may respond to pituitary irradiation. In some patients, medical therapy or total adrenalectomy will be necessary. Because of the effectiveness of pituitary microsurgery, radiotherapy is usually not recommended as primary treatment for Cushing disease.

B. Adrenalectomy

Compared with patients with other adrenal tumors, those with severe Cushing syndrome are at a higher risk for postoperative complications such as wound infection, hemorrhage, peptic ulceration, and pulmonary embolism. Adrenalectomy, however, is usually successful in reversing the devastating effects of hypercortisolism.

Laparoscopic adrenalectomy causes less morbidity than open adrenalectomy and is preferred for benign hyperplasia or adenomas. Laparoscopic adrenalectomy for adrenocortical carcinoma is technically challenging. Local recurrence may be more common after laparoscopic resection for large and invasive cancer, especially if the capsule is breached during dissection.

Unilateral adrenalectomy is indicated for adrenal adenomas or carcinomas that secrete cortisol. The contralateral adrenal gland and the hypothalamic-pituitary-adrenal axis will usually recover from the suppression 1–2 years after the operation.

Total bilateral adrenalectomy is indicated for selected patients with Cushing disease or ectopic ACTH syndrome in whom the ACTH-secreting tumor cannot be found or resected. It is also indicated for patients with bilateral primary adrenal disease, such as pigmented micronodular hyperplasia or massive macronodular hyperplasia.

Bilateral adrenalectomy can almost always be accomplished by the laparoscopic approach.

Subtotal resection is not recommended in patients with Cushing syndrome, because it usually leaves inadequate adrenocortical reserve initially, and the disease frequently recurs with continuing ACTH stimulation. Total bilateral adrenalectomy with adrenal gland autotransplantation is rarely successful and offers little advantage over pharmacologic replacement.

C. Medical Treatment

Drugs are mainly used as adjuvant therapy. Hypercortisolism may be controlled with ketoconazole, metyrapone, or aminoglutethimide, all of which inhibit steroid biosynthesis. Ketoconazole is usually the first choice. A combination of drugs may be necessary to control hypercortisolism and to decrease dose-related side effects. Mifepristone (RU 486), a progesterone and glucocorticoid receptor antagonist, is also effective, but it raises cortisol and ACTH levels, making it difficult to monitor the patient. Experience with the medication is still limited.

Mitotane is a dichlorodiphenyltrichloroethane (DDT) derivative that is toxic to the adrenal cortex. It has been used with modest success in the treatment of adrenal hypersecretory states, especially adrenocortical carcinoma. Unfortunately, serious side effects are common at effective doses.

D. Postoperative Maintenance Therapy

For patients who require total adrenalectomy, lifelong corticosteroid maintenance therapy becomes necessary after total adrenalectomy. The following schedule is commonly used: No cortisol is given until the adrenals are removed during surgery. On the first day, give 100 mg of hydrocortisone intravenously every 8 hours. On the second day, give 50 mg every 8 hours. Thereafter, the dose should be tapered as tolerated. The same tapering process is used after excision of a unilateral cortisol-secreting adenoma, because the remaining adrenal may not function normally for months.

As the hydrocortisone dose is reduced below 50 mg/d, it is often necessary to add fludrocortisone (a mineralocorticoid), 0.1 mg daily orally. The usual maintenance doses are about 15–30 mg of hydrocortisone and 0.1 mg of fludrocortisone daily. More than half the hydrocortisone dose is given in the morning.

Patients who have had a total bilateral adrenalectomy and are on maintenance therapy can develop addisonian crisis when under stress, such as general anesthesia or infection. Adrenal insufficiency causes fever, hyperkalemia, abdominal pain, and hypotension and should be promptly recognized and treated with saline infusion and cortisol.

▶ Prognosis

The prognosis is good after resection of benign adrenal adenomas, pituitary adenomas, or benign ACTH-secreting tumors. Symptoms and signs of hypercortisolism resolve, usually over months. Short-term adrenal insufficiency after surgery requires cortisol replacement. Cushing disease can recur after excision of a pituitary adenoma. An occult ACTH-secreting tumor may become apparent later and require removal.

Residual adrenal tissue or embryonic rests are present in up to 10% of patients after total adrenalectomy. Cushing syndrome can then recur if stimulation with ACTH continues.

The prognosis is extremely poor in patients with adrenocortical carcinoma and in those with malignant tumors causing ectopic ACTH syndrome.

Biller BMK et al. Treatment of ACTH dependent Cushing's syndrome: a consensus statement. J Clin Endocrin Metab 2008; 93:2454.

Findling JW, Raff H: Newer diagnostic techniques and problems in Cushing's disease. Endocrinol Metab Clin North Am 1999; 28:191.

Hall WA et al: Pituitary magnetic resonance imaging in normal human volunteers: occult adenomas in the general population. Ann Intern Med 1994;120:817.

Hawn MT et al: Quality of life after bilateral adrenalectomy for Cushing's disease. Surgery 2002;132:1064.

Kemink L et al: Residual adrenocortical function after bilateral adrenalectomy for pituitary-dependent Cushing's syndrome. J Clin Endocrinol Metab 1992;75:1211.

Liu C et al: Cavernous and inferior petrosal sinus sampling in the evaluation of ACTH-dependent Cushing's syndrome. Clin Endocrinol (Oxf) 2004;61:478.

Nieman LK et al: The diagnosis of Cushing's syndrome: an Endocrine Society Clinical Practice Guideline. J Clin Endocrinol Metab 2008;93:1526.

Raff H et al: Late-night salivary cortisol as a screening test for Cushing's syndrome. J Clin Endocrinol Metab 1998;83:2681.

Tyrrell JB et al: Cushing's disease. Therapy of pituitary adenomas. Endocrinol Metab Clin North Am 1994;23:925.

Walz MK: Extent of adrenalectomy for adrenal neoplasm: cortical sparing (subtotal) versus total adrenalectomy. Surg Clin North Am 2004;84:743.

VIRILIZING ADRENAL TUMORS

In adults, hormonally active benign adrenal adenomas usually secrete aldosterone or cortisol. Virilizing tumors in women are more likely to be caused by ovarian tumors. Virilizing adrenal tumors are rare, and virilization is usually due to hypersecretion of adrenal androgens, mainly dehydroepiandrosterone (DHEA), its sulfate derivative (DHEAS), and androstenedione, all of which are converted peripherally to testosterone and 5-dihydrotestosterone. Very rarely, virilizing adrenal tumors secrete only testosterone.

The differentiation of benign from malignant adrenocortical tumors may be difficult when based on histologic features; some patients with histologically benign tumors may develop metastases, and others with histologically malignant tumors may never have recurrent disease. Malignancy is only definitely diagnosed from local or distant spread. Seventy percent of virilizing adrenal tumors exhibit malignant behavior. Adrenocortical carcinomas are usually large tumors with local spread or distant metastases. They often secrete multiple steroids, most commonly cortisol and androgens, leading to Cushing syndrome and virilization.

In children, adrenocortical tumors are rare, but virilization with or without hypercortisolism is the most frequent feature. Virilizing adrenal tumors are less likely to be malignant in children than in adults. Histologic features of malignancy do not always predict malignant behavior. Large tumors (> 100 g) have a worse prognosis.

Signs and symptoms of virilization include hirsutism, male-pattern baldness, acne, deep voice, male musculature, irregular menses or amenorrhea, clitoromegaly, and increased libido. Rapid linear growth with advanced bone age is common in children.

CT and MRI are used to image virilizing adrenal tumors. Resection is the only successful treatment.

Virilization can also be caused by congenital adrenal hyperplasia, an autosomal recessive disorder. The mutated genes encode enzymes essential for cortisol and mineralocorticoid synthesis. 21-Hydroxylase deficiency accounts for 90% of cases. The inhibition of cortisol synthesis leads to stimulated ACTH secretion, accumulation of precursors, and overproduction of androgens. Administration of glucocorticoids is the mainstay of treatment in patients with classic congenital adrenal hyperplasia. Mineralocorticoid replacement is also required. Corrective surgery is needed in female infants born with ambiguous genitalia. The combination of antiandrogens, aromatase inhibitors, and lower-dose glucocorticoid replacement to minimize the effect of excess androgen is being investigated. Adrenalectomy with lifelong steroid replacement is another approach in the most severely affected patients.

Cordera F et al: Androgen-secreting adrenal tumors. Surgery 2003;134:874.

Latronico AC et al: Extensive personal experience: adrenocortical tumors. J Clin Endocrinol Metab 1997;82:1317.

Liou LS et al: Adrenocortical carcinoma in children. Review and recent innovations. Urol Clin North Am 2000;27:403.

Merk DP et al: NIH conference. Future directions in the study and management of congenital adrenal hyperplasia due to 21-hydroxylase deficiency. Ann Intern Med 2002;136:320.

Michalkiewicz EL et al: Clinical characteristics of small functioning adrenocortical tumors in children. Med Pediatr Oncol 1997;28:175.

Moreno S et al: Profile and outcome of pure androgen-secreting adrenal tumors in women: experience of 21 cases. Surgery 2004;136:1192.

FEMINIZING ADRENAL TUMORS

Estrogens are not normally synthesized by the adrenal cortex. Feminizing adrenal tumors are extremely rare and are almost always carcinomas. They are usually seen in men with feminization or in girls with precocious puberty. Vaginal bleeding may be the presenting symptom in adult women. Feminizing adrenal carcinomas frequently hypersecrete other hormones. The diagnosis is based on a finding of increased plasma estrogens. Ovarian tumors and administration of exogenous estrogen should be ruled out.

Definitive treatment is by excision of the tumor. The prognosis is guarded.

Goto T et al: Oestrogen producing adrenocortical adenoma: clinical, biochemical and immunohistochemical studies. Clin Endocrinol 1996;45:643.

ADRENOCORTICAL CARCINOMA

Adrenocortical carcinomas are rare. Fifty percent of patients have symptoms related to hypersecretion of hormones, most commonly Cushing syndrome and virilization. Feminizing and purely aldosterone-secreting carcinomas are rare. In some cases, hormone hypersecretion is subclinical and only found by biochemical studies. A palpable abdominal mass is common. The mean diameter of adrenal carcinoma is 12 cm (range, 3–30 cm). Adrenocortical carcinoma invades the surrounding tissues, and about half of the patients have metastases (lung, liver, and elsewhere) at the time of diagnosis. In those without local spread or distant metastases, a diagnosis of carcinoma based on cytologic features may be wrong.

The median survival is 25 months, and 5-year actuarial survival is 25%. Tumor stage at the initial operation predicts the prognosis. Surgery is the only treatment that potentially provides a cure; however, beneficial outcomes are confined to patients with localized disease. When grossly complete resection is possible, the 5-year survival is 50%. Thus, recurrence is common despite apparent complete resection due to micrometastases at initial presentation. Laparoscopic adrenalectomy is technically more difficult for adrenocortical carcinomas than for other adrenal tumors because the tumor is fragile and adjacent organs may have to be removed. Where the adrenal tumor is small, malignancy is uncertain, and the surgeon is technically capable, starting the operation laparoscopically is acceptable, but the abdomen should be opened if there is any question about whether a better operation could be accomplished that way. For local recurrent disease, reoperation is indicated and may prolong life. Patients with distant metastases at initial presentation usually die within 1 year. Resecting the adrenal tumor in these patients does not improve survival.

Mitotane, an adrenolytic agent, has been used as an adjuvant to surgery in patients with advanced adrenocortical carcinoma. It controls endocrine symptoms in 50% of patients, and the tumor regresses in some. Nevertheless, survival is not generally affected, though a few cases of prolonged remission have been reported.

In patients who underwent complete primary resection, older reports of routine adjuvant mitotane therapy postoperatively did not confer definitive benefits. However, a recent large retrospective study showed that mitotane improved recurrence-free survival.

Dose-related side effects (eg, gastrointestinal symptoms, weakness, dizziness, and somnolence) may limit its use. A variety of other chemotherapeutic agents have been tried with limited success. The role of radiation is limited and usually is for palliation, especially for bony metastases.

Abiven G et al: Clinical and biological features in the prognosis of adrenocortical cancer: poor outcome of cortisol-secreting tumors in a series of 202 consecutive patients. J Clin Endocrinol Metab 2006;91:2650.

Allolio B et al: Management of adrenocortical carcinoma. Clin Endocrinol (Oxf) 2004;60:273.

Bellantone R et al: Role of reoperation in recurrence of adrenal cortical carcinoma: results from 188 cases collected in the Italian National Registry for Adrenal Cortical Carcinoma. Surgery 1997;122:1212.

Dackiw AP et al: Adrenal cortical carcinoma. World J Surg 2001;25:914.

Icard P et al: Adrenocortical carcinomas: surgical trends and results from a 253-patient series from the French Association of Endocrine Surgeons study group. World J Surg 2001;25:891.

Kirschner LS: paradigms for adrenal cancer: think globally, act locally. J Clin Endocrinol Metab 2006;91:4250.

Schteingart ED et al: Management of patients with adrenal cancer: recommendations of an international consensus conference. Endocr Relat Cancer 2005;12:667.

Stratakis CA et al: Adrenal cancer. Endocrinol Metab Clin North Am 2000;29:15.

Terzolo et al: Adjuvant mitotane treatment for adrenocortical carcinoma. N Engl J Med 2007;356:2372.

INCIDENTALOMAS

Adrenal tumors have traditionally been diagnosed after presentation with clinical symptoms of excess hormone secretion. However, the increased use of ultrasonography, CT, and MRI for various diseases in the abdomen has led to the discovery of what are referred to as adrenal incidentalomas. Most are small nonfunctioning adrenal cortical adenomas; some are functioning adenomas or pheochromocytomas with subclinical secretion of hormones; and some are adrenocortical carcinomas or metastases.

Incidentalomas are found in 1–4% of CT scans and 6% of random autopsies. The incidence increases with age. Subclinical Cushing syndrome, pheochromocytoma, and adrenocortical carcinoma each account for about 5% of cases, metastatic carcinoma for 2%, and aldosteronoma for 1% (Table 33–2). Thus, over 80% of patients have presumed nonfunctioning cortical adenomas. Simple adrenal cysts, myelolipomas, and adrenal hemorrhages can be identified by the CT characteristics alone. Adrenal cysts can be large but are rarely malignant. Adrenal hemorrhage may occur in preexisting adrenal tumors.

The major issues in managing a patient with an incidentaloma is to determine whether the tumor is hormonally active and whether it is a cancer; either would be an indication for resection. Since most incidentalomas are nonfunctioning adenomas, the workup should be selective to avoid unnecessary expense and procedures.

Table 33–2. Adrenal Incidentalomas.[1]

Tumor Types	Percentage
Subclinical Cushing	5%
Pheochromocytoma	5%
Adrenocortical carcinoma	5%
Metastatic carcinoma	2%
Aldosterone-producing adenoma	1%
Presumed nonfunctional adenoma	82%
Total	100%

[1]Based on data reported in Endocrinol Metab Clin North Am 2000;29:159.

The workup should include a complete history and physical examination with specific reference to a history of previous malignancy and signs and symptoms of Cushing syndrome or pheochromocytoma. Hyperaldosteronism, pheochromocytoma, and virilizing or feminizing adrenocortical carcinoma should be investigated. Further laboratory studies may be indicated depending on the clinical presentation.

The management of an incidentaloma depends on its functional status and the size and imaging characteristics of the tumor. All functioning tumors should be excised. Large nonfunctioning tumors also should be excised because of the increased risk of cancer. Small nonfunctioning tumors are almost always benign adenomas; they can be followed with serial CT scans checking for changes in size.

All patients—even those who do not have hypertension—should have a 24-hour urine collection for fractionated catecholamines and metanephrines or fractionated plasma metanephrines to search for pheochromocytoma; the risk of unrecognized pheochromocytoma is high, and the hypertension may be absent or episodic. Most pheochromocytomas are over 2 cm in diameter and characteristically bright on T2-weighted MRI. *Forty percent of pheochromocytomas are found incidentally because of CT or MRI scans obtained for other indications.*

Subclinical Cushing syndrome refers to autonomous cortisol secretion in patients without typical signs and symptoms of Cushing syndrome. Autonomous cortisol secretion is best assessed by overnight 1 mg dexamethasone suppression test.

Patients with subclinical Cushing syndrome may experience an addisonian crisis if the tumor is resected and glucocorticoid replacement is not adequate.

Patients who are hypertensive should also have plasma aldosterone and plasma renin activity measured to screen for primary hyperaldosteronism.

If the above studies show that the tumor is nonfunctional, the size and imaging characteristics of the tumor and the patient's overall medical condition should determine the appropriate treatment. Nonfunctioning adrenal tumors larger than 5 cm in diameter should usually be removed because of higher risk of cancer. Nonfunctioning adrenal tumors smaller than 3 cm that are homogeneous and have low density on CT or MRI are unlikely to be cancers and can be safely followed. The patient's age and overall medical condition and the CT scan findings will usually determine whether a tumor 3–5 cm in size should be resected. High density, delayed wash out of contrast, irregular borders, and heterogeneity make pheochromocytoma, adrenocortical carcinoma, and metastases more likely.

In patients with a previously treated malignancy such as lung or breast cancer, an adrenal mass larger than 3 cm is very likely a metastasis. Once the possibility of pheochromocytoma is excluded, a CT-guided fine-needle aspiration biopsy can be used to diagnose metastatic cancer if it will change management of the patient. Fine-needle aspiration of an adrenocortical cancer may not be diagnostic, and breaching the capsule risks local spread of cancer. Resection of a solitary adrenal metastasis from a primary lung cancer may improve long-term survival (to about 25% at 5 years) if there are no other clinically obvious metastases. Patients with a metachronous solitary adrenal metastasis are more likely to benefit from adrenalectomy than are those with a synchronous metastasis. Patients with adrenal metastases from melanoma or renal cell carcinoma also benefit from resection. Adrenal metastasis can be resected laparoscopically with minimal risk of local recurrence.

Bulow B et al: Adrenal incidentaloma: follow-up results from a Swedish prospective study. Eur J Endocrinol 2006;154:419.

Grumbach MM et al: NIH Conference. Management of the clinically inapparent adrenal mass ("incidentaloma"). Ann Intern Med 2003;138:424.

Lee JA et al: Adrenal incidentaloma, borderline elevations of urine or plasma metanephrine levels, and the "subclinical" pheochromocytoma. Arch Surg 2007;142:870.

Quayle FJ et al: Needle biopsy of incidentally discovered adrenal masses is rarely informative and potentially hazardous. Surgery 2007;142:497.

Sippel RS, Chen H: Subclinical Cushing's syndrome in adrenal incidentalomas. Surg Clin North Am 2004;84:875.

Young WF: The incidentally discovered adrenal mass. N Engl J Med 2007;356:601.

Arteries

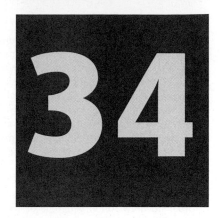

Joseph H. Rapp, MD

Jason MacTaggart, MD

Arterial disease can be broadly classified into two categories: occlusive and aneurysmal. The major sequelae of arterial obstruction are tissue ischemia and necrosis, while those of aneurysmal disease are rupture and hemorrhage in the aortic position and thrombosis and embolization in the peripheral arteries.

ARTERIAL OCCLUSIVE DISEASE

Although atherosclerosis is the dominant cause of arterial occlusive disease, other etiologies such as congenital and anatomical anomalies, arterial dissection, and remote thromboembolism can also result in arterial obstruction. Symptoms of occlusive vascular disease primarily are end-organ dysfunction and, in the muscle beds, pain with exercise and tissue necrosis.

ATHEROSCLEROSIS

Atherosclerosis can be seen in any artery, with plaques most commonly developing in areas of low shear stress, such as at arterial branch points. Lesions are usually symmetrically distributed, although the rate of progression may vary. Early lesions are confined to the intima. In advanced lesions, both intima and media are involved, but the adventitia is spared. Preservation of the adventitia is essential for the vessel's structural integrity and is the basis for all cardiovascular interventions.

The hemodynamic circuit consists of the diseased major artery, a parallel system of collateral vessels, and the peripheral runoff bed. Collateral vessels are smaller, more circuitous, and always have a higher resistance than the original unobstructed artery. The stimuli for collateral development include abnormal pressure gradients across the collateral system and increased flow velocity through intramuscular channels that connect to reentry vessels. Adequate collateral vessels take time to develop but often maintain tissue viability in patients with chronic major arterial occlusions.

Generally, arterial insufficiency occurs in medium-sized and large arteries with a 50% reduction in arterial diameter. This correlates with a 75% narrowing of cross-sectional area and enough resistance to decrease downstream flow and pressure. Compensatory dilation of the vessel wall may preserve lumen diameter as the atherosclerotic lesion develops, but with continued growth, lesions overcome this adaptation and result in flow limiting stenoses.

Atherosclerosis develops over decades. Significant luminal narrowing with reduced flow may produce ischemia with increased demand (exercise), or the presenting event may be sudden thrombosis. If there is adequate collateral flow, single stenoses or even occlusions are reasonably well tolerated. Severe ischemia is usually associated with multiple levels of disease.

Libby P: Atherosclerosis: the new view. Sci American 2002;286:46.
Davì G, Patrono C: Platelet activation and atherothrombosis. N Engl J Med 2008;358:1638.

CHRONIC LOWER EXTREMITY OCCLUSIVE DISEASE

 ESSENTIALS OF DIAGNOSIS

General:

► Decreased pulses.
► Low ankle-brachial index.
► Intermittent claudication.
► Cramping calf pain with walking.

Critical limb Ischemia:

► Rest pain of the foot relieved by dependency.
► Ulceration of the foot or ankle.
► Pallor of foot on elevation, rubor on dependency.
► Gangrene and atrophy.

General Considerations

Peripheral arterial insufficiency is predominantly a disease of the lower extremities. Upper extremity arterial lesions are uncommon and confined mostly to the subclavian arteries. Even when present, upper extremity atherosclerosis rarely produces symptoms due to abundant collateral pathways. In the lower extremities, however, obstructive lesions are distributed widely, with lesions of the superficial femoral and iliac arteries the most common (Figure 34–1). Symptoms are related to the location and number of obstructions.

Peripheral arterial disease affects at least 20% of individuals older than 70 years. Although most patients with this disorder do not develop gangrene or require amputations, adverse outcomes of systemic atherosclerosis, including death, are common. Even after adjustment for known risk factors, individuals with peripheral arterial disease exhibit a several-fold higher risk of mortality than the nonaffected population. A low ankle-brachial index is one of the strongest risk factors for all-cause mortality. Peripheral arterial disease is more a marker of a more virulent form of atherosclerosis and early death from cardiovascular or cerebrovascular disease than an indicator of imminent limb loss; thus, identifying and treating associated atherosclerotic risk factors is essential (Figure 34–2).

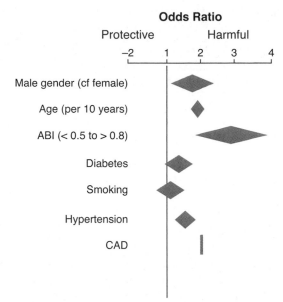

▲ **Figure 34–2.** Odds ratios for risk factors for all-cause mortality. ABI, ankle-brachial index; CAD, coronary artery disease. (Reproduced, with permission, from TASC Working Group: Management of peripheral arterial disease: epidemiology, natural history, risk factors. J Vasc Surg 2000;31 [1 Suppl]:S22. © 2000 Society for Vascular Surgery. Reprinted with permission from Elsevier.)

Clinical Findings

A. Symptoms

1. Intermittent claudication—Intermittent claudication refers to pain in muscles of the lower extremity associated with walking and relieved by rest. Because tissue perfusion is adequate at rest, tissue loss is not present and the risk of amputation is low unless there is progression of disease. Claudication is derived from the Latin word meaning "to limp"; therefore, the term should be used only for symptoms in the lower extremities. The pain is a deep-seated ache usually in the calf muscle, which gradually progresses until the patient is compelled to stop walking. Patients occasionally describe "cramping" or "tiredness" in the muscle. Typically, symptoms are completely relieved after 2–5 minutes of inactivity. Claudication is distinguished from other types of pain in the extremities in that it does not occur at rest and some period of exertion is always required before it appears, it generally occurs after a relatively consistent distance traveled, and it is relieved by cessation of walking. Relief of symptoms is not dependent upon sitting or other positional change. The severity of claudication is traditionally expressed in terms of city blocks.

Regardless of which arterial segment is involved, claudication most commonly involves the calf muscles because of their

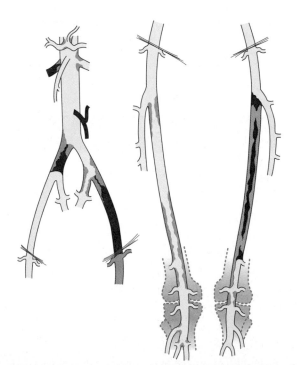

▲ **Figure 34–1.** Common sites of stenosis and occlusion of the visceral and peripheral arterial systems.

high workload with the mechanics of normal walking. Occlusions proximal to the origin of the profunda femoris can extend the pain to involve the thigh. Gluteal pain indicates lesions in or proximal to the hypogastric arteries and is often accompanied by impotence. **Leriche syndrome** occurs in men with aortoiliac disease and includes claudication of calf, thigh, and buttock muscles; impotence; and diminished or absent femoral pulses. Occasionally, patients describe transient numbness of the extremity accompanying the pain and fatigue of claudication as nerves as well as muscles become ischemic.

The two conditions that most often mimic claudication are osteoarthritis of the hip or knee and neurospinal compression due to congenital or osteophytic narrowing of the lumbar neurospinal canal (spinal stenosis). Osteoarthritis can be differentiated from claudication because pain occurs predominantly in joints, the amount of exercise required to elicit symptoms varies, symptoms are characteristically worse in the morning and upon initiating exercise, rest does not relieve symptoms promptly, the severity of symptoms changes from day to day, and anti-inflammatory agents may relieve the pain. Impingement on the spinal canal or nerve root produces neurospinal compression symptoms; therefore, the pain is typically burning in nature and symptoms may occur with sitting or standing. Neurospinal pain may follow a dermatomal distribution.

Uncommon conditions such as coarctation of the aorta, chronic compartment syndrome, popliteal artery entrapment, and vasculitis can mimic symptoms of atherosclerotic arterial insufficiency. Age at presentation and associated findings may aid in diagnosing these conditions.

The correct diagnosis of vascular claudication should be easily established by determining the location of pain with exercise (calf), the quality of the pain (aching or cramping), the length of time required for relief of symptoms after stopping exercise (immediate), and the reproducibility of the distance walked before symptoms begin (initial claudication distance).

2. Critical limb ischemia—With extensive disease, patients develop ischemic rest pain and/or ulceration. Ischemic rest pain, a grave symptom caused by ischemic neuritis, indicates advanced arterial insufficiency that carries a risk of gangrene and amputation if arterial reconstruction cannot be performed. The pain is severe and burning, usually confined to the forefoot distal to the metatarsals. It may be localized to the vicinity of an ischemic ulcer or pregangrenous toe. It is aggravated by elevation of the extremity or by bringing the leg to the horizontal position. Thus, it appears at bed rest (hence the name) and may prevent sleep. Because gravity aids the delivery of arterial blood, classically, the patient with rest pain can obtain relief by simply hanging the leg over the side of the bed. This simple maneuver will not relieve pain caused by peripheral neuropathy, the most common cause of foot pain at rest. If the foot is constantly kept dependent to relieve pain, the leg and foot may be swollen, causing some confusion in diagnosis. The ischemic neuritis of rest pain is severe and resistant to opioids for relief.

Patients with rest pain may give a history of claudication, but rest pain also may occur de novo in diabetics with distal tibial disease, embolic occlusion of the distal tibial arteries, and patients whose walking is limited by other conditions. Differentiating ischemic rest pain from neuropathy in diabetics may be difficult and require vascular testing.

3. Nonhealing wounds or ulcers—Patients with severe lower extremity arterial insufficiency often develop ulcers or wounds on the feet even from seemingly trivial trauma. These lesions are most commonly located on the distal foot and toes, but on occasion they can be in the upper foot or ankle. Typically, the wounds are excruciatingly painful, deep, and devoid of any evidence of healing such as contraction or formation of granulation tissue.

4. Erectile dysfunction—Inability to attain or maintain an erection may be produced by lesions that obstruct blood flow through both hypogastric arteries and is commonly found in association with narrowing of the terminal aorta or common iliac arteries. Vasculogenic erectile dysfunction is less common than that due to other causes.

5. Sensation—Although the patient may report numbness in the extremity, sensory abnormalities are generally absent on examination. If decreased sensation is found in the foot, peripheral neuropathy should be suspected.

B. Signs

Physical examination is of paramount importance in assessing the presence and severity of vascular disease. The physical findings of peripheral atherosclerosis are related to changes in the peripheral arteries and to tissue ischemia.

1. Arterial palpation—Decreased amplitude of the pulse denotes proximal obstructions to flow. The pulse examination can help localize disease. For example, an absent femoral pulse usually signifies aortoiliac disease. It is unusual for collateral flow to be sufficient to produce a pulse distal to an occluded artery.

2. Bruits and thrills—A bruit is the sound produced by dissipation of energy as blood flows through a stenotic arterial segment. With extremely high flows, the energy may vibrate the artery, creating a "thrill." The bruit or thrill is transmitted distally along the course of the artery. Thus, when a bruit is heard through a stethoscope placed over a peripheral artery, stenosis is present at or proximal to that level. The pitch of the bruit rises as the stenosis becomes more marked, until a critical stenosis is reached or the vessel becomes occluded, when the bruit may disappear. Thus, absence of a bruit does not indicate insignificant disease.

3. Response to exercise—Exercise in a normal individual increases the pulse rate without producing arterial bruits or reduction in pulse amplitude. In an individual who complains of claudication, there may be minimal findings at rest, but exercise will produce decreased pulse strength, distal arterial pressure, and possibly an audible bruit unmasking a significant stenosis. Exercise is best used in conjunction with noninvasive vascular testing.

4. Integumentary changes—Chronic ischemia commonly produces loss of hair over the dorsum of the toes and foot and may be associated with thickening of the toenails (onychomycosis) due to slowed keratin turnover. With more advanced ischemia, there is atrophy of the skin and subcutaneous tissue so that the foot becomes shiny, scaly, and skeletonized. Hence, a quick glance at a foot usually can identify the presence or absence of serious arterial insufficiency.

5. Pallor—Pallor of the foot on elevation of the extremity with a complete absence of capillary refill indicates advanced ischemia. Pallor on elevation does not occur unless advanced ischemia is present.

6. Reactive hyperemia—When pallor is produced with elevation, the ischemia results in maximum cutaneous vasodilation. When the extremity is returned to a dependent position, blood returning to the dilated vascular bed produces an intense red or possibly ruborous color in the foot, called reactive hyperemia, and denotes advanced disease. The delay in the appearance of color when the extremities return to a dependent position is proportionate to the impairment in circulation.

7. Rubor—In advanced atherosclerotic disease, the skin of the foot displays a characteristic dark red/cyanotic color on dependency. Because of low inflow, the blood in the capillary network of the foot is relatively stagnant, oxygen extraction is high, and the capillary blood becomes the color of the venous blood. The concurrent vasodilation due to ischemia causes blood to suffuse the cutaneous plexus, imparting a purple color to the skin. The purple discoloration due to severe chronic venous insufficiency does not develop pallor on elevation.

8. Skin temperature—With chronic ischemia, the temperature of the skin of the foot decreases. Coolness can best be detected by palpation with the back of the examiner's hand with comparison to the contralateral foot.

9. Ulceration—Ischemic ulcers are usually very painful and accompanied by rest pain in the foot. They occur in toes or at a site where minor trauma from a shoe or bedding can initiate the injury. The margin of the ulcer is sharply demarcated or punched-out, and the base is devoid of healthy granulation tissue. The surrounding skin is pale and mottled, and signs of chronic ischemia are invariably present

10. Atrophy—Moderate to severe degrees of chronic ischemia produce gradual soft tissue and muscle atrophy and loss of strength in the ischemic zone. Joint mobility may be reduced in the forefoot as atrophy of the muscles of the foot produces increasing prominence of the interosseous spaces. Subsequent changes in foot structure and gait increase the possibility of developing foot ulceration.

11. Necrosis—Tissue necrosis first becomes apparent in the most distal portions of the extremity or at an ulcer site. Necrosis halts proximally at a line where the blood supply is sufficient to maintain viability and results in dry gangrene. If the necrotic portion is infected (wet gangrene), necrosis may extend into tissues that would normally remain viable.

C. Noninvasive Vascular Laboratory Tests

Noninvasive assessment is helpful to determine the severity of hypoperfusion and the sites of hemodynamically significant stenoses or occlusions.

The **ankle-brachial index (ABI)** is a quick screening test and the cornerstone of the diagnosis of peripheral vascular disease. The ABI is determined by dividing the systolic pressure obtained by Doppler insonation at the ankle by the brachial arterial pressure. Normally, the ABI is 1.0 or greater; a value below 1.0 indicates occlusive disease proximal to the point of measurement. The ABI correlates roughly with the degree of ischemia (eg, claudication occurs with a value less than 0.7 and rest pain usually appears when the ratio is 0.3 or lower). Patients with diabetic vascular disease may have artificially elevated ABI values due to calcified, noncompressible arteries, and toe-to-brachial pressure ratios should be substituted.

Blood pressures can be measured at rest and after exercise in the ankle, and the effect of exercise can be monitored. **Exercise testing** confirms and quantitates the diagnosis of claudication. To perform exercise testing, the patient walks on a treadmill at a standard speed and grade until claudication pain is experienced or a time limit is reached. With significant arterial occlusive disease, there will be a decrease in the ABI with exercise, usually measured 1 minute after cessation of walking. If the pain is not due to arterial stenosis, no fall in pressure will occur. This test is particularly useful in differentiating neurogenic pain with walking from claudication.

D. Imaging Studies

Color duplex ultrasound imaging is a mainstay of vascular imaging. It is a painless, relatively inexpensive, and (in experienced hands) accurate method for acquiring anatomic and functional information (eg, velocity gradients across stenoses). Although the accuracy of this study is operator dependent, it can supply sufficient information to permit intervention in selected cases.

CT angiography (CTA) is useful for imaging the arterial tree and has the advantage of visualizing cross sections of the vessel lumen. In many instances, this allows for more accurate determination of vessel diameter and stenosis severity than conventional angiography. It does require the administration of nephrotoxic contrast dye, and its images may be obscured by the presence of calcification or metallic implants. **MR angiography (MRA)** also can be used to obtain images similar in quality to angiography in most cases. MRA does not show calcifications and gives better visualization of tibial vessels than CTA. MRA also can reveal details of composition of atherosclerotic plaque. Gadolinium-associated nephrogenic fibrosing dermopathy limits its use in patients with renal insufficiency. The integrated use of computer workstations with CT and MR image data can provide 3D images that can be useful in visualizing patient anatomy and planning interventional procedures.

Conventional arteriography provides detailed anatomic information about peripheral arterial disease. It is reserved for patients warranting invasive intervention such as percutaneous transluminal angioplasty (often shortened to PTA) or vascular surgery. Complications of angiography are related to technique and contrast media. Technical complications such as puncture site hematomas, arteriovenous fistulas, and false aneurysms are rare (1%). Contrast agents may precipitate allergic reactions (0.1%). Patients with renal failure, proteinuria, diabetes, and dehydration are at increased risk for contrast-induced renal failure. Adequate hydration of patients before and after angiography, acetylcysteine, and periprocedural infusions of sodium bicarbonate infusions may reduce the incidence of this complication.

▶ Treatment & Prognosis

The objectives of treatment for lower extremity occlusive disease are relief of symptoms, prevention of limb loss, and maintenance of bipedal gait.

A. Nonoperative Treatment

In general, patients with peripheral vascular disease have shortened life expectancies because of their severe atherosclerotic disease. Nondiabetic patients with ischemic disease of the lower extremity have a 5-year survival rate of 70%. The survival rate is 60% in patients with associated ischemic heart disease or cerebrovascular insufficiency. Patients with peripheral vascular disease and renal failure have a 2-year survival rate of less than 50%. Most deaths are due to myocardial infarctions and strokes. Only 20% of deaths are due to nonatherosclerotic causes.

Nonoperative treatment consists of (1) medical management of cardiovascular risk factors, (2) exercise rehabilitation, (3) foot care, and (4) pharmacotherapy.

1. Reduction of cardiovascular risk factors—See Table 34–1. Cigarette smoking is the single most important risk factor for peripheral vascular disease, and all patients should stop smoking. At high levels of consumption, 2–3 packs per day, claudicants will experience immediate improvement in walking distance.

In the past, elevated lipids were not usually associated with peripheral vascular disease. Hyperlipidemia, however, is often present, especially in patients with early onset of disease. Elevated triglyceride levels and low high-density lipoprotein (HDL) cholesterol levels are more prevalent than elevated levels of low-density lipoprotein (LDL) cholesterol. Reduction of elevated lipid levels is associated with stabiliza-

Table 34–1. Summary of Risk Factor Modification in Peripheral Vascular Disease.

Risk Factor	Therapy	Clinical Effect
Tobacco use	Counseling Pharmacotherapy Nicotine replacement Bupropion, varenicline	Reduced overall mortality Reduced cardiovascular events
Antiplatelet	Aspirin Clopidogrel (Plavix)	Antiplatelet therapy gives > 20% reduction in MI, stroke, or vascular death
Hyperlipidemia	Statin Lipid goals in PAD patients: LDL < 100 mg/dL	20–30% reduction in cardiovascular and all-cause mortality in CAD patients
Hypertension	Target BP < 140/90 in PAD patients Beta-blocker ACE inhibitor	Beta-blocker and ACE inhibitors each associated with > 20% reduction in cardiovascular mortality
Diabetes	Goal hemoglobin A1c < 7%	Benefits in vascular disease unproven
Lifestyle	Daily aerobic exercise Weight loss Healthy, low-fat diet	Reduced lipid levels Reduced cardiovascular events

BP, blood pressure; CAD, coronary artery disease; LDL, low-density lipoprotein; MI, myocardial infarction; PAD, peripheral artery disease.

tion or regression of arterial plaques. Statins are extremely effective in reducing LDL cholesterol, and goals of therapy for patients with peripheral vascular disease are to maintain cholesterol levels at less than 100 mg/dL (2.6 mmol/L). Statins have other pleiotropic effects that may reduce inflammation, stabilize plaques, and independently increase walking distance in claudicants. Other antihyperlipidemic medications, including niacin and fibrates (gemfibrozil), may be used to lower hypertriglyceridemia, which can increase HDL cholesterol.

Both type 1 and type 2 diabetes increase the prevalence and severity of cardiovascular disease. Intensive glycemic control reduces the incidence of nephropathy, neuropathy, and retinopathy in diabetes, but it does not correlate with the severity or progression of peripheral arterial disease. In order to reduce all-cause mortality, however, it is recommended that fasting blood sugars should be controlled with hemoglobin A1c levels less than 7%.

2. Exercise rehabilitation—For claudicants, exercise ranging from unsupervised walking to formal supervised exercise on a treadmill significantly improves walking ability. A 21-study meta-analysis of exercise programs showed an average

180% increase in initial claudication distance and a 120% increase in maximal walking distance achieved through exercise. The precise mechanism behind this improvement is not firmly established. Collateral development seems unlikely because ankle pressures and limb flow do not increase substantially. Possible explanations include improved metabolic capacity and conditioning of the muscles.

Since patients with claudication are at a twofold to fourfold greater risk of dying from complications of generalized atherosclerosis than people without claudication, an additional benefit of exercise in these patients is that an improvement in walking distance as part of an aggressive risk factor modification regimen results in an overall decrease in cardiovascular risk.

3. Foot care—The feet of patients with neuropathy or with critical limb ischemia should be inspected and washed daily and kept dry. Mechanical and thermal trauma to the feet should be avoided. Toenails should be trimmed carefully, and corns and calluses should be attended to promptly. Even minor foot infections or injuries should be treated aggressively. Educating the patient to understand neuropathy, peripheral vascular insufficiency, and the importance of foot care is a central aspect of treatment.

4. Pharmacotherapy—The Antiplatelet Trialists Collaboration found an overall 25% decrease in fatal and nonfatal myocardial infarctions, strokes, and vascular deaths in those treated with antiplatelet agents. Aspirin at dosages ranging from 75 to 350 mg/d is the first-line antiplatelet agent recommended, though clopidogrel, which blocks the activation of platelets by adenosine diphosphate (ADP), may be useful in aspirin-intolerant patients. Clopidogrel is also an important adjunctive therapy in reducing thrombogenicity at locations of endovascular arterial treatment. All patients with cardiovascular disease, whether symptomatic or asymptomatic, should be considered for antiplatelet therapy to reduce the risk of cardiovascular morbidity and mortality.

Two drugs have been approved by the FDA for treatment of intermittent claudication. Pentoxifylline produces a small improvement in both initial claudication distance (about 20%) and absolute claudication distance (about 10%). Cilostazol is a phosphodiesterase III inhibitor with vasodilator, antiplatelet, and antilipid activity. Randomized, placebo-controlled, blinded trials have shown an increase of about 50% in absolute claudication distance in patients treated with cilostazol. Quality-of-life assessments also improved significantly. Gene therapy for cardiovascular disease is being investigated, but conclusions regarding safety and efficacy are premature.

Baigent C et al: Efficacy and safety of cholesterol-lowering treatment: prospective meta-analysis of data from 90,056 participants in 14 randomised trials of statins. Lancet 2005;366:1267.

Clagett P et al: Antithrombotic therapy in peripheral arterial disease: the seventh ACCP conference on antithrombotic and thrombolytic therapy. Chest 2004;126:S609.

Critchley JA, Capewell S: Mortality risk reduction associated with smoking cessation in patients with coronary heart disease: a systematic review. JAMA 2003;290:86.

Dormandy JA, Murray GD: The fate of the claudicant–a prospective study of 1969 claudicants. Eur J Vasc Surg 1991;5:131.

Fowkes F, Lee A, Murray G: Ankle-brachial index as an independent indicator of mortality in fifteen international population cohort studies. ABI Collaboration. Circulation 2005;112:3704.

McCullough PA: Contrast-induced acute kidney injury. J Am Coll Cardiol 2008;51:1419.

Rehring TF, Stolcpart RS, Hollis HW Jr: Pharmacologic risk factor management in peripheral arterial disease: a vade mecum for vascular surgeons. Society for Vascular Surgery. J Vasc Surg 2008;47:1108.

Stewart K et al: Exercise training for claudication. N Engl J Med 2002;347:1941.

Yusuf S et al: Effects of an angiotensin-converting-enzyme inhibitor, ramipril, on cardiovascular events in high-risk patients. Heart Outcomes Prevention Evaluation Study Investigators. N Engl J Med 2000;342:145.

B. Operative Treatment

Interventional procedures, open or endovascular, are performed both for limb salvage and for incapacitating claudication. The choice of operative procedure depends on the location and distribution of arterial lesions and the patient's comorbidities. Recognition of coexistent cardiopulmonary disease is particularly relevant, because many patients with peripheral vascular disease also have ischemic heart disease and/or chronic lung disease associated with tobacco use. Preoperative cardiac functional assessment is sometimes necessary, but preoperative myocardial revascularization is not beneficial in patients with reasonable cardiac reserve. All patients undergoing vascular surgery should have preoperative risk assessment. Randomized trials have shown that perioperative beta-blocker, angiotensin-converting enzyme (ACE) inhibitor, and statins may reduce cardiac morbidity in patients undergoing vascular surgery. Evidence is also emerging demonstrating the importance of maintaining statin therapy throughout the perioperative period.

1. Endovascular therapy—Endovascular therapy consists of image-guided techniques to treat diseased arterial segments from within the lumen of the vessel. Access to the arterial system is established by the insertion of valved sheaths, usually percutaneously, into the access vessel, often the common femoral artery. Steerable wires and catheters are then passed through the vasculature under fluoroscopic guidance to the target lesion (Figure 34–3). Once the target lesion is accessed, therapeutic maneuvers, such as angioplasty, or devices, such as stents, can be delivered. In many arterial beds, endovascular therapy is more commonly utilized than open surgical therapy because of its minimally invasive nature and reduction of short-term morbidity and mortality. However, many questions remain concerning the long-term durability of endovascular repairs, and open surgery still plays a major role in the treatment of patients with arterial disease.

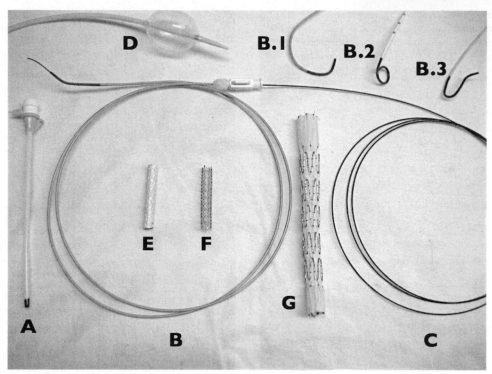

▲ **Figure 34–3.** Endovascular gear. **A:** Sheath. Inserted using Seldinger technique into access vessel. Wires, catheters, and devices pass through the sheath. Sheaths provide stable working access points and protect artery. **B:** Catheter. Variable length, stiffness, coating, and shape (examples: B.1, cobra; B.2, pigtail; B.3, mesenteric selective). Catheters help steer wires through vasculature and also maintain access in vessel. **C:** Guidewire. Variable diameter, length, stiffness, and shape. Used to gain access into vasculature, cross lesions, and deliver devices. **D:** Balloon catheter. **E:** Peripheral stent graft. **F:** Peripheral nitinol self-expanding stent. **G:** Aortoiliac stainless steel/Dacron stent-graft.

Percutaneous transluminal angioplasty, with or without placement of an intravascular stent, is often the treatment of choice when stenoses or even occlusions are relatively short and localized. As the angioplasty balloon expands, it stretches the adventitia, fracturing and compressing plaque, expanding the artery to widen the lumen. Energy losses associated with a stenosis are inversely proportionate to the fourth power of the radius; therefore, even small increases in radius can result in substantial increases in blood flow, although durability of the procedure is improved with the reestablishment of a normal lumen. Concomitant stenting is frequently performed to improve luminal expansion and the arteriographic appearance of the lesion. Stent grafts (stents with fabric covering) may also be used in selected cases or to repair the inadvertent rupture of an artery during angioplasty (Figure 34–4).

Both stents and stent grafts are commonly used from the aortic bifurcation to the distal popliteal artery. Stenting is rarely performed below the knee, but angioplasty of tibial disease is now common with the use of small catheters and wires. Percutaneous mechanical and laser atherectomy are other options in removing obstructing lesions in lower extremity atherosclerotic occlusive disease. Mechanical atherectomy removes plaque by shaving with a cutting or rotating catheter.

For short, stenotic segments in larger, more proximal vessels, the results of endovascular therapies are good with 1-year success rates of 85% in common iliac disease and 70% in external iliac disease. The results with superficial femoral and popliteal lesions are lower (Figure 34–5). The success of endovascular therapy for lower extremity occlusive disease is inversely related to the complexity of the lesion, defined by the number and length of stenoses treated.

Since disease may recur more frequently after angioplasty than after bypass surgery, the patient should be closely followed up using noninvasive tests. Repeat angioplasty or stenting may be indicated for recurrent disease, but the improvement in morbidity and mortality of endovascular interventions may be offset by the need for multiple repeat procedures. In general, minimally invasive percutaneous treatment of lower extremity occlusive disease is best used in patients of high operative risk and severe, limb-threatening ischemia (Figure 34–6).

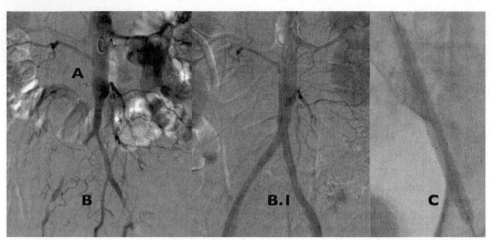

▲ **Figure 34–4.** Aortoiliac occlusive disease. **A:** Aorta. **B:** Severely stenotic/occluded iliac arteries. **B.1:** Widely patent iliac arteries following balloon angioplasty and stenting (**C**).

2. Surgical treatment

A. AORTOILIAC RECONSTRUCTION—Open operations are indicated for aortoiliac occlusive disease in younger patients with low operative risk or patients with severe disease not amena-ble to endovascular therapy. To completely bypass the aor-toiliac segment, an inverted Y-shaped prosthesis is interposed between the infrarenal abdominal aorta and the femoral arteries, creating an **aortofemoral bypass**. The goal of operation is restoration of blood flow to the common

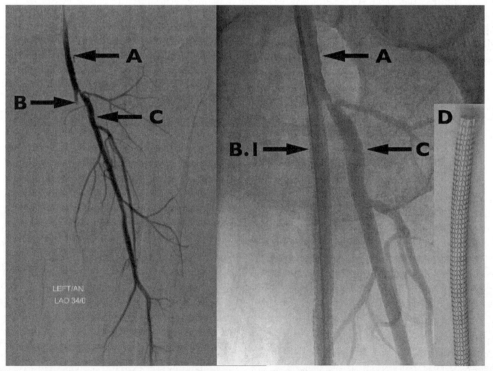

▲ **Figure 34–5.** Superficial femoral artery occlusion, angioplasty and stent-graft. **A:** Common femoral artery. **B:** Occluded superficial femoral artery. **B.1:** Recannulized, stent-grafted superficial femoral artery. **C:** Profunda femoris artery. **D:** Stent-graft.

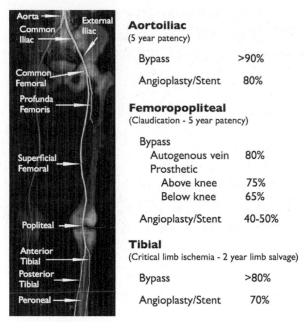

Aorta
Common Iliac
External Iliac
Common Femoral
Profunda Femoris
Superficial Femoral
Popliteal
Anterior Tibial
Posterior Tibial
Peroneal

Aortoiliac
(5 year patency)

Bypass	>90%
Angioplasty/Stent	80%

Femoropopliteal
(Claudication - 5 year patency)

Bypass	
Autogenous vein	80%
Prosthetic	
Above knee	75%
Below knee	65%
Angioplasty/Stent	40-50%

Tibial
(Critical limb ischemia - 2 year limb salvage)

Bypass	>80%
Angioplasty/Stent	70%

▲ **Figure 34-6.** Comparison of outcomes for surgical and endovascular intervention in lower extremity occlusive disease.

femoral artery or, when occlusive disease of the superficial femoral artery is present, to the profunda femoris artery. The clinical results of aortofemoral reconstruction are excellent, although the mortality and morbidity clearly are higher than for endovascular therapy. The operative death rate is 5%; early patency rate, 95%; and late patency rate (5–10 years postoperatively), about 80%. Late complications may be as high as 10% and include graft-intestinal fistula formation, anastomotic aneurysm formation, renal failure, and erectile dysfunction.

Lower risk procedures may be preferable in high-risk patients. If the clinically important lesions are confined to one side, a femoral-femoral or iliofemoral bypass graft can be used. A graft from the axillary to the femoral artery (ie, axillofemoral graft) can be used for bilateral disease. Unfortunately, these "extra-anatomic" methods of arterial reconstruction are more prone to late occlusion than are direct reconstructions.

B. FEMOROPOPLITEAL RECONSTRUCTION—When disease is confined to the femoropopliteal segment, **femoropopliteal bypass** is used. The principal indication for these operations is limb salvage. In patients with claudication alone, the indications for femoropopliteal bypass are more difficult to define but must include substantial disability from claudication. For limited lesions of the superficial femoral artery, endovascular therapy is often attempted first, with surgery reserved for extensive disease or angioplasty failure.

The best graft for femoropopliteal bypass is an autologous greater saphenous vein. The saphenous vein may be left in situ or removed and reversed. In the former instance, the venous tributaries are ligated, and special instruments are used to render the valves incompetent. Expanded polytetrafluoroethylene (PTFE) may also be used as a conduit, particularly for bypass to the suprageniculate popliteal artery. Below the knee, PTFE conduits produce much lower patency rates than saphenous veins. Operative death rates are low (2%), and 5-year patency rates range from 60% to 80%. Limb salvage rates are higher than graft patency rates.

The profunda femoris artery perfuses the thigh and acts as an important source of collateral flow when the superficial femoral artery is diseased. When there is a stenosis of the profunda, **profundoplasty** alone can be performed for limb salvages with success rates of 80% when the suprageniculate popliteal artery is patent and 40–50% when the popliteal artery is occluded. Isolated profundoplasty is rarely helpful for treating claudication.

C. TIBIOPERONEAL ARTERIAL RECONSTRUCTION—Reconstruction of tibial arteries (ie, **distal bypass** to the tibial, peroneal, or pedal vessels) is performed only for limb salvage. Advancing technology allows better endovascular therapy in the tibial vessels, with decreased short-term morbidity and mortality, and similar gains in limb salvage when compared to bypass surgery. However, endovascular techniques are not as widely used in the tibial vessels, and bypass still remains the primary mode of therapy for these patients. Autogenous saphenous veins are preferred because prosthetic conduits have high failure rates. Due to smaller vessel size, extensive disease, and probably the length of the bypass conduit, these grafts are not as durable as femoropopliteal bypass, so the limb salvage rate is substantially higher than graft patency. The operative death rate for these procedures is about 5%.

D. AMPUTATION—Amputation of the limb is necessary within 5–10 years in only 5% of patients presenting with claudication. Amputation is more common if patients continue to smoke cigarettes. Patients with multiple risk factors for atherosclerosis and short-distance claudication are also at increased risk for eventual limb loss. Of patients who present with ischemic rest pain or ulceration, 5–10% require amputation as initial therapy, and most eventually will require amputation if not revascularized. Successful revascularization results in lower costs than primary amputation and an infinite improvement in quality of life. Occasionally, primary amputation may be preferable to revascularization if the likelihood of successful bypass is low, extensive foot infection is present, or the patient is nonambulatory. Amputation levels, options, and the special needs of amputees are covered in the section on Lower Extremity Amputation.

Hirsch AT et al: ACC/AHA 2005 guidelines for the management of patients with peripheral arterial disease (lower extremity, renal, mesenteric, and abdominal aortic): a collaborative report from the American Association for Vascular Surgery/Society for Vascular Surgery, Society for Cardiovascular Angiography and Interventions, Society for Vascular Medicine and Biology, Society of Interventional Radiology, and the ACC/AHA Task Force on Practice Guidelines (Writing Committee to Develop Guidelines for the Management of Patients with Peripheral Arterial Disease) endorsed by the American Association of Cardiovascular and Pulmonary Rehabilitation; National Heart, Lung, and Blood Institute; Society for Vascular Nursing; TransAtlantic Inter-Society Consensus; and Vascular Disease Foundation. J Am Coll Cardiol 2006;47:1239.

Norgren L et al: Inter-Society consensus for the management of peripheral arterial disease (TASC II). TASC II Working Group. J Vasc Surg. 2007;45(Suppl S):S5.

ACUTE LOWER EXTREMITY OCCLUSIVE DISEASE

ESSENTIALS OF DIAGNOSIS

▶ Sudden onset of diffuse limb pain with absent pulses.

General Considerations

Sudden occlusion of a previously patent artery is a dramatic event characterized by the abrupt onset of severe pain and absent pulses in the involved extremity. Tissue viability depends on the extent to which flow is maintained by collateral circuits or surgical intervention. When ischemia persists, motor and sensory paralysis and muscle infarction become irreversible in a matter of hours. If left untreated, a line of demarcation will develop between viable and nonviable tissue.

Acute major arterial occlusion may be caused by an embolus, primary arterial thrombosis, trauma, or dissection. The heart is the source of embolus in 80–90% of episodes, with the remainder from proximal arterial lesions. Aortic aneurysms often contain thrombus, but this material rarely causes symptomatic emboli. In contrast, femoral and particularly popliteal aneurysms embolize frequently. Ulceration in atherosclerotic plaques also can lead to formation of thrombus, which may fragment. Miscellaneous infrequent sources of emboli include cardiac tumors (including cardiac myxoma) and paradoxical emboli (venous thrombi migrating through a patent foramen ovale). Up to 5–10% of spontaneous emboli originate from a source that remains unidentified despite thorough diagnostic interrogation.

It may be difficult to differentiate between sudden thrombosis of an atherosclerotic peripheral artery and embolic occlusion. The former patients usually have preexisting atherosclerotic stenosis and low blood flow, which predisposes to stagnation and thrombosis. One should also keep in mind the clinical setting and a history of preexisting symptoms such as atrial fibrillation (embolus) or claudication (primary thrombosis).

▶ Clinical Findings

The Five Ps

    Pain

    Pallor

    Pulselessness

    Paresthesias

    Paralysis

Acute arterial occlusion is characterized by the five Ps: pain, pallor, pulselessness, paresthesias, and paralysis. Severe sudden pain is present in 80% of patients, and its onset usually indicates the time of vessel occlusion. Pain is absent in some patients because of prompt onset of anesthesia and paralysis and portends a poor prognosis.

On examination, the key finding is a lack of palpable pulses in a diffusely painful extremity. It is important to determine if sensitivity to light touch is maintained. These fibers are highly susceptible to ischemia, and their dysfunction heralds the beginning of irreversible ischemic changes. The onset of motor paralysis implies impending gangrene. Early intervention is critical. Swelling with acute tenderness of a muscle belly—usually in the calf following acute femoral artery occlusion—generally denotes irreversible muscle infarction. Skin and subcutaneous tissues have greater resistance to hypoxia than nerves and muscles, which may demonstrate irreversible histological changes after 3–4 hours or less of ischemia.

▶ Treatment & Prognosis

A. Embolism and Thrombosis

Immediate anticoagulation by intravenous heparin slows the propagation of thrombus and allows time for assessment of adequacy of collateral flow and preparation for operation. If light touch is intact, arteriography may be performed to define the anatomy and assist in planning the operation. Diagnosis of acute embolic occlusion is based on an abrupt block of the artery with little accompanying arterial disease; conversely, acute in situ thrombosis is associated with extensive atherosclerosis and a well-established collateral network. The operative treatment for an embolus, embolectomy, differs from that of preexisting atherosclerosis, which may require bypass. Nonoperative management is rarely indicated except in debilitated patients and patients with emboli to major arteries in the upper extremities, which generally have good collateral circulation.

Therapeutic options include catheter-directed thrombolysis, percutaneous mechanical thrombectomy, and surgical embolectomy. For patients with severe acute ischemia, operative therapy is preferable because it is usually associated with the least delay in reestablishing perfusion. Surgical embolectomy may be performed through an arteriotomy at the site of the embolic occlusion or, most commonly, by clot extraction with a balloon (Fogarty) catheter inserted through a remote arteriotomy. Successful embolectomy requires removal of the embolus and the "tail" of thrombus that extends distally or proximally from it. If operation is not performed within the first few hours, the clot may become adherent, and subsequent revascularization is less successful. Intraoperative infusion of thrombolytic agents is often a useful adjunct to embolectomy.

In patients who will tolerate a delay in revascularization (ie, those who do not have neural changes on examination), intra-arterial thrombolysis should be considered. The usual regimen involves selective intra-arterial infusion of low doses of thrombolytic agent (eg, tissue plasminogen activator) directly into the clot. This activates thrombus plasminogen more efficiently, allows high concentrations in the clot while limiting systemic effect, and has acceptable complication rates. In cases of thrombosis on preexisting atherosclerotic lesions, thrombolysis reveals the underlying lesions that will require treatment to prevent recurrent thrombosis.

Fasciotomy is normally required after prolonged acute ischemia to treat the compartment syndrome that may accompany the reperfusion injury. Renal insufficiency from myoglobin release should be anticipated after reperfusion of ischemic muscle. Treatment consists of vigorous hydration and alkalinization of the urine. Administration of free radical scavengers such as Mannitol may be helpful in this disorder.

Patients with clearly irreversible limb ischemia should undergo amputation without an attempt at revascularization, as revascularization may expose the patient to the serious hazards of reperfusion caused by release of acidic and hyperkalemic venous blood from the dying extremity.

B. Traumatic Arterial Occlusion

Traumatic arterial occlusion must be corrected within a few hours to avoid development of gangrene. Repair of arterial injury is usually performed in conjunction with repair of other injuries. Occasionally, temporary shunts are used to restore flow to the injured extremity while other injuries are addressed and repaired.

Berridge DC, Kessel D, Robertsson I: Surgery versus thrombolysis for initial management of acute limb ischemia. Cochrane Database Syst Rev 2002;1:CD000985.

Blaisdell FW, Steele M, Allen RE: Management of acute lower extremity arterial ischemia due to embolism and thrombosis. Surgery 1978;84:822.

Eliason J et al: A national and single institutional experience in the contemporary treatment of acute lower extremity ischemia. Ann Surg 2003;238:382.

Kasirajan K et al: Rheolytic thrombectomy in the management of acute and subacute limb-threatening ischemia, J Vasc Interv Radiol 2001;12:413.

Results of a prospective randomized trial evaluating surgery versus thrombolysis for ischemia of the lower extremity. The STILE trial. Ann Surg 1994;220:251.

Two randomised and placebo-controlled studies of an oral prostacyclin analogue (Iloprost) in severe leg ischemia. The Oral Iloprost in Severe Leg Ischemia Study Group. Eur J Vasc Endovasc Surg 2000:358.

PERIPHERAL MICROEMBOLI

Microemboli are most damaging when they occlude a digital artery. This causes sudden pain, cyanosis, and coldness or numbness in the affected digit. These changes characteristically improve over several days. If there are multiple emboli, these symptoms may reappear in a different area of the hand or foot. In the lower extremity, this clinical entity has been called **blue toe syndrome** or trash foot. The sudden onset of pain and purple discoloration of a toe in the presence of palpable pulses is recognized as a potentially limb-threatening arterial problem. With each succeeding episode, recovery is slower and less complete.

The most common source of microembolization is cardiac valvular disease. However, if no cardiac valvular lesions are found, a careful examination of the proximal arterial tree must be done to identify an arterial source shedding atheroemboli.

Sudden onset may differentiate peripheral microembolism from other causes of blue toes, such as vasculitis, thromboangiitis obliterans, trauma, or chronic ischemia. If a single toe is affected, it is more likely to be the result of emboli, while multiple cyanotic toes are more likely to be vasculitis or chronic ischemia. It is important to remember that a patent proximal artery is required to serve as a conduit for the embolus, so pulses are intact. Furthermore, a normal blood supply is present in adjacent tissue segments. The appearance of a normally perfused foot with a cyanotic toe is characteristic. However, the waxing and waning symptoms of repeated emboli can make the diagnosis difficult. Unless the syndrome is recognized, alternative diagnoses investigated, and the lesion of origin corrected, survival of the foot or hand may be in peril.

Farooq MM et al: Penetrating ulceration of the infrarenal aorta: case reports of an embolic and an asymptomatic lesion. Ann Vasc Surg 2001;15:255.

Matchett WJ et al: Blue toe syndrome: treatment with intra-arterial stents and review of therapies. J Vasc Interv Radiol 2000;11:585.

Sharma PV et al: Changing patterns of atheroembolism. Cardiovasc Surg 1996;4:573.

DIABETIC VASCULAR DISEASE

Atherosclerotic arterial disease in patients with diabetes mellitus is more diffuse and more severe than in nondiabetics. In diabetic patients, the tibioperoneal vessels frequently contain atherosclerotic changes, and the vessels are often heavily calcified. The degree of ischemia may be severe and extensive, and noninvasive tests (ABIs) may be falsely normal. Fortunately, in many diabetics, the small arteries in the foot are relatively spared, making distal bypass to these arteries possible and allowing foot salvage in cases of threatened limb loss.

Diabetic patients also have a high incidence of neuropathy and are more apt to ignore minor foot injuries, which can develop into ulcerations. Daily foot inspections are essential to avoid progression of minor injuries. Neuropathy is also responsible for loss of tone of intrinsic foot muscles that leads to subluxation of the metatarsal phalangeal joints, resulting in a "rocker-bottom" foot and ultimately producing complete joint destruction termed a Charcot foot. These architectural changes also make skin breakdown more likely to occur and require referral to a foot and ankle clinic.

Akbari CM et al: Diabetes and peripheral vascular disease. J Vasc Surg 1999;30:373.

LoGerfo FW, Coffman JD: Current concepts. Vascular and microvascular disease of the foot in diabetes. Implications for foot care. N Engl J Med 1984;311:1615.

Nehler MR et al: Intermediate-term outcome of primary digit amputations in patients with diabetes mellitus who have forefoot sepsis requiring hospitalization and presumed adequate circulatory status. J Vasc Surg 1999;30:509.

Prompers L et al: Predictors of outcome in individuals with diabetic foot ulcers. Diabetologia 2008;51:747.

NONATHEROSCLEROTIC DISORDERS CAUSING LOWER LIMB ISCHEMIA

▶ Thromboangiitis Obliterans

Thromboangiitis obliterans (Buerger disease) is characterized by multiple segmental occlusions of obliterating tibial and pedal arteries. The most distal arteries are affected making bypass impossible. Migratory phlebitis may be present. In contrast to atherosclerosis, which involves the intima and media, thromboangiitis obliterans is manifested by infiltration of round cells in all three layers of the arterial wall. The disease occurs almost exclusively in young male smokers. It is essential that the patient stop smoking to avoid progression of the disease. Patients with Buerger disease may have specific cellular immunity against arterial antigens, specific humoral antiarterial antibodies, and elevated circulatory immune complexes, but a precise diagnosis can be made only by tissue histology. Arteriographic findings are distinctive but not pathognomonic. Sympathectomy decreases arterial spasm and is useful in some patients. Amputation is indicated for persistent pain or gangrene and can be performed adjacent to the line of demarcation with satisfactory primary healing.

The disease may become dormant if the patient can stop smoking. Unfortunately, smoking cessation seems particularly difficult in these patients, and many ultimately require multiple amputations.

▶ Popliteal Artery Entrapment Syndrome

This rare cause of popliteal artery stenosis or occlusion occurs as a result of an anomalous course of the popliteal artery. The popliteal artery normally passes between the two heads of the gastrocnemius muscle as it enters the lower leg. In the entrapment syndrome, the artery passes medial to both heads of the gastrocnemius, causing compression of the popliteal artery when the knee is extended. There are five anatomic variants of popliteal artery entrapment, but all produce similar clinical effects. Fibrous thickening of the intima occurs at the site of compression and gradually progresses to total occlusion. Symptoms vary from calf claudication to those of more severe ischemia depending on lesion severity and embolization. Popliteal artery entrapment should be considered when a young, otherwise healthy patient presents with calf claudication. Until the artery becomes occluded, the only finding is a decrease in strength of the pedal pulses, most evident when using provocative maneuvers like foot dorsiflexion and plantar flexion. MRI and CT studies are most useful in confirmation of the diagnosis. Atherosclerotic changes are notably absent. Treatment consists of returning the popliteal artery to its normal anatomic course or bypass with saphenous vein.

▶ Cystic Degeneration of the Popliteal Artery

Arterial stenosis is produced by a mucoid cyst in the adventitia, usually located in the middle third of the artery. Calf claudication is the most common symptom, and the only finding is a decrease in the strength of the peripheral pulses. Rarely, a mass can be palpated. Arteriography shows a sharply localized zone of popliteal stenosis with a smooth concentric tapering. Ultrasound or CT scans can be used to demonstrate the cyst within the vessel wall. The stenosis may be missed on conventional anteroposterior films and may appear only on lateral exposures. The cyst and the affected artery should be excised because of the possibility of recurrence with evacuation of the cyst only.

▶ Abdominal Aortic Coarctation

Coarctations of the thoracic or abdominal aorta are rare. They may be congenital or may result from an inflammatory large vessel arteritis such as Kawasaki or Takayasu disease. These rare disorders may produce symptoms of lower extremity, mesenteric, or renal ischemia depending on the location of the constriction. The congenital variant of this condition is best managed surgically when it is recognized; autogenous repair may be preferable to the use of prosthetic grafts. Surgical repair in the presence of ongoing inflammation is not recommended because those patients do poorly. However, if the disease is quiescent with a normal sedimentation rate, standard surgical operations appear to produce satisfactory results.

LOWER EXTREMITY AMPUTATION

▶ General Considerations

More than 90% of the 110,000 amputations performed in the United States each year are for ischemic disease or infective gangrene. More than half of lower extremity amputations are performed for complications of diabetes mellitus, and 15–50%

of diabetic amputees will lose a second leg within 5 years. This risk is about two times higher for men than for women. Other indications for amputations are nondiabetic infection with ischemia (15–25%), ischemia without infection (5–10%), osteomyelitis (3–5%), trauma (2–5%), and frostbite, tumors, neuromas, and other miscellaneous causes (5–10%).

Many patients facing amputation are near the end of life because of systemic cardiovascular disease. Approximately 20–30% of patients undergoing major amputation (below-knee or above-knee) will be dead within 2 years. The prevalence of many comorbidities in this population is also reflected in the perioperative mortality rates for major amputation, ranging from 5% to 10% for below-knee amputations to 10% or higher for above-knee amputations.

The level of amputation is determined by assessing the likelihood of healing of the limb in association with the functional potential of the patient. Compared with normal walking, energy expenditure is increased 10–40% with a below-knee prosthesis, 50–70% with an above-knee prosthesis, and 60% with crutches. The clinical conundrum in patients with limb ischemia is twofold: (1) determining which limbs have adequate blood supply to heal at the below-knee level and (2) determining which patients with vascular disease have reasonable rehabilitation potential. The best predictions are based on clinical assessment by an experienced surgeon, assisted by one of the several techniques for determining amputation level.

▶ Determination of Amputation Level

Technical decisions regarding amputation level are based on adequacy of blood flow and extent of tissue necrosis.

A. Clinical Examination

The presence of palpable pedal pulses in a warm, pink limb is a reliable indicator that arterial flow is adequate to support healing of a below-knee amputation. In general, the presence of a palpable pulse in the major artery immediately above the amputation site (eg, femoral pulse for above-knee, popliteal pulse for below-knee) indicates a high probability of amputation primary healing, and absence of a palpable pulse in these locations significantly reduces the likelihood of amputation healing.

B. Measurement of Blood Pressure

Segmental blood pressures are fallible, and blood pressure measured by Doppler in the ankle is an unreliable guide to healing in the foot if the tibial vessels are calcified and cannot be compressed by the cuff, a condition reported in at least 20–25% of diabetics.

C. Oxygen Tension Measurements

Transcutaneous measurement of oxygen tension (using a modified Clark-type oxygen electrode) is another guide to healing. A transcutaneous PaO_2 of zero indicates a high probability that healing will be unsatisfactory at that site, whereas a PaO_2 above 40 mm Hg indicates that good healing is likely. Intermediate values do not correlate closely with the degree of healing. Transcutaneous PaO_2 measurement is noninvasive and very reproducible. It may not be accurate in the presence of edema.

D. Lower Extremity Amputation Levels

Lower extremity amputations are done most commonly at one of the following levels: toe (called digit amputations, which may be extended to include resection of the metatarsal and called ray amputations), transmetatarsal, below-knee, and above-knee. Amputations at other levels (Syme amputation, Chopart amputation, knee disarticulation, and hip disarticulation) are infrequently performed, usually to treat conditions other than vascular disease.

1. Toe and ray amputations—Toe amputations are the most frequently performed amputation (Figure 34–7). Over two thirds of amputations in diabetics involve the toes and forefoot. A guiding principle is midphalangeal or metatarsal resection to assure that all cartilaginous articular surface is removed because this material has no blood supply. The indications include gangrene, infection, neuropathic ulceration, frostbite, and osteomyelitis limited to the middle or distal phalanx. Good blood flow is required. Contraindications to digit amputation include indistinct demarcation, infection at the metatarsal level, pallor on elevation, or dependent rubor indicating ischemia of the forefoot.

For dry, uninfected gangrene of one or more toes, autoamputation may be allowed to occur. During this process, epithelialization occurs beneath the eschar, and the toe spontaneously detaches, leaving a clean residual limb at the most distal site. Although preferable in many patients (and especially frostbit patients), autoamputation sometimes requires months to complete.

Ray, or wedge, amputation includes removal of the toe and metatarsal head; occasionally, two adjacent toes may be amputated by this method. As with toe amputation, there is modest cosmetic deformity and a prosthesis is not required. Ray amputation of the great toe leads to unstable weight bearing and some difficulty with ambulation resulting from loss of the first metatarsal head.

Complications that may require amputation at higher levels include infection, osteomyelitis of remaining bone, and nonhealing of the incision. These complications have been reported in up to one third of diabetic patients.

2. Transmetatarsal amputation—Transmetatarsal forefoot amputations preserve normal weight bearing. The principal indication is gangrene of several toes or the great toe, with or without soft tissue infection or osteomyelitis. Good blood supply is needed because the incision creates a generous plantar flap. There is no dorsal flap. On the plantar surface, the incision is continued medially to laterally just

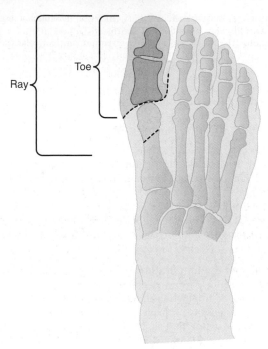

▲ Figure 34–7. Toe and ray amputations.

proximal to the metatarsophalangeal crease. The metatarsal bones are divided with the medial and lateral shafts cut shorter than those in the middle to preserve the normal architecture of the foot and assist with orthotic fitting postoperatively, and the tendons are pulled down and transected as high as possible.

Transmetatarsal amputation produces an excellent functional result. Walking requires no increase in energy expenditure, and the gait is usually smooth. A prosthesis is not mandatory, but to achieve optimal gait, the shoes must be modified.

3. Major leg amputations—An attempt at performing a below-knee amputation is warranted in almost any patient who appears to be a potential candidate for rehabilitation. This may explain why up to one third of patients having below-knee amputations require reamputation.

A. BELOW-KNEE AMPUTATION—The most common procedure for below-knee amputation is the Burgess technique, which utilizes a long posterior flap (Figure 34–8). The blood supply to a posterior flap is generally better than the supply to an anterior flap or to sagittal flaps, because the sural arteries (which supply the gastrocnemius and soleus muscles) arise high on the popliteal artery, an area not often diseased. The use of rigid dressings and immediate postoperative prostheses has proved advantageous. Application of a rigid cast bandage has several potential advantages: (1) It controls postoperative edema, which may reduce pain; (2) it protects

the stump from trauma, particularly when a patient falls during attempts at mobilization; and (3) it allows the patient to be ambulatory with a temporary prosthesis much sooner.

B. ABOVE-KNEE AMPUTATION—Absolute indications for primary above-knee amputation include contracture at the knee joint (observed in debilitated patients with longstanding extremity pain who have been in a prolonged withdrawal posture with the knee flexed) and nonviable calf muscle or skin for creation of the below-knee flap. The frequent failure of healing of below-knee amputation, the higher perioperative morbidity and mortality in this population (making secondary operations more dangerous), and the modest functional benefit of preserving the knee joint are the major arguments in favor of primary above-knee procedures in nonambulatory patients.

Above-knee amputation may be performed at several levels, including knee disarticulation. Although it is advantageous to preserve as long a lever arm as possible, knee disarticulation is technically more demanding than transfemoral amputation at a higher level. The technique is straightforward. Short anterior and posterior flaps, sagittal flaps, or a circular incision may be used. The bone is divided substantially higher than the skin and soft tissue to avoid tension when the wound is closed and later when the muscles of the thigh atrophy. A simple dressing is then applied.

SPECIAL PROBLEMS OF AMPUTEES

▶ Thromboembolism

The amputee is at great risk for deep venous thrombosis (15%) and pulmonary embolism (2%) postoperatively because (1) amputation often follows prolonged immobilization during treatment of the primary disease, and (2) the operation involves ligation of large veins, causing stagnation of blood, a situation that predisposes to thrombosis. If immediate-fit prosthetic techniques are not employed, an additional period of inactivity follows the operation, further increasing the risk of thromboembolism.

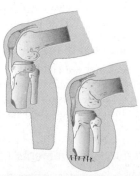

▲ Figure 34–8. Below knee amputation.

Rehabilitation after Amputation

The rehabilitation goals following amputation are highly variable. Younger patients universally want to regain ambulatory status and frequently return to work. Elderly patients with significant comorbid conditions may remain wheelchair-bound, and much of their rehabilitation is focused on providing wheelchair access in their living situations and working on independent transfers. It is important to understand that amputation in an elderly patient is frequently an event that occurs near the end of life. For these people, relief of pain and provision for modest function may be the most appropriate outcome in the limited amount of time they have left.

The length of the residual limb correlates well with regaining the ability to walk. Cardiopulmonary disease and physical weakness make walking an overwhelming effort for some patients; this emphasizes the importance of preserving a below-knee amputation if possible, so that walking will require the least possible amount of energy.

Pain & Flexion Contracture

Flexion contractures of the knee or hip occur rapidly in the painful limb because of the natural tendency to assume a flexed posture. Measures to prevent contracture are indicated preoperatively, and application of a rigid dressing postoperatively decreases the incidence of this complication.

Phantom Pain

Persistent sensations in a residual limb are almost universal. Unfortunately, phantom limb pain also is common. Treatment is difficult; improvement has been reported using tricyclic antidepressants, transcutaneous electrical nerve stimulation (TENS), and calcitonin. The incidence and severity of phantom limb pain are increased if there was prolonged ischemia before amputation and decreased if postoperative rehabilitation is rapid.

Ischemia in the Residual Limb

Progressive vascular disease results in ischemia of about 8% of above-knee amputations and 1% of below-knee amputations. Operations are often required to improve arterial flow when gangrene develops in a residual limb. The mortality rate of this condition is high.

Adunsky A et al: Non-traumatic lower limb older amputees: a database survey from a geriatric center. Disabil Rehabil 2001; 20:80.

Fletcher DD et al: Rehabilitation of the geriatric vascular amputee patient: a population-based study. Arch Phys Med Rehabil 2001;82:776.

Huang ME, Levy CE, Webster JB: Acquired limb deficiencies. 3. Prosthetic components, prescriptions, and indications. Arch Phys Med Rehabil 2001;82:S17.

Kent R, Fyfe N: Effectiveness of rehabilitation following amputation. Clin Rehabil 1999;13(Suppl I):43.

Levy CE et al: Acquired limb deficiencies. 4. Troubleshooting. Arch Phys Med Rehabil 2001;82:S25.

Manord JD et al: Management of severe proximal vascular and neural injury of the upper extremity. J Vasc Surg 1998;27:43.

Mayfield JA et al: Trends in lower limb amputations in the Veterans Health Administration, 1989–1998. J Rehabil Res Dev 2000;37:22.

Nehler MR et al: Intermediate term outcome of primary digit amputations in diabetic patients with forefoot sepsis and adequate circulatory status. J Vasc Surg 1999;30:509.

Sewell P et al: Developments in the trans-tibial prosthetic socket fitting process: a review of past and present research. Prosthet Orthot Int 2000;24:97.

Trautner C et al: Incidence of lower limb amputations and diabetes. Diabetes Care 1996;19:1006.

CEREBROVASCULAR DISEASE

 ESSENTIALS OF DIAGNOSIS

- ▶ Sudden-onset unilateral cortical motor and sensory dysfunction.
- ▶ Unilateral vision loss (amaurosis fugax), aphasia, or dysarthria.
- ▶ Cervical arterial bruits.
- ▶ Duplex ultrasound confirmation of carotid stenosis.

General Considerations

Unlike in the other vascular beds, symptoms of extracranial carotid disease are most often not the result of hypoperfusion but are caused by emboli. Arterial emboli account for approximately one quarter of strokes in Europe and North America, and 80% of these originate from atherosclerotic lesions in a surgically accessible artery in the neck. The most common lesion is at the bifurcation of the carotid artery. Transcranial Doppler (TCD) studies have shown that emboli are seen in approximately 20% of patients with moderate (> 50% stenosis) lesions at the carotid bifurcation and even higher rates with more than 70% stenoses. The incidence and frequency of emboli is increased in recently symptomatic patients. It would appear that transient deficits and strokes from emboli may not be single events but the result of multiple small emboli that temporarily or permanently obliterate the collateral reserve of the cerebral cortex.

The neurologic dysfunction associated with microemboli may appear as sudden "short-lived," or transient, neurologic symptoms that may include unilateral motor and sensory loss, aphasia (difficulty finding words), or dysarthria (difficulty speaking due to motor dysfunction). These are termed **transient ischemic attacks** (TIA). Most TIAs are brief (minutes). By convention, 24 hours is the arbitrary limit of a TIA. If the symptoms persist, it is a stroke, or **cerebrovascular accident** (CVA). An embolus to the ophthalmic artery, the first branch of the internal carotid artery, produces a temporary monocular loss of vision called amaurosis fugax or permanent blindness. Atherosclerotic emboli may be visible as small bright flecks (Hollenhorst plaques) lodged in arterial bifurcations in the retina.

Characteristically, lesions of atherosclerosis in the internal carotid artery occur along the wall of the carotid bulb opposite to the external carotid artery origin (Figure 34–9). The enlargement of the bulb just distal to this major branch point creates an area of low wall shear stress, flow separation, and loss of unidirectional flow. Presumably this allows greater interaction of atherogenic particles and the vessel walls at this site and accounts for the localized plaque at the carotid bifurcation.

The accessibility of this localized atheroma allows effective removal of the plaque and a dramatic reduction in stroke risk. Without treatment, 26% of patients with TIAs and more than 70% with carotid stenosis will eventually develop permanent neurologic impairment (CVA) from continued embolization. The risk of CVA is lower for patients presenting with amaurosis fugax.

▶ Clinical Findings

A. Symptoms

Patients with cerebrovascular disease can be grouped into five categories based on symptoms at presentation.

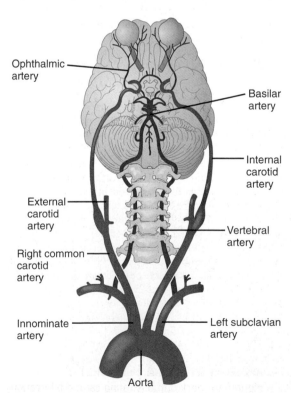

▲ Figure 34–9. Cerebrovascular circulation anatomy.

Ophthalmic artery

Basilar artery

Internal carotid artery

External carotid artery

Vertebral artery

Right common carotid artery

Innominate artery

Left subclavian artery

Aorta

1. Asymptomatic disease—An audible bruit heard in the neck may be the only manifestation of cerebrovascular disease. Severe carotid stenosis may also occur in the absence of a bruit with markedly reduced blood flow. Ultrasound screening also can identify these patients.

2. Transient neurologic episodes—Sudden onset of a neurologic deficit in the distribution of the anterior or middle cerebral arteries requires investigation of the carotid arteries. Symptoms depend on the ischemic area of the brain, the size of the embolus, and the condition of collaterals to the affected area. Hypoperfusion rarely causes transient neurologic and visual attacks. In symptomatic patients, stroke risk after TIA correlates with the severity of internal carotid artery stenosis.

3. Acute unstable neurologic deficits—Patients in this category have multiple (crescendo) TIAs, stroke in evolution, or waxing and waning neurologic deficits and high-grade stenoses. These patients must be treated urgently, because even with anticoagulation, their deficits may become permanent within hours.

4. Stroke (CVA)—Intervention is indicated for patients after stroke that have either complete recovery or mild to moderate deficits, because up to one half will suffer another stroke with further loss of neural function. The timing of intervention is controversial. If the infarct is large and the stenosis severe, a healing period prior to revascularization may be advisable to prevent hemorrhage into the necrotic area with restoration of systemic pressure. In stroke patients, the perioperative risk of additional neurologic deficit is higher than in patients post-TIA.

5. Vertebrobasilar disease—In the posterior circulation, emboli are less common and hypoperfusion is the dominant pathology. Reduction of flow in the vertebral and basilar arteries may cause drop attacks, clumsiness, and a variety of sensory phenomena. Frequently, the symptoms are bilateral. Vertigo, diplopia, or dysequilibrium occurring individually is rarely due to vertebrobasilar disease, but when these symptoms occur in combination, the diagnosis becomes more likely. It is unusual for dizziness alone to be due to cerebrovascular disease.

B. Signs

Auscultation of the carotid and subclavian arteries may delineate the sites of hemodynamically significant disease. However, bruits are nonspecific findings correlating more with overall risk for cardiovascular disease than with stroke.

C. Imaging

1. Doppler ultrasound—The most useful test for the diagnosis of extracranial carotid artery disease is the duplex ultrasound. As the stenosis encroaches on the lumen of the vessel, the velocity of blood increases in the area of the stenosis to maintain distal flow. Doppler spectral velocity analysis determines the flow rate rapidly and with reasonable accurately and thereby gives an estimate of the degree of stenosis. Ultrasound can also display plaque morphology but with less reproducibility than stenosis.

2. CTA and MRA—CTA and MRA are often used for confirmation of duplex findings and planning interventional procedures (Figure 34–10). Both types of angiography can assess the degree of stenosis at the carotid bifurcation, providing information on the configuration of the aortic arch and identifying additional disease in the proximal supra-aortic trunk and intracerebral vessels. These studies also delineate regions of ischemic damage in the brain. Diffusion-weighted MRI is particularly sensitive and will define areas of injury as well as areas of infarction.

3. Arteriography—Cerebral arteriography is occasionally performed in patients with symptomatic or asymptomatic cerebrovascular disease. It is most useful for cases in which noninvasive studies are in disagreement or in those patients who are candidates for carotid angioplasty and stenting. Cerebral diagnostic arteriography is invasive and has a low but significant risk of stroke (0.5–1.0%).

▶ Treatment

Stroke risk is highest immediately after a TIA, returning to baseline at approximately 6 months. Consequently, in symptomatic patients with carotid stenosis, early intervention is mandatory. Antiplatelet therapy, usually in the form of aspirin or clopidogrel, is particularly important in cerebrovascular patients, although clopidogrel should not be initiated in a patient who is scheduled to have a carotid endarterectomy because of the increased risk of bleeding. Cardiovascular risk factor modification is also imperative in reducing stroke and overall mortality. After a completed stroke, caution must be exercised when planning an intervention.

A. Carotid Endarterectomy

Carotid endarterectomy, the removal of the atherosclerotic lesion at the carotid bifurcation, is the primary operation performed (Figure 34–11). In the North American Symptomatic Carotid Endarterectomy Trial (NASCET), carotid endarterectomy was shown to reduce incidence of ipsilateral stroke from 26% to 9% at 2 years in patients presenting with either TIA or stroke and carotid lesions of 70% stenosis or greater. The results also favored surgery in patients with moderate carotid stenosis (50–69%), but less dramatically. The 5-year risk of ipsilateral stroke was 15.7% among patients treated surgically ($n = 1108$) and 22.2% among those treated medically ($n = 1118$; $P = .045$). Patients with stenoses of less than 50% did not benefit from surgery.

Large clinical trials have also shown a benefit of surgery for asymptomatic carotid stenosis. Both the Asymptomatic Carotid Atherosclerosis Study (ACAS) in North America and the Asymptomatic Carotid Surgery Trial in Europe showed that stroke incidence is halved (12% to 6%) by carotid endarterectomy versus best medical therapy, which included antiplatelet agents, in patients with substantial carotid narrowing at 5 years of follow-up. While ACAS did not show a benefit for endarterectomy in women, the larger European study did.

Carotid endarterectomy cannot be performed when the internal carotid artery is completely occluded, because complete thrombectomy is not possible and residual clot has been shown to embolize.

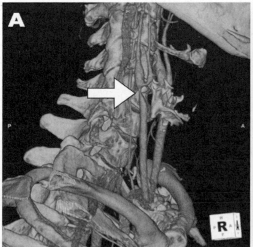
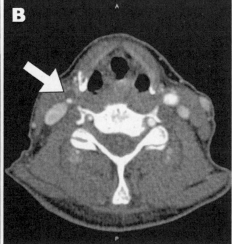

▲ **Figure 34–10.** Carotid bifurcation occlusive disease. **A:** 3-D CT angiogram of neck demonstrating carotid bifurcation stenosis. **B:** Axial CT view demonstrating the lesion.

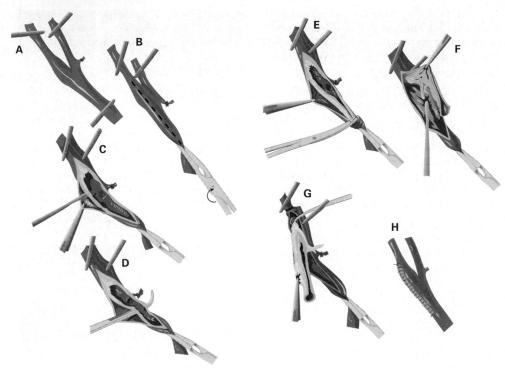

▲ **Figure 34–11.** Technique of carotid endarterectomy.

B. Carotid Angioplasty and Stenting (CAS)

Early studies of carotid angioplasty and stenting (CAS; Figure 34–12) have shown promise with similar morbidity and mortality rates to carotid endarterectomy. Because of the higher rate of emboli with stenting, cerebral protection devices, either filters placed in the internal carotid or devices that allow a washout of atherosclerotic debris, should always be used. Poststenting, clopidogrel is prescribed for 6 weeks to limit late embolization from the stent.

CAS has already become the primary treatment option for occlusive lesions of the origins of the arch vessels and for recurrent stenosis after treatment. It is also chosen over endarterectomy in patients with hostile neck anatomy due to prior radiation or distal lesions not accessible via a neck incision. There is a large randomized trial (CREST) comparing the benefits of CAS to carotid endarterectomy that will determine the role of CAS in patients currently judged to be candidates for endarterectomy.

C. Treatment Results

The main complication of cerebrovascular interventions is stroke, which occurs in 2–7% of patients depending on the operative indications and cerebrovascular anatomy. Higher stroke rates occur in the setting of symptomatic stenosis or contralateral carotid occlusion. Lower stroke rates occur with asymptomatic stenosis. The operative death rate for all extracranial cerebrovascular interventions is less than 1%.

Transient cranial nerve injury occurs in about 10% of cases after endarterectomy and may cause tongue weakness, hoarseness, mouth asymmetry, earlobe numbness, and dysphagia. Less than 2% of peripheral nerve deficits are permanent, although this number goes up with surgery for recurrent disease, making stenting attractive for this indication.

Restenosis or occlusion is uncommon after carotid endarterectomy (5–10% at 5 years) and appears to be equally uncommon after carotid stenting. For endarterectomy, using a prosthetic patch for closure of the arteriotomy can reduce restenosis.

▶ Subclavian Steal Syndrome

The subclavian steal syndrome is characterized by reversal of flow through the vertebral artery due to a more proximal occlusion or stenosis of the subclavian artery (ie, the vertebral artery serves as a collateral to supply blood to the arm). While this anatomic arrangement is often demonstrated on angiograms, clinical sequelae are rare. Symptoms of effort fatigue in the involved extremity are more common than neurologic complaints. When necessary, treatment consists of bypass grafting from the common carotid to the subclavian artery distal to the lesion or transposition of the subcla-

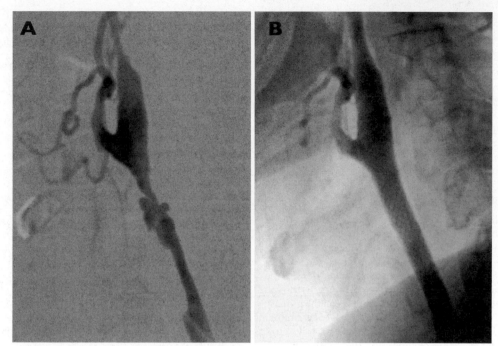

▲ **Figure 34–12.** Carotid angioplasty and stenting. **A:** Conventional arteriogram demonstrating diffuse occlusive disease of common and internal carotid arteries. **B:** Completion arteriogram following angioplasty and stenting of the lesions.

vian artery beyond the lesion to the side of the nearby common carotid artery.

Concomitant Coronary and Cerebrovascular Disease

When patients have coexistent severe coronary and carotid atherosclerosis requiring treatment, there has been controversy as to which lesion should be addressed first. Since most strokes during cardiac procedures are from atheromatous emboli from the aortic arch, not from low flow through a carotid stenosis, our policy has been to perform combined procedures only in patients with simultaneous symptomatic carotid and coronary disease, with critical bilateral asymptomatic stenoses, or with extremely high-grade (99%) unilateral stenosis. We have initiated a program of stenting the carotid stenoses 1 day prior to coronary artery bypass graft and have found this to be quite satisfactory.

Other Causes of Cerebrovascular Symptoms

Other than atherosclerosis, primary disease of the extracranial arteries is rare.

A. Takayasu (Giant Cell) Arteritis

Takayasu arteritis is an obliterative arteriopathy principally involving the aortic arch vessels that often affects young women. The pararenal abdominal aorta and pulmonary arteries also may be affected. High-dose corticosteroids and cyclophosphamide have been shown to arrest and in some cases reverse the progress of the disease. Operative treatment of nonspecific arteritis should be avoided when the arteritis is active, but it may be successful in quiescent disease.

B. Dissecting Aortic Aneurysms

Dissecting aortic aneurysms may extend into the arch branches, producing obstruction and cerebral symptoms. These are discussed in Chapter 19, Part I.

C. Internal Carotid Dissection

Classically occurring in exercising young adults, dissection originating in the internal carotid artery and localized to its extracranial segment occurs as an acute event that may narrow or obliterate the internal carotid lumen. The primary lesion is an intimal tear at the distal end of the carotid bulb. It may also follow various types of neck trauma or severe hypertension.

Cerebral symptoms are the result of ischemia in the ipsilateral hemisphere. Acute neck pain in association with localized cervical tenderness adjacent to the angle of the mandible is a frequent finding.

Arteriography shows a characteristic pattern of tapered narrowing at or just beyond the distal portion of the carotid bulb. The lumen beyond this point may be obliterated or may persist as a barely visible narrow shadow. If the lumen persists, it resumes a normal caliber beyond the bony foramen.

Because thrombus tends to form in and around the dissected vessel, anticoagulation is the treatment of choice for this disorder. In many patients, the intramural clot will be resorbed, restoring a normal lumen. Intervention is indicated for patients with recurrent TIAs. Stenting is the procedure of choice and will restore the normal carotid contour. If stenting is not successful and symptoms persist, ligation can be performed if the carotid back-pressure exceeds 65 mm Hg. Extracranial to intracranial bypass will be needed if the pressure is low.

D. Fibromuscular Dysplasia

Fibromuscular dysplasia is a nonatherosclerotic angiopathy of unknown cause that affects specific arteries chiefly in young women. Symptoms of cerebrovascular disease can occur when the carotid artery is affected. It is usually bilateral and involves primarily the middle third of the extracranial portions of the internal carotid artery. Several pathologic variants of the disease have been described, but in most of them, the primary lesion is overgrowth of the media in a segmental distribution, producing irregular zones of arterial narrowing. The most common result is a series of concentric rings, producing the radiologic appearance of a string of beads in a long internal carotid artery. Approximately one third of patients are also hypertensive due to renal artery involvement.

The prevalence of fibromuscular dysplasia and the portion of patients who develop symptoms are not known. Once symptoms develop, transient neurologic events are the most common manifestation. However, more than 20% of patients have had a stroke by the time of presentation. Because of the high incidence of neurologic disability, the lesion should be corrected by angioplasty with distal protection when patients develop symptoms. Surgery with dilation of the carotid with graduated dilators or balloon dilation has given excellent results.

Baker WH et al: Effect of contralateral occlusion on long-term efficacy of endarterectomy in the asymptomatic carotid atherosclerosis study (ACAS). ACAS Investigators. Stroke 2000;31:2330.

Barnett HJJM et al: Benefit of carotid endarterectomy in patients with symptomatic moderate or severe stenosis. N Engl J Med 1998;339:1415.

Beneficial effect of carotid endarterectomy in symptomatic patients with high-grade stenosis. North American Symptomatic Carotid Endarterectomy Trial Collaborators. N Engl J Med 1991;325:445.

Darling RC 3rd et al: Analysis of the effect of asymptomatic carotid atherosclerosis study on the outcome and volume of carotid endarterectomy. Cardiovasc Surg 2000;8:436.

Endarterectomy for asymptomatic carotid artery stenosis. Executive Committee for the Asymptomatic Carotid Atherosclerosis Study (ACAS). JAMA 1995;273:1421.

Ferguson GG et al: The North American Symptomatic Carotid Endarterectomy Trial: surgical results in 1415 patients. Stroke 1999;30:1751.

Halliday A et al: Prevention of disabling and fatal strokes by successful carotid endarterectomy in patients without recent neurological symptoms: randomized controlled trial. Lancet 2004;363:1491.

Hobson RW: Carotid angioplasty-stent: clinical experience and role for clinical trials. J Vasc Surg 2001;33:5117.

Kresowik TF et al: Improving the outcomes of carotid endarterectomy: results of a statewide quality improvement project. J Vasc Surg 2000;31:918.

Moore WS et al: Indications, surgical technique, and results for repair of extracranial occlusive lesions. In: *Vascular Surgery,* 5th ed. Rutherford RB (editor). Saunders, 2000.

A randomised, blinded, trial of clopidogrel versus aspirin in patients at risk of ischemic events (CAPRIE). CAPRIE Steering Committee. Lancet 1996;348:1329.

Rothwell PM et al: Interrelation between plaque surface morphology and degree of stenosis on carotid angiograms and the risk of ischemic stroke in patients with symptomatic carotid stenosis. On behalf of the European Carotid Surgery Trialists' Collaborative Group. Stroke 2000;342:1693.

Rothwell PM et al: Prediction and prevention of stroke in patients with carotid stenosis. Eur J Vasc Endovasc Surg 2008;35:255.

Roubin GS et al: Immediate and late clinical outcomes of carotid artery stenting in patients with symptomatic and asymptomatic carotid artery stenosis: a 5-year prospective analysis. Circulation 2001;103:532.

Schievink WI: Spontaneous dissection of the carotid and vertebral arteries. N Engl J Med 2001;344:898.

Theiss W et al: Predictors of death and stroke after CAS. Stroke 2008;39:2325.

Yadav JS et al: Stenting and angioplasty with protection in patients at high risk for endarterectomy investigators. Protected carotid-artery stenting versus endarterectomy in high-risk patients. N Engl J Med 2004;351:1493.

RENOVASCULAR HYPERTENSION

 ESSENTIALS OF DIAGNOSIS

▶ Severe hypertension.

▶ Declining renal function.

▶ Renal insufficiency with ACE inhibitor use.

▶ Flank bruits.

▶ General Considerations

More than 23 million people in the United States have hypertension, and renovascular disease is a causative factor in 2–7% of cases. Atherosclerosis of the aorta and renal artery (two thirds of cases) and fibromuscular dysplasia are the two primary causes of renovascular hypertension. Less common causes of hypertension include renal artery emboli, renal artery aneurysms, renal artery dissection, hypoplasia of the renal arteries, and stenosis of the suprarenal aorta.

Atherosclerosis characteristically produces stenosis at the orifice of the main renal artery. The lesion usually consists of aortic atheroma that protrudes over the renal artery orifice. Less commonly, the atheroma arises in the renal artery itself. Renal artery stenosis is more common in males over age 45 years and is bilateral in about 95% of cases.

Fibromuscular dysplasia usually involves the middle and distal thirds of the main renal artery and may extend into the branches. Medial fibroplasia is the most common variety of fibromuscular dysplasia, accounting for 85% of these lesions. It is bilateral in 50% of cases. Concentric rings of hyperplasia that project into the arterial lumen cause the arterial stenoses. Renal artery aneurysms frequently coexist. Fibromuscular dysplasia occurs mainly in young women, with onset of hypertension usually occurring before age 45 years. It is the causative disorder in 10% of children with hypertension. Developmental renal artery hypoplasia, coarctation of the aorta, and Takayasu aortitis are other vascular causes of hypertension in childhood.

Hypertension due to renal artery stenosis results from the kidney's response to reduced blood flow. Cells of the juxtaglomerular complex secrete renin, which acts on circulating angiotensinogen to form angiotensin I, which is rapidly converted to angiotensin II by ACE. This octapeptide constricts arterioles, increases aldosterone secretion, and promotes sodium retention. Due to the excess aldosterone, hypertension becomes volume-dependent. Over time, pathologic changes occur in the uninvolved kidney, and the hypertension may not be sensitive to ACE inhibition. With sodium restriction and volume reduction (diuretics), the hypertension may once again become sensitive to ACE inhibition. If both kidneys have renal artery stenoses, or if the disease exists in a solitary kidney, renal insufficiency may occur with ACE inhibitor administration with a loss of pressure in the glomerulus due to a reduction of angiotensin II constriction of the efferent arteriole.

▶ Clinical Findings

A. Symptoms and Signs

Most patients are asymptomatic, but irritability, headache, and emotional depression are seen in a few. Persistent elevation of the diastolic pressure is usually the only abnormal physical finding. A bruit is frequently audible to one or both sides of the midline in the flank or upper abdomen. Other signs of atherosclerosis may be present when this is the cause of the renal artery disease.

Other clues to the presence of renovascular hypertension include absence of a family history of hypertension, early onset of hypertension (particularly during childhood or during early adulthood), marked acceleration of the degree of hypertension, resistance to control with antihypertensive drugs, and rapid deterioration of renal function. One should suspect renovascular hypertension if initial diastolic pressure is greater than 115 mm Hg or if renal function deteriorates while a patient is being given ACE inhibitors. Sudden onset of pulmonary edema with severe hypertension also is highly suggestive of renovascular hypertension.

B. Diagnostic Studies

In the past, several diagnostic tests were devised to diagnose renovascular hypertension. Divided urinary excretion studies, selective renin determinations from renal vein samples, and captopril renal scintigraphy are now rarely used.

Noninvasive or minimally invasive imaging of the renal arteries is justified when the patient has a precipitous drop in blood pressure, decreased renal function with an ACE inhibitor, difficult-to-control hypertension, or unexplained deteriorating renal function.

C. Imaging Studies

In experienced hands, duplex ultrasound scanning has an overall agreement with angiography of over 90%. Renal artery stenosis is characterized by peak systolic velocities in the range of 180–200 cm/s, and the ratio of these velocities to those in the aorta approaches 3.5. CTA or MRA may provide high-resolution images of diseased renal arteries, although must be used with caution in patients with renal insufficiency. The contrast required with CTA is nephrotoxic and gadolinium has been associated with systemic nephrogenic fibrosis in patients with reduced renal clearance.

Renal arteriography is the most accepted method for delineating the obstructive lesion. Since atherosclerotic disease most often involves the origins of the renal arteries, a midstream aortogram should be obtained in addition to selective renal artery catheterization. The presence of collateral vessels circumventing a renal artery stenosis suggests a hemodynamically significant renal artery lesion.

Nonionic contrast agents should be used, and the patient should be prepared with overnight hydration. Administration of N-acetylcysteine and periprocedural sodium bicarbonate infusion dramatically reduces the incidence of acute tubular necrosis with angiography and should used routinely.

▶ Treatment

A. Medical Management

Patients with renovascular hypertension require aggressive management of modifiable risk factors. If hypertension responds well to medical therapy and the renal function is stable, no intervention on the renal artery stenosis is needed.

B. Percutaneous Transluminal Angioplasty and Stenting

Percutaneous transluminal angioplasty and stenting is the preferred procedure for most patients (Figure 34–13). Although clearly valuable for some patients, the overall results of percutaneous interventions for renal artery stenosis have been mixed, and large randomized clinical trials are underway to clarify its role in this disease. Patients with fibromuscular dysplasia typically respond to angioplasty alone.

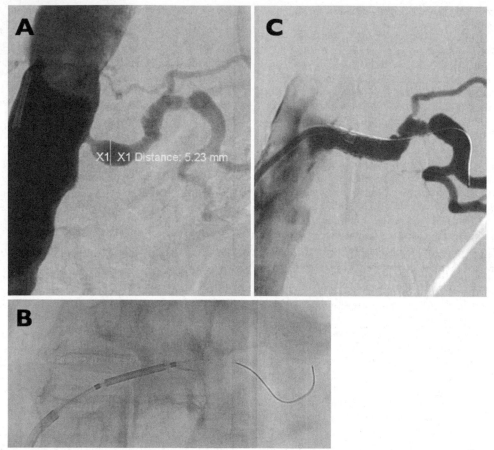

▲ **Figure 34–13.** Renal artery occlusive disease. **A:** Aortogram demonstrating ostial lesion in left renal artery. **B:** Renal stent constrained on delivery catheter over wire positioned across lesion. **C:** Arteriogram demonstrating widely patent renal artery following balloon angioplasty and stent placement.

C. Surgical Treatment

In the very young, surgery is still the primary mode of treatment due to concern regarding the long-term durability of angioplasty and stenting. Surgical repair also is required for failed angioplasty and stenting, renal revascularization during a procedure on the aorta, and lesions that are in branch vessels. As with any operation, the indications for arterial reconstruction are influenced by the extent of disease, the patient's life expectancy, and the anticipated morbidity associated with operation. Nephrectomy may be considered when arterial repair is impossible or especially hazardous and the disease is unilateral.

Options include endarterectomy, which is most easily accomplished through an incision into the adjacent aorta, or bypass using prosthetic or autogenous conduits. An alternative is "nonanatomic" bypass such as a hepatorenal or splenorenal procedure. The celiac and splenic arteries often have coexistent occlusive atherosclerotic disease that mandates preoperative arteriographic assessment of these vessels.

Extracorporeal techniques have been developed for distal branch aneurysms or extensive fibromuscular dysplasia. These require removal of the kidney from the abdomen (ex vivo arterial reconstruction), continuous cold perfusion of its vascular tree, and microvascular techniques for arterial replacement. The kidney is then either returned to a site near its original position or transplanted to the ipsilateral iliac fossa.

▶ Prognosis

Procedures for revascularization of the renal artery are successful in lowering blood pressure in over 90% of patients with fibromuscular hyperplasia. Operation for atherosclerotic stenosis results in improvement or cure of hypertension in about 60%. The results for angioplasty and stenting are not as good, perhaps because of atheroembolization to the kidney during angioplasty.

The results of intervention for salvage of renal function are better than those for treatment of hypertension. The procedural mortality rate of operative renovascular surgery in children is almost nil, whereas it increases to 2–8% in adults with diffuse atherosclerosis. Stenting of the renal arteries is also very well tolerated.

Airoldi S et al: Angioplasty of atherosclerotic and fibromuscular renal artery stenosis time course and predicting factors of the effects on renal function. Am J Hypertens 2000;13:1210.

Cherr GS et al: Surgical management of atherosclerotic renovascular disease. J Vasc Surg 2002;35:236.

Chobanian AV et al: The seventh report of the Joint National Committee on Prevention, Detection, Evaluation, and Treatment of High Blood Pressure (JNC 7 report). JAMA 2003;289:2560.

Clair DG et al: Safety and efficacy of transaortic renal endarterectomy as an adjunct to aortic surgery. J Vasc Surg 1995;21:926.

Hansen KJ et al: Prevalence of renovascular disease in the elderly a population-based study. J Vasc Surg 2002;36:443.

Hollenberg NK: Medical therapy of renovascular hypertension efficacy and safety of captopril in 269 patients. Cardiovasc Rev Rep 1983;4:852.

Piercy KT et al: Renovascular disease in children and adolescents. J Vasc Surg 2005;41:973.

Plouin PF: Stable patients with atherosclerotic renal artery stenosis should be treated first with medical management. Am J Kidney Dis 2003;42:851.

Scolari F et al: Cholesterol crystal embolism a recognizable cause of renal disease. Am J Kidney Dis 2000;36:1089.

Sos TA et al: Percutaneous transluminal renal angioplasty in renovascular hypertension due to atheroma or fibromuscular dysplasia. N Engl J Med 1983;309:274.

MESENTERIC ISCHEMIA SYNDROMES

ESSENTIALS OF DIAGNOSIS

Chronic mesenteric ischemia:

▶ Postprandial pain.

▶ Fear of eating.

▶ Weight loss.

▶ Epigastric bruit.

Acute mesenteric ischemia:

▶ Abdominal pain out of proportion to physical findings.

▶ Metabolic acidosis.

▶ General Considerations

The celiac axis and the superior and inferior mesenteric arteries are the principal sources of blood supply to the stomach and intestines, with the inferior mesenteric artery and internal iliac arteries supplying flow to the distal colon (Figure 34–14). The anatomic collateral interconnections between these arteries are numerous. Single or even multiple visceral artery lesions are generally well tolerated, because collateral flow is readily available (Figure 34–15).

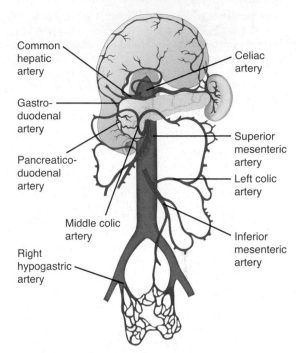

▲ **Figure 34–14.** Visceral arterial circulation and interconnections.

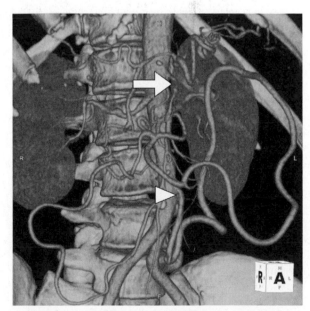

▲ **Figure 34–15.** Three-dimensional CT angiogram demonstrating a critical superior mesenteric artery stenosis (arrow) and collateral vessel enlargement originating at the inferior mesenteric artery (arrowhead).

Atherosclerosis is the cause of obstructive lesions in the visceral arteries in the vast majority of cases. Vasculitis (eg, lupus erythematosus, Takayasu disease) is much less common. When atherosclerosis is the cause, the usual lesion is a collar of plaque spilling over from the aorta that creates a proximal stenosis or occlusion. Associated atherosclerosis in the aorta and its other branches is common.

CHRONIC MESENTERIC ISCHEMIA

▶ Clinical Findings

The principal complaint is postprandial abdominal pain, which has been labeled abdominal or visceral angina. Pain characteristically appears 15–30 minutes after the beginning of a meal and lasts for an hour or longer. Pain is occasionally so severe and prolonged that opiates are required for relief. Pain occurs as a deep-seated, steady ache in the epigastrium, occasionally radiating to the right or left upper quadrant. Weight loss results from reluctance to eat. Although mild degrees of malabsorption can occur, gastrointestinal absorption studies are not helpful. Diarrhea and vomiting have been described. An upper abdominal bruit may be heard.

Arteriography in the anteroposterior and especially the lateral projections demonstrates both the arterial lesion and the patterns of collateral blood flow. Patients should be well hydrated before angiography because this procedure can precipitate hypercoagulability and osmotic diuresis with dehydration, vascular occlusion, and bowel infarction. Duplex scanning, CTA, and MRA are used with increasing frequency because they are less invasive methods of screening.

▶ Treatment

Percutaneous transluminal angioplasty and stenting has gained acceptance as a first line of therapy for mesenteric ischemia. Results are best for focal, nonorificial stenoses. Embolization to the gut is a rare but potentially fatal complication of instrumentation of these lesions.

Surgical revascularization of the superior mesenteric and celiac axes may be performed by either endarterectomy or graft replacement. During endarterectomy, a sleeve of aortic intima and the orifice lesions in the celiac or superior mesenteric arteries are removed. The operation is performed by a retroperitoneal approach to the aorta through a left thoracoabdominal incision. Alternatively, Dacron grafts may be brought antegrade from the lower thoracic aorta or retrograde from the iliac arteries to the celiac axis or superior mesenteric artery—operations that are performed from within the abdomen. Operation should be avoided in patients with acute vasculitis as the underlying cause of mesenteric ischemia; high-dose steroids and immunosuppressive agents are indicated instead.

▶ Prognosis

Opening flow to the mesenteric vascular bed almost always results in relief of symptoms. The limited durability of endovascular therapy necessitates close follow-up and reintervention if symptoms recur.

ACUTE MESENTERIC ISCHEMIA

Acute mesenteric ischemia is a highly morbid disorder. Patients classically present with excruciating diffuse abdominal pain with a surprising absence of physical findings such as abdominal tenderness or distention—unless actual bowel perforation produces a surgical abdomen. Symptoms of chronic mesenteric ischemia may precede this catastrophic event, or the onset may be sudden if the cause is embolic occlusion of the superior mesenteric artery. The diagnosis can be difficult, and its recognition is often delayed, resulting in irreversible bowel ischemia. The mortality rate from acute mesenteric ischemia remains high. Patients who require massive bowel resection rarely survive or, if they survive, can develop incapacitating short-gut syndrome. The prognosis improves dramatically if revascularization can be achieved prior to intestinal infarction. This obviously requires early diagnosis, which will only occur if the practitioner has a high index of suspicion.

CELIAC ARTERY COMPRESSION

External compression of the celiac artery, or median arcuate ligament syndrome, is an unusual cause of visceral ischemia. It generally affects young adults, with women more often affected than men, and is commonly associated with rapid weight loss. The classic sign is a loud epigastric bruit with exhalation as the crus of the diaphragm descends to compress the artery. The artery is scarred and must be repaired in conjunction with release of the compressing ligament. The diagnosis is difficult to make with certainty because some compression of the celiac artery by the arcuate ligament is common. Surgery should be advised only after a search for other causes of postprandial pain.

Patients with median arcuate ligament compression respond favorably to operation in most cases; however, some of these patients are not improved even though a technically adequate operation is performed.

Fisher DF Jr, Fry WJ: Collateral mesenteric circulation. Surg Gynecol Obstet 1987;164:487.

Foley MI et al: Revascularization of the superior mesenteric artery alone for treatment of intestinal ischemia. J Vasc Surg 2000; 32:37.

Herbert GS, Steele SR: Acute and chronic mesenteric ischemia. Surg Clin North Am 2007;87:1115.

Jimenez JG et al: Durability of antegrade synthetic aortomesenteric bypass for chronic mesenteric ischemia. J Vasc Surg 2002;35:1078.

Johnston KW et al: Mesenteric arterial bypass grafts early and late results and suggested surgical approach for chronic and acute mesenteric ischemia. Surgery 1995;118:1.

Moneta GL et al: Duplex ultrasound criteria for diagnosis of splanchnic artery stenosis or occlusion, J Vasc Surg 1991;14:511.

Sarac TP et al: Endovascular treatment of stenotic and occluded visceral arteries for chronic mesenteric ischemia. J Vasc Surg 2008;47:485.

Schoenbaum SW et al: Superior mesenteric artery embolism treatment with intra-arterial urokinase. J Vasc Interv Radiol 1992;3:485.

ARTERIAL ANEURYSMS

ESSENTIALS OF DIAGNOSIS

Abdominal aortic aneurysm:

▶ Pulsatile midabdominal mass.

▶ Severe abdominal pain radiating to the lower back, with hypotension.

Peripheral arterial aneurysms:

▶ Pulsatile mass in groin or behind knee.

▶ Sudden onset of lower extremity ischemia.

▶ General Considerations

An aneurysm is defined as a localized dilation of an artery to at least 1.5 times its normal diameter. The expanding vessel elongates as well as dilates. A true aneurysm involves primary dilation of the artery, including all vessel wall layers (intima, media, and adventitia). A false aneurysm, also called pseudoaneurysm, is characterized by a disruption of the artery wall, does not include all layers of the wall, and may actually be a pulsatile hematoma not contained by the artery wall but by a fibrous capsule. A false aneurysm caused by infection is called a mycotic aneurysm.

False aneurysms of the femoral artery secondary to catheterization are the most numerous of all aneurysms. Infrarenal abdominal aortic aneurysms are the most common of the true aneurysms. In descending order, other arteries affected are the iliac arteries, the popliteal artery, the arch and descending portions of the thoracic aorta (including dilation after aortic dissection), the common femoral artery, the carotid arteries, and other peripheral arteries. Other rare causes of true aneurysms include Marfan syndrome, Ehlers-Danlos syndrome, Behçet disease, and cystic medial necrosis.

ABDOMINAL AORTIC ANEURYSMS

Abdominal aortic aneurysms (AAAs) are found in 2% of the elderly male population, and the incidence may be increasing. In selected groups, the incidence is higher—5% of patients with coronary artery disease and as many as 50% of patients with femoral or popliteal aneurysms have aortic aneurysms. Males are four times as likely to be affected as females. Ruptured aortic aneurysms are the 13th leading cause of death in the United States, resulting in 15,000 deaths per year.

Numerous mechanisms have been proposed for the cause of AAA. Structural issues may contribute; reductions in the number of elastic lamellae and virtual absence of vasa vasorum in the media of the distal abdominal aorta compared with the thoracic aorta may favor aneurysmal degeneration. Excessive protease activity or local reductions in the concentration of protease inhibitors have been implicated in aneurysm formation, allowing for the enzymatic destruction of the two principle structural elements of the aorta, elastin, and collagen. There may be hemodynamic factors as well, owing to large pulsatile stresses because of tapering geometry, increased stiffness, and reflected pressure waves from branch vessels in the infrarenal aorta. Genetic factors influencing connective tissue metabolism and structure also have been associated with AAA development. Indeed, a positive family history of aortic aneurysms infers a 20% chance that a first-degree family member will have an aneurysm.

In terms of risk factors, cigarette smoking has a powerful influence on developing an aortic aneurysm, with an 8:1 preponderance of AAAs in smokers compared with non-smokers. The excess prevalence associated with smoking accounted for 78% of all AAAs that were 4 cm or larger in the Veterans Administration ADAM study sample. Hypertension is present in 40% of patients with AAAs but did not correlate with enlargement in the ADAM study. Surprisingly, diabetics appear to have a lower incidence of aortic aneurysm formation.

Ninety percent of aneurysms of the abdominal aorta occur between the takeoff of the renal arteries and the aortic bifurcation but may include variable portions of the common iliac arteries. Rupture with exsanguination is the major complication of AAAs. Unfortunately, neither the expansion rate nor the rupture risk is predictable. Tension on the aneurysm wall is governed by the law of Laplace. Thus, rupture risk is related to diameter. While relating this to an individual's risk is not possible, population-wide risks have been established. Because most aneurysms cause no symptoms prior to rupture, the number of deaths due to ruptured AAAs has not changed significantly in the past 20 years. This has prompted a recommendation for ultrasound screening of smoking males over the age of 65 years.

▶ Clinical Findings

A. Symptoms and Signs

The vast majority of unruptured aneurysms are asymptomatic. Rarely, intact AAAs produce back pain due to pressure on nerves or erosion into vertebral bodies. Severe pain in the absence of rupture characterizes the rare inflammatory aneurysm that is surrounded by 2–4 cm of perianeurysmal retroperitoneal inflammatory reaction.

Eighty percent of 5 cm AAAs are palpable as a **pulsatile abdominal mass** in the midabdomen just above and to the left side of the umbilicus. Physical examination for an AAA is less reliable in obese patients. The aneurysm may be slightly tender to palpation. Extreme tenderness suggests a "symptomatic aneurysm" and is found in inflammatory aneurysms or if the aneurysm has recently expanded. A truly noninflammatory, symptomatic aneurysm demands urgent surgery.

B. Imaging Studies

Plain films of the abdomen reveal calcification in the outer layers of only 20% of abdominal aneurysms.

Ultrasound is the least expensive method for measuring the size of infrarenal aortic aneurysms. Repeated ultrasound examinations are cost effective for observing small AAAs and may be used to follow resolution of the aneurysm after endovascular repair. However, ultrasound examinations do not delineate adjacent structures as well as CT or MR.

CT scan or MRI with 3D reconstructions are both accurate methods for assessing aneurysm diameter, although the ADAM trail showed that there can be substantial interreader variability in size determinations (Figure 34–16). An important source of error occurs when the course of the aneurysmal aorta is diagonal to the cross-sectional image. This creates an elliptical image of the AAA and a falsely elevated diameter in the larger dimension. CT scans provide valuable information about aneurysm location and size as well as important adjacent structures that affect AAA repair, such as horseshoe kidneys or other renal abnormalities, and venous anomalies, including retroaortic renal veins, circumaortic renal veins, and left-sided or duplicated vena cavae. If the patient has a multiplanar CT scan, aortograms, once routine studies in planning operative management of AAAs, are rarely needed.

C. Natural History

Most aneurysms continue to enlarge and will eventually rupture if left untreated. The average expansion rate for an AAA is 0.4 cm per year. The rate of expansion correlates with continued smoking, initial aneurysm diameter, and the degree of obstructive pulmonary disease. An expansion of 0.5 cm in 6 months or 1 cm over 12 months qualifies as rapid enlargement and suggests the aneurysm is unstable and should be repaired.

Aneurysm size is currently the best determinant of rupture risk. About 40% of aneurysms 5.5–6 cm or larger in diameter will rupture within 5 years if untreated, and the average survival of an untreated patient is 17 months. In contrast, the ADAM study found a 0.5% per year rupture rate in AAAs 4–5.4 cm, an overall rate remarkably similar to a comparable trial in the United Kingdom. Thus, *surgery is recommended for aneurysms 5.5 cm or more in size,* but small aortic aneurysms can be safely followed. Regardless of size, repair is mandatory for an aneurysm that is symptomatic or enlarging rapidly.

D. Treatment

1. Endovascular repair—Endovascular repair, introduced in 1991, is achieved with a synthetic graft to which metal stents have been attached (Figure 34–17). Endovascular repair requires that the aorta proximal to the aneurysm have a cylindrical configuration for at least 1.5 cm to allow for adequate sealing and iliac arteries of sufficient size and limited tortuosity so that the device can be introduced from the femoral arteries. Devices for endovascular repair of AAAs are

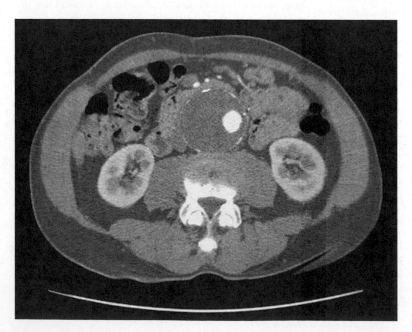

▲ **Figure 34–16.** CT showing the typical position of a 5.5 cm abdominal aortic aneurysm and its proximity to the abdominal wall.

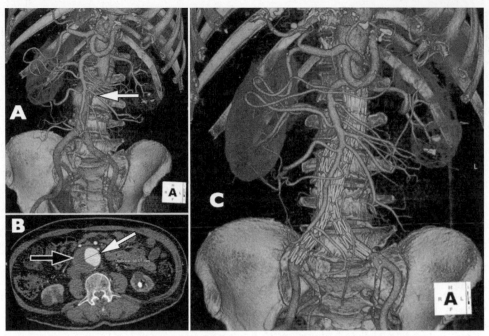

▲ **Figure 34–17. A:** Three-dimensional CT angiogram reconstruction of abdominal aortic aneurysm. White arrow points to aortic flow lumen at same level as that in panel B. **B:** Axial CT view. White arrow points to flow lumen, black arrow points to thrombus within aneurysm sac. Notice only aortic flow lumen visualized on CT angiogram, just as in conventional angiography. Total diameter of the aorta, including area containing thrombus, is used in predicting rupture risk and determining need for intervention. **C:** Three-dimensional CT angiogram following aortic stent graft repair.

delivered using a system of guidewires and delivery systems with large-bore sheaths. Several devices are available with unique design features. The authors have the most experience with the Zenith Endograft (Cook), which guards against migration by aggressive fixation of the graft with bare metal stents extending above the renal arteries. In series of comparable patients, patients with endovascular repair have less operative blood loss, shorter hospital stays, and reduced operative morbidity compared to those undergoing conventional repair.

The most important intermediate or long-term adverse outcome is persistent perfusion of the aneurysm ("endoleak"). These are divided into types denoting clinical importance. A type 1 endoleak denotes ineffective proximal or distal sealing with pressurization of the aneurysm sac and should be fixed immediately. A type 2 endoleak results in persistent flow through the aneurysm between small aortic branches, usually from the inferior mesenteric artery to a patent lumbar artery. These have relatively low pressures and, unless the aneurysm is enlarging, are not treated. Pressurization of the aneurysm through the graft itself is a type 3 endoleak. The graft should be repaired or replaced if the aneurysm continues to enlarge over time.

Rupture has occurred after endovascular aortic aneurysm repair. The rate of late ruptures is low but underscores that patients need extended follow-up to ensure the durability of

endovascular aneurysm repair. Endograft repair is more expensive than open repair in spite of the lower periprocedural morbidity and shorter hospital stays. The devices are expensive ($10,000–15,000), and there is further cost due to the extended follow-up with imaging studies to identify graft movement or endoleak.

2. Open repair—Conventional open operative AAA repair consists of replacing the aneurysmal segment with a synthetic fabric graft (Figure 34–18). Tubular or bifurcation grafts of Dacron or PTFE are preferred. The proximal anastomosis is made to the aorta above the aneurysm. The site of the distal anastomosis is determined by the extent of aneurysmal involvement of the iliac arteries. Traditionally, a transperitoneal approach via midline laparotomy has been used for AAA repair, but retroperitoneal operations via flank incision may decrease perioperative pulmonary and gastrointestinal complications.

Elective infrarenal abdominal aneurysmectomy has a 2–4% operative death rate and a 5–10% rate of complications, such as bleeding, renal failure, myocardial infarction, graft infection, limb loss, bowel ischemia, and erectile dysfunction. Paraplegia is a very rare complication due to involvement of an abnormally low artery of Adamkiewicz, a major collateral of the anterior spinal artery. Malignant tumors are

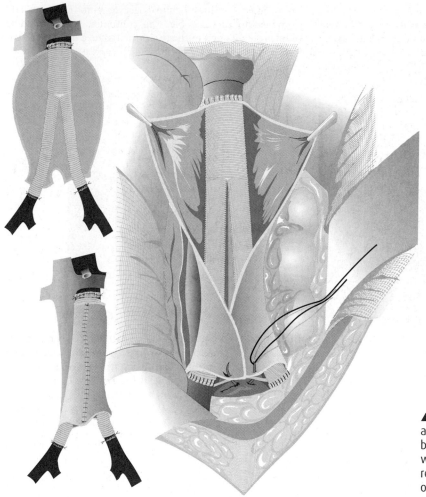

▲ **Figure 34–18.** Replacement of an aortic aneurysm with a synthetic bifurcation graft. The laminated clot within the aneurysm has been removed, and the outer wall is closed over the graft.

encountered unexpectedly in about 4% of cases, although that rate is now dwindling with the routine use of multiplanar CT scans. If gastrointestinal malignancy is encountered during an aneurysm resection, the aneurysm repair should be done first unless there is impending bowel obstruction.

Long-term results of open aneurysmectomy are excellent: The graft failure rate is low, and false aneurysm formation at the anastomoses is rare. The long-term survival of these patients is determined principally by their extent of coronary artery disease.

ILIAC ANEURYSMS

Iliac artery aneurysms generally occur in conjunction with AAAs. Isolated iliac aneurysms are unusual, but in some cases the iliac segment of the aneurysmal artery may enlarge at a greater rate than the aortic segment and is the primary reason for repair. As with aortic aneurysms, most iliac aneurysms are asymptomatic. However, they may present with symptoms related to compression or erosion of surrounding structures, such as obstructive uropathy with ureteral obstruction, neuropathy from compression of local nerves, and unilateral leg swelling from compression of the adjacent iliac vein.

Physical examination can suggest the diagnosis of large (> 4 cm) iliac artery aneurysms if the physician is alert to that possibility. Most symptomatic iliac aneurysms can be palpated as pulsatile masses on abdominal or rectal examinations. However, iliac aneurysms are usually found incidentally on ultrasound or CT.

Similar to aortic aneurysms, iliac aneurysms tend to enlarge and rupture unpredictably, but size is the most important determinant of rupture risk. Iliac aneurysms that are less than 3.5 cm in size should be followed up with serial imaging. Those that enlarge to 4 cm should be repaired in patients without serious operative risk factors.

The challenge of iliac aneurysm repair is in preserving flow to the pelvis through at least one internal iliac artery to prevent pelvic ischemia that can present as buttock claudication, impotence, or ischemia of the distal colon. Open repair of isolated iliac arteries is well tolerated and can be done through a retroperitoneal approach. If the ipsilateral hypogastric artery is also aneurysmal, repair will require opening the sac and ligating the branches from within the aneurysm, taking care not to injure the iliac veins surrounding the aneurysm.

SUPRARENAL AORTIC ANEURYSMS

Aneurysms of the segment of aorta between the diaphragm and the renal arteries account for only 10% of AAAs, with 6% being pararenal and 4% involving the visceral vessels. Resection and graft replacement of the upper abdominal aorta is an operation of far greater magnitude and risk than operations on the infrarenal aorta. Involvement of the renal arteries doubles operative mortality with additional risk for involvement of the visceral vessels. Renal failure and bowel ischemia are much more common after repair of these aneurysms than after repair of infrarenal aortic aneurysms. There is also a risk of paraplegia if flow is interrupted to the artery of Adamkiewicz. An extended incision is usually necessary, and provisions must be made for revascularization of the celiac axis and the superior mesenteric and renal arteries. The use of perfusion catheters for the visceral and renal arteries has improved results, and left heart bypass is used in true thoracoabdominal aneurysms. Because of the mortality and morbidity of repair of suprarenal aneurysms, there has been considerable interest in endovascular repair of these aneurysms using branched systems. Initial experience from selected centers, including our own, have shown dramatic reduction in morbidity and mortality from these technically demanding endovascular procedures.

RUPTURED AORTIC ANEURYSMS

▶ General Considerations

With increasing aneurysm size, lateral pressure within the aneurysm will eventually lead to spontaneous rupture of the aneurysm wall. Although immediate exsanguination may ensue, there is often an interval of several hours between the first episode of bleeding and death from exsanguination when the initial bleed is contained in the retroperitoneal tissues, a "contained rupture." When the periaortic tissue can no longer contain the expanding hematoma, "free rupture" occurs with exsanguination into the free peritoneal cavity.

▶ Clinical Findings

The patient presents with sudden, severe abdominal pain that usually radiates into the back and occasionally into the inguinal region. Lightheadedness or syncope results from blood loss. Pain may lessen and lightheadedness may disap-pear after the first hemorrhage, only to reappear and progress to shock if bleeding continues. When bleeding remains contained in the periaortic tissue, a discrete, pulsatile abdominal mass may be felt. In contrast with an intact aneurysm, the ruptured aneurysm at this stage is painful to palpation. Signs of an acute abdomen may be present. As bleeding continues, usually into the retroperitoneum, the discrete mass is replaced by a poorly defined midabdominal fullness, often extending toward the left flank.

Shock can be profound, manifested by peripheral vasoconstriction, hypotension, and anuria. Unfortunately, the classic triad of pain, a pulsatile abdominal mass, and hypotension is not always present, and precious time may be lost while confirming the diagnosis. An abdominal ultrasound performed in the emergency room will confirm the presence of an aortic aneurysm but may not disclose hemorrhage. CT scans reliably confirm hemorrhage from an aneurysm, but in unstable patients, the delay in progressing to the operating room precludes their use. It is best to follow the adage that a patient with an AAA, signs of an acute abdomen, and hypotension belongs in the operating room.

▶ Treatment & Prognosis

Repair should be performed as soon as intravenous fluids have been started, the airway has been secured, and blood has been sent for crossmatching. Surgical control of the aorta proximal and distal to the aneurysm must be obtained immediately and should be attempted from the abdomen. Attempts to control the proximal aorta through the chest have been associated with poor outcomes. A successful outcome of the operation is related to the patient's condition on arrival, the promptness of diagnosis, and the speed of operative control of bleeding and blood replacement. The operative death rate is between 30% and 80%, with an average of approximately 50%. Because many patients with ruptured aneurysms die before reaching the hospital, the overall death rate approaches 80%. Without operation, the outcome is uniformly fatal. Many centers are now treating ruptured AAA using endovascular stent grafts; however, morbidity and mortality remain high.

INFLAMMATORY ANEURYSMS

Inflammatory aneurysms are degenerative aneurysms that elicit a unique inflammatory response adjacent to the external calcified layer of the aneurysm wall. Although similar to retroperitoneal fibrosis, the inflammation is usually confined to the anterior aorta and iliac arteries. The aneurysm may be responsible to chronic abdominal pain and is tender to palpation. One fourth of patients have some degree of ureteral obstruction. CT scanning reliably demonstrates the characteristic thickened wall and confirms the diagnosis. Characteristic pathologic changes include infiltration of the aortic wall by lymphocytes, plasma cells, occasional multinucleated giant cells, and lymphoid follicles with germinal centers. Inflammation resolves in most cases after successful repair. Inflammatory aneurysms are easily recognized at operation by the dense, shiny, white, fibrotic material that envelops the adjacent viscera, especially the duodenum, left renal vein, and inferior vena cava. Those structures therefore are especially vulnerable to operative injury. Endovascular repair is ideal and is the procedure of choice for inflammatory aneurysms.

INFECTED (MYCOTIC) ANEURYSMS

The confusing term "mycotic aneurysm" is commonly used to denote infected aneurysms in general, which are rarely fungal. The aneurysm is secondary to a microbial aortitis in which virulent bacteria infect the aorta and destroy the aortic wall. Historically, salmonella infection was the most common cause. In the current era, staphylococcus is the more common infection due to intravenous drug use. These organisms may involve every major artery, but aortic involvement predominates.

The typical patient presents with a rapidly enlarging, tender pulsatile mass that may feel warm, if palpable. Fever is present, and half the patients have positive blood cultures. Alternatively, the aneurysm may be discovered late, after successful treatment of the infection. Angiography of these patients may show a saccular false aneurysm. Treatment consists of excision and remote bypass grafting if possible. Liberal application of muscle flap coverage techniques facilitates healing. Direct repair has been successful when done after a course of antibiotics. A prolonged course of antibiotics should be given to guard against recurrence.

PERIPHERAL ARTERIAL ANEURYSMS

▶ General Considerations

Popliteal artery aneurysms account for 70% of peripheral arterial aneurysms. Like aortic aneurysms, they are silent until critically symptomatic. However, unlike aortic aneurysms, they rarely rupture. The presenting manifestations are due to peripheral embolization and thrombosis. Popliteal aneurysms may embolize repetitively over time and occlude distal arteries. Due to the redundant parallel arterial supply to the foot, ischemia does not occur until a final embolus occludes flow to the remaining tibial/peroneal artery. Acute ischemia caused by popliteal aneurysms has a poor prognosis because of the chronicity of the process. The results of both chemical and mechanical thrombolysis may be disappointing because of clot age and adherence to the artery wall. After presentation with acute ischemia, approximately one third of patients will require an amputation. To prevent embolization and thrombosis, popliteal artery aneurysms should be repaired electively if greater than 2 cm in diameter or at any size if lined with thrombus.

Primary aneurysms of the femoral artery are much less common than aneurysms of the popliteal artery. However, pseudoaneurysms of the femoral artery following arterial punctures for arteriography and cardiac catheterization occur with an incidence ranging from 0.05% to 6%. Thrombosis and embolization are the main risks of femoral true or false aneurysms and, like popliteal aneurysms, should be repaired when greater than 2 cm in diameter.

▶ Clinical Findings

A. Symptoms and Signs

Until progressive embolization or thrombosis occurs, peripheral artery aneurysms are usually asymptomatic. The patient may be aware of a pulsatile mass when the aneurysm is in the groin, but popliteal aneurysms are often undetected by the patient and physician. Peripheral aneurysms may produce symptoms by compressing the local vein or nerve, but this is unusual. In most patients, the first symptom is due to ischemia of acute arterial occlusion. The pathologic findings range from rapidly developing gangrene to moderate ischemia that slowly lessens as collateral circulation develops. Symptoms from recurrent embolization to the leg are often transient if they occur at all. Sudden ischemia may appear in a toe or part of the foot, followed by slow resolution, and the true diagnosis may be elusive. The onset of recurrent episodes of pain in the foot, particularly if accompanied by cyanosis, suggests embolization and requires investigation of the heart and proximal arterial tree.

Because popliteal pulses are somewhat difficult to palpate even in normal individuals, a particularly prominent or easily felt pulse is suggestive of aneurysmal dilation and should be investigated by ultrasound. Since popliteal aneurysms are bilateral in 60% of cases, the diagnosis of thrombosis of a popliteal aneurysm is often aided by the palpation of a pulsatile aneurysm in the contralateral popliteal space. Approximately 50% of patients with popliteal aneurysms have an aneurysmal abdominal aorta.

B. Imaging Studies

Duplex color ultrasound is the most efficient investigation to confirm the diagnosis of peripheral aneurysm, to measure its size and configuration, and to demonstrate mural thrombus.

Arteriography may not demonstrate aneurysms accurately, because mural thrombus reduces the apparent diameter of the lumen. Three-dimensional imaging by CTA or MRA is required—especially when operation is considered—to define the anatomy and plan intervention.

C. Treatment

Early operation is indicated for an aneurysm that is associated with any peripheral embolization greater than 2 cm in size or an aneurysm with mural thrombus. Urgent operation is indicated when acute embolization or thrombosis has caused acute ischemia. Intra-arterial thrombolysis may be done in the setting of acute ischemia if examination (light touch) suggests that immediate surgery is not imperative to prevent tissue loss. Bypass with saphenous vein may include either excision or exclusion, depending on location. If exclusion rather than resection is performed, the geniculate "feeder" arteries within the aneurysm must be ligated or progressive enlargement can still occur.

Endovascular repair with covered stents can be used but are less durable than open repair and should be reserved for high-risk patients.

Acute pseudoaneurysms of the femoral artery due to arterial punctures can be successfully treated using ultrasound-guided compression and thrombin injections if the aneurysm is not large. Open surgery with prosthetic interposition grafting is preferred for primary aneurysms of the femoral artery and vein graft for the popliteal arteries. Endovascular repair with small stent-grafts has been done but is reserved for patients who are at prohibitive risk for an open operation.

D. Prognosis

The long-term patency of bypass for femoral and popliteal aneurysms is generally excellent but depends on the adequacy of the outflow tract. Late graft occlusion is less common than in similar operations for occlusive disease.

UPPER EXTREMITY ANEURYSMS

▶ Subclavian Artery Aneurysms

Subclavian artery aneurysms are less common than aneurysms of the lower extremity, and most supraclavicular pulsatile masses represent tortuous vessels, not aneurysms. Pseudoaneurysms due to injections by drug addicts are becoming increasingly frequent. An anomaly, the aberrant right subclavian artery (incidence 0.5%), arises from the aorta distal to the left subclavian and courses behind the esophagus. As found in other aberrant arteries, enlargement is common and may compress the esophagus against the trachea, causing difficulty swallowing (termed dysphagia lusoria). This anomaly also is the most common cause of a nonrecurrent laryngeal nerve.

A true subclavian artery aneurysm is usually due to poststenotic dilation in a patient with thoracic outlet syndrome or a large callous from a fractured clavicle. As with popliteal aneurysms, the most common manifestation is embolization with episodic hand ischemia and Raynaud phenomenon. The diagnosis is often missed. Sudden onset Raynaud, particularly with a history of waxing and waning digital ischemia, is indication for proximal arterial imaging. Treatment consists of resection of the restricting structures at the time of arterial replacement.

▶ Radial Artery False Aneurysms

The incidence of radial artery false aneurysms has increased as a result of increasing use of radial artery catheters. Occasionally, the aneurysm is infected. If the Allen test is normal and adequate collateralization is confirmed with imaging, treatment consists of excision and ligation. If the ulnar

collaterals are insufficient to preserve viability of the hand, excision and replacement with vein should be performed.

Small aneurysms of the palmer arch may be due to repetitive trauma. These aneurysms can be responsible for emboli to the digital arteries. The adage that hand ischemia requires angiography should be applied to ensure that all potentially reversible causes of hand ischemia, including these unusual aneurysms, be identified.

Anderson PL et al: A statewide experience with endovascular abdominal aortic aneurysm repair rapid diffusion with excellent early results. J Vasc Surg 2004;39:10.

Baxter BT, Terrin MC, Dalman RL: Medical management of small abdominal aortic aneurysms. Circulation 2008;117:1883. Review.

Chuter TA et al: Endovascular treatment of thoracoabdominal aortic aneurysms. J Vasc Surg 2008;47:6.

Cinà CS et al: Kommerell's diverticulum and right-sided aortic arch: a cohort study and review of the literature. J Vasc Surg 2004;39:131. Review.

Curi MA et al: Mid-term outcomes of endovascular popliteal artery aneurysm repair. J Vasc Surg 2007;45:505.

Ganchi PA et al: Ruptured pseudoaneurysm complicating an infected radial artery catheter: case report and review of the literature. Ann Plast Surg 2001;46:647. Review.

Katz DJ, Stanley JC, Zelenock GB: Operative mortality rates for intact and ruptured abdominal aortic aneurysms in Michigan an eleven-year statewide experience. J Vasc Surg 1994;19:804.

Kazmers A et al: Nonoperative therapy for postcatheterization femoral artery pseudoaneurysms. Am Surg 1997;63:199.

Lederle FA, Simel DL: The rational clinical examination. Does this patient have abdominal aortic aneurysm? JAMA 1999;281:77.

Lederle FA et al: Immediate repair compared with surveillance of small abdominal aortic aneurysms. N Engl J Med 2002; 346:1437.

Lederle FA et al: Rupture rate of large abdominal aortic aneurysms in patients refusing or unfit for elective repair. JAMA 2002;287:2968.

Lindholt JS, Norman P: Screening for abdominal aortic aneurysm reduces overall mortality in men. A meta-analysis of the mid- and long-term effects of screening for abdominal aortic aneurysms. Eur J Vasc Endovasc Surg 2008;36:167.

Parodi JC, Palmaz JC, Barone HD: Transfemoral intraluminal graft implantation for abdominal aortic aneurysms. Ann Vasc Surg 1991;5:491.

Thompson RW, Geraghty PJ, Lee JK: Abdominal aortic aneurysms: basic mechanisms and clinical implications. Curr Probl Surg 2002;39:110.

UK Small Aneurysm Trial Participants, Mortality results for randomised controlled trial of early elective surgery or ultrasonographic surveillance for small abdominal aortic aneurysms. Lancet 1998;352:1649.

Wain RA, Hines G: A contemporary review of popliteal artery aneurysms. Cardiol Rev 2007;15:102. Review.

VISCERAL ARTERY ANEURYSMS

▶ General Considerations

The etiology of this interesting group of aneurysms is generally unknown. Most often they occur as single lesions in a younger age group than those at risk for aortic aneurysms. Rupture is the primary danger and is one cause of "abdominal apoplexy."

Splenic Artery Aneurysms

Aneurysms of the splenic artery account for more than 60% of splanchnic artery aneurysms. Women are affected four times more commonly than men and often during childbearing years. Arterial fibrodysplasia and portal hypertension predispose to formation of splenic artery aneurysms. Rupture, the major complication, has been reported in less than 2% of splenic aneurysms; it rarely occurs with lesions smaller than 2–3 cm in diameter. Rupture during pregnancy tends to occur in the third trimester and is associated with a 75% maternal death rate and 90% fetal death rate. Diagnosis is most often made from plain x-ray films of the abdomen, showing concentric calcification in the upper left quadrant.

Intervention is indicated for patients with symptomatic aneurysms, aneurysms in pregnant women, and patients who have a low operative risk profile with aneurysms greater than 3 cm in diameter. Endovascular repair with covered stent grafts is ideal with the use of microcatheters developed for intracranial work, improving the ability to negotiate the often tortuous splenic artery. Laparoscopic ligation of the artery is also feasible.

Hepatic Artery Aneurysms

Hepatic artery aneurysms account for 20% of splanchnic artery aneurysms. There is a 2:1 male-to-female ratio, and the frequency of reported rupture is about 20%. Aneurysm rupture is associated with a 35% mortality rate. Rupture into the biliary tree producing hemobilia is as frequent as intraperitoneal rupture. The symptom triad of intermittent abdominal pain, gastrointestinal bleeding, and jaundice strongly suggests the diagnosis and is present in about one third of patients. Surgery is usually required to control bleeding. If the common hepatic artery is involved, the artery may be safely ligated if collateral flow through the gastroduodenal artery has been demonstrated. Aneurysms in other portions of the artery usually require vascular reconstruction. Endovascular placement with a covered stent is preferred if the anatomy is suitable.

Superior Mesenteric Artery Aneurysms

Aneurysms of the proximal superior mesenteric artery account for 5% of all splanchnic artery aneurysms. Unlike splenic or hepatic aneurysms, 60% of superior mesenteric artery aneurysms are mycotic. The aneurysm may involve the origin or branches of the artery. Symptoms include nonspecific abdominal pain. The diagnosis can be made on CT scan.

Operative therapy for mycotic superior mesenteric artery aneurysms includes ligation if there are adequate collaterals or replacement with a segment of autogenous vessel. Endovascular stent graft placement is not advisable in an acute infection. However, it is valuable for true aneurysms as long as critical branches can be avoided. For distal branch aneurysms, bowel resection may be necessary.

RENAL ARTERY ANEURYSMS

This uncommon aneurysm occurs in less than 0.1% of the population and is often associated with hypertension. The aneurysm is usually saccular and located at a primary or secondary bifurcation of the renal arteries. Women are affected slightly more frequently than men. There are three principal categories: (1) idiopathic, (2) aneurysms associated with medial fibrodysplastic disease, and (3) arteritis-related microaneurysms.

Renovascular hypertension may occur because of distortion of the involved or nearby vessels by the aneurysm. Spontaneous rupture of renal artery aneurysms is rare except during pregnancy. CT scans or digital subtraction angiography should be performed to monitor enlargement. Operation is indicated in women of childbearing age or in patients with associated renal artery disease, uncontrolled hypertension, or large aneurysms. Most renal artery aneurysms can be repaired in situ, but ex vivo repair is occasionally required. Endovascular options are usually limited due to the involved vessel size and the aneurysm's proximity to artery branch points.

Carr SC et al: Current management of visceral artery aneurysms. Surgery 1996;120:627.

Martin RS et al: Renal artery aneurysm: selective treatment for hypertension and prevention of rupture. J Vasc Surg 1989;9:26.

Pasha SF et al: Splanchnic artery aneurysms. Mayo Clin Proc 2007;82:472. Review.

VASOCONSTRICTIVE DISORDERS

General Considerations

Vasoconstrictive disorders are characterized by abnormal activity of the sympathetic nervous system that reduces peripheral blood flow, causing tissue ischemia.

Raynaud Disease/Phenomenon

Raynaud disease/phenomenon consists of sequential pallor, cyanosis, and rubor of fingers or toes after exposure to cold. Excessive vasoconstriction, sluggish flow, and reflex vasodilation produce the characteristic white-blue-red color changes. In Raynaud disease, this response, due to spasm alone without underlying arterial lesions, is quite common and benign.

Sudden onset or progression of symptoms suggests underlying arterial lesions that exaggerate the normal reduction in blood flow caused by vasoconstriction. This is termed Raynaud phenomenon, a more virulent entity associated primarily with immunologic and connective tissue disorders (eg, scleroderma, systemic lupus erythematosus, polymyositis, or drug-induced vasculitis). However, repeated embolization, occupational trauma (vibration injury, cold injury), and other disorders (cold agglutinins, chronic renal failure, and neoplasia) also have been reported.

Hyperreactivity to cold stimuli may be the initial presentation of arterial pathology. In new onset or severe cases of Raynaud-type symptoms, a search for underlying pathology is required. All patients with Raynaud syndrome should avoid cold exposure, tobacco, oral contraceptives, β-adrenergic blocking agents, and ergotamine preparations. Calcium-channel blockers are generally prescribed but may cause hypotension. Transdermal prostaglandins, ketanserin, and cilostazol also have been used, with relief of symptoms in some patients. In rare cases, symptoms progress to tissue loss. Finger amputation is necessary once gangrene has developed.

Acrocyanosis

Acrocyanosis is a common, chronic, benign vasoconstrictive disorder related to Raynaud syndrome that is largely restricted to young females. It is characterized by persistent cyanosis of the hands and feet. The changes disappear with exposure to a warm environment. Examination in a cool room shows diffuse symmetric cyanosis, coldness, and occasionally hyperhidrosis of the hands and feet. Cyanosis of the skin of the calf, thigh, or forearm usually displays a reticulated pattern and has been called livedo reticularis and cutis marmorata. The peripheral pulses may diminish in the cold but return to normal with rewarming.

THORACIC OUTLET SYNDROME

General Considerations

Thoracic outlet syndrome refers to the variety of disorders caused by abnormal compression of arterial, venous, or neural structures in the base of the neck. Numerous mechanisms for compression have been described, including cervical rib, anomalous ligaments, hypertrophy of the anterior scalene muscle, and positional changes that alter the normal relation of the first rib to the structures that pass over it. Patients may describe a history of cervical trauma.

Symptoms rarely develop until adulthood. For this reason, it has been assumed that an alteration of normal structural relationships that occurs with advancing years is the primary factor. Even anomalous cervical ribs seem well tolerated during childhood and adolescence.

Transient circulatory changes may occur, but the primary cause of symptoms in most patients is intermittent compression of one or more trunks of the brachial plexus. Thus, neurologic symptoms predominate over those of ischemia or venous compression. When present, compression of the subclavian artery and vein in the thoracic outlet also can produce severe sequelae. Compression of the subclavian artery can produce stenosis and poststenotic dilation of the artery, leading to arterial occlusion or emboli, as discussed earlier. Compression of the vein can produce thrombosis, which can result in severe upper extremity pain and swelling. Compression may be exaggerated with exercise precipitating an occlusion. This syndrome is termed effort thrombosis or **Paget-Schroetter syndrome**.

Clinical Findings

A. Symptoms and Signs

Neural symptoms consist of pain, paresthesias, or numbness in the distribution of one or more trunks of the brachial plexus (usually in the ulnar distribution). Most patients associate their symptoms with certain positions of the shoulder girdle. These may occur from prolonged hyperabduction, as in house painters, hairdressers, and truck drivers. Others may relate their symptoms to the downward traction of the shoulder girdle produced by carrying heavy objects. Numbness of the hands often wakes the patient from sleep. On physical examination, motor deficits are rare and usually indicate severe compression of long duration. Muscular atrophy may be present in the hand. Pulses can be weakened by abduction of the arm with the head rotated to the opposite side (Adson test), though pulse reduction by this maneuver often occurs in completely asymptomatic persons. Light percussion over the brachial plexus in the supraclavicular fossa may reproduce the symptoms in patients with chronic neurologic impingement.

Arterial symptoms are less common and often the result of emboli. A bruit may be heard over the subclavian artery with abduction of the arm, but this is not a specific finding. Venous occlusion results in unilateral arm swelling. There are good collaterals around the shoulder girdle, but symptoms may be debilitating in young active patients.

B. Diagnosis

Neurogenic thoracic outlet compression must be differentiated from other disorders that mimic this condition (eg, carpal tunnel syndrome and cervical disk disease). Cervical x-rays and peripheral nerve conduction studies are not diagnostic but are valuable to eliminate other possibilities. Unfortunately, there is no recognized objective study to unequivocally confirm the diagnosis of neurogenic thoracic outlet syndrome. Arteriograms may demonstrate subclavian or axillary artery stenosis when the arm is in abduction. This finding is not diagnostic, but poststenotic dilation of the artery is distinctly abnormal and indicates a definite lesion.

Treatment

Most patients benefit from postural correction and a physical therapy program directed toward restoring the normal relation and strength of the structures in the shoulder girdle. Surgical techniques for decompression of the thoracic outlet are reserved for patients who have not responded after 3–6 months of conservative treatment. Some surgeons prefer transaxillary first rib resection, while others prefer a supraclavicular approach. With either operation, the anterior scalene muscle and any associated fibrous bands should be excised.

Symptomatic arterial stenoses require decompression of the thoracic outlet in combination with arterial reconstruction. Effort thrombosis of the subclavian vein is usually best treated by catheter-directed thrombolysis of the venous occlusion followed by thoracic outlet decompression with or without operative venous reconstruction or intraluminal stent placement. Insertion of intraluminal venous stents without rib resection is ineffective because the stents themselves are compressed and narrowed by the underlying anatomy.

Sanders RJ, Hammond SL, Rao NM: Diagnosis of thoracic outlet syndrome. J Vasc Surg 2007;46:601. Review.

Schneider DB et al: Combination treatment of venous thoracic outlet syndrome: open surgical decompression and intraoperative angioplasty. J Vasc Surg 2004;40:599.

ARTERIOVENOUS FISTULAS

Arteriovenous fistulas may be congenital, often called "malformations," or acquired. Abnormal communications between arteries and veins occur in many diseases and affect vessels of all sizes and in many locations. In congenital fistulas, the systemic effect is often not great, because although the communications may be multiple, they are small. When a limb is involved, extensive arteriovenous communications may exist with increased flow and increased muscle mass and bone length.

Acquired fistulas are usually the result of trauma, violent or iatrogenic. These communications can have considerable flow, and high-output heart failure can occur. The third class of fistulas is surgically created fistulas for hemodialysis access.

Arteriovenous malformations in the gastrointestinal tract may cause hemorrhage. Osler-Weber-Rendu disease or syndrome (also termed hereditary hemorrhagic telangiectasia) is an autosomal dominant disorder characterized by gastrointestinal bleeding and epistaxis due to large arteriovenous anomalies in the gastrointestinal tract and lungs. Pulmonary lesions cause recirculation with lower PO_2, polycythemia, clubbing, and cyanosis.

Penetrating injuries either from trauma or iatrogenic ones from arterial punctures are the most common causes of acquired fistulas. Blunt trauma, erosion of an atherosclerotic or mycotic arterial aneurysm into adjacent veins, communication with an arterial prosthetic graft, or neoplastic invasion can all cause arteriovenous fistulas as well. When large vessels are involved, the presentation may be dramatic. For example, if an aortic aneurysm ruptures into the inferior vena cava, the fistula enlarges rapidly and can result in cardiac dilation and failure.

ARTERIOVENOUS FISTULA FOR HEMODIALYSIS

General Considerations

A successful arteriovenous fistula for hemodialysis access requires a large vein (> 5 mm) that lies close to the skin for at least 20 cm. The cephalic vein is ideal for this purpose, and radial artery to cephalic vein arteriovenous fistula (Cimino fistula) is the classic hemodialysis access fistula. If no suitable vein is available for an autogenous fistula, prosthetic grafts are used, most commonly PTFE. These are most commonly placed in a loop configuration. The poor patency rates of these grafts, 40% at 2 years, and potential for infection have driven national guidelines to encourage a higher rate of autogenous fistula formation. To maximize autogenous vein utilization, current practice includes transposing deep veins such as the basilic vein in the upper arm to the subcutaneous tissue. All veins used for access require "arterialization" of the wall, which takes at least 6 weeks prior to cannulization for dialysis. Transposed veins may take even longer to mature.

Flow rates of 300 cc/min or greater are necessary for efficient dialysis. Patients with a newly created arteriovenous access should be watched carefully for arterial steal and distal ischemia. Diabetics are the most vulnerable to this complication because of calcified proximal arteries or intrinsic arterial lesions of the arm. High-output cardiac failure does not occur.

Clinical Findings

A. Symptoms and Signs

A typical continuous machinery murmur can be heard over the arteriovenous fistulas and is often associated with a palpable thrill and locally increased skin temperature. Proximally, the arteries and veins dilate, and the pulse distal to the lesion diminishes. There may be signs of venous insufficiency, coolness, and hypertrophy distal to the communication on the involved extremity. Tachycardia occurs in some patients as a feature of increased cardiac output. The pulse rate slows (Branham sign) when the fistula is occluded by compression.

In contrast, venous malformations rarely produce hemodynamic effects. In this disorder, the presence of a mass, which may or may not be tender, is the principal finding. Because flow rates are low, bruits and thrills are absent.

B. Imaging Studies

MRI has become the imaging study of choice for the evaluation and follow-up of peripheral arteriovenous malformations, but CTA also gives excellent anatomic information. Precise delineation of arteriovenous fistulas can be done with selective arteriograms.

Treatment

Not all arteriovenous connections require treatment. Most venous malformations should be treated conservatively. In addition, small peripheral fistulas may be observed and will often remain asymptomatic. Some are surgically inaccessible.

The indications for intervention include hemorrhage, local expansion, severe venous or arterial insufficiency, cosmetic deformity, and, rarely, heart failure. Most fistulas are now managed by embolization under radiographic control.

The embolic material used includes blood clot, glass beads, and Gelfoam. Arteriovenous malformations of the head and neck and of the pelvis appear particularly well suited for this form of therapy. Direct injection of sclerosant compounds into venous malformations under fluoroscopic control also has been successful.

Surgical options are generally reserved for large acquired fistulas. When the fistulous connections involve substantial portions of an extremity, local ligation is invariably followed by recurrence, and only temporary palliation can be expected. Covered stent grafts are now being used for a variety of traumatic fistulas.

▶ Prognosis

The results of therapy vary according to the extent, location, and type of fistula. In general, traumatic fistulas have the most favorable prognosis. Congenital fistulas are more difficult to eradicate because of the numerous arteriovenous connections present.

Hisamatsu K et al: Peripheral arterial coil embolization for hepatic arteriovenous malformation in Osler-Weber-Rendu disease. Intern Med 1999;38:962.

Jacobowitz GR et al: Transcatheter embolization of complex pelvic vascular malformations: results and long-term follow-up. J Vasc Surg 2001;33:51.

Mattle HP et al: Dilemmas in the management of patients with arteriovenous malformations. J Neurol 2000;247:917.

Maya ID et al: Vascular access core curriculum 2008. Am J Kidney Dis 2008;51:702.

Mulliken JB et al: Vascular anomalies. Curr Probl Surg 2000;37:517.

White RI Jr et al: Long-term outcome of embolotherapy and surgery for high-flow extremity arteriovenous malformations. J Vasc Interv Radiol 2000;11:1285.

Veins & Lymphatics

35

Thomas W. Wakefield, MD

John R. Rectenwald, MD

Louis M. Messina, MD

I. THE VEINS

VENOUS ANATOMY

Veins of the lower extremity (Figure 35–1) consist of superficial and deep systems joined by venous perforators. The greater and lesser saphenous veins are superficial—veins, the name "saphenous" aptly derived from the Greek word for "manifest, clear," or "visible." They contain many valves and show considerable variation in their location and branching points. The greater saphenous vein may be duplicated in up to 10% of patients. Typically, it originates from the superficial arch of the foot and is found anterior to the medial malleolus at the ankle. As it ascends in the calf just beneath the superficial fascia, it is joined by two major tributaries: an anterior vein, which crosses the tibia; and a posterior arch vein, which arises posterior to the medial malleolus beside the posterior tibial artery. The greater saphenous vein then enters the fossa ovalis in the groin to empty into the deep femoral vein.

The saphenofemoral junction is marked by four or five prominent branches of the greater saphenous vein: the superficial circumflex iliac vein, the external pudendal vein, the superficial epigastric vein, and the medial and lateral accessory saphenous veins. Another important anatomic landmark is the relationship of the greater saphenous vein to the saphenous branch of the femoral nerve; as it emerges from the popliteal space, the nerve follows a course parallel to the vein. Injury during saphenous vein stripping or saphenous vein harvest for bypass produces neuropathic pain or numbness along the medial calf and foot. The lesser saphenous vein arises from the superficial dorsal venous arch behind the lateral malleolus at the ankle and curves toward the midline of the posterior calf, ascending to join the popliteal vein behind the knee.

Deep veins of the leg parallel the courses of the arteries. Two or three venae comitantes accompany each tibial artery. At the knee, these paired high-capacitance veins merge to

form the popliteal vein, which continues proximally as the femoral vein. At the inguinal ligament, the femoral and deep (profunda) femoral veins join medial to the femoral artery to form the common femoral vein. Proximal to the inguinal ligament, the common femoral vein becomes the external iliac vein. In the pelvis, external and internal iliac veins join to form common iliac veins that empty into the inferior vena cava (IVC). The right common iliac vein ascends almost vertically to the IVC while the left common iliac vein takes a more transverse course. For this reason, the left common iliac vein may be compressed between the right common iliac artery and lumbosacral spine, a condition known as May-Thurner (Cockett) syndrome when thrombosis of the left iliac vein occurs.

Muscular sinusoids represent another component of the deep veins of the leg. These thin-walled, nonvalved venous lakes run longitudinally within soleus muscle bellies and then coalesce to join the posterior tibial and peroneal veins. Blood empties from these sinusoids during muscle contraction; inactivity leads to stasis and may contribute to the development of deep venous thrombosis.

Blood flow is directed from superficial to deep veins of the leg via valved perforating (communicating) veins. Perforators are located below the medial malleolus (inframalleolar perforator), in the medial calf (Cockett perforators), at the level of the adductor canal (Hunterian perforator), and just above (Dodd perforator) and below (Boyd perforator) the knee.

Delicate bicuspid venous valves prevent reflux and direct the flow of blood from the foot and leg toward the heart and generally against gravity. Valves are more numerous in the distal part of the extremity, decrease in number proximally, and are virtually absent in the IVC itself.

The IVC ascends in the abdomen and ends at the right atrium. It lies to the right of the midline, lateral to the aorta, and receives a number of lumbar veins that connect with the vertebral and paravertebral venous plexuses. The IVC and its tributaries are derived in the 6th to 10th week of life from the fusion and obliteration of several paired embryonic veins:

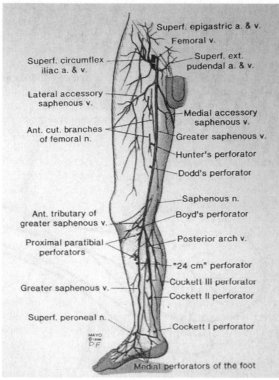

the anterior and posterior cardinal veins, the subcardinal veins, the supracardinal veins, and the sacrocardinal veins. Because of this complex embryonic development, anomalies in the venous system are not uncommon. The most common abnormality is a circumaortic left renal vein (1.5–8.7% incidence), followed by a retroaortic left renal vein (1.2–2.4% incidence), duplication of the IVC (0.2–3% incidence), and left-sided IVC (0.2–0.5% incidence). An unsuspected retroaortic or circumaortic renal vein can be inadvertently injured during aortic cross-clamping. Most unusual is the congenital absence of the suprarenal IVC, which results from failure of the right subcardinal vein branches to join the veins of the embryologic liver. This ultimately results in the infrarenal segment of the IVC joining the azygos-hemiazygos veins to drain into the superior vena cava. The hepatic veins drain directly into the right atrium in patients with this unusual anomaly.

Veins of the upper extremity are also divided into superficial and deep groups, though direction of flow from superficial to deep is not as distinct as in the lower extremity. Dorsal veins of the hand empty into the cephalic vein ("intern vein") on the radial aspect and into the basilic vein

on the ulnar aspect of the forearm. The cephalic vein ascends lateral to the biceps muscle into the deltopectoral groove, where it passes through the clavipectoral fascia to join the axillary vein. The cephalic vein is useful for arteriovenous fistulas, both at the wrist and in the upper arm, because it is superficial and lateral in the arm, allowing easy access for hemodialysis needles. The basilic vein, which runs medially in the arm to become the axillary vein, is deeper and thicker-walled than the cephalic vein. Its many branches make it tedious to harvest, but it can be used for a bypass conduit or for a laterally tunneled upper-arm dialysis fistula (basilic vein transposition). The median cubital vein links the cephalic and basilic veins in the antecubital space.

Paired brachial veins comprise the deep system of veins. They accompany the brachial artery and join the basilic vein as it becomes the axillary vein. The axillary vein continues medially as the subclavian vein, which passes through a tight space anterior to the first rib and anterior scalene muscle and posterior to the clavicle. The subclavian vein and the internal jugular vein join behind the clavicular head to form the brachiocephalic vein, which empties into the superior vena cava.

Caggiati A et al: Nomenclature of the veins of the lower limbs: an international interdisciplinary consensus statement. J Vasc Surg 2002;36:416.
Giordano JM et al: Anomalies of the vena cava. J Vasc Surg 1986;3:924.
Scultetus AH et al: Facts and fiction surrounding the discovery of venous valves. J Vasc Surg 2001;33:435.

VENOUS PHYSIOLOGY

Knowledge of lower extremity venous anatomy is essential to understanding the physiology of venous flow. The volume of blood in the lower extremities may increase by one-half liter when an individual moves from a reclining to an erect position (Figure 35–2). Increased blood volume is accommodated by increased venous capacitance, which is regulated by smooth muscle contractility in the vein walls. Erect posture creates a vertical column of blood, exerting a hydrostatic pressure equal to the distance from the toes to the right atrium (about 100–120 mm Hg). The hydrostatic pressure must be overcome to avoid pooling of blood in the legs and to provide venous return to the heart. Several aspects of the venous system make it possible to move blood against the force of gravity. Because the circulation is a closed system, venous return is affected by arterial inflow and by the negative intrathoracic pressure created during inspiration. Valves assure unidirectional movement of blood from superficial to deep systems and from the foot back to the heart. Hydrostatic pressure is dissipated by lack of simultaneous opening of the valves. Soleal venous sinusoids are another central component to the system. When the muscle contracts during exercise, blood empties from the sinusoid into the deep veins of the calf and leg. This high-velocity flow siphons

▲ **Figure 35–1.** Anatomy of the superficial and perforating veins of the lower extremity. (From Rutherford RB, Cronenwett JL, Gloviczki P: *Vascular Surgery*. Philadelphia: Saunders, 2000. Reproduced by permission from Elsevier.)

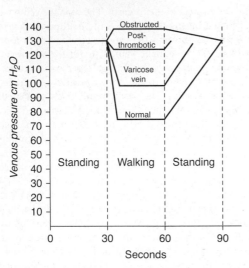

▲ **Figure 35–2.** Pedal venous pressure measurements with exercise. The normal drop in pressure associated with ambulation is impaired by deep vein incompetence and proximal venous obstruction. (Reproduced, with permission, from DeWeese JA: Venous and lymphatic disease. In: *Principles of Surgery,* 4th ed. Schwarz S [editor]. McGraw-Hill, 1983.)

blood from deep veins of the foot upward into the calf, analogous to smoke being drawn up a smokestack by wind blowing past the chimney (Venturi effect).

DISEASES OF THE VENOUS SYSTEM

VARICOSE VEINS

 ESSENTIALS OF DIAGNOSIS

▶ Dilated, tortuous superficial veins in the lower extremities, usually bilateral.

▶ May be asymptomatic or may be associated with localized pain, nocturnal cramps, aching discomfort and "heaviness" with prolonged standing, and bleeding.

▶ Pigmentation, ulceration, and edema suggest concomitant venous stasis disease.

▶ Increased frequency after pregnancy.

▶ General Considerations

Varicose veins are very common, afflicting 10–20% of the world's population. Abnormally dilated veins occur in several locations in the body: the spermatic cord (varicocele),

esophagus (esophageal varices), and anorectum (hemorrhoids). Varicosities of the legs were described as early as 1550 BC and in the 1600s AD were correlated with trauma, childbearing, and "standing too much before kings." Modern studies identify female sex, pregnancy, family history, prolonged standing, and a history of phlebitis as risk factors for varicose veins. In the Framingham Study, the highest incidence was found in women between 40 and 49 years of age.

Varicose veins are classified as either primary or secondary. Primary varicose veins are thought to be due to genetic or developmental defects in the vein wall that cause diminished elasticity and valvular incompetence. Most cases of isolated superficial venous insufficiency are primary varicose veins. Secondary varicose veins arise from destruction or dysfunction of valves caused by trauma, deep venous thrombosis, arteriovenous fistula, or nontraumatic proximal venous obstruction (pregnancy, pelvic tumor). When valves of the deep and perforating veins are disrupted, chronic venous stasis changes may accompany superficial varicosities. It is important to recognize that untreated, longstanding venous dysfunction from either primary or secondary varicose veins may cause chronic skin changes that lead to infection, non-healing venous ulceration, and chronic disability. To define the optimal method of treatment, the etiologic factors and distribution of disease must be clearly identified.

▶ Clinical Findings

The clinical presentation of patients with varicose veins can be quite variable. Many varicose veins are asymptomatic and come to medical attention because of aesthetic concerns. If symptomatic, varicose veins may be associated with localized pain, a burning sensation over the vein, a diffuse ache or "heaviness" in the calf (particularly with prolonged standing), or phlebitis. Mild ankle edema may occur. Symptoms generally improve with leg elevation.

The varicosities appear as dilated, tortuous, elongated veins predominantly on the medial aspect of the lower extremity along the course of the greater saphenous vein. Overlying skin changes may be absent even in the presence of extensive large varicosities. Smaller flat, blue-green reticular veins, telangiectasias, and spider veins may accompany varicose veins and are further evidence of venous dysfunction. A cluster of telangiectasias below the inframalleolar perforator is termed a corona phlebectatica paraplantaris. Secondary varicose veins can cause symptoms characteristic of chronic venous insufficiency, including edema, hyperpigmentation, stasis dermatitis, and even venous ulcerations.

Physical examination begins with inspection of all extremities to determine the distribution and severity of the varicosities. Bimanual circumferential palpation of the thighs and calves is helpful. Palpation of a thrill or auscultation of a bruit indicates the presence of an arteriovenous fistula as a possible etiologic factor. Today, tourniquet tests have been virtually replaced by venous duplex ultrasound imaging, identifying points of venous reflux.

Differential Diagnosis

Ulceration, brawny induration, and hyperpigmentation often indicate accompanying chronic deep venous insufficiency. This is important to recognize because the changes generally do not resolve with saphenous vein stripping alone.

If extensive varicose veins are encountered in a young patient, especially if unilateral and in an atypical distribution (lateral leg), Klippel-Trenaunay syndrome must be considered. The classic triad is varicose veins, limb hypertrophy, and a cutaneous birthmark (port wine stain or venous malformation). Because the deep veins are often anomalous or absent, saphenous vein stripping can be hazardous. Standard treatment for patients with Klippel-Trenaunay syndrome is graduated support stockings, limited stab avulsion of symptomatic varices after thorough duplex ultrasound vein mapping, and occasional surgery for correction of limb length discrepancy.

Treatment

A. Nonsurgical Treatment

Treatment for both primary and secondary varicose veins initially involves a program directed at management of venous insufficiency, including elastic stocking support, periodic leg elevation, and regular exercise. Prolonged sitting and standing are discouraged. For most patients, knee high or thigh-high gradient compression stockings of 20–30 mm Hg are sufficient, although some patients require 30–40 mm Hg pressure. The compression stockings are worn all day to diminish venous distention during standing and are removed at night.

B. Surgical Treatment

Indications for surgical treatment (Figure 35–3) include persistent or disabling pain, recurrent superficial thrombophlebitis, erosion of the overlying skin with bleeding, and manifestations of chronic venous insufficiency (particularly ulceration).

The operative plan is dependent on determination of the competency of the deep and perforating veins and the location of sites of venous reflux. Surgery can then be tailored to the pattern of disease. High ligation and stripping of the saphenous system is performed for patients with an incompetent valve at the saphenofemoral junction and varicosities throughout the length of the greater saphenous vein. This was traditionally performed by ligating the saphenofemoral junction and the major proximal saphenous vein branches through a small incision in the groin. Then the saphenous vein was removed to the point of clusters of varicosities. Today, the saphenous vein is ablated by either radiofrequency ablation (RFA) or endovenous laser treatment (EVLT). These clusters of varicose veins are then removed by the stab-avulsion technique, or if they are small, they may be observed to determine if they get smaller just by the saphenous vein ablation. Stab incisions 1.5–2 mm long

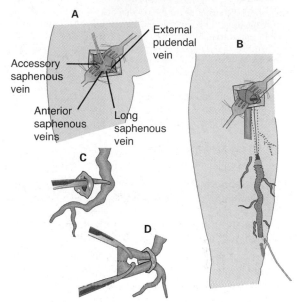

▲ **Figure 35–3.** Technique of varicose vein stripping. (From Bergan JJ, Kistner RL: *Atlas of Venous Surgery.* Saunders, 1992. Reproduced by permission from Elsevier.)

are made along premarked varicosities, and specially designed vein hooks are then used to loop the vein segments, which are then delivered through the incisions. With careful patient selection and properly selected operative techniques, the recurrence rate should be approximately 10%. Complications include hematoma formation, infection, and saphenous nerve irritation.

C. Compression Sclerotherapy

Compression sclerotherapy is usually applied to telangiectasias, spider veins, and small varicosities that persist after vein stripping. With the patient supine, a small volume of sclerosing solution (0.2–3% sodium tetradecyl sulfate or hypertonic saline) is injected into a varix isolated by proximal and distal digital venous occlusion. Direct pressure with compression stockings is maintained for 1 week afterward. The goal is to obliterate the abnormal vein by inducing localized endothelial destruction and fibrosis. More than one treatment is often required. Complications, including allergic reactions, thrombophlebitis, neoangiogenesis, and skin necrosis or hyperpigmentation, are rare.

Belcaro G et al: Endovascular sclerotherapy, surgery, and surgery plus sclerotherapy in superficial venous incompetence: a randomized, 10 year follow-up trial: final results. Angiology 2000;51:529.

Bradbury A et al: The relationship between lower limb symptoms and superficial and deep venous reflux on duplex ultrasonography: the Edinburgh Vein Study. J Vasc Surg 2000;32:921.

Dwerryhouse S: Stripping the long saphenous vein reduces the rate of reoperation for recurrent varicose veins: five year results of a randomized trial. J Vasc Surg 1999;29:589.

Merchant RF et al: Long-term outcomes of endovenous radiofrequency obliteration of saphenous reflux as a treatment for superficial venous insufficiency. Closure Study Group. J Vasc Surg 2005;42:502.

Puggioni A et al: Endovenous laser therapy and radiofrequency ablation of the great saphenous vein: analysis of early efficacy and complications. J Vasc Surg 2005;42:488.

DEEP VEIN THROMBOSIS

 ESSENTIALS OF DIAGNOSIS

▸ Pain in the thigh or calf sometimes accompanied by edema. Half of patients are asymptomatic.

▸ History of recent surgery, trauma, cancer, prolonged immobilization, or oral contraceptive use.

▸ Clinical impression is accurate in 50% of cases.

▸ Venous duplex ultrasound is the diagnostic modality of choice.

▸ General Considerations

Deep venous thrombosis (DVT) and pulmonary embolism (PE) affect up to 900,000 people per year in the United States, and their incidence increases with age. Treatment is estimated to cost billions of dollars per year, not even including expenditures associated with long-term sequelae of this disease.

The Virchow triad (stasis, vascular injury, and hypercoagulability) should be the cornerstone for assessment of risk factors for DVT. In most cases, the cause is multifactorial.

Acquired risk factors include older age, cancer, surgery, trauma, immobilization, hormone replacement therapy, oral contraceptive use, pregnancy, neurologic disease, cardiac disease, and antiphospholipid antibodies. Approximately 30–40% of patients with a new DVT (both upper and lower extremity) have been found to present with malignancy within 5 years. In men, pancreatic and colorectal cancers are most frequently associated with thrombotic risk, while hematological malignancies carry a lower risk. Cancers of the pancreas, ovary, and brain are mostly associated with thrombotic complications. Breast cancer, especially during its chemotherapy treatment, is also a risk factor. Most of these malignancies are associated with increased fibrinogen or thrombocytosis.

Endothelial injury can result from direct trauma (severed vein, venous cannulation, or transvenous pacing) or local irritation secondary to infusion of chemotherapy, previous DVT, or phlebitis. Damaged endothelium leads to platelet aggregation, degranulation, and formation of thrombus as well as vasoconstriction and activation of the coagulation cascade. Thrombin activation from release of tissue factor

and diminished fibrinolysis mediated by plasminogen activator inhibitor are intraoperative events that may be related to endothelial disruption.

Hypercoagulable states may also be inherited. Genetic causes include deficiencies of natural coagulation inhibitors (antithrombin III, protein C, protein S), factor V Leiden, prothrombin 20210A gene variant, blood group non-O, elevated homocysteine levels, plasminogen abnormalities, elevated levels of coagulation factors (such as factor VIII), and reduced heparin cofactor II activity. Hematologic disorders associated with DVT include disseminated intravascular coagulation, heparin-induced thrombocytopenia, antiphospholipid antibody syndrome, thrombotic thrombocytopenic purpura, hemolytic uremic syndrome, polycythemia vera, and essential thrombocythemia. Inflammatory bowel disease, systemic lupus erythematosus, and obesity are additionally associated with DVT.

DVT occurs most frequently in the calf veins, though it may arise in the femoral or iliac veins. Thrombi originate in soleal sinusoids or in valve sinuses, where there are flow eddies. Treatment of isolated calf vein thrombosis is controversial, as it is associated with a low risk of pulmonary embolism. However, if untreated, up to 25% may progress to proximal deep veins of the leg, where the incidence of chronic venous insufficiency is 25% and that of pulmonary embolism is 10%. These observations and the improved safety profile of low-molecular-weight heparin (LMWH) are compelling practitioners to treat isolated calf DVTs aggressively.

▸ Clinical Findings

A. Symptoms and Signs

The diagnosis of DVT cannot be made solely on the basis of presenting symptoms and signs, as up to half of patients with acute thromboses have no abnormality detectable in the involved extremity. Homans sign (pain on passive dorsiflexion of the ankle) is positive in only half of cases and is so nonspecific that it is not useful and should no longer even be performed. Some patients present with acute pulmonary embolism unaccompanied by leg edema or pain.

Symptomatic patients most often complain of a dull ache or pain in the calf or leg associated with mild edema. With extensive proximal DVT, there can be massive edema, cyanosis, and dilated superficial collateral veins. Low-grade fever and tachycardia occasionally occur. Iliofemoral venous thrombosis can result in phlegmasia. In phlegmasia alba dolens, the leg is pulseless, pale, and cool, which may progress to phlegmasia cerulea dolens, characterized by cyanosis of the limb and a precursor to gangrene.

B. Imaging Studies

Because DVT is difficult to diagnose on the basis of physical signs or symptoms, some objective diagnostic study is required before treatment is started. Historically, the standard for diagnosis was ascending phlebography, accomplished by fluoroscopic imaging during contrast injection into an intravenous line on the dorsum of the foot. The patient stands but is non-weight-bearing on the extremity studied. An abrupt cutoff of the contrast column indicates DVT. The complications of this procedure include risk of contrast allergy, contrast-induced nephropathy, and phlebitis.

Duplex ultrasound has now become the test of choice. It is a noninvasive examination, does not expose the patient to radiation, is easily reproducible, and has specificity and sensitivity of greater than 95%. It is also useful to detect other potential pathologic processes such as Baker cyst. The examination includes both a B-mode image and Doppler flow analysis. Each venous segment is assessed for the presence of thrombosis, indicated by venous dilation and incompressibility during probe pressure. Doppler findings suggestive of acute DVT are absence of spontaneous flow, loss of flow variation with respiration, and failure to increase flow velocity after distal augmentation. The criteria for the presence of chronic venous thrombosis are less well established. The chronically occluded vein is often narrowed, and there are prominent nearby collaterals. Chronic thrombi are highly echogenic, while acute thrombi are anechoic (and therefore not visible) on the B-mode image. Duplex ultrasound is less accurate in detection of calf thromboses and is highly operator dependent.

Magnetic resonance venography shows promise as a diagnostic study for this disorder. The sensitivity and specificity of magnetic resonance venography are 100% and 96%, respectively. The injection of gadolinium is useful for determining the age of the thrombus. CT imaging, especially as part of a pulmonary embolism protocol CT image, may also be a good alternative to establish the diagnosis.

Measurement of D-dimer levels is too nonspecific for use alone and, when combined with a negative risk assessment, may be useful to rule out DVT but not to rule in the diagnosis of DVT. Radiolabeled fibrinogen is too sensitive in the pelvis for use in the acute clinical setting and carries with it a risk of transmission of infectious disease. It is no longer used. Older tests such as impedance plethysmography and venous pressure measurements do not achieve the same accuracy as duplex ultrasound and have been largely abandoned.

▶ Differential Diagnosis

Localized muscle strain, contusion, or Achilles tendon rupture can often mimic the symptoms of DVT. Cellulitis may cause edema, localized pain, and erythema. Unilateral leg swelling can also result from lymphedema, obstruction of the popliteal vein by Baker cyst, or obstruction of the iliac vein by retroperitoneal mass or idiopathic fibrosis. Bilateral leg edema suggests heart, liver, or kidney failure or IVC obstruction by tumor or pregnancy.

▶ Treatment

Treatment is aimed at reducing the incidence of complications associated with DVT. Short-term complications include recurrent DVT or pulmonary thromboembolism, while long-term complications include the development of varicose veins and chronic venous insufficiency. The primary treatment of DVT is systemic anticoagulation. This reduces the risk of pulmonary embolism and extension of venous thrombosis and also decreases the rate of recurrent DVT by 80%. Systemic anticoagulation does not directly lyse thrombi but stops propagation and allows natural fibrinolysis to occur. Heparin is initiated immediately and dosed to a goal partial thromboplastin time (PTT) of 1.5–2.5 times normal, or, more currently, LMWH, weight-based without monitoring. Achieving therapeutic heparinization within the first 24 hours after diagnosis is shown to reduce the rate of recurrent DVT.

Warfarin is started after therapeutic heparinization. The two therapies should overlap to diminish the possibility of a hypercoagulable state, which can occur during the first few days of warfarin administration, because warfarin also inhibits the synthesis of natural anticoagulant proteins C and S. The recommended treatment for a first episode of uncomplicated DVT is 3–6 months of warfarin, maintained at a goal international normalized ratio (INR) of 2.0–3.0. After a second episode of DVT, the usual recommendation is prolonged or lifelong warfarin. The risk for recurrent venous thrombosis is increased markedly in the presence of homozygous factor V Leiden mutations, antiphospholipid antibody, and antithrombin III and protein C or protein S deficiencies, so lifelong anticoagulation is usually recommended for these conditions as well.

LMWH has been shown to be as safe and effective as standard unfractionated heparin in the treatment of DVT. It is administered once or twice daily by subcutaneous injection. LMWH does not require monitoring of its anticoagulant effect because of its predictable dose-response relationship, and this feature of the drug has made feasible the outpatient treatment of DVT. Standard unfractionated heparin inhibits thrombin because it is large enough to make a three-way complex between thrombin, antithrombin, and itself. LMWHs are much smaller than standard heparin molecules and do not inhibit thrombin; their main therapeutic effect comes from inhibition of factor Xa activity. The advantages of LMWHs over standard heparin preparations include a lower risk of bleeding complications and thrombocytopenia, less interference with proteins C and S, less complement activation, and a lower risk of osteoporosis. Moreover, recent randomized trials have shown regression of thrombus with LMWH. In many situations, standard heparin is being replaced by LMWH.

Two new areas of treatment that have demonstrated significant promise are direct thrombin inhibitors and specific factor Xa inhibitors. Regarding direct thrombin inhibitors, oral ximelagatran/melagatran had shown considerable promise for both the prophylaxis and treatment of DVT. However, this drug was not approved by the FDA because of problems with hepatic toxicity. A relative, dabigatran, also an oral direct thrombin inhibitor, has shown promise and is currently undergoing evaluation. The specific factor Xa inhibitor pentasaccharide has also shown significant promise for the prophylaxis and treatment of DVT. This drug potentiates by approximately 300-fold the neutralization of factor Xa by antithrombin III without inactivating thrombin. In orthopedic surgical indications, this agent has shown superiority to the best currently available DVT prophylaxis using LMWH. Regarding DVT treatment, large prospective randomized studies for both DVT and pulmonary embolism have been conducted. For DVT, in 154 centers, 23 countries, and with 2205 patients (> 30% outpatients), the recurrent DVT rate/major hemorrhage rate was 3.9%/1.1% for pentasaccharide versus 4.1%/1.2% for LMWH. For pulmonary embolism, in 214 centers, 20 countries, and with 2213 patients (with 15% outpatients), the recurrent pulmonary embolism/major hemorrhage rate was 3.8%/1.3% for pentasaccharide and 5%/1.1% for standard unfractionated heparin. Mortality rates were equal. Other oral factor Xa inhibitors are undergoing testing. These agents, along with others in development, likely will revolutionize the prophylaxis and treatment (acute and chronic) of DVT.

The prevention of chronic venous insufficiency after DVT can be divided into those measures that are useful with traditional anticoagulant treatment of DVT and measures that involve more aggressive interventions to lyse thrombus. Certain LMWHs decrease indices of chronic venous insufficiency compared to standard therapy when used over an extended period of time. Associated with this traditional therapy, the rate and severity of the postthrombotic syndrome after proximal DVT can be decreased by approximately 50% by the use of surgical compression stockings and ambulation without increasing the risk of pulmonary embolism.

The clinical outcome after DVT can be thought of as resulting in either valvular reflux, persistent venous obstruction, or their combination. Patients with both obstruction and valvular reflux often have the most severe postthrombotic symptoms. In order to limit these consequences, thrombus removal should be the best solution. The longer a thrombus is in contact with a vein valve, the more likely the valve will no longer function. Additionally, the thrombus initiates an inflammatory response in the vein wall, which may lead to vein wall and valve dysfunction.

Venous thrombectomy produces long-term improvements in venous patency and rates of chronic venous insufficiency, compared to standard heparin, both at 6 months and at 10 years. Thrombolysis has been evaluated with validated quality-of-life scales and is associated with a decrease in long-term postthrombotic symptoms. Three studies have demonstrated that excellent venous patency can result from intrathrombus administration of thrombolytic agents, while a small prospective randomized trial of catheter-directed thrombolysis confirmed this observation. Additionally, new devices have been developed or are being developed that can be combined with the thrombolytic agents and/or ultrasound to aid in thrombus removal.

▶ Prevention

Surgery increases the risk of DVT 21-fold. This disorder is a reported complication for approximately 20–25% of patients admitted for a general surgical procedure, 20–30% of those undergoing an elective neurosurgical procedure, and 50–60% of those undergoing hip or knee arthroplasty. These statistics emphasize the need for routine DVT prophylaxis in the surgical patient. The most commonly used measures are elastic stockings, pneumatic sequential compression devices (PCD), low-dose unfractionated heparin (5000 units given by subcutaneous injection), or LMWH given at a prophylactic dose subcutaneously (either once or twice daily).

For general surgical patients, the incidence of DVT is high without prophylaxis, and the risk of pulmonary embolism is 1.6%, 0.9% fatal. Patients have been categorized into levels of risk. In low-risk patients undergoing a minor procedure, 40 years old with no additional risk factors, no specific thromboembolism prophylaxis is indicated other than early ambulation. In moderate-risk patients, prophylaxis includes low-dose standard unfractionated heparin (LDH), LMWH, PCD, or elastic stockings. For higher-risk patients, LDH, LMWH, or PCD should be used, whereas for very high-risk patients, LDH or LMWH plus PCD is recommended. Full-dose warfarin may also be used, but few general surgeons use full-dose warfarin during surgery because of the risk of significant bleeding. Aspirin alone is not recommended for general surgery patients. In selected high-risk general surgery patients, including those undergoing cancer surgery, posthospital prophylaxis with LMWH is recommended.

For orthopedic patients without prophylaxis, the incidence of DVT is as high as 45–57% for total hip replacement, 40–84% for total knee replacement, and 35–60% for hip fracture surgery patients. For these groups, total pulmonary embolism incidence is 0.7–30%, 1.8–7%, and 4.3–24%, respectively, and fatal pulmonary embolism incidence is 0.1–0.4%, 0.2–0.7%, and 3.6–12.9%, respectively. For total hip replacement, LMWH, adjusted-dose warfarin, or fondaparinux has been recommended. Adjuvant physical modalities may provide additional benefit. For total knee replacement, LMWH, adjusted-dose warfarin, or fondaparinux again should be used. For both total hip and knee surgery, mechanical measures are indicated when anticoagulation cannot be used due to the risk of bleeding, although isolated usage of mechanical prophylaxis is not recommended as sole therapy for total hip surgery. For hip fracture surgery, preoperative or postoperative LMWH or adjusted-dose warfarin is suggested, along with fondaparinux or LDH. Again, mechanical prophylaxis may be indicated in times of high risk for bleeding. Prolonged posthospital prophylaxis may improve both total DVT and pulmonary embolism rates, as studies suggest that up to one third of these episodes occur after discharge.

For trauma patients, evidence is lacking, and randomized studies are needed. Without DVT prophylaxis, DVT may occur in more than 50% of cases. Pulmonary embolism is the third-most common cause of death in trauma patients surviving past the first day. Trauma risk factors include lower extremity or pelvic fractures, surgical procedures, advanced age, femoral vein lines or major venous repairs, prolonged immobility, spinal cord injury, and prolonged duration of hospital stay. Acceptable prophylaxis includes LMWH and PCD (when bleeding risk is high). Duplex ultrasound screening is appropriate when standard methods cannot be used. IVC filters are recommended in patients when anticoagulation is contraindicated.

In neurosurgery, DVT and pulmonary embolism occur equivalent to rates in general surgery patients, and risk factors include intracranial surgery, prolonged surgery, malignant tumors, the presence of leg weakness, and increased age. PCD with or without elastic stockings is recommended when anticoagulation cannot be used, although combining LDH or postoperative LMWH with PCD with or without stockings may be more effective than either technique alone. Overall rates of DVT and proximal DVT are reduced approximately 50% by combined treatment. For those with spinal cord injury, pulmonary embolism is a frequent cause of death. LMWH with or without mechanical measures is recommended for 3 months or at least until the completion of rehabilitation. LDH, PCD, and elastic stockings are inadequate alone, whereas adjusted-dose warfarin or LMWH has been suggested in the rehabilitation phase. Although IVC filters have been recommended in high-risk trauma and orthopedic patients to prevent pulmonary embolism with good results in small series, no large randomized prospective studies comparing prophylactic filters with more standard methods is available.

Bates SM, Ginsberg JS: Clinical practice. Treatment of deep-vein thrombosis. N Eng J Med 2004;351:268.
Bauer KA, Rusendaal FR, Heit JA: Hypercoagulability: too many test, too much conflicting data. Hematology 2002;1:353.
Bergqvist D et al: Venous thromboembolism and cancer. Curr Prob Surg 2007;44:145.
Breddin HK et al: Effects of a low-molecular-weight heparin on thrombus regression and recurrent thromboembolism in patients with deep-vein thrombosis. N Engl J Med 2001;344:626.
Comerota A and Gravett MH: Iliofemoral venous thrombosis. J Vasc Surg 2007;46:1065.
Douglas MG, Sumnar DS: Duplex scanning for deep vein thrombosis: has it replaced both phlebography and non-invasive testing? Sem Vasc Surg 1996;9:3.
Ferrari E et al: Travel as a risk factor for venous thromboembolic disease: a case-control study. Chest 1999;115:440.
Forster A et al: Tissue plasminogen activator for the treatment of deep venous thrombosis of the lower extremity: a systematic review. Chest 2001;119:572.
Geerts WH et al: Prevention of venous thromboembolism. Chest 2001;119:132S.
Heit JA et al: The epidemiology of venous thromboembolism in the community. Thromb Haemost 2001;86:452.
Heit JA et al: Estimated annual number of incident and recurrent, non-fatal and fatal venous thromboembolism (VTE) events in the US. Blood 2005;106:abstract #910, 267a.
Hirsh J et al: Clinical trials that have influenced the treatment of venous thromboembolism: a historical perspective. Ann Intern Med 2001;134:409.
Hyers TM et al: Antithrombotic therapy for venous thromboembolic disease. Chest 2001;119(Suppl):176S.
The Matisse Investigators: Subcutaneous fondaparinux versus intravenous unfractionated heparin in the initial treatment of pulmonary embolism. N Engl J Med 2003;349:1695
Prandoni P et al: The long-term clinical course of acute deep venous thrombosis. Ann Intern Med 1996;125:1.

AXILLARY-SUBCLAVIAN VENOUS THROMBOSIS

 ESSENTIALS OF DIAGNOSIS

▶ History of strenuous, repetitive upper extremity activity or recent venous cannulation.

▶ Arm swelling, pain, heaviness, upper limb cyanosis.

▶ Prominent distended venous collaterals.

▶ Subclavian vein obstruction at the thoracic outlet.

▶ General Considerations

Thrombosis of the axillary or subclavian vein is a relatively uncommon event, accounting for less than 5% of all cases of DVT. Only 12% result in clinically apparent pulmonary thromboembolism, but the incidence is higher if all patients undergo diagnostic testing. Besides pulmonary embolism, the most common consequence of axillary-subclavian vein thrombosis is chronic edema and resultant disability.

There are two major etiologies. Primary axillary-subclavian thrombosis, also known as Paget-Schroetter syndrome or "effort thrombosis," occurs as a result of intermittent transient obstruction of the vein in the costoclavicular space during repetitive or strenuous activities involving the upper extremity (Figure 35–4). This condition was first described in independent reports by Paget and von Schroetter in the late 19th century. During strenuous repetitive movements of the upper extremity, the subclavian vein is compressed between the first rib and the anterior scalene muscle posteriorly and the clavicle—with underlying subclavius muscle and fibrous costocoracoid ligament—anteriorly. Primary subclavian vein thrombosis can also occur in patients with hypercoagulable states such as antiphospholipid antibody syndrome or factor V Leiden mutation. Secondary subclavian vein thrombosis, which is increasing in incidence, results from venous injury by indwelling central venous catheters, external trauma, or pacemaker wires.

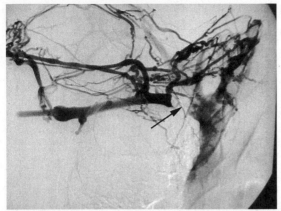

A

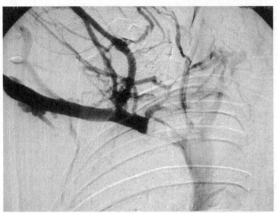

B

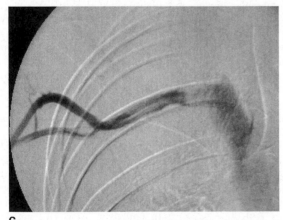

C

▲ **Figure 35–4. A:** Effort thrombosis in a 13-year-old wrestler. Arrow marks subclavian vein thrombosis refractory to rt-PA thrombolysis. **B:** Arm in abduction. Note disappearance of prominent venous collaterals. **C:** Immediate postoperative venogram following scalenectomy, first rib resection, and thrombectomy.

▶ Clinical Findings

A. Symptoms and Signs

Primary axillary-subclavian vein thrombosis usually occurs in healthy young athletes and people who perform repetitive activities that involve hyperabduction of the upper extremities. Most patients present with edema of the affected extremity, diffuse aching pain, prominent chest wall venous collaterals, and cyanosis of the upper extremity.

Paget-Schroetter syndrome may also be accompanied by symptoms of neurogenic thoracic outlet syndrome, often causing tingling, numbness, and pain in the hand and arm, sometimes in an ulna distribution indicating compression of the C-8/T-1 roots of the brachial plexus between hypertrophied or anomalous anterior and middle scalene muscles. Some patients may have a positive Adson test, signifying impingement of the subclavian artery in the thoracic outlet. This test is positive when the radial pulse disappears after abducting and externally rotating the arm while turning the head away from the arm being examined.

B. Imaging Studies

Upper extremity venous duplex ultrasound is a sensitive and reliable modality to diagnose axillary-subclavian vein thrombosis. If this study is positive, upper extremity venography and thrombolysis should be undertaken using newer techniques such as power-pulse spray thrombectomy. After successful venolysis, the patient undergoes positional venography, abducting the arm 120 degrees to confirm extrinsic compression of the subclavian vein at the thoracic outlet. Venous compromise is further evidenced on venography by the simultaneous appearance of prominent collateral veins.

Chest x-ray should be obtained on all patients to exclude the presence of cervical rib, which can also contribute to compression of the subclavian vein.

▶ Treatment

For patients with secondary axillo-subclavian thrombosis, any indwelling central venous lines or pacemaker wires in the thrombosed vein should be removed if possible. If not contraindicated, anticoagulation should be considered as well as arm elevation and pain control.

Patients who have primary venous thrombosis secondary to thoracic outlet compression should be considered for decompression because, if left untreated, the patients have a 35–65% risk of postthrombotic syndrome characterized by recurrent episodes of pain, swelling, and chronic venous insufficiency secondary to venous hypertension and valvular damage.

Previously, it was advocated that patients who were to undergo thoracic outlet decompression should be maintained on anticoagulation to allow the vein endothelium to heal. Because a significant number of patients can rethrombose their vein during this waiting period, immediate decompression is often recommended.

Because the etiology of venous thoracic outlet syndrome is compression of the vein between the first rib–anterior scalene muscle origin and the clavicle, surgery consists of anterior scalenectomy, first rib resection, and venolysis (release of the vein from any externally constricting scar). It is particularly important to resect the entire medial portion of the rib to the sternal junction. Management of any residual stenosis should be addressed, but the options are controversial. One approach is to perform intraoperative positional venography and, if a stenosis is seen, undertake balloon angioplasty. Should this not prove successful, venotomy, resection of scar, and vein patch angioplasty can be performed. Others advocate direct reconstruction under all circumstances (thrombectomy with interposition graft, internal jugular turndown, or jugular-subclavian bypass). If neurogenic thoracic outlet syndrome symptoms are present, radical anterior and middle scalenectomy with neurolysis should be undertaken. If the uncomplicated cases in which the decompression is straightforward, we have not advocated postoperative anticoagulation and this has been accompanied by a patency greater than 90%. Warfarin is continued for 1–3 months for patients who undergo some form of venous reconstruction or who have more than one episode of venous thrombosis preoperatively.

All patients who present with primary venous thrombosis should undergo a work up for a hypercoagulable state, the most common of which are mutations in coagulation factor V, protein C and S deficiencies, and antithrombin III. Because of a 40–60% rate of recurrent thrombosis, these patients are maintained indefinitely on warfarin.

▶ Prognosis

The prognosis after axillary-subclavian vein thrombosis is dependent on the cause of the condition. Most patients experience fairly rapid resolution of their initial presenting symptoms. For patients with secondary forms of this disease, the outcome is dependent on resolution of the underlying condition, such as a malignancy. For patients with Paget-Schroetter syndrome who undergo thoracic outlet decompression, excellent outcomes, characterized by continued venous patency and absence of symptoms of chronic venous insufficiency, are typical. In contrast, chronic axillary-subclavian vein thrombosis with symptoms persisting for over 3 months does not often respond to thrombolysis, mechanical thrombolysis, or prolonged anticoagulation and may cause significant long-term disability.

Kreinenberg P et al: Long-term results in patients treated with thrombolysis, thoracic inlet decompression, and subclavian vein stenting for Paget-Schroetter syndrome. J Vasc Surg 2001; 33:S100.

Molina JE et al: Paget-Schroetter syndrome treated with thrombolytics and immediate surgery. J Vasc Surg 2007;45:328.

Schneider DB et al: Combination treatment of venous thoracic outlet syndrome: open surgical decompression and intra-operative angioplasty. J Vasc Surg 2004;40:599.

PULMONARY THROMBOEMBOLISM

ESSENTIALS OF DIAGNOSIS

▶ Acute onset of dyspnea, chest pain, and hemoptysis.

▶ Tachypnea and a widened arterial-alveolar oxygen difference.

▶ Abnormal findings on a ventilation-perfusion lung scan, spiral CT scan, or magnetic resonance angiogram.

▶ General Considerations

Pulmonary thromboembolism is responsible for up to 50,000 deaths each year in the United States. It is the third-leading cause of death among hospitalized patients, yet only 30–40% of those with pulmonary thromboembolism have suspected DVT at the time of diagnosis. Efforts directed at reduction in the mortality rate of pulmonary thromboembolism demand an aggressive approach to the prevention of DVT and diagnosis of pulmonary thromboembolism in patients identified to be at high risk.

Pulmonary thromboemboli arise from a number of sources. Air embolism can occur during the placement or removal of central venous catheters intraoperatively during operation on large venous vessels. Amniotic fluid emboli may occur during active labor. Fat emboli from long bone fractures cause a syndrome characterized by respiratory insufficiency, coagulopathy, encephalopathy, and an upper body petechial rash. Other less common causes of pulmonary emboli include septic emboli, tumor emboli from atrial myxoma or IVC extension of renal cell carcinoma, and parasitic emboli. However, DVT remains the most common source of pulmonary thromboemboli. Up to 60% of patients with untreated proximal lower extremity DVT may develop pulmonary thromboembolism.

Fewer than 10% of pulmonary thromboemboli will produce pulmonary infarction. The pathophysiology of pulmonary embolism depends on the size and frequency of the emboli as well as the condition of the underlying lung. Obstruction of large pulmonary arteries results in increases in pulmonary artery pressure and acute right-ventricular failure, but many of the clinical manifestations of pulmonary thromboembolism result from release of vasoactive amines that cause severe pulmonary vasoconstriction. Vasoconstriction leads to increased physiologic dead space and systemic hypoxia from a right-to-left shunt. Reflex bronchial vasoconstriction is also common.

▶ Clinical Findings
A. Symptoms and Signs

Signs and symptoms associated with pulmonary embolism are notoriously vague. Dyspnea and chest pain are present in up to 75% of patients with pulmonary thromboembolism. However, these symptoms are nonspecific, especially in patients who may have underlying cardiopulmonary disease. Tachycardia, tachypnea, and altered mental status are highly suggestive findings in an at-risk population. The classic triad of dyspnea, chest pain, and hemoptysis is present in only 15% of patients with pulmonary thromboembolism. Pleural friction rub and the S1Q3T3 morphology on electrocardiography are even less common findings.

B. Imaging and Other Diagnostic Studies

Chest x-ray is most often normal but may show a pleural cap. Electrocardiography may reveal new-onset atrial fibrillation, evidence of right-heart strain, or ischemic changes, but in most cases only acute sinus tachycardia and nonspecific ST and T wave changes are identified. Arterial blood gas determination reveals hypoxia and often a respiratory alkalosis or increased arterial-alveolar oxygen gradient. Plasma D-dimer levels are elevated in the presence of both pulmonary thromboembolism and acute DVT, but this test lacks sufficient specificity to be of primary diagnostic value.

Until recently, the most common studies used to diagnose pulmonary embolism were ventilation-perfusion (VQ) scan and pulmonary angiogram (Figure 35–5). Ventilation-perfusion scans have sensitivity and specificity that approach 90% if results of the scan correlate with clinical risk factor assessment. For example, treatment can be started in a patient with a high-probability scan and a highly suggestive examination. Unfortunately, two thirds of studies are inconclusive. Pulmonary angiography remains the most reliable test for diagnosis, but it is invasive, time-consuming, and expensive.

Two newer modalities have improved the accuracy and safety of the diagnosis of pulmonary thromboembolism. Spiral CT scan has virtually replaced VQ scan in the diagnosis of pulmonary thromboembolism. Accuracy supersedes that of VQ scan and does not require clinical correlation, although clinical assessment is important when false-negative and false-positive spiral CT scan studies were recently retrospectively evaluated. Magnetic resonance angiography has also demonstrated excellent sensitivity and specificity and is now being used in many institutions.

▶ Treatment

A. Anticoagulation

Rapid anticoagulation remains the mainstay of treatment of pulmonary embolism. Heparin or LMWH anticoagulation is started as soon as the diagnosis is made after initial stabilization with ventilatory support and vasopressor medications. Thrombolysis is considered for large clot burden, severe respiratory compromise, hemodynamic instability, or right-heart failure. When compared with heparin alone, thrombolytic therapy speeds the resolution of pulmonary emboli in the first 24 hours. The disadvantages of lytic therapy include its greater cost and higher risk of significant bleeding complications.

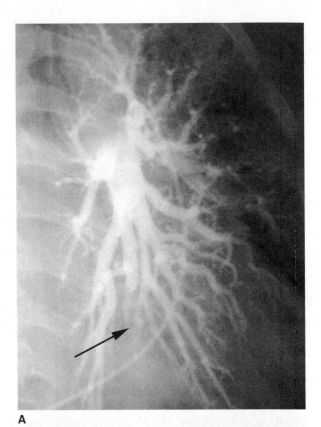

A

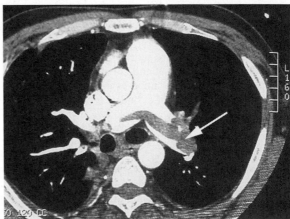

B

▲ **Figure 35–5.** Pulmonary embolism. **A:** Pulmonary angiogram. Arrow marks location of left lower lobe emboli. **B:** Spiral CT. Arrow marks location of large embolus in left main pulmonary artery.

B. Inferior Vena Cava Interruption

IVC interruption is considered in patients who have extension of venous thrombus on adequate heparin therapy, patients in whom heparin anticoagulation is contraindicated, patients who have had a complication of anticoagulation, or patients who have had recurrent DVT or pulmonary embolism despite *therapeutic* anticoagulation. More recently, temporary or permanent IVC filters have been placed prophylactically in high-risk patients such as those with unresectable cancer or major trauma.

Historically, IVC interruption was performed as an open surgical procedure, involving ligation or plication of the infrarenal vena cava or placement of a serrated clip to "strain" blood returning to the right atrium. The Greenfield filter, developed in 1973, was initially deployed by venous cutdown. Multiple devices are now available for fluoroscopically guided percutaneous placement through a range of sheath sizes from 6F to 12F and are introduced into the common femoral vein or, in cases of femoral thrombus, into the internal jugular vein. Diagnostic inferior venacavogram is essential prior to placing the filter to exclude the presence of a duplicated IVC because lower extremity DVT might still serve as a source of emboli. The presence of thrombus within the IVC, the diameter of the IVC, and identification of the level of the renal veins are also important to evaluate.

Newer devices being developed today include those used for only a temporary period of time (retrievable filter). Both the development and placement of retrievable filters has largely been driven by the PREPIC study. This study remains the only prospective randomize study comparing subject with DVT treated with anticoagulation alone to those treated with IVC filters and concurrent anticoagulation. At 8 years, the study has shown a statistically higher incidence of recurrent DVT in patients treated with IVC filters compared to patients treated with anticoagulation alone. There was a corresponding increase in the number of recurrent pulmonary emboli in patients treated with anticoagulation alone compared to patients who had filters placed.

Additionally, alternative imaging modalities (other than venography) are successfully being used to place filters. Specifically, devices are being successfully and safely deployed under ultrasound guidance, both intravascular and transabdominal ultrasound. The use of CT and MRI to place filters, although largely impractical, has also been described in the literature.

C. Surgical Treatment

Hemodynamically unstable patients in whom thrombolytic therapy has failed or cannot be instituted require percutaneous or open surgical extraction of the thrombus. Open surgical pulmonary embolectomy is reserved for patients who develop intractable hypotension, those who fail transcatheter pulmonary embolectomy, and those who have tumor or foreign body emboli. Catheter techniques involve mechanical thrombolysis or removal of intact pulmonary emboli using a suction embolectomy device.

Prognosis

Pulmonary embolism is one of the most frequent causes of preventable hospital death. Prevention by use of DVT prophylaxis and early diagnosis by selective testing of high-risk patients are essential steps to reducing the morbidity of this disease. The placement of IVC filters in selected patients can aid in prevention of pulmonary embolus but does nothing to treat the underlying disease process (venous thromboembolic disease) or prevent the long-term sequelae of DVT-postthrombotic syndrome.

Anderson FA et al: A population-based perspective of the hospital incidence and case-fatality rates of deep vein thrombosis and pulmonary embolism: the Worcester DVT Study. Arch Intern Med 1991;151:933.

Cross JJ et al: A randomized trial of spiral CT and ventilation perfusion scintigraphy for the diagnosis of pulmonary embolism. Clin Radiol 1998;53:177.

Dalen JD et al: Thrombolytic therapy for pulmonary embolism. Is it effective? Is it safe? When is it indicated? Arch Intern Med 1997;157:2550.

Greenfield LJ, Proctor MC: Vena caval filters for the prevention of pulmonary embolism. N Engl J Med 1998;339:47.

Hull RD: Low-molecular-weight heparin vs. heparin in the treatment of patients with pulmonary embolism: American-Canadian Thrombosis Study Group. Arch Intern Med 2000;160:229.

Meaney JF: Diagnosis of pulmonary embolism with magnetic resonance angiography. N Engl J Med 1997;336:1422.

Mohan CR et al: Comparative efficacy and complications of vena caval filters. J Vasc Surg 1995;21:235.

The PREPIC study group: Eight-year follow-up of patients with permanent vena cava filters in the prevention of pulmonary embolism. Circulation 2005;112:416.

Stein PD et al: Spiral computed tomography for the diagnosis of acute pulmonary embolism. Thromb Haemost 2007;98:713.

Value of the ventilation/perfusion scan in acute pulmonary embolism: results of the prospective investigation of pulmonary embolism diagnosis (PIOPED). The PIOPED Investigators. JAMA 1990;263:2753.

SUPERFICIAL THROMBOPHLEBITIS

 ESSENTIALS OF DIAGNOSIS

► Erythema, induration, and tenderness along the superficial vein.

► Usually spontaneous but can follow venous cannulation.

General Considerations

Superficial thrombophlebitis may appear spontaneously in patients with varicose veins, in pregnant or postpartum women, or in patients with thromboangiitis obliterans or Behçet disease. It may also occur after intravenous therapy or in an area of localized trauma. The presence of superficial phlebitis, particularly if it occurs in a migratory manner, suggests the presence of an abdominal cancer such as carcinoma of the pancreas (Trousseau thrombophlebitis). The most common vein affected is the greater saphenous vein and its branches. In up to 20% of cases, a simultaneous DVT exists, and duplex imaging is a must in these situations. Pulmonary emboli are rare unless extension into the deep venous system occurs.

Clinical Findings

The patient usually presents complaining of localized extremity pain and redness. Areas of induration, erythema, and tenderness correspond to dilated and often thrombosed superficial veins. Over time, a firm cord may develop. Generalized edema is absent unless the deep veins are involved. The presence of fever and shaking chills suggests septic or suppurative phlebitis, which occurs most commonly as a complication of intravenous cannulation.

Differential Diagnosis

Superficial thrombophlebitis must be distinguished from ascending lymphangitis, cellulitis, erythema nodosum, erythema induratum, and panniculitis. Unlike these other disorders, superficial phlebitis tends to be well localized over a superficial vein.

Treatment

The primary treatment of superficial venous thrombophlebitis is the administration of nonsteroidal anti-inflammatory drugs, local heat, elevation, and support stockings or elastic wraps. Ambulation is encouraged. In most cases, symptoms will resolve within 7–10 days. Excision of the involved vein is recommended for symptoms that persist over 2 weeks despite treatment or for recurrent phlebitis in the same vein segment. If there is progressive proximal extension with involvement of the saphenofemoral junction or cephalic-subclavian junction, ligation and resection of the vein at the junction should be performed. Alternatively, full-dose anticoagulation can be utilized. Ligation and resection is most effective treating pain, while anticoagulation is most effective treating thrombus extension/embolization.

Septic thrombophlebitis requires treatment with broad-spectrum intravenous antibiotics. If rapid resolution of the cellulitis occurs, no treatment beyond a short course of antibiotics is required. However, if the patient becomes septic, excision of the entire infected vein is required. With positive blood cultures, an extended course of antibiotics specific for the identified organism is indicated.

Prognosis

Most episodes of uncomplicated superficial thrombophlebitis respond to conservative management. Cases in which extension into the deep venous system occurs can be associated with thromboembolism.

Belcaro G et al: Superficial thrombophlebitis of the legs: a randomized, controlled, follow-up study. Angiology 1999;50:523.

Di Nisio M et al: Treatment for superficial thrombophlebitis of the leg. Cochrane Database of Syst Rev 2007;2:CD004982.

Lucia MA et al: Images in clinical medicine: superficial thrombophlebitis. N Engl J Med 2001;344:1214.

Sullivan V et al: Ligation versus anticoagulation: treatment of above-knee superficial thrombophlebitis not involving the deep venous system. J Am Coll Surg 2001;193:556.

CHRONIC VENOUS INSUFFICIENCY

Chronic venous insufficiency can result from congenital venous valvular insufficiency or can result from previous venous thrombosis. In the former circumstance, it is called chronic venous insufficiency (CVI) while in the latter circumstance, it is called the postthrombotic syndrome (PTS). Varicose veins (also a manifestation of venous insufficiency), CVI, and PTS occur in 76/100,000 person-years, and it has been estimated that 6–7 million Americans suffer from stasis pigmentation changes in the legs with another 400,000–500,000 patients with skin ulceration. Treatment costs are in the billion dollar range. The basic physiologic abnormality in patients with chronic venous insufficiency is chronic elevation of venous pressure. The normal venous capacitance can accommodate large-volume changes that occur during exercise with only minimal changes in venous pressure. However, with calf muscle pump dysfunction and valvular reflux, blood pools in the lower extremities and venous hypertension occurs, leading to venous hypertension. Outflow obstruction from proximal obstruction can also produce venous hypertension, resulting in "venous claudication" as the deep venous system fills with blood during exercise. The leg becomes painful, swollen, and heavy (especially with exercise), mimicking arterial insufficiency.

Valvular incompetence of the deep veins can be congenital or result from damage following phlebitis, varicose veins, or DVT. The best estimate for the incidence of chronic venous insufficiency is approximately 30% after 8-year follow-up. Chronic venous stasis changes are centered in the "gaiter areas" around the ankles. This is the location of the commonly affected perforator veins and is a region with sparse soft tissue support to withstand elevated venous pressures. Brawny edema is produced by extravasation of plasma fluid, red blood cells, and plasma proteins. Lysis of red blood cells results in deposition of hemosiderin, which creates a brownish discoloration. Leukocytes become sequestered in the microcirculation, leading to capillary occlusion and release of superoxide radicals, proteolytic enzymes, and growth factors. Macrophages and T lymphocytes are primary mediators of this inflammatory response, which results in fibroblast activation and scarring and fibrosis of the subcutaneous tissues. Ultimately, this fibrosis results in compromised skin perfusion and ulceration.

Clinical Findings

A. Symptoms and Signs

Both isolated saphenous vein incompetence and deep venous insufficiency can lead to venous varicosities and chronic venous stasis changes. One of the first symptoms to develop is usually ankle and calf edema. Involvement of the foot and toes suggests lymphedema. Typically, the edema is worse at the end of the day and improves with leg elevation. Longstanding disease is characterized by stasis dermatitis, hyperpigmentation, brawny induration, and ulceration. Venous stasis ulcers are large, painful, and irregular in outline. They have a shallow, moist granulation bed, occur in the gaiter area on the medial or lateral aspects of the ankle, and are often accompanied by stasis dermatitis and stasis pigmentation changes.

B. Imaging and Other Diagnostic Studies

Duplex ultrasound can identify the presence and location of incompetent perforating veins and has been used to evaluate the function of individual venous valves. Duplex imaging has become the most important test of venous pathophysiology today and should be performed in every patient with CVI and PTS. However, it does not easily assess calf muscle pump function or the presence of proximal obstruction. These concerns are addressed with use of other tests, such as air plethysmography, which gives a quantitative assessment of venous reflux (by the venous filling index), calf muscle pump function (by the ejection fraction), and overall venous function (by residual volume function). These measurements help to stratify patients into treatment groups.

Determination of functional outflow obstruction requires venography with or without pressure measurement, although intravascular ultrasound is also very useful to determine the presence or absence of venous obstruction. Descending phlebography involves injection of contrast media into the common femoral vein to test the valves during normal breathing and with a forced Valsalva maneuver. Using this technique, pathologic reflux can be identified in patients with postthrombotic damage. Such testing is reserved in anticipation of surgical correction of the venous pathology.

▷ Differential Diagnosis

Congestive heart failure and chronic liver and kidney disease must be considered in the differential diagnosis of bilateral lower extremity edema. Lymphedema is characterized by nonpitting edema of the dorsum of the foot and toes as well as the calf and generally is not associated with skin pigment changes, dermatitis, or ulceration. Severe arterial insufficiency produces ulcers that are painful, well circumscribed, and located over pressure points on the distal end of the extremity and foot. Ulcers due to autoimmune diseases, erythema nodosum, and fungal infections are distinguished by appearance and distribution.

▷ Treatment

Venous insufficiency is an incurable but manageable problem. Most patients respond well to a conservative treatment program composed of intermittent leg elevation, regular exercise to improve calf muscle pump function, and the use of surgical elastic graduated compression stockings. Although the mechanism by which elastic compression improves the symptoms of chronic venous insufficiency has not been clearly established, recent work suggests that external compression may restore competency of dilated valve cusps and affect venoarterial reflex. Most venous ulceration will improve with leg elevation, external compression, and local wound care. Compression can be achieved with an inelastic bandage such as an Unna boot, an occlusive wound dressing covered by elastic bandage wrapping, or surgical support stockings.

Surgery is indicated for a small percentage of patients with nonhealing ulcers or disabling symptoms refractory to conservative management. The three main categories of procedures include those ablative procedures on the superficial venous system in the face of superficial venous reflux, antireflux procedures, and bypass operations for obstruction. If superficial venous reflux is a significant component of the total venous reflux present, then superficial ablation is appropriate. Such ablation has been found successful in preventing recurrent venous ulceration and has also been found to improve patients' symptoms of both varicose veins and venous reflux. Ablation may be performed with traditional open surgical ligation and stripping or the more recent endovenous procedures such as radiofrequency ablation or endovenous laser therapy. The pathology must be accurately characterized so that an appropriate operative strategy can be developed. The most common abnormality in patients with chronic venous insufficiency is incompetence of the popliteal or tibial veins; 50–60% of patients have incompetent perforators.

Perforating vein ligation is used in patients with recurrent or recalcitrant venous ulcers with demonstrated incompetence of perforating veins under the area of ulceration. It is performed to reverse the local wound complication of venous ulceration and does nothing to change the underlying deep venous hemodynamics of the leg. Therefore, patients must understand that for maximal effectiveness after perforator ligation, standard treatment for chronic venous insufficiency must be continued. Patients who have proximal venous obstruction should have this problem corrected prior to perforator interruption. The incidence of ulcer recurrence after perforator ligation is 15–20%, but the wound complication rate secondary to impaired incisional healing with severe stasis disease ranges from 12% to 55%. Wound complications have been reduced to 5% with the introduction of subfascial endoscopic perforator surgery, which achieves an ulcer recurrence rate of 12–28% at 2 years, equal to the rate following open surgery. Perforator interruption may now be performed using endovenous techniques.

Direct venous reconstructive surgery is indicated for (1) venous reflux not amenable to a conservative treatment regimen, (2) failure to relieve symptoms after vein stripping or perforator ligation, or (3) intractable, disabling venous claudication associated with venous outflow obstruction.

Procedures for reflux include valvuloplasty, valvular transplantation, and venous segment transposition. The best results with valvuloplasty are achieved when it is combined with perforator ligation. The reported success rate is approximately 80% in one recent study of 155 extremities with a 1-year to 13-year follow-up. Valvuloplasty can be performed by placement of external cuffs or bands, vein wall plication, angioscopic repair, or open valve repair. Venous valve transplantation involves replacing a refluxing segment of vein with a healthy segment of autologous axillary vein with functional valves. Transplantation of individual valves at the level of the popliteal vein is a technique with reported good clinical results in 60–70% of cases and an improvement in venous hemodynamics by air plethysmography. Alternatively, a competent segment of profunda vein can be used to replace an incompetent segment of superficial femoral or greater saphenous vein in a vein transposition. Although initial results of these procedures are good, the effect may not be long lasting as the competent valve becomes incompetent.

Bypasses and angiographic procedures can be performed for venous obstruction. The Palma procedure is a cross-femoral bypass first described in 1958 for iliac vein obstruction. In this procedure, the proximal saphenous vein from the contralateral leg is tunneled suprapubically to the femoral vein on the side of the iliac obstruction. This allows for venous flow to bypass across the pelvis and empty through the patent contralateral iliac vein. Prosthetic material has also been used. Overall 5-year graft patency averages 75–80%. Historically, distal femoral arteriovenous fistulas were constructed to improve iliofemoral vein graft patency, but more current experience does not support their continued use in many cases. Patients with short-segment iliac vein obstruction from May-Thurner syndrome (left iliac vein compression) have also been successfully treated by angioplasty and stenting. Factors associated with a poor response include male sex, a history of recent trauma causing the compression, and young age under 40 years.

Saphenopopliteal bypass (May-Husni procedure) can be considered for patients with occlusion of the superficial femoral vein. In this procedure, calf blood flow is shunted around the obstructed superficial femoral vein through the patent saphenous vein. Approximately 75% of patients are reported to show clinical improvement postoperatively.

Criado E et al: The role of air plethysmography in the diagnosis of chronic venous insufficiency. J Vasc Surg 1998;27:660.

DePalma RG et al: Target selection for surgical intervention in severe chronic venous insufficiency: comparison of duplex scanning and phlebography. J Vasc Surg 2000;32:913.

Gloviczki P et al: Mid-term results of endoscopic perforator vein interruption for chronic venous insufficiency: Lessons learned from the North American Subfacial Endoscopic Perforator Surgery registry. J Vasc Surg 1999;29:489.

Gohel MS et al: Randomized clinical trial of compression plus surgery versus compression alone in chronic venous ulceration (ESCHAR study): haemodynamic and anatomical changes. Br J Surg 2005;92:291.

Gruss JD, Heimer W: Bypass procedures for venous obstruction. In: *Surgical Management of Venous Disease.* Raju S, Villavicencio JL (editors). Williams & Wilkins, 1997.

Heit JA et al: Trends in the incidence of venous stasis syndrome and venous ulcer: a 25-year population based study. J Vasc Surg 2001;33:1022.

Knipp BS et al: Factors associated with outcome after interventional treatment of symptomatic iliac vein compression syndrome. J Vasc Surg 2007;46:743.

Prandoni P et al: The long-term clinical course of acute deep venous thrombosis. Ann Intern Med 1996;125:1.

▼ II. THE LYMPHATICS

LYMPHEDEMA

ESSENTIALS OF DIAGNOSIS

▶ Can be developmental or acquired.

▶ Painless edema of an extremities, usually lower extremity starting at the ankle, the dorsum of the foot, and the toes.

▶ Edema is usually pitting at first and then becomes firm, rubbery, and nonpitting due to fibrosis.

▶ Frequent episodes of lymphangitis and cellulitis may occur.

▶ General Considerations

Much less is known about the fluid dynamics of the lymphatic system than of the venous or arterial system. Most energy for lymph propulsion arises from the intrinsic lymphatic smooth muscle contractions that occur rhythmically. Lymphatic luminal pressures are usually 30–50 mm Hg and can exceed arterial pressure under special circumstances. The lymphatic system carries interstitial fluid and macromolecular proteins lost from the capillaries, as well as infectious agents and foreign material, back into the central circulation. Two to 4 liters a day of lymph drain into the subclavian vein.

The fundamental mechanism responsible for lymphedema formation is impaired lymph flow out of the extremity. Primary lymphedema is caused by abnormal lymphatic development, most often hypoplasia resulting in severe reduction in the number of lymphatics and the lymphatic diameters. It is classified by age at onset of the disease. Congenital lymphedema develops before 1 year of age, is usually bilateral, and affects males more than females; if familial, it is known as Milroy disease. More often, lymphedema develops during adolescence (lymphedema praecox) and is unilateral; there is a 10:1 female predominance. Lymphedema occurring after age 35 is referred to as lymphedema tarda.

Secondary lymphedema results from a wide variety of disease processes that cause obstruction to the lymphatic system. The most common of these is surgical excision and radiation to the axillary or inguinal lymph nodes as part of the treatment of breast cancer, cervical cancer, prostate cancer, melanoma, and soft tissue tumors. Less common causes of secondary lymphedema are bacterial and fungal infections, trauma, and lymphoproliferative diseases. In many developing countries, lymphatic obstruction due to filariasis is caused by three different parasites: *Wuchereria bancrofti, Brugia malayi,* and *Brugia timori.*

▶ Clinical Manifestations

A. Symptoms and Signs

The history of the disease process will usually define the cause of the lymphedema. Development of painless edema in an adolescent girl with a family history of lymphedema would indicate primary lymphedema as a diagnosis. A history of lymph node dissection, irradiation, or the presence of a parasitic infection suggests secondary lymphedema.

Lymphedema development is usually slowly progressive and painless. In the early stages the edema is pitting, but as the disease progresses, chronic fibrosis occurs and the edema becomes nonpitting. The distribution of edema is also characteristic. It is usually centered on the ankle (Figure 35–6) and is most pronounced on the dorsum of the foot, producing a buffalo hump appearance. Unlike edema of venous stasis disease, lymphedema also often involves the toes. In the early stages, the skin is normal, but skin thickening and hyperkeratosis occurs with long-standing disease. A chronic eczematous dermatitis may ensue.

Rarely, lymphangiosarcoma or angiosarcoma may develop as a complication of chronic lymphedema. This neoplastic transformation of blood vessels and lymphatics is called Stewart-Treves syndrome.

B. Imaging Studies

Venous duplex scans are performed to rule out venous insufficiency. Lymphangiography is rarely used now, because it can further damage the lymphatics and is unnecessary to establish the diagnosis. Lymphoscintigraphy is a specialized test that may be used to confirm the diagnosis. CT and MRI are useful tests in patients with suspected secondary lymphedema from unknown malignancy.

▶ Differential Diagnosis

A variety of diseases can result in bilateral lower extremity edema. These include congestive heart failure, chronic renal or hepatic insufficiency, and hypoproteinemia. In patients with unilateral leg edema, differential diagnosis includes congenital vascular malformations, chronic venous insufficiency, and reflex sympathetic dystrophy.

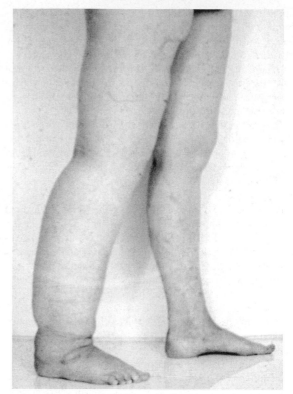

▲ **Figure 35–6.** Acquired lymphedema. Edema is centered at the ankle and involves the foot and toes.

▶ Treatment

Lymphedema is a chronic disease for which there is no complete cure. However, a variety of conservative measures can substantially reduce the risk of further complications and disability.

No drug therapy is effective. Use of benzopyrones (to increase lymphatic transport by macrophages) have shown some benefit. Diuretics can be useful for acute exacerbation of edema secondary to infection or for coexisting venous stasis disease, but these agents are not recommended for long-term use in lymphedema.

The mainstay of treatment is external compression and meticulous skin care. Mechanical reduction of lymphedema can best be achieved with a program of frequent leg elevation, manual lymphatic drainage massage, low-stretch wrapping techniques, and intermittent pneumatic compression. Sequential pneumatic compression devices are traditionally the first line of treatment. Many different devices are available for use on the leg, and sleeves can be custom fit for patients with postmastectomy arm lymphedema. Graduated compression stockings maintain the limb after reduction by pneumatic compression. Good skin care is imperative in order to prevent infection. Moisturizing lotions should be applied regularly, especially after showering or bathing. Drying and cracking of the skin can create portals of entry for bacteria. Infection is difficult to eradicate because of disordered lymphatic drainage and can be limb threatening.

The psychologic impact of chronic lymphedema cannot be underestimated. However, with appropriate patient education that results in the prevention of chronic infection or massive edema, this problem can be manageable.

Operation may be considered in rare cases of severe functional impairment and recurrent lymphangitis. The primary goals of these operations are to reduce limb bulk, either by ablative techniques (excision of excess tissue) or physiologic techniques (lymphatic reconstruction). The Charles procedure involves excision of all skin and subcutaneous tissue from the tibial tuberosity to the lateral head of the fibula and wound coverage by a split-thickness skin graft. This has been largely replaced by the Sistrunk procedure, which is a staged subcutaneous tissue excision. Wide skin flaps are raised for excision of subcutaneous tissues in the medial leg and then 3 months later in the lateral leg. Ablative techniques have been less successful in the upper extremity than in the lower extremity.

The Thompson procedure is an indirect lymphatic reconstruction. A flap of dermis is buried in the muscle compartment to promote formation of communications between subdermal and deep lymphatics. Omental free flaps are similarly designed to encourage new lympholymphatic channels. Direct lymphatic reconstruction by creation of lymphovenous anastomoses or lymphatic interposition grafting is achievable by microsurgical techniques and has had limited success in some centers. Long-term efficacy is not yet known. Again, the use of any of these operative procedures for lymphedema is limited to rather rare situations.

Pain SJ et al: Lymphoedema following surgery for breast cancer. Br J Surg 2000;87:1128.

Singh I, Burnand KG: Lymphoedema. Surgery 2002;20:42.

Tiwari A et al: Differential diagnosis, investigation, and current treatment of lower limb lymphedema. Arch Surg 2003;138:152.

LYMPHANGITIS

 ESSENTIALS OF DIAGNOSIS

▶ Red streaks traveling longitudinally up an extremity toward regional lymph nodes.

▶ Shaking chills, fever, and malaise.

▶ General Considerations

Lymphangitis is usually caused by a hemolytic streptococcal or staphylococcal infection that arises in an area of cellulitis near an open wound. Multiple long red streaks can be seen coursing toward the regional lymph nodes. Severe systemic manifestations include tachycardia, fever, chills, and malaise, which untreated can lead to sepsis and death.

▶ Clinical Findings

A. Symptoms and Signs

Pain at the site of the initial wound is present. High fevers develop rapidly. The streaks may be faint in appearance initially, especially in dark-skinned patients. Regional lymph nodes are often enlarged and tender.

B. Laboratory Findings

An elevated white blood cell count associated with a left shift is almost universally present. Blood and wound cultures should be obtained routinely.

▶ Differential Diagnosis

Lymphangitis should be distinguished from superficial thrombophlebitis, which is usually localized to a single venous segment often with a palpable cord. Patients with thrombophlebitis usually do not appear toxic, as do patients with lymphangitis. Cat-scratch fever should always be considered when lymphadenitis is present. It is also important to differentiate cellulitis and severe soft tissue infections from lymphangitis. In general, lymphangitis is characterized by its superficial location and the linear pattern of erythema.

▶ Treatment

The extremity should be elevated and warm compresses applied. Analgesics and intravenous antibiotics should be instituted immediately. Examination of the wound should be made to determine the need for debridement or incision and drainage of an abscess.

▶ Prognosis

Delayed or inadequate therapy can lead to overwhelming sepsis and death. Aggressive institution of appropriate antibiotic therapy and wound care will usually control the infection within 48–72 hours.

Neurosurgery

John A. Cowan Jr., MD
B. Gregory Thompson, MD

▼ DIAGNOSIS & MANAGEMENT OF DEPRESSED STATES OF CONSCIOUSNESS

Sheron Beltran, MD, & George Mashour, MD

DEFINITIONS

Consciousness is usually described as having two components: arousal and awareness. Many terms are used to describe the continuum of consciousness ranging from alert to comatose. The **alert** patient is awake and immediately responsive to all stimuli. **Stupor** is a condition in which the patient is less alert but still responds with stimulation. An **obtunded** patient appears to be asleep much of the time but still responds to noxious stimuli. The **comatose** patient appears asleep and does not respond to stimuli. A **vegetative state** is a state of arousal without awareness in which the patient may open his or her eyes, track objects, chew and swallow, but not respond to auditory stimuli or appear to sense pain. Often, terms used to describe states of consciousness lack consistent definitions, and a clear description of a patient's state of arousal and awareness results in more precise communication.

THE NEUROLOGIC EXAMINATION

The neurologic examination includes assessment of level of consciousness, brainstem reflexes, and motor activity. The **Glasgow Coma Scale (GCS)** (Table 36–1) was designed to assess level of consciousness in patients with head injury. A patient with a GCS of 8 or lower is generally considered to be comatose. Brainstem reflexes, including pupillary response to light, corneal reflexes, oculocephalic reflex (doll's eyes), vestibuloocular reflex (cold calorics), breathing patterns, and cough and gag reflexes, are further used to accurately describe the level of consciousness and localize the level of brainstem dysfunction. Motor responses may be described as spontaneous or induced by noxious stimuli, purposeful or nonpurposeful, unilateral or bilateral, and upper or lower extremity. The patient may display withdrawal from a stimulus, abnormal flexion (decorticate rigidity), abnormal extension (decerebrate rigidity), or absence of motor activity.

ETIOLOGY

The differential diagnosis of altered states of consciousness is broad (Table 36–2), and while the etiology may be obvious, as in trauma, a history, physical examination, laboratory studies, and imaging studies may be required to establish a diagnosis. Metabolic etiologies (eg, sodium or glucose abnormalities) and pharmacologic causes (eg, sedatives or illicit drugs) should be excluded. Onset and progression of symptoms may provide important clues; for example, neoplasms often present with a progressive course, while vascular occlusions often present with abrupt changes. Associated symptoms and conditions such as recent fevers or a history of diabetes may also aid in diagnosis.

DIAGNOSTIC TOOLS

Laboratory studies should, at a minimum, include serum electrolytes, glucose, blood urea nitrogen, complete blood count, platelet count, coagulation studies, and serum osmolality. Blood gas analysis, urinalysis, and urine and blood toxicology screening may also be helpful. Cerebrospinal fluid (CSF) analysis should be performed on the basis of the clinical scenario; it may disclose meningitis, neoplastic cells or subarachnoid hemorrhage.

Neuroimaging studies should be ordered on the basis of patient history and examination. Patients with trauma or a suspected structural lesion should undergo emergent computed tomography (CT) scanning. Although magnetic resonance imaging (MRI) may provide images of superior quality, it may not always detect acute intracerebral bleeding and usually takes longer to perform than CT. In patients with bilateral hemispheric dysfunction, emergent CT scan is seldom of benefit.

Table 36–1. Glasgow Coma Scale.

Eye opening:	
Spontaneous	4
To Voice	3
To pain	2
None	1
Verbal response:	
Oriented	5
Confused, disoriented	4
Inappropriate words	3
Incomprehensible sounds	2
None	1
Best motor response:	
Obeys	6
Localizes	5
Withdraws (flexion)	4
Abnormal flexion posturing	3
Extension posturing	2
None	1

An electroencephalogram may disclose patterns consistent with encephalopathy or nonconvulsive status epilepticus. After structural lesions have been excluded, electroencephalogram should be performed in most patients with altered consciousness at some point during the course of their care.

MANAGEMENT

The initial treatment of a patient with an alteration in consciousness must employ management of the ABCs: **airway, breathing,** and **circulation**. Patients who are not responsive

Table 36–2. Etiology of Altered State of Consciousness.

Physiologic	Neurologic	Pharmacologic
Hypoxia, hypercarbia	Trauma	Sedatives
Hypotension	Tumor	Narcotics
Hypoglycemia, hyperglycemia	Infection	Ethyl alcohol, illicit substances
Hypothyroidism	Vascular (stroke)	Poisoning
Hypothermia, hyperthermia	Seizures	
Electrolyte abnormalities		
Uremia		
Hyperammonemia		

enough to protect their own airway require intubation to reduce the risk of aspiration of gastric contents. During intubation, hypoxia and hypotension should be avoided in patients with brain injury, and a high suspicion of cervical spine injury should be maintained. A patient presenting with a GCS of 8 or lower should be intubated. Mechanical ventilation should be used if necessary to provide adequate oxygenation and ventilation as guided by arterial blood gases. Patients presenting with hypotension and shock must be aggressively treated with fluids and vasopressors to maintain adequate perfusion. Sources of shock (septic, cardiogenic, hypovolemic) should be investigated and treated appropriately.

ELEVATED INTRACRANIAL PRESSURE (ICP)

The skull has three major components: brain parenchyma, CSF, and blood. The volumetric sum of these components is maintained at a constant; an increase in one component must be offset by a decrease in another. This is normally accomplished by displacement of CSF into the contiguous subarachnoid space of the spinal cord, termed *spatial compensation*. This delicate balance, however, has physiologic limits. Once these compensatory limits are met, an increase in the volume of any component will lead to an exponential increase in intracranial pressure as illustrated by the intracranial compliance curve (Figure 36–1).

Normal intracranial pressure (ICP) in adults is less than 10 to 15 mm Hg. The presence of tumor or blood, the impedance of CFS drainage (hydrocephalus), cerebral edema, or increased cerebral blood flow (hyperemia as a response to head injury or hypoventilation causing hypercarbia and vasodilation) may raise the intracranial pressure to a dangerous level. The increased intracranial pressure may lead to impedance of

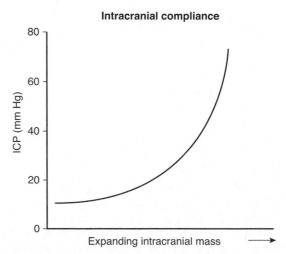

▲ **Figure 36–1.** Intracranial compliance curve demonstrating the approximate relationship between intracranial pressure and an expanding intracranial mass.

cerebral perfusion and ischemia or a mass effect progressing to shifting of the brain substance and devastating herniation.

SIGNS & SYMPTOMS OF INCREASED INTRACRANIAL PRESSURE

Increased intracranial pressure is often accompanied by altered mental status, headache, vomiting (without nausea), and papilledema on funduscopic examination. The Cushing triad may be seen in patients with increased intracranial pressure and consists of hypertension, bradycardia, and respiratory irregularity. Obtundation, focal neurologic findings including unilateral pupillary dilation from pressure or traction exerted on the third cranial nerve, and hemodynamic instability are late findings and indicate pending uncal herniation.

HERNIATION SYNDROMES

Herniation occurs when increased intracranial pressure results in a portion of the brain shifting from one intracranial compartment to another. These shifts may lead to ischemia to portions of the brain, disruption of white matter pathways, and pressure on structures such as cranial nerve III.

▶ Subfalcine Herniation

Subfalcine herniation occurs in patients with a frontal lobe mass as the cingulated gyrus herniates beneath the falx. Symptoms are often related to the mass or increased intracranial pressure.

▶ Lateral Mass Herniation

Lateral mass herniation occurs in patients with an expanding lateral mass. Symptoms include contralateral hemiparesis, diminished consciousness, and an ipsilateral cranial nerve III palsy. Compression of pupillary fibers also causes a dilation of the pupil, and as lateral displacement of the midbrain continues, ipsilateral hemiplegia occurs. Late in the process, the uncus and hippocampus may herniate transtentorially.

▶ Cerebellar Tonsillar Herniation

Posterior fossa masses cause symptoms by compressing the brainstem and obstructing the flow of CSF (hydrocephalus). As pressure increases, the cerebellar tonsils may be pushed into or through the foramen magnum. As the medulla is compressed, apnea results from dysfunction of the medullary respiratory center.

▶ Upward Transtentorial Herniation

Posterior fossa masses may cause obstructive hydrocephalus. If these patients undergo ventriculostomy, there is a possibility of upward herniation of posterior fossa contents into the diencephalic region.

METHODS OF INTRACRANIAL PRESSURE MONITORING

Intracranial pressure cannot accurately be estimated on the basis of clinical findings or imaging. Several methods of direct intracranial pressure measurement exist, but the two most commonly employed in clinical practice are ventricular catheters and intraparenchymal microtransducer systems. Other methods, such as subarachnoid and epidural devices, have much lower accuracy.

The gold standard of intracranial pressure monitoring is via an intraventricular catheter connected to a standard pressure transducer. These catheters are usually placed into the lateral ventricle by a small frontal burr hole. The advantages of intraventricular catheters are that they measure global intracranial pressure, allow for therapeutic drainage of CSF, and are amenable to external calibration. Disadvantages are risk for infection, hematoma, and difficult insertion.

Microtransducer-tipped intracranial pressure monitors are placed in the brain parenchyma or subdural space either through a skull bolt, a burr hole, or intraoperatively. They are almost as accurate as intraventricular catheters and have the advantages of lower infection and complication rates. The major disadvantages are an inability to drain CSF, no in vivo calibration, and a small zero drift over time.

MANAGEMENT OF INCREASED INTRACRANIAL PRESSURE

Although there are various cutoff values at which elevated intracranial pressure should be treated, many centers regard an intracranial pressure of more than 20 mm Hg as the upper limit. Treatment should include the following:

Positioning: Elevate the head of bed 30 to 45 degrees to promote venous drainage and displacement of CSF into the spinal compartment.

Hyperventilation: Cerebral blood flow is governed in part by $PaCO_2$. Hyperventilation and the subsequent decrease in $PaCO_2$ to the range of 30 to 35 mm Hg can be used for short periods during acute neurologic deterioration.

Mannitol: Mannitol draws fluid from the cerebral parenchyma by osmotic effect.

Furosemide: Furosemide may reduce cerebral edema and slow the production of CSF. It works synergistically with mannitol.

Control fever: Hyperthermia increases the cerebral metabolic rate.

Steroids: Delayed effect (after 6–8 hours). *Not recommended for patients with severe traumatic brain injury.*

CFS drainage: Ventriculostomy or shunt is necessary for patients with chronic conditions.

Bony decompression: Bony decompression allows for expansion of tissue.

Barbiturates: Barbiturate "coma" (burst suppression on electroencephalogram) allows for near maximal reductions in cerebral metabolism and cerebral blood flow. Hypotension is often a limiting factor.

Duff D: Altered states of consciousness, theories of recovery, and assessment following a severe traumatic brain injury. Axon 2001;23:18. Review.

Giacino JT: The minimally conscious state: defining the borders of consciousness. Prog Brain Res 2005;150:381.

Goetz CG, Pappert EJ: *Textbook of Clinical Neurology,* 3rd ed. Saunders, 1999.

Heegaard W et al: Traumatic brain injury. Emerg Med Clin N Am 2007;25:655.

Smith M: Monitoring intracranial pressure in traumatic brain injury. Anesth Analg 2008;106:240.

▼ IMAGING OF THE CENTRAL NERVOUS SYSTEM

Douglas J. Quint, MD, & Shawn L. A. Hervey-Jumper, MD

Imaging has become central to medical care in the past 25 years and is currently the fastest-growing component of medical care expenditures in this country. In no field of medicine has imaging made more of an impact than in the neurosciences. Our ability to demonstrate anatomy and pathology noninvasively and to treat many pathologic central nervous system (CNS) processes minimally invasively has grown immensely with improvements in imaging technology in the last few years.

Thirty-five years ago, the only way to image the central nervous system was to replace CFS with contrast material (dye) or air via a lumbar puncture and take x-rays—a painful technique called pneumoencephalography; normal and abnormal CNS structures could be crudely outlined in this manner. Injecting dye directly into major blood vessels of the neck (cerebral angiography) could also be performed, permitting exquisite delineation of intrinsic vascular pathology, but the procedure still did little to directly visualize the brain or spinal cord. While angiography is still performed today for both diagnostic and therapeutic purposes, the catheter is now placed via cannulation of a femoral artery instead of directly into a neck blood vessel. Pneumoencephalography was abandoned in the late 1970s.

With the advent of CT scanning in the early 1970s, direct visualization of the brain was finally possible, although resolving different brain structures and some pathologic processes remained difficult. MRI first became available for clinical use in the early 1980s and has been the standard for evaluation of most CNS processes since the mid-1980s.

CT and MRI have continued to mature through the 1990s and into the 21st century. By using extremely rapid scanning techniques on the latest generation (2007) CT scanners (*multislice* or *multidetector* scanners), useful data reflecting blood perfusion of the brain can now be collected during a 5-minute study. Similarly, such state-of-the-art scanners can be used to generate models of the major blood vessels of the brain (CT angiograms) without intra-arterial catheterization. MRI advances have been even more dramatic. The sensitivity of some of the newer MRI scanning techniques developed over the last 5 years enables identification of physiologic changes in the brain minutes after ischemia occurs, a time frame that can potentially permit pharmacologic interventions that can affect clinical outcomes (eg, stroke). Functional MRI can assess eloquent areas of the brain near pathologic lesions (eg, tumors) that must be avoided during surgery. Magnetic resonance (MR) spectroscopy can identify lesion metabolites that can help discriminate among pathologic processes (eg, among tumors, necrosis, ischemia, inflammation, and infections). MR spectra can identify metabolites accumulating in the brain in patients with congenital metabolic disorders. MRI can also be used to generate magnetic resonance angiographic (MRA) images to evaluate blood vessels without injection of dye or the use of ionizing radiation. The new, higher field-strength MRI scanners (3.0 Tesla) released for clinical use in 2005 have further improved and expanded imaging capabilities.

Catheter (endovascular) angiography, which has been available in various forms for 80 years, has also continued to evolve in the last decade. Endovascular surgery—treating blood vessel abnormalities such as aneurysms or arteriovenous malformations (AVMs) through a catheter instead of open surgery—is now commonly performed and has become the treatment of choice for the management of many lesions. Similarly, in the setting of an acute stroke due to an obstructing thromboembolus, a catheter can be placed in the obstructing lesion, a clot resected or clot-dissolving (eg, thrombolytic) agents injected, and a vessel reopened.

BASIC CNS IMAGING TECHNIQUES

▶ Plain Radiographs

Plain radiographs (x-rays) are relatively inexpensive, universally available, and can demonstrate osseous abnormalities such as fractures or gross destructive lesions (Figure 36–2). The main disadvantage of plain x-rays is that essentially all normal soft tissues (eg, all intracranial and spinal canal structures) and pathologic processes (eg, hemorrhage, infarctions, tumors, abscesses, herniated disks) are undetectable. Even many intrinsic osseous lesions are difficult to delineate. In fact, until 30% of a bone is replaced by a pathologic process (eg, tumor, infection), no osseous abnormality will be seen on a plain radiograph.

Plain radiographs superimpose all structures on an image as the x-ray beam passes through the entire head or spine (rather than tomograms demonstrating "slices" of the tissue scanned)

There is little role for plain radiographs for the evaluation of CNS disease because the interior of the head or spinal canal is not imaged. One exception is in patients with suspected child abuse. In these patients, in addition to other cross-

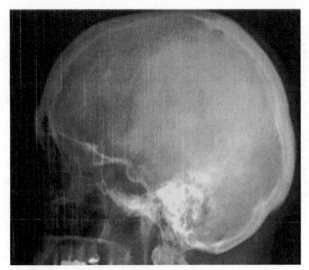

▲ **Figure 36–2.** Lateral plain radiograph (x-ray) of the skull (ionizing radiation). Note the excellent delineation of the osseous structures but poor delineation of soft tissues; specifically, no portion of the brain is imaged. Also, this study is not tomographic (ie, is not a slice), and therefore, both the left and right sides of the head are superimposed.

sectional imaging (such as CT and MRI, which are performed to assess for intracranial injuries), plain radiographs should be obtained because they may show subtle nondisplaced fractures not readily identified on other imaging tests.

Other roles for plain radiographs include assessing spinal motion (ie, lateral flexion/extension radiographs of the cervical or lumbosacral spine to assess spinal stability) and assessing intracranial or spinal structures where internal fixation hardware or other radiodense/ferromagnetic foreign material is present, limiting the use of CT or MRI scanning.

Ultrasound

Ultrasound of the central nervous system is predominantly used in the intraoperative setting to evaluate ventricular morphology and underlying parenchymal pathology. Intraoperative ultrasound can be used to help position ventricular catheters during placement of shunts. It can also be used to guide intracranial and intraspinal tumor resections.

Outside of the operative setting, ultrasound has growing applications because it is noninvasive, portable, and does not involve radiation. However, an "acoustic window" is necessary for viewing the intracranial and intraspinal tissues, so overlying osseous structures usually must be removed before scanning can be performed (ie, portions of the skull or posterior spinal elements must be removed before the desired regions of the brain or spinal cord, respectively, can be evaluated).

Ultrasound has multiple applications in infants (usually such infants still have open fontanelles, so no additional

acoustic window to the brain must be created). It has become the imaging study of choice for the evaluation of premature infants to assess for intraventricular hemorrhage and/or hydrocephalus. In adults, intracranial Doppler examinations can be performed by scanning through sutures. For example, scanning through the temporal suture allows access to the circle of Willis. These examinations can be performed at the bedside for assessment of arterial vasospasm (eg, in the setting of subacute subarachnoid hemorrhage).

Computed Tomography

CT scanning without or with intravenous contrast material injection is performed with a thin fanlike band of x-rays (ionizing radiation) generated by an x-ray tube that literally moves around the patient in about 1 second. The resultant imaged sections (slices) of tissue can be obtained with imaging thickness as thin as 1 mm. "Reformatted" submillimeter images can also be generated from the axially obtained primary CT scan data reformatted by the CT computer in any plane (sagittal, coronal, off-axis, etc). Three-dimensional images can also be created in this manner.

CT demonstrates better than any other imaging test most osseous abnormalities with the possible exception of nondisplaced, nondistracted fractures, which are still often better seen on plain x-rays (Figure 36–3). Soft tissue lesions can also be detected with much better sensitivity than is possible with plain x-rays. However, distinguishing some similar but not identical normal soft tissues from one another, delineating normal from pathologic soft tissue, and evaluating certain areas of the brain that are limited by scanning artifacts can still be difficult with CT scanning, which is why CT remains inferior to MRI for evaluation of most brain and spinal canal abnormalities.

When discussing CT images, *density* and *attenuation* refer to the same process: absorption of the x-ray beam. Areas of increased density have greater attenuation of the x-ray beam and result in more whitish areas on the CT scan image (eg, bones, iodine-based contrast material, acute blood, areas of calcification, and some foreign bodies appear white on a CT scan). Areas of lower density have lower attenuation because they absorb less of the x-ray beam as it passes through the patient, resulting in darker areas on the CT scan image (eg, fluid in the ventricles, fat).

CT image contrast can be adjusted to highlight differences in the densities of different tissues.

Myelography

Myelography involves performing a lumbar subarachnoid puncture (or a lateral C1–2 subarachnoid puncture) and instilling less than an ounce of contrast material to opacify the subarachnoid space in the spinal canal, effectively outlining cauda equina nerve roots, the spinal cord, and any process that impinges on the opacified subarachnoid space. Such processes include tumors, infections, herniated disk material, degenerative spinal changes, and processes that

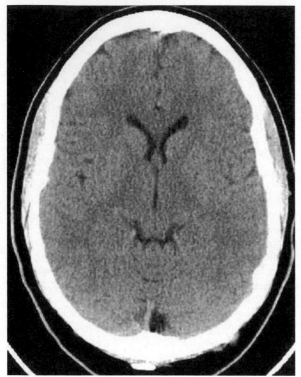

▲ **Figure 36–3.** CT scan (ionizing radiation). This image represents a single section ("slice") through the head (ie, it is a tomographic image; the left and right sides of the head can be separately delineated). The brain is directly imaged, though resolving differences in intracranial structures can be difficult (eg, resolving gray and white matter structures).

directly involve the intrathecal structures (spinal cord tumors, vascular malformations, metastases, etc).

Myelography is no longer a primary imaging technique for evaluating the spinal canal, having been replaced by MRI. It is currently reserved for problem solving: when the results of an MRI scan are not clear or when MRI is not possible (contraindications to MRI scanning, internal fixation hardware limits evaluation by MRI, etc).

Myelography is always followed immediately (within hours) by CT scanning to better delineate relationships of pathologic processes to the subarachnoid space.

▶ Magnetic Resonance Imaging

MRI is an imaging technique that does not use ionizing radiation. The physics of creating an MRI scan are quite complex. Briefly, a patient is placed in a strong magnetic field (30,000 times that of the earth's magnetic field). Radiofrequency pulses are transiently (milliseconds) applied to the patient to briefly perturb the patient's water molecules (by raising them to a slightly higher energy level). When the radiofrequency pulse is turned off, these water molecules rapidly return to their respective baseline states by giving off their recently absorbed energy. The rate at which these perturbed water molecules return to their respective baseline states can be measured by using extremely sensitive receiver coils in the MRI scanner. Because the rates at which these molecules return to their respective baseline states vary by local magnetic environment (eg, the local magnetic environment is different in the ventricular system than in the lentiform nucleus, white matter, eyeball, muscles, tumors, etc), these measurable differences among tissues can be localized in 3D space and used to create an image.

MR images can be obtained that highlight various magnetic field differences among tissues. In general, most MRI studies include *T1-weighted* and *T2-weighted* scans as part of the overall evaluation of the patient. MRI scans take longer to perform than CT scans in part because T1-weighted and T2-weighted scans must be obtained separately. T1-weighted images are distinguishable by the black color of the CSF over the surface of the brain and in the ventricles. In contrast, on a T2-weighted scan, the CSF over the surface of the brain and in the ventricles is white (Figure 36–4).

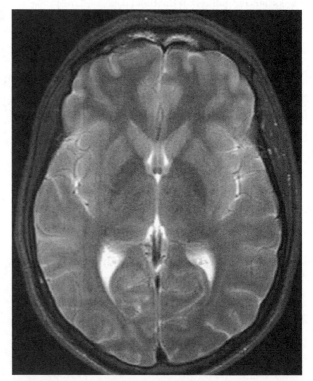

▲ **Figure 36–4.** MR scan (no ionizing radiation). Similar to CT, this image represents a single section ("slice") through the head. The white matter and gray matter structures are more easily resolved than on a CT scan, and even some gray matter structures can be resolved (eg, putamina and globus pallidae).

In general, T1-weighted scans are best for delineating anatomy and areas of contrast enhancement. T2-weighted scans are exquisitely sensitive to subtle changes in water concentrations (in both normal and pathologic tissues). These changes identify most pathologic processes (eg, strokes, tumors, infections). These subtle changes are manifested as increased signal (more whiteness) on T2-weighted scans.

Most MRI studies done in the past 5 years include *FLAIR* (fluid-attenuated inversion recovery) scans. In general, FLAIR scans can be considered super T2-weighted scans on which normal fluid (eg, in the ventricles and subarachnoid spaces) has no signal (is black), and subtle pathologic processes (which still appear white as on standard T2-weighted scans) are therefore easier to identify.

A gadolinium-based contrast agent can be injected intravenously to enhance imaging of some pathologic processes.

MRI best delineates soft tissues both intrinsic and immediately extrinsic to the brain, can be performed in any plane (including nonorthogonal planes), and has no known side effects at the field strengths used for clinical studies. In addition to demonstrating tissues better than CT, MRI is not limited by many of the artifacts that limit evaluation by CT, particularly in the posterior fossa and spinal canal regions where CT can be severely limited. While not ideal for directly visualizing dense osseous structures (where many fractures, cortical erosions, and degenerative changes occur), MRI is superb for detecting intrinsic (eg, bone marrow) osseous abnormalities (eg, metastatic disease, diskitis/osteomyelitis).

▶ Cerebral Angiography

Cerebral angiography is performed by directly placing a catheter into the femoral artery, passing it cephalad in a retrograde manner up the aorta to the level of the aortic arch, and manipulating it into either a vertebral or carotid artery and then further cephalad into the neck and even intracranially (Figure 36–5). The catheter is moved under fluoroscopic guidance with small amounts of dye injected at selected intervals to confirm the location of the catheter. When in position, larger amounts of dye are injected and serial plain x-rays are rapidly exposed as the injected dye passes through the intracranial vessels in the distribution of the injected blood vessel. Over 100 images might be obtained during a single 8-second injection of contrast material. This procedure is associated with a 0.1% to 0.5% chance of causing a stroke.

This technique best delineates intrinsic blood vessel pathology such as atherosclerosis, vasculitis, aneurysms, AVMs, dural venous sinus thromboses, fistulas, blocked vessels, and other intrinsic vascular disorders. It can be used to inject drugs into specific blood vessel territories for diagnostic or therapeutic purposes. Catheters can be placed directly into aneurysms, vascular malformations, and recently occluded vessels for definitive therapy.

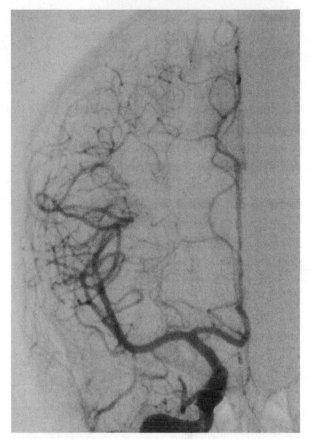

▲ **Figure 36–5.** Angiogram (ionizing radiation). A catheter was placed in the right carotid artery in the neck and dye injected while imaging was performed in a front-to-back projection of the right side of the head. The bones are then digitally "subtracted" from the image. The exquisite delineation of the blood vessels of the right carotid territory are demonstrated, but intra-axial (ie, brain soft tissues) structures are not.

Diagnostic endovascular (catheter) angiography is risky and expensive, requires complex equipment, and must be performed by highly trained personnel. Several alternatives to catheter angiography exist to evaluate for vascular lesions such as atherosclerotic vascular narrowing and aneurysms. Ultrasound (in the neck), CT angiography, and MRA are each useful alternatives in many situations (Figure 36–6).

ADVANCED CNS IMAGING TECHNIQUES

▶ Magnetic Resonance Imaging

A. Magnetic Resonance Angiography

MR data can be collected using software that images only moving tissues (ie, extravascular stationary soft tissue does

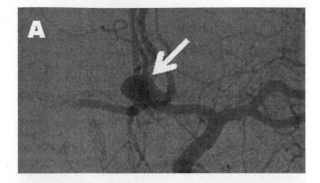

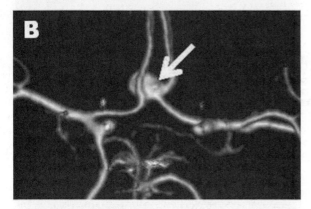

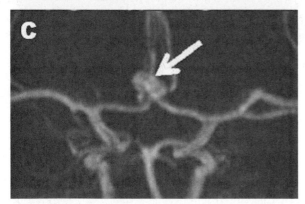

▲ **Figure 36–6.** Aneurysm demonstrated by multiple imaging techniques. **A:** Catheter angiogram (ionizing radiation). **B:** CT angiogram (ionizing radiation). **C:** MR angiogram (no ionizing radiation). Note that the catheter angiogram **(A),** an imaging modality associated with a risk of causing a stroke, best defines this anterior communicating artery region aneurysm (arrow). However, the aneurysm is still well seen on the CT angiogram **(B),** an imaging technique not associated with any risk of causing a stroke, and is also well seen on the MR angiogram **(C),** an imaging technique not associated with any risk of causing a stroke and that does not employ ionizing radiation.

not generate any MR signal on these images, while moving blood does generate signal). Using these techniques, images of blood vessels can be created with a sufficient level of detail that, in many cases, formal endovascular catheter angiography can be avoided (eg, to demonstrate significant atherosclerotic disease in the region of the carotid artery bifurcation or to monitor a known aneurysm at intervals).

B. Diffusion MRI and Perfusion MRI

Using rapidly applied magnetic field gradients, random molecular motion of water molecules can be converted to images and can be presented as diffusion MR images. Steep MR gradients can also be used to assess cerebral blood perfusion.

Diffusion MRI is sensitive to early changes of cerebral ischemia, often on the order of minutes. In the setting of acute cerebral ischemia, MR diffusion imaging changes (which usually reflect acute ischemic change) and MR perfusion imaging changes (which reflect cerebral brain perfusion) can be performed. The MR perfusion and diffusion images can be compared. Because diffusion images usually represent permanent injury (infarction) and perfusion (blood flow) deficits are potentially reversible, if a perfusion deficit is more extensive than an associated diffusion deficit, it is possible that an area of perfusion abnormality without diffusion abnormality represents viable brain that is at risk to go on to permanent injury but is not yet irreversibly injured (the "ischemic penumbra") and might benefit from aggressive therapy. Alternatively, if a diffusion deficit (usually representing a region of irreversible brain injury) is similar in extent to a perfusion deficit, then the ischemic changes may be permanent and there is no remaining at-risk penumbra brain, so no aggressive therapy is warranted.

C. MR Spectroscopy

Using standard MR hardware, MR spectroscopy can be performed to evaluate brain metabolites. Normal brain tissue includes many metabolites, the most important of which are N-acetyl-aspartate (which is found in normally functioning neurons and decreases with irreversible neuronal injury), choline (a component of cell membranes that increases in any process that increases cellular turnover, such as tumors, acute infections, etc), and creatine (a marker of cellular energy). Lactic acid can also be seen in ischemic cells, as a byproduct of anaerobic glycolysis, but is not present in normal brain tissue.

▶ Computed Tomography
A. Biopsy

CT can be used for guidance to percutaneously (through the skin) biopsy lesions that previously required an open surgical procedure.

B. Perfusion CT

While rapidly infusing contrast material through a peripheral vein, using a high-speed multisection CT scanner, data can be collected that reflects how well different portions of the brain are being perfused. In some patients, there are areas of underperfused brain that may manifest clinically with transient symptoms (eg, transient ischemic attacks); these regions might benefit from revascularization before the patient suffers irreversible injury (ie, a stroke).

C. CT Angiography

While rapidly infusing contrast material through a peripheral vein, using a high-speed multisection CT scanner, data can be collected that can be "reconstructed" with background data removed such that images similar to a catheter angiogram can be created without risk of stroke. While intrinsic vascular detail is not as good as detail shown by endovascular catheter angiography, in many patients, it is adequate to address the relevant clinical issue.

▶ Angiography

A. Coiling of Aneurysms

Instead of open surgery to place a clip around an aneurysm neck, small wires can be passed through endovascular (ie, within a blood vessel) catheters and directly deposited into aneurysms; an aneurysm can be filled with wires, obliterating the aneurysm lumen, eliminating the chance that such an aneurysm might rupture in the future, and obviating the need for a craniotomy for placement of an aneurysm clip.

B. Stenting

Instead of open surgery to address a narrowed atherosclerotic or dissected blood vessel, affected blood vessels can be treated with an intravascular catheter that first uses a balloon to dilate the narrowed blood vessel and then releases a mesh stent to maintain the patency of the newly dilated vessel.

C. Treating Intraluminal Thrombus

An acute (within 6 hours of onset of symptoms) intraluminal occluding thrombus (clot) or thromboembolus can be treated with intra-arterial catheter placement within the blood clot with injection of a clot lysing agent (eg, tissue plasminogen activator [t-PA]) to reestablish blood flow to an affected vascular territory before permanent brain damage occurs. Alternatively, some intravascular clots can be captured and removed from the vascular system using specialized catheters.

▶ Radionuclide Imaging

PET (positron emission tomography) and SPECT (single photon emission computed tomography) scans are molecular imaging techniques. Unlike other imaging techniques, they provide information beyond the structural appearance of normal and pathologic tissues. These techniques can provide physiologic information reflecting the functional state of tissues.

Low doses of radiotracers (positron emitters for PET scanning and single photon–emitting isotopes in SPECT scanning) are used to radiolabel molecules or drugs to image molecular interactions of biological processes in vivo. The nanomolar concentration of the radiotracer allows in vivo assessment of biologic processes without interfering with the process itself.

PET and SPECT cameras can measure the regional distribution of radioactivity within the brain. CT techniques (such as filtered backprojection or iterative reconstruction) allow the 3D reconstruction of the imaged brain.

The main advantage of PET imaging over SPECT imaging is that PET utilizes "coincidence" detection, which is the ability to detect the simultaneous emission of 2 gamma rays that are generated as positrons annihilate when encountering negative electrons. This results in greater spatial resolution of PET compared to SPECT. Both techniques can be used to study the same biologic processes.

The biological significance of measured radioactivity on PET and SPECT scans will depend on the biological function of the molecule that is attached to the radioisotope. For example, radioligands are available to measure cerebral blood flow, blood-brain barrier permeability, neurotransmitter synthesis, enzyme activity, receptor density, glucose metabolic rates, and gene expression, among other physiologic processes. Analysis of regional brain functions can be more specific by performing repeated imaging before and after specific pharmacological interventions, specialized motor or mental tasks ("activation" studies), or therapeutic interventions, such as stem cell or gene therapy.

PET or SPECT imaging can also be used in the clinical arena for localization of epileptogenic foci, diagnosis of dementing disorders, and distinction between tumor recurrence and radionecrosis, and to provide a chronologic record of disease progression or remission.

Finally, the same SPECT radioligands that are used for cerebral blood flow imaging, such as technetium-99m hexamethyl propyleneamine oxime (HMPAO), can also be used for bedside brain death studies using a regular planar gamma camera. Radioligands such as [111]Indium diethylenetriamine pentaacetic acid can be used intrathecally for radioisotope cisternograms for the clinical evaluation of patients with hydrocephalus or suspected CSF leaks. Radioisotope shunt studies can be performed to evaluate patency of CSF shunts.

Gibby WA: Basic principles of magnetic resonance imaging. Neurosurg Clin N Am 2005;16:1.

Johnson MH, Chiang VL, Ross DA: Interventional neuroradiology adjuncts and alternatives in patients with head and neck vascular lesions. Neurosurg Clin N Am 2005;16:547.

Waldron JS, Cha S: Radiographic features of intramedullary spinal cord tumors. Neurosurg Clin N Am 2006;17:13.

CRANIOCEREBRAL TRAUMA

Hugh J. L. Garton, MD, MHSC, & Emily Lehmann, MD

OVERVIEW & EPIDEMIOLOGY

Head injury (traumatic brain injury) is a leading cause of morbidity and mortality. The incidence of hospitalization for traumatic brain injury is 75–200/100,000 population. Traumatic brain injury occurs among all ages, peaking in 15- to 24-year-old males. Head injury is very frequent in polytrauma patients managed by trauma surgeons or emergency physicians. Thorough familiarity of the basics of care is therefore highly desirable.

Motor vehicle accidents are the most frequent cause of traumatic brain injury in the developed world, accounting for 30% to 50% of all serious head injuries. Falls and recreational injuries account for about 10% to 15% of traumatic brain injury. Inflicted injury (assault) accounts for about 10% to 20% of injuries in adult patients. Age and mechanism of injury are related: assaults occur mostly to very young infants (child abuse) and to young adults ages 18 to 24. Falls are the most common source of head injury in patients over 80 years of age. Response to injury also appears to be age dependent. Young people, particularly young males, are more likely to suffer a brain injury, but the chances of dying from that injury are much higher in the elderly. Head injury is the leading cause of death among all patients suffering traumatic injury.

Head injury can be divided on clinical grounds into mild, moderate, and severe forms. About 80% of injuries are mild, including most concussions. Many patients with these injuries do not require hospitalization. Moderate and severe injuries account for about 10% each of the total injury burden, and all of these patients are hospitalized. The death rate from head injury is estimated as 20–30/100,000.

Because recovery from moderate and severe injury is often incomplete, survivors of head injury and their care providers often must manage lifelong disability.

PATHOPHYSIOLOGY

▶ Classifications & Definitions

Brain injury literature groups injury in several different and unrelated ways, which may cause confusion. First, injury can be divided into primary and secondary types. Primary injury occurs at the time of the brain injury or immediately thereafter. It includes the immediate deformative or concussive forces applied to the brain. Clinically, primary injuries include skull fractures, lacerations of the brain, and hemorrhage in and around the brain (which may take some time to fully accumulate). In contrast to primary brain injury, secondary brain injury denotes the brain's response to injury, including, for example, loss of regulation of cerebral blood flow, cellular ischemic injury, and brain edema. Most of head injury research involves identification and interruption of these secondary injury pathways. Primary injuries can be induced by either *focal* or *diffuse* force application and by either *linear* or *angular* changes in momentum. The brain is much more sensitive to a diffuse, angular application of force than a focal, linear one. Experimentally, concussions occur at much lower total acceleration when an angular force is applied than when a linear one is applied.

Penetrating injury to the brain results in trauma both from the direct disruption of the brain caused by the projectile and from compression/decompression injury caused by the passage of the bullet or other device. The energy that a projectile imparts to the head is directly proportional to the projectile mass and to the square of the velocity. Velocity therefore is usually the stronger determinant of the extent of projectile injury, and the distinction between low-velocity and high-velocity injuries is important.

Secondary brain injury describes the processes that occur in the brain in response to the primary brain injury. These occur from the subcellular to the macroscopic level. Calcium-dependent mechanisms, oxidative stresses from free radicals, and apoptotic mechanisms are all likely involved. Tissue ischemia clearly occurs after severe traumatic brain injury, and in most cases, cerebral blood flow (a marker for tissue perfusion) drops considerably in the early phases after severe traumatic brain injury. The consequence of the microscopic injury cascade at a more macroscopic level is an increase in brain water content: cerebral edema. This occurs both through cytotoxic (cell injury and cell swelling) and vasogenic (incompetent vasculature) mechanisms, although the former mechanism is probably the more important. Brain edema acts as additional mass within the cranial vault that must be accommodated in managing intracranial pressure. The skull forms a rigid, protective covering for the brain. Any increase in the amount of material within the skull, such as a hematoma or edema, must be accommodated within the fixed volume of the skull and will generally increase the intracranial pressure (Figure 36–1). The intracranial compartment is subdivided into compartments by folds in the dura. The tentorium divides the cranial vault into supratentorial and infratentorial compartments, while the falx cerebri divides the supratentorial compartment into right and left halves. This compartmentalization is of benefit after trauma by helping restrict the consequences of injury from impacting the other compartments. However, the compartmentalization and the protections that occur because of it are incomplete, and in severe injuries, brain material will herniate out from its compartment of origin, often producing specific clinical herniation syndromes.

▶ Clinical Assessment

The basics of management for patients with brain injury can be divided into initial resuscitation, primary neurologic survey, a search for lesions requiring immediate surgical management, and identification and management of cerebral edema and increased intracranial pressure. These steps are often applied recursively because the patient condition may change frequently during injury course. The processes required to resuscitate, triage, and manage a concussion are less involved than for a severe brain injury, but the basic steps are similar.

Initial resuscitation for patients suffering brain injury is similar to that for all trauma victims. Management of the airway, breathing, and circulation (the ABCs) is paramount. While patients sustaining isolated mild traumatic brain injury will usually maintain these functions, patients with multiple injuries or patients with severe brain injuries often cannot maintain these critical functions without assistance. For example, hypoxia occurs in 30% of patients presenting with severe traumatic brain injury, who often, because of their injury, cannot protect their airway. In addition to its obvious primary deleterious effects on the brain, hypoxia is also a strong stimulus to increase cerebral blood flow through vasodilatation of the cerebral vasculature. The additional volume of blood in the cerebral vasculature then adds measurably to the intracranial pressure after injury. Early endotracheal intubation to secure an airway and provide adequate ventilation is essential. All patient with severe brain injuries and many patients with more serious moderate brain injuries may require intubation purely on the basis of a reduced ability to protect the airway and maintain ventilation. Intubation of a patient with brain injury should be performed with short-acting pharmacologic agents. It is best to avoid the use of long-acting sedating medications and even the reflexive repetitive use of shorter-acting agents in the prehospital and trauma bay settings. The loss of the neurological examination that results can impair or delay critical management decisions. Adequate analgesia and sedation are necessary for many trauma patients at intubation and during early resuscitation, but the goal should be use the minimum necessary with repeated doses based on reassessment of patient status.

Restoring and maintaining an adequate blood pressure is also of critical importance. This should be accomplished by using intravenous fluids and blood as needed to restore a normal circulating blood volume and by control of active hemorrhage. The use of pressor agents to support blood pressure may also be appropriate if hypotension persists despite an adequate circulating blood volume. Brain injury, unless it has progressed past a herniation event, is rarely the cause of hypotension, so a standard search for the source of hemorrhage should accompany resuscitation as for any traumatic injury. Scalp injuries, which often accompany traumatic brain injury, can be a significant source of blood loss especially in children. Database research demonstrates that a single episode of hypotension following a brain injury doubles the risk of dying compared to patients who never have such an episode.

The Glasgow Coma Scale

Once the ABCs have been addressed, the goal of the primary neurologic survey is a rapid, accurate categorization of the severity of the brain injury and a search for clinical evidence of large intracerebral hematomas that could require immediate evacuation. The Glasgow Coma Scale, a 3-component scoring system, is the main tool of the primary neurological survey (Table 36–1). To apply the scale, patients are asked to give their name or description of what happened and to follow a simple command. Patients who are unresponsive to verbal requests should receive a brief, firm, noxious stimuli. An effective approach is to apply digital pressure to the trapezius muscle and observe for the response. Additional stimuli may be needed elsewhere to confirm the motor response. Patients can localize when their actions are purposeful and they attend specifically to a noxious stimuli in an attempt to remove it. Patients are withdrawing when they do not attend to stimuli but do act to move away from noxious stimuli in a nonstereotypic fashion. Decorticate and decerebrate posturing are stereotypic movements. The possible scores range from 3 to 15. Patients receive the better score when the left and right sides are different. Intubated patients may be given a score of "T," or their verbal score may be estimated from other communicative efforts that they make. The power of this grading scheme is that it is quick and accurate in terms of long-term prognosis, assuming the examination is not clouded by sedatives or other confounding factors. A score between 3 and 8 indicates severe traumatic brain injury, 9 to 12 indicates moderate brain injury, and 13 to 15 indicates mild closed head injury.

In addition to determining the GCS scale, the primary neurological survey includes an assessment of the pupils and gross motor function to assess for the presence of lateralizing signs of a large intracranial hemorrhage. These examinations can also alert to the potential presence of a concomitant spinal cord injury. The mass of hematoma, depending on size and location, may produce uncal herniation with unilateral pupillary dilation and contralateral hemiparesis. These findings may indicate that a life-threatening intracranial hemorrhage is present, which can be amenable to urgent evacuation. Depending on the situation, it may be appropriate to assess other brainstem responses during the primary survey, but more often these are deferred until after an initial head CT scan is obtained. These brainstem reflexes can help to localization injuries (Table 36–3). Two additional brainstem reflexes, the oculocephalic (doll's eyes) and oculovestibular (caloric), are not usually tested initially in traumatic settings because of potential exacerbation of cervical spine injuries (doll's eyes) or basilar skull fractures (caloric testing).

▶ Diagnostic Imaging

Once the patient's ABCs are safe, the severity of the head injury is determined, and the primary neurological survey is completed, all patients with moderate and severe brain injuries should have a CT scan of the head. Rapid use of the head CT is also appropriate in many cases of mild closed head injury, especially when other risk factors, such as the use of anticoagulants, are present. Although the presence of

Table 36-3. Common Brainstem Reflexes Evaluated in Patients with Traumatic Brain Injury.

Reflex	Afferent	Brainstem Level	Efferent	How Tested
Pupillary	CN II	Midbrain	CN III	Light shined in the eye, observed for pupillary constriction
Corneal	CN V	Pontine	CN VII	Saline dropped into the eye, observed for blink
Gag	CN IX	Medulla	CN XI	Pharynx stimulated with endotracheal tube or probe, observed for swallow/cough or aversion

a skull fracture significantly increases the chances of finding a lesion on a head CT, plain skull x-rays are not advised as a substitute for the head CT. MRI may at some point replace CT as the primary imaging tool for traumatic brain injury, but this has not yet occurred. CT is quicker, safer for management of uncooperative patients, and safer for the environmental issues of loose ferromagnetic materials near, on, or in the patient. MRI may be useful in assessing cervical and intracranial vasculature, and it may be helpful in more accurate prognostication of injury outcome.

The head CT is reviewed for the presence of surgically significant intracranial hemorrhage. In addition, specific radiographic markers can predict increased intracranial pressure (Figure 36-7). These include effacement of the basal and convexity subarachnoid spaces (cisternal effacement), mass effect (compression or deformation of adjacent brain structures), and shifting of the brain contents from one side to the other, causing midline shift. Patients with certain facial, skull base, and cervical fractures are at risk for cervical intracranial vascular injury, and dedicated vascular imaging

may be indicated. Conventional angiography, CT angiography, and MRA are all potential considerations in these situations. Conventional angiography is the gold standard for injury detection and offers the option of endovascular treatment; however, it is also time intensive and may separate the patient from the optimal critical care environment for a protracted period. CT angiography is convenient and rapid but may miss some injuries. MRA may be more sensitive but has the same downsides as MRI in other trauma settings. No highly regarded predictive tool exists, but risk factors that should prompt consideration of a vascular injury and subsequent vascular imaging include an unexplained neurological deficit, massive facial bleeding or epistaxis, and fracture involving the foramen lacerum of the skull base or foramen transversarium of the cervical vertebrae.

After the head CT scan, the clinical and radiographic information should be synthesized to formulate a plan either to operate to evacuate an intracranial lesion, to evaluate for intracranial hypertension with monitoring technology and clinical examination, or to observe clinically for worsening of

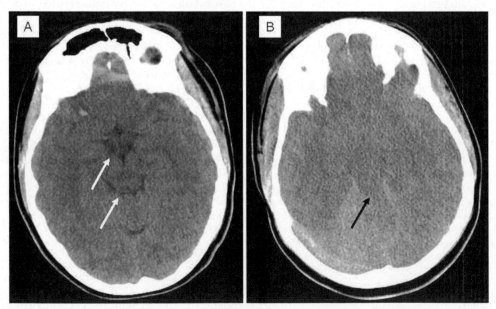

▲ **Figure 36-7. A:** Normal head CT demonstrating normal basal cisterns (white arrows). **B:** A head CT demonstrating effacement of basal cisterns (black arrow) and global edema after head trauma.

neurological status with clinical examinations alone. Radiographic assessments, similar to clinical assessments, are often iterative with repeat imaging used regularly to assess for an alteration in status and optimal management plan.

CLINICAL INJURY PATTERNS & HERNIATION SYNDROMES

Several important clinical syndromes herald herniation events within the brain. Each has both an imaging and clinical correlate. Immediate recognition and treatment of these syndromes is essential for patient survival. Herniation is the decompensated response to an increasingly large intracranial mass or unchecked cerebral edema. When the intracranial pressure or regional compartment pressure reaches a sufficiently high level, the brain tissue is displaced out of the compartment into the adjacent one. If all the intracranial compartments are under equally high pressure, the brain seeks to exit the calvarium through the foramen magnum. **Subfalcine herniation** occurs when part of the cerebrum is forced from one side to the other under the falx cerebri. This is evident radiographically by the degree of *midline shift* present on head CT or MRI. Usually, the falx itself is shifted to some extent with the brain. In trauma, there is a general correlation between the degree of midline shift, the depression in the level of consciousness, and the severity of the injury. Rarely, the anterior cerebral artery can be pinched by the falx when there is subfalcine herniation. **Uncal herniation** occurs when the uncus (Latin for "hook") of the temporal lobe is shifted medially by a mass or swelling in the ipsilateral hemisphere. This is most likely to happen with temporal lobe masses because of the close proximity of the mass or swelling to the uncus. Anatomically, the uncus compresses the adjacent subarachnoid space, wherein lies cranial nerve III (oculomotor), resulting in loss of its parasympathetic fiber function to the ipsilateral eye and pupillary dilatation from unopposed sympathetic tone. With more severe or prolonged compression, the extraocular muscle function of cranial nerve III is lost also, leading to an eye that is deviated interiorly and laterally (unopposed lateral rectus and superior oblique function). If the uncus is forced further medially, it compresses the cerebral peduncle, producing contralateral hemiparesis. The clinical syndrome associated with these events therefore is an initial restlessness, then somnolence followed by a dilated ipsilateral pupil, and then contralateral hemiparesis. A somewhat confusing variation is the *Kernohan notch phenomenon*, wherein the entire brainstem is shifted by the uncus and the contralateral peduncle comes into contact with the opposite tentorial edge, leading to weakness that appears clinically on the same side as the pupillary dilation. This is relevant clinically, because if faced with the clinical contradiction of left pupillary dilatation and left hemiparesis, the left pupillary dilation is a stronger predictor of the ipsilateral nature of the cranial problem than the left hemiparesis, which would otherwise predict a right-sided problem. Uncal herniation can have the secondary complication of compression of the posterior cerebral artery which runs near cranial nerve III. Patients are at risk for a posterior cerebral artery–distribution stroke. **Tonsillar herniation** occurs when the intracranial contents, particular the contents of the posterior fossa, are forced out of the foramen magnum at the base of the skull. The tonsils of the cerebellum are pushed downward and compress the medulla oblongata, leading to respiratory depression and death. Radiographically, this is identified by the loss of CSF spaces around the brainstem and foramen magnum as brain tissue is pushed into these spaces.

The **Cushing triad** is the constellation of bradycardia, hypertension, and respiratory irregularity that often occupies a herniation event clinically. It is likely due to brainstem compression. The hypertension can be conceptualized as an attempt to protect the brain's perfusion pressure from the high intracranial pressure. Intubation and mechanical ventilation often obscure the respiratory part of the triad, but the other two are observed regularly.

SPECIFIC INJURIES & SURGICAL MANAGEMENT

Skull fractures are usually the result of focal application of force to the head. They are usually categorized as open or closed, depressed or nondepressed, and basilar or convexity varieties. Depressed fractures can tear the dura or lacerate the cortex of the brain. Depressed fractures greater than the width of the bone are usually considered for operative repair, particularly if there is an associated laceration of the skin. Skull fractures that are not depressed usually do not usually require repair. *Basilar skull fractures* (those fractures involving the bones at the base of the brain: parts of the sphenoid, temporal, occipital bones, and clivus) can damage the vasculature and cranial nerves and can lead to a CSF leak and meningitis. Clinically, one may suspect a basilar skull fracture in the presence of Battle sign, which is retroauricular ecchymosis, or "raccoon eyes," which is bilateral periorbital ecchymosis. Basilar and nondepressed calvarial vault fractures are usually managed conservatively, although their presence should prompt consideration of vascular and cranial nerve injury. Controversy exists as to the best management of fractures involving the inner table of the frontal sinus or extending from the skull base into the ethmoid or other skull base sinus. There is the potential for the spread of infection through sinus communication with the epidural space. However, many such fractures heal spontaneously without complications, and management must be individualized.

An **epidural hematoma (EDH)** can occur with a skull fracture that lacerates an artery in the dura (Figure 36–8). The classic example is laceration of the middle meningeal artery by the temporal bone. The bleeding occurs on the outside of the dura and collects in and expands the potential epidural space between bone and dura. Because the source of bleeding is an artery, the hematoma can compress the

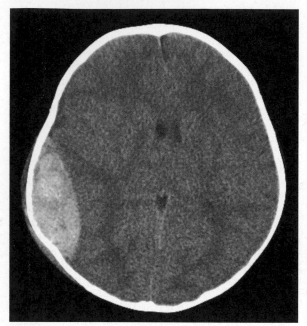

▲ **Figure 36–8.** Acute epidural hematoma after head trauma in a 5-year-old patient.

adjacent brain to the point of serious injury or death. Not all epidural hematomas are caused by an arterial injury in the dura. Blood from a skull fracture or dural venous sinus can sometimes collect in the epidural space. These *venous epidural hematomas* are much less likely to produce life-threatening compression of the brain. Distinguishing between the two types is largely a matter of location (temporal vs nontemporal), size (small vs large), and rate of change (slow vs fast). Because the primary injury in an isolated epidural hematoma does not involve the brain, the neurological outcome is excellent if the diagnosis and treatment are prompt. The classic presentation of a temporal epidural hematoma is a patient suffering a blow to the temple and a brief loss of consciousness. This is followed by a lucid interval during which the patient appears to be neurologically well because there has been little primary brain injury. During this time, either the epidural hematoma expands slowly enough for the compensatory mechanisms of the brain to maintain consciousness or the hemorrhage stops temporarily. Subsequently, either due to rebleeding or exhaustion of the compensatory mechanisms, a rapid decline in level of consciousness follows from the mass of hematoma associated with the other elements of uncal herniation, including an ipsilateral cranial nerve III palsy and contralateral hemiparesis. However, this classic sequence is present only in about 25% of patients with epidural hematoma. Many patients have no loss of consciousness with injury, while conversely, about 20% decline after injury without the

lucid interval. Epidural hematomas are usually diagnosed from CT imaging and have a lens-shaped (lentiform) appearance, as the dura is attached firmly to the skull at nearby sutures, tapering each end of the hematoma. CT images are also helpful to judge the impact of the hematoma on the brain, such as the degree of shift of the midline or compression of adjacent structures. Management of an epidural hematoma is determined by lesion size, location, and time from injury to diagnosis. Generally, an epidural hematoma more than 1 cm in depth is considered for surgical removal, as are lesions in the temporal fossa where there is less room for further expansion before brain injury occurs. In some cases, an epidural hematoma is diagnosed 2 or more days after the injury that caused it. Since the bulk of hematoma expansion occurs within the first 24 to 36 hours, it is considered safe to observe patients with epidural hematoma of modest size (about 1 cm deep) when the diagnosis has been delayed. The hematomas in many of these cases will reabsorb spontaneously. In contrast, a 1-cm-thick temporal epidural hematoma in a patient only 30 minutes out from injury should be strongly considered for emergent surgical removal of the hematoma prior to care of other injuries not immediately threatening to the ABCs. The operative approach involves positioning the patient to gain access to the site of the hematoma. For a temporal epidural hematoma, a skin incision is made from the root of the zygoma extending into the ipsilateral frontal region in a reverse question mark fashion. As circumstances dictate, a burr hole can be placed in the temporal region after incising the temporalis muscle before the skin incision is completed to allow blood to escape from the epidural space. However, in most instances, the blood is clotted, and rapid completion of craniotomy must follow. The temporalis muscle is elevated and retracted anteriorly. Additional burr holes are placed as needed, and a bone flap is elevated. The hematoma is removed. Lacerated dural vessels can be controlled with bipolar cautery or suture depending on size. The dural surface is inspected for an associated subdural hematoma, and intraoperative ultrasound may be useful as needed. The dura is then sutured to the bony margins of the craniotomy to prevent reaccumulation. When a hematoma has collected in the vicinity of a major dural venous sinus, such as the transverse or sigmoid, the sinus itself may be torn, and the resulting hemorrhage is very difficult to control. The outcome for a patient suffering even from a large epidural hematoma can be quite good if managed promptly.

Acute subdural hematoma (ASDH) results from trauma to the brain causing rupture of veins over the surface of the brain that transit from the cortical surface to the inner surface of the dura to reach the dural sinuses. When these vessels are injured, the blood collects between the dura matter and the arachnoid membrane, in the potential subdural space. The force required to shear vessels in this fashion can occur with a focal blow to the head but is more common with diffuse, rotational force applications to the brain, as often occur in motor vehicle accidents. Except in the elderly, acute subdural hematoma generally occurs in conjunction with fairly severe associated brain injury. Focal bruising of the brain is often present beneath the subdural hematoma. Most patients present with a significantly depressed level of consciousness and may have other findings related to the compressive mass of the hematoma. A subdural hematoma has more of a crescent shape to it on imaging studies, because there is no barrier to its spreading over the hemispheric surface of the brain. Associated intracerebral hemorrhage and edema is often evident beneath the acute subdural hematoma (Figure 36–9).

Management of the acute subdural hematoma involves emergent operative removal by craniotomy for lesions more than 1 cm thick. A large craniotomy is generally required, and acute brain swelling during the surgical procedure must be expected. Unlike the situation in an epidural hematoma, the bleeding source in an acute subdural hematoma is often difficult to discern. Diffuse hemorrhage arising from under the margins of the bone flap adjacent to dural venous sinuses is often best managed with gentle packing of hemostatic materials rather than aggressive exploration. Medical management of elevated intracranial pressure and the underlying brain injury is an essential part of the patient's care. Outcomes are often poor, with a mortality of 50% to 90%. Survivors often have significant disabilities. Outcomes can be predicted by the admission GCS score, and in certain cases, medical care is likely to be futile and offered only with reservations.

In the elderly, the atrophy of the brain places the transiting veins under stretch, and injury can occur with much less force. Subdural hematomas can present more chronically in such elderly patients, even several months after injury, with a collection several centimeters thick. Such **chronic subdural hematomas** should be thought of as a different injury from the acute subdural hematoma (Figure 36–10).

In cases of chronic subdural hematoma, drainage of the hematoma either through a burr hole in the skull or via a craniotomy is indicated. Outcomes are much better than for acute subdural hematoma, although recurrence and reoperation are common.

Coagulopathy, whether from anticoagulant medications or as a complication of severe trauma, presents a special risk to patients with traumatic brain injury who are prone to sudden deterioration from hematoma expansion. Immediate, aggressive correction of coagulopathy is indicated for such patients.

Intraparenchymal contusions are common after trauma. These are hemorrhage mixed with brain and usually occur either at the site of a direct blow to the head or at a point opposite the point of impact. This latter phenomena is called

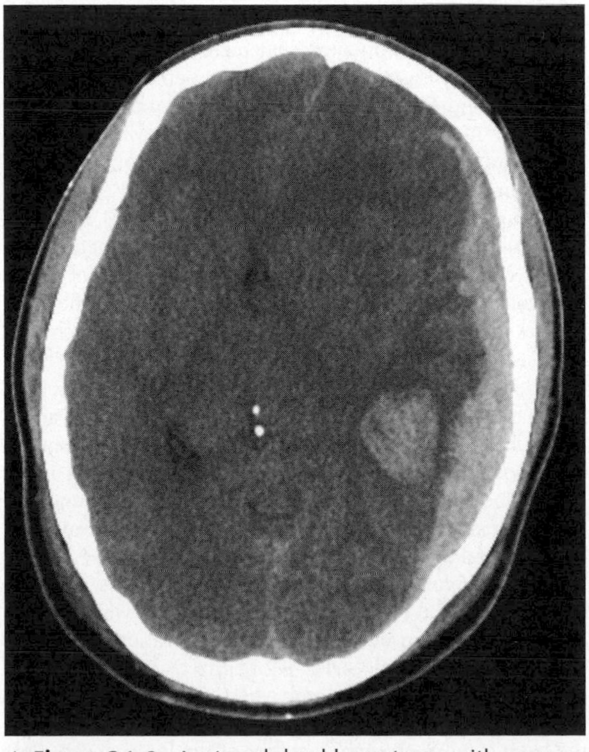

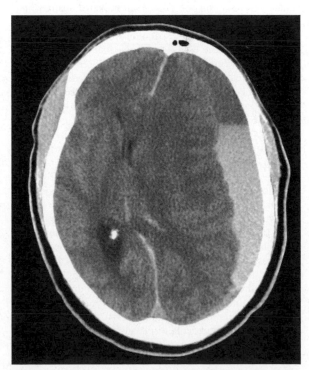

▲ **Figure 36–9.** Acute subdural hematoma with an associated intraparenchymal hemorrhage after head trauma in a 25-year-old patient.

▲ **Figure 36–10.** Chronic subdural hematoma with acute blood layering in fluid in a 55-year-old patient.

a *contrecoup* injury and is the result of the pressure wave of force moving through the brain and impacting and rebounding from the skull opposite the impact site. Contusions often occur in anterior temporal lobes after frontal impact as the temporal lobes impact into the sphenoid wing anteriorly. The base of the frontal and temporal lobes is also a common site for contusions caused by the brain moving roughly over the irregular bony surfaces of the frontal and middle fossae. Posteriorly, such contusions do not occur because the brain moves over the smoother tentorium. The clinical presentation of contusions is specific to their location in the brain, but they can also produce more widespread symptoms through their mass effect, as discussed in the section on Elevated Intracranial Pressure. Intraparenchymal contusions should be distinguished from smaller hemorrhages associated with **diffuse axonal injury,** discussed in the next section. There is certainly overlap in terms of size and location, but the typical intraparenchymal hemorrhages are large than 0.5 cm in diameter and relate to either bony anatomy or force vector, as described earlier. Management for these lesions is generally as conservative as the situation will allow because the hematoma is often intimately mixed with brain, some of which may still be functional. Lesions larger than 25 mL are often considered for resection, but the relative eloquence of brain and the response to attempted medical management are often important considerations.

Penetrating brain injury usually produces a focal injury pattern specific to the site of penetration. High-velocity injuries such as those from a gunshot produce, in addition to the focal injury, a large area of cavitation and hemorrhagic injury from the blast effect. Gunshot wounds that pass through the ventricular system, as a marker for the "middle" of the brain, are most often fatal. Management of less severe penetrating injury revolves around managing the potential infectious complications of injury and repairing the breach to the skull.

DIFFUSE BRAIN INJURY DIAGNOSES NOT TYPICALLY REQUIRING IMMEDIATE SURGICAL MANAGEMENT

Concussion is an immediate and transient loss of consciousness or normal mentation after head trauma, often associated with a period of amnesia. It is a very common injury. Sport injuries are a common source of concussions, and young patients appear to be at highest risk. Concussion is most easily induced by sudden rotation of the head. The presumption is that the cerebral cortex is rotating around the more fixed midbrain and diencephalon, producing disruption of input and outflow from the reticular activating system. Presentation after concussion can be surprisingly varied, with some patients displaying no loss of consciousness but rather confusion and amnesia. The severity of concussion appears to be proportional to the duration of amnesia, particularly the anterograde (since injury) amnesia. Relying on consensus and expert opinion, several different

criteria for diagnosis and grading systems for severity have been proposed. These systems use the duration of the confusion or amnesia and the presence or absence of a loss of consciousness to form a 3-tiered scale of severity and are primarily designed to assist with return-to-play decisions for athletes. To the surgeon, the more typical concern is to decide whether a patient presenting with a concussion needs a CT scan of the head. Validated clinical decision rules stress that all patients with a GCS of less than 15, those that are vomiting, and those older than 60 to 65 years are at high enough risk to warrant a CT scan. Other factors warranting a CT scan are severe headache, intoxication, persistent anterograde amnesia, a seizure with the injury, evidence of trauma to bone or soft tissue above the clavicle, and severe mechanism of injury such as auto-pedestrian or ejection injury.

Management for isolated concussions presenting for emergency department evaluation usually includes a period of observation for at least 2 hours, assuming the individual is neurologically normal. Dependent on any other injuries, the patient may be discharged to a responsible adult with written instructions to return for specific symptoms (as listed for obtaining a head CT). Patients with abnormal CT scans are usually admitted for care. Long-term outcome is generally good, with most patients experiencing no long-term sequelae. However, up to 25% of patients report an increased incidence of headaches and memory difficulties even several months later. **Postconcussive syndrome** is a more severe version of this phenomenon that includes these and other symptoms, such as depression, anxiety, emotional lability, insomnia, and fatigue. Treatment is largely one of reassurance and management of individual symptoms. Because athletes are often concussed, questions arise around when it is reasonable to return to play.

Traumatic subarachnoid hemorrhage is a relatively common finding in patients suffering severe traumatic brain injury. Following injury, a relatively small amount of blood may collect in the subarachnoid space, often over the convexities of the brain but also in the basal cisternal arachnoid spaces. Trauma, not rupture of an aneurysm, is the most common cause of subarachnoid hemorrhage, so the report of subarachnoid hemorrhage after trauma should not automatically prompt a search for a ruptured aneurysm. A history of a neurological collapse before the trauma or more dense blood collecting in the basal cisterns or around the larger intracranial vasculature should prompt more concern for a cerebral aneurysm.

Diffuse axonal injury occurs when axons become sheared off at the boundary between gray and white matter during rapid brain acceleration or deceleration. The substance of the cerebral cortex is organized in to a series of alternating layers of gray and white matter (gray cortical mantle, subcortical white matter, deep gray matter nuclei of the basal ganglia, and white matter of the internal capsule). These layers have different tissue densities and behave differently when subjected to force in trauma. The border between these two tissues is often a site of injury because the two layers accelerate or decelerate at rates according to their tissue properties. Diffuse axonal injury is a common finding in severe injury, occurring in up to 50% of patients. Clinically, diffuse axonal injury can occur in varying degrees of severity. In minimal cases, a prolonged, mildly concussive state of confusion and memory loss might occur. In more severe cases, the presentation is a depressed level of consciousness. Focal findings can occur if there are diffuse axonal injury hemorrhages in specific locations such as the internal capsule or brainstem. The appearance on head CT is of multiple small (< 1 cm) hemorrhages scattered throughout the brain at the junction of gray and white matter. Grading schemes that relate the severity of the CT findings to the eventual neurological outcome exist. Effacement of the basal cisterns and midline shift are examples of radiographic prognosticators of poor outcome after diffuse axonal injury. Management for patients suffering from diffuse axonal injury is primarily medical and focuses on prevention and management of secondary brain injury, discussed later.

MEDICAL MANAGEMENT AFTER TRAUMATIC BRAIN INJURY

Medical management after traumatic brain injury is largely directed at detecting and preventing secondary brain injury from seizures, systemic phenomena such as hypotension and hypoxia, and intracranial hypertension.

▶ Seizure Management

The incidence of seizures following traumatic brain injury is estimated at between 5% and 15%. Most of these events occur within the first 7 days after trauma. A seizure has the possibility of increasing brain demand for oxygen and nutrients at a point when the injury may limit the ability of the brain to respond in this fashion. Prophylactic anticonvulsants, usually phenytoin (Dilantin), or more recently levetiracetam (Keppra), are reasonably used to prevent seizures after a moderate and severe traumatic brain injury when there is evidence of nontrivial brain injury on CT scans. However, experimental evidence supports their use for only the first 7 days after a traumatic brain injury, and there does not appear to be benefit to continuing the prophylaxis beyond 7 days. Patients experiencing seizures outside of the immediate point of impact are candidates for therapeutic anticonvulsant use extending beyond the 7-day time frame, usually for several months or more, depending on whether the seizures recur.

▶ Homeostatsis

Just as in the initial resuscitation, ongoing care of acute brain injury requires careful protection against hypoxia, hypotension, and hyperthermia. Each of these conditions has the potential to increase intracranial pressure or further deprive the brain of adequate glucose or oxygen, or both.

▶ Physiology of Increased Intracranial Pressure

Other than its impact on the neurological examination, secondary brain injury manifests itself clinically as cerebral edema and an increase in intracranial pressure. The **Monro-Kellie doctrine** states that given a fixed intracranial volume, consisting of brain, CSF, and arterial and venous blood, any additional material must be accommodated by a decline in the amounts of the others or a rise in pressure due to the increase in total intracranial material (Figure 36–1). When a mass is introduced into the cranial vault, CSF and, later, venous blood are displaced to make room for the mass while initially allowing relatively normal intracranial pressures. However, these mechanisms are overcome, and eventually the rise in pressure with increasing volume becomes exponential. The compensatory phase is very important clinically, because a patient may harbor a clinically important lesion while showing only modest symptoms of increased pressure in the brain. This model works well in trauma but is overly simplistic and does not explain clinical phenomena that occur over a longer time frame, such as might occur with chronic hydrocephalus or a brain tumor. In such cases, the compressibility of the brain, usually described as its compliance (change in volume for a given change in pressure), matters a great deal, and brain pressures may be normal even in the face of a mass that, if it occurred acutely, would overwhelm the compensatory mechanisms. Despite these limitations, the compartment model is very useful for managing cerebral edema and increased intracranial pressure. Left unchecked, these consequences of secondary injury lead to increased cerebral edema, increased intracranial pressure, compression, and finally injury of adjacent brain and its vasculature, producing additional brain ischemia and tissue injury, cyclically generating more brain edema, and further increasing intracranial pressure. Intracranial pressure is both a surrogate measure of the presence of cerebral edema and a primary actor in ongoing secondary brain injury. Increased intracranial pressure, like hypoxia and hypotension, is a strong predictor of mortality and morbidity after head injury.

The concept of **cerebral perfusion pressure** highlights the ability of elevations in intracranial pressure to reduce tissue perfusion:

$$CPP = MAP - ICP$$

where CPP is cerebral perfusion pressure, MAP is mean arterial pressure, and ICP is intracranial pressure. In adult patients, cerebral perfusion pressure lower than 70 mm Hg is associated with worsened outcome. The equation also illustrates the importance of maintaining an adequate blood pressure in traumatic brain injury management. Hypotension is among the strongest predictors of poor neurological outcome after traumatic brain injury.

Detection of cerebral edema and intracranial hypertension is based on suspicion, radiographic features, and direct measurement of intracranial pressure. In severe head injury, as measured by the GCS score, the incidence of increased intracranial pressure is 50% to 60%. Radiographic findings of concern include the presence of mass effect, midline shift, loss of the evident pattern of sulci and gyri from displacement of CSF, loss of distinction of the gray/white matter junction, and effacement of the basal CSF cisterns. Increased intracranial pressure can occur in the absence of any of these findings, so in patients with severe head injury, direct measurement of the intracranial pressure can still be indicated without concerning radiographic features. At present, it is unproven whether treatment directed by intracranial pressure is preferable to one based on CT and clinical examination. Nevertheless, current guidelines from the Brain Trauma Foundation recommend intracranial pressure monitoring for all patients

1. with GCS score of 3 to 8 and abnormal head CT;

2. with GCS score of 3 to 8 with normal head CT but with hypotension or age over 40;

3. in whom the neurological examination cannot be assessed because of sedation or need for general anesthesia if the suspicion of increased intracranial pressure is high.

Intracranial pressure is measured in trauma by either introduction of a transducer into the brain parenchyma or placement of a catheter into the ventricles of the brain to measure the pressure of the cerebrospinal fluid in a minor surgical procedure. Complication rates of intracranial hemorrhage (2% vs < 1%) and infection (10% vs 2%) are higher for catheter-based measurement systems over parenchymal transducers, but only a catheter-based system can drain CSF, a distinct treatment advantage. Parenchymal monitors are subject to drift in accuracy and may be inaccurate by 3 to 4 mm Hg after 4 to 5 days. Catheter-based systems may occlude or be unreliable in the face of very compressed ventricles. In trauma, intracranial pressure is not measured by lumbar puncture because of the risk of brain herniation from higher cranial versus lumbar pressures. Normal intracranial pressures range between about 5 and 15 mm Hg at rest and vary with position and activity. Treatment thresholds after brain injury are typically greater than 20 mm Hg in adult patients, while children and infants likely require treatment at a lower intracranial pressure, although the precise numbers are not yet established. Measurement of the intracranial pressure allows calculation of the cerebral perfusion pressure. Managing brain injury based on cerebral perfusion pressure rather than intracranial pressure holds interest because a sufficiently high blood pressure should be able to perfuse the brain despite the intracranial pressure. However, clinical research suggests that while cerebral perfusion pressures lower than 70 mm Hg in adult patients are associated with poor outcome, artificially raising blood pressure to supraphysiologic levels in an effort to overcome an increase in intracranial pressure worsens rather than improves outcomes. Cerebral perfusion pressure measure-

ments currently focus care on avoiding relative hypotension during management.

Treatment options for intracranial hypertension and cerebral edema are most easily understood with reference to the 4-compartment model of the brain (brain, venous, arterial blood, CSF). When patients present with elevated intracranial pressure, treatments aim to manipulate the volume of one of these compartments. At present, the selection and style of intracranial hypertension management is as much art as science. Few well-designed studies exist to directly compare different management strategies. Each treatment has risks associated with its use. General strategies include employing less risky strategies first and escalating as needed, and applying methods directed at each of the compartments before applying multiple methods to the same compartment, although many therapies work on multiple parts of the model. The following sections cover the treatment options in general but not rigid order of preference. A therapy from the end of the list would very rarely be used before one at the beginning, but adjacent items in the list might be interchanged.

A. Improve Venous Drainage

If blood is restricted from exiting the central nervous system, intracranial pressure is increased as the venous compartment size becomes larger. In trauma patients, tight-fitting cervical collars, a supine body position, and fighting against the ventilator all increase venous pressures. Loosening collars, elevating the head of the bed 30 degrees, and minimizing ventilator pressures all improve venous drainage and lower intracranial pressures. These measures have very little risk and can be employed widely.

B. CSF Drainage

Reducing the size of the CSF space can make more room for brain edema and lower intracranial pressure. This is done by draining CSF from the same ventricular catheter used to measure intracranial pressure. The risks of this therapy are infection and hemorrhage, and a capable surgeon must be available to place the catheter.

C. Sedation/Paralysis

Besides caring for the patient's comfort after an injury, sedation and/or chemical paralysis are important in reducing excessive brain metabolism that accompanies agitation from brain injury. This metabolism can be directly toxic in an injured brain and obligates increased arterial and venous blood volume to supply the tissue with nutrients. In addition, sedatives and paralytic agents reduce fighting against the ventilator, reducing venous congestion. However, these agents reduce the ability to follow the neurological examination and have the side effect of hypotension when given in excess. Typically, agents such as morphine and lorazepam are used for analgesia and sedation, while muscular paralytics such as vecuronium are used to facilitate ventilation, but little evidence supports the use of specific regimens with the exception of propofol, which should not be used in children. In general, shorter-acting agents are preferable to long-acting ones because of the desire to periodically examine the patient without their influence.

D. Osmotic Agents and Diuretics

In theory, excessive brain water can be removed directly in some cases by establishing a favorable osmotic gradient for diffusion of fluid back into the bloodstream. Mannitol, a sugar, and concentrated saline solutions (3% NaCl), do not cross the blood-brain barrier and therefore provide such a gradient. Their effect appears to require an intact blood-brain barrier. Experimentally, they draw water from less injured areas of the brain rather than from the more injured areas. This reduces the overall brain volume and can decrease the intracranial pressure in the 4-compartment model. In addition, experimental evidence suggests that a significant part of the intracranial pressure–reducing effect of osmotic agents comes from reducing the viscosity of blood by altering red blood cell morphology. This allows delivery of more blood through smaller channels, permitting safe reduction in vessel caliber and therefore in total intracranial blood volume. The adverse effects of these therapies include dehydration (and hypotension) in the case of mannitol and nephrotoxicity from increased osmolarity for all agents. In addition, some of the osmolar particles do make it across the blood-brain barrier and can pull water back into the brain if the therapy is withdrawn too quickly. Dosing regimens for these agents are variable but mannitol is usually used at 0.5 to 1 gm/kg per dose as often as every 2 to 3 hours. Doses of 1 gm/kg are given for impending herniation. NaCl 3% may be dosed either continuously at 1 to 3 mL/kg per hour or as bolus doses of similar amounts. Serum sodium and osmolarity measurements should be assessed frequently. For mannitol, a serum osmolarity above 320 mOsm/L appears to threaten toxicity and limit efficacy, while for hypertonic saline, serum osmolarities of 360 mOsm/dl or more have been reported without renal injury. In this area, the medical literature is limited.

E. Hyperventilation

The autoregulatory mechanisms of the brain rely in part on CO_2 (or perhaps pH) concentrations in the blood. A high metabolic rate leads to increased CO_2 production and acidosis. The natural response to this event is vasodilatation to remove waste products and increase the supply of metabolites. Clinically, artificially increasing the respiratory rate (and dropping the CO_2) significantly decreases the intracranial blood volume by vasoconstriction. The downside risk is that if done to excess, the vasoconstriction produces ischemia. While hyperventilation was once widely practiced, it is now reserved for situations in which the brain injury has produced an excessive, as opposed to reduced degree of

blood flow. This is relatively rare. However, it is import to manage ventilator settings to avoiding elevated CO_2 levels (and reduced O_2 levels). This avoids unnecessary vasodilation and the increased intracranial pressure that results. Arterial CO_2 levels of 35 mm Hg and O_2 levels of 100 mm Hg are the common therapy targets.

F. Barbiturates

High doses of barbiturates reduce cerebral metabolism and experimentally protect against brain injury from the regional ischemia common in secondary brain injury (the "induced coma"). This reduced demand for metabolites decreases the blood flow requirements for adequate cell nutrition and thus can decrease intracranial pressure. However, no clinical experiment has clearly shown that barbiturates improve outcome. The risk is that these agents can profoundly lower blood pressure. They must used very carefully if at all.

G. Hypothermia

In experimental settings, hypothermia appears to slow the destructive secondary injury pathways at a cellular level. This reduces the edema that comes from cell death. However, randomized trials in adult head injury have not shown benefit, and pediatric trials are ongoing. In the published trial protocols, cooling is typically begun early in the hospital course, if not immediately, with target temperatures of 32 to 33 °C maintained for several days after the initial injury. Complications associated with the therapy in the adult clinical trials have been an increase in infection rate and serious electrolyte disturbances, particularly hyperkalemia.

H. Surgical Decompression

Surgical management of cerebral edema involves enlarging the space available for swelling by removing a portion of the calvarium. The surgical technique is to remove a large portion of the skull over the more effected side (hemicraniectomy) or to remove large portions of both frontal bones (bifrontal craniectomy). The dura is generally opened and patched with either allograft or native periosteum. Clinical studies suggest that surgical decompression is effective in lowering intracranial pressure, but data regarding neurological outcomes are varied.

OUTCOMES AFTER TRAUMATIC BRAIN INJURY

While many patients with mild traumatic brain injury return to their preinjury level of function, a significant number develop chronic symptoms of fatigue, memory impairment, headaches, and difficulty with concentration. In one study of prospectively followed injury victims, Thornhill and colleagues reported that over 50% had some identifiable disability 1 year after injury, including both physical and mental impairments. These were severe enough to impact activities of daily living in one third to one fourth of patients. Predictors for poor outcome included age over 40, and preinjury disability. The medical literature is mixed with regard to the longer-term outcome. In a separate study by Whitnall and coauthors, the overall rates of disability were similar at 1 year and 5 years from injury, but about 25% of patients had exchanged categories from good to disabled, and vice versa. Changes in depression, anxiety, and reported stress appeared to correlate strongly with category change, and only 7% reported the use of rehabilitation services by the 5-year postinjury point. Patients with moderate closed head injuries have more varied outcomes. Most recover to maintain their activities of daily living and even return to work or school. Detailed neurocognitive testing, however, often reveals deficits in executive function and memory. There are more consistent reports of chronic fatigue and headaches. Severe traumatic brain injury is often a life-altering event for both patient and family. The prognostic implications of injury are often vitally important for family members making decisions about what degree of aggressive care to provide. As an average, perhaps 15% to 20% of all patients with severe injury will make a good recovery, while more than 50% will either die or be severely disabled. Sadly, for some patients, the degree of injury and the poor likelihood of meaningful recovery make the provision of aggressive care an exercise in futility. Elderly patients older than 80 years with severe head injuries have a very poor prognosis. For patients with the worst prognostic features (eg, older age; very low GCS; or GCS of 3 to 5 without improvement with resuscitation, with lack of pupillary response to light, and with associated chest or abdominal injuries with hypotension), the prognosis for meaningful recovery is very poor. Once the diagnosis and injury severity are confirmed by examination and imaging studies and the condition is unchanged despite resuscitation and withdrawal of all pharmacologic agents likely to be affecting the examination, a gentle but frank discussion of the situation is necessary and appropriate. However, generally, the younger the patient is, and the higher the presenting GCS score, particularly the motor GCS scores, even within the severe injury group, the better the chances of some degree of recovery. The physician would do well to remember that prognostic information represents a probability of an outcome, not a certainty of it. While some families may appreciate knowing these details, others will more appreciate whatever kernels of hope can be provided under the circumstances.

Adelson PD et al: Guidelines for the acute medical management of severe traumatic brain injury in infants, children, and adolescents. Chapter 5. Indications for intracranial pressure monitoring in pediatric patients with severe traumatic brain injury. Pediatr Crit Care Med 2003;4(3 suppl):S19.

Bullock MR et al: Surgical management of traumatic parenchymal lesions. Neurosurgery 2006;58(3 suppl):S25.

Crutchfield JS et al: Evaluation of a fiberoptic intracranial pressure monitor. J Neurosurg 1990;72:482.

Eisenberg HM et al: Initial CT findings in 753 patients with severe head injury. A report from the NIH Traumatic Coma Data Bank. J Neurosurg 1990;73:688.

Gelabert-Gonzalez M et al: Chronic subdural haematoma: surgical treatment and outcome in 1000 cases. Clin Neurol Neurosurg 2005;107:223.

Guidelines for the management of severe traumatic brain injury. J Neurotrauma 2007;24(suppl 1):S14.

Hawley CA et al: Use of the functional assessment measure (FIM+FAM) in head injury rehabilitation: a psychometric analysis. J Neurol Neurosurg Psychiatry 1999;67:749.

Haydel MJ et al: Indications for computed tomography in patients with minor head injury. N Engl J Med 2000;343:100.

Levy ML: Outcome prediction following penetrating craniocerebral injury in a civilian population: aggressive surgical management in patients with admission Glasgow Coma Scale scores of 6 to 15. Neurosurg Focus 2000;8:E2.

Miller MT et al: Initial head computed tomographic scan characteristics have a linear relationship with initial intracranial pressure after trauma. J Trauma 2004;56:967.

Nirula R, Gentilello LM: Futility of resuscitation criteria for the "young" old and the "old" old trauma patient: a national trauma data bank analysis. J Trauma 2004;57:37.

Nonfatal traumatic brain injuries from sports and recreation activities—United States, 2001–2005. Morb Mortal Wkly Rep 2007;56:733.

Ommaya AK, Goldsmith W, Thibault L: Biomechanics and neuropathology of adult and paediatric head injury. Br J Neurosurg 2002;16:220.

Park P et al: Risk of infection with prolonged ventricular catheterization. Neurosurgery 2004;55:594.

Rothman MS et al: The neuroendocrine effects of traumatic brain injury. J Neuropsychiatry Clin Neurosci 2007;19:363.

Schootman M, Fuortes LJ: Ambulatory care for traumatic brain injuries in the US, 1995–1997. Brain Inj 2000;14:373.

Schootman M, Buchman TG, Lewis LM: National estimates of hospitalization charges for the acute care of traumatic brain injuries. Brain Inj 2003;17:983.

Stiell IG et al: Comparison of the Canadian CT Head Rule and the New Orleans Criteria in patients with minor head injury. JAMA 2005;294:1511.

Stiell IG et al: The Canadian CT Head Rule for patients with minor head injury. Lancet 2001;357:1391.

Surgical management of penetrating brain injury. J Trauma 2001;51(2 suppl):S16.

Teasdale G, Jennett B: Assessment of coma and impaired consciousness. A practical scale. Lancet 1974;2:81.

Temkin NR et al: A randomized, double-blind study of phenytoin for the prevention of post-traumatic seizures. N Engl J Med 1990;323:497.

Thornhill S et al: Disability in young people and adults one year after head injury: prospective cohort study. Br Med J 2000;320:1631.

Thurman DJ et al: Traumatic brain injury in the United States: a public health perspective. J Head Trauma Rehabil 1999;14:602.

Timofeev I et al: Effect of decompressive craniectomy on intracranial pressure and cerebrospinal compensation following traumatic brain injury. J Neurosurg 2008;108:66.

Wakai A, Roberts I, Schierhout G: Mannitol for acute traumatic brain injury. Cochrane Database Syst Rev 2007;1:CD001049.

Werner C, Engelhard K: Pathophysiology of traumatic brain injury. Br J Anaesth 2007;99:4.

Whiteneck G et al: Population-based estimates of outcomes after hospitalization for traumatic brain injury in Colorado. Arch Phys Med Rehabil 2004;85(4 suppl 2):S73.

Whitnall L et al: Disability in young people and adults after head injury: 5-7 year follow up of a prospective cohort study. J Neurol Neurosurg Psychiatry 2006;77:640.

Wood RL: Long-term outcome of serious traumatic brain injury. Eur J Anaesthesiol Suppl 2008;42:115.

SPINAL CORD INJURY

John Ziewacz, MD, & Frank La Marca, MD

General Considerations

Traumatic spinal cord injury (SCI) is devastating. It primarily affects young people and often results in significant disability or death. The median age at diagnosis of SCI is 37.6 years. The main causes in order of incidence are motor vehicle collision, fall, violence, and sport injuries. Despite maximal medical and surgical therapy, the prognosis for significant recovery of a complete lesion is poor. Recent research into stem cell technology and other new modalities of therapy have not yet been effective in human clinical trials.

The cost to the health care system and to society is significant. A 25-year-old with a high cervical cord injury (C1–4) is estimated to incur $741,425 in medical costs in the first year following SCI and $132,807 for each year survived thereafter. In addition, the loss of wages and productivity for patients with SCI averages $57,000 annually. With 12,000 to 14,000 Americans suffering SCI per year, the social and economic costs are significant.

The demographics of SCI have changed in the last 30 years. The median age of 37.6 years is an increase from 28.7 years in the 1970s, largely due to an increase in the incidence of falls causing SCI in patients over 60 years of age. Although the relative incidence of both sport injuries and violent injuries has declined over the last 30 years, the larger decrease in sport injuries has placed it below violent injuries as a cause of SCI.

Treatment for SCI consists of acute and chronic management. Acutely, the ABCs must be secured and the spine immobilized to prevent extension of injuries. Compressive lesions must be identified and the need for urgent surgical management determined. Methylprednisolone is currently a treatment option used widely in the initial phases of SCI, though it is associated with side effects that may sometimes outweigh the potential benefits of its use. Chronic management includes physical and occupational therapy designed to maximize functionality. Specific therapy and improvement depends on the level and completeness of the injury.

Clinical Findings

Clinical findings in SCI depend on the level, mechanism, and severity of injury. Injuries can be classified as either complete or incomplete. A complete SCI refers to the lack of motor or sensory function below the level of the lesion. Incomplete lesions spare some degree of sensory and/or motor function below the level of the lesion. Incomplete lesions often result in recognized SCI syndromes based on the region of the spinal cord affected. The American Spinal Injury Association publishes a scale to further classify the severity of SCI (Table 36–4).

Table 36–4. The ASIA Classification of Spinal Cord Injury.

A	Complete: No sensory or motor function preserved in the lowest sacral segments (S4-5).
B	Sensory incomplete: Sensory but no motor function preserved below the neurologic level including the sacral segments S4-5.
C	Motor incomplete: Motor function is preserved below the neurologic level, and more than half of the key muscles below the neurologic level have a muscle grade less than 3; there must be some sparing of sensory and/or motor function in the segments S4-5.
D	Motor incomplete: Motor function is preserved below the neurologic level, and more than half the key muscles below the neurologic level have a muscle grade ≥ 3. There must be some sparing of sensory and/or motor function in the segments S4-5.
E	Normal: Sensory and motor functions are normal. Patient may have abnormalities on reflex examination.

Adapted from American Spinal Injury Association: *Standards for Neurological Classification of Spinal Cord Injury* (rev. 2000). Chicago: ASIA, 2002.

Initial clinical findings include motor deficit, sensory deficit, and hyporeflexia. Initially, all reflexes below the lesion are lost, including the bulbocavernosus, cremasteric, and abdominal cutaneous reflex. Over time, these reflexes may return, and the deep tendon reflexes become hyperreflexive due to the loss of descending tonic inhibition of the reflex arc. Initially, paralysis is flaccid, but eventually upper motor neuron signs develop, and a spastic paralysis results. If the lesion is in the high cervical region (C1–5), respiratory effort may be compromised due to the loss of innervation to the phrenic nerve. Loss of bowel or bladder function often occurs, and loss of rectal tone and sensation, as well as priapism, may result. The loss of bladder control manifests as urinary retention, and developing urinary incontinence is typically overflow incontinence. Loss of anal sphincter tone and sensation results in leakage of stool and lack of awareness of bowel movements.

An important early finding that can occur in SCI is spinal shock, which is a drop in the systolic blood pressure with accompanying bradycardia, often to a level of 80 mm Hg systolic following SCI. This pressure drop is due to the loss of sympathetic tone to the regions below the lesion and causes venous pooling and decreased venous return to the heart.

Chronic clinical findings in SCI are related to the long-term need for ventilatory support, immobilization, and catheterization. Pneumonia, urinary tract infections, and decubitus ulcers are common findings and are often the cause of death in patients with SCI.

Incomplete SCIs may demonstrate a variable pattern of sensory or motor preservation, though they can often be categorized into recognizable clinical syndromes, depending on the mechanism of injury and the portion of the cord affected:

A. Central Cord Syndrome

Central cord syndrome refers to a pattern of injury that affects the motor strength in the upper extremities more severely than in the lower extremities. Sensory function is variable below the level of the lesion, and sphincter control is often affected. This usually occurs in older patients with spinal stenosis following a hyperextension injury. The central cervical cord is a watershed vascular territory that is thought to be disrupted in this syndrome. The spinal cord is somatotopically organized such that cervical fibers are more medial compared to fibers traveling to the lower extremities, resulting in the more severely affected upper extremities.

B. Anterior Cord Syndrome

Anterior cord syndrome results from the compression of the anterior portion of the cord by a herniated disk or bone fragment or from occlusion of the anterior spinal artery. The corticospinal tracts and spinothalamic tracts are preferentially affected because of their more anterior location. The posterior columns are relatively spared. This results in loss of motor function and loss of pain and temperature sensation below the level of the lesion, with preserved proprioception, vibration, and pressure sensation. It is important to distinguish surgical from nonsurgical (ie, anterior spinal artery occlusion) etiologies in this condition.

C. Brown-Séquard Syndrome

Brown-Séquard syndrome occurs after spinal cord hemisection. It is usually the result of penetrating trauma occurring in 2% to 4% of SCIs. Motor function and posterior column function (proprioception, vibration sense) is disrupted on the side of the lesion. Pain and temperature sensation is diminished on the contralateral side due to the crossing of the spinothalamic tract in the spinal cord at or 1 to 2 levels above the entrance of the fibers into the cord.

D. Conus Medullaris Syndrome

Conus medullaris syndrome results from injury to the sacral spinal cord. Symptoms include saddle anesthesia, loss of bowel/bladder function, and lower extremity weakness. It includes a combination of both upper and motor neuron signs.

E. Cauda-Equina Syndrome

Cauda-equina syndrome refers to compression and dysfunction of the lumbosacral nerve roots. It is not a true SCI because it affects only the nerve roots, not the cord itself. The clinical syndrome is similar to conus medullaris syndrome with saddle anesthesia, loss of bowel/bladder function, and lower extremity weakness, but findings are all lower motor neuron.

▶ Physical Examination

Initial physical examination in SCI focuses on the ABCs. The spine should be immobilized to prevent further injury.

Special attention must be focused on the airway in high cervical injuries because patients may require endotracheal intubation given injury to the nervous supply to the diaphragm. Blood pressure must be closely monitored given the possibility of spinal shock, which manifests as a drop in the systolic blood pressure and must be addressed immediately in order to prevent further cord ischemia.

In the awake patient after the ABCs have been attended to, a history focusing on mechanism of injury and detailed neurologic examination is undertaken to determine the level and completeness of the injury. Motor strength should be tested in all muscle groups, and sensation should be tested with pinprick and proprioception. Rectal tone and sensation should be tested with digital examination. Reflexes, including the bulbocavernosus, cremasteric, and abdominal cutaneous reflexes, should be examined. Careful palpation of the spine is important to evaluate for obvious step-offs or tenderness to palpation at all levels. The examination must be carefully documented and a neurologic level and evaluation of completeness of the lesion determined.

In the comatose patient, a complete neurologic examination is often difficult. In this situation, observation of spontaneous movements or movements to painful stimuli is important. Deep tendon reflexes should be examined, and palpation of the spine should be undertaken to observe for obvious step-offs. Radiologic imaging is often required to adequately determine a level of injury and its etiology.

▶ Differential Diagnosis

After a complete history and physical examination is performed, with the addition of radiographic imaging, the diagnosis of SCI is usually apparent. Radiographic imaging can help determine the mechanism of the injury, which is usually due to a fracture or subluxation of the bony spinal elements.

Some peripheral nerve lesions may resemble SCI, but these can usually be distinguished after careful examination and with knowledge of the anatomy of the spinal cord and the peripheral nervous system. Peripheral injuries are typically unilateral and affect only lower motor neurons. Sometimes malingering and conversion disorders may mimic SCI. Serial examinations and inconsistencies in examination in the setting of unremarkable imaging usually permits differentiation.

▶ Radiologic Examination

In the asymptomatic patient with no spinal tenderness, no distracting injury (eg, long-bone fracture), and no evidence of disturbed consciousness or intoxication, no radiographic imaging is necessary. Patients with spine tenderness, numbness, tingling, or obvious signs of SCI (eg, weakness, loss of bowel/bladder control) require radiographic imaging. The hallmark of radiographic imaging has been 3-view cervical spine x-rays with anteroposterior/lateral films of the thoracic and lumbar spine. The American Association of Neurological Surgeons/Congress of Neurological Surgeons (AANS/CNS) recommends 3-view cervical spine x-rays in conjunction with CT scanning of the cervical spine in patients with suspected SCI. With the advent of CT scanning with detailed coronal and sagittal reconstructions, CT scanning alone has replaced x-ray examination as the initial diagnostic study of choice in many centers (Figure 36–11). This obviates the need for multiple x-rays and diagnostic and treatment delay in the case of inadequate plain films. MRI is listed as an option in the diagnosis of SCI by the AANS/CNS because it can better detect ligamentous/soft tissue injury, though it often "overcalls" injuries that do not cause instability and may lead to prolonged and unnecessary immobilization. MRI is often reserved for patients for whom SCI signs and symptoms are present and no clear evidence is found on x-ray imaging or CT or in whom a herniated disk or other soft-tissue abnormality is suspected. MRI (particularly T2-weighted sequences) also clearly demonstrates compression of and/or signal change within the spinal cord (Figure 36–12).

In awake patients, clearance of the cervical spine consists of normal x-rays (or CT with reconstructions), CT scan, and flexion/extension views or MRI obtained within 48 hours of injury. At this point, cervical immobilization may be discontinued.

Under current recommendations in obtunded patients, cervical spine clearance may be obtained following normal x-rays, CT, and dynamic flexion/extension films performed under fluoroscopic guidance, normal MRI obtained within 48 hours of injury, or at the discretion of the treating

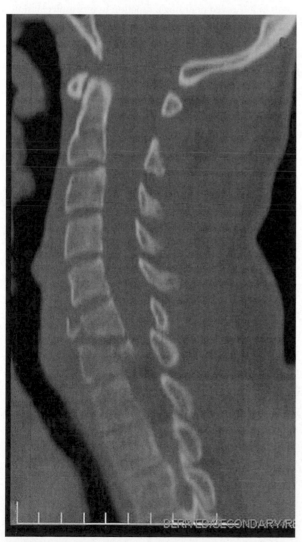

▲ **Figure 36–11.** Sagittal reconstruction of a cervical CT scan demonstrating a C6-7 traumatic fracture.

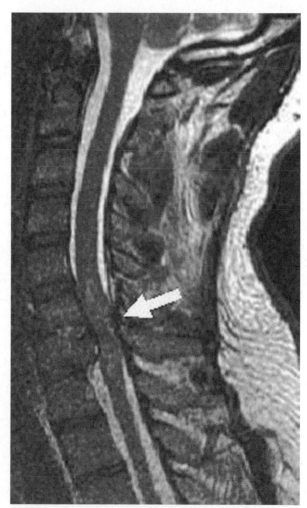

▲ **Figure 36–12.** Sagittal T2-weighted magnetic resonance image of a C6-7 traumatic fracture demonstrating spinal cord compression and signal change within the spinal cord (arrow).

physician. However, with the advent of CT with sagittal and coronal reconstruction providing greater sensitivity for the detection of injury, and the propensity of MRI to overcall injuries, some centers clear the cervical spine in obtunded patient with normal x-rays and CT scans. Clearance of the cervical spine in this population is still cause for debate, and recommendations are in flux. Further studies will elucidate the necessary and sufficient studies to definitively clear the cervical spine in this population.

In patients with SCI, the combination of x-rays with CT scanning has high sensitivity and identifies the vast majority of lesions causing SCI.

► Treatment

Initial treatment of SCI consists of securing the ABCs and immobilizing the spinal column. In the case of high cervical spine injury, the need for endotracheal intubation must be identified, and if it is not immediately necessary, serial arterial blood gas assessments should be monitored to evaluate for hypocapnia and progressive ventilatory failure. Spinal shock and the resultant decrease in blood pressure must be treated aggressively if it occurs. Volume expansion should be initiated promptly, and decreased systolic blood pressure refractory to volume expansion should be treated with pressor therapy. The choice of pressors has not been conclusively defined, but typically a beta-agonist is followed by an alpha-agonist given the possibility of bradycardia in spinal shock.

Patients should be placed in a hard cervical collar, and cervical immobilization should be ensured until clearance of the cervical spine or definitive treatment has occurred. Patients should be placed on a board for transfers and log-rolled for movement until the thoracic and lumbar spine is cleared.

Other initial management considerations include placement of an arterial line to monitor blood pressure on a constant basis and placement of a Foley catheter to decompress the bladder.

Methylprednisolone has been used in the acute phase of SCI based on studies that demonstrated motor improvement in patient groups that received methylprednisolone in the early period after SCI. However, due to the lack of demonstrated clinical significance of any improvement and studies demonstrating side effects of high-dose methylprednisolone, it is offered as an option by the AANS/CNS current guidelines with the knowledge that "evidence suggesting harmful side effects is more consistent than any suggestion of clinical benefit."

Following initial stabilization and imaging studies, the need for surgical intervention is assessed. Surgery has two main goals: decompression and stabilization. Surgery is employed on an emergent basis for incomplete lesions in the hopes of preserving or improving neurologic function and on a nonemergent basis for complete lesions because there is no demonstrated improvement in neurologic function for emergent surgery for complete lesions. Goals of surgery in this setting are to prevent cranial extension of injury and to prevent progressive deformity. Choice of surgical approach for SCI is not standardized and is dependent on the location of the pathology. Current stabilization procedures typically involve instrumented fusion techniques and may be approached via an anterior, posterior, or combined approach.

Cervical traction may be employed either alone or as an adjunct to surgical therapy to attempt realignment of the spinal column. This is accomplished by fixing a halo ring or specialized devices (ie, Gardner-Wells tongs) to the head, connecting the fixture to a rope-and-pulley system, and adding weight to adjust the spine in the desired vector.

Chronic treatment of SCI focuses on rehabilitation and adaptation to permanent injury. Rehabilitation can often result in improved neurologic function in incomplete lesions and can help those with complete injuries become as functional as possible. Patients may require ventilatory support, tracheostomy, intermittent catheterization, frequent turning (to prevent decubitus ulcers), and functional accommodations such as wheelchairs and other devices aimed at improving functionality. Attention to long-term care issues can prolong the life and productivity of SCI patients.

► Prognosis and Outcome

Despite exciting research into novel treatments, SCI remains a devastating injury. Death in the acute trauma setting from SCI is 20%. Complete lesions that remain so at 72 hours are unlikely to improve beyond one level above the lesion in the long term. Patients with quadriplegia who have initial ventilator dependency have 5-year survival rates of approximately 33%. Incomplete lesions have a more favorable outcome. Among recognized SCI syndromes, central cord syndrome and Brown-Séquard syndrome have the most favorable outcomes: Up to 90% of patients with these syndromes are able to ambulate independently at 1 year. Patients with anterior cord syndrome have a worse prognosis, with 10% to 20% recovering functional motor control. Death in long-term SCI patients is usually due to cardiac, respiratory, or infectious causes, often related to the sequelae of SCI.

Current multidisciplinary approaches, including emergency department, medical, surgical, and rehabilitation staff, provide the best therapy for patients with SCI. Nevertheless, SCI remains a devastating injury with high rates of mortality and permanent disability. Novel research and innovations will hopefully provide better outcomes for SCI in the future.

American Spinal Injury Association: *Standards for Neurological Classification of Spinal Cord Injury* (rev. 2000). Chicago: ASIA, 2002.

Bracken MB et al: Administration of methylprednisolone for 24 or 48 hours or tirilazad mesylate for 48 hours in the treatment of acute spinal cord injury. Results of the Third National Acute Spinal Cord Injury Randomized Controlled Trial. National Acute Spinal Cord Injury Study. JAMA 1997;277:1597.

Garshick E et al: A prospective assessment of mortality in chronic SCI. Spinal Cord 2005;43:408.

Hadley MN et al: Guidelines for the management of acute cervical spine and spinal cord injuries. Clin Neurosurg 2002;49:407.

Ho CH et al: Spinal cord injury medicine. 1. Epidemiology and classification. Arch Phys Med Rehabil 2007;88(suppl 1):S49.

Jackson AB et al: A demographic profile of new traumatic spinal cord injuries: change and stability over 30 years. Arch Phys Med Rehabil 2004;85:1740.

Matsumoto T et al: Early complications of high-dose methylprednisolone sodium succinate treatment in the follow-up of acute cervical spinal cord injury. Spine 2001;26:426.

McKinley W et al: Incidence and outcomes of spinal cord injury clinical syndromes. J Spinal Cord Med 2007;30:215.

National Spinal Cord Injury Statistical Center: Spinal cord injury: facts and figures at a glance. J Spinal Cord Med 2005;28:379.

Priebe MM et al: Spinal cord injury medicine 6. Economic and societal issues in spinal cord injury. Arch Phys Med Rehabil 2007;88(suppl 1):S84.

Soden RJ et al: Causes of death after spinal cord injury. Spinal Cord 2000;38:604.

Wicks AB, Menter RR: Long-term outlook in quadriparetic patients with initial ventilator dependency. Chest 1986;90:406.

PERIPHERAL NERVE LESIONS

Cheerag Upadhyaya, MD, Linda Yang, MD, & John McGillicuddy, MD

Peripheral nerves are composed of varying combinations of sensory and motor axons. An axon is a long projection from a nerve cell body that is bounded by a cell membrane as well as a basement membrane. Some axons are surrounded by sheaths of myelin, a fatty substance secreted by Schwann cells. Myelin insulates the axon, thereby increasing the velocity of neurotransmission. The axon is, in turn, surrounded by a layer of connective tissue called endoneurium. Axons travel together in bundles called fascicles, each of which is covered by another layer of connective tissue called perineurium. Fascicles are grouped together to form a peripheral nerve, which is surrounded by a final layer of connective tissue called epineurium.

ACUTE PERIPHERAL NERVE INJURIES

General Considerations

Common etiologies of acute peripheral nerve injury include penetrating trauma, blunt trauma, traction, fractured bones, and compression from hematomas. Minor peripheral nerve injuries arise from blunt trauma that temporarily compresses or stretches a nerve but leaves its axons intact. In such cases, axonal transport may be temporarily impaired, but wallerian degeneration, or the death of axons distal to the point of injury, does not occur. These injuries generally recover spontaneously over the course of days to weeks. Slightly more severe injuries may interrupt axons and their myelin sheaths while leaving endoneurium intact. In these cases, wallerian degeneration inevitably follows. Axonal regeneration may occur spontaneously, however, guided to areas of previous innervation by intact endoneurial tubes. With this type of injury, there is a good prognosis for spontaneous functional recovery, with axonal regeneration occurring at a rate of about 1 mm per day, or 1 inch per month.

Peripheral nerves may be severed cleanly, as in the case of iatrogenic scalpel injuries during surgery. If the divided ends of the nerve remain in proximity, regeneration can occur via axonal sprouting from the proximal stump. These axonal sprouts may bridge the gap to the distal stump, propagating through preserved endoneurial tubes at a rate of 1 mm per day. Severe crush injuries may create internal damage to a peripheral nerve without completely transecting it. Such injuries disrupt axons and their endoneurium and disturb the organization of fascicles within the nerve. In these cases, fibrous scar tissue may form within the macerated nerve, which can block the regeneration of axonal sprouts. A tangle of axonal sprouts contained in fibrous scar tissue is called a neuroma. Neuroma formation acts as a barrier to spontaneous peripheral nerve regeneration.

Clinical Findings

A careful clinical history and a meticulous neurological examination are paramount in determining which peripheral nerves have been injured and the type of injury present. The type of trauma will generally suggest whether or not the nerve is in continuity. A penetrating injury with a sharp object, such as a knife, suggests a clean transection that is amenable to immediate surgical repair. Nonpenetrating trauma or a stretch injury is more suggestive of nerve continuity.

The sensory and motor findings associated with acute peripheral nerve injury vary widely, depending on which particular nerve is injured. Pain may also be a symptom, but it usually develops in a delayed fashion. Pain can occur as a result of neuroma formation, where it is often associated with a tender lump in the area of injury. Neurogenic pain may also develop because of a disturbance in the processing of pain signals. This type of pain, when associated with autonomic hyperfunction, is referred to as complex region pain syndrome (formally known as causalgia or reflex sympathetic dystrophy); it is notoriously difficult to treat. When neurogenic pain is associated with nerve root avulsion, it is known as deafferentation pain. Deafferentation pain often responds well to surgical intervention via dorsal root entry zone ablation.

In the diagnosis of acute peripheral nerve injury, electromyogram and nerve conduction studies are generally not useful until at least 3 weeks after injury. Nevertheless, it is important to obtain baseline electrodiagnostic studies because they are important for monitoring recovery. In the case of brachial plexus injury, it is useful to obtain an MRI scan or CT myelogram to look for pseudomeningoceles in the vicinity of the nerve roots, which would indicate nerve root avulsion.

Certain peripheral nerve injuries are associated with traumatic fractures of specific bones. For example, the radial nerve is particularly vulnerable to injury from fractures of the humerus. Traumatic injuries of the radial nerve classically occur with fractures of the shaft of the humerus at the level of the spiral groove. Such injuries result in weakness of wrist extension, finger extension, and thumb extension, as well as numbness over the radial aspect of the dorsal surface of the hand. In this type of injury, elbow extension is not affected, since muscular branches to the triceps are given off proximal to the spiral groove.

Trauma to the brachial plexus can cause a wide array of neurological signs and symptoms. Clinical manifestations are determined by the location of the lesion within the brachial plexus as well as the severity of the injury. Erb-Duchenne palsy is a well-described condition involving injury primarily to the upper trunk of the brachial plexus (derived from C5 and C6 nerve roots). It typically results from a stretch injury such as traction on the arm at the time of birth or a fall that forcefully separates the head from the shoulder. The resulting deficits to the deltoid, biceps, rhomboids, brachioradialis, supraspinatus, and infraspinatus leave the arm hanging to the side, internally rotated and extended at the elbow. This posture is often called the "waiter's tip" position.

▶ Differential Diagnosis

In acute trauma, when unilateral limb findings are present, it is important to rule out acute radiculopathy from peripheral nerve injury. A thorough neurological examination is critical. Several general principles should be considered. Radiculopathy is often accompanied by neck or back pain, which tends to radiate down an arm or a leg. Also, the sensory findings of radiculopathy tend to be blurred, reflecting the overlapping nature of dermatomes, while sensory findings in peripheral nerve injuries are sharply demarcated. Weakness from radiculopathy occurs in muscles innervated by one spinal nerve, but by more than one peripheral nerve. Thus, it is often only partial weakness, since nearly all muscles are innervated by more than one spinal nerve.

One crucial task in diagnosing acute peripheral nerve trauma is to rule out ongoing neural compression. Acute trauma to a peripheral nerve usually results in maximal deficits at the time of injury. A peripheral nerve deficit that progresses should raise a red flag and initiate further workup. Immediate surgical exploration should be considered in order to address compressive lesions such as expanding hematomas or growing traumatic pseudoaneurysms. Sources of ongoing neurologic compression should be removed as soon as possible.

▶ Treatment & Prognosis

Sharp nerve transections with clean ends (eg, knife wounds) should be repaired within 3 days. The repair should be performed in an end-to-end fashion, with no tension across the repair site. Transections from penetrating trauma that do not have clean edges or where significant tissue loss is present should be repaired in a delayed fashion. During exploration of the wound, transected nerve stumps should

be identified and tagged. The tagged nerve endings should be attached to fascia to reduce the possibility of retraction. After 3 weeks, the lesion should be reexplored and the injured nerve repaired. At that time, areas of axonal damage and neuroma formation are easier to visualize. Better visualization of damaged axons reduces the possibility of subsequent neuroma formation at the site of repair.

In the case of nonpenetrating injury, where stretch or temporary compression is the likely etiology of the problem, recovery often occurs spontaneously, without the need for surgery. In these cases, nonoperative management with serial neurological examinations, including electrophysiologic testing, should be the initial treatment modality. If, after 3 months, there is no sign of clinical recovery, the injured nerve should be explored. Intraoperative electrophysiologic nerve mapping should be performed to determine if there is conduction across the site of injury. If there is no conduction of evoked potentials, the neuroma should be resected. The stubs should be trimmed and brought together primarily if it can be done without creating tension. If primary anastomoses of the two nerve ends would result in tension across the repair, then a nerve graft should be employed (usually sural). If intraoperative stimulation reveals conduction across an area of injury, than the nerve should be left intact and allowed to regenerate on its own. A well-known mnemonic for remembering the appropriate timing of operative repair for traumatic nerve injuries is the rule of 3s: 3 days for a sharp transection, 3 weeks for an open ragged transection, and 3 months for a closed stretch injury.

Peripheral nerve repair is generally performed under the microscope using 8-0 or 9-0 suture for coaptation. Many surgeons now use tissue glue rather than suture to coapt the nerve endings. In the case of nerve root avulsions, which cannot be repaired directly, nerve transfer procedures may be employed, such as coapting a fascicle from an intact ulnar nerve to a nonfunctioning musculocutaneous nerve in order to restore elbow flexion.

Prognosis for recovery depends on the type of injury as well as the treatment. Axonal regeneration occurs at a rate of 1 inch per month, proximally to distally. Thus, clinical recovery may proceed slowly. Maximal recovery occurs over the course of approximately 1 to 2 years. Rehabilitation and physical therapy is important for avoiding the development of muscle contractures that may limit mobility when nerve function has returned. Tendon transfers may be of assistance if neural function does not completely recover.

PERIPHERAL ENTRAPMENT NEUROPATHIES

▶ General Considerations

Peripheral nerves are subjected to chronic mechanical forces, such as compression, stretching, and friction. These forces, when applied over time, may lead to peripheral nerve entrapment syndromes, such as carpal tunnel syndrome, or ulnar nerve entrapment. Both static and dynamic factors may contribute to chronic peripheral nerve injury. Static factors include musculotendinous anomalies or inflexible anatomic tunnels that compress peripheral nerves. Dynamic factors include mobile joints, muscular contraction, or nerve mobility that leads to stretching of a peripheral nerve or increased friction along its course during movement. Peripheral entrapment neuropathies occur more frequently in upper than in lower limbs, probably because of the greater mobility of the arms.

► Clinical Findings

Entrapment neuropathies are characterized by weakened muscles as well as sensory disturbances in the distribution of a single peripheral nerve. In general, any given individual muscle is supplied by one peripheral nerve. Thus, entrapment of a peripheral nerve can lead to severe motor findings in a muscle it innervates. Muscle atrophy and fasciculations are not uncommon in peripheral nerve entrapment. Marked atrophy on clinical examination should raise the surgeon's suspicion that a peripheral nerve lesion is present. Sensory complaints associated with entrapment neuropathy generally include paresthesias, rather than pain, in the distribution of the involved nerve. Percussion over the nerve may result in an electric sensation radiating along the nerve and its territory. In the clinical setting, this is known as Tinel sign. Electrodiagnostic testing is also useful in the diagnosis of peripheral nerve entrapment. The finding of a nerve conduction delay at the site of compression on nerve conduction studies is common to all compression neuropathies.

The most common peripheral nerve entrapment syndrome is median nerve entrapment at the wrist. This condition generally arises from compression of the median nerve by the transverse carpal ligament and is therefore referred to as carpal tunnel syndrome. Carpal tunnel syndrome occurs with higher frequency in patients with conditions leading to connective tissue thickening: rheumatoid arthritis, acromegaly, hypothyroidism, and pregnancy. It may be related to repetitive hand or wrist movements. Common presenting symptoms include dysesthetic pain in the hands that is worse at night, often awaking the patient from sleep. This occurs because many people sleep with flexed wrists, a position which exacerbates median nerve compression at the wrist. The pain sometimes radiates upwards, into the forearm. Patients also complain of numbness on the palmar side of the hand as well as in the first 3 digits, including the thumb, and sometimes extending to the ring finger. When the ring finger is involved, the sensory disturbance "splits" the finger, involving the radial side of the digit only. The intrinsic hand muscles innervated by the median nerve in the hand are sometimes referred to as the LOAF muscles, stemming from a commonly used mnemonic device: lumbricals (first and second only), opponens pollicis, abductor pollicis brevis, and flexor pollicis brevis. Patients with carpal tunnel syndrome may complain of decreased grip strength and difficulty grasping small objects. Atrophy of the abductor pollicis

brevis at the lateral base of the thumb may be present. There is often a positive Tinel sign at the wrist. The Phalen test is a clinical maneuver that is sometimes used in the diagnosis of carpal tunnel syndrome. The patient's wrists are held in forced flexion for at least 30 seconds. The test is considered positive if this maneuver produces symptoms of median neuropathy in the hand.

Ulnar nerve entrapment is the second-most common peripheral nerve entrapment syndrome, behind carpal tunnel syndrome. The most common site of ulnar nerve entrapment is at the elbow. Patients typically present with upper extremity pain that localizes to the medial aspect of the elbow. Paresthesias and numbness of the small finger and the ulnar half of the ring finger are also common. A Tinel sign is often present at the medial aspect of the elbow: tapping the patient over this area sends electric sensations into the fourth and fifth digits. The ulnar nerve innervates most of the intrinsic hand muscles, including the adductor pollicis, the first dorsal interosseous, and the hypothenar muscles. Patients complain of hand weakness, leading to reduced grip strength and pinch strength. They complain of dropping things or of trouble opening jars. Atrophy of hand intrinsic muscles may be marked, particularly the first dorsal interosseous and the muscles of the hypothenar eminence. When nerve dysfunction is severe, the hand may take on a "claw hand" appearance. The patient may also exhibit a Froment sign: when asked to hold a piece of paper between the thumb and index finger, the distal interphalangeal joint will flex because the patient fires the flexor pollicis longus muscle, innervated by the median nerve, to compensate for lack of abductor pollicis function.

► Differential Diagnosis

The differential diagnosis for peripheral nerve dysfunction includes neuropathies of infectious origin (both bacterial and viral), hereditary conditions (such as Charcot-Marie-Tooth disease), neuropathy associated with nutritional deficiency (such as vitamin B_{12} deficiency), metabolic or endocrinologic conditions (such as diabetes), inflammatory or immune-mediated conditions (such as polyarteritis nodosa), and toxic conditions (such as lead poisoning.) When more than one peripheral nerve is involved, the surgeon should be wary of the diagnosis of generalized neuropathy, which is typically symmetrical and bilateral. Decreased amplitude on electrodiagnostic studies (which suggests axonal loss) is characteristic of neuropathy of hereditary or metabolic origin. Peripheral nerve entrapment, on the other hand, causes damage to the myelin surrounding an axon, thereby slowing conduction velocity but not affecting amplitude.

Chronic cervical or lumbar radiculopathy must also be ruled out. Several features that distinguish radiculopathy from peripheral nerve dysfunction were outlined in the section on acute peripheral nerve injuries. It is important to recognize that sensory changes that "split" the ring finger suggest ulnar nerve dysfunction rather than C8 radiculopathy.

Treatment & Prognosis

Surgical management of peripheral nerve entrapment generally involves decompressing the involved nerve. In the case of carpal tunnel syndrome, the transverse carpal ligament is divided, thus relieving compression on the median nerve as it passes from the wrist into the hand. In the case of ulnar neuropathy, simply freeing the nerve from surrounding scar tissue or hypertrophied connective tissue (external neurolysis) is usually sufficient; however, most surgeons will also transpose the nerve anterior to the medial epicondyle.

Surgical management of peripheral nerve entrapment should be strongly considered when patients present with significant motor weakness or muscle atrophy. Surgical intervention should also be considered when patients fail to improve with medical treatments. Nonoperative management strategies include avoidance of repetitive activities that precipitate symptoms or the use of immobilization braces that hold joints in positions that avoid compression.

Carpal tunnel release results in excellent relief of symptoms in 80% of patients and partial relief in another 10%. Similar results are observed for surgical management of ulnar neuropathy.

PERIPHERAL NERVE TUMORS

General Considerations

Peripheral nerve tumors can be divided into nonneoplastic masses, benign masses, and malignant masses. The nonneoplastic masses include traumatic neuromas, Morton neuromas, and nerve sheath ganglion cysts. Benign masses include neurofibromas, schwannomas (also know as neurilemmoma), perineuriomas, lipofibromatous hamartoma (also known as neural fibrolipoma), nerve sheath myxoma, and granular cell tumors. Malignant masses include the malignant peripheral nerve sheath tumor.

Neurofibromas can be subdivided into solitary, diffuse, and plexiform varieties. The solitary neurofibroma is the most common benign peripheral nerve tumor. Axons are incorporated within the neurofibroma along with Schwann cells, collagen matrix, perineurial cells, and fibroblasts. Because the axons are intermixed within the tumor, the tumor cannot be excised without resecting a portion of the involved nerve. Diffuse neurofibromas and plexiform neurofibromas are less common than the solitary variety. The diffuse neurofibroma typically involves the skin and subcutaneous tissues. Plexiform neurofibroma are large, irregular expansions of nerves ranging from small cutaneous nerves to large trunks. Neurofibromas are commonly found in patients with neurofibromatosis type 1 (NF1, or von Recklinghausen disease).

Schwannomas are slow-growing lesions made up of Schwann cells in a collagen matrix. Differentiating schwannomas from neurofibromas is that the nerve fascicles run alongside the tumor rather than through the tumor as in neurofibromas. Schwannomas are the second-most com-

mon peripheral nerve tumor. Generally, only mild neurologic deficits occur, and operative resection can be considered in the setting of pain, paresthesias, or weakness in the distribution of the nerve.

Malignant peripheral nerve sheath tumor is the most common malignant peripheral nerve tumor. Nearly two thirds arise from neurofibromas in the setting of von Recklinghausen disease. The remainder arise either de novo or in patients with history of prior external beam radiation.

Clinical Findings

The symptoms of peripheral nerve tumors are generally related to the nerve involved and include weakness, numbness, paresthesias, and pain. MRI with gadolinium contrast can be useful in imaging the tumors.

Differential Diagnosis

The differential diagnosis of peripheral nerve tumors include entrapment neuropathies, nonneoplastic masses, radiculopathies, and neuropathies associated with infection, malnutrition, metabolic, endocrinologic, inflammatory, immune-mediated, and toxic conditions. Generally, a symptomatic peripheral nerve tumor will be palpable. Further, the peripheral nerve tumor can occur anywhere along the course of the nerve, whereas entrapment neuropathies typically occur in defined locations, and the various other neuropathies listed are often diffuse processes. Finally, a radiculopathy will be symptomatic in the distribution of the nerve root, likely involving several peripheral nerves.

Treatment & Prognosis

Schwannomas can generally be resected without any neurologic deficit, since the nerve fascicles run alongside the tumor. The fascicles can generally be dissected free. Operative resection is curative. Neurofibromas generally cannot be resected without neurologic deficit because the axons run within the substance of the tumor. Indications for surgical resection of solitary neurofibromas are large tumor mass, accelerated growth, neurologic deficit, and pain. Plexiform neurofibromas (excluding superficial ones) can rarely be totally resected and should generally be followed.

The prognosis for benign peripheral nerve sheath tumors generally is very good with improvement in pain, weakness, paresthesias noted after resection of solitary lesions. Malignant peripheral nerve sheath tumors require aggressive surgical treatment. The expected 5-year survival is 15% to 20% in patients with von Recklinghausen disease and 56% in patients with de novo disease.

Grant GA, Goodkin R, Kliot M: Evaluation and surgical management of peripheral nerve problems. Neurosurgery 1999;44:825.
Mondelli M et al: Mononeuropathies of the radial nerve: clinical and neurographic findings in 91 consecutive cases. J Electromyogr Kinesiol 2005;15:377.

Russell SM, Kline DG: Complication avoidance in peripheral nerve surgery: preoperative evaluation of nerve injuries and brachial plexus exploration—part 1. Neurosurgery 206;59(ONS suppl 4):ONS-441.

▼ BRAIN TUMORS

Daniel Orringer, MD, & Shawn Hervey-Jumper, MD

▶ Clinical Presentation

Whenever possible, the evaluation of a brain tumor patient begins with a detailed history focusing on the most common symptoms observed in patients bearing intracranial mass lesions. Headaches are the most common symptom in brain tumor patients, occurring in at least 50% of patients at some point. Classically, brain tumor patients present with headaches that are worse upon waking in the morning or severe enough to wake a patient from sleep. This type of headache is thought to occur as a result of temporary increases in intracranial pressure caused by physiologic elevations in P_{CO_2} common during sleep. Normally, transient increases in P_{CO_2} that occur during sleep do not result in headache. However, in the patient with brain tumor, during sleep, the combination of elevated intracranial pressure due to mass effect from the presence of the tumor and cerebral vasodilation due to increased P_{CO_2} causes an additive increases in intracranial pressure, ultimately resulting in headache. Headaches related to elevated intracranial pressure can also occur throughout the day as a result of maneuvers that raise intracranial pressure, such as straining, coughing, and bending over.

More commonly, headaches seen in patients with brain tumor are not related to elevations in intracranial pressure. Headaches typically caused by brain tumors occur as the neoplastic process involves intracranial structures containing pain fibers. Unlike the brain parenchyma, the dura is richly innervated with pain fibers and is likely the most common source of headaches in patients with brain tumor. Dural irritation is also involved in the pathogenesis of other types of headaches. This pathophysiologic overlap may explain the clinical observation that brain tumor–associated headaches may lack any distinguishing characteristics. Patients often describe their headaches as deep and aching, but these features are highly variable and may have been previously misdiagnosed as sinus, tension, or migraine headaches. Headaches in patients with brain tumor may also be due to vision difficulties in the setting of tumor involvement with the optic pathways and oculomotor nerves.

A number of attributes of the headaches associated with brain tumors can provide useful diagnostic information. First, brain tumors in patients who present with headaches are more likely to be found in noneloquent or functionally silent areas of the central nervous system. Second, headaches occur more frequently in patients with rapidly growing brain tumors. Rapidly growing brain tumors commonly cause severe head-aches from meningeal irritation, hemorrhage within the tumor, and/or obstructive hydrocephalus. Obstructive hydrocephalus is a neurosurgical emergency that must be considered in any brain tumor patient presenting with the acute onset of severe headache. In addition, the location of headache commonly provides localizing information. Brain tumors are usually located ipsilateral to the most severe pain.

Seizures are another common presenting finding in patients with brain tumors. Interestingly, seizures are more common with low-grade gliomas than with high-grade gliomas. The incidence of seizures in patients with low-grade glioma is estimated as high as 85%. Seizures are the initial presenting symptom in 9% of patients with metastatic brain tumors and 18% of patients with high-grade glioma. Moreover, 25% to 50% of all patients with brain tumors experience seizures at some point in their disease course. While seizures associated with brain tumors can be disabling, they can also lead to early diagnosis and therefore early treatment.

The nature of seizure activity may hold diagnostic significance. Subcortical and cortical tumors are more likely to cause seizures than are those of deeper structures. Focal seizures with primarily motor phenomena, such as tonic-clonic seizures, often affect the primary motor cortex within the frontal lobe. Focal temporal lobe seizures typically have variable manifestations that may make it difficult to localize a lesion. Focal seizures due to parietal lesions may present with aphasia, sensory abnormalities, or vestibular symptoms. Focal seizures caused by brain tumors may be secondarily generalized and may ultimately affect multiple cortical regions, causing variable symptomatology. Status epilepticus also can occur as a presentation of brain tumors.

Syncope, another common presentation of brain tumor, must be distinguished from seizure. There are multiple pathophysiologic mechanisms underlying syncope in patients with brain tumor. In patients with tumor burden resulting in chronically elevated intracranial pressure and decreased brain compliance, a sudden additional rise in intracranial pressure may compromise cerebral blood flow, resulting in syncope. Transient increases in intracranial pressure that may result from sneezing, coughing, vomiting, or straining are tolerated in patients with normal physiology but may cause syncope in patients with brain tumor. Syncope caused by transient increases in intracranial pressure may represent impending herniation and requires urgent neurosurgical attention.

A number of additional symptoms commonly present in association with headache, seizure, or syncope. Nausea and vomiting are present at the initial encounter with at least 40% of patients with brain tumors. Nausea and vomiting may be caused by elevations in intracranial pressure and/or direct tumor involvement of the area postrema in the dorsal surface of the fourth ventricle.

Cognitive decline is common especially in the elderly patient and is often misdiagnosed as Alzheimer disease. Cognitive decline may easily be confused with depression and is thought to result from generalized fatigue, loss of appetite, and lack of interest in everyday activities. Frontal tumors are commonly associated with cognitive decline. Frontal masses, especially those affecting both frontal lobes, may also result in apraxia and urinary retention.

A key component of the interview of the patient with brain tumor is the past medical and family history. The incidence of CNS metastases is increasing due to improved survival in patients with the most common types of solid organ cancers. A family history of brain tumors may suggest a familial cancer syndrome. Among the most common familial syndromes predisposing to brain tumor occurrence include von Hippel Lindau syndrome, tuberous sclerosis, neurofibromatosis 1 and 2, Turcot syndrome (familial adenomatous polyposis), and Lynch syndrome (hereditary nonpolyposis colorectal cancer).

▶ Physical Findings

Physical findings are highly variable depending on tumor location and extent of disease. Nonspecific physical findings, including papilledema (edema of the head of the optic nerve associated with engorgement of retinal veins) and oculomotor palsy (due to uncal herniation), can occur with elevated intracranial pressure. However, the most helpful physical findings are those that assist in localizing the lesion (Table 36–5). Focal neurologic signs such as muscle weakness are common and, when caused by peritumoral edema, may be rapidly reversible with the administration of steroids.

Aphasia suggests involvement with cortical language centers located in the dominant frontal or parietal lobe. Aphasic patients may be misdiagnosed with dementia or psychiatric disorders. The diagnosis of brain tumor should be considered in patients without psychiatric history who develop a psychiatric disorder.

▶ Imaging

Radiographic imaging is performed to confirm the clinical diagnosis of brain tumor. Imaging provides information regarding localization, tumor type, and the effect of a lesion on surrounding structures. Due to its wide availability, speed, and affordability, noncontrast CT is commonly the initial screening test for patients with brain tumors. CT is also the test of choice for evaluating the extent of tumor invasion into adjacent bony structures. CT angiography can be helpful in evaluating blood supply to tumors and the relationship of blood vessels to the tumor.

Whenever possible, MRI of the brain with and without gadolinium-based contrast is performed. Traditional morphologic MRI assesses tumor location, size, cellularity, associated cystic components, associated edema or hemorrhage, necrosis, margins and invasion into surrounding structures, vascularity, and enhancement. Morphologic data can be used to estimate the World Health Organization (WHO) grade and suggest the tissue diagnosis of a lesion. However,

Table 36–5. Brain Tumor Localizing Signs and Symptoms.

Location	Sign(s)
Frontal lobe[a]	Impaired intellectual function
	Language impairment,[b] specifically abulia
	Impaired gait
	Personality changes
	Hemiparesis[c]
Dominant temporal lobe	Aphasia
	Impaired auditory discrimination
	Memory loss
	Contralateral superior quadrantanopia
Nondominant temporal lobe	Seizures
	Visual, auditory, olfactory hallucinations
	Contralateral superior quadrantanopia
Uncus	CN III palsy
Parietal lobe	Impaired sensory perception
	Contralateral inferior quadrantanopia
	Aphasia
	Anosoagnosia[d]
Occipital lobe	Visual deficits
Posterior fossa	Posterior headache
	Neck stiffness
	Opisthotonos
Brainstem	Cranial nerve palsies
	Long-tract signs
Cerebellopontine angle	Unilateral hearing loss
	Tinnitus
	Vertigo
	Facial palsy
	Facial anesthesia
	Cerebellar signs
Sellar region	Endocrine abnormalities
	Bitemporal hemianopsia
	CN III palsy
Pineal region	Parinaud syndrome:
	upgaze palsy
	ptosis
	loss of pupillary light reflex
	retraction-convergence nystagmus
Meningeal infiltration	Cranial nerve palsies
	Diffuse headache
	Meningeal reaction

[a]Usually occurs only if both frontal lobes involved.
[b]Occurs only when dominant hemisphere is involved.
[c]When motor cortex is involved.
[d]When nondominant temporal lobe is involved.

the gold standard for brain tumor diagnosis remains tissue histology. High-quality contrast MRI images are vital for defining the relationship of tumor tissue to eloquent cortical areas and, consequently, for developing an operative plan. In addition, MRI images can be reconstructed to create 3D models that can be used during surgery.

Metabolic MRI or MR spectroscopy can be used to supplement information obtained from traditional morphologic MRI. MR spectroscopy is used to compare the small molecule content of tumor tissue and normal surrounding brain tissue. MR spectroscopy improves the accuracy of brain tumor diagnosis by differentiating brain tumors from lesions that appear similar on routine MRI, such as abscesses. In addition, MR spectroscopy detects subtle changes in small molecule content that correlate with tumor grade. In treated brain tumors, MR spectroscopy enables differentiation between radiation necrosis and residual tumor.

A number of alternative MR techniques have clinical application in the imaging of brain tumors. These can enable clinicians to make more accurate preoperative diagnoses and provide information about interaction of tumor tissue with adjacent functional cortical structures. Diffusion MRI characterizes brain tumors on the basis of measurement of molecular mobility and is useful in differentiating tumors from similar-appearing lesions, estimating cellularity, and measuring response to treatment. Perfusion MRI is useful for evaluating tumor angiogenesis, endothelial permeability, and response to treatment. Functional MRI maps functional cortical areas and can be used to create an operative corridor or plan for resection that minimizes risk to eloquent surrounding structures. Similarly, diffusion tensor imaging defines the integrity of white matter tracts surrounding a tumor and is commonly used in the planning of both surgical and radiation therapy.

Traditional catheter-based cerebral angiography has both historical and contemporary significance in brain tumor imaging. Cerebral angiography was once used to infer tumor location and morphology by measuring displacement of blood vessels by a tumor. Currently, angiography is used in the context of highly vascular lesions, including some meningiomas and hemangiomas, for preoperative embolization. Embolization of vascular tumors diminishes operative risk and difficulty.

▶ Tumor Types

A. Gliomas

Fifty percent of newly diagnosed brain tumors are primary tumors of glial origin (astrocytes and oligodendrocytes). Glial tumors are stratified in a scale of increasing aggressiveness. Grades 1 and 2 are classified as low-grade gliomas; grades 3 and 4 are high-grade. High-grade gliomas grow faster and consequently carry a worse prognosis than low-grade gliomas.

1. Low-grade gliomas: astrocytes, oligodendroglio-mas, and mixed gliomas—Approximately 26% of newly diagnosed glial tumors are astrocytomas, and 2% are oligo-

dendrogliomas. Between 1500 and 1800 new low-grade gliomas are diagnosed in the United States each year. WHO grade 1 gliomas are reserved for pilocytic tumors. Pilocytic astrocytomas represent 6% of all primary intracranial tumors and 20% of all brain tumors in children younger than 15 years of age. WHO grade 2 lesions are diagnosed on the basis of their infiltration and tendency to progress to higher-grade lesions over time. The most common subtypes of low-grade gliomas include juvenile astrocytomas, diffuse astrocytomas, oligodendrogliomas, and mixed gliomas.

The etiology of low-grade gliomas is unknown. Genetic studies suggest that mutation or deletion of the tumor suppressor gene *TP53* plays a role in the tumorigenesis of low-grade gliomas. While oligodendrogliomas rarely show a mutation in *TP53*, there is often a loss of the long arm of chromosome 1 and the short arm of chromosome 19.

Low-grade astrocytomas occur with peak incidence in the young adult population (most commonly in the 20s to 40s age range). They originate in white matter regions within the central nervous system, grow slowly, and distort surrounding brain structures. Histologically, there is a modest increase in cellularity, disruption of the normal orderly pattern of glial cells, and elongated nuclei. There is no endothelial proliferation or tissue necrosis. Three histologic subtypes of low-grade astrocytomas include fibrillary, gemistocytic, and protoplasmic.

Oligodendrogliomas occur predominantly within the gray matter of the cerebral hemispheres, are well circumscribed and calcified, and have a slight predominance for the frontal lobes. Like astrocytomas, they occur predominantly in younger patients with most frequent diagnosis in the third decade of life. Histologically, oligodendrogliomas are characterized by uniform cell density and round nuclei with perinuclear halos having a classic "fried egg" appearance.

Radiographically, low-grade gliomas are isodense or hypodense to brain on CT scan and do not enhance with contrast. Calcification is common in oligodendrogliomas. On MRI, low-grade glioma are isointense to hypointense on T1-weighted imaging and typically hyperintense on T2-weighted imaging and are not contrast enhancing.

2. High-grade gliomas—*Malignant gliomas* include anaplastic astrocytoma (AA), glioblastoma multiforme (GBM), gliosarcoma, and malignant oligodendroglioma (Figure 36–13). There is wide difference in the prognosis, aggressiveness, and response to therapy among the different tumors in this group.

Malignant astrocytoma, the most common type of adult brain tumor, makes up 15% of all intracranial tumors and 50% to 60% of primary brain tumors. While relatively rare, malignant astrocytoma is the fourth most common cause of cancer-related deaths. The incidence of anaplastic astrocytomas and glioblastoma multiforme increases with age. There is little difference in incidence among nations, but in the United States, these tumors are less common among Africans and African Americans.

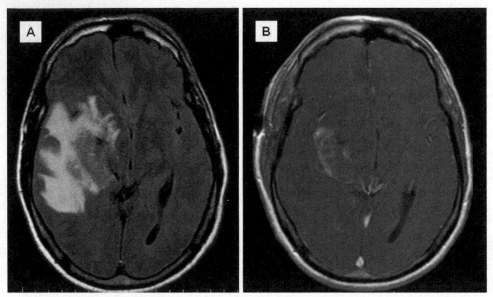

▲ **Figure 36–13.** MRI of a deep right temporal mass proven to be a high-grade glioma. **A:** Fluid-attenuated inversion recovery imaging demonstrating a mass with significant surrounding white matter edema. **B:** T1-weighted contrast-enhanced image demonstrating smaller enhancing portion of the mass.

Most malignant gliomas occur sporadically. However, patients with the autosomal recessively inherited Turcot syndrome have a high rate of malignant glioma (usually medulloblastomas and astrocytomas) in combination with familial adenomatous polyposis. Similarly, patients with tuberous sclerosis and neurofibromatosis types 1 and 2 often develop brain tumors, including gliomas.

Several tumor suppressor genes have been identified in malignant gliomas. Mutations of *TP53* have been identified in the autosomal dominantly inherited Li-Fraumeni syndrome, which results in malignant gliomas in addition to tumors involving breast, blood, bone, and the adrenal cortex. Loss of *TP53* function occurs in approximately 30% of gliomas. Another 33% of malignant gliomas exhibit an amplification of the gene encoding for the epidermal growth factor receptor *(EGFR)*. Growing evidence suggests that stem cells give rise to astrocytes with neoplastic potential and promote tumor growth and recurrence.

A hallmark of malignant gliomas is the propensity to invade and migrate along white matter tracts. Invasion increases with increased grade, and growth factors such as epidermal growth factor (EGF) increase this invasion. Autopsy studies show that malignant glioma cells spread through the CSF and extend into and beyond areas on MRI with T2 signal change. Histologically, grade 3 gliomas show mitotic activity and nuclear atypia but no necrosis, while grade 4 tumors have nuclear atypia, mitoses, endothelial proliferation, and areas of necrosis. The radiologic hallmarks of glioblastoma multiforme are ring enhancement and areas of central necrosis detected on CT and MRI.

3. Gangliogliomas—Gangliogliomas are rare tumors found most commonly in patients between the ages of 15 and 20 with a history of seizures. They can be found in any region of the central nervous system but seem to occur predominantly in the temporal lobes. Gangliogliomas are distinguished histologically from pure gliomas by their mixture of neuronal and glial elements. Calcification is common. Macroscopically, they may appear solid or cystic. They are generally well-circumscribed, cystic tumors that may display a mural nodule projecting into the cyst cavity. Imaging characteristics vary in their enhancement and signal qualities on MRI. Lesions can exhibit cystic or solid components or a combination of both. Tumor calcification is a common imaging feature.

4. Brainstem gliomas—Brainstem gliomas represent 10% to 20% of all CNS tumors in children. Brainstem gliomas are a heterogeneous group with diverse clinical presentations, prognoses, and patterns of growth. They are described as focal, diffuse, cervicomedullary, and dorsally exophytic. Focal tumors are less than 2 cm in size with a well-circumscribed appearance on MRI and no surrounding edema. They are most prevalent in the midbrain and medulla but can occur at any level in the brainstem. Children with brainstem gliomas typically present with focal cranial nerve deficits and contralateral hemiparesis. Diffuse tumors account for the majority of brainstem gliomas (80%) and commonly arise in the pons. These patients typically present with bilateral cranial nerve deficits, ataxia, and long-tract signs. Cervicomedullary brainstem gliomas originate in the upper cervical cord and extend rostrally into the cervicomedullary junction and often present with lower cranial nerve deficits and long-tract signs. Dorsal exophytic tumors account for 20% of brainstem gliomas and arise from the floor of the fourth ventricle. They are typically sharply delineated from surrounding structures. These patients typically present with cranial nerve deficits, elevated intracranial pressure, and failure to thrive.

MRI scan has allowed for the recognition of the four classes of brainstem glioma. Even though MRI contrast signal poorly correlates with histologic grade, MRI provides adequate anatomic visualization. Focal tumors are classically well circumscribed and small without infiltration or a significant amount of surrounding edema. Dorsal exophytic tumors arise in the floor of the fourth ventricle and are typically hypointense on T1-weighted imaging, hyperintense on T2-weighted imaging, and homogenously enhance with gadolinium contrast. Diffuse brainstem tumors are hypointense on T1-weighted images and hyperintense on T2 sequences. Because the MRI characteristics for diffuse tumors are highly specific, biopsy is not generally necessary for diffuse brainstem tumors.

B. Primitive Neuroectodermal Tumors

Primitive neuroectodermal tumors (PNETs) originate in cells from the primitive neural crest. PNETs include medulloblastomas, pinealoblastomas, ependymoblastomas, esthesioneuroblastomas, and neuroblastomas. They are more common in children than in adults. Medulloblastomas are PNETs within the posterior fossa and account for 20% of childhood brain tumors and 1% of all adult tumors. Medulloblastomas are the most common primary CNS tumor in children younger than 18 years.

Several syndromes express an increased incidence of medulloblastomas, including tuberous sclerosis, neurofibromatosis, Gorlin syndrome, and Turcot syndrome. Loss of portions of chromosome 17 either through deletions or unbalanced translocation is associated with over 50% of medulloblastomas.

Grossly, medulloblastomas typically occur within the cerebellar vermis and are poorly demarcated, purplish, soft, and friable. Histologically, these tumors are highly cellular, composed of homogenous fields of small, round, blue-cell tumors with hyperchromatic nuclei, minimal cytoplasm, and occasional calcification. Other histologic characteristics include varying degrees of neuronal and glial differentiation, Homer Wright rosettes (nuclei surround a clear central area of cell processes indicative of neuroblastic differentiation) are often present, and mitotic figures are numerous.

Meduloblastomas are PNETs within the posterior fossa. Histologically similar tumors within the pineal gland are pinealoblastomas, and within the supratentorial space, are neuroblastomas. Retinoblastomas are histologically similar tumors within the eye; PNETs originating from olfactory epithelium are termed esthesioneuroblastomas; and intraventricular PNETs are ependymoblastomas.

On CT scan, medulloblastomas are typically hyperdense, homogenously enhancing, and occasionally cystic. Small areas of calcification can be appreciated on CT. Scattered areas of hemorrhage, necrosis, and calcification can occur. On MRI, medulloblastomas are isointense or hypointense to brain on T1-weighted imaging, hyperintense to brain on T2-weighted imaging, and intensely contrast enhancing. If medulloblastoma is suspected, MRI of the spine is obtained to rule out metastases. Lumbar puncture should be performed with extreme caution because the majority of children have associated obstructive hydrocephalus.

C. Pineal Tumors

The pineal gland is bounded ventrally by the quadrigeminal plate and midbrain tectum, dorsally by the splenium of corpus callosum, rostrally by the posterior aspect of the third ventricle, and caudally by the cerebellar vermis. Tumors in this region are usually found incidentally on MRI and are most common in children, making up 3% to 8% of pediatric brain tumors. The pineal region has several diverse cell types, including glial cells, arachnoid cells, pineal glandular tissue, ependymal lining, sympathetic nerves, germ cells, and remnants of ectoderm. Tumors within this area can therefore be grouped into 4 categories: germ cell tumors, pineal parenchymal cell tumors, glial cell tumors, and other miscellaneous tumors and cysts. In the pediatric population, germinomas and astrocytomas are the most common tumor type. Germ cell tumors and pineal cell tumors occur primarily during childhood. In the adult population, pineal tumors are more commonly gliomas and meningiomas.

Germ cell tumors, ependymomas, and pineal cell tumors can metastasize through the CSF, causing myelopathic or radiculopathic symptoms. Pineal tumors typically present with symptoms of increased intracranial pressure from obstructive hydrocephalus, direct brainstem and cerebellar compression, and endocrine dysfunction. In addition, Parinaud syndrome (upgaze paralysis, convergence-retraction nystagmus, pseudo-Argyll Robertson pupils, eyelid retraction, and conjugate downgaze in the primary position) is associated with pineal tumors.

MRI is the primary diagnostic imaging modality for pineal tumors, but it does not reliably predict tumor histology. In contrast, tumor markers may be useful in the diagnostic process, to determine response to treatment, or as an indicator of early recurrence. Elevation of serum or CSF α-fetoprotein or human chorionic gonadotropin suggests a germ cell tumor. Mildly elevated α-fetoprotein suggests the presence of a fetal yolk sac tumor. Marked elevation of α-fetoprotein suggests endodermal sinus tumors, while smaller elevations suggest embryonal cell carcinoma or immature teratoma. Human chorionic gonadotropin is often markedly elevated with choriocarcinomas.

D. Ependymoma

Ependymomas arise from the ependymal cells lining the ventricles and central canal of the spinal cord. They occur in both children and adults, and 65% occur within the posterior fossa (most commonly in children). Ependymomas are quite rare, representing only 6% of all gliomas and 10% of all primary tumors found in children. Three cases per 100,000 children younger than 15 are diagnosed each year with this tumor type.

The etiology of most ependymomas is unknown. Familial cases have been identified. As with several other primary CNS tumors, these tumors often have loss of heterozygosity of chromosome 22q, which contains the neurofibromatosis 2 (NF2) gene. Patients with neurofibromatosis have an increased incidence of gliomas, including ependymomas.

A histologic grading system that correlates with tumor aggressiveness is used to classify ependymomas. Histologically, ependymomas are often characterized by epithelium-like cells in a rosette pattern formed by a ring of polygonal cells surrounding a central cavity. Tumors may also exhibit perivascular pseudorosettes, intranuclear inclusions, calcifications, and papillary clusters.

The imaging characteristics of ependymomas are variable, but they are typically isodense to cerebral cortex on noncontrast head CT. Calcifications and cystic components within the tumor are frequent. On MRI, the solid portion is typically isointense to gray matter on T1-weighted imaging and isointense to hyperintense on T2-weighted imaging.

E. Cerebral Lymphoma

Cerebral lymphoma involving the brain, spinal cord, or ocular structures can occur either primarily or as a metastasis. The source of premalignant lymphocytes is controversial because the central nervous system lacks lymphoid tissue. CNS lymphoma represents 1% of intracranial tumors with a steady increase in prevalence over the past 20 years. The increase in CNS lymphoma is likely secondary to the increased number and longer lifespan of patients with acquired immunodeficiency syndrome (AIDS) and immunosuppression after organ transplantation. While no clear genetic factors predispose to CNS lymphoma, this typically occurs in the context of acquired immunodeficiency, congenital immunodeficiency, autoimmune diseases, and Epstein-Barr virus infection. Deletions of DKN2A are frequently reported in CNS lymphoma.

Macroscopically, primary CNS lymphomas occur within the parenchyma, subependyma, or meninges and can be either circumscribed or irregular. Microscopically, they exhibit diffuse perivascular distribution and infiltrate the walls of blood vessels (perivascular cuffing). The tumor cells are similar in histology to systemic non-Hodgkin's lymphoma cells. Primary CNS lymphomas are usually monoclonal B-cell lymphomas of diffuse large cell or large cell immunoblastic variant. Anti-CD45 antibody staining differentiates CNS lymphoma from other tumor types.

On CT, CNS lymphomas are typically hyperdense or isodense to brain with strong contrast enhancement. On MRI, these tumors are usually isointense or hypointense on T1-weighted imaging, hyperintense on T2-weighted imaging, and display varying degrees of gadolinium enhancement. Low-volume lumbar puncture performed during the workup of CNS lymphoma may reveal high-protein, low-glucose pleocytosis. While CSF cytology may be diagnostic, stereotactic brain biopsy is often needed for definitive diagnosis.

F. Choroid Plexus Tumors

The most common tumors of the choroid plexus include choroid plexus papillomas. Choroid plexus carcinomas are rare. Choroid plexus papillomas are most prevalent in patients under age 2 and account for less than 1% of all intracranial tumors. Presenting symptoms result from elevated intracranial pressure due to hydrocephalus and mass effect from tumor growth.

G. Meningiomas

Meningiomas are typically benign, slow-growing extra-axial tumors arising from the arachnoid cap cells of the meninges (Figure 36–14). They can originate wherever arachnoid is present. They are characterized by either location or histopathology and are commonly located along the falx, cortical convexity, and sphenoid bone.

Meningiomas account for 15% to 19% of primary brain tumors, and as many as 3% of the population older than 60 years of age have an intracranial meningioma on autopsy. Their incidence increases with age and peaks by 45 years of age. There is a female-to-male ratio of 2:1.

Alterations in the long arm of chromosome 22 (22q12.3) likely have a role in the development of meningiomas. Loss of one copy of chromosome 22 occurs in up to 50% of

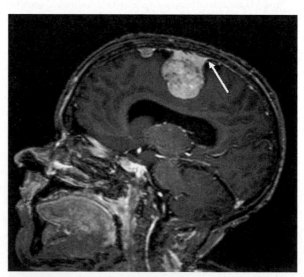

▲ **Figure 36–14.** Sagittal MRI image demonstrating a contrast-enhancing dural-based lesion (arrow) proven to be a meningioma at time of resection.

patients with meningioma. Chromosome 22q contains the *NF2* tumor suppressor gene, encoding Merlin, which is mutated in neurofibromatosis 2. Consequently, patients with neurofibromatosis 2 are more likely to develop intracranial meningioma of varying types.

There are multiple histologic subtypes of meningioma, but they are typically characterized by the presence of densely packed sheets of cells (similar to appearance of normal arachnoid cells), psammoma bodies (whorls of calcium and collagen), intranuclear cytoplasmic pseudoinclusions, and Orphan Annie nuclei (nuclei with central clearing from peripheral migration of chromatin). Radiographically, meningiomas are hyperdense to brain, and a broad dural attachment can often be identified. On T2-weighted MRI, most meningiomas are hyperintense and are typically contrast-enhancing on both CT and MRI.

H. Nerve Sheath Tumors and Acoustic Neuromas

Nerve sheath tumors are benign tumors of Schwann cell origin that predominantly involve cranial nerves V, VII, VIII, and X. The most common vestibular schwannomas (or *acoustic neuromas*) originate in the internal auditory canal from the inferior or superior portion of the vestibular nerve at the junction of the central and peripheral myelin. The three most common presenting symptoms include insidious hearing loss, high-pitched tinnitus, and disequilibrium.

Acoustic neuromas account for 8% to 10% of all intracranial tumors in adults. Most are unilateral; however, patients with neurofibromatosis 2 commonly have bilateral acoustic neuromas. Acoustic neuroma is believed to result from the loss of a tumor suppressor gene located on the long arm of chromosome of 22.

Macroscopically, acoustic neuromas are lobular, encapsulated, and solid with grayish colored material. Surrounding cranial nerves are often stretched over the capsule of the tumor. Microscopically, these tumors are identical to peripheral schwannomas. They are composed of Antoni A and Antoni B fibers. Antoni A fibers are dense, narrow, elongated bipolar cells with numerous nuclei and firm cytoplasm. Antoni B fibers are a loose, reticulated, semipalisading arrangement of Schwann cells.

CT is useful for distinguishing tumor extension into the bony internal auditory canal. On MRI, acoustic neuromas are isointense on T1-weighted imaging without contrast. With gadolinium enhancement, they are often homogenously enhancing. The lack of a dural tail differentiates acoustic neuromas from cerebellopontine angle meningiomas.

I. Pituitary Tumors

Pituitary adenomas are benign tumors originating from the anterior pituitary gland and represent 10% of intracranial tumors diagnosed. They are most commonly diagnosed in patients between 40 and 50 years of age. They are classified according to their endocrine function or histological staining. Secreting tumors release supraphysiologic levels of hormones that result in distinct clinical syndromes. Hypersecretion of prolactin causes amenorrhea-galactorrhea syndrome in women and impotence in men. Hypersecretion of adrenocorticotropic hormone causes Cushing disease. Hypersecretion of growth hormone causes acromegaly in adults and gigantism in children. Pituitary adenomas can hypersecrete thyrotropin (producing hyperthyroidism) or gonadotropins (luteinizing hormone and follicle-stimulating hormone).

Pituitary tumors may exert mass effect on adjacent structures. Optic chiasm compression results in bitemporal hemianopsia. Compression of the pituitary gland itself results in varying degrees of hypopituitarism. Compression on the cavernous sinus causes ptosis, facial pain, and diplopia from pressure on cranial nerves III, IV, V1, V2, and VI. Occlusion of the cavernous sinus may cause proptosis and chemosis.

J. Metastatic Brain Tumors

Metastatic brain tumors originate from malignancies outside of the central nervous system that have spread to the brain or spinal cord (Figure 36–15). They are the most common brain tumor with a yearly incidence of 100,000 to 200,000 cases per year in the United States. Autopsy studies show that 20% to 25% of patients with cancer have brain metastasis. Metastases occur more frequently in adults in their fifth to seventh decades of life. The most common primary tumors in adults giving rise to CNS metastases are lung, breast, skin, renal, and colon cancers. In children, leukemia and lymphoma, osteogenic sarcoma, and rhabdomyosarcoma are the most common primary tumors that spread to the central nervous system.

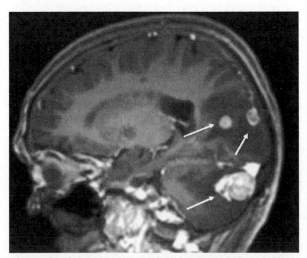

▲ **Figure 36–15.** Sagittal MRI image demonstrating multiple contrast-enhancing lesions (arrows) in the infratentorial and supratentorial spaces. Biopsy demonstrated metastatic adenocarcinoma.

Histopathology of metastases mirrors that of the primary tumor. MRI is more sensitive than CT in detecting metastases. Metastases are typically seen at the gray-white junction and show varying degrees of contrast enhancement.

Differential Diagnosis

The differential diagnosis of intracranial masses is narrowed through a detailed history and physical examination. Important considerations include patient demographics, chronology of symptoms, medical history, and specific neurologic deficits. Once imaging is obtained, the list of possible diagnoses can be further refined, as the location of a lesion can suggest its nature. For example, the three most common posterior fossa tumors of childhood include astrocytoma, medulloblastoma, and ependymoma. The most common tumors of the cerebellopontine angle include meningioma, acoustic neuroma, and epidermoid cyst. In addition, the pattern of contrast enhancement and whether the lesion appears to arise from within the brain parenchyma or meninges are important considerations in generating an accurate differential diagnosis.

Treatment

A. Preoperative Medical Management

With few exceptions, surgery is the backbone of the current treatment of brain tumors. The success of surgical intervention depends on adequate preoperative medical management and surgical planning. Steroids are commonly used preoperatively to reduce the symptoms of mass effect and edema caused by the tumor. The timing and dose of steroids varies according to surgeon preference. A common regimen for adults is dexamethasone, 6 mg intravenously or orally every 6 hours. If mass effect is profound, doses as high as 20 mg every 4 hours may be considered. Some surgeons believe it is easier to resect a tumor when peritumoral edema is minimized by preoperative dexamethasone (Decadron) administration.

The use of anticonvulsants in brain tumor patients at presentation, preoperatively, and postoperatively is somewhat controversial. Without question, patients presenting with seizures attributed to a brain tumor should be initiated on an anticonvulsant. However, with few exceptions, there is no data to suggest prophylactic use of anticonvulsants reduces the risk of new-onset seizures in patients with brain tumor. Among the exceptions are (1) tumor involvement in highly epileptogenic areas such as the motor cortex; (2) low-grade gliomas, which carry a high risk of seizures; (3) patients with metastatic lesions that commonly invade the cortex; and (4) patients with both metastases and leptomeningeal spread.

Because of a favorable toxicity profile and cost, phenytoin is the first-line antiepileptic agent. Phenytoin may cause gastrointestinal upset and should be administered with an H_2-blocker or proton-pump inhibitor. Phenytoin levels must be monitored to ensure a therapeutic serum drug concentration. Levetiracetam is an alternative used for patients if there is potential for drug interactions related to induction of the P450 system by phenytoin. In contrast to phenytoin, levels of levetiracetam need not be monitored.

B. Surgical Considerations

The surgeon must decide whether the goal of intervention is obtaining biopsy only, subtotal resection, or attempting gross total resection. With few exceptions, gross total resection offers the best chance of survival and is the preferred treatment. Tumor resection requires careful consideration of a number of key factors, including (1) tumor size; (2) location; (3) gross, radiographic, and pathologic characteristics; (4) sensitivity to radiation; and importantly, (5) the medical and neurologic status of the patient.

The timing of surgery is important in preoperative planning. Patients who present with rapid deterioration usually require prompt intervention. Tumor growth can be brisk in patients with large, high-grade tumors, and small increases in tumor volume can cause a profound increase in intracranial pressure. Rapid intervention may also be necessary in the setting of obstructive hydrocephalus. CSF diversion (typically via ventriculostomy) is an alternative to urgent tumor resection in patients with obstructive hydrocephalus secondary to tumor growth. In most cases, tumor resection can be arranged as an elective procedure.

Once in the operating room for brain tumor resection, a number of important principles of positioning are vital to a successful resection. Most tumor resections require immobilization of patient's head in a Mayfield head holder. The position should be selected to create the most direct access to the lesion while avoiding risk to other bodily structures. Positioning should promote venous drainage from the lesion and the cranial compartment by ensuring the jugular veins are not compressed and that the head is elevated. Some surgeons prefer to position the patient with the operative corridor perpendicular to the floor. This approach generally minimizes brain retraction and is the most ergonomic for the surgeon. Pressure points of the remainder of the patient should be padded especially thoroughly given the lengthy nature of some tumor resections.

The shape of the skin incision and bone flap is dependent on the desired approach, size of the lesion, and surgeon preference. Small tumors can be adequately exposed and resected via linear or curvilinear incisions with a small bone flap. Resection of deep lesions, especially those involving the skull base, often require creation of a sizable scalp flap and removal of a large window of bone. Whenever possible, incisions should be planned behind the hairline, minimizing the amount of hair removal in deference to cosmetic concerns. The placement of the incision is largely determined by the location of the lesion. Frameless stereotaxy can enable accurate tumor localization based on preoperative imaging and can be helpful in minimizing the size of the incision. Standard approaches to intracranial lesions minimize the morbidity of exposure by limiting the risk to key neural and vascular structures.

The central goal of brain tumor surgery is maximizing the removal of neoplastic tissue while minimizing collateral damage to surrounding normal brain and vascular structures. Standards for achieving this goal vary according to tumor type. For example, the goal of the resection of a high-grade glioma is to remove all enhancing portions of the tumor; the goal for the resection of a low-grade glioma is to remove the tissue that appears abnormal on T2-weighted MRI. The goal for resection of meningioma is to remove both the tumor and its dural origin. Metastatic tumors are typically well demarcated and often encapsulated, and the goal is to remove the entire tumor.

Neoplastic tissue that is easily detected on imaging is often virtually indistinguishable from normal brain. Several studies evaluating the extent of brain tumor resection emphasize that in many cases, especially in diffusely invasive brain tumors, a significant amount of residual tumor remains even after gross total resection. Stereotactic navigation and intraoperative MRI have been utilized to improve extent of resection, but their impact on outcome is still controversial. Fluorescent and visible dyes have been proposed as a means of identifying tumor margins intraoperatively. Early clinical studies on fluorescent dyes suggest that they may improve the extent of resection. Dye-loaded nanoparticles are currently under investigation as a possible means of tumor margin delineation.

Intraoperative monitoring of brain activity is often used in tumors within eloquent cortex to determine a safe route for exposure of tumor and the effects of resection. The electrical activity of the cortex can be recorded by placing grids on the surface of exposed cortex. Differences in electrical activity can be observed in adjacent cortical areas that suggest their function. Motor and sensory cortices are often mapped in this way. Awake craniotomies are commonly used in tumor resections that may involve cortical regions necessary for language function and motor function. During an awake craniotomy, the function of specific cortical areas can be deduced by using electrical currents to disrupt cortical activity while evaluating neurologic function.

Following resection, meticulous attention is paid to closure of the operative corridor. Whenever possible, to diminish the risk of CSF leak, a watertight dural closure is performed. The bone flap is replaced, and the galea is reapproximated. Scalp closure that omits closure of the galea provides little strength and raises the risk of dehiscence.

C. Postoperative Management

Following resection, patients are observed closely in an intensive care setting, typically overnight, where serial neurological examination is carried out. Depending on the extent of resection, steroids may be tapered over the days following surgery. Anticonvulsants are continued in patients who have a history of seizures, and when there has been

extensive brain dissection, they may be continued for 1 to 4 weeks following surgery. Many surgeons prefer to obtain postoperative MRI imaging with contrast to evaluate for residual tumor within 24 hours of resection, especially for gliomas because of the difficulty of delineating tumor margins during resection. When there is a low suspicion of residual tumor, postoperative imaging may be deferred during recovery.

D. Adjuvant Therapies

Surgical resection is the cornerstone of brain tumor therapy, but it rarely eradicates all tumor cells. Furthermore, resection may not be favored when eloquent structures are likely to be damaged. Adjuvant radiation and chemotherapy regimens have been developed to address the inability of current surgical techniques to reliably eradicate residual or unresectable tumor.

1. Radiation—Radiation kills tumor cells by directly damaging cellular structures, inducing lethal mutations in cellular DNA, and by activating pathways for programmed cell death. Radiation can be delivered to brain tumors in a fractionated manner, which allows normal tissue repair between treatments and increases the toxicity of the radiation to tumor tissue.

Regimens for radiation therapy of brain tumors vary with tumor type. The optimal dose and timing of adjuvant radiation therapy for low-grade glioma is controversial. Several recent clinical trials have informed the current recommendations of the European Organization for Research and Treatment of Cancer and the Radiation Therapy Oncology Group to deliver 54 Gy in 30 fractions. Early radiation therapy is suggested in elderly patients who have had subtotal resection because of their high risk of recurrence. Because of the cognitive consequences of radiation therapy, it may be delayed in younger patients until there is suspicion of recurrence

For high-grade glioma, the findings of a study conducted by the Brain Tumor Cooperative Group demonstrated an increase in survival in patients with high-grade glioma undergoing radiation therapy plus surgery compared to surgery alone from 14 to 31 weeks. This is currently the standard recommendation.

Two important clinical trials have established the standard therapy for metastatic lesions. Currently, acceptable care of patients with brain metastases consists of (1) resection followed by whole-brain radiation therapy or (2) stereotactic radiosurgery, in which a high dose of radiation is administered to the tumor bed, in addition to whole-brain radiation therapy. The use of radiation therapy has been extensively investigated. Currently, radiation therapy is indicated as an adjunct to surgery in the setting of recurrent meningioma or subtotal resection. Occasionally in a poor surgical candidate or if a meningioma is in a location carrying high surgical risk, radiation therapy may be used in isolation.

2. Chemotherapy—Clinical trials of chemotherapy for low-grade glioma have been limited, and the use of chemotherapy remains experimental. In contrast, a recent landmark clinical trial in patients with proven glioblastoma multiforme comparing radiation alone to radiation in combination with the oral alkylating agent temozolomide demonstrated a modest but significant increase in survival from 12.1 to 14.6 months. The current standard of care for patients with glioblastoma multiforme combines radiation therapy with oral temozolomide. Chemotherapy has not shown any benefit in the treatment of brain metastases and meningiomas. Future efforts in the development of chemotherapeutic agents are focused on developing novel inhibitors of signaling pathways that are active only in brain tumor cells. Developing novel methods for the delivery of traditional chemotherapeutic agents is also an area of active research.

► Complications

Patients with primary and metastatic brain tumors are at risk of developing postoperative medical as well as surgical complications. Sawaya proposed the most common classification scheme for complications associated with brain tumor surgery in 1998. In a case series of 400 craniotomies for treatment of brain tumors, complications were classified as neurological, regional, and systemic. Neurologic complications are outcomes that produce visual field, motor, sensory, or language deficits; they result from injury to normal brain structures, cerebral edema, hematoma, or vascular injury. In most series, the risk of a new neurologic deficit after craniotomy for resection of an intrinsic brain tumor ranges from 10% to 25%. The risk factors for adverse neurologic outcomes include older age (> 60 years), deep tumor location, tumor proximity to eloquent regions, and low functional performance score (Karnofsky score < 60%). Neurologic complications can be minimized by individualizing the surgical approach for each patient, cortical mapping techniques, minimizing excessive brain retraction, meticulous hemostasis, and early identification of major venous structures.

Regional complications are those related to the surgical wound or brain parenchyma, without neurologic deficit. They occur in 1% to 5% of patients undergoing craniotomy for resection of an intrinsic brain tumor. Regional complications include wound infections, pneumocephalus, CSF fistula, hydrocephalus, seizure, brain abscess or cerebritis, meningitis, and pseudomeningocele. These complications occur more readily in the elderly. Posterior fossa location and reoperations are associated with a higher rate of pseudomeningocele, CSF fistula, hydrocephalus, and wound infections. Postoperative wound infections and cellulitis occur in 1% to 2% of patients after supratentorial craniotomy. They typically result from skin bacterial contamination (staphylococcus aureus and staphylococcus epidermidis). The risk of postoperative seizures following supratentorial craniotomy is 0.5% to 5%. Prophylactic antiepileptic drugs can be routinely used in the postoperative period; however, their dose and duration is an area of controversy.

Systemic complications include all generalized adverse events, including deep vein thrombosis, pulmonary embolus, pneumonia, urinary tract infections, myocardial infarction, and sepsis. These medical complications occur in 5% to 10% of patients undergoing craniotomy for removal of an intrinsic brain tumor and are more prevalent in older patients (> 60 years) and neurologically impaired patients (Karnofsky score less than 60%). Deep vein thrombosis is the most common complication, occurring in 1% to 10% of patients within the first month after a craniotomy. Patients with systemic cancer, glioblastoma multiforme, meningiomas, lower extremity paralysis, bed rest, and prolonged surgery are at particularly increased risk of developing a deep vein thrombosis or pulmonary embolus. Early postoperative mobilization, intermittent compression devices, and postoperative anticoagulation with low-molecular-weight heparin have decreased the incidence of postoperative deep vein thrombosis.

Craniotomy for resection of brain tumor can be performed safely, and most complications can be prevented with careful preoperative planning, meticulous surgical technique, and attentive postoperative care.

► Prognosis

The prognosis of brain tumor patients varies depending on a number of factors, including but not limited to general functional status at the time of diagnosis, tumor type, location, and age.

A. Glioma

The prognosis of patients with glioma is determined by tumor grade, age, Karnofsky performance status, and treatment response. The extent of resection is also likely a key factor in prognosis. Improvement in survival when radiographically complete resection is achieved is greatest for those with low-grade lesions. Patients with high-grade glioma with radiographically complete resection also have survival improvement (though more modest) compared to those incomplete resection. Achieving gross total resection improves survival by lowering the risk of recurrence and reducing tumor cell burden to levels that can be eradicated or controlled with adjuvant therapy.

B. Meningioma

In general, the prognosis of patients with meningioma is more favorable than that of glioma patients. The prognosis is determined by the extent of resection and tumor grade. The Simpson classification system stratifies patients into outcome groups based on extent of resection. Patient age, extent of surrounding structure invasion, male gender, genetic factors, and tumor grade are among the factors linked to prognosis.

Metastases

The survival of patients with untreated brain metastasis is quite poor (1–2 months), but survival can be prolonged by 4 or more months with optimal surgical and radiation therapies. Extent of extracranial disease is a key prognostic factor in patients with brain metastases. Age and Karnofsky performance status have an important bearing on overall survival.

Davis F et al: Survival rates in patients with primary malignant brain tumors stratified by patient age and tumor histologic type: an analysis based on surveillance, epidemiology, and end results (SEER) data, 1973–1991. J Neurosurg 1998;88:1.

Kleihues P, Burger PC, Scheithauer BW: The new WHO classification of brain tumors. Brain Pathol 1993;3:255.

Lemort M et al: Progress in magnetic resonance imaging of brain tumors. Curr Opin Oncol 2007;19:616.

Truong MT: Current role of radiation therapy in the management of malignant brain tumors. Hematol Oncol Clin North Am 2006;20:431.

TUMORS OF THE SPINE & SPINAL CORD

Anthony C. Wang, MD, Khoi D. Than, MD, & Paul Park, MD

Neoplastic pathology affecting the spinal cord is uncommon in the general population, but it is an important consideration in the evaluation of patients presenting with neck and/or back pain with or without associated radicular symptoms, sensorimotor deficits, and bowel or bladder dysfunction. An estimated 15% of primary CNS tumors are intraspinal, and most of these are benign. Since the first resection of a spinal cord tumor was reported in 1888, surgery has remained a mainstay of treatment in the majority of spinal tumors, though radiotherapy and chemotherapy have demonstrated benefit in a growing number of instances.

Spinal tumors are differentiated on the basis of their locations within three anatomic compartments. Extradural tumors are located outside of the thecal sac, typically arising from tissues of the osseous spine, paravertebral soft tissues, or epidural space. Intradural-extramedullary tumors occur within the thecal sac but are outside of the spinal cord. These tumors are thought to develop from the leptomeninges or nerve roots. Intramedullary tumors are found within the spinal cord and originate from either the spinal cord parenchyma or pia mater.

In addition to gender and age of presentation, localization of the lesion to the cervical, thoracic, lumbar, or sacrococcygeal spine aids in refining the differential diagnosis because certain tumors demonstrate a predilection for particular regions of the spinal column.

Clinical Presentation

Symptoms experienced by patients presenting with spinal tumors are more commonly produced by compression than by direct invasion or ischemia of the spinal cord and/or nerves. Classically, the pain associated with neoplasms is unremitting, worse in the supine position, and more noticeable at rest or in bed. Hence, the patient may wake up at night due to pain. Although the progression of symptoms can be insidious, radicular pain, motor weakness, as well as paresthesias, hyperesthesia, or anesthesia, can frequently occur as a result of nerve compression. Long-tract findings such as ataxia, hyperreflexia, extensor plantar response, spasticity, sensorimotor loss, and/or sphincter dysfunction can be caused by anterior or posterior horn cell dysfunction due to spinal cord compression. Unusual findings include muscle wasting or hyporeflexia, referred pain, autonomic changes such as in Horner syndrome and Brown-Séquard hemicord syndrome. Fracture and deformity causing axial pain often occur as well and may be the presenting complaint.

Extradural tumors frequently involve the osseous spine and so most typically present with axial pain, often increased by motion or Valsalva maneuver. Signs and symptoms of neural compression occur secondarily. Intradural-extramedullary tumors present most commonly with motor deficits, while also frequently causing radicular pain and long-tract disturbances. Sphincter dysfunction is often found in these cases as well. Intramedullary tumors can demonstrate an insidious succession of symptoms starting with neuralgic pain that can progress to a Brown-Séquard syndrome and finally to complete spinal cord dysfunction.

Diagnosis

A. Radiographic Evaluation

MRI is currently the primary mode of assessment of spinal tumors (Figure 36–16). Gadolinium-enhanced and noncontrasted MR sequences are the standard initial imaging modality for the evaluation of suspected extradural, intradural-extramedullary, and intramedullary lesions. Nearly all intramedullary lesions demonstrate contrast uptake, and the resolution that MRI provides is typically sufficient for determination of margins and infiltration. The addition of MRA is indicated for the suspicion of a vascular pathology.

If unable to obtain MRI, more invasive methods are used. Myelography, which was once the modality of choice for imaging the spinal canal, provides excellent structural detail. Fusiform cord widening, a dumbbell-shaped deformity, or complete blockage are classic findings suggesting the presence of a tumor. Plain, contrast-enhanced, and postmyelography CT imaging is commonly done in conjunction with MRI to assess the spinal bony anatomy and to help differentiate identified masses. Nuclear scintigraphy is used primarily in the characterization of skeletal metastases. Catheter angiography can be employed in the evaluation of suspected vascular lesions. Plain x-rays of the spine have limited utility in the assessment of spinal tumors. Findings such as enlarged intervertebral foramina and interpedicular spaces or bony erosion with scalloped edges suggest the presence of an enlarging mass.

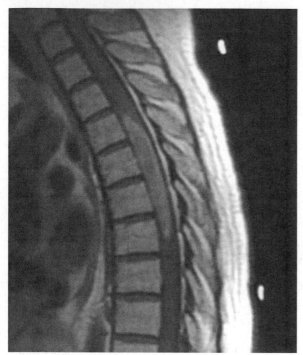

▲ **Figure 36–16.** Sagittal T1-weighted image with contrast of the upper thoracic spinal cord demonstrating an intradural, intramedullary lesion found on biopsy to be a high-grade glioma.

B. Laboratory Analysis

Lumbar puncture can provide additional clues to the presence of a spinal cord tumor. Elevated CSF protein is present in approximately 95% of cases, though CSF glucose is normal. Xanthochromia and the presence of fibrinogen causing clotting can also occur. Specific serum immunohistochemical tests can aid the diagnosis of specific neoplasms.

C. Differential Diagnosis

In 2000, the WHO created a comprehensive classification of neoplasms affecting the central nervous system based on the specific cell type from which each tumor arises, which guides therapy and prognosis; many of these neoplasms can occur in the spinal column (Table 36–6). Approximately 0.5% of tumors involving the spinal column are primary neoplasms.

Among all spinal tumors, extradural lesions are discovered with the greatest frequency, comprising an estimated 55% to 60%. A vast majority of these are metastatic lesions via hematogenous dissemination along the Batson plexus. The most common primary sources of vertebral metastases are lung, breast, and prostate. Patients with primary epidural spinal neoplasms, both malignant and benign, typically present similarly to those with metastases, with pain being the most prominent initial complaint and with radicular symptoms and/or myelopathy secondarily.

Of the intradural tumors, an estimated 70% are extramedullary. The nerve sheath tumors (schwannoma and neurofibroma) and meningiomas comprise the bulk of these

Table 36–6. Spinal Tumor Characteristics.

Compartment	Tumor	Predilection	Treatment Options	Comments
Extradural	Vertebral hemangioma	Thoracic	Preoperative embolization + resection (+ XRT) for progressive symptoms	Honeycomb radiographic appearance
	Giant cell tumor	Sacral	Resection (+ XRT)	Aggressive spread, often biopsy for diagnosis before treating
	Plasmacytoma	Thoracic	(XRT + steroids + surgical stabilization)	Precursor to multiple myeloma
	Osteoid osteoma	Lumbar	Resection of nidus (+ fusion)	Peak incidence in adolescence
	Osteoblastoma	Lumbar	En bloc resection (+ XRT)	Similar to osteoid osteoma but > 1.5 cm
	Osteochondroma	Cervical	Resection (+ fusion) to treat symptoms	Often causes spinal deformity
(nonneoplastic)	Eosinophilic granuloma	Cervical	Spine stabilization	Classic vertebra plana in children
(nonneoplastic)	Aneurysmal bone cyst	Thoracic and lumbar	GTR (+ fusion)	Aggressively expansile, peak incidence in adolescence
(nonneoplastic)	Angiolipoma	Thoracic	Resection to treat symptoms	Onset of symptoms often during pregnancy
	Metastasis		XRT + steroids	

(continued)

Table 36–6. Spinal Tumor Characteristics. *(Continued)*

Compartment	Tumor	Predilection	Treatment Options	Comments
Extradural *(continued)*	Chordoma	Sacral, cervical	En bloc resection (+ XRT)	Most common primary bone malignancy of the spine
	Ewing sarcoma	Sacral	Resection + XRT + chemotherapy	Usually metastatic from another site, HBA-71 Ag
	Multiple myeloma		Chemotherapy + XRT (+ steroids + surgical stabilization)	Pathological fractures seen in 50% at presentation
	Lymphoma		Chemotherapy	Hodgkin and non-Hodgkin
	Chondrosarcoma	Thoracic	En bloc resection	Second-most common primary bone malignancy
	Osteosarcoma		Chemotherapy + en bloc resection (+ XRT)	Bimodal age distribution, potentially curable
	Paravertebral sarcomas		En bloc resection + XRT + chemotherapy	Often painless, presents with neurological deficits
Intradural-extramedullary	Schwannoma	Thoracic	GTR	Associated with dorsal root origin
	Neurofibroma	Thoracic	Resection	Associated with ventral root origin
	Meningioma	Thoracic	GTR (+ XRT for recurrence)	Extension common
	Metastasis		XRT + steroids	Drop metastases from GBM, AA, ependymoma, and MB
	Myxopapillary ependymoma	Conus	Resection + XRT	Dissemination common
	Lymphoma		Chemotherapy	
	Lipoma	Lumbosacral	Resection	Congenital, can cause tethered cord
	Paraganglioma	Conus	GTR	Can secrete hyperadrenergic state
	Neuroganglioma			Rare nerve sheath tumor
	Dermoid and epidermoid		GTR (+ steroids for chemical meningitis)	Commonly in children
	Teratoma	Sacral	GTR	Can be in any compartment
Intramedullary	Ependymoma	Cervical	GTR	Strongly enhancing, well-circumscribed
	Astrocytoma	Cervical	Biopsy ± resection + XRT	Infiltrative, common in children
	Lipoma	Cervical and thoracic	Debulking	
	Hemangioblastoma	Thoracic and cervical	GTR	Cystic with mural nodule, associated with von Hippel-Lindau syndrome
	Metastasis	Cervical and conus	XRT + steroids	Most commonly small-cell lung cancer
	Ganglioglioma	Thoracic	GTR + XRT	Commonly in children
	Oligodendroglioma	Thoracic	GTR + XRT	Spinal deformity, syrinx common
	Neuroblastoma	Cervical	GTR	

AA, anaplastic astrocytoma; GBM, glioblastoma multiforme; GTR, gross total resection; MB, medulloblastoma; XRT, radiation therapy.

cases. Of similar origin, nerve sheath tumors are usually benign and can demonstrate a typical dumbbell-shaped appearance caused by the neuroforamina through which they pass. They are an important consideration when deviation of the pleural reflection is noted with suspicion of a posterior mediastinal mass. Schwannomas are well differentiated and typically grossly resectable; however, neurofibromas consist of both Schwann cells and fibroblasts and cannot be resected completely from the parent nerve. In the setting of von Recklinghausen neurofibromatosis, suspicion of multiple neurofibromas, meningioma, and ependymoma should be heightened. Schwannoma, neurofibroma, and meningioma multiplicity is associated with type 2 neurofibromatosis. Meningiomas are seen most often in the thoracic spines of middle-aged women and arise from persistent arachnoid cells. They frequently have calcifications and can have irregular contrast enhancement.

Intramedullary tumors comprise only approximately 10% of all spinal tumors and arise most commonly in the cervical segment of the spinal cord. Gliomas are the most common of these, with ependymomas occurring twice as frequently as astrocytomas in adults. In children, the relationship is reversed, with astrocytomas being twice as common as ependymomas. Myxopapillary ependymomas form from the conus medullaris and filum terminale and are a very common tumor to be found at this location.

▶ Treatment

Treatment options are tailored to the patient. Some patients present with axial pain absent of radiculopathy; others present with mild or stable evidence of spinal cord compression causing myelopathy. Still others present with a rapidly progressive course of neurologic deterioration. Overall, outcome of therapy depends heavily on severity and duration of symptoms at the time of presentation. The Enneking system provides oncologic staging for primary bone tumors, has been successfully applied to the spine, and is helpful in guiding treatment. Generally, primary tumors of the spinal column are best treated by complete resection if possible. In the vertebral column, en bloc resection is frequently the goal of surgery, whereas with any involvement of the spinal cord, gross total resection is most commonly the desired treatment. Symptomatic deformity or spinal instability warrants immediate consideration of surgical fixation.

Extradural metastases are the most frequently seen tumors of the spinal column, and their treatment is complicated by many factors. Until recently, these lesions were generally treated with radiation therapy, often in conjunction with corticosteroids. More recently, surgical resection, decompression of the spinal cord, and surgical stabilization followed by radiation have shown promising results in the setting of neurologic deficits caused by spinal metastatic disease.

Intradural tumors are generally best treated by surgical resection; the outcome depends heavily on the extent of resection. There has been no conclusive association between extent of resection and tumor control, and the preservation of preexisting neurologic function remains the primary objective in surgery. Determination of a dissection plane between tumor and spinal cord is the initial aim of any resection procedure. For example, complete removal of attached dura in spinal meningiomas assures a more favorable prognosis in terms of recurrence when compared with incomplete resection. Overall, prognosis is excellent in nearly all cases of spinal meningioma unless paraplegia is the presenting condition. In contrast, recurrence of infiltrative gliomas is very common,

and progression to paralysis is inevitable if malignant. Progressive neurologic deterioration demands particular focus on facilitating appropriate surgical therapy.

Binning M et al: Spinal tumors in children. Neurosurg Clin N Am 2007;18:631.

Kim MS et al: Intramedullary spinal cord astrocytoma in adults: postoperative outcome. J Neurooncol 2001;52:85.

Koeller KK, Rosenblum RS, Morrison AL: Neoplasms of the spinal cord and filum terminale: radiologic-pathologic correlation. Radiographics 2000;20:1721.

Loblaw DA, Laperriere NJ: Emergency treatment of malignant extradural spinal cord compression: an evidence-based guideline. J Clin Oncol 1998;16:1613.

Lonser RR et al: Surgical management of spinal cord hemangioblastomas in patients with von Hippel-Lindau disease. J Neurosurg 2003;98:106.

Ozawa H et al: Spinal dumbbell tumors: an analysis of a series of 118 cases. J Neurosurg Spine 2007;7:587.

Patchell RA et al: Direct decompressive surgical resection in the treatment of spinal cord compression caused by metastatic cancer: a randomized trial. Lancet 2005;366:643.

Schwartz TH, McCormick PC: Intramedullary ependymomas: clinical presentation, surgical treatment strategies and prognosis. J Neurooncol 2000;47:211.

Van Goethem JW et al: Spinal tumors. Eur J Radiol 2004;50:159.

▼ PITUITARY TUMORS

John Ziewacz, MD, Stephen Sullivan, MD,
& William Chandler, MD

▶ Clinical Considerations

The pituitary gland, involved in the regulation of the major hormonal axes of the body, is located in the sella turcica ("Turkish saddle") of the sphenoid bone and is comprised of the anterior pituitary (adenohypophysis), posterior pituitary (neurohypophysis), and functionally insignificant pars intermedia separating the two lobes. The anterior pituitary secretes prolactin, adrenocorticotropic hormone, thyroid-stimulating hormone, luteinizing hormone, follicle-stimulating hormone, and growth hormone. The posterior lobe is a repository of the hypothalamic hormones oxytocin and antidiuretic hormone (vasopressin).

Pituitary tumors are typically benign adenomas that arise from the anterior lobe of the pituitary gland. They comprise approximately 10% of CNS tumors. They are classified by both their secretory status (secreting or nonsecreting) and their size. Microadenomas have diameters less than 1 cm, while tumors greater than 1 cm are termed macroadenomas (Figure 36–17). Secreting (endocrine-active) tumors are further classified by which hormone is being hypersecreted and the resulting clinical syndrome.

▶ Clinical Findings

Clinical findings in patients with pituitary adenomas are caused by compression of surrounding structures, decrease in

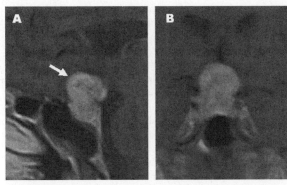

▲ **Figure 36–17.** MRI. Sagittal plane **(A)** and coronal plane **(B)** of a pituitary macroadenoma.

pituitary function, hypersecretion of pituitary hormones, and, rarely, acute pituitary failure (apoplexy). Pituitary tumors can also be asymptomatic and discovered incidentally.

A. Compression

Compression caused by slowly expanding adenomas causes a variety of findings, which include headache, bitemporal hemianopsia (decreased perception of the lateral visual fields), diplopia, and hypopituitarism (decreased secretion of pituitary hormone).

Bitemporal hemianopsia results from the upward extension of the tumor with associated compression of the decussating nasal fibers of the optic chiasm, which lie directly above the pituitary gland. This can be detected on examination as red color desaturation in the temporal visual fields. Without treatment, changes in vision can progress to loss of visual acuity and eventual blindness.

Hypopituitarism results from compression and injury of the normal pituitary cells by the expanding mass. Diminished secretion of growth, luteinizing, and follicle-stimulating hormones occurs early, while diminished secretion of thyroid-stimulating and adrenocorticotropic hormones occurs later.

Symptoms related to decreased production of luteinizing and follicle-stimulating hormones manifest as a loss of libido and amenorrhea. In men, this is often overlooked and only recognized in retrospect. The decreased production of luteinizing hormone and follicle-stimulating hormone can be due to either direct compression of the gland or compression of the stalk, which releases the tonic inhibition of prolactin secretion by dopamine from the hypothalamus. This results in a mild increase in prolactin (usually less than 150 ng/dl), which inhibits gonadotropin release. This can cause galactorrhea as well and is the mechanism of the amenorrhea/galactorrhea syndrome.

Decreased production of thyroid-stimulating hormone causes classic findings of hypothyroidism, including cold intolerance, weight gain, fatigue, coarse hair, and myxedema. Decreased production of adrenocorticotropic hormone causes hypocortisolism, resulting in fatigue, slow return to health after minor illness, orthostatic hypotension, and, rarely, cardiovascular collapse when the body is under extreme stress.

B. Hypersecretion

Functional adenomas that produce hormone manifest symptoms related to hypersecretion of the specific hormone. They can also produce findings related to compression, but this is less common given that they are often discovered at an earlier stage because of the clinical findings caused by hypersecretion.

Prolactinomas are the most common pituitary tumor, accounting for nearly 30% of pituitary tumors. Prolactinomas cause hypersecretion of prolactin. Interruption of the pituitary stalk can cause hyperprolactinemia as well, but levels are typically more modest ($\leq$ 150 ng/dl). Levels greater than 300 ng/dl are virtually always associated with prolactin-secreting tumors. Symptoms of hyperprolactinemia include galactorrhea, amenorrhea (via suppression of gonadotropins), diminished libido, and infertility.

Growth hormone–secreting tumors are the next most common endocrine-active tumors. They cause gigantism in children or acromegaly in adults. Acromegaly is characterized by skeletal overgrowth, prognathism, widely spaced teeth, macroglossia, cardiomyopathy, arthropathy, glucose intolerance, sleep apnea, nerve entrapment syndromes, and cardiomyopathy. It is insidious in onset and is often not noticed by the patient's friends or family. Patients often note a change in shoe size as an adult, an inability to wear a wedding ring, or a striking physical change when comparing a recent to a past photograph.

Tumors that secrete adrenocorticotropic hormone are the cause of Cushing disease, which refers specifically to hypercortisolism caused by a functional pituitary tumor. The resultant signs and symptoms of hypercortisolism from any etiology are termed Cushing syndrome. Characteristic findings include weight gain (with centripetal fat distribution), "buffalo-hump" redistribution of fat to the posterior neck, purple abdominal striae, thin skin with easy bruising, hypertension, round "moon" facies, glucose intolerance, hypertension, osteoporosis, poor wound healing, psychiatric disturbance (depression, mood lability), amenorrhea, impotence, and hyperpigmentation (only with elevated adrenocorticotropic hormone).

Gonadotropin-producing tumors are rare and result in the hypersecretion of luteinizing and follicle-stimulating hormones. They are often clinically silent, especially in men. In women, they can produce amenorrhea and infertility.

Thyroid-stimulating hormone–producing tumors are very rare, accounting for less than 1% of secretory tumors. Clinical findings are those of classic hyperthyroidism, including weight loss, tachycardia, heat intolerance, anxiety, and tremor.

C. Acute Pituitary Failure (Apoplexy)

Acute pituitary failure is usually the result of hemorrhage and/or necrosis in a preexisting adenoma. Symptoms are abrupt and result in headache, vision disturbance, ophthalmoplegia, and change in mental status. Pituitary hormonal failure almost always accompanies an apoplectic event, and rapid administration of corticosteroids is necessary to avoid cardiovascular collapse. Urgent decompression is warranted for acute or continuing neurologic decline in order to prevent untoward neurologic consequences, especially blindness.

D. Stalk Compression

Symptoms related to stalk compression are rare in the setting of pituitary adenomas and consist of diabetes insipidus and the effects of prolactin elevation. Diabetes insipidus results from the diminished release of antidiuretic hormone, which causes an inability to concentrate the urine, resulting in hypernatremia. Symptoms include frequent high-volume urination and excessive thirst. This can be very dangerous in the setting of a patient with an impaired thirst mechanism.

Mild prolactin elevation results from blocking the inhibitory effect of dopamine on prolactin-producing cells. This release of tonic inhibition results in a modest elevation of prolactin (usually < 150 ng/dl), which is called the "stalk effect" and may result in amenorrhea and galactorrhea.

▶ Differential Diagnosis

The differential diagnosis for sellar and parasellar masses is broad. The hallmarks of distinguishing among the multiple possibilities are a detailed history and physical examination, MRI scan, and pituitary hormone testing. The history and physical examination should be aimed at symptoms related to pituitary hypersecretion or hyposecretion and compression of surrounding structures. A detailed visual field examination should be included in the evaluation of any potential pituitary mass. MRI should be obtained with and without contrast, with thin cuts through the sellar region in coronal and sagittal planes. This will identify the size, configuration, and extent of invasion of a pituitary tumor. Laboratory testing should include evaluation of anterior pituitary hormones, directly or indirectly, in order to establish a hypersecretory or hyposecretory state. Testing should include prolactin, 8:00 am cortisol, free thyroxine (T4), thyroid-stimulating hormone, insulinlike growth factor I, growth hormone, luteinizing hormone, follicle-stimulating hormone, and testosterone (in men). If symptoms of diabetes insipidus are present, serum sodium, osmolality, and urine osmolality should be obtained to confirm the diagnosis.

If a hypersecretory state is not detected on detailed laboratory testing, the lesion is likely a nonfunctional pituitary adenoma or other entity. Other possibilities include craniopharyngioma, Rathke cleft cyst, or meningioma. A number of other less common lesions are in the differential, including metastasis and chordoma.

If a hypersecretory state is discovered, the diagnosis depends on the hormone being hypersecreted. It is important to distinguish a primary pituitary lesion causing hypersecretion from a lesion in another location in the hormonal axis.

Prolactin levels greater than 200 ng/dl indicate the presence of a prolactinoma. Modest elevations in prolactin, less than 150 ng/dl, can be caused by compression of the pituitary stalk, antidopaminergic drugs, estrogen excess (usually from oral contraceptives), chest wall lesions, primary hypothyroidism, and hypothalamic damage. In evaluating prolactin, it is important to include a diluted sample (1:100 or 1:1000) in addition to the undiluted serum value in order to obviate a false-negative value in cases of extremely elevated prolactin levels caused by the so-called hook effect. False-negative values result from excess prolactin binding to both antibodies of the assay, causing a lack of formation of the complexes identified in the current assays. If the diluted level is still elevated, one can conclude there is a truly elevated prolactin level.

Evaluation of hypercortisolism includes an 8:00 am serum cortisol after taking 1 mg of dexamethasone at 11:00 the night before. If the cortisol level does not suppress to less than 5 mcg/dl, hypercortisolism is strongly suspected. A 24-hour urinary free cortisol should be obtained to confirm hypercortisolism. If this value is clearly elevated, then hypercortisolism is definite and search is initiated to find the etiology of the hypercortisolism. If the level is equivocal and suspicion of hypercortisolism is still strong, then a low and high dose dexamethasone suppression test (Liddle test) may be employed.

Once hypercortisolism is confirmed, the location of the pathology must be identified. Tests useful in confirming a pituitary etiology include a 4:00 pm serum adrenocorticotropic hormone, which would be elevated in a pituitary adenoma and decreased with adrenal pathology. The Liddle test can also help to confirm a pituitary etiology. In Cushing disease, serum cortisol is not suppressed with the low dose of 0.5 mg dexamethasone every 6 hours for 2 days, but does suppress with the higher dose of 2.0 mg every 6 hours for 2 days. In cases of proven hypercortisolism in which a pituitary tumor is not seen on MRI, inferior petrosal sinus sampling is required to confirm a pituitary etiology as well as to help localize the side of the tumor.

Laboratory diagnosis of growth hormone–secreting tumors is often indirect because the secretion of growth hormone is pulsatile and levels in those without a hypersecreting tumor can often be elevated at certain times during the day. Insulinlike growth factor I (somatomedin-C) is the gold standard for diagnosing growth hormone–secreting tumors. Insulinlike growth factor I is produced in the liver and other organs and is dependent on growth hormone for its production. Serum levels of insulinlike growth factor I are relatively stable and provide a better confirmatory test than the more volatile growth hormone.

Luteinizing hormone–secreting and follicle-stimulating hormone–secreting tumors are diagnosed by serum elevated levels in the setting of a pituitary mass diagnosed on MRI.

Thyroid-stimulating hormone–secreting tumors are rare and must be distinguished from other pathologic entities on the hypothalamic-pituitary-thyroid axis. Secondary hyperthyroidism (that produced by a pituitary tumor) is diagnosed by an elevated thyroid-stimulating hormone level as well as an elevated free thyroxine level. In primary hyperthyroidism, free thyroxine would be elevated, and thyroid-stimulating hormone would be suppressed via a negative feedback mechanism.

Findings of pituitary stalk dysfunction in a pituitary adenoma are rare and should prompt search for another cause. Diabetes insipidus caused by stalk compression can be confirmed by a high serum osmolality in the setting of a low urine osmolality, with associated hypernatremia. The differential diagnosis for lesions of the stalk includes germ cell tumors, Langerhans granulomatosis (histiocytosis X), lymphocytic hypophysitis, and sarcoidosis.

▶ Treatment

Treatment of pituitary tumors depends on their size, hormonal characteristics, and level of invasiveness. Microadenomas or macroadenomas that are nonsecreting and are not causing symptoms of compression may be treated conservatively and followed with serial imaging.

Nonsecreting macroadenomas that cause signs of compression are currently treated surgically. The typical surgical approach is a transsphenoidal route, generally performed transnasally, usually with the operating microscope and sometimes with endoscopic assistance. Recent advances in frameless stereotactic guidance and endoscopic techniques have allowed a greater ability to localize lesions intraoperatively and provide a more minimally invasive approach to treatment of pituitary adenomas. There is evidence that the transnasal approaches, compared with previous techniques, are tolerated better with less pain, less morbidity, and shorter hospital stays, but transsphenoidal resection via any approach carries a low risk of morbidity and mortality.

Occasionally, if an adenoma has an unusual amount of suprasellar extension or lateral extension, a craniotomy may be necessary. In some cases, lesions that invade the cavernous sinus or have a significant amount of extrasellar extension are not surgically accessible by any approach, and radiation therapy is often necessary to provide tumor control.

Patients with hypopituitarism due to compression who do not experience return of pituitary function postoperatively require hormone replacement on a chronic basis. If chronic steroid replacement is necessary, it is important that patients be provided with a medic-alert bracelet for the possibility of trauma or illness.

Treatment for hypersecreting tumors depends on the hormone being secreted. It is therefore very important to establish the hormonal profile of a tumor prior to treatment.

Currently, prolactinomas are treated first with a dopamine agonist. The most common medications used to treat prolactinomas are cabergoline and bromocriptine. Cabergoline is a selective D-2 dopamine receptor agonist that is widely considered first-line therapy for prolactinomas. It is favored over bromocriptine because of its selectivity, twice weekly dosing, better tumor control, effective lowering of prolactin levels, greater return of gonadal function/menstrual cycles, and possibility of obviating the need for life-long therapy. Recently, association of cabergoline with cardiac valvular disease has prompted a reexamination of the initial treatment of prolactinoma, but currently, medical treatment as first line is still favored. If medical therapy fails to reduce the tumor or sufficiently control prolactin levels, surgery via the transsphenoidal approach is offered.

Other hypersecreting tumors are treated via the transsphenoidal approach, as with nonsecreting adenomas. Postoperative laboratory testing confirms the efficacy of therapy. As with nonsecreting tumors, craniotomy and/or radiation are sometimes necessary depending on the extent and location of tumor growth. Pituitary replacement may be necessary postoperatively as well.

In the case of pituitary apoplexy, treatment consists of urgent transsphenoidal decompression to prevent further vision deficit and prompt initiation of stress-dose steroid replacement in order to avoid a pituitary crisis.

▶ Summary

Pituitary adenomas are largely benign tumors that are either secreting or nonsecreting. Diagnosis is established with history, physical examination, MRI, and hormonal testing. Treatment consists of conservative therapy for nonsecreting microadenomas and macroadenomas without symptoms of compression, medical therapy for prolactinomas, and transsphenoidal surgery for symptomatic macroadenomas and other hypersecreting tumors. Occasionally, craniotomy and/or radiation may be necessary for further tumor control. Depending on hormonal status, chronic pituitary replacement may be necessary postoperatively. Successful treatment of pituitary tumors can often be achieved with the combined effort of a medical endocrinologist and pituitary neurosurgeon.

Adrogue HJ, Madias NE: Hypernatremia. N Engl J Med 2000;20:1493.

Barkan AL, Chandler WF: Giant pituitary prolactinoma with falsely-low serum prolactin: the pitfall of the "high-dose hook effect": case report. Neurosurgery 1998;42:913.

Cabergoline for Hyperprolactinemia. Med Letter 1997;39:58.

Chandler WF, Barkan AL, Schteingart DE: Management options for persistent functional tumors. Neurosurg Clin N Am 2003;14:139. Review.

Dumont AS et al: Post-operative care following pituitary surgery. J Intensive Care Med 2005;20:128.

Koc K et al: The learning curve in endoscopic pituitary surgery and our experience. Neurosurg Rev 2006;29:298.

Mayernecht J et al: Comparison of low and high dose corticotrophin stimulation tests in patients with pituitary disease. J Clin Endocrinol Metab 1998;83:2350.

Neal JG et al: Comparison of techniques for transsphenoidal pituitary surgery. Am J Rhinol 2007;21:203.

Oelkers W: Adrenal insufficiency. N Engl J Med 1999;335:1206.

Park P et al: The role of radiation therapy after surgical resection of nonfunctional pituitary macroadenomas. Neurosurgery 2004;55:100.

Sandeman D, Moufid A: Interactive image-guided pituitary surgery. An experience of 101 procedures. Neurochirurgie 1998;44:331.

Semple PL et al: Clinical relevance of precipitating factors in pituitary apoplexy. Neurosurgery 2007;61:956.

Webster J et al: A comparison of cabergoline and bromocriptine in the treatment of hyperprolactinemic amenorrhea. N Engl J Med 1994;331:904.

Zada G et al: Endonasal transsphenoidal approach for pituitary adenomas and other sellar lesions: an assessment of efficacy, safety, and patient impressions. J Neurosurg 2003;98:350.

PEDIATRIC NEUROSURGERY

Debbie K Song, MD, Cormac O. Maher, MD, & Karin M. Muraszko, MD

CONGENITAL MALFORMATIONS

▶ Craniospinal Dysraphism

Craniospinal dysraphism results from improper formation and closure of the neural tube during development. These malformations may be classified on the basis of whether they are open or closed neural tube defects, the location of the lesion, or the embryological basis for the malformation. Open neural tube defects are those in which neural elements are exposed or covered by a dysplastic membrane, while closed neural tube defects are skin covered.

Myelomeningocele, the most common type of spinal dysraphism compatible with life, occurs with an incidence of 1 in every 1200 to 1400 live births. It is due to a local failure of neural tube closure during primary neurulation. Fusion of the lateral cutaneous ectoderm and the process of disjunction also fail to occur in myelomeningocele, resulting in a midline cutaneous defect over exposed neural tissue called the neural placode. Therefore, myelomeningoceles are considered open neural tube defects. Myelomeningoceles occur most commonly in the lumbar spine, and the anatomic level of the spinal cord lesion approximates the patient's neurologic deficits. The diagnosis of a neural tube defect can be suspected prenatally with an elevated maternal serum α-fetoprotein and confirmed by in utero imaging such as a maternal-fetal MRI or ultrasound. Pregnant mothers who have inadequate folate intake or who have other children with neural tube defects are at increased risk for giving birth to a child with a myelomeningocele. A Chiari II malformation is found in most patients with myelomeningocele.

Eighty percent of patients with myelomeningocele have associated hydrocephalus. Other CNS abnormalities that can be found with increased incidence among patients with myelomeningocele include lipomas, syringomyelia, and diastematomyelia. Patients with myelomeningocele commonly have orthopedic problems that include scoliosis, hip dislocation, and knee and foot deformities. Besides a neurogenic bladder, patients with myelomeningocele are at increased risk of genitourinary abnormalities as well as intestinal, cardiac, esophageal, and renal abnormalities. Workup for the newborn child with myelomeningocele includes a cranial and spinal ultrasound and orthopedic and urology consults. The neonate should be placed in the prone position with pressure off of the myelomeningocele. The myelomeningocele should be covered in moist dressings. Surgical closure of the myelomeningocele is performed soon after birth. The Management of Myelomeningocele Study (MOMS) is an ongoing trial examining the utility of in utero myelomeningocele repair.

Closed neural tube defects, also called occult spinal dysraphisms, can arise from problems with disjunction, secondary neurulation, or postneurulation events. Types of closed neural tube defects include dermal sinus tracts, spinal lipomas, neurenteric cysts, sacral dysgenesis, and diastematomyelia. Spina bifida occulta, which is characterized by a defect in the posterior elements of the spine, is often a harbinger of an underlying closed neural tube defect. These malformations can tether the spinal cord in an abnormally low position and produce excessive tension on the neural elements. Neuronal dysfunction may ensue with symptoms of a clinical tethered cord syndrome such as back or leg pain, worsening lower extremity motor and sensory function, decline in bladder and bowel function, worsening lower extremity orthopedic deformities, and progressive scoliosis. Early surgical repair of occult spinal dysraphisms is often recommended at the time of diagnosis in order to prevent the onset or halt the progression of neurological symptoms.

Dermal sinus tracts are epithelial-lined tracts that originate in the midline skin, usually in the caudal lumbosacral region above the S2 level. The sinus tract extends from a pinhole opening in the skin, through bifid spinous processes, and into the dura to communicate with the spinal cord. The lining of the dermal sinus tract contains normal skin appendages that can shed and communicate with the intradural space, and recurrent episodes of meningitis and arachnoiditis may ensue. They appear as dimples above the gluteal crease and must be differentiated from pilonidal cysts, which are closer to the anus. Both entities may drain from the skin. The skin around the ostium of a dermal sinus tract may be discolored or have a hairy tuft. Dermal sinuses can be associated with lipomas, dermoid tumors, or epidermoid cysts at any point along the tract or within the spinal canal. Examination of the child with a suspected dermal sinus tract should include assessment of sphincter function, lower extremity reflexes, and motor and sensory function. Treatment should be performed in an expeditious fashion after diagnosis in order to reduce the risk of CNS infection and prevent the development of neurological deficit. Less commonly, dermal sinus tracts can occur in the cranial region. The most common cranial locations are in the occipital or nasal region. Children may present with a midline dimple at the tip of the nose or in the occipital region and with a history of recurrent meningitis. Cranial dermal sinus tracts can be associated with intracranial dermoid cysts.

Spinal lipomas are the most common closed neural tube defects and include three separate entities: intradural lipomas, lipomyelomeningoceles, and lipomas derived from the caudal cell mass, including fibrolipomas of the filum terminale. A lipomyelomeningocele consists of an intradural lipoma that is attached to the spinal cord and extends through defects in the dura, bony spine, and fascia to become continuous with the subcutaneous fat. Seventy percent of lipomyelomeningoceles are associated with subcutaneous fatty masses. Lipomyelomeningoceles present as skin-covered lumbosacral masses above the gluteal crease. The overlying skin may be discolored from a port-wine stain or hemangioma, have a hairy tuft, or contain an ostium of a dermal sinus tract. The caudal end of the spinal cord is usually tethered in a low-lying position in cases of lipomyelomeningocele, with the conus medullaris positioned below the normal L1–2 level. Filum terminale fibrolipomas and distal conus lipomas, in contrast to lipomyelomeningoceles, are malformations of secondary neurulation. Intradural lipomas, lipomyelomeningoceles, and filum terminale lipomas can all tether the spinal cord. The neurological examination in such children may be normal, or patients may present with symptoms of a clinical tethered cord syndrome. Symptoms may become more prominent and neurological deficits can worsen during growth spurts. As a child gains weight, intraspinal lipomas will also undergo fat deposition, which can compress or tether neural elements. Treatment of lipomyelomeningoceles includes cord untethering with resection or debulking of the intraspinal lipoma.

Diastematomyelia, also known as a split cord malformation, occurs when the spinal cord is split into 2 hemicords. The hemicords may be contained within separate dural sleeves separated by a bony septum, or both hemicords may be contained within a single dural sac and separated by a fibrous septum. The 2 hemicords reunite below the level of the lesion. Diastematomyelia is most commonly found in the lumbar spine and has a gender predilection for females. Children with diastematomyelia often have cutaneous stigmata such a nevus or a hairy tuft (hypertrichosis) at the level of the malformation. Bony anomalies including spina bifida occulta, hemivertebrae, butterfly vertebrae, bony spurs at the level of the lesion, scoliosis, and orthopedic foot deformities are associated with split cord malformations. Clinically, diastematomyelia presents with symptoms of a tethered cord. Surgical treatment involves resection of any bony spurs and/or septum, untethering of the spinal cord, and reconstitution of a single dural sac.

Encephaloceles occur when there is a herniation of brain tissue and meninges through defects in the cranial vault. The tissue contained within an encephalocele consists of dysplastic and nonfunctional neural tissue with variable amounts of blood vessels, choroid plexus, dura, and ventricular tissue. The prognosis in children with encephaloceles is dependent on the amount of neural tissue contained within the encephalocele. Encephaloceles can be categorized as either posterior or anterior cranial fossa malformations depending on their location, and they are further classified according to the bone through which the herniation of tissue occurs. Posterior encephaloceles are associated with other midline congenital anomalies, including myelomeningocele, Dandy-Walker malformation, Klippel-Feil anomaly, dorsal interhemispheric cysts, abnormalities of the corpus callosum, and neuronal migration disorders. For occipital and parietal encephaloceles, it is important to delineate the relationship of the lesion with adjacent venous sinuses. The goals of operative repair include removal of the encephalocele sac, preservation of any possible functional neural tissues, and closure of the dura in a water-tight fashion and of the wound with nondysplastic skin. Up to 50% of infants will develop hydrocephalus within 1 month of encephalocele repair; thus, surveillance with serial cranial ultrasounds is warranted in this group.

▶ Arachnoid Cysts

Arachnoid cysts are developmental anomalies that form between separated layers of the arachnoid membrane. The walls of an arachnoid cyst may thicken with collagen deposition over time or hemorrhage. These cysts most commonly occur in the middle cranial fossa and suprasellar region. The brain may be shifted by the arachnoid cyst, but the overall brain volume is normal. Arachnoid cysts may be asymptomatic incidental findings, or they may present with symptoms specific to the location of the lesion. Headaches and developmental delay may also result. Arachnoid cysts are associated with hydrocephalus in more than 50% of cases. The natural history of an arachnoid cyst is quite variable, as cysts may remain static, enlarge, or even regress with time. Treatment is typically recommended only if the arachnoid cyst is symptomatic, enlarging, or causing significant mass effect. There are various surgical treatment options available, including endoscopic or open fenestration of the cyst. If the arachnoid cyst does not reduce in size following fenestration, then a cyst-to-peritoneal shunt is considered the definitive treatment.

▶ Chiari Malformations

Chiari malformations consist of 4 types of congenital hindbrain abnormalities. Chiari I malformations are characterized by the herniation of the cerebellar tonsils to at least 5 mm below the foramen magnum (Figure 36–18). The tonsils assume a pointed peg shape instead of the normal rounded shape. The tonsillar herniation creates crowding at the foramen magnum, which limits CSF flow through the craniover-

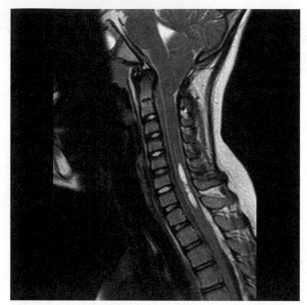

▲ **Figure 36–18.** Sagittal T2-weighted MRI scan of a Chiari showing typical peglike appearance of cerebellar tonsils and associated syringomyelia.

tebral junction. Other CNS abnormalities associated with Chiari I malformation include syringomyelia (cavitation within the spinal cord), basilar invagination, platybasia, and Klippel-Feil anomaly. Children with Chiari I malformations may be asymptomatic or present with (occipital) headaches exacerbated by straining or coughing, weakness, numbness, progressive scoliosis,; long-tract signs, central sleep apnea, or hydrocephalus. Workup should include imaging of the brain and spine to assess for the presence of a syrinx and CSF flow studies to evaluate flow at the foramen magnum. For children with a Chiari I malformation and syrinx, surgical treatment is recommended. The decision to proceed with surgical intervention in a child with radiographic tonsillar ectopia, headaches, but no syrinx must be made carefully. Surgical treatment entails a suboccipital craniectomy, C1 laminectomy, and duraplasty. Syringomyelia associated with Chiari I malformation often resolves or improves significantly after posterior fossa decompression. Chiari II malformations are found in patients with myelomeningocele, and they consist of inferior herniation of the cerebellar vermis below the foramen magnum; elongation, kinking, and displacement of the medulla below the foramen magnum and around the cervical spinal cord; abnormal lamination of the cerebral cortex; and upward displacement of the rostral cerebellum through a low-lying tentorium. Additional MRI characteristics of Chiari II malformations include hydrocephalus, fusion of the inferior colliculi of the brainstem, a large thalamic massa intermedia, a high-riding third ventricle, an elongated fourth ventricle, and a disproportionately small posterior fossa with asymmetric and flattened cerebellar folia. This can manifest as apnea and other respiratory abnormalities secondary to compression of the medullary respiratory control center. Long-tract signs, headache, ataxia, and gait instability may also be evident. In addition to myelomeningocele, other CNS abnormalities associated with Chiari II malformations include basilar impression, corpus callosum abnormalities, and cortical malformations. Surgical treatment consists of a posterior fossa decompression. Chiari III and IV malformations are rare. Chiari III malformations include features of Chiari II malformation plus an occipital encephalocele. Chiari IV malformations are characterized by severe cerebellar hypoplasia without an encephalocele.

► Craniosynostosis

Craniosynostosis refers to the premature fusion of one or more cranial sutures. When this occurs, bone growth is restricted in a direction perpendicular to the fused suture, and there is compensatory growth at other sites. The result is a misshapen head, which may take one of several forms depending on which of the cranial sutures is involved. One or multiple sutures may be affected. The incidence of craniosynostosis is approximately 5 per 10,000 live births, and males are affected more than females.

Sagittal synostosis, the most common type of single-suture synostosis, results in an elongated, boat-shaped skull referred to as scaphocephaly. In scaphocephaly, the biparietal diameter is reduced, while the anteroposterior diameter is increased. Frontal bossing is common in this condition. Patients with sagittal synostosis have a palpable keel-like prominence over the fused sagittal suture.

Coronal synostosis may be either unilateral or bilateral. Unilateral coronal synostosis produces an asymmetric head shape known as plagiocephaly. The forehead on the affected side is flattened, while the forehead on the unaffected appears to bulge abnormally. Bilateral coronal synostosis results in brachycephaly, characterized by a broad, flattened forehead. The anteroposterior diameter is reduced, while the bitemporal and biparietal diameters are increased. When bilateral coronal synostosis occurs in combination with sagittal synostosis, turricephaly results. Turricephaly is characterized by a high, towerlike head shape with a vertical forehead.

Metopic synostosis is associated with trigonocephaly, a head shape that is characterized by a triangular-shaped forehead and hypotelorism. The bitemporal diameter is narrowed, and there is often a bony ridge in the midline of the forehead over the fused metopic suture.

True unilateral lambdoid craniosynostosis is rare with an incidence of 1 in 300,000 live births, and it must be differentiated from positional posterior plagiocephaly, an increasingly common diagnosis. In unilateral lambdoid synostosis, there may be slight prominence of the forehead on the unaffected side. The ear on the affected side will be posteriorly and inferiorly displaced relative to the contralateral ear of the unaffected side. The head shape is trapezoidal when viewed from above.

While most cases of craniosynostosis are sporadic and involve a single suture, multiple-suture craniosynostosis occurs in certain genetic syndromes. Crouzon syndrome is an autosomal dominant disorder characterized by the premature fusion of the bilateral coronal, frontosphenoid, and fronto-ethmoid sutures. Clinically, the condition is characterized by brachycephaly, maxillary hypoplasia, shallow orbits, proptosis, and a beaked nose. Apert syndrome is an autosomal dominant condition characterized by pansynostosis. Clinically, patients have hypertelorism, midface hypoplasia, and shallow orbits in addition to their craniosynostosis. Symmetric syndactyly and short thumbs are also characteristic of Apert syndrome. Hydrocephalus is common in this condition.

Operative repair of craniosynostosis is often improving cosmesis. Operative approaches vary from endoscopic strip craniectomies of the involved suture to more extensive cranial vault reconstruction.

HYDROCEPHALUS

Disturbances in CSF circulation or absorption result in hydrocephalus. Hydrocephalus can be classified into 2 types: obstructive or communicating. In obstructive hydrocephalus, CSF circulation is blocked within the ventricular system, and there is enlargement in the ventricles proximal to the obstruction. In communicating hydrocephalus, CSF absorption is blocked at the level of the arachnoid granulations. Rarely, hydrocephalus may be due to the overproduction of CSF, as is the case in certain choroid plexus tumors.

The incidence of congenital hydrocephalus ranges from 0.9 to 1.8 per 1000 births. Neonatal hemorrhages of the germinal matrix and choroid plexus, as well as infections, can cause adhesions to form in the cerebral aqueduct or at the foramen of Magendie and Luschka, interfering with CSF absorption.

Hydrocephalus can cause elevations in intracranial pressure, which may manifest in different ways depending on the age of the child. In neonates and infants whose anterior fontanelle is still open, untreated hydrocephalus will present with a tense or bulging fontanelle, apneic and bradycardic episodes, engorgement of the scalp veins, upward gaze palsy, gaps between the cranial sutures, rapid increases in head circumference, irritability, poor head control, and poor oral intake. In children with a closed cranial vault whose fontanelle has closed, untreated hydrocephalus will present with symptoms of intracranial hypertension including lethargy or excessive sleepiness, papilledema, headache, nausea, vomiting, gait disturbance, increased fussiness, or upgaze or lateral gaze palsy.

Several surgical options can be considered in the treatment of hydrocephalus. The most common CSF diversionary procedure is ventriculoperitoneal shunting, creating a shunt between the cerebral ventricles and the peritoneal cavity. Other types of shunts may drain into other locations, including the right atrium (ventriculoatrial shunt) or pleural cavity (ventriculopleural shunt). In children with certain types of obstructive hydrocephalus, an endoscopic third ventriculostomy may be considered, which involves fenestration of the floor of the third ventricle, thereby creating an alternative CSF pathway.

Shunt failure or infection may manifest with signs and symptoms of acute intracranial hypertension. Ventricular enlargement may or may not be present in shunt failure. Prompt treatment of acute hydrocephalus and/or shunt failure is indicated to prevent irreversible neurologic injury, including herniation, blindness, or death.

PEDIATRIC CNS TUMORS

Brain tumors are the most common solid tumors of childhood. The locations and types of tumors in the pediatric population differ from those in adults. Approximately two thirds of brain tumors in children between 2 and 12 years of age occur in the infratentorial space. Brain tumors present in varying manners among different age groups. In neonates and infants, brain tumors may manifest with nonspecific findings, and mass effect from a tumor may not be clinically evident initially due to a compliant skull and an open fontanelle. In young children, a primary brain tumor may present with symptoms related to intracranial hypertension such as headache, nausea, and vomiting. Papilledema may be evident on funduscopic examination. Older children more often present with focal neurological signs and symptoms. The most common pediatric posterior fossa brain tumors are medulloblastoma, juvenile pilocytic astrocytoma, and ependymoma. When a posterior fossa brain tumor is diagnosed, preoperative imaging of the entire neuraxis should be performed whenever possible to evaluate for drop metastases in the spinal canal.

▶ Medulloblastoma

Medulloblastomas comprise approximately 20% of all pediatric brain tumors and 30% of all posterior fossa tumors in children. They appear as hyperdense lesions in the region of the fourth ventricle on CT imaging and enhance following contrast administration (Figure 36–19). Complete or near-complete surgical resection is the goal, as the extent of residual tumor is related to prognosis. Patients with medulloblastoma are stratified into either a standard-risk or high-risk group. Children under 3 years old who have greater than 1.5 cm^2 residual tumor on postoperative imaging or have dissemination of tumor away from the primary site as deemed by either imaging studies or positive CSF cytology have a worse prognosis and are classified as high risk. Postoperative craniospinal radiation with a boost to the posterior fossa is indicated in children older than 3 years. Those patients who are classified as high risk are typically treated with chemotherapy as well. Because of the increased

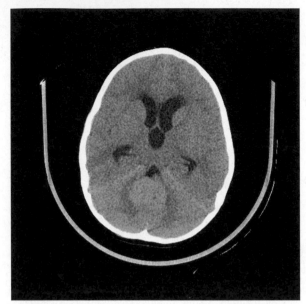

▲ **Figure 36-19.** Head CT demonstrating large mass (medulloblastoma) within the fourth ventricle causing ventricular dilation.

morbidity of radiation in children under 3 years old, chemotherapy is used to delay the radiation dose in such young patients. Recurrences, if they occur, typically occur within 3 years. The 5-year survival in standard-risk patients is 70%, while that in high-risk patients is approximately 40%. Up to 25% of patients with a posterior fossa medulloblastoma may require a CSF diversionary procedure due to persistent postoperative hydrocephalus.

Cerebellar Astrocytoma

Cerebellar astrocytomas account for approximately 20% of all pediatric brain tumors. The peak age of presentation is 10 years. The characteristic appearance on imaging studies is an enhancing mural nodule with a surrounding cyst. The goal of treatment is complete surgical resection, as patients with a gross total resection have a 90% long-term survival rate without any additional adjuvant therapies.

Ependymoma

Ependymomas can arise anywhere along the neuraxis in relation to an ependymal surface. In the pediatric population, 90% of ependymomas are intracranial, and of these, two thirds are located in the posterior fossa. Ependymomas commonly arise from the floor of the fourth ventricle in close proximity to the brainstem. When located in the fourth ventricle, ependymomas may extend out the foramina of Luschka and Magendie into the surrounding CSF subarachnoid cisterns. Dissemination of ependymoma tumor cells in

the CSF can occur in up to 10% of cases, underscoring the importance of full neuraxis imaging to properly stage the disease. Treatment usually consists of tumor resection and postoperative focal radiation.

Brainstem Glioma

Brainstem gliomas are a heterogeneous group of tumors of varying histology, biological behavior, and prognosis. Brainstem gliomas are typically subdivided into 4 groups based on imaging characteristics: diffuse brainstem gliomas, focal brainstem gliomas, dorsally exophytic brainstem gliomas, and cervicomedullary gliomas. Diffuse brainstem gliomas represent up to 80% of all brainstem gliomas and carry the worst prognosis. They most commonly occur in the pons and can extend into the medulla or midbrain. The majority of children who are affected are between 6 and 10 years of age, and they present with a relatively short clinical history of unilateral or bilateral cranial neuropathies, progressive ataxia, gait abnormality, and long-tract signs. On MRI studies, diffuse brainstem gliomas appear as nonenhancing, hypointense masses that expand the pons (Figure 36–20). They appear hyperintense on T2-weighted sequences, and with disease progression, the tumor may completely encase the basilar artery. Histologically, they are malignant (WHO grade III or IV) astrocytomas. Diagnosis of a diffuse brainstem tumor can be made on the basis of imaging alone, and biopsy is usually not recommended. Radiation therapy and steroids may improve symptoms but have not been shown to prolong survival. These tumors are universally fatal, with a median survival of 8 to 10 months.

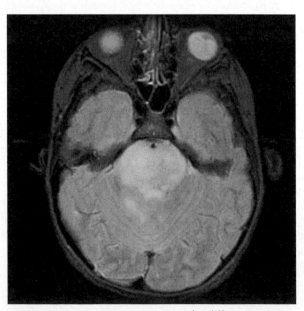

▲ **Figure 36-20.** MRI appearance of a diffuse pontine glioma.

Other types of brainstem gliomas are associated with a better prognosis. Dorsally exophytic brainstem tumors grow from the subependymal surface into the fourth ventricle, away from the brainstem. They are characterized by slow growth with gradual onset of symptoms. Eventually, they may obstruct CSF outflow from the fourth ventricle and result in hydrocephalus. Surgical excision should be performed when the predicted morbidity is not prohibitive. Histologically, focal intrinsic and dorsally exophytic brainstem gliomas are usually lower grade (WHO grade I or II) lesions. Cervicomedullary brainstem gliomas have behavior and histology similar to that of intramedullary spinal cord gliomas. These tumors may cause symptoms including weakness and lower cranial neuropathies. They should be resected.

Tumors of Infancy

Brain tumors are present in 1.1 newborns per 100,000 births. Infantile tumors include medulloblastoma, central neuroblastoma, supratentorial primitive neuroectodermal tumor (PNET), pineoblastoma, and atypical teratoid/rhabdoid tumor (AT/RT). These are all high-grade tumors with a propensity to spread throughout the CSF. Medulloblastoma, central neuroblastoma, supratentorial PNET, and pineoblastomas are all considered primitive neuroectodermal tumors with similar histologies. The combination of bilateral retinoblastomas and a midline pineoblastoma is referred to as *trilateral neuroblastoma* and carries a dismal prognosis. Atypical teratoid/rhabdoid tumors are usually found in the posterior fossa and are associated with deletions on chromosome 22 in over 90% of cases. Atypical teratoid/rhabdoid tumors have a poor prognosis, and most children die within 1 year of diagnosis.

Pineal Region Tumors

Tumors arising in the region of the pineal gland comprise 3% to 8% of pediatric brain tumors. Histologically, pineal region tumors are most often germ cell tumors such as germinomas, teratomas (mature and immature), embryonal cell carcinomas, choriocarcinomas, and endodermal sinus tumors. Germinomas are the most common pineal region tumors and demonstrate a gender predilection for males. Pineal parenchymal tumors such as pineocytoma or pineoblastomas occur less frequently. Pineal tumors can compress the cerebral aqueduct and cause hydrocephalus. Patients may present with a Parinaud syndrome consisting of impaired upgaze, convergence-retraction nystagmus, lid retraction, convergence paralysis, pupillary dilatation, and light-near dissociation. Complete neuraxis imaging should be performed because drop metastases can occur via CSF pathways. Serum and CSF should be tested for tumor markers that may be secreted by germ cell tumors, including placental alkaline phosphatase, α-fetoprotein, and β-human chorionic gonadotropin. Radiation therapy with or without chemotherapy is the mainstay of treatment for germ cells tumors.

Dysembryoplastic Neuroepithelial Tumor

Dysembryoplastic neuroepithelial tumor is a low-grade cortical-based tumor with a median age of presentation of 7 years. They appear as superficial cystic tumors in the temporal or frontal lobes. On MRI, they are hypointense on T1-weighted sequences, hyperintense on T2-weighted sequences, and do not enhance. The affected cortical gyrus often has a bubbly appearance. There is no edema or mass effect associated with dysembryoplastic neuroepithelial tumors. Patients with these tumors typically present with a long history of intractable complex partial seizures and have a normal neurological examination. Gross total resection of the tumor is curative and usually eliminates seizures.

Sellar Tumors

Tumors that arise in the region of the sella turcica and pituitary gland in children include pituitary adenomas and craniopharyngiomas. Pituitary adenomas are relatively rare among children. Craniopharyngiomas, however, represent 6% to 9% of all pediatric brain tumors and are the most common nonglial intracranial masses in children. On imaging, craniopharyngiomas appear as cystic tumors that originate from a suprasellar location. Calcification within these tumors is common. Craniopharyngiomas are hyperintense on T1-weighted and T2-weighted sequences due to fat, cholesterol, and proteinaceous contents within the cystic tumor. Craniopharyngiomas may cause symptoms attributable to intracranial hypertension and hydrocephalus, or they may present with vision disturbances. Also, craniopharyngiomas may cause endocrine disturbances such as growth failure, diabetes insipidus, hypothyroidism, or menstrual dysfunction. A thorough endocrine workup is warranted in patients with suspected craniopharyngioma. The surgical approach depends on the location and extent of the craniopharyngioma. Potential surgical complications include diabetes insipidus or hypothalamic insufficiency.

Hypothalamic Optic Gliomas

Gliomas of the optic pathway are more common in the pediatric population. Included in this category are optic nerve gliomas and chiasmatic/hypothalamic astrocytomas. Histologically, these tumors are most often pilocytic astrocytomas. Optic nerve gliomas are associated with neurofibromatosis 1. Gliomas of the optic chiasm and hypothalamus are cystic, globular tumors that enhance and rarely calcify. They may cause hydrocephalus due to compression at the foramen of Monro. Infants with hypothalamic/chiasmal gliomas present with vision loss, macrocephaly, and a diencephalic syndrome consisting of failure to thrive, cachexia, motor hyperactivity, and hyperalertness. Children 2 to 5 years of age may present with vision loss and endocrine dysfunction, including short stature or precocious puberty. Symptoms in older children include vision loss and hypopituitarism. The goals of surgical treatment for chiasmatic/

hypothalamic tumors are to obtain a tissue diagnosis and reestablish patent CSF pathways. Radiation has a clear benefit in extending progression-free survival. The 10-year relapse-free rate is approximately 55% with radiation versus 14% with biopsy alone. Chemotherapy is reserved for patients younger than 5 years in order to delay radiation. The 10-year survival following surgical biopsy and radiation for chiasmatic/hypothalamic gliomas ranges from 48% to 55%; however, these tumors and their treatments are associated with significant morbidity, including vision impairment, endocrine dysfunction, obesity, and neurocognitive decline.

Choroid Plexus Tumors

Choroid plexus tumors include choroid plexus papillomas and choroid plexus carcinomas. They represent 2% to 4% of all pediatric brain tumors. Choroid plexus papillomas occur in the atrium of the lateral ventricle in children and are attached to normal choroid plexus. These tumors avidly enhance and may calcify. If a gross total resection of the tumor is achieved, no adjuvant therapy is required. Choroid plexus papillomas are WHO grade I or II tumors and have a good prognosis. Choroid plexus carcinomas are malignant tumors for which the average age of diagnosis is 2 years. Like choroid plexus papillomas, these tumors are usually located in the lateral ventricles. Forty-five percent of choroid plexus carcinomas demonstrate dissemination at diagnosis. These tumors contain necrosis and can hemorrhage. Treatment consists of surgical resection, radiation therapy, and possibly chemotherapy. For children younger than 3 years, multiagent chemotherapy is used to delay the onset of radiation therapy. The prognosis is poor.

Spinal Cord Tumors

Spinal cord tumors in children account for 15% of all pediatric CNS tumors. Spinal cord tumors typically present with progressive back and leg pain, neurologic deficit, gait instability, torticollis, or bowel and bladder dysfunction. The most common intradural-intramedullary spinal cord tumors are low-grade glial tumors, including astrocytomas. Treatment consists of early surgery, because postoperative morbidity is worse if preoperative neurologic deficits exist. Near-total resections of low-grade spinal cord gliomas in children can confer long-term progression-free survival. High-grade gliomas are treated with surgical debulking followed by adjuvant therapies. Intradural-extramedullary tumors in children include dermoid cysts, teratomas, and neurofibromas. Extradural primary spinal tumors that occur in childhood can present with myelopathy and spinal cord compression; such tumors include aneurysmal bone cysts, osteoid osteomas, osteoblastomas, eosinophilic granulomas, and, rarely, metastatic disease.

Phakomatoses

Phakomatoses are neurocutaneous syndromes that manifest with skin lesions and CNS tumors. Most of the phakomatoses are inherited conditions. Neurofibromatosis 1 is an autosomal dominant inherited condition caused by a mutation on chromosome 17. Optic nerve gliomas are associated with neurofibromatosis 1 and, in affected children, usually occur before 6 years of age. Neurofibromatosis 2 is an autosomal dominant syndrome that results from a mutation on chromosome 22. Typical CNS tumors associated with neurofibromatosis 2 include bilateral acoustic neuromas, meningiomas, schwannomas, and intramedullary spinal cord ependymomas.

Tuberous sclerosis is an autosomal dominant syndrome that arises from mutations in chromosomes 9, 11, or 16. Children with tuberous sclerosis can get periventricular hamartomas known as subependymal nodules near the foramen of Monro and adjacent to the caudate nucleus. In 15% of patients with tuberous sclerosis, subependymal nodules can transform into a subependymal giant cell astrocytoma, a WHO grade I lesion. These are benign, enhancing tumors that arise at the foramen of Monro and cause obstructive hydrocephalus. These tumors typically occur prior to the end of the second decade of life. They can enlarge with time, and gross total resection of the subependymal giant cell astrocytoma is considered curative. The CNS lesions in tuberous sclerosis frequently cause seizures.

Von Hippel-Lindau disease is an autosomal dominant disease due to a mutation on chromosome 3. Patients with von Hippel-Lindau disease can get hemangioblastomas, most commonly in the posterior fossa and spinal cord. Although hemangioblastomas are considered benign tumors, they may recur in multiple locations in patients with this disease.

CEREBROVASCULAR DISEASE IN CHILDREN

Aneurysms & Vascular Malformations

Children may present with a variety of intracranial vascular malformations such as AVMs, venous angiomas, capillary telangiectasias, and cavernous malformations. AVMs may present with seizures or focal deficits from a hemorrhage. Without treatment, patients are at risk for recurrent hemorrhages. AVMs are usually treated with surgery in the pediatric age group but may occasionally be treated with stereotactic radiation or embolization techniques. In patients with an autosomal dominant inherited cavernous malformation syndrome, the cavernous malformations may be multiple and hemorrhage at an earlier age. Cavernous malformations are treated with surgical resection. Intracranial saccular aneurysm rupture is rare in the pediatric population. Depending on the size and configuration of the aneurysm, these lesions may be treated by surgical clipping, endovascular coiling, or managed conservatively.

Vein of Galen Malformations

Vein of Galen malformations are congenital vascular malformations characterized by extensive arterial feeders draining into an enlarged vein of Galen. Although these malformations are also known as vein of Galen aneurysms, they represent arteriovenous fistulae. Newborns can present with high-output cardiac failure due to the arteriovenous shunting. Hydrocephalus is common from compression of the cerebral aqueduct by the malformation. Seizures are also associated with these lesions. The extensive arteriovenous shunting can produce a steal effect and result in cerebral ischemia and infarction. The prognosis may be poor for patients diagnosed in early infancy with heart failure. The prognosis is better for those diagnosed later in life. Treatment usually involves endovascular embolization of feeding arteries.

▶ Moyamoya Disease

Moyamoya disease is an idiopathic vasculopathy that leads to progressive occlusion of one or both internal carotid arteries with secondary formation of a collateral capillary network at the base of the brain. The disease can also involve the proximal middle and anterior cerebral arteries. On angiography, the collateral vessels have a characteristic "puff-of-smoke" appearance. Children with Moyamoya disease present with ischemic events that may be provoked by straining or hyperventilation. Refractory headaches, seizures, and alternating hemiplegia are also associated with Moyamoya disease. Moyamoya is treated with surgical revascularization to improve blood flow via direct or indirect bypass procedures.

SPASTICITY

Spasticity in children is most often due to cerebral palsy, and several surgical options are available for treatment. In determining whether a child with hypertonia will benefit from surgical intervention, it is important to assess if dystonia is also present and, if so, its contribution to the hypertonia; the ambulatory potential of the child; and to what extent the underlying spasticity is useful for the child in terms of providing strength and allowing them to support their own weight. In addition to medication, orthopedic procedures, and periodic injections that are used to treat spasticity, the neurosurgical treatments for spasticity include placement of an intrathecal baclofen pump and selective dorsal rhizotomy. An intrathecal baclofen pump entails inserting a catheter into the intrathecal space and connecting it to a subcutaneous pump so that the antispasticity drug baclofen may be continuously delivered. Depending on at what spinal level the catheter tip is placed, upper and lower extremity spasticity may be treated. Intrathecal baclofen pumps are useful if the upper extremities are affected by severe hypertonia, if the tone conferred by spasticity is required for standing or walking, or if the lower extremity spasticity in nonambulatory patients is disabling and hinders care of the patients. Those patients who are ambulatory and whose spasticity primarily affects their lower extremities may be candidates for a selective dorsal rhizotomy. It is thought that inputs entering the spinal cord through the dorsal roots have a net excitatory effect on the anterior roots, thus contributing to spasticity. The premise of a selective dorsal rhizotomy is to intraoperatively stimulate lumbosacral dorsal nerve rootlets and record responses from the anterior nerve roots and muscles. This allows for the identification of those nerve rootlets that are relatively more involved into maintaining hypertonia, and such nerve rootlets are sectioned. Selective dorsal rhizotomy has been shown to improve ambulation, but the procedure does not confer previously nonambulatory patients the ability to walk.

PEDIATRIC TRAUMA AND BIRTH INJURIES

▶ General Principles

Head injury and its management are discussed elsewhere, and treatment principles used in the management of adult trauma also apply to the pediatric patient. Certain aspects of trauma that are unique to the pediatric population are highlighted. Head injuries are 30 times more common than spinal cord injuries in children, and they represent the most common cause of mortality and morbidity in children. In infants and young children, the brain and head are disproportionately large compared to the trunk and torso, and the neck and paraspinal musculature are incompletely developed. In children younger than 4 years of age, the skull is soft, unilaminar, and without diploë; as a result, it provides less protection to the brain for absorbing a traumatic impact and is more prone to fracture. Skull fractures in children can be linear, depressed, or ping-pong ball fractures. Ping-pong ball fractures occur in newborns and appear as a focal area of caved in skull that resembles a crushed ping-pong ball. No surgical intervention is required for ping-pong ball fractures in the temporoparietal region, as the growing skull will correct the deformity. Surgical elevation of a frontal ping-pong ball fracture may be considered for cosmetic purposes.

▶ Nonaccidental Trauma

Nonaccidental head trauma is the leading cause of death and morbidity in children under 2 years of age. In shaken baby syndrome, there may be few signs of external trauma with significant neurological injury. Alternatively, the child may present with lethargy, irritability, poor feeding, apneic episodes, or seizures. Multiple skull fractures that are associated with underlying brain injury, bilateral chronic subdural hematomas or subdural hematomas of varying ages, subarachnoid hemorrhage, and retinal hemorrhages should raise the index of suspicion for child abuse. Subdural hemorrhages commonly occur along the bilateral convexities or in the posterior interhemispheric fissure. MRI is best at evaluating subdural hematomas of varying ages as well as the extent of diffuse axonal injury that occurs with the acceleration-deceleration and rotational forces in shaken baby syndrome. A workup should include imaging of the brain and possibly spine, a skeletal survey to assess for long-bone or rib fractures, a funduscopic examination to check for retinal hemorrhages, and a thorough external examination to assess for bruising. Death from nonaccidental trauma is most often due to refractory intracranial hypertension.

Spine Trauma

Spinal cord injury is relatively rare in the pediatric population and accounts for 5% of all spinal cord injury. The pediatric spine continues to develop throughout the first 2 decades of life. Ligamentous injury is more common than bony injury, owing to ligamentous laxity, immature supporting musculature, and the developing bony joints of the spine. The cervical spine is most commonly injured in children, and in children under 9 years of age, two thirds of cervical spine injuries occur between the C1 and C3 levels.

Bulsara KR et al: Clinical outcome differences for lipomyelomeningoceles, intraspinal lipomas, and lipomas of the filum terminale. Neurosurg Rev 2001;24:192.

Cunningham ML, Heike CL: Evaluation of the infant with an abnormal skull shape. Curr Opin Pediatr 2007;19:645.

Dias MS, Partington M: Embryology of myelomeningocele and anencephaly. Neurosurg Focus 2004;16:E1.

Lew SM, Kothbauer KF: Tethered cord syndrome: an updated review. Pediatr Neurosurg 2007;43:236.

Maher CO, Raffel C: Neurosurgical treatment of brain tumors in children. Pediatr Clin N Am 2004;51:327.

Nield LS, Brunner MD, Kamat D: The infant with a misshapen head. Clin Pediatr 2007;46:292.

Pang D: Spinal cord injury without radiographic abnormality in children, 2 decades later. Neurosurgery 2004;55:1325.

Shu HG et al: Childhood intracranial ependymomas. Twenty-year experience from a single institution. Cancer 2007;110:432.

Steinbok P: Selection of treatment modalities in children with spastic cerebral palsy. Neurosurg Focus 2006;21:E4.

CEREBRAL ARTERY ANEURYSMS

John A. Cowan, Jr., MD, & B. Gregory Thompson, MD

General Considerations

Cerebral artery aneurysms (CAAs) represent an abnormal dilation or expansion of an artery within the cranial vault. Autopsy studies suggest that CAAs are present in 1% to 5% of the population. Most epidemiologic studies suggest that CAAs are more common in females (3:2) and result in the clinical presentation of approximately 30,000 to 35,000 people annually in the United States. Aneurysms are categorized as saccular, fusiform, or mycotic and can be ruptured, expanding, or unruptured. Aneurysms can be located anywhere within the cerebral artery tree but are most commonly located in the circle of Willis. The specific type, status, and location of a CAA can drastically effect a patient's clinical presentation, treatment options, and outcome. CAA can be detected with a variety of imaging modalities, including cerebral angiography (Figure 36–21), CT angiography, or MRA. Patients with any type of CAA should be referred to a neurosurgeon who specializes in the treatment of neurovascular diseases.

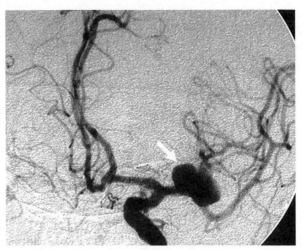

▲ **Figure 36–21.** Anterior view of left carotid artery cerebral angiogram demonstrating a large cerebral artery aneurysm (arrow) at the middle cerebral artery bifurcation.

Clinical Findings

A ruptured CAA typically presents as a sudden, severe headache associated with nuchal rigidity and lethargy. Patients often describe the headache as the "worst headache of my life"; however, sentinel (or smaller) bleeds may not present with such severity. Other features at presentation can include vomiting, seizure, focal neurologic deficit (eg, hemiparesis, oculomotor palsy), or coma. The Hunt-Hess grading scale is commonly used to convey the severity of symptoms and is often used to stratify risk (Table 36–7). Approximately 10% to 20% of patients die before reaching a hospital, and the overall mortality rate approaches 30% to 50%. The peak age of rupture is between 45 and 55 years. The rebleed rate of a ruptured CAA is approximately 25% at 2 weeks and 50% by 6 months. The mortality of a rebleed approaches 80%.

Since the cerebral arteries course within the subarachnoid space, ruptures result in subarachnoid hemorrhages. Sub-

Table 36–7. Hunt-Hess Scale.

Grade	Findings
I	Mild headache or nuchal rigidity
II	Severe headache, nuchal rigidity, possible cranial nerve deficit
III	Lethargic, confused, mild focal deficit
IV	Stuporous, moderate to severe hemiparesis, early decerebrate posturing
V	Deep coma, decerebrate posturing, moribund

From Hunt WE, Hess RM: Surgical repair as related to time of intervention in the repair of intracranial aneurysms. J Neurosurg 1968;28:14.

arachnoid hemorrhages have a classic appearance on CT scans, where the blood fills the normal CSF spaces surrounding the cortex, brainstem, and cerebellum (Figure 36–22). When presented with subarachnoid hemorrhages, the clinician must exclude the following diagnoses (before exploring more obscure causes): aneurysm rupture, trauma, coagulopathy, pretruncal (or perimesencephalic) venous bleed, cranial/spinal AVM, and dural venous sinus thrombosis. More severe aneurysm ruptures can present as intracerebral hemorrhage, subdural hemorrhage, and/or intraventricular hemorrhage.

Expanding CAAs may or may not present with symptoms of subarachnoid hemorrhages. Patients with an expanding CAA may exhibit neurologic symptoms consistent with focal compression. Although often not as dramatic as a ruptured CAA, expanding CAAs should be treated as emergencies. The specific deficit at presentation depends on the location of the aneurysm. Aneurysms along the posterior communicating artery classically present with a third nerve palsy (pupil dilation, eye abducted and downward in position). Aneurysms along the posterior cerebral artery, although rarer, can have such a presentation. Aneurysms on the anterior communication artery can present with signs of optic chiasm/tract compression. Cavernous carotid aneurysms can lead to oculomotor palsies with retroorbital pain. Ophthalmic artery aneurysms can lead to unilateral vision loss. Giant aneurysms (> 2.5 cm) can lead to more pronounced symptoms, including hemiparesis, obstructed hydrocephalus, hypothalamic dysfunction, seizures, and brainstem compression.

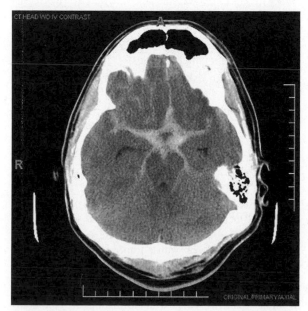

▲ **Figure 36–22.** Classic appearance of a large subarachnoid hemorrhage. Notice the hemorrhage pattern fills the cerebrospinal fluid spaces at the base of the brain and around the brainstem.

With the increasing availability and resolution of neuroimaging modalities, the detection of unruptured (and often asymptomatic) aneurysms is increasing. Although controversial, the estimated rupture rate of an unruptured CAA is 0.1% to 2% per year. Given the potentially devastating consequences of CAA rupture, however, treatment of an unruptured CAA should be considered in almost all cases.

▶ Treatment

A. Initial Management

A rapid history and physical examination of the patient, including determination of the ABCs, should be performed in patients with suspected CAAs. Patients with unstable or unprotected airways or poor respiratory effort should immediately be intubated and placed on mechanical ventilation. If symptoms of herniation are present, maintenance of P_{CO_2} values between 28 and 32 mm Hg can help acutely lower intracranial pressure. Blood pressure elevation beyond 160/90 mm Hg should be immediately controlled with intravenous medications. Prophylactic anticonvulsant and gastrointestinal (H_2-blocker or proton-pump inhibitor) should be given as well. Arterial and central venous lines should be placed to further assist in management. Basic laboratory values needed include blood gas, complete blood count, coagulation function, sodium level, blood urea nitrogen, and creatinine. An electrocardiogram and chest x-ray should also be performed. Occasionally, a patient presenting with subarachnoid hemorrhage can exhibit signs and symptoms of pulmonary edema and/or heart failure requiring further intervention. Determination of the type and status of the CAA, via cerebral imaging, is paramount in dictating the remainder of the treatment algorithm. Demonstration of subarachnoid hemorrhage on the initial head CT in patients with suspected CAA should be immediately followed by an assessment of the cerebral vascular tree (conventional angiography, CT angiography, etc). If the head CT does not demonstrate subarachnoid hemorrhage and suspicion is high, a lumbar puncture can be performed. Typically, in the setting of CT-negative subarachnoid hemorrhage, a lumbar puncture will reveal xanthochromia or high red blood cell counts that do not decrease (or "clear") across serial CSF samples. CSF diversion, typically through ventriculostomy, can be performed if the patient presents with hydrocephalus or has signs or symptoms of elevated intracranial pressure.

B. Surgical Management

Currently, two main modalities exist for treating CAAs: surgical clip occlusion and endovascular coiling. Surgical clip occlusion requires an open craniotomy and microsurgical dissection to the base of a CAA in order to apply a surgical clip around the neck of the aneurysm. Endovascular coiling utilizes as approach similar to that of conventional angiography and is thus less invasive. The endovascular surgeon navigates a microcatheter to the aneurysmal defect and inserts detachable coils into the aneurysm dome. These coils promote thrombus formation and thus exclude the aneurysm from the native circulation.

The decision between clipping or coiling a CAA is complex and beyond the scope of this text. Factors considered in this decision include a patient's age, overall medical condition, and preference as well as the aneurysm's size, location, and morphology. To date, one trial has attempted to compare the two approaches for a very select group of ruptured CAAs. The study concluded that endovascular coiling resulted in slightly less morbidity and mortality at 1 year follow-up. Case series with long-term follow-up have demonstrated some increase in rebleeding and/or the need for further treatment with endovascular coiling as compare to clip occlusion.

C. Medical Management

The medical management of patients who undergo either surgical clip occlusion or endovascular coiling for a ruptured CAA is particularly challenging. Patients require recovery in an intensive care setting that has particular expertise in neurological conditions. Once an aneurysm has been secured, the blood pressure parameters are loosened and "permissive" hypertension is allowed (typically not treated unless systolic blood pressure is > 200 mm Hg). Early tracheostomy and enteral feeding tubes are placed in patients who have neurologic deficits affecting respiratory or swallowing function. Patients are typically placed on nimodipine, which has been demonstrated to slightly decrease postoperative vasospasm. Magnesium sulfate infusions are used in some centers for prevention of vasospasm, although the data for this practice, while promising, is emerging.

Vasospasm is an idiopathic response of cerebral blood vessels to subarachnoid blood whereby the vessel constricts, thus limiting distal blood flow. The peak time for vasospasm occurs between 4 to 14 days postbleed. Approximately 20% to 40% of patients experience symptomatic vasospasm with 30% of those suffering a permanent neurologic deficit. Vasospasm can occur anywhere along a vessel and in vessels distant from the treated aneurysm. Patients can exhibit significant neurologic sequelae from vasospasm, such as hemiparesis, aphasia, and vision disturbance depending on the particular vessel affected. Subtle findings such as elevated temperature and mental status changes can be harbingers of vasospasm. Vasospasm is typically treated using a regimen referred to as *triple H* therapy, which involves hypertension (using vasopressors if needed to achieve systolic pressure > 180), hemodilution (achieve hematocrit ~30%), and hypervolemia (using albumin or hypertonic solutions to achieve central venous pressure of 8–14 mm Hg). Cerebral angioplasty is an effective means for treating proximal constriction and is a first-line treatment for symptomatic patients. Distal or diffuse spasm can respond to injection of calcium-channel blockers (eg, verapamil) or papaverine through a superselective microcatheter.

Outcomes and Prognosis

For elective surgical clip occlusion or endovascular coiling, mortality rates (1–2%) and morbidity rates (5–10%) are relatively low. Risk factors for poor outcome include aneurysm location and size and presence of intraoperative rupture as well as other comorbid conditions (eg, coronary artery disease, diabetes, age). In patients presenting with subarachnoid hemorrhage, patient age, comorbid conditions, and Hunt-Hess grade are the strongest predictors of outcome. Overall, for patients stable enough for surgical intervention, mortality rates range from 10% to 20% with morbidity rates of 20% to 40%.

Douglas C, Porterfield R: Nuances of middle cerebral artery aneurysm microsurgery. Neurosurgery 2001;48:339.

Kassell NF et al: The International Cooperative Study on the Timing of Aneurysm Surgery. Part 1: Overall management results. J Neurosurg 1990;73:18.

Molyneux A et al: International Subarachnoid Aneurysm Trial (ISAT) Collaborative Group. Lancet 2002;360:1267.

Unruptured intracranial aneurysms—risk of rupture and risks of surgical intervention. International Study of Unruptured Intracranial Aneurysms Investigators. N Engl J Med 1998;339:1725.

ARTERIOVENOUS MALFORMATIONS

W. Christopher Fox, MD, & B. Gregory Thompson, MD

KEY CONCEPTS

▶ Congenital, abnormal connections of arteries and veins without intervening capillaries.

▶ Annual rupture risk of brain arteriovenous malformation is 2% to 4% per year.

▶ Treatment may be surgical, endovascular, or radiosurgical and is performed to prevent intracranial hemorrhage.

▶ In some instances, observant management may be appropriate.

General Considerations

AVMs are tangles of congenital, abnormal connections between artery and vein with no normal intervening capillary bed. Ninety percent of AVMs are found in the supratentorial space with the remainder found in the brainstem and spine. AVMs can present at any time but are more common in younger patients. Vascular malformations are commonly seen in neurosurgical practice, and with modern imaging techniques, they are increasingly diagnosed in asymptomatic patients being evaluated for headaches or after minor head trauma. Because of their risk of rupture and the high morbidity associated with intracranial hemorrhage, it is important that all acute care physicians be aware of the presentation, initial management, and treatment of these lesions.

Epidemiology & Presentation

Because many AVMs are asymptomatic, it is difficult to absolutely determine their prevalence. Autopsy data estimate that AVMs occur in less than 1% to 4% of the population. A limited number of population-based studies have examined the natural history and bleeding risks in patients with AVM. In counseling patients, the following formula has been used to estimate lifetime of intracranial hemorrhage due to AVM rupture:

Lifetime risk (%) = 105 − patient age in years

Hemorrhage is the most common presentation, occurring in over 50% of patients. Consequently, many patients with AVM are initially evaluated in the emergency department. Seizures and headaches are also frequent, especially with larger lesions. Spinal AVMs may cause back or radicular pain, lower extremity weakness, gait disturbance, or incontinence. Large AVMs with high-volume venous drainage can cause steal phenomena; focal neurologic deficits may result from decreased tissue perfusion of surrounding brain. Increasingly, patients are referred after AVMs are found incidentally by CT or MRI.

Initial Evaluation & Care

The initial evaluation of AVMs depends on the patient's presentation. Many patients who present with rupture are neurologically and medically stable. Most intracranial bleeding from AVM rupture is intraparenchymal. Although there may be an aspect of subarachnoid hemorrhage, it is rare to see isolated subarachnoid hemorrhage in the setting of AVM rupture. In contrast to aneurysmal subarachnoid hemorrhage, where the presence of clot in the subarachnoid space is often immediately devastating, AVM bleeds are less likely to cause death. Also in contrast to aneurysmal subarachnoid hemorrhage, vasospasm is a relatively rare event with AVM-associated hemorrhage. This is not to suggest a ruptured AVM is a minor problem—mortality associated with a single hemorrhage is estimated at 10% and morbidity at 30%. However, the heterogeneous nature of presenting complaints in patients with AVM helps explain why the initial approach varies from those with aneurysms, especially in the acute setting.

In patients with AVM rupture, after the ABCs are addressed, a complete neurological evaluation should be performed. Neurosurgical consultation is appropriate. Blood pressure should be maintained in the normal range. In any patient with suspected intracranial hemorrhage, a noncontrast head CT should be obtained as soon as possible. Depending on physician and institutional preferences, CT angiography or conventional diagnostic angiography (Figure 36–23) may then be performed to further evaluate the

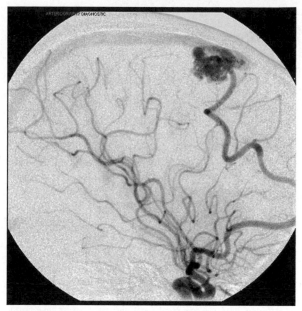

▲ **Figure 36–23.** Cerebral angiogram demonstrating a frontal arteriovenous malformation filling from the left anterior cerebral artery.

angiographic architecture of the AVM and to guide treatment. MRA takes longer to obtain than CT angiography, and the angiographic image quality, in our opinion, is suboptimal when compared to CT angiography; it is not routinely used in the acute setting.

With an initial CT scan that appears consistent with AVM rupture, a standard approach includes conventional angiography, which provides the neuroendovascular team the potential to proceed with AVM embolization during the same procedure as the diagnostic angiogram. Alternatively, for small or deep AVMs, CT angiography may be appropriate because these types of lesions are often treated with radiosurgery and the risks of diagnostic angiography may be avoided. In some instances, CT angiography may not provide a sufficiently clear picture of the AVM, and conventional angiography will need to be performed. In this case, it is important to closely monitor renal function because of the multiple contrast dye loads. Adequate hydration with intravenous fluids is important, and in patients with renal insufficiency, bicarbonate infusion and Mucomyst are useful for renal protection. Any patient with intracranial hemorrhage, even those who are neurologically intact, should initially be admitted to the neurosurgical intensive care unit for close monitoring with hourly neurologic examinations.

In patients presenting with seizures or those with large bleeds and mass effect, treatment with antiepileptic medication is appropriate. Phenytoin or Keppra are effective in the acute setting for seizure prophylaxis.

An important concept when discussing brain AVM treatment options and prognosis with patients and the multiple physicians who may care for patients with these lesions is AVM grade. Grading is most often performed using the Spetzler-Martin (Spetzler) scale (Table 36–8). Points are assigned according to size (< 3 cm, 1 point; 3–6 cm, 2 points; > 6 cm, 3 points), venous drainage (superficial, 0 points; deep, 1 point), and eloquence (absent, 0 points; present, 1 point) of the surrounding brain, yielding grades of I to V. The size and venous drainage categories are straightforward; eloquent areas are defined as the sensorimotor, language, and visual cortex; the thalamus and hypothalamus; the internal capsule; the brainstem; the cerebellar peduncles; and the deep cerebellar nuclei. AVM grade correlates with surgical results.

▶ Treatment

Four options currently exist for the treatment of AVMs. They are endovascular embolization, microsurgical resection, stereotactic radiosurgery, and observant management. Treatment often employs a combination of these approaches. AVMs should be treated in referral centers with significant experience. There is no treatment algorithm for these complex lesions. Multiple variables intrinsic to the AVM or the patient have been implicated as making certain lesions higher risk for bleeding; most of these are controversial. It is important to evaluate each patient individually, preferably with a multidisciplinary team of vascular neurosurgery, interventional neuroradiology, and radiation oncology. Multiple factors must be considered prior to recommending treatment, including AVM grade and location (for surgical safety), angiographic architecture and presence of reachable arterial pedicles (for endovascular safety), and the ability of the patient to safely tolerate an invasive procedure. Patient preference is also important, especially when considering

Table 36–8. Spetzler-Martin AVM Grading Scale.

Graded Feature	Points Assigned
Size of AVM	
3 cm	1
3-6 cm	2
> 6 cm	3
Eloquence* of adjacent brain	
Noneloquent	0
Eloquent	1
Venous drainage	
Superficial	0
Deep	1

*Eloquent areas include visual, language, and sensorimotor cortex; the thalamus and hypothalamus; the internal capsule; the brainstem; the cerebellar peduncles; and the deep cerebellar nuclei.

radiosurgery. Treatment is primarily performed because of intracranial hemorrhage—to prevent an initial or recurrent hemorrhage or to evacuate the intracranial clot that occurs after AVM rupture. Secondary treatment goals include the relief of mass effect causing headache or seizures.

A. Endovascular Embolization

The goal of endovascular embolization for AVMs is usually to reduce the size of the nidus and risk of bleeding during microsurgical resection or to reduce the size of the AVM prior to radiosurgery. However, in some cases (10–20%) complete cure can be achieved with embolization alone. It is important to appropriately counsel patients prior to AVM embolization that if complete occlusion of the AVM cannot be achieved, further treatment with surgery or radiosurgery is necessary because incompletely embolized AVMs may have a higher risk of bleeding.

B. Microsurgical Resection

Because complete obliteration is the only way to cure an AVM, microsurgical resection for small, superficial lesions is the gold standard by which all other treatment modalities are measured. Most neurosurgeons agree that Spetzler-Martin grade I to III AVMs on the cerebral convexity should be surgically resected. Complication rates associated with these lesions are low when they are operated on by neurosurgeons with significant experience. Spetzler and Martin retrospectively reported the risk of minor and major neurologic deficit and death in a series of 100 patients with grade I to V AVMs. For grade I AVMs, risk of minor and major deficit was 0%; grade II AVMs carried a 5% risk of minor deficit and 0% risk of major deficit; grade III lesions had a 12% risk of minor deficit and 4% risk of major deficit. There were no deaths. Complication rates are higher for grade IV and V AVMs. Grade IV AVMs carried a 20% risk of minor deficit and 7% risk of major deficit. With grade V lesions, risk of minor and major deficit were 19% and 12%, respectively. The prospective application of the Spetzler-Martin scale in 120 patients revealed permanent major neurological deficits in 0% of patients with grade I to III AVMs, 21.9% of patients with grade IV AVMs, and 16.7% of those with grade V AVMs. The relatively high risk of neurological deficit in patients with grade IV and V lesions makes recommending surgery for these patients a difficult decision. As endovascular technology has improved, however, some of these lesions may be approached endovascularly first, with the goal of attempting to reduce the size of the AVM prior to surgical resection.

C. Stereotactic Radiosurgery

Radiosurgery is an excellent treatment modality for many AVMs, especially those located in deep locations of the cortex or lesions of the basal ganglia, thalamus, or brainstem that are not easily approachable from a microsurgical or endovascular standpoint. Stereotactic radiosurgery is also indicated for patients with significant medical comorbidities and can be used if an AVM is subtotally resected. In general, stereotactic radiosurgery works best for AVMs less than 3 cm in size. In patients with AVMs larger than 3 cm, preradiosurgical embolization may be used to reduce the size of the nidus. The complete obliteration rate after stereotactic radiosurgery is 90% with small AVMs. The primary disadvantage of stereotactic radiosurgery is the 2 to 3 years it takes for the AVM to involute. During that period, the patient remains at baseline risk of hemorrhage (~4%) from AVM rupture.

D. Observant Management

Although this is not the opinion of the vast majority of neurosurgeons and neurointerventionalists, there are occasions when conservative management is indicated. Older patients with comorbid conditions may not benefit from aggressive management. Because of the risk of complications during open or endovascular operations with grade IV and V AVMs, and because of the reduced rate of complete obliteration after radiosurgery for large lesions, some surgeons advocate conservative treatment for these AVMs. A prospective randomized clinical trial is currently underway that should help address this issue.

▶ Postoperative Care

Patients who have undergone endovascular or open operations should be observed postoperatively in an intensive care setting until it is certain they are neurologically stable. Typically, patients are sent to the ward on postoperative day 1 from microsurgical resection. Postembolization patients are usually discharged home after an overnight stay. Complications after microsurgical resection include the usual postcraniotomy difficulties such as bleeding and seizures. Hydrocephalus can also occur, especially in patients who present with ventricular blood as part of an initial intracranial hemorrhage. Complications to keep in mind after embolization include stroke, renal insufficiency, and groin hematoma. Creatinine and hematocrit should be monitored. Any patient with unstable vital signs or decreasing hematocrit after embolization should be assumed to have a retroperitoneal hematoma and should undergo abdominal CT scanning and be treated aggressively.

After AVM resection, a phenomenon known as normal perfusion pressure breakthrough can occur. As the pathological shunting of blood through the AVM nidus is removed, relative increases in blood flow to the surrounding blood vessels and brain occur. Because these blood vessels are often chronically dysregulated by the relative lack of blood flow caused by the AVM, hemorrhage can result when blood flow returns to normal. One similarly dangerous potential complication after partial embolization is AVM rupture. In general, endovascular neurosurgeons and interventionalists do not embolize more than one third of an AVM at a time because with larger embolizations, dramatic changes in

blood flow to the AVM can occur, effectively overwhelming the remaining pathologic vessels and causing hemorrhage. Therefore, in both instances, patients must be carefully observed postoperatively. Also, it is critical that blood pressure remain in the normotensive range for at least 24 hours posttreatment.

▶ Spinal AVMs

Spinal AVMs are divided into 4 types: (1) dural arteriovenous fistulas, (2) glomus AVMs, (3) juvenile intradural AVMs, and (4) intradural, extramedullary arteriovenous fistulas. Types 1 and 4 have high blood flow but low pressure; types 2 and 3 have high blood flow, high pressure, and are more likely to hemorrhage. Dural arteriovenous fistulas (type 1) are the most common spinal vascular malformation seen. They typically occur near the thoracolumbar junction and consist of a single transdural arterial feeding vessel that directly connects to an intradural arterialized vein. Embolization of the feeding artery or clip placement across the artery is curative. Symptoms from spinal AVMs may be due to hemorrhage or venous congestion. Acute or subacute lower extremity neurological deficit, gait difficulties, myelopathy, or loss of bladder or bowel control may result. Initial diagnostic evaluation should include spinal MRI/MRA. Patients with spinal vascular malformations should also undergo cranial imaging to ensure vascular abnormalities of the brain are not present. In patients with negative imaging, spinal angiography is performed.

▶ Summary

AVMs within the central nervous system are rare. However, with advances in imaging, an increasing number of these lesions are being diagnosed. AVMs are congenital tangles of direct arteriovenous connections that annually place approximately 2% to 4% of patients with AVM at risk of hemorrhage. The morbidity and mortality associated with intracranial hemorrhage is high, and most patients with AVM are young. Therefore, treatment is often recommended to prevent intracranial hemorrhage or to relieve mass effect causing seizures, headaches, or other neurologic deficits. Treatment options include endovascular embolization, surgical resection, stereotactic radiosurgery, or a combination of these. With an experienced team of neurosurgeons, interventionalists, and radiation oncologists, treatment can be accomplished with minimal risk. In a minority of cases, observant management may be appropriate.

AVM Study Group: Arteriovenous malformations of the brain in adults. N Engl J Med 1999;340:1812.

Fiorella D et al: The role of endovascular therapy for the treatment of brain arteriovenous malformations. Neurosurgery 2006; 59:163.

Kondziolka D, McLaughlin MR, Kestle JR: Simple risk predictions for arteriovenous malformation hemorrhage. Neurosurgery 1995;37:851.

Ledezma CJ et al: Complications of cerebral arteriovenous malformation: multivariate analysis of predictive factors. Neurosurgery 2006;58:602.

Ogilvy CS et al: AHA Scientific Statement: Recommendations for the management of intracranial arteriovenous malformations. A statement for healthcare professionals from a special writing group of the stroke council, American stroke association. Stroke 2001;32:1458.

Spetzler RF, Hamilton MG: The prospective application of a grading system for arteriovenous malformations. Neurosurgery 1994;34:2.

SURGICAL MANAGEMENT OF MEDICALLY INTRACTABLE REFRACTORY EPILEPSY

Arnold B. Etame, MD, & Oren Sagher, MD

KEY CONCEPTS

▸ Understand the prevalence, varied etiologies, and broad classification of epilepsy.

▸ Describe the various diagnostic modalities for epilepsy.

▸ Recognize that focal and lateralizing epilepsy is more amenable to surgery.

▸ Recognize that mesial temporal sclerosis is highly epileptogenic with very favorable outcomes following surgical resection.

▸ Appreciate palliative and curative surgical treatments for epilepsy.

A seizure is an abnormal synchronization of electrical neuronal activity that can manifest as an alteration in mental state, tonic or clonic movements, or convulsions. The medical syndrome of recurrent, unprovoked seizures is termed epilepsy. Epilepsy is a common neurological disorder with a prevalence of 0.5% in the general population. The multiple etiologies of epilepsy include strokes, trauma, genetic disorders, tumors, vascular lesions, infections, and systemic and metabolic diseases. In most cases, epilepsy is primarily managed with anticonvulsant medications. However, despite optimal medical management, approximately 30% of patients continue to have disabling seizures. Such patients are candidates for surgical therapy. This section focuses on the surgical management of these patients.

CLASSIFICATION

Seizure types are organized according to whether the source of the seizure within the brain is localized (partial or focal onset seizures) or nonlocalized (generalized seizures). Partial seizures are further divided on the extent to which consciousness is affected. If conscious awareness is unaffected, then a seizure is said to be *simple*; otherwise it is a *complex*

seizure. A partial seizure may spread within the brain, a process known as secondary generalization. Primary generalized epilepsy is usually secondary to a genetic derangement in cell membrane function and is characterized by diffuse onset with involvement of both cerebral hemispheres. In partial epilepsy, seizure onset is focal and typically secondary to structural abnormalities in the brain.

DIAGNOSIS

Several modalities are employed in the diagnosis of epilepsy, including clinical examination, neurophysiology, imaging, and neuropsychologic assessments.

▸ Clinical Examination & Laboratory Assessment

The clinical symptomatology associated with epilepsy is a critical component of the diagnosis and is called its *semiology*. Symptoms during the time of seizure may provide localizing clues to the region of onset. For example, seizures starting with motor twitching of the upper extremity are likely to be caused by a lesion in the vicinity of the primary motor cortex. Past medical history of febrile seizures or encephalitis are associated with risk of epilepsy. In addition, family history of epilepsy appears to be a strong risk factor in the development of epilepsy. Finally, serum metabolic studies should be undertaken in order to rule out potentially reversible entities. Such studies include fasting blood glucose, serum electrolyte panel, complete blood count, erythrocyte sedimentation rate, and renal and hepatic functional assays. In patients for whom historical data and the clinical examination point to an intoxicating entity, applicable urine and serum toxicology assays should be obtained.

▸ Electrophysiology

The standard modality for recording brain activity is the scalp electroencephalograph (EEG). EEG recordings are usually obtained both between and during seizures. In some instances, patients undergo long-term monitoring with video EEG whereby seizure semiology can be assessed together with EEG pattern. Generally, the presence of lateralized or localized seizures suggests a focus that may be amenable to surgical resection. In patients whose seizure localization cannot be demonstrated convincingly by scalp EEG, intracranial EEG electrodes may be placed. These electrodes can be placed either on the surface of the brain (subdural electrodes) or within the substance of the brain (depth electrodes). Subdural electrodes register surface cortical activity, while depth electrodes can provide information related to deep structures such as the hippocampus.

▸ Imaging Studies

MRI is the usual imaging study of choice for evaluating patients with epilepsy. Structural lesions such as tumors, vascular malformations, or dysplastic cortex can be easily identified on MRI. Highly epileptogenic entities such as mesial temporal sclerosis with hippocampal atrophy can also be detected with high-resolution MRI scans, as demonstrated in Figure 36–24.

Nuclear medicine studies such as positron emission tomography (PET) and single photon emission computed tomography (SPECT) scans can serve as complementary diagnostic tests. These tests are especially useful when the MRI and EEG do not correlate. PET studies demonstrate metabolic activity within the brain, while SPECT studies reflect regional blood flow patterns at the time of tracer injection. SPECT studies performed at the beginning of a seizure often demonstrate increased flow to areas involved in seizure onset. Alternatively, PET studies performed between seizures are more likely to demonstrate hypometabolism within epileptogenic foci. Both studies are useful for patients with focal epilepsy who have normal MRIs or in whom the site of seizure origine is uncertain.

Magnetoencephalography is a functional imaging technique that can accurately provide information on synchronized electrical activity in the brain. Magnetoencephalography detects the magnetic dipole equivalents of electrical current. In addition, it has the advantage of providing a 3D localization of neuronal activity. Finally, there is accumulating data to suggest a high correlation between magnetoencephalography and intracranial seizure localization.

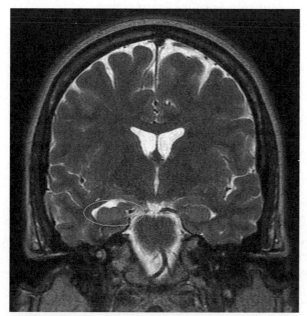

▲ **Figure 36–24.** Coronal MRI of the brain demonstrating right mesial temporal sclerosis with associated atrophy of the right hippocampus and prominence of the temporal horn of the right lateral ventricle.

Neuropsychological evaluation is an important component of the epilepsy workup. Patients should undergo a battery of standardized neuropsychological tests assessing verbal and nonverbal intelligence, memory, executive functions, and behavioral functions. These tests often point to subtle deficiencies that accompany the presence of a seizure focus. In addition to these tests, patients may undergo more invasive neuropsychological tests such as the **Wada test,** which involves selective injection of a fast-acting barbiturate such as amobarbital into each hemisphere via the carotid artery while memory and language functions are tested. The goal of the Wada test is to assess language and memory dominance. If the Wada test suggests that a significant amount of language function is subserved by the diseased hemisphere, then surgical resection may result in significant deficits.

SURGICAL SELECTION

In general, patients with structural lesions such as tumors and vascular malformations should be managed primarily with surgical resection. In addition, those patients with a localized epileptogenic focus who have failed medical management should be considered for surgery. The most common surgical lesion amenable to surgery is mesial temporal sclerosis. This entity is very epileptonic and accounts for the majority of cases of partial epilepsy.

There is evidence to suggest that early surgical intervention improves outcome. With surgical success, patients can be gradually weaned off anticonvulsants, thereby sparing them of the deleterious long-term effects of these medications. However, in patients with epileptonic foci within the eloquent cortex, the risk of postsurgical deficits must be considered against the probability of rendering the patients seizure free. Ultimately, the decision to recommend surgery is made by a multidisciplinary team consisting of epileptologists, neurosurgeons, radiologists, neuropsychologists, and social workers.

GOALS OF SURGERY

Surgical procedures can be viewed as either curative or palliative. Curative procedures are designed for patients with seizures convincingly localized to a specific cortical region that is safe to remove. The goal in curative surgery, therefore, is complete resection of the affected cortex. Procedures such as anterior temporal lobectomy, selective amygdalohippocampectomy, neocortical resections, and hemispherectomy would be considered potentially curative. Palliative surgery, on the other hand, is employed in situations in which a seizure focus is either not identified or cannot be safely removed. For example, patients with congenital syndromic epilepsies such as Lennox-Gastaut syndrome experience life-threatening generalized seizures for which an identifiable focus is not possible. The goal of palliative surgery, therefore, is reduction of seizure frequency and severity. Common palliative procedures include placement of a vagus nerve stimulator and corpus callosotomy.

SURGICAL TECHNIQUES

Temporal Lobectomy

Patients with temporal lobe epilepsy secondary to mesial temporal sclerosis are often candidates for temporal lobectomy. The surgical technique involves a temporal craniotomy with subsequent resection of the amygdala, hippocampus, and variable amounts of the neocortex. The long-term seizure-free outcomes are around 60% to 80%. Potential complications include minor visual field deficits and deficits with short-term memory.

Temporal lobectomy can also be used for other structural pathologies of the temporal lobe. However, for circumscribed lesions, a lesionectomy might suffice. Seizure-free outcomes with lesionectomy are estimated at 70% to 90%.

When temporal lobectomy is performed in the nondominant hemisphere, intraoperative mapping and language localization is not necessary. Language mapping might be necessary with dominant temporal lobe resections, where language-bearing structures may be at risk.

Selective Amygdalohippocampectomy

This procedure is a modified, minimalistic version of the temporal lobectomy. It involves resection of the amygdala and hippocampus via a temporal craniotomy, sparing the temporal cortex. The approach to these structures is either through a slit in the temporal lobe cortex or via the sylvian fissure. The procedure is utilized in individuals with language-dominant mesial temporal lobe epilepsy in whom resection of the neocortex would risk significant language deficits. Seizure-free outcomes are quite similar to those with temporal lobectomy. Potential complications include deficits with short-term memory as well as mild naming deficits.

Extratemporal Resections

These procedures are performed in patients with focal epilepsy arising outside the temporal lobe. The frontal lobe is the most common location for such resections. In light of the potential overlap with functional areas, resection is often limited, and seizure-free outcome is not as favorable as that seen in temporal lobe epilepsy, averaging approximately 50%. Surgery entails a craniotomy with resection of cortex, at times guided by intraoperative electroencephalograph recordings. Complications are contingent upon associated eloquent areas involved.

Hemispherectomy

This procedure involves surgical resection or disconnection of one hemisphere from the other. Patients with fixed or progressive neurological deficits in the context of diffuse unilateral hemispheric seizures from conditions such as Sturge-Weber syndrome or Rasmussen encephalitis. The affected brain lacks normal function, and as a result, patients are often hemiplegic prior to surgery. Hemispherectomy can control seizures in about 70% to 90% of patients. In properly selected cases, function is preserved with associated improvements in cognitive, behavioral, and motor domains.

As originally described, hemispherectomy entailed complete removal of half of the brain. This was fraught with progressive postoperative neurological deficits secondary to deposition of iron over the brain (superficial cerebral hemosiderosis). In light of these problems, a modified functional hemispherectomy has replaced the anatomic hemispherectomy. This procedure involves disconnecting the corpus callosum and the various interhemispheric commissures. The major risks include hemorrhage, damage to functioning cortex, persistent seizures, disseminated intravascular coagulation, and transient decrease in contralateral muscle tone.

Corpus Callosotomy

This procedure is palliative and is utilized in situations in which patients have diffuse epileptonic foci involving both hemispheres. Sectioning the corpus callosum prevents interhemispheric propagation of seizures. Seizures that cause drop attacks such as atonic seizures are often amenable to corpus callosotomy. The procedure typically involves resection of the anterior two thirds of the corpus callosum, with the option of further resections if seizures persist. Approximately 5% of patients are seizure free, while over half experience improvements in seizure outcome and severity.

Multiple Subpial Transection

This procedure is indicated for patients with seizure foci within functionally important cortex (eg, primary motor cortex). The procedure is palliative, with over half of patients experiencing a significant improvement in short-term seizure control. The surgical technique involves creating shallow vertical transections across cortical gyri. The rationale underlying this procedure is that the interruption of horizontal fibers caused by the transection prevents seizure recruitment, spread, and hence progression of the seizures.

Vagus Nerve Stimulation (VNS)

The vagus nerve stimulation is a relatively low-risk surgical procedure that decreases seizure frequency in patients whose disease is not safely amenable to resection. The exact mechanism by which this technique treats epilepsy is unknown. Surgery involves placement of a stimulator electrode along the vagus nerve in the neck, which is then connected via leads to a generator implanted on the anterior chest wall. Current data suggests seizure-free outcomes are close to 2%. In addition, approximately 40% of patients experience at least a 50% decline in seizure frequency. The main risks of the procedure include injury to the vagus nerve, carotid artery, and jugular vein. Patients may develop hiccups secondary to overstimulation. Nonetheless, this remains a low-risk intervention in comparison to other surgical modalities.

Stereotactic Radiosurgery

The application of highly focused irradiation to specific brain regions, known as *radiosurgery*, has been used to treat a wide variety of brain lesions such as tumors and vascular lesions. The role of radiosurgery in seizure control has been fairly limited. However, it has been proposed as a potential treatment of deep-seated seizure foci, such as hypothalamic hamartomas. Hypothalamic hamartomas are benign malformations in the hypothalamus associated with intractable seizures and encephalopathy *(gelastic epilepsy)*. Surgical resection in this location is fraught with risk, and it appears that radiosurgery may be used more safely in a subset of patients with gelastic seizures.

Benifla M et al: Temporal lobe surgery for intractable epilepsy in children: an analysis of outcomes in 126 children. Neurosurgery 2006;59:1203.

Devlin AM et al: Clinical outcomes of hemispherectomy for epilepsy in childhood and adolescence. Brain 2003;126:556.

Hennessy MJ et al: Predictors of outcome and pathological considerations in the surgical treatment of intractable epilepsy associated with temporal lobe lesions. J Neurol Neurosurg Psychiatry 2001;70:450.

Holmes MD et al: Outcome after surgery in patients with refractory temporal lobe epilepsy and normal MRI. Seizure 2000;9:407.

Iida K et al: Characterizing magnetic spike sources by using magnetoencephalography-guided neuronavigation in epilepsy surgery in pediatric patients. J Neurosurg 2005;102(2 suppl):S187.

Kuzniecky R, Devinsky O: Surgery insight: surgical management of epilepsy. Nat Clin Pract Neurol 2007;42:829.

Kwan P, Brodie MJ: Early identification of refractory epilepsy. N Engl J Med 2003;42:314.

Mulligan LP et al: Multiple subpial transections: the Yale experience. Epilepsia 2001;42:226.

Regis J et al: Gamma knife surgery for epilepsy related to hypothalamic hamartomas. Neurosurgery 2000;47:1343.

Roberts DW et al: Investigation of extra-temporal epilepsy. Stereotact Funct Neurosurg 2001;77:216.

Spencer S et al: Predicting long-term seizure outcome after resective epilepsy surgery. Neurology 2005;65:912.

Tecoma ES, Iragui VJ: Vagus nerve stimulation use and effect in epilepsy: what have we learned? Epilepsy Behav 2006;8:127.

van Empelen R et al: Functional consequences of hemispherectomy. Brain 2004;127:2071.

SURGICAL MANAGEMENT OF PAIN

Arnold Etame, MD, & Parag G. Patil, MD, PhD

The subjective, emotional, and physical components of pain make its management complex. Hence, pain management is an interdisciplinary endeavor encompassing medical, surgical, and psychological treatment modalities. Surgery for pain should be reserved for patients who have been unresponsive to therapies directed toward the inciting processes and to oral pain medications.

Pain may be classified as *nociceptive* or *neuropathic*. Nociceptive pain results from tissue injury. Common characteristics include constant aching or throbbing and responsiveness to opiate medications. Neuropathic pain is initiated or caused by a primary lesion or dysfunction in the nervous system. Common characteristics include burning, allodynia, and paresthesias. Neuropathic pain responds poorly to opiate medications. Pain surgeons should be familiar with these concepts to assess medical intractability.

The aim of surgery is to interrupt pain signaling pathways. Ablative surgical techniques involve physical interruption through the destruction of neural tissue. Nonablative procedures involve functional interruption through the modulation of pain transduction mechanisms.

ABLATIVE PROCEDURES TO INTERRUPT AFFERENT PAIN PATHWAYS

Neurosurgical procedures to physically interrupt pain signaling have been directed toward the nerves (neurectomy), spinal roots (rhizotomy), dorsal root ganglia (ganglionectomy), dorsal root entry zone (DREZ lesioning), spinal cord (cordotomy, myelotomy), and cerebral cortex (cingulotomy). Ablative surgery for pain is most often utilized in the treatment of cancer-related, nociceptive pain, as long-term analgesia is less commonly observed for these procedures.

Neurectomy

Neurectomy involves cutting an injured nerve or the nerve to a painful region. Target nerves are identified on the basis of local anesthetic blockade. Denervation of joints, distal sensory nerves, and neuroma surgery are examples of peripheral neurectomy. Neurectomy is not typically utilized for cancer-related pain because of the changing pain distribution with tumor growth. Reported success rates for pain control with neurectomy vary widely between 40% and 90%.

Rhizotomy & Ganglionectomy

Rhizotomy and ganglionectomy target the dorsal sensory rootlets or ganglia, respectively. Spinal cord segments are identified through paraspinal local anesthetic blockade, with placebo controls. The procedures are utilized most commonly for cancer-related regional pain or occipital neuralgia. These procedures are rarely utilized in the treatment of extremity pain because of functional impairment resulting from the loss of proprioception. Successful longer-term pain control has been reported in 40% to 70% of patients.

Dorsal Root Entry Zone Lesioning

Dorsal root entry zone surgery targets the superficial dorsal horn region, where sensory fibers enter the spinal cord. Levels including and flanking the region of interest, as defined by imaging studies or pain distribution, are typically ablated. A knife or radiofrequency heating is used to make the lesion. Dorsal root entry zone surgery is most effective in the treatment of neuropathic pain following nerve root avulsion and at-level spinal cord injury pain. Risks of surgery include injury to descending motor pathways and decreased sensory function in the territory of the ablated region. In carefully selected patients, rates of successful pain control range from 70% to 90%.

Cordotomy & Myelotomy

Cordotomy is a spinal procedure to interrupt pain transmission along the lateral spinothalamic tract. Cordotomy is most commonly performed in patients with intractable, unilateral, nociceptive cancer pain at the level of the chest or below. The procedure may be performed either with a knife or with radiofrequency heating. Risks of surgery include lower extremity weakness, ataxia, and respiratory or urinary dysfunction. These risks are significantly increased when cordotomy is performed bilaterally.

Midline myelotomy involves destruction of the mesial dorsal columns at a single spinal level to treat midline, bilateral, or visceral pain. The procedure typically preserves dorsal column and spinothalamic signal transmission. Risks include transient lower extremity paresthesias and weakness.

Rates of successful pain control with cordotomy and myelotomy are initially high (> 80%) but decline over time (40% at 2 years).

Cingulotomy

Unlike procedures directed along pathways of pain neurotransmission, cingulotomy is directed toward alteration of the experience of pain. Because the cingulate gyrus is part of the limbic system, radiofrequency ablation of the anterior cingulate gyrus reduces the affective, unpleasant aspects of pain, particularly in patients with obsessive and affective components to their pain. Cingulotomy is performed in relatively few centers and only in carefully selected patients. Following cingulotomy for intractable, cancer-related pain, over 50% of patients have been reported to have moderate to complete pain relief.

PROCEDURES TO MODULATE AFFERENT PAIN PATHWAYS

Intrathecal Analgesic Delivery Pumps

When compared to oral narcotics, intrathecal administration of morphine provides more potent analgesia with reduced side effects, such as nausea, constipation, and sedation. To benefit from intrathecal delivery, patients should have significant reduction in pain level with oral opiates, limited by intolerable side effects.

Analgesics such as morphine are delivered through a catheter placed into the cerebrospinal fluid of the spinal canal. The catheter tubing is then connected to an external or surgically implanted pump. External pumps are utilized in patients with cancer-related pain and expected survival of less than 3 months. Principal complications of intrathecal drug delivery include the side-effects of the medication, mechanical failure of the system, and infection.

Intrathecal drug delivery may be effective in either nociceptive or neuropathic pain syndromes. However, as with oral opiate administration, long-term tolerance to medications can develop. Hence, these devices are most beneficial for patients with cancer-related pain syndromes and limited life expectancy.

Peripheral Nerve & Spinal Cord Stimulation

Peripheral nerve and spinal cord stimulators deliver pulses of electricity to injured nerves or the dorsal columns of the spinal cord, respectively. According to the gate theory of pain, such stimulation blocks the flow of pain signals from the periphery to the brain.

Peripheral nerve stimulation is most effective in neuropathic peripheral nerve syndromes such as occipital neuralgia and complex regional pain syndrome. More recently, peripheral stimulation has been used to treat headaches and fibromyalgia. Spinal cord stimulation is most effective in patients with lumbosacral radiculopathy due to scar tissue formation following back surgery as well as in patients with complex regional pain syndrome.

Patient candidates typically undergo an initial trial with a temporary electrode applied to the spinal cord or nerve. After the 1-week trial, permanent placement is performed if benefit is demonstrated. Benefit is measured as a reduction in pain as well as an increase in daily activities. Complications of the therapy are most commonly stimulating lead migration, breakage, and infection.

Deep Brain Stimulation

Deep brain stimulation involves the precise surgical placement of electrodes into the deep nuclei of the brain. Common targets of deep brain stimulation for pain include the thalamus, which is the sensory relay of the brain, and the periaqueductal grey region, which results in the upregulation of endogenous opiates. Once electrodes are implanted, trial stimulation is performed for 1 to 2 weeks. A successful trial is characterized by the experience of pain-relieving and tolerable paresthesias in the treated region during thalamic stimulation, a sense of warmth and ocular movement during periaqueductal stimulation, a poststimulatory pain-relieving effect, and the absence of an analgesic effect during sham stimulation. Following the trial, a pulse generator is connected to the wires and implanted in the chest. Long-term results in patients with a successful trial are variable, ranging from 19% to 79%.

Motor Cortex Stimulation

Electrical stimulation of the region of the motor cortex results in analgesia in neuropathic pain syndromes such as hemibody poststroke pain and trigeminal deafferentation pain. The mechanism of motor cortex stimulation is unknown.

The surgical procedure involves placement of a stimulating electrode under the skull in the region of the motor cortex. Patients undergo a trial of stimulation. Stimulus intensity is typically set to 80% of the level needed to produce motor cortical responses. Following a successful trial, the electrodes are connected to an implantable pulse generator in the chest. Motor cortex stimulation has a success rate of 70% in facial pain syndromes and of 50% in central neuropathic pain.

Burchiel KJ (editor): *Surgical Management of Pain*. Thieme, 2002.

Melzack R, Wall PD: Pain mechanisms: a new theory. Science 1965;150:171.

Patil PG, Campbell JN: Peripheral and central nervous system surgery for pain. In: *Wall and Melzack's Textbook of Pain*, 5th ed. McMahon SB, Koltzenburg M (editors). Elsevier, 2006.

Simpson BA (editor): *Electrical Stimulation and the Relief of Pain*. Elsevier, 2003.

SURGICAL MANAGEMENT OF MOVEMENT DISORDERS

Arnold Etame, MD, & Parag G. Patil, MD, PhD

Neurosurgical procedures for movement disorders have evolved considerably in recent years. Formerly popular stereotactic tissue-destructive procedures, such as pallidotomy and thalamotomy, have been superseded by nonlesional deep-brain stimulation (DBS). Careful, prospective and well-controlled studies have demonstrated significant benefits of DBS in the treatment of Parkinson disease, essential tremor, and dystonia.

PARKINSON DISEASE

Clinical Considerations & Pathophysiology

James Parkinson was the first to describe the "shaking palsy" in 1817. The clinical signs of Parkinson disease (PD) are tremor, bradykinesia (slowness of movement), rigidity (increased muscle tone), and postural instability. The tremor of PD occurs at rest, has a "pill-rolling" character, and typically decreases with voluntary movement. The rigidity of PD has a "cogwheel" ratchetlike quality during passive movement. Postural instability results from a loss of reflexes, leading to impaired balance. Other signs of PD include a shuffling gait, decreased voice volume, slowed reaction time, and dementia. A popular scale for the measurement of parkinsonism is the Unified Parkinson Disease Rating Scale (UPDRS).

PD is accompanied by a loss of dopaminergic neurons in the substantia nigra pars compacta. According to a well-accepted model of basal-ganglia function, the loss of dopamine results in activation of the subthalamic nucleus and the globus pallidus pars interna (GPi). The GPi inhibits motor regions of the thalamus, resulting in decreased cortical excitation and the symptoms of PD. The central role of the GPi and subthalamic nucleus in this scheme provides the impetus for the surgical therapies for PD.

Idiopathic PD must be distinguished from other parkinsonian syndromes that have similar signs and symptoms. These syndromes include multiple system atrophy, progressive supranuclear palsy, corticobasal degeneration, and dementia with Lewy bodies. There are no laboratory or blood tests that help in the diagnosis of PD. CT and MRI studies of patients with PD are typically normal. For each patient, the diagnosis is based entirely on the history and physical examination as well as responsiveness to medication. As a result, only 75% of patients with a clinical diagnosis of PD are confirmed at autopsy.

Medical Management

Medical management strategies for the treatment of PD center upon manipulation of the dopaminergic system. L-dopa, which was introduced in 1967, crosses the blood-brain barrier and is converted by dopaminergic neurons into dopamine. L-dopa is often compounded with carbidopa, an inhibitor of dopamine metabolism in the bloodstream, to increase the efficiency of L-dopa delivery to the brain. Other medications that are useful in the treatment of PD include inhibitors of the COMT and MAO-B enzymes, which metabolize dopamine, as well as direct agonists of dopamine receptors in the brain. Patients with non-PD, atypical parkinsonian syndromes do not respond well to L-dopa therapy.

Over 5 to 10 years, PD patients develop several troublesome side effects of L-dopa. Dyskinesias are involuntary writhing movements of the face and extremities that occur at peak dopamine levels. In addition, after chronic therapy, patients may develop on-off fluctuations in which their parkinsonian symptoms oscillate in an unpredictable manner. Finally, patients may develop involuntary freezing during movement. The presence of such side effects of L-dopa should prompt surgical evaluation.

Surgical Management

Lesional stereotactic surgery for PD has been performed since the 1950s. Principal targets for ablation include the thalamus (thalamotomy) and the GPi (pallidotomy). With the introduction of L-dopa, these lesional surgical therapies declined. However, with the appearance of L-dopa side effects in the 1980s and with the development of DBS techniques in the 1990s, surgery for PD has increased significantly. At present, DBS of the subthalamic nucleus or GPi is favored over lesional surgery because of its heightened safety and reversibility. Since FDA approval in 1997, over 10,000 patients with PD have been treated with DBS.

Surgical indications for the treatment of PD are well established. Guidelines defined by the Core Assessment Program for Surgical Interventional Therapies in PD (CAPSIT-PD) include the following:

- A diagnosis of idiopathic PD for a period of 5 years.

- Exclusion by history and MRI of atypical parkinsonism.

- Dopaminergic responsiveness (33% reduction in UPDRS motor score with L-dopa).

- No significant cognitive deterioration or depression.

The goal of surgery for PD is an improvement in motor symptoms. DBS results in significant improvements in tremor, rigidity, bradykinesia, postural stability, freezing, and gait, compared to the *off*-L-dopa state. DBS is not expected to provide improvement to patients with PD beyond their best *on*-L-dopa state. However, as doses of L-dopa are typically lowered after DBS surgery, DBS provides relief from the dyskinesias and on-off fluctuations associated with chronic L-dopa therapy.

A recent study has determined that DBS results in a significant improvement in quality of life for patients with PD. Compared to medication alone, DBS provides increased ability to perform activities of daily living, improved emotional well-being, decreased stigma of disease, and reduced bodily discomfort. Benefits are likely to be reduced, however, in patients over 70 or with significant cognitive deficits in whom motor improvements alone are unlikely to alter quality of life significantly.

ESSENTIAL TREMOR

▶ Clinical Considerations & Pathophysiology

Essential tremor (ET) is the most common movement disorder, affecting an estimated 2% to 4% of the population. ET can be present in adolescence but most often appears in middle age or later life and is slowly progressive. There is a strong genetic component, with 25% to 60% of patients reporting a family history of tremor, typically with an autosomal dominant pattern of inheritance.

The tremor of ET occurs during maintenance of posture against gravity and with action. ET can occur in any part of the body but is most commonly observed in the hand (90–100%), head (40–60%), and voice (25–35%). The tremor of ET is distinguished from rest tremors, which occur when a limb is fully supported against gravity, and from intention tremors, which occur during visually guided movement as the limb approaches the target. However, in severe cases, patients with ET may experience either rest or intention tremor in addition to action tremor.

The pathophysiology of ET is not well understood, though cerebellar function appears to be involved. In addition to tremor, patients with ET may have mildly ataxic or dysmetric gait, oculomotor deficits, and disordered eye-hand movements, reminiscent of cerebellar dysfunction. In addition, PET studies have demonstrated increased cerebellar activity in patients with ET. It is thought that disruption to olivocerebellar rhythmicity may be central to the development of essential tremor.

ET must be differentiated from other tremor disorders. Disease processes resulting in action tremor may include PD, enhanced physiological tremor, dystonia, and Wilson disease. Other tremor disorders may include cerebellar (intention) tremors, Holmes (rubral) tremor, toxic/metabolic disorders, and psychogenic disorders.

▶ Medical Management

In many cases, ET begins late in life, progresses slowly, and is neither physically disabling nor psychologically burdensome. Some patients may experience reduced tremor by restricting or eliminating caffeine from the diet or by wearing small weights about their wrists. Some patients may experience reduced tremor with moderate alcohol consumption. However, alcohol is not typically recommended as a treatment because of risks of resulting chemical dependence in susceptible individuals.

For patients with disabling tremor, first-line therapies include beta-blockers, such as propranolol, and the antiepileptic primidone. Approximately 50% to 70% of patients obtain benefit from beta-blockade. Primidone is a medication related to phenobarbital, with similar efficacy to beta-blockade in the treatment of ET. In some patients, the two therapies may be combined for an additive effect. Additional pharmacological agents for ET include gabapentin, topiramate, and long-acting benzodiazepines, such as clonazepam. Finally, a subset of patients with ET may be treated by local botulinum toxin injection.

▶ Surgical Management

As in the treatment of PD, lesional surgery for ET has been largely superseded by DBS. The targets of ablation and DBS are the same, the ventralis intermedius nucleus of the thalamus. The ventralis intermedius nucleus receives inputs from the deep cerebellar nuclei, including the dentate nucleus, which may account for its importance in the treatment of ET. A unilateral procedure is favored for patients with disabling unilateral extremity tremor, while a bilateral procedure may be required to control bilateral or axial tremors.

Thalamotomy of the ventralis intermedius nucleus is highly effective in the treatment of ET, with over 80% of patients experiencing effective long-term tremor suppression. Complications of thalamotomy occur in some 25% of patients and primarily include hemorrhage, weakness, dysarthria, and ataxia.

Ventralis intermedius nucleus DBS has largely replaced thalamotomy in the surgical treatment of ET. In a prospective, randomized study comparing DBS to thalamotomy, both therapies achieve similar tremor control. However, DBS results in fewer adverse effects. DBS may have more favorable effects on patient functional status, including activities of daily living. Complications of thalamotomy and DBS are more pronounced in patients following a bilateral procedure.

PRIMARY DYSTONIA

▶ Clinical Considerations & Pathophysiology

Dystonia is the sustained cocontraction of opposing muscle groups. Patients with dystonia exhibit abnormal and awkward postures, engage in repetitive movements, and often experience significant pain. Dystonia may affect muscles throughout the body (eg, generalized dystonia) or muscles in a region (eg, torticollis), or it may have a specific focus (eg, blepharospasm). Like tremor, dystonia may be an isolated finding or a manifestation of a more generalized neurological condition.

The pathophysiology of dystonia is not known. Some cases of dystonia have been shown to result from dopamine deficiency or disordered function of dopamine receptors in the basal ganglia. One model suggests that decreased or dysregulated activity in GPi results in disinhibition of motor cortical areas.

Dystonia often occurs as an idiopathic condition, without a clear etiology. Alternatively, dystonia may occur as a secondary condition, resulting from birth injury, stroke, drug toxicity, or a hereditary degenerative neurological condition. Recently, over a dozen hereditary forms of previously idiopathic dystonia have been identified, including mutations of the *DYT1* gene on chromosome 9. The distinction between primary and secondary dystonia is important, as secondary dystonias respond less well to surgical interventions.

▶ Medical Management

Primary dystonia may be treated with anticholinergic drugs such as trihexyphenidyl, benzodiazepine muscle relaxants such as valium, or the injection of botulinum toxin into affected muscle groups. In addition, some dopamine-blocking medications have been utilized in the treatment of dystonia, although use of such medications also may worsen some forms of dystonia. Physical therapy is also an important component of dystonia treatment to prevent the formation of fixed muscle contractures.

▶ Surgical Management

Patients who fail to respond to oral medications and who fail to achieve adequate relief with botulinum toxin injections should be referred for surgical management. Dystonia has been treated with either ablation or stimulation of the GPi. Pallidotomy improves dystonia by 60% to 70% when measured by standard rating scales. Bilateral pallidal DBS is also highly effective in the treatment of primary dystonia. By comparison to sham stimulation, DBS significantly improved motor symptoms, pain, and quality of life. The most common side effect of pallidal DBS is dysarthria.

TECHNIQUES OF STEREOTACTIC NEUROSURGERY

Stereotactic neurosurgery involves the ablation of tissue or the placement of electrodes deep into the brain. Both the clinical efficacy and risks of surgery depend on submillimeter accuracy, requiring specialized techniques. Patients are typically placed in a stereotactic frame. This frame is affixed to the skull, under local anesthetic. The patient then undergoes an MRI or CT scan. Performance of a scan while in the frame allows a precise coordinate system to be defined within the brain.

In the operating room, a small hole is drilled into the skull, allowing the introduction of microelectrodes along a trajectory leading to the target. The microelectrodes record extracellular neuronal activity. Each region of the brain has a specific electrophysiological signature. Depending on the surgery, the patient may be examined for motor or sensory responsiveness of cellular activity.

Once electrophysiology has confirmed the target for surgery, DBS electrodes are placed into the same location along the same trajectory. With the electrode in position, stimulation is applied and the patient is examined for undesirable clinical effects. Once a desirable effect is confirmed, the electrodes are secured. As a second stage, the electrodes are tunneled under the skin to an implantable stimulation generator placed under the skin, just below the clavicle. This generator may be precisely tuned to the requirements of each patient.

In lesional surgery, a radiofrequency or cryoprobe is placed into the location following microelectrode recording, and a temporary lesion is created. When the absence of undesired effects is confirmed, a permanent lesion is created.

Coubes P et al: Treatment of *DYT1*-generalized dystonia by stimulation of the internal globus pallidus. Lancet 2000;355:2220.

Eltaway HA et al: Primary dystonia is more responsive than secondary dystonia to pallidal interventions: outcome after pallidotomy or pallidal deep brain stimulation. Neurosurgery 2004;54:613.

Gill SS et al: Direct brain infusion of glial cell line-derived neurotrophic factor in Parkinson disease. Nat Med 2003;9:589.

Krack P et al: Five year follow-up of bilateral stimulation of the subthalamic nucleus in advanced Parkinson's disease. N Engl J Med 2003;349:1925.

Kupsch A et al: Pallidal deep-brain stimulation in primary generalized or segmental dystonia. N Engl J Med 2006;355:1978.

Shuurman PR et al: Comparison of continuous thalamic stimulation and thalamotomy for suppression of severe tremor. N Engl J Med 2000;342:461.

Vidailhet M et al: Bilateral deep-brain stimulation of the globus pallidus in primary generalized dystonia. N Engl J Med 2006;352:459.

INTERVERTEBRAL DISK DISEASE

Cheerag Upadhyaya, MD, Hunter Brumblay, MD,
& Paul Park, MD

▶ General Considerations

The human spinal column is composed of 33 longitudinally stacked bone segments called vertebrae: 7 cervical, 12 thoracic, 5 lumbar, 5 sacral (fused), and 2 to 4 coccygeal (fused). A typical vertebra is composed of a rounded body anteriorly and a protective boney arch posteriorly, which together form a canal through which the spinal cord passes. Vertebral bodies articulate anteriorly via intervertebral disks and posteriorly via synovial joints formed by the articular facets of adjoining vertebrae. They are also connected by several ligaments: the anterior and posterior longitudinal ligaments, which traverse the vertebral bodies from top to bottom; the supraspinous and interspinous ligaments, which run between the posterior projecting spinous processes of each vertebra; and the ligamentum flavum, which connects the lamina (part of the posterior arch) at each vertebral level.

In a normal adult, the spinal cord extends from the craniocervical junction to the lumbar level, where it tapers and typically ends at L1–2 as the conus medullaris. Eight sets of nerve roots exit the spine in the cervical region, though there are only seven cervical vertebrae. The C1 nerve root exits above the C1 vertebra, while the C2 nerve root exits between the C1 and C2 vertebrae. The C8 nerve root exits between the C7 and T1 vertebral bodies, and the T1 nerve root exits between the T1 and T2 vertebral bodies. This relationship continues downward to the level of the sacrum. Thus, the nerve root that emerges at the L5–S1 level is the L5 nerve root. In the case of lumbar disk herniation, the affected nerve root is typically the root that is passing by to exit at the next level. As an example, a disk herniation at the L4–5 level would typically compress the L5 nerve root. Conversely, in the cervical spine, the nerve that is affected is at the level of the disk herniation. A C5–6 disk herniation would therefore impact the C6 nerve root.

Intervertebral disks act as pads separating the vertebral bodies of the spine. They also function as shock absorbers, helping to cushion and distribute downward forces on the spine. Additionally, intervertebral disks allow a limited amount of movement to occur between different spinal levels so that the spine may bend and rotate. The intervertebral disk is composed of a gellike, elastic fibrocartilaginous central nucleus (the nucleus pulposus) surrounded by a fibrous outer ring (the annulus fibrosis) composed of 15 to 25 concentric layers of parallel fibers. Vertebral body endplates less then 1-mm thick and composed of hyaline cartilage form an interface between the bone of the vertebral bodies and the disk, sandwiching the nucleus pulposus superiorly and inferiorly.

Intervertebral disks degenerate over time. At birth, the nucleus pulposus contains 80% water. As people age, however, disks gradually lose their water and elasticity, becoming less gellike. The process of disk degeneration is common and may even be "normal" as people age. About 20% of teenagers have signs of mild disk degeneration, whereas, by age 70, approximately 60% of disks are severely degenerated. Degenerated disks do not distribute load in the same way as healthy, well-hydrated disks. They do not maintain their height under load-bearing conditions, and as a consequence, more load is placed on vertebral bodies and adjacent facet joints. This promotes the formation of osteophytes. If osteophytes form in the spinal canal or within the neural foramina, neurologic compression may develop over time. With loss of disk height, the tensional forces on the ligamentum flavum are reduced, causing the ligamentum to remodel, thicken, and bulge into the canal. Degenerative disk disease occurs at all levels of the spine; however, because the lumbar spine and cervical spine have greater mobility, pathology is more common in these regions.

CERVICAL SPINE

▶ General Considerations

Degenerative disk disease of the cervical spine may occur chronically, leading to bulging of intervertebral disks, hypertrophy of facet joints, and osteophyte formation. Chronic degeneration initially manifests as neck pain. As osteophytes enlarge and ligamentous hypertrophy progresses, neurologic symptoms may develop. Compression of nerve roots leads to radiculopathy, while compression of the spinal cord itself leads to myelopathy. Alternatively, disk degeneration may occur acutely when the nucleus pulposus of a disk is extruded through a tear in the annulus. If an acute disk herniation occurs centrally, the spinal cord may become compressed, causing severe neurologic injury. This may result in paraplegia or quadriplegia, depending on the level and severity of the herniation. More commonly, however, disk rupture results in compression of a nerve root by the extruded disk fragment, causing radiculopathy. This is typically manifest as pain radiating down the arm, sensory disturbance, and sometimes weakness in the distribution of the involved nerve root.

▶ Clinical Findings

A. Symptoms and Signs

Degenerative disease of the cervical spine often presents with a history of neck pain, which may either be abrupt, in the case of disk rupture, or slowly progressive. There is often a loss of cervical lordosis (the normal, backward curvature of the neck), which may be related to muscle spasm or to deformity from chronic degeneration. In addition to neck pain, which often abates over time, compression of a single nerve root by an osteophyte or disk fragment (radiculopathy) often causes an aching pain along the medial border of the scapula on the side of the lesion. This scapular pain tends to be longer lasting than the neck pain. The characteristic finding in radiculopathy is a sharp, burning pain that radiates down the arm, following the distribution of the involved spinal nerve. This pain may be exacerbated when the patient tilts the head toward the side of the pain, crowding the neural foramina on the effected side. Indeed, the patient may habitually tilt the head to the opposite side to reduce the pain. Hyperextension of the neck (with or without compression of the head) may worsen the pain. In the clinical setting, reproducing the patient's pain by tilting the head toward the side of the pain is called the Spurling maneuver. Sensory disturbances (paresthesias, numbness, or decreased sensation) tend to occur in the terminal distribution of the involved dermatome, in the fingers rather than the proximal arm. Hypersensitivity of the skin in the distal distribution of the dermatome is also common. A decrease or loss of deep tendon reflexes is a frequent and early finding in radiculopathy from a herniated disk or a compressive cervical osteophyte. Weakness from radiculopathy occurs in muscles innervated by one spinal nerve (but by more than one peripheral nerve); that is, it is myotome based. Thus, weakness from radiculopathy is often partial or incomplete, since nearly all muscles are innervated by more that one spinal nerve. Profound weakness, atrophy, and muscle fasciculations are rare in radiculopathy except in very longstanding cases. The presence of these findings should generate suspicion of a peripheral nerve lesion.

C5 radiculopathy (typically resulting from pathology at the C4–5 level) involves pain radiating into the shoulder, with sensory disturbances crossing over the top of the shoulder and extending to the mid portion of the upper arm (following the distribution of the C5 dermatome). Patients may exhibit weakness of shoulder abduction and arm flexion. The biceps reflex may be attenuated. C6 radiculopathy (as from a C5–6 herniated disk) typically involves pain radiating from the neck into the lateral aspect of the arm, with sensory disturbance in the dorsum of the hand and, in particular, the thumb. Patients may present with weakness of arm flexion (biceps). The biceps reflex as well as the brachioradialis reflex may be attenuated. C7 nerve root compression (from C6–7 pathology) often involves pain radiating from the neck into the back of the shoulder, the triceps, and the dorsolateral surface of the forearm. Sensory disturbance typically involves the middle finger. Weakness of arm extension (triceps) is generally noticed in a delayed fashion, perhaps because day-to-day extension of the arm occurs with the assistance of gravity. The triceps reflex is often attenuated.

In advanced cases of degenerative disk disease of the cervical spine, signs of myelopathy may develop, including hyperreflexia, spasticity leading to gait disturbance, and sensory disturbance in the upper and lower extremities. Patients with myelopathy from cervical stenosis often complain of difficulty manipulating objects with their hands (for example, problems buttoning their shirt).

B. Diagnostic Studies

Plain films are useful in determining the degree of degenerative change present in the cervical spine. In cases of cervical deformity, plain films are used for evaluating the alignment of the cervical spine. Flexion-extension plain films are important when there is a question of instability of the cervical spine (for example, when a patient is having positional symptoms). Likewise, CT scans may offer detailed views of the bony anatomy and are often useful for preoperative planning, especially in cases of severe deformity. CT also offers good resolution of boney anatomy when bone spurs are suspected as the cause of neural compression. The major disadvantage of CT scanning is the lack of resolution of soft tissue structures; it is difficult to detect compression from a herniated disk on a normal CT scan. CT myelography solves the problem of resolving soft tissue compressive lesions; however, its main disadvantage is its invasiveness: cervical puncture of the thecal sac (required for dye injection) carries a small risk of neurologic injury. In the era of MRI scanning, CT myelography is often reserved for cases in which the spine has been previously instrumented, which may cause significant artifact on MRI.

MRI allows the resolution of neural structures in a noninvasive manner and has become the most common imaging method for evaluating potentially compressive pathology of the cervical spine. MRI can resolve soft tissue disk herniations and detect nerve root compression. It is also useful in detecting chronic or acute changes in the spinal cord that may be associated with myelopathy. MRI findings should be carefully correlated with clinical findings, as false positives are frequently generated. MRI reveals degenerative disk disease of the cervical spine in 25% of asymptomatic people under 40 years of age and in 60% of people over 40.

Electrodiagnostic studies, particularly electromyogram, may be useful in diagnosing radiculopathy. Nerve conduction studies alone are of little value in identifying radiculopathy and are generally normal, even with severe compression of a nerve root. Electromyogram, on the other hand, is highly sensitive. Classic electromyogram findings in radiculopathy are fibrillations at rest in muscles supplied by a single nerve root (ie, a myotome) along with denervation in the corresponding paraspinal muscles. Unfortunately, electromyogram will not reliably detect fibrillations in muscles until at least 3 to 4 weeks following the onset of radiculopathy. This may lead to false-negative studies if the test is performed too soon. Electromyogram findings may be normal in upwards of 50% of cases of spinal nerve compression in patients with radicular symptoms but no signs of weakness, numbness, or decreased reflexes.

▶ Differential Diagnosis

Neck pain associated with a history of malignancy, unexplained weight loss, pain unrelieved by bedrest, or age older than 50 with cancer risk factors should raise suspicion of a metastatic tumor invading the cervical spine. Similarly, infectious etiologies such as diskitis, osteomyelitis, or abscess should be considered when there is a history of fever, immunosuppression, or recent infection. Peripheral nerve entrapment syndromes such as carpal tunnel syndrome or ulnar nerve compression may mimic cervical radiculopathy. In general, severe weakness and muscle atrophy suggest a peripheral nerve lesion, while early loss of a reflex (biceps, triceps) suggests radiculopathy. Other conditions that may mimic cervical degenerative disk disease include myocardial infarction, idiopathic brachial plexitis (Parsonage-Turner syndrome), or inflammatory conditions such as ankylosing spondylitis or sarcoidosis. Local conditions affecting the shoulder (rotator cuff tears, acromial bursitis, etc) must also be ruled out.

▶ Treatment & Prognosis

Most conditions that cause pain in the cervical spine, such as exacerbations of degenerative arthritis, muscle spasm, and minor trauma, are self-limiting and ultimately do not require operation. Acute neck pain may be treated with gentle exercise or a mobilization program, moist heat, or a soft collar to help muscle relaxation. Anti-inflammatory medications are also useful in this regard. For persistent neck pain, intermittent traction is sometimes helpful, either through physical therapy or with a home traction kit. Roughly 80% to 90% of patients improve with medical management alone, though many continue to have mild symptoms they ultimately learn to manage.

Neck pain itself responds poorly to operative management. Even in cases of radiculopathy where imaging reveals a clear-cut disk herniation compressing a nerve root, surgical management is most likely to improve only arm pain rather than neck pain. Surgical management of cervical degenerative disk disease should be reserved for cases failing medical management in which there is neurologic compression (leading to either myelopathy or radiculopathy). Operative management of the cervical spine involves decompression of the spinal cord or nerve roots with or without fusion. The cervical spine may be approached either anteriorly or posteriorly. The choice depends on many factors, including the age of the patient, the number of levels involved, whether the compressive lesion is predominantly anterior or posterior, and any concurrent deformity of the cervical spine. Both anterior and posterior approaches may be used to decompress nerve roots and/or the spinal cord. For complicated cases involving extensive degenerative change, particularly with severe deformity, a combined anteroposterior approach may be employed.

Disk herniations and osteophytes may be addressed anteriorly either by removing just the disk (anterior cervical diskectomy) or by drilling away the vertebral body (a procedure known as corpectomy). Posterior cervical laminectomy is useful for decompression of multiple levels, as in the case

of multilevel cervical stenosis. Because there is a risk of subsequent deformity (progressive kyphosis related to loss of the posterior tension band following operation), some patients who are approached posteriorly may need to be fused. The decision to fuse should be made on a case-by-case basis. Posterior keyhole foraminotomy is ideally suited for soft disk herniations that occur laterally (it cannot be used for central disk bulges) and may be done in a minimally invasive fashion using tubular retractors.

In the case of cervical radiculopathy, symptoms improve in approximately 80% of patients following operative management. Where surgical decompression is performed for myelopathy, neurologic improvement occurs in approximately 70% of cases.

THORACIC DISK DISEASE

Thoracic disk herniations are rare, with an incidence between 0.25% and 0.75% of all disk herniations. The majority of disk herniations occur below the level of the midthoracic spine. Often there is a delay in diagnosis because of poorly defined symptoms and the lack of objective findings on physical examination. If the disk herniation is secondary to trauma and results in severe cord compression, paralysis may be the result. If the disk herniation is secondary to degenerative changes, the cord compression occurs more slowly and is associated with a variety of presentations.

Patients may present with symptoms of axial pain, radiculopathy, myelopathy, or some combination of the three. The axial pain may be dull, aching, burning, stabbing, or cramping. Load bearing, activity, or Valsalva will often exacerbate the pain. Radicular symptoms generally present in the appropriate dermatomal band. Myelopathy can present as paraparesis but more often presents with a vague history of lower extremity weakness, heaviness, stiffness, or numbness. Bowel and bladder complaints are common.

Treatment is surgical and is directed at alleviating pain or preventing progression of a neurologic deficit. There are a variety of surgical options, including laminectomy, as well as a variety of approaches (thoracotomy, costotransversectomy, lateral extracavitary, transpedicular) to pathology that occurs in the anterior spine, such as a disk herniation. In cases of a thoracic disk herniation, a strictly dorsal midline approach (laminectomy) offers poor exposure of the disk and has a high risk of neurologic injury.

LUMBAR SPINE

▶ General Considerations

One must understand the anatomy of the lumbosacral roots to appreciate the clinical syndromes associated with a displaced lumbar intervertebral disk. An extruded lumbar intervertebral disk can lead to loss of reflexes (ankle jerk, patellar reflex), motor loss, sensory loss, and pain in a dermatomal distribution. A central disk herniation can lead to a variety of presentations up to paraplegia below the level of the lesion along with urinary symptoms. A typical disk herniation will generally spare the exiting nerve root but impinge on the traversing nerve root of the level below. A more rare far-lateral disk herniation, however, will impinge on the exiting nerve root.

With age, the disk will degenerate. Autopsy specimens have noted disk degeneration starting as early as the second decade of life, and nearly all individuals have some degree of degeneration by the sixth decade. Osteophytes may then form around the disk space and cause stenosis of the spinal canal and neuroforamina.

Ninety-five percent of lumbar disk herniations occur at the L5–S1 and L4–5 levels. Only 4% of lumbar disk herniations occur at the L3–4 levels and are infrequent at the upper lumbar levels.

▶ Clinical Findings

A. Symptoms and Signs

The symptoms and signs of lumbar disk herniation are variable. Generally, patients complain of symptoms of radiating leg pain with a minor component of back pain. Valsalva maneuvers (coughing, sneezing, etc) generally exacerbate the pain, as can movement. Alternatively, rest often improves the pain. The pain itself can be described as a constant burning, aching pain with an intermittent sharp, shooting pain that radiates down into the level.

Straight-leg raise and crossed straight-leg raise may support the diagnosis of lumbar disk herniation. The straight-leg raise is 80% sensitive but only 40% specific. The crossed straight-leg raise is only 25% sensitive and 90% specific. It should be noted that patients with a high lumbar disk herniation or a far-lateral disk herniation may not have these signs. Examination of the paravertebral musculature may reveal tenderness and/or muscle spasm.

Motor findings may be helpful in predicting the involved lumbar level. Compression of the L4 nerve root (L3–4 herniation) may cause weakness of knee extension (quadriceps). Compression of the L5 nerve root (L4–5 herniation) may precipitate weakness of the extensor hallucis longus and dorsiflexion. Finally, compression of the S1 nerve root (L5–S1 herniation) may lead to weakness of the plantar flexion (gastrocnemius). Reflexes may also be diminished. The ankle jerk (Achilles) reflex is diminished with S1 nerve root compression, and the patellar reflex is diminished with L4 nerve root compression.

Sensory examination is often variable and the least helpful in predicting the involved lumbar level. L4 nerve root compression can be associated with anterior thigh to medial ankle sensory findings. L5 nerve root compression can present with findings along the dorsum of the foot and the first web space. Finally, S1 nerve root compression may present with sensory findings along the lateral and plantar regions of the foot.

A large central disk herniation can present with cauda equina syndrome. In these cases, patients may present with saddle anesthesia, urinary dysfunction, diminished rectal tone, and leg weakness.

B. Imaging Studies

If symptoms are limited to pain and the patient does not have risk factors for other diseases, it is reasonable to delay imaging workup for 4 weeks, since improvement in pain over time is not uncommon. Persistent symptoms, however, are an indication for imaging. Plain radiographs have limited utility in the diagnosis of disk herniation. However, they are useful in evaluating trauma, infection, or neoplastic process. Myelography may identify extradural filling defects and can be particularly helpful when combined with CT scanning. Indeed, CT myelography remains useful in the setting when an MRI scan is not possible.

MRI has become the gold standard for the diagnosis of herniated disks. MRI is noninvasive and does not involve radiation exposure. MRI provides detailed images of the disk spaces, surrounding soft tissue, and thecal sac. It can help exclude tumors, cysts, and postoperative scar as etiologies of the patient's symptoms. It is important to correlate the patient's symptoms and the imaging findings precisely, since MRI imaging can generate a significant number of false positives. For example, nearly 20% of healthy individuals under age 40 and over 50% of individuals over 40 were noted to have imaging abnormalities.

C. Special Examinations

Electromyography can be useful for diagnosing radiculopathy, but its utility is rather limited. Electromyography classically has findings of fibrillations at rest in the muscles supplied by a single nerve root and denervation of corresponding paraspinal muscles. Unfortunately, fibrillations require at least 3 to 4 weeks from the onset of the radiculopathy to be evident on electromyograph examination. Nerve conductions studies are of minimal utility in diagnosing radiculopathy.

▶ Differential Diagnosis

It is important to obtain a complete history and physical examination because the differential diagnosis for patients with back pain and radicular symptoms is broad. A history of trauma can point to fractures, especially in the setting of osteoporosis and/or steroid use. Tumors that often metastasize to the spine include prostate, breast, kidney, thyroid, and lung cancer. Patients with metastatic disease often have nighttime pain and pain that persists even with rest and a supine position. Inflammatory disorders, infections, bony abnormalities (spondylolisthesis), peripheral neuropathies, degenerative spinal cord lesions, peripheral vascular occlusive disease, and peripheral nerve lesions should all be considered in the differential diagnosis.

▶ Treatment

A. Medical Measures

The natural history of the radicular pain associated with lumbar disk disease is that of improvement over time. Therefore, conservative measures are recommended for patients who present with a new radiculopathy without neurologic impairment. Conservative measures are directed toward initially limiting physical activity, including a brief period of bed rest followed by a gradual exercise program. It is also important for patients to modify their types of movement (eg, to limit heavy lifting, twisting, or bending). Physical therapy can be useful after the acute period for instruction in abdominal and back musculature–strengthening exercises.

    The core of medical treatment is nonsteroidal antiinflammatory drugs (NSAIDs). Oral steroids (ie, Medrol dose pack) also may be useful in the acute setting to help alleviate radicular pain. Epidural steroid injections and narcotic pain medications can also be useful in helping alleviate pain.

B. Surgical Treatment

Patients who present with acute neurologic deterioration warrant immediate surgical attention. Surgery can also be indicated in patients who fail conservative measures outlined previously and continue to suffer from debilitating pain.

    The microdiskectomy is the gold-standard surgical intervention for patients with a herniated lumbar disk. A microdiskectomy involves a laminotomy to gain access to the disk space. The nerve root and the thecal sac are protected while the disk fragment is identified and removed. A fusion can sometimes be recommended in the setting of recurrent disk herniations at the same level or pain associated with joint instability. Another procedure that has been utilized with mixed results is chemonucleolysis using an intradiskal injection of chymopapain.

▶ Prognosis

Overall, patients who have symptoms of radicular pain without neurologic deterioration have an excellent prognosis with improvement in symptoms over time.

Kanpolat Y: The surgical treatment of chronic pain: destructive therapies in the spinal cord. Neurosurg Clin N Am 2004;15:307.
Wallace BA, Ashkan K, Benabid AL: Deep brain stimulation for the treatment of chronic, intractable pain. Neurosurg Clin N Am 2004;15:343.

▼ CSF DIVERSION FOR HYDROCEPHALUS

Hugh J. L. Garton, MD, MHSC, & Jason Sack, BS

OVERVIEW, EPIDEMIOLOGY, & PATHOPHYSIOLOGY

Hydrocephalus is a common diagnosis in both adult and pediatric patients. Most often, this disease is chronically treated with an implanted catheter system to divert CSF from the brain to an alternative absorptive space such as the pleural or peritoneal space. Children and adults with CSF shunts can require surgical treatment for other associated conditions. The presence of the shunt may thus complicate the surgical management of various intra-abdominal processes. For example, a child with the distal portion of his shunt within the peritoneal may develop appendicitis. What management steps should be taken with regard to the management of the potentially contaminated CSF shunt catheter? In addition, CSF shunt failure is common, occurring in up to 30% to 35% of individuals within 1 year of initial shunt placement. About 1% of all shunt failures are fatal. Familiarity with the diagnosis and treatment of shunt failure is therefore desirable for providers caring for patients in whom a CSF shunt is present.

    In pediatric patients, hydrocephalus is commonly seen in patients with a history of premature birth or intraventricular hemorrhage, after meningitis, in patients with myelomeningocele or other congenital cranial malformations, and in patients with brain tumors. In adults, patients suffering from subarachnoid hemorrhage, brain tumor, or head injury may develop hydrocephalus. In older adults, "normal pressure" hydrocephalus is a potentially treatable cause of dementia. CSF shunt management is also used in the management of idiopathic intracranial hypertension (also know as pseudotumor cerebri).

    Among children, the prevalence of hydrocephalus is estimated at about 1 to 2 per 1000 children. Among adult patients, the incidence of idiopathic intracranial hypertension and the shunt treatment for it appear to be increasing in accordance with increasing obesity rates.

    Pathophysiologically, hydrocephalus results from an interruption in CSF circulation. The choroid plexus of the brain's ventricular system generates about 80% of the total adult CSF production of about 20 mL/hr by an active ion pump–dependent process. The remainder is thought to be generated by more general metabolic processes of the brain and arachnoid. Importantly, the production of CSF is independent of the intracranial pressure over a wide range of physiologic values. Thus, the increase in intracranial pressure that typically results from the increasing CSF volumes within the nervous system does not act to check the further production of spinal fluid. Once produced, spinal fluid moves in an oscillatory fashion out of the ventricular system and into the subarachnoid space around the brain. From there it is reabsorbed by passive, pressure-dependent mechanisms into the cerebral venous sinuses and possibly into lymphatic systems adjacent to the dura. The vast majority of hydrocephalus results from interruption of the egress of CSF. Traditionally, hydrocephalus has been classified as either *obstructive*, if the blockage to CSF outflow prevents egress from the ventricular system, or *communicating*, if reabsorption is interrupted beyond the ventricular system at the dural venous and/or lymphatic absorption sites. The determination of the site of obstruction is usually radiographic and may require invasive studies. To the nonneurosurgeon, this distinction is mostly important in determining the safety of lumbar puncture. If a patient has obstructive hydrocephalus, a lumbar puncture may be unsafe because of the potential for differential pressures between the cranial and spinal spaces after the puncture. Radiographically, hydrocephalus is sometimes assumed to be communicating when all four ventricles, as opposed to only the first second, and third ventricles, are dilated. However, blockage at the outflow of the fourth ventricle to the subarachnoid space could produce the same CT or MRI picture despite obstructive physiology. Consultation with a neurosurgeon or neurologist may be helpful if the situation is unclear.

CLINICAL PRESENTATION & ASSESSMENT

The relative difference between the volume of CSF produced and reabsorbed, along with the relative compressibility of the brain, determine the severity and type of clinical symptoms and signs at presentation. Slower buildup of CSF or a brain more compliant to compression, such as might occur at the extremes of age, produce a more protracted course of symptoms compared to rapid CSF accumulation in a poorly compressible brain. Whether presenting initially or after treatment failure, the symptoms of hydrocephalus can be grouped into three broad categories: those related to acute increased intracranial pressure, usually seen with a more rapid accumulation of CSF or a poorly compliant brain; those related to more chronic deformation of the nervous system by more slowly accumulating CSF; and those symptoms that are specific to treatment complications, including CSF shunt infection.

Acute, rapidly progressive hydrocephalus presents with headaches, nausea and vomiting, and as it progresses, a deterioration in level of consciousness. The headaches associated with hydrocephalus and/or CSF shunt failure may have morning predominance or worsen with a Valsalva maneuver. The patient may be lethargic or difficult to arouse or awaken with ordinary stimuli. Some patients may present with a loss of upgaze or Parinaud syndrome, others with cranial nerve VI palsy from increased intracranial pressure. In young children with an open fontanelle, this area may be tense and raised. Hydrocephalus of a more slowly progressive nature may present with more subtle signs of cognitive impairment. In the elderly, normal pressure hydrocephalus presents with the triad of dementia, gait disturbance, and incontinence. Other signs include papilledema, and in young children, an inappropriately expanding head size. If the patient has already undergone treatment for hydrocephalus with a CSF shunt, then additional symptoms and signs to consider include those of device infection, including a stiff neck, fever, and redness around the device. If the device has broken or malfunctioned, then CSF may accumulate around the shunt. If the distal cavity into which a shunt is placed fails

to absorb spinal fluid, there may be related symptoms such as abdominal pain with a large intraperitoneal fluid collection (a *pseudocyst*). Some CSF shunt devices possess diagnostic chambers that can be manually compressed and observed for response. However, the utility of such tests is questionable and best left to a neurosurgeon.

Patients presenting with clinical features described above, especially with a history of a CSF shunt in place for prior treatment of hydrocephalus, must be promptly evaluated with imaging studies, usually a CT or MRI scan of the brain. In the setting of a possible shunt failure, it is critical to have previous images available for comparison. Patients with working shunts may have ventricles that are smaller than normal; "normal ventricular size" or "no evidence of shunt failure" in a radiology report has been demonstrated to correlate poorly with final diagnosis. Additional studies that can be useful include plain radiographs of the shunt and imaging of the cavity into which the CSF shunt is draining, such as by ultrasound of the abdomen. Other invasive diagnostic studies may be necessary, usually as directed by a neurosurgical consultant. These can include a CSF shunt tap, in which a portion of the shunt that sits under the scalp is accessed percutaneously, similarly to a vascular access port. It is helpful to know that a high percentage of shunt failures occur within the first 2 years after shunt placement, with a reduction in failure rates thereafter. In children, young age at presentation also appears to be a risk factor for repeated shunt failure. Similarly, most shunt infections occur within 1 year from shunt placement. However, despite these epidemiologic data, a perfectly predictive clinical decision algorithm remains elusive, and a low threshold for obtaining imaging studies and appropriate expert consultations is warranted.

MANAGEMENT

Progressive hydrocephalus must be dealt with in a timely manner to minimize neurologic deterioration. As noted previously, the rate of pathologic CSF accumulation may vary and produce different clinical symptoms. However, because of the potential for acute and fatal deterioration from hydrocephalus, the initial presumption should be that rapid intervention is needed, subject to reconsideration after all the data are available.

Medical management of hydrocephalus may be appropriate in the management of idiopathic intracranial hypertension (pseudotumor cerebri) and, in some patients, after subarachnoid hemorrhage. It is also used in the initial management of hydrocephalus in neonates after an intraventricular hemorrhage. The diuretics acetazolamide and furosemide are used in this context. Both decrease CSF production by inhibiting carbonic anhydrase, albeit by slightly different mechanisms, thus producing an additive effect when used in combination. However, randomized control trials of diuretic therapy in newborns demonstrated no reduction in the need for subsequent shunt placement for patients on diuretic regimens. If diuretics are utilized, patients must be closely monitored for electrolyte imbalances and acetazolamide toxicity (acute gastritis, paresthesias, and drowsiness.). It should be noted that with the exception of idiopathic intracranial hypertension, protracted use of diuretics to manage hydrocephalus is rarely successful, and in most cases, surgical therapy is indicated without a trial of diuretics.

Intraventricular administration of fibrinolytic agents (eg, streptokinase) has also been investigated as a treatment for newborns with posthemorrhagic hydrocephalus. However, a systematic review of randomized trials failed to show any benefit in terms of reducing shunt requirement or death. Furthermore, secondary intraventricular hemorrhage is a potential complication of this treatment.

Temporary drainage methods include serial lumbar punctures, ventricular taps, placement of an external ventriculostomy catheter, or implanted reservoir in communication with the ventricular system for periodic aspiration. These techniques are used when natural history suggests possible resolution of the hydrocephalus, as may occur in intraventricular hemorrhage in the newborn and in subarachnoid hemorrhage. In addition, temporary diversion is appropriate when the patient's condition precludes definitive treatment.

Endoscopic third ventriculostomy is an alternative to CSF shunt placement for the treatment of some forms of hydrocephalus. During the endoscopic procedure, a perforation is made in the floor of the third ventricle, communicating it to the subarachnoid space. Endoscopic third ventriculostomy is currently used as the initial treatment of choice in cases of obstructive hydrocephalus and is curative in 80% of properly selected patients, avoiding the need for shunt placement. Patients who undergo endoscopic third ventriculostomy may suffer recurrent hydrocephalus if the fenestration closes. The vast majority of such failures have occurred within the first year after the procedure, and failures beyond 5 years are exceedingly rare.

CSF shunt treatment is indicated in most cases of progressive hydrocephalus, when conservative management and endoscopic third ventriculostomy are not indicated or have previously failed. This procedure involves placement of a mechanical shunt as a means to divert excess CSF from the ventricles into other body cavities. CSF shunts have a ventricular catheter, a valve that regulates unidirectional flow, and distal tubing to distribute the CSF to its absorption site. Many shunts also have reservoirs that can be percutaneously tapped for diagnostic purposes or as a temporizing measure in shunts in which the distal tubing or valve becomes blocked. Most often, the proximal catheter of the shunt system is placed into one of the lateral ventricles, either in the frontal horn via a frontal approach or via the atrium of the lateral ventricle via a parietal approach. Shunt systems are used to treat a variety of other conditions, such as intracranial cysts and chronic subdural hematomas/hygromas. The

proximal catheter placement in such cases is dictated by the location of the pathology to be treated. Shunt valve mechanics regulate the amount of drainage. Most are differential pressure systems that respond to increasing fluid pressure by allowing more CSF through the valve. Various shunts are designed to open in different pressure ranges (eg, low: 4–7 cm H_2O; medium: 8–12 cm H_2O; high: 13–15 cm H_2O), and some valves can be externally adjusted to different performance levels using a magnet. These adjustable ("programmable") valves may be inadvertently reprogrammed by other external magnets, and while all systems approved for sale in the United States as of this writing are MRI compatible to 1.5 Telsa, the patient must have the valve setting checked and reset as necessary following an MRI. Alternative systems are designed to produce a constant flow through the valve over a range of physiological intracranial pressures. Valve systems may incorporate devices that prevent excessive drainage from the siphoning effect of a long run of distal tubing running inferiorly when patients assume an upright posture. The distal end of the system consists of a catheter that terminates in a body cavity, wherein the fluid can be adequately absorbed. A ventriculoperitoneal shunt, in which the catheter terminates into the abdominal cavity and fluid is absorbed by the peritoneum, is the most commonly used shunt at present. Other common distal sites include the pleural space (V-pleural shunt) and the cardiac ventriculoatrial shunt. These two sites are chosen when extensive scarring or adhesions, recent abdominal infection, peritonitis, or morbid obesity preclude peritoneal catheter placement. Other less common options for distal placement of a ventricular shunt include gall bladder and ureter/bladder. Immediate complications from shunt placement are fortunately rare but include misplacement of the ventricular catheter with inadequate shunt function. Much more rarely, a patient may suffer intracranial hemorrhage or perforated abdominal viscus.

Complications that are not encountered intraoperatively but may nonetheless present in the early postoperative period include inguinal hernia and/or hydrocele; ascites; pseudocyst formation; septicemia, pulmonary thromboembolism, and cardiac tamponade with ventriculoatrial placement; subcutaneous CSF collections and fistulas; hemorrhage; shunt obstruction/occlusion; and infection (shunt and/or incisional).

CSF SHUNT FAILURE

While the surgical procedure of CSF shunt placement is generally an uncomplicated process, the long-term management of shunted hydrocephalus is more problematic. Multiple clinical studies in both adult and pediatric patients attest to the high rate of device failure from tubing obstruction, catheter fracture, infection, and excessive drainage and compartmentalization of the ventricular system (with a catheter draining part of the ventricular system but with another part expanding because of noncommunication). In young children undergoing first shunt placement, roughly one third of shunts will require reoperation in the first year following surgery. Shunt infection rates in these children are as high as 10% to 12%. Adult patients fair somewhat better, but 20% will still require reoperation within the first year after shunt failure. Analysis of the "shunt survival" curves shows that failure rates for devices drops considerably after the first year or two from surgery, but the threat of failure remains present to some degree as long as the device remains in place.

In evaluating a patient for potential CSF shunt failure, the epidemiological data above provide a baseline estimate of the probability of the diagnosis. Other risk factors for shunt failure include young age at shunt placement and recent previous shunt surgery. A history and physical examination along with images compared to previous findings, as described previously, should allow for a reasonably accurate diagnosis. However, several pitfalls deserve mention. First, not all patients with CSF shunt failure will show significant expansion of the ventricular system. Some patients, particularly those with a long history of shunted hydrocephalus, may present with "slit-ventricle" syndrome. The radiographic finding of slit ventricles is relatively common for patients with a functioning shunt. The clinical slit-ventricle syndrome presents with episodic severe headaches that appear to be due to intermittent occlusion of the shunt in a small ventricular system that does not dilate despite an increase in CSF pressures because change in ventricular size is too small to be noted on standard radiographs. The diagnosis is often confirmed by direct intracranial pressure measurements obtained from a separately placed intracranial pressure monitor.

A second group that deserves special attention is children and adults with myelomeningocele. Given a frequent need for both urological and plastic surgical care, these patients are frequently encountered on surgical services. About 70% of patients with this spinal dysraphism will require treatment for hydrocephalus, most with a CSF shunt. Myelomeningocele is associated with a number of abnormalities of the brainstem and foramen magnum. These abnormalities allow CSF shunt failure to produce a much wider array of clinical symptoms than would otherwise be the case. As intracranial CSF and pressure build because of CSF shunt failure, downward pressure on the brainstem can produce lower cranial nerve palsies, including swallowing and breathing irregularities. The death rate from shunt failure may be higher in this population, and more precipitous, related to the susceptibility of the hindbrain to herniation. In additional, CSF shunt failure may precipitate or exacerbate a preexisting syrinx in these patients, producing symptoms related to spinal cord dysfunction.

Shunt contamination may occur during unrelated intra-abdominal procedures, in the case of a ventriculoperitoneal shunt, or from repeated bacteremia in ventriculoatrial shunts. Infections of this sort can obviously occur at any time and are not temporally restricted to the year or so following the most recent shunt surgery. Clinically, the presentation of infection may lack an overt inflammatory response with fever and redness around the shunt. Rather, the presentation may be more insidious, with failure of the CSF to absorb and development of a pseudocyst. The presence of a large intra-abdominal fluid collection in a patient with a ventriculoperitoneal shunt should raise suspicion of shunt infection, although sterile fluid collections are not uncommon.

Abdominal surgical procedures in patients with ventriculoperitoneal shunts raise the issue of the best management of an intraperitoneal distal shunt catheter during and after the procedure. While no validated guideline exists, the literature and the authors' experience suggest that the infection risk is low during clean and clean contaminated cases. If an enterotomy or open bladder procedure is to be performed, it is reasonable to relocate the shunt away from this area once the tubing is identified intraperitoneally and/or to protect it with gauze sponges during the procedure. Other than routine preoperative antibiotics, expectant management for shunt infection and failure can be practiced, and the shunt does not require externalization. When there is frank contamination of the shunt catheter in the abdomen, externalization of the shunt appears prudent. Laparoscopic procedures have been demonstrated to transiently increase intracranial pressure, but there is no body of literature to suggest that this produces identifiable complications, presumably because of its transient nature. Constipation and ileus, conversely, have been suggested to be a source of at least transient shunt dysfunction due to increased abdominal pressure.

Shunt externalization, when necessary, involves palpation of the shunt proximal to its entry into the peritoneum, followed by a sterile prep and, if the patient is awake, local anesthesia. If the shunt has been in place for several years, it may be quite adherent to the surrounding tissues, and the procedure is then best performed in the operating room with anesthesia. For recently placed shunts, this is less of an issue, and the procedure can be performed at the bedside, assuming a cooperative patient. A cut down is made over the shunt tract, avoiding laceration of the underlying tubing. The catheter is often encased in a thick sheath of scar that must be teased open to gain access to the catheter. If a specimen of fluid is required from a peritoneal fluid collection, the tubing is withdrawn slightly, then cut and aspirated distally. In a large pseudocyst, a liter or more of fluid may be withdrawn. The distal catheter is then withdrawn from the patient and discarded. The remaining tubing should be observed for CSF drainage and connected to a sterile, enclosed CSF drainage system. Neurosurgical consultation is advisable before embarking on the procedure. Patients with externalized shunts are draining isotonic CSF and may suffer hyponatremia if appropriate fluid and electrolyte replacement are not performed, particularly in young children.

ONGOING CARE

Patients with ventriculoperitoneal or ventriculopleural shunts do not require prophylactic antibiotics for surgical or dental procedures in which the shunt is outside the operative field. Prophylactic antibiotics may be helpful when the shunt is in the operative field or during a planned CSF shunt revision. For patients with ventriculoatrial CSF shunts in place, an argument can be made for antibiotic prophylaxis before procedures likely to result in bacteremia, including dental procedures. Dental practice guidelines suggest antibiotic prophylaxis. American Heart Association guidelines for endocarditis prophylaxis recommend Amoxicillin, 2 gm 30 to 60 minutes before the procedure for adults and 50 mg/kg for pediatric patients, or Clindamycin, 600 mg for adults and 20 mg/kg for children who are allergic to penicillin.

Shunt independence has been reported for children with a prior history of shunt placement. In this situation, a child previously dependent on a CSF shunt becomes once again able to drain CSF independently. Clinically, this issue is often raised when a CSF shunt has gone without a revision for many years or even decades, or a CSF shunt is found disconnected in the absence of clinical symptoms. One series reported that 3% of children with hydrocephalus became shunt independent later in life. However, in the setting of a shunt found to be fractured on x-ray without ventricular enlargement or clinical symptoms of shunt failure, it is clinical experience that CSF can often drain between the fractured catheter segments through the tube of scar tissue that forms around the catheter initially after shunt placement. Such a scarred tract can subsequently close over, even several years after the catheter fracture and separation of the fractured tubing ends. Therefore, caution should be exercised in the presumption of shunt independence unless it has been verified by invasive testing. Patients incidentally found to have broken shunt catheters may reasonably be referred to a neurosurgeon for evaluation.

Shunted hydrocephalus during pregnancy frequently raises concerns over management of headaches during pregnancy, mechanism of delivery, and the potential impact of hydrocephalus on the pregnancy outcome. Pregnancy, particularly in the third trimester, increases intra-abdominal pressures. For patients with ventriculoperitoneal shunts, this can lead to a relative decrease in CSF shunt function. In case series of pregnant patients with hydrocephalus, headaches are commonly reported, particularly during the third trimester. These may herald shunt failure, the evaluation of which may be complicated by a desire to avoid radiation administration during pregnancy. MRI may be a useful option in these circumstances. In the absence of radiographic manifestations of shunt failure or additional clinical symptoms, safe observation of headaches has been successfully practiced, but treatment decisions must be individualized, and other diagnoses, particularly eclampsia and preeclampsia, must be considered. There is little evidence to suggest that the presence of a CSF shunt is a contraindication to labor and vaginal delivery. It has been argued that patients who are suspected of being symptomatic from increased intracranial pressure may benefit from avoiding protracted labor, but no comparative studies exist to provide a clear answer. Hydrocephalus and the presence of a CSF shunt does not appear to impact pregnancy outcome. However, recalling that hydrocephalus is coincident with other diagnoses, such as epilepsy and myelomeningocele, that do have a significant impact on the potential for birth defects, the importance of prenatal care can be emphasized.

Bradley NK et al: Maternal shunt dependency: implications for obstetric care, neurosurgical management, and pregnancy outcomes and a review of selected literature. Neurosurgery 1998; 43:448.

Clinical Affairs Committee: Guideline on antibiotic prophylaxis for dental patients at risk for infection. 1990 (rev. 2008). American Academy Council on Clinical Affairs. Available at: http://www.aapd.org/media/policies_guidelines/g_antibioticprophylaxis.pdf. Accessed February 20, 2009.

Curry WT Jr, Butler WE, Barker FG 2nd: Rapidly rising incidence of cerebrospinal fluid shunting procedures for idiopathic intracranial hypertension in the United States, 1988–2002. Neurosurgery 2005;57:97.

Ein SH, Miller S, Rutka JT: Appendicitis in the child with a ventriculo-peritoneal shunt: a 30-year review. J Pediatr Surg 2006;41:1255.

Farin A et al: Endoscopic third ventriculostomy. J Clin Neurosci 2006;13:763.

Garton HJ, Piatt JH Jr: Hydrocephalus. Pediatr Clin North Am 2004;51:305.

Garton HJ, Kestle JR, Drake JM: Predicting shunt failure on the basis of clinical symptoms and signs in children. J Neurosurg 2001;94:202.

Iannelli A, Rea G, Di Rocco C: CSF shunt removal in children with hydrocephalus. Acta Neurochir (Wien) 2005;1475:503.

Jackman SV et al: Laparoscopic surgery in patients with ventriculoperitoneal shunts: safety and monitoring. J Urol 2000; 164:1352.

Johnston M et al: Evidence of connections between cerebrospinal fluid and nasal lymphatic vessels in humans, non-human primates and other mammalian species. Cerebrospinal Fluid Res 2004;1:2.

Li G, Dutta S: Perioperative management of ventriculoperitoneal shunts during abdominal surgery. Surg Neurolog 2008;70:492.

Patwardhan RV, Nanda A: Implanted ventricular shunts in the United States: the billion-dollar-a-year cost of hydrocephalus treatment. Neurosurgery 2005;56:139.

Powers CJ, George T, Fuchs HE: Constipation as a reversible cause of ventriculoperitoneal shunt failure. Report of two cases. J Neurosurg 2006;105(3 suppl):227.

Tuli S, Drake J, Lamberti-Pasculli M: Long-term outcome of hydrocephalus management in myelomeningoceles. Childs Nerv Syst 2003;19:286.

Tuli S et al: Risk factors for repeated cerebrospinal shunt failures in pediatric patients with hydrocephalus. J Neurosurg 2000; 92:31.

Whitelaw A, Kennedy CR, Brion LP: Diuretic therapy for newborn infants with posthemorrhagic ventricular dilatation. Cochrane Database Syst Rev 2001;2:CD002270.

Whitelaw A, Odd DE: Intraventricular streptokinase after intraventricular hemorrhage in newborn infants. Cochrane Database Syst Rev 2007;4:CD000498.

Wilson W et al: Prevention of infective endocarditis: guidelines from the American Heart Association: a guideline from the American Heart Association Rheumatic Fever, Endocarditis, and Kawasaki Disease Committee, Council on Cardiovascular Disease in the Young, and the Council on Clinical Cardiology, Council on Cardiovascular Surgery and Anesthesia, and the Quality of Care and Outcomes Research Interdisciplinary Working Group. Circulation 2007;116:1736.

Wu Y et al: Ventriculoperitoneal shunt complications in California: 1990 to 2000. Neurosurgery 2007;61:557.

CNS INFECTIONS

Khoi D. Than, MD, Anthony C. Wang, MD, Jean-Christophe A. Leveque, MD, & Stephen E. Sullivan, MD

BRAIN ABSCESS

Brain abscesses are an uncommon entity, with approximately 2000 cases reported in the United States each year. There is a higher incidence in developing countries, and men are affected slightly more often than women. Classically, these abscesses arise locally from otorhinolaryngeal infections or hematogenously from distant infections, though opportunistic infections have become an important consideration upon initial presentation as well. The pathogenic organisms most commonly implicated are of the *Streptococcus* family; *Klebsiella, Staphylococcus aureus,* and anaerobes are also frequent. In immunocompromised patients, it is important to include *Toxoplasma, Listeria,* and *Nocardia* as possible etiologic agents, as well as fungal pathogens.

A patient with a brain abscess can present with nonspecific symptoms. Headache, nausea, vomiting, and altered mental status can occur due to increased intracranial pressure, while unilateral headache, seizures, and many focal neurological deficits occur due to the presence of a mass lesion. Fever and nuchal rigidity are also seen in many cases. Additional findings in the newborn patient may include cranial enlargement, meningeal signs, irritability, and failure to thrive.

Risk factors for brain abscess include sinus, ear, or dental infections. These sources usually lead to formation of frontal or temporal lobe abscesses through direct spread. Hematogenous spread from intra-abdominal, pelvic, pulmonary, or cardiac seeding occurs most commonly via the middle cerebral artery, leading to microembolic infarcts at the gray-white junction. Risk factors for these types of abscesses include infectious lung processes or congenital cyanotic heart disease. In these conditions, the lungs have a decreased filtering capability, and the associated relative hypoxia promotes abscess formation. Head trauma—blunt, penetrating, or surgical—can introduce a nidus for infection with delayed abscess formation. Parasitic infections such as cysticercosis should be considered more likely in recent foreign travelers.

The differential diagnosis for brain abscess includes subdural empyema, septic emboli, dural sinus thrombosis, mycotic aneurysm, meningitis, focal necrotizing encephalitis (HSV), and tumor, as all of these conditions can present with headaches and altered mental status. In the initial evaluation of brain abscess, blood work that can be drawn includes a white blood cell count, cultures, erythrocyte sedimentation rate, and C-reactive protein; however, normal test results do not rule out the diagnosis. The key to diagnosing brain abscess is correlating the clinical scenario with an imaging study, such as contrast-enhanced CT or MRI. The classic finding on CT or MRI is a circular lesion with a strongly contrast-enhancing surround rim. CT images are typically the first obtained on admission, although MRI is the imaging modality of choice, as it can provide greater anatomic detail. MRI evaluation for brain abscess should always include diffusion-weighted images, which can differentiate between ring-enhancing lesions of infectious and neoplastic origin, as abscesses are typically hyperintense on diffusion-weighted images, while neoplastic lesions are hypointense.

One general warning is to avoid immediate lumbar puncture, because CSF results are often nondiagnostic and this procedure is associated with a worsened outcome in patients with brain abscesses. Less than one quarter of patients have positive CSF cultures, and with a large enough abscess, there is a real risk for transtentorial or brainstem herniation. CSF sampling should be considered only if parasitic pathogens are suspected. A definitive diagnosis is made by biopsy sampling of the abscess through surgical means.

The treatment of brain abscesses involves both surgical and medical therapy. Treatment should also be aimed at correcting the primary source of infection (ie, draining a pulmonary empyema or repairing a correctable heart defect). Initial surgical treatment usually consists of needle aspiration of the abscess. A total excision can be performed if the abscess is in its chronic, encapsulated form. It is advisable to perform surgery before starting antibiotics in order to confirm the diagnosis as well as to identify the organisms and their antibiotic sensitivities. Antibiotic therapy typically consists of 6 to 8 weeks of intravenous treatment followed by 4 to 8 weeks of oral treatment. Patients should receive routine follow-up imaging and should also be started on an antiepileptic medication. Glucocorticoids should be considered to counteract symptomatic intracranial hypertension, although their role is less important than in the treatment of brain tumors.

In certain situations, medical therapy can suffice without the need for surgery. These situation include an abscess in its early stages (ie, symptoms for less than 2 weeks), a small (< 2 cm) abscess, or a definite clinical improvement after 1 week of antibiotics only. Medical treatment without surgery should also be considered in poor surgical candidates, patients with multiple abscesses and/or concomitant meningitis, patients with abscesses in eloquent locations, or patients with hydrocephalus and ventricular shunts.

Patients with brain abscess have a reported mortality risk of 0% to 30% depending on etiology and presentation. An overall 50% morbidity risk of permanent neurological deficits is conferred, which depends heavily on the severity of presenting symptoms.

SUBDURAL EMPYEMA

A subdural empyema is a collection of pus that forms in the subdural space. It is less common than brain abscess, but like abscesses, it is more commonly found in males. Subdural empyema is an emergent condition because, unlike the brain parenchyma, the subdural space does not pose much of a barrier to prevent the spread of infection. Additionally, antibiotics have poor penetration into the subdural space.

The most common cause of subdural empyema (70%) is paranasal sinusitis, especially in cases involving the frontal sinus. Chronic otitis media accounts for another 15% of cases. As such, the organisms typically cultured from a subdural empyema include *Streptococcus* (aerobic and anaerobic) and *Staphylococcus*. Symptoms present in the majority of patients with subdural empyema include fever, headache, nuchal rigidity, hemiparesis, and altered mental status. Other common symptoms include seizures and sinus tenderness.

CT or MRI imaging will typically diagnose a subdural empyema. Three fourths of empyemas are located over the convexity, while 15% are parafalcine (ie, adjacent to the falx cerebri). Just as with brain abscesses, lumbar puncture should be avoided due to the risk of herniation.

Almost all cases of subdural empyema will require surgical drainage, preferably emergently. The two surgical options are burr-hole drainage and craniotomy. Although burr-hole drainage is less invasive, it is also less effective; thus, craniotomy is the preferred surgical option. Antibiotics are used for a course of 4 to 6 weeks, and patients are put on therapeutic or prophylactic antiseizure medication. Medical treatment alone can be effective if the empyema is small, there is minimal neurologic involvement, and antibiotics have an early efficaciousness.

Subdural empyema carries a 15% mortality rate. Half of patients have residual neurological deficits at the time of hospital discharge. Factors known to be associated with poor prognosis include age over 60 years, obtunded or comatose state at presentation, and empyema formation secondary to surgery or trauma.

OSTEOMYELITIS

Osteomyelitis can affect the skull or the vertebrae. Osteomyelitis of the skull usually results from contiguous spread from an infected sinus or from penetrating trauma (ie, postoperative). The infectious agents are typically *Staphylococcus aureus* or *epidermidis,* and treatment consists of surgery followed by 6 to 12 weeks of antibiotics (intravenously for the first 1 to 2 weeks). Surgical treatment is aimed at removing all infected bone. A cranioplasty or other hardware is not placed until several months later in order to minimize the risk of reseeding an infection.

Vertebral osteomyelitis represents 3% of all cases of osteomyelitis and is more common than skull osteomyelitis because of the spine's rich vascular supply. Both anterograde arterial seeding as well as retrograde venous plexus spread have been implicated in vertebral osteomyelitis, with *S aureus* as the most common organism. Vertebral osteomyelitis caused by *Mycobacterium tuberculosis* is known as Pott disease. Those at higher risk for developing vertebral osteomyelitis include intravenous drug users, diabetics, sickle cell patients, patients on hemodialysis, and the elderly.

The most common symptom at presentation in patients with vertebral osteomyelitis is back pain (> 90%), usually unaffected by activity. Other typical presenting symptoms include fever, weight loss, radicular pain, and myelopathy. The nervous symptoms are usually a result of destruction of the vertebral body and subsequent retropulsion of bone into the spinal canal or neural foramen. The most commonly affected segment of the spine is the lumbar region followed by, in order, the thoracic, cervical, and sacral segments. Any source of infection can theoretically put one at risk for developing vertebral osteomyelitis, although important sources include infections of the urinary tract, respiratory system, and mouth. Vertebral osteomyelitis also develops at sites of previous spine surgeries.

Definitive diagnosis of vertebral osteomyelitis is made with positive cultures, either from biopsy of the tissue itself or via blood cultures in the setting of suggestive radiographic findings. MRI has demonstrated excellent diagnostic accuracy of over 90% of cases and is the preferred diagnostic modality. When unable to obtain MRI, bone scintigraphy with SPECT has also demonstrated excellent sensitivity.

The treatment of vertebral osteomyelitis is nonsurgical in the vast majority of cases, with disease resolution being accomplished via antibiotics and immobilization. The goals of therapy should be to minimize neurologic involvement and to maintain structural stability of the spine. Surgical treatment is indicated to obtain a tissue diagnosis if closed-needle biopsy is unfeasible. In patients with a worsening neurologic deficit, the onset of structural instability, or a failure of medical management, surgery may be warranted for abscess drainage, alleviation of compression, and stabilization.

SPINAL EPIDURAL ABSCESS

Spinal epidural abscesses are often associated with vertebral osteomyelitis, with the majority of cases arising from *S aureus. Streptococcus* species are the second-most commonly implicated organism (Figure 36–25). Spinal epidural abscesses are located most often in the thoracic region (50%), followed by the lumbar (35%) and cervical (15%) regions. The vast majority of abscesses (80%) are located posterior to the cord.

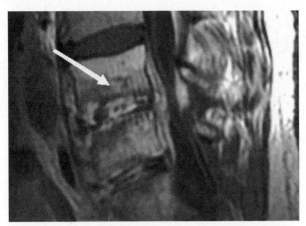

▲ **Figure 36–25.** Sagittal MRI T1-weighted image with contrast of the lumbar spine demonstrating diskitis/osteomyelitis associated with a spinal epidural abscess.

The primary infection leading to spinal epidural abscess can be from hematogenous spread or direct extension. Hematogenous spread is more common, with skin infections being the usual originating source. Other mechanisms of hematogenous spread include nonsterile intravenous injections, bacterial endocarditis, urinary tract infections, respiratory infections, and oropharyngeal abscesses. Spinal epidural abscesses caused by direct extension can be from decubitus ulcers or penetrating trauma, including following spinal procedures.

Patients with spinal epidural abscess are typically middle aged. Risk factors for developing spinal epidural abscess include diabetes, intravenous drug use, chronic renal failure, and alcoholism. Patients often present with back pain, spine tenderness, fever, sweats, and rigors. When motor weakness ensues, there is a very rapid progression to paraplegia, usually within 1 day! Thus, the diagnosis and treatment of spinal epidural abscess is emergent.

The workup of spinal epidural abscesses should include a complete blood count, erythrocyte sedimentation rate, and blood cultures. A lumbar puncture can be helpful but is unnecessary with good diagnostic imaging; it is also somewhat risky given the potential to spread infection. The imaging modality of choice is MRI, although CT and myelography may also be used to arrive at a diagnosis.

The treatment of spinal epidural abscess, as with most infections of the central nervous system, is surgery plus antibiotics. Surgery is used to drain pus, débride any granulation tissue, and provide stability (usually in cases where there is bony destruction secondary to vertebral osteomyelitis). Antibiotics are given intravenously for 3 to 4 weeks and then orally for another 4 weeks. In addition, patients are typically immobilized for 6 weeks. Nonsurgical management with antibiotics only is rare and reserved only for very poor surgical candidates, abscesses that are very extensive in length, or cases in which complete paralysis has been present for at least 3 days with irreversible neurologic injury.

The overall prognosis for patients with spinal epidural abscess is relatively poor, with a mortality rate of 20%. In patients who survive, restoration of baseline neurological function is rare.

Sampath P, Rigamonti D: Spinal epidural abscess: A review of epidemiology, diagnosis, and treatment. J Spinal Disord 1999;12:89.

Tattevin et al: Bacterial brain abscesses: a retrospective study of 94 patients admitted to an intensive care unit (1980 to 1999). Am J Med 2003;115:143.

Tay BKB, Deckey J, Hu SS: Spinal Infections. J Am Acad Orthop Surg 2002;10:188.

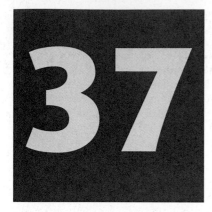

The Eye & Ocular Adnexa

Linda M. Tsai, MD

Stephen A. Kamenetzky, MD

EXAMINATION OF THE EYE

Evaluation of the eye and its adnexa requires a good history, physical examination of the eyes, and assessment of visual function. The history should include general information about the patient's age, occupation, and health status as well as ocular complaints. Occasionally, special examinations may be required to identify specific ocular disorders or to establish the presence of associated systemic disease.

The basic office equipment required for a routine eye examination by a nonophthalmologist includes the following: (1) a handheld flashlight, (2) a binocular magnifying loupe, (3) an ophthalmoscope, (4) a visual acuity chart, and (5) a tonometer.

The basic medications required for an eye examination are (1) a local anesthetic such as proparacaine 0.5% or tetracaine 0.5%; (2) fluorescein strips; and (3) dilating drops, such as phenylephrine 2.5% or tropicamide 0.5–1%.

▶ Visual Acuity Testing

Determination of central visual acuity should be part of the routine examination of the eye in all patients. The Snellen chart is most commonly used. The patient faces the test chart at a distance of 6 meters (20 feet). The patient is tested by occluding one eye and measuring the vision in the opposite eye. Visual acuity corresponds to the smallest line the patient can read and is recorded as 20/20, 20/30, 20/40, 20/50, and so on. The patient who is unable to read the large letters at the top of the chart (typically a 20/200 letter) should be moved progressively closer until the characters can be read, with the distance between the patient and the chart recorded as the numerator. If the patient wears eyeglasses for distance, the visual acuity should be repeated with the glasses on and the results recorded as uncorrected vision and corrected vision.

Preschool children or illiterates can be tested with the illiterate E chart or Allen picture chart.

▶ Visual Field Testing

Confrontation visual fields can be used to detect gross visual field defects such as quadrantanopia, hemianopia, or severe visual field constriction. With one eye occluded, the patient is asked to fixate on the examiner's face and detect finger count or hand motion in each quadrant. Formal visual field testing (perimetry) is used to more carefully examine the central and peripheral visual fields. The technique is performed separately for each eye and measures the function of the retina, the optic nerve and intracranial visual pathway. Perimetry relies on subjective patient responses so results will depend on the patient's alertness and cooperation. Several methods are used to assess visual field functions, including the tangent screen, Goldmann perimetry, and computerized automated perimetry.

▶ Tonometry

Tonometry measures intraocular pressure. The most common instruments used are the Tono-Pen and the Goldmann applanation tonometer. The normal intraocular pressure varies between 10 mm Hg and 20 mm Hg. Intraocular pressure (IOP) measurements can vary slightly with corneal thickness.

▶ Inspection of Anterior Segment & Adnexa

Evaluation of the external ocular structures—lids, conjunctiva, cornea, sclera, and lacrimal apparatus—should include everting the upper eyelid with the patient looking down to enable inspection of the hidden conjunctival surface. The conjunctiva is inspected for anatomic defects, foreign bodies, lacerations, inflammation, discharge, tearing, dryness, or other abnormalities. In patients who are unconscious or in coma, the presence or absence of Bell phenomenon—upward rotation of the cornea during sleep—may be an important measure of neurological function. Corneal sensation and reflex in each eye should be noted before any anesthetic drops are used.

A direct ophthalmoscope focused on the ocular surface may provide some magnification. In addition, considerable detail of the ocular surface can be observed using a magnifying glass and a handheld flashlight. Shining a light across the eye from the lateral to medial aspects and noting whether or not the nasal iris is shadowed can assess the depth of the anterior chamber. The presence of shadowing may indicate a narrow anterior chamber angle requiring special precautions if dilating drops are to be used.

Assessment of Pupillary Functions

Examination of the pupils should be performed before any dilating drops are instilled. Both the direct and consensual light reflex should be assessed. The reaction of the pupils with accommodation should be noted. The size of the pupils should be noted, and any difference in size (anisocoria) should be recorded. Irregular pupils may indicate traumatic, postsurgical, neurological, or congenital defects. In hospitalized patients and those with neurological disorders requiring monitoring of pupillary reaction to assess clinical status, pupils should be dilated with discretion and only with short-acting mydriatics.

Eye Movements

Ocular motility should be assessed in all positions of gaze. One should also observe the patient for random movements and assess the alignment of the eyes when the patient is looking straight ahead. The position of the light reflection from a penlight ("reflex") on the cornea is at the same point in each eye when the eyes are properly aligned. The oculocephalic reflex (doll's head reflex) may be tested, and the upward rotation of the cornea in response to resistance to forced eyelid closure (Bell phenomenon) should be noted when clinically appropriate.

Ophthalmoscopy

Ophthalmoscopy is important for the diagnosis of both ocular and systemic conditions. It can provide critical information in neurologic and neurosurgical contexts. In most instances, the optic nerve head can be clearly seen without dilating the pupils. As noted earlier, in hospitalized patients with neurologic and neurosurgical disorders, dilation of the pupils should be avoided unless absolutely necessary.

SYMPTOMS & SIGNS OF OCULAR DISORDERS

Decrease in Visual Acuity

Efforts should be made to determine if the decrease in visual acuity is unilateral or bilateral, painful or painless, persistent or transient, recent or chronic, isolated or associated with other symptoms. Unilateral acute painful loss of vision may be due to angle-closure glaucoma, endophthalmitis, or uveitis. Painless unilateral loss of vision is often caused by ischemic optic neuropathy, optic neuritis, central retinal artery or vein occlusion, retinal detachment, vitreous hemorrhage, or retinal hemorrhages. Transient painless unilateral loss may be due to retinal migraine or amaurosis fugax. Hemispheric strokes are often responsible for visual field loss with preservation of the central visual acuity.

Disturbances in Vision

Disturbances in vision are transient, varied, and suggest different etiologies. They may consist of image distortion, light sensitivity (photophobia), color change, spots before the eyes, visual field defects, night blindness, momentary loss of vision, or halos around lights. Distortion of normal shape (metamorphopsia) is most commonly caused by macular lesions. Photophobia can be due to corneal inflammation, iritis, ocular albinism, or aniridia. Toxicity from systemic medications such as digoxin and certain retinal conditions can cause the patient to complain of abnormally colored vision (chromatopsia). Patients with vitreous opacities or intraocular inflammation may report floating spots in their vision, although retinal tears and detachment have to be ruled out. Visual field defects may be due to lid edema, retinal and optic nerve lesions, visual pathway lesions, or cortical abnormalities. Night blindness may be genetic, as in patients with retinitis pigmentosa, or acquired with vitamin A deficiency, glaucoma, optic atrophy, cataract, or retinal degeneration being important causes. Transient loss of vision may imply impending cerebrovascular accident or partial occlusion of the internal carotid artery. Colored halos around lights can be caused by elevated intraocular pressure, most commonly due to acute angle-closure glaucoma. Incipient cataract or incorrect refractive error may also cause colorless halos around point light sources.

Fortification images or scintillating scotomas are common in ocular migraine. Patients often describe these as occurring in one eye but they are actually a bilateral phenomenon, distinguishing them from the flashing caused by retinal detachment.

Double Vision (Diplopia)

Diplopia can be constant or intermittent, sudden or gradual, painful or painless, horizontal or vertical. It may occur only in certain gaze positions. Binocular double vision is most often due to misalignment of the eyes from extraocular muscle dysfunction or neurologic abnormalities. Monocular diplopia (multiple images in a single eye) occurs with refractive error, lenticular changes, macular lesions, malingering, or conversion reactions.

Ocular & Orbital Pain

Ocular pain may result from corneal lesions, inflammation, sudden increase in intraocular pressure, anterior uveitis, cyclitis, scleritis, or optic neuritis. Other causes of pain include inflammation of the orbital contents or tumors in the orbit. Dacryocystitis (lacrimal sac inflammation) may also cause severe pain. Eyelid pain and irritation may also arise from infections of the meibomian glands and the glands of Zeis and Moll.

Redness of the Eye

Acute redness (injection) of the eye not associated with trauma may be due to conjunctivitis, acute anterior uveitis, acute angle-closure glaucoma, corneal infection, or corneal abrasion (Table 37–1). Subconjunctival hemorrhage may also present as a red eye, but this is usually painless and otherwise asymptomatic. Conjunctivitis is the most frequent cause of red eye and can be due to bacterial, chlamydial, viral, or allergic causes. Nonspecific irritation from exogenous agents or a foreign body may also cause redness of the eye. Chemical and thermal injuries cause similar findings. "Dry eye" or ocular surface anomalies will cause redness, a foreign body sensation, and variable degrees of decreased vision.

Discharge

Ocular discharge may be described as watery, mucopurulent, purulent, or simply as chronic crusting of the lid margins. When watery discharge is not associated with redness or pain, it may be due to excessive tear production or obstruction of the lacrimal outflow passages. Watery discharge with photophobia, pain, or irritation indicates possible keratitis or keratoconjunctivitis. Purulent or mucopurulent discharge is a sign of bacterial infection, severe inflammation of the conjunctival surface, or bacterial infection of the lacrimal sac or canaliculus. Pseudomonas or haemophilus species involve-

ment are common. When the discharge forms mucoid strings, it is characteristic of allergic disorders involving the conjunctiva (vernal conjunctivitis) or dry eye syndrome.

Swelling of the Eyelids

Swelling of the eyelids may be unilateral or bilateral. In unilateral swelling, the cause is often a sty or chalazion. Bilateral swelling may indicate blepharitis or allergic dermatitis. Systemic diseases associated with water retention, hyperthyroidism, or hypothyroidism can also cause swelling or puffiness of the eyelids.

Displacement of the Eyes

The most common cause of both unilateral and bilateral exophthalmos (proptosis) is hyperthyroidism. Other etiologies include tumors of the orbit.

Strabismus

Strabismus results from misalignment of the eyes due to muscle imbalance and may be in the form of tropia (manifest deviation) or phoria (latent deviation). Ocular deviations may be lateral (exotropia) or medial (esotropia) and upward (hypertropia) or downward (hypotropia).

Leukocoria

A white pupil in a child indicates a serious eye disorder. The most frequent cause of leukocoria is congenital cataract, which requires urgent management to prevent amblyopia. Other causes include retinoblastoma, retrolental fibroplasia (retinopathy of prematurity), toxocariasis, persistent hyperplastic primary vitreous, vitreous hemorrhage, retinal

Table 37–1. Differential Diagnosis of Common Causes of Inflamed Eye.

	Acute Conjunctivitis	Acute Iritis[1]	Acute Glaucoma[2]	Corneal Trauma or Infection
Incidence	Extremely common	Common	Uncommon	Common
Discharge	Moderate to copious	None	None	Watery or purulent
Vision	No effect on vision	Slightly blurred	Markedly blurred	Usually blurred
Pain	None	Moderate	Severe	Moderate to severe
Conjunctival injection	Diffuse; more toward fornices	Mainly circumcorneal	Diffuse	Diffuse
Cornea	Clear	Usually clear	Steamy	Change in clarity related to cause
Pupil size	Normal	Small	Moderately dilated and fixed	Normal
Pupillary light response	Normal	Poor	None	Normal
Intraocular pressure	Normal	Normal	Elevated	Normal
Smear	Causative organisms	No organisms	No organisms	Organisms found only in corneal ulcers due to infection

[1]Acute anterior uveitis.
[2]Angle-closure glaucoma.

detachment, retinal dysplasia, incontinentia pigmenti, Coats disease, and Norrie disease.

▶ Other Symptoms

Patients may present with other symptoms such as burning, itching, gritty and foreign body sensations, or a "sandy" feeling. These symptoms in elderly patients are suggestive of dry eye syndrome. Itching is frequently associated with allergic disorders.

▼ DISEASES OF THE EYE & ADNEXA

ACUTE HORDEOLUM

Acute hordeolum (sty) is a common infection of the glands of the eyelids. External hordeolum involve the glands of Zeis or Moll. Internal hordeolum is an infection of the meibomian glands. The usual causative agent is *Staphylococcus aureus*. Acute hordeolum is characterized by pain, swelling, and redness of the eyelid. A large hordeolum is infrequently associated with a preauricular lymph node.

If pus is localized and pointing out to the skin or conjunctiva, treatment consists of making a local horizontal (skin) or vertical (conjunctiva) incision. If there is no abscess formation, treatment with warm compresses three times daily and topical broad-spectrum antibiotic drops such as tobramycin or sulfacetamide 10% three or four times daily for 5–7 days usually suffices. Ophthalmic ointments such as erythromycin or bacitracin may alternatively be used twice daily for 5–7 days. Oral antibiotics, especially tetracycline derivatives, may be required as an adjunct in patients with acne rosacea.

CONJUNCTIVITIS

Acute conjunctivitis is the most frequent cause of red eye. Infectious causes include bacterial, viral, chlamydial, fungal, and parasitic agents. Noninfectious causes of conjunctivitis include chemical irritation, allergy, hypersensitivity to topical medications, vitamin A deficiency, dry eye syndrome, and injury.

▶ Clinical Findings

A. Symptoms and Signs

Patients with conjunctivitis complain of redness, irritation, foreign body sensation, and conjunctival discharge. One or both eyes may be affected. The eyelids are often stuck together in the morning. Bacterial conjunctivitis has conjunctival hyperemia with purulent or mucopurulent discharge and variable degrees of lid swelling. In viral conjunctivitis, follicles are present in the inferior conjunctival fornix, and preauricular lymph nodes are often involved. The hallmark symptom of allergic conjunctivitis is itching.

B. Laboratory Findings

If bacterial conjunctivitis is suspected, conjunctival swabs and scrapings can be cultured on blood agar and chocolate agar and for staining with Gram and Giemsa stains.

▶ Treatment

In patients with suspected bacterial conjunctivitis, topical broad-spectrum antibacterial agents can be prescribed (eg, sulfacetamide 10% eye drops or ciprofloxacin 0.3% eye drops four times daily during the day), with the addition of erythromycin or bacitracin ophthalmic ointment at bedtime if clinical indications warrant.

Viral conjunctivitis is usually self-limited and does not require treatment. However, if the diagnosis is unclear, topical antibiotics are often used. Contact precautions are useful in all situations of suspected bacterial and viral conjunctivitis because spread of disease occurs through contact with contaminated tears, either directly or through fomites.

Treatment of patients with allergic conjunctivitis consists of topical decongestants (naphazoline 0.1%), and H_1 receptor blocker (levocabastine) or a mast cell stabilizer (cromolyn). Combination mast cell and antihistamine drops such as olopatadine are also available. In severe cases of allergic conjunctivitis, topical corticosteroids may be required but should be initiated only with the assistance of an ophthalmologist.

CORNEAL ULCERS

Corneal infections leading to ulceration may be due to bacteria (including chlamydia), viruses, fungi, or protozoa. The most serious infection of the cornea is caused by pseudomonas species.

▶ Clinical Findings

A. Symptoms and Signs

Patients with corneal ulcers complain of pain, photophobia, and blurring of vision. Patients develop conjunctival hyperemia and chemosis, with ulceration of the cornea and whitish or yellowish infiltrate. Hypopyon (pus in the anterior chamber) may be present in cases due to bacterial or fungal infections.

B. Laboratory Findings

Laboratory studies include culture and cytologic inspection of corneal scrapings.

▶ Treatment

Corneal ulceration is a serious condition that should be managed carefully and followed closely. The most severe and devastating infection of the cornea is caused by *Pseudomonas aeruginosa*. Topical and subconjunctival antibiotics should be given on an empirical basis until the results of culture and sensitivity tests are obtained. Organism-specific antimicrobial treatment should then be given. Central corneal ulcers may leave corneal scars, causing loss of vision. Patients severely affected may require penetrating keratoplasty (corneal transplant).

Patients wearing contact lenses, especially extended-wear contacts, are at higher risk of corneal ulcers. As with any corneal infection, patients should be advised to stop wearing them. Patients using topical corticosteroids should stop using them.

HERPES SIMPLEX

Herpes simplex is a DNA virus that can affect the eye in a primary ocular reaction as well as in a reactivated state when latent virus travels down the axon of the sensory nerve to its target tissue. Herpes simplex virus (HSV) is extremely common, and about 90% of the population is seropositive for HSV antibodies. HSV-1 predominantly causes infection above the waist (face, lips, and eyes), and HSV-2 typically causes infection below the waist. Very occasionally, HSV-2 is transmitted to the eye through infected genital secretions during birth, but most ocular infections are HSV-1.

▶ Clinical Findings

A. Symptoms and Signs

Primary infections usually occur in children between ages 6 months and 5 years and may be associated with generalized symptoms of a viral illness. HSV is usually self-limited, and the most common symptoms are blepharoconjunctivitis and keratitis, which is classically in a dendritic pattern.

B. Laboratory Findings

A clinical diagnosis can be made with the classic dendritic presentation. However, definitive diagnosis is made using viral culture or Giemsa-stained smears of corneal scrapings that reveal mononuclear cells, polymorphonuclear neutrophil leukocytes, multinucleated giant epithelial cells, and eosinophilic Lipschutz inclusion bodies in the cell nuclei. Enzyme-linked immunosorbent assay (ELISA) can be used to detect whether live viral particles are present.

▶ Treatment

The mainstays of treatment are topical and oral antiviral medications. Antibiotic ointment may be used at night to help prevent bacterial superinfection. Topical trifluorothymidine (Viroptic), 1%, or acycloguanosine (Vira-A) ointment is used to treat keratitis. Oral acyclovir (400 mg five times a day) or valacyclovir (500 mg three times a day) is used. Topical steroids may be used to treat corneal scarring or uveitis, but must be used carefully with concurrent topical or systemic antiviral therapy or both. Cost effectiveness of prophylaxis with valacyclovir or acyclovir has been analyzed, but currently they are rarely used unless significant visual loss has occurred from previous herpetic episodes.

Miserocchi E et al: Efficacy of valacyclovir versus acyclovir for the prevention of recurrent herpes simplex virus eye disease: a pilot study. Am J Ophthalmol 2007;144:547.

HERPES ZOSTER

Herpes zoster is caused by a reactivation of latent varicella (chickenpox) virus dormant in the dorsal root ganglion. Approximately 15% of herpes zoster cases arise from the ophthalmic division of the trigeminal nerve, which is then referred to as herpes zoster ophthalmicus. Hutchinson sign (involvement of the nasociliary nerve, which supplies the tip of the nose) occurs in about one third of patients with herpes zoster ophthalmicus; if present, it suggests intraocular involvement. Reactivation is associated with decreased cell-mediated immunity, and patients with HIV, blood dyscrasias, neoplasms, or other forms of immunosuppression are more at risk.

▶ Clinical Findings

Herpes zoster ophthalmicus can involve virtually all ocular and adnexal tissues. Reactivation often starts with headache, malaise, fever, and ocular pain, followed within 24–48 hours by the classic vesicular lesions in a dermatomal, unilateral pattern. Corneal involvement may occur with the acute event or may follow it by months or years. A corneal pseudodendritic pattern is common. Conjunctivitis, keratitis, episcleritis/scleritis, and uveitis can also occur.

▶ Treatment

Treatments of skin lesions include warm compresses and topical antibiotic ointment. Dry eye and poor corneal sensation are common. Oral antiviral medication is the standard of care. Oral acyclovir (800 mg five times a day) or valacyclovir (1000 mg three times a day), initiated within 72 hours of symptoms, has been demonstrated to accelerate the resolution of skin rash and the healing of skin lesions; reduce lesion formation and viral shedding; and reduce the incidence of episcleritis, keratitis, and iritis. Oral antiviral medication also appears to reduce acute zoster-associated pain and may decrease postherpetic neuralgia. Topical antiviral medication and steroids may be indicated in certain situations to treat corneal lesions or uveitis. See Table 37–2.

DRY EYE

Dry eye is a disorder of the tear film due to either deficiency of production or excess tear evaporation. The tear film is composed of mucin, aqueous, and lipid components. Abnormalities of any layer lead to a wide variety of symptoms.

Table 37-2. Herpes Simplex Virus (HSV) versus Herpes Zoster Virus (HZV).

	HSV	HZV
Rash	Clear vesicles on erythematous base; crusting	Vesicular rash along dermatomal distribution, not crossing midline; Hutchinson sign (nasociliary branch of V1) may be present
Epithelial lesion	Dendritic epithelial lesions with heaped edges	Pseudodendrites (mucous plaques without true terminal bulbs)
Staining	Edges stain with rose bengal; central ulceration stains with fluorescein	Minimal fluorescein staining
Patient population	Young	Older or immunocompromised

Primary lacrimal deficiency from disease such as Riley-Day syndrome and hypoplastic lacrimal glands is rare. Most lacrimal deficiency is secondary to postradiation or related to lymphoma, sarcoidosis, graft-versus-host disease, HIV, hemochromatosis, and amyloidosis. Systemic medications such as anticholinergics (including antihistamines and anti-depressants), antiadrenergics, and diuretics can also cause decreased tear production. Dry eye has also been associated with menopause, presumably due to decreased androgens, and women have a much higher incidence of symptomatic dry eye. Dry eye has become one of the most common reasons for visits to ophthalmologists. Symptoms are often exacerbated by weather, climate, reading, and computer use.

Evaporative dry eye problems are most often associated with meibomian gland dysfunction. The protective lipid and mucin layers that normally keep the aqueous layer of tears stable are reduced, leading to a poor-quality tear film that breaks up easily. These symptoms are often associated with rosacea and treated conservatively with warm compresses. Occasionally, oral tetracycline medications may be used. Oral flax or fish oil supplements may help.

▶ Clinical Findings

Symptoms of tear deficiency often include foreign body sensation, redness, decreased vision, and even reflex tearing. These symptoms tend to vary with time and eye usage; symptoms are usually worse at the end of the day.

Symptoms of evaporative tear loss include a chronic "film" over the vision, redness, burning, and itching of the eyelid margin; these symptoms are often worse in the morning. The quick breakup time of the tear film leads to difficulty reading and prolonged eye usage.

Post-LASIK (laser in-situ keratomileusis) patients have decreased corneal sensation, lower tear production, and diminished blink rate, which may cause dry eye symptoms for 6–18 months or more postoperatively.

▶ Treatment

Treatment for aqueous deficiency includes lubricant tear supplementation. In meibomian gland disease, eyelid hygiene is extremely important. Hot compresses with eyelid scrubs can improve tear quality and prevent evaporative tear loss. Mild topical corticosteroids or systemic tetracycline may also be used, especially if the patient has associated signs of acne rosacea. Recently, topical cyclosporine A, because of its anti-inflammatory action, has been found to dramatically improve dry eye symptoms, although it may take up to 6 weeks for symptomatic improvement. Punctal occlusion may be used in eyes shown to have decreased tear production.

DACRYOCYSTITIS

Dacryocystitis is a common infection of the lacrimal sac. Acute or chronic, it occurs most often in infants and in persons over age 40 years. It is usually unilateral and always secondary to obstruction of the nasolacrimal duct. In rare instances, the nasolacrimal duct may be obstructed by a tumor.

Normally, the nasolacrimal duct opens spontaneously during the first month of life. Failure of canalization leads to obstruction of the sac and secondary dacryocystitis.

The cause of acquired nasolacrimal duct obstruction is usually unknown, but trauma to the nose or infection may be responsible. In infants, dacryocystitis leading to obstruction may be due to *Haemophilus influenza*, staphylococci, or streptococci. In patients with trachoma, nasolacrimal and canalicular obstruction is common. The cause of acute dacryocystitis in adults is usually *Staphylococcus aureus* or β-hemolytic streptococci. In chronic dacryocystitis, *Streptococcus pneumoniae* is a common pathogen.

▶ Clinical Findings

A. Symptoms and Signs

Acute dacryocystitis is characterized by pain, swelling, tenderness, and redness in the tear sac area; pus may be expressed. In chronic dacryocystitis, tearing and discharge are the principal signs. Mucus or pus may be expressed from the tear sac.

B. Laboratory Findings

Pus can be expressed from the upper or lower puncta and can be examined by Gram stain and culture and sensitivity testing.

▶ Treatment

A. Adults

Acute dacryocystitis responds well to systemic antibiotic therapy, but recurrences are common if the obstruction is not surgically relieved.

B. Infants

When ductal obstruction is due to failure of canaliculization in the first month of life, daily forceful massage of the tear sac is indicated, and topical antibiotics should be instilled in the conjunctival sac four or five times daily. If this is not successful, probing of the nasolacrimal duct is indicated. Most ophthalmologists postpone probing until the age of 6 months because in most cases the ducts that will open spontaneously have opened by that time. The probe should be passed through both the upper and the lower canaliculi. In cases of previous failure or in children older than the age of 2, balloon dacryocystoplasty at the time of probing may increase chances of success.

> Luchtenberg M et al: Clinical effectiveness of balloon dacryocysto-plasty in circumscribed obstructions of the nasolacrimal duct. Ophthalmologica 2007;221:434.

ORBITAL CELLULITIS

Orbital cellulitis is manifested by an abrupt onset of swelling and redness of the lids, accompanied by proptosis, decreased vision, diplopia, and fever. It is usually caused by staphylococci or streptococci. Immediate treatment with intravenous antibiotics is indicated to prevent abscess formation and rapid increase in the orbital pressure, which may interfere with the blood supply to the eye. The response to antibiotics is usually excellent, but surgical drainage may be required if an abscess forms. CT is indicated to rule out abscess formation. Preseptal cellulitis is limited to the area anterior to the orbital septum and may be treated with oral antibiotics while monitoring closely for progression to full-blown orbital infection.

PTERYGIUM

Pterygium is a fleshy, triangular growth from the conjunctiva that is usually associated with excessive exposure to wind, sun, sand, and dust. It is often on the nasal side of the cornea. It may be either unilateral or bilateral. There may be a genetic predisposition, but no hereditary pattern has been described. Excision is indicated if the growth threatens vision by approaching the visual axis, though recurrence is common.

Treatment is by superficial excision. After excising large or recurrent pterygia, autologous conjunctival tissue or amniotic membrane transplantation is indicated. A thin layer of conjunctiva is obtained from the upper bulbar conjunctiva and sutured to the area from which the pterygium was removed. This leads to rapid restoration of ana-tomic integrity of the epithelial surface and may prevent further recurrences. Patients should be advised to wear UV protection outdoors. Topical mitomycin eye drops have been used to prevent recurrences of the disease, but serious complications such as scleral thinning and keratitis have been reported.

CATARACT

Cataract is opacity of the lens and is the leading cause of curable blindness in the world. There are three types of cataracts: (1) congenital, (2) those associated with other disorders, and (3) age-related. Some cataracts are rapidly progressive, while others may show slow progression. Indications for surgical removal occur when patients have difficulty with daily activities or if visual development is at risk.

1. Congenital Cataract

Congenital cataract may be genetically determined or may be caused by intrauterine factors that interfere with normal development of the lens. Intrauterine viral infections (most commonly rubella), for example, can lead to congenital cataract.

Congenital cataract may be unilateral or bilateral and complete or incomplete. Dense cataract present at birth is an indication for urgent surgical management to prevent amblyopia.

Phacoemulsification or simple aspiration with central posterior capsulotomy and limited anterior vitrectomy is recommended for congenital cataract. Preservation of the peripheral posterior capsule and zonules is important for future implantation of intraocular lenses. If the cataract is aspirated, leaving the posterior capsule intact, the posterior capsule becomes opaque, requiring capsulotomy at a later stage. Correction with soft contact lenses can be started immediately after surgery. Posterior chamber intraocular lenses may be implanted when the child is older, although children as young as 2 years are being given primary intraocular lens implants. Restoration of true binocular vision in very young children is seldom achieved after removal of unilateral congenital cataracts.

2. Cataracts Associated with Other Disorders

Many systemic conditions may be associated with cataracts, including diabetes mellitus, galactosemia, hypocalcemia, myotonic dystrophy, Down syndrome, and cutaneous disorders such as atopic dermatitis. Certain systemic medications and eye drops containing corticosteroids can also cause cataracts. Other disorders of the eye, such as retinal detachment or chronic uveitis, may also be associated with cataracts. Eyes that have undergone retinal surgical procedures, particularly vitrectomy, have increased risk of cataract development. Physical trauma to the lens as well as injury from thermal and ionizing radiation can cause cataract formation.

The indication for surgical intervention and surgical treatment of such cataracts is similar to that of senile cataract, discussed next.

3. Age-Related (Senile) Cataract

This is the most common type of cataract. The rate of progression is variable. Diagnosis is by slit-lamp examination. Nuclear changes of the lens produce a brunescent color and often affect distance vision. In advanced cortical cataracts, a white opacity may be seen in the pupillary area upon gross inspection. Diplopia can occur. Posterior subcapsular cataracts are often in younger patients, causes glare, and affects near reading.

▶ Treatment

Once the cataract leads to visual impairment, treatment is by surgical removal of the lens. Clinical trials of agents that may delay or prevent the formation of cataracts are under way, but no pharmacologic means of prevention is available at present.

Phacoemulsification of the cataract is the procedure of choice in most developed countries. Primary lens implant is preferred unless there is a contraindication to their use. In that situation, optical correction can be achieved with eyeglasses or contact lenses.

A. Intracapsular Lens Extraction

Intracapsular extraction, rarely used today, removes the lens entirely with its capsule either by forceps or a cryoprobe. This procedure cannot be performed on children or young adults because of the adhesion between the lens and the vitreous.

B. Extracapsular Extraction

For standard extracapsular cataract extraction, the anterior capsule of the lens is removed, the nucleus of the cataract is expressed, and the residual cortical material is aspirated from the eye through a 9–11 mm incision. Smaller incision techniques with fracturing the lens nuclei are available. The posterior capsule is left intact, and an intraocular lens is placed in the capsular bag. The incision is then sutured with 10-0 nylon. In 25–35% of patients undergoing extracapsular cataract extraction, the posterior capsule may become opacified. This is treated by Nd:YAG laser capsulotomy. If such a laser is not available, surgical incision of the opaque posterior capsule is required.

C. Phacoemulsification

See Figure 37–1. Phacoemulsification is the most common form of extracapsular cataract extraction and involves technology that fragments the nucleus of the lens using a high-frequency ultrasonic probe while simultaneously aspirating these fragments from the eye. The advantage of phacoemulsification is that incision size is reduced, there is less astigmatism induced from the surgery, and the patient can be more quickly rehabilitated. Remaining cortical material is removed by irrigation and aspiration, and an intraocular lens implanted. The use of foldable or injectable intraocular lenses is now possible through small incisions, and in many

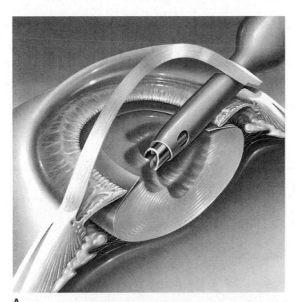 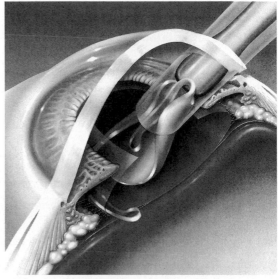

A   **B**

▲ **Figure 37–1.** Phacoemulsification. **A:** Phacoemulsification probe removing lens nucleus through a clear corneal incision. **B:** Implantation of an injectable intraocular lens implant into the capsular bag through a small incision. (Photos, Courtesy of Alcon Laboratories, Inc.)

cases, no suture is required. Retrobulbar anesthesia used to be the standard method of anesthesia used, but both injection of subtenon through a blunt canula and topical anesthesia are safer, widely used methods.

Srinivasan S et al: Randomized double-blind clinical trial comparing topical and sub-Tenon's anaesthesia in routine cataract surgery. Br J Anaesth 2004;93:68.
Studholme S: Comparison of methods of local anesthesia for cataract extraction. J Periop Pract 2008;18:17.

ANGLE-CLOSURE GLAUCOMA

About 1% of people over age 35 have anatomically narrow anterior chamber angles. In such patients, if the pupil dilates spontaneously or is dilated with a mydriatic or cycloplegic agent, the angle may close and an attack of acute glaucoma may be precipitated. For this reason, it is a wise precaution to estimate the depth of the anterior chamber angle before instilling these drugs.

Acute angle-closure glaucoma is manifested by sudden onset of pain, headache, and blurring of vision. Some patients develop nausea and vomiting. The eye is red, the cornea is hazy, and the pupil is mid-dilated and does not react to light. Intraocular pressure is elevated.

The attack is aborted by use of topical pilocarpine, beta-blockers, apraclonidine and latanoprost drops, systemic acetazolamide, and, if necessary, an intravenous hyperosmotic agent such as mannitol. Definitive treatment consists of peripheral iridotomy, which establishes a communication between the posterior and anterior chambers and reopens the angle. This is usually done with an argon or Nd:YAG laser. Rarely, surgical peripheral iridectomy is required.

OPEN-ANGLE GLAUCOMA

In open-angle glaucoma, the intraocular pressure is elevated, causing, over a number of years, segmental atrophy of the optic nerve. The damage to the nerve results in loss of vision, ranging in severity from slight constriction of the upper nasal peripheral visual field to complete blindness. The cause of the

decreased rate of aqueous outflow that characterizes open-angle glaucoma has not been fully determined. The disease is bilateral but can be asymmetric and is probably genetically influenced. African Americans are particularly at risk.

▶ Clinical Findings

Open-angle glaucoma is painless, so patients may be unaware of damage until late in the course of the disease. On examination, there may be slight cupping (segmental atrophy) of the optic disk. There is loss of peripheral visual field, but central vision acuity usually remains unaffected even in patients with severe visual field loss. Absolute glaucoma is the total loss of peripheral and central vision, often with decreased light perception. Tonometry, evaluation of the optic nerve, and visual field testing are the three principal tests used for the diagnosis and continued clinical evaluation of glaucoma. Central corneal thickness should be assessed and included in risk calculations for glaucoma.

The normal intraocular pressure ranges from 10–20 mm Hg. The diagnosis should never be made on the basis of a single tonometric measurement. Transient elevations of intraocular pressure do not constitute glaucoma for the same reason that periodic or intermittent elevations of blood pressure do not constitute hypertensive disease. All persons over age 20 should have tonometric and ophthalmoscopic examinations every 3–5 years. If there is a family history of glaucoma or other risk factors, annual examination is indicated. Low-tension glaucoma is an uncommon condition characterized by visual field changes and optic nerve cupping in the presence of intraocular pressure that remains in the normal range.

▶ Treatment

See Table 37–3. Most patients can be controlled with topical medications including beta-blockers (eg, timolol maleate 0.25–0.5%, 1 drop twice daily), α-adrenergic agonists (eg, brimonidine 0.2%, 1 drop twice daily), carbonic anhydrase inhibitors (eg, dorzolamide 2%, 1 drop twice daily), or prostaglandins (eg, latanoprost 0.005%, 1 drop once daily). Oral carbonic anhydrase inhibitors (eg, acetazolamide) can

Table 37–3. Types of Glaucoma Medications and Side Effects.

Class	Mechanism	Side Effects	Pregnancy Class
Beta-blockers (eg, timolol)	Decrease aqueous production	Hypotension, bradycardia, asthma exacerbation	C
α_2-adrenergic agonist (eg, brimonidine, Propine)	Decrease aqueous production	Allergy, tachyphylaxis, CNS depression	B
Cholinergics (eg, pilocarpine)	Increase outflow	Brow ache, cataract formation, retinal detachment	C
Carbonic anhydrase inhibitors (eg, acetazolamide, dorzolamide)	Decrease aqueous production	Sulfa allergy, systemic metabolic acidosis, tingling, aplastic anemia, metallic taste	C
Prostaglandin analogues (eg, latanoprost)	Increase outflow	Bitter taste, iris color change, red eye	C

be used in patients with persistent elevation of intraocular pressures despite topical treatment. Miotics (eg, pilocarpine 1–4%, 1 drop four times daily) and epinephrine eye drops (0.5–2.0%, 1 drop twice daily) are less commonly used today.

Argon laser trabeculoplasty can be helpful in decreasing the intraocular pressure in some patients, and if successful can be performed on each eye twice. Selective laser trabeculoplasty is a newer laser treatment similar to argon laser trabeculoplasty, but studies suggest it can be repeated multiple times in each eye. In those with persistent pressure elevation, surgery is indicated to create an alternate drainage passage for fluid from the eye. The most common procedure is trabeculectomy. The success of this procedure has been improved by the use of intraoperative application of mitomycin or 5-fluorouracil to inhibit the fibrosis and closure of the newly created filtering channel. In certain types of glaucoma, such as neovascular glaucoma or aphakic glaucoma, or for those with who have failed previous surgery, insertion of prosthetic drainage valves or shunts can be used.

Damji KF et al: Selective laser trabeculoplasty versus argon laser trabeculoplasty: results from a 1-year randomized clinical trial. Br J Ophthalmol 2006;90:1490.
Juzych MS et al: Comparison of long-term outcomes of selective laser trabeculoplasty versus argon laser trabeculoplasty in open-angle glaucoma. Ophthalmology 2004;11:1853.

OCULAR MIGRAINE

Migraine is a disorder with multiple clinical presentations. Recurrent headaches are classic, and ocular symptoms are often associated. The pathophysiology of migraine is uncertain, and there may be a genetic component. The differential diagnosis for migraine headaches includes stress-tension headache, cluster headache, sinus congestion/pathology, elevated intracranial pressures, orbital inflammation, orbital neoplasia, and, rarely, temporal arteritis. A thorough headache history and neurologic examination are important diagnostic tools.

In patients with ocular migraine, visual symptoms are present initially, and headache and nausea, if present at all, follow. The ocular symptoms can mimic retinal disease, and a dilated ocular examination is needed to rule out retinal pathology when the symptoms are atypical. The flashing lights from retinal disease are primarily unilateral, while migraine presents with bilateral visual distortion. Asking the patient to cover each eye and see if the symptoms are unilateral or bilateral may assist in clarifying the situation. Prophylaxis to prevent migraine with oral β-adrenergic blockers, calcium-channel blockers, and tricyclic antidepressants may be used. Triptans such as sumatriptan (Imitrex) are often used to treat the acute episodes. Acephalgic migraine typically is not treated with systemic agents because of the self-limited nature of the disease.

Classical Migraines

Classical migraine is characterized by throbbing headaches preceded by visual auras lasting about 20 minutes. The aura may consist of bright or dark spots, zigzag lines (fortification scotoma), heat haze distortions, scintillating scotomas, and tunnel vision. Homonymous or altitudinal hemianopia may rarely occur. The headaches that follow may vary in intensity. Ocular symptoms without subsequent headache (acephalgic migraine) also occur.

Retinal Migraine

Retinal migraine is characterized by acute, transient unilateral loss of vision that can be identical to that seen in amaurosis fugax. Vascular etiologies must be ruled out with thorough ocular and medical examination before attributing symptoms to be migraine. Amaurosis is often shorter in duration and has a more "curtainlike" quality.

Ophthalmoplegic Migraine

Ophthalmoplegic migraine is very rare and typically starts before the age of 10 years. It is characterized by a recurrent transient third nerve palsy that is associated with a typical migraine headache.

Complicated Migraine

Complicated migraine is associated with neurologic deficits such as tingling in the extremities, hemisensory disturbance, or partial visual loss, and rarely, the deficit persists after the headache has resolved. Antiplatelet therapy with aspirin is often recommended.

DIABETIC RETINOPATHY

Diabetes is the number-one cause of new blindness in most industrialized countries. Diabetic retinopathy eventually develops in almost half of all diabetics and is a major cause of blindness. There are two clinical classifications: (1) **nonproliferative or background diabetic retinopathy** and (2) **sight threatening proliferative diabetic retinopathy.** The prevalence of retinopathy increases with the duration of diabetes. Patients who have had type 1 for 5 years or less are at low risk of retinopathy. However, 27% of those with diabetes for 5–10 years and 71–90% of those with diabetes for longer than 10 years have some form of diabetic retinopathy. After 20–30 years, the prevalence rises to 95%, with 30–50% of those patients having proliferative changes.

Diabetes can have other effects on the eye. Poor corneal healing and decreased corneal sensation have been noted. Neovascular glaucoma caused by iris neovascularization, which blocks the outflow passage in the anterior chamber angle, is seen in some patients with proliferative retinal disease. There is thought be an association between diabetes and primary open-angle glaucoma. Optic neuropathy and cranial neuropathies may occur.

Clinical Findings

Microaneurysms, intraretinal hemorrhages, cotton wool spots, and lipid deposits due to vascular leakage are the retinal changes seen in early diabetic retinopathy. Later stages include retinal ischemia and neovascularization with subsequent vitreous hemorrhage often associated with traction or rhegmatogenous retinal detachment. Diabetic retinopathy may be asymptomatic until vision decreases, usually from macular edema or vitreous hemorrhage. The presence of renal microvascular disease (microalbuminuria, elevated blood urea and creatinine levels) correlates well with the presence of diabetic retinopathy.

Treatment

Careful control of blood sugar and blood pressure appears to reduce the incidence and severity of diabetic retinopathy. Recent epidemiologic studies show that many diabetics fail to have the recommended yearly eye examinations. However, if patients are followed up closely and retinopathy is detected early and treated according to the guidelines of the Early Treatment Diabetic Retinopathy Study (ETDRS), the risk of severe visual loss is less than 5%. Treatment consists of photocoagulation, either of the macula to reduce edema or of the retinal periphery to reduce ischemic neovascular changes. Adjunctive intravitreal injection of triamcinolone with laser treatment has been suggested for macular edema and proliferative retinopathy. Results seem promising, but long-term studies are necessary. Complications such as endophthalmitis or steroid-induced glaucoma are possible.

Kang SW et al: Macular grid photocoagulation after intravitreal triamcinolone acetonide for diffuse macular edema. Arch Ophthalmol 2006;124:653.

Zein WM et al: Panretinal photocoagulation and intravitreal triamcinolone acetonide for the management of proliferative diabetic retinopathy with macular edema. Retina 2006;26:137.

AGE-RELATED MACULAR DEGENERATION (AMD)

Age-related macular degeneration (AMD) is the leading cause of central visual loss among individuals aged 65 and older. The cause of AMD is unknown, although recent research documents a genetic component. Regardless of the mechanism, the disease appears to affect the retinal pigment epithelium at the level of Bruch membrane. Drusen, yellowish deposits in the retina caused by the thickening, hyalinization, and calcification of the retinal pigment epithelium are characteristic of AMD.

1. Atrophic ("Dry") Macular Degeneration

Atrophic ("dry") macular degeneration is the most common form of AMD, occurring in approximately 80% of those with the disease. Drusen, pigment changes, and atrophy are present, but there is no leakage of fluid into the subretinal space. Usually, only minimal to moderate visual loss is present.

2. Exudative ("Wet") Macular Degeneration

Exudative ("wet") macular degeneration is characterized by the development of a choroidal neovascular membrane that leaks fluid and blood. This causes a serous detachment of the central fovea that can lead to profound vision loss.

Clinical Findings

Visual loss is caused by geographical atrophy, serous detachment of the retinal pigment epithelium, or choroidal neovascularization. Central visual acuity is primarily affected with the peripheral vision remaining intact. Metamorphopsia, distortion of the central vision, is a classic patient complaint. Patients can follow their own progression of disease with an Amsler grid. Certain racial predispositions, those with cardiovascular risk factors, and smokers have been suggested to be associated with a higher incidence of advanced AMD.

Treatment

The Age-Related Eye Disease Study (AREDS) is the first large, prospective clinical trial to show the benefit of antioxidant and zinc supplementation on the progression of AMD and associated visual loss. In evaluating the rate of progression to advanced visual loss, nutritional supplements statistically significantly benefited only patients who had moderate to severe disease. Supplements were not found to prevent the development of AMD or to prevent progression in patients with mild disease.

Treatment of exudative AMD is more difficult. Standard laser photocoagulation can be useful in treating certain neovascular complexes. Photodynamic therapy (PDT) is a method of more selective laser therapy using verteporfin to enhance treatment success in destroying the subretinal neovascular membrane that is producing the fluid leakage. Both methods reduce the rate of visual loss when compared to controls.

Recently, the use of intravitreal injections of anti–vascular endothelial growth factor agents to treat exudative AMD has led to major improvement in visual outcomes. The most promising agent that has been evaluated in a controlled clinical trial (ranibizumab [Lucentis]) actually leads to an increase in visual acuity in a significant number of patients with exudative AMD. A structurally similar drug (bevacizumab [Avastin]) has shown similar results and is much less expensive. A head-to-head trial is being developed to see which is superior.

Smoking cessation is extremely important. Exercise and control of other systemic diseases such as hypertension and hypercholesterolemia may also help.

Andreoli CM, Miller JW: Anti-vascular endothelial growth factor for ocular neovascular disease. Curr Opin Ophthalmol 2007; 18:502.

Bashsur ZF et al: Intravitreal bevacizumab for the management of choroidal neovascularization in age-related macular degeneration. Am J Ophthalmol 2006;142:1.

Fraser-Bell S et al: Cardiovascular risk factors and age-related macular degeneration: the Los Angeles Latino Eye Study. Am J Ophthalmol 2008;145:308.

Klein R et al: Further observations on the association between smoking and the long-term incidence and progression of age-related macular degeneration: the Beaver Dam Eye Study. Arch Ophthalmol 2008;126:115.

Rosenfeld PJ et al: Ranibizumab for neovascular age-related macular degeneration. N Eng J Med 2006;355:1419.

RETINAL DETACHMENT

Detachment of the retina is usually spontaneous but may be secondary to trauma. Spontaneous detachment occurs most frequently in persons over 50 years of age.

▶ Clinical Findings

Retinal tears or holes are the most important predisposing factors. Increased risk of retinal detachment is also associated with cataract surgery and high myopia. In the presence of a retinal tear or hole, fluid from the vitreous cavity enters the defect and transudation from choroidal vessels and detaches the retina from the pigment epithelium (rhegmatogenous). These small retinal holes may need to be lasered to prevent detachment by sealing small retinal tears before detachment occurs.

The superior temporal area is the most common site of detachment. The area of detachment rapidly increases, causing progressive visual loss. Central vision remains intact until the macula becomes detached. On ophthalmoscopic examination, the detached retina is seen as an elevated gray membrane. One or more retinal tears may be seen.

▶ Treatment

All cases of retinal detachment should be referred immediately to an ophthalmologist. If the patient must be transported a long distance, the head should be positioned to try to minimize the progression of the detachment. If the upper retina is detached, the head should be kept flat. Patients with an inferior detachment should be kept upright.

Retinal detachment is a true ophthalmic emergency if the macula is threatened. If the macula is detached, permanent loss of central vision may occur even though the retina is eventually successfully reattached by surgery. Treatment consists of drainage of subretinal fluid and closure of retinal tears by cryosurgery, laser, or scleral buckling. This produces an inflammatory reaction that causes the retina to adhere to the choroid. The creation of an inflammatory adhesion between the choroid and the retina helps to prevent future redetachment by sealing small retinal tears.

In uncomplicated retinal detachment with a superior retinal tear and healthy vitreous, pneumoretinopexy may be performed. The procedure consists of injection of air or certain gases into the vitreous cavity through the pars plana and positioning the patient to allow the gas bubble to seal the retinal hole and permit spontaneous reabsorption of the subretinal fluid.

About 85% of uncomplicated cases can be reattached with one operation. About 10% will need more than one procedure, and the remainder never reattach. The prognosis is worse if the macula is detached, if the vitreous is not healthy, or if the detachment is of long duration.

Without treatment, retinal detachment almost always becomes total in 1–6 months. Spontaneous detachments are ultimately bilateral in 20–25% of cases.

STRABISMUS IN CHILDREN

Any child under age 7 (and especially infants and young children) with obvious strabismus should be seen without delay to allow prompt treatment to prevent amblyopia. About 3% of children are born with or develop strabismus. In descending order of frequency, the eyes may deviate inward (esotropia), outward (exotropia), upward (hypertropia), or downward (hypotropia).

▶ Clinical Findings

Children with manifest strabismus suppress the visual image from the deviating eye to avoid diplopia, and the vision in that eye fails to develop normally. This is the first stage of amblyopia. Most cases of strabismus are obvious, but if the angle of deviation is small or if the strabismus is intermittent, the diagnosis may be missed.

Fortunately, amblyopia due to strabismus can be detected by routine visual acuity testing of all preschool children. Those who cannot be tested with a standard eye chart can use visual acuity testing with an illiterate E card or Allen picture chart.

▶ Treatment

The objectives in the surgical treatment of strabismus in children (Figure 37–2) are to achieve good visual acuity in each eye and align the eyes so that normal binocular vision with fusion can occur. Surgery can be performed in infants, and the earlier the problem is detected and corrected, the better the chance of getting a good result. Correcting the problem in children above age 7–8 often fails to result in visual improvement.

If the child is under age 6 years and has an amblyopic eye and strabismus, patching of the better eye should be instituted to improve the vision before any surgery for strabismus is performed. At age 1 year, patching may be successful within 1 week; at 6 years, it may take a year to achieve the same result. Surgery to align the eye is usually performed after the visual acuity has been equalized.

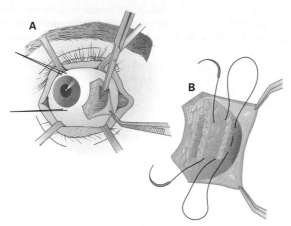

▲ **Figure 37–2. A:** Exposure of an extraocular muscle in surgery for strabismus. **B:** Recession of the muscle behind its original insertion followed by suturing to the sclera with absorbable suture.

Surgery for correction of strabismus in both adults and children consists of weakening or strengthening the extraocular muscles. To weaken the action of a muscle, it is recessed by detaching it from its insertion site and resuturing it to a more posterior location of the sclera. To strengthen a muscle's action, it is separated at the insertion site from the globe, and a portion of it is resected and then resutured to its original insertion site. Muscles should not be recessed more than 8 mm or resected more than 6 mm.

For correction of exotropia, the lateral rectus muscles in both eyes can be recessed. Alternatively, the lateral rectus muscle may be recessed and the medial rectus muscle resected in the same eye. The amount of recession and resection and the number of extraocular muscles resected or recessed is determined by the degree of ocular deviation. The decision to involve one or both of the eyes is influenced by the visual acuity and potential of each eye. In patients with esotropia, the options are to recess the medial recti of both eyes or to recess the medial rectus in combination with resecting the lateral rectus in the same eye.

For vertical deviation, the vertical muscles are recessed, resected, tucked, or weakened by myectomy (usually the inferior oblique).

STRABISMUS IN ADULTS

In adults with mature visual systems, development of strabismus usually produces double vision. Strabismus can be arise from head trauma, microvascular infarct as in diabetes, intracranial hemorrhage or elevated intracranial pressure, brain tumor, or orbital disease.

▶ Treatment

Surgical management of strabismus is the same as described for children. Since visual pathways have already been formed, the indications for surgery are for cosmetic reasons or because of diplopia. Changes in visual acuity or potential after alignment of the eyes are not common in adults. Care must be taken not to induce diplopia after surgery.

▼ OCULAR BURNS

CHEMICAL BURNS

Apart from the history, the diagnosis of chemical eye burns is usually based on the presence of swelling of the eyelids and marked conjunctival hyperemia and chemosis. The limbal area may show blanched patchy areas and conjunctival sloughing, especially in the interpalpebral area. There is usually corneal stromal haze and diffuse edema, with wide areas of epithelial cell loss and corneal ulcerations. Defects in the corneal epithelium can be better visualized with the instillation of fluorescein dye.

Alkali burns of the eye are particularly serious because the agents tend to rapidly penetrate intraocularly and damage the tissue. Retained particles in the conjunctival fornices may continue to release alkaline material and must be promptly removed. Patients are managed by instilling a topical anesthetic agent and then promptly irrigating copiously with isotonic saline or other immediately available irrigating solution, including water. Double eversion of the upper eyelid should be performed to look for and remove material lodged in the superior fornix. This can be easily done by using a forceps or moist cotton applicator. A lid speculum is placed after the instillation of tetracaine 0.5% eye drops, and the eye is irrigated with saline until a neutral pH is reached. This may require hours of flushing. Topical dilating drops such as atropine 1% or homatropine 5% are instilled, and a topical antibiotic ointment such as ophthalmic erythromycin and bacitracin should be applied. Severe injuries that result in eyelid destruction require hospitalization and specialized care.

Acid burns cause rapid damage but are in general less serious than alkali burns because of lack of intraocular penetration. Management consists of immediate irrigation with sterile isotonic saline solution, water, or whatever safe liquid is available. A topical anesthetic agent is instilled to minimize pain during irrigation. The patient is then given an analgesic and the eye is patched. Topical antibiotic ointment may also be used.

THERMAL BURNS

The treatment of thermal burns of the eyes is similar to the treatment of burns elsewhere on the body. Adequate systemic analgesia should be provided. A topical anesthetic agent such as proparacaine 0.5% or tetracaine 0.5% is used to minimize pain during manipulation. In cases of burns involving the cornea, topical dilating drops such as atropine 1% or homatropine 5% are instilled. Antibiotic drops are often prescribed for 3–5 days.

BURNS DUE TO ULTRAVIOLET RADIATION

Injuries to the corneal epithelium by ultraviolet rays vary in severity. They are described as actinic keratitis, snow blindness, welder's arc burn, or flash burn, depending on the source of ultraviolet radiation. Patients present with severe pain, tearing, and photophobia. The examination reveals diffuse punctate staining of the cornea, best seen with fluorescein staining, proper magnification, and a cobalt blue light.

A topical antibiotic such as ophthalmic erythromycin or bacitracin ointment is instilled. Topical nonsteroidal drops such as diclofenac or ketorolac tromethamine may be used for pain.

OCULAR TRAUMA

Eye injuries are common in spite of the protection afforded by the bony orbit. Blunt trauma is the most common injury, but penetrating injuries of the globe, although less frequent, are often more serious. The use of protective eyewear at work helps prevent most serious occupational injuries.

Clinical Evaluation

A careful history of the injury should be obtained from the patient or someone who knows what happened. Visual acuity should be measured with and without glasses. The eyelids, conjunctiva, cornea, anterior chamber, iris, lens, vitreous, and fundus should be inspected for lacerations, breaks, or hemorrhage. Detection of corneal damage (such as abrasions) can be performed by instilling fluorescein dye and examining the eye using a cobalt blue light under magnification. CT scan or x-ray examination is helpful in looking for fractures of the orbital bones and trying to rule out radiopaque foreign bodies. Patients with severe injuries should have immediate ophthalmic consultation.

PENETRATING OR PERFORATING INJURIES

Penetrating or perforating ocular injuries require immediate treatment and prompt surgical care to maximize chances for preservation of vision.

Many facial injuries—especially those occurring in automobile accidents—are associated with penetrating ocular trauma. Some injuries may be undetected because of eyelid swelling or because the patient's other injuries have demanded the attention of the emergency room staff. Accurate records and a description of how the injury occurred should be obtained. The eye and ocular adnexa should be examined, including vision testing and testing of ocular motility. *Do not apply pressure on the globe.* X-ray examination and CT scan are performed to rule out fractures of orbital bones or the presence of intraocular foreign bodies.

Careful repair and approximation of corneal and scleral lacerations should be performed in the operating room. Mag-

netic metallic intraocular foreign bodies can be extracted with a magnet in the operating room. The major objectives in management of ocular penetrating or perforating injuries are to relieve pain, preserve or restore vision, and achieve good cosmetic results. Pain relief may be achieved by the administration of morphine, 2–4 mg intravenously or subcutaneously, or meperidine, 50–75 mg intramuscularly as needed. Sedatives such as diazepam, 5 mg, may be given orally as required.

An eye with a penetrating injury should be protected from further injury with a Fox or similar shield and light dressing. Parenteral broad-spectrum antibiotics such as cefazolin or gentamicin should be given. Antiemetics—ondansetron, 4 mg intravenously—should be given to the patient when needed to prevent vomiting, which can lead to extrusion of the intraocular contents.

LACERATIONS OF THE OCULAR ADNEXA

Lacerations of the eyelids and the periorbital skin should be carefully evaluated and inspected. Small linear skin lacerations can be easily sutured and the wound secured with interrupted 6-0 nylon sutures. Because of the good blood supply in the eyelid, the sutures may be removed in 3–5 days. In cases of deep eyelid lacerations, intraocular or orbital damage should be ruled out before the repair is performed. The skin of the eyelids has good elasticity, is loosely attached to underlying tissue, and in adults is frequently present in surplus quantities. This facilitates the development of flaps and grafts. In deep lacerations of the eyelids, if the wound divides the orbicularis muscle parallel to its fibers, only skin sutures are generally required. When the muscle fibers are transversely divided, they should be approximated with 6-0 absorbable synthetic sutures. The skin can be approximated with nylon sutures. In patients with lacerations resulting in round or oval losses of skin, the skin is undermined and the laceration approximated. In larger defects, reconstruction with flaps may be required. Flaps used in reconstruction of the eyelids are advancement flaps, rotational flaps, transposition flaps, island flaps, and Z-plasty flaps.

In large defects, when flaps cannot be used, free skin grafts may be obtained from behind the ear or from the skin of the inner upper arm. Special care should be taken with repair of lacerations of the lower lid to be certain that the lid is not closed under tension to prevent eversion and distortion of the lid margin.

BLUNT TRAUMA TO THE OCULAR ADNEXA & ORBIT

See Table 37–4. Contusions of the eyeball and ocular adnexa may result from blunt trauma. The significance of such an injury cannot always be determined, and the extent of damage to the vision may not be obvious upon initial examination. A careful dilated eye examination is needed for all patients with this type of injury.

Table 37–4. Types of Ocular Injury Associated with Blunt Trauma.

Eyelids	Ecchymosis, swelling, laceration, abrasions, conjunctival or subconjunctival hemorrhages
Cornea	Edema, lacerations
Anterior chamber	Hyphema, recession of angle, secondary glaucoma
Iris	Iridodialysis, iridoplegia, rupture of iris sphincter
Ciliary body	Hyposecretion of aqueous humor
Lens	Cataract, dislocation
Vitreous	Vitreous hemorrhage
Ciliary muscle	Paralysis
Retina	Commotio retinae, retinal edema, choroidal breaks in Bruch membrane, choroidal hemorrhage

BLOWOUT FRACTURE OF THE FLOOR OF THE ORBIT

Blowout fracture of the floor of the orbit can be associated with enophthalmos, double vision in primary position or upgaze, restriction of ocular movement, hypotropia, and decreased or absent sensation over the maxillary area in the distribution of the infraorbital nerve. CT scan of the orbit will document the extent of the orbital injury that can involve the medial wall as well as the floor. There may be air noted in the sinuses.

The initial evaluation and management of patients with blowout fractures may involve both an ophthalmologist and an otolaryngologist because of potential associated fractures of the maxilla or zygoma. Patients are usually treated with a systemic antibiotic (cephalothin or amoxicillin/potassium clavulanate), told not to blow their nose, and reassessed within 1 week by an ophthalmologist. Many blowout fractures do not require surgical correction. Operative management is recommended if there is significant enophthalmos, continued diplopia in primary gaze, or significant instability of the orbital floor.

CORNEAL & CONJUNCTIVAL FOREIGN BODIES

Patients may give a history of working with high-speed tempered steel tools, or drilling, or hammering against a hard object. There may be no history of trauma to the eye, and the patient may not be aware of a foreign body. In most cases, however, the patient complains of foreign body sensation in the eye or under the eyelid, with associated pain, tearing, and photophobia.

A corneal foreign body can be seen with the aid of a loupe and diffuse light. Conjunctival foreign bodies often become embedded in the conjunctiva on the inner surface of the upper lid, which must be everted to facilitate inspection and removal. A topical anesthetic such as proparacaine 0.5% or tetracaine 0.5% is applied. Sterile fluorescein should be instilled to assist in the visualization of small foreign bodies. Some loose foreign bodies can be removed with a moist cotton applicator, while superficial foreign bodies can be removed with the tip of a hypodermic needle. Topical antibiotic ointment should be instilled (eg, erythromycin or bacitracin), and the eye may be patched for a short while. Continued foreign body sensation, pain, or decreased vision needs to be referred to an ophthalmologist for the possibility of corneal ulceration.

Use of the topical anesthetic by the patient will decrease healing and increase risk of corneal ulceration. Topical anesthetics should be used only for examination purposes, *never* for treatment. **Note:** If there is any suspicion of penetrating trauma or history consistent with that type of injury, appropriate ultrasound and radiologic tests should be performed.

▼ OCULAR TUMORS

Tumors of the adnexal structures can often be recognized and diagnosed early because they are usually visible and cause local disfigurement, interference with vision, or displacement of the globe. Intraocular tumors are more difficult to diagnose, but in children, ocular tumors such as retinoblastoma that affect visual function may present with strabismus or leukocoria. Tumors of the eye may be primary, affecting only the ocular or adnexal tissues, or secondary to metastasis of tumors from other organs. In the eye, the most frequent site of metastasis is the choroid, due to its high vascularity. The tumors that most frequently metastasize to the eye are carcinoma of the breast and lung.

The history of growth of the lesion is extremely important, as well as recent changes in its size or appearance. Excisional biopsy of lesions of the skin or conjunctiva is indicated if cancer is suspected.

LID TUMORS

▶ Benign Tumors of the Eyelids

The most frequent benign tumors of the eyelids are **melanocytic nevi.** Excision is indicated primarily for cosmetic reasons (Figure 37–3). Xanthelasmas represent lipid deposits in histiocytes in the dermis of the skin of the eyelid. In such patients, serum lipid and serum cholesterol levels should be determined. Treatment is indicated for cosmetic reasons and consists of simple excision. The lesions tend to be larger than the surface size would indicate, and recurrences are common. Care must be taken not to foreshorten the eyelid skin and cause decreased eyelid closure.

Hemangiomas of the eyelids consist of two types: capillary and cavernous. **Capillary hemangiomas** consist of dilated capillaries and proliferation of endothelial cells. The

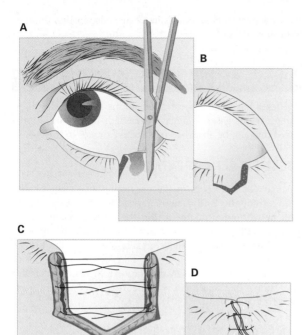

▲ Figure 37–3. Tumor of the left lower eyelid involving the lid margin. **A:** Two vertical incisions are made. **B:** The defect after removal of the tumor. **C:** Suturing of the tarsus and orbicularis with absorbable sutures. **D:** Approximation of the eyelid margin. Skin is approximated with 6-0 silk sutures.

lesions appear as bright red spots. They may show rapid growth in early childhood but later often undergo involution and subside spontaneously. Treatment of hemangiomas in infancy and early childhood is not indicated unless the lesion causes interference with vision that may lead to amblyopia. Low-dose oral steroids or local injection of steroids may cause rapid involution of capillary hemangiomas. **Cavernous hemangiomas,** on the other hand, are venous channels in the subcutaneous tissue. They appear bluish in color and are distended. Surgical excision may be required. Radiation is not recommended because it leads to excessive scarring of the eyelid.

Other benign tumors of the eyelids include verrucae and molluscum contagiosum. These lesions are caused by viruses.

Malignant Tumors of the Eyelids

Squamous cell carcinoma has a tendency to grow slowly and painlessly. It begins as a small lesion covered by a layer of keratin. The lesion may erode, causing an ulcer with hypere-mic edges. It may enlarge to form a fungating mass and may invade the orbital cavity. Early excision may result in cure. If early treatment is not provided, squamous cell carcinoma may spread via the lymphatic system to the preauricular and submandibular lymph nodes.

Basal cell carcinoma begins as a slowly growing, locally invasive tumor forming the so-called rodent ulcer with raised nodular borders. Inner canthal basal cell carcinoma may invade locally and extend into the orbit. Treatment should include complete excision to prevent recurrence. Mohs is usually performed to assure clean margins prior to eyelid reconstruction. Often, the lesions are more extensive than they appear visually. Systemic metastasis is rare.

Malignant melanomas of the eyelids are similar to malignant melanomas of the skin elsewhere on the body.

CONJUNCTIVAL TUMORS

Benign tumors of the conjunctiva include melanocytic nevi (pigmented or nonpigmented), papillomas, granulomas, dermoids, and lymphoid hyperplasia. Malignant tumors of the conjunctiva include carcinoma, malignant melanoma, and, rarely, lymphoma. Carcinoma of the conjunctiva arises frequently at the limbus or the inner canthus in the exposed area of the bulbar conjunctiva. Early in the course of the disease, the lesion may resemble a pterygium. The tumor is slightly elevated, with a gelatinous surface, and may spread over the corneal surface. The growth of this lesion is slow. Treatment is by wide excisional biopsy. Topical mitocmycin-C therapy has been used.

INTRAOCULAR TUMORS

▶ Benign Intraocular Tumors

Melanocytic nevi of the iris, ciliary body, or choroid is common. No treatment is required for these lesions. Retinal angioma may be seen in patients with phacomatoses (eg, Bourneville disease). Choroidal hemangioma is another less frequently encountered benign intraocular tumor.

▶ Malignant Intraocular Tumors

Malignant intraocular tumors include malignant melanoma of the uvea, retinoblastoma, and a rare tumor of the ciliary body known as diktyoma or medulloepithelioma.

Malignant melanoma of the uvea is the most common primary intraocular tumor in adults. It typically occurs in the fifth or sixth decade and is almost always unilateral. The most frequent site is the choroid, but malignant melanoma may occur also in the ciliary body or iris. Malignant melanomas of the choroid may cause decrease in vision and may undergo necrosis, leading to intraocular inflammation. Histopathologic examination shows spindle-shaped cells with or without prominent nuclei and large epithelioid tumor cells. Intraocular malignant melanomas may spread directly through the sclera by local invasion or directly into the central nervous system via optic nerve extension.

Malignant melanomas can be detected by ophthalmoscopy after pupillary dilation.

Treatment of malignant melanoma consists of enucleation or radiotherapy, using radioactive plaques or charged particles. Extension outside the eye may require exenteration of the orbit. Patients with small melanomas—less than 10 mm in diameter—can be followed with serial fundus photos. Similarly, small melanomas of the iris that have not invaded the iris root can be safely followed and observed until growth is documented. If there is growth of the iris tumor, treatment is by local iridectomy. If the iris malignant melanoma invades the root and ciliary body, it can be removed surgically by iridocyclectomy.

Retinoblastoma is a rare but life-threatening condition in childhood. It is the most frequent intraocular malignant tumor in children arising from embryonic cone cells of the photoreceptor layer. Most patients with retinoblastoma present in the first or second year of life. Patients may present with leukocoria or strabismus. Retinoblastoma may be unilateral or bilateral and is often multifocal. There are both sporadic and inherited forms of the disease. It may grow slowly to fill the intraocular space and undergo necrosis, leading to calcific deposits. Tumor cells may seed on the iris and in the anterior chamber, causing fluffy whitish exudates.

Spontaneous remission of retinoblastoma has been reported. Treatment options include radiotherapy, cryotherapy, chemotherapy, and enucleation.

Chintagumpala M et al: Retinoblastoma: review of current management. Oncologist 2007;12:1237.

ORBITAL TUMORS

Orbital tumors may be of two types: those arising from orbital tissues (primary orbital tumors) and those invading the orbit from adjacent structures (secondary orbital tumors). Primary orbital tumors include benign tumors such as dermoid cysts, hemangiomas, lipomas, fibromas, osteomas, chondromas, neurofibromas, and lacrimal gland tumors. Malignant tumors of the orbit include rhabdomyosarcoma, adenocarcinoma of the lacrimal gland, and lymphomas. In children, rhabdomyosarcoma often presents with acute, painless, unilateral proptosis and needs to be evaluated immediately.

Invading tumors include malignant melanoma and retinoblastoma from the intraocular structures and malignant melanomas and carcinomas from the skin of the eyelids and conjunctiva. Metastatic lesions may reach the orbit from the lung or breast. Neuroblastoma may also metastasize to the orbit in children. Meningiomas of the cranial nerves may invade the orbit through the optic canal.

Treatment and prognosis in all cases depend on the type of tumor.

LASER TREATMENTS FOR OCULAR DISEASE

The laser has many useful applications in ophthalmology. Using various gases, a single-wavelength beam can be produced that can be absorbed by selective tissues in the eye.

FOCAL DIABETIC TREATMENT

Macular edema occurs in the preproliferative stage of diabetic retinopathy and is characterized by retinal thickening with or without exudates within the central macular area. This procedure is performed with a slit-lamp laser delivery system with a contact lens and is aided by fluorescein angiography. Improvement may take up to 3 months to occur. Long-term studies by the National Institutes of Health have shown that treatment with an argon laser may improve visual outcome by up to 50%.

PANRETINAL PHOTOCOAGULATION

Panretinal photocoagulation is indicated for treatment of proliferative diabetic retinopathy. Using a contact lens and a slit-lamp delivery system, extensive destruction of peripheral retina is undertaken to decrease production of vasoproliferative factors and increase retinal oxygenation, thus causing regression of abnormal blood vessels that lead to hemorrhage, scarring, and retinal detachment.

LASER SURGERY FOR CORRECTION OF REFRACTIVE ERROR

Laser in-situ keratomileusis (LASIK) is a lamellar refractive surgical procedure, which involves creation of a partial-thickness corneal flap under high suction. The flap is then lifted and an ArF (argon-fluoride) excimer beam is used to ablate stromal tissue with minimal damaging thermal effect. The flap is then replaced and allowed to heal. The combination of accuracy, precision, minimal postoperative discomfort, and quick visual recovery make this the most popular refractive technique. Newer technology of flap creation with laser instead of microkeratome blades is becoming more popular.

Laser epithelial keratomileusis (LASEK) is used mostly for people with corneas that are too thin or too flat for LASIK. A finer trephine may be used to create a thinner flap, or, more commonly, alcohol can be used to devitalize corneal epithelium to remove it prior to laser treatment. LASEK often has a slower rehabilitation, and bandage contact lenses are required after the procedure, but it may be a better option for some patients.

PHOTODYNAMIC THERAPY

Photodynamic therapy is a laser procedure that allows selective treatment for wet exudative AMD in patients who have subfoveal choroidal neovascularization. The choroidal lesion must be predominantly "classic" in nature, which means more than half of it must be evident on fluorescein angiography. The procedure involves intravenous infusion of a photosensitizer, verteporfin, which collects only in abnormal vascular tissue and is then photoactivated by a nonthermal laser light applied through a slit-lamp delivery system. The theory is that photoactivation leads to cellular damage and subsequent vessel occlusion and regression of abnormal blood vessels without damage to surrounding normal tissue.

Mennel S et al: Ocular photodynamic therapy—standard applications and new indications. Ophthalmologica 2007;221:282.

Urology

Christopher S. Cooper, MD

Fadi N. Joudi, MD

Richard D. Williams, MD

EMBRYOLOGY OF THE GENITOURINARY TRACT

A basic understanding of genitourinary embryology facilitates learning many aspects of urology. Embryologically, the genital and urinary systems are intimately related. Associated anomalies of the two systems are commonly encountered.

The Kidneys

The kidneys pass through three embryonic phases (Figure 38–1): (1) The **pronephros** is a vestigial structure without function in human embryos that, except for its primary duct, disappears completely by the fourth week. (2) The pronephric duct gains connection to the **mesonephric tubules** and becomes the mesonephric duct. While most of the mesonephric tubules degenerate, the mesonephric duct persists bilaterally; from where it bends to open into the cloaca, the ureteral bud grows cranially to interact with the metanephric blastema. (3) This forms the **metanephros,** which is the final phase. The metanephros develops into the kidney. During cephalad migration and rotation, the metanephric tissue progressively enlarges, with rapid internal differentiation into the nephron and the uriniferous tubules. Simultaneously, the cephalad end of the ureteral bud expands and divides within the metanephros to form the renal pelvis, calices, and collecting tubules.

The Bladder & Urethra

Subdivision of the cloaca (the blind end of the hindgut) into a ventral (urogenital sinus) and a dorsal (rectum) segment is completed during the seventh week and initiates early differentiation of the urinary bladder and urethra. The urogenital sinus receives the mesonephric duct and absorbs its caudal end, so that by the end of the seventh week, the ureteral bud and mesonephric duct have independent openings. The ureteral orifice migrates upward and laterally. The mesonephric duct orifice moves downward and medially, and the structure in between (the trigone) is formed by the absorbed mesodermal tissue, which maintains direct continuity between the two tubes (Figure 38–2).

The fused müllerian ducts also meet the urogenital sinus at Müller's tubercle. The urogenital sinus above Müller's tubercle differentiates to form the bladder and the part of the prostatic urethra proximal to the seminal colliculus in the male or the bladder and the entire urethra in the female (Figure 38–3). Below Müller's tubercle, the urogenital sinus differentiates into the distal part of the prostatic urethra and the membranous urethra in the male or the distal vagina and vaginal vestibule in the female. The rest of the male urethra is formed by fusion of the urethral folds on the ventral surface of the genital tubercle. In the female, the genital folds remain separate and form the labia minora.

The prostate develops at the end of the 11th week as several groups of outgrowths of urethral epithelium both above and below the entrance of the ejaculatory duct (distal vas deferens). The developing glandular element (seminal colliculus) incorporates the differentiating mesenchymal cells surrounding it to form the muscular stroma and capsule of the prostate. The seminal vesicles form as duplicate buds from the distal end of the mesonephric duct (vas deferens).

The Gonads

The potential to differentiate along male or female lines is present in every embryo initially. The development of one set of sex primordia and the gradual involution of the other are determined by the genetic sex of the embryo and differential secretion of numerous hormones. The *SRY* gene—or testis-determining factor—on the Y chromosome drives the gonad to differentiate into a testicle. Gonadal differentiation begins during the seventh week (Figure 38–3). If the gonad develops into a testis, the germinal epithelium progressively grows into radially arranged, cordlike seminiferous tubules. The production of müllerian-inhibiting factor (MIF) by the testicle causes regression of the müllerian duct and acts in a local (paracrine) fashion so that only the ipsilateral müllerian duct

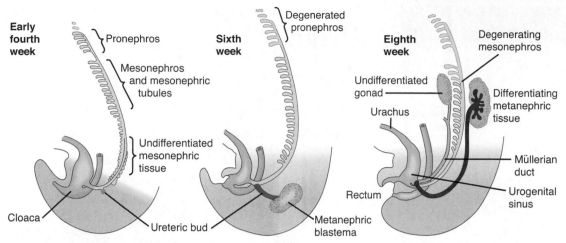

▲ **Figure 38–1.** Schematic of the development of the nephric system. Only a few of the tubules of the pronephros are seen early in the fourth week, while the mesonephric tissue differentiates into mesonephric tubules that progressively join the mesonephric duct. The first sign of the ureteral bud from the mesonephric duct is seen at 4 weeks. At 6 weeks, the pronephros has completely degenerated and the mesonephric tubules start to do so. The ureteral bud grows dorsocranially and has met the metanephric blastema. At the eighth week, there is cranial migration of the differentiating metanephros. The cranial end of the ureteral bud expands and starts to show multiple successive outgrowths (renal calices).

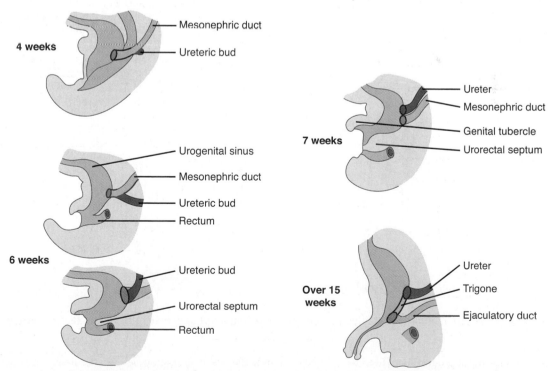

▲ **Figure 38–2.** The development of the ureteral bud from the mesonephric duct and their relationship to the urogenital sinus. The ureteral bud appears at the fourth week. The mesonephric duct distal to this ureteral bud is gradually absorbed into the urogenital sinus, resulting in separate endings for the ureter and the mesonephric duct. The mesonephric tissue that is incorporated into the urogenital sinus expands and forms the trigonal tissue. The mesonephric duct forms the vas deferens in the male and Gartner's duct (if present) in the female.

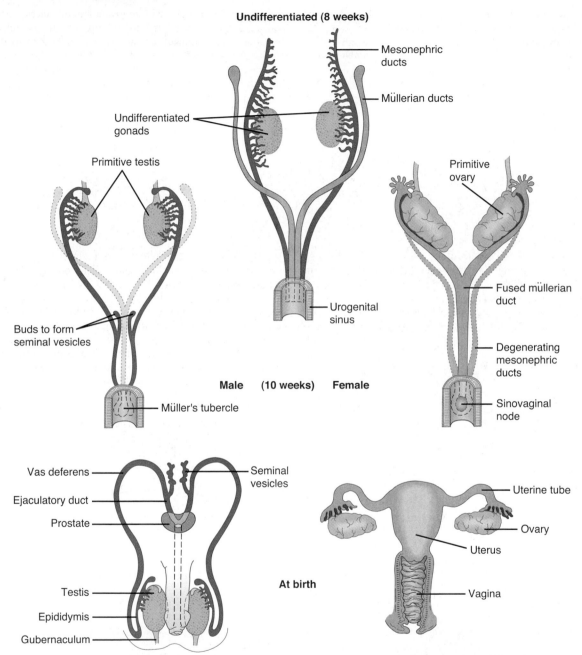

Undifferentiated (8 weeks)

Mesonephric ducts

Müllerian ducts

Undifferentiated gonads

Primitive testis

Primitive ovary

Fused müllerian duct

Buds to form seminal vesicles

Urogenital sinus

Degenerating mesonephric ducts

Male   (10 weeks)   Female

Müller's tubercle

Sinovaginal node

Vas deferens

Seminal vesicles

Ejaculatory duct

Prostate

Uterine tube

Ovary

Uterus

At birth

Testis

Epididymis

Vagina

Gubernaculum

▲ **Figure 38–3.** Transformation of the undifferentiated genital system into the definitive male and female systems.

is affected. The subsequent production of testosterone by the testicle leads to masculinization of the mesonephric (wolffian) duct structures (ie, epididymides, vas deferens, seminal vesicles, and ejaculatory duct). If the gonad develops into an ovary, it becomes differentiated into a cortex and a medulla; the cortex later differentiates into ovarian follicles containing ova. The lack of testosterone leads to the disappearance of the mesonephric duct.

The testes remain in the abdomen until the seventh month and then pass through the inguinal canal to the scrotum, following the path of the gubernaculum. The mechanism of descent remains uncertain. Lack of complete testicular descent is known as cryptorchidism; descent to an abnormal site beyond the external inguinal ring is known as testicular ectopia.

The ovary, which is attached to ligaments, undergoes internal descent to enter the pelvis.

In the female, the genital duct system develops from the müllerian ducts, which fuse at their caudal ends and differentiate into the uterine tubes, the uterus, and the proximal two thirds of the vagina.

The external genitalia start to differentiate by the eighth week. The genital tubercle and genital swellings develop into the penis and scrotum in the male and the clitoris and labia majora in the female. The external genitalia are masculinized by dihydrotestosterone (DHT), which is created from testosterone under the influence of 5α-reductase.

With the breakdown of the urogenital membrane in the seventh week, the urogenital sinus achieves a separate opening on the undersurface of the genital tubercle. The expansion of the infratubercular part of the urogenital sinus forms the vaginal vestibule and the distal third of the vagina. The two folds on the undersurface of the genital tubercle unite in the male to form the penile urethra; in the female, they remain separate to form the labia minora.

ANATOMY OF THE GENITOURINARY TRACT: GROSS & MICROSCOPIC

▶ The Kidneys

The kidneys lie retroperitoneally in the posterior abdomen and are separated from the surrounding renal fascia (Gerota's fascia) by perinephric fat. The renal vascular pedicle enters the renal sinus; the vein is anterior to the artery, and both are anterior to the renal pelvis. The renal artery divides just outside the renal sinus into anterior and posterior branches that undergo further subdivisions with variable extents of distribution. They are end arteries and thus result in segmental infarction when occluded. The venous tributaries anastomose freely and usually drain into one renal vein.

▶ The Renal Parenchyma

The renal parenchyma consists of more than 1 million functioning units (nephrons) and is divided into a peripheral cortex containing secretory elements and a central medulla containing excretory elements. The nephron starts as Bowman's capsule, which surrounds the glomerulus and leads to elongated proximal and distal convoluted tubules with the loop of Henle in between, ending in a collecting duct that opens into a minor calix at the tip of a papilla.

▶ The Renal Pelvis & Calices

The renal pelvis and calices are within the renal sinus and function as the main collecting reservoir. The pelvis, which is partly extrarenal and partly intrarenal (but occasionally is totally extrarenal or intrarenal), branches into three major calices that in turn branch into several minor calices. These calices are directly related to the tips of the medullary pyramids (the papillae) and act as a receiving cup to the collecting tubules. The pelvicaliceal system is a highly muscular structure; the fibers run in many directions and are directly continuous from the calices to the pelvis, allowing synchronization of contractile activity.

▶ The Ureter

The ureter connects the renal pelvis to the urinary bladder. It is a muscularized tube; its muscle fibers lie in an irregular helical arrangement and function primarily in peristaltic activity. Ureteral muscle fibers are directly continuous from the renal pelvis cranially to the vesical trigone distally.

The blood supply to the renal pelvis and ureters is segmental, arising from multiple sources, including the renal, gonadal, and vesical arteries, with rich subadventitial anastomoses.

▶ The Bladder

The bladder is primarily a reservoir with a meshwork of muscle bundles that not only change from one plane to another but also branch and join each other to constitute a synchronized organ. Its musculature is directly continuous with the urethral musculature and thus functions as an internal urethral sphincteric mechanism in spite of the lack of a true circular sphincter.

The ureters enter the bladder posteroinferiorly through the ureteral hiatus; after a short intravesical submucosal course, they open into the bladder and become continuous with the trigone, which is superimposed on the bladder base though deeply connected to it.

▶ The Urethra

The adult female urethra is about 4 cm long and is muscular in its proximal four fifths. This musculature is arranged in an inner longitudinal coat that is continuous with the inner longitudinal fibers of the bladder and an outer circular coat that is continuous with the outer longitudinal coat of the bladder. These outer circular fibers comprise the sphincteric mechanism. The striated external sphincter surrounds the middle third of the urethra.

In the male, the prostatic urethra is heavily muscular and sphincteric. The membranous urethra is within the urogenital diaphragm and is surrounded by the striated external sphincter. The penile urethra is poorly muscularized and traverses the corpus spongiosum to open at the tip of the glans.

▶ The Prostate

The prostate surrounds the proximal portion of the male urethra; it is a fibromuscular, cone-shaped gland about 2.5 cm long and normally weighing about 20 g in the adult. It is traversed from base to apex by the urethra and is pierced posterolaterally by the ejaculatory ducts from the seminal vesicles and vas deferens that converge to open at the verumontanum (seminal colliculus) on the floor of the urethra.

The prostatic glandular elements drain through about 12 paired excretory ducts that open into the floor of the urethra above the verumontanum. The prostate is surrounded by a thin capsule, derived from its stroma, which is rich in musculature, and part of the urethral musculature and the sphincteric mechanism. A rich venous plexus surrounds the prostate, especially anteriorly and laterally. Its lymphatic drainage is into the hypogastric, sacral, obturator, and external iliac lymph nodes.

▶ The Testis, Epididymis, & Vas

The testis is a paired organ surrounded by the tunica albuginea and subdivided into numerous lobules by fibrous septa. The extremely convoluted seminiferous tubules gather to open into the rete testis, where they join the efferent duct and drain into the epididymis. The epididymis drains into the vas deferens, which courses through the inguinal canal into the pelvis and is joined by the duct from the seminal vesicle to form the ejaculatory duct, which opens before opening into the prostatic urethra on either side of the verumontanum.

Arterial supply is via the spermatic, vas deferential, and external cremasteric arteries. Venous drainage is through the pampiniform plexus, which drains into the internal spermatic veins; the right spermatic vein joins the vena cava, and the left joins the renal vein.

Testicular lymphatics drain into the retroperitoneal lymph nodes; the right primarily into the interaortocaval area, the left into the para-aortic area, both just below the renal vessels.

PHYSIOLOGY OF THE GENITOURINARY TRACT

▶ The Kidneys

The kidneys maintain and regulate homeostasis of body fluids by glomerular filtration, tubular reabsorption, and tubular secretion.

A. Glomerular Filtration

This mechanism is dependent on glomerular capillary arterial pressure minus plasma colloid osmotic pressure plus Bowman's capsular resistance. The resultant glomerular filtration pressure (about 8–12 mm Hg) forces protein-free plasma through the capillary filtering surface into Bowman's capsule. Normally, about 130 mL of plasma is filtered every minute through the renal circulation; the entire volume of plasma recirculates through the kidney and is subjected to the filtration process once every 27 minutes.

B. Tubular Reabsorption

About 99% of the filtered volume is reabsorbed through the tubules, together with all the valuable constituents of the filtrate (chlorides, glucose, sodium, potassium, calcium, and amino acids). Urea, uric acid, phosphates, and sulfates are also reabsorbed to varying degrees. The process of reabsorption is a combination of active and passive transport mechanisms. Reabsorption of water and electrolytes is under the control of adrenal, pituitary, and parathyroid hormones.

C. Tubular Secretion

Tubular secretion helps (1) to eliminate certain substances and thus maintain their plasma levels and (2) to exchange valuable ions from the filtrate for less desirable ions in the plasma (eg, a sodium ion from the urine for a hydrogen ion in the plasma). Failure of adequate secretory function leads to the acidosis commonly encountered in chronic renal disease.

▶ The Ureteropelvicaliceal System

This system is one continuous tubular structure with a syncytial type of smooth musculature that is imperceptibly in motion from one segment to the other. Waves of peristaltic contractions start from the calices and are propagated along the smooth muscle cells to the renal pelvis. At normal urine flow rates, many of these contraction waves are terminated at the ureteropelvic junction; however, some are transmitted to the ureter and down toward the urinary bladder. These peristaltic waves occur at a rate of about 5–8/min, involve a 2-cm to 3-cm segment at a time, and usually proceed at the velocity of 3 cm/s. Frequency, amplitude, and velocity are influenced by urine output and flow rate. In a state of diuresis, there may be a 1:1 relationship between caliceal contractions and ureteral contractions. Ureteral filling is primarily passive and occurs by reception of a bolus of urine from a renal pelvis contraction. The ureteropelvic junction closes after passing a bolus of urine, preventing back-pressure and back-flow of urine into the renal pelvis secondary to the elevated ureteral contraction pressure. A contraction ring forms in the proximal ureter, and as it migrates down the ureter, it pushes the bolus of urine antegrade. In states of diuresis, the size of the bolus increases and the pressure in the bolus may be greater than the pressure in the contraction ring ahead of it. In this case, the ureteral walls cannot coapt, and urine is transported as an uninterrupted column of fluid.

▶ The Ureterovesical Junction

The ureterovesical junction allows flow of urine from the ureter to the bladder and at the same time prevents retrograde flow. The continuity and the specific muscular arrangement of the intravesical ureter and the trigone provide a muscularly active valvular mechanism that can efficiently adapt itself to the variable phases of bladder activity during filling and voiding.

The normal resting pressure of the ureterovesical junction (10–15 cm H_2O) is greater than the more cephalad ureteral resting pressure (0–5 cm H_2O). Progressive bladder filling leads to firm occlusion of the intravesical ureter against retrograde urine flow and to increased resistance to antegrade flow resulting from trigonal stretching. During voiding, trigonal contraction completely seals the intravesical ureter against any antegrade or retrograde flow of urine.

The Urinary Bladder

The urinary bladder functions primarily as a reservoir that can accommodate variable volumes without increasing its intraluminal pressure. When the bladder reaches full capacity, the detrusor muscle voluntarily contracts following relaxation of the external sphincter and maintains its contraction until the bladder is completely empty. Funneling of the bladder outlet with progressive downward movement of the dome ensures complete emptying.

The vesical sphincteric mechanism is primarily a smooth muscle sphincter in the bladder neck and male prostatic urethra and in the proximal four fifths of the female urethra. There is no purely circular sphincteric entity, but there are abundant circularly oriented smooth muscle fibers that are directly continuous with the outer coat of the detrusor muscles. The sphincter has an abundance of alpha receptors that respond to sympathetic neural input from the pelvic nerve to maintain urethral closure. Parasympathetic input from the pelvic nerve facilitates bladder contracture and voiding.

There is a voluntary striated muscle sphincter that is part of the urogenital diaphragm and surrounds the mid urethra in the female and the membranous urethra in the male. It responds to somatic neural input from the pudendal nerve. It is essential for continence when the internal sphincter is nonfunctional. Its pathologic irritability or spasticity can lead to obstructive manifestations.

DEVELOPMENTAL ANOMALIES OF THE GENITOURINARY TRACT

Genitourinary tract anomalies constitute about one third of all congenital abnormalities and occur in over 10% of the population. The severity varies from lesions incompatible with life to insignificant findings detected during diagnostic studies for unrelated reasons. The anatomic abnormalities are often not intrinsically harmful, yet they may predispose to infection, stone formation, or chronic renal failure.

RENAL ANOMALIES

Bilateral absence of the kidneys is rare and is associated with oligohydramnios, Potter facies, and pulmonary hypoplasia. It occurs more often in males and results in death shortly after birth. Unilateral renal agenesis is seen more often but is not usually associated with illness. **Renal agenesis** is thought to be due to both lack of a ureteral bud and lack of subsequent development of the metanephric blastema. The trigone is absent on the affected side. Because adrenal gland development is unrelated to kidney development, both adrenals are usually present in the normal position. Rarely, more than two kidneys are seen, a condition clearly dissimilar to ureteral duplication, as described later.

Abnormal ascent of the metanephros leads to an **ectopic kidney,** which may be unilateral or bilateral. Lumbar, pelvic, and the less common thoracic and crossed ectopic varieties are seen. Ectopic kidneys are associated with genital anomalies in 10–20% of cases. Fusion abnormalities are also associated with failure of normal ascent and include fused pelvic kidneys and **horseshoe kidneys** (the most common), which are typically fused at the lower poles. Intravenous urography typically establishes the diagnosis. The relationship of the kidneys to the psoas muscles is abnormal: Instead of an oblique orientation with the medial border of the kidney parallel to the psoas muscle, the kidneys are vertical and the medial border intersects and crosses the psoas muscle. Horseshoe kidneys have an elevated incidence of vesicoureteral reflux and are at increased risk of ureteropelvic junction obstruction. The latter may be related to a high ureteral insertion in the renal pelvis, crossing of the ureter over the isthmus, or compression by one of many anomalous arteries. Failure of rotation during ascent results in "malrotated" kidneys and is rarely significant.

Polycystic Kidneys

Parenchymal anomalies include a variety of cystic and dysplastic lesions. Polycystic kidney disease is hereditary and bilateral. The autosomal recessive polycystic kidney disease (ARPKD), previously called infantile PKD, has numerous small cysts that arise only from the collecting ducts and result in bilateral symmetrical enlargement of the kidneys. The autosomal dominant ADPKD, previously called adult PKD, has cysts arising from all areas of the nephron, which are usually larger and more variable in size than the ARPKD cysts. ARPKD occurs in 1 in 40,000 births and may be detected in utero by the presence of enlarged hyperechogenic kidneys and oligohydramnios. Infants usually die of respiratory failure rather than renal problems; however, the 1-year survival probability after the first month is over 85%. These children have declining renal function as well as severe hypertension and hepatic periportal fibrosis with portal hypertension leading to hypersplenism and esophageal varices.

The genes mutated in ADPKD may include the *PKD1* gene (located on chromosome 16p13.3) in 85% of patients or the *PKD2* gene (on chromosome 4q21-23) in 12% to 15% of patients. These genes code for the polycystin-1 and polycystin-2 proteins, respectively. ADPKD occurs in 1 in 1000 individuals and is a major cause of end-stage renal disease in adults. Cysts may also be present in the liver, pancreas, and spleen, and cerebral arterial aneurysms may occur. Renal cystic enlargement exerts pressure on normal parenchyma, leading to its gradual destruction and glomerulosclerosis.

The diagnosis is often made during a workup for hypertension or uremia discovered in the third to sixth decades.

Hematuria with or without flank pain is a common finding. An intravenous urogram reveals the enlarged kidneys, with marked elongation of the calices, which are compressed by large cysts. Ultrasonography or CT scan readily makes the diagnosis.

Surgery is rarely warranted. Therapy is medical and ultimately includes dialysis. The median age for reaching end-stage renal disease is 54 years in PKD1 and 74 years in PKD2. Renal transplantation is often indicated, though potential family donors must be carefully screened to determine whether they have the same disorder. The leading cause of death in ADPKD is cardiovascular disease, which may relate to early untreated hypertension.

Medullary Sponge Kidney

Medullary sponge kidney results from collecting tubular ectasia (see section on Polycystic Kidneys) and is associated with recurrent urolithiasis and an increased incidence of infection in 50% of patients. The lesion is often bilateral and may involve all of the calices. Intravenous urograms reveal dilated collecting tubules as a "blush" in the renal papilla. Microscopic hematuria is common. Specific antibiotics should be given for documented infections, and prophylactic therapy for renal stones should be recommended on the basis of metabolic stone evaluation.

Simple Renal Cysts

Simple renal cysts are common (approximately 50% after age 50) and are thought to arise from tubular dilation. They may be solitary or bilateral and multiple. They rarely have pathologic significance except in the differentiation from solid renal masses. (See the section on Renal Adenocarcinoma.)

Multicystic Dysplastic Kidney

Multicystic dysplastic kidney is a congenital abnormality consisting of macroscopic cysts of variable sizes compressing dysplastic renal parenchyma. It is usually associated with an atretic proximal ureter. The disorder occurs in about 1 in 3000 live births and is frequently noted on prenatal ultrasound. Rarely, it may occur bilaterally and is associated with oligohydramnios and renal failure. It may be distinguished from other causes of hydronephrosis by the absence of any renal function on renal scan. There is an increased incidence of contralateral ureteropelvic junction obstruction (5–10%) and reflux (18–43%), either of which increases the patient's risk of subsequent chronic renal insufficiency.

The chance of developing a malignancy in multicystic dysplastic kidney appears to be no greater than 1 in 2000. There may also be an increased incidence of hypertension. These two factors constitute a rationale for treatment by nephrectomy. However, conservative management with routine ultrasound examinations at intervals of 6 to 12 months is reasonable practice, since about half involute within 5 years.

Renal Vascular Abnormalities

Multiple renal arteries occur in 15% to 20% of patients and are significant only when they cause ureteropelvic junction obstruction. Congenital **renal artery aneurysms** are infrequent; they are differentiated from acquired lesions by their location at the bifurcation of the main renal artery or at a distal branch point. The lesions are usually asymptomatic, but they can cause hypertension. They require surgical treatment only if hypertension is uncontrolled, if they are incompletely calcified, or if they have a diameter of more than 2.5 cm. **Congenital arteriovenous fistulas** are rare but may result in hematuria, hypertension, or cardiac failure necessitating operative treatment.

Renal Pelvis Anomalies

Ureteropelvic junction obstruction is the most common cause of antenatal hydronephrosis. The condition may be associated with compression by anomalous renal arteries or intrinsic stenosis of the junction. The diagnosis is not uncommonly made when gross hematuria follows minor trauma. Renal ultrasound provides a safe screening technique in patients suspected of having ureteropelvic junction obstruction. Diuretic renal scan may confirm the diagnosis and suggest functional significance. Intravenous pyelogram or retrograde pyelography may further define the anatomy. Bilaterality is not uncommon, and the condition requires surgical repair if symptomatic or severe. Percutaneous incision of the obstruction with short-term stenting has been successful in adults. Symptoms include intermittent flank pain, particularly with orally induced diuresis.

Cooper CS et al: Antenatal hydronephrosis: evaluation and outcome. Curr Urol Rep 2002;3:131.
Hateboer N: Clinical management of polycystic kidney disease. Clin Med 2003;3:509.
Winyard P, Chitty L: Dysplastic and polycystic kidneys: diagnosis, associations and management. Prenat Diagn 2001;21:924.

URETERAL ANOMALIES

Congenital Obstruction of the Ureter

Congenital obstruction of the ureter may be due to ureterovesical and ureteropelvic junction obstruction or to neurologic deficits such as sacral agenesis or myelomeningocele. Functional ureteral obstruction—also known as **primary obstructive megaureter**—is not uncommon. Symptoms are renal pain during diuresis or resulting from pyelonephritis. Excretory urograms depict dilation above the obstruction. Vesicoureteral reflux is uncommonly associated with megaureter. Milder forms without symptoms or significant hydronephrosis are the rule and do not require treatment if renal function is normal. When treatment is necessary, it consists of division of the ureter proximal to the obstruction and reimplantation of the ureter into the bladder, often involving ureteral tapering or plication.

Duplication of Ureters

Bifurcation of the ureteral bud before it interacts with the metanephric blastema results in incomplete ureteral duplication, commonly in the mid or upper ureter. A second ureteral bud from the metanephric duct leads to complete ureteral duplication (Figure 38–4; right kidney) draining one kidney. This represents the most common ureteral anomaly, occurring in 1 in 125 people. It occurs twice as often in females. The presence of more than two ureters on each side is not common, but bilaterality of ureteral duplication occurs in 40%. Usually, all of the duplicated ureters enter the bladder; the ureter draining the upper pole of the kidney enters closest to the bladder neck (due to its later reabsorption into the bladder). Because of this relationship, the ureter draining the lower pole often has a short intramural tunnel and an inadequate surrounding musculature and is thus prone to vesicoureteral reflux. The ureter draining the upper pole may be ectopic (because of its late absorption) and thus empty into the bladder neck, urethra, or genital structures (vagina or vestibule in the female and seminal vesicle or vas deferens in the male [Figure 38–4; left kidney]). The ureter draining the upper pole is prone to obstruction and may be associated with a ureterocele, which is a common cause of obstruction. Duplication becomes significant when hydronephrosis or pyelonephritis occurs. The diagnosis is made by intravenous urography. Ureteral reimplantation to prevent recurrent infection is necessary in some cases. An anastomosis between the upper pole renal pelvis and the lower pole ureter or a low ureteroureterostomy are alternatives in selected cases. The upper pole of the kidney and its ureter may require removal if obstruction is severe and renal function of that segment is poor.

Ectopic Ureteral Orifice

Ureteral ectopia can occur in the absence of duplication and drain into any of the abnormal positions mentioned previously. If the orifice lies proximal to the external urinary sphincter, no incontinence ensues, but vesicoureteral reflux is common. In contradistinction to the female, the ectopic orifice in the male never lies distal to the external sphincter, making incontinence an extremely rare presentation. Should the ectopic orifice in the female drain into the vagina or at the vestibule, there may be continuous leakage of urine apart from voiding. Most ectopic orifices involve the ureter draining the upper pole of a duplicated system, and most are observed in females. Hydroureteronephrosis of the involved segment frequently occurs due to ureteral obstruction as it traverses the muscle of the bladder neck.

An ectopic orifice may be seen beside the urethral orifice or in the roof of the vagina on endoscopy. Renal ultrasound or intravenous urograms often demonstrates hydroureteronephrosis of the upper renal segment. Cystography may

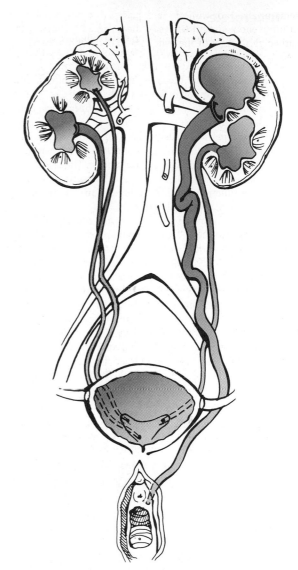

▲ **Figure 38–4.** Duplication of ureters and ectopic ureteral orifice. Complete duplication with obstruction to one ureter with ectopic orifice on left. The ureter with the ectopic opening always drains the upper pole of the kidney.

show reflux into the ectopic orifice but may require cyclic voiding first to decompress the obstructed segment with bladder neck relaxation and subsequently to permit reflux. In the rare case when there is significant upper pole renal function, the ureter can be divided and reimplanted into the bladder or lower pole ureter. Usually, however, heminephroureterectomy is necessary.

▶ Ureterocele

A ureterocele is a ballooning of the distal submucosal ureter into the bladder. This structure commonly has a pinpoint orifice and therefore leads to hydroureteronephrosis. If large enough, it may obstruct the vesical neck or the contralateral ureter. It is most common in females with ureteral duplication and always involves the ureter draining the upper renal pole.

Most ureteroceles are now detected by prenatal ultrasound. Symptoms are usually those of pyelonephritis or obstruction. Intravenous urograms may show a negative shadow in the bladder cast by the ureterocele. The ureter and renal calices may be normal or may reveal marked dilation or no excretory function at all. A cystogram may show reflux into the ipsilateral lower pole ureter.

Treatment of ureteroceles depends on multiple factors, including the presence or absence of reflux in any or all of the ureters as well as whether or not the ureterocele is completely contained within the bladder (intravesical/orthotopic) or if a portion is at the bladder neck or urethra (extravesical/ectopic). A simple method of establishing drainage involves cystoscopy and puncture of the ureterocele. Associated reflux, if present, can be managed with prophylactic antibiotics until the child has grown larger, at which time a technically easier ureteral reimplant may be performed with a decompressed ureter. In the relatively uncommon situation when there is no associated reflux, an upper pole heminephrectomy is considered. Minimally obstructive ureteroceles within the bladder in adults do not require treatment.

Cooper CS et al: Long-term follow-up of endoscopic incision of ureteroceles: intravesical versus extravesical. J Urol 2000; 164:1097.

Fretz PC et al: Long-term outcome analysis of Starr plication for primary obstructive megaureters. J Urol 2004;172:703.

VESICOURETERAL REFLUX

The main function of the ureterovesical junction is to permit free drainage of the ureter and simultaneously prevent urine from refluxing back from the bladder. Anatomically, the ureterovesical junction is well equipped for this function, because the ureteral musculature continues uninterrupted into the base of the bladder to form the superficial trigone. Additionally, the terminal 4 to 5 cm of ureter are surrounded by a musculofascial sheath (Waldeyer's sheath) that follows the ureter through the ureteral hiatus and continues in the base of the bladder as the deep trigone (Figure 38–5).

Direct continuity between the ureter and the trigone offers an efficient, muscularly active, valvular function. Any stretch of the trigone (with bladder filling) or any trigonal contraction (with voiding) leads to firm occlusion of the intravesical ureter, thus increasing resistance to flow from above downward and sealing the intravesical ureter against retrograde flow (Figure 38–6).

▶ Etiology & Classification

Vesicoureteral reflux may be classified as primary reflux due to developmental ureterotrigonal weakness or associated with ureteral anomalies such as ectopic orifice or ureterocele, and secondary reflux due to bladder outlet or urethral obstruction, neuropathic dysfunction, iatrogenic causes, and inflammation, especially specific infection (eg, tuberculosis). Primary reflux is associated with some degree of congenital muscular deficiency in the trigone and terminal ureter.

Reflux is associated with an increased incidence of pyelonephritis and renal damage. It also allows bacteria free access from the bladder to the kidney.

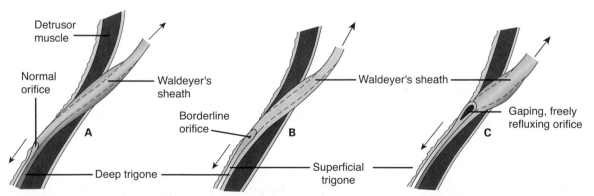

▲ **Figure 38–5.** Vesicoureteral reflux. The length and fixation of the intravesical ureter and the appearance of the ureteral orifice depend on the muscular development and efficiency of the lower ureter and its trigone. **A:** Normal structures. **B:** Moderate muscular deficiency. **C:** Marked deficiency results in a golf hole distortion of the submucosal ureter.

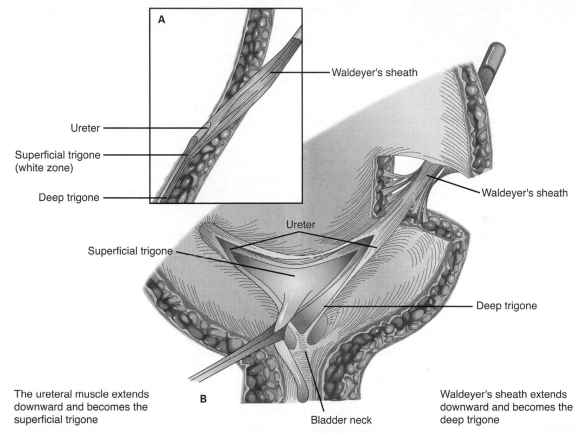

▲ **Figure 38–6.** Normal ureterotrigonal complex. **A:** Side view of ureterovesical junction. The Waldeyer muscular sheath invests the juxtavesical ureter and continues downward as the deep trigone, which extends to the bladder neck. The ureteral musculature becomes the superficial trigone, which extends to the verumontanum in the male and stops just short of the external meatus in the female. **B:** Waldeyer's sheath is connected by a few fibers to the detrusor muscle in the ureteral hiatus. This muscular sheath, inferior to the ureteral orifices, becomes the deep trigone. The musculature of the ureters continues downward as the superficial trigone. (Adapted from Tanagho EA, Pugh RCB: The anatomy and function of the ureterovesical junction. Br J Urol 1963:35;151. Reproduced with permission of Blackwell Publishing, Ltd.)

Reflux is the most common cause of pyelonephritis and is found in 30% to 50% of children presenting with urinary tract infection. It is present in over 75% of patients with radiologic evidence of chronic pyelonephritis and is responsible for end-stage renal disease in a large percentage of patients requiring chronic dialysis or renal transplantation.

In primary reflux, the child (on average, between 2 and 3 years of age) usually presents with symptoms of pyelonephritis or cystitis. Vague abdominal pain is not uncommon. Renal pain and pain with voiding are relatively uncommon. On rare occasions, the patient may present with advanced renal failure with bilateral renal parenchymal damage. Significant reflux and its sequelae are more common in females

and are usually detected after a urinary tract infection. About one third of the siblings of a child with reflux will also have reflux, and one half of the children of a mother with reflux will also have reflux.

In secondary reflux, manifestations of the primary disease (neuropathic, obstructive, etc) are usually the presenting symptoms.

▶ **Clinical Findings**

A. Symptoms and Signs

With acute pyelonephritis, fever, chills, and costovertebral angle tenderness may be present. Children usually do not have renal pain but may complain of vague abdominal pain. Occasionally, daytime frequency, incontinence, or enuresis may be caused by infection associated with reflux. In cases of obstruction or neuropathic deficit, a palpable hydronephrotic kidney or a distended bladder may be found. The diagnosis may be elusive in infants who present with ill-defined symptoms.

B. Laboratory Findings

Urinalysis usually reveals evidence of infection (pyuria and bacteriuria). Urine cultures are mandatory when infection is suspected. Renal function tests may be abnormal if reflux and infection have caused renal scarring.

C. Imaging Studies

The most useful study for conclusive diagnosis of reflux continues to be voiding cystourethrography (Figure 38–7). This study demonstrates the grade of reflux as well as the urethral anatomy. Radionuclide voiding studies are extremely sensitive at detecting reflux but do not demonstrate the anatomic detail seen with a voiding cystourethrogram. Radionuclide voiding studies are often performed as follow-up after an initial voiding cystourethrogram because they offer the advantage of decreased radiation exposure.

Radioisotopic renal scanning provides accurate differential renal function data and detection of renal scars. Ultrasound can provide accurate measurement of renal size and may demonstrate the presence of renal scarring and ureteral or caliceal dilation. In many cases, there may be no abnormality visible in the upper urinary tract, or only mild distal ureteral dilatation may be seen.

D. Urodynamic Considerations

A significant number of children with dysfunctional voiding present with urinary tract infections and are subsequently found to have reflux. These children contract the bladder against a closed external sphincter. Elevated voiding pressures associated with dysfunctional voiding may increase renal damage with an associated urinary tract infection and may also lessen the chance for either spontaneous or surgical resolution of reflux. When the history suggests the possibility of voiding dysfunction (incontinence, frequency, urgency), urodynamic studies are conducted to evaluate the voiding dynamics. Treatment of voiding dysfunction may result in resolution of the reflux.

▶ Treatment

Although some children with lower grades of reflux may not require antibiotics, traditionally any child with reflux was maintained on prophylactic antibiotics to attempt to decrease the incidence of urinary tract infections. Several recent studies suggest that the practice of daily antibiotic prophylaxis in all children with reflux may be of limited benefit in preventing urinary tract infection. Prompt treatment of pyelonephritis prevents renal scar formation. Factors causing secondary reflux—such as dysfunctional voiding or obstruction—should be corrected.

In many children, reflux resolves with time. Reflux is graded as seen on voiding cystourethrography as follows:

Grade I: Contrast enters ureter

Grade II: Contrast enters the renal collecting system

Grade III: Slight dilation of the calices or ureter

Grades IV and V: Progressively increased amounts of caliceal dilation and ureteral dilation or tortuosity

Reflux most likely to resolve is of lower grade or detected at a younger age. Over 70% of children with grades I, II, or unilateral grade III reflux will have resolution within 5 years. Resolution in children with grade V or bilateral grade IV reflux can be anticipated in less than 10% of cases. Other factors that appear to negatively affect the chance for reflux resolution include early reflux during bladder filling, presentation with a febrile urinary tract infection, renal scars, and voiding dysfunction.

In obstructive secondary reflux (eg, posterior urethral valves), release of obstruction may cure reflux. Occasionally, surgical reimplantation is still required. In neuropathic reflux, intermittent catheterization for control of infection may allow return of valvular competence. However, many cases require bladder augmentation for a noncompliant bladder and ureteral reimplantation. In reflux associated with ectopic orifices,

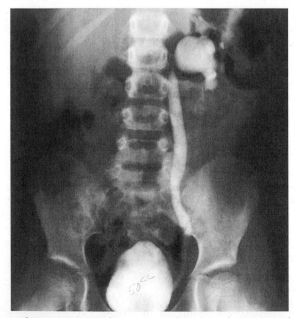

▲ **Figure 38–7.** Voiding cystourethrogram showing total (grade IV) left vesicoureteral reflux.

duplication with ureterocele, and other congenital malformations, reimplantation is generally required.

The aim of surgery is to correct the reflux. This is accomplished by the creation of a longer submucosal tunnel for the ureter. With bladder filling and increased pressure, the ureter is compressed between the mucosa and underlying detrusor muscle. This flap valve prevents reflux of urine. The necessary length of the tunnel to stop reflux depends on the diameter of the ureter, with a 5:1 length-to-diameter ratio being ideal. One of three methods is used in most cases: (1) In suprahiatal repair (Politano-Leadbetter procedure), a new ureteral hiatus is developed about 2.5 cm above the original one, and the ureter—after passing through a submucosal tunnel—is sutured to the cut edge of the trigone at the level of the original orifice. (2) In the cross-trigonal repair (Cohen procedure), the original hiatus is maintained, and the ureter is advanced through a submucosal tunnel, extending across the trigone to the contralateral bladder wall. (3) A totally extravesical ureteral advancement procedure (extravesical ureteroplasty) achieves results similar to those achieved with the intravesical methods, with a shorter hospital stay and shorter convalescence.

Injections of subureteric bulking agents have also been used to increase submucosal support of the ureter. With proper placement beneath the ureteral orifice under endoscopic vision, these injections act to bolster the deficient antireflux mechanism. Concern regarding late sequelae of Teflon injections (eg, particle migration) has prevented use of this approach in the United States. Currently, hyaluronic acid/dextranomer (NASHA/Dx) gel (Deflux) is the only FDA-approved material for endoscopic injection to manage vesicoureteral reflux in children. Short-term success in stopping reflux with the injection techniques appears to be around 75%. The long-term success rates with agents other than Teflon remain to be determined.

▶ Prognosis

The long-term prognosis is excellent for patients with mild to moderate reflux successfully treated with antibiotic prophylaxis. There are few instances of recurrent infection or renal insufficiency. Patients with more significant reflux or persistent urinary tract infections may benefit from subureteric injection or surgical reimplantation; the success rate is approximately 95% with the open surgical technique (cessation of reflux, clearance of renal infection, and absence of obstruction). Unfortunately, for patients with advanced disease (irreversible ureteral decompensation and severe bilateral scars), the prognosis is less favorable. These patients account for a significant proportion of patients with end-stage renal disease who ultimately require chronic dialysis, renal transplantation, or both.

Austin JC, Cooper CS: Vesicoureteral reflux: surgical approaches. Urol Clin North Am 2004;31:543.

Cooper CS, Austin JC: Vesicoureteral reflux: who benefits from surgery? Urol Clin North Am 2004;31:535.

Cooper CS et al: The outcome of stopping prophylactic antibiotics in older children with vesicoureteral reflux. J Urol 2000; 163:269.

Elder JS et al: Pediatric Vesicoureteral Reflux Guidelines Panel summary report on the management of primary vesicoureteral reflux in children. J Urol 1997;157:1846.

Garin EH et al: Clinical significance of primary vesicoureteral reflux and urinary antibiotic prophylaxis after acute pyelonephritis: a multicenter, randomized, controlled study. Pediatrics 2006;117:626.

Jodal U et al: Infection pattern in children with vesicoureteral reflux randomly allocated to operation or long-term antibacterial prophylaxis: the international reflux study in children. J Urol 1992;148:1650.

Knudson MJ et al: Predictive factors of early spontaneous resolution in children with vesicoureteral reflux. J Urol 2007; 178:1684.

BLADDER ANOMALIES

Anomalies of the bladder are infrequent and include the following: (1) **agenesis,** or complete absence, which results in a persistent cloaca; (2) bladder **duplication,** which may be complete, with separate ureteral openings drained by duplicated urethras, or incomplete, with a septum or hourglass deformity; and (3) **urachal anomalies,** which in the most severe forms appear as a patent opening at the umbilicus and are usually associated with some form of bladder outlet obstruction. In less severe forms, a **urachal diverticulum** may be present at the dome of the bladder or a **urachal cyst** along the course of the partially obliterated urachus. These latter conditions may cause abdominal pain and umbilical or bladder infection requiring surgical treatment. Occasionally, adenocarcinoma develops in a urachal remnant (see section on Tumors of the Bladder).

Failure of cloacal division results in a persistent cloaca. Incomplete division is more frequent (though still rare) and results in a rectovesical, rectourethral, or rectovestibular fistula (usually with imperforate anus or anal atresia).

▶ Exstrophy of the Bladder

Exstrophy of the bladder is the most severe bladder anomaly—the result of a complete ventral defect of the urogenital sinus and the overlying inferior abdominal wall musculature and integument. The lower central portion is devoid of skin and muscle. The anterior bladder wall is absent, and the posterior wall is contiguous with surrounding skin. Urine drains onto the abdominal wall, the rami of the pubic bones are widely separated, and the open pelvic ring may affect gait. In males, the penis is shortened and the urethra is epispadiac. The exposed bladder mucosa tends to be chronically inflamed.

Currently, the favored treatment is bladder salvage, which includes closure of the bladder in the newborn period. Urethral closure and penile reconstruction have also been advocated at the time of the initial bladder closure.

Ureteral obstruction or vesicoureteral reflux may develop and require ureteral reimplantation. The closed bladder may have a small capacity, and incontinence is often a complication. Patients frequently require multiple operations, including bladder augmentation and bladder neck reconstruction. Good results have been observed in more than half of all patients treated, with preservation of renal function and continence.

Cooper CS et al: Pediatric reconstructive surgery. Curr Opin Urol 2000;10:195.

Prune Belly Syndrome

Prune belly syndrome consists of a triad of abnormalities: deficient abdominal wall musculature, bilateral cryptorchidism, and variable amounts of dilation of the urogenital tract. The cause is not known. Almost all children with prune belly syndrome have reflux. The incidence of eventual renal failure is 25% to 30%. Risk factors for renal failure include bilateral abnormal kidneys on ultrasound or renal scan, a serum creatinine that never falls below 0.7 mg/dL, and clinical pyelonephritis. These children are managed with prophylactic antibiotics and frequent urine cultures, followed by prompt treatment of any urinary tract infections. Abdominoplasty may be performed to help correct the abdominal wall defect.

Noh PH et al: Prognostic factors of renal failure in children with prune belly syndrome. J Urol 1999;162:1399.

Congenital Neurovesical Dysfunction

Congenital neurovesical dysfunction frequently accompanies a posterior myelomeningocele or sacral agenesis, with associated spinal abnormalities. Both conditions may result in incontinence and recurrent urinary infection with late sequelae (ureteral reflux, pyelonephritis, and renal failure). These children require frequent evaluation of their kidneys and kidney function because high bladder storage pressures may harm the kidneys.

PENILE & URETHRAL ANOMALIES

Hypospadias

Hypospadias results from failure of fusion of the urethral folds on the undersurface of the genital tubercle. The urethral meatus is ventrally displaced on the glans on the shaft of the penis or more proximal at the level of the scrotum or perineum. With more proximal displacement, chordee (ventral curvature of the penile shaft) frequently occurs and requires treatment, or it precludes straight erections and normal intercourse (Figure 38–8). The midscrotal hypospadiac penis may resemble female external genitalia with an enlarged clitoris and labia. Sexual assignment in these latter infants requires hormonal and chromosomal analysis.

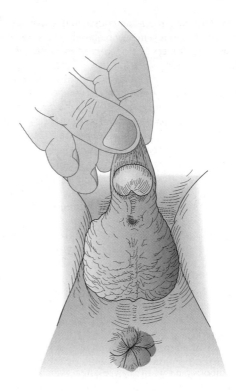

▲ **Figure 38–8.** Hypospadias, penoscrotal type. Redundant dorsal foreskin that is deficient ventrally; ventral chordee.

In hypospadias with the meatus positioned proximal to the corona, the prepuce is abnormal—not forming a complete cylinder due to a ventral defect. Circumcision should not be done in these patients, as the prepuce can be used later in surgical repair.

The degree of hypospadias dictates the need for repair. If the opening is glandular or coronal (85% of patients), the penis is usually functional both for micturition and procreation, and repair is done primarily for cosmetic reasons. Openings that are more proximal on the shaft require correction to allow voiding while standing, normal erection, and proper sperm deposition during intercourse. Surgical plastic repair of hypospadias is currently accomplished by a variety of highly successful one-stage operations and is routinely performed between 6 and 18 months of age. The most common complications of hypospadias surgery include meatal stenosis and fistula formation; however, improved techniques have decreased the incidence of these complications.

Epispadias

Epispadias is a rare congenital anomaly that is commonly associated with bladder exstrophy. When it occurs alone, it is considered a milder degree of the exstrophy complex.

The urethra opens on the dorsum of the penis, with deficient corpus spongiosum and loosely attached corpora cavernosa. If the defect is extensive, it may extend to the bladder neck, causing incontinence because of deficient sphincter muscles. The pubic bones are separated, as in exstrophy. Marked dorsiflexion of the penis is usually present.

Treatment consists of correction of penile curvature, reconstruction of the urethra, and reconstruction of the bladder neck in incontinent patients.

▶ Urethral Strictures

Congenital urethral strictures are rare but when present are most common in the fossa navicularis (just proximal to the meatus) and in the bulbomembranous urethra. Commonly, these strictures are thin diaphragms that may respond to simple dilation or to direct vision internal urethrotomy. Rarely is open surgical repair necessary. Congenital urethral strictures in girls and meatal stenosis in boys are uncommon. When the latter does occur, it appears to be acquired, as it is seen only in circumcised boys.

▶ Urethral Diverticulum

In males, urethral diverticula are nearly always in the pendulous or bulbous urethra. They are often associated with an obstructive flap of the urethral mucosa (anterior urethral valve), thought to represent incomplete closure of the urethral folds. Treatment by endoscopic unroofing is usually successful, though most diverticula are small and require no therapy. In females, they occur in adult life and are usually manifested by irritative symptoms and recurrent infection. The cause is unknown, but the disorder is most likely congenital. Treatment is usually by transvaginal excision. Diverticula may occasionally harbor stones or tumors.

▶ Posterior Urethral Valves

Posterior urethral valves are the most common obstructive urethral lesion in newborn and infant males and the most common cause of end-stage renal disease in boys. They consist of obstructive folds of mucosa, which originate at or are attached at some point to the verumontanum in the prostatic urethra. The embryologic derivation is indefinite. They are partially obstructive and thus lead to variable degrees of back-pressure damage to the urinary bladder and upper urinary tract. Dilation and obstruction of the prostatic urethra are always present. Spontaneous urinary ascites from the kidneys is often seen in neonates. This clears when the obstruction is relieved.

About one third of children with posterior urethral valves are now diagnosed by prenatal ultrasound. Another one third are diagnosed in the first year of life, with the remaining third presenting later. Clinical manifestations consist of difficult voiding, a weak urinary stream, and a midline lower abdominal mass that represents a distended bladder. In some cases, the kidneys are palpable and the child may have signs and symptoms of uremia and acidosis. Urinary incontinence and urinary tract infection may occur. Laboratory findings include elevated serum urea nitrogen and creatinine and evidence of urinary infection. Ultrasound shows evidence of bladder thickening and trabeculation, hydroureter, and hydronephrosis. Demonstration of urethral valves on a voiding cystourethrogram establishes the diagnosis, as does endoscopic identification of valves. Up to 70% of children with valves may have vesicoureteral reflux.

Treatment consists of destruction of the valves by endoscopic incision. In a premature infant with a small urethra prohibiting transurethral resection, a temporary cutaneous vesicostomy may be required to provide drainage and improve impaired kidney function.

The prognosis depends on the original degree of kidney damage and the success of efforts to prevent or treat infection. Rates of chronic renal failure or end-stage renal disease range from 25% to 67% of boys with valves. Poor prognostic factors include the presence of bilateral reflux or an elevated nadir serum creatinine in the first year of life. Many of these children have delayed development of urinary continence due to bladder changes and impaired urinary concentration.

Grady RW et al: Complete repair of exstrophy. J Urol 1999; 162:1415.

Snodgrass W: Snodgrass technique for hypospadias repair. Br J Urol (Int) 2005;95:683.

Ylinen E, Ala-Houhala M, Wikström S: Prognostic factors of posterior urethral valves and the role of antenatal detection. Pediatr Nephrol 2004;20:874.

SCROTAL & TESTICULAR ANOMALIES

▶ Testicular Torsion

Neonatal testicular torsion (extravaginal torsion) is an extremely rare condition. The entire testicle and the tunica vaginalis are twisted. No trigger mechanism associated with the torsion has been identified. Although the vast majority are necrotic and nonsalvageable, several studies have reported salvage of testicular tissue when torsion is detected immediately following birth. Any scrotal swelling in the neonate requires close follow-up. Intravaginal testicular torsion in adolescents is described later in this chapter.

Cooper CS et al: Bilateral neonatal testicular torsion. Clin Pediatr 1997;36:653.

▶ Scrotal Lesions

Congenital scrotal lesions include hypoplasia of the scrotum (unilateral or bilateral) in association with cryptorchidism and bifid scrotum with extensive hypospadias. Midline inclusion cysts may also occur.

CRYPTORCHIDISM

Etiology & Classification

True undescended testicles stop along the normal path of descent into the scrotum. They may remain in the abdominal cavity (least common), in the inguinal canal (canalicular), or just outside the external ring (suprascrotal, most common). Testes may also pass through the external ring and then be located ectopically, most commonly in a superficial inguinal pouch. The incidence of undescended testicles increases from 3% to 5% in full-term infants to 30% in premature infants. Most undescended testicles descend within the first 6 months of life, and by 1 year of age the prevalence is 1%. The left testicle is affected more often, and 1% to 2% of children with cryptorchidism will have both testicles affected. Twenty percent of boys who present with cryptorchidism have one nonpalpable testis. Of nonpalpable testes, 20% are intra-abdominal; 40% are canalicular, scrotal, or ectopic testes; and 40% are atrophic or absent.

Clinical Findings

The diagnosis of cryptorchidism relies on physical examination. Absence of an identifiable testicle with ultrasound, computed tomography, or magnetic resonance imaging does not prove testicular agenesis and therefore does not alter the need for surgical exploration. Testicular examination in the infant and young child requires two hands, with the first hand being swept from the anterior iliac spine along the inguinal canal to gently express any retained testicular tissue into the scrotum, which is palpated with the other hand. A true undescended or ectopic inguinal testis may slip or "pop" under the examiner's fingers. To distinguish a retractile testicle, the testicle is brought into the scrotal position, holding it in place for a minute to fatigue the cremaster muscle. After this, a retractile testicle remains in the scrotum, whereas an ectopic or undescended testis immediately snaps back out of the scrotum. If a testis cannot be palpated in the inguinal canal or the scrotum, or in the typical ectopic sites, evaluation for a nonpalpable testis must be performed.

A child with bilateral nonpalpable testes should undergo hormonal evaluation for testicular absence. Elevations in luteinizing hormone (LH) and follicle-stimulating hormone (FSH) and absence of detectable müllerian-inhibiting substance suggest testicular absence. Testicular absence is confirmed by a negative human chorionic gonadotropin (hCG) stimulation test. The hCG stimulation test is performed by the administration of intramuscular hCG (2000 IU/day for 3–4 days). Raised gonadotropin levels (FSH and LH) *and* a lack of a testosterone rise from hCG indicate bilateral absent testes, and a formal surgical exploration is unnecessary. When one or both components are lacking or there is detectable müllerian-inhibiting substance, surgical exploration is warranted.

Surgical Therapy

Treatment of the undescended testicle offers the possibility of improved fertility, correction of patent processus vaginalis, prevention of testis torsion, and improvement in body image. There is controversy whether orchidopexy decreases the risk of malignancy, but placement of an undescended testicle in the scrotum assists physical examination of the testis. Histologic changes related to infertility occur in the undescended testicle as young as 1 year of age, and spontaneous descent rarely occurs after 6 months of age, making this the optimal time for surgical correction.

Almost 90% of undescended testes have an associated patent processus vaginalis, which predisposes to formation of a hydrocele or hernia. Occult inguinal hernia in patients with untreated undescended testis can present at any time with the typical symptoms or complications, including incarceration.

Prior to any surgical intervention, the patient is reexamined while under anesthesia because on occasion a retractile testicle descends under anesthesia or a previously nonpalpable testicle becomes palpable. For a palpable testicle, an open inguinal approach is performed. For the nonpalpable testicle in a child, a laparoscopic approach is preferred, but an open inguinal approach may be performed.

Outcomes

Success rates following orchidopexy are 74% for the abdominal testis, 87% for canalicular, and 92% for those distal to the external ring. The most significant complication is testicular atrophy, which occurs in 1% to 2% of cases of orchidopexy, while complete devascularization of the testis is rare. Paternity rates have been reported at 65%, 90%, and 93% in men with bilateral cryptorchidism, unilateral cryptorchidism, and normally descended testicles, respectively. If only one testis is undescended, the sperm count is subnormal in 25% to 33% patients, and serum FSH concentration is slightly elevated. These abnormalities suggest that both testes are abnormal, perhaps congenitally, although only one fails to descend. If both testes are undescended, sperm count usually is severely subnormal, and serum testosterone may be reduced.

Alternative Therapy

Hormonal therapy is an option in the treatment of cryptorchidism because the condition may be related to hypogonadotropic hypogonadism. hCG is the only hormone approved for use in the treatment of cryptorchidism in the United States. Side effects of hCG treatment include enlargement of the penis, growth of pubic hair, increased testicular size, and aggressive behavior during administration. The likelihood of success with hormonal therapy is greatest for the most distal undescended testes or for testes that have been previously descended. Some suggest that hormonal therapy is effective only for retractile and not truly undescended testes. Although hormonal therapy may not be effective in achieving testicular descent, it may improve fertility in cryptorchid boys.

Hutcheson JC et al: The anatomical approach to inguinal orchiopexy. J Urol 2000;164:1702.

Lee MM et al: Measurements of serum müllerian inhibiting substance in the evaluation of children with nonpalpable gonads. N Engl J Med 1997;336:1480.

Lee PA et al: Fertility after bilateral cryptorchidism. Evaluation by paternity, hormone, and semen data. Hormone Res 2001;55:28.

ACQUIRED LESIONS OF THE GENITOURINARY TRACT

OBSTRUCTIVE UROPATHY

Obstruction is one of the most important abnormalities of the urinary tract, since it eventually leads to decompensation of the muscular conduits and reservoirs, back-pressure, and atrophy of renal parenchyma. It also invites infection and stone formation, which cause additional damage and can ultimately end in complete unilateral or bilateral destruction of the kidneys.

Both the level and the degree of obstruction are important to an understanding of the pathologic consequences. Any obstruction at or distal to the bladder neck may lead to back-pressure affecting both kidneys. Obstruction at or proximal to the ureteral orifice leads to unilateral damage unless the lesion involves both ureters simultaneously. Complete obstruction leads to rapid decompensation of the system proximal to the site of obstruction. Partial obstruction leads to gradual progressive muscular hypertrophy followed by dilation, decompensation, and hydronephrotic changes.

▶ Etiology

Acquired urinary tract obstruction may be due to inflammatory or traumatic urethral strictures, bladder outlet obstruction (benign prostatic hyperplasia or cancer of the prostate), vesical tumors, neuropathic bladder, extrinsic ureteral compression (tumor, retroperitoneal fibrosis, or enlarged lymph nodes), ureteral or pelvic stones, ureteral strictures, or ureteral or pelvic tumors.

▶ Pathogenesis

Regardless of its cause, acquired obstruction leads to similar changes in the urinary tract, which vary depending on the severity and duration of obstruction.

A. Urethral Changes

Proximal to the obstruction, the urethra dilates and balloons. A urethral diverticulum may develop, and dilation and gaping of the prostatic urethra and ejaculatory ducts may occur.

B. Vesical Changes

Early detrusor and trigonal thickening and hypertrophy compensate for the outlet obstruction, allowing complete bladder emptying. This change leads to progressive development of bladder trabeculation, cellules, saccules, and, finally, diverticula. Subsequently, bladder decompensation occurs and is characterized by the above changes plus incomplete bladder emptying (ie, postvoid residual urine). Trigonal hypertrophy leads to secondary ureteral obstruction owing to increased resistance to flow through the intravesical ureter. With detrusor decompensation and residual urine accumulation, there is stretching of the hypertrophied trigone, which appreciably increases ureteral obstruction. This is the mechanism of back-pressure on the kidney in the presence of vesical outlet obstruction (while the ureterovesical junction maintains its competence). Catheter drainage of the bladder relieves trigonal stretch and improves drainage from the upper tract.

A very late change with persistent obstruction (more frequently encountered with neuropathic dysfunction) is decompensation of the ureterovesical junction, leading to reflux. Reflux aggravates the back-pressure effect on the upper tract by transmitting abnormally high intravesical pressures and favors the onset or persistence of urinary tract infection.

C. Ureteral Changes

The first change noted is a gradual increase in ureteral distention. This increases ureteral caliber and stimulates hyperactive ureteral contraction and ureteral muscular hypertrophy. Because the ureteral musculature runs in an irregular helical pattern, stretching of its muscular elements leads to lengthening as well as widening, causing the dilated ureter to assume a tortuous, serpiginous course, weaving back and forth across the relatively straight course of the ureteral vessels, which are unaffected by the ureteral obstruction. This is the start of ureteral decompensation, where tortuosity and dilation become apparent. These changes progress until the ureter becomes atonic, with infrequent, ineffective, or completely absent peristalsis.

D. Pelvicaliceal Changes

The renal pelvis and calices, subjected to increased volumes of retained urine, distend. The pelvis shows evidence first of hyperactivity and hypertrophy and then of progressive dilation and atony. The calices show similar changes to a variable degree, depending on whether the renal pelvis is intrarenal or extrarenal. In the latter, caliceal dilation may be minimal in spite of marked pelvic dilation. In the intrarenal pelvis, caliceal dilation and renal parenchymal damage are maximal. The successive phases seen with obstruction are rounding of the fornices, followed by flattening of the papillae and finally clubbing of the minor calices.

E. Renal Parenchymal Changes

With continued pelvicaliceal distention, there is parenchymal compression against the renal capsule and, more importantly, compression of the arcuate vessels results in a marked drop in renal blood flow leading to parenchymal ischemic atrophy. With increased intrapelvic pressure, there is progressive dilation of the collecting and distal tubules, with compression and atrophy of tubular cells.

Clinical Findings

A. Symptoms and Signs

The findings vary according to the site of obstruction.

1. Infravesical obstruction—Infravesical obstruction (eg, due to urethral stricture, benign prostatic hypertrophy, bladder neck contracture) leads to difficulty in initiation of voiding, a weak stream, and a diminished flow rate with terminal dribbling. Burning and frequency are common associated symptoms. A distended or thickened bladder wall may be palpable. Urethral induration due to stricture, benign prostatic hypertrophy, or cancer of the prostate may be noted on rectal examination. Meatal stenosis and impacted urethral stones are readily diagnosed by physical examination.

2. Supravesical obstruction—Renal pain or renal colic and gastrointestinal symptoms are commonly associated. Supravesical obstruction (eg, due to ureteral stone, ureteropelvic junction obstruction) may be completely asymptomatic when it develops gradually over a period of months. An enlarged kidney may be palpable. Costovertebral angle tenderness may be present.

B. Laboratory Findings

Evidence of urinary tract infection, hematuria, or crystalluria may be seen. Impaired renal function may be noted in cases of bilateral obstruction. Postrenal azotemia (serum changes reflecting impaired renal function due primarily to obstruction) is suggested by elevation of serum urea nitrogen and serum creatinine with a ratio greater than 10:1.

C. Imaging Studies

Radiologic examination is usually diagnostic in cases of stasis, tumors, and strictures. Dilation and anatomic changes occur above the level of obstruction, whereas distal to the obstruction, the configuration is usually normal. This helps in localizing the site of obstruction. Combined antegrade imaging by intravenous urograms and retrograde imaging by ureterograms or urethrograms is sometimes needed to demonstrate the obstructed segment. In supravesical obstruction, demonstration of stasis and delayed drainage is essential to establish and quantitate the severity of obstruction.

1. Ultrasonography—Ultrasonography reveals the degree of dilation of the renal pelvis and calices and allows for diagnosis of hydronephrosis even in the prenatal period. Color Doppler ultrasound can reveal blood flow and restrictive indices to help determine functional impairment.

2. Isotope studies—A technetium-99m DTPA scan or MAG-3 scan portray the degree of hydronephrosis as well as

renal function. Use of diuretics during the scan can provide specific data on the significance of the obstruction and the need for treatment. Multiple studies can reveal ongoing functional changes.

3. CT scan—CT scan is of particular value in revealing the degree and site of obstruction as well as the cause in many cases. The use of contrast (CT urogram) agents allows estimation of residual renal function.

4. MR urogram—Magnetic resonance imaging provides anatomic images and identification of the site of obstruction. With dynamic contrast-enhanced MR urography, functional information is also obtained without the use of ionizing radiation.

5. Antegrade urography—Antegrade urography via percutaneous needle or tube nephrostomy is valuable when the obstructed kidney fails to excrete the radiopaque material on excretory urography. The Whitaker test requires percutaneous catheter access to the collecting system above the site of suspected obstruction. This permits fluid introduction into the renal pelvis and simultaneous measurement of urine flow rate and pressures in the bladder and renal pelvis, thus providing a quantitative assessment of the degree and severity of obstruction. The fluid transport can be measured and the degree of obstruction estimated by the use of a pressure monitor.

Complications

The most important complication of urinary tract obstruction is renal parenchymal atrophy as a result of backpressure. Obstruction also predisposes to infection and stone formation, and infection occurring with obstruction leads to rapid kidney destruction.

Treatment

The first goal of therapy is relief of the obstruction (eg, catheterization for relief of acute urinary retention). Definitive therapy often requires surgery, but minimally invasive techniques are becoming utilized more often. Simple urethral stricture may be managed by dilation or internal urethrotomy (incision of the stricture under direct vision through the resectoscope). However, urethroplasty (open surgical graft or flap of skin or buccal mucosa to replace urethral diameter) may be required and have better long-term success. Benign prostatic hyperplasia classically requires excision, but laser techniques are providing satisfactory outcomes with less morbidity. Impacted ureteral stones may either be removed or bypassed by a catheter unless it is thought that they may pass spontaneously.

Ureteral or ureteropelvic junction obstruction requires surgical repair; however, endoscopic approaches within the ureter or by laparoscopy may be equal to open repair. Renal stones may be removed instrumentally via retrograde or antegrade percutaneous approach by direct extraction with baskets or by ultrasonic or laser lithotripsy or by irrigation through a tube placed directly into the kidney.

Preliminary drainage above the obstruction is sometimes needed to improve kidney function. Occasionally, intestinal urinary diversion or permanent nephrostomy is required. If damage is advanced, nephrectomy may be indicated.

▶ Prognosis

The prognosis depends on the cause, site, duration, and degree of kidney damage and renal decompensation. In general, relief of obstruction leads to improvement in kidney function except in seriously damaged kidneys, especially those destroyed by inflammatory scarring.

Grattan-Smith JD et al: MR imaging of kidneys: functional evaluation using F-15 perfusion imaging. Pediatr Radiol 2003; 33:293.
Padmanabhan P, Nitti VW: Primary bladder neck obstruction in men, women, and children. Curr Urol Rep 2007;8:379.

URETEROPELVIC JUNCTION OBSTRUCTION

Stenosis of the renal pelvis outlet is commonly due to congenital narrowing of the junction or compression by anomalous vessels. However, the lesion may be acquired. Presentation in adults often includes the abrupt onset of flank pain usually following ingestion of large amounts of fluids. Presentation in childhood is now most often made following the diagnosis of hydronephrosis by prenatal ultrasonography.

The diagnosis may be confirmed with a diuretic nuclear renal scan or intravenous urography, which reveals hydronephrosis with a dilated renal pelvis and slow drainage of either radiotracer or contrast medium. Occasionally, patients present with intermittent hydronephrosis and normal urograms, except during attacks of pain, when x-rays show typical obstruction. These patients generally have normal renal parenchyma. Retrograde ureteropyelography is usually needed in patients with chronic moderate to severe obstruction to determine the extent of the lesion and to provide assurance that the distal ureter is normal. Marked obstruction may make it difficult to determine whether kidney function is surgically salvageable. In these cases, it may be necessary to perform either (1) differential radioisotope renography with use of a diuretic during the study or (2) percutaneous nephrostomy and creatinine clearance by 24-hour urine collection.

Severe obstruction with minimal remaining renal function is best treated by unilateral nephrectomy. If renal function is adequate (> 10% of total renal function or > 10 mL/min creatinine clearance), surgical repair of the stenosis, either by creation of a renal pelvis flap or by resection of the stenotic area and reanastomosis, is warranted. The use of ureteroscopy or percutaneous nephroscopy with endopyelotomy, incising the strictured ureteropelvic junction, offers an alternative method of therapy. This approach appears less successful in the presence of a crossing vessel, poor renal function, and significant hydronephrosis. Laparoscopic repair has proponents as well. The surgical results of these methods are excellent in terms of functional preservation, improvement of urine flow, and relief of symptoms, but dilation of the calices may persist.

Tan BJ, Smith AD: Ureteropelvic junction obstruction repair: when, how, what? Curr Opin Urol 2004;14:55.

URETERAL STENOSIS

Ureteral stenosis can be secondary to congenital or acquired lesions. Congenital causes can include compression by an anomalous vessels such as a lower pole renal artery in ureteropelvic junction obstruction or a retroperitoneal vein or primary megaureter where the distal ureter is partially obstructed. More commonly, the ureter is secondarily obstructed due to acquired conditions such as inflammation from chronic ureteral stones, trauma secondary to gynecologic or vascular surgery, or external penetrating trauma from a knife or gunshot wound. Enlarged pelvic lymph nodes or an iliac artery aneurysm or retroperitoneal fibrosis may obstruct the ureter, as can intrinsic ureteral cancer or bladder cancer infiltrating the ureter at its insertion into the bladder. Finally, infection such as urinary tuberculosis can cause distal ureteral strictures, and bilateral ureteral obstruction can occur from bladder neck obstruction with urinary retention secondary to benign prostatic hyperplasia.

Chronic conditions with slow development may not cause symptoms, whereas acute obstruction such as that from a stone will cause severe flank pain that may radiate to the groin or testes/labia. Diagnosis is most often made by a CT urogram with contrast that will show delayed function and a dilated renal pelvis and ureter down to the site of the obstruction. This is often an unsuspected finding on a CT done for other reasons in an asymptomatic patient.

Treatment depends entirely on the cause. Severe stenosis may require resection of the lesion and spatulated end-to-end anastomosis of the ureter. Less severe obstruction may be managed by cystoscopy and ureteral or balloon dilation of the narrowed area under direct vision via a ureteroscope. Placement of an indwelling ureteral stent may dilate the stenosis over time and be a useful treatment as well in selected patients.

RETROPERITONEAL FIBROSIS

See also Chapter 22.

One or both ureters may be compressed by a chronic inflammatory process, usually of unknown cause, which involves the retroperitoneal tissues of the lumbosacral area. Patients treated for migraine with methysergide may develop this fibrosis. Sclerosing Hodgkin disease and fibrosis from metastatic cancer have also been implicated. Symptoms include renal pain, low backache, and those associated with uremia. Some patients present with complete anuria. Urinary infection is unusual. If both ureters are obstructed, the serum creatinine is elevated.

Excretory urograms show hydronephrosis and a dilated ureter down to the point of obstruction. The ureters are displaced medially in the lumbar area. Retrograde ureterograms show a long segment of ureteral stenosis, though a catheter passes easily through the ureter. Sonograms and CT scans may demonstrate fibrous plaques with proximal hydroureteronephrosis. If the patient is anuric, indwelling ureteral catheters or percutaneous nephrostomy should be done. When the patient's condition has improved, definitive therapy can be accomplished. If methysergide is suspected to be the causative agent, fibrosis may subside when the drug is discontinued. These patients may benefit from administration of corticosteroids. Chronic indwelling ureteral stents have also been used successfully. If these methods fail, ureterolysis must be performed to free the ureter from the fibrous plaque. The involved ureter should be dissected from the plaque, moved to a lateral position, and wrapped with omentum to prevent recurrent entrapment. This has been accomplished quite successfully with a laparoscopic approach.

BENIGN PROSTATIC HYPERPLASIA

ESSENTIALS OF DIAGNOSIS

▶ Prostatism: nocturia, hesitancy, slow stream, terminal dribbling, frequency.

▶ Residual urine.

▶ Acute urinary retention.

▶ Uremia in advanced cases.

▶ General Considerations

The cause of benign prostatic enlargement is not known but is probably related to hormonal factors. The mechanism for opening and funneling the vesical neck at the time of voiding is altered by hyperplasia of the prostate, which causes increased outflow resistance. Consequently, a higher intravesical pressure is required to accomplish voiding, causing hypertrophy of the vesical and trigonal muscles. This may lead to the development of bladder diverticula—outpocketings of vesical mucosa between the detrusor muscle bundles. Hypertrophy of the trigone causes excessive stress on the intravesical ureter, producing functional obstruction and resulting in hydroureteronephrosis in late cases. Stagnation of urine can lead to infection; the onset of cystitis exacerbates the obstructive symptoms. The periurethral and subtrigonal prostate enlargement produces the most significant obstruction.

The prostate in young men has an anatomic capsule like an apple peel. In men with prostatic enlargement, there is a thick "surgical" capsule similar to an orange peel, composed of peripherally compressed true prostatic tissue ("peripheral zone"). The hyperplastic benign periurethral glands correspond to the "transition zone" and are the cause of the obstruction (Figure 38–9).

▶ Clinical Findings

A. Symptoms and Signs

Typically, the patient has lower urinary tract symptoms and notices hesitancy and loss of force and caliber of the stream. The urgent need to void when the bladder is nearly full may be an early sign. He may also be awakened by the urge to void several times at night (nocturia). Postvoid dribbling ("terminal dribbling") is particularly disturbing. The complication of infection increases the degree of obstructive symptoms and is often associated with burning on urination. Acute urinary retention may supervene. This is associated with severe urgency, suprapubic pain, and a distended, palpable bladder.

The size of the prostate rectally is not of primary diagnostic importance, since there is a poor correlation between the size of the gland and the degree of symptoms and amount of residual urine. The American Urological Association (AUA) developed a 7-item, self-administered questionnaire (AUA

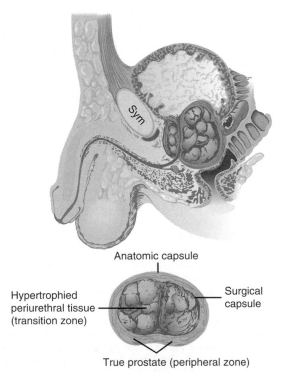

Anatomic capsule

Hypertrophied periurethral tissue (transition zone)

Surgical capsule

True prostate (peripheral zone)

▲ **Figure 38–9.** Benign prostatic hyperplasia. The enlarged periurethral glands are enclosed by the surgical capsule. The true prostate has been compressed.

symptom score) that can assist the patient and physician in evaluating the patient's lower urinary tract symptoms.

B. Laboratory Findings

Urinalysis may reveal evidence of infection. Residual urine is commonly increased (> 50 cc), and a timed urinary flow rate is decreased (< 10–15 cc/s). The serum creatinine may be elevated in cases with prolonged severe obstruction.

C. Imaging Studies

Excretory urograms are often normal and not diagnostic and are thus not required. In late-stage cases, the study may show hydroureteronephrosis if severe obstruction is present. This almost always resolves after prostatectomy. The enlarged gland may cause an indentation in the inferior surface of the bladder, which may result in a J-hook deformity of the distal ureter. The postvoiding film may reveal varying amounts of residual urine. Renal ultrasound examination may obviate the need for urograms; however, imaging is not required to make the diagnosis or to determine the need for or method of treatment. Pelvic ultrasound in the office setting accurately predicts the amount of residual urine and thus obviates bladder catheterization.

D. Cystoscopic Examination

Bladder cystoscopy reveals secondary vesical changes (eg, trabeculation) and enlargement of the periurethral prostatic glands; however, cystoscopy is not required to make the diagnosis. It may identify other conditions such as bladder stones or tumors in selected cases.

E. Urodynamic Studies

Simultaneous physiologic monitoring of bladder filling and emptying, urethral sphincter activity, abdominal pressure, and pelvic floor muscle activity (electromyography) can be extremely useful in documenting whether bladder outlet obstruction, poor bladder function, or other causes are responsible for lower urinary tract symptoms. While urodynamic studies are not required for diagnosis in all cases, they are helpful in cases with large postvoid residual volumes or underlying neurologic disease to help determine appropriate management.

▶ Differential Diagnosis

Neuropathic bladder may produce a similar syndrome. A history suggesting a neuropathic difficulty, such as diabetes mellitus, stroke, or spinal cord injury or compression, may be obtained. Neurologic deficit involving S2-4 is particularly significant.

Cancer of the prostate also causes symptoms of vesical neck obstruction. Serum prostate-specific antigen may be elevated in patients with benign prostatic hypertrophy, and the level increases as the volume of the prostate increases.

Thus, an absolute value is not diagnostic, but in general, if it is over 10 ng/mL, the possibility of cancer should be evaluated.

Acute prostatitis may cause symptoms of obstruction, but the patient is septic and has infected urine. The prostate is exquisitely tender.

Urethral stricture diminishes the caliber of the urinary stream. There is usually a history of gonorrhea or local trauma. A retrograde urethrogram shows the stenotic area. A stricture blocks the passage of an instrument or catheter.

▶ Complications

Obstruction and residual urine lead to vesical and prostatic infection and occasionally pyelonephritis; these may be difficult to eradicate.

The obstruction may lead to the development of bladder diverticula. Infected residual urine may contribute to the formation of calculi.

Functional obstruction of the intravesical ureter, caused by the hypertrophic trigone, may lead to hydroureteronephrosis.

▶ Treatment

The indications for operative management are impairment of or threat to renal function and bothersome symptoms. Because the degree of obstruction progresses slowly in most patients, conservative treatment may be adequate. Drugs that relax the prostatic capsule and internal sphincter (α-adrenergic blocking agents) or decrease the volume of the prostate (5α-reductase inhibitors or antiandrogens) have been tried with considerable success.

A. Conservative Measures

Treatment of chronic prostatitis may reduce symptoms. The resolution of a complicating cystitis usually affords some relief. In order to protect vesical tone, the patient should be cautioned to void as soon as the urge develops. Forcing fluids over a short time causes rapid vesical filling and decreasing vesical tone; this is a common cause of sudden acute urinary retention and thus should be avoided. Patients with urinary obstructive symptoms should avoid the use of cold remedies, including antihistamines, because they are also a common cause of urinary retention. These conservative measures are of only temporary help—if any—in patients with prostatic hyperplasia. There has been recent great interest, particularly by patients, in the use of phytotherapy for treatment of lower urinary tract symptoms, including saw palmetto, pumpkin seeds, and other plant extracts. Despite the claim of efficacy, however, adequate scientific studies have not been done.

Controversy surrounds choices in the treatment of benign prostatic hyperplasia. No treatment (watchful waiting) may be appropriate in patients who complain of mild to moderate symptoms and thus have low AUA symptom scores and residual urine less than 70 cc to 100 cc. Interest has also focused on nonoperative medical therapy for those with more significant symptoms. α-Adrenergic blocking agents relax the internal (bladder neck) sphincter and prostatic capsule. Selective agents that are long-acting and preferentially work for this purpose include doxazosin and tamsulosin. 5α-Reductase inhibitors block conversion of testosterone to dihydrotestosterone (the androgen active in promoting prostate growth) and are useful for large glands, particularly in combination with an alpha-blocker, which has been shown to best prevent urinary retention and other common progressive symptoms of prostatic obstruction.

Catheterization is mandatory for acute urinary retention. Spontaneous voiding may return, but a catheter should be left indwelling for 3 days while detrusor tone returns. If this fails, treatment is indicated.

B. Surgical Measures

There are four classic approaches used in prostatectomy: transurethral, retropubic, suprapubic, and perineal. The transurethral route is preferred in patients with glands weighing under 50 g to 70 g because morbidity rates are lower and the hospital stay is shorter. Larger glands may require open surgery, depending on the preference and experience of the urologist. The death rate is low in each procedure (1–2%). Potency is at greatest risk when the transperineal exposure is used, but impotence occasionally results following transurethral resection of the prostate.

An alternative approach to the treatment of benign prostatic hyperplasia is transurethral incision of the prostate. This procedure consists of incision of the prostate at the bladder neck up to the verumontanum, allowing expansion of the entire prostatic urethra. It is especially effective when the primary point of obstruction is caused by a "median bar" or high posterior lip of the bladder neck without lateral lobe obstruction.

Additional alternative treatments are transurethral vaporization, laser prostatectomy, transurethral microwave thermotherapy, transurethral needle ablation, and high-intensity focused ultrasound ablation of the prostate. Laser prostatectomy seems to have the most promise at present, and recent data suggest that Holmium and KTP (potassium titanyl phosphate) laser may have nearly the same efficacy as transurethral resection of prostate, with less morbidity. However, long-term results of randomized trials are pending.

▶ Prognosis

Most patients with marked symptoms receive considerable relief and substantial improvement in urine flow following surgical treatment; however, those with milder forms may benefit from drug therapy.

American Urological Association: Clinical guidelines. Management of BPH. Available at www.auanet.org. Accessed February 23, 2009.
Lam JS, Cooper KL, Kaplan SA: Changing aspects in the evaluation and treatment of patients with benign prostatic hyperplasia. Med Clin North Am 2004;88:281.

Tan A et al: Meta-analysis of holmium laser enucleation versus transurethral resection of the prostate for symptomatic prostatic obstruction. Br J Surg 2007;94:1201.

URETHRAL STRICTURE

Acquired urethral strictures in men may be due to external trauma or to prior instrumentation (most common). Strictures may be inflammatory, due to gonorrhea, tuberculous urethritis, or schistosomiasis, or may rarely be a complication of cancer. The common presenting symptoms are dysuria, weak stream, splaying of the urinary stream, urinary retention, and urinary tract infection. Evidence of scarring due to trauma or induration and perineal fistula may be seen. Urethroscopy reveals the degree of narrowing. A retrograde urethrogram delineates the site and degree of stricture.

Urethral stricture must be differentiated from bladder outlet obstruction due to prostatism, impacted urethral stones, urethral foreign bodies, and tumors.

Initial treatment consists of transurethral direct-vision internal urethrotomy (incision of the stricture). Successful results are obtained in 75% of patients. For long, dense strictures or those failing to respond to an initial internal urethrotomy, open surgical repair is indicated. This is probably best achieved by the transpubic or perineal route if the lesion involves the membranous urethra. If the mid urethra is involved, the perineal approach is indicated; if the distal urethra is involved, the ventral penile approach is appropriate. End-to-end anastomosis is satisfactory, but a 1-stage inlay patch graft, tube, or pedicle flap of preputial skin is currently favored for most strictures.

Andrich DE et al: Urethral strictures and their surgical treatment. Br J Urol (Int) 2000;86:571.
Kessler TM et al: Long-term results of surgery for urethral stricture: a statistical analysis. J Urol 2003;170:840.
McAninch JW: Reconstruction of external urethral strictures: circular fasciocutaneous penile flap. J Urol 1993;149:488.
Wessels H et al: Current controversies in anterior urethral stricture repair: free-graft versus pedicled skin-flap reconstruction. World J Urol 1998;16:175.

HEMATURIA

Hematuria, gross or microscopic, is a common urologic consult because it can be a presenting sign for underlying urologic malignancies. Red-colored urine may not necessarily include blood, and microscopic examination looking for red blood cells is prudent. Microscopic hematuria is defined as 3 or more red blood cells per high-powered field on urine microscopy in 2 out of 3 properly collected specimens. The degree of hematuria bears no relation to the seriousness of the underlying cause. Urine dipstick test is the simplest method to check for blood and has a sensitivity of 91% to 100% and a specificity of 65% to 99%. Caution should be taken because false positives (menstrual blood, myoglobin, and hemolysis, among others) and false negatives (dipstick exposed to moisture and presence of reducing agents like ascorbic acid) can lead to confusing results. Knowledge of the medical history and medications can help rule out other causes of colored urine. Beets, rifampin, and phenazopyridine, among other substances, can cause urine discoloration. Anticoagulation at normal therapeutic levels does not predispose to hematuria, and patients should be evaluated for the hematuria, because 13% to 45% of these patients may have significant urologic disease.

Ideally, a clean-catch midstream sample should be collected. If that is not possible, a catheterized specimen is indicated. It is important to note that hematuria can be due to urologic or renal parenchymal disease. The differential diagnosis thus includes benign causes like renal or bladder stones, papillary necrosis, urinary tract infections, prostatitis, or instrumentation, and malignant causes like renal, renal pelvis, bladder, prostate, or urethral cancer. Renal parenchymal causes of hematuria include glomerular and interstitial renal disease. These patients may have proteinuria and casts on the urinalysis, and the red blood cells are typically dysmorphic.

Patients with hematuria referred to urology are classified into low-risk and high-risk groups. High-risk groups include smokers, age older than 40 years, history of exposure to pelvic radiation or cyclophosphamide, occupational exposure to chemicals or dyes, and history of urinary tract infections or other urological disorders. It is recommended that a complete workup be performed for all patients with symptomatic hematuria, all patients with gross hematuria, and high-risk patients with microscopic hematuria. The workup includes history and physical examination, serum creatinine, upper tract imaging (typically CT urogram), cystoscopy, and urine cytology. Asymptomatic patients younger than 40 years who have microscopic hematuria and have no risk factors can be evaluated with upper tract imaging and either cystoscopy or voided cytology, as the risk of significant pathology in this population is very low. If the workup is negative, it is recommended that the patient be evaluated with urinalysis, voided cytology, and blood pressure check at 6, 12, 24, and 36 months.

Culclasure TF et al: The significance of hematuria in the anticoagulated patient. Arch Int Med 1994;154:649.
Grossfeld GD et al: Evaluation of asymptomatic hematuria in adults: the American Urological Association best practice policy—part II: patient evaluation, cytology, voided markers, imaging, cystoscopy, nephrology evaluation, and follow-up. Urology 2001;57:604.
Van Savage JG, Fried FA: Anticoagulant associated hematuria: a prospective study. J Urol 1995;153:1594.

URINARY TRACT INFECTIONS

Urinary tract infection is the second-most common type of infection in humans and is frequently encountered by primary care physicians as well as urologists.

These infections are caused by a variety of pyogenic bacteria that typically produce a nonspecific tissue response. The most common organisms are gram-negative bacteria, particularly *Escherichia coli*. Less common are *Enterobacter aerogenes, Proteus vulgaris, Proteus mirabilis, Pseudomonas aeruginosa,* and *Enterococcus faecalis.*

Owing to the short length of the female urethra and bacterial colonization of the introitus, ascending infection is a common occurrence in young girls and in sexually active women. In men, ascending infection is often a consequence of urethral instrumentation.

Although relatively uncommon, descending or hematogenous urinary tract infection is usually associated with local urinary tract disorders—most commonly, obstruction and stasis; less commonly, trauma, foreign bodies, or tumors.

Lymphatic spread occasionally occurs from the large bowel or from the cervix and adnexa in the female through the perivesical and periureteral lymphatics.

Direct extension to the urinary bladder of nearby inflammatory processes (eg, appendiceal abscess, enterovesical fistula, or pelvic abscess) may occur.

► Predisposing Factors

Infection is usually initiated or sustained by predisposing factors. Predisposing systemic factors include diabetes mellitus, immunosuppression, and malnutrition; these disorders likely interfere with normal bladder and body defense mechanisms. Predisposing local factors include incontinence, constipation, organic or functional obstruction, stasis (residual urine), foreign bodies (especially catheters and stones), tumors, or necrotic tissue. Vesicoureteral reflux facilitates transport of bacteria from the bladder to the kidney, which subsequently predisposes to pyelonephritis.

► Classification of Urinary Tract Infection

Urinary tract infection is classified as (1) upper urinary tract infection (most commonly acute or chronic pyelonephritis or infection due to renal abscess), (2) lower urinary tract infection (cystitis or urethritis), or (3) genital infection (prostatitis, epididymitis, seminal vesiculitis, or orchitis).

► Urologic Instrumentation or Surgery & Urinary Tract Infection

In the absence of urinary tract infection, surgery of the upper urinary tract should require only short-term prophylactic antibacterial therapy. In the presence of infection, one attempts to sterilize the system before operation. If stenting or tube drainage is required and there are no symptoms of infection, colonization does not call for antibacterial therapy until the stent or tube is to be changed or removed. Broadspectrum antibacterial prophylaxis is started at that time.

With lower urinary tract surgery, antibacterial therapy is advised before operations involving the urethra and the bladder, especially for women in whom contamination from vaginal organisms is likely. Men undergoing prostatectomy for obstructive prostatism often have urinary tract infection, particularly when catheter drainage is used preoperatively. In these cases, antimicrobial therapy is necessary before and after surgery to prevent bacteremia.

In the presence of urinary tract infection, any urethral instrumentation poses a threat of bacteremia—more apt to occur in men than in women. Appropriate antibacterial coverage should be instituted before manipulation.

A. Principles of Catheterization

After a short-term single catheterization, the rate of infection is 1% to 5%. However, in certain patients—pregnant women, elderly or debilitated patients—and in the presence of urologic disease, the risk is much higher. An indwelling catheter often leads to colonization, especially in women. The incidence is proportionate to the duration of catheterization and reaches approximately 95% after 5 days.

Strict aseptic technique is of critical importance in catheterization. Proper cleansing of the genitalia is essential. Iodophor preparations may be used for cleaning the vaginal introitus or the glans penis. Many common urinary tract pathogens are present in normal colonic flora, and these organisms often gain access to the urinary tract of catheterized patients. Cross-contamination of urinary catheters (passive transmission of bacteria from patient to patient on the hands of hospital personnel) is a frequent mode of transfer of resistant organisms. Measures directed to the prevention of catheter cross-contamination are essential. Closed catheter drainage is probably the best way to reduce cross-contamination.

With sterile technique during catheterization and a closed drainage system, most catheters can be kept sterile for 48–72 hours. In a closed drainage system, an added airlock or one-way valve preventing reflux of urine from the collecting bag to the draining tubes also helps prevent infection. The general principles are as follows: (1) Indwelling catheters should be used only when absolutely necessary. (2) Catheters should be inserted with strict aseptic technique. (3) A closed drainage system, preferably with a one-way valve, is advisable. (4) Nonobstructed dependent drainage is essential. (5) Unnecessary irrigation of the system should be avoided. (6) If the catheter is needed for a prolonged period, it should be changed every 2–3 weeks to minimize encrustation and stone formation. (7) Catheterized patients with asymptomatic catheter colonization should be given antibiotics just before the catheter is changed or removed—not during the period of catheterization unless symptomatic infection occurs.

B. Evaluation

Imaging of the urinary tract is recommended in every febrile infant or young child following the first urinary tract infection. Imaging includes a renal and bladder ultrasound and a voiding cystourethrogram. The renal ultrasound may detect hydronephrosis, duplication anomalies, stones, or abnor-malities of the bladder wall and should be obtained at the earliest convenient time. A cystogram may be obtained by instillation of contrast medium with fluoroscopy or by instillation of a radionuclide. Radionuclide cystography has the advantage of decreased radiation, while the contrast-voiding cystourethrogram has the advantage of providing better anatomic detail, which may help detect bladder or urethral abnormalities. Either method should include a voiding phase because reflux is the most likely abnormality to be detected and may only occur with voiding. The cystogram should be obtained once the child is free of infection. Imaging recommendations in adults with a urinary tract infection vary depending on the patient's past history and present symptoms.

C. Antibacterial Therapy

The choice of antibiotics depends on the type of organism and its sensitivity, as determined by urine cultures. For uncomplicated infection, adequate urine concentrations of the antibiotic determine efficacy, but in cases of bacteremia and septic shock, serum concentrations are crucial. Commonly used oral medications are sulfonamides, nitrofurantoin, ampicillin, trimethoprim-sulfamethoxazole, fluoroquinolones, and oxytetracycline. For parenteral therapy, aminoglycosides and cephalosporins are effective against the most common organisms (ie, *P mirabilis*, *E aerogenes*, and *P aeruginosa*).

ACUTE PYELONEPHRITIS

 ESSENTIALS OF DIAGNOSIS

▶ Chills, fever, and flank pain.

▶ Frequency and urgency of urination; dysuria.

▶ Pyuria and bacteriuria.

▶ Bacterial growth on urine cultures.

▶ General Considerations

Except in the presence of stasis, foreign bodies, trauma, or instrumentation, pyelonephritis is an ascending type of infection. Pathogenic organisms usually reach the kidney from the bladder, often via an incompetent ureterovesical junction.

▶ Clinical Findings
A. Symptoms and Signs

In acute attacks, pain is present in one or both flanks. Diagnosis in infants requires a high index of suspicion, since they may present with nonspecific symptoms such as fever and failure to thrive. Young children commonly present with poorly localized abdominal pain; irritative lower urinary tract symptoms may be present. Chills and fever are common. Severe infection may produce hypotension, peripheral vasoconstriction, and acute renal failure. Gross hematuria is not common.

B. Laboratory Findings

Pyuria and bacteriuria are consistent findings. Leukocytosis with a shift to the left is common. Urine culture identifies the organism.

C. Imaging Studies

In acute attacks, only minimal changes such as delayed visualization and poor concentrating ability are noted on intravenous urography. CT scans may demonstrate zones of decreased enhancement in the renal parenchyma as well as perinephric fat stranding. Renal or ureteral calculi may be seen on plain abdominal x-rays or nonenhanced CT scans. Chest x-ray may show a small ipsilateral pleural effusion.

► Differential Diagnosis

Pneumonia, acute cholecystitis, or splenic infarction can be confused with pyelonephritis. Acute appendicitis sometimes causes pyuria and microhematuria. Any acute abdominal illness such as pancreatitis, diverticulitis, or intestinal angina can simulate pyelonephritis. Appropriate chest x-rays and urinalysis usually makes the distinction.

► Complications

If the diagnosis is missed in the acute stage, the infection may become chronic. Both acute and chronic pyelonephritis lead to progressive renal damage.

► Treatment

Specific antibiotic therapy should be given for at least 7 days to eradicate the infecting organism after proper identification and sensitivity determination. Symptomatic treatment is indicated for pain and irritative voiding symptoms. Adequate fluid intake to assure optimum urinary output is required. Failure to simultaneously identify and treat predisposing factors (eg, obstruction) is the principal cause of failure to respond to therapy, leading to chronic pyelonephritis.

► Prognosis

The prognosis is good with adequate treatment of both the infection and its predisposing cause, depending on the degree of preexisting renal parenchymal damage.

EMPHYSEMATOUS PYELONEPHRITIS

Emphysematous pyelonephritis is a form of acute necrotizing pyelonephritis secondary to a gas-producing bacteria (*E coli*

in 66% of cases and *Klebsiella* in 26%). It is commonly seen in patients with poorly controlled diabetes (over 90% of cases) or in patients with upper urinary tract obstruction. The diagnosis is made by the usual signs of acute pyelonephritis and by the presence of gas in the renal collecting system and parenchyma seen on plain films, ultrasound, or CT. The condition is life threatening, with a mortality rate of 40% to 80% with intravenous antibiotics alone. Obstruction requires drainage either percutaneously or by stent placement. Operative treatment, including nephrectomy and drainage along with antibiotics, decreases the mortality rate to less than 20%.

CHRONIC PYELONEPHRITIS

Chronic pyelonephritis is the result of inadequately treated or recurrent acute pyelonephritis. The diagnosis is primarily made by x-ray, since patients rarely have signs or symptoms until late in the course, when they develop chronic flank pain, hypertension, anemia, or renal failure. Pyuria is not a consistent finding. Because chronic pyelonephritis may be a progressive, localized immune response initiated by bacteria long since eradicated, urine cultures are usually sterile. Early cases may have no findings on intravenous urography, whereas in late cases it may reveal small kidneys with typical caliceal deformities (clubbing), with evidence of peripheral scarring and a thin cortex. Voiding cystourethrography may document vesicoureteral reflux as the cause. Complications include hypertension, stone formation, and chronic renal failure.

Antibiotic treatment is not helpful in these patients unless ongoing infection can be documented. The prognosis depends on the status of renal function but is generally not good, particularly when the disease is contracted in childhood. Progressive deterioration of renal function usually occurs.

Xanthogranulomatous pyelonephritis is a form of chronic pyelonephritis seen most frequently in middle-aged diabetic women and rarely in children. The disease is usually unilateral and is associated with prolonged obstructing nephrolithiasis. Patients often have nonspecific symptoms similar to those of acute pyelonephritis but have an enlarged kidney with calculi and a mass often indistinguishable from tumor. Proteus species are common causative agents. Nephrectomy is usually the treatment of choice, though a partial nephrectomy may be performed for focal disease. Histologic examination confirms the diagnosis following nephrectomy by the demonstration of foamy lipid-laden macrophages.

PAPILLARY NECROSIS

This disorder consists of ischemic necrosis of the renal papillae or of the entire pyramid. Excessive ingestion of analgesics, sickle cell trait, diabetes, obstruction with infection, and systemic conditions decreasing renal blood flow are common predisposing factors.

The symptoms are usually those of chronic cystitis with recurring exacerbations of pyelonephritis. Renal pain or renal colic may be present. Azotemic manifestations may be the presenting symptoms. In acute attacks, localized flank tenderness and generalized toxemia may occur. Laboratory findings consist of pyuria, hematuria, occasionally glycosuria, and acidosis. Impaired kidney function is shown by elevated serum creatinine and urea nitrogen. Intravenous urography usually shows impaired function and poor visualization in advanced cases. Evidence of ulceration, cavitation, or linear breaks in the base of the papillae and radiolucent defects due to sloughed papillae may be seen; the latter may become calcified. Retrograde urograms may be needed for proper imaging if kidney function is markedly impaired.

Preventive measures consist of proper management of diabetic patients with recurrent infections and avoidance of chronic use of analgesic compounds containing phenacetin and aspirin.

Intensive antibacterial therapy may be needed, though it is commonly unsuccessful in eradicating infection. Little can be done surgically except to remove obstructing papillae and correct predisposing factors (eg, reflux, obstruction) if identified.

In severe cases, the prognosis is poor. Renal transplantation may be required.

RENAL ABSCESS

While renal abscess is occasionally due to hematogenous spread of a distant staphylococcal infection, most abscesses are secondary to chronic nonspecific infection of the kidney, often complicated by stone formation. The onset may be acute, with high fever, but occasionally low-grade fever and general malaise are the presenting symptoms. Localized costovertebral angle tenderness and a palpable flank mass may be present. A mass may be evident on intravenous urograms, DTPA scans, sonograms, CT scans, or renal angiograms. If the abscess is due to hematogenous spread, the urine does not contain bacteria unless the abscess has broken into the pelvicaliceal system. More frequently, gram-negative organisms are found, as would be expected in light of the preponderance of ascending infection.

If organism sensitivity can be established by appropriate tests (blood and urine cultures and sensitivity tests), treatment with the proper antibiotic is indicated. Many infections have responded to percutaneous drainage and irrigation with antibiotic solutions, especially in cases of unilocular abscess cavity seen on either ultrasound or CT examination. In multilocular abscess or persistent bacteremia despite percutaneous drainage, surgical drainage or even heminephrectomy may be necessary.

When the abscess is found to be secondary to chronic renal infection, nephrectomy is usually indicated because of advanced destruction of the kidney.

PERINEPHRIC ABSCESS

Abscess between the renal capsule and the perirenal fascia most often results from rupture of an intrarenal abscess into the perinephric space. *E coli* is the most common causative organism. The pathogenesis usually begins with severe pyonephrosis secondary to obstruction, as with renal or ureteral calculi. Clinical findings are similar to those of renal abscess. A pleural effusion on the affected side and signs of psoas muscle irritation are common. Abdominal plain films may show obliteration of the psoas muscle shadow, and an intravenous urogram may show poor concentration of contrast medium and hydronephrosis. CT scan is the current study of choice for diagnosis.

Treatment involves prompt drainage of the abscess and use of appropriate systemic antibiotics, including coverage of anaerobes. Percutaneous drainage is often successful; however, open surgical drainage is necessary if percutaneous drainage is incomplete. Mortality ranges between 20% and 50% with antibiotics and drainage, whereas treatment with antibiotics alone increases this rate to 75% to 100%.

CYSTITIS

Cystitis is more common in females and is usually an ascending infection. In males, it usually occurs in association with urethral or prostatic obstruction, prostatitis, foreign bodies, or tumors. The urinary bladder is normally capable of clearing bacterial inoculation unless an underlying pathologic process interferes with its defensive mechanisms.

In the acute phase, the principal symptoms of cystitis are dysuria, frequency, urgency, and hematuria; low-grade fever and suprapubic, perineal, and low back pain may be present. In chronic cystitis, irritative symptoms are usually milder.

Evidence of prostatitis, urethritis, or vaginitis may be present. Laboratory findings, in addition to hematuria, consist of bacteriuria and pyuria. Leukocytosis is not common. Urine culture identifies the organism. Cystoscopy is not advisable in the acute phase. In chronic cystitis, evidence of mucosal irritation may be present.

In any documented recurrent lower urinary tract infection (particularly in males), a complete urologic workup is indicated. Instrumentation is contraindicated in the acute phase, but cystoscopy is essential to identify the predisposing factor in chronic or recurrent bacterial cystitis.

Specific antibacterial therapy is given according to sensitivity testing of recovered organisms (*E coli* in > 80% of cases). Sterilization of urine should usually be followed by a variable period of continuous antibiotic therapy (depending on the predisposing factor or the chronicity and recurrence of the disease). Prolonged suppressive medication is usually indicated in cases associated with voiding dysfunction.

In females with recurrent postcoital cystitis, premedication (eg, sulfonamides, nitrofurantoin) on the night of intercourse and the following day in addition to immediate postcoital voiding decreases recurrences.

PROSTATITIS

Acute Bacterial Prostatitis

Acute bacterial prostatitis is a severe acute febrile illness caused by ascending coliform bacteria, which frequently colonize the male urethra. Symptoms include high fever, chills, low back and perineal pain, and urinary frequency and urgency with diminished stream or retention. On examination, the prostate is extremely tender, swollen, and warm to the touch. A fluctuant abscess may be palpable. The prostate must be examined cautiously, because vigorous palpation may cause acute septicemia. Laboratory findings include pyuria, bacteriuria, and leukocytosis.

Transurethral manipulation by catheter or cystoscopy should be avoided; urinary retention should be treated by introducing a percutaneous suprapubic tube. Treatment with systemic antibiotics (fluoroquinolones or aminoglycosides and ampicillin-cephalosporin) should be started immediately and should be adjusted later when results of urine culture or blood culture (or both) and sensitivity tests are known. E coli is found in 80% of cases. Treatment with oral antibiotics for several weeks after the initial phase has subsided is necessary to eradicate the bacteria completely. A prostatic abscess usually requires open perineal drainage or transurethral unroofing. The prognosis is good if treatment is thorough and prompt.

Chronic Prostatitis

Chronic prostatitis is a common and complex problem. With differential diagnosis including urethritis, bacterial and nonbacterial prostatitis, prostatodynia (chronic pelvic pain syndrome [CPPS]), and seminal vesiculitis, assigning the correct diagnosis may challenge even the expert. The symptoms are varied and include suprapubic pain, low back pain, orchialgia, dysuria at the tip of the penis, and urinary frequency and urgency. The urinalysis may be normal. There may be a clear white urethral discharge. Prostate examination may reveal a soft, boggy prostate.

Expressed prostatic secretions may contain numerous leukocytes (> 10 per high-power field) in clumps as well as macrophages. Cultures of urine are usually sterile, but cultures of expressed prostatic secretions and urine obtained after prostatic massage are usually positive in bacterial prostatitis. Chlamydia or Ureaplasma may be an offending organism, particularly in men under age 35. Determination of the site of infection may require differential cultures. The first part of the voided urine stream is collected as VB_1 and the midstream specimen as VB_2. The prostate is then massaged to obtain expressed prostatic secretions, and the postmassage urine is collected as VB_3. The differential leukocyte and bacterial counts from each of these specimens can help localize the site of infection. If VB_1 has high levels of leukocytes and bacteria relative to the other specimens, urethritis is likely; if VB_2 has high levels, a site above the bladder neck is likely; and if the expressed prostatic secretions, VB_3, or both have high counts, prostatitis is likely.

Treatment depends on culture results, but if there is no bacterial growth on culture, tetracycline, 250 mg to 500 mg four times a day for 14 days, may be curative. For chronic bacterial prostatitis, at least a 6-week course of a fluoroquinolone or trimethoprim-sulfamethoxazole is often given. Surgical treatment for prostatitis is rarely indicated or helpful. Some patients improve following discontinuation of caffeine and alcohol, and a few respond to repeated prostatic massage. Patients with no evidence of bacterial infection or obstructive findings, and those who have recurrent pelvic pain in association with voiding dysfunction (eg, intermittent or weak urinary stream) may be treated with α-adrenergic blocking agents or biofeedback to decrease the internal and external sphincter tone. 5α-Reductase inhibitors may be helpful, and phytotherapy has proponents but needs further study.

Nickel JC: Recommendations for the evaluation of patients with prostatitis. World J Urol 2003;21:75.

Schaeffer AJ: Etiology and management of chronic pelvic pain syndrome in men. Urology 2004;63(suppl 3A):75.

ACUTE EPIDIDYMITIS

Acute epididymitis is most commonly a disease of young males, caused by bacterial infection ascending from the urethra or prostate. The disease is less common in older males, but when it does occur, it is most often due to infection secondary to urinary tract obstruction or instrumentation.

The symptoms are sudden pain in the scrotum, rapid unilateral scrotal enlargement, and marked tenderness that extends to the spermatic cord in the groin and may be relieved by scrotal elevation (**Prehn's sign**). Fever is present. An acute hydrocele may result, and secondary orchitis with a swollen, painful testicle may occur. Laboratory studies reveal pyuria, bacteriuria, and marked leukocytosis.

Epididymitis must be differentiated from torsion of the testis, testicular tumor, and tuberculous epididymitis. A technetium-99m pertechnetate scan reveals increased uptake with epididymitis but decreased uptake with torsion. Scrotal ultrasound distinguishes between the solid mass of a testicular tumor and an enlarged, inflamed epididymis and can also identify epididymal or testicular abscess, which requires operative treatment. Increased blood flow on Doppler ultrasound also helps distinguish epididymitis from torsion, though it is not completely reliable.

Cultured aspirates from inflamed epididymides of males under age 35 tend to show gonococci and chlamydiae; in men older than 35, E coli is most common. Epididymal aspiration for culture is not required routinely, however. Pyuria with a negative urine culture suggests the presence of chlamydial infection in both prostate and epididymis. (See also section on Tuberculosis.)

Treatment consists of antibiotics, usually ceftriaxone and doxycycline in males under age 35 and fluoroquinolones in those over age 35. In some patients, pain is relieved by scrotal hypothermia, and consideration should be given to infiltration of the spermatic cord by 1% bupivacaine. Nonsteroidal anti-inflammatory drugs are recommended to aid in pain relief. In most instances, prompt treatment results in rapid resolution of pain, fever, and swelling. Patients must refrain from exertion for 1 to 3 weeks.

Exacerbations can be controlled by treating the predisposing factor. Chronic epididymitis rarely resolves completely; it has no consequences except, occasionally in bilateral cases, sterility due to scarring and obstruction of the delicate epididymal tubules. Rarely, epididymectomy is necessary.

TUBERCULOSIS

Tuberculosis is a commonly missed genitourinary infection that should be considered in any case of pyuria without bacteriuria or in any case of urinary tract infection that does not respond to treatment.

Genitourinary tuberculosis is always secondary to pulmonary infection, though in many cases, the primary focus has healed or is quiescent. Infection occurs via the hematogenous route. The kidneys and (less commonly) the prostate are the principal sites of urinary tract involvement, though any part of the genitourinary system can be affected.

▶ Pathology

Renal tuberculosis usually starts as a tuberculoma that gradually enlarges, caseates, and finally ulcerates, breaking into the pelvicaliceal system. Caseation and scarring are the principal pathologic features of renal tuberculosis. In the ureter, tuberculosis usually leads to distal strictures, periureteritis, and mural fibrosis.

In the bladder, the infection is characterized by areas of hyperemia and a coalescent group of tubercles, followed by ulcerations. Bladder wall fibrosis and contraction are the end results.

Urethral involvement in the male is uncommon but when present leads to urethral stricture, usually in the bulbous portion. Periurethral abscess and fistula are possible complications.

Genital tuberculosis may involve the prostate, seminal vesicles, and epididymides, either separately or in association with renal involvement. Tubercle formation with later caseation and fibrosis is the basic pathologic feature. The prostate becomes enlarged, with palpable nodules and an irregular consistency. The affected seminal vesicle is fibrotic and distended. Induration and thickening of the epididymis and beading of the vas deferens are characteristic findings. The testicles are rarely involved.

▶ Clinical Findings
A. Symptoms and Signs

The patient commonly presents with lower urinary tract irritation, usually with pyuria. Less common manifestations are hematuria, renal pain, and renal colic.

B. Laboratory Findings

"Sterile" pyuria is the rule, but 15% of cases have secondary bacterial infection (eg, *E coli*). *Mycobacteria* can be identified on an acid-fast stain of the centrifuged sediment of the first morning urine collected on 3 successive days (positive in 90% of cases). Culture of the sediment should yield the mycobacteria, which may then be speciated by niacin and nitrate tests, both of which must be positive for a diagnosis of Mycobacterium tuberculosis.

C. Imaging Studies

Radiologic findings that suggest genitourinary tuberculosis include moth-eaten, caseous renal cavities or bizarre, irregular calices. Strictures in straight, rigid, moderately dilated ureters and a contracted bladder with vesicoureteral reflux are all suggestive evidence.

▶ Treatment
A. Medical Treatment

Tuberculosis must be treated as a systemic disease. Once the diagnosis is established, medical treatment is indicated regardless of the need for surgery. Whenever possible, medical treatment should be continued for at least 3 months before surgery is considered.

Active medications against tuberculosis include rifampin, isoniazid, pyrazinamide, ethambutol, and streptomycin. Standard initial treatment is with rifampin, isoniazid, and pyrazinamide for 8 weeks. Pyridoxine, 100 mg/d, is given in divided doses to counteract the vitamin B_6 depletion effect of isoniazid. In patients with more severe infections, ethambutol or streptomycin may be added to the initial treatment. Following the initial 8 weeks of therapy, rifampin and isoniazid are continued in combination three times per week for another 8 weeks. Liver function tests must be followed in view of the hepatotoxicity of rifampin, isoniazid, and pyrazinamide.

B. Surgical Measures

If medical therapy fails to cure a unilateral lesion, nephrectomy may be necessary. However, this is rare. In bilateral disease that has seriously damaged one kidney and is in an early stage in the other, unilateral nephrectomy may be considered; in localized polar lesions, partial nephrectomy may be done.

In unilateral epididymal involvement, epididymectomy plus contralateral vasectomy is indicated to prevent descent of the infection to the prostate; bilateral epididymectomy should be done if both sides are involved.

For a severely contracted bladder, augmentation enterocystoplasty increases vesical capacity following eradication of the infection.

Prognosis

In a high percentage of cases, cure is obtained by medical means. Unilateral renal lesions have the best prognosis.

Cooper CS et al: The outcome of stopping prophylactic antibiotics in older children with vesicoureteral reflux. J Urol 2000; 163:269.

Hodson EM, Willis NS, Craig JC: Antibiotics for acute pyelonephritis in children. Cochrane Database Syst Rev 2007; 4:CD003772.

Smaill F, Vazquez JC: Antibiotics for asymptomatic bacteriuria in pregnancy. Cochrane Database Syst Rev 2007;2:CD000490.

Wise GJ, Marella VK: Genitourinary manifestations of tuberculosis. Urol Clin North Am 2003;30:111.

▼ CALCULI

RENAL STONE

ESSENTIALS OF DIAGNOSIS

- ▶ Flank pain, hematuria (gross or microscopic), pyelonephritis, previous stone passage.
- ▶ Costovertebral angle tenderness.
- ▶ Stone visualized on urography, ultrasonography, or noncontrast spiral CT scan.

General Considerations

Stone disease is common, with the lifetime risk of stone formation in the United States exceeding 12% in males and 6% in females. Prevalence of stone disease varies by racial background and geographic location within the United States, with older white males and southeastern states having the highest prevalence. Seventy-five percent of most stones are composed of calcium salts (oxalate, phosphate), while uric acid and struvite stones (magnesium-ammonium phosphate stones that form secondary to urea-splitting organisms) constitute 10% each. Formation of calcium stones can be due to one or multiple factors that include hypercalciuria, hypocitraturia, hyperoxaluria, and hyperuricosuria. In patients with hyperparathyroidism or those who ingest large amounts of calcium or vitamin D or in patients who are dehydrated or immobilized, hypercalciuria promotes stone formation.

Uric acid stones form in acidic urine. Cystine stones, which make up 1% of all stones, usually form secondary to impaired renal reabsorption of cystine. Owing to the radiodensity of sulfur, cystine stones are radiopaque (albeit less so than calcium stones), whereas uric acid stones are radiolucent. Stones that obstruct the ureteropelvic junction or ureter lead to hydronephrosis and possibly infection.

Clinical Findings

A. Symptoms and Signs

If the stone acutely obstructs the ureteropelvic junction or a calix, moderate to severe renal pain is noted, often accompanied by nausea, vomiting, and ileus. The pain starts in the upper lateral back and may radiate anteriorly and inferiorly toward the groin. Gross or microscopic hematuria is common. Symptoms of infection, if present, are exacerbated. Nonobstructing calculi are usually painless. This includes staghorn calculi, which may form a cast of all calices and the pelvis. In the symptomatic patient, there may be costovertebral angle tenderness and a quiet abdomen. Infection secondary to obstruction may lead to high fever and a rigid abdomen.

B. Laboratory Findings

With acute infection, leukocytosis is to be expected. Urinalysis may reveal red and white blood cells and bacteria. A pH of 7.6 or higher implies the presence of urea-splitting organisms. A pH consistently below 5.5 is compatible with the formation of uric acid or cystine stones. If the pH is fixed between 6.0 and 7.0, renal tubular acidosis should be considered as a cause of nephrocalcinosis. Crystals of uric acid (rhomboid) or cystine (hexagonal) in the urine are suggestive. A 24-hour urine collection can help identify the metabolic effect that predisposes to stone formation (hypercalciuria, hypocitraturia, hyperoxaluria). Hypercalciuria can be resorptive (due to hyperparathyroidism), absorptive (increased gastrointestinal absorption), or renal (increased urine loss of calcium). Citrate is a stone inhibitor and hypocitraturia predisposes to stone formation.

Increases in urine calcium and phosphate plus hypercalcemia (and hypophosphatemia) suggest the presence of hyperparathyroidism, and measurement of serum parathyroid hormone is helpful. Excessive urinary uric acid is compatible with uric acid stone formation.

A qualitative test for urinary cystine should be part of the routine evaluation. If levels are elevated, a 24-hour quantitative measurement should be made. Hyperchloremic acidosis suggests distal renal tubular acidosis with secondary renal calcifications. Total renal function is impaired only if the stones are bilateral, and particularly if chronic infection complicates the clinical presentation.

C. Imaging Studies

About 90% of calculi are radiopaque; the majority are calcium stones and can be seen on plain x-ray. Excretory urography is necessary to verify their location within the urinary tract and also affords a qualitative measure of renal function. An acutely obstructed kidney may show only increasing density of the renal shadow without significant radiopaque material in the calices. A nonopaque stone (uric acid) is identified as a radiolucent defect in the opaque contrast media. Calculi larger than 1 cm cast a specific acoustic shadow on ultrasonography. Spiral (helical) CT has become the first study of choice, because the entire urinary tract can be scanned rapidly and without contrast injection (Figure 38–10). Calculi can be readily identified and distinguished from clot or tumor. Plain x-ray of the skeletal system may identify Paget's disease, sarcoidosis, or osteoporosis due to prolonged immobilization responsible for hypercalciuria.

D. Stone Analysis

If a stone has previously been passed or if one is recovered, its chemical composition should be analyzed. Such information may be useful when planning a preventive program.

▶ Differential Diagnosis

Acute pyelonephritis may begin with acute renal pain mimicking that of renal stone. Urinalysis reveals pyuria, and urograms or CT fails to reveal a calculus.

Renal adenocarcinoma may bleed into the tumor, causing acute pain mimicking that of an obstructing stone. Imaging can make the differentiation.

Transitional cell tumors of the renal pelvis or calices mimic uric acid stone; both are radiolucent. CT scan without contrast or ultrasound reveal the stone by virtue of increased density compared with adjacent soft tissues.

Renal tuberculosis is complicated by stone formation in 10% of cases. Pyuria without bacteriuria is suggestive. Urography reveals the moth-eaten calices typical of tuberculosis.

Papillary necrosis may cause renal colic if a sloughed papilla obstructs the ureteropelvic junction. Imaging (particularly CT) settles the issue.

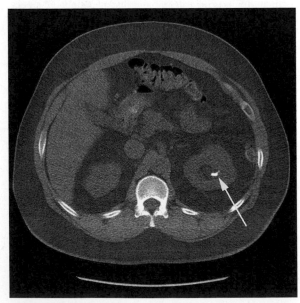

▲ **Figure 38–10.** CT scan without intravenous contrast demonstrating a left renal calculus (arrow).

Renal infarction may cause renal pain and hematuria. Evidence of a cardiac lesion, nonfunction of the kidney on urography, and exclusion of a calculus help in differentiation. Infarction is confirmed by angiography, radioisotopic renography, or color Doppler ultrasound.

Other conditions to be considered in the differential diagnosis include ureteropelvic junction obstruction, obstruction due to blood clots, ureteral strictures or fungal bezoars, and renal abscess.

▶ Complications

Acting as a foreign body, a stone increases the probability of infection. However, primary infection may incite stone formation. A stone lodged in the ureteropelvic junction leads to progressive hydronephrosis. A staghorn calculus, as it grows, may destroy renal tissue by pressure, and the infection that is usually present also contributes to renal damage. The presence of an obstructed renal unit should be considered and is a urologic emergency. Drainage of the kidney should be performed promptly with insertion of a ureteral stent or percutaneous nephrostomy tube.

▶ Prevention

An effective preventive regimen depends on stone analysis and chemical studies of the serum and urine.

A. General Measures

Ensure a high fluid intake (3–4 L/d) to keep solutes well diluted. This measure alone may decrease stone-forming potential by 50%. Treat infection, relieve stasis or obstruction, and advise the patient to avoid prolonged immobilization.

B. Specific Measures

1. Calcium stones—Remove the parathyroid tumor, if present. High dietary sodium promotes renal calcium absorption, and restriction to 100 meq/d may be helpful. Limitation of proteins and carbohydrates may also reduce hypercalciuria. Recent randomized trials have shown that in men with recurrent calcium oxalate stones and hypercalciuria, restricted intake of animal protein and salt, combined with a normal calcium intake, provides greater protection than the traditional low-calcium diet. Potassium citrate can decrease stone formation by increasing urine levels of citrate, which is a stone inhibitor.

Oral orthophosphates are effective in reducing the stone-forming potential of urine by decreasing urine calcium and increasing inhibitor activity. Thiazide diuretics such as hydrochlorothiazide, 50 mg twice daily, decrease the calcium content in urine by 50%. If hyperuricosuria is coincident with calcium urolithiasis, then allopurinol and urinary alkalinization can reduce the formation of urate crystals, which may act as a nidus for calcium crystallization.

For a patient with primary absorptive hypercalciuria, cellulose sodium phosphate can be given. This substance combines with calcium in the gut to prevent absorption.

2. Oxalate stones (calcium oxalate)—Prescribe phosphate or a thiazide diuretic (see above). Elimination of excessive oxalate in coffee, tea, colas, leafy green vegetables, and chocolate may also be helpful. Excess vitamin C can be metabolized to oxalate and thus should be avoided.

3. Magnesium-ammonium-phosphate stones—These stones are usually secondary to urinary tract infection due to bacteria that produce urease (primarily proteus species). Eradication of the infection prevents further stone formation but is impossible when stones are present. Acetohydroxamic acid, a urease inhibitor, can be used for oral chemolysis and can potentiate antibiotic action. After all calculi have been removed, prevention of stone growth is best accomplished by urinary acidification and long-term use of antibiotics.

4. Metabolic stones (uric acid, cystine)—These substances are most soluble at a pH of 7.0 or higher. Give potassium citrate, 10 meq to 20 meq by mouth three times a day, and monitor the urine pH with a litmus paper indicator. For uric acid stone formers, limit purines in the diet and give allopurinol if they have hyperuricemia. Patients with mild cystinuria may need only urinary alkalinization, as described previously. For severe cystinuria, penicillamine, 30 mg/kg/d orally, reduces urinary cystine to safe levels. Penicillamine should be supplemented with pyridoxine, 50 mg/d orally. Tiopronin, which has fewer side effects than D-penicillamine and captopril, can be used as well.

▶ Treatment

A. Conservative Measures

Intervention is not required for small, nonobstructive, asymptomatic caliceal stones. Hydration and dietary management may be sufficient to prevent growth of existing or new calcium stones in patients without metabolic abnormalities. Those with identifiable metabolic disorders may benefit from the specific measures described previously. Patients with known uric acid stones can be treated with hydration and urinary alkalinization, which can help dissolve the stone. Patients with active infection, obstruction, or intractable nausea or pain may need definitive treatment. In the acute setting, a ureteral stent can be inserted endoscopically under intravenous sedation.

B. Ureteroscopic Intervention

Patients with small stones can be managed with ureteronephroscopy and laser lithotripsy or basketing of the stones. The presence of a ureteral stent several days prior helps passively dilate the ureter and makes the ureteroscopy easier. This is done under general anesthetic and as an outpatient procedure.

C. Percutaneous Intervention (Endourology)

In selected patients with symptomatic or large pelvic stones, percutaneous stone removal may be successful. A percutaneous tract enters the renal collecting system through an appropriate calix (**percutaneous nephrostomy**). The tract is subsequently dilated, and endoscopic extraction of the stones (**percutaneous nephroscopy** and **percutaneous nephrolithotomy**) is done. Pulverization of the fragments by means of ultrasonic, electrohydraulic, or laser probes passed through the nephrostomy tract can be done. Residual stones after infection may be dissolved by percutaneous irrigation with hemiacidrin. For cystine and uric acid stones, alkaline or other irrigants that increase the specific crystal solubility may be used (eg, *N*-acetyl-L-lysine or propionyl glycine for cystine stones). Specific antibiotic treatment for infection must be given before irrigation to prevent sepsis.

Success with these endourologic methods approaches 100%. The advantages over surgical procedures include no incision and rapid recovery and return to full activity. Disadvantages include the occasional need for multiple treatments to completely remove the calculi and the uncommon occurrence of significant hemorrhage.

C. Extracorporeal Shock Wave Lithotripsy (ESWL)

With this technique, patients are positioned in the path of shock waves focused on the renal calculi with the aid of fluoroscopy or ultrasound. General or regional anesthesia is required in selected patients, but sedation is sufficient in most cases. The shock waves (more than 1500 are usually given) pulverize the stones, and the small particles pass spontaneously over 2 to 5 days. Results are excellent. Calcium stones and magnesium-ammonium-phosphate stones have been treated successfully. Because of the physical properties of the crystal lattice, ESWL is not as effective in fragmenting cystine stones. Radiolucent uric acid stones, which can be visualized using contrast medium via intravenous pyelography or retrograde ureteropyelography, are amenable to ESWL treatment. Patients with low-volume staghorn calculi can be managed with ESWL, though percutaneous nephrolithotomy remains the treatment of choice for most staghorn calculi.

A variety of devices now effectively pulverize stones using less energy and thus can be used with only intravenous sedation; an increased number of pulses are required to obtain the same results as with previous higher-energy devices. Some instruments use ultrasound instead of x-ray for stone localization.

D. Open Surgical Removal of Stones

Endourologic intervention and ESWL have markedly decreased the indications for open surgery. Rarely, both percutaneous nephrolithotomy and ESWL are contraindicated, and open nephrolithotomy is necessary. The goal of any approach is to remove all stone fragments, and the approach chosen must allow for intraoperative localization by radiography or ultrasonography. Incisions into the renal pelvis (pyelolithotomy) or the renal parenchyma (radial nephrotomy or anatrophic nephrolithotomy) may be required for complete stone removal. Instillation of a mixture of thrombin and calcium into the kidney causes the fragments to become trapped in a dense clot, which is removed through a pyelotomy incision (coagulum pyelolithotomy). Operative nephroscopy allows a full view of all the calices and removal of all fragments. "Bench" surgery with autotransplantation of the kidney may be required in very few instances. Rarely, poorly functioning kidneys containing symptomatic stones require nephrectomy.

▶ Prognosis

The recurrence rate of renal stone can be as high as 40% and can be decreased with sufficient attention to measures for prevention of stone formation. The danger of recurrent stone is progressive renal damage due to obstruction and infection.

URETERAL STONE

ESSENTIALS OF DIAGNOSIS

- ▶ Severe ureterorenal colic.
- ▶ Hematuria.
- ▶ Nausea, vomiting, and ileus.
- ▶ Stone visible on excretory urography or spiral CT.

▶ General Considerations

Ureteral stones originate in the kidney. When symptoms occur, ureteral obstruction is implicit and renal function endangered. Complicating infection may occur. Most ureteral stones pass spontaneously, especially if they are less than 0.5 cm in greatest dimension.

▶ Clinical Findings

A. Symptoms and Signs

The onset of pain is usually abrupt. Pain is felt in the costovertebral angle and radiates to the ipsilateral lower abdominal quadrant. Nausea, vomiting, abdominal distention, and gross hematuria are common. When the stone approaches the bladder, symptoms mimic cystitis, with frequency and urgency. If the kidney is infected, acute ureteral obstruction exacerbates the infection.

The patient is usually in such agony that only parenteral opioids will give relief. Costovertebral angle tenderness and guarding may be evident. Absence of bowel sounds and abdominal distention signify ileus. Fever may occur as a result of complicating renal infection.

B. Laboratory Findings

Laboratory findings are the same as for renal stone.

C. Imaging Studies

Excretory urograms or spiral CT is essential. Plain films may reveal an opacity in the region of the ureter. Confirmation of ureteral location requires demonstration of confluence of stone and ureteral contrast. Spiral CT is diagnostic and is currently used as the first-line imaging modality (Figure 38–11). This procedure depicts the degree of obstruction and the size and position of the stone, information that permits selection of appropriate treatment. A radiolucent stone appears as a filling defect within a proximally dilated ureter—indistinguishable from a ureteral tumor or blood clot by intravenous urography. CT scan discriminates between stone and tumor or clot density. Cystoscopy, ureteral catheterization, retrograde urography, and ureteroscopy may also be helpful.

▶ Differential Diagnosis

A tumor of the kidney or renal pelvis may bleed, and passage of a blood clot may cause ureteral colic. Urograms may reveal a radiolucent area in the ureter surrounded by the radiopaque urine. A CT scan with and without contrast agents reveals no radiopacity in the ureter and helps define the renal parenchymal or renal pelvis tumor.

A primary tumor of the ureter may cause obstructing pain and hematuria. The urogram reveals the ureteral filling defect, often with secondary obstruction. A CT scan can differentiate a stone from tumor. Urinary cytologic study may reveal malignant urothelial cells.

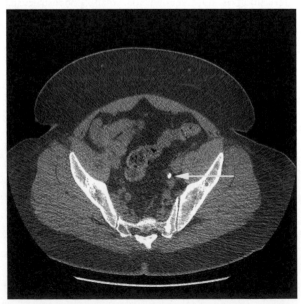

▲ **Figure 38–11.** CT scan without intravenous contrast demonstrating a left ureteral calculus (arrow).

Acute pyelonephritis may cause pain as severe as that seen with stone. Pyuria and bacteriuria are found but do not rule out stone. Stone is absent on noncontrast CT or urography.

A sloughed papilla (consequent to conditions such as diabetes mellitus) traversing the ureter may cause colic and produces a urogram compatible with uric acid stone. Papillary sloughs should be evident, however.

▶ Complications

If obstruction from the ureteral stone is prolonged, progressive renal damage may ensue. Bilateral stones may cause anuria, requiring immediate drainage of the proximal collecting system with indwelling ureteral catheters or percutaneous nephrostomy.

Infection may supervene, but many renal infections are iatrogenic (ie, introduced at the time of stone manipulation).

▶ Prevention

See Renal Stone.

▶ Treatment

A. General Measures

Most ureteral stones pass spontaneously—particularly those less than 0.5 cm in diameter. Once the diagnosis has been established, analgesics should be given and the patient hydrated. Recent reports have found alpha-blocker therapy useful in expulsion of distal ureteral stones by relaxing smooth muscle. Periodic plain films should be taken to follow the progress of the stone and interval renal ultrasound studies obtained to assess the degree of hydronephrosis. The urine should be strained until the stone passes in order to recover the calculus for analysis. With larger stones, acute obstruction can be temporarily relieved by inserting an indwelling ureteral stent.

B. Specific Measures

If the stone causes intractable pain, progressive hydronephrosis, or acute infection, it should be removed. Obstructing stones in the upper two thirds of the ureter can often be successfully treated by ureteroscopy or ESWL, with or without ureteral stent insertion to help facilitate stone passage. Ureteroscopy permits ultrasonic or laser fragmentation or stone basket retrieval under direct vision. Retrograde basket extraction under fluoroscopic control may be used to remove small distal ureteral stones. Open surgical removal (ureterolithotomy) is only very rarely required for ureteral stones. ESWL has been applied to ureteral stones in the proximal ureter but is more problematic in the distal ureter owing to bone interference by surrounding pelvis, which interferes with imaging and attenuates shock wave force.

▶ Prognosis

About 80% of ureteral stones pass spontaneously. Periodic plain films of the abdomen or excretory urograms portrays progress of the stone and warn of ensuing renal damage that would prompt operative intervention.

VESICAL STONE

Primary vesical calculi are rare in the United States but are common in Southeast Asia and the Middle East. The cause is probably dietary. Secondary stones usually complicate vesical outlet obstruction with residual urine and infection; 90% of those affected are men. Other causes of bladder stasis such as neurogenic bladder, and bladder diverticula also promote vesical stone formation. They are common in vesical schistosomiasis or in association with radiation cystitis. Foreign bodies in the bladder may act as a nidus for the precipitation of urinary salts. Most stones contain uric acid or struvite (in infected urine).

▶ Clinical Findings

A. Symptoms and Signs

Symptoms of bladder neck obstruction are elicited. There may be sudden interruption of the stream and urethral pain if a stone occludes the bladder neck during voiding. Hematuria is common. Vesical distention may be noted; evidence of urethral stricture or an enlarged prostate is usually found.

B. Laboratory Findings

Pyuria and hematuria are almost always present.

C. Imaging Studies

Vesical calculi may be missed on plain x-rays due to the high component of radiolucent uric acid. Excretory urograms reveal a filling defect in the bladder; residual urine is usually depicted on the postvoiding film. CT scan or ultrasound differentiates between stones and vesical tumors or blood clots, but direct vision endoscopically is preferred.

D. Instrumental Examination

Inability to pass a catheter into the bladder signifies urethral stricture. Catheterization may demonstrate residual urine. Cystoscopy visualizes the stones and may reveal an obstructing prostate.

▶ Differential Diagnosis

A pedunculated vesical tumor may suddenly occlude the vesical neck during voiding. Excretory urograms, pelvic ultrasound, CT scan, or cystoscopy leads to definitive diagnosis.

Extravesical opacifications may simulate stones on a plain film.

▶ Complications

Acting as foreign bodies, bladder stones exacerbate urine infection and foil antibiotic therapy given for the purpose of sterilizing the urine. Stones obstructing the urethra must be removed.

Prevention

Prevention requires relief of the primary obstruction, removal of the stones, and sterilization of the urine.

Treatment

A. General Measures

Analgesics should be given for pain and antimicrobials for control of infection until the stones can be removed.

B. Specific Measure

Small stones can be removed or crushed transurethrally (**cystolithalopaxy**). Larger stones are often disintegrated by transurethral electrohydraulic lithotripsy (shock wave–generating probe) or laser destruction, or they may require suprapubic transvesical removal (vesicolithotomy). Suprapubic prostatectomy helps address the cause of obstruction and provides access for open stone removal.

Prognosis

Recurrent vesical stone is uncommon if the obstruction and infection are treated.

NEPHROCALCINOSIS

Nephrocalcinosis is a precipitation of calcium in the tubules, parenchyma, and, occasionally, the glomeruli. It always causes renal functional impairment, often severe. Stones may be found in the calices and pelvis. The common causes are primary or secondary hyperparathyroidism, excessive milk-alkali or vitamin D intake, or they may be found with severe renal damage associated with renal tubular acidosis, or sarcoidosis. Calcifications may also be seen in the skin, lungs, stomach, spleen, and corneas, or around the joints.

Clinical Findings

A. Symptoms and Signs

There are no specific symptoms. In childhood, the patient may merely fail to thrive. Stones or sand may be passed. The complaints are usually those of the primary disease. Physical examination may reveal an enlarged parathyroid gland, corneal calcifications, and pseudorickets.

B. Laboratory Findings

The urine may be infected. In renal tubular acidosis, the pH is fixed between 6.0 and 7.0. Urinary calcium is high in hyperparathyroidism, both primary and secondary. Tests of renal function are depressed; uremia is common. Hypercalcemia and hypophosphatemia are seen with primary hyperparathyroidism; secondary hyperparathyroidism may be associated with a low serum calcium and an elevated serum phosphate. Hyperchloremic acidosis and hypokalemia accompany renal tubular acidosis.

C. Imaging Studies

A plain x-ray reveals punctate calcifications in the papillae of the kidneys. Caliceal or pelvic stones may also be noted. The pattern of calcification may have to be differentiated from renal tuberculosis and medullary sponge kidney.

Complications

Complications include renal damage caused by the calcifications and renal and ureteral calculi. Chronic renal infection may complicate the primary disease.

Treatment & Prognosis

The primary cause should be treated if possible (eg, parathyroidectomy). Hydration with isotonic saline along with furosemide can help enhance calcium excretion. Discontinue vitamin D and milk-alkali producers if the primary cause was due to excessive intake. With hyperchloremic acidosis, alkalinize the urine with potassium citrate. Osteomalacia requires administration of vitamin D and calcium even though nephrocalcinosis is present.

If nephrocalcinosis is secondary to primary renal disease, the outlook is poor. If the cause is correctable and renal function is fairly good, the prognosis is more favorable.

Borghi L et al: Comparison of two diets for the prevention of recurrent stones in idiopathic hypercalciuria. N Engl J Med 2002;346:77.

Borghi L et al: Medical treatment of nephrolithiasis. Endocrinol Metab Clin North Am 2002;31:1051.

Curhan GC: Epidemiology of stone disease. Urol Clin North Am 2007;34:287.

Park S, Pearle MS: Pathophysiology and management of calcium stones. Urol Clin North Am 2007;34:323.

Parsons JK et al: Efficacy of alpha-blockers for the treatment of ureteral stones. J Urol 2007;177:983.

Shine S: Urinary calculus: IVU vs. CT renal stone? A critically appraised topic. Abdom Imaging 2007;33:41.

Wen CC, Nakada SY: Treatment selection and outcomes: renal calculi. Urol Clin North Am 2007;34:409.

Wolf JS: Treatment selection and outcomes: ureteral calculi. Urol Clin North Am 2007;34:421.

GENITOURINARY TRACT TRAUMA

INJURIES TO THE KIDNEY

 ESSENTIALS OF DIAGNOSIS

- ▶ History or evidence of trauma, usually localized.
- ▶ Hematuria.
- ▶ Flank mass.
- ▶ Failure to opacify the kidney or extravasation of urine on excretory urography.

General Considerations

Renal injury is uncommon but potentially serious and often accompanied by multisystem trauma. The most common causes are athletic, industrial, or automobile accidents. The degree of injury may range from contusion to laceration of the parenchyma or disruption of the renal pedicle.

Clinical Findings

A. Symptoms and Signs

Gross hematuria following trauma means injury to the urinary tract. Pain and tenderness over the renal area may be significant but could be due to musculoskeletal injury. Hemorrhagic shock may result from renal laceration and lead to oliguria. Nausea, vomiting, and abdominal distention (ileus) are the rule. Physical examination may reveal ecchymosis or penetrating injury in the costovertebral angle or flank. Extravasation of blood or urine may produce a palpable flank mass. Other injuries should be sought.

B. Laboratory Findings

Serial hematocrit determinations will give clues to persistent bleeding. Hematuria is to be expected, but the absence of hematuria does not exclude renal injury (as in renal vascular injury).

C. Imaging Studies

A plain film may reveal obliteration of the psoas shadow; this suggests the presence of a retroperitoneal hematoma or urinary extravasation. Bowel gas may be displaced from the area. Evidence of transverse vertebral process or rib fractures may be noted. In the past, the excretory urogram was used for evaluating renal trauma. Excretory urograms may show a normal kidney if it is mildly contused or may show extravasation of contrast medium if the kidney is lacerated. Nonfunction suggests injury to the vascular pedicle. The excretory urogram should demonstrate that the contralateral kidney is normal. CT scan with intravenous contrast medium is now the method of choice for staging a patient with hemodynamically stable renal trauma. CT scans may miss urinary extravasation if performed too rapidly following intravenous contrast administration—before the contrast is excreted into the collecting system and ureter. If renal vascular damage is suspected and the patient's condition is stable, preoperative renal angiography may facilitate planning of renovascular reconstruction or permit arterial stenting. In special circumstances, selective renal artery embolization may control segmental arterial bleeding. Renal imaging is indicated in any adult with gross hematuria or microscopic hematuria with shock. Imaging is also required with deceleration injuries and is indicated in children with any hematuria of less than 50 red blood cells per high-power field.

Differential Diagnosis

Bony fractures or contusion of soft tissues in the region of the kidney may cause confusion. Hematuria might be secondary to vesical injury. The absence of a perirenal mass (ie, hematoma or urinoma) or contrast extravasation on urograms or CT scan would rule out significant trauma.

Complications

A. Early

The most serious complication is continued perirenal hemorrhage, which may be fatal. Serial hematocrit, blood pressure, and pulse determinations are essential. Serial CT scans may also be useful. Evidence of an enlarging flank mass implies persistent bleeding. In most cases, bleeding stops spontaneously, probably as a result of tamponade by the perirenal fascia. Delayed bleeding 1 or 2 weeks later is rare. Infection of the perirenal hematoma may occur.

B. Late

Ultrasound should be obtained 1 to 3 months after management of renal trauma to look for progressive hydronephrosis from ureteral obstruction. The blood pressure should be checked at regular intervals, because hypertension may be a late sequela.

Treatment

Treat shock and hemorrhage with fluids and transfusion. Most patients with blunt renal trauma stop bleeding and heal spontaneously. Bed rest is indicated until hematuria resolves. If bleeding persists, laparotomy is indicated.

Penetrating renal trauma requires exploration. Lacerations may be sutured, the collecting system closed, and urinary extravasation drained. Nephrectomy or partial nephrectomy may be necessary to remove devitalized tissue and secure the collecting system.

Late complications may occur. Perinephric abscess should be drained. Hypertension due to renal ischemia requires vascular reconstruction or nephrectomy.

Prognosis

Most injured kidneys heal spontaneously, though the patient must be examined at intervals for the onset of hypertension due to renal ischemia or progressive hydronephrosis due to secondary ureteral stricture. Many patients with genitourinary trauma have associated injuries. In most cases, death is due to associated injury rather than renal injury.

INJURIES TO THE URETER

ESSENTIALS OF DIAGNOSIS

► Anuria or oliguria; prolonged ileus or flank pain following pelvic operation.

► Onset of urinary drainage through wound or vagina.

► Demonstration of urinary extravasation or ureteral obstruction by urography.

General Considerations

Most ureteral injuries are iatrogenic in the course of pelvic surgery. Ureteral injury may occur during transurethral bladder or prostate resection or ureteral manipulation for stone or tumor. Ureteral injury is rarely a consequence of penetrating trauma. Unintentional ureteral ligation during operation on adjacent organs may be asymptomatic, though hydronephrosis and loss of renal function results. Ureteral division leads to extravasation and ureterocutaneous fistula.

Clinical Findings

A. Symptoms

If the ureteral injury is not recognized at surgery, the patient may complain of flank and lower abdominal pain on the injured side. Ileus and pyelonephritis may develop. Later, urine may drain through the wound (or through the vagina following transvaginal surgery). Wound drainage may be evaluated by comparing creatinine levels found in the drainage fluid with serum levels: Urine exhibits very high creatinine levels when compared with serum. Intravenous administration of 5 mL of indigo carmine causes the urine to appear blue-green; therefore, drainage from a ureterocutaneous fistula becomes blue, compared to serous drainage. Anuria following pelvic surgery not responding to intravenous fluids means bilateral ureteral ligation until proved otherwise. Peritoneal signs may occur if urine leaks into the peritoneal cavity.

B. Laboratory Findings

Microscopic hematuria is usually found but may be absent. Tests of renal function may be normal unless both ureters are occluded.

C. Imaging Studies

Excretory urograms may show evidence of ureteral occlusion. Extravasation of radiopaque fluid may be seen in the region of the ureter. Retrograde ureterography depicts the site and nature (occlusion or division) of the injury.

Ultrasonography may reveal hydroureter and hydronephrosis or a fluid mass representing urinary extravasation. Radionuclide scanning shows delayed excretion, with an accumulation of counts in the pelvis and renal parenchyma resulting from ureteral obstruction; although urinary extravasation is detected, anatomic specificity for site of injury is not clearly defined.

Differential Diagnosis

Ureteral injury may mimic peritonitis if urine leaks into the peritoneal cavity. Excretory urography reveals the ureteral involvement.

Oliguria may be due to dehydration, transfusion reaction, or bilateral incomplete ureteral injury. A survey of fluid and electrolyte intake and output, including serial body weights,

should prove definitive. Total anuria implies bilateral ureteral injury and indicates the need for immediate urologic investigation.

Vesicovaginal and ureterovaginal fistulas may be confused. Methylene blue solution instilled into the bladder stains the drainage of a vesicovaginal fistula. Cystoscopy may show the vesical defect. Retrograde ureterography should reveal a ureteral fistula. The presence of both injuries occurring simultaneously should also be considered and evaluated.

Complications

These include urinary fistula, ureteral obstruction or stenosis with hydronephrosis, renal infection, peritonitis, and uremia (with bilateral injury).

Prevention

Before operation for large pelvic masses, which may cause displacement of the ureters, catheters should be placed in the ureters to facilitate their identification at surgery. Although the catheters may not prevent injury, they facilitate recognition of a ureteral injury.

Treatment

A. Injury Recognized at Surgery

1. Ureteral division—Repair of a ureter inadvertently cut during surgery consists of anastomosis of the ends over an indwelling stent (**ureteroureterostomy**), reimplanting the ureter into the bladder if the injury is juxtavesical (**neoureterocystostomy**), or anastomosing the proximal segment of divided ureter to the side of the contralateral ureter (**transureteroureterostomy**). The anastomosis must be tension free, and the area of repair must be drained.

2. Ureteral resection—Repair of a ureter from which a substantial segment has been removed requires interposition of a ureteral substitute or mobilization of the proximal and distal ureter to provide a tension-free anastomosis. With loss of the distal ureter, the bladder may be hitched cephalad to the psoas muscle, or a bladder flap may be created to facilitate a ureteral implant. In extreme cases, autotransplant of the kidney to the pelvis may be necessary.

B. Injury Discovered after Surgery

Early reoperation is recommended. Depending on the findings, any of the procedures noted above may be utilized. If a long segment of ureter is not viable, an intestinal ureter may be constructed. If hydronephrosis is advanced or if sepsis develops, percutaneous nephrostomy should precede repair. When the patient's condition is stable, definitive repair can be accomplished. Nephrectomy may be indicated if the contralateral kidney is normal and there is a contraindication to transureteroureterostomy (such as calculi or upper tract transitional cell carcinoma).

Prognosis

In cases of iatrogenic injury, the results are best if the injury is recognized at the time of surgery. Late repair, if severe periureteral fibrosis has developed, is less likely to afford a good outcome.

INJURIES TO THE BLADDER

 ESSENTIALS OF DIAGNOSIS

▶ History of trauma (including surgical or endoscopic).
▶ Fracture of the pelvis.
▶ Suprapubic pain and abdominal muscle rigidity.
▶ Hematuria.
▶ Extravasation shown on cystogram.

General Considerations

The most common cause of vesical injury is an external blow over a full bladder. Rupture of the organ is seen in 15% of patients with pelvic fracture. The bladder may be inadvertently opened during pelvic surgery or injured by cystoscopic maneuvers (eg, transurethral resection of bladder tumor). If the injury is intraperitoneal (40% of all bladder ruptures), blood and urine will extravasate into the peritoneal cavity, producing signs of peritonitis. If it is extraperitoneal (54% of all bladder ruptures), a mass develops in the pelvis. About 6% of all bladder ruptures have a combination of both intraperitoneal and extraperitoneal extravasation.

Clinical Findings

A. Symptoms and Signs

There is usually a history of hypogastric or pelvic trauma. Hematuria and suprapubic pain and an inability to void are expected. Associated injury may cause hemorrhagic shock. There is suprapubic tenderness and guarding. Intraperitoneal extravasation causes peritoneal signs, while extraperitoneal extravasation results in formation of a pelvic urinoma.

B. Laboratory Findings

A falling hematocrit reflects continued bleeding. Hematuria is expected in patients who are able to void. A patient who cannot void should be catheterized unless pelvic fracture (and urethral injury) is suspected or blood is noted at the urethral meatus.

C. Imaging Studies

A plain film may reveal fracture of the pelvis. An extraperitoneal collection of blood and urine may displace the bowel gas laterally or out of the pelvis. If bladder trauma is suspected, cystography should precede excretory urography. Extravasation is most reliably demonstrated by a postdrainage cystogram film. If one suspects urethral trauma, a retrograde urethrogram should precede catheter insertion. The excretory urogram may suggest the diagnosis of bladder perforation but by itself is insufficient to exclude bladder injury. A CT cystogram can be used, but images of the bladder obtained by passive bladder filling after catheter clamping are not sufficient to exclude a bladder injury. The bladder should be filled to capacity by gravity with diluted contrast (350–400 mL), a pelvic x-ray taken, and then the bladder should be emptied and another pelvic x-ray taken. This method should identify even subtle leaks.

Differential Diagnosis

Renal injury is also associated with bladder trauma and usually presents with hematuria. Excretory urograms show changes compatible with renal trauma; the cystogram is negative.

Injury to the membranous urethra can mimic extraperitoneal rupture of the bladder. A urethrogram reveals the site of injury. Urethral disruption is a contraindication to urethral catheterization.

Complications

Extraperitoneal extravasation may lead to pelvic abscess. Intraperitoneal extravasation causes delayed peritonitis, oliguria, and azotemia.

Treatment

Treat shock, hemorrhage, and other life-threatening injuries. Marked extraperitoneal extravasation should be drained, the bladder decompressed by either a suprapubic or urethral catheter, and appropriate antibiotics administered. Small extraperitoneal extravasations are treated nonoperatively by urethral catheter.

Intraperitoneal extravasation of bladder urine requires exploratory laparotomy, midline cystotomy, bladder closure, and bladder catheter drainage. Penetrating injuries (ie, gunshot, stabbing) require exploration and closure of the bladder. The ureters should also be evaluated in all cases of bladder injury by preoperative imaging or intraoperative assessment, which may be done by injecting indigo carmine and looking for ureteral extravasation or by retrograde passage of 5F feeding tubes through the ureteral orifice.

Prognosis

Early diagnosis minimizes morbidity and mortality rates. The prognosis depends chiefly on the severity of associated injuries.

INJURIES TO THE URETHRA

Membranous Urethra

Injury to the membranous urethra is usually a consequence of pelvic fracture and thus is associated with hemorrhage and multiorgan injury. The mechanism of injury is blunt trauma and deceleration resulting in shearing forces applied to the prostate and urogenital diaphragm. Penetrating injuries result from external missiles or laceration by bone fragments acting as secondary projectiles.

If the urethral disruption is incomplete, the patient may be able to void, and hematuria would be inevitable. Urethral injury is suspected if blood is expressed from the urethral meatus. In cases of complete avulsion, extravasation causes a suprapubic mass. Rectal examination may reveal a nonpalpable or upwardly displaced prostate.

X-ray reveals a fractured pelvis; urethrography delineates any extravasation, and cystography identifies an associated bladder injury. An immediate excretory urogram or CT scan should be obtained in all cases to assess kidney and ureteral function.

Treatment must be coordinated with care of associated injury. Once a membranous urethral injury with urinary extravasation has been identified, suprapubic cystostomy should be performed either at the time of laparotomy or percutaneously before placement of external pelvic fixation. Definitive urethral repair may be delayed until the patient has recovered from the acute injury and pelvic fractures have healed. Occasionally, when urethral disruption is incomplete, late repair is unnecessary. Primary repair may be indicated in cases of severe prostatomembranous dislocation, major bladder neck laceration, or concomitant pelvic vascular or rectal injury.

Late sequelae are urethral stricture, impotence, and incontinence. Urethral stricture must be identified by retrograde urethrography and may be treated by transurethral incision of the stricture or urethroplasty. Impotence due to injury of nerves to the corpora cavernosa that course adjacent to the membranous urethra may resolve without treatment during the year following injury. Vascular injury of the hypogastric or pudendal arteries may cause impotence following trauma. Cavernosometry and arteriography confirms the diagnosis; appropriate treatment may include vascular reconstruction. Incontinence depends on the neurologic status of the patient. Medical or surgical therapy is utilized to increase bladder capacity and bladder outlet resistance.

Bulbous Urethra

The bulbous urethra may be injured as a result of instrumentation or, more commonly, falling astride an object (straddle injury). Urethral contusion may cause a perineal hematoma without injury to the urethral wall. Laceration leads to urinary extravasation.

Perineal pain and some urethral bleeding are to be expected. Sudden swelling in the perineum may develop following attempted urination. Examination reveals a perineal mass; swelling due to extravasation of blood and urine involves the penis and scrotum and may spread onto the abdominal wall.

If the patient can void well and the perineal hematoma is small, no treatment is necessary. If urethrography reveals significant extravasation, suprapubic cystostomy should be performed. Minor injury without extravasation (contusion, compression by hematoma) may be managed by careful insertion of a urethral catheter.

The only serious complication is stricture, which requires subsequent internal urethrotomy or surgical repair.

Pendulous Urethra

External injury to this portion of the urethra is not common, since the penis is so mobile. The erect organ, however, is vulnerable. Most trauma to this area is secondary to instrumentation or sex play. As a rule, these injuries are mild, although a few may be complicated by stricture.

Urethral bleeding and penile swelling are to be expected. A urethrogram reveals the site and severity of injury.

If voiding is normal, no treatment is required. A large hematoma may require drainage. If significant injury is present, a suprapubic tube should be inserted and delayed surgical repair performed after swelling and inflammation have resolved.

INJURIES TO THE PENIS

Mechanisms of penile injury include penetration, blunt trauma to the erect penis during sexual activity (eg, fracture of corpora cavernosa), avulsion of skin, and amputation.

Tourniquet injury is also uncommon; the circumferential compression may be due to a rubber band, a steel ring, string, or a hair and may be exacerbated by subsequent erection. The tourniquet may have been applied unintentionally, but child abuse cases have been reported in which the penis has been ligated as punishment for enuresis.

Treatment includes assessment and care of urethral injuries if present. Removal of tourniquet, split-thickness skin grafting of avulsion injuries, and primary closure of corporal lacerations are principles of therapy. The penis may be acutely reimplanted up to 16 hours following amputation using microsurgical techniques.

INJURIES TO THE SCROTUM & TESTIS

Avulsion of the scrotal skin may require a meshed split-thickness skin graft. If the avulsion is severe, involving the skin and dartos muscle, then the testes may be implanted in the subcutaneous tissue of the thigh and dressed outside the wound with 0.25% acetic acid-soaked gauze. Scrotal reconstruction is performed at a later time, frequently by using skin grafts.

Penetrating trauma rarely injures the mobile testes. Lacerations should be explored, debrided, and closed primarily.

If hemorrhage into the tunica vaginalis is noted, drainage is indicated.

Blunt trauma to the testes may cause contusion or rupture. Rupture of the tunica albuginea may be demonstrated by ultrasonography as abnormal echotexture of the parenchyma. In cases of rupture, scrotal exploration allows debridement and closure of the tunica albuginea. The testes may ultimately undergo atrophy despite these efforts.

Gomez RG et al: Consensus statement on bladder injuries. Br J Urol 2004;94:27.

Morey AF et al: Reconstruction of posterior urethral disruption injuries: outcome analysis in 82 patients. J Urol 1997;157:506.

Santucci RA et al: Evaluation and management of renal injuries: statement of the Renal Trauma Subcommittee. Br J Urol (Int) 2004;93:937.

Wessels H et al: Criteria for nonoperative treatment of significant penetrating renal lacerations. J Urol 1997;157:24.

▼ TUMORS OF THE GENITOURINARY TRACT

Tumors of the genitourinary tract are among the most common neoplastic diseases found in adults. Prostate cancer, for example, is the most common cancer in men (33%), and renal and bladder cancer account for nearly 10% of all malignant tumors in men, but only about 3% in women. Even though excellent diagnostic methods are available, one third of all genitourinary tumors are not found until regional or distant spread has occurred. Advances in diagnosis and treatment of genitourinary tract tumors have occurred in recent years, and the prognosis has improved in conditions such as Wilms' tumor, testicular cancer, and bladder cancer. The mainstay of diagnosis continues to be physical examination, complete urinalysis, intravenous urography or CT, and cystoscopy whenever indicated. Curative treatment of these tumors continues to be surgical in most instances.

RENAL ADENOCARCINOMA (RENAL CELL CARCINOMA)

ESSENTIALS OF DIAGNOSIS

▶ Painless gross or microscopic total hematuria.

▶ Solid renal parenchymal mass on intravenous urography with nephrotomograms, renal ultrasound, or abdominal CT scan.

▶ Paraneoplastic syndromes common.

▶ General Considerations

Malignant tumors of the kidney account for approximately 3% of all tumors in adults. Often, the diagnosis is suspected because of microscopic hematuria or manifestations of

metastases such as pathologic fractures or superficial skin nodules. The cause is unknown, though risk factors include cigarette smoking, obesity, and hypertension. The disease occurs in men three times more commonly than in women. A suppressor gene on chromosome 3p has been shown to be present in von Hippel-Lindau renal cancers as well as in most sporadic renal adenocarcinomas. The most common cell type is clear cell (also called conventional) carcinoma, accounting for 70% to 80% of renal carcinomas. The cell of origin is in the proximal convoluted tubule. Other cell types include papillary (10–15%), chromophobe (3–5%), and collecting duct renal carcinoma (1%). The tumor metastasizes commonly to the lungs (50–60%), adjacent renal hilar lymph nodes (25%), ipsilateral adrenal (12%), opposite kidney (2%), and lytic lesions in mainly long bones (30–40%).

Numerous conditions predispose to renal cell cancer, including von Hippel-Lindau syndrome (cerebellar hemangioblastomas, retinal angiomatosis, and bilateral renal cell carcinoma), tuberous sclerosis, and acquired renal cystic disease developing in patients with end-stage renal disease. Paraneoplastic syndromes are common in renal cell carcinoma and are often what suggests the diagnosis, yet they rarely have prognostic significance. These syndromes include hypercalcemia, erythrocytosis, hypertension, fever of unknown origin, anemia, and hepatopathy (**Stauffer's syndrome**). Renal cell carcinoma has a predilection for producing occlusive tumor thrombi in the renal vein and the inferior vena cava (particularly from the right), manifested by signs of lower extremity edema and acute scrotal varicocele when occluding the left renal vein. This phenomenon of inferior vena cava thrombus occurs in approximately 5% to 10% of patients. Occasionally, the tumor thrombus reaches up through the inferior vena cava to the right atrium.

▶ Clinical Findings

A. Symptoms and Signs

Painless gross or microscopic hematuria throughout the urinary stream ("total hematuria") occurs in 60% of patients. The degree of hematuria is not necessarily related to the size or stage of the tumor. Although a triad of hematuria, flank pain, and a palpable flank mass suggests renal cell carcinoma, fewer than 10% of patients will so present. Both pain and a palpable mass are late events occurring only with tumors that are very large or invade surrounding structures or when hemorrhage into the tumor has occurred. Symptoms due to metastases may be the initial complaint (eg, bone pain, respiratory distress).

B. Laboratory Findings

Microscopic urinalysis reveals hematuria in most patients. The erythrocyte sedimentation rate may be elevated but is nonspecific. Elevation of the hematocrit and levels of serum calcium, alkaline phosphatase, and aminotransferases occur in less than 10% of patients. These findings nearly always resolve with curative nephrectomy and thus are not usually signs of metastases. Anemia unrelated to blood loss occurs in 20% to 40% of patients, particularly those with advanced disease.

C. Imaging Studies

The diagnosis of renal cell carcinoma is often made by CT (and, less frequently, by intravenous urography) performed as an initial step in the workup of hematuria, an enigmatic metastatic lesion, or suspicious laboratory findings (Figure 38–12). Ultrasonography and CT scan often reveal incidental renal masses, which now account for 50% of the initial diagnoses of renal cancer in patients without manifestations of renal disease. Plain abdominal x-rays may reveal a calcified renal mass, but only 20% of renal masses contain demonstrable calcification. (Twenty percent of masses with peripheral calcification are malignant; over 80% with central calcification are malignant.) The initial technique for workup of hematuria is currently CT urography; intravenous urography alone defines only 75% of renal mass lesions. Differentiation of the most common renal mass (ie, a simple benign cyst) can be made by the finding of a radiolucent center with a thin wall and a sharp interface between the mass and the renal cortex (the typical "beak sign" of a cortical cyst).

1. Ultrasonography—Further definition of all renal masses seen on intravenous urography is required. Occasionally, some masses detected on CT require further characterization by ultrasound. Abdominal ultrasonography can define the mass as a benign simple cyst or a solid mass in 90% to 95% of cases. Abdominal ultrasound can also identify a vena caval tumor thrombus and its cephalad extent in the cava.

2. Isotope scanning—Occasionally, a renal mass is suspected on intravenous urography but is equivocal or not seen on ultrasound. In these cases, a renal cortical isotope scanning agent such as technetium-99m DMSA is helpful. Isotope scans of a renal tumor or cyst show an area of decreased uptake, whereas an area of increased uptake indicates a renal "pseudotumor" or a hypertrophied column of Bertin.

3. CT scan—CT scan is the diagnostic procedure of choice when a solid renal mass is noted on ultrasound. CT scan accurately delineates renal cell carcinoma in over 95% of cases. Over 80% of tumors are enhanced by iodinated contrast medium, reflecting their high vascularity.

CT scan is also helpful in local staging and can reveal tumor penetration of perinephric fat; enlargement of local hilar lymph nodes, indicating metastases; or tumor thrombi in the renal vein or inferior vena cava. CT angiography can delineate the renal vasculature, which is helpful in surgical planning for partial nephrectomies.

4. MRI—MRI is not more accurate than CT and is much more expensive. It is, however, the most accurate noninvasive means of detecting renal vein or vena caval thrombi. With the further refinement of pulse sequencing and the use

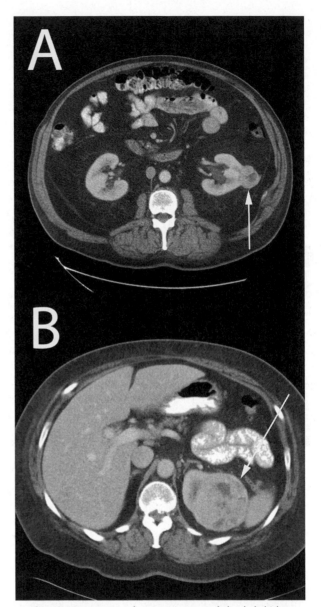

▲ **Figure 38–12. A:** Adenocarcinoma of the left kidney. CT scan of the abdomen shows an exophytic lesion from the midpolar kidney (arrow). **B:** CT scan showing a large left renal mass (arrow) incidentally found on imaging done to evaluate nonspecific abdominal pain. Final pathology revealed clear cell renal carcinoma.

of paramagnetic contrast agents, MRI has become one of the primary techniques for staging solid renal masses. Magnetic resonance angiography (MRA) has become particularly useful for mapping the blood supply and the relationship to adjacent structures in candidates for partial nephrectomy.

D. Other Diagnostic or Staging Techniques

Isotopic bone scanning is useful in patients with bone pain, elevated alkaline phosphatase, or known metastases. Chest x-ray is sufficient if negative, but if equivocal, then CT scan of the chest can be used to detect metastases. There are currently no tumor markers specific for renal cell carcinoma. Occasionally, aspiration cytology of the mass can be useful in an enigmatic case. Previously, such procedures were discouraged because of fear of disseminating the tumor along the needle tract, but this has proved to be rare, and the technique is safe. The diagnosis is most often made by noninvasive means, and needle aspiration is required only in indeterminate cases ($< 10\%$).

▶ Differential Diagnosis

A variety of lesions in the retroperitoneum and kidney other than renal cysts may simulate renal cancer. These include lesions due to hydronephrosis, adult polycystic kidney disease, tuberculosis, xanthogranulomatous pyelonephritis, metastatic cancer from another primary cancer, angiomyolipoma or other benign renal tumors, or adrenal cancer and retroperitoneal lipomas, sarcomas, or abscesses. In general, the radiographic, MRI, or ultrasonographic techniques described previously should make the differentiation. Hematuria may be caused by renal, ureteral, or bladder calculi; renal pelvis, ureteral, or bladder tumors; or many other benign conditions usually delineated by the studies described. Cystoscopy is obligatory in hematuric patients with a normal CT scan or intravenous urogram to rule out disease of the bladder and to determine the source of the hematuria.

▶ Complications

Occasionally, patients may present with acute flank pain secondary to hemorrhage within a tumor or colic secondary to obstructing ureteral clots. Tumor in the renal vein or vena cava may cause an acute left varicocele or lower extremity edema associated with proteinuria. Pathologic fractures due to osteolytic metastases in long bones are common, as are symptomatic brain metastases.

▶ Treatment

Staging is the key to designing the treatment plan (Table 38–1). Patients with disease confined within the renal fascia (Gerota's fascia) or limited to nonadherent renal vein or vena caval tumor thrombi (stages T1, T2, and T3a) are best treated by radical nephrectomy. This involves en bloc removal of the kidney and surrounding Gerota fascia (including the ipsilateral adrenal), the renal hilar lymph nodes, and the proximal half of the ureter. Para-aortic node dissection has not been proven beneficial and is not routinely performed. In patients with very large tumors and a normal contralateral kidney, radical nephrectomy is recommended. Recent reports have advocated including the ipsilateral adrenal gland in the resection only in

Table 38–1. TNM Staging Classification and Prognosis of Renal Cell Cancer.

Robson Stage	T	N	M	5-Year Survival (%)
I. Tumor confined by renal capsule	T1 (< 7.0 cm tumor) T2 (> 7.0 cm tumor)	N0 (nodes negative)	M0 (no distant metastases)	80–100
II. Tumor extension to perirenal fat or ipsilateral adrenal but confined by Gerota's fascia	T3a	N0	M0	50–60
IIIa. Renal vein or inferior vena cava involvement	T3b (renal vein involvement) T3c (renal vein and caval involvement below the diaphragm) T4b (caval involvement above the diaphragm)	N0	M0	50–60 (renal vein) 25–35 (vena cava)
IIIb. Lymphatic involvement	T1–3	N1 (single regional node involved) N2 (multiple regional, contralateral, or bilateral nodes involved)	M0	15–35
IIIc. Combination of IIIa and IIIb	T3–4	N1–2	M0	15–35
IVa. Spread to contiguous organs except ipsilateral adrenal	T4	N1–2	M0	0–5
IVb. Distant metastases	T1–4	N0–2	M1	0–5

cases where the mass is large or involving the upper pole of the kidney. Patients with tumors in solitary kidneys, those with diabetes mellitus or renal insufficiency, and those with tumors under 4 cm (even with a normal opposite kidney) should be considered for partial nephrectomy because the prognosis in such cases (if negative surgical margins are obtained) is the same as that of radical nephrectomy. Laparoscopic radical or partial nephrectomy has been advocated as a method equal to the open approach with the advantages of less blood loss, shorter hospitalization, and earlier return to normal function. It is the gold standard in institutions with appropriate expertise. Laparoscopic or percutaneous cryoablation of renal cancer has also shown considerable promise. Alternatively, radiofrequency ablation has been utilized for small renal tumors, but this procedure requires more definitive study and longer follow-up in treated patients.

Nephrectomy has not been associated with improved survival rates in patients with multiple distant metastases (stage IV), and the procedure is not recommended unless patients are symptomatic or a promising therapeutic protocol is being studied. Flanigan and others have shown, however, that up to a 6-month improvement in survival can be achieved with nephrectomy—even with soft tissue metastasis—in selected patients who also receive interferon alfa. Patients with solitary pulmonary metastases have benefited from joint surgical removal of both the primary lesion and the metastatic lesion (30% survival at 5 years). Preoperative arterial embolization in patients with or without metastases does not improve survival rates, though it may be helpful as a single treatment measure in patients with symptomatic but nonresectable primary lesions. Radiation therapy is of little benefit except as treatment for symptomatic bone metastases. Medroxyprogesterone for metastatic renal cell carcinoma has given an equivocal 5% to 10% response rate of short duration. Vinblastine has also had a response rate of approximately 20%, again of minimal duration. There are no other cytotoxic chemotherapeutic agents of benefit.

Immunotherapy with interferon alfa has had a 15% to 20% response rate. Other interferons, alone (interferon beta, interferon gamma) or in combination with chemotherapeutic agents, have been less effective than interferon alfa. Adoptive immunotherapy—using lymphocytes (lymphokine-activated killer cells) from exposure of the patient's own peripheral blood lymphocytes to interleukin-2 (IL-2) in vitro followed by reinfusion into the patient along with systemic IL-2 infusion—has shown up to 33% objective response rates. High-dose intravenous IL-2 causes a profound capillary leak syndrome and substantial toxicity. Subsequent studies have shown only a 16% response rate.

Recent advances in research on the von Hippel-Lindau tumor suppressor gene has led to identification of growth factors including vascular endothelial growth factor (VEGF) and platelet-derived growth factor as molecular targets in treating advanced renal cancer. Initial studies using bevacizumab, an anti–vascular endothelial growth factor antibody, have shown promising results. Sorafenib, a tyrosine kinase inhibitor that blocks the pathway leading to the production of several growth factors, has been studied in patients with metastatic renal cancer and shown longer median progression-free survival than placebo (24 weeks vs 6 weeks). Sunitinib, another tyrosine kinase inhibitor, has shown longer progression-free survival and higher response rates than interferon alfa in patients with metastatic renal cancer. These oral agents are currently used as first-line therapy in this group of patients.

Temsirolimus is another targeted agent that is a specific inhibitor of the mammalian target of rapamycin kinase (mTOR inhibitor) and has shown promising results. It is now used as first-line therapy in poor prognosis patients. Many other agents are currently being studied.

▶ **Prognosis**

Patients with localized renal cancer (stages T1, T2, and T3a) treated surgically have 5-year survival rates of approximately 70% to 80%, whereas rates for those with local nodal extension or distant metastases are 15% to 25% and less than 10%, respectively. Most patients who present with multiple distant metastases succumb to disease within 15 months (Table 38–1). The advent of new agents for renal cancer may improve the outcome in these patients.

RENAL SARCOMA

Renal sarcomas include rhabdomyosarcoma, liposarcoma, fibrosarcoma, and leiomyosarcoma; the latter is the most common, though all are very uncommon. Sarcomas are highly malignant and are usually detected at a late stage and thus have a poor prognosis. The diagnostic approach is similar to that of renal cell carcinoma. The histology of the lesion is rarely suspected preoperatively. These tumors have a tendency to surround the renal vasculature and do not exhibit neovascularity on MRA.

Treatment is surgical, with wide local excision; however, local recurrence and subsequent distant metastases are the rule. There is no therapy of proved benefit for metastatic disease.

SECONDARY MALIGNANT RENAL TUMORS

Metastatic tumors to the kidney are more common than primary renal tumors and often develop from primary tumors of distant sites, most commonly the lung, stomach, and breast. It is rare for the diagnosis to be made before autopsy; this suggests that renal metastasis is a late event. There are usually no symptoms, though microscopic hematuria occurs in 10% to 20% of cases. Intravenous urograms may be normal, since the tumors are located peripherally in the parenchyma. Contiguous spread of a tumor adjacent to the kidney is not infrequent (eg, tumors of the adrenal, colon, and pancreas and retroperitoneal sarcomas). Tumors such as lymphoma, leukemia, and multiple myeloma may also infiltrate the kidney.

Routine radiologic, hematologic, and chemical examinations should demonstrate the primary tumor in most cases.

BENIGN RENAL TUMORS

▶ Renal Adenoma

Renal adenoma is the most common benign solid parenchymal lesion. Tumors less than 3 cm in diameter have been considered benign and those larger than 3 cm malignant; however, small lesions are not histologically distinguishable from renal adenocarcinomas, and the biology cannot be predicted preoperatively. These tumors should be considered potentially malignant and should be treated aggressively.

▶ Renal Oncocytoma

Renal oncocytomas are benign renal neoplasms. The tumors are generally asymptomatic and not associated with the paraneoplastic syndromes. The finding of a central stellate scar on CT or a spoke-wheel pattern of feeding arteries on angiography may suggest the diagnosis, although these findings have been found to be unreliable. Oncocytomas can coexist with renal carcinoma in the same lesion or in other lesions in the same kidney (7–30%). This finding, along with difficulty differentiating oncocytoma from clear cell or chromophobe renal cancers on fine-needle aspirates, make it difficult to make a definitive diagnosis preoperatively. Consequently, definitive treatment of these lesions with radical or partial nephrectomy or with thermal or cryoablation have been recommended.

▶ Mesoblastic Nephroma

Mesoblastic nephroma is a benign congenital renal tumor seen in early childhood, which must be distinguished from the highly malignant nephroblastoma, or Wilms' tumor. Unlike Wilms tumor, mesoblastic nephroma is commonly diagnosed within the first few months of life. Histologically, it is distinguished from Wilms tumor by cells resembling fibroblasts or smooth muscle cells and by the lack of epithelial elements. The prognosis is excellent; complete surgical resection is curative, and neither chemotherapy nor radiotherapy is required.

▶ Angiomyolipoma

Angiomyolipoma is a benign hamartoma seen most often bilaterally in adults with tuberous sclerosis (which also includes adenoma sebaceum, epilepsy, and mental retardation). The tumor is also common in middle-aged women, but only unilaterally. These tumors can be detected following spontaneous retroperitoneal hemorrhage, though 50% of these lesions are currently diagnosed incidentally. CT scan can be diagnostic, with negative Hounsfield units detected in the fat-containing area of the tumor. Occasionally, an angiomyolipoma eludes diagnosis preoperatively and requires nephrectomy (especially the lipid-poor angiomyolipoma). Asymptomatic patients with small (< 4 cm) tumors and typical findings on CT scan of fat within the tumor do not require surgery, as the prognosis is excellent without treatment. These patients can be followed with serial imaging. Those presenting with a retroperitoneal hemorrhage or a size greater than 4 cm should have the tumor removed surgically or with partial nephrectomy or via angioinfarction, which has been shown to be effective.

▶ Other Benign Renal Tumors

Other benign renal tumors include (1) **fibroma,** a renal parenchymal capsular or perinephric fibrous mass; (2) **lipoma,** an adipose deposit within or around the kidney, often perihilar or within the renal sinus; (3) **leiomyoma,** a common retroperitoneal tumor that may arise from the renal capsule or renal vascular walls; and (4) **hemangioma,** which is occasionally found to be the elusive cause of hematuria. Hemangiomas are generally quite small, and the diagnosis can be confirmed by direct vision of the lesion in the renal collecting system on ureteroscopy.

Hudes G et al: Temsirolimus, interferon alfa, or both for advanced renal-cell carcinoma. New Eng J Med 2007;356:2271.

Jemal A et al: Cancer statistics, 2007. CA Cancer J Clin 2007;57:43.

Klingler HC: Kidney cancer: energy ablation. Curr Opin Urol 2007;17:322.

Motzer RJ, Bukowski RM: Targeted therapy for metastatic renal cell carcinoma. J Clin Oncol 2006;24:5601.

Motzer RJ et al: Sunitinib versus interferon alfa in metastatic renal-cell carcinoma. New Eng J Med 2007;356:115.

Pantuck AJ et al: Incidental renal tumors. Urology 2000;56:190.

Parton M et al: Role of cytokine therapy in 2006 and beyond for metastatic renal cell cancer. J Clin Oncol 2006;24:5584.

Portis AJ, Clayman RV: Should laparoscopy be the standard approach used for radical nephrectomy? Curr Urol Rep 2001;2:165.

Ratain MS et al: Phase II placebo-controlled randomized discontinuation trial of sorafenib in patients with metastatic renal cell carcinoma. J Clin Oncol 2006;24:2505.

Siemer S et al: Adrenal metastases in 1635 patients with renal cell carcinoma: outcome and indication for adrenalectomy. J Urol 2004;171:2155.

Thiel DD, Winfield HN: State-of-the-art surgical management of renal cell carcinoma. Expert Rev Anticancer Ther 2007;7:1285.

Van Poppel H: Partial nephrectomy: the standard approach for small renal cell carcinoma? Curr Opin Urol 2003;13:431.

Yang JC et al: A randomized trial of bevacizumab, an anti-vascular endothelial growth factor antibody, for metastatic renal cancer. New Eng J Med 2003;349:427.

TUMORS OF THE RENAL PELVIS & CALICES

ESSENTIALS OF DIAGNOSIS

▶ Gross or microscopic hematuria.

▶ Radiolucent filling defect in the renal pelvis or the calices on intravenous urography or CT.

▶ Malignant cells on urine cytologic study.

General Considerations

In over 90% of cases, tumors involving the collecting system of the kidney are urothelial (or transitional cell) carcinomas. Less than 5% of tumors in this location are squamous carcinomas (often in association with chronic inflammation and stone formation) or adenocarcinomas. The cause of urothelial carcinoma of the upper urinary tract is similar to that of epithelial tumors in the ureter or bladder; there is a strong association with cigarette smoking and exposure to industrial chemicals. Excessive use of phenacetin-containing analgesics and the presence of Balkan nephritis are also predisposing factors.

Clinical Findings

A. Symptoms and Signs

Gross or microscopic painless hematuria occurs in over 70% of patients. The lesions are usually asymptomatic unless bleeding causes acute flank pain secondary to obstructing clots. Presenting symptoms can often be due to metastases to bone, the liver, or the lungs. Physical examination is usually negative for any positive findings.

B. Laboratory Findings

Microscopic hematuria on urinalysis is the rule. Pyuria is not seen. Cytologic examination of voided urine specimens may be diagnostic in high-grade tumors. Urine obtained from the ureter by retrograde catheterization or by brushing with specialized ureteral instruments can improve the diagnostic accuracy of cytologic examinations. Direct biopsy during ureteroscopy is the most accurate. There are no commonly associated paraneoplastic syndromes or diagnostic serum tumor markers in urothelial carcinoma. A large number of urine markers are currently being studied, but only in situ hybridization studies identifying abnormalities in chromosomes 3, 7, 17 and 9p21 can be recommended at present.

C. Imaging Studies

The diagnosis is commonly made on CT urography or intravenous urography and confirmed by retrograde pyelography, which reveals a radiolucent filling defect in the renal pelvis or calices. Renal ultrasound or CT scan can be used to rule out calculus. CT scan is also useful in local staging of the tumor. The tumors metastasize to the lungs, liver, and bone, so chest x-ray, CT scan of the lungs and liver, and a bone scan are useful to determine the presence of metastases. Urothelial carcinoma tends to be multifocal in the urinary tract, involving the opposite kidney (1–2%), ipsilateral ureter, or bladder (38–50%). Surveillance of these potential sites is important.

D. Endoscopic Findings

Cystoscopy is necessary when gross hematuria is present to determine the location of the bleeding. Retrograde pyelography and ureteral cytologic studies or brushing, as described previously, can be useful, though mildly abnormal cytologic findings may occur in patients with upper tract inflammation or calculi. Rigid or flexible ureteroscopes can be used to view the upper ureter and renal pelvis directly. Biopsy of upper tract lesions is possible through these instruments. Although percutaneous approaches to the renal collecting system have been perfected, their use for diagnosis or treatment of suspected urothelial carcinoma in routine cases is not recommended, because of the possibility of spreading tumor cells outside the kidney.

Differential Diagnosis

A variety of conditions may mimic transitional cell carcinoma of the renal pelvis, including calculi, sloughed renal papillae, tuberculosis, and renal cell carcinoma with pelvic extension of the tumor. These can usually be ruled out by the diagnostic studies described previously.

Complications

Occasionally, bleeding may be severe enough to require immediate nephrectomy. Infection may develop, particularly when there is obstruction and hydronephrosis, requiring prompt use of systemic antibiotics.

Treatment

Renal urothelial carcinoma is treated by nephroureterectomy (perifascial nephrectomy and removal of the entire ureter, down to and including the ureteral orifice within the bladder). Transureteral or percutaneous endoscopic techniques for resection of selected low-grade lesions have been successful. Upper tract instillation of bacille Calmette-Guérin (BCG) or mitomycin C have been reported with modest results. High recurrence rates and the potential for local tumor spread would argue against this approach in high-grade or extensive lesions. Laparoscopic nephroureterectomy has become common practice, but management of the distal ureter and bladder cuff by this technique has been the subject of controversy. Regional lymph node dissections have not been traditionally performed, although recent reports have shown some benefit for patients with aggressive disease. Because 50% of these patients will develop urothelial carcinoma of the bladder, cystourethroscopy must be performed postoperatively; it is usually done quarterly during the first year, twice the second year, and then annually.

Prognosis

Because most of these tumors are low grade and noninvasive, the 5-year tumor-free survival rate is higher than 90% for lesions treated with complete removal of the ipsilateral upper urinary tract. Survival rates are much lower for lesions that invade the renal parenchyma or are of high histologic grade.

A poor prognosis is associated with tumors having histologic features of squamous carcinoma or adenocarcinoma. These tumors are mildly radiosensitive, but preoperative or postoperative radiotherapy has not been particularly helpful. Metastatic lesions are particularly problematic, and survivors are rare. Chemotherapy combinations, which have shown benefit in urothelial carcinoma of the bladder (methotrexate, vinblastine, Adriamycin, and cisplatin [MVAC] or gemcitabine and cisplatin), are also efficacious in urothelial carcinoma of the upper urinary tract.

TUMORS OF THE URETER

 ESSENTIALS OF DIAGNOSIS

▶ Gross or microscopic hematuria.
▶ Radiolucent filling defect in the ureter on CT urography, intravenous urography, or retrograde pyelography.
▶ Malignant cells on urine cytologic study.

General Considerations

Ureteral tumors are rarely benign, but benign fibroepithelial polyps do occasionally occur within the ureter. More than 90% of ureteral tumors are urothelial carcinomas. The cause is unknown, but tobacco smoking and exposure to industrial chemicals are known to be associated. Ureteral urothelial carcinoma is often found in association with renal pelvis urothelial carcinoma and slightly less often with bladder urothelial carcinoma. The lesions develop in persons aged 60 to 70 years and are twice as common in men as in women. More than 60% of these tumors occur in the lower ureter.

Clinical Findings

A. Symptoms and Signs

Gross or microscopic hematuria is the rule (80% of cases). Because ureteral tumors grow slowly, they may not cause symptoms even though they completely obstruct the kidney. Occasionally, gross hematuria may cause acute obstruction because of clots. The initial presentation may be due to symptomatic metastases to bone, lungs, or liver.

B. Laboratory Findings

Urinalysis commonly reveals hematuria. There are no biochemical markers specific to the diagnosis, though patients with metastases may have abnormal liver function tests or anemia. Serum creatinine levels may be elevated with complete unilateral obstruction in elderly patients. Cytologic studies of voided urine or ureteral urine or brush biopsy studies may be diagnostic.

C. Imaging Studies

The diagnosis may be made on CT or intravenous urography, though the tumor often obstructs the ureter completely, so that cystoscopy and retrograde pyelography are required for definition of the lesion. These studies often reveal a filling defect in the ureter (classically described as a goblet sign). The ureter is dilated proximal to the lesion. CT scan is useful in ruling out nonopaque calculi and in abdominal tumor staging. Chest x-ray, CT scans, and bone scans are helpful in determining the presence of metastases.

D. Endoscopic Findings

Cystoscopy is necessary when gross hematuria is present to determine the site of bleeding. Retrograde pyelography may then be necessary. Ureteroscopy may provide a direct view of the tumor and access for biopsy.

Differential Diagnosis

Nonopaque calculi, sloughed renal papillae, blood clots, or extrinsic compression by retroperitoneal masses or nodes may all produce signs, symptoms, and x-ray findings similar to those with ureteral tumors. The radiographic, cytologic, and endourologic studies listed above should make the distinction, but surgical exploration is required occasionally.

Treatment

Most ureteral transitional cell carcinomas are not associated with metastases and can be definitively treated with nephroureterectomy. Selected patients with noninvasive low-grade lesions may be treated by segmental ureteral resection with end-to-end anastomosis (ureteroureterostomy). In some patients carefully selected with low-grade noninvasive tumors, resection or laser ablation can be considered. Regional lymph node dissections have not been traditionally performed, although recent reports have shown some benefit. Preoperative or postoperative radiation therapy appears to be of no benefit. As with renal pelvis and bladder urothelial carcinoma, cystoscopy should be performed periodically postoperatively. Patients with metastases are rarely helped by removal of the primary tumor. These tumors are responsive to chemotherapy. Traditional agents that have been used include cisplatin with gemcitabine or MVAC. These have shown reasonable response rates but poor long-term outcomes.

Prognosis

The 5-year survival rate for patients with low-grade noninvasive lesions treated surgically approaches 100%. Those with high-grade or invasive lesions have a poorer prognosis, and those with metastases have a 5-year survival rate of less than 10%.

TUMORS OF THE BLADDER

ESSENTIALS OF DIAGNOSIS

▶ Gross or microscopic hematuria.

▶ Malignant cells on urine cytologic study.

▶ Cystoscopic visualization of the tumor.

▶ Histologic confirmation of the lesions.

▶ General Considerations

Vesical neoplasms account for nearly 6% of all cancers in men and are the second-most common cancer of the genitourinary tract in men. In women, these tumors account for 2% of all cancers and are the most common cancer of the genitourinary tract. Men are affected twice as often as women. More than 90% of tumors are urothelial carcinomas, while a few are squamous cell carcinomas (associated with chronic inflammation, as in bilharziasis) or adenocarcinomas (often seen at the dome of the bladder in patients with a urachal remnant).

Most urothelial carcinomas (70–80%) are superficial (not invasive into the bladder wall) when recognized. Only 10% to 15% of recurrent tumors become invasive.

The cause of urothelial carcinoma is unknown; there is a strong association with chronic cigarette smoking and exposure to chemicals prevalent in dye, rubber, leather, paint, and other chemical industries. Common use of artificial sweeteners such as cyclamates and saccharin was thought to be related to bladder tumor development, but evidence to substantiate this claim has not been forthcoming.

The treatment and prognosis depend entirely on the degree of anaplasia (grade) and the depth of penetration of the bladder wall or beyond (Table 38–2). Most of these tumors develop on the trigone and the adjacent posterolateral wall; thus, ureteral involvement with obstruction is common. Tumors tend to be multifocal within the bladder.

Approximately 5% of patients develop upper urinary tract urothelial carcinoma as well.

▶ Clinical Findings

A. Symptoms and Signs

Gross hematuria is a common finding, though microscopic hematuria often leads to the diagnosis. Patients with diffuse superficial tumors, particularly carcinoma in situ, may have urinary frequency and urgency. Occasionally, large necrotic tumors become secondarily infected, and patients exhibit symptoms of cystitis. Pain secondary to clot retention, tumor extension into the bony pelvis, or ureteral obstruction may occur but are not frequent presenting complaints. When both ureters are obstructed, azotemia with attendant secondary symptoms may be the finding that requires diagnostic studies.

External physical examination is not generally revealing, though occasionally a suprapubic mass may be palpable. Rectal examination may reveal large tumors, particularly when they have invaded the pelvic side walls. Thus, bimanual examination is a necessary part of staging evaluation.

B. Laboratory Findings

Microscopic hematuria is the only consistent diagnostic finding. Patients with bilateral ureteral obstruction may have azotemia and anemia. Liver metastases may cause elevation of serum transaminases and alkaline phosphatase. There are no paraneoplastic syndromes or tumor markers consistently present in patients with urothelial carcinoma. Urinary markers currently being studied are various tumor-associated antigens, growth factors, and nuclear matrix proteins, but none are proved to be accurate enough to obviate cystoscopy for diagnosis.

C. Imaging Studies

Small bladder tumors are not seen on intravenous urography but may be seen on CT. Larger tumors usually produce filling defects in the bladder on both urography or CT (Figure 38–13). Ureteral obstruction with hydrouretero-

---

Table 38–2. Treatment and Prognosis of Bladder Tumors Related to Stage of Disease.

Conventional Stage	TNM Stage	Tumor Involvement	Treatment	5-Year Survival (%)
0	Ta	Mucosa only	Transurethral resection	85–90
A	T1	Submucosal invasion (lamina propria)	Transurethral resection and intravesical chemoimmunotherapy	60–80
B1	T2a	Superficial muscle invasion	Total cystectomy and pelvic lymphadenectomy	50–55
B2	T2b	Deep muscle invasion	Total cystectomy and pelvic lymphadenectomy	30–50
C	T3	Perivesical fat invasion	Total cystectomy and pelvic lymphadenectomy	30–40
D1	T3–4N+	Regional lymph node invasion	Systemic chemotherapy	6–35
D2	T3–4M1	Distant metastases	Systemic chemotherapy	0–10

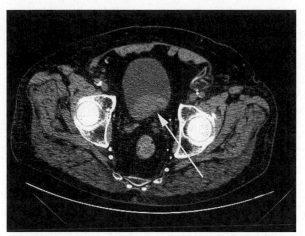

▲ **Figure 38–13.** Noncontrast CT scan showing space-occupying lesion (transitional cell carcinoma) on the posteroinferior of the bladder (arrow).

nephrosis may occur as well. Invasion of the bladder wall may be predicted in patients with asymmetry or marked irregularity of the bladder wall. Noninvasive lesions seen on CT or intravenous urography tend to be exophytic within the bladder, without evidence of bladder wall distortion.

Ultrasonography by external, transrectal, or transurethral routes can accurately define moderate-sized bladder tumors and can often depict deep invasion.

CT scan can be useful for staging, but the depth of bladder wall penetration and delineation of tumor deposits in adjacent nonenlarged lymph nodes are not accurately defined. In patients with nodal metastases suspected on CT scans, fine-needle aspiration and cytologic studies may confirm the diagnosis and eliminate the need for surgical exploration. MRI is helpful in the pelvis, where motion artifacts are minor and the scant pelvic fat is just enough to provide organ differentiation. However, the information is not superior to that obtained with CT.

D. Urinary Cytologic Studies

Urothelial tumors shed neoplastic cells into the urine in large numbers. Low-grade tumor cells may not appear abnormal on cytologic examination, but higher-grade tumor cells can be detected by cytologic study. These studies are most useful in checking for recurrence of urothelial carcinoma. Flow cytometry (differential staining of DNA and RNA within urine cells to measure the amount of nuclear protein and thus the relative number of aneuploid [abnormal] cells) has been used to screen patients with some success. This technique may be useful for early diagnosis of recurrence. The urinary fluorescence in situ hybridization (FISH) assay is more sensitive and comparably specific for bladder cancer cells as compared to cytology.

E. Endoscopic Findings

Cystoscopy is mandatory in any adult patient with unexplained hematuria and a normal CT or intravenous urogram. Many urothelial carcinomas are not identified on CT or intravenous urography. Cystoscopic examination should detect nearly all tumors in the bladder (Figure 38–14). Only a few patients will have carcinoma in situ (high-grade noninvasive tumor) that is not visible. Any tumor seen should be biopsied. Superficial-appearing tumors can be diagnosed and removed transurethrally at the same time. The entire bladder, including the bladder neck, should be routinely scrutinized in all patients with microscopic hematuria. In patients without visible tumor and no other causes of hematuria, random biopsies may be diagnostic of carcinoma in situ. A bimanual examination should be done during cystoscopy in all patients with urothelial carcinoma to be certain that the bladder is not fixed, signifying extensive extravesical extension.

F. Staging

Therapy depends on the stage of the tumor as seen on histologic sections and examinations for metastases. Table 38–2 sets forth the stage, treatment, and prognosis of patients with urothelial carcinoma of the bladder. The histologic grade of the tumor is also important in determining treatment and prognosis, but in general, low- and high-grade histologic characteristics tend to occur in low- and high-stage tumors, respectively.

As previously discussed, CT scan, MRI, or both may be helpful in predicting the stage of the tumor. Isotope bone scanning, chest x-ray, and chest CT scan evaluate the possibility of bone or pulmonary metastases and should be done before determining therapy in patients with invasive lesions.

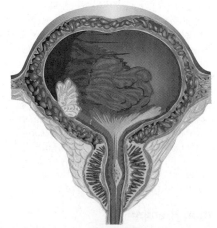

▲ **Figure 38–14.** Transitional cell (papillary) carcinoma of the bladder with minimal invasion of the bladder wall.

▶ Treatment

A. Transurethral Resection, Fulguration, and Laser Therapy

Endoscopic transurethral resection of superficial and submucosally invasive low-grade tumors can be curative. Nevertheless, because the tumor recurs in more than 50% of patients, cystoscopy should be performed periodically. Quarterly examinations are recommended during the first year following tumor resection, every 6 months during the second year, and annually thereafter. Periodic urinary cytologic examinations can be helpful as well. CT or intravenous urography is recommended yearly for the first 3 to 5 years but is not mandatory. Recurrent small tumors without obvious invasion may be treated by fulguration only, though biopsy is recommended to document the stage and grade.

Neodymium:YAG lasers have been used for desiccation of low-grade, low-stage tumors. There is as yet no proven advantage to this approach except that patients can be treated under local anesthesia as outpatients and perhaps that tumor cells are rendered nonviable and thus incapable of reimplantation elsewhere in the bladder or urethra. Biopsies for diagnosis and staging are still required.

B. Intravesical Chemotherapy

A variety of chemotherapeutic agents have been used in patients with recurrent low-grade, low-stage tumors. Mitomycin C is instilled into the bladder by catheter (40 mg in 40 mL of water) and left indwelling for 2 hours. Patients are treated once a week for 1 month and then monthly for up to 2 years. Treatment results in decreased frequency of recurrence or no recurrence in nearly 50% of patients. Other agents include thiotepa and doxorubicin. Immunotherapeutic drugs, which include BCG, are effective in prophylaxis (60%) of recurrent papillary tumors and curative (70%) in carcinoma in situ, a highly malignant lesion less responsive to the cytotoxic agents described earlier. Side effects of BCG include vesical irritability (90%) and systemic BCG-osis (1%). Although the mechanism of action of BCG is not entirely known, it is suspected to induce T-cell recruitment and subsequent cytokine release locally at the tumor site. It is the most effective agent currently used. Interferon alfa has also been studied and is effective (nearly 50% of cases) for carcinoma in situ, with less toxicity than BCG; however, its durability as a single agent is poor. The combination of BCG and interferon alfa has shown nearly 50% response rates and is occasionally used in patients who have failed BCG. Immediate posttransurethral resection intravesical chemotherapy with mitomycin C has shown a substantial decrease in recurrence rates and is now standard of care.

C. Radiation Therapy

Definitive radiation therapy should be reserved for patients who have inoperable muscle-invasive bladder cancer localized to the pelvis or who refuse surgical treatment, as the 5-year survival rate is only 30%. In some patients with recurrence after radiation therapy, salvage cystectomy can be curative (in at least 30% of cases), though surgical morbidity rates are high.

Much controversy surrounds the use of radiation therapy preoperatively. Some authors have claimed a down-staging effect with 2000 cGy given over 1 week or 4000 cGy given over 3 to 4 weeks. The studies were poorly controlled, however, and subsequent reports have not confirmed these findings. Currently, urologic oncologists rarely use preoperative radiation therapy.

D. Surgical Therapy

Occasional patients are seen with muscle-invasive lesions (T2) localized to an area in the bladder well away from the bladder base or orifices and without tumor in other sites of the bladder (proved by multiple biopsies) or beyond. Partial cystectomy (removal of the tumor and a 3-cm surrounding margin of normal bladder) is appropriate in these patients. Such tumors are rare, and patients must be selected carefully for partial cystectomy. All other patients with high-grade or invasive (T2 and T3) lesions without distant spread or a fixed pelvis on bimanual examination are best treated by cystectomy and pelvic lymph node dissection. This includes removal of the bladder and the prostate in men. Removal of the entire urethra may be necessary in selected patients with tumors at the bladder neck or in the prostate or in those with diffuse carcinoma in situ in the bladder. In women, the uterus, the urethra, and the anterior vaginal wall are usually removed. Urinary diversion is required and is commonly accomplished by creation of an ileal diversion. Continent cutaneous urinary diversions requiring intermittent cutaneous catheterization rather than cutaneous bag drainage became popular in the late 1980s. The basic principles are large-volume reservoirs with detubularization of bowel to maintain low intrapouch pressures and construction of an intussuscepted or plicated ileal segment to provide cutaneous continence. Orthotopic reservoirs also have been devised using bowel configurations similar to those described above to connect directly to the membranous urethra in men and in the distal two thirds of the female urethra, permitting the patient to void normally. These procedures are appropriate in both men and women and have been shown to be safe, with minimal increase in morbidity over cutaneous diversions. Recently, laparoscopic and robotic cystectomy and urinary diversion has been done in a few centers in the United States and Europe.

E. Systemic Chemotherapy

Chemotherapy in the form of CMV (cisplatin, methotrexate, vinblastine) or MVAC (CMV plus doxorubicin [Adriamycin]) has been used precystectomy (neoadjuvant) or postcystectomy (adjuvant) for muscle-invasive tumors or as treatment of metastatic urothelial cancer. More recently, gemcitabine and cisplatin have become standard of care after a randomized trial showed similar efficacy to MVAC with fewer side effects. A recent randomized trial showed improved survival in patients with locally advanced bladder cancer who received neoadjuvant chemotherapy and cystectomy compared to those who underwent cystectomy alone. Adjuvant chemotherapy has been shown in randomized trials to help patients with locoregional disease but not patients with localized disease (stage T1–T2). Several reports of efficacy with either CMV or MVAC for treatment of metastatic disease have shown a 60% overall objective response rate with a 30% complete response rate. A few long-term survivors with apparent cure have been reported (10–15%), and either of these regimens thus appears to be a definite advance in the treatment of urothelial cancer. Other chemotherapeutic agents used in urothelial cancer include paclitaxel and carboplatin in various regimens that appear to have similar efficacy with less toxicity. These results have caused a few investigators to study chemotherapy alone or in combination with radiation to attempt bladder salvage in patients with invasive bladder cancer, and this has become a viable alternative to cystectomy in selected patients.

Prognosis

Approximately half of the low-grade superficial tumors are controlled by transurethral surgery or intracavitary use of chemotherapeutic agents (Table 38–2). Following radical cystectomy, the 5-year survival rate varies with the extent, stage, and grade of the tumor, but with T2N0M0 tumors averages about 50% to 70%. The complications of urinary diversion (ureteral obstruction with hydronephrosis, pyelonephritis, and nephrolithiasis) also influence the outcome.

CARCINOMA OF THE PROSTATE

ESSENTIALS OF DIAGNOSIS

▶ Palpable rock-hard nodule in the prostate on rectal examination.

▶ Serum prostate-specific antigen elevation.

▶ Histologic confirmation on needle biopsy.

▶ Osteoblastic bone metastases in advanced cases.

General Considerations

In adult men, prostate cancer is the most common neoplasm (after skin cancer) and the second-most common cause of death due to cancer. The tumor is more prevalent in black men than in any other group in the United States. The tumor rarely occurs before age 40, and the incidence increases with age such that more than 75% of men older than age 85 have prostate cancer on autopsy. In most of these older men,

however, the disease is not clinically apparent; only 10% of men over age 65 develop clinical evidence of the disease. Ninety-five percent of tumors are adenocarcinomas. The tumor arises primarily in the peripheral zone (85%), an area that differs in embryologic derivation from the periurethral (transition) zone, which is the site of formation of benign prostatic hyperplasia. The cause of prostate cancer is unknown, but many factors appear to be involved, including genetic, hormonal, dietary (particular high-fat diets), and perhaps environmental carcinogenic influences.

Screening

Although screening with annual prostate-specific antigen (PSA) monitoring and digital rectal examination has been controversial due to lack of evidence that it affects mortality, it is recommended by the American Cancer Society and the American Urological Association and is widely implemented. It has been shown that the combination of digital rectal examination and serum PSA monitoring is better than either alone as a screening method. There are two ongoing randomized trials that will address whether screening affects mortality from prostate cancer (the Prostate, Lung, Colon and Ovarian Cancer Screening Trial [National Cancer Institute] and the European Randomized Study of Screening for Prostate Cancer). Screening is recommended for most men age 50 or older, for black men 45 or older, and for those with first-degree relatives diagnosed with prostate cancer. Each patient should receive detailed information prior to screening so they understand the possible benefits and risks of screening (shared decision making).

Clinical Findings

A. Symptoms and Signs

Incidental or stage A (T1) carcinoma of the prostate presents no physical signs (it is nonpalpable) and is only diagnosed by the pathologist when prostate tissue is removed as treatment for symptomatic bladder outlet obstruction presumed to be caused by benign prostatic hyperplasia or is found by an elevated PSA (T1c). Patients with stage B (T2) or higher disease have a hard nodule on the prostate that can be felt during rectal examination (Table 38–3). Previously, 50% of patients presented with evidence of metastases, including weight loss, anemia, bone pain (commonly in the lumbosacral area), or acute neurologic deficit in the lower limbs. Today, however, fewer than 20% of patients present in this way because of earlier diagnosis due to wide use of PSA screening (stage migration).

B. Laboratory Findings

Patients with extensive metastases may have anemia due to bone marrow replacement by tumor. Those with bilateral ureteral obstruction secondary to trigonal compression by tumor may exhibit azotemia and uremia. Serum alkaline

Table 38–3. Treatment and Prognosis of Prostate Cancer Related to Tumor Stage.

Conventional Stage	TNM Stage 1997	Clinical Findings	Treatment	15-Year Recurrence-Free Survival (%)
A1	T1a	Nonpalpable tumor; incidental finding at transurethral prostatectomy (low-grade cancer seen in < 5% of prostate).	Observation	100
A2	T1b	Same as above except tumor is high-grade, or > 5% of prostate is involved, or both.	Radical prostatectomy with pelvic lymphadenectomy OR	70–80
B1	T2a	Tumor involves 1 lobe or less	External beam radiation OR	85
B2	T2b	Tumor involves more than 1 lobe	Brachytherapy	60–70
C	T3a	Unilateral extraprostatic extension		20–60
C2	T3b	Bilateral extraprostatic extension	Hormonal therapy (orchiectomy or LHRH/ antiandrogen) plus external beam radiation	0–10
	T3c	Seminal vesicle invasion		
	T4a	Invades bladder neck or rectum		
	T4b	Invades levator muscle and/or fixed to pelvic sidewall		
D	N+ or M+	Pelvic lymph node involvement or distant metastases	Hormonal therapy (orchiectomy or LHRH/ antiandrogen) when symptomatic; irradiation for isolated bone pain	0–10

LHRH, luteinizing hormone–releasing hormone.

phosphatase is often elevated in patients with bone metastases but not in those with localized disease.

PSA is elevated in the serum of approximately 60% of men with prostate cancer. Levels above 4 ng/mL are considered abnormal but rise normally with age and volume of benign prostatic hypertrophy and can be falsely elevated due to cystoscopy, prostate biopsy, or urethral catheterization but *not* by normal digital rectal examination.

Methods for enhancing PSA specificity include the following: (1) age-specific PSA (younger men [< age 50 years], normal < 2.5 ng/mL; older men [> age 70 years], normal > 6.5 ng/mL); (2) PSA density (PSA divided by prostate volume), where less than 0.15 ng/mL suggests cancer; (3) percent-free PSA (total PSA minus complexed PSA), where when less than 10%, the risk of prostate cancer is 60% (only useful with total PSA 2–10 ng/mL) While total PSA is useful for staging, it is not absolute. PSA appears to be most helpful in following up on patients after treatment, as levels fall to almost nil with complete response. There are several new prostate cancer markers currently being investigated, but none are thought to be more sensitive and specific than PSA at present.

C. Imaging Studies

Transrectal ultrasound has become very useful for evaluating prostate volume and guiding biopsy needles into the periph-eral zone and other specific areas, such as the base, the apex, and the transition zone of the prostate. The study can also reveal typical hypoechoic peripheral zone lesions in 70% of patients with palpable lesions. Because many prostate cancers are not hypoechoic and not all hypoechoic lesions are cancer, transrectal ultrasound alone for screening for prostate cancer is not recommended. An intravenous urogram or CT may reveal urinary retention or distal ureteral obstruction. Extensive lesions may exhibit a ragged-edged filling defect in the bladder base. A chest x-ray may help in identifying the uncommon lung metastases but more often shows typical osteoblastic metastases in the thoracic spine or ribs. An abdominal x-ray may reveal metastases in the lumbosacral spine or ilium. A CT scan of the pelvis may show an enlarged prostate and large pelvic or para-aortic lymph nodes; however, the study is rarely accurate for staging and is not routinely recommended unless the PSA is higher than 20 ng/mL or the Gleason sum of the tumor is 7 or more, or the tumor is palpable outside of the prostate (stage C/T3). Fine-needle aspiration and cytologic studies or laparoscopic dissection of abnormal nodes may provide important staging data. Endorectal and pelvic MRI appear to be more helpful than CT scan in pelvic staging of prostate cancer. A monoclonal antibody, Cyt-356 (which identifies the *intra*cellular epitope of prostate-specific membrane antigen), has been coupled with a radioisotope for diagnosis of soft tissue metastases. Results show that the Prostascint scan is 60% accurate but that it has a relatively high false-positive rate, which limits its usefulness.

D. Biopsy

The diagnosis is established by transrectal ultrasound–guided biopsies in most instances. Because the great majority of patients have biopsies due to an elevated serum PSA (stage T1c) and no abnormal findings on transrectal ultrasound, biopsies of the base, middle, and apex of the prostate—concentrating on the peripheral zone with 6 biopsies per side of the prostate—are required for accurate diagnosis.

Differentiation of the tumor is graded by the pathologist using the Gleason scale, which assigns a grade of 1 to 5 (low to high grade) for both the primary and secondary forms of the tumor. The two numbers are added, and the cancer can thus be Gleason sum 2 to Gleason sum 10, with 10 being the most poorly differentiated cancer. The likelihood of metastasis can be inferred from the Gleason sum: 7 (4 + 3) or more is an aggressive cancer.

E. Staging

Rectal examination can provide initial staging in patients with palpable tumors (Table 38–3). Needle biopsy is confirmatory, and histologic grading can fairly accurately predict the metastatic potential of the tumor. A normal isotopic (technetium 99m) bone scan rules out bone metastases but is not necessary if Gleason score is less than 7 and/or PSA is less than 20 ng/mL. A pelvic CT scan may be useful to define pelvic lymphadenopathy in patients with high-grade lesions, PSA over 20 ng/mL, or both. The laparoscopic approach to pelvic lymph node dissection has provided the same prognostic information as an open surgical procedure with less morbidity and a markedly reduced hospital stay. This approach is useful in patients with high-grade or high-stage lesions and those considered for radical perineal prostatectomy. Cystoscopy is not required except in large lesions suspected to involve the bladder neck and trigone.

▶ Differential Diagnosis

Nodules caused by benign prostatic hyperplasia may be difficult to distinguish from cancer; benign nodules are usually rubbery, whereas cancerous nodules have a much harder consistency. Fibrosis following a prior prostatectomy for benign disease or secondary to chronic prostatitis or prior biopsies may be associated with lesions indistinguishable from cancerous nodules and require biopsy for definition. Occasionally, phleboliths or prostatic calculi on the surface of the prostate may be confusing; however, transrectal ultrasound can be helpful in the differentiation and for biopsy guidance.

▶ Treatment

A. Curative Therapy

Curative treatment for localized prostate cancer includes radical prostatectomy, external beam radiation therapy, and transperineal radioactive seed placement (brachytherapy with ^{125}I, ^{103}Pd, or ^{192}Ir). Complete staging is important so that appropriate candidates will be selected. Patients with localized prostate cancer are stratified into three risk groups (Table 38–4). Low-risk patients have similar 5-year recurrence survival rates irrespective of the curative treatment modality. Intermediate-risk and high-risk patients have better recurrence-free rates with prostatectomy or external beam radiation compared to brachytherapy. None of these modalities have been compared in randomized trials. The only reported randomized trial compared watchful waiting to radical prostatectomy and that showed improved disease-free as well as overall survival in the prostatectomy group. Studies have shown that neoadjuvant androgen deprivation and external beam radiation improve survival in patients with localized prostate cancer, especially patients in the intermediate and high-risk groups. Patients with grossly positive pelvic lymph nodes are not candidates for curative therapy. Recent advances in surgical technique have led to a low incidence of incontinence (1–4%) and preservation of potency in up to 70% of patients. Alternative procedures include external beam pelvic irradiation plus interstitial radiation. Recently, laparoscopic and robotic-assisted laparoscopic radical prostatectomy has been shown to have decreased blood loss and length of hospital stay and more rapid return to normal activity than open surgery. It is as yet uncertain if long-term complications and efficacy will be improved as well.

B. Palliative Therapy

Patients with metastatic disease cannot be cured, but significant palliation can be offered. Androgen deprivation therapy in the form of luteinizing hormone–releasing hormone (LHRH agonist or bilateral orchiectomy) is effective in 70–80%

Table 38–4. Localized Prostate Cancer Risk Groups.

Low risk	• PSA ≤ 10 ng/ml
	• Clinical stage T1c–T2a
	• Gleason score 2–6
Intermediate risk	• PSA 10–20 ng/ml
	• Clinical stage T2b
	• Gleason score 7
High risk	• PSA > 20 ng/ml
	• Clinical stage ≥ T2c
	• Gleason score 8–10

PSA, prostate-specific antigen.

of symptomatic patients. Estrogen-based treatments are less commonly used due to the numerous side effects (in about 25% of patients), including congestive heart failure, thrombophlebitis, and myocardial infarction, and thus should not be used except in selected patients. These hormonal treatments are not additive, and use of both treatments simultaneously has no advantages over use of either alone. LHRH agonists have shown efficacy comparable to that of estrogen or orchiectomy, with reduced side effects, and are preferred by patients who find bilateral orchiectomy unacceptable. The drug must be given by injection every 3 to 4 months and is expensive. Studies have also shown that if an LHRH agonist is used, concomitant administration of an antiandrogen (flutamide or bicalutamide) slightly improves survival. Studies to determine if orchiectomy plus an antiandrogen is more effective than orchiectomy alone have not shown an advantage to the combination. Osteoporosis is a long-term side effect of either orchiectomy or LHRH agonist.

Controversy continues concerning whether to treat asymptomatic patients at the time of diagnosis or to wait until symptoms develop. Because either approach is palliative only and there are no definitive studies showing survival advantages with early treatment, it is recommended that treatment be withheld until PSA is relatively high (> 20 ng/ml) or symptoms occur except in patients who cannot accept a no-treatment philosophy. Recent studies do show that patients who have had a radical prostatectomy and have node-positive disease do have a slight survival advantage with early hormonal treatment.

Patients whose prostate cancer becomes hormone refractory (median of 18 months after starting treatment) can be treated by ketoconazole (which inhibits adrenal androgen production) with oral corticosteroids for short-term response. Radiation therapy for symptomatic bone lesions can be helpful, as can local irradiation for an obstructing or bleeding prostate tumor. On occasion, transurethral prostatectomy is required to relieve bladder outlet obstruction. Chemotherapy with docetaxel and prednisone has recently shown a slight survival advantage in phase III trials.

▶ Prostate Cancer Prevention

Because the etiology of prostate cancer is not known, prevention is difficult to determine. However, there is evidence that a low-fat diet and lycopene (found in processed tomatoes) decrease the growth of prostate cancer cells in vitro and in vivo in animals. Further large-scale epidemiologic studies suggest a decrease in prostate cancer in humans who consumed vitamin E and selenium. However, these studies were not planned specifically for this purpose, and thus the results were questionable. A current randomized trial comparing selenium and vitamin E (SELECT) was recently halted due to the lack of evidence of prostate cancer prevention. The largest chemoprevention trial (Prostate Cancer Prevention Trial [PCPT]), with over 18,000 men, compared finasteride (5α-reductase) to placebo and found a 25% reduction in

prostate cancer with finasteride but also showed an increased risk of high-grade cancer in the finasteride-treated patients. While this is thought to be an artifact of the study, these results have limited enthusiasm for recommending prevention therapy with finasteride routinely.

▶ Prognosis

Radical prostatectomy cures 70% to 80% of the patients suitable for that operation, but its use should be limited to those with a reasonable life expectancy (Table 38–3). Currently, about 60% to 70% of patients with prostatic cancer are amenable to curative therapy when their disease is discovered.

SARCOMA OF THE PROSTATE

Sarcoma of the prostate is rare. Half of all cases occur in boys under age 5. The tumor is highly malignant and metastasizes to the pelvic and lumbar lymph nodes, lungs, liver, and bone. Symptoms of urinary tract obstruction are present. The prostate is enlarged. Cystography or excretory urography may show superior displacement of the bladder or encroachment of the tumor into the bladder. Endoscopy reveals the mass and allow biopsy.

Total prostatocystectomy, postoperative radiotherapy, and chemotherapy have cured a few cases in adults. In children, combination chemotherapy with surgery for residual tumor has shown increasing success. The tumor is relatively radioresistant.

Bill-Axelson A et al: Radical prostatectomy versus watchful waiting in early prostate cancer. New Eng J Med 2005;352:1977.

Bolla M et al: Long-term results with immediate androgen suppression and external irradiation in patients with locally advanced prostate cancer (an EORTC study): a phase III randomised trial. Lancet 2002;360:103.

Chu KC et al: Trends in prostate cancer mortality among black men and white men in the United States. Cancer 2003;97:1507.

D'Amico AV et al: Biochemical outcome after radical prostatectomy, external beam radiation therapy, or interstitial radiation therapy for clinically localized prostate cancer. JAMA 1998;280:969.

Grönberg H: Prostate cancer epidemiology. Lancet 2003;361:859.

Leman ES et al: EPCA-2: a highly specific serum marker for prostate cancer. Urology 2007;69:714.

Moul JW: Population screening for prostate cancer and emerging concepts for young men. Clin Prostate Cancer 2003;2:87.

Tannock IF et al: Docetaxel plus prednisone or mitoxantrone plus prednisone for advanced prostate cancer. New Eng J Med 2004;351:1502.

Thompson IM: Chemoprevention of prostate cancer: agents and study designs. J Urol 2007;178:S9.

TUMORS OF THE URETHRA

Malignant tumors of the urethra are rare. The disease is more common in women than in men (4:1). Squamous cell types are seen most often in both sexes.

In women, urethral bleeding is the most common symptom. Distal urethral lesions of low grade and without extension can be treated by radiotherapy or wide local excision. Advanced disease is best treated by combination radiotherapy, chemotherapy, and surgery to achieve good local and distant disease control. Surgery includes anterior exenteration (removal of the bladder, uterus, adnexa, and urethra with the anterior vaginal wall), including pelvic lymphadenectomy and urinary diversion. The prognosis is excellent for distal lesions without extension, but 5-year survival rates are less than 50% for those with proximal lesions.

In men, the lesion is most commonly in the bulbomembranous urethra and is associated with a history of chronic urethral strictures, often secondary to gonorrheal infection. Patients present with urethral bleeding, a weak urinary stream, and a perineal mass. The diagnosis is made by urethroscopy and biopsy. Distal penile urethral lesions can be treated by partial or total penectomy. Lesions in the bulbous urethra or more proximal lesions require extensive surgical resection, including en bloc removal of the penis, urethra, prostate, bladder with overlying pubis, pelvic lymph nodes, and urinary diversion. In both men and women with distal lesions, groin lymphatics may be involved, but node dissection is required only when gross disease is palpable. Prophylactic node dissection is controversial. Five-year survival rates are 60% for distal urethral tumors but less than 40% for the more common proximal lesions.

Primary irradiation—other than to distal lesions in the female—is rarely helpful. Patients with metastatic disease may respond to methotrexate or cisplatin alone or in combination, but objective remissions are usually of short duration.

TUMORS OF THE TESTIS

ESSENTIALS OF DIAGNOSIS

▶ Painless, firm mass within the testicle in a man aged 18 to 40.

▶ Elevated serum levels of the beta subunit of human chorionic gonadotropin (β-hCG), α-fetoprotein, lactic dehydrogenase, or all three.

▶ Enlarged retroperitoneal nodes on abdominal CT scan.

▶ Palpable abdominal mass in advanced cases.

▶ General Considerations

Most testicular tumors are malignant germ cell tumors. Non–germ cell tumors such as Sertoli cell tumors and Leydig cell tumors are rare and usually benign. Germ cell tumors are categorized as either seminomatous (35%) or nonseminomatous (embryonal, 20%; teratocarcinoma, 38%; teratoma, 5%; choriocarcinoma, 2%). Cryptorchidism predisposes to testicular cancer, with the incidence increasing inversely with the level of testicular descent (ie, testicles remaining in the abdomen have a much higher incidence of cancer). Metastases first develop in the retroperitoneal nodes; right-sided tumors metastasize primarily to the interaortocaval region just below the renal vessels and left-sided tumors primarily to the left para-aortic area at the same level. Distant spread is to supraclavicular areas (left, primarily) and the lungs. Just under 50% of patients have metastases when first seen.

▶ Clinical Findings

A. Symptoms and Signs

Testicular tumors present as a painless firm mass within the testicular substance. They often have been present for several months before the patient seeks consultation. Occasionally (10%), a hydrocele is present, obscuring palpation of the mass. A few patients have spontaneous bleeding into the mass, causing pain. Patients with high serum levels of hCG may have gynecomastia. Patients with extensive abdominal metastases may present with abdominal pain, anorexia, and weight loss. Examination may reveal palpable retroperitoneal nodes when spread is extensive or palpable supraclavicular nodes, particularly on the left side.

B. Laboratory Findings

In general, testicular tumors do not alter the usual laboratory parameters, but serum tumor markers are diagnostically helpful. Patients with extensive retroperitoneal metastases may have bilateral ureteral obstruction that causes azotemia and anemia.

Serum lactic dehydrogenase, particularly isoenzyme I, is elevated in approximately 60% of patients. β-HCG, a particularly sensitive marker, is a glycoprotein produced by 65% of nonseminomatous testicular tumors but only 10% of seminomas. The alpha subunit of the molecule is identical to LH, but the beta subunit is unique to testicular tumors in adult men. There is cross-reactivity in some assays between the alpha and beta subunits; treated patients who develop modest elevations should have simultaneous assay of LH to be certain the marker detected is β-hCG.

α-Fetoprotein is elevated in 70% of patients with nonseminomatous testicular cancer but is *not* elevated in patients with seminoma. Patients in whom histologic study has shown seminoma but in whom serum AFP is elevated should be suspected of having nonseminomatous elements in the primary specimen or metastatic lesions.

Approximately 85% of patients demonstrate elevation of one of these markers at presentation. Serum levels decrease when the tumor is completely removed or regresses. Markers are used mainly to follow tumor regression or predict recrudescence, as even minute amounts of tumor may cause serum elevations; however, tumor may be present without elevation of serum markers.

C. Imaging Studies

Abdominal CT scan defines enlarged lymph nodes in approximately 90% of cases when they are present. Chest x-ray and CT scan will detect most pulmonary metastases.

Scrotal ultrasound is useful for identifying the typical hypoechoic lesion in the testicle. Regardless of the findings on ultrasound, however, a young man with an intratesticular mass on palpation requires surgical definition of the mass.

▶ Differential Diagnosis

Testicular masses in men aged 18 to 40 are frequently malignant and should be treated accordingly. Confusion can occur with scrotal hydroceles, cord hydroceles, epididymal masses or cysts, or epididymitis. Most of these can be differentiated from masses within the testicle by palpation, but if not, scrotal ultrasound is usually helpful.

▶ Treatment

See also Table 38–5.

Inguinal orchiectomy with high ligation of the cord at the internal ring is proper initial treatment for all subtypes of testicular cancer. Rarely is incisional biopsy of the testicle advisable. Recommendations for further therapy (retroperitoneal node dissection, chemotherapy, radiation therapy) are then based on the pathologic findings. A staging workup, including postoperative measurement of serum markers, chest x-ray, and chest and abdominal CT scan, is conducted to determine the extent of disease.

A. Nonseminomatous Tumors

Following orchiectomy, retroperitoneal lymph node dissection is recommended for all patients with nonseminomatous testicular cancer except in the presence of bulky abdominal or distant metastases. Patients with pure choriocarcinoma are an exception and do not usually require retroperitoneal surgery, because the disease in such cases is invariably systemic and requires multiagent chemotherapy. The extent of lymphadenectomy depends on the testicle involved but in general includes para-aortic and paracaval nodes from the renal vessels down to the aortic bifurcation and along the external iliac artery to the internal inguinal ring on the involved side. Seminal emission can be preserved; loss of this function was previously a complication of retroperitoneal lymph node dissection because of interruption of autonomic nerves crossing the aorta and near the aortic bifurcation.

Because of the associated morbidity, some have proposed that retroperitoneal lymph node dissection be withheld after orchiectomy in patients with normal serum markers and no evidence of retroperitoneal nodal disease on abdominal CT scan and who have no findings of distant metastases on chest x-ray and CT scan. The rationale was that only 20% of these patients will develop recurrent disease, which could then be treated when it appeared. This approach should be discussed at length with the patient to ensure his reliable compliance with a program for frequent follow-up.

Patients with any nonseminomatous cell type who have extensive retroperitoneal or chest metastases are best treated after orchiectomy by multiagent chemotherapy followed by excision of persistent masses. Combination chemotherapy with bleomycin, etoposide, and cisplatin achieves over a 90% cure rate in stage II patients and a 70% cure rate in stage III patients. Patients who do not respond may be treated with ifosfamide, doxorubicin, or both, with some expectation of success.

B. Seminoma

In the absence of extensive distant spread, patients with pure seminoma should be treated with external beam radiation therapy (2500 cGy) to the abdomen following orchiectomy. A recent study showed that one cycle of carboplatin is

Table 38–5. Treatment and Prognosis of Testicular Cancer Related to Tumor Stage.

Conventional Stage	TNM Stage	Clinical Findings	Treatment	5-Year Survival (%)
I	T1	Confined to testicle	Nonseminoma: RPLND vs. surveillance; seminoma: irradiation	> 95
IIA	N1	Regional nodes < 2 cm	Adjuvant chemotherapy	> 90
			Nonseminoma: RPLND or chemotherapy; seminoma: XRT or chemotherapy	
IIB	N2	Nodes 2–5 cm	Adjuvant chemotherapy	> 85
			Nonseminoma; RPLND or adjuvant chemotherapy; seminoma: XRT or chemotherapy	
IIC	N3	Nodes > 5 cm	Chemotherapy followed by resection of residual disease	~70
III	M+	Distant metastases	Chemotherapy followed by resection of residual disease	~70

Note: All patients undergo inguinal orchiectomy.
RPLND, retroperitoneal lymph node dissection.

equivalent to radiation therapy for stage I seminoma. In the presence of bulky abdominal disease or more distant metastases, survival rates are better with multiagent chemotherapy (described earlier) given initially in lieu of radiation therapy. Patients with substantial residual retroperitoneal tumor (> 3 cm) after chemotherapy may benefit from surgical removal of the remaining tumor.

▶ Prognosis

Even in the presence of metastases, many of these patients can be cured. The only exception is patients with choriocarcinoma, who still have a poor survival rate (35% at 5 years) despite extensive chemotherapy.

TUMORS OF THE PENIS

Cancer of the penis is a rare disease occurring in the fifth to sixth decades. The cause is uncertain. The disease is rarely seen in circumcised men. The lesion commonly is on the glans penis or foreskin. Early cases may exhibit a painless red, velvety lesion, but most often the lesion is an exophytic nodular or wartlike growth with secondary infection. The initial diagnosis is made by a generous incisional biopsy of the lesion, which reveals squamous cell carcinoma in over 95% of cases. The tumors tend to metastasize to superficial or deep inguinal nodes, though the attendant infection may cause enlarged, tender nodes, which may be difficult to differentiate from metastatic cancer.

The differential diagnosis includes syphilitic chancre, soft chancre due to *Haemophilus ducreyi* infection, and simple or giant condyloma. Biopsy usually differentiates among these conditions.

Small, noninfiltrating lesions can be treated with fluorouracil cream, external beam radiation, or laser therapy. However, close follow-up is mandatory in patients so treated. Larger lesions not involving deep structures are treated by partial penile amputation at least 2 cm proximal to the lesion, leaving enough of the penis for adequate direction of the urinary stream. Deeply infiltrating lesions require total penectomy, with formation of a perineal urethrostomy.

Patients with high-risk features (high T stage, high grade, or presence of lymphovascular invasion) are at risk of inguinal nodal metastases. Prophylactic node dissection has been associated with improved survival.

Palpable inguinal nodes should be treated by antibiotics for 6 weeks following treatment of the primary lesion to eliminate infection. Persistently palpable nodes require bilateral ilioinguinal lymphadenectomy. An alternative would be fine-needle aspiration of the palpable nodes and node dissection if positive for metastases. Even those who undergo delayed node dissection when the nodes become palpable can be cured, though this is a lower percentage. Radiation therapy for palpable nodes or as prophylaxis for nonpalpable nodes has been occasionally effective.

Patients with distant metastases (to the lungs or bone) have a poor prognosis, though cisplatin and methotrexate have shown objective but not durable responses. Five-year survival rates for patients with noninvasive lesions localized to the penis are 80%; for those with inguinal node involvement, 50%; and for those with distant metastases, nil.

Flanigan RC et al: Cytoreductive nephrectomy in patients with metastatic renal cancer: a combined analysis. J Urol 2004;171: 1071.

Glas AS et al: Tumor markers in the diagnosis of primary bladder cancer. A systematic review. J Urol 2003;169:1975.

Grossman HB et al: Neoadjuvant chemotherapy plus cystectomy compared with cystectomy alone for locally advanced bladder cancer. N Engl J Med. 2003;349:859. Erratum in: N Engl J Med. 2003;349:1880.

Gschwend JE et al: Radical cystectomy for invasive bladder cancer: contemporary results and remaining controversies. Eur Urol 2000;38:121.

Han M et al: Prostate-specific antigen and screening for prostate cancer. Med Clin North Am 2004;88:245.

Hernandez J, Thompson IM: Diagnosis and treatment of prostate cancer. Med Clin North Am 2004;88:267.

Jewett MA, Groll RJ: Nerve-sparing retroperitoneal lymphadenectomy. Urol Clin North Am 2007;34:149.

Jewett MAS et al: Management of recurrence and follow-up strategies for patients with nonseminoma testis cancer. Urol Clin North Am 2003;30:819.

Joudi FN, Crane CN, O'Donnell MA: Minimally invasive management of upper tract urothelial carcinoma. Curr Urol Rep 2006;7:23. Review.

Joudi FN, Smith BJ, O'Donnell MA: National BCG-Interferon Phase 2 Investigator Group Final results from a national multicenter phase II trial of combination bacillus Calmette-GuÈrin plus interferon alpha-2B for reducing recurrence of superficial bladder cancer. Urol Oncol 2006;24:344..

Kirkali Z, Tuzel E: Transitional cell carcinoma of the ureter and renal pelvis. Crit Rev Oncol Hematol 2003;47:155.

Kondagunta GV, Motzer RJ: Adjuvant chemotherapy for stage II nonseminomatous germ cell tumors. Urol Clin North Am 2007;34:179.

Lotan Y, Roehrborn CG: Sensitivity and specificity of commonly available bladder tumor markers versus cytology: results of a comprehensive literature review and meta-analyses. Urology 2003;61:109.

Matlaga BR et al: Radiofrequency ablation of renal tumors. Curr Urol Rep 2004;5:39.

Meuillet E et al: Chemoprevention of prostate cancer with selenium: an update on current clinical trials and preclinical findings. J Cell Biochem 2004;91:443.

Michaelson MD et al: Selective bladder preservation for muscle-invasive transitional cell carcinoma of the urinary bladder. Br J Cancer 2004;90:578.

Moinzadeh A, Gill IS: Laparoscopic radical cystectomy with urinary diversion. Curr Opin Urol 2004;14:83.

Nanus DM et al: Clinical use of monoclonal antibody HuJ591 therapy: targeting prostate specific membrane antigen. J Urol 2003;170:S84.

Neill M et al: Management of low-stage testicular seminoma. Urol Clin North Am 2007;34:127.

O'Donnell MA: Combined bacillus Calmette-Guérin and interferon use in superficial bladder cancer. Expert Rev Anticancer Ther 2003;3:809.

O'Donnell MA: Practical applications of intravesical chemotherapy and immunotherapy in high-risk patients with superficial bladder cancer. Urol Clin North Am 2005;32:121. Review.

Oliver RT et al: Radiotherapy versus single-dose carboplatin in adjuvant treatment of stage I seminoma: a randomised trial. Lancet 2005;366:293.

Pentyala SN et al: Prostate cancer: a comprehensive review. Med Oncol 2000;17:85.

Raghavan D: Testicular cancer: maintaining the high cure rate. Oncology 2003;17:218.

Roberts JT et al: Long-term survival results of a randomized trial comparing gemcitabine/cisplatin and methotrexate/vinblastine/doxorubicin/cisplatin in patients with locally advanced and metastatic bladder cancer. Ann Oncol 2006;17(suppl 5):v118.

Rosenberg JE, Carroll PR, Small EJ: Update on chemotherapy for advanced bladder cancer. J Urol 2005;174:14. Review.

Saisorn I et al: Fine needle aspiration cytology predicts inguinal lymph node metastasis without antibiotic pretreatment in penile carcinoma. Br J Urol (Int) 2006;97:1225.

Sarosdy MF et al: Use of a multitarget fluorescence in situ hybridization assay to diagnose bladder cancer in patients with hematuria. J Urol 2006;176:44.

Secin FP et al: Evaluation of regional lymph node dissection in patients with upper urinary tract urothelial cancer. Int J Urol 2007;14:26.

Sonpavde G, Sternberg CN: Treatment of metastatic urothelial cancer: opportunities for drug discovery and development. Br J Urol (Int) 2008;102:1354. Review.

Stenzl A, Höltl L: Orthotopic bladder reconstruction in women—what we have learned over the last decade. Crit Rev Oncol Hematol 2003;47:147.

Studer UE et al: Orthotopic ileal neobladder. Br J Urol (Int) 2004;93:183.

Sylvester RJ, Oosterlinck W, van der Meijden AP: A single immediate postoperative instillation of chemotherapy decreases the risk of recurrence in patients with stage Ta T1 bladder cancer: a meta-analysis of published results of randomized clinical trials. J Urol 2004;171:2186, quiz 2435.

Vaughn DJ: Chemotherapy for good-risk germ cell tumors: current concepts and controversies. Urol Clin North Am 2007;34:171.

NEUROPATHIC (NEUROGENIC) BLADDER

A neuropathic bladder has abnormal activity secondary to a neurologic condition. To understand the variety of neuropathic bladder conditions, a basic understanding of the normal innervation and myoneurophysiology is required.

Myoneural Anatomy

The urinary bladder and its involuntary sphincter develop and differentiate from the tubular urogenital sinus. The differentiation of the encasing mesenchymal cells forms the musculature of the detrusor and urethral sphincter.

Innervation

The innervation of the bladder and its involuntary sphincter is via the autonomic nervous system. The parasympathetic supply to the bladder and the sphincter is via the pelvic nerves, which arise from S2–4. These fibers also carry the stretch sensory receptors to the same spinal cord center (S2–4).

The sensory supply for pain, touch, and temperature is carried via the sympathetic fibers arising from the thoracolumbar segments (T11-L2).

Motor and sensory supply of the trigone is via the thoracolumbar sympathetic fibers.

The striated external sphincter, as well as the entire urogenital diaphragm, receives its motor and sensory innervation from the somatic fibers arising from S2–4 (via the pudendal nerve).

It is clear that the S2–4 segment is the origin of the motor supply to the bladder musculature, to the involuntary sphincter, and to the striated external sphincter. The trigone is the only structure that is partly independent in its innervation. This is why segment S2–4 is called the spinal cord center for micturition. It is located at the level of the T12 and L1 vertebral bodies. There are connections between the spinal reflex center and the midbrain and cerebral cortex. Through these connections, inhibition and control of the spinal cord reflexes can be maintained. The micturition reflex is coordinated in the pontine micturition center.

Myoneurophysiology

The primary functions of the urinary bladder are to store and empty urine at a safe pressure and in a continent fashion. Intact myoneural elements are essential for these functions. The primary reservoir function is possible because of the specialized detrusor muscle arrangement and because of the bladder compliance phenomenon. The normal adult bladder can accommodate volumes up to 400 mL without increasing intravesical pressure. Bladder fullness is perceived through increases in stretching of bladder mechanoreceptors.

Distention and stretch initiate detrusor activity that can be controlled and inhibited by the high cortical centers or can be allowed to progress to active detrusor contraction and voiding. Normally during voiding, detrusor contraction continues until the bladder is completely empty unless voiding is voluntarily interrupted or inhibited.

Before voiding begins, the pelvic floor and the striated external sphincter relax, the bladder base descends, and the bladder outlet assumes a funnel shape. As a result, urethral resistance decreases. This is followed by detrusor muscle contraction and a rise in intravesical pressure to 20 to 40 cm of water, which results in a urine flow of about 15 to 30 mL/s. When the bladder is completely empty, the pelvic floor and striated external sphincter contract, elevating the bladder base, increasing urethral pressure, and ending voiding. Intact nerve pathways are essential for these synchronized activities to occur.

Cystometry

Cystometry is a simple method for testing the bladder's storage function and gives the following information: bladder capacity, extent of accommodation or compliance, the ability to sense bladder filling and temperature, and the presence of an appropriate detrusor muscle contraction. In addition, postvoid residual urine can be measured at the same time. A normal cystometrogram is shown in Figure 38–15A.

Uroflowmetry

Uroflowmetry is the measurement of urine flow rate. If detrusor contraction is properly coordinated with sphincter relaxation, then the outlet resistance falls as the bladder pressure increases, and the flow rate is adequate. Normally, the flow rate changes with age but is more than 20 mL/s in men under 60 and more than 25 mL/s in women under 50 years of age. Any flow rate below 15 mL/s suggests obstruction or detrusor dysfunction. A flow rate under 10 mL/s strongly suggests underlying pathology.

Urodynamics

Urodynamic studies require measurement of bladder pressure during micturition. The pressure measured within the bladder (intravesical pressure) is a combination of the intra-abdominal pressure and the pressure generated by the detrusor. To determine the detrusor pressure, the intra-abdominal pressure is measured with a rectal catheter, and this pressure is subtracted from the total intravesical pressure (measured by the bladder catheter). The urine flow rates may then be assessed in light of the detrusor pressure. No consensus exists on a critical value for pressure and flow that is diagnostic of obstruction. Nomograms have been developed for evaluating the pressure-flow relationship and thus to categorize these values as obstructed, equivocal, or unobstructed.

Electromyographic Recording

Needle or patch electrodes may be employed to record the activity of the external sphincter. This information is useful when obtained during micturition. Increased activity in the sphincter after voiding begins suggests detrusor-sphincter dyssynergia.

Classification & Clinical Findings

Several classification systems exist that describe the variety of pathologic bladder conditions that develop secondary to neuropathies. Many bladder conditions are predictable on the basis of the neurologic lesion. A lesion above the brain stem (ie, stroke) affecting micturition frequently results in involuntary bladder contractions (detrusor hyperreflexia) with coordinated (synergistic) sphincter relaxation. These patients have urge incontinence.

A complete lesion of the spinal cord (ie, trauma) above the T12 vertebral body may leave the spinal reflex center intact. This often leads to what has been categorized as an upper motor neuron lesion. These patients have detrusor hyperreflexia and uncoordinated sphincter activity (detru-

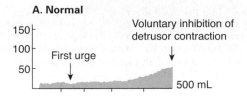

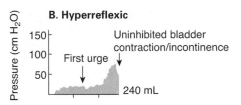

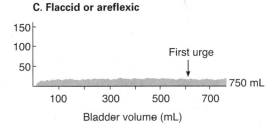

▲ **Figure 38–15.** Cystometrograms. **A:** Normal cystometrogram. **B:** Cystometrogram in a patient with hyperreflexic bladder caused by transection of the spinal cord above S2. **C:** Cystometrogram in a patient with an areflexic flaccid neuropathic bladder caused by a myelomeningocele.

sor-sphincter dyssynergia). Although detrusor contractions can generate abnormally high intravesical pressure, they are not effective in producing adequate urine flow because of the spastic external sphincter. Thus, there is residual urine. Bladder capacity is reduced. Detrusor contraction and mass reflexes can be initiated from certain trigger areas.

Figure 38–15B is a typical cystometrogram of a hyperreflexic bladder.

An injury to the spinal reflex center or below often leads to what has been categorized as a lower motor neuron lesion. These patients often develop detrusor areflexia. Trauma is the most common cause, but tumors, ruptured intervertebral disks, and meningomyelocele may also cause this type of neuropathic bladder. Both motor and sensory fibers are usually affected, and there is loss of sense of fullness (Figure 38–15C). These contractions are usually weak and unsustained, and bladder emptying is incomplete, resulting in large amounts of residual urine.

The bladder dynamics in a person with a neuropathic bladder often change over time. This may occur secondary to changes in innervation (ie, tethering of spinal cord, multiple sclerosis, recovery from spinal shock) or changes in the bladder. For example, a patient with a hyperreflexic bladder and dyssynergic sphincter often develops a trabeculated, noncompliant bladder over time. These changes require periodic reevaluation of all patients with neuropathic bladders regardless of the initial classification.

Differential Diagnosis

Cystitis, interstitial cystitis, and organic obstruction are occasionally confused with neuropathic bladder, but associated neurologic lesions usually make the diagnosis of neuropathic bladder easy. Psychosomatic disturbances can cause spasm of the external sphincter, incomplete voiding, retention, or incontinence.

Complications

Common complications include urinary tract infection, stone formation, and incontinence. The most serious consequences of these lesions are the hydrodynamic back-pressure on the kidneys, hydronephrosis, infection, decompensation of the ureterovesical junction, and loss of renal function.

Treatment

Immediately following spinal cord injury, there is a shock phase that may last a few weeks to 2 to 3 years. The average time is 2 to 3 months. The bladder is completely dissociated from nervous control and thus has no sensation and is areflexic.

Treatment is aimed at avoiding the aforementioned complications in the hope of partial or complete recovery. During the shock phase, continuous closed drainage or, preferably, clean intermittent (every 4–6 hours) catheterization should be instituted until bladder activity is restored.

A. Hyperreflexic Bladder

In the hyperreflexic bladder, attaining a functional bladder depends on mobilizing residual urine and increasing the bladder capacity. Residual urine volume can be decreased by reducing urethral resistance by several methods: transurethral prostatectomy, division of the external sphincter, pudendal nerve manipulation (ablation or electrical stimulation), or alpha-blocker pharmacologic therapy. Clean intermittent catheterization may also be required to evacuate the residual urine.

Functional capacity can be increased by decreasing detrusor instability with anticholinergic-parasympatholytic drugs (ie, oxybutynin or tolterodine) or by operative augmentation. This is often performed with small or large intestine (enterocystoplasty).

Conversion to a flaccid areflexic bladder can be achieved by cord rhizotomy. The storage function of the bladder is preserved, and the patient can be managed by clean intermittent catheterization.

Supravesical urinary diversion may be called for in patients with upper tract deterioration due to elevated storage pressures or female incontinence. Male incontinence may be controlled by a condom catheter.

B. Areflexic Bladder

Function of the flaccid bladder can be improved by measures that facilitate complete emptying; these include voiding by the Credé maneuver (suprapubic pressure), transurethral resection of the bladder neck to reduce outlet resistance, and timed voiding or timed clean intermittent catheterization. An indwelling urethral catheter or suprapubic cystostomy is required in a few cases, but chronic intubation should be avoided if possible.

Suprapubic urinary diversion (ileal or colon conduit, etc) can circumvent deterioration of upper tracts. Implantable prosthetic sphincters, periurethral bulking agent injections, or urethral slings may also improve urinary control.

A new technique of microanastomosis of a lumbar ventral nerve root to the S3 ventral root has generated promising results in children with spina bifida. This technique is reported to result in improved bladder function in children with an areflexic bladder as well as those with a hyperreflexic bladder.

Prognosis

Renal injury from elevated bladder pressure and infection are the most serious consequences of neuropathic bladder. When diversion or bladder augmentation is required, proper timing of the operation is essential for preservation of kidney function. Patients with a neuropathic bladder require close follow-up of their kidneys with renal ultrasound and serum creatinine determinations.

Cooper CS et al: Pediatric reconstructive surgery. Curr Opin Urol 2000;10:195.

Van Arendonk KJ et al: Improved efficacy of extended release oxybutynin in children with daytime urinary incontinence converted from regular oxybutynin. Urology 2006;68:862.

OTHER DISEASES & DISORDERS OF THE GENITOURINARY TRACT

SIMPLE RENAL CYST

A simple renal cyst is usually unilateral and solitary but may be multiple and bilateral. The cause of this disorder is unclear. The cyst can compress and destroy adjacent parenchyma. Cysts contain fluid that resembles (but is not) urine. Most are diagnosed in patients after the fourth decade. Occasionally, what appears to be a simple cyst may in fact be a papillary cystadenocarcinoma—an uncommon form of renal cancer with both solid and cystic components. In those cases, however, ultrasound usually demonstrates a complex mass with both cystic and solid components.

Flank pain may be a presenting symptom, though most renal cysts are found incidentally on urography done for other purposes. A mass may be felt in the flank or upper quadrant and must be distinguished from tumor. Urinalysis and tests of renal function are normal. Excretory urograms reveal a mass that distorts adjacent calices. Nephrotomography shows a radiolucent mass (in contradistinction to tumor). If the CT scan or ultrasound reveals an equivocal cystic mass, cyst aspiration may be performed, the fluid submitted for cytologic examination, and the cyst filled with contrast material to delineate its wall. A simple cyst must be distinguished from adenocarcinoma of the kidney; ultrasonography or CT scan usually makes that distinction.

Complications are rare, but bleeding into or infection of a cyst may occur.

If the diagnosis of cyst is established, surgery is not necessary unless the lesion causes pain or endangers renal function. Simple percutaneous aspiration with instillation of 95% ethanol may suffice. If sclerosis fails, laparoscopic or open excision may be performed.

RENAL ARTERY ANEURYSM

Aneurysm of the renal artery is relatively rare. It results from weakening of the artery wall by arteriosclerosis, poststenotic dilation, intimal or perimedial fibroplasia, or trauma. If the aneurysm causes stenosis of the artery, hypertension may ensue secondary to ischemia and activation of the renin-angiotensin system. A plain abdominal x-ray may reveal a ringlike calcification in the wall. Angiography or CT scan is diagnostic.

Surgery is indicated in the following situations: (1) secondary renal ischemia and hypertension, (2) dissecting aneurysm, (3) aneurysm associated with pain or hematuria, (4) anticipation of pregnancy, (5) aneurysm coincident with significant stenosis, (6) radiographic evidence of incomplete calcification or increase in size on serial films, and (7) aneurysm containing thrombus with evidence of distal embolization. If the aneurysm ruptures, emergency nephrectomy may be necessary.

RENAL INFARCTION

The common causes of renal artery occlusion include emboli due to subacute infective endocarditis, atrial or ventricular thrombi, arteriosclerosis, polyarteritis nodosa, trauma, and, in the neonate, umbilical artery catheterization. Multiple emboli are common and lead to patchy renal ischemia. Occlusion of a main renal artery causes renal total infarction.

The patient may suffer from severe flank pain, or the lesion may be silent. Hematuria is common. Excretory urograms may reveal no excretion of radiopaque material or may only opacify a portion of the kidney. With complete acute occlusion of the main renal artery, a ureteral catheter drains no urine, yet the retrograde urogram reveals normal anatomy. Renal angiography, color Doppler ultrasound, or magnetic resonance angiography makes the diagnosis by revealing occlusion of the artery or arterioles; a renal scan shows similar findings. CT scan after the intravenous injection of radiopaque medium shows no concentration in the ischemic area. Ureteral stone may mimic renal infarction, but urograms, CT scan, or angiograms distinguish one from the other. Following renal infarction, hypertension may develop secondary to renal ischemia; it may later resolve spontaneously.

If the diagnosis is made promptly (within 5–8 hours), thrombectomy or endarterectomy should be considered. Otherwise, anticoagulation therapy should be instituted (eg, heparin). Thrombolytic therapy (eg, streptokinase) may be used to lyse the clot. If permanent hypertension develops, definitive treatment of the arterial occlusion or nephrectomy (preferably laparoscopic) should be performed.

RENAL VEIN THROMBOSIS

Thrombosis of the renal vein affects both infants and adults and can be either acute or chronic. In children, thrombosis may be caused by severe dehydration (eg, due to ileocolitis and diarrhea or the nephrotic syndrome). In adults, it may be secondary to renal infection, ascending thrombosis of the vena cava, or caval occlusion due to tumor thrombus. There is usually flank pain and a palpable distended kidney. If renal vein thrombosis is secondary to infection, the patient is septic and urinalysis reveals pus cells and bacteria. In noninfectious cases, the urine may reveal microhematuria and mild proteinuria. The patient with bilateral involvement is azotemic. Nephrotic syndrome may develop. Excretory urograms show delayed opacification in an enlarged kidney. The calices are elongated. Later, the kidney may become atrophic. Renal angiography reveals stretching and bowing of arterioles. Selective renal venography demonstrates the thrombus, as does renal ultrasound.

Treatment should attempt to eliminate the underlying cause whenever possible. If the diagnosis of unilateral infected renal vein thrombosis can be established, nephrectomy should be performed. In bilateral disease, anticoagulant or thrombolytic therapy (or both) is required.

VESICAL FISTULAS

Vesical fistulas may be congenital or acquired. Congenital fistulas usually involve the urachus. Acquired fistulas may be iatrogenic or due to trauma, tumor, or inflammation.

The most common types of vesical fistulas are vesicovaginal, vesicointestinal, and vesicocutaneous. Vesicovaginal fistulas are commonly secondary to gynecologic or birth trauma; rarely, they occur as a complication of infiltrating cervical carcinoma. Vesicointestinal fistulas are most often due to inflammatory bowel disease: Crohn disease, diverticulitis, and appendicitis. Cystostomy in the presence of bladder outlet obstruction, bladder cancer, or foreign body may result in vesicocutaneous fistula.

Diagnostic maneuvers include cystoscopy, conventional cystography, barium enema or barium swallow, and CT scan with contrast infusion. Oral charcoal may be useful for detecting a urinary intestinal fistula, as the granules can be seen in spun urine under the microscope.

Therapy for vesicovaginal fistula requires surgical closure, with placement of an omental flap between the bladder and the vagina. For vesicointestinal fistula, the primary intestinal lesion must be resected and the bladder closed. An indwelling urethral catheter is necessary during the healing period.

INTERSTITIAL CYSTITIS

This lesion is most commonly found in middle-aged women. Urinary frequency both day and night is most often accompanied by suprapubic pain with bladder distention. The cause is uncertain, though some suggest an autoimmune collagen disease, while others have documented the presence of mast cells and mast cell mediators (histamine and prostaglandin) in bladder biopsy specimens of affected patients.

The diagnosis is based on the history and the results of cystoscopy under general anesthesia. Cystoscopy reveals a small-capacity bladder and punctate hemorrhage following forceful distention. (Studies suggest this is a nonspecific finding.) Biopsy may reveal lymphocytic infiltration, mast cell infiltration, and submucosal fibrosis. In patients suspected of having interstitial cystitis, one must rule out carcinoma in situ; urine cytologic study at the time of cystoscopy and random bladder biopsy.

Treatment of established cases of interstitial cystitis often fails. Response has been obtained with hydraulic bladder overdistention, intravesical treatment with 50% dimethyl-sulfoxide, 0.4% oxychlorosene sodium, or sodium pentosan-polysulfate. Systemic corticosteroids have their proponents as well, and BCG has been tried with some success. Some patients require operative augmentation of bladder capacity by enterocystoplasty or, rarely, cystourethrectomy and permanent urinary diversion.

URINARY STRESS INCONTINENCE

Involuntary loss of urine during stress (coughing, sneezing, or physical strain) is a common complaint of postmenopausal women. The cause is related to pelvic relaxation with age, resulting in descent of the trigone and proximal urethra. There is obliteration of the urethrovesical angle, which normally provides resistance at the bladder outlet. The diagnosis is made by the history and physical examination and urodynamic evaluation. When the bladder is full, the patient should be asked to cough while in both the supine and upright positions, producing incontinence. Digital pressure applied to the paraurethral tissues in an anterior direction through the vagina reestablishes the urethrovesical angle and prevents stress incontinence (Marshall test).

Treatment in patients with normal bladder function and low residual urine is initiated with behavioral therapy and perineal exercises; if unsuccessful, pharmacologic methods include oxybutynin and ephedrine. Definitive management is surgical. Currently, the most effective surgical approach is a sling procedure with a piece of autologous or synthetic fascia attached to the rectus muscle or os pubis and surrounding the urethra at the bladder neck. Newer approaches include the use of collagen injection into the periurethral tissues, resulting in increased urethral outflow resistance.

FEMALE URETHRITIS & PERIURETHRITIS

Urethritis in the female may be acute or chronic. Acute urethritis can be gonorrheal in origin. Chemical urethritis is occasionally acquired from exposure to soap or bath oils. Chronic urethritis is a common problem in women, since the female urethra is exposed to pathogenic bacteria because of its anatomic location. Urethral trauma, instrumentation, and increase in the number of pathogenic organisms lead to infection and overt urethritis. Urethritis usually precedes cystitis.

Hormonal changes associated with menopause cause vaginal and urethral mucosal changes, leading to irritative symptoms and increased susceptibility to inflammation.

Urethritis usually causes irritative voiding symptoms similar to those of cystitis and, occasionally, functional obstructive symptoms. Examination may reveal urethral discharge, marked tenderness, or congested everted mucosa at the external meatus. Induration of the urethra may be associated with vaginitis and cervicitis. Endoscopy may reveal obstruction, mucosal congestion, and inflammatory polyps. Urethral calibration rarely reveals obstruction. Spasm of the external sphincter may be noted.

Treatment is directed to the underlying cause. Estrogen cream is indicated for senile vaginitis. Surgical treatment consists of urethral dilation and opening and draining infected periurethral ducts. Alpha-blockers given orally may also help decrease urethral resistance. Correction of vaginitis, cervicitis, and cervical erosions helps in ameliorating symptoms.

FEMALE URETHRAL CARUNCLE

Urethral caruncle, commonly seen after menopause, represents granulomatous overgrowth of the posterior lip of the external meatus. The caruncle is tender and causes pain with intercourse and urination. The primary concern is exclusion of urethral cancer. Treatment is complete excision.

FEMALE URETHRAL DIVERTICULUM

Urethral diverticulum in the female commonly presents as recurrent lower urinary tract infection. It should be suspected whenever urinary infection fails to resolve with treatment. Symptoms are urinary dribbling and cystic swelling in the anterior vaginal wall during voiding. If diverticulum is suspected, it can usually be identified during panendoscopy and opacified by contrast medium on a voiding cystourethrogram while occluding the external meatus. These lesions occasionally contain stones or tumors. Treatment consists of transvaginal diverticulectomy.

Brubaker L: Surgical treatment of urinary incontinence in women. Gastroenterology 2004;126:S71.

Chancellor MB, Yoshimura N: Treatment of interstitial cystitis. Urology 2004;63(suppl 3A):85.

Diokno AC: Medical management of urinary incontinence. Gastroenterology 2004;126:S77.

Nickel JC: Interstitial cystitis. A chronic pelvic pain syndrome. Med Clin North Am 2004;88:467.

SPERMATOCELE

Spermatocele is a retention cyst of a tubule of the rete testis or the head of the epididymis. The cyst is distended with a milky fluid that contains sperm. Located at the superior pole of the testis and caput epididymidis, the spermatocele is soft and fluctuant and can be transilluminated. No treatment is needed unless the spermatocele is painful, in which case surgical excision may be performed.

VARICOCELE

Varicocele is due to incompetent valves in the testicular vein, permitting transmission of hydrostatic venous pressure; distention and tortuosity of the pampiniform plexus results. Varicocele is found in 15% of male adolescents with left-sided predominance (90%), presumably because of venous drainage of the left testes to the left renal vein, causing increased retrograde venous pressure. Bilateral varicoceles are palpable in less than 2% of male adults.

Mild varicoceles are commonly asymptomatic, but a dragging scrotal sensation may be noted. Varicocele may lead to infertility in some men.

Asymptomatic varicocele is best untreated unless it is a suspected factor in male infertility. Treatment then consists of operative ligation of the spermatic vein at or above the internal inguinal ring. In recurrent varicocele, transfemoral catheterization and occlusion or ablation of the spermatic vein may be performed with a detachable balloon or sclerosing agents. The technical success rate is high.

TORSION OF THE SPERMATIC CORD

Torsion of the spermatic cord (intravaginal torsion or torsion within the space of the tunica vaginalis) is most common in adolescent boys. A twist in the spermatic cord interferes with testicular blood supply. If torsion is complete, testicular infarction may occur within 4 to 6 hours. The cause is unknown, but an underlying anatomic abnormality (spacious tunica vaginalis, loose epididymotesticular connection, undescended testis) is usually present.

Clinical findings consist of precipitous onset of lower abdominal and scrotal pain and scrotal swelling. There may be a history of previous trauma in young adolescents. The testis is swollen, tender, and retracted. The pain is not relieved by testicular support. The cord above the swelling is normal. The cremasteric reflex is usually absent on the affected side.

Torsion must be differentiated from orchitis, epididymitis, and pain due to testicular trauma. Technetium 99m pertechnetate scan *may* differentiate orchitis-epididymitis from testicular torsion if performed early in the course of symptoms: The former demonstrates increased blood flow, in contrast to the ischemic pattern of torsion. Color Doppler ultrasound is more definitive and less time consuming and can delineate the lack of testicular blood flow. No radiologic study is completely accurate, and imaging should be used to confirm the clinical decision that the cause of the acute scrotum is not torsion. If the diagnosis cannot be established by examination, history, and imaging, exploration is required.

Torsion of the spermatic cord is a surgical emergency! Contralateral orchiopexy is always necessary because of frequent bilateral involvement (ie, the "bell clapper" deformity: lack of fixation of the cord structures by the testicular mediastinum) and the high incidence of recurrent torsion and infertility in bilateral cases.

TORSION OF TESTICULAR APPENDAGES

The epididymis and the testicle often have a vestigial remnant of embryologic ducts known as an appendix testis or appendix epididymis. These structures can undergo spontaneous infarction usually in young boys, causing acute testicular pain and swelling that may be difficult to differentiate from testicular torsion. With torsion of the appendix testis or epididymis, physical examination often demonstrates point tenderness at the site of the torsed appendage. Occasionally, the infarcted appendage can be seen through the scrotal wall as a "blue dot" sign on the scrotum. This sign is only visible early in the course, prior to hydrocele formation and onset of scrotal edema. Scrotal ultrasound occasionally delineates the enlarged appendage and a normal testicle, establishing the diagnosis. In most cases—and certainly in equivocal ones—immediate scrotal exploration and removal of the infarcted appendage is required to rule out testicular torsion. Although the appendages often occur bilaterally, appendiceal torsion does not; thus, removal of the opposite appendage is not indicated.

MALE INFERTILITY

Male infertility accounts for 30% to 50% of infertile couples (10–15% of marriages). Both partners should be evaluated for causes of infertility.

The causes of male infertility include the following: congenital anomalies (genetic, such as Klinefelter's syndrome, or developmental, such as absent vas deferens); trauma (both testicular, resulting in atrophy, and neurologic, resulting in erectile or ejaculatory dysfunction); infections (either systemic or reproductive organ specific); endocrine disorders (pituitary insufficiency, androgen deficiency); acquired anatomic abnormalities (varicocele, vasectomy); or drug side effects (nitrofurantoin, estrogens, antineoplastic agents).

Diagnosis

The most important aspect of infertility evaluation is the history, which uncovers the cause in many patients. The physical examination is no less important and may reveal small testicles, a varicocele, or absence of the vas deferens.

A. Semen Analysis

Semen analysis is essential in evaluation of male factor infertility. At least two samples should be analyzed, since values may vary over time and with the method of collection. The specimen is produced by masturbation after 3 days of ejaculatory abstinence and collected in a clean wide-mouth container and examined within 2 hours. Determination of the volume, pH, liquefaction, sperm count, viability, abnormal forms, and motility constitutes a complete analysis. Normal values include volume of more than 2.0 mL, concentration greater than 20 million sperm per mL, more than 50% motile sperm, and 75% or more viable sperm (World Health Organization criteria).

B. Hormone Studies

Patients with no sperm in the ejaculate (azoospermia) or very low counts (oligospermia, < 10 million sperm/ml) should have serum FSH, LH, and testosterone levels measured. Patients with low testosterone should have prolactin levels checked and, if elevated, should be investigated for pituitary tumor. A significant elevation of FSH represents a problem with spermatogenesis.

C. Testicular Biopsy

Testicular biopsies are indicated in azoospermic patients to distinguish obstructive versus parenchymal disease. Testicular biopsy should be performed in patients with unexplained oligospermia to establish a histologic diagnosis, to assess prognosis, and to direct treatment. If the serum FSH is more than two times normal, one may presume the presence of severe and irreversible testicular damage without confirmatory testis biopsy.

Vasography requires injection of contrast material into the vas. The purpose of this study is to delineate obstruction of the vas, epididymis, seminal vesicle, or ejaculatory duct. Vasography is used in patients who are azoospermic and have no evidence of retrograde ejaculation while demonstrating normal spermatogenesis on testicular biopsy. Seminal fructose levels should be obtained before operative exposure of the vas. Absence of fructose would indicate obstruction of the ejaculatory duct, and if this diagnosis is confirmed by vasography, the obstructing tissue may be resected by transurethral methods.

D. Other Diagnostic Studies

The **sperm penetration assay,** performed by incubation of sperm with hamster eggs whose zona pellucida has been enzymatically removed, offers an objective method of determining the ability of sperm to penetrate the ovum. The **cervical mucus penetration test** compares sperm motility in cervical mucus with a known standard. Although these two important parameters of sperm function can be evaluated, neither test alone can establish the cause of male factor infertility.

Antisperm antibodies can be measured in the serum of either the male or female partner or in the seminal fluid. This assessment is indicated when spontaneous sperm agglutination or decreased sperm motility is noted on semen analysis. If antisperm antibodies are found, immunosuppressive therapy in the form of steroids may be effective in reducing agglutination (clumping) and increasing motility. Another method of treating antisperm antibodies is in vitro sperm washing with immunobeads coated by antihuman antibody. The sperm not bound by antibody remain in the supernatant and can be used for intrauterine insemination.

Studies to detect a nonpalpable varicocele are not recommended except in cases in which the physical examination is inadequate. Physical examination is the most effective method of detecting clinically significant varices. Venography is reserved for patients with recurrent varices, since identification of collateral venous channels would direct choice of therapy.

Transrectal ultrasound is used to support the diagnosis of ejaculatory duct obstruction in the azoospermic patient. Absence of the seminal vesicles or distention due to distal obstruction can be identified. This study should be preceded by measurement of fructose in the ejaculate (lack of fructose suggests obstruction of the ejaculatory duct) and examination of postejaculate urine (to determine the presence of sperm, suggesting retrograde ejaculation).

Treatment

A. Nonoperative Treatment

Primary male infertility may be caused by hypogonadotropic hypogonadism, diagnosed by demonstrating low serum levels of FSH, LH, and testosterone. Spermatogenesis may be stimulated by administration of hCG followed by FSH. Isolated absence of either FSH or LH is rare; the LH deficiency is overcome by administration of testosterone, and lack of FSH is treated by administration of menotropins. Hyperprolactinemia may contribute to male infertility and would be treated with bromocriptine.

Infection of the reproductive organs should be treated when found during evaluation of male infertility. Infection may cause infertility immediately by several mechanisms: decreased spermatogenesis due to hyperthermia, immune interaction with sperm causing agglutination and decreased motility, as well as later sequelae such as obstruction of the ejaculatory tract. Pyospermia suggests the diagnosis, and treatment should be designed to eliminate the common pathogens: *Neisseria gonorrhoeae, Chlamydia trachomatis,* and *Ureaplasma urealyticum* (all are sensitive to tetracycline).

If antisperm antibodies are found in either partner, steroids may be used to suppress the immune system. One must use steroids with caution and after thorough discussion of possible side effects with the patient; acne, hypertension, gastrointestinal bleeding, and avascular necrosis of the hip have been reported with steroid administration. Response to treatment is assessed by repeat semen analysis and measurement of antisperm antibodies in the patient's serum. Sperm washing in an attempt to remove cytotoxic antibodies may improve motility and decrease clumping; washed semen may then be instilled into the uterus (artificial insemination of the husband's semen) or used in conjunction with in vitro fertilization techniques.

Retrograde ejaculation or lack of seminal emission— usually due to spinal cord injury or sympathetic nerve injury during retroperitoneal surgery leading to bladder neck (ie, internal sphincter) incompetence—can be treated with α-adrenergic drugs or antihistamines to reestablish internal sphincter function and antegrade ejaculation. Alternatively, alkalinized postejaculate urine can be collected and centrifuged and the concentrated sperm instilled into the female partner's uterus.

Clomiphene and tamoxifen are antiestrogens that are currently used in patients with idiopathic oligospermia, though the efficacy of these medications has been doubted.

B. Operative Therapy

Ligation of varicocele yields pregnancy in 30% to 50% of patients. Several approaches are available, including inguinal and retroperitoneal. Transvenous occlusion of the spermatic vein by balloon is useful especially in cases of recurrent varicocele.

Obstruction of the epididymis-vas system may be amenable to vasovasostomy or vasoepididymostomy. Currently, these procedures are performed with the aid of the operating microscope, and patency is established in 50% to 90% of cases.

Obstruction of the ejaculatory ducts is rare. When this diagnosis is made, transurethral resection of the ducts may establish patency.

C. Assisted Reproductive Techniques

These include the following: artificial insemination with husband's sperm (AIH), gamete intrafallopian transfer (GIFT), and in vitro fertilization (IVF) using intracytoplasmic sperm injection (ICSI) after retrieving eggs by transvaginal ultrasound guidance and sperm by testicular aspiration in selected partners. In cases of male factor infertility not amenable to treatment, artificial insemination by donor sperm is also available.

Bong GW, Koo HP: The adolescent varicocele: to treat or not to treat. Urol Clin North Am 2004;31:509.

Brugh VM III, Lipshultz LI: Male factor infertility. Evaluation and management. Med Clin North Am 2004;88:367.

Carlsen E et al: Effects of ejaculatory frequency and season on variations in semen quality. Fertil Steril 2004;82:358.

Hopps CV et al: The diagnosis and treatment of the azoospermic patient in the age of intracytoplasmic sperm injection. Urol Clin North Am 2002;29:895.

Jarow JP: Endocrine causes of male infertility. Urol Clin North Am 2003;30:83.

Siddiq FM, Sigman M: A new look at the medical management of infertility. Urol Clin North Am 2002;29:949.

Wald M et al: Therapeutic testis biopsy for sperm retrieval. Curr Opin Urol 2007;17:431.

PRIAPISM

Priapism is a rare disorder in which prolonged, painful erection occurs, usually not associated with sexual stimulation. The blood in the corpora cavernosa becomes hyperviscous but not clotted. About 25% of cases are associated with leukemia, metastatic carcinoma, sickle cell anemia, or trauma. In most cases, the cause is uncertain.

If the erection does not subside, needle aspiration of the sludged blood of the corpora followed by lavage with alpha-adrenergic agents such as phenylephrine should be performed. Delayed or unsuccessful treatment may result in impotence. Unsuccessful treatment calls for the Winter procedure, in which a biopsy needle is passed through the glans into one of the corpora, creating a fistula between corpora cavernosa and corpus spongiosum. If this procedure is successful, then potency is usually maintained. Other procedures include excising the tunica albuginea at the tip of the corpora cavernosum, proximal cavernosal-spongiosum shunt, and saphenous vein-cavernous shunt. If priapism persists, impotence results.

In sickle cell anemia, hydration and hypertransfusion often give relief and should constitute initial therapy.

PEYRONIE'S DISEASE (PLASTIC INDURATION OF THE PENIS)

Fibrosis of the dorsal covering sheaths of the corpora cavernosa occasionally occurs without known cause in men over age 45. Trauma to the penis during intercourse has been implicated in the etiology of Peyronie's disease. The fibrosis does not permit the involved surface to lengthen with erection, thus leading to dorsal chordee. The disorder may be due to vasculitis in the connective tissues. Palpation of the penile shaft reveals a raised, firm plaque dorsally. There is an association with Dupuytren contracture.

Controversy exists regarding treatment. Expectant therapy or medical treatment, including vitamin E, para-aminobenzoic acid, colchicine, and intralesional verapamil may limit progression of disease. Operative therapy is necessary for patients who do not respond or for impotent patients. In the potent patient, either plication of the tunica albuginea on the opposite side of the plaque or a Nesbit procedure—excision of an ellipse of the tunica albuginea from the ventral convex aspect of the shaft and suture closure—or plaque excision and dermal grafting have been used successfully. If the patient is impotent, insertion of a penile prosthesis is the procedure of choice.

Taylor FL, Levine LA: Peyronie's disease. Urol Clin North Am 2007;34:517.

PHIMOSIS & PARAPHIMOSIS

Phimosis—inability to retract the foreskin to expose the glans—may be congenital but is more often acquired. At birth, the foreskin cannot be easily retracted, but by age 3, the prepuce becomes pliant and the glans can be exposed and cleansed. If the foreskin is then retractable, circumcision is not necessary. Acquired phimosis is usually a result of chronic and recurrent bacterial balanitis (infection of the prepuce), common in patients with diabetes or balanitis xerotica obliterans. These patients are best treated by circumcision.

Paraphimosis is the inability to reduce a previously retracted foreskin. The prepuce becomes fixed in the retracted position proximal to the corona. With prolonged retraction, lymphedema of the prepuce exacerbates the condition and increases the circumferential pressure of the shaft proximal to the glans. Manual reduction can usually be accomplished using the index fingers to pull the prepuce distally while pushing the glans into the prepuce. If this measure fails, the preputial cicatrix may be incised (dorsal slit) and the foreskin reduced with relative ease. Circumcision may be performed as an elective procedure once the edema has subsided.

CONDYLOMATA ACUMINATA

Condylomata acuminata are wartlike lesions that occur on the penis, scrotum, urethra, and perineum in men and the vagina, cervix, and perineum in women. They are caused by human papillomavirus and are usually transmitted by sexual contact. Pain and bleeding are common presenting complaints. Warts outside the urethra can be treated with excision, application of podophyllum resin, liquid nitrogen, or CO_2 laser. Urethroscopy is needed to determine the proximal extent of lesions in the urethra. Intraurethral fulguration, CO_2 laser treatment, injection of fluorouracil solution, or interferon-α can be therapeutic.

IMPOTENCE

Impotence is the inability to obtain and sustain an erection satisfactory for sexual intercourse.

▶ Causes of Impotence

Causes can be grouped into the following categories: neurologic, vascular, endocrine, systemic, pharmacologic, and psychologic. Treatment is directed accordingly.

A. Neurologic

Reflex erections are mediated by the afferent fibers of the pudendal nerve and efferent fibers of the parasympathetic outflow (S2–4). Psychogenic erections are initiated via cerebral centers. Specific neurologic diseases that may cause impotence may be congenital (spina bifida), acquired (cerebrovascular accident, Alzheimer disease, multiple sclerosis), iatrogenic (electroshock therapy), neoplastic (pituitary or hypothalamic tumors), traumatic (cord compression), infectious (tabes dorsalis), and nutritional (vitamin deficiency).

B. Vascular

Vascular causes of impotence may be cardiac (anginal syndromes, congestive failure), aortoiliac disease (Leriche syndrome, atherosclerosis, other embolic phenomena), microangiopathy (diabetes, radiation injury), and abnormal venous drainage.

C. Endocrine

The accepted endocrine causes of impotence are hypogonadism, hyperprolactinemia, pituitary tumors, hypothyroidism, Addison disease, Cushing syndrome, acromegaly, and testicular feminizing syndrome.

D. Pharmacologic

Impotence is a common and often unsuspected complication of many therapeutic and illicit drugs. Major groups that may cause sexual dysfunction are the following: tranquilizers, antidepressants, antianxiety agents, anticholinergic drugs, antihypertensives, and many drugs with abuse potential. One should recognize that virtually all antihypertensives (including diuretics) can be associated with impotence or ejaculatory dysfunction. Drugs with abuse potential include alcohol (both as a direct affect and secondary to cirrhosis) and cocaine.

E. Psychogenic

Up to 50% of cases of impotence are related to psychogenic factors. Establishing an organic cause of impotence is important in choosing appropriate therapy. Factors that indicate a psychogenic cause are the following: selective erectile dysfunction (episodic, normal nocturnal erections, normal erections with masturbation), sudden onset, associated anxiety or external stress, affect disturbances (anger, anxiety, guilt, fear), and patient convinced of an organic cause.

▶ Diagnosis

The history and physical examination suggest the cause in most cases. Confirmatory tests are necessary to ensure an appropriate choice of therapy.

In investigating a possible neurologic cause of impotence, the neurologic examination should include review of systems with respect to bladder and bowel function. More invasive studies include a cystometrogram with bethanechol supersensitivity testing, electromyography of the external urethral sphincter, and bulbosphincteric reflex latency.

Vascular impotence is suggested by signs of peripheral vascular disease as well as a history of atherosclerotic heart disease. Noninvasive diagnostic testing is performed by Doppler penile-brachial index. A penile blood pressure to brachial blood pressure ratio less than 0.6 suggests a vascular cause. Venous leak requires cavernosography and cavernosometry. Arteriography is rarely required but may be indicated in patients with a history of pelvic trauma.

Endocrine evaluation mandates measurement of serum testosterone and prolactin; many investigators include assessment of FSH and LH. Routine automated chemical screening may suggest other hormonal abnormalities that require additional testing. These studies should also detect systemic disease capable of causing impotence: cirrhosis, renal failure, scleroderma, and diabetes.

Psychogenic impotence may be established by nocturnal penile tumescence monitoring or outpatient snap-gauge cuffs. Additional testing includes one of the following: Minnesota Multiphasic Personality Inventory, DeRogatis Sexual Function Inventory, and Walker Sex Form.

▶ Treatment

A. Nonoperative Treatment

First-line treatment includes oral phosphodiesterase inhibitors (sildenafil, vardenafil, tadalafil). These medications are contraindicated in men with heart disease who are taking nitroglycerin. These medications work in patients who have normal blood flow and neurologic innervation. In patients without arterial-vascular causes of impotence, intracorporal injections of papaverine, phentolamine, or prostaglandin E_1 (or all three) offer a nonoperative means of restoring sexual function. Intractable psychogenic impotence may also respond to this treatment. Intraurethral pellets of alprostadil (prostaglandin E_1) can also be used; however, they often cause pain and are not favored by most patients. Finally, a vacuum erection device can be used to sustain erection.

Endocrine disturbances responsible for impotence include hypotestosteronemia and hyperprolactinemia. Testosterone deficiency is treated by replacement therapy using a once-daily topical testosterone gel or depot testosterone intramuscular injection every 2 to 3 weeks. Hyperprolactinemia is treated by bromocriptine therapy; the patient should be evaluated to assess the presence of a pituitary tumor.

Pharmacologic causes of impotence require altering medical treatment to ameliorate or eliminate secondary impotence. The ability to change medications depends on the severity of the underlying disease.

Psychogenic impotence is treated by a trained sex therapist, and response may be anticipated in most cases. The importance of eliminating organic causes of impotence before embarking on psychological therapy is obvious: The best psychological methods applied to organic impotence do not resolve the dysfunction but serve to frustrate both the therapist and patient.

B. Operative Treatment

Penile prosthesis insertion is currently the most common operative method for treatment of impotence. Two categories of prosthesis are in use: semirigid and inflatable. The semirigid prostheses are composed of a rigid shaft and a flexible hinge at the penile-pubic junction or a malleable soft metal case within the prosthesis; the erection is constant and is satisfactory to effect vaginal penetration, but the penile circumference is not equal to that of a natural erection.

Inflatable prostheses offer erections more similar in size to those experienced by the patient prior to the onset of impotence when compared to those achieved by semirigid prostheses. Two types of inflatable prostheses are available: The standard inflatable prosthesis consists of two corporal inflatable rods, a reservoir situated in the retropubic space, and a pump placed in the scrotum; the new inflatable rods combine the simplicity of two corporal rods with the sophistication of a self-contained pump and reservoir system (FlexiFlate and Hydroflex), permitting the convenience of inflation and deflation without tubing and multiple components.

Satisfactory results are achieved in 85% of patients. Complications common to both types of prostheses are infection and erosion of skin or urethra. The inflatable prostheses are also at risk for mechanical failure of the pump, tubing or reservoir leak, and aneurysm or rupture of the corporal cylinders.

Arterial revascularization of the penile arteries has met with limited success. Aortoiliac reconstruction improves erectile function in only 30% of cases. Microsurgical revascularization of the penile arteries (dorsal artery of the penis or deep corporal arteries) is successful in 60% of patients. While these methods avoid the risks of prosthetic infection and offer the advantage of reestablishing the natural physiologic mechanisms of erection, the mediocre success rate (when compared with the results of prosthetic insertion) would suggest that microsurgical penile revascularization be reserved for carefully selected cases.

Seftel AD et al: Office evaluation of male sexual dysfunction. Urol Clin North Am 2007;34:463.

Gynecology

R. Kevin Reynolds, MD
Paul V. Loar III, MD

PERTINENT HISTORY & PHYSICAL EXAMINATION FOR GYNECOLOGIC DISEASES

Accurate diagnosis and treatment of gynecologic disease begins with obtaining a complete history and physical examination. A thorough history should include the following:

- First day of the most recent menstrual cycle.
- Current genital tract symptoms.
- Age at first menses (menarche).
- Interval from starting one menses to the next (cycle length).
- Duration and amount of menstrual flow.
- Presence or absence of irregular or unexplained bleeding.
- Symptoms associated with each menstrual cycle such as cramping before or during menses.
- Other genital tract symptoms such as urinary or fecal incontinence, prolapse, dyspareunia, discharge, or pruritus.
- Sexual history, including assessment of risk factors such as knowledge of safe sex practices, age of first intercourse (coitarche), number and gender of partners, and presence of any history of abuse.
- Number of pregnancies and subsequent outcome, including term delivery, mode of delivery, preterm delivery, miscarriage, or abortion.
- Contraceptive use, including type, duration.
- History of sexually transmitted disease such as infection with human papillomavirus, gonorrhea, or chlamydia.
- Adequacy of cervical cancer screening with Pap tests, including date of most recent screen and any prior history of abnormal screens.
- History of any gynecologic surgery, including type, date, and indication.
- Age of menopause.

- Presence of postmenopausal bleeding, regardless of amount of flow.
- Hormone therapy of any type, including oral contraceptives, postmenopausal estrogen replacement therapy, hormone therapy of breast cancer, and so on.
- Family history of pertinent cancer sites, including ovarian cancer, endometrial cancer, breast cancer, and colorectal cancer. Determine the age at time of cancer diagnosis and relationship of the affected individual to the patient.
- Determine the ethnicity of the patient regarding potential for hereditary diseases.

Perform a complete pelvic examination. Inspect external genitalia, including vulva and urethra, for development, symmetry, and visible lesions. Place a vaginal speculum to inspect the vagina and cervix for symmetry or visible lesions, and perform Pap test, cultures, or wet mount tests as indicated to evaluate symptoms or update screening. Bimanual examination is then performed with careful compression of pelvic viscera between the examiner's hand on the abdominal wall and the finger(s) in the vagina. The process is repeated with the rectovaginal examination whereby one finger is placed in the vagina and one is inserted into the rectum. The rectovaginal examination allows the examiner to feel higher into the pelvis and may improve the ability to feel the cardinal and uterosacral ligaments, cul-de-sac peritoneum, ovaries, rectocele, and sphincter integrity. The rectovaginal examination is particularly important for assessing pelvic masses or malignancies, rectocele, and fecal incontinence.

EMBRYOLOGY & ANATOMY

Development of the reproductive tract in the female fetus results from fusion and differentiation of the müllerian ducts and the urogenital sinus. Fusion defects may result in duplication, malformation, or absence of genital tract structures. The most common defects are imperforate hymen, presence of longitudinal or transverse septae within the vagina, congenital absence of the vagina, and duplication defects of the uterus (see Figure 39–1). The etiology of most of these congenital defects is idiopathic, but some cases arise as a result of teratogens such as androgen exposure to the developing fetus during the first and second trimesters.

Careful examination of the newborn is necessary. Cursory examination of the genital structure of the newborn may result in errors of gender assignment. Ultrasound and/or MRI, examination under anesthesia, and possible laparoscopy or hysteroscopy provide information for accurate diagnosis. One third or more of children diagnosed with genital tract anomalies will have associated anomalies of the urinary tract, such as absent kidney, horseshoe kidney, and duplication of ureters.

The pelvis is a space constrained by bony architecture and filled with gastrointestinal, urologic, and gynecologic viscera. The blood supply is rich, including the external and internal ileac arteries and veins and numerous branches within the pelvis. Motor nerves, including the sciatic, obturator, and femoral nerves, transit the pelvis along the pelvic sidewall. Sensory nerves, including the genitofemoral nerve, are superficially located and easily injured. The ureter is closely placed to the uterine artery and is at risk for injury during hysterectomy procedures. See Figure 39–2A and B. A pelvic surgeon must be intimately familiar with the close spacing of critical pelvic structures to minimize risk of injury.

THE LOWER GENITAL TRACT: VULVA, VAGINA, & CERVIX

SCREENING & TREATMENT OF PREMALIGNANT LOWER GENITAL TRACT NEOPLASIA

As recently as 1945, cervical cancer and related lower genital tract cancers were the most common cancers in women. With the advent of the Pap test in the 1940s, cervical cancer incidence began to fall with more than an 80% reduction of risk of mortality in the ensuing six decades. It is now understood that virtually all cervical cancers and some vaginal and vulvar cancers are caused by persistent infection with oncogenic strains of the human papillomavirus (HPV). There are more than 75 HPV types identified, with types 6 and 11 most commonly associated with condyloma and types 16 and 18 associated with preinvasive and invasive carcinoma. Prevalence of HPV infection is as high as 80% of the population, but most infections are transient in nature. With appropriate screening and treatment to detect individuals with persistent high-risk HPV infection, the risk of developing invasive cervical cancer is low. In parts of the world without screening, cervical cancer remains prevalent and is the second-most common cancer diagnosis for unscreened women. Recent FDA approval of vaccination effective for the prevention of oncogenic HPV strains has the potential to greatly reduce HPV-mediated lower genital tract cancers in women.

A number of professional groups have issued guidelines for cervical cancer screening, including initiation of screen-

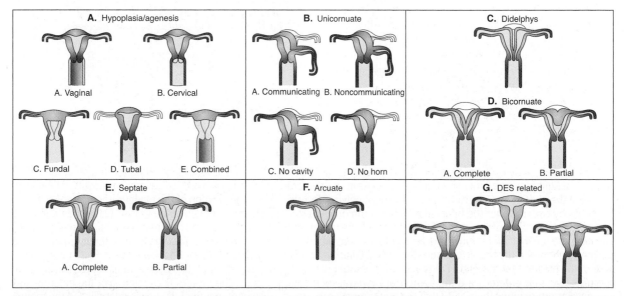

▲ **Figure 39–1.** Classification of müllerian anomalies. DES, diethylstilbestrol. (From Schorge JO, Williams JW: *Williams Gynecology,* Figure 18–13. McGraw-Hill Medical, 2008.)

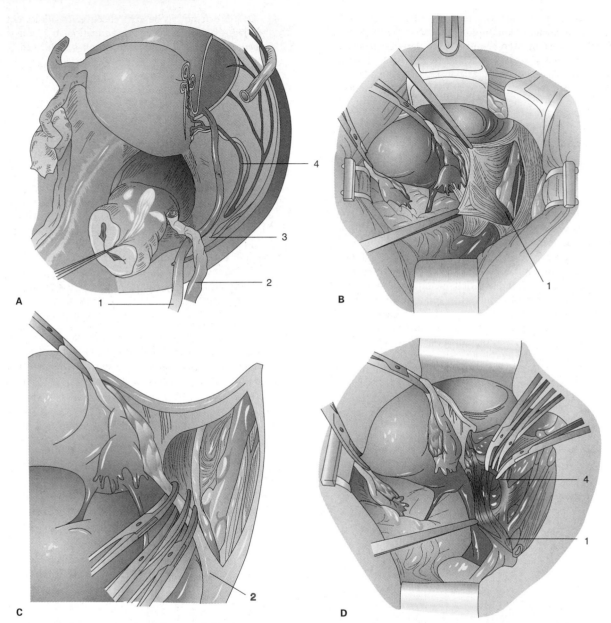

▲ **Figure 39–2.** Pelvic retroperitoneal anatomy. **A:** Dissected right retroperitoneal space illustrating the course of the pelvic ureter. The right uterine adnexa are transected adjacent to the uterus, the ovarian vessels are severed just distal to the pelvic brim, and the peritoneum is removed from the right pelvic sidewall and the right portion of the bladder. The ureter (1) enters the pelvis by crossing over the bifurcation of the common iliac artery just medial to the ovarian vessels (2). It then descends medial to the branches of the internal iliac artery (3). The ureter then courses through the cardinal ligament and passes under the uterine artery (4, "water under the bridge") approximately 1–2 cm lateral to the cervix at the level of the internal cervical os. The origin of the uterine artery from the internal iliac artery (3) is shown. The ureter then courses medially toward the base of the bladder. The distal part of the ureter is associated with the upper portion of the anterior vaginal wall. **B:** The retroperitoneal space is entered, and the peritoneum is retracted medially to show the ureter (1) crossing over the external and internal iliac artery bifurcation. Note that the ureter remains attached to the peritoneum of the pelvic sidewall and the medial leaf of the broad ligament. **C:** The ovarian vessels (2) are clamped and transected after visualization of the ureter. **D:** The uterine artery (4) is being clamped and transected. Note the ureter (1) crossing under this vessel lateral to the cervix.

ing, screening interval, and discontinuation of screening. The American Society for Colposcopy and Cervical Pathology (ASCCP) has issued the most up-to-date, evidence-based guidelines for screening and subsequent management. Similar recommendations are also issued by the American Cancer Society, National Comprehensive Cancer Network, and the American College of Obstetricians and Gynecologists.

When to initiate screening

1. Begin 3 years after coitarche or by age 21
2. Begin earlier if patient has history of diethylstilbestrol (DES) exposure, HPV, or cervical cancer or is immunocompromised

When to discontinue screening

1. Age 70 or older with three consecutive negative Pap tests and no cervical intraepithelial neoplasia (CIN) for 10 years
2. Hysterectomy without CIN-2, CIN-3 or cancer as indication
3. Comorbid or life-threatening illness

Screening interval

1. Initial interval
   a. Every year with conventional Pap smear, or
   b. Every 2 years with liquid-based thin film cytology due to higher sensitivity than the glass-slide method
2. At age 30 or older, screening interval may be increased to
   a. Every 2–3 years if three consecutive, satisfactory, negative Pap tests and no high-risk factors such as cancer, DES exposure, or immunocompromised status is present, or
   b. Every 3 years using hybrid-capture DNA testing for high-risk HPV types combined with either Pap method as long as both tests are negative

If the Pap test detects an abnormality or if the hybrid capture assay for high-risk HPV DNA types is positive, the patient requires further evaluation based on the severity of the abnormality and the age of the patient. Key points from the ASCCP's comprehensive guidelines are as follows:

1. Pap tests are reported using standard nomenclature defined by the Bethesda system. Key preinvasive diagnoses with which the clinician should be familiar include the following:
   a. Atypical squamous cells (ASC). The report will indicate either "uncertain significance" (ASC-US), or "cannot rule out high-grade dysplasia" (ASC-H). ASC-US should be further tested via a reflex hybrid capture assay for high-risk HPV DNA unless the patient is an adolescent. ASC-H has a high risk of high-grade dysplasia and must be evaluated with colposcopy.
   b. Low-grade squamous intraepithelial lesion (LSIL) is virtually always caused by HPV, and HPV testing has been shown not to be cost effective. In adolescent patients, a repeat cytology examination in 1 year is recommended. In adults, colposcopy is performed.
   c. High-grade squamous intraepithelial lesion (HSIL) has a high likelihood of high-grade dysplasia on biopsy, and invasive cancer will sometimes be detected. Patients with HSIL, regardless of age, are evaluated with colposcopy.
   d. Glandular abnormalities are diseases in the endocervical canal. These lesions are difficult to see and may therefore be detected in later stages. Skip lesions occur in 10–15% of patients, indicating the importance of evaluating the entire canal with curettage or similar sampling methods. All three glandular lesions reported have a high likelihood of high-grade dysplasia and a moderate likelihood of associated invasive cancer. Colposcopy and endocervical gland sampling with curettage with possible endometrial sampling is required. Glandular lesions within this category are reported as
      i. Atypical glands, not otherwise specified (AGC-NOS)
      ii. Atypical glands, favor neoplasia
      iii. Adenocarcinoma in situ (AIS)
2. Adolescents (people 20 years of age and younger) have a very high prevalence of HPV infection and a very low likelihood of cervical cancer. Because the disease often regresses in this age range, management guidelines have become progressively more conservative.
3. The colposcope is a binocular microscope (see Figure 39–3) that allows close inspection of the squamocolumnar junction (SCJ) on the cervix where most squamous cervical cancers arise. High-grade lesions have a characteristic appearance, including white light reflection after staining with acetic acid in areas of dysplasia (acetowhite change), abnormal vascular patterns (punctation, mosaic, and atypical vessels), and altered contours. Small biopsies are obtained with colposcopic guidance using cervical biopsy forceps designed for this task. Treatment decisions are based on biopsy results. See Figure 39–4 for details.
4. Biopsy-proven low-grade CIN-1 has a high likelihood of spontaneous regression with a median time of 2 years and very little likelihood of progressing to cancer. Management is conservative in order to minimize treatment morbidity that has been shown to adversely effect fertility. Disease persisting longer than 2 years may be treated or surveillance may be continued.
5. Biopsy-proven high-grade CIN-2–3 has a much higher risk of progressing to invasive disease if left untreated. Treatment options are discussed in the section on Surgery for Malignant Cervical Disease.
6. HPV-mediated disease may also affect the vagina and vulva. Colposcopic examination and directed biopsies allow triage of lesions into low-grade and high-grade lesions that are managed either by surveillance or removal, respectively.

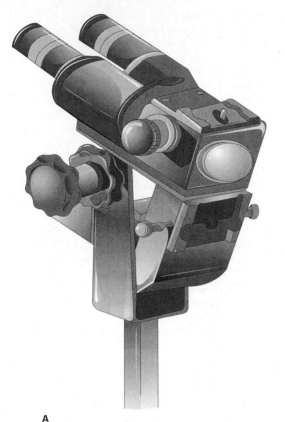

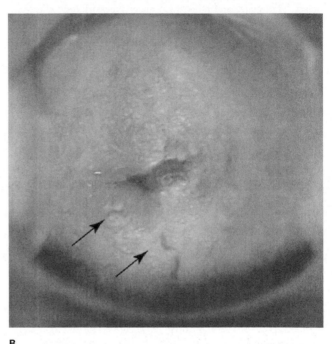

A   B

▲ **Figure 39–3.** Colposcopy. **A:** Zeiss colposcope. (From *Current Diagnosis & Treatment Obstetrics and Gynecology,* Figure 33–13. McGraw-Hill Medical, 2007.) **B:** Mosaic vascular pattern with atypical vessels (arrows). (From Schorge JO, Williams JW: *Williams Gynecology,* Figure 29–10. McGraw-Hill Medical, 2008.)

Wright TC Jr et al: 2006 consensus guidelines for the management of women with cervical intraepithelial neoplasia or adenocarcinoma in situ. Am J Obstet Gynecol 2007;197:340.

Wright TC Jr et al: 2006 consensus guidelines for the management of women with cervical screening tests. J Lower Genital Tract Dis 2007;11:201.

SURGERY FOR BENIGN VULVAR DISEASE

There are a large number of possible masses and benign neoplasms of the vulva. This section discusses HPV, Bartholin abscess, benign tumors, pigmented lesions, and hidradenitis suppurativa. The clinical approach is to rule out potential malignancy and to treat symptomatic lesions. Biopsy or excision of small masses is usually performed in the office setting under a local anesthetic with either a punch biopsy instrument or scalpel. Punch biopsy sites are usually left open, while elliptical excisions are closed with fine, interrupted, absorbable sutures. The differential diagnosis for benign lesions is as follows:

1. Solid lesions

   A. Leiomyoma

      Natural history: Uncommon on vulva. Benign, smooth-muscle tumor that arises from deep connective tissues. Occurs at any age, predominating in fourth and fifth decades. May become very large. Rarely undergoes malignant degeneration.

      Appearance: Slow-growing, firm, usually mobile subcutaneous nodule.

      Diagnosis: Excisional biopsy.

      Treatment: Local complete excision.

   B. Lipoma

      Natural history: Uncommon on vulva. Benign tumor of histologically normal-appearing adipose cells. Large lesions may ulcerate. Usually asymptomatic. Rarely associated with family lipoma syndrome, an autosomal dominant disease. Rarely undergoes malignant degeneration.

Management of the abnormal Pap test in adult women

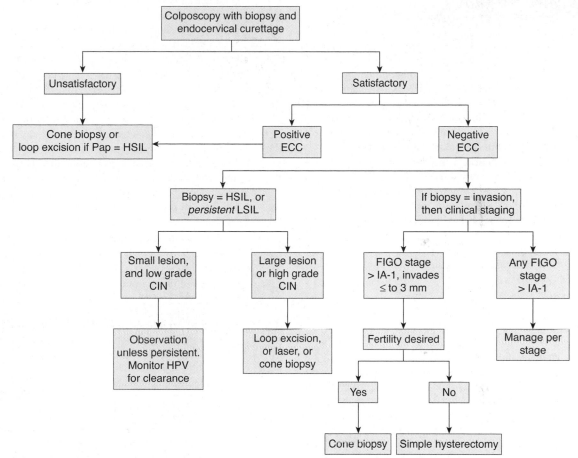

▲ **Figure 39–4.** Colposcopy triage. Satisfactory colposcopy is defined as complete visualization of the squamocolumnar epithelium, which comprises the cervical region most likely to develop invasive disease. Endocervical curettage (ECC) is used to obtain tissue from the endocervix above the area that may be inspected with the colposcope. Colposcopically directed biopsies are taken. Low-grade dysplasia usually resolves, and the preferred treatment is observation with periodic retesting for high-risk HPV DNA on 12-month intervals. Persistent low-grade cervical intraepithelial neoplasia (CIN) or any high-grade CIN must be treated. New guidelines treat adolescent patients differently. See text for details.

Appearance: Soft, rounded, slow-growing sessile or pedunculated mass ranging widely in size.
Diagnosis: Excisional biopsy if symptomatic.
Treatment: Local excision if symptomatic.
C. Syringoma
Natural history: Benign tumor of eccrine ductal origin within fibrous stroma. Occurs mostly after puberty.
Appearance: Multiple, 1–2 mm, flesh-colored or yellow papules on lateral labia major.
Diagnosis: Biopsy.
Treatment: Local excision.

D. Trichoepithelioma
Natural history: Rare benign tumor on vulva, derived from hair follicle without hair development.
Appearance: Single or multiple small, pink or flesh-colored nodules that can mimic basal cell carcinoma.
Diagnosis: Biopsy.
Treatment: Local excision.
E. Granular cell tumor
Natural history: Rare benign tumor of nerve sheath. Occurs in adults and children. Usually asymptomatic and solitary in 85%.

Appearance: Slow-growing subcutaneous nodule, usually on labia majora, clitoris, or mons pubis.

Diagnosis: Biopsy.

Treatment: Wide local excision.

F. Neurofibroma

Natural history: Rare on vulva. Benign tumor of nerve sheath. Half occur in patients with von Recklinghausen disease, an autosomal dominant heritable disease affecting skin, nervous system, bone, and endocrine glands. Rare before puberty. Rarely undergoes malignant degeneration.

Appearance: Solid, cutaneous nodules usually less than 3 cm but reported as large as 25 cm.

Diagnosis: Clinical appearance of von Recklinghausen disease or biopsy.

Treatment: In asymptomatic patients with von Recklinghausen disease, no treatment for a vulvar lesion is needed. For symptomatic patients, local excision.

G. Schwannoma

Natural history: Rare benign tumor of neuroectodermal nerve sheath.

Appearance: Usually solitary.

Diagnosis: Biopsy.

Treatment: Local excision.

2. Glandular lesions

A. Papillary hidradenoma

Natural history: Benign tumor of apocrine sweat glands. Contains both glandular and myoepithelial elements. Occurs after puberty. Usually asymptomatic. Virtually always in Caucasian women.

Appearance: Hemispherical in shape, measuring less than 2 cm in diameter. Usually located in labia majora or lateral labia minora.

Diagnosis: Biopsy.

Treatment: Local excision.

B. Nodular hidradenoma

Natural history: Benign tumor of eccrine sweat glands. Probably arises from embryonic rests. Clear cells on biopsy. Rare on vulva.

Diagnosis: Biopsy.

Treatment: Local excision.

C. Ectopic breast or nipple

Natural history: Rare. May occur on the vulva with or without underlying glands, and lactation has been reported. Rarely undergoes malignant degeneration.

Appearance: Amorphous swelling of the labia most often detected with pregnancy. Pigmented vestigial nipple may or may not be present.

Diagnosis: Biopsy.

Treatment: Local excision if symptomatic.

D. Endometriosis

Natural history: Rare on vulva. Benign ectopic endometrial tissue. May cause cyclic pain and may ulcerate or bleed.

Appearance: Nodule with blue or red-brown appearance. Cyclic tenderness.

Diagnosis: Biopsy.

Treatment: Local excision.

3. Cysts

A. Bartholin cysts or masses

Natural history: Cysts are common, arising in 1–2% of women. Cysts often occur after gland abscesses, although the duct may become occluded any time. Small cysts are usually asymptomatic. Large or infected cysts are painful.

Appearance: Spherical cyst or nodule in subcutaneous tissue of posterior labia majora.

Diagnosis:

i. Incise and drain abscesses.

ii. Biopsy recurrent cysts or solid nodules.

Treatment:

i. Incise and drain abscesses using a small balloon-tip catheter (Word catheter) introduced through a stab incision in the medial aspect of the cyst cephalad to the hymen. The catheter should remain in place for 2 weeks to allow tract epithelialization. In the event of surrounding cellulitis, antibiotic therapy can be added.

ii. Marsupialize or resect recurrent cysts.

iii. Resect solid nodules since these may be malignant.

B. Epithelial inclusion cyst (sebaceous cyst)

Natural history: Common. Usually on labia majora. Can occur at any age and may be solitary or multiple. Usually asymptomatic. Caused by trauma to skin or occlusion of pilosebaceous duct.

Appearance: Single or multiple round cysts usually ranging from 2–3 mm to 1–2 cm in diameter. Often have yellow color.

Diagnosis: Clinical appearance.

Treatment: No treatment if asymptomatic. If symptomatic, local excision.

C. Wolffian cyst (mesonephric cyst)

Natural History: Uncommon. Benign, thin-walled cysts on lateral vagina at the introitus.

Appearance: Round cysts with thin, smooth walls.

Diagnosis: Clinical appearance or biopsy.

Treatment: No treatment if asymptomatic. If symptomatic, local excision.

D. Cyst of canal of Nuck (mesothelial cyst)

Natural history: Uncommon. Benign cyst.

Appearance: Smooth cysts usually located in anterior labia majora or inguinal canal. Thought to be due to peritoneal inclusions. May become large. Differential diagnosis includes inguinal hernia.

Diagnosis: Clinical appearance or excisional biopsy.

Treatment: No treatment if asymptomatic. If symptomatic, local excision.

4. Vascular lesions

A. Angiokeratoma

Natural history: Very common. A clinically insignificant variant of hemangioma that occurs almost exclusively on vulva (and scrotum in men). Occurs during reproductive years. Contains dilated vessels and may have hyperkeratotic overlying epithelium. May resemble Kaposi sarcoma or angiosarcoma. Some forms associated with inborn errors of glycosphingolipid metabolism.

Appearance: Red to purple to brown-black 2–5 mm papules usually in large numbers anywhere on the vulva.

Diagnosis: Clinical appearance. Occurrence of multifocal lesions in childhood may indicate inborn errors of glycosphingolipid metabolism.

Treatment: None, if asymptomatic. Symptomatic lesions treated with laser ablation, electrodesiccation, or local excision.

B. Capillary hemangioma

Natural history: Capillary hemangioma (strawberry hemangioma) occurs in infants and young children. Usually regresses spontaneously over time. May ulcerate or bleed.

Appearance: Well demarcated, red, slightly raised lesion.

Diagnosis: Clinical appearance.

Treatment: None if asymptomatic.

C. Cavernous hemangioma

Natural history: Rare on vulva. Dilated vessels that may be associated with underlying pelvic hemangioma. Usually regresses spontaneously over time. May ulcerate or bleed.

Appearance: Dilated vessels.

Diagnosis: Clinical appearance.

Treatment: None if asymptomatic.

5. Nevi and pigmented skin lesions

A. Vitiligo

Natural history: Inherited disorder with loss of melanocytes. Asymptomatic.

Appearance: Depigmented skin in well-circumscribed macular pattern.

Diagnosis: Clinical appearance.

Treatment: None.

B. Fibroepithelial polyp (skin tag, acrochordon)

Natural history: Very common. Single or multiple. Hormonal factors are implicated in development, and lesions are more common in obese or diabetic patients. Also common in axilla.

Appearance: Multiple soft, skin-colored or pigmented lesions. Usually painless unless inflamed or torsed.

Diagnosis: Gross recognition. Biopsy or excision if symptomatic.

Treatment: Excise, electrodesiccate, or freeze with liquid nitrogen if symptomatic.

C. Seborrheic keratosis

Natural history: Common on body but uncommon on vulva. Usually occur after age 30. Probably autosomal dominant inheritance. Multiple lesions occurring over a short period of time may indicate internal malignancy (Leser-Trelat syndrome).

Appearance: Lesions appear "stuck on" and are brown to black in color. Most are asymptomatic but can be pruritic. Occur on hair-bearing skin.

Diagnosis: Gross appearance, biopsy, or excision.

Treatment: If asymptomatic, no treatment. If symptomatic, excise, electrodesiccate, curette, or freeze with liquid nitrogen.

D. Lentigo simplex

Natural history: Most common hyperpigmentation lesion on vulva. Occurs on skin and mucous membranes.

Appearance: Usually small, less than 4 mm, flat, uniformly pigmented. Often resemble junctional nevi.

Diagnosis: Clinical appearance. Biopsy only if clinical morphology is worrisome. Remember ABCDE criteria: asymmetry, border irregularity, color variations, diameter larger than 6 mm, enlargement or elevation.

Treatment: None required.

E. Vulvar melanosis

Natural history: Hyperpigmented macules or freckles are benign and asymptomatic. They are usually acquired, beginning between ages 30 and 40.

Appearance: Asymptomatic brown to black irregular macular patches on vulva.

Diagnosis: Clinical appearance. Biopsy only if clinical morphology is worrisome. Remember ABCDE criteria: asymmetry, border irregularity, color variations, diameter larger than 6 mm, enlargement or elevation.

Treatment: None required.

F. Acquired melanocytic nevocellular nevus

Natural History: Common, especially in Caucasians. Tend to develop in childhood and early adulthood, followed by gradual involution by age 60. Lesions are usually asymptomatic.

Classification:

i. Junctional nevus: Melanocytes at the dermal-epidermal junction above the basement membrane. First stage of nevus evolution. Least common type on vulva.

ii. Compound nevus: Melanocytes in both the dermis and above the basement membrane. Second stage of nevus evolution.

iii. Intradermal nevus: Melanocytes exclusively in the dermis below the basement membrane. Final stage of evolution after which many nevi involute.

iv. Other types include halo nevus and blue nevus.

Appearance:

i. Junctional nevus: Pigmented macule with smooth border and uniform tan, brown, or dark brown pigmentation.

ii. Compound nevus: Papule with dome shape or macule. Dark brown or black color. May have hairs.

iii. Intradermal nevus: Papule with dome shape or macule. Skin colored, tan, or light brown.

Diagnosis: Clinical appearance. Biopsy if clinical morphology is worrisome. Remember ABCDE criteria: asymmetry, border irregularity, color variegations, diameter larger than 6 mm, enlargement or elevation.

Treatment: None required if asymptomatic and if ABCDE criteria are benign. All others, local excision.

G. Dysplastic nevus

Natural history:

i. Rare on the vulva.

ii. Lesions arise later in childhood than nevi in general and continue to develop throughout life.

iii. Sun exposure contributes to development of these lesions on other areas of the body. Several genetic loci have been implicated for development of melanoma.

iv. Risk of melanoma doubles with one dysplastic nevus and increases 12-fold if 10 or more dysplastic nevi are present.

v. Dysplastic nevi are sometimes associated with a hereditary propensity for melanoma.

Appearance:

i. On biopsy, atypical cells are superficial, and the deeper cells are without atypia. Pagetoid spread of cells is noted in lower third of epithelium.

ii. Tend to be larger in size than nevi (> 10 mm vs. < 5 mm, respectively)

iii. Dysplastic nevi are asymmetrical, with variegation of color.

Diagnosis: A Wood lamp accentuates pigmentation, and margins are more easily delineated. Remember ABCDE criteria: asymmetry, border irregularity, color variegations, diameter larger than 6 mm, enlargement or elevation. Excisional biopsy.

Treatment: Excisional biopsy. Careful longitudinal skin surveillance examinations.

Fisher BK, Margesson LJ: *Genital Skin Disorders.* Mosby, 1998.
Fitzpatrick TB et al: *Color Atlas and Synopsis of Clinical Dermatology,* 4th ed. McGraw Hill, 2001.

Jenison EL: Surgery for benign and indolent growths of the vulva. Operat Tech in Gynecol Surg 1998;3:241.

SURGERY FOR MALIGNANT VULVAR DISEASE

Vulvar cancer accounts for about 5% of gynecologic malignancies. At least 90% of vulvar cancers are of squamous cell type. Etiology of vulvar carcinoma is grouped into the HPV-associated basaloid-warty histological group and the non-HPV-associated keratinizing squamous cancers. The age distribution is bimodal, with younger women more likely to develop HPV-associated disease and older women more likely to develop keratinizing squamous cell carcinoma. The latter group is often associated with lichen sclerosis of the vulva. Vulvar intraepithelial neoplasia (VIN) is a preinvasive form of HPV-associated neoplasia and is often associated with persistent pruritus. Uncommon histological types of vulvar cancer include melanoma (6%), Bartholin gland adenocarcinoma (4%), basal cell carcinoma (< 2%), extramammary Paget disease of the vulva (< 1%), and rare sarcomas found arising primarily in the soft tissues or metastasizing from other tumor sites.

Lesions arise in the labia majora in about 50% of cases, and about 25% of cases occur on the labia minora. Clitoral lesions and Bartholin gland adenocarcinomas are less common. The natural history of vulvar carcinoma includes spread to inguinal lymph nodes. Lesion depth and diameter are of prognostic value for assessing risk of metastasis and, to a lesser degree, histological type and presence of lymphatic involvement. Lesions of 1 mm or less in depth have less than a 1% risk of nodal metastasis and define a category of microinvasive disease that may be treated more conservatively by omitting the inguinal node dissection. Lymph node status is the most significant predictor of survival.

In patients with HPV-mediated disease, multifocal involvement of the vagina and cervix predisposes to a significantly higher risk of cancer at these sites. Smoking is a cofactor for the development of HPV-mediated disease. Smoking cessation may reduce risk of persistent or progressive disease. For women with extramammary Paget disease and those with in situ apocrine adenocarcinoma related to breast tissue developed along the milk line in utero, there is a significant risk of a second, underlying adenocarcinoma elsewhere. Sites that require evaluation include the colon (especially for perianal lesions), Bartholin gland, cervix, endometrium, ovary, and breast.

Cancer of the vulva is staged by the International Federation of Gynecology and Obstetrics (FIGO) criteria, which is a surgical staging system. Melanoma is staged using AJCC staging rules.

▶ Appearance

Vulvar intraepithelial neoplasia occurs in women 15–20 years before the average age of invasive disease. Incidence has risen strongly, and the average age at time of incidence has fallen from 52.7 years in 1961 to 35 years in 1992. One third of lesions are solitary, and two thirds are multifocal. Lesions are widely variable in size and may be slightly raised or papillary. Color variation ranges from white to red to brownish patches on the skin or mucosa. Ulcerated lesions or underlying subcutaneous induration may indicate invasion. Larger lesions have a higher probability of lymph node involvement, but metastatic disease in the lymph nodes may not be palpable. Local spread may involve the urethra, vagina, anus, and, rarely, the symphysis pubis or other pelvic bones.

▶ Diagnosis

Biopsy is necessary to establish the correct diagnosis. The differential diagnosis is large and includes benign lesions discussed earlier in addition to infections that mimic neoplasms and also vulvar dystrophies. Granulomatous infections such as lymphogranuloma venereum and granuloma inguinale of the vulva may be clinically suspicious, and biopsy of the involved tissue may need to be supplemented with cultures for documentation of infection. These infections are rare unless a patient has traveled internationally. Vulvar intraepithelial neoplasia is best diagnosed by colposcopic examination techniques, including use of magnification and staining of the epithelium with 5% acetic acid. Lesions usually appear acetowhite.

▶ Treatment

Focal vulvar intraepithelial neoplasia may be treated by wide excision or CO_2 laser photoablation. Excision is preferred for lesions in the hair-bearing skin, and laser is generally less prone to cause scarring in the mucosal surfaces. Laser ablation is contraindicated if there is any suspicion of invasion. A skinning vulvectomy with split-thickness skin grafting is effective for widely multifocal disease. Extramammary Paget disease requires wide but superficial excision because the tumor cells often spread far wider than is visible to the surgeon. Local recurrences are common, but invasion is rare.

Vulvar cancer is staged using the international system developed by FIGO. See Table 39–1 for details. Microinvasive lesions of less than or equal to 1 mm of invasion are adequately treated by wide and deep local excision with 1 cm margins due to the low likelihood of nodal spread. Stage I lesions are generally treated with radical local excision with a 2 cm margin. If the lesion is lateral, unilateral ipsilateral inguinal lymphadenectomy is performed. Contralateral groin dissection is performed if ipsilateral positive nodes are found or if the primary lesion is central, such as occurs with clitoral or perineal body tumors. More advanced stages are treated with radical vulvectomy and bilateral inguinal lymphadenectomy. Current clinical trials are evaluating whether sentinel node-mapping techniques are valid for treating vulvar malignancies. The trials are still accruing patients, and conclusions may take several years. Radiation therapy with

Table 39–1. FIGO Staging for Vulvar Cancer.

TNM Class	Description
T1	Tumor confined to vulva, ≤ 2 cm in largest diameter
T1a	Tumor invades $\leq$ 1mm
T1b	Tumor invades > 1mm
T2	Tumor confined to vulva, > 2 cm in largest diameter
T3	Tumor of any size with spread to urethra, vagina, or anus
T4	Tumor of any size infiltrating bladder or rectal mucosa and/or fixed to bone
N0	No lymph node metastases
N1	Unilateral regional node metastases
N2	Bilateral regional node metastases
M0	No clinical metastases
M1	Spread to pelvic nodes or distant metastases
FIGO stage grouping	
Stage I	T1a-b, N0, M0
Stage II	T2, N0, M0
Stage III	T3-2-1, N0-1, M0
Stage IVa	T3-2-1, N2, M0; T4, N(any), M0
Stage IVb	T(any), N(any), M1

AJCC and FIGO staging systems are identical TNM systems, revised in 1995. This system applies for all tumor types other than melanoma. Melanoma should be staged using the AJCC melanoma staging system. Staging assessment may require cystoscopy, sigmoidoscopy, and chest X-ray for locally advanced lesions.

concurrent chemosensitization is required for inoperable lesions and for patients with positive nodes or involved resection margins.

▶ Prognosis

Following radical resection with negative nodes and margins, a 5-year rate of 90% is anticipated. If nodes are involved, survival is linked to number of nodes involved, unilaterality versus bilaterality, and bulk of disease.

Creasman WT et al: The National Cancer Data Base report on early stage invasive vulvar carcinoma. American College of Surgeons Commission on Cancer and the American Cancer Society. Cancer 1997;80:505.

Grendys EC Jr et al: Innovations in the management of vulvar carcinoma. Curr Opin Obstet Gynecol 2000;12:15.

Trimble CL et al: Heterogeneous etiology of squamous carcinoma of the vulva. Obstet Gynecol 1996;87:59.

Wechter ME et al: Vulvar melanoma: a report of 20 cases and review of the literature. J Am Acad Dermatol 2004;50:554.

SURGERY FOR BENIGN VAGINAL DISEASE

▶ Imperforate Hymen

Diagnosis of imperforate hymen is often delayed until puberty, when either a workup for primary amenorrhea has ensued or the patient presents with menstrual symptoms such as cramping without associated menses. If the patient has obstructed flow of her menses, defined as hematocolpos, examination will reveal a bulging imperforate hymen. Confirmatory rectal examination will detect a bulging, cystic mass. In younger girls, the finding is more subtle due to the absence of swelling. Delay of diagnosis may result in back-pressure causing a cystically enlarged uterus (hematometra) and possible retrograde menstruation leading to endometriosis. In the presence of a tightly distended hematocolpos, compression of the bladder and ureters may result in urinary obstruction.

Imperforate hymen is treated with a hymenotomy, whereby the obstructed hymen is incised or resected with either a scalpel or laser.

▶ Longitudinal Vaginal Septum

Duplication of the vagina resulting in a septum may occur with or without similar defects in the uterus depending on where the defect of müllerian duct fusion occurred. The duplication may take the form of a partial longitudinal septum or complete duplication of the vagina. Patients will occasionally report bleeding despite placing a tampon during menses, indicating the possibility of a second passage for menstrual flow. Excision is performed transvaginally for symptomatic patients, including those with dyspareunia, obstruction of labor, or similar problems.

▶ Transverse Vaginal Septum

Occasionally, the vagina fails to communicate with the urogenital sinus at the introitus. This may result in formation of a transverse septum, most of which are partial. If the septum is imperforate, hematocolpos will develop following menarche. Marsupialization or excision of the septum restores vaginal patency.

▶ Vaginal Agenesis

Vaginal agenesis, or absence of the vagina, is associated with absence of the uterus in most cases. The lower vagina, derived from the urogenital sinus, may be present, but müllerian ductal structures comprising the upper two thirds of the vagina and the uterus are absent or deficient. Diagnosis is usually made at time of evaluation for primary amenorrhea.

Vaginal agenesis is treated by reconstruction of a functional vagina. Treatment is usually deferred until the patient wishes to become sexually active. In a motivated patient, the vagina may be created by nonoperative dilation and elongation of the vulvar vestibule or vaginal introitus. This method,

called the Frank nonoperative technique, requires up to 2 hours of dilating per day for 4–6 months. Success has been reported with vaginal dilators, vaginal molds, modified bicycle seat, and with intercourse alone. If there is failure to progress, or if the anatomy does not favor dilation alone, surgical construction using a skin graft (McIndoe procedure), interposed bowel, or myocutaneous flaps from the perineum are effective.

▶ Gartner Duct Cyst

Gartner duct cysts are derived from mesonephric (wolffian) duct remnants and contain a serous fluid. They are usually located in the lateral walls of the upper vagina and are generally asymptomatic. These cysts are detected most often during a routine physical examination. Small asymptomatic cysts require no treatment. Gartner duct cysts may occasionally reach 5–6 cm in diameter. Larger or symptomatic cysts should be excised.

American Fertility Society classifications of adnexal adhesions, distal tubal occlusion, tubal occlusion secondary to tubal ligation, tubal pregnancies, müllerian anomalies and intrauterine adhesions. Fertil Steril 1988;49:944.

SURGERY FOR MALIGNANT & PREMALIGNANT VAGINAL DISEASE

Vaginal intraepithelial neoplasia (VAIN) is the preinvasive neoplastic changes that arise in the vagina. VAIN is frequently present whenever carcinoma in situ or invasive carcinoma of the cervix or vulva is present, and it may develop in the vagina years after completion of treatment for cancers of these two sites. Carcinoma in situ, or VAIN-3, of the vagina is most often detected with a Pap test. Subsequent evaluation with colposcopy, staining with 5% acetic acid, and directed biopsies provide an accurate assessment of grade and location of disease.

Low-grade dysplasia (VAIN-1) has a low probability of progression and may be managed with surveillance using the same principles as for management of low-grade cervical dysplasia. High-grade dysplasia (VAIN-2–3) should be treated by local excision of involved areas or with CO_2 laser photoablation. The irregular surface topography of the vagina caused by rugae make successful visualization of lesions for treatment challenging. Recurrence rates for dysplasia are higher for vaginal dysplasia than for similarly treated cervical dysplasia, with a failure rate in the 25% range. Intravaginal placement of topical 5-fluorouracil is an off-label indication that has been reported in the literature, and failure rates are higher than for resection or ablation. Topical 5-fluorouracil has been reported to cause painful vaginal ulcers that heal poorly, limiting the utility of this treatment to carefully selected patients. Extensive involvement of the vagina may require subtotal or complete vaginectomy with skin grafting for maintenance of sexual function. For the elderly, sexually inactive patient, colpocleisis, whereby the vagina is resected and closed permanently, is an option.

Invasive carcinoma of the vagina is rare, accounting for less than 2% of gynecologic malignancies. Most vaginal cancers involve extension from either cervical or vulvar cancers, both of which are more common than lesions arising in the vagina. By convention, if the cancer involves the cervix or vulva in addition to the vagina, the tumor is categorized as either cervical or vulvar cancer, respectively. True vaginal cancer arises only in the vagina. About 85% of vaginal cancers are of squamous type. The next most common type is adenocarcinoma, usually with clear cell type. Rare primary tumors of the vagina include mixed mesodermal tumors, sarcoma botryoides (embryonal rhabdomyosarcoma), sarcoma, adenocarcinoma arising from Gartner duct or müllerian duct remnants, embryonal carcinoma, and malignant melanoma.

The most common presenting symptoms of vaginal cancer include postmenopausal bleeding in about 65% of patients and persistent vaginal discharge in about 30%. Most tumors arise in the upper third of the vagina along the anterior and posterior surfaces. These sites are usually covered by the vaginal speculum and can easily be missed unless the physician observes all vaginal surfaces upon insertion and withdrawal of the speculum. Diagnosis is confirmed by biopsy.

Staging of carcinoma of the vagina is defined by FIGO and is clinical rather than surgical. See Table 39–2. Squamous cancers are most commonly found in postmenopausal patients, although they may occur even in adolescent patients. Clear cell adenocarcinoma of the vagina is more likely to occur in women under 25, generally arising in vaginal adenosis. Diethylstilbestrol has been implicated in increasing the incidence of clear cell carcinoma from 1:50,000 in the unexposed population to 1:1000 in women exposed to DES in utero. Although DES is no longer produced or prescribed in this country, DES and similar substances have been detected in the environment and in some food supplies.

Treatment of vaginal cancer is most often a combination of radiation therapy and chemosensitization using treatment plans similar to cervical cancer. Radical surgery such as radical hysterectomy with vaginectomy is possible for selected, small, upper vaginal lesions, favoring lesions on the posterior wall because of the improved likelihood of attaining adequate margins. Surgery is preferred for young patients with clear cell carcinoma as long as negative margins can be attained. In over 50% of patients, tumor has penetrated the vaginal wall at the time of the initial examination. Involvement of the bladder and rectum is common. Survival for stage I disease is about 70% but falls to about 40% for stage II and stage III disease.

Fine BA et al: The curative potential of radiation therapy in the treatment of primary vaginal carcinoma. Am J Clin Oncol 1996;19:39.

Manetta A et al: Primary invasive carcinoma of the vagina. Obstet Gynecol 1990;76:639.

Table 39–2. FIGO Staging for Vaginal Cancer.

FIGO Stage	Description	TNM Class
Stage 0	Carcinoma in situ; intraepithelial neoplasia grade 3	Tis, N0, M0
Stage I	The carcinoma is limited to the vaginal wall	T1, N0, M0
Stage II	The carcinoma has involved the subvaginal tissue but has not extended to the pelvic wall	T2, N0, M0
Stage III	The carcinoma has extended to the pelvic wall	T1, N1, M0
		T2, N1, M0
		T3, N0, M0
		T3, N1, M0
Stage IV	The carcinoma has extended beyond the true pelvis or has involved the mucosa of the bladder or rectum; bullous edema as such does not permit a case to be allotted to stage IV	
IVA	Tumor invades bladder and/or rectal mucosa and/or directly extends beyond the true pelvis	T4, N(any), M0
IVB	Spread to distant organs	T(any), N(any), M1

Benedet JL, Hacker NF, Ngan HYS (editors): Staging classifications and clinical practice guidelines of gynaecologic cancers. Int J Gynaecol Obstet 2000;70:207. http://www.figo.org/content/PDF/staging-booklet.pdf.

SURGERY FOR MALIGNANT CERVICAL DISEASE

Cervical cancer is the 12th-most common cancer of women in the United States, but remains the second-most common cancer of women worldwide. Almost all cervical cancers arise because of persistent infection with high-risk HPV types, most commonly types 16, 18, and 45. Low-risk HPV types such as types 6 and 11 are usually associated with condyloma and rarely, if ever, with cancer. This cancer can therefore be considered a sexually transmitted disease, since most HPV infections are transmitted via sexual contact. Early sexual debut and multiple partners greatly increase the risk of exposure to high-risk HPV types. HPV infections are common, and about 80% of the population will have detectable HPV antibodies indicating prior infection. In most infected individuals, the immune system will mount a successful response, with a median time to regression of infection of about 2 years. Persistent infection with a high-risk HPV type after age 30 increases the relative risk of cervical cancer more than 400-fold over the population at large. Persistent infections and progression to cancer may be more likely in women who smoke or those with dietary deficiency of folate and betacarotene. Progression to cancer is usually gradual, allowing development of effective screening strategies with Pap tests and testing for high-risk HPV DNA in addition to effective triage with colposcopy. Low-grade lesions usually regress, making potentially destructive treatments that have an adverse effect on fertility unnecessary. In 2006, the FDA approved the first vaccine for primary prevention of HPV infection. The vaccine is targeted for adolescent girls prior to their sexual debut. Widespread vaccination may largely eradicate cervical cancer in the future, although the vaccines are selective only for the most common of high-risk HPV types, raising the possibility of shifting prevalence of HPV types.

About 75% of cervical cancers are squamous type; the remainder consist of adenocarcinomas, mixed carcinomas (adenosquamous), and rare sarcomas (mixed mesodermal tumors, lymphosarcomas). The relative prevalence of cervical adenocarcinoma has risen in recent years and now accounts for about 25% of cases.

Most cervical cancers arise from a preinvasive dysplastic lesion through a process that generally lasts for years. Carcinoma in situ occurs most frequently in the fourth decade, whereas invasive carcinoma is encountered most often in perimenopausal women between ages 40 and 50. Once invasion occurs, spread is by direct extension to the vagina and the parametrium in addition to lymphatic channels to the iliac and obturator nodes, with occasional direct spread to para-aortic nodes. Staging is clinical, since not all stages will require surgery. The staging system defined by FIGO is used internationally and is included in Table 39–3. Probability of lymph node metastasis increases according to the extent of the primary lesion, being approximately 12% in stage I, 30% in stage II, and 45% in stage III. About 80% of patients with stage IV cancer have lymph node involvement.

▶ Dysplasia & Carcinoma In Situ

Successful screening has greatly reduced the incidence and mortality of cervical cancer and its precursors over the last 50 years. Current screening recommendations for lower genital tract cancers of the vulva, vagina, and cervix are discussed earlier in this chapter. When a neoplastic lesion is detected by screening, proper and timely triage is needed. High-grade squamous intraepithelial lesions and carcinoma in situ are typically asymptomatic.

Colposcopic examination of the cervix is the gold standard for assessing dysplasia, carcinoma in situ, and early invasive disease. Application of Lugol iodine can be a useful adjunct to the colposcopic examination. Normal mature squamous epithelium of the cervix and vagina contains glycogen and stains a dark brown color, whereas dysplastic cells lack glycogen and stain a light yellow color.

Colposcopically directed biopsy is performed for visible abnormalities, including acetowhite change, abnormal vessels, ulceration, and papillary lesions. Biopsy-confirmed low-

Table 39–3. FIGO Staging for Cervical Cancer.

FIGO Stage	Description	TNM Class
Stage 0	Carcinoma in situ	Tis
Stage I	Cervical carcinoma confined to uterus (extension to corpus should be disregarded)	T1
IA	Invasive carcinoma, diagnosed only by microscopy; all macroscopically visible lesions, even with superficial invasion, are TIB-1	T1a
IA-1	Measured stromal invasion 3 mm or less and 7 mm or less in horizontal spread	T1a1
IA-2	Measured stromal invasion more than 3 mm and not more than 5 mm with a horizontal spread of 7 mm or less	T1a2
IB	Clearly visible lesion confined to the cervix or microscopic lesion greater than TIA2	T1b
IB-1	Clearly visible lesion 4 cm or less in greatest dimension	T1b1
IB-2	Clearly visible lesion more than 4 cm in greatest dimension	T1b2
Stage II	Tumor invades beyond uterus but not to pelvic wall or to the lower third of vagina	T2
IIA	Tumor without parametrial invasion	T2a
IIB	Tumor with parametrial invasion	T2b
Stage III	Cervical carcinoma extends to the pelvic wall and/or involves lower third of vagina or causes hydronephrosis or nonfunctioning kidney	T3
IIIA	Tumor involves lower third of the vagina, no extension to pelvic wall	T3a
IIIB	Tumor extends to pelvic wall or causes hydronephrosis or nonfunctioning kidney	T3b
Stage IV	Cervical carcinoma involving the mucosa of adjacent organs, or distant metastases	
IVA	Tumor invades mucosa of bladder or rectum and/or extends beyond true pelvis	T4
IVB	Distant metastasis	M1

Benedet JL, Hacker NF, Ngan HYS (editors): Staging classifications and clinical practice guidelines of gynaecologic cancers. Int J Gynecol Obstet 2000;70:207. http://www.figo.org/content/PDF/staging-booklet.pdf.

grade cervical intraepithelial neoplasia (CIN-1) is managed conservatively because most of these lesions regress spontaneously and there is very little risk of progression to cancer.

Biopsy showing a high-grade dysplastic lesion, including moderate dysplasia (CIN-2), severe dysplasia (CIN-3), and carcinoma in situ (CIN-3), are treated with either ablative therapy or resection using cryotherapy or electrosurgical loop excision, respectively. Treatment is directed to either ablation or removal of the entire transformation zone, defined as the area bounded by the original and current squamocolumnar junction. These two treatment modalities are usually performed in the office setting and are well tolerated. There are some exceptions when treating adolescent patients, so the clinician must be familiar with current guidelines. Some dysplastic lesions, including squamous lesions and most glandular lesions, may extend into the endocervical canal. The preferred treatment for lesions extending out of colposcopic view into the endocervical canal is excision with a cold-knife cone biopsy in the operating room. Both electrosurgical loop excision and cold-knife cone biopsy significantly increase future risk of preterm delivery, mandating careful triage of only those individuals truly requiring an excisional therapy.

▶ Invasive Carcinoma

Early stromal lesions defined as microinvasion are usually asymptomatic. Larger lesions frequently cause postmenopausal bleeding (46%), intermenstrual bleeding (20%), or postcoital bleeding (10%). A watery or malodorous vaginal discharge may be the only symptom. Pain is a manifestation of advanced-stage disease typically extending to the pelvic sidewall with entrapment of the sciatic nerve or femoral nerve. Inspection of the cervix typically reveals an ulcerated or papillary lesion of the cervix that bleeds on contact. The cytologic examination almost always demonstrates exfoliated malignant cells, although the false-negative rate for Pap tests approaches 50% for invasive lesions due to obscuration of malignant cells by inflammation and necrotic debris.

▶ Differential Diagnosis

Chronic cervicitis may appear similar to cancer of the cervix. Polyps of the cervix are often benign, but malignancy can only be ruled out with biopsy. Nabothian cysts are benign, common, and can appear bizarre to the untrained eye but are readily distinguished from cancer by biopsy.

▶ Natural History

Spread of cervical cancer into the parametrium may cause obstruction of the ureter, resulting in hydroureter, hydronephrosis, and uremia. Bilateral obstruction of the ureters leads to failure of kidney function and death. Involvement of the iliac and obturator lymph nodes may lead to lymphatic obstruction resulting in lymphedema. Pelvic sidewall nerves, especially the sciatic nerve, may become compressed, causing sciatica or pain in the low back, hip, and leg. Tumor invasion into the bladder or rectum sometimes causes vesicovaginal or rectovaginal fistula, especially following radiation therapy. Widespread metastases to lung, liver, brain, and bone may occur.

▶ Treatment

Treatment of cervical cancer is stratified by stage. Microinvasive disease, defined as FIGO stage IA-1, has less than a 1% chance of lymphatic metastasis and may be managed conservatively with cone biopsy for preservation of fertility or with simple hysterectomy when preservation of fertility is not desired or relevant. Radical hysterectomy with bilateral pelvic lymph node dissection is the preferred treatment for FIGO stage IA-2, IB, and IIA lesions. Radical hysterectomy results is resection of much wider margins than is performed with a simple hysterectomy, including removal of cardinal and uterosacral ligaments and the upper third of the vagina, in addition to pelvic, obturator, and para-aortic nodes. Radical hysterectomy procedures may be performed either via laparotomy or laparoscopy. The radical hysterectomy is a completely different type of hysterectomy from the simple or total hysterectomy. Procedural details for the most commonly used hysterectomy types are described in Table 39–4.

Complications of radical surgery include hemorrhage, infection, thromboembolism, and less than 1% risk of ureterovaginal, vesicovaginal, or rectovaginal fistula. Early-stage lesions may also be treated with radiation therapy and concurrent chemosensitization with cisplatin with equal likelihood of cure but higher potential morbidity.

The recently developed radical vaginal trachelectomy with laparoscopic lymphadenectomy procedure offers carefully selected individuals with stage IA-2 or stage IB-1 lesions of 2 cm diameter or less a fertility-sparing option. The cervix, upper vagina, and supporting ligaments are removed as with a radical hysterectomy, but the uterine corpus is preserved. In the more than 300 subsequent pregnancies currently reported, there is a 10% likelihood of second trimester loss, but 72% of patients carry their gestation to 37 weeks or more.

Advanced-stage disease, including FIGO stage IIB and above, requires treatment with external radiation, brachytherapy implants, and concurrent chemosensitization. At least five randomized trials have confirmed a survival advantage for cisplatin-based therapy given weekly during radiation therapy. Delayed complications of radiation therapy affect quality of life and include cystitis and proctitis, but are uncommon and usually manageable. Severe radiation cystitis or proctitis may result in hemorrhage, fistula, or strictures, typically arising several years after treatment in about 1% to 3% of patients. Radiation necrosis of the cervix and diffuse radiation pelvic fibrosis are rare complications. Radiating the reproductive tract destroys the function of the uterus, and unless the ovaries have been surgically transposed out of the pelvis, ovarian failure is unavoidable. Recurrent or persistent disease in the central pelvis following radiation therapy may potentially be cured with the ultraradical pelvic exenteration procedure.

Table 39–4. Types of Hysterectomy.

Anatomic Structure	Extrafascial Type 1	Modified Radical Type 2	Radical Type 3
Uterus	Removed	Removed	Removed
Ovaries	Optional removal	Optional removal	Optional removal
Cervix	Removed	Removed	Removed
Vaginal margin	None	1–2 cm margin	Upper third of vagina
Ureters	Not mobilized	Dissected through broad ligament	Dissected through broad ligament
Cardinal ligaments	Divided at uterine border	Divided where ureter transits the broad ligament	Divided at pelvic sidewall
Uterosacral ligaments	Divided at cervical border	Partially resected	Divided near sacral origin
Bladder	Mobilized to base of cervix	Mobilized to upper vagina	Mobilized to middle vagina
Rectum	Not mobilized	Mobilized below cervix	Mobilized below middle vagina

▶ Prognosis

Survival is strongly linked to stage at time of diagnosis. Properly treated stage I disease averages 90% survival at 5 years and approaches 96% in radical hysterectomy cases with negative margins and negative nodes. For stage II, 5-year survival is about 65%, dropping to about 45% for stage III and to less than 10% for stage IV.

Morris M et al: Pelvic radiation with concurrent chemotherapy compared with pelvic and para-aortic radiation for high-risk cervical cancer. N Engl J Med 1999;340:1137.

Rose PG et al: Concurrent cisplatin-based radiotherapy and chemotherapy for locally advance cervical cancer. N Engl J Med 1999;340:1144.

Wright TC Jr et al: 2006 consensus guidelines for the management of women with cervical intraepithelial neoplasia or adenocarcinoma in situ. Am J Obstet Gynecol 2007;197:340.

SURGERY FOR PELVIC FLOOR DEFECTS

1. Cystocele, Rectocele, & Incontinence

An understanding of pelvic support defects requires a thorough knowledge of the anatomic relationship of the pelvic viscera and their supporting tissues. These conditions were originally thought to result from stretching and tearing of the muscles, nerves, and connective tissues of the pelvis during vaginal childbirth. The current understanding is that many pelvic floor defects arise from site-specific tears or breaks of pelvic connective tissue. Causes can include stretching, compression, or tearing during parturition as well as behaviors that increase intra-abdominal pressure such as chronic constipation, heavy lifting, obesity, and chronic cough. Smoking, poor nutrition, and lack of pelvic floor exercise may exacerbate pelvic floor defects. The symptoms of pelvic floor defects may include pelvic pressure or a sensation of "falling out" of the pelvic organs, a mass protruding from the vagina (which may be a cystocele, rectocele, cervix, or all of these), stress incontinence, fecal incontinence, and other difficulties with defecation.

Complete examination generally requires evaluating the patient in the lithotomy and standing position and asking her to valsalva or cough. Vaginal support is described with three different levels and formed by the muscles and fascia illustrated in Figure 39–5. Level I includes the cervix and upper third of the vagina. Level I support is provided superiorly by uterosacral ligaments, endopelvic fascia, and smooth muscle; laterally by the cardinal ligaments; and anteriorly by the pubocervical fascia. Level II defines mid-vaginal support and is provided laterally by attachments to the arcus tendineus fascia pelvis, anteriorly by the pubocervical fascia, and posteriorly by Denonvillier fascia. Level III is support of the lower vagina and urethra and is provided anteriorly by attachment of the urogenital membrane to the symphysis pubis, laterally to the levator ani muscle, and posteriorly to the perineal body. A pelvic organ prolapse quantification (POPQ) profile was defined by the International Continence Society, the American Urogynecology Society, and the Society of Gynecologic Surgeons (see Figure 39–6). Use of the POPQ quantitates the extent and location of defects such that subsequent therapy is directed more specifically. Descent and bulging of the anterior vagina is usually a cystocele, a paravaginal defect, or an anterior enterocele. An anatomic defect in the posterior vagina is usually a rectocele or enterocele.

Additional testing that may be necessary for elucidation of the site-specific defect includes assessment of urethral mobility with the so-called Q-tip test, cystourethroscopy, cystometrogram, anoscopy, colonoscopy, anal manometry, and transanal ultrasound. Chronic urinary tract infections must be ruled out prior to deciding upon surgical repair. For fecal incontinence, gastrointestinal disorders such as irritable bowel syndrome, infections such as *Clostridium difficile* or other causes of diarrhea, or malabsorption must be ruled out before proposing surgery.

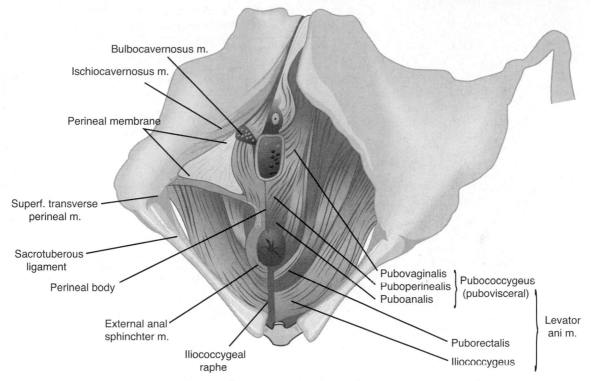

▲ Figure 39–5. Anatomy of pelvic support. (From Schorge JO, Williams JW: *Williams Gynecology,* Figure 38–8. McGraw-Hill Medical, 2008.)

Repair of pelvic floor defects is based on identification of the specific site of injury leading to site-specific repair. Pelvic support defects are often treated nonsurgically. For example, postmenopausal woman with mild to moderate defects as determined by the POPQ score may experience improvement of symptoms after the administration of a topical estrogen, initiation of Kegel exercises, or by fitting a pessary to support pelvic structures. Pessaries are inert material manufactured in many different sizes and shapes that can be fitted to the patient. When inserted in the vagina, a pessary mechanically supports pelvic structures, resulting in temporary correction of the underlying symptoms. A pessary is a good option for patients who choose not to undergo surgery or for those who cannot have surgery.

▶ Differential Diagnosis

Urethral diverticulae may mimic cystocele and produce a bulge of the anterior vaginal wall. A discrete mass is usually palpable. Pressure or massage of the mass may result in turbid or purulent urethral drainage. Vaginal cysts such as Gartner duct or Skene duct cysts are occasionally mistaken for bladder support defects.

▶ Treatment

Categories of pelvic floor defects include anterior compartment, vault prolapse, uterine prolapse, enterocele, posterior compartment, urinary incontinence, and fecal incontinence.

A. Anterior Compartment

Anterior compartment defects, including cystocele and paravaginal defects, often are associated with concurrent urinary incontinence. **Stress incontinence** is involuntary loss of urine. Stress incontinence is associated with leakage caused by increases in intra-abdominal pressure resulting from coughing, heavy lifting, or Valsalva maneuver in the absence of detrusor contraction. Stress incontinence is usually demonstrated during examination by asking the patient to cough. Stress incontinence should be distinguished from other common types of urinary incontinence, including urge and overflow incontinence. With **urge incontinence,** the detrusor muscle contracts or spasms, resulting in leakage with associated urgency. **Mixed incontinence** is defined as a combination of stress and urge incontinence. **Overflow incontinence** is often a continual slow leak of urine but may present with symptoms of any of the other types of incontinence. It can be ruled out by detecting large residual urine volume following voiding. Surgical

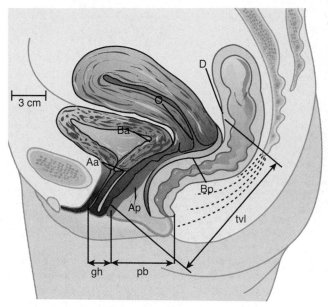

The Nine Point POPQ and Staging Definitions		
Point	Description	Range
Aa	Anterior wall 3 cm from hymen	-3 to +3
Ba	Most dependent part of the rest of the anterior wall	-3 to +TVL
C	Cervix or vaginal cuff	+/- TVL
D	Posterior fornix (if no prior total hysterectomy)	+/- TVL
Ap	Posterior wall 3 cm from hymen	-3 to +3
Bp	Most dependent part of the rest of the posterior wall	-3 to +TVL
GH	Genital hiatus (mid-urethra to PB)	No limit

▲ **Figure 39–6.** Pelvic organ prolapse quantification table. Six sites (points Aa, Ba, C, D, Bp, and Ap), genital hiatus (GH), perineal body (PB), and total vaginal length (TVL) are used for quantification of pelvic organ support. Each point is described with respect to position relative to the hymen in centimeters. Positive values represent distance outside the hymen, and negative numbers represent distance superior to the hymen. (Schwartz SI, Brunicardi F: *Schwartz's Principles of Surgery: Self-Assessment and Board Review,* 8th ed. McGraw-Hill Medical, 2007.)

correction of stress incontinence occasionally produces urge incontinence that may persist in 10–15 % of patients.

Normally, the proximal urethra is supported above the urogenital diaphragm and is subjected to the same intra-abdominal pressure changes as those applied to the bladder. In patients with anterior vaginal compartment defects, increased intra-abdominal pressure causes the hypermobile proximal urethra and bladder base to descend into the vagina. Pressure in the bladder thereby exceeds the sphincter pressure, resulting in leakage of urine. Intrinsic sphincter deficiency is a second mechanism of stress incontinence. Risk factors include previous incontinence surgery, prior radiation therapy, and age over 50.

Site-directed repair of anterior compartment defects may include anterior colporrhaphy, or repair of paravaginal defect. Repair or stress urinary incontinence often involves retropubic colposuspension using either the Burch or Marshall-Marchetti-Kranz procedures. Success of these two procedures is approximately 85% at 5 years. Recurrent or difficult cases of stress urinary incontinence are often surgically treated with use of slings or grafts to augment support. Grafts may be created from endogenous fascia, usually harvested from the rectus fascia, or

from exogenous sources, including allografts, xenografts, and synthetic mesh. Procedures utilizing the grafts may include sling procedures or the tension-free vaginal tape (TVT) procedure, which has significantly reduced the morbidity of graft procedures compared to historical controls. For patients with intrinsic sphincter deficiency or who are not candidates for more involved surgical procedures, a minimally invasive treatment involves injection of collagen at the urethrovesical junction as a bulking agent to increase outlet resistance.

B. Prolapse

Prolapse, in which the level I support involving the upper vagina or uterus is deficient, results in symptomatic descent of the upper vaginal tissues and/or uterus. Prolapse may also be associated with anterior and posterior compartment defects.

Repair of vaginal prolapse is generally performed with a unilateral sacrospinous ligament suspension (SSLS) procedure performed transvaginally or with an abdominal sacro-colpopexy procedure performed via laparotomy or laparos-copy. In the SSLS procedure, the upper vagina is sutured to the uterosacral ligament. In the abdominal sacrocolpopexy procedure, a retroperitoneal mesh is sutured from the upper vagina to the anterior longitudinal sacral ligament. Treatment of uterine prolapse sometimes involves hysterectomy combined with SSLS or with abdominal sacrocolpopexy procedures. Uterine preservation is permissible, combined with plication of uterosacral ligaments or the other procedures described previously. Results of surgical correction of prolapse are not optimal: Up to one third of patients require reoperation for recurrent disease. Sacrocolpopexy outcomes appear to be more durable.

C. Enterocele

Enterocele is a hernia that develops between the vagina and the rectum. Diagnosis is confirmed by palpation on pelvic examination and can also be documented on transvaginal ultrasound. Surgical repair requires reapproximation of the fascial defect at the apex of the rectovaginal septum via laparotomy, laparoscopy, or vaginal approach depending on other planned combined procedures such as hysterectomy.

D. Posterior Compartment

Posterior compartment defects, including rectocele and anal sphincter defects often are associated with concurrent fecal incontinence or difficulty with defecation. Fecal incontinence is involuntary loss of stool or flatus.

Etiology of fecal incontinence is associated with diarrhea; increased bowel motility; neurological disorders such as diabetes, spinal cord injury, or multiple sclerosis; and pelvic support defects including injury to the anal sphincter. Testing includes careful examination of level II and level III structures, anal sphincter tone, and voluntary anal sphincter contraction. Additional test that may be needed to elucidate the etiology of the lesion include anal manometry, transanal ultrasound, MRI, colonoscopy, defecography, and electromyography. Diarrheal illness and gastrointestinal disorders such as irritable bowel syndrome are treated prior to consideration of surgery.

Nonsurgical treatment may include use of medication to slow transit time, bulking agents, biofeedback, and electrical stimulation therapy.

Site-directed repair of posterior compartment defects may include posterior colporrhaphy, whereby posterior fascial defects are repaired primarily or with grafts, sphincteroplasty, or repair of rectal prolapse.

In patients for whom sexual activity is not an issue, closure (colpocleisis) or removal (colpectomy) of the vagina is an option.

Black NA et al: The effectiveness of surgery for stress incontinence in women: a systematic review. Br J Urol 1996;78:497.

Bump RC et al: Epidemiology and natural history of pelvic floor dysfunction. Obstet Gynecol Clin North Am 1998;25:723.

Bump RC et al: The standardization of terminology of female pelvic organ prolapse and pelvic floor dysfunction. Am J Obstet Gynecol 1996;175:10.

DeLancey JOL: Anatomic aspects of vaginal eversion after hysterectomy. Am J Obstet Gynecol 1992;166:1719.

DeLancey JOL: Structural support of the urethra as it relates to stress urinary incontinence: the hammock hypothesis. Am J Obstet Gynecol 1994;170:1713.

Nygaard IE et al: Abdominal sacrocolpopexy: a comprehensive review. Obstet Gynecol 2004;104:805.

Olsen AL et al: Epidemiology of surgically managed pelvic organ prolapse and urinary incontinence. Obstet Gynecol 1997; 89:501.

2. Urinary Tract Fistula

Urinary tract fistulae to the vagina include vesicovaginal, ureterovaginal, and urethrovaginal types. Vesicovaginal fistula is the most common type. Most urinary tract fistulae occur following pelvic surgery with unrecognized injury or because of ischemia. Potential causes of ischemic change include effects of radiation therapy upon vasculature of pelvic organs. Less common in this country, but much more frequent in other parts of the world, is ischemic injury following prolonged or obstructed labor. Fistulae may also occur as a result of tumor invasion, retained foreign bodies, and chronic inflammation.

Most urologic fistulae arise following gynecologic surgery rather than urologic or colorectal surgery. Total abdominal hysterectomy is the procedure most often complicated by the development of vesicovaginal fistula. A skillful surgeon using a technique of careful identification of anatomic structures can greatly minimize the risk of causing fistula formation. Injuries recognized at the time of primary surgery should be repaired immediately. Development of postoperative fistulae may require a waiting period to allow inflammation to subside before undertaking repair.

► Symptoms & Signs

Vaginal leakage of urine or constant urinary leakage are symptoms of a urologic fistula. If the fistula involves the distal urethra, the patient may experience vaginal leakage only at the time of voiding. Vesicovaginal and ureterovaginal fistulae almost always develop near the vaginal vault. A urethrovaginal fistula opens into the anterior vagina.

On speculum examination, urine will usually be seen pooling at the vaginal apex. Most fistulae in nonradiated patients are small and may not be readily seen with the naked eye. Confirmation of a suspected vesicovaginal fistula may be demonstrated by instilling dilute methylene blue dye or sterile milk into the bladder with a catheter while inspecting the vaginal vault. A small fistula may leak very little and is often better seen by placing a tampon in the vagina when methylene blue dye is instilled and then removing the tampon to inspect for blue staining after 15 to 20 minutes. If a vesicovaginal fistula is not detected, intravenous methylene blue or indigo carmine blue dye will be excreted through the ureters. This is best detected by placement of a tampon for about 30 minutes followed by inspection for staining.

Other useful diagnostic tests include cystoscopy, cystogram, and intravenous pyelogram to assess for the site of injury.

▶ Treatment

In nonradiated, noninfected tissue, many small fistulae will close spontaneously if the bladder is drained with an indwelling catheter. Larger fistulae or small fistulae that fail conservative management must be repaired surgically. Approximately 8 to 12 weeks must be allowed for resolution of edema and inflammatory reactions prior to undertaking repair. Premature repair has a high likelihood of being unsuccessful. Urinary tract infections should be treated, and skin integrity should be protected with an occlusive barrier cream before surgical correction is attempted.

Repair of vesicovaginal fistulae involves a number of techniques, including layered closure with the Latzko procedure via the vaginal approach or via laparotomy with omental interposition. Principles of repair include meticulous and atraumatic technique using fine suture material, approximation without tension, and bladder decompression postoperatively. Ureterovaginal fistulae are repaired with ureteroneocystostomy if the ureteral injury is in the lower pelvis and with ureteroureterostomy for injury sites higher in the pelvis. These are usually performed via laparotomy, but the laparoscopic approach is also used. Fistulae in radiated tissue cannot be repaired primarily because of chronic tissue ischemia. These fistulae require a nonradiated blood supply provided by bulbocavernosus or gracilis myocutaneous flaps for successful repair or permanent diversion.

3. Rectovaginal Fistula

Rectovaginal fistulae may occur following obstetrical injury, pelvic surgery, cervical or rectal cancer, radiation therapy, inflammatory bowel disease, or diverticular disease. The patient will report vaginal passage of flatus or feces or foul vaginal discharge, sometimes associated with bleeding. The fistula can often be demonstrated upon speculum examination or by palpation on rectovaginal examination. Diagnostic studies such as barium enema or sigmoidoscopy may be useful for smaller lesions.

To reduce the risk of infection and breakdown of a planned fistula repair, the bowel should be prepared with a low-residue diet, antibiotics, and a cathartic bowel regimen preoperatively. A rectovaginal fistula in the lower third of the vagina should be repaired after the surrounding inflammation and edema have resolved, usually requiring a delay of about 12 weeks. Rectovaginal fistulae in the upper two thirds of the vagina are best treated with a preliminary diverting colostomy followed by fistula repair and subsequent colostomy takedown 2 to 3 months after the repair.

Fistulae caused by inflammatory bowel disease such as Crohn disease have a high likelihood of recurrence unless the disease is clearly in remission. Ileostomy and abdominoperineal resection are necessary in patients whose symptoms are unacceptable despite medical management. Fistulae associated with radiation therapy can rarely be repaired, and those associated with cancer are not amenable to surgical repair. A diverting colostomy provides considerable relief of symptoms.

Tancer ML et al: Genital fistulas secondary to diverticular disease of the colon: a review. Obstet Gynec Surv 1996;51:67.
Woo HH et al: The treatment of vesicovaginal fistulae. Eur Urol 1996;29:1.

▼ THE UPPER GENITAL TRACT

SURGERY FOR BENIGN UTERINE DISEASE

1. Congenital Uterine Anomalies

Congenital duplication defects of the uterus are rare, with a reported incidence of 0.4% to 1% and are usually diagnosed following investigation for recurrent spontaneous abortions, premature labor, fetal malpresentation, retained placenta and postpartum hemorrhage (see Figure 39–1). Anomalies include septate uterus consisting of a simple midline septum; bicornuate uterus, which is a duplication of the uterine horns; and uterus didelphys consisting of complete duplication of the corpus and cervix. These anomalies are often detected with physical examination, especially during or after pregnancies complicated by malpresentation, or preterm labor. Testing with MRI or hysterosalpingogram will usually confirm the diagnosis, and tests are combined with ultrasonography or laparoscopy if the diagnosis remains uncertain. Combined laparoscopy and hysteroscopy is useful for planning surgical correction.

Surgical correction of uterine anomalies is indicated for prevention of documented or anticipated pregnancy-related complications. A septate uterus is twice as likely to cause spontaneous abortion than a bicornuate uterus, with an overall loss rate of 88% reported for patients with a complete septum. The septate uterus is treated with a septoplasty, completed in most cases by hysteroscopic division or resection of the septum with up to an 86% success rate for subsequent pregnancy. Alternatively, the abdominal metroplasty is indicated for a large or thick septum or for the bicornuate uterus. A wedge of myometrium is resected, allowing the two horns of the uterus to be reconstructed. This procedure results in measurable loss of uterine volume. Pregnancies occurring after abdominal metroplasty should be delivered by cesarean section because the risk of uterine rupture is increased.

American Fertility Society classification of müllerian anomalies. Fertil Steril 1988;49:944.
Grimbizis G et al: Hysteroscopic septum resection in patients with recurrent abortions or infertility. Hum Reprod 1998;13:1188.
Heinonen PK: Reproductive performance of women with uterine anomalies after abdominal or hysteroscopic metroplasty or no surgical treatment. J Am Assoc Gynecol Laparosc 1997;4:311.

Hensle TW et al: Vaginal reconstruction. Urol Clin North Am 1999;26:39.

Li S et al: Association of renal agenesis and müllerian duct anomalies. J Comput Assist Tomogr 2000;24:829.

2. Abnormal Uterine Bleeding

Abnormal uterine bleeding may occur at any age. It is not unusual for a female infant to have a small amount of self-limited vaginal bleeding attributable to the decline of circulating estrogen from maternal sources after delivery.

Abnormal uterine bleeding during the reproductive years is described according to the chronicity and amount of bleeding because this information is often useful in elucidating the etiology. Hypermenorrhea, also called menorrhagia, is excessive or prolonged bleeding at the normal time of menstruation. Polymenorrhea is bleeding that occurs more frequently than every 3 weeks, and metrorrhagia is intermenstrual bleeding that occurs in the interval between menses.

Hypermenorrhea may be due to physical disease of the uterus such as uterine leiomyoma, adenomyosis, and endometrial polyp. Dysfunctional uterine bleeding is abnormal uterine bleeding related to functional response of a normal uterus to extrauterine causes such as abnormal cycling of estrogen and progesterone in patients with anovulation, oligoovulation, or persistence of the corpus luteum. This condition is seen most often in adolescents and in perimenopausal women. Polymenorrhea is sometimes related to a shortened proliferative phase secondary to hypothyroidism. Causes of metrorrhagia include endometrial polyps, submucous leiomyoma, coagulopathy, granulomatous infections such as tuberculosis, and cancer of the cervix or uterine corpus. Complications of pregnancy should not be overlooked as a cause of abnormal bleeding in women of reproductive age.

Postmenopausal bleeding is any vaginal bleeding occurring a year or more after menopause and is of concern because it may be a symptom of endometrial cancer. When postmenopausal bleeding is fully evaluated, including biopsy and hormone studies, the majority will be attributed to benign etiologies such as atrophic change, benign polyp, cervicitis, and physiologic withdrawal from exogenous hormones. Endometrial cancer is detected in about 15% of cases of postmenopausal bleeding but is also linked to the age of the patient: a 50-year-old woman has about a 2% chance of cancer, while an 80-year-old woman with the same symptom has about a 60% chance of malignancy. Cervical cancer may also present with postmenopausal bleeding. The exogenous administration of estrogenic substances, including hormone replacement therapy, and use of estrogen analogs such as tamoxifen cause postmenopausal bleeding. Much less likely are estrogen-producing tumors of the ovary, coagulopathy, or environmental sources of estrogenic substances. Postmenopausal bleeding in any amount ranging from scant brown vaginal discharge to frank, profuse, bright red bleeding should prompt further workup. Cancer should be considered the likely cause until proven otherwise.

▶ Clinical Findings

Obtain a complete history and perform a careful pelvic examination including a Pap test. The examination will often reveal vaginal, cervical, uterine, or adnexal disease. A complete blood count and measurement of red cell indices will ascertain the degree of chronic blood loss. Additional blood studies, including thyroid function and coagulopathy testing, may be necessary in some cases.

Abnormal bleeding in women over the age of 35 or with Pap test results showing atypical glandular cells of any type, or in women of any age with a Pap test showing atypical glandular cells, or in women with risk factors for gynecologic cancer, endometrial biopsy is required to confirm a diagnosis. The biopsy should be timed at an appropriate point in the menstrual cycle, such as after the 16th day of the cycle if anovulatory bleeding is suspected, but may be performed at any time to evaluate for hyperplasia or carcinoma. Endometrial sampling with a disposable suction device can be accomplished in an office setting in most patients. Obese patients or patients with cervical stenosis may require dilatation and curettage in the operating room. Pregnancy should always be ruled out before performing a biopsy in a woman of reproductive age.

Hysteroscopy, involving insertion of a narrow-diameter videoscope through the cervix while distending the uterine cavity, allows inspection of the endometrium and directed biopsy of suspicious features. Hysteroscopy is very useful for determining the cause of bleeding and offers the opportunity for simultaneous treatment such as hysteroscopic resection of a polyp. Hysteroscopy can be accomplished in an office or outpatient surgical setting and is recommended when bleeding is recurrent or resistant to therapy or when structural abnormalities of the endometrium, such as polyps or submucous leiomyomata, are suspected.

Transvaginal ultrasound is useful to measure endometrial thickness and structural abnormalities of the uterus, such as a polyp or leiomyoma. In the postmenopausal patient, an endometrial strip of less than or equal to 4 mm virtually excludes the likelihood of cancer. Biopsy is still preferable unless it is unable to be performed for technical reasons. The sonohysterogram, where saline is introduced into the endometrial cavity during ultrasound, increases diagnostic accuracy for defects in the endometrial cavity.

▶ Treatment

Dilation and curettage is both diagnostic and therapeutic for many causes of uterine bleeding. Definitive treatment, however, will be targeted toward the etiology of the abnormal uterine bleeding.

Medical management of most nonneoplastic causes of abnormal uterine bleeding is generally prescribed before considering surgery because many symptoms will resolve or can be managed without surgical intervention. Chronic blood loss due to hypermenorrhea produced by leiomyoma or hyperplasia can be reduced by the administration of a progestin. A gonadotropin-releasing hormone agonist will result in amenorrhea and is sometimes prescribed prior to planned surgery for leiomyomata. The antiprogestin mifepristone may significantly shrink leiomyomata, but a side effect includes increased risk of endometrial hyperplasia. Dysfunctional bleeding due to chronic anovulation is treated with cyclic progestin therapy, or oral contraceptives. For women who wish to conceive, ovulation induction with drugs such as clomiphene is prescribed. Control of acute heavy bleeding may be achieved through the use of higher doses of combination oral contraceptives prescribed as 1 pill four times a day for 3 or 4 days, tapered to 1 pill a day over 1 week. Alternatively, intravenous conjugated estrogen, 25 mg every 4 hours, has been used also to control acute bleeding. Such a regimen must be followed by a progestin to prevent additional irregular bleeding at a later time. Following control of acute bleeding, maintenance therapy with an oral contraceptive is recommended. Another strategy for maintenance is to place an intrauterine device (IUD) containing levonorgestrel, resulting in amenorrhea in about 25% of women and light menses in the remainder. In the absence of identified intrauterine pathology, hypermenorrhea associated with ovulatory cycles can be ameliorated with nonsteroidal anti-inflammatory drugs.

Persistence of symptoms will generally require surgical intervention. Surgical treatment of bleeding caused by uterine leiomyoma is discussed later in this chapter. Severe and intractable dysfunctional uterine bleeding may rarely require hysterectomy. Endometrial ablation by hysteroscopic Nd:YAG laser or electrosurgery or use of proprietary endometrial ablation devices (eg, Novasure, ThermaChoice) may preclude hysterectomy in the premenopausal patient with bleeding that cannot be managed medically. Ablation generally requires normal size and shape of the uterine cavity. Only about 20% of women report amenorrhea following endometrial ablation, and about one third will undergo eventual hysterectomy. Placement of a levonorgestrel-containing IUD is nearly as effective as hysteroscopic endometrial ablation.

Postmenopausal bleeding due to atrophic changes may resolve with estrogen therapy administered with progestin in either a cyclic or continuous fashion. Postmenopausal bleeding attributed to physiologic withdrawal bleeding from prescribed estrogen-based therapy is treated by discontinuing therapy or converting to a continuous regimen. Curettage for removal of benign endometrial polyps is often curative, although polyps may recur. Endometrial carcinoma is a contraindication to estrogen therapy and is treated surgically with possible postoperative adjuvant therapy based on stage and grade of the tumor. Well-differentiated endometrial adenocarcinoma in young women who desire to maintain fertility has been successfully treated using high-dose progestins in about three fourths of cases.

Randall TC: Progestin treatment of atypical hyperplasia and well-differentiated carcinoma of the endometrium in women under age 40. Obstet Gynecol 1997;90:434.

A randomized trial of endometrial ablation versus hysterectomy for the treatment of dysfunctional uterine bleeding: outcome at four years. Aberdeen Endometrial Ablation Trials Group. Br J Obstet Gynaecol 1999;106:360.
Smith-Bindman R et al: Endovaginal ultrasound to exclude endometrial cancer and other endometrial abnormalities. JAMA 1998;280:1510.
Stewart A: The effectiveness of the levonorgestrel-releasing intrauterine system in menorrhagia: a systematic review. Br J Obstet Gynaecol 2001;108:74.

3. Adenomyosis

Extension of endometrial glands and stroma into the myometrium is defined as adenomyosis. Symptomatic adenomyosis is most prevalent in women between age 35 and menopause. Symptoms include dysmenorrheal, hypermenorrhea, polymenorrhea, metrorrhagia, and dyspareunia. Concurrent endometriosis is common. Symptoms typically improve after menopause supports.

Upon pelvic examination, the uterus is slightly to moderately enlarged and is frequently tender to palpation, particularly in the secretory phase of the menstrual cycle. Preoperative confirmation of adenomyosis is challenging. Neither ultrasound nor endometrial biopsy are useful for making the diagnosis. The T2-weighted sequences on MRI is more effective, with sensitivity of 70% and specificity of 86%. Definitive diagnosis is confirmed after hysterectomy.

▶ Differential Diagnosis

Leiomyomata of the uterus are common and cause many symptoms similar to adenomyosis. Low-grade endometrial stromal sarcoma is rare but can be mistaken adenomyosis. This is an indolent malignancy with a significant likelihood of local recurrence. Distant metastases to the ovary, peritoneal surfaces, and lung are occasionally seen. Tumors of this type should not be morcellated. Subsequent treatment may include pelvic radiation therapy and hormone therapy based on stage at time of diagnosis and presence of estrogen and progesterone receptors.

▶ Treatment

Total hysterectomy with or without bilateral salpingo-oophorectomy is the only clearly effective treatment. Hormonal approaches may be successful in treating symptoms, particularly if the patient is nearing menopause. Menopause causes symptoms to regress.

Fedele L et al: Treatment of adenomyosis-associated menorrhagia with a levonorgestrel-releasing intrauterine device. Fertil Steril 1997;68:426.
Vercellini P et al: Transvaginal ultrasonography versus uterine needle biopsy in the diagnosis of diffuse adenomyosis. Hum Reprod 1998;13:2884.
Vercellini P et al: Treatment with a gonadotropin releasing hormone agonist before endometrial resection: a multicentre, randomised controlled trial. Br J Obstet Gynaecol 1996;103:562.

4. Leiomyomata

Uterine leiomyomata, or fibroids, are present in 20–30% of women of reproductive age. The true prevalence is unknown because many fibroids are asymptomatic. Black women have a threefold higher incidence than white, Asian, and Hispanic women. Other risk factors include obesity, nulliparity, and early menarche or infertility. Myomas arise from monoclonal proliferation and are stimulated by estrogen, progesterone, and growth factors. Fibroids increase growth rate during pregnancy and regress after menopause. Fibroids are usually multifocal and vary hugely in size, ranging from a few millimeters to masses that fill the abdomen. Location of leiomyomata can be nearly anywhere within the uterus. Descriptive terms for location include intramural for fibroids arising within the myometrium, subserosal for lesions below the exterior surface of the uterus, and submucosal for fibroids below or adjacent to the endometrium. Other types of leiomyomata include pedunculated lesions connected with a narrow vascular stalk to the uterus, intraligamentous lesions within the broad ligament, and parasitic leiomyomata, detached from the uterus and deriving blood supply from adjacent organs.

▶ Clinical Findings

Symptoms are determined by location, number, and size of the lesions. Common symptoms include hypermenorrhea, prolonged menses, pelvic pressure, increased abdominal girth, urinary frequency, dyspareunia, low back pain, and constipation. Infertility may occur secondary to fibroids, particularly if the uterine cavity is enlarged or distorted by a submucous lesion. Adverse pregnancy outcomes such as abnormal placentation, malpresentation, abruption, and dysfunctional labor are recognized complications associated with fibroids. Degenerative changes may spontaneously occur, potentially causing significant pain that requires treatment. Submucous leiomyomata are more likely to cause hypermenorrhea, polymenorrhea, and metrorrhagia.

Palpation of the uterus during bimanual examination detects a lobular and enlarged structure with a characteristic rubbery consistency. Soft and tender lesions are characteristic of degenerating fibroids. Larger lesions may be felt on abdominal examination.

Anemia may result from acute or chronic abnormal uterine bleeding. Endometrial biopsy should be performed in women with abnormal uterine bleeding to rule out endometrial cancer. Pelvic ultrasound is the most useful study for diagnosis. Sonohysterogram or hysteroscopy are useful for confirmation of submucous leiomyomata. MRI is expensive and should be utilized selectively for evaluation of atypical lesions that could represent sarcoma or for localization of lesions prior to a myomectomy. Hydronephrosis may be apparent on imaging studies, arising as a result of external compression of the by the mass.

▶ Differential Diagnosis

Uterine leiomyosarcoma is a rare but aggressive neoplasm. Among women undergoing surgery for fibroids, only 0.23% are found to harbor sarcoma. The rapidly growing leiomyoma, defined as 6 cm growth in 1 year, is malignant in less than 0.1% of cases. In a postmenopausal woman with an enlarging uterine mass, sarcoma is more likely. Most sarcomas are not detected prior to surgery, although a high T1/high T2 pattern on MRI has been reported to be predictive of sarcoma. On cut section, leiomyomata are well-circumscribed, solid tumors with a pseudocapsule and an off-white, whorled appearance. If a lesion lacks an apparent capsule, appears necrotic, or is soft or friable, then a frozen section should be submitted. These findings are likely to represent a sarcoma.

Other potential diagnoses to consider include solid ovarian tumors. Enlargement of the uterus may arise due to adenomyosis or could represent an undiagnosed pregnancy. A pregnancy test should be done in all suspected cases.

▶ Treatment

Asymptomatic fibroids require no therapy. Women with hypermenorrhea or polymenorrhea often benefit from a trial of cyclic or continuous oral contraceptives or progestins. GnRH agonists decrease myoma size and stop menstruation prior to surgery. Long-term use of GnRH agonists causes osteoporosis. Treatment with the antiprogestin mifepristone may result in significant shrinkage of fibroids but may cause endometrial hyperplasia. In premenopausal women, leiomyomata grow soon after medication is discontinued.

For women with symptoms unresponsive to medical management, several treatment options are available. Myomectomy is a procedure for removal of leiomyomata with subsequent repair of resultant defects in the uterine wall in order to preserve the uterus. Myomectomy is usually offered to women who desire to retain their fertility. Some women who do not desire pregnancy also choose this option. Myomectomy is performed via laparotomy, laparoscopy, or hysteroscopy depending on the location, number, and size of the leiomyomata. Women who have completed childbearing and desire an alternative to hysterectomy may choose uterine artery embolization or guided focused ultrasound surgery, both of which are designed to decrease the size of lesions. Embolization involves diminishing blood flow to the uterus by occluding vessels to the lesion using angiography. Uterus and fibroids have been reported to decrease in size by one third to one half. Bleeding and pelvic pressure improve in 80–90% of women. Hysterectomy is definitive treatment for women with symptomatic myomas. Alternatives to total abdominal hysterectomy include vaginal hysterectomy, supracervical hysterectomy, and laparoscopic hysterectomy.

▶ Prognosis

Myomectomy results in improvement of symptoms in 80% of women. Ten percent of women undergoing myomectomy require additional surgery for recurrent lesions, and 50% will develop recurrent leiomyomata.

American College of Obstetricians and Gynecologists: ACOG practice bulletin #16, surgical alternatives to hysterectomy in the management of leiomyomas. May 2000 (replaces educational bulletin number 192, May 1994). Int Gynaecol Obstet 2000;73:285.

Hanafi M: Predictors of leiomyoma recurrence after myomectomy. Obstet Gynecol 2005;105:877.

Hurst BS et al: Uterine artery embolization for symptomatic uterine myomas. Fertil Steril 2000;74:855.

Lefebvre et al: The management of uterine leiomyomas. J Obstet Gynaecol Can 2003;25:396.

SURGERY FOR MALIGNANT UTERINE DISEASE

1. Endometrial Cancer

Endometrial carcinoma is the most common gynecologic malignancy in the United States. It is primarily a disease of postmenopausal women. Tumors are grouped into type I and II categories based on their underlying etiology. The more common type I tumors arise from prolonged estrogen stimulation of the endometrium. The estrogen is most commonly endogenously produced estrone arising by aromatase conversion of androstenedione in peripheral adipocytes. Obese women produce much more estrogen and are at much higher risk for developing this cancer. Exogenous estrogens prescribed without accompanying progestin in postmenopausal women greatly increases the risk of endometrial cancer as does treatment with other estrogen receptor agonists such as tamoxifen when prescribed for treatment or prevention of breast cancer. Other risk factors for development of endometrial cancer include diabetes, early menarche, late menopause, and low parity. Oral contraceptives are protective against this cancer. Also at risk are premenopausal women with chronic anovulation such as with polycystic ovary syndrome.

Complex hyperplasia with atypia is a precursor lesion for type I endometrial cancer. These tumors usually express estrogen and progesterone receptors. Type II endometrial cancers include anaplastic or high-grade, papillary serous, clear cell, and squamous carcinomas. These tumors rarely express estrogen or progesterone receptors and are not thought to arise as a result of estrogen stimulation. Adverse prognostic factors include grade, histology, depth of myometrial invasion, cervical extension, tumor size, and extension beyond the uterus.

Endometrial cancer surgical staging is listed in Table 39–5.

▶ Clinical Findings

Postmenopausal bleeding is the presenting symptom in about 90% of cases and should be considered to be cancer until proven otherwise. Common etiologies of postmenopausal bleeding include physiologic bleeding from hormone

Table 39–5. FIGO Staging for Endometrial Cancer.

FIGO Stage	Description	TNM Class
Stage 0	Carcinoma in situ	Tis
Stage I	Tumor limited to corpus uteri	T1
IA	Tumor limited to endometrium	T1a
IB	Invasion to less than half the myometrium	T1b
IC	Invasion to more than half the myometrium	T1c
Stage II	Tumor invades cervix but does not extend beyond uterus	T2
IIA	Endocervical glandular involvement only	T2a
IIB	Cervical stromal invasion	T2b
Stage III	Local and/or regional spread	T3 and/or N1
IIIA	Tumor invades serosa and/or adnexa and/or positive cytologic findings	T3a
IIIB	Vaginal involvement (direct or metastases)	T3b
IIIC	Metastases to pelvic and/or para-aortic lymph nodes	T(any), N1
Stage IVA	Tumor invades bladder or bowel mucosa	T4
Stage IVB	Distant metastases, including intra-abdominal and/or inguinal lymph nodes	M1
Grade 1	≤ 5% of nonsquamous solid growth pattern	
Grade 2	6–50% of nonsquamous solid growth pattern	
Grade 3	> 50% of nonsquamous solid growth pattern	

Benedet JL, Hacker NF, Ngan HYS (editors): Staging classifications and clinical practice guidelines of gynaecologic cancers. Int J Gynecol Obstet 2000;70:207. http://www.figo.org/content/PDF/staging-booklet.pdf.

replacement therapy (27%), benign polyps (7–23%), cervicitis (6–14%), endometrial carcinoma (13–16%), atrophy (10%), and cervical carcinoma (1–4%). Despite workup, up to 20–23% of cases will have no identified etiology. Cervical stenosis with pyometrium or hematometrium is highly suggestive of endometrial carcinoma. Pain is not a common symptom. Vaginal cytology is positive in 40–80% of cases but is entirely unreliable as a diagnostic tool for endometrial cancer. Endometrial biopsy performed in the office using a disposable biopsy instrument is highly sensitive. If endometrial biopsy fails to provide a definitive diagnosis, dilatation and curettage of endocervix and endometrium is definitive.

Type II endometrial carcinoma consisting of poorly differentiated or adverse histological types may disseminate relatively early in the course of the disease. Metastatic spread may occur to the vagina, regional pelvic and para-aortic lymph nodes, ovaries, lungs, brain, and bone. The most frequent site of recurrence following treatment for endometrial carcinoma is the vaginal vault.

Prevention

Oral contraceptives have been shown to reduce the risk of endometrial cancer by up to 50% depending on duration of treatment. Progestin therapy reduces the possibility of endometrial carcinoma in the anovulatory patient as well as in postmenopausal women receiving estrogen replacement therapy. Progestins in both oral contraceptives and hormone replacement regimens cause downregulation of estrogen receptors and atrophy of endometrium.

Treatment

Endometrial cancer is staged surgically. The route of surgical approach for the staging procedure can be via either laparotomy or laparoscopy. Definitive therapy includes total hysterectomy, bilateral salpingo-oophorectomy, pelvic and para-aortic lymphadenectomy, and pelvic washings for type I cancers. For type II lesions, mastectomy is usually added. Lymphadenectomy is occasionally omitted for patients with type I lesions with low risk, such as small, grade-1 cancers without myometrial invasion.

If the cervix is grossly involved, patients should receive preoperative radiation followed by total hysterectomy, bilateral salpingo-oophorectomy, pelvic and para-aortic lymphadenectomy, and pelvic washings. Alternatively, a radical hysterectomy, bilateral salpingo-oophorectomy, pelvic and para-aortic lymphadenectomy may be performed without preoperative radiation. The radical hysterectomy includes removal of the upper third of the vagina and the cardinal and uterosacral ligaments.

Adjuvant pelvic radiation therapy is administered to patients with cervical extension (stage II); deep myometrial invasion with a grade 3, type I lesion; or vaginal extension (stage IIIB). A randomized clinical trial comparing radiation to chemotherapy with cisplatin and doxorubicin showed a survival benefit for patients with positive nodes (stage IIIC) treated with chemotherapy. Type II lesions such as papillary serous carcinomas are very likely to recur after surgery regardless of stage. These tumors are usually treated with multimodal therapy using a combination of radiation and chemotherapy.

Metastatic or recurrent disease is usually treated with multimodal therapy using surgery, radiation, and/or chemotherapy based on the location, size, and histology of lesions. Chemotherapy combinations usually include either a doublet of cisplatin with paclitaxel or doxorubicin or a triplet regimen combining all three drugs. Metastatic cancer of type I may be treated with progestin therapy.

Prognosis

Survival at 5 years is about 70–90% for stage I disease, depending on grade and myometrial invasion. Survival declines to about 60% in stage II. Anaplastic tumors, deep myometrial penetration, and absence of estrogen and progesterone receptors all worsen the prognosis.

American College of Obstetricians and Gynecologists: ACOG practice bulletin #65, clinical management guidelines for obstetrician-gynecologists. August 2005: management of endometrial cancer. Obstet Gynecol 2005;106:413.
Rose PG: Endometrial carcinoma. N Engl J Med 1996;335:640.

2. Uterine Sarcoma

Uterine sarcomas fall into three histological groups: leiomyosarcoma, endometrial stromal sarcoma, and carcinosarcoma. These tumors are rare, accounting for about 3% of uterine neoplasms. Sarcomas of the uterus spread via hematogenous and lymphatic pathways in addition to direct extension. Lung and liver are frequent sites of metastases and recurrence.

In patients in whom the tumor is confined to the pelvic organs, treatment consists of total hysterectomy, bilateral salpingo-oophorectomy, pelvic and para-aortic lymphadenectomy, omentectomy, and pelvic washings. There are no randomized trials documenting survival benefit for adjuvant therapy with either chemotherapy or radiation. However, individualized postoperative radiation and/or chemotherapy may be offered based on the poor prognosis of these tumors. Radiation reduces pelvic recurrences but does not appear to improve overall survival.

The outlook for patients with uterine sarcoma is dependent on grade and stage of the tumor. Leiomyosarcomas with more than 10 mitoses per 10 high-power fields carry a poor prognosis, with recurrence within 5 years in about two thirds of patients. About 40% of patients with malignant mixed müllerian tumors survive. Isolated, late recurrence of leiomyosarcoma in the lung is treated by resection of the affected lobe with generally good salvage rates of about 50% at 2 years.

Gemcitabine and Taxotere is the combination with the highest likelihood of response for metastatic or recurrent leiomyosarcoma. High-dose progestin therapy is very effective for treatment of metastatic low-grade endometrial sarcoma. Carcinosarcoma is most effectively treated with combination of either cisplatin and ifosfamide or ifosfamide and paclitaxel.

Gonzalez-Bosquet E et al: Uterine sarcoma: a clinicopathological study of 93 cases. Eur J Gynaecol Oncol 1997;18:192.
Levenback CF et al: Uterine sarcoma. Obstet Gynecol Clin North Am 1996;23:457.

3. Gestational Trophoblastic Disease

Gestational trophoblastic disease refers to tumors arising from placental tissue. They are unique among all neoplasms in that their genetic complement is provided by the father, thereby resulting in a tumor with genetic material and markers foreign to the patient. Gestational trophoblastic diseases may be divided into preinvasive and invasive types. The preinvasive types include complete and partial hydatidiform moles.

The frequency of hydatidiform mole is about 1:700 to 1:2000 pregnancies in the United States, Canada, and Western Europe and about 1:85 to 1:520 pregnancies in Asia. Hydatidiform mole is more common in women over 40. A prior history of gestational trophoblastic disease significantly increases the risk of recurrence with a future gestation.

The gross appearance of a hydatidiform mole is related to the hydropic villi in the absence of a fetal circulation. The histological appearance reveals varying degrees of trophoblastic proliferation. Hydatidiform moles can be classified as either complete or partial based on cytogenetics and histopathology. These features are compared in Table 39–6. Most complete moles carry a 46XX karyotype, with chromosomes exclusively of paternal origin. Partial moles are typically triploid with 69XXX or 69XXY, where 2 or 3 sets of chromosomes are paternal in origin. Complete moles are not associated with a developing fetus, and partial moles may include a fetus that is typically small and with multiple anomalies.

Invasive gestational trophoblastic disease is categorized as invasive mole, choriocarcinoma, or placental site trophoblastic tumor. Invasive mole is diagnosed after 15% of complete moles and 3.5% of partial moles. Metastases occur following 4% of complete moles and 0.6% of partial moles. Choriocarcinoma occurs following 3–7% of hydatidiform moles and 1:40,000 term pregnancies. Out of all choriocarcinoma cases, 50% are preceded by a mole, 25% by spontaneous abortion, and 25% by term pregnancy. Placental site trophoblast tumor (PSTT) is a very rare variant with only 55 cases reported in the literature by 1991.

Invasive mole is composed of hyperplastic trophoblasts with villi invading myometrium. Choriocarcinoma involves sheets of syncytiotrophoblasts with no villi and demonstrates invasion into myometrium or other tissues. Necrosis and hemorrhage are common. Placental site trophoblast tumor is composed of intermediate cytotrophoblasts.

Beta-human chorionic gonadotropin (β-hCG) is a clinically useful tumor marker for all types of preinvasive and invasive gestational trophoblastic disease except placental site trophoblast tumor, in which human placental lactogen (hPL) can be elevated.

Clinical Findings

The most common presenting symptom with hydatidiform mole is vaginal bleeding, occurring in 97% of complete moles and 73% of partial moles. On pelvic examination, about 50% of complete moles and 8% of partial moles will reveal uterine size greater than expected for a given estimated gestational age. Theca lutein cysts are physiologic ovarian cysts resulting from hyperstimulation by very high levels of β-hCG produced by 50% of complete moles. These cysts typically resolve once the β-hCG level regresses following appropriate treatment. Pre-

Table 39–6. Features of Hydatidiform Moles.

Characteristic	Complete Mole	Partial Mole
Karyotype	46XX (90%)	Triploid (90%)
	46XY (10%)	69XXX or 69XXY
	All paternal chromosomes	Diploid (10%)
		46 paternal chromosomes
Fetus	Absent	Often present
Villous edema	Prominent and diffuse	Focal if at all
Fetal RBC	None	Usually present
Proliferation of trophoblast	Prominent	Mild to moderate
Likelihood of local invasion	15%	3.5%
Likelihood of metastasis	4%	0.6%

eclampsia may develop in 27% of women with complete moles and virtually never with partial moles. Clinical hyperthyroidism can develop in about 7% of women with complete moles with very high β-hCG levels due to cross-reactivity of this hormone with thyroid-stimulating hormone. A rare but potentially fatal complication is trophoblastic embolization to the lung during or after evacuation of large complete moles.

Diagnosis is usually confirmed with either ultrasound or β-hCG values. Serum β-hCG levels are above 100,000 mIU/mL in 46% of women with complete moles, and these values persist beyond the 12th week gestation, neither of which should be observed in a normal pregnancy. Ultrasound will usually demonstrate multiple small sonolucencies due to the hydropic villi. In a partial mole, the fetus, if present, will usually be small and afflicted with multiple anomalies.

Differential Diagnosis

Threatened abortion or missed abortion will often present with similar symptoms of bleeding, and both are more likely than gestational trophoblastic disease. A multiple gestation must be considered because it may produce unusually high levels of β-hCG in addition to uterine size greater than the gestational date.

Complications

Metastasis is most common with choriocarcinoma but may occur with any of the invasive types of gestational trophoblastic disease. The most common sites of spread include lung (80%), vagina (30%), pelvis (20%), brain or liver (10%), bowel or kidney or spleen (< 5%). Unlike virtually any other tumor, metastatic disease is still potentially curable in many patients.

Treatment

Once the diagnosis of a molar pregnancy has been established, the uterus should be emptied by suction curettage. All specimens are submitted for histology and cytogenetics. Theca lutein cysts of the ovaries regress following treatment of the mole and should not be surgically excised.

Following evacuation of the uterus, weekly serum β-hCG levels should be monitored until normalized for 3 weeks, followed by monthly testing for 6–12 months depending on assessment of pretreatment risk factors. If the β-hCG value plateaus for 3 weeks or rises for 2 weeks, invasive gestational trophoblastic disease, including either invasive mole or choriocarcinoma, should be suspected. Effective contraception during the surveillance phase is important in order not to complicate interpretation of the β-hCG.

Patients with invasive or persistent gestational trophoblastic disease should be evaluated with a metastatic workup including pelvic examination; CT scan of the head, chest, abdomen, and pelvis; a complete blood count; and renal and liver function tests. Lumber puncture to detect occult central nervous system metastases is sometimes necessary.

Staging of gestational trophoblastic tumors is outlined in Table 39–7. Unlike most neoplasms, gestational trophoblastic disease is staged using a nonanatomic staging system based on prognostic factors. Current FIGO staging combines anatomic staging with the modified World Health Organization (WHO) prognostic scoring system. For anatomic stage I disease, risk is usually low, and for anatomic stage IV disease, risk is usually high. Stage II and III disease is best stratified with the modified WHO prognostic scoring sys-

tem. Stage is recorded as anatomic stage and FIGO modified WHO score, separated by colon.

Single-agent chemotherapy is the preferred treatment for patients with stage I or low-risk disease who wish to maintain reproductive options. If future childbearing is not an issue, patients with invasive mole may be treated with a hysterectomy and possible adjuvant chemotherapy. Preferred regimens for single-agent therapy include methotrexate or dactinomycin. Both of these regimens can be toxic and should be administered under the guidance of a gynecologic oncologist or medical oncologist. Intermediate and high-risk gestational trophoblastic disease should receive aggressive combination chemotherapy. The most effective regimen reported is etoposide, methotrexate, dactinomycin, cyclophosphamide, and vincristine (EMACO). There is occasionally a role for surgery or radiation for selected metastatic disease sites, and intrathecal methotrexate is sometimes needed for treatment of central nervous system disease.

▶ Prognosis

The prognosis for cure of gestational trophoblastic tumors is excellent, including cases with pulmonary metastases, which are still considered low risk. Five-year survival of up to 85% is reported in cases with high-risk metastatic disease. The risk of recurrence of gestational trophoblastic disease in a future pregnancy has a relative risk of 20–40%, but in

Table 39–7. FIGO Anatomic Staging for Gestational Trophoblastic Neoplasia (GTN).

FIGO Staging	Description			
Stage I	Disease confined to the uterus			
Stage II	GTN extends outside of uterus but is limited to genital structures, including adnexa, vagina, broad ligament			
Stage III	GTN extends to lungs with or without genital tract involvement			
Stage IV	All other metastatic sites			

Modified WHO Prognostic Scoring System as adapted by FIGO

Description	Score			
Factor	0	1	2	4
Age (years)	< 40	≥ 40		
Antecedent pregnancy type	Mole	Abortion	Term	
Pregnancy to treatment interval (months)	< 4	$4 \leq 7$	7–13	≥ 13
Pretreatment β-hCG (mIU/L)	< 10^3	10^3–10^4	10^4–10^5	≥ 10^5
Tumor size including uterus (cm)	—	3–5	≥ 5	—
Site of metastases	Lung	Spleen Kidney	GI	Brain Liver
Number of metastases	0	1–4	5–8	> 8
Previous failed chemo regimens			Single	≥ 2

Total: If score is ≥ 7, then patient is high risk and requires intensive, multiagent chemotherapy. Current staging combines anatomic staging with the modified WHO prognostic scoring system. Stage is recorded as anatomic stage and FIGO modified WHO score, separated by colon. Example of format: Stage IV: 8.

absolute terms, this translates to a recurrence risk of less than 5%. During any subsequent pregnancy, ultrasound is recommended. The placenta should be examined after delivery, and β-hCG should be monitored until normalization.

American College of Obstetricians and Gynecologists: ACOG practice bulletin #53, diagnosis and treatment of gestational trophoblastic disease. Obstet Gynecol 2004;103:1365.

Berkowitz RS et al: Chorionic tumors. N Engl J Med 1990;335:1740.

Bower M et al: EMA/CO (etoposide, methotrexate, dactinomycin, cyclophosphamide, vincristine) for high-risk gestational trophoblastic tumours: results from a cohort of 272 patients. J Clin Oncol 1990;15:2636.

Newlands ES et al: Recent advances in gestational trophoblastic disease. Hematol Oncol Clin North Am 1999;13:225.

SURGERY FOR BENIGN FALLOPIAN TUBE DISEASE

1. Infertility Attributed to Fallopian Tube Disease

Infertility is failure to conceive after 1 year of normal coital activity without use of contraceptives. About 15% of couples are infertile within this definition. When the etiology of infertility is evaluated, approximately 40% will be attributable to male factor infertility, including low sperm count, impaired motility, or abnormal morphology of sperm. Anatomic abnormality of the pelvic organs is the single-most common cause of infertility in women, and tubal factor infertility is the most common cause of infertility.

Common causes for tubal factor infertility include acute and chronic salpingitis, endometriosis, and adhesions from previous appendicitis with rupture or surgery. Chlamydia and gonorrhea infections are the most common causes of tubal damage causing infertility. Desire to reverse previous tubal sterilization may also be a reason for tubal surgery. One third of infertile couples have more than one problem.

▶ History

It is important to elicit any history of sexually transmitted disease, pelvic inflammatory disease, pelvic surgery, cyclic pain, or dyspareunia.

▶ Clinical Findings

The size and mobility of the uterus should be assessed. Adnexae should be palpated for masses consistent with endometrioma or hydrosalpinx in particular. Cul-de-sac or uterosacral ligament nodularity and tenderness suggests endometriosis. Ultrasound may reveal the presence of iso-echoic masses, suggesting endometriosis or a tubular mass consistent with hydrosalpinx. Hysterosalpingogram, a test that involves fluoroscopic assessment of tubal patency by transcervical injection of the uterus with radiocontrast, may reveal an obstruction and its location. Use of a water-based dye is indicated for the first attempt, and if occlusion is noted, an oil contrast medium may be used subsequently. The oil-based hysterosalpingogram is reported to have therapeutic benefit.

Laparoscopy is warranted if the evaluation for anatomic abnormalities is inconclusive. Therapeutic interventions including lysis of adhesions or ablation of endometrial implants may be efficacious. If laparoscopy is performed following a normal hysterosalpingogram, 24% will have mild endometriosis and 6% of patients will have adhesions.

▶ Treatment

Tuboplasty procedures restore tubal patency. Successful outcomes are more likely if the tube is minimally affected by extrinsic adhesions than if it is intrinsically scarred. Improvement of surgical technique to minimize tissue trauma and inflammation also improves outcomes. These techniques include atraumatic tissue handling, microsurgical techniques, laparoscopy, and use of adhesion barriers. Hydrosalpinx is usually treated by salpingectomy in order to optimize subsequent in vitro fertilization. Other factors of prognostic significance include age of the couple and presence of other causes of infertility, including ovulatory dysfunction or male factor infertility.

In vitro fertilization has become a much more popular intervention in recent years for treatment of infertility attributed to tubal occlusion or when multiple infertility factors affect the couple. Heterotopic pregnancies and multiple gestation pregnancies are much more likely for patients undergoing in vitro fertilization than for the general population.

▶ Prognosis

Age and severity of tubal disease are predictors of success. Women with mild adhesive disease and age less than 35 have the highest success rates, approaching 70%. For severe tubal disease, success is less than 15%. Ectopic pregnancy is 20 times more likely with a history of fallopian tube surgery or preexisting scar resulting in a 10% incidence. In vitro fertilization success rates vary by program and have generally been improving steadily in recent years. Decisions regarding planned tubal surgery versus in vitro fertilization should take into account the relative costs and success rates.

Benadiva CA et al: In vitro fertilization versus tubal surgery: is pelvic reconstructive surgery obsolete? Fertil Steril 1995;64:1051.

Bildirici I et al: A prospective evaluation of the effect of salpingectomy on endometrial receptivity in cases of women with communicating hydrosalpinges. Hum Reprod 2001;16:2422.

Marcoux S, Maheux R, Berube S: Laparoscopic surgery in infertile women with minimal or mild endometriosis. Canadian Collaborative Group on Endometriosis. N Engl J Med 1997;337:217.

Spielvogel K et al: Surgical management of adhesions, endometriosis, and tubal pathology in the woman with infertility. Clin Obstet Gynecol 2000;43:916.

Watson A et al: Liquid and fluid agents for preventing adhesions after surgery for subfertility. Cochrane Database Syst Rev 2000;2:CD001298.

Watson A et al: Techniques for pelvic surgery in subfertility. Cochrane Database Syst Rev 2000;2:CD000221.

2. Ectopic Pregnancy

Ectopic pregnancy is implantation of a viable pregnancy in a location other than within the endometrium lining the uterus. Risk factors for ectopic pregnancy include prior tubal surgery, previous ectopic pregnancy, history of pelvic inflammatory disease or chlamydia infection, and pregnancy arising from assisted reproduction techniques. Smoking and history of infertility are also associated with increased risk of ectopic pregnancy. Over 95% of ectopic pregnancies occur in the fallopian tube, generally within the ampullary portion. A less common location includes interstitial pregnancy within the tubal lumen where it passes through the myometrium. Rare sites include cervix, ovary, omentum, pelvis, and abdomen. Heterotopic pregnancy is the rare occurrence of an intrauterine pregnancy with a synchronous ectopic pregnancy. The incidence of heterotopic pregnancy has increased from a spontaneous rate of 1:30,000 pregnancies to 0.1–1% for pregnancies arising from assisted reproductive technology.

The incidence of ectopic pregnancy has been reported to occur in approximately 2% of pregnancies, although the true incidence is difficult to ascertain due to the potential for spontaneous resolution of some ectopic pregnancies resulting in unrecognized disease in addition to underreporting of early ectopic pregnancies treated medically rather than surgically. Pregnant women with pain or bleeding have a fourfold higher incidence of ectopic pregnancy. The primary potential morbidity of ectopic pregnancy is the potential rupture of the fallopian tube or other implantation site resulting in hemorrhage. Failure to make a timely diagnosis can result in hemorrhagic shock and death.

Symptoms & Signs

Patients usually present with amenorrhea and a diagnosis of pregnancy. Subsequent irregular bleeding occurs in many but not all cases. In the early evolution of the ectopic pregnancy, patients may be asymptomatic. Presence of pain is also variable. Classic symptoms of a ruptured ectopic pregnancy include severe abdominal pain, referred pain to the shoulder, and hemodynamic instability. Upon pelvic examination an adnexal mass may or may not be present. The uterus is usually slightly enlarged and softened secondary to hormonal influence of the ectopic pregnancy.

Diagnostic Studies

Trophoblastic cells of the blastocyst produce β-hCG that may be detected shortly after implantation. The rise of β-hCG is logarithmic, with a doubling time of about 48 hours. The β-hCG should rise at least 66% every 48 hours in 85% of normal pregnancies and plateaus in normal pregnancy late in the first trimester. Ectopic pregnancies show a slower rise of β-hCG in all but 15% of cases. An absolute β-hCG does not permit distinction between an ectopic and a nonviable intrauterine pregnancy.

Transvaginal ultrasound has almost 100% sensitivity for detection of intrauterine pregnancy as long as care is taken to discriminate between an actual pregnancy and the pseudosac, defined as intrauterine fluid that can be mistaken for an intrauterine pregnancy. A true gestational sac is located eccentrically in the uterus and should demonstrate a fetal pole. The absence of an intrauterine pregnancy in the setting of a positive β-hCG is strongly suggestive of an ectopic pregnancy if the β-hCG value is above the discriminatory threshold of transvaginal ultrasound to detect a gestational sac. The discriminatory threshold has been reported to occur with β-hCG values above 1500–3000 mIU/mL, although variables such as body mass index, quality of ultrasound equipment, and experience of the sonographer all impact on the threshold value. Diagnosis of the ectopic pregnancy by direct ultrasound localization of the pregnancy is much less accurate than detection of intrauterine implantation.

Other tests that are of value include obtaining a blood count to assess for anemia in addition to serum progesterone levels. Variability of progesterone values in normal pregnancy limits the utility of this test for diagnosis of ectopic pregnancy.

Treatment

If the β-hCG shows an abnormal rate of rise, including plateau, slow rise, or declining values, then ultrasound is warranted. However, if the β-hCG value is below the discriminatory threshold, suction curettage is useful to distinguish between a nonviable intrauterine pregnancy and an ectopic gestation. The absence of chorionic villi in the curettage specimen in the presence of an elevated β-hCG is predictive of an ectopic pregnancy, though in early gestation the curettage may be falsely negative for villi.

Treatment of ectopic pregnancy is either surgical or medical depending on several variables. The surgical approach is definitive but invasive and more costly than medical management. Medical management results in successful treatment for 90% of appropriately selected patients. Methotrexate is utilized for medical management. Appropriate indications for medical management require a hemodynamically stable patient who is compliant and has no medical contraindication to methotrexate. Relative contraindications include a gestational sac larger than 3.5 cm, presence of fetal cardiac motion, or a β-hCG value higher than 15,000 mIU/mL. Administration of a single dose of methotrexate has reported efficacy of 84%. Use of multidose regimens increases the rate of success. Failure of the β-hCG value to fall by at least 15% within 4–7 days after treatment indicates that additional methotrexate or surgery is indicated. Patients who are Rh negative are given RH$_o$(D) immune globulin whether treated medically or surgically. Other developments in medical management include the use of other agents such as potassium chloride, prostaglandins, and mifepristone, but these have not been studied as well as methotrexate.

Surgical options for treatment of ectopic pregnancy are intended to remove the ectopic gestation and preserve a functional fallopian tube, if possible. If the patient is hemodynamically stable, the laparoscopic approach is usually preferred. If she is in shock or if the abdomen is distended with blood, emergent laparotomy is necessary. If the fallopian tube is generally healthy, a salpingostomy is possible whereby the involved section of the fallopian tube is removed through an incision in the antimesenteric portion of the tube, while leaving the remainder of the tube intact. If the tube is more extensively damaged, complete or partial salpingectomy is recommended. If conservative approaches to preserve the fallopian tube are utilized, the β-hCG value should be monitored postoperatively until normalization occurs.

Expectant management of a documented ectopic pregnancy may be an option in stable patients if the β-hCG value is less than 200 mIU/mL and declining. Patients must be counseled regarding the risks of rupture and hemorrhage, and emergency management must be readily available.

American College of Obstetricians and Gynecologists: ACOG practice bulletin #3, medical management of ectopic pregnancy. December 1998.
Practice Committee of the American Society for Reproductive Medicine: Early diagnosis and management of ectopic pregnancy. Fertil Steril 2004;82:S146.

▶ Contraception

Contraception to prevent unwanted pregnancy may be attained using either reversible or permanent methods. Reversible methods include hormonal contraceptives via oral, transcutaneous, or subcutaneous routes; injectable, long-acting progestins; IUDs; and condoms, to name a few. Modern IUD contraceptives contain progestational hormones or copper, delivered in low doses to the uterine cavity where they inhibit sperm motility and block fertilization. They are inserted as an office procedure without requiring local anesthetic or cervical dilation in most cases. Both copper and progestin devices are highly effective and long lasting. Contemporary IUD contraceptives do not increase the risk of pelvic infection. Progestin-releasing IUDs decrease menstrual flow by about 50% and have been shown to be as effective for control of abnormal uterine bleeding, prevention of hyperplasia during estrogen replacement therapy, and treatment of hyperplasia.

Subdermal implant contraception uses low serum concentrations of contraceptive progestins found in birth control pills to thicken cervical mucus and inhibit ovulation. These actions result in failure rates comparable to those reported following sterilization and intrauterine contraception. Their duration of action ranges from 1 year to 7 years depending on the number of implants, the progestin employed, and the delivery system. As with intrauterine contraceptives, the principal side effect is change in menstrual bleeding; the majority of users experience a diminution in blood loss but an increase in number of days of bleeding, sometimes at unpredictable intervals.

Contraceptive implants require subdermal insertion with a disposable trocar with local anesthetic and are removed under local anesthetic through a small incision. These procedures take only a few minutes, and pain and infections are rare. Contemporary systems utilize a single rod and are easier to use, have a shorter life, and are associated with somewhat more acceptable bleeding patterns than the now-discontinued multirod implants.

Unintended pregnancies result in about 1 million abortions per year in the United States. Uterine aspiration using either manual or electric vacuum pumps allow safe elective abortion in the first trimester, with a mortality rate of less than 1:200,000 procedures. Morbidity and mortality of abortion rises substantially as the length of gestation increases.

Permanent sterilization options are available for both men and women. Prior to performing any permanent sterilization procedure, the physician must carefully counsel and determine whether a permanent method of contraception is appropriate for the patient. Reversal of permanent sterilization is costly and often ineffective. Permanent male sterilization via vasectomy is safe, effective with reported failure rates of 1.5 per 1000, and minimally invasive. For women, there are several permanent sterilization options. Most of the procedures for women are designed to occlude or remove the fallopian tube via laparotomy or laparoscopy. These include Pomeroy, Irving, Uchida, and Madelener laparotomy operations in addition to laparoscopic procedures using unipolar or bipolar electrosurgical coagulation of the fallopian tubes and application of silastic bands or proprietary clips (Filshie clips, Hulka clips). Mini laparotomy for Pomeroy-type tubal occlusion is often utilized for postpartum sterilization. There are now a limited number of proprietary methods of transcervical tubal occlusion based on intrauterine access to the tubal ostia using a hysteroscope.

The observed failure rate for tubal ligation procedures ranges from 0.7% to 3.6%, which is comparable to the failure rate of IUD and subdermal implants.

Darney P et al: *Protocols for Ambulatory Gynecologic Surgery.* Blackwell Science, 1996.
Speroff L et al: *A Clinical Guide for Contraception,* 3rd ed. Lippincott Williams & Wilkins, 2001.

SURGERY FOR MALIGNANT FALLOPIAN TUBE DISEASE

Benign and malignant tumors of the fallopian tubes are very rare. Adenocarcinoma of the fallopian tube accounts for less than 1% of female reproductive tract cancers. Women with

BRCA12 mutations are at increased risk for fallopian tube cancer concordant with their increased risk for ovarian cancer.

The most common presenting symptoms for cancer of the fallopian tubes are postmenopausal vaginal bleeding or history of intermittent and profuse, watery vaginal discharge. The latter symptom is referred to as hydrops tubae perfluens. An adnexal mass sometimes, but not always, is palpable. Tumor markers such as CA-125 are usually elevated, although early-stage disease may result in elevation of the CA-125 in less than half of patients with fallopian tube or ovarian cancers. The diagnosis of the fallopian tube carcinoma is usually not made preoperatively.

The differential diagnosis for fallopian tube cancer includes disorders that may result in enlargement or obstruction of the distal fallopian tube. The most common example is hydrosalpinx whereby obstruction of the fallopian tube results in accumulation of fluid within the lumen and causes distension of the tube. Common causes of hydrosalpinx include prior infection or endometriosis. Another potential confounding diagnosis is the presence of paratubal cysts, which are simple cysts arising in the mesosalpinx or loosely attached to the exterior of the tube. Paratubal cysts are nearly always benign and arise from müllerian and wolffian duct remnants.

Fallopian tube cancer is staged using the FIGO staging rules for ovarian cancer.

Treatment for fallopian tube cancer is essentially identical to treatment for the much more common diagnosis of ovarian cancer. Multimodal therapy including a primary surgery for staging and debulking of disease is followed by adjuvant chemotherapy based on the stage and grade of the disease. A more detailed discussion of the surgery and postoperative adjuvant therapy considerations is described in the section on Surgery for Malignant Ovarian Disease. If the disease is confined to the tube, the prognosis is good. Like ovarian cancer, most fallopian tube cancers are of advanced stage at the time of diagnosis, and the subsequent survival is much lower.

Nikrui N et al: Fallopian tube carcinoma. Surg Oncol Clin N Am 1998;7:363.

SURGERY FOR BENIGN OVARIAN DISEASE

▶ Adnexal Masses

Adnexal masses are abnormal structures arising in the ovary, fallopian tube, or broad ligament. Preoperative assessment can narrow the differential diagnosis, but definitive diagnosis usually requires surgical resection or biopsy.

The differential diagnosis of adnexal masses is complex (see Table 39–8). Every structure native to the pelvis can potentially present as a detectable adnexal mass. Most are benign, but the probability of malignancy increases with age. About 10% of persistent adnexal masses attributable to the ovary are malignant in premenopausal women, rising to nearly 50% in postmenopausal women.

Table 39–8. Differential Diagnosis of Adnexal Masses.

Ovarian Etiology	Fallopian Tube Etiology
Functional ovarian cyst	Non-neoplastic Fallopian tube conditions
Corpus luteum cyst	
Follicular cyst	Ectopic pregnancy
Theca lutein cyst	Tubo-ovarian abscess / PID
Endometrioma	Hydrosalpinx
Polycystic ovaries	Paraovarian or paratubal cyst
Benign ovarian neoplasm	Malignant Fallopian tube neoplasms
Germ cell	
Mature cystic teratoma	**Uterine Etiology**
Epithelial	Benign conditions
Serous cystadenoma	Pedunculated leiomyoma
Mucinous cystadenoma	Uterine anomalies
Stromal	Undiagnosed pregnancy
Adenofibroma	Malignant neoplasms
Fibroma	Endometrial carcinoma
Thecoma	Uterine sarcoma
Malignant ovarian neoplasm	**Nongynecologic Etiology**
Germ cell	Diseases of appendix or colon
Dysgerminoma	Diseases of bladder
Immature teratoma	Vascular anomalies
Endodermal sinus (yolk sac)	Bony deformation
Embryonal	
Choriocarcinoma	
Epithelial	
Invasive	
Papillary serous	
Endometrioid	
Mucinous	
Clear cell	
Transitional cell	
Low malignant potential	
Serous	
Mucinous	
Stromal	
Sertoli-Leydig	
Granulosa cell, adult	
Granulosa cell, juvenile	

Functional Cysts

Functional cysts are relatively common in women of reproductive age but are also reported in postmenopausal women. These cysts are usually larger than 3 cm in order to be diagnosed and may attain diameters of up to 10 cm. Histological examination reveals no pathologic features such as atypia, necrosis, or invasion. Follicular cysts produce estrogen until resolution of the cyst, and the corpus luteum cyst produces progesterone until resolution. Because of the hormone production by these types of cysts, menses may be delayed or irregular, often leading to an incorrect clinical diagnosis of ectopic pregnancy. The least common type of functional cyst is the theca lutein cyst, which arises as a physiologic response to hyperstimulation by elevated β-hCG values produced by complete hydatidiform moles. Functional cysts usually regress spontaneously within 1–3 months or, in the case of theca lutein cysts, when the β-hCG value normalizes following treatment.

Correct identification of functional cysts prevents many unnecessary surgical procedures. The functional cyst is typically a smooth, unilateral cyst on pelvic examination. Transvaginal ultrasound will show a simple, sonolucent morphology, and β-hCG is not elevated. Follow-up examination with ultrasound after 4–6 weeks will generally demonstrate resolution without treatment. About 85% of functional cysts smaller than 6 cm regress, but larger masses may be more likely to persist. Feedback inhibition on pituitary gonadotropin production by hormonal suppression with oral contraceptives may prevent development of additional functional cysts and is advocated by some clinicians to assist in the regression of existing cysts. Hormonal suppression is by no means required, however, since the majority of functional cysts will regress without intervention.

Most functional cysts remain asymptomatic, but they occasionally rupture or undergo torsion, resulting in acute colicky abdominal or flank pain. Torsion requires prompt surgical intervention, usually with laparoscopy, in order to restore the vascular supply to the ovary by untwisting the pedicle before significant ischemia or necrosis of the ovary can occur. If the functional cyst ruptures, pain of varying levels may occur. In rare cases, bleeding from the ovary leads to hemodynamic instability requiring surgery. Hospitalization for observation for 24 hours, allowing serial examinations and blood counts, is appropriate for patients with symptomatic cyst rupture.

Persistent Adnexal Masses

Adnexal masses that persist are likely to be neoplasms. Benign masses can generally be removed effectively by the general gynecologic surgeon, while malignancies are more effectively treated by gynecologic oncologists with expertise for surgical staging, debulking, and administration of adjuvant therapies to optimize outcome. Triage of adnexal masses provides the best opportunity to serve the patient's interest by having the correct surgical team involved in care of the patient.

The most useful test for assessment of the newly diagnosed adnexal mass is transvaginal ultrasound. Ultrasound is particularly well suited for delineation of the morphologic features of adnexal masses. Medical literature abounds with descriptions of morphology that correlates with benign and malignant neoplasms of the ovary. Figure 39–7 illustrates the morphologic features used to distinguish possible cancers from likely benign lesions. The reported sensitivity for identifying a malignant ovarian neoplasm is 90–94%, but specificity is only about 60%. Specificity can be improved to about 85% without reducing sensitivity by evaluating Doppler waveforms in the tumor vessels. Vessels arising in malignant lesions have lower resistance to flow than those in normal tissues: the ratio of diastolic to systolic flow is therefore higher than in normal tissue (see Figure 39–8), and this can be quantitated by reporting the pulsatility index. This test is more specialized, costly, and time consuming, limiting its effective use to selected lesions. MRI appears to have a promising role in the characterization of adnexal masses, but its sensitivity is somewhat less than that of ultrasound, particularly for early-stage tumors of low-malignant potential. In addition, MRI is much more costly than ultrasonography.

In addition to ultrasound, tumor markers can be very useful for triage of the palpable adnexal mass. The ideal tumor marker is elevated only in the presence of cancer and should correlate with the burden of disease. In reality, no marker is perfect. There are identified markers for ovarian malignancies arising from germ cell, epithelial, and stromal origins. Optimal use of tumor markers involves ordering markers most likely to be clinically useful based on clinical presentation rather than to order all of them. Commonly used tumor markers are listed in Table 39–9. Many new markers will likely be validated in the next few years, including panels of multiple markers using gene chip technology. For example, malignant germ cell neoplasms usually arise in women younger than 35, are almost always unilateral, and typically demonstrate solid morphology on ultrasound evaluation. In this setting, it would be appropriate to order tumor markers including α-fetoprotein (AFP), β-hCG, and lactate dehydrogenase (LDH). Epithelial tumors are more often complex cystic and solid bilateral lesions. In this circumstance, CA-125, CA-19-9, and CEA are better markers. Interpretation of CA-125 is difficult in premenopausal women because benign diseases such as endometriosis, which is much more common than ovarian cancer, will cause false-positive test results. In addition, many tumor markers are normally elevated in pregnancy, thereby complicating evaluation of masses diagnosed during pregnancy.

The American College of Obstetricians and Gynecologists has issued a committee opinion regarding triage of adnexal masses that recommends referral of individuals with high-risk characteristics to gynecologic oncology subspecialists. For postmenopausal women, referral is warranted for patients with a pelvic mass and at least one of the following: CA-125 above 35 U/mL, ascites, nodular or fixed mass,

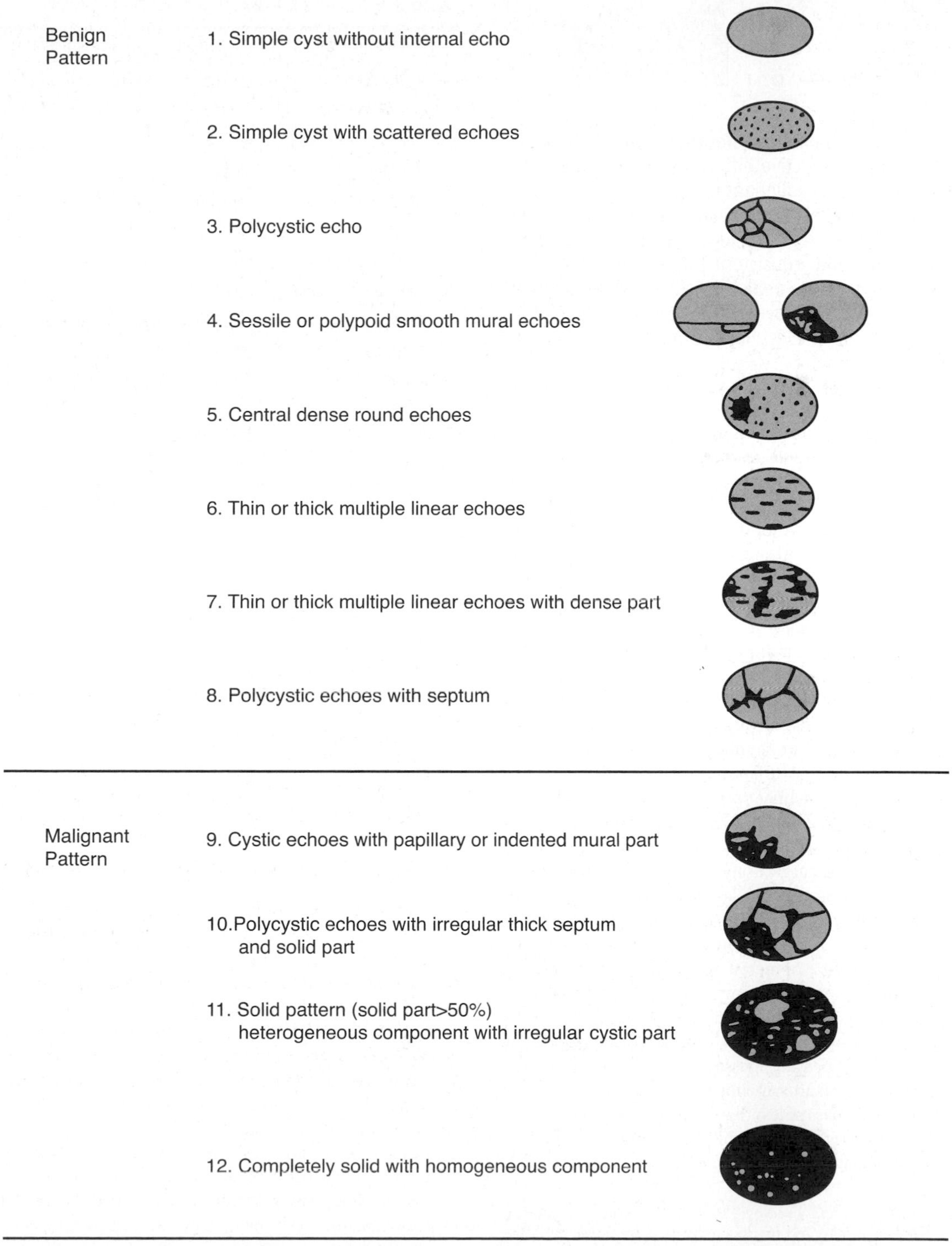

Benign
Pattern

1. Simple cyst without internal echo

2. Simple cyst with scattered echoes

3. Polycystic echo

4. Sessile or polypoid smooth mural echoes

5. Central dense round echoes

6. Thin or thick multiple linear echoes

7. Thin or thick multiple linear echoes with dense part

8. Polycystic echoes with septum

Malignant
Pattern

9. Cystic echoes with papillary or indented mural part

10. Polycystic echoes with irregular thick septum
    and solid part

11. Solid pattern (solid part>50%)
    heterogeneous component with irregular cystic part

12. Completely solid with homogeneous component

▲ **Figure 39–7.** Differential diagnosis of adnexal masses by ultrasound morphology. (From Kawai M et al: Transvaginal Doppler ultrasound with color flow imaging in the diagnosis of ovarian cancer. Obstet Gynecol 1992;79:163.)

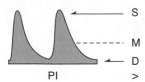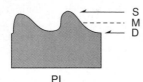

▲ **Figure 39–8.** Doppler waveform and pulsatility index (PI) indicating the objective differences between perfusion in normal versus malignant tissue. If the ratio of 1/PI is greater 0.8, the likelihood of cancer is 96% ($p < 0.01$). The waveform on the right has high diastolic flow, and the pulsatility index is low, consistent with a cancer diagnosis. PI = (peak systolic flow − peak diastolic flow)/mean flow. (From Kawai M et al: Transvaginal Doppler ultrasound with color flow imaging in the diagnosis of ovarian cancer. Obstet Gynecol 1992;79:163.)

evidence of abdominal or distant metastasis, or family history of one or more first-degree relatives with ovarian or breast cancer. In premenopausal women, the recommendations are identical except the threshold for CA-125 is raised to higher than 200 U/mL to account for diseases such as endometriosis in this age group. Motivation for referral is based on data showing higher staging accuracy and improved outcome when subspecialists treat ovarian cancer patients.

Low-risk masses thought to be functional cysts are managed expectantly. A mass that persists or demonstrates worrisome features on examination, imaging studies or tumor marker measurement should be resected. A basic principle of surgical resection for ovarian neoplasms is not to allow spill or rupture of cyst contents into the abdomen. It is never appropriate to needle-aspirate an ovarian mass that may harbor malignancy because of the potential to spread disease intra-abdominally. The surgical procedure to be performed is oophorectomy for high-risk lesions and ovarian cystectomy for low-risk lesions. The route of surgical approach may be with either laparoscopy or laparotomy. The laparoscopic approach is better suited for cystic masses that are small enough to be placed in a specimen retrieval bag without spill or rupture. Large or solid masses or evidence of metastatic disease such as ascites or omental caking require laparotomy for removal. Ovarian conservation is chosen after a balanced assessment of relative risk for cardiac disease versus ovarian cancer. Women under 60 who have benign-appearing masses can expect some cardioprotective benefit even after menopause.

A simple cystic mass of less than 5 cm with normal CA-125 is considered low risk even in the postmenopausal woman. Conservative management is reasonable.

ACOG Committee on Gynecologic Practice: American College of Obstetricians and Gynecologists committee opinion #280. The role of the generalist obstetrician-gynecologist in the early detection of ovarian cancer. December 2002 (issued jointly by the SGO). Obstet Gynecol-NY 2002;100:1413.

Table 39–9. Tumor Markers for Ovarian Cancer.

Tumor Histology	Commonly Used Serum Markers
Epithelial tumors	CA-125, CA-19-9, CEA
Papillary serous	CA-125
Endometrioid	CA-125
Mucinous	CA-19-9, CEA
Germ cell tumors	AFP, β-hCG, lactate dehydrogenase (LDH)
Dysgerminoma	LDH
Endodermal sinus	AFP
Immature teratoma	None
Mixed type	AFP, β-hCG, lactate dehydrogenase (LDH)
Choriocarcinoma	β-hCG
Sex-cord stromal tumors	Testosterone, estradiol, inhibin A & B
Sertoli-Leydig	Testosterone
Granulosa cell	Estradiol, inhibin A & B

Aslam N et al: Prospective evaluation of three different models for the pre-operative diagnosis of ovarian cancer. Br J Obstet Gynaecol 2000;107:1347.

Dottino PR et al: Laparoscopic management of adnexal masses in premenopausal and postmenopausal women. Obstet Gynecol 1999;93:223.

Kawai M et al: Transvaginal Doppler ultrasound with color flow imaging in the diagnosis of ovarian cancer. Obstet Gynecol 1992;79:163.

Kinkel K et al: US characterization of ovarian masses: a meta-analysis. Radiology 2000;217:803.

Sassone AM et al: Transvaginal sonographic characterization of ovarian disease: evaluation of a new scoring system to predict ovarian malignancy. Obstet Gynecol 1991;78:70.

SURGERY FOR MALIGNANT OVARIAN DISEASE

Ovarian cancer is stratified into three histological groups based on the cellular origin of the tumor. Epithelial tumors, germ cell tumors, and sex-cord stromal tumors comprise the primary lesions, and the fourth category is from disease arising elsewhere that metastasizes to ovary. Epithelial carcinoma accounts for about 85% of ovarian cancers, and about 5% arise from each of the remaining categories of germ cell, sex-cord stromal and metastatic disease from other sites. The peak incidence of epithelial ovarian cancer is in the fifth and sixth decades of life, while malignant germ cell tumors are more likely to occur under the age of 30. Stromal tumors have a bimodal distribution with peaks around ages 25 and 55 years. Malignant ovarian disease spreads by primary extension in the peritoneal cavity in addition to lymphatic and hematogenous spread.

Epithelial ovarian cancer etiology can be either sporadic or hereditary. The sporadic cases appear to be strongly related to number of lifetime ovulations or chronicity of gonadotropin stimulation. There are also data to suggest environmental impact with the observation that tubal ligation results in reduction of risk, and diets with high lipids relative to omega-3 fatty acids increase risk. Up to 10% of ovarian cancers are hereditary. Three pedigrees account for most hereditary cases, including ovary site-specific cancer, breast–ovary cancer, and hereditary nonpolyposis colorectal cancer (HNPCC). Genetic inheritance of a mutation in the *BRCA1* or *BRCA2* gene imparts up to a 40% lifetime risk of developing ovarian cancer and an 80% lifetime risk of developing breast cancer. Ethnic groups including Ashkenazi Jews and Icelandic peoples have increased incidence of founder mutations that increase risk. Other reproductive factors associated with an increased risk include infertility, including use of ovulation induction agents.

Epithelial tumors are divided into invasive and low malignant potential (borderline) types. The invasive type accounts for 80% of epithelial cancer and is usually detected in advanced stages. The low malignant tumors occur in women with an average age 10 to 15 years younger than for invasive disease, and up to 80% are stage I at diagnosis. Destructive stromal invasion is absent in low malignant potential tumors, but they are considered to be malignant and have the potential to metastasize. Epithelial tumors are subcategorized by histology as serous, mucinous, endometrioid, clear cell, transitional cell, or undifferentiated types. Serous tumors are the most common, accounting for about 50% of epithelial carcinomas. Endometrioid carcinomas are the second-most frequent variety, accounting for 24% of ovarian cancers, and are sometimes associated with endometriosis. Clear cell tumors, accounting for less than 5% of epithelial tumors, are also associated with endometriosis and have a more virulent natural history. Mucinous tumors account for 15% of epithelial cancers and may become very large. Epithelial ovarian cancer commonly involves both ovaries.

Germ cell cancer types include dysgerminomas, immature teratoma, endodermal sinus tumor, mixed types, and rare nongestational choriocarcinoma. Germ cell cancers are almost always unilateral and are commonly detected while in stage I. Germ cell cancers are three times more common in women of Asian or African descent. A separate entity is adult-type cancer arising in an otherwise benign mature cystic teratoma. This can occur in up to 1% of mature cystic teratomas and is most commonly a squamous carcinoma.

The most common sex-cord stromal tumors include Sertoli-Leydig, adult granulosa, and juvenile granulosa cell tumors. These are frequently hormonally active tumors. Sertoli-Leydig cell tumors occur most often in the third decade and arise from wolffian duct remnants. They are rare and usually produce testosterone, resulting in manifest defeminization (amenorrhea, atrophy of the breast) and virilization (deepening of the voice, hirsutism, clitoral hypertrophy). Adult granulosa cell tumors arise in the sixth decade and are estrogen-producing tumors in most instances. Because of the estrogen production, postmenopausal bleeding is common, and endometrial cancer may arise in up to 15%. Juvenile granulosa cell tumors are similar but arise in younger patients. Like germ cell tumors, the sex-cord stromal tumors are unilateral in most cases, and detection is typically at early stages.

Metastatic carcinoma from other primary sites occurs frequently. Common sites include the gastrointestinal tract (Krukenberg tumor), breast, pancreas, lymphoma, and kidney. These tumors are classically solid and bilateral. Prognosis for these tumors is especially poor.

▶ Clinical Findings

Almost 90% of stage I patients have symptoms, and only 5% are asymptomatic. The symptoms usually include gastrointestinal complaints that persist for an average of 12 days per month for 3 months. Less often, pelvic pain or metrorrhagia may be present. On examination, any mass should prompt further evaluation. An ovarian mass should be regarded as potentially malignant until proven otherwise. Smooth, mobile masses on examination indicate low risk; solid, irregular, or fixed pelvic masses suggest malignancy. Triage of the pelvic mass should include transvaginal pelvic ultrasound and selective tumor markers as described previously in the discussion of adnexal masses. CA-125 may be negative in half of early-stage ovarian cancers. If an ovarian malignancy is suspected preoperatively, referral to a gynecologic oncologist is recommended.

Occasionally, ovarian cancer is discovered during an operation for different indication or when triage has not been properly performed. If ascites, carcinomatosis, or papillary excrescences are noted, the tumor should be removed intact and submitted for frozen section. If cancer is diagnosed, a gynecologic or surgical oncologist should be consulted for surgical staging and debulking.

▶ Treatment

Ovarian cancer is staged surgically (see Table 39–10). When a complex adnexal mass is to be removed, the procedure should begin with obtaining washings for cytology, and the mass should subsequently be removed intact. Upon removal of the mass, a frozen section should be obtained for definitive diagnosis. If an ovarian malignancy is confirmed, complete staging requires assessment and biopsy of the pelvic and para-aortic nodes, omentum, and peritoneum. All peritoneal surfaces are inspected, and any suspicious lesions are biopsied. If no suspicious lesions are noted, a predetermined pattern of biopsies is taken from the pelvic sidewalls, cul-de-sac, bladder peritoneum, pericolic gutters, and both hemidiaphragms. A decision must be made about possible resection of the uterus and contralateral ovary. If the patient is young and desires to retain her fertility, criteria to identify candidates for conservation of fertility should be applied. Factors that favor preservation of fertility include germ cell and sex-cord stromal tumors because they are usually unilateral, and

Table 39–10. FIGO Staging for Ovarian Cancer.

FIGO Staging	Description	TNM Class
Stage I	Tumor limited to the ovaries	T1
IA	Limited to one ovary, no tumor on external surface, capsule intact; negative peritoneal cytology	T1a
IB	Limited to both ovaries, no tumor on external surface, capsule intact; negative peritoneal cytology	T1b
IC	IA or IB tumor but with surface tumor, ruptured capsule, or positive ascites or peritoneal cytology	T1c
Stage II	Tumor extending to the pelvis	T2
IIA	Metastasis to the uterus or tubes	T2
IIB	Metastasis to other pelvic tissues	T2b
IIC	IIA or IIB tumor, both with surface tumor, ruptured capsule, or positive ascites or peritoneal cytology	T2c
Stage III	Tumor extending outside the pelvis and/or retroperitoneal or inguinal nodes; extension to small bowel, omentum, or superficial liver	T3 and/or N1
IIIA	Histologically confirmed microscopic disease of abdominal peritoneal surfaces; lymph nodes negative	T3a
IIIB	Implants of abdominal or peritoneal surfaces not exceeding 2 cm in diameter; lymph nodes negative	T3b
IIIC	Implants of abdominal or peritoneal surfaces greater than 2 cm in diameter, or positive retroperitoneal or inguinal lymph nodes	T3c and/or N1
Stage IV	Distant metastasis beyond the peritoneal cavity	M1

Benedet JL, Hacker NF, Ngan HYS (editors): Staging classifications and clinical practice guidelines of gynaecologic cancers. Int J Gynecol Obstet 2000;70:207. http://www.figo.org/content/PDF/staging-booklet.pdf.

subsequent chemotherapy, if needed, has curative potential. Low malignant potential tumors affecting one ovary or in select cases where extraovarian disease can be completely resected are also candidates. Patients with invasive epithelial tumors are poor candidates for conservative surgery because of the high likelihood of bilateral involvement and the primarily palliative role of chemotherapy for all but early stages of disease. If preservation of fertility is not appropriate, then hysterectomy and removal of the contralateral tube and ovary is completed.

When the disease spread into the pelvis or abdomen is documented, debulking of all resectable macroscopic disease is critically important. Numerous randomized clinical trials have demonstrated the concept of debulking and consistently show survival advantage for patients with maximal cytoreduction. Intraoperative decision making for debulking focuses effort on the biggest tumor, wherever it may be. If the largest lesion can be resected, attention is directed to the next largest lesion. This process continues until either all measurable disease is removed or a lesion that is unresectable is encountered. In order to resect the disease at each decision point of this algorithm, the surgeon may need to perform intestinal resection, splenectomy, modified posterior exenteration, culdectomy, diaphragm resection, and other upper abdominal procedures. In two prospective Gynecologic Oncology Group clinical trials, survival for microscopically debulked ovarian cancer was 65% at 4 years and fell to about 35% if less than 1 cm of macroscopic residual disease remained after surgery. If greater than 2 cm of residual disease remained, the 4-year survival was only 20%. Optimal debulking can be attained in up to 70% of patients who are operated on by subspecialists trained in ovarian cancer surgery.

Patients with stage IA grade 1 or grade 2 epithelial tumors have a very good prognosis and usually are not treated with additional chemotherapy. For more advanced stages of epithelial cancer, chemotherapy is very effective for inducing clinical remission, but relapses are very common with an average progression interval between 2 and 3 years. The best chemotherapy combination for treating advanced stage epithelial cancer includes both taxane and platinum agents, administered either intravenously or intraperitoneally for at least 6 cycles. Intraperitoneal chemotherapy has been demonstrated to induce longer progression free intervals, but acute toxicity is much higher, and only 40% of patients are able to complete planned therapy on this regimen. The CA-125 tumor marker is useful as a marker for assessing the effectiveness of therapy.

The best current regimen for malignant germ cell tumors is cisplatin, etoposide, and bleomycin, administered as a 5-day treatment that is continued until at least one cycle after normalization of elevated tumor markers. Sex-cord stromal tumors are treated similarly.

▶ Prognosis

The prognosis for epithelial ovarian carcinoma is related primarily to stage and histological grade. Because most ovarian cancers are of advanced stage at the time of initial diagnosis, the long-term survival rate for ovarian cancer is only 50%. Five-year survival rates for patients with stage III or stage IV disease are around 20–35%. Prolonged disease-free intervals can be achieved by combining comprehensive surgical staging, aggressive debulking, and adjuvant chemotherapy.

▶ Prevention

Oral contraceptives reduce the risk of ovarian epithelial carcinoma. The magnitude of risk reduction is based on dose and duration of therapy. The protective effects are durable, lasting for a decade or more after discontinuation of the medication.

Any woman with a strong family history should be considered for genetic counseling and testing. Patients with a confirmed hereditary risk of ovarian cancer based on careful pedigree analysis or genetic testing will benefit from prophylactic removal of ovaries and fallopian tubes. The current recommendation is for removal after completion of childbearing at age 35 or 10 years younger than the earliest incidence of disease in the family. Prophylactic removal of ovaries and tubes reduces the risk of ovarian cancer at least 95%, but a small number of individuals may still develop primary peritoneal carcinoma.

To date, no screening test for ovarian cancer has proven to be sufficiently sensitive or specific to have earned the recommendation of the US Preventive Services Task Force, ACOG, or the American Cancer Society. Prospective ultrasound screening studies and combined CA-125/ultrasound studies show a trend toward earlier stage at time of diagnosis on screened patients, resulting in prolongation of progression-free intervals, but not survival.

Armstrong DK et al: Intraperitoneal cisplatin and paclitaxel in ovarian cancer. N Engl J Med 2006;354:34.

Bomalaski JJ: The treatment of recurrent ovarian carcinoma: balancing patient desires, therapeutic benefit, cost containment and quality of life. Curr Opin Obstet Gynecol 1999;11:11.

Goff BA et al: Ovarian carcinoma diagnosis. Cancer 2000;89:2068.

Lynch HT et al: Genetics and ovarian carcinoma. Semin Oncol 1998;25:265.

Marsden DE et al: Current management of epithelial ovarian carcinoma: a review. Semin Surg Oncol 2000;19:11.

Ozols RF: Update of the NCCN ovarian cancer practice guidelines. Oncology 1997;11:95.

Scully RE et al: *Tumors of the Ovary, Maldeveloped Gonads, Fallopian Tube, and Broad Ligament*. Armed Forces Institute of Pathology, 1998.

Van Nagell JR et al: Ovarian cancer screening with annual transvaginal sonography. Cancer 2007;109:1887.

SURGERY FOR MULTIORGAN DISEASE

1. Chronic Pelvic Pain

Chronic pelvic pain is generally defined as 6–12 months of pain below the umbilicus producing a significant impact on quality of life. Evaluation and treatment of chronic pelvic pain accounts for up to 40% of all referrals to gynecologists, leading to up to 40% of all laparoscopies and 12% of all hysterectomies.

▶ Diagnosis

The differential diagnosis of chronic pelvic pain is complex. While many patients attribute their pain to a gynecologic cause, the physician must consider nongynecologic diagnoses of the gastrointestinal, urinary, and musculoskeletal systems in addition to psychological and psychosomatic problems. The most common nongynecologic diagnoses include irritable bowel syndrome, inflammatory bowel disease, nephrolithiasis, interstitial cystitis, ventral or inguinal hernia, muscle strain, nerve injury, depression, and somatization. Of note, patients are more likely to have suffered sexual assault as an adult or child.

The gynecologic causes of chronic pelvic pain are classified as cyclic or continuous in nature. Sources of cyclic pain include primary dysmenorrhea, defined as painful menses without identifiable pelvic pathology; and secondary dysmenorrhea attributable to pathologic conditions such as endometriosis or adenomyosis. Midcycle ovulatory pain may occur that produces unilateral pain at midcycle that resolves after a day or two. Continuous pain sources include endometriosis and adenomyosis and pelvic organ prolapse, both discussed earlier in this chapter, in addition to chronic salpingitis and pelvic adhesions. Another cause of continuous pain is ovarian remnant syndrome, which occurs when residual ovarian tissue after oophorectomy becomes retroperitoneal location. Pain may occasionally be caused by degenerating fibroids or by mass effect from large fibroids.

▶ Clinical Findings

The pelvic examination requires careful communication with the patient to understand where and when her pain occurs. Identification of palpable abnormalities and localization of focal tenderness is important. If a pelvic mass is detected, it should be triaged as discussed previously in the section on Adnexal Masses. An abnormal pelvic examination has about an 80% predictive value for pelvic abnormalities noted at laparoscopy.

▶ Treatment

Nongynecologic causes of pain are treated according to the diagnosis. Gynecologic pain etiology is also treated according to the diagnosis. Women of reproductive age with cyclic pain are offered treatment consisting of nonsteroidal anti-inflammatory drugs and ovulation suppression, usually with oral contraceptives if appropriate for the age and medical risk factors of the patient. Continuous pain attributable to endometriosis or adenomyosis is treated similarly. Other causes of continuous pain include spasm or tension in pelvic floor musculature. Physical therapy and "reverse Kegel" exercises to relax the muscles often result in improvement. An antibiotic may be prescribed if a chronic infection is suspected, but care should be taken to treat documented infection and not to overprescribe antibiotics. Concurrent depression is common, usually arising as a secondary effect of the pain rather than as the primary etiology. Treatment with antidepressant medication is often beneficial. The tricyclic antidepressant class is often more effective that serotonin reuptake inhibitors for this indication. Severe and refractory pain may require narcotics to attain control. The physician must use careful judgment regarding initiation of narcotics in a chronic setting due to the potential for dependence and addiction. It is often useful to manage these patients with a narcotic contract between the patient and her physician to regulate drug use. Referral to a multidisciplinary pain service is often useful for difficult or refractory cases.

If the pain is refractory to medical management or if the physical examination is abnormal, then diagnostic laparoscopy is indicated. During the laparoscopic procedure, upper abdominal structures, pelvic organs and peritoneum, appendix, rectum, and sigmoid colon are carefully inspected. The most commonly identified pathology is endometriosis occurring in one third of patients and adhesions in one third of cases. Most of the remaining cases will have no identified pathology. The presence of abnormalities may not explain the pain, and treatment of disease such as endometriosis may not resolve the pain.

The evidence for therapeutic benefit of laparoscopy for treatment of pelvic pain is tenuous at best. Procedures that remove or ablate adhesions or endometriosis may or may not relieve pain. If pain is attributed to the uterus or cervix and cannot be controlled with lesser procedures or medical management, options include hysterectomy, or if fertility preservation is desired, interruption of the autonomic nerve tracts with a presacral neurectomy. Pain attributed to degenerating or large fibroids may be relieved either with uterine artery embolization procedures or surgical removal of the leiomyomata with either hysterectomy or myomectomy. Severe dysmenorrhea that is refractory to medical management may be significantly improved with endometrial ablation.

Published data indicate that laparoscopic treatment will produce a short-term reduction of pain in about 60–80% of patients, but long-term benefits are not well documented. In patients who have completed their childbearing or who wish definitive treatment, hysterectomy has reported success rates of up to 95% if uterine pathology such as degenerating fibroids is present. If no pelvic pathology is noted, 50–91% experience improvement. The success rate is poor if the patient has symptoms of depression. Patients with endometriosis should also be offered bilateral salpingo-oophorectomy to minimize pain from residual implants.

American College of Obstetricians and Gynecologists: ACOG practice bulletin #51, chronic pelvic pain. Obstet Gynecol 2004;103:589.

Jamieson DF et al: The prevalence of dysmenorrhea, dyspareunia, pelvic pain, and irritable bowel syndrome in primary care practices. Obstet Gynecol 1996;87:55.

Mathias SD et al: Chronic pelvic pain: prevalence, health-related quality of life, and economic correlates. Obstet Gynecol 1996;87:321.

2. Endometriosis

Endometriosis is defined as extrauterine, functional endometrial tissue. The most common sites include ovaries, uterosacral ligaments, and the cul-de-sac. Less commonly, fallopian tubes, uterine serosa, sigmoid colon and rectum, peritoneum, and small intestine or mesentery are involved.

Ectopic endometrium is occasionally detected at distant sites such as the lung, lymph nodes, surgical incision sites, umbilicus, perineum, and breasts.

The etiology of endometriosis is thought to occur from any of three potential mechanisms: (1) retrograde menstruation with implantation, (2) metaplasia of müllerian duct remnants or coelomic epithelium, and (3) lymphatic or venous dissemination. Retrograde menstruation through the uterine tubes is common and yet rarely causes endometriosis. It is not known what factors contribute to implantation and growth of endometriosis. Uterine outflow obstruction from cervical stenosis or congenital anomalies such as imperforate hymen increase the likelihood of developing endometriosis.

Endometriosis may develop at any time after onset of menarche and will virtually regress after menopause. Prevalence of endometriosis is difficult to determine because many women with the disease are asymptomatic. The estimated prevalence of endometriosis is about 15–20%. Endometriosis may cause scarring that impairs fertility. As a consequence, diagnosis of endometriosis during a workup for infertility is higher, with up to 20–47% of patients affected. Conversely, women with proven fertility who elect tubal sterilization are found to have endometriosis on only 1–5% of cases. The incidence of endometriosis is higher in women who choose to delay childbearing and in women with a family history of the disease. Environmental toxins, such as dioxin, may predispose to endometriosis. Pregnancy and hormonal contraceptive hormones are protective.

Carcinoma may arise in endometriosis at any site and is most commonly of endometrioid histology. Clear cell carcinoma is rare and more aggressive.

► Classification

The American Society of Reproductive Medicine developed an anatomic staging system for endometriosis (see Figure 39–9). The Revised AFS classification system is accepted worldwide. The staging system is broadly predictive of outcome with treatment. The stage of endometriosis does not correlate well with pain symptoms. Alternative systems that recognize the varied presentation of endometriosis in addition to development of serum markers have been proposed.

► Symptoms & Signs

Endometriosis frequently causes pain. The pain often begins shortly before menses and continues during menstruation. The presence of pain and its severity is highly variable. Some patients with extensive disease are asymptomatic, while others with small peritoneal implants may be incapacitated. Unexplained infertility may be present in asymptomatic endometriosis. Symptoms may occur at any time during reproductive years but are most common in the third and fourth decades of life. Symptoms usually resolve with menopause unless the patient is prescribed a hormone replacement regimen. Patients may also complain of dyspareunia,

American Society for Reproductive Medicine
Revised Classification of Endometriosis

Patient's Name _____ Date _____

Stage I	(Minimal)	- 1-5
Stage II	(Mild)	- 6-15
Stage III	(Moderate)	- 16-40
Stage IV	(Severe)	- >40
Total _____		

Laparoscopy_____ Laparotomy_____ Photography_____
Recommended Treatment _____
_____
Prognosis _____

PERITONEUM	ENDOMETRIOSIS		<1cm	1-3cm	>3cm
	Superficial		1	2	4
	Deep		2	4	6
OVARY	R	Superficial	1	2	4
		Deep	4	16	20
	L	Superficial	1	2	4
		Deep	4	16	20

	POSTERIOR CUL-DE-SAC OBLITERATION		Partial		Complete
			4		40

	ADHESIONS		<1/3 Enclosure	1/3-2/3 Enclosure	>2/3 Enclosure
OVARY	R	Filmy	1	2	4
		Dense	4	8	16
	L	Filmy	1	2	4
		Dense	4	8	16
TUBE	R	Filmy	1	2	4
		Dense	4*	8*	16
	L	Filmy	1	2	4
		Dense	4*	8*	16

*If the fimbriated end of the fallopian tube is completely enclosed, change the point assignment to 16.
Denote appearance of superficial implant types as red [(R), red, red-pink, flamelike, vesicular blobs, clear vesicles], white [(W), opacifications, peritoneal defects, yellow-brown], or black [(B) black, hemosiderin deposits, blue]. Denote percent of total described as R ___%, W___% and B ___%. Total should equal 100%

Additional Endometriosis:_____
_____
_____

Associated Pathology: _____
_____
_____

L	To be used with normal tubes and ovaries	R

L	To be used with abnormal tubes and/or ovaries	R

▲ **Figure 39–9.** Staging of endometriosis. (American Society for Reproductive Medicine: Revised American Society for Reproductive Medicine classification of endometriosis. Fertil Steril 1997;67:817.)

tenesmus, back pain, or sciatica. Rare manifestations may include ureteral obstruction or bowel obstruction.

Pelvic Examination

Bimanual pelvic examination, including the rectovaginal examination, should be performed. Common findings include pelvic tenderness, adnexal masses, and soft nodularity in the cul-de-sac or along the uterosacral ligaments. Adnexal masses attributable to endometriosis are often bilateral and are frequently immobile because of adhesions along the posterior broad ligament.

Testing

Ultrasound description of isoechoic masses within the ovaries is highly suggestive of endometrioma. Serum concentrations of CA-125 are elevated above 35 U/mL in about one third of patients with advanced disease, which complicates triage of adnexal masses that may be either benign (endometriosis) or malignant. Following surgical and medical treatment, measurement of the CA-125 trend is a useful marker of treatment efficacy and disease recurrence, similar to its use for monitoring treatment of ovarian cancer.

Definitive diagnosis requires biopsy, usually obtained with a laparoscopic procedure. The biopsy diagnosis requires the presence of both glands and stroma. Location and extent of disease is noted at the time of surgery to complete disease staging. Characteristic peritoneal implants include the "powder-burn" marks of darkly colored endometrium in addition to red, blue, and white lesions. Peritoneal disease may be flat or raised, including nodular or vesicular appearance. Laparotomy is occasionally necessary for large ovarian masses or bowel and ureteral obstructions that may be present.

Treatment

Treatment should be tailored to severity of symptoms, age of the patient, desire for fertility, and stage of disease. Therapeutic options range from observation to medical management with hormones and analgesics to hysterectomy with bilateral salpingo-oophorectomy. A conservative approach is preferred for patients with minimal symptoms or minimal measurable disease on pelvic examination. Surveillance examinations should be regularly performed, with the interval determined by severity of symptoms, age of the patient, desire for fertility, and stage of disease. If symptoms or physical finding worsen, the management plan may be changed accordingly.

A. Medical Treatment

The goal of medical therapy is to control disease by inducing a remission. There are no known medical therapies that result in a cure. Hormonal therapy is not administered for patients actively attempting to conceive. Upon treatment discontinuation, symptoms commonly recur. Long-term suppression with hormonal contraceptive regimens should be considered.

B. Progestins

Norethynodrel, norethindrone acetate, and medroxyprogesterone acetate are commonly used. Continuous progestins induce amenorrhea, resulting in decreased symptoms in more than three quarters of patients. Progestin therapy causes downregulation of estrogen receptors in endometrial tissue, resulting in atrophic change in both endometriosis and endometrium. Breakthrough bleeding is not unusual. Side effects include weight gain secondary to appetite stimulation, fluid retention, headaches, and mood swings.

C. Oral Contraceptives

Oral contraceptives induce a pseudopregnancy state. Formulations with a low estrogen dose and a high potency progestin are preferred and may be administered either as cyclic or as continuous regimens without withdrawal intervals each month. Symptoms are relieved in up to 80% of patients. Oral contraceptive may be continued long term as a maintenance therapy in healthy women. Women over 35 who smoke or individuals with hypertension are at increased risk of thromboembolic complications. Side effects include headaches, fluid retention, breast tenderness, breakthrough bleeding, and occasional nausea.

D. GnRH Analogs

Gonadotropin-releasing hormone analogs act by negative feedback inhibition on the pituitary resulting in prevention of follicle-stimulating hormone and luteinizing hormone secretion. The consequence of low gonadotropin levels is absence of follicle development and low estrogen production. This treatment strategy induces the medical equivalent of the postmenopausal state. Endometrial implants atrophy in the hypoestrogenic environment, and about 80% of patients report clinical improvement. Side effects mimic menopause with vasomotor symptoms, vaginal dryness, and mood swings. Long-term treatment causes osteopenia and osteoporosis. To prevent bone loss, "add-back" therapy with either norethindrone acetate or combined hormone replacement therapy concurrent with GnRH analog may be prescribed and does not interfere with treatment of the endometriosis.

E. Surgical Treatment

Indications for surgery include treatment of current infertility, treatment to preserve future fertility, or control of symptoms. Medical therapy is unlikely to result in reduction of symptoms for bulky disease, and surgery is recommended for any endometrioma larger than 4 cm. Options for preservation of fertility in symptomatic women who have failed medical therapy include laparoscopic procedures for resection or ablation of implants, lysis of adhesions, or presacral neurectomy. When definitive therapy is necessary and preservation of fertility is not an issue, total hysterectomy and bilateral salpingo-oophorectomy is indicated. Endometriosis is dependent upon estrogen. Preservation of an ovary in this setting causes symptoms sufficient to prompt additional surgery in 20% of cases. Bowel implants can be locally resected by appropriately trained surgeons.

Postoperative estrogen replacement therapy usually does not lead to exacerbation of endometriosis. The use of estrogen-progestin combinations is generally not required.

American Society for Reproductive Medicine: Revised American Society for Reproductive Medicine classification of endometriosis. Fertil Steril 1997;67:817.

Henzl MR et al: Administration of nasal nafarelin as compared with oral danazol for endometriosis: a multicenter double-blind comparative clinical trial. N Engl J Med 1988;318:485.

Hoeger KM et al: An update on the classification of endometriosis. Clin Obstet Gynecol 1999;42:611.

Hughes E et al: Ovulation suppression for endometriosis. Cochrane Database Syst Rev 2000;CD000155.

Lebovic DI et al: Immunobiology of endometriosis. Fertil Steril 2001;75:1.

Moore J et al: Modern combined oral contraceptives for pain associated with endometriosis. Cochrane Database Syst Rev 2000;CD001019.

Reddy S et al: Treatment of endometriosis. Clin Obstet Gynecol 1998;41:387.

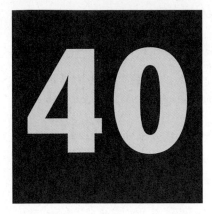

Orthopedic Surgery

Ramesh C. Srinivasan, MD

Stephen Tolhurst, MD

Kelly L. Vanderhave, MD

Orthopedic surgery has evolved substantially during the last decade. Improvements in implant design and materials have been responsible for significant advances in our ability to treat patients with complex orthopedic problems. Like all medical fields, orthopedic surgery has become a group of subspecialized fields in recent years. This chapter reflects this trend, divided into the following sections: Orthopedic Trauma, Pediatric Orthopedics, Sports Medicine, Joints, Orthopedic Spine, Orthopedic Oncology, and Foot and Ankle.

TERMINOLOGY

Varus and **valgus** are frequently used to describe angular musculoskeletal deformities. They refer to the direction of the apex of the deformity in relation to the midline of the body. When the apex points away from the midline, the deformity is termed varus; when the apex points toward the midline, the deformity is termed valgus. Knock-knees is an example of a valgus deformity: The apex is defined by the patient's knees pointing toward the body's midline. Conversely, bow-leggedness is a varus deformity. These terms can also be applied to fractures such that the apex of the deformity is the fracture itself. **Comminution** describes a fracture that is significantly fragmented. A fracture is **displaced** when the main bony fragments are translated or separated from each other. Displacement can further be subcategorized into minimally, moderately, or completely displaced.

Open fractures define fractures with overlying wounds such that the fracture is exposed to the external environment. Open fractures can be obvious in significant trauma with substantial degloving of the soft tissues, or they can be more subtle with only a small poke hole visible when draining fracture hematoma. As a result, when patients are transferred from other hospitals or urgent care facilities, all splints should be removed, and the skin overlying all fractures must be carefully inspected for open injury. Open fractures are orthopedic emergencies and must be addressed with prompt surgical debridement and irrigation to mini-

mize the subsequent development of infection and associated fracture nonunions.

Joint dislocations also warrant immediate treatment. **Reduction** is the maneuver used to restore proper alignment of a joint or fracture. Vascular structures spanning the joint or fracture may be damaged at the time of injury. Alternatively, these structures may be compressed or kinked due to the resulting deformity. Arterial pulses should always be assessed distal to a musculoskeletal injury and carefully documented. Often, absent pulses are restored with reduction of a joint or fracture. If reduction does not successfully return pulses, the vessels are likely torn; early repair and reconstruction is often required to restore distal circulation to the limb. Vascular injuries repaired prior to fracture or joint reduction and stabilization may be in danger of subsequent failure due to bony instability. Orthopedists can quickly stabilize fractures and dislocations using external fixation, providing a stable scaffold onto which necessary vascular repairs can be made.

Joint or fracture reduction may be treated by **open** or **closed** techniques. A dislocation or fracture is described as **unstable** if there is a high likelihood of subsequent deformation after reduction is performed. Following reduction, unstable fractures or dislocations may be stabilized by closed or open means. Closed treatment may involve traction, casts, splints, or braces; open techniques involve surgical exposure of the fracture or joint and reduction followed by maintenance of the reduction with internal or external fixation devices. The surgical treatment of an unstable fracture or dislocation is therefore described as open reduction with internal or external fixation.

SPLINTING & CASTING

Splinting and casting are noninvasive ways of stabilizing fractures and maintaining reductions. **Splints** are typically made of plaster and are not circumferential, while **casts** are circumferential and can be made of either plaster or fiberglass. Splints are best used for a short period of time (days up to 1 or 2 weeks) in acute scenarios shortly after injury or after an operation when swelling is a concern to avoid compartment syndrome. Casts are sturdier, used to maintain bones in appropriate alignment for extended periods of time (weeks to a few months). For example, a distal radius fracture may be reduced and placed in a sugar-tong splint with follow-up in clinic. At clinic follow-up, if the reduction is adequate and swelling has subsided, the splint can be overwrapped in a cast or transitioned to a new cast for continued closed treatment. After ankle fractures are surgically fixed with open reduction and internal fixation (ORIF), they are often placed in a short-leg splint with stirrups postoperatively, followed by transitioning to a short-leg cast for 4–6 weeks to protect the operative repair. There are many types of splints and casts depending on the type of injury being treated. Examples of splints include the volar forearm, sugar-tong, long-arm posterior, double sugar-tong, coaptation, short-leg posterior with or without stirrups, and long-leg posterior. Splints can be augmented with a thumb spica or foot plate depending on the injury. Examples of casts include short-arm, long-arm, with or without thumb spica, as well as short-leg, long-leg, and spica.

ORTHOPEDIC HISTORY TAKING & PHYSICAL EXAMINATION

Key elements of the history taking include the demographics of the patient (age, sex, and race), comorbidities, hand dominance (if there is an upper extremity injury), mechanism of injury, allergies to medication, and smoking or drinking history.

Examination begins with visualization of the injured extremity, noting deformity, swelling, and bruising. Careful skin examination is crucial to rule out wounds and the presence of open fracture. Neurovascular examination should document motor and sensory function as well as strength of pulses (palpable, 1+, 2+, or identifiable by Doppler). Finally, careful secondary examination should be performed on all other joints and extremities, testing for tenderness to palpation as well as range of motion. Distracting pain from the primary injury can often prevent a patient from realizing they have an injury elsewhere. Secondary examinations should be performed multiple times during the treatment course of the patient. As the pain from the primary injury subsides, patients may begin to appreciate additional injuries.

ORTHOPEDIC EMERGENCIES

The following conditions require immediate orthopedic evaluation and treatment: compartment syndrome, open fractures, septic arthritis, and acute dislocations. Other injuries, such as femoral neck fractures, depending on the age of the patient and choice of treatment, require intervention as soon as possible.

▶ Compartment Syndrome

Compartment syndrome is caused by increased pressure in a closed fascial space that initially leads to compromised perfusion followed by severe tissue damage. Nerves and muscles in the affected area can be significantly compromised in a matter of hours. Severe ischemia for 6–8 hours leads to muscle and nerve death, resulting in chronic debilitating dysfunction of the affected extremity. Compartment syndrome is therefore an orthopedic emergency requiring immediate evaluation and treatment. Compartment syndrome can occur after fracture, limb compression or crush, vigorous exercise, or burns.

Although it most commonly occurs in the forearm and leg, it can occur in the foot, thigh, and arm. Compartment syndrome typically presents as a painful, swollen, tense extremity. Pain with passive range of motion of the digits and pain out of proportion are considered to be the most reliable early indicators of compartment syndrome. Clinical signs of compartment syndrome include the 5 P's: pain, poikilothermia, pallor, paresthesias, and pulselessness. A change in pulses is a very late sign occurring after significant damage has already occurred. Of note, compartment syndrome can occur at intracompartmental pressures well below arterial pressure. Therefore, compartment syndrome can occur in a pink limb with normal pulses.

Compartment syndrome is a clinical diagnosis; many authors advocate that if compartment syndrome is suspected, immediate fasciotomy should be carried out. In patients who are obtunded, intubated, or otherwise unable to express having pain, compartment pressure can be evaluated using a commercially available self-contained pressure monitor. If a commercial pressure monitor is not available, a large-bore catheter can be inserted in the compartment under sterile technique. The catheter is connected to a pressure monitor via intravenous tubing filled with sterile saline solution. Absolute pressure greater than 30 mm Hg in any compartment, or a pressure within 30 mm Hg of the diastolic blood pressure in hypotensive patients, are indications for surgical compartment release.

Fasciotomy should be carried out with complete release of the skin and fascia of the involved compartments. Adjacent compartments in the same limb are typically released as well. Compartment pressures are rechecked after release to ensure adequate decompression. The wounds are left open and covered with sterile dressings or a vacuum-assisted closure (VAC) and are subsequently treated with delayed primary closure or skin grafting days later.

▶ Open Fractures

An open fracture is a defined as an osseous disruption with a break in the overlying skin and soft tissues resulting in communication between the fracture, its hematoma, and the external environment. Any wound occurring on the same limb as a fracture must be carefully inspected to prove that it is not an open fracture. Open fractures have important soft tissue consequences: (1) contamination of the wound and fracture by the external environment, (2) crushing, stripping, and devascularization that results in soft tissue devitalization and subsequent increased infection susceptibility, (3) disruption of the soft tissue envelope that may affect the type of fracture immobilization as well as adversely affect fracture healing due to the loss of osteoprogenitor cell contribution from overlying soft tissues, and (4) loss of function from damaged muscle, tendon, nerve, vascular, and ligamentous structures.

Open fractures are typically high-energy injuries. One third of patients with open fractures have multiple injuries. As a result, initial evaluation of the patient with an open fracture follows the ABCDEs: airway, breathing, circulation, disability, and exposure. Initial resuscitation is performed along with immediate treatment for any potential life-threatening injuries. The head, chest, abdomen, pelvis, and spine are individually evaluated for injury. Injuries to the other extremities should be identified. Neurovascular examination of the injured limb should be carefully documented; the skin and soft tissues should be assessed as well. Wound hemorrhage should be managed with direct pressure rather than limb tourniquets or clamping, which may disrupt perfusion to the rest of the limb. Due to risk of further contamination and precipitation of additional hemorrhage, exploration of the wound in the emergency department setting is not indicated if operative intervention is planned. If surgical delay is anticipated, gentle irrigation with sterile normal saline may be undertaken. Only obvious foreign fragments that are easily accessible should be removed. Bone fragments should not be removed and disregarded, regardless of apparent nonviability. Sterile injection of joints can be performed to determine if there is communication with a nearby wound. The wound should be covered with a sterile normal saline–soaked piece of gauze (iodine has fallen out of favor due to reports of tissue toxicity). Provisional reduction and splinting should be performed, followed by neurovascular examination to confirm no additional damage. Standard trauma survey includes radiographic evaluation of the spine, chest, abdomen, and pelvis. The injured extremity, including the joint above and below, along with any other extremities suspected of injury, should be evaluated with x-rays in anticipation of operative intervention.

Angiogram should be performed if vascular injury is suspected in the following scenarios: knee dislocation; cool, pale hand or foot with poor distal capillary refill; high-energy injury in an area of susceptible vessels (eg, popliteal fossa); and documented ankle brachial index (ABI) lower than 0.9 in an extremity with an associated injury. Of note, evaluation of the contralateral limb may reveal underlying vascular disease rather than acute injury as the cause of decreased ABI.

Open fractures can be characterized using the Gustilo and Anderson classification: grade I, clean skin opening smaller than 1 cm; grade II, laceration larger than 1 cm but smaller than 10 cm, soft tissue damage without significant fracture comminution or crush component; grade IIIA, extensive soft tissue damage; grade IIIB, extensive soft tissue injury with periosteal stripping or bone exposures requiring flap coverage; grade IIIC, concomitant vascular injury requiring repair.

Antibiotic treatment and tetanus prophylaxis should be addressed as soon as possible in the emergency department setting. Grade I and II fractures require treatment with a first-generation cephalosporin. Previously, grade III fractures mandated the addition of an aminoglycoside to cephalosporin; however, the most recent recommendations entail treatment with ceftriaxone. For farm injuries with gross contamination, add a penicillin in addition to ceftriaxone.

Operative intervention should be carried out for open fractures as soon as possible. Intervention less than 8 hours after injury has been reported to result in a lower incidence of infection and subsequent osteomyelitis. In the operating room, the wound should be extended proximally and distally to examine the zone of injury. Soft tissues, including the skin, subcutaneous fat, and surrounding muscle, should be meticulously debrided. Large skin flaps should be avoided because their development risks further devitalization. The fracture surfaces should be exposed and debrided. Fractures can be stabilized provisionally or definitively with external or internal fixation depending on the scenario and surgeon expertise. Pulsatile lavage irrigation should be performed, followed by meticulous hemostasis. Fasciotomy should be considered as treatment for or prophylaxis against impending compartment syndrome. Historically, only the surgically extended portions of the wound were closed, followed by dressing the open wound with saline-soaked gauze or by VAC. Serial debridements should be performed every 24–48 hours until there is no evidence of remaining necrotic soft tissue and bone. Bone grafting and wound coverage using delayed primary closure, skin graft, or rotational or free muscle flaps can be performed at this time.

Bucholz et al: *Rockwood and Green's Fractures in Adults,* 6th ed. Lippincott Williams & Wilkins, 2006.
Fischgrund JS: *OKU 9: Orthopedic Knowledge Update.* American Academy of Orthopaedic Surgeons, 2008.
Koval KJ, Zuckerman JD: *Handbook of Fractures,* 3rd ed. Lippincott Williams & Wilkins, 2002.

▼ ORTHOPEDIC TRAUMA: FRACTURES & JOINT INJURIES

FRACTURES & DISLOCATIONS OF THE SPINE

▶ Demographics

Approximately 11,000 new spinal cord injuries occur each year. The ratio of male to female patients sustaining vertebral fractures is 4:1. For patients with spinal cord injury, the overall mortality rate is 17% during the initial hospital stay. Unfortunately, delayed diagnosis happens frequently due to loss of consciousness secondary to trauma or intoxication with alcohol or drugs. As a result, suspicion for spinal cord injury should remain high in trauma patients who are unable to provide an accurate history.

Anatomy

The spinal cord occupies 35–50% of the spinal canal depending on the vertebral level. The remainder of the canal is filled with cerebrospinal fluid (CSF), dura mater, and epidural fat. The caudal termination of the spinal cord, located dorsal to the L1 vertebral body and L1–L2 intervertebral disk, is called the conus medullaris. The conus medullaris gives off motor and sensory nerve rootlets, also known as the cauda equina, or horse's tail.

The spinal column consists of four major components that contribute to its stability: (1) the vertebral bodies, (2) the posterior elements (pedicles, laminae, spinous process, and interlocking paired facets at each level), (3) the intervertebral disk, and (4) attached ligamentous tissues (interspinous ligaments, facet capsules, ligamentum flavum).

The atlas is the first cervical vertebra (C1). Although it does not have a vertebral body, it has two large lateral masses that serve as weightbearing articulations between the skull and the vertebral column. The tectorial membrane and the alar ligaments are key contributors to normal craniocervical stability. The axis is the second cervical vertebra, whose body is the largest in the cervical spine. The transverse atlantal (aka cruciform) ligament is the primary stabilizer of the atlantoaxial joint, with the alar ligaments providing secondary stability. There are five additional cervical vertebra: C3–C7.

The thoracolumbar spine consists of 12 thoracic vertebrae and 5 lumbar vertebrae. The thoracic region is naturally kyphotic (apex of bow is posterior), while the lumbar region is lordotic (apex of bow is anterior). The thoracic spine is much stiffer than the lumbar spine in flexion-extension and lateral bending because of the additional stability provided by the rib cage as well as thinner intervertebral disks. As a result of its transition zone status, the thoracolumbar junction (T11–L1) is more susceptible to injury.

The spinal column can also be conceptualized as three columns with regard to its stability: (1) the anterior column (anterior half of the vertebral body, anterior half of the intervertebral disk, anterior longitudinal ligament), (2) the middle column (posterior half of the vertebral body, posterior half of the intervertebral disk, posterior longitudinal ligament), and (3) the posterior column (facet joints, lateral masses, intraspinous ligaments, supraspinous ligaments, spinous processes). In general, a one-column injury is relatively stable, while a three-column injury is significantly unstable with increased risk of injury to the spinal cord.

The spinal cord roots exit the spinal canal through the intervertebral foramina. In the cervical spine, the C1 root exits above the C1 vertebral body; the C2 root exits below the C1 vertebral body. This pattern continues for the other cervical nerve roots ending with the C8 root exiting below the C7 body. In the thoracic and lumbar spine, each root exits under the pedicle with the same number. For example, the L4 nerve root exits under the L4 pedicle.

Clinical Evaluation

Clinical evaluation of the spine injury patient begins with the ABCDEs. All victims of trauma are suspected of having a spinal column injury until it is proven otherwise. Initially, patients are placed in a c-collar and on a backboard until the patient's spine can be assessed. A special backboard with head cutout should be used for children (6 years old or younger) to prevent unintended neck flexion due to their proportionally larger head size and resulting prominent occiput.

The head-tilt-chin-lift maneuver should be avoided because of possible further disruption of the cervical spine. Airway and breathing are ensured by intubation and mechanical ventilation. Nasotracheal intubation is the safest method of airway control in the acute setting because it leads to less cervical spine motion compared with direct oral intubation.

Neurogenic shock with hypotension and bradycardia can occur in the setting of spinal cord injury. Initial resuscitation of the patient entails administering isotonic fluids as well as evaluating injuries to the head, chest, abdomen, pelvis, and extremities. The diastolic pressure should be kept above 70 mm Hg to maximize spinal cord blood flow. However, once the diagnosis of neurogenic shock is established, the blood pressure should be managed with vasopressors to prevent fluid overload.

If within 8 hours of injury, administer methylprednisolone for complete or incomplete spinal cord injuries. An initial bolus of 30 mg/kg is administered over the first 15 minutes and followed by 5.4 mg/kg/h over the following 24 hours (if steroids were started within 3 hours after injury) or 48 hours (if steroids were started within 3–8 hours after injury). Treatment with methylprednisolone has been shown to improve long-term motor recovery.

Sensory deficits caused by either cord-level or root-level injuries can result in the rapid development of decubitus ulcers over insensate skin over high-pressure areas of the body (eg, the heels and ischium). As a result, timely assessment and removal of the patient from the spine board and onto an appropriate bed is critical.

Evaluating the spine includes logrolling the patient for visual inspection, palpating the spinous processes for tenderness or diastasis, and performing a rectal examination to assess resting tone, perianal sensation, and the bulbocavernosus reflex (squeeze of the glans penis or pull on urethral catheter results in contraction of the anal sphincter). Neurologic examination should also be performed to assess motor strength and dermatomal sensation. The motor strength testing and motor nerve roots correspond as follows: shoulder abduction (C5), elbow flexion and wrist extension (C6), elbow extension and wrist flexion (C7), wrist extension and finger flexion (C8), finger abduction (T1), hip flexion (L2), knee extension (L3), ankle dorsiflexion (L4), long toe extensors (L5), and ankle plantar flexors (S1). Careful evaluation and documentation of the patient's neurologic status will allow the physician to determine the appropriate treatment plan and estimate the prognosis for functional recovery

The cervical spine can be cleared clinically in patients if the following criteria are met: (1) no posterior midline tenderness, (2) full pain-free range of motion, (3) no focal neurologic deficit, (4) normal level of alertness, (5) no evidence of intoxication, and (6) no distracting injury. Radiographic evaluation is not required. The process of clearing the thoracolumbar spine is similar; however, anteroposterior and lateral radiographs of the thoracolumbosacral spine should be routinely obtained for evaluation. If any of the above criteria are not met for clearing the cervical spine, CT scan with sagittal reconstructions of the cervical spine to rule out injury has become the standard of care because of its increased sensitivity compared to radiographs.

In addition to spinal trauma, other injuries should be assessed, since they may influence the treatment of the patient. Suspicion of associated injuries depends on the mechanism and location of injury. Cervical spine injuries can be associated with injuries to the vertebral artery. Flexion-distraction injuries (seat-belt injuries) of the thoracolumbar spine are associated with intra-abdominal injuries. Axial-loading injury mechanisms that often result in burst fractures of the lumbar spine are also responsible for axial-loading injury patterns in the lower lumbar spine and lower extremities. These include fractures of the pars interarticularis of the L5 vertebra, the tibial plafond, and the calcaneus.

It is important to note that any injury associated with progressive neurologic deficit warrants surgical intervention.

Neurologic injury can be described as complete (no sensation/motor caudal to the level of the spinal cord pathology) or incomplete (some neurologic function persists caudal to the level of injury). Five major patterns of incomplete spinal cord injury can occur: (1) **Brown-Séquard syndrome** (hemicord injury with ipsilateral muscle paralysis, loss of proprioception, and light touch sensation), (2) **central cord syndrome** (flaccid paralysis of the upper extremities and spastic paralysis of the lower extremities with sacral sparing), (3) **anterior cord syndrome** (motor and pain/temperature loss controlled by the corticospinal and spinothalamic tracts with preserved light touch and proprioception controlled by the dorsal columns), (4) **posterior cord syndrome** (rare, involves loss of deep pressure, deep pain, and proprioception with full voluntary power, pain, and temperature sensation), and (5) **conus medullaris syndrome** (T12–L1 injuries resulting in loss of voluntary bowel and bladder control with preserved lumbar root function).

Nerve root lesions can occur at any level accompanying spinal cord injury. These lesions may be partial or complete, resulting in radicular pain, sensory dysfunction, weakness, hyporeflexia, or areflexia.

Cauda equina syndrome is caused by multilevel lumbosacral root compression within the lumbar spinal canal. Clinical presentation can include saddle anesthesia, bilateral radicular pain, numbness, weakness, hyporeflexia or areflexia, and loss of voluntary bladder or bowel function.

▶ Classification of Neurologic Injury

The motor and sensory examination outlined by the American Spinal Injury Association (ASIA) is one system to assess the impact on the patient of spinal cord injury. This grading system allows the patient to be assessed through scales of impairment and functional independence, evaluating remaining sensory and motor function. A thorough neurologic examination should be performed and documented when the patient is initially seen and at frequent intervals thereafter both to ensure that there is no further neurologic deterioration and to document the resolution of spinal shock.

Spinal shock is a spinal cord dysfunction due to physiologic disruption, resulting in hypotonia, areflexia, and paralysis distal to the level of injury. Resolution usually occurs within 24 hours with the return of reflex arcs caudal to the level of injury; the bulbocavernosus reflex is usually the first one to come back.

If a patient has a complete neurologic deficit after spinal shock has resolved, the chance for recovery of neurologic function below the level of injury is extremely poor. In contrast, patients with root level injuries (at or below the cauda equina) will recover from functionally complete injuries if they have not been transected and if initial compression by bone fragments, malalignment, or disk material has been relieved.

▶ Determination of Sensory Levels

The sensory level is determined by the patient's ability to perceive pinprick (using a disposable needle or safety pin) and light touch (using a cotton ball). Testing of a key point in each of the 28 dermatomes on the right and left sides of the body as well as evaluation of perianal sensation is necessary. The variability in sensation for each individual stimulus is graded on a 3-point scale:

0 = Absent
1 = Impaired
2 = Normal
NT = Not testable

In the cervical spine, the C3 and C4 nerve roots supply sensation to the entire upper neck and chest in a capelike distribution from the tip of the acromion to just above the nipple line. The next adjacent sensory level is the T2 dermatome. The brachial plexus (C5–T1) supplies the upper extremities.

ASIA also recommends testing of pain and deep pressure sensation in the same dermatomes as well as evaluation of proprioception by testing the position sense of the both index fingers and both great toes.

Determination of Motor Levels

The motor level is determined by manual testing of a key muscle in the 10 paired myotomes from cephalad to caudal. The strength of each muscle is graded on a 6-point scale:

0 = Complete paralysis

1 = Palpable or visible contraction

2 = Full range of motion of the joint powered by the muscle with gravity eliminated

3 = Full range of motion of the joint powered by the muscle against gravity

4 = Active movement with full range of motion against moderate resistance

5 = Normal strength

NT = Not testable

ASIA Impairment Scale

The grading system is as follows: (1) grade A (complete impairment; no motor or sensory function is preserved below the neurologic injury level), (2) grade B (incomplete; sensory but not motor function is preserved below the neurologic level and extends through the sacral segment S4–S5), (3) grade C (incomplete; motor function is preserved below the neurologic level with key muscles having a muscle grade lower than 3), (4) grade D (incomplete; motor function is preserved below the neurologic level of injury; most key muscles below the neurologic level have a muscle grade higher than 3), and (5) grade E (normal; motor and sensory function is normal).

Imaging Studies

A. Cervical Spine

Plain radiographs can be used as the first imaging modality for the cervical spine, although CT scan of the cervical spine is becoming the initial test of choice because of its increased sensitivity and consistent ability to visualize the occipitocervical and cervicothoracic junctions. The standard series of radiographs includes an anteroposterior, a lateral, and an open-mouth "odontoid" view. Eighty-five percent of all significant injuries to the cervical spine will be detected on the lateral view of the cervical spine. Radiographic markers of cervical spine instability include the following: compression fractures with more than 25% loss of height, angular displacement greater than 11 degrees between adjacent vertebrae, translation greater than 3.5 mm, and intervertebral disk space separation greater than 1.7 mm. If the standard lateral view does not adequately visualize the C7–T1 junction, further studies such as a swimmer's view, oblique views, or CT of this area are necessary. Flexion-extension views of the cervical spine can be performed if instability is still suspected in a patient with otherwise normal radiographic

findings. Performance of these radiographs should be delayed in a patient with neck pain, as muscle spasm can mask instability.

B. Thoracolumbar Spine

All patients with significant injury and pain in the spinal area require anteroposterior and lateral x-rays of symptomatic regions of the thoracic and lumbar spine. CT can be used to evaluate canal compromise, and for preoperative planning, MRI is useful for assessing the degree of neural injury and prognosis.

Complications

Patients with cervical spine injury may have impaired pulmonary function secondary to intercostal nerve paralysis. Mobilization of secretions by chest physical therapy and frequent suctioning are critical for preventing atelectasis and pulmonary infections. All patients with sensory deficits and paralysis are at high risk of developing pressure ulcers. Padding and suspension of high-risk pressure points (heels), frequent turning, and vigilant nursing care are necessary.

Patients with thoracolumbar spine fractures with or without spinal cord injury may have paralytic ileus secondary to sympathetic chain dysfunction. Oral intake should be limited to clear fluids initially, and gastric suction may be necessary if the degree or duration of ileus is significant.

The stress caused by the injury itself—in combination with systemic corticosteroid therapy—can increase the incidence of gastrointestinal ulceration and bleeding. High-dose corticosteroids can also contribute to the development of pancreatitis and infections.

Venous thromboembolic disease remains a significant problem in the management of patients with spinal injury. Pulmonary embolism is the most common cause of preventable death in hospitalized patients. Heparin can be used for deep vein thrombosis prophylaxis until the patient's mobility improves.

CERVICAL SPINE INJURIES

Injuries to the Occiput-C1–C2 Complex

A. Occipital Condyle Fractures

Occipital condyle fractures can be classified as follows: (1) type I (impaction of condyle, stable), (2) type II (shear injury associated with basilar or skull fractures; potentially unstable), and (3) type III (condylar avulsion fracture, unstable). Treatment involves rigid cervical collar immobilization for 8 weeks for stable injuries and halo immobilization or surgical stabilization for unstable injuries.

B. Occipitoatlantal Dislocation

Also known as craniovertebral dislocation, occipitoatlantal dislocation is almost always fatal. Postmortem studies show this injury to be the leading cause of death in motor vehicle accidents. Rare survivors usually have severe neurologic deficits. Immediate treatment includes halo vest application with strict avoidance of traction. Long-term stabilization is done surgically with occipitocervical fusion.

C. Atlas Fractures

Atlas fractures are rarely associated with neurologic injury. Instability due to transverse alar ligament insufficiency should be suspected with identification of bony avulsion or widening of the lateral masses on radiographic evaluation. These injuries can be classified as follows: (1) isolated bony apophysis fracture, (2) isolated posterior arch fracture, (3) isolated anterior arch fracture, (4) comminuted lateral mass fracture, and (5) burst fracture (anterior and posterior fractures of the pelvic ring). Stable fractures (posterior arch or nondisplaced fractures) may be treated with rigid cervical orthosis; unstable fractures require prolonged halo immobilization. Chronic instability or pain may be treated with C1–C2 fusion.

D. Transverse Ligament Rupture

This injury is rare but usually fatal when it occurs. Transverse ligament rupture is diagnosed by visualizing the avulsed lateral mass fragment, an atlantodens interval (ADI) greater than 3 mm in adults, atlantoaxial offset greater than 6.9 mm on an odontoid radiograph, or direct visualization of the rupture on MRI. Survivors are treated with halo or C1–C2 fusion.

E. Fractures of the Odontoid Process (Dens)

There is a significant association of dens fracture with other cervical spine fractures and a 5–10% incidence of neurologic injury. The vascular supply to the odontoid arrives through the apex and the base of this bone with a watershed area in the neck. Odontoid fractures are classified as follows: (1) type I (oblique avulsion fracture of the apex), (2) type II (fracture at the junction of the body and the neck; high nonunion rate, which can lead to myelopathy), (3) type IIa (highly unstable comminuted injury extending from the waist of the odontoid to the vertebral body), and (4) type III (fracture extending in the cancellous body of C2 and possibly involving the lateral facets). Treatment entails cervical orthosis for type I fractures and halo immobilization for type III fractures. Treatment of type II fractures is controversial because of the high incidence of nonunion related to poor vascularity; halo or surgical intervention is advocated depending on patient factors.

F. C2 Lateral Mass Fractures

These injuries are usually diagnosed via CT scan. Treatment varies from collar immobilization to late fusion for chronic pain.

G. Traumatic Spondylolisthesis of C2

Also known as the hangman's fracture, this injury may be associated with cranial nerve, vertebral artery, or craniofacial injuries. Type I injuries are nondisplaced fractures without angulation, with less than 3 mm of translation, and with the C2–C3 disk is intact. Type II injuries are displaced fractures of the pars. Type IIa is a displaced pars fracture with disruption of the C2–C3 disk. Type III is a dislocation of the C2–C3 facet joints in addition to the pars fracture. Type I injuries are treated with rigid cervical orthosis, type II injuries are treated with halo immobilization, and type III injuries are usually treated initially with halo immobilization followed by surgical stabilization.

▶ Injuries to C3–C7

Injuries for the remaining vertebrae from C3–C7 include teardrop fractures of the anterior portion of the vertebral body due to compression flexion, vertical compression (burst fractures), anterior dislocations due to distractive flexion, vertebral arch and lamina fractures due to compressive extension, distractive extension injuries resulting in posterior dislocations, and lateral flexion injuries resulting in translational dislocations.

Clay shoveler's fracture is an avulsion fracture of the spinous processes of the lower cervical and upper thoracic vertebra. Sentinel fracture is a fracture through the lamina on either side of the spinous process.

Treatment for each of these fractures includes the use of cervical orthoses, halo immobilization, traction, and surgery. Soft cervical orthosis does not provide any significant immobilization. It is used as needed for the patient's comfort. Rigid cervical orthoses do not provide complete immobilization; this treatment mainly limits range of motion in the flexion-extension plane. Cervicothoracic orthoses are effective in flexion-extension and rotational control but do not limit lateral bending very effectively. Halo immobilization offers rigid immobilization in all planes, as does surgical treatment. Traction can be used to reduce unilateral or bilateral facet dislocations with neurologic deficits or to stabilize and indirectly compress the canal in patients with neural deficits from burst-type fractures. Traction is contraindicated in type IIa spondylolisthesis injuries of C2 and distractive cervical spine injuries.

Choice of treatment depends on the type of injury and individual patient characteristics. In general, stable fractures can be managed with bracing, while unstable fractures require more rigid stabilization via halo application or surgical treatment.

The halo apparatus includes the metal ring and halo vest. The halo ring should be applied approximately 1 cm above the ears. Anterior pin sites should be placed above the supraorbital ridge, anterior to the temporalis muscle over the lateral two thirds of the eyebrow to avoid the supraorbital nerve. Posterior sites are variable and are placed to maintain the horizontal orientation of the halo. Pin pressure should be

6–8 lbs in the adult. Pin care is essential. The halo vest relies on a tight fit that should be carefully maintained.

▶ Thoracolumbar Spinous Injuries

Anteroposterior and lateral radiographs of the thoracolumbosacral spine are the standard initial evaluation. Abnormal interpedicular distance, height loss, and canal compromise should all be noted. Minor spine injuries include articular process fractures, transverse process fractures, spinous process fractures, and pars interarticularis fractures. Generally, these injuries can simply be observed. Six significant injury patterns requiring treatment are described: (1) wedge compression fracture, (2) stable burst fracture, (3) unstable burst fracture, (4) Chance fracture, (5) flexion-distraction injury, and (6) translational injuries.

A. Compression Fractures

Based on the 3-column theory of instability, compression fractures are fractures that affect only the anterior column. Compression fractures can be anterior or lateral. In general, these fractures are stable injuries and are rarely associated with neurologic injury. Fractures are considered unstable if there is more than 50% loss of vertebral body height, angulation greater than 20–30 degrees, or multiple adjacent compression fractures. Four subtypes are described on the basis of endplate involvement: type A (fracture of both endplates), type B (fracture of superior endplate), type C (fracture of inferior endplate), and type D (both endplates are intact). Stable fractures are treated with Jewett brace or thoracolumbosacral orthosis. Unstable fractures can be treated with hyperextension casting or with surgery.

B. Burst Fractures

Burst fractures are fractures that involve the anterior and middle columns of the spinal cord. Radiographs may show loss of posterior vertebral body height and splaying of the pedicles on the anteroposterior view. It is important to note that no direct relationship exists between the amount of canal compromise and the degree of neurologic injury. Treatment can entail thoracolumbosacral orthosis bracing or hyperextension in casting for stable fracture patterns without neurologic compromise. If the thoracolumbosacral orthosis fails to restore appropriate alignment on radiographs, surgery should be considered. Early surgical intervention restoring sagittal and coronal alignment should also be considered for fractures with more than 50% loss of vertebral height, angulation of more than 20–30 degrees, scoliosis greater than 10 degrees, and concomitant neurologic deficit. Surgical treatment options include decompression via a posterior or anterior approach with or without instrumentation.

C. Flexion-Distraction Injuries

Also known as Chance fractures, flexion-distraction injuries involve all three columns of the spinal cord. These fractures,

also called "seat-belt type injuries" due to the most common mechanism by which they occur, often are associated with abdominal injuries. Radiographically, one may appreciate increased interspinous distance on the anteroposterior and lateral views. Four types of Chance fractures are recognized: (1) type A (1-level bony injury), (2) type B (1-level ligamentous injury), (3) type C (2-level injury through the bony middle column), and (4) type D (2-level injury through the ligamentous middle column). Treatment for type A fractures may entail thoracolumbosacral orthosis; however, surgical stabilization should be considered for the other three fractures given their innate lack of stability.

D. Fracture Dislocations

Fracture dislocations involve injury to all three columns with translational deformity. These injuries are often associated with neurologic injury and require surgical stabilization because of their unstable nature. There are three types of fracture dislocations: (1) flexion-rotation, (2) shear, and (3) flexion-distraction. Patients without neurologic injury do not require emergent surgery; however, patients whose fractures are stabilized within 72 hours of injury have a lower incidence of complications such as pneumonia and undergo a shorter hospital stay than patients whose fractures are stabilized outside this time frame.

E. Gunshot Wounds

Fractures associated with low-velocity gunshot wounds are usually stable when a handgun is the weapon. These injuries are typically associated with a low infection rate and can be prophylactically treated with broad-spectrum antibiotics for 48 hours.

Any present neural injury is usually secondary to "blast effect" in which the energy of the bullet is absorbed and transferred to the soft tissues. As a result, decompression is usually not indicated. An exception to this rule is if the bullet fragment is found in the spinal canal between levels T12 and L5. Steroids after gunshot wounds to the spine are not recommended.

F. Spine Fractures or Dislocations with Neurologic Deficit

1. Incomplete neurologic deficit—If there is a neurologic deficit, surgical decompression is indicated. This can be done through an anterior approach with bone graft and internal fixation, a posterior costotransversectomy approach, or a combined anterior and posterior approach. The operative plan is individualized to the patient.

Patients with incomplete neurologic deficits and unstable fractures or fracture dislocations have the same stability requirements as patients without neurologic deficits. They are best managed with open reduction, instrumentation, and spinal fusion. Neural canal compromise should be managed as in the preceding paragraph.

2. Complete neurologic deficit—No operative procedure has been devised that will achieve recovery in cases of complete neurologic deficit that has persisted beyond the stage of spinal shock. However, surgical stabilization is often necessary (1) because spinal instability may interfere with early mobilization and rehabilitation training and (2) because it may result in loss of function at a higher level by causing mechanical injury on the root or cord segment just above the level of injury.

Daffner RH et al: Expert Panel on Musculoskeletal and Neurologic Imaging. Suspected spine trauma. American College of Radiology, 2007. Available at http://www.acr.org/SecondaryMainMenu Categories/quality_safety/app_criteria/pdf/ExpertPanelonMusculo skeletalImagingSuspectedCervicalSpineTraumaDoc22.aspx. Accessed February 14, 2009.

Outcomes Following Traumatic Spinal Cord Injury: A Clinical Practice Guideline for Health-Care Professionals. Paralyzed Veterans of America, 1999. Available at http://www.pva.org. Accessed February 14, 2009.

FRACTURES & DISLOCATIONS OF THE PELVIS

Pelvic fractures are among the most serious injuries and account for 3% of all fractures. The mechanism is often high energy in nature; 60% result from vehicular trauma (eg,, automobile, motorcycle, bicycle), 30% from falls, and 10% from crush injuries, athletic injuries, or penetrating trauma. Pelvic fractures are the third-most commonly seen injury in fatalities due to motor vehicle accidents.

Life-threatening hemorrhage, deformity, neurologic injury, and genitourinary injury are all potential complications that must be identified and treated early in the setting of a pelvic fracture. Pelvic fractures pose a formidable clinical challenge. Hemodynamically unstable patients who present to the emergency department with pelvic fracture have a mortality rate of 40–50%.

▶ Anatomy

An understanding of pelvic anatomy is essential for identifying fracture patterns and complications. The pelvis is made up of three bones: two innominate bones joined anteriorly at the symphysis and posteriorly at the paired sacroiliac joints. The innominate bones are further subdivided into the ilium, ischium, and pubis.

The acetabulum is the portion of the pelvic bone that articulates with the femoral head to form the hip joint. It results from closure of the triradiate cartilage and is covered with hyaline cartilage. The innominate bone support of the acetabulum can be thought of as an inverted Y formed by two columns. The anterior column (iliopubic component) extends from the iliac crest to the pubic symphysis, including the anterior wall of the acetabulum. The posterior column (ilioischial component) extends from the superior gluteal notch to the ischial tuberosity. including the posterior wall. The acetabular dome is the superior weightbearing portion of the acetabulum at the junction of the anterior and posterior columns, including contributions from both.

The stability of the pelvis is dependent on its ligamentous attachments. A thick fibrocartilaginous disk joins the anterior aspects of the innominate bones to form the pubic symphysis. This joint acts as a supporting strut for the pelvis because the stability of the ring depends mostly upon the sacroiliac joints.

The posterior ligamentous structures supporting the sacroiliac joints can be divided into anterior and posterior complexes. The anterior sacroiliac joint ligaments are broad and flat and connect the iliac wing and the sacral ala. These ligaments primarily resist external rotation and torsional forces. The sacroiliac ligaments provide most of the stability. Composed of the interosseous sacroiliac ligaments within the joint and the posterior sacroiliac ligaments spanning the sacrum between the posterior iliac spines, the posterior complex is considered to be the strongest ligament in the human body. The posterior sacroiliac complex resists shear forces between the sacrum and the ilium, clinically preventing displacement of the ilium onto the sacrum.

The pelvic floor contains two additional strong ligaments, the sacrospinous and the sacrotuberous ligaments. The sacrospinous ligament maintains rotational control, and the sacrotuberous ligament is especially important in maintaining vertical stability of the pelvis. Additional stability is conferred by ligamentous attachments between the spine and the pelvis. The iliolumbar ligaments originate from L4 and L5 transverse processes and insert onto the posterior iliac crest. The lumbosacral ligaments originate from the transverse process of L5 and insert onto the sacrum ala.

▶ Stability

Pelvic stability can be defined as the ability of the pelvic ring to withstand physiologic forces without abnormal deformation. Pathologically, the pelvic ring fails under one or more of three basic modes. External rotation strains the pubic symphysis and the sacrotuberous, sacrospinous, and anterior sacroiliac joint ligaments. After roughly 2.5 cm of diastasis, the pelvic floor ligaments and the anterior sacroiliac ligaments begin to fail, giving rise to gross rotatory instability. Because the posterior ligament complex is largely intact, superior or posterior displacement of the involved hemipelvis does not occur. Combined external and shear forces are necessary to completely disrupt pelvic stability. Conversely, internal rotation places the pubic rami under compression and the posterior ligament complexes under tension. The rami often fail in their midportions with transverse fractures and sacral alar impaction. The pelvic floor ligaments remain intact, and gross posterior stability is maintained. Therefore, fractures involving torsional forces on the pelvis often have partial instability in the rotatory plane only, with maintenance of stability to other displacement.

Complete instability, however, occurs with disruption of both the anterior and the posterior ligamentous restraints.

These injuries often present with widely displaced sacroiliac joints and multiaxial instability of the involved hemipelvis. Such fractures have components of superior and posterior displacement relative to the sacrum in addition to rotational displacement in the sagittal and horizontal planes.

Clinical Evaluation

Physical examination includes palpation of the pelvic bony landmarks, compression maneuvers to assess stability, rectovaginal examination looking for bony spikes protruding through the mucosa representing an open fracture, and looking for blood at the urethral meatus or a high-riding prostate on rectal examination, which may indicate genitourinary injury. If bladder or urethral injury is suspected, retrograde urethrogram should be considered. The mortality rate of open pelvic fractures is as high as 50%—compared with 8–15% for closed fractures. A secondary musculoskeletal survey examining each of the other four limbs, including distal vascular status, and a thorough neurologic examination should be performed as well.

Radiographic Examination

The anteroposterior radiograph required in all patients with blunt trauma rapidly identifies the major pelvic injury. The anteroposterior pelvis radiograph can be looked at in a systematic way: the pubic rami, the pubic symphysis (looking for widening > 2.5 cm), the iliopectineal lines (represents limit of the anterior column of the acetabulum), the ilioischial lines (represents limit of the posterior column of the acetabulum), the anterior lip of the acetabulum, the posterior lip of the acetabulum, the radiographic roof of the acetabulum, the pelvic wings, the sacroiliac joints, the femoral head position (rule out concomitant hip dislocation), associated fracture of the femoral head or femoral neck, and the lumbar spine. Disruption of the iliopectineal line, ilioischial line, anterior lip, posterior lip, or radiographic roof may be indicative of acetabular fracture. Suspected acetabular fractures should be further evaluated with **Judet views** (iliac oblique and obturator oblique). The **iliac oblique** (45-degree external rotation view) view better delineates the anterior column and posterior wall of the acetabulum, while the **obturator oblique** (45-degree internal rotation view) characterizes the posterior column and anterior wall of the acetabulum in greater detail. Inlet and outlet radiographs are often required to supplement the anteroposterior film. The **inlet view** (patient supine, tube directed 60 degrees caudal) can be used to evaluate for any anterior-posterior instability, while the **outlet view** (patient supine, tube directed 45 degrees cephalad) will best show any vertical displacement. CT scan is recommended for any suspected pelvis fracture; this modality is especially good for evaluation of the acetabulum and posterior pelvis, including the sacrum and sacroiliac joints.

Acute Management

Immediate care of the polytrauma patient with a pelvic fracture must address associated retroperitoneal hemorrhage, pelvic ring instability, and injuries to the genitourinary system and rectum as well as fractures open to the peritoneum. Cessation of blood loss, minimization of septic sequelae, and stabilization of the fracture, allowing early and safe patient mobilization, are the immediate treatment goals. Hemorrhage is the leading cause of death in patients with pelvic fracture, accounting for 60% of the deaths. Most of the blood loss is from the fracture site or injured retroperitoneal veins; only 20% of the deaths are associated with major arterial injury. An average blood replacement of 5.9 units has been reported.

General resuscitative principles are applied to stabilize the patient and provide adequate tissue perfusion. Once other sites of hemorrhage have been ruled out, active bleeding from a pelvic fracture may be controlled by wrapping a pelvic binder or sheet circumferentially around the pelvis. The sheet should enclose the bilateral anterior superior iliac spines and greater trochanters and can be fixed in placed by clipping the two ends with a hemostat. Wrapping the pelvis in this way stabilizes major fracture fragments and closes down the volume of the pelvis, dramatically reducing active blood loss. If this fails to control hemorrhage, angiography or arterial embolization is indicated. Definitive internal fixation is usually required after hemorrhage has been controlled and the patient has been stabilized.

Fracture dislocations of the pelvis should be treated with immediate closed reduction of the hip. Stability should be assessed by ranging the hip through a full arc of motion. Unstable hips should be re-reduced and placed in skeletal traction. An irreducible hip or new-onset sciatic nerve palsy after closed hip reduction requires immediate operative treatment.

Classification & Treatment

Fractures of the pelvis may be classified according to the Young and Burgess system based on mechanism of injury. Anteroposterior compression (APC) injuries result from anteriorly applied force. APC-I characterizes less than 2.5 cm of symphyseal diastasis; vertical fractures of one or both pubic rami occur, but the sacroiliac ligaments are intact imparting rotational and vertical stability. In an APC-II injury, disruption of the anterior sacroiliac ligaments results in greater than 2.5 cm of symphyseal diastasis that is rotationally unstable but vertically stable due to intact posterior sacroiliac ligaments. APC-III injury occurs with complete disruption of the symphysis, sacrotuberous, sacrospinous, and anterior and posterior sacroiliac ligaments, resulting in a pelvis that is rotationally and vertically unstable. Lateral compression (LC) injury results from a laterally applied force to the pelvis that leads to shortening of the anterior sacroiliac and the sacrospinous and sacrotuberous ligaments with resulting transverse or oblique fractures of the pubic rami. LC-I injuries are transverse fractures of the pubic rami with sacral compression on the side of injury without rotational or vertical instability. LC-II injuries include the addition of a crescent iliac wing fracture on the side of impact with variable disruption of the posterior ligamentous structures, resulting in rotational instability. LC-III is an LC-I or LC-II injury on the side of impact with continuation of the force producing an external rotation or open-book (APC) type injury on the contralateral side. Vertical shear injury due to vertical or longitudinal forces caused by falls onto an extended lower extremity, impacts from above, or motor vehicle accidents with a lower extremity impacted against the dashboard or floorboard typically results in complete ligamentous disruption, rotational and vertical instability, with a high incidence of neurovascular injury and hemorrhage. Combined mechanical injury is a combination of injuries often due to crush mechanism.

Pelvic fractures may also be classified according to instability using the Tile classification: type A (rotationally and vertically stable), type B (rotationally unstable and vertically stable), or type C (rotationally and vertically unstable). Common radiographic signs of pelvic instability include (1) displacement of the posterior sacroiliac complex more than 5 mm in any plane, (2) the presence of a posterior fracture gap rather than an impaction, and (3) the presence of an avulsion fracture of the transverse process of the fifth lumbar vertebra or the sacroischial end of the sacrospinous ligaments. Type A fractures involve the pelvic ring in only one location and are considered stable. Type A1 fractures are avulsion fractures that usually occur at muscle origins such as the anterosuperior iliac spine, anteroinferior iliac spine, and ischial apophysis. These fractures most often occur in adolescents, and conservative treatment is usually sufficient. Rarely, symptomatic nonunions develop and can be best treated surgically. Type A2 fractures are isolated fractures of the iliac wing without involvement of the hip or sacroiliac joints and are usually a result of direct trauma. Even with significant displacement, bony healing is expected and treatment is therefore symptomatic. Healing may be accompanied by ossification of the hematoma with exuberant new bone formation. Type A3 fractures are isolated fractures of the obturator foramen and usually involve minimal displacement of the pubic or ischial rami. The posterior sacroiliac complex is intact, and the pelvis remains stable. Treatment is symptomatic, with early ambulation and weightbearing as tolerated.

Type B fractures involve breaks in the pelvic ring in two or more sites. This creates a pelvic fracture that is rotationally unstable but vertically stable. Type B1 fractures are open-book fractures that occur from anteroposterior compression. Unless the anterior separation of the pubic symphysis is severe (> 6 cm), the posterior sacroiliac complex is usually intact and the pelvis is relatively stable to vertical forces. Significant associated injuries to the perineal and urogenital structures are often present and should always be looked for. For minimally displaced symphysial injuries (< 2.5 cm), only symptomatic

treatment is needed. However, if conservative treatment is pursued, serial radiographs are required after mobilization is begun to monitor for subsequent increased displacement that may require surgery. For more displaced fracture dislocations, reduction is done by lateral compression using the intact posterior sacroiliac complex as the hinge on which the "book is closed." Reduction can be maintained with the use of an external fixator; however, internal fixation with a symphyseal plate is currently favored. "Closing the book" decreases the space available for hemorrhage and increases patient comfort.

Type B2 and B3 fractures involve a lateral force applied to the pelvis, causing inward displacement of the hemipelvis through the sacroiliac complex and ipsilateral (B2) or, more often, contralateral (B3) pubic rami fractures. The degree of involvement of the posterior sacroiliac ligament complex will determine the degree of instability. The hemipelvis is infolded, with overlapping of the pubic symphysis. Reduction can be accomplished with external fixation, with internal fixation, or with both. External fixation facilitates nursing care but is not strong enough for ambulation. Definitive care usually is accomplished with internal fixation of both the anterior and posterior aspects of the pelvic ring. Major hemorrhage is associated with these fracture types.

Type C fractures are both rotationally and vertically unstable. They often result from a vertical shear injury such as a fall from a height. Anteriorly, the pubic symphysis or pubic rami may be disrupted. Posteriorly, the sacroiliac joint may be disrupted and dislocated, or there may be a fracture through the sacrum or adjacent iliac wing. The hemipelvis is completely unstable, and there may be associated massive hemorrhage and injury to the lumbosacral pelvis. External fixation is insufficient to maintain reduction, but it may help to control hemorrhage and ease nursing care in the acute stage. Internal fixation is usually required as definitive treatment.

SACRAL FRACTURES

Fractures of the sacrum can be described using the Denis classification according to the location of the fracture in relation to the sacral foramen: Denis I, lateral to the foramen; Denis II, through the foramen; Denis III, medial to the foramen. The incidence of neurologic injury increases with higher classification.

FRACTURES OF THE ACETABULUM

Fractures of the acetabulum (Figure 40–1) occur through direct trauma on the trochanteric region or indirect axial loading through the lower limb. The position of the limb at the time of impact (rotation, flexion, abduction, or adduction) will determine the pattern of injury. Comminution is common.

▶ Classification

Letournel has classified acetabular fractures into 10 different types: 5 simple patterns (1 fracture line): posterior wall,

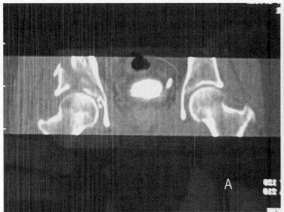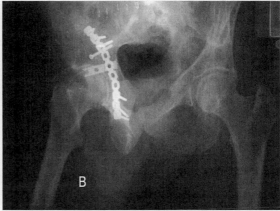

▲ **Figure 40–1.** Forty-year-old man who fell from a height, sustaining a posterior hip dislocation and an acetabular fracture of the weightbearing dome. **A:** Coronal CT reconstructions showing large fragment of the superior dome of the right acetabulum. **B:** Oblique radiograph demonstrating concentric reduction of the hip and restoration of the articular surface after open reduction and internal fixation.

posterior column, anterior wall, anterior column, and transverse; and 5 complex patterns (the association of 2 or more simple patterns): T-shaped, posterior column and posterior wall, transverse and posterior wall, anterior column/posterior hemitransverse, and both columns. This is the most widely used classification system because it allows the surgeon to choose the most appropriate surgical approach.

▶ Treatment

The goal of treatment is to achieve a spherical congruency between the femoral head and the weightbearing acetabular dome and to maintain it until the bones are healed. As with other pelvic fractures, acetabular fractures are frequently associated with abdominal, urogenital, and neurologic injuries, which should be systematically sought and treated. Significant bleeding is often present and should be stopped as soon as possible.

The stabilized patient with **protrusion** (the femoral head is impacted through the fracture of the acetabulum into the pelvis) or unstable fracture dislocation should be put in longitudinal skeletal traction through a distal femoral or proximal tibial pin pulling axially in neutral position. Postreduction x-rays are obtained. Operative indications for acetabular fractures include displacement (> 2–3 mm), large posterior wall fragments, interposed intra-articular loose fragment, femoral head fractures, unstable reductions, and an irreducible fracture dislocation by closed methods. The choice of approach is of primary importance, and more than one approach will sometimes prove necessary. Acetabular surgery uses extensile approaches and sophisticated reduction and fixation techniques and is best performed by pelvic surgeons.

▶ Complications

Complications inherent to the injury include posttraumatic degenerative joint disease, heterotopic ossification, femoral head osteonecrosis, deep vein thrombosis, and other complications related to conservative treatment. Surgery is performed to prevent or delay osteoarthritis, but it increases the possibility of complications such as infection, iatrogenic neurovascular injury, and increased heterotopic ossification. When the reduction is stable and fixation is solid, the patient can be mobilized after a few days with nonweightbearing ambulation, and weightbearing may begin as early as 6 weeks. Prophylactic anticoagulation and aggressive pulmonary toilet are key elements of postoperative care.

Holevar M et al: *Practice Management Guidelines for the Evaluation of Genitourinary Trauma.* Eastern Association for the Surgery of Trauma, 2003.

Shuman WP et al: Expert Panel on Gastrointestinal Imaging. Blunt abdominal trauma. American College of Radiology, 2005. Available at http://www.acr.org/SecondaryMainMenuCategories/quality_safety/app_criteria/pdf/ExpertPanelonGastrointestinalImaging/BluntAbdominalTraumaDoc3.aspx. Accessed February 14, 2009.

SHOULDER INJURIES

1. Clavicular Fractures

▶ Epidemiology, Mechanism, Anatomy, & Clinical Evaluation

Clavicle fractures are relatively common, accounting for 2–12% of all fractures. Clavicle fractures are characterized by location: medial, lateral, and middle third of the clavicle, which is the most common type (80%). The most common mechanism of injury is fall onto the ipsilateral shoulder (87%); direct impact (7%) and falls onto an outstretched hand cause the rest. The clavicle is an S-shaped bone that serves as a strut bracing the shoulder in relation to the trunk, allowing the shoulder to function at maximum strength. The clavicle is stabilized by the acromioclavicular and coracoclavicular ligaments. The acromioclavicular ligaments prevent horizontal displacement, while the coracoclavicular ligaments provide vertical stability. The middle one third of the clavicle protects the brachial plexus, superior lung, and subclavian and axillary arteries. As a result, it is critical to document a thorough neurovascular examination and rule out concomitant injuries such as brachial plexus palsy, vascular injury, and pneumothorax. It is also important to note the appearance of the skin: Tenting may be an indication for surgery. Clavicle fractures are most often incidentally seen on the anteroposterior radiograph of the chest. Proximal third clavicle fractures can be further evaluated with CT to differentiate sternoclavicular dislocations from epiphyseal injury.

▶ Classification

Clavicle fractures are classified into three groups: group I, middle third fracture; group II, distal third; and group III, proximal third. Group II fractures are subclassified into three types according to the location of the coracoclavicular ligaments relative to the fracture. Type I fractures are interligamentous, either between the conoid and trapezoid ligaments or between the coracoclavicular and acromioclavicular ligaments, with the ligaments still intact. Because ligaments are attached to both the proximal and distal fracture segments, the fracture is typically nondisplaced or minimally displaced. Group II, type II fractures occur medial to the coracoclavicular ligaments or between the conoid and trapezoid ligaments, with the conoid ligament torn such that the proximal fracture segment is predisposed to significant displacement. Group II, type III is a distal third fracture of the articular surface of the acromioclavicular joint without ligamentous injury.

▶ Treatment

Clavicle fractures are typically treated conservatively with a sling or figure-of-8 brace for 4–6 weeks until healing is appreciated radiographically and clinically (area no longer tender with palpation). Sling is typically preferred because of lower incidence of skin problems and increased patient comfort. Some degree of shortening and deformity is expected with closed treatment. However, shoulder dysfunction is rare, and there is no scar. Strict indications for surgery include open clavicle fractures, associated neurovascular injury, and skin tenting concerning for impending open fracture. Some authors advocate fixing significantly displaced (> 1–2cm) middle third clavicle fractures and group II, type II distal clavicle fractures because of predisposition to

nonunion, which may result in cosmetic deformity and shoulder dysfunction.

The Diagnosis and Management of Soft Tissue Shoulder Injuries and Related Disorders. New Zealand Guidelines Group, 2004.
Steinbach LS et al: Expert Panel on Musculoskeletal Imaging. Shoulder trauma. American College of Radiology, 2005. Available at: http://www.acr.org/SecondaryMainMenuCategories/quality_safety/app_criteria/pdf/ExpertPanelonMusculoskeletalImaging/ShoulderTraumaDoc18.aspx. Accessed February 14, 2009.

2. Acromioclavicular Dislocation

The acromioclavicular joint is diarthrodial with fibrocartilage-covered articular surfaces between the medial acromion and the lateral end of the clavicle. The acromioclavicular ligaments blend with fibers from the deltoid and trapezius to provide strength to the joint and provide horizontal stability, while the coracoclavicular ligaments provide vertical stability. The mechanism for dislocation of the acromioclavicular joint is most commonly direct impact caused by a fall on the tip of the shoulder. Thorough neurovascular examination along with standard trauma series of the shoulder (anteroposterior, scapular-Y, and axillary views) completes the standard workup. Stress radiographs, in which 10–15 lb weights are strapped to the wrists, and an anteroposterior radiograph are taken of both shoulders comparing coracoclavicular distances to differentiate between partial grade I–II injuries and grade III acromioclavicular separations.

▶ Classification

Type I injury is a strain of the acromioclavicular ligament. **Type II** injury involves rupture of the acromioclavicular ligament and strain of the coracoclavicular ligament complex, with slight superior displacement of the superior clavicle. **Type III** injury involves rupture of both the acromioclavicular and the coracoclavicular ligaments, which causes marked superior migration of the lateral end of the clavicle. **Types IV, V,** and **VI** injuries involve detachment of the deltoid and trapezius from the distal clavicle in addition to disruption of the acromioclavicular and coracoclavicular ligaments with marked posterior, superior, and inferior displacement of the clavicle, respectively.

▶ Treatment

Type I, II, and III acromioclavicular joint injuries are typically managed nonoperatively with a sling for approximately 4 weeks followed by gradual return to full activity. Most patients do not have significant dysfunction or any need to modify their activities. Surgical reconstruction may be indicated for type IV, V, and VI acromioclavicular joint injuries. Type III injuries in young athletes or laborers who perform a lot of overhead work may be treated surgically.

The Diagnosis and Management of Soft Tissue Shoulder Injuries and Related Disorders. New Zealand Guidelines Group, 2004.

3. Sternoclavicular Joint Dislocation

Dislocation of the sternoclavicular joint is rare. The mechanism of injury is usually a motor vehicle accident or sporting injury. Physical examination and anteroposterior and anteroposterior-cephalic tilt x-rays may demonstrate asymmetry. However, computed tomography is the diagnostic test of choice because it can distinguish fractures of the medial clavicle from sternoclavicular dislocation and can show minor subluxation. Anterior dislocation is more common, but posterior dislocation can cause injury to the esophagus, trachea, great vessels, subclavian artery, carotid artery, and pneumothorax. Dislocations of the sternoclavicular joint in children are often associated with physeal fractures.

▶ Treatment

Most injuries to the sternoclavicular joint may be treated with ice for the first 24 hours and immobilization with a sling, sling and swathe, or figure-of-8 bandage. Posterior dislocations may require emergent reduction if there is associated vascular compression or injury to the trachea, esophagus, or lungs. Closed reduction of posterior dislocations has been described using shoulder retraction and a towel clip. Rarely, open reduction may be necessary.

The Diagnosis and Management of Soft Tissue Shoulder Injuries and Related Disorders. New Zealand Guidelines Group, 2004.

4. Scapular Fracture

Scapular fractures are classified by anatomic location: scapula body, neck, spine, acromion, coracoid, and glenoid. Scapular body fractures are often associated with other injuries, such as subclavian vessel injury, aortic rupture, pneumothorax, rib fractures, brachial plexus injuries, and other soft tissue injuries associated with high-energy trauma. Fractures of the acromion and coracoid are rare. Glenoid fractures must be carefully evaluated for articular surface step-off and associated glenohumeral instability. These fractures may be caused by a blow on the shoulder or by a fall on the outstretched arm. Diagnosis with anteroposterior x-ray in the plane of the scapula and axillary x-ray may be supplemented by an axial view of the scapular body and transscapular Y-view. CT scan may also be helpful if surgery is being considered.

▶ Treatment

Most scapular fractures are treated nonoperatively in a sling for 4–6 weeks. Associated injuries may need to be treated emergently and should not be overlooked. Surgical indications are controversial but may include displaced intra-articular fractures involving more than 25% of the articular surface, scapular neck fractures angulation greater than 40 degrees or 1 cm of medial translation, scapula neck fractures with an associated displaced clavicle fracture, acromion fractures that cause subacromial impingement, and coracoid fractures that cause functional acromioclavicular separation.

Steinbach LS et al: Expert Panel on Musculoskeletal Imaging. Shoulder trauma. American College of Radiology, 2005. Available at: http://www.acr.org/SecondaryMainMenuCategories/quality_safety/app_criteria/pdf/ExpertPanelonMusculoskeletalImaging/ShoulderTraumaDoc18.aspx. Accessed February 14, 2009.

5. Dislocation of the Shoulder Joint

The shoulder (glenohumeral) joint is the most commonly dislocated joint in the body because of its freedom of motion and mobility in multiple planes. Diagnosis and management of this injury is presented in detail in the section on Sports Medicine.

6. Proximal Humerus Fracture

Fractures of the proximal humerus occur most commonly in elderly individuals with osteoporosis after a fall. Initial assessment should seek to determine the cause of any related fall as well as the fracture pattern. Prodromal symptoms related to a syncopal episode, myocardial infarction, stroke, transient ischemic attack, or seizure are possible etiologies that should be investigated. Associated injuries include neurovascular injuries, dislocation, and rotator cuff tears. Axillary nerve function should be assessed, testing sensation over the lateral aspect of the shoulder and overlying deltoid muscle (motor testing is usually not possible because of pain).

Diagnosis is established by standard shoulder trauma series (anteroposterior, lateral scapular Y, and axillary views). The axillary view is the best view for evaluating glenoid articular fractures and dislocations. If axillary view cannot be obtained because of pain, another option is a Velpeau axillary view in which the patient is left in a sling leaned obliquely backward 45 degrees over the cassette with the beam directed caudally. CT can be used to further evaluate articular involvement, fracture displacement, impression fractures, and glenoid rim fractures.

▶ Classification & Treatment

Proximal humerus fractures can be classified according to the system developed by Neer. There are four major parts of the proximal humerus: humeral head, humeral shaft, and greater and lesser tuberosities. A part is defined as displaced if there is more than 1 cm of fracture displacement or more than 45 degrees of angulation. Most proximal humerus fractures are minimally displaced (< 1 cm and < 45 degrees of angulation) and can be treated in a sling with early gentle range-of-motion exercises. Displaced fractures usually require surgery. Surgical options include closed reduction and percutaneous fixation, ORIF, and prosthetic arthroplasty (Figures 40–2 and 40–3). Other indications for surgery include superior displacement of the greater tuberosity fragment of 5 mm or more, which can lead to subacromial impingement, and

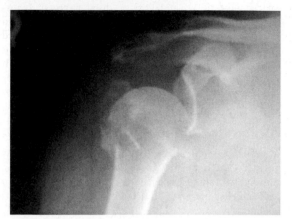

▲ **Figure 40–2.** Four-part proximal humerus fracture, impacted on inferior glenoid rim.

lesser tuberosity fractures that block internal rotation. Patients often lose some range of motion, but excellent pain relief and function can be attained. Long-term complications include shoulder stiffness and avascular necrosis of the humeral head (due to disruption of the arcuate branch off of the anterior circumflex humeral artery).

Shrader MW: Proximal humerus and humeral shaft fractures in children. Hand Clin 2007;23:431.

Zlotolow DA et al: Surgical exposures of the humerus. J Am Acad Orthop Surg 2006;14:754.

FRACTURES OF THE SHAFT OF THE HUMERUS

Most fractures of the shaft of the humerus result from direct trauma; indirect mechanism from fall on an outstretched arm is also a possibility. A careful neurovascular examination is required (radial nerve injury is most common). Anteroposterior and lateral radiographs of the humerus, as well as shoulder and elbow series, are mandatory to rule out the possibility of fracture or dislocation involving adjacent joints. Humerus fractures can be described descriptively: open or closed; location (proximal, middle, and distal third); nondisplaced or displaced; transverse, oblique, spiral, segmental, or comminuted fracture; intrinsic condition of bone (osteopenic or not); and articular extension if present.

▶ Treatment

Most midshaft humeral fractures can be treated nonoperatively in a cast, splint, or brace. Alignment should be verified using anteroposterior and lateral x-rays with the patient standing. Twenty degrees of anterior angulation, 30 degrees of varus angulation, and up to 3 cm of bayonet apposition are acceptable for continued closed treatment. Other surgical indications include open fractures, concomitant vascular injury, pathologic fracture, "floating elbow" (concomitant

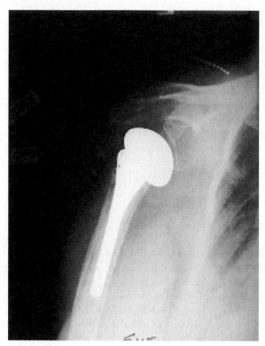

▲ **Figure 40–3.** Surgical reconstruction with hemiarthroplasty.

fracture of the forearm bones), segmental fracture, intra-articular extension, and bilateral humeral fractures. Radial nerve injury most commonly occurs with middle third fractures. Most radial nerve injuries are the result of stretching or contusion; function usually returns in 3–4 months. Delayed surgical exploration is warranted if there is no evidence of recovery on electromyogram or nerve conduction velocity studies.

Bhandari M et al: Compression plating versus intramedullary nailing of humeral shaft fractures: a meta-analysis. Acta Orthop 2006;77:279.

FRACTURES & DISLOCATIONS ABOUT THE ELBOW

▶ Anatomy & Biomechanics

The elbow is a modified hinge joint consisting of three separate articulations: ulnohumeral, radiohumeral, and proximal radioulnar. The elbow joint is intrinsically stable with bony and soft tissue contributions. The trochlea-olecranon fossa, coronoid fossa, radiocapitellar joint, biceps, triceps, and brachioradialis provide anterior-posterior stability during flexion and extension. On the medial side of the elbow, the anterior bundle of the medial collateral ligament is the primary stabilizer to valgus stress, while the lateral ulnar collateral ligament is the primary stabilizer on the opposite side of the elbow, preventing posterolateral instability. Normal elbow range of motion entails 0–150 degrees of flexion, 85 degrees of supination, and 80 degrees of pronation. Functional range of motion requires 30–130 degrees of flexion and 50 degrees of pronation and supination. Elbow injury mandates careful examination of the entire upper extremity, including shoulder and wrist, with thorough neurovascular examination. Anteroposterior, lateral, and oblique radiographs are required to adequate visualize the elbow joint.

Distal Humerus Fractures

The distal humerus can be conceptualized as medial and lateral columns, each roughly triangular in shape and composed of a condyle articulating with the bones of the forearm and an epicondyle (distal part of the humerus that flares just above the elbow joint at the level of the supracondylar ridge) connecting to the shaft of the humerus. These fractures can be classified descriptively: intercondylar (most common), supracondylar (extension or flexion type), transcondylar, condylar, capitellum, trochlea, lateral epicondyle, medial epicondyle, or supracondylar process fractures. They can also be classified using the AO system based on the concept of column integrity and articular involvement. Type A fractures are extra-articular (epicondylar, supracondylar, transcondylar) fractures. Type B fractures involve only a portion of the articular surface (unicondylar or intercondylar). Type C fractures involve the entire distal articular surface.

Radiographic Evaluation

Standard anteroposterior, lateral, and oblique radiographs should be obtained. Traction radiographs or CT scans may provide better fracture pattern visualization for preoperative planning. On the lateral radiograph, the anterior or posterior **"fat pad sign,"** representing displacement of the adipose layer over the joint capsule, may be the only indication of a nondisplaced distal humerus fracture. The anteroposterior radiograph should be carefully scrutinized for an intercondylar split. If an intercondylar split is present, the amount of rotation, in addition to displacement and fracture comminution, should be noted.

Management

The patient can be initially managed with a posterior long-arm splint with the elbow flexed at 90 degrees and the forearm neutral. Nonoperative treatment is indicated for nondisplaced or minimally displaced fractures. Surgery is indicated for displaced fractures, vascular injury, or open fracture.

SPECIFIC FRACTURE TYPES

Supracondylar Fractures of the Humerus

Supracondylar fractures are much more common in children. There are two types: extension (distal fragment is displaced posteriorly) and flexion (distal fragment is displaced anteriorly). Nondisplaced, minimally displaced, and severely comminuted fractures in the elderly with limited functional needs may be treated nonoperatively. Posterior splint immobilization is continued for 1–2 weeks after which gentle range-of-motion exercises are begun. The splint may be discontinued and weightbearing advanced after 6 weeks if signs of radiographic healing are appreciated. Surgical options include ORIF with plates and screws. Total elbow replacement may be considered in elderly patients who were otherwise active with good preinjury function with severely comminuted fractures not amenable to ORIF.

Transcondylar Fractures

Nonoperative treatment is indicated for nondisplaced or minimally displaced fractures or for debilitated elderly patients with poor function preinjury. Range-of-motion exercises should be initiated as soon as the patient is able to tolerate therapy. Surgical options include ORIF or total elbow arthroplasty.

Intercondylar Fractures

Intercondylar fractures are the most common type of distal humerus fracture in adults. Fracture fragments are often displaced due to opposing muscle forces on the medial (flexor mass) and lateral (extensor mass) epicondyles, causing rotation of the articular surfaces (Figure 40–4). Fractures can be classified as type I (nondisplaced), type II (slight displacement with no rotation between the condylar fragments), type III (displacement with rotation), and type IV (comminution of the articular surface). Nonoperative treatment with 2 weeks of immobilization followed by range-of-motion exercises is indicated for nondisplaced fractures. Type IV fractures in the elderly with osteopenic bone can be treated with the "bag of bones" technique, which entails very short-term immobilization with early range of motion. ORIF with dual plates is the preferred surgical treatment. Early range of motion is critical to prevent stiffness unless fixation is tenuous. Total elbow arthroplasty is another option.

Condylar Fractures

Medial or lateral condyle fractures are rare in adults (Figure 40–5). Type I (Milch classification) fractures do not traverse the lateral trochlear ridge. Involvement of the lateral trochlear ridge (type II) leads to medial-lateral instability. Nonoperative treatment, entailing a posterior splint, with elbow flexed to 90 degrees and the forearm supinated for lateral condyle fractures or pronated for medial epicondyle fractures, may be pursued for nondisplaced or minimally displaced fractures. Open or displaced fractures can be treated surgically with screw fixation with or without collateral ligament repair as needed.

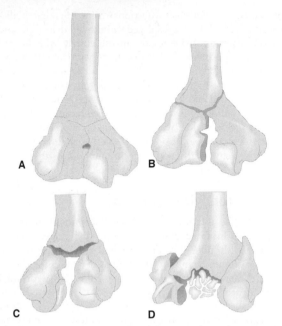

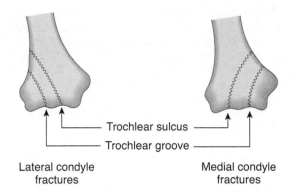

Lateral condyle
fractures

Medial condyle
fractures

▲ **Figure 40–5.** Condyle fractures. Milch classification. The type II fracture involves the lateral lip of the trochlea—thus its inherent instability. (Reproduced, with permission, from Milch H: Fractures and fracture dislocation of the humeral condyles. J Trauma, 1964.)

▲ **Figure 40–4.** Intercondylar fractures. **A:** Type I undisplaced T-condylar fracture of the elbow. **B:** Type II displaced but not rotated T-condylar fracture. **C:** Type III displaced and rotated T-condylar fracture. **D:** Type IV displaced rotated and comminuted T-condylar fracture.

Capitellum Fractures

Capitellum fractures are rare, representing less than 1% of all elbow fractures. Because of lack of significant soft tissue attachments, these fractures may result in a free articular fragment that may displace anteriorly into the coronoid or radial fossa, causing a block to elbow flexion. These fractures typically result from a fall on an outstretched arm with the force transmitted through the radial head to the capitellum. Occasionally, radial head fracture may also be present. Capitellum fractures can be classified as follows (Figure 40–6): type I, Hahn-Steinthal fracture, large osseous fragment with or without trochlear involvement; type II, Kocher-Lorenz fracture, fragmented articular cartilage with minimal subchondral bone attached; and type III, significant comminution. Nonoperative treatment, reserved for nondisplaced fractures, consists of immobilization in a posterior splint followed by elbow range-of-motion exercises. Surgical treatment entails ORIF with screws or excision for type II fractures, severely comminuted type I fractures, or chronic missed fractures with limited range of motion.

Trochlea Fractures

These fractures are extremely rare and associated with elbow dislocation. Nondisplaced fractures can be treated with posterior splint for 3 weeks, followed by elbow range-of-motion exercises. Displaced fractures are treated with ORIF; fragments not amenable to internal fixation can be excised.

Epicondylar Fractures

Lateral epicondyle fractures can be treated with symptomatic immobilization with early range of motion. Nondisplaced or minimally displaced medial epicondyle fractures can be treated with immobilization in posterior splint with the forearm pronated, wrist and elbow flexed for 10–14 days. ORIF is indicated for displaced fractures, especially in the presence of ulnar nerve symptoms, valgus stress instability, wrist flexor weakness, and symptomatic nonunion.

Supracondylar Process Fractures

The supracondylar process is osseous or cartilaginous projection arising from the anteromedial surface of the humerus. The ligament of Struthers, which connects the supracondylar process to the medial epicondyle, is a fibrous arch through which the median nerve and brachial artery passes. Most of these fractures are amenable to closed treatment with symptomatic posterior splint immobilization followed by early range of motion. Median nerve or brachial artery compression are indications for surgical exploration and release.

Elbow Dislocation

Elbow dislocation most commonly results from a fall on an outstretched hand. A careful neurovascular examination along with anteroposterior and lateral radiographs of the

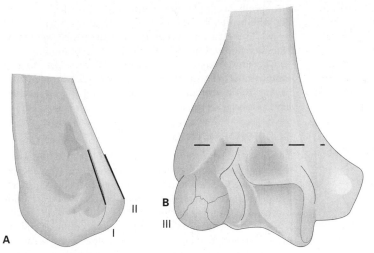

▲ **Figure 40–6.** Fractures of the capitellum. The type I fracture involves a large portion of bone, often the entire structure. Type II is a shear fracture, often with minimal subchondral bone, and may displace posteriorly **(A)**. A type III fracture is a comminuted fracture with varying amounts of displacement of the fracture fragments **(B)**.

elbow are required. Simple elbow dislocations (no associated fracture) are classified according to the direction of displacement of the ulna relative to the humerus: posterior (most common type), posterolateral, posteromedial, lateral, medial, and anterior (Figure 40–7). Acute elbow dislocations should undergo closed reduction with patient under sedation and adequate anesthesia as soon as possible. For posterior dislocation, the reduction maneuver entails longitudinal traction with elbow flexion. Postreduction range-of-motion examination, neurovascular examination, and radiographs should be performed, followed by placement in a posterior splint with 90 degrees of flexion. A block to full range of motion may indicate an incarcerated fracture fragment or inadequate reduction. If reduction does not restore arterial flow, angiography and immediate operative intervention are warranted. Postreduction films should be carefully evaluated for concentric reduction and associated fractures (medial or lateral epicondyle, radial head, coronoid process). Elbow dislocation with radial head and coronoid process fractures is known as the "terrible triad" because of associated instability. Surgical intervention is indicated if the elbow cannot be held in a concentrically reduced position, if it re-dislocates,

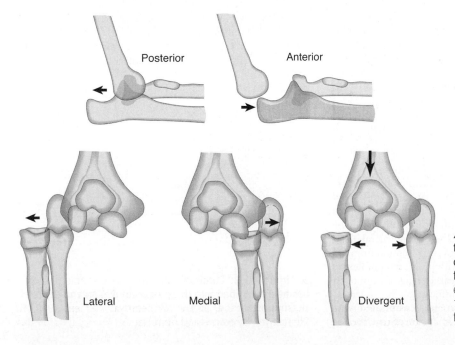

▲ **Figure 40–7.** Elbow dislocations. An elbow dislocation is defined by the direction of the forearm bones. (From Browner B et al: *Skeletal Trauma*. Saunders, 1992. Reproduced by permission from Elsevier.)

or if the dislocation is deemed unstable (if the elbow dislocates prior to reaching 30 degrees of flexion from a fully flexed position). Recovery of motion and strength may take 3–6 months. The most common complication is stiffness associated with prolonged immobilization. Recently, the trend has been to immobilize elbows for 1 week postinjury and then start range-of-motion exercises. If symptomatic heterotopic ossification is present, excision can be pursued 6 months or longer after injury.

FRACTURES OF THE PROXIMAL ULNA

▶ Olecranon Fractures

The olecranon is the most proximal palpable portion of the ulna. The subcutaneous position of the olecranon causes it to be especially susceptible to direct trauma. Posteriorly, the triceps tendon envelops the articular capsule before it inserts on to the olecranon. As a result, displaced fractures of the olecranon represent a functional disruption of the triceps mechanism, resulting in loss of active elbow extension. Anteriorly, the olecranon forms the greater sigmoid (semilunar) notch of the ulna, which articulates with the trochlea. The most proximal anterior portion of the ulna is the coronoid process, which lends stability to the elbow joint.

Olecranon fractures may result from a direct blow (fall on to the tip of the elbow), resulting in a comminuted olecranon fracture, or fall onto an outstretched arm accompanied by a strong, sudden triceps contraction, resulting in a transverse or oblique fracture. Careful neurovascular examination followed by anteroposterior and lateral radiographs should be part of the initial evaluation. A true lateral radiograph should be carefully scrutinized for the extent of the fracture, any displacement of the radial head (the radial head should point toward the capitellum in all views; otherwise, subluxation or dislocation is present), degree of comminution, and articular surface involvement. Olecranon fractures are classified on the basis of fracture pattern (transverse, transverse-impacted, oblique, comminuted, oblique-distal, fracture dislocation) or according to the Mayo classification: type I (nondisplaced or minimally displaced), type II (displacement without elbow instability), type III (fracture with features of elbow instability). The goals of treatment are to restore articular congruity, restore and preserve the elbow extensor mechanism, and restore range of motion.

Nondisplaced fractures or displaced fractures in the elderly with poor preinjury function can be managed with closed treatment in a long-arm splint or cast with the elbow flexed 45–90 degrees. Careful follow-up with radiographs should be done at weekly intervals for at least 2 weeks. In general, there is sufficient stability at 3 weeks to allow early motion from full extension to 90 degrees of flexion, with progression of flexion at 6 weeks. Some authors advocate earlier range of motion at 1 week out from injury to prevent stiffness.

Indications for surgery include any disruption of the extensor mechanism (any displaced fracture) or articular incongruity. Multiple surgical options are available, including intramedullary fixation, tension band wiring, plate and screws, and excision. Postoperatively, the patient should be placed in a posterior splint with early range of motion.

The most frequent complication of these fractures is prominent implants that subsequently require removal after healing has occurred. Elbow stiffness and loss of fixation have also been reported.

▶ Coronoid Fractures

The coronoid process is the anterior beak-shaped portion of the ulna, forming the buttress anteriorly of the greater sigmoid notch. The anterior portion of the medial collateral ligament attaches here, as well as a portion of the anterior capsule, contributing to elbow stability.

Isolated fractures of the coronoid are uncommon and are more frequently associated with posterior elbow dislocations or other fractures about the elbow. The mechanism of injury is usually forced posterior displacement of the proximal ulna, as with a dislocation, or hyperextension force of the elbow. Oblique radiographs may aid evaluation of these fractures, since they are sometimes difficult to see on lateral and anteroposterior views.

These fractures have been classified by Regan and Morrey based on the size of the fracture fragment (Figure 40–8): type I (coronoid process tip avulsion), type II (single or comminuted fragment involving 50% or less of the coronoid process), and type III (a single or comminuted fragment involving > 50% of the process). Type I fractures can be treated with immobilization in flexion for 3 weeks (or less if the fragment and elbow are stable). Associated fractures should be treated as appropriate in each case with the goal of fracture stability for early range of motion. Isolated coronoid fractures without elbow instability can be treated in the same way as type I fractures. Unstable type II fractures and type III fractures usually require operative intervention.

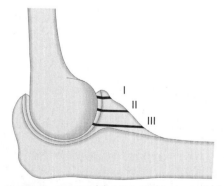

▲ **Figure 40–8.** Coronoid fractures. The coronoid fracture has been classified into three types by Regan and Morrey. (From Browner B et al: *Skeletal Trauma.* Saunders, 1992. Reproduced by permission from Elsevier.)

FRACTURES OF THE PROXIMAL RADIUS

▶ Radial Head Fractures

Radial head fractures typically result from a fall on an outstretched arm causing an axial load collision between the radial head and capitellum. Patients typically present with limited elbow and forearm motion, along with pain with passive range of motion of the forearm. The forearm and wrist should be examined for any tenderness, which may indicate an Essex-Lopresti type injury (radial head-fracture dislocation with associated interosseous ligament and distal radioulnar joint disruption). After documentation of neurovascular status, anteroposterior, lateral, and radial head view radiographs should be evaluated for fracture. Nondisplaced fractures should be suspected if a fat pad sign is present without obvious fracture. If Essex-Lopresti injury is suspected, additional radiographs of the forearm and wrist are indicated as well.

The Mason classification system is used to describe these fractures (Figure 40–9): type I (nondisplaced fractures), type II (marginal fractures with displacement), type III (comminuted fractures involving the entire radial head), and type IV (fracture associated with elbow dislocation).

Assessment of range of motion and stability to valgus stress is critical and can be performed after aspiration of the hemarthrosis and injection of lidocaine. This can be done through direct lateral needle insertion at the "soft spot" of the olecranon, radial head, and capitellum junction. Any mechanical block to motion should be carefully documented because it can affect treatment decision making.

Most isolated radial head fractures are treated with a brief period of immobilization in a sling followed by early range of motion 24–48 hours after the injury. Surgery is indicated for mechanical block to range of motion and type III fractures. A relative indication for surgery is displacement of a large fragment (> 2 mm); however, this treatment is controversial. Surgical treatment options include ORIF and fragment excision with or without prosthetic replacement. Type IV injuries should be treated with closed reduction, followed by additional treatment based on the previously outlined criteria.

Evidence-based care guideline for loss of elbow motion following surgery or trauma in children aged 4 to 18. Cincinnati Children's Hospital Medical Center, 2007. Available at: http://www.cincinnatichildrens.org/svc/alpha/h/health-policy/ev-based/elbow.htm. Accessed February 14, 2009.

Lee DH: Treatment options for complex elbow fracture dislocations. Injury 2001;32:SD41.

Ring D, Jupiter JB: Fracture-dislocation of the elbow. Hand Clin 2002;18:55.

FRACTURES OF THE FOREARM

Forearm fractures are more common in men than women, secondary to a higher incidence of motor vehicle collisions,

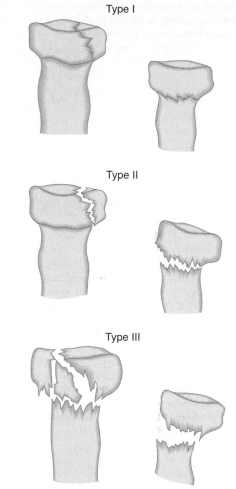

▲ **Figure 40–9.** Radial head fractures. The modified Mason classification system for radial head fractures. (From Browner B et al: *Skeletal Trauma.* Saunders, 1992. Reproduced by permission from Elsevier.)

athletic injury, altercations, and falls from height experienced by men. The forearm acts as a ring: a fracture that significantly shortens the radius or ulna will cause disruption of the proximal radioulnar joint or distal radioulnar joint (DRUJ). The ulna acts as an axis around which the laterally bowed radius rotates during supination and pronation. The interosseous membrane occupies the space between the radius and ulna; it provides a significant contribution to forearm stability.

Clinical assessment includes careful neurovascular examination (median, radial, ulnar nerves) and assessment of any open wounds (even superficial wounds can expose an ulna fracture to the outside world because of its subcutaneous position). Practitioners should have a high index of suspicion for compartment syndrome if pain out of proportion, tense compartments, or pain on passive stretch are present. Both-bone forearm fractures or fracture of one bone with concomitant injury to the elbow or wrist joint are more common than a fracture to either bone in isolation. It is therefore crucial to obtain anteroposterior and lateral radiographs of the forearm that include both the wrist and elbow joints. The radial head must be aligned with the capitellum on all views to rule out subluxation or dislocation.

Forearm fractures can be classified from a descriptive standpoint: closed or open, location, comminuted, segmental, multifragmented, displacement, angulated, and rotational alignment.

FRACTURES OF THE SHAFT OF THE RADIUS

► Isolated Radial Shaft Fractures

Radial shaft fractures can result from direct trauma or indirect trauma such as a fall on an outstretched hand. Although isolated fractures of the proximal two thirds of the radius are possible, a fracture of the distal one third should raise high suspicion for concomitant injury to the DRUJ. Nondisplaced fractures can be managed closed in a long arm cast. Any displacement, loss of radial bow, or concomitant injury to the DRUJ are surgical indications. Fractures of the radius are typically fixed with ORIF with 3.5 mm DCP plates.

This is a fracture of the shaft of the radius (most commonly the distal third) in conjunction with a DRUJ injury. Wrist pain on physical examination should arouse suspicion. The diagnosis should be confirmed radiographically. DRUJ disruption is suggested by the following radiographic findings: fracture at the base of the ulnar styloid, widening of the DRUJ space on the anteroposterior radiograph, subluxation of the ulna, and radial shortening greater than 5 mm relative to the distal ulna.

In adults, these injuries should always be treated surgically with ORIF, along with intraoperative evaluation of the DRUJ. After fixing the radius, if the joint is stable through full pronation and supination, only short-term immobilization in a splint is required to protect the incision. If the joint can be reduced but is unstable with rotation, additional surgical treatment is necessary. If there is a repairable ulnar styloid fracture, then ORIF of this piece will result in a stable DRUJ. If there is no ulnar styloid fracture but the DRUJ is reducible but unstable with rotation, then two 0.0625-inch Kirschner wires are used to pin the distal ulna to the radius in a reduced position (usually supination). With both ORIF of the ulnar styloid and the use of transfixing pins, the forearm should be immobilized in full supination in an above-elbow cast or brace for 4–6 weeks. The transfixing pins are removed prior to allowing forearm range of motion. Rarely, the DRUJ cannot be reduced. In this instance, a dorsal approach to the joint is used to extract interposed tissues (extensor carpi ulnaris is most common) blocking reduction.

FRACTURES OF THE SHAFT OF THE ULNA

► Isolated Ulnar Shaft Fractures (Nightstick Fractures)

Ulna nightstick fractures usually result from a direct blow to the ulna along its subcutaneous border. Careful neurovascular examination and radiographs of the forearm including the wrist and elbow are essential. Radiographs should be carefully scrutinized for elbow dislocation; the radial head should point to the capitellum in all views or a Monteggia variant may be present. Nondisplaced or minimally displaced fractures may be treated acutely in a sugar-tong splint. When swelling has subsided (after 7–10 days), the patient's arm can be transitioned to a long-arm cast or functional brace. Displaced fractures (> 10 degrees of angulation or > 50% displacement of the shaft) are best treated surgically with ORIF.

► Monteggia Fracture

Monteggia fracture is a fracture of the proximal ulna with a radial head dislocation. Thorough neurovascular examination is necessary; injuries to the radial nerve or posterior interosseous nerve have been described. The Bado classification is based on the direction of the radial head dislocation: type I (anterior), type II (posterior), type III (lateral or anterolateral), type IV (anterior dislocation with a fracture of the radius and ulna) (Figure 40–10).

Closed reduction and casting of Monteggia fractures should be attempted only in children. These injuries are typically treated with ORIF with plates and screws. Failure of the ulna to reduce may indicate annular ligament interposition. If open reduction of the radial head is necessary, consideration should be given to repairing the annular ligament. Postoperatively, if the repair is considered stable, the patient can be placed in a posterior splint for 7–10 days, followed by beginning range-of-motion exercises.

► Both-Bone Forearm Fractures

Fractures of both radius and ulna are usually the result of high-energy mechanisms (motor vehicle accidents or fall from a height). The fractures are most often displaced. Careful examination to rule out neurovascular injury and compartment syndrome should be performed. Radiographs of the entire forearm including the elbow and wrist are necessary.

Treatment for both-bone forearm fractures in adults consists of ORIF with compression plating using 3.5 mm dynamic plates. The goal of plate fixation is to restore the normal ulnar and radial length, rotational alignment, and radial bow (which have been shown to be essential for rotation of the arm). With solid fixation, active range of motion of the forearm and elbow can be started at 10–14 days. Open fractures can also be treated successfully with these methods. However, if there is excessive soft tissue damage or wound contamination, the use of an external fixator may be a preferable option.

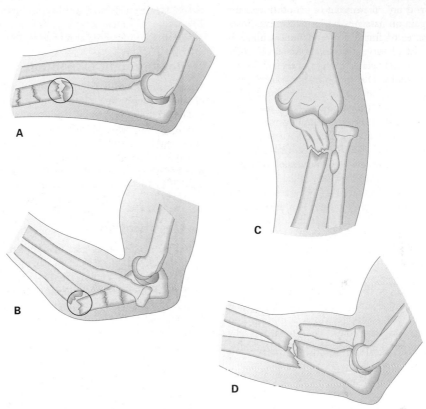

▲ **Figure 40–10.** Monteggia fractures. The classification of Monteggia lesions by Bado. **A:** Type I: anterior angulation of the ulnar fracture and anterior dislocation of the radial head. **B:** Type II: posterior angulation of the ulnar fracture and anterior dislocation of the radial head. **C:** Type III: fracture of the proximal ulna metaphysis and lateral dislocation of the radial head. **D:** Type IV: anterior dislocation of the radial head and fracture of the radial and ulnar shafts. (From Browner B et al: *Skeletal Trauma.* Saunders, 1992. Reproduced by permission from Elsevier.)

Complications of this fracture include nonunion, malunion, infection, neurovascular injury, compartment syndrome, synostosis, and loss of motion.

INJURIES OF THE WRIST REGION

▶ Anatomy

The distal radius has three articulations: the sigmoid notch, which articulates with the ulna, and facets for the scaphoid and lunate bones. The base of the ulna styloid serves as an insertion point for the triangular fibrocartilage complex (TFCC), which is the primary stabilizer of the DRUJ. Normally, 80% of the axial load is supported by the distal radius and 20% by the ulna and TFCC. There are six dorsal compartments of the wrist that contain wrist and digital extensor tendons. On the volar surface, the pronator quadratus lies across the distal radius and ulna. Just anterior to the pronator quadratus are the contents of the carpal canal, containing 9 digital flexor tendons and the median nerve. Anterior to the

transverse carpal ligament lie the flexor carpi radialis, flexor carpi ulnaris, and palmaris longus muscles. The Guyon canal contains the ulnar nerve and artery. It is bounded by the volar retinacular ligament and flexor retinacular ligament, the hook of the hamate radially, and the pisiform ulnarly.

Extrinsic ligaments connect the radius to the carpus and the carpus to the metacarpals. The proximal row of carpal bones consisting of the scaphoid, lunate, triquetrum, and pisiform bones, are attached to the distal radius via two sets of radiocarpal ligaments (volar and distal). The volar radiocarpal ligaments (radioscaphocapite, radioscapholunate, radiolunate, and radiolunotriquetral) are stronger and confer more stability to the radiocarpal articulation when compared to the dorsal radiocarpal ligaments. The radiocarpal joint is the primary joint for wrist motion (70 degrees of flexion/extension, 20 and 40 degrees of radial and ulnar deviation, respectively).

Intrinsic ligaments connect carpal bone to carpal bone (eg, scapholunate). The trapezium, trapezoid, capitate, and hamate of the distal carpal row are connected to each other and the base of the metacarpals with strong, extrinsic ligaments. As a result, the distal carpal row is relatively immobile. The lunate is the key to carpal stability; injury to the scapholunate or lunotriquetral ligaments leads to unstable motion of the lunate and generalized carpal instability. Disruption of the scapholunate ligament or scaphoid fracture can lead to excessive dorsiflexion of the lunate and triquetrum (dorsal intercalated segmental instability [DISI]). Injury to the lunotriquetral ligament leads to volar flexion of the lunate (volar intercalated segmental instability [VISI]). The space of Poirier (ligament-free area between the capitate and lunate) is a potential area of weakness.

Normal anatomic relationships include radial inclination of 23 degrees, 11 mm of radial length, 11–12 degrees of palmar tilt, a 0-degree capitolunate angle (straight line drawn from the shaft of the third metacarpal through the capitate and lunate with the wrist in a neutral position), a 47-degree scapholunate angle, and less than 2 mm of scapholunate space.

The vascular supply to the wrist consists of the radial, ulnar, and anterior interosseous arteries intertwining to form a network of arterial arches on the volar and dorsal surfaces of the carpal bones. The radial artery gives off branches that supply the scaphoid volarly (supplies distal scaphoid) and dorsally (supplies proximal scaphoid). The lunate typically receives blood supply from dorsal and volar surface branches.

1. Distal Radius Fracture

▶ Epidemiology

More than 450,000 distal radius fractures occur annually in the United States, representing one sixth of all fractures treated in emergency departments. The incidence of distal radius fractures increases with old age and osteopenia.

▶ Mechanism

The most common mechanism for a distal radius fracture is fall onto an outstretched dorsiflexed hand. High-energy mechanisms such as motor vehicle collisions and falls from height can result in highly displaced or significantly comminuted fractures in younger patients.

▶ Clinical Evaluation

Patients typically present with a swollen, ecchymotic, tender wrist. Deformity of the wrist is variable with dorsal displacement of the distal segment (Colles fracture) being more common than volar (Smith-type fracture). The ipsilateral elbow and shoulder should be carefully evaluated for concomitant injury. Careful neurovascular examination is paramount and should include the motor and sensory median, ulnar, and radial nerve distributions (motor: A-OK, finger spread, and thumbs-up signs; sensory: volar aspect of the thumb, index, middle fingers, volar aspect of the small finger, and dorsal aspect of the thumb). Particular attention should be given to median nerve function because carpal

tunnel syndrome is a relatively common complication (13–23%) due to traction injury, fracture fragment trauma, hematoma, or increased compartment pressure.

▶ Radiographic Evaluation

Posteroanterior and lateral views of the wrist should be obtained. Elbow and shoulder symptoms should also be evaluated radiographically. Contralateral wrist views may be used for comparison of ulnar variance and the DRUJ. CT scan can be useful for further characterization of intra-articular involvement and for preoperative planning. Normal radiographic relationships include the following averages: 23 degrees of radial inclination, 11 mm of radial length, and 11 degrees of palmar or volar tilt.

▶ Classification

Distal radius fractures can be characterized descriptively: open or closed, displacement, angulation, comminution, and loss of radial length. The Frykman classification organizes these fractures based on the degree of articular involvement as well concomitant fracture of the distal ulna (Figure 40–11). Higher classification fractures have worse prognoses.

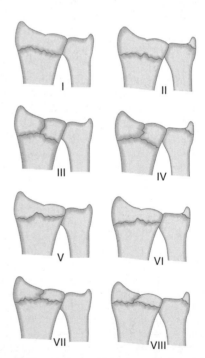

▲ **Figure 40–11.** Frykman classification of distal radius fractures. Types I, III, V, and VII do not have an associated fracture of the distal ulna. Fractures III–VIII are intra-articular fractures. Higher-classification fractures have worse prognoses. (From Green D, Hotchkiss R, Pederson W: *Green's Operative Hand Surgery.* Churchill Livingstone, 1993.)

AO/ASIF CLASSIFICATION OF DISTAL RADIUS FRACTURES

Type A: Extra-articular fractures

1. Isolated distal ulnar fracture
2. Simple radius fracture
3. Radial fracture with metaphysial impaction

Type B: Intra-articular complex fracture

1. Radial styloid fracture
2. Dorsal rim fracture
3. Volar rim fracture

Type C: Intra-articular complex fracture

1. Metaphysial fracture with radiocarpal congruity preserved
2. Articular displacement
3. Diaphysial-metaphysial involvement

The AO/ASIF classification separates distal radius fractures into three groups as shown in the accompanying box.

▶ Treatment

Emergent operative management is indicated for open fractures. Acute surgical intervention should be considered for distal radius fractures complicated by carpal tunnel syndrome that is not relieved with closed reduction.

A. Nonoperative Treatment

All distal radius fractures should undergo closed reduction, even if surgical intervention is expected. The benefits of fracture reduction include limiting postinjury swelling, pain relief, and median nerve decompression. Although casting may be considered for nondisplaced or minimally displaced fractures with minimal swelling, a sugar-tong splint encompassing the dorsal and volar aspects of the wrist and limiting subsequent forearm rotation and possible fracture displacement is generally preferred. One week postinjury, the patient may be transitioned to a long-arm cast. If closed treatment is planned, radiographic evaluation should be done on a weekly basis for the first 2–3 weeks to monitor for displacement. Acceptable radiographic parameters for continued closed treatment include radial length within 2–3 mm of the contralateral wrist, neutral palmar tilt (0 degrees), intra-articular step-off less than 2 mm, and less than 5-degree loss of radial inclination. Surgery is indicated if reduction with respect to these parameters cannot be achieved or maintained.

B. Closed Reduction Technique

Hematoma block, Bier block, or conscious sedation can be used to provide analgesia. Hematoma block offers the benefit of speed and does not require that the patient have been without oral intake for a significant amount of time. Conscious sedation offers the benefit of muscle relaxation facilitating reduction. Initially, manual or fingertrap-assisted traction is applied to facilitate reduction via ligamentotaxis. For dorsally tilted fractures, volar-directed pressure is applied to the distal fracture segment. C-arm, if available, can be used to assess fracture reduction. Once reduction is adequate, a well-molded long-arm (sugar-tong) splint can be applied with the wrist in neutral and the metacarpophalangeal joints free.

C. Techniques of Surgical Management

Many surgical options are available. Choice of operation is determined by several factors, including the fracture pattern, bone quality, and surgeon preference.

D. Closed Reduction Percutaneous Pinning

Reduction is achieved via closed means, followed by fixation typically with 0.0625-inch Kirschner wires. Interfragmentary technique entails wires used to stabilize a fracture and prevent collapse after reduction is achieved. With intrafocal technique, these wires are driven into the fracture site and used to lever the pieces, achieving reduction, and are then driven through the opposite cortex to maintain reduction. Postoperatively, patients are placed in a splint or cast. The wires are typically removed after 6 weeks once bone healing is appreciated radiographically.

E. External Fixation

This technique uses ligamentotaxis to restore radial length and radial inclination, but it rarely restores palmar tilt. It is especially useful for treating very comminuted or intra-articular fractures in which there are several small pieces. External fixation is also useful for treating open fractures with severe tissue compromise or as a temporizing measure when a patient has other critical medical issues that need immediate attention.

F. Open Reduction and Internal Fixation

In recent years, volar plating has become much more popular than dorsal plating because of its advantages when treating distal radius fractures with significant dorsal comminution and because of the extensor tendon complications associated with dorsal plating of the distal radius.

▶ Complications

Stiffness of the wrist and digits is common. Patients should be instructed to begin range-of-motion exercises for the digits immediately after the fracture is initially treated. Complications include median nerve dysfunction; malunion; nonunion; stiffness; posttraumatic arthritis; tendon rupture; and finger, wrist, and elbow stiffness. Articular congruity after surgical fixation is critical for avoiding the development of posttraumatic arthritis.

2. Isolated Radial Styloid Fracture

Also called a chauffeur's fracture, backfire fracture, or Hutchinson fracture, isolated radial styloid fracture is an avulsion fracture with extrinsic ligaments remaining attached to the styloid fragment. This injury is often associated with intercarpal ligamentous injuries such as scapholunate dislocation and perilunate dislocation. It often requires ORIF.

FRACTURES OF THE ULNAR STYLOID

Fractures of the ulnar styloid are commonly seen in conjunction with distal radius fractures and but can also be seen in isolation. Fractures of the tip of the ulnar styloid are often too small to fix. However, large fragments (the entire styloid from its base) may be indicative of a TFCC disruption that can lead to DRUJ instability. As a result, these displaced fractures should be treated with ORIF.

DISTAL RADIOULNAR JOINT DISLOCATION

DRUJ dislocation is discussed in the section on Pediatric Orthopedics. DRUJ dislocation can also occur with a simple distal radius fracture. Careful examination of radiographs and the DRUJ will keep the clinician from missing this injury in the face of a distal radius fracture.

FRACTURES & DISLOCATIONS OF THE CARPUS

Most carpal bone fractures occur in the proximal carpal row, with the scaphoid being the carpal bone most commonly fractured. Carpal bone fractures usually occur in younger people, often from high-energy falls on an outstretched hand. Wrist radiographs can be difficult to interpret, and careful scrutiny is necessary so as not to miss these injuries. In addition to the standard anteroposterior, lateral, and oblique views of the wrist, special radiographic views such as a scaphoid view (anteroposterior radiograph with the wrist supinated 30 degrees and in ulnar deviation), clenched fist view (to evaluate for carpal instability), or carpal tunnel view can often be helpful. CT scan is also useful to identify fractures if radiographs are inconclusive; MRI is sensitive for detecting occult fractures, osteonecrosis of carpal bones, and soft injuries including disruption of the scapholunate ligament or TFCC.

1. Fracture of the Scaphoid

The scaphoid is the carpal bone most commonly fractured. Anatomically, the scaphoid is divided into proximal and distal poles, a tubercle, and a waist. The blood supply for the scaphoid comes largely from branches of the radial artery traveling from a distal to proximal location. As a result, fractures of the scaphoid at the waist or more proximal are particularly prone to nonunion or avascular necrosis.

Fractures of the scaphoid most commonly occur as a result of a fall on an outstretched hand. Patients typically present with pain on the radial side of their wrist and tenderness to palpation over the anatomic snuffbox. Physical examination maneuvers include the scaphoid lift test (reproduction of pain with dorsal-volar shifting of the scaphoid) and the Watson test (painful dorsal scaphoid displacement as the wrist is moved from ulnar to radial deviation with compression of the tuberosity). Radiographic evaluation includes a scaphoid view in addition to the standard wrist series. Initial radiographs are nondiagnostic in up to 25% of cases. As a result, if clinical examination suggests a scaphoid fracture, it is appropriate to employ a trial of immobilization with repeat radiographs in 1–2 weeks. Additionally, technetium bone scan, MRI, or CT scan can be used to diagnose occult scaphoid fractures. Scaphoid fractures can be classified according to pattern (horizontal oblique, transverse, vertical oblique), displacement (nondisplaced fractures with no step-off [considered stable], displaced fractures > 1 mm, scapholunate angulation > 60 degrees, radiolunate angulation >15 degrees), and location (tuberosity, distal pole, waist, and proximal pole). Nondisplaced fractures should be treated in a long-arm thumb spica cast for 6 weeks. After 6 weeks, the patient's wrist can be placed in a short-arm spica cast until the fracture is united. Expected time to union for distal third fractures is 6–8 weeks, 8–12 weeks for middle third fractures, and 12–24 weeks for proximal third fractures. Surgical indications include fracture displacement greater than 1 mm, radiolunate angle greater than 15 degrees, scapholunate angle greater than 60 degrees, and humpback deformity, or nonunion.

Complications of scaphoid fractures include fracture nonunion or avascular necrosis (Figure 40–12). Patients with longstanding scaphoid nonunions develop early arthritis of the radioscaphoid joint secondary to altered mechanics of the wrist.

2. Fracture of the Lunate

The lunate is the carpal bone most likely to dislocate, but fractures are rare. Fractures usually result from a fall on an outstretched hand. Patients typically present with tenderness to palpation over the volar wrist overlying the distal radius and lunate with painful range of motion. Radiographs are usually not helpful because of overlapping densities of multiple bones; CT, MRI, or bone scan are usually required to make the diagnosis. Nondisplaced fractures can be treated in a short-arm or long-arm cast. Displaced or angulated fractures require surgical treatment. Osteonecrosis (Kienböck disease) can complicate this injury, leading to advanced collapse and radiocarpal degeneration. Several surgical treatments are available for this sequela.

3. Fracture of the Hamate

This fracture generally occurs from a direct blow to the area such as occurs when swinging a baseball bat or golf club that suddenly comes to an abrupt stop as it encounters a firm surface. Patients present with ulnar-sided hand pain over the

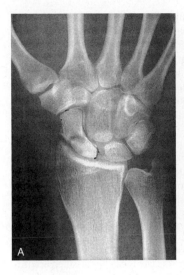 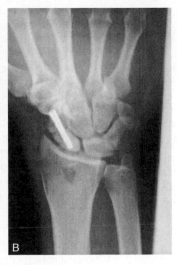

▲ **Figure 40–12.** Scaphoid fracture. **A:** Scaphoid fracture nonunion. **B:** Open reduction and internal fixation of scaphoid nonunion.

hamate. Fracture will often not be seen on routine wrist and hand radiographs. A carpal tunnel view (20-degree supination oblique view of the wrist) should be obtained if this fracture is suspected. If the diagnosis is suspected clinically but the radiographs show no fracture, a CT scan may be helpful. Nondisplaced fractures may be treated in a short-arm cast for 6 weeks. Displaced fractures of the body can be treated with ORIF with screws or wires.

4. Other Carpal Bone Fractures

Fractures can occur in any of the other carpal bones as well, but much less commonly. Triquetral avulsion or dorsal impaction fractures can occur from falls on the outstretched hand. Isolated fractures of the remaining carpal bones are rare and generally occur with high-energy trauma and other injuries.

5. Traumatic Carpal Instability

Severe injury to the wrist causing damage to the complex ligamentous structures may lead to carpal bone dissociation, carpal dislocations, and fracture dislocations. The lunate is often called the carpal keystone; its ligamentous attachments to the radius and other carpal bones make a significant contribution to radiocarpal stability. A sequence of progressive perilunate instability starts with scapholunate disruption (stage I), then midcarpal or capitolunate disruption (stage II), lunotriquetral disruption (stage III), ending in disruption of the radiolunate joint leading to volar lunate dislocation (stage IV).

Scapholunate dissociation secondary to disruption of the scapholunate and the radioscapholunate ligament leads to altered kinematics of the wrist and early degenerative arthritis. Clinical findings include volar wrist tenderness/bruising, positive Watson test, pain with grasping, and decreased grip strength. Radiographically, widening of the scapholunate space more than 3 mm (Terry Thomas sign), or scapholunate angle greater than 70 degrees on the lateral are indicative of scapholunate disruption. Closed reduction with an audible, palpable click followed by thumb spica immobilization for 8 weeks is the first line of treatment. Inability to obtain or maintain reduction is a surgical indication.

Lunotriquetral dissociation occurs as a result of disruption of the radiolunotriquetral ligament. Patients typically present with swelling over the peritriquetral area and tenderness dorsally, typically 1–2 cm distal to the ulnar head. Radiographs may show disruption of the normal proximal carpal row contour; frank gapping of the lunotriquetral space is rarely seen. Treatment with a short-arm cast for 6–8 weeks or closed reduction with pinning of the lunate to the triquetrum is warranted.

Carpal dislocations represent a continuum of perilunate ligamentous injury with frank lunate dislocation being the final stage. Patients present with severe wrist pain and swelling after trauma. Most dislocations can be diagnosed with adequate anteroposterior and lateral views of the wrist. With a perilunate dislocation, the lunate remains in its normal position, articulating with the distal radius, but is angled in a volar direction, and the rest of the carpus is dislocated. With lunate dislocation, on the lateral radiograph the lunate will be volar to the rest of the carpus and not in alignment with the distal radius. Treatment of carpal dislocations is accomplished with closed reduction of the midcarpal joint via traction combined with direct manual pressure over the capitate and lunate. Irreducible dislocations or unstable injuries should be treated surgically with ORIF.

Ulnocarpal dissociation may result from disruption of the TFCC, where the lunate and triquetrum assume a supinated and palmar flexed position while the distal ulna subluxes dorsally. Radiographs may show ulnar styloid avulsion or dorsal displacement of the ulna; MRI may demonstrate TFCC tear. Treatment requires operative repair of the TFCC and/or ORIF of large displaced ulnar styloid fragments.

Even with the best care, carpal bone and ligament injuries can be devastating, with long-term sequelae of pain, stiffness, and early arthritis.

Bond CD et al: Percutaneous screw fixation versus cast immobilization for nondisplaced scaphoid fractures. J Bone Joint Surg Am 2001;83:483.

Cassidy C et al: Traumatic wrist disorders—what's in and what's out. AAOS 68th Annual Meeting Instructional Course, 2001.

Jupiter JB et al: Update on the management of traumatic and reconstructive problems of the scaphoid. AAOS 68th Annual Meeting Instructional Course, 2001.

Kozion SH: Peri-lunate injuries: diagnosis and treatment. J Am Acad Orthop Surg 1998;6:114.

Shin AY, Bishop AT, Berger RA: Vascularized pedicled bone grafts for disorders of the carpus. THUES 1998;2:94.

Trumble TE et al: Intra-articular fractures of the distal aspect of the radius. AAOS Instructional Course Lecture, Vol 48, 1999.

FRACTURES & DISLOCATIONS ABOUT THE HAND

Metacarpal and phalangeal fractures are relatively common, comprising a significant portion of emergency department visits. The significant variation in mechanism of injury accounts for the large number of different types of fracture patterns seen in hand injuries. Axial load or "jamming" injuries often result in shearing articular fractures or metaphyseal compression fractures, sometimes with concomitant injury to the carpus, forearm, elbow, and shoulder due to force transmission. Injury mechanisms with a bending component result in diaphyseal fractures or joint dislocations. Individual digits or joints caught in clothing or equipment can result in spiral fractures or complex dislocations. Industrial settings with heavy objects predispose to crushing mechanisms of injury. The direction of fracture angulation depends on the deforming forces caused by attached muscle. The palmar and dorsal interosseous muscles arise from the metacarpal shafts, usually flexing the fracture and causing apex-dorsal angulation. Proximal phalanx fractures typically angulate in the opposite direction, apex-volar. Middle phalanx fractures angulate variably, while distal phalanx fractures are usually comminuted tuft fractures resulting from crush injuries. Clinical evaluation includes documentation of the patient's age, hand dominance, occupation, mechanism of injury, time of injury, exposure to contamination, and financial issues (worker's compensation). Physical examination should document neurovascular status and pay particular attention range of motion, angulation, and malrotation (best evaluated when the intervening joint is flexed to 90 degrees). Radiographic evaluation includes anteroposterior, lateral, and oblique radiographs of the hand and the specific injured digit. Fractures can be classified descriptively: open or closed, location, fracture pattern (comminuted, transverse, spiral, vertical split), extraarticular or intraarticular, stable or unstable, and angulational or rotational deformity. Fractures of the small bones of the hand heal more rapidly than fractures of larger bones, and prolonged immobilization can cause stiffness and loss of motion that can be difficult or impossible to regain. As a result, fractures of the metacarpals and phalanges should not be immobilized for more than 3 weeks, except under rare circumstances, to avoid subsequent development of stiffness. The safe position for splinting or casting of the hand is with slight wrist extension, the metacarpophalangeal joints flexed 60–90 degrees, and the proximal interphalangeal and distal interphalangeal joints extended. This "intrinsic plus" position puts the ligaments of the hand on maximum stretch, avoiding posttreatment stiffness.

1. Open Fractures, Fight Bite, Animal Bites

These types of fractures require special consideration. Open fractures of phalanges or metacarpals can be classified according to the Swanson, Stabo, and Anderson classification: type I (clean wound without significant contamination or delay in treatment), type II (contamination with gross dirt/debris, human or animal bite, lake/river injury, barnyard injury, or accompanied by significant systemic illness such as diabetes, hypertension, rheumatoid arthritis, hepatitis, or asthma). Type I injuries can be treated with primary internal fixation and immediate wound closure. Although type II injuries can be treated with primary internal fixation (no increase in infection rate), these injuries should not be closed primarily. Delayed closure is preferred to decrease infection risk.

Any laceration overlying a joint in the hand, particularly the metacarpophalangeal joint, must be suspected as being caused by a human tooth. Also known as a "fight bite," these injuries should be assumed to have been contaminated with oral flora and should be treated aggressively with broad-spectrum antibiotics, including anaerobic coverage. Animal bites require antibiotic treatment that covers *Pasteurella* and *Eikenella*.

2. Metacarpal Fractures
▶ Metacarpal Head Fractures

Fractures of the metacarpal can be subclassified as follows: epiphyseal fractures; collateral ligament avulsion fractures; oblique, vertical, and horizontal head fractures; comminuted fractures; and fractures with joint loss. Most of these fractures require anatomic reduction to reestablish joint congruity and avoid posttraumatic arthritis. Stable reductions of fractures may be splinted in the intrinsic plus position. If unstable, percutaneous pinning, ORIF, or external fixation are options.

▶ Metacarpal Neck Fractures

Metacarpal neck fractures are typically caused by direct trauma with volar comminution and dorsal apex angulation. The most common metacarpal neck fracture is the boxer's fracture of the fifth metacarpal, usually caused by the fist striking a stationary object. These fractures can typically be closed reduced successfully. The degree of acceptable deformity varies according to the metacarpal injured: less than 10 degrees for the second and third metacarpal, less than 30–40 degrees for the fourth and fifth metacarpals. Unstable fractures require surgical intervention with percutaneous pinning or ORIF.

▶ Metacarpal Shaft Fractures

Nondisplaced or minimally displaced metacarpal shaft fractures can be reduced and splinted. Surgical indications include rotational deformity (all fingers should point toward the scaphoid when flexed) and dorsal angulation greater than 10 degrees for second and third metacarpals and greater than 40 degrees for fourth and fifth metacarpals.

▶ Metacarpal Base

Fractures of the base of the second, third, and fourth metacarpals are typically minimally displaced and treated with splinting and early range of motion. A reverse Bennett fracture is a fracture dislocation of the fifth metacarpal and hamate bones. This injury often requires ORIF.

Fractures of the thumb metacarpal base can be extra-articular or intra-articular. Extra-articular fractures are usually transverse or oblique and amenable to closed reduction and casting. Unstable fractures may require percutaneous pinning. Intra-articular fractures come in two types: type I or **Bennett Fracture** in which a single fracture line separates the majority of the metacarpal from the volar lip fragment and type II, also known as a **Rolando fracture,** which is a comminuted intra-articular fracture usually with a Y or T pattern including dorsal and palmar fragments. Both type I and type II fractures are treated with closed reduction and percutaneous pinning or ORIF.

3. Proximal & Middle Phalanx Fractures

Intra-articular fractures can be classified as condylar fractures or fracture dislocations. There are three types of condylar fractures: unicondylar, bicondylar, and osteochondral. Each requires anatomic reduction; ORIF should be performed for displacement of more than 1 mm. Comminuted intra-articular fractures not amenable to surgical treatment can be treated closed with early protected mobilization.

Fracture dislocations come in two varieties: volar lip fracture and dorsal lip fracture. Volar lip fracture (dorsal fracture dislocation) treatment is controversial; if less than 35% of the articular surface is involved, the injury may be treated with buddy taping. However, for more than 35% involvement, some clinicians recommend ORIF or volar plate arthroplasty if the fracture is comminuted, while others recommend extension block splint if the joint is not subluxed. Dorsal lip fracture (volar fracture dislocation) with less than 1 mm of displacement may be treated closed with splinting, while more than 1 mm of displacement requires operative intervention.

Extra-articular fractures of the phalanges should be initially treated with closed reduction with fingertrap traction and splinting. Unstable fractures should be treated surgically.

▶ Distal Phalanx Fractures

Intra-articular dorsal lip fractures may be complicated by an extensor tendon disruption resulting in a "mallet finger." Mallet finger may also result from purely tendinous disruption, without fracture. For either scenario, treatment is controversial. Some recommend full-time extension splinting for 6–8 weeks, while others recommend surgical intervention. For professionals who work extensively with their hands, such as surgeons, full-time extension splinting is not practical. Closed reduction with percutaneous pinning is a good option.

Intra-articular volar lip fractures can be associated with a flexor digitorum profundus rupture resulting in a "jersey finger," often seen in football or rugby players and most commonly involving the ring finger. Treatment is typically surgical, especially if large, displaced bony fragments are present.

Extra-articular fractures can be transverse, longitudinal, or comminuted (nail matrix injury very common). These fractures are usually treated with closed reduction and splinting that traverses the distal interphalangeal joint, leaving the proximal interphalangeal joint free. Because of the increased risk of nonunion, surgery is indicated for fractures with wide irreducible displacement.

▶ Nailbed Injuries

Nailbed injuries are easily missed in the context of distal phalanx fractures. When untreated, these injuries result in nail growth disturbances. Subungual hematomas are often indicative of nailbed injury. The nail plate should be removed and the hematoma drained. Nailbed disruptions should be carefully sutured with 6-0 chromic catgut under magnification. The nail plate should be replaced to keep the nail fold open; alternatively, a piece of aluminum foil or Xeroform gauze can be used.

4. Dislocations of the Digits

Carpometacarpal dislocations are usually high-energy injuries. Careful neurovascular examination is essential. These injuries usually require surgical intervention for maintenance of a stable reduction.

Metacarpophalangeal joint dislocations are usually dorsal in direction, presenting with a hyperextended posture. Simple dislocations can be reduced by flexion of the joint without traction. Wrist flexion, causing the flexor tendons to relax, can be used to facilitate the reduction maneuver. Complex metacarpophalangeal dislocations with the volar plate interposed in the joint are irreducible. The pathognomonic radiograph finding is the appearance of the sesamoid in the joint space. Complex dislocations require surgery. Traction during reduction of simple dislocations should be avoided because simple dislocations can be converted into complex ones. Volar dislocations are rare; however, because they are particularly unstable, they often require surgical intervention.

Thumb metacarpophalangeal dislocations are unique because of the multiplanar motion of the thumb metacarpophalangeal joint. With a one-sided collateral ligament injury, the phalanx tends to sublux volarly, rotating around the opposite intact ligament. The ulnar collateral ligament of the thumb metacarpophalangeal joint is the most commonly injured ligament in the digits. If the injury is acute, it is called a "skier's thumb," whereas chronic injury from repetitive trauma is known as a "gamekeeper's thumb." Nonoperative treatment with reduction and thumb spica splinting or casting is usually sufficient. A Stener lesion occurs when the ulnar collateral ligament avulses and comes to rest dorsal to the adductor aponeurosis. The ulnar collateral ligament cannot return to its normal insertion, preventing healing. As a result, Stener lesions and irreducible metacarpophalangeal dislocations require surgical intervention.

Proximal interphalangeal joint dislocations include dorsal dislocation, pure volar dislocation, and rotatory volar dislocation. Once reduced, rotatory volar dislocations, collateral ligament ruptures, and dorsal dislocations congruent in full extension on the lateral radiographs can all begin active range-of-motion exercises immediately with adjacent digit strapping. Dorsal dislocations that continue to sublux on lateral radiograph can be treated with a few weeks of extension block splinting. Volar dislocations with central slip disruptions are treated with 4–6 weeks of proximal interphalangeal extension splinting, followed by an additional 2 weeks of nighttime splinting. Irreducible dislocations or unstable reductions may require surgical intervention.

Distal interphalangeal dislocations and thumb interphalangeal joint dislocations can present late. Injuries are considered chronic after 3 weeks. Acute reduced dislocations may begin immediate active range of motion. Unstable dislocations should be immobilized in 30 degrees of flexion for 3 weeks. Complete collateral ligament injury should be protected from lateral stress for at least 4 weeks. Recurrent stability can be treated with Kirschner wire fixation. Chronic dislocation may be treated with open reduction to resect scar tissue, allowing for a tension-free reduction. Transverse open wounds in the volar skin crease are not infrequent. Open dislocations require debridement to prevent infection.

Rubin DA et al: Expert Panel on Musculoskeletal Imaging. Acute hand and wrist trauma. American College of Radiology, 2005. Available at http://www.acr.org/SecondaryMainMenuCategories/quality_safety/app_criteria/pdf/ExpertPanelonMusculoskeletal Imaging/AcuteHandandWristTraumaDoc1.aspx. Accessed on February 14, 2009.

Freiberg A et al: Management of proximal interphalangeal joint injuries. Hand Clin 2006;22:235.

Freeland AE, Orbay JL: Extraarticular hand fractures in adults: a review of new developments. Clinical Orthop Relat Res 2006; 445:133.

INJURIES OF THE HIP REGION

1. Hip Dislocations

▶ Epidemiology

Hip dislocations of the native hip are relatively rare, usually due to high-energy injury such as a motor vehicle accident. Posterior hip dislocations (85–90%) are more common than anterior (remaining 10–15%). Sciatic nerve injury may complicate 10–20% of posterior hip dislocations. Anterior hip dislocations are associated with a greater incidence of femoral head injury. Up to 50% of patients with a hip dislocation will sustain a concomitant fracture elsewhere (most commonly of the ipsilateral femur or pelvis).

▶ Anatomy

The hip articulation is a ball-and-socket joint, formed by the femoral head and acetabulum. Forty percent of the femoral head is covered by the acetabulum. The labrum surrounding the acetabulum has the effect of deepening the hip joint, increasing its stability. The medial and lateral circumflex femoral arteries from the profunda femoral artery form an extracapsular vascular ring at the base of the femoral neck; ascending branches provide the primary blood supply to the femoral neck and head, along with a minor contribution from the ligamentum teres off of the obturator artery. The contribution of the medial and lateral circumflex arteries is often disrupted with hip dislocation, leading to long-term complications including avascular necrosis. The sciatic nerve exits the pelvis at the greater sciatic notch, traveling deep to the piriformis muscle, down the posterior aspect of the thigh.

▶ Clinical Evaluation

A full trauma survey is essential because of the high-energy nature of this injury. Patients typically present with severe discomfort and inability to move the injured extremity. The classic appearance of a posterior hip dislocation is shortened extremity with the hip flexed, internally rotated and adducted (Figure 40–13). Patients with an anterior dislocation hold their hip with marked external rotation, mild flexion, and abduction. Careful neurovascular examination is key. If the sciatic nerve is injured, the tibial nerve is often preserved with the peroneal portion of the nerve showing the effects of injury. Radiographic evaluation includes an anteroposterior view of the pelvis as well as radiographs of the entire ipsilateral femur. Evaluate the femoral neck and acetabulum to rule out concomitant fractures.

▶ Treatment

The hip should be reduced emergently to avoid osteonecrosis from associated vascular disruption. Regardless of the direction of the dislocation, the hip can be reduced with inline longitudinal traction with the patient supine. The key to successful reduction is relaxation of the patient's muscles,

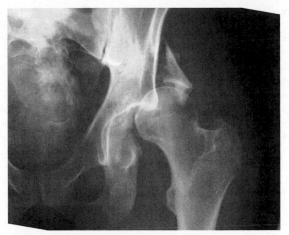

▲ **Figure 40–13.** Posterior hip dislocation with concomitant fracture of the posterior wall and weightbearing dome of the acetabulum.

which is accomplished with adequate sedation (ideally via general anesthesia, or intravenous sedation if general anesthesia is not available) and fatiguing of the patient's muscles that occurs with time. Following closed reduction, the hip should be examined for stability by flexing the hip to 90 degrees in neutral position and applying a posteriorly directed force. If any subluxation is detected, the hip is deemed unstable and will require surgery or traction. Postreduction radiographs should be obtained to confirm reduction. Careful comparison should be made with the contralateral side to determine if the reduction is concentric. Even slight asymmetry or subluxation may indicate the presence of a concomitant fracture or incarcerated piece of bone in the joint. Additionally, postreduction CT should be performed to investigate the presence of other fractures or an incarcerated bony fragment. If closed reduction is unsuccessful, open reduction should be performed as soon as possible.

Fractures of the Femoral Head

Fractures of the femoral head are extremely rare. Most are secondary to motor vehicle accidents and are associated with hip dislocations. Clinical evaluation includes careful neurovascular examination, anteroposterior view of the pelvis, as well as anteroposterior and lateral radiographs of the injured hip. Femoral head fractures can be classified according to the Pipkin classification: type I (hip dislocation with fracture of the femoral head inferior to the fovea capitis femoris), type II (hip dislocation with fracture of the femoral head superior to the fovea capitis femoris), type III (type I or type II injury with femoral neck fracture), and type IV (type I or type II injury with associated fracture of the acetabular rim). Type I fractures involve the nonweightbearing surface of the femoral head. As a result, closed treatment can be

pursued if reduction is adequate (< 1 mm step-off). Type II fractures involve the weightbearing surface. Thus, if the reduction is not anatomic as seen on CT, surgical treatment should be pursued. Type III and type IV injuries usually require surgical treatment. Complications include osteonecrosis and posttraumatic arthritis.

The Femoral Neck

Approximately 350,000 fractures of the femoral neck occur each year. This number is expected to double by the year 2050 due to the aging demographics of the American population. Fractures of the femoral neck occur most often in elderly patients with osteopenic bone after a fall. Femoral neck fractures in patients under 50 years old are rare, usually due high-energy trauma. Patients with displaced fractures usually present with inability to walk, severe pain, and an externally rotated and shortened extremity. Patients with nondisplaced fractures may present with mild, persistent hip pain (for several days or couple of weeks); these patients often will have been walking, and index of suspicion should be high. A careful secondary survey should be performed because 10% of elderly patients have associated upper extremity injuries. Radiographic evaluation includes anteroposterior pelvis radiograph, anteroposterior and lateral radiographs of the hip, and internal rotation or traction view, which can further delineate the fracture pattern. If no fractures are detected in an elderly patient with persistent hip pain, one should consider MRI or bone scan to look for a nondisplaced or incomplete fracture.

Fractures of the femoral neck may be classified according to location (subcapital, transcervical, and basocervical) or based on stability of the fracture pattern. The Pauwels classification describes increasing instability of the increasing fracture angle from the horizontal: type I (30 degrees), type II (50 degrees), and type III (70 degrees). The garden classification describes four patterns: type I (incomplete fracture/valgus impacted), type II (complete fracture, nondisplaced), type III (complete fracture with partial displacement; the trabecular bone pattern of the femoral head does not line up with the acetabulum), and type IV (completely displaced fracture; the trabecular bone pattern of the head does line up with the acetabulum).

Some authors advocate nonoperative treatment with limited weightbearing for type I or valgus impacted fractures. Others advocate internal fixation with multiple screws to prevent fracture displacement. Type II (nondisplaced) fractures are treated with internal fixation regardless of the patient's age. Treatment of type III and type IV (displaced) fractures is more controversial. For patients under 60 years old, with good bone quality and little fracture comminution, ORIF is the usual choice. For patients over 60 years old, with osteopenic bone and comminuted fractures, arthroplasty is the treatment of choice. Unipolar hemiarthroplasty is most commonly used. If the patient has evidence of preexisting acetabular arthritis, total hip arthroplasty may be offered. Recent studies have suggested that in the elderly, previously active patient with intact mental status, total hip arthroplasty may be the best treatment option for displaced femoral neck fracture. Although, bipolar arthroplasty theoretically reduces the risk of prosthetic arthritis compared with unipolar hemiarthroplasty, this has not been borne out in the literature. As a result, given the higher cost, most authors do not advocate the use of bipolar hemiarthroplasty.

2. Trochanteric Fractures

▶ Fracture of the Lesser Trochanter

Isolated fractures of the lesser trochanter are quite rare. This fracture occurs most commonly in the adolescent patient secondary to forceful iliopsoas contracture. In the elderly patient, this fracture may be secondary to metastatic disease.

▶ Fracture of the Greater Trochanter

Like isolated fractures of the lesser trochanter, isolated fracture of the greater trochanter is rare. The typical mechanism is direct blow due to fall in an elderly patient. Treatment is typically nonoperative. In a young, active patient with a widely displaced greater trochanter, surgery may be considered.

▶ Intertrochanteric Fractures

Intertrochanteric fractures are fractures that occur in the region between the greater and lesser trochanters of the proximal femur. These fractures are extracapsular, occurring in cancellous bone with abundant blood supply. Unlike displaced femoral neck fractures, these fractures are not predisposed to nonunion and osteonecrosis. These fractures are relatively common, accounting for nearly 50% of all fractures of the proximal femur (Figure 40–14). The typical presentation occurs in an elderly individual after a fall. Clinical evaluation includes neurovascular check, secondary survey, and appropriate x-rays (anteroposterior pelvis, anteroposterior and lateral of injured hip). One may consider an internal rotation or traction view for improved delineation of the fracture. Consider MRI or technetium bone scan in a patient with persistent hip pain despite negative radiographs; these two studies may be useful for delineating nondisplaced or incomplete fractures.

It is important to evaluate the location of fracture line (proximal to distal), obliquity of the fracture line, the degree of comminution (paying specific attention to the posteromedial cortex, which determines stability), and magnitude of displacement. Basocervical neck fractures are located just proximal to or along the intertrochanteric line. These fractures are usually extracapsular; however the proximity to the blood supply of the femoral neck can result in a higher incidence of osteonecrosis. Typically, intertrochanteric fractures have an oblique fracture line that extends from the lateral cortex proximally to the medial cortex distally; this "standard obliquity" fracture pattern is considered stable, amenable to standard surgical treatment. "Reverse obliquity" intertrochanteric fractures (oblique fracture line extending from the medial cortex proximally to the lateral cortex distally) are considered unstable. Significant posteromedial comminution indicates an unstable fracture. Finally, subtrochanteric extension of the fracture should be noted, as it may affect treatment choice.

Nonoperative treatment is associated with a higher mortality rate when compared to operative treatment. As a result,

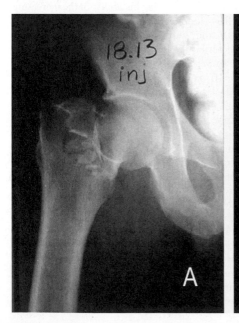
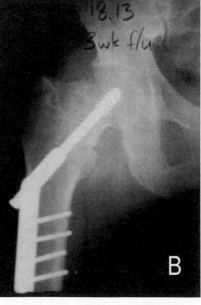

▲ **Figure 40–14.** Comminuted intertrochanteric hip fracture. **A:** Anteroposterior radiograph. **B:** Anteroposterior radiograph after fixation with a compression hip screw and sideplate.

it may be considered for patients who carry high surgical risk or demented/nonambulatory patients with mild hip pain. Early bed-to-chair mobilization is crucial to avoid the risks and complications of prolonged recumbency (atelectasis, deep venous thrombosis, and ulcers).

Treatment is usually surgical, with the goal being early ambulation with full weightbearing status. Dynamic hip screw (large screw and side plate) is the typical surgical implant of choice. Intramedullary hip screws are used for unstable fracture patterns, including reverse obliquity intertrochanteric fractures, fractures with significant posteromedial comminution, and fractures with subtrochanteric extension. Finally, arthroplasty may be chosen in patients for whom previous ORIF has failed or as primary treatment for comminuted, unstable fractures.

▶ Subtrochanteric Fracture

The subtrochanteric femur fracture is located between the lesser trochanter and a point 5 cm distal to the lesser trochanter. This stretch of bone is subjected high biomechanical stresses. The medial and posteromedial cortices are sites of high compressive forces, while the lateral cortex experiences high tensile forces. Additionally, this area of bone is composed mainly of cortical bone. Because it has less vascularity than cancellous bone, the potential for healing is diminished.

The mechanism of injury may be low energy, such as a fall in an elderly person, or high energy in patients involved in motor vehicle accidents, falls from heights, or gunshot wounds. Additionally, fractures in this region may be pathologic in nature due to bone metastases.

Clinical evaluation includes standard trauma evaluation for patients involved in high-energy injury mechanisms. Field dressings or splints should be completely removed to examine for soft tissue injury and rule out open fracture. Neurovascular status should be documented. Secondary survey should be performed. Blood loss can be significant in the thigh compartments, representing a potential source for hypovolemia. Traction pin should be considered until definitive fixation can be performed to limit further soft tissue damage and bleeding. Radiographic evaluation includes the anteroposterior pelvis, anteroposterior, and lateral views of the hip and femur down to the knee.

The fracture may be classified according to its distance from the lesser trochanter, fracture line characterization, number of bone fragments, and involvement of the piriformis fossa.

Open fractures should be treated with immediate surgical debridement and fracture stabilization. Surgical treatment can involve the use of an intramedullary nail or fixed-angle plates depending on the fracture pattern (Figure 40–15).

The fracture is typically healed by 3–4 months postoperatively, but delayed union and nonunion are not uncommon. Hardware failure can occur in these cases, requiring repeat internal fixation and bone grafting.

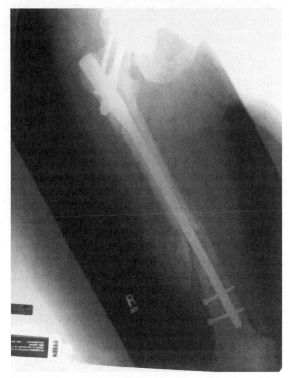

▲ **Figure 40–15.** Subtrochanteric femur fracture with fracture of the distal third of the ipsilateral femoral shaft treated with a reconstruction type intramedullary nail.

Acute Management and Immediate Rehabilitation after Hip Fracture amongst People Aged 65 Years and Over. New Zealand Guidelines Group, 2003.

DeSmet AA et al: Expert Panel on Musculoskeletal Imaging. Avascular necrosis of the hip. American College of Radiology, 2005. Available at http://www.acr.org/SecondaryMainMenu Categories/quality_safety/app_criteria/pdf/ExpertPanelon MusculoskeletalImaging/AvascularNecrosisoftheHipDoc3.aspx. Accessed February 14, 2009.

Geerts WH et al: Prevention of venous thromboembolism: 7th ACCP Conference on Antithrombotic and Thrombolytic Therapy. Chest 2004;126:338S.

FRACTURE OF THE SHAFT OF THE FEMUR

A femoral shaft fracture is a fracture of the femoral diaphysis that occurs between 5 cm distal to the lesser trochanter and 5 cm proximal to the adductor tubercle. Femoral shaft fractures typically occur in young men after high-energy trauma, such as motor vehicle accidents. This injury can occur in the elderly after a fall, although less commonly. Fractures that are inconsistent with the level of trauma should be suspected for pathologic fracture.

The vascular supply to the femoral shaft is derived mainly from the profunda femoral artery. Due to the large volume of the three fascial compartments of the thigh (anterior, medial, and posterior), significant blood loss and hemodynamic instability can occur. In one series, blood loss was greater than 1200 ml, with 40% of patients ultimately requiring blood transfusion.

Clinical evaluation includes careful neurovascular examination and secondary survey looking for concomitant injury to other joints and extremities. Specific attention should be paid to the ipsilateral hip and knee joints. Knee ligament injuries are common and easily missed. Radiographic evaluation should include anteroposterior and lateral views of the femur as well as the ipsilateral hip and knee. Anteroposterior pelvis should also be obtained. Ipsilateral femoral neck and intertrochanteric fractures have been reported in up 10% of patients with femur fractures.

Femoral shaft fractures can be classified descriptively: open or closed, location (proximal, middle, distal one third), pattern (spiral, oblique, transverse), degree of comminution, angulation, rotational deformity, displacement, and amount of shortening. Winquist and Hansen described a classification based off amount of comminution: type I (minimal or no comminution), type II (cortices of both fragments at least 50% contact), type III (50–100% cortical comminution), and type IV (circumferential comminution with no cortical contact).

In the acute setting, femoral shaft fractures can be stabilized with skeletal traction. Traction provides pain relief and can help minimize soft tissue injury and blood loss. Ideally, surgical stabilization should occur within 24 hours of injury (Figure 40–16). If surgery is delayed because of an unstable patient, traction has the added benefit of pulling the fracture fragments out to length, making subsequent fracture reduction and operative treatment more manageable.

Open fractures constitute a surgical emergency. Fractures should be debrided and stabilized as soon as possible. The most frequently used surgical treatment for femoral shaft fractures is intramedullary nailing. Compared with plate fixation, intramedullary nailing offers the following benefits: lower infection rate; less extensive exposure/dissection of the fracture, promoting healing; less quadriceps scarring; and lower tensile and shear stresses on the implant. Other advantages include early functional use of the extremity (the surgeon may allow immediate weightbearing depending on strength of surgical management), restoration of length and alignment, rapid and high union rate, and low refracture rates.

Intramedullary nailing can be performed in an antegrade or retrograde fashion. Indications for retrograde nailing include ipsilateral injuries (fracture of the femoral neck, pertrochanteric, patella, acetabulum, or tibia), bilateral femoral shaft fractures, morbidly obese patient, pregnant woman, ipsilateral knee amputation, or when speed of surgi-

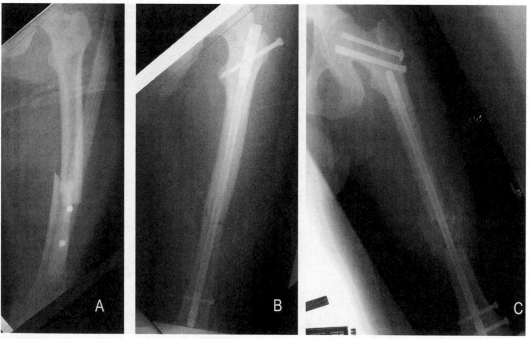

▲ **Figure 40–16.** Femoral shaft fracture. **A:** Anteroposterior x-ray showing fracture of the midshaft of the femur. **B:** Anteroposterior x-ray after closed reduction and intramedullary fixation using an antegrade titanium locked nail. **C:** Anteroposterior x-ray showing fixation of a midshaft femoral fracture and ipsilateral femoral neck fracture with a retrograde intramedullary nail.

cal treatment is essential (unstable patient). Contraindications to retrograde nailing include restricted knee motion (< 60 degrees), patella baja, and presence of associated open traumatic wound increasing the risk of intra-articular knee sepsis. One major disadvantage to retrograde nailing is the postoperative incidence of anterior knee pain.

Other surgical options include plating and external fixation. External fixation may be used acutely as a temporary bridge in the severely injured, unstable patient. Plating may be indicated in patients whose femoral canals are not amenable to intramedullary nailing (medullary canal too narrow, medullary canal obliterated due to infection, previous closed fracture management, etc).

Postoperatively, early patient mobilization and knee range of motion is recommended. Weightbearing status is dependent on multiple factors, including the strength of operative fixation, patient's other injuries, soft tissue status, and location of fracture. Later complications are those of prolonged recumbency, joint stiffness, malunion, nonunion, leg-length discrepancy, and infection.

Baker RP et al: Total hip arthroplasty and hemiarthroplasty in mobile, independent patients with a displaced intracapsular fracture of the femoral neck. A randomized, controlled trial. J Bone Joint Surg Am 2006;88:2583.

Olsson O, Ceder L, Hauggaard A: Femoral shortening in intertrochanteric fractures. A comparison between the Medoff sliding plate and the compression hip screw. J Bone Joint Surg Br 2001;83:572.

INJURIES OF THE KNEE REGION

1. Fractures of the Distal Femur

Distal femur fractures account for about 7% of all femur fractures. Incidence follows a bimodal age distribution with the first peak occurring in young adults as a result of high-energy trauma and the second peak occurring in the elderly after a fall. Distal femur fractures can be subclassified as supracondylar or condylar fractures.

The supracondylar region of the femur is the area between the femoral condyles and the junction of the metaphysic with the femoral shaft. The distal femur widens from the cylindrical shaft to form two curved condyles separated by an intercondylar groove. The medial condyle extends more distally and is more convex than the lateral condyle, producing the normal valgus position of the distal femur. The proximal fracture fragment is typically pulled superiorly by the quadriceps and hamstrings; the distal fragment is typically displaced and angulated posteriorly due to the pull of the gastrocnemius muscle.

Neurovascular examination is key as the distal fragment may impinge on the popliteal fossa, causing a loss or marked decrease of pedal pulses. Immediate reduction is indicated. If reduction of the fracture fragment fails to restore pulses, immediate arteriogram and vascular operative intervention is indicated. Secondary survey should be performed, with concomitant injury to the ipsilateral hip, knee, leg and ankle ruled out. If a distal femoral fracture is associated with an overlying laceration or wound, the ipsilateral knee should be injected with 50 ml of sterile normal saline to rule out continuity with the wound.

Radiographic evaluation includes anteroposterior, lateral, and oblique radiographs of the distal femur as well as the entire length of the femur (Figure 40–17). Traction views and CT scan may be helpful for preoperative planning. MRI may be used to evaluate injuries to the meniscus and ligaments of the knee. Arteriography should be considered in the setting of knee dislocation (up to 40% associated vascular disruption reported in the literature).

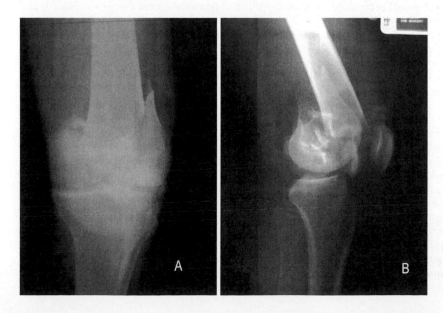

▲ **Figure 40–17. A:** Anteroposterior radiograph demonstrating a comminuted supracondylar femur fracture with intra-articular extension. **B:** Lateral radiograph.

Distal femur fractures may be classified descriptively: open or closed, location (supracondylar, intercondylar, condylar), fracture pattern (spiral, oblique, transverse), intra-articular or extra-articular, degree of comminution, angulation, rotational deformity, displacement, and amount of shortening.

Nonoperative treatment may be pursued for stable nondisplaced fractures. Treatment involves immobilization of the extremity in a hinged knee brace with partial weightbearing.

Displaced distal femur fractures are best treated surgically. If operative treatment is delayed more than 8 hours, a tibial traction pin should be considered. Plates and screws are the typical choice of implant. A variety of plates are available, including the 95-degree condylar blade plate, nonlocking periarticular plates, and locking periarticular plates. Because of the advantage of increased stability, locking periarticular plates are becoming more popular.

▶ Dislocation of the Knee Joint

Traumatic knee dislocation is extremely rare. However, this injury can be limb threatening because of disruption of the vasculature. The knee is a hinge joint consisting of three articulations: patellofemoral, tibiofemoral, tibiofibular. Normal range of motion of the knee is from 10 degrees of extension to 140 degrees of flexion. Significant soft tissue injury, including disruption of three out four major ligaments of the knee (anterior cruciate, posterior cruciate, medial collateral, and lateral collateral ligaments), is necessary for knee dislocation to occur. During knee dislocation, the popliteal vascular bundle may be injured or tethered. Associated fractures of the tibial eminence, tibial tubercle, fibular head or neck, and capsular avulsions should be ruled out. The mechanism is typically high energy.

If the knee remains dislocated at presentation, immediate reduction should be performed without waiting for radiographs. Postreduction neurovascular status should be carefully documented. Isolated ligament examination may be difficult to perform because of patient discomfort. Standard ligament examination includes Lachman testing for the anterior cruciate ligament, posterior drawer for the posterior cruciate ligament, and varus and valgus stress to assess the lateral collateral ligament and medial collateral ligament respectively. Due to the incidence of delayed ischemia resulting from vasospasm or thrombosis occurring hours or even days after reduction, serial neurovascular exams should continue to be performed.

If a limb remains ischemic (absent pulses) after reduction, emergent surgical exploration is indicated; do not wait for an arteriogram. If the limb continues to display abnormal vascular status (diminished pulses, decreased capillary refill or ABI < 0.9), then arteriogram is indicated. Normal vascular status should be followed closely with serial exams.

Radiographic evaluation includes anteroposterior, lateral, and notch views of the knee as well as a "sunrise" view of the patella. Arteriography is indicated as described previously. MRI is used to evaluate the ligaments and menisci of the knee, as well as articular cartilage lesions.

Knee dislocations can be classified according to the displacement of the proximal tibia in relation to the distal femur (anterior, posterior, lateral, medial, and rotational).

Immediate closed reduction is achieved with axial traction followed by placement of a splint with the knee in 20–30 degrees of flexion. Of note, posterolateral dislocation usually requires open reduction. Surgery is indicated for unsuccessful closed reduction, residual soft tissue interposition, open injuries, and vascular injuries. External fixation may be necessary for grossly unstable knees and dislocations that required vascular repair. Prophylactic fasciotomy of the leg compartments should be considered at the time of vascular repair to eliminate the compartment syndrome caused by postischemic edema. Ligamentous repair is controversial; timing of surgery is dependent on the status of both the patient and the limb.

2. Fracture of the Patella

Patella fractures represent only 1% of all skeletal injuries, occurring most commonly in the 20–50-year-old age group. The patella is the largest sesamoid bone in the body, with the quadriceps tendon inserting at its superior pole and the patellar ligament originating from the inferior pole. The patella has seven articular facets; the lateral facet is the largest (accounting for 50% of the articular surface). The medial and lateral extensor retinacula are strong longitudinal expansions of the quadriceps that envelop the patella and insert on the tibia. If the retinacula are intact, active extension will be preserved despite patella fracture.

The function of the patella is to increase the lever arm and mechanical advantage of the quadriceps tendon. The blood supply originates from the geniculate arteries, which form anastomoses circumferentially around the outer border of the patella. Fractures of the patella may result from direct trauma or, more commonly, from forceful quadriceps contraction while the knee is semiflexed during a stumble or fall.

Open lacerations associated with patella fracture should be investigated with 50 ml of sterile saline solution instilled into the knee joint to rule out communication and open fracture. Active knee extension should be assessed; decompression of hemarthrosis and intra-articular lidocaine injection may facilitate testing.

Radiographic examination should include anteroposterior, lateral, and sunrise views of the knee. Of note, bipartite patella (8% of the population) may be confused with fracture. Bipartite patella usually occurs in the superolateral portion of the patella and has smooth margins. Interestingly, it is bilateral in 50% of patients; thus, contralateral knee x-rays may facilitate diagnosis.

Patella fractures may be classified descriptively: open or closed, degree of displacement, fracture pattern (stellate, comminuted, transverse, vertical, polar, or osteochondral).

Nondisplaced or minimally displaced (2 mm) with minimal articular disruption (1 mm or less) can be treated nonoperatively in a knee immobilizer for 4–6 weeks if the extensor mechanism remains intact.

Surgical treatment for displaced fractures includes tension band wires, cerclage wiring, screws, or combination thereof. Retinacular disruption should also be repaired at the time of surgery. Postoperatively, the patient should be placed in a splint to protect the skin; knee motion should be instituted early, 3–6 days postoperatively, with progression to full weightbearing by 6 weeks. Severely comminuted or marginally repaired fractures may be immobilized longer. Partial patellectomy may be performed in the setting of a large, salvageable fragment with a smaller, comminuted polar fragment not amenable to stable surgical fixation. Total patellectomy is rarely indicated, reserved for extensive patella fractures with severe comminution.

▶ Dislocation of the Patella

Patella dislocation is more common in women and in patients with connective tissue disorders (Ehlers-Danlos or Marfan) due to increased soft tissue laxity. Dislocation of the patella can be acute (traumatic) or chronic (recurrent).

Patients with an unreduced patella dislocation will present with inability to flex the knee, hemarthrosis, and palpably displaced patella. Patients with reduced or chronic patella dislocation may demonstrate a positive apprehension test whereby laterally directed force applied to the patella with the knee in extension reproduces pain and sensation of impending patella dislocation.

Radiographic evaluation includes anteroposterior and lateral views of the knee along with sunrise views of bilateral patellae for comparison. Assessment of patella alta (high-riding patella) or patella baja should also be performed using the Insall-Salvati ratio (the ratio of the patellar ligament length compared to the length of the patella, normal is 1.0; a ratio of 1.2 indicates patella alta, while 0.8 indicates patella baja).

Patella fractures may be classified descriptively: reduced or unreduced, congenital or acquired, acute (traumatic) or chronic (recurrent), and direction of dislocation (lateral, medial, intra-articular, superior [lateral is most common]).

These injuries are typically treated closed with reduction and casting or bracing with the knee in extension. Operative intervention is generally reserved for recurrent dislocation.

▶ Tear of the Quadriceps Tendon

Quadriceps tendon tears occur most commonly in patients over 40 years old. The tendon usually ruptures within 2 cm of the superior pole of the patella. Location of rupture is associated with the patient's age: for patients over 40, the tear usually occurs at the bone-tendon junction; however, patients under 40, often have midsubstance tears. Risk factors for quadriceps tendon rupture include anabolic steroid use, local steroid injection, diabetes mellitus, inflammatory arthropathy, and chronic renal failure. Typically, patients present with a history of a sudden "pop" while stressing the extensor mechanism. Patients have pain at the site of injury,

difficulty with weightbearing, knee joint effusion, tenderness at the upper pole of the patella, and a palpable defect proximal to the superior pole of the patella. Complete tears result in loss of active knee extension; partial tears can still have knee extension.

Radiographic examination includes anteroposterior, lateral, and sunrise views of the knee. Nonoperative treatment includes immobilization with the knee in extension for 4–6 weeks followed by progressive physical therapy. Complete ruptures should be surgically repaired. Choice of surgical technique varies depending on location of the tear: Complete ruptures near bone require reapproximation of the tendon to bone using nonabsorbable sutures passed through bone tunnels. Midsubstance tears may undergo end-to-end repair.

▶ Tear of the Patellar Ligament

Patella tendon ruptures are less common than quadriceps tendon ruptures. This injury typically occurs in patients under 40. Rupture commonly occurs at the inferior pole of the patella; risk factors include rheumatoid arthritis, lupus, diabetes, renal failure, systemic corticosteroid treatment, local steroid injection, and chronic patella tendonitis. Patients typically provide a history of an audible pop after forceful quadriceps contraction. Physical examination may show a palpable defect, hemarthrosis, painful passive range of motion, and partial or complete loss of active extension. Radiographic examination includes anteroposterior and lateral x-rays of the knee. Nonoperative treatment is reserved for partial tears with intact extensor mechanism. Early repair (within 2 weeks of injury) is preferred to delayed repair (> 6 weeks from injury), which is technically more demanding because of quadriceps contraction, patellar migration, and adhesions.

Dursun N, Dursun E, Kilic Z: Electromyographic biofeedback-controlled exercise versus conservative care for patellofemoral pain syndrome. Arch Phys Med Rehabil 2001;82:1692.

Veselko M, Kastelec M: Inferior patellar pole avulsion fractures: osteosynthesis compared with pole resection. Surgical technique. J Bone Joint Surg Am 2005;87:113.

FRACTURES OF THE TIBIA & FIBULA

Fractures of the Tibial Plateau

Tibial plateau fractures account for 1% of all fractures. Isolated lateral tibial plateau fractures are most common, although isolated fractures of the medial tibial plateau and bicondylar fractures happen as well.

▶ Anatomy

The tibia is the primary weightbearing bone in the leg, supporting 85% of the transmitted load. The tibial plateau consists of the articular surfaces of the medial and lateral tibial plateaus. The medial plateau is larger and concave in shape, while the lateral plateau extends higher and is convex in shape. Normally, the plateau has a 10-degree posteroinferior slope. The two plateaus are separated by the intercondylar eminence, which serves as the tibial attachment for the anterior and posterior cruciate ligaments. There are three bony prominences 2–3 cm distal to the tibial plateau that serve as important insertion sites for tendinous structures: The tibial tubercle is located anteriorly and serves as the insertion for the patellar ligament; the pes anserinus is located medially and serves as attachment for semitendinosus, sartorius, and gracilis muscles; and the Gerdy tubercle, which is the insertion site for the iliotibial band, is located laterally. The peroneal nerve travels around the neck of the fibular head, splitting into the superficial peroneal nerve, which travels down the lateral aspect of the leg anterior to the fibula, and the deep peroneal nerve, which dives deep and travels down through the anterior compartment. The trifurcation of the popliteal artery is located posteriorly between the adductor hiatus proximally and the soleus complex distally. These structures are all at risk with a tibial plateau fracture.

Mechanism of Injury

Tibial plateau fractures are usually the result of axial loading coupled with varus or valgus force. There is a bimodal age distribution where fractures can occur in young people after a high-impact injury (eg, motor vehicle collision) and in the elderly after a simple fall.

Clinical Evaluation

Neurovascular examination to document the function of the deep peroneal, superficial peroneal, and medial and lateral plantar nerves distally is crucial. Documentation of the popliteal artery, dorsalis pedis, and posterior tibial artery is also required. Associated injuries include meniscal tears as well as injuries to the collateral and cruciate ligaments, although initial swelling and pain may prevent examination

of these ligaments. When the swelling has reduced, ligamentous testing should be carried out. Consider intra-articular injection of the knee in the acute setting in order to perform a ligamentous examination.

The skin should be carefully examined for any breaks to rule out open fracture. Intra-articular injection of 50 ml sterile normal saline can be performed to rule out communication of the fracture and overlying skin lacerations.

Radiographic Examination

Anteroposterior and lateral x-rays of the knee are part of the standard evaluation (Figure 40–18). Additionally, 40-degree internal or external rotation oblique views can be used to better assess the lateral and medial tibial plateaus, respectively. A 5–10 degree caudally tilted plateau view can be used to evaluate articular step-off. CT scan is best for assessing the articular surface and is often used for preoperative planning. Associated ligamentous injury may be indicated by avulsion of the fibular head (lateral collateral ligament injury) and Segond sign (lateral capsular avulsion off of the lateral tibial plateau, indicating anterior cruciate ligament disruption). MRI should be considered if ligamentous injury is suspected. Arteriography should be performed if vascular injury is suspected.

Classification

Tibial plateau fractures are most commonly classified according to the Schatzker classification: type I (lateral plateau, split fracture), type II (lateral plateau, split depression fracture), type III (lateral plateau, depression fracture), type IV (medial plateau fracture), type V (bicondylar plateau fracture), and type VI (plateau fracture with extension into the metaphysis. Of note, types IV–VI are higher-energy fractures. Type I split fractures usually occur in younger individuals and are often associated with injury to the medial collateral ligament. Type III depression fractures usually occur in older individuals with osteoporotic bone.

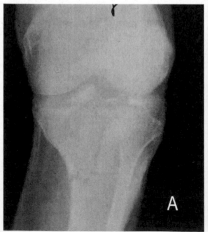
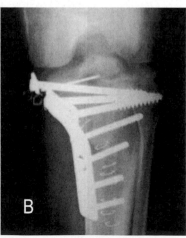

▲ **Figure 40–18.** Schatzker II tibial plateau fracture. **A:** Anteroposterior radiograph. **B:** Radiograph after fixation with lateral plate and bone grafting.

Treatment

Initial treatment for lower-energy fractures usually entails placement in a knee immobilizer locked in full extension and nonweightbearing status with crutches. For higher-energy fractures with significant displacement, placement in a posterior splint or external fixation should be considered.

Nondisplaced or minimally displaced fractures can be treated with protected weightbearing and early knee range of motion in a hinged brace. Radiographs should be taken at regular intervals to ensure no further displacement. Progression to full weightbearing can occur at 8–12 weeks from injury if no further displacement occurs and fracture healing is appreciated radiographically.

Surgical indications include displacement of the articular surface, open fractures, compartment syndrome, or associated vascular injury. A variety of operative methods are used, including external fixation and ORIF with plates or screws depending on fracture type and surgeon preference.

The postoperative course usually entails nonweightbearing with continuous passive motion and progressive active range of motion. Progression to full weightbearing is usually allowed by 8–12 weeks after surgery.

Dirschl DR, Del Gaizo D: Staged management of tibial plateau fractures. Am Orthop 2007;36:12.
Lubowitz JH, Elson WS, Guttmann D: Part I: arthroscopic management of tibial plateau fractures. Arthroscopy 2004;20:1063.
Lubowitz JH, Elson WS, Guttmann D: Part II: arthroscopic treatment of tibial plateau fractures: intercondylar eminence avulsion fractures. Arthroscopy 2005;21:86.

FRACTURE OF THE SHAFTS OF THE TIBIA & FIBULA

Fractures of the tibia and fibula are the most common long bone fractures. Mechanism of injury can be low energy due to twisting/rotation or high energy related to motor vehicle accidents. Isolated fractures of the tibia and/or fibula are rare; these fractures most often occur together.

Anatomy

The tibia is a tubular bone with a triangular cross section. The tibia has a subcutaneous anteromedial border and is otherwise enveloped by four tight fascial compartments (anterior, lateral, posterior, deep posterior). The fibula is responsible for 10–15% of the weightbearing load. The common peroneal nerve is located subcutaneously, traveling around the fibular neck, making it particularly vulnerable to direct blows or traction injuries at this level.

Clinical Evaluation

Neurovascular status, including the deep peroneal, superficial peroneal, and medial and lateral plantar nerves, as well as the posterior tibial artery and dorsalis pedis artery, should

be documented carefully. Thorough skin examination should be performed to rule out open fracture. Additionally, the examiner should have a high suspicion for compartment syndrome in the acute setting. Pain out of proportion, pain with passive stretch, tense compartments, numbness, tingling, and cool toes are all signs of compartment syndrome. For obtunded or intubated patients who cannot relate an accurate history or their symptoms (pain level, presence of numbness/tingling), a monitor can be used to measure pressures in each of the four compartments. Greater than 30 mm Hg or pressure within 30 mm Hg of the diastolic pressure are accepted indications for fasciotomy.

Radiographic Evaluation

Radiographic investigation begins with anteroposterior and lateral x-rays of the tibia and fibula (Figure 40–19). X-rays of the joint above and below should also be performed to rule out other injury. Radiographs should be examined carefully to determine the location and morphology of the fracture and to detect the presence of any secondary fracture lines that could displace during operative management. CT scan and MRI are rarely necessary. Technetium bone scans and MRI can be used in patients with persistent pain to diagnose stress fractures in tibial shafts that were not visible on radiographs.

Classification

Fractures of the tibia shaft can be classified descriptively: open or closed, anatomic location (proximal, middle, distal third), fragment number and position (comminution, butterfly fragments), configuration (transverse, spiral, oblique), angulation (varus/valgus, anterior/posterior), shortening, displacement (percentage of cortical contact), rotation, and associated injuries.

Open fractures are classified according to the Gustilo and Anderson classification, described at the beginning of this chapter.

Treatment

Fracture reduction and closed treatment in a long-leg cast with the knee in 0–5 degrees of flexion may be attempted for isolated, closed, low-energy fractures with minimal displacement and comminution. Protected weightbearing with crutches with advancement to full weightbearing after 2–4 weeks is usually tolerated. After 4–6 weeks, the long-leg cast may be exchanged for a short leg cast or fracture brace. Regular radiographic follow-up is crucial to ensure no further displacement of the fracture. Acceptable parameters for continued closed treatment include less than 5 degrees of varus/valgus angulation, less than 10 degrees of anterior/posterior angulation, less than 10 degrees of rotational deformity (external rotation is tolerated better than internal rotation), less than 1 cm of shortening, and more than 50% cortical contact.

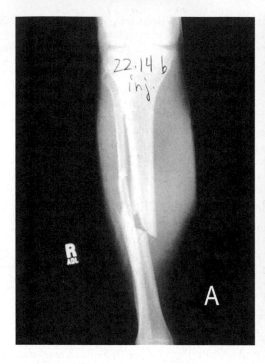

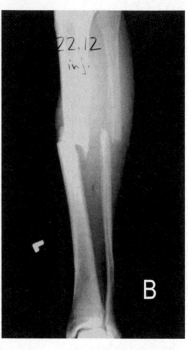

▲ **Figure 40-19. (A)** Antero-posterior and **(B)** lateral radiographs of a displaced midshaft tibia fracture.

Fractures with significant displacement or comminution that requires operative intervention can be treated acutely with a posterior long-leg splint or external fixation if significant shortening is noted. Definitive surgical treatment includes several options: intramedullary nailing, external fixation, plates and screws. Intramedullary nailing is by far the most popular technique because it preserves the periosteal blood supply, optimizing conditions for fracture healing. Compartment syndrome should be treated emergently with 4-compartment fasciotomies. Concomitant fractures of the fibula do not require surgical treatment once the tibia has been stabilized.

Fracture of the Shaft of the Fibula

Isolated fracture of the shaft of the fibula is uncommon, though it can occur with a direct blow to the side of the lower leg. Particular attention should be given to clinical and radiographic examination of the ankle and knee to rule out ligamentous or other subtle bony injuries. If no other injury is present, immobilization is for comfort only. Three weeks or a month in a walking cast or removable cast boot is usually sufficient, and complete healing can be expected.

Mashru RP, Herman MJ, Pizzutillo PD: Tibial shaft fractures in children and adolescents. JAAOS 2005;13:345.
Papadokostakis G et al: The role and efficacy of retrograding nailing for the treatment of diaphyseal and distal femoral fractures: a systematic review of the literature. Injury 2005; 36:813.

INJURIES OF THE ANKLE REGION

1. Ankle Fracture

The incidence of ankle fractures has increased significantly since the 1960s. Most ankle fractures are isolated malleolar fractures; however, bimalleolar and trimalleolar fractures make up approximately one third of the total. Open fractures are rare.

▶ Anatomy

The ankle is a hinge joint composed of the fibula, tibia, and talus articulations along with several important ligaments. Specifically, the distal tibial articular surface is often referred to the plafond, which, combined with the medial and lateral malleoli, forms the mortise, which is a constrained articulation with the talar dome.

The talar dome is trapezoidal in shape and almost entirely covered with articular cartilage. The anterior portion of the talus is wider than the posterior portion. The tibial plafond is also wider anteriorly in order to accommodate the shape of the talus, conferring intrinsic stability to the ankle joint.

The medial malleolus, which articulates with the medial facet of the talus, can be divided into the anterior colliculus and posterior colliculus, which serve as attachments for the superficial and deep deltoid ligaments, respectively. The deltoid ligament provides ligamentous support to the medial aspect of the ankle. The superficial portion of the deltoid is composed of three ligaments: tibionavicular ligament (prevents inward displacement of the talar head), tibiocalcaneal ligament (prevents valgus displacement), and superficial tibiotalar ligament.

The lateral malleolus is the distal portion of the fibula, articulating with the lateral aspect of the talus. The distal fibula is attached to the distal tibia via soft tissue constraint known as the syndesmosis. The syndesmosis, which is made up of four ligaments (anterior inferior tibiofibular, posterior inferior tibiofibular, transverse tibiofibular, and interosseous ligaments), resists axial, rotational, and translational forces, making it critical for ankle stability. The fibular collateral ligament, composed of the anterior talofibular ligament, posterior talofibular ligament, and calcaneofibular ligament, provides additional stability to the lateral aspect of the ankle.

▶ Clinical Evaluation

Neurovascular status (deep peroneal, superficial peroneal, medial and lateral plantar nerves, posterior tibial artery, and dorsalis pedis artery) should all be documented. The skin should be examined for open injury and blistering. The entire length of the fibula, including the proximal portion (head and neck), should be palpated to rule out additional fractures. The "squeeze test" performed approximately 5 cm to the intermalleolar axis can be used to assess for syndesmotic disruption.

▶ Radiographic Evaluation

Initial workup includes anteroposterior, lateral, and mortise (15–20 degrees of internal rotation) x-rays of the ankle. Radiographs of the full tibia and fibula, including the knee joint, should be obtained to identify additional injuries. The dome of the talus should be centered under the tibia in all three views. Tibiofibula overlap of less than 10 mm, tibiofibula clear space greater than 5 mm, and medial clear space between the medial malleolus and talus all indicate syndesmotic disruption. If initial mortise views do not indicate medial clear space widening, an external rotation or gravity stress can be applied to the ankle. If widening of more than 4 mm is noted with this stress, then significant syndesmotic injury is likely. Additionally, talar shift is indicative of ligamentous disruption. CT scan, MRI, and bone scan can be used to further investigate ankle injuries.

▶ Classification

Ankle fractures can be classified according to the Lauge-Hansen system which focuses on four patterns of ankle injury that are the result of different mechanisms. The supination-adduction (SA) fracture pattern usually results in medial displacement of the talus and a transverse or avulsion-type fracture of the fibula distal to the joint and/or a vertical medial malleolus fracture. The supination-external rotation (SER) injury is the most common, producing variable disruption of the anterior talofibular ligament, spiral fracture of the distal fibula, posterior malleolus fracture, and fracture of the medial malleolus or deltoid ligament disruption. The pronation-abduction (PA) and pronation-external rotation (PER) injuries result in variable injury or fracture to the medial malleolus, deltoid ligament, syndesmotic ligament, and distal fibula fractures.

Ankle fractures can also be classified according to the Weber classification based on the level of fibula injury: Weber A (fracture of the fibula below the tibia plafond), Weber B (oblique or spiral fracture of the fibula occurring at or near the level of the syndesmosis), and Weber C (fracture of the fibula above the level of the syndesmosis). The two classification systems correlate as follows: Weber A (SA injury pattern), Weber B (SER), and Weber C (PA or PER).

Other fracture variants include Maisonneuve fracture (ankle injury with fracture of the fibula proximal third) and various avulsion fractures due to disrupted ligaments.

▶ Treatment

The goal of treatment is anatomic restoration of the ankle joint with preservation of fibular length and rotation. Initial treatment includes closed reduction and placement in a well-padded posterior splint with stirrups. Postreduction radiographs should be obtained to ensure correct position of the talus under the tibia. The injured limb should be elevated to the level of the heart at all times.

Nondisplaced, stable fracture patterns (isolated malleolus fractures) without disruption of the syndesmosis can be treated closed—transitioned from the splint to a long-leg cast for 4–6 weeks with serial radiographic examination to ensure no subsequent displacement. After this time, the patient can be transferred to a short-leg cast. Weightbearing is restricted until fracture healing is demonstrated.

Surgical treatment is indicated for displaced medial malleolus fractures and lateral malleolar fractures with displacement greater than 2 mm or any loss of fibular length. Isolated lateral malleolus fractures with minimal displacement and no loss of length should be investigated for syndesmotic injury. Medial-sided tenderness or medial clear-space widening noted radiographically is indicative of additional injury resulting in what is likely an unstable ankle fracture; as a result, surgery is usually recommended.

Surgical treatment includes plates and/or screws. For bimalleolar and trimalleolar fractures, the fibula is initially fixed with a plate and screws. If the medial malleolus fracture remains unreduced, it should be stabilized with screws or tension band construct. Indications for surgical fixation of the posterior malleolus fracture include involvement of more than 25% of the articular surface, persistent displacement greater than 2 mm, or persistent posterior subluxation of the talus. Bimalleolar equivalent fractures (fibula fractures with medial ligament injury or syndesmotic disruption) may require syndesmotic screws. Proximal fibula fractures with syndesmotic disruption can be stabilized with syndesmotic screws once correct fibula length and rotation are achieved via reduction maneuvers.

Postoperative course usually entails nonweightbearing in a splint, cast, or removable boot for 4–6 weeks until fracture healing is appreciated radiographically. Ankle range-of-motion exercises should be started early to prevent postoperative stiffness.

2. Ankle Sprain

Ankle sprain is common, usually the result of forced inversion or eversion of the foot. Pain is usually maximal over the anterolateral aspect or medial aspects of the joint depending on the mechanism of injury. Ankle sprain is a diagnosis of exclusion. If no fractures, dislocations, or widening (> 4 mm) is appreciated between either malleolus and the talus, then ankle sprain is a reasonable diagnosis.

Ankle sprains are usually treated with RICE (rest, ice, compression with elastic bandage, and elevation), nonsteroidal anti-inflammatory drugs (NSAIDs), and nonweightbearing or protected weightbearing with crutches for 3–5 days. Splinting or use of an air cast is optional. Continued pain and/or swelling that have not improved require further work-up.

Ankle Sprain. Institute for Clinical Systems Improvement, 2006.
Dalinka MK et al: Expert Panel on Musculoskeletal Imaging. Suspected ankle fractures. American College of Radiology, 2005. Available at http://www.acr.org/SecondaryMainMenu Categories/quality_safety/app_criteria/pdf/ExpertPanelon MusculoskeletalImaging/SuspectedAnkleFracturesDoc21.aspx. Accessed February 14, 2009.

3. Syndesmosis Injuries

Syndesmotic injuries account for approximately 1% of all ankle ligament injuries. Many of these injuries go undiagnosed and can lead to chronic ankle pain and instability if not treated appropriately.

▶ Clinical Evaluation & Diagnosis

Patients often present late, several hours or even days after a twisting injury to ankle, with persistent swelling, pain, and difficulty bearing weight. The fibula should be palpated along its entire length, proximally and distally. Two clinical tests have been used to evaluate for isolated syndesmotic injury: (1) The squeeze test indicates injury if squeezing the fibula at mid calf reproduces distal tibiofibular pain. (2) For the external rotation test, the patient is seated with knee flexed to 90 degrees, the examiner stabilizes the patient's leg and externally rotates the foot; if pain is reproduced at the syndesmosis, then injury is likely.

▶ Radiographic Evaluation

Radiographic evaluation starts with anteroposterior, lateral, and mortise views of the ankle looking for widening of the medial clear space between the medial malleolus and the medial border of the talus or widening of the tibiofibular clear space (interval between the medial border of the fibula and the lateral border of the posterior tibial malleolus). If no injury is appreciated, external rotation stress view (mortise

view with an external rotation stress applied to the foot with the leg stabilized) should be performed.

▶ Classification

Syndesmotic injuries can be organized according to the Edwards and DeLee classification: type 1 (diastasis involving lateral subluxation without fracture), type 2 (lateral subluxation with plastic deformation of the fibula), type 3 (posterior subluxation/dislocation of the fibula), and type 4 (superior subluxation/dislocation of the talus).

▶ Treatment

Patients can be initially immobilized in a nonweightbearing cast for 2–3 weeks, followed by use of an ankle-foot orthosis that eliminates external rotation of the foot for an additional 3 weeks. Operative intervention with syndesmotic screws from the fibula to the tibia is considered for patients with an irreducible diastasis. These patients are often kept nonweightbearing for 6 weeks with screw removal at 12–16 weeks.

4. Pilon Fractures

▶ Epidemiology

Tibial plafond, or "pilon," fractures involve the weightbearing surface of the distal tibia that articulates with the talus (Figure 40–20). Pilon fractures account for 7–10% of all tibia fractures. Most occur in men aged 30–40 years from high-energy mechanisms such as motor vehicle collisions or falls from significant height. As a result, extra care should be taken to rule out concomitant injuries. Specifically, tibial plateau, calcaneus, and pelvis and vertebral fractures should be ruled out.

▶ Mechanism of Injury

A fall from significant height results in an axial compression force directed through the talus into the tibial plafond, causing impaction and comminution of the articular surface. Shear injuries, such as can occur in a skiing accident, will result in a fracture with two or more large fragments and minimal comminution. Combined compression and shear result in fracture pattern that is somewhere in between.

▶ Clinical Evaluation

Examination of the patient includes documentation of a neurovascular examination and secondary survey to rule out other injuries. Careful skin examination should be performed to exclude open fracture. Swelling is often rapid and considerable, potentially resulting in skin necrosis and blistering depending on fracture displacement. As a result, these fractures should be reduced provisionally and placed in a splint as soon as possible. The amount of swelling should be noted; some authors advocate delaying operation for 7–10 days to allow swelling to subside or until "skin wrinkling" is appreciated to avoid postoperative wound complications.

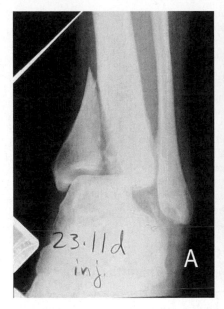 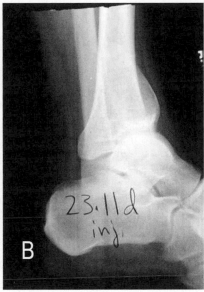

▲ **Figure 40–20.** Axial loading injury to the ankle joint with the foot in dorsiflexion leading to a fracture of the tibial plafond. Anteroposterior **(A)** and lateral **(B)** radiographs.

▶ Radiographic Evaluation

Initial radiographic evaluation includes anteroposterior, lateral, and mortise views of the ankle joint. CT scan with thin-cut coronal and sagittal reconstructions is useful for preoperative evaluation of the fracture pattern and articular surface. Radiographs of the contralateral side, which can be used for preoperative templating, should be considered.

▶ Classification

The Ruedi and Algower classification is most commonly used: type 1 (nondisplaced fracture), type 2 (displaced fracture with minimal impaction and comminution), and type 3 (displaced fracture with significant comminution and/or metaphyseal impaction).

▶ Treatment

Choice of treatment is based on multiple factors, including the fracture pattern; age of patient; patient's functional status; severity of injury to soft tissues, bone, and cartilage; degree of comminution and/or osteoporosis; other injuries to the patient; and comfort level of the surgeon.

Nonoperative treatment, which involves long-leg cast for 6 weeks followed by bracing and range-of-motion exercises with progressive weightbearing, is reserved for the nondisplaced fracture or severely debilitated patients.

Displaced fractures are usually treated surgically. Surgery may be delayed for 7–14 days to allow the soft tissues to calm down in an effort to avoid postoperative wound complications. Skin wrinkling may indicate that enough swelling has subsided for operative intervention to occur. Spanning external fixation should be considered initially to provide stabiliza-

tion, partial fracture reduction, and restoration of length while waiting for final surgical management. Associated fibula fractures may undergo ORIF at the time of fixator application.

The goals of operative fixation of pilon fractures include restoration of fibula length and stability, restoration of the tibial articular surface, buttressing of the distal tibia, and bone grafting metaphyseal defects as needed. Definitive surgical management may involve plates and screws, external fixation, or a combination thereof.

5. Achilles Tendon Rupture

▶ Epidemiology

Achilles tendon problems are often related to overuse injury. In the setting of trauma, acute rupture can occur. Delayed or missed diagnosis is common, so caregivers should therefore have a high index of suspicion for this injury.

▶ Anatomy

The Achilles tendon is the largest tendon in the body. It has a paratenon with visceral and parietal layers instead of a true synovial sheath, allowing approximately 1.5 cm of tendon glide. There are three sources for the tendon's blood supply: (1) musculotendinous junction, (2) osseous insertion, and (3) multiple mesosternal vessels on the tendon's anterior surface.

▶ Clinical Evaluation

Complete rupture often results in a palpable defect in the tendon that is not present with an incomplete injury. In the setting of complete rupture, the Thompson test (plantar flexion with calf squeeze) is positive (no plantar flexion occurs) and the patient is unable to perform a single heel-raise.

▶ Treatment

Surgical treatment compared with nonoperative management results in lower recurrent rupture rates, improved strength, and a higher percentage of patients returning to sports activities. However, significant complication rates are associated with surgery, including wound infection, skin necrosis, and nerve injuries. As a result, surgery is usually reserved for the young, athletic patient looking to return to playing sports.

Nonoperative treatment usually entails 2 weeks of immobilization in a plantar-flexed splint, followed by 6–8 weeks of cast immobilization with progressive dorsiflexion to neutral and slow advancement of weightbearing. Cast removal is followed by the use of a heel-lift with eventual transition back to normal shoes. Progressive resistive exercises are started at 8–10 weeks from injury, with return to sports at 4–6 months. Maximal recovery can take up to 1 year; some residual weakness is often present.

Operative treatment can be done percutaneously or through a medial longitudinal approach. Postoperative management is similar to that used for closed treatment.

6. Peroneal Tendon Subluxation

Subluxation or frank dislocation of the peroneal tendon is rare, usually resulting from injury sustained during sports activities such as skiing. Clinical evaluation reveals lateral ankle swelling and tenderness posterior to the lateral malleolus. Radiographs may show a small fleck of bone off of the posterior aspect of the lateral malleolus indicating avulsion injury. MRI can be used for evaluation if diagnosis remains unclear. Treatment involves reduction of the tendon and placement in a well-molded cast with foot in slight plantar flexion and mild inversion. If dislocation of the tendon continues, operative intervention may be considered.

INJURIES OF THE FOOT

1. The Talus
▶ Anatomy

Sixty percent of the talus is covered by articular cartilage, including the superior surface, which is the weightbearing portion. The cartilage extends medially and laterally in a plantar direction allowing articulation with the medial and lateral malleoli. The inferior surface of the talar body articulates with the calcaneus. The anterior aspect of the talus is wider than the posterior aspect, conferring inherent stability to the ankle joint. The neck of the talus extends from the body proximally and posteriorly, deviates medially, and join the talar head anteriorly and distally. The talar neck is most vulnerable to fracture. The head of the talus meets with the navicular bone anteriorly, the spring ligament inferiorly, the sustentaculum tali posteroinferiorly, and the deltoid ligament medially. The lateral process of the talus meets the posterior calcaneal facet inferiorly and the lateral malleolus superolaterally. The posterior process of the talus has a medial and lateral tubercle separated by a groove for the flexor hallucis longus tendon. An os trigonum, which can be mistaken for fracture, is present just posterior to the lateral tubercle in up to 50% of normal feet. The blood supply to the talus is composed of arteries to the sinus tarsi (originating from the peroneal and dorsalis pedis artery), an artery of the tarsal canal (posterior tibial artery), and the deltoid artery (posterior tibial artery). The vascular supply reaches the talus through various fascial structures; when these structures are disrupted (eg, with dislocation), avascular necrosis of the talus can result.

▶ Fractures of the Talus
A. Epidemiology and Mechanism of Injury

Fractures of the talus represent approximately 2% of all lower extremity injuries. These injuries most commonly occur from high-energy mechanisms such as falls from significant height or motor vehicle accidents, resulting in hyperdorsiflexion and causing the talar neck to impact the anterior portion of the tibia.

B. Clinical Presentation and Radiographic Examination

Patients typically present with foot pain and diffuse swelling of the hindfoot. Associated fractures of the ankle and foot are common.

Initial radiographs include anteroposterior, lateral, and mortise views of the ankle as well as anteroposterior, lateral, and oblique views of the foot. A Canale view with the ankle in maximum equinus (plantar-flexion), pronated 15 degrees and the radiograph machine directed 15 degrees from the vertical, provides optimal visualization of the talar neck. Additionally, a CT scan should be considered for better fracture characterization and to assess for any articular involvement. Bone scan and/or MRI should be considered for patients with persistent hindfoot pain despite negative radiographs to look for occult fractures of the talar neck.

C. Classification

Fractures of the talus are classified initially according to their anatomic location: talar neck fractures, talar body fractures, talar head fractures, lateral process fractures, and posterior process fractures.

Fractures of the talar neck are further subclassified according to the Hawkins classification: I (nondisplaced), II (with associated subtalar dislocation), III (with associated subtalar and tibiotalar dislocation), and IV (associated subtalar, tibiotalar, and talonavicular dislocations).

D. Treatment

Truly nondisplaced fractures with no signs of articular comminution on CT scan can be treated nonoperatively initially in a short-leg cast, no weightbearing for at least 6 weeks until radiographic signs of healing are noted, followed by progressive weightbearing.

Displaced fractures should be treated with closed reduction and splint placement. Open or irreducible fractures require immediate operative treatment. Surgery entails ORIF with plates and screws.

Other Fractures of the Talus

Lateral process fractures of the talus are commonly seen in snowboarders. These fractures are often misdiagnosed as ankle sprains upon initial presentation. If the fracture is displaced less than 2 mm, then it can be treated closed with a short leg cast. Greater than 2 mm of displacement requires operative intervention.

Posterior process fractures of the talus can be difficult to diagnose due to the presence of the os trigonum. Nondisplaced or minimally displaced fractures of the posterior process can be treated with a nonweightbearing short-leg cast. Displaced fractures require surgical treatment with ORIF.

Talar head fractures may be associated with fractures of the navicular bone or talonavicular disruption. Nondisplaced or minimally displaced fractures can be treated for 6 weeks in a partial weightbearing short-leg cast molded to preserve the longitudinal arch. After discontinuation of the cast, an arch support should be worn in the shoe to reduce stress on the talonavicular articulation for an additional 4–6 months. Displaced fractures are treated with ORIF and/or primary excision of small fragments.

Complications

The most common complication is posttraumatic arthritis. Avascular necrosis occurs as well and correlates with initial fracture displacement: Hawkins I (0–15%), Hawkins II (20–50%), Hawkins III (20–100%), and Hawkins IV (100%). Other complications include delayed union or nonunion, malunion, and wound complications.

Subtalar Dislocation

Subtalar dislocation is defined by the simultaneous dislocation of the distal articulations of the talocalcaneal and talonavicular joints. Inversion of the foot results in medial subtalar dislocation, while eversion causes lateral subtalar dislocation. The large majority of these dislocations (approximately 85%) are medial. All subtalar dislocations should be reduced as soon as possible with knee flexion and accentuation of the deformity to unlock the calcaneus and longitudinal traction. Subtalar dislocations are often stable once closed reduction is achieved. CT scan should be performed postreduction to assess for other associated fractures or continued subluxation. Failed closed reduction may be due to interposed extensor digitorum brevis muscle in the case of a medial dislocation or posterior tibial tendon for lateral dislocation. Unsuccessful closed reduction requires operative intervention.

Total Dislocation of the Talus

Total dislocation of the talus is rare and usually an open injury. In general, ORIF is required. Complications including infection, osteonecrosis, and posttraumatic arthritis.

2. The Calcaneus

Fracture of the Calcaneus

A. Epidemiology

The calcaneus is the most frequently fractured tarsal bone, constituting approximately 2% of all fractures. The large majority of calcaneus fractures occur in men aged 21–45 years.

B. Mechanism

Most intra-articular calcaneus fractures are the result of axial loading where the talus is driven into the calcaneus during a fall from significant height or a motor vehicle accident. Extra-articular calcaneus fractures may be the result of twisting injuries. For diabetic patients, there is an increased incidence of calcaneus tuberosity fractures resulting from Achilles avulsion injuries.

C. Clinical Presentation

Patients often present with significant heel pain, swelling, and ecchymosis. When open fractures occur, they most often occur on the medial side of the foot. Compartment syndrome should be carefully ruled out. Associated injuries to rule out include lumbar spine injuries and other lower extremity fractures. Of note, bilateral calcaneus fractures occur approximately 10% of the time.

D. Radiographic Evaluation

Initial radiographs include a lateral radiograph of the hindfoot, anteroposterior of the foot, a Harris axial view, and standard ankle series. The lateral radiograph should be examined to determine the Böhler tuber joint angle (intersection of the line drawn from the anterior process to the highest point of the posterior facet and the line drawn from the superior aspect of the calcaneal tuberosity to the highest point of the posterior facet). The Böhler angle is usually 20–40 degrees. A decrease in this angle indicates significant depression of the weightbearing posterior facet. The anteroposterior radiograph should be examined for extension of the fracture into the calcaneocuboid joint. A Harris axial view can be taken with the foot maximally dorsiflexed and the radiograph beam directed 45 degrees cephalad to better visualize the articular surface. However, dorsiflexion may be difficult because of patient discomfort. CT scan with 3–5 mm cuts offers the best characterization of the articular surface and as a result is most useful for preoperative planning (Figure 40–21).

E. Classification

Extra-articular fractures of the calcaneus include fractures of the anterior process, calcaneal tuberosity, medial process, sustentaculum tali, and body fractures outside of the articular surface. Anterior process and calcaneal tuberosity fractures are best seen on lateral radiographs. Fractures of the medial process, sustentacular, or body fractures are best investigated on axial views or CT scan. Intra-articular fractures can be classified according to the Sanders classification, which is based on the coronal cuts of CT scans showing the number and location of articular fracture fragments. The posterior facet of the calcaneus is divided into three fractures lines (A, B, C) moving from lateral to medial. There can be a total of four pieces: lateral, central, medial, and sustentaculum tali. The classification is as follows: type I (all nondisplaced fractures regardless of number of fracture lines), type II (2-part fracture, with further subclassification based on the location of the fracture line IIA, IIB, IIC), type III (3-part fractures, subtypes IIIAB, IIIAC, IIIBC), and type IV (4-part articular fractures).

F. Treatment

Treatment remains controversial—even with adequate reduction, fractures of the calcaneus often result in chronic pain and functional disability. Nonoperative indications include nondisplaced or minimally displaced extra-articular fractures, nondisplaced intra-articular fractures, anterior process fractures with less than 25% involvement of the calcaneocuboid articulation, fractures in patients with severe peripheral vascular occlusive disease or diabetes (due to frequent wound complications associated with surgery), fractures in patients with other severe medical comorbidities, and fractures associated with significant soft tissue compromise. Initial treatment involves placement in a bulky Jones splint or dressing with avoidance of pressure on the heel. The splint is converted to a prefabricated boot locked in neutral to prevent equinus contracture and elastic compression stocking to prevent dependent edema. Early subtalar and ankle joint range of motion is started; nonweightbearing is instituted for approximately 10–12 weeks until radiographic healing is appreciated.

Operative indications include displaced intra-articular fractures, fractures of the anterior process with more than 25% involvement of the calcaneocuboid joint, displaced calcaneal tuberosity fractures, fracture dislocations of the calcaneus, open fractures of the calcaneus, tuberosity fractures that are displaced resulting in prominence through the skin, incompetence of the gastrocnemius-soleus complex, and/or fractures extending into the articular surface. Surgery should only be attempted 7–14 days after the injury, allowing enough time for swelling to subside. Fracture fixation depends on the type of fracture. Anterior process fractures are typically fixed with small or minifragment screws. Calcaneal tuberosity fractures usually require lag screw fixation with or without cerclage wire. Intra-articular posterior facet fractures may be fixed with lag screws into the sustentaculum tali and a thin lateral plate providing a lateral buttress. Postoperatively, the patient is kept nonweightbearing for 8–12 weeks with early subtalar range-of-motion exercises.

3. Fractures of the Midfoot

▶ Epidemiology, Mechanism of Injury, & Anatomy

Fractures of the midfoot are relatively rare, most often resulting from direct impact during a motor vehicle accident or a combination of axial loading and torsion during fall from a significant height. The midfoot consists of five bones: navicular, cuboid, medial, middle, and lateral cuneiforms. The midtarsal joint consists of the calcaneocuboid and talonavicular articulations, which act together with the subtalar joint during eversion and inversion of the foot. The cuboid extends distal to the three naviculocuneiform joints, minimizing motion at this level.

▶ Clinical & Radiographic Evaluation

Patient presentation is variable, ranging from a limp with mild swelling and dorsal foot tenderness to a grossly swollen, painful midfoot resulting in nonambulatory status. Initial radiographs include anteroposterior, lateral, and oblique x-rays of

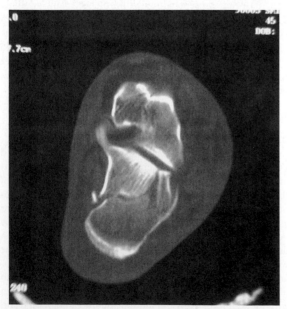

▲ **Figure 40–21.** Axial CT section showing a fracture of the calcaneus caused by an axial loading mechanism.

the foot. Stress views and weightbearing x-rays can provide additional detail, including detection of any ligamentous instability. CT scan is best for characterizing fracture dislocations or discovering injuries that are otherwise undetected on x-ray. MRI may be used to evaluate ligamentous injury.

Navicular Bone

The navicular is the keystone bone of the foot's medial longitudinal arch, transmitting motion from the subtalar joint to the forefoot. The talonavicular articular surface is concave and has a significant arc of motion. The distal articular surface has three separate facets for the three cuneiforms. Not much motion occurs at these joints. The navicular tuberosity is the medial prominence located on the inferior aspect of the navicular bone; it provides an attachment point for the posterior tibial tendon. Anatomic variants include the shape of the tuberosity and the presence of an accessory navicular bone (occurs up to 15% of the time and is bilateral in 70–90% of cases).

Patients typically present with painful foot and dorsomedial swelling and tenderness. Radiographic evaluation can include medial and lateral oblique x-rays of the midfoot, in addition to the standard foot series, to assess the lateral pole of the navicular as well as the medial tuberosity.

Classification

There are three basic types of navicular fractures with a subclassification of the body type fractures. Avulsion-type fractures can involve the talonavicular or naviculocuneiform ligaments. Tuberosity fractures usually involve disruption of the tibialis posterior tendon insertion without damage to the joint surface. Type I body fractures divide the navicular into dorsal and plantar pieces. Type II body fractures split the navicular into medial and lateral pieces. Type III body fractures are comminuted and often have significant displacement of the medial and lateral poles.

Treatment

Nondisplaced fractures without instability may be treated closed in a cast or boot, nonweightbearing for 6–8 weeks. Disruption of the articular surface of more than 2 mm requires operative intervention. Small fragments may be excised if symptomatic. Larger fragments (> 25% of the articular surface) require ORIF with lag screw fixation. If more than 40% of the talonavicular joint cannot be reconstructed, acute talonavicular fusion should be considered. Isolated dislocation or subluxation of the navicular bone without fracture requires surgical stabilization.

Cuboid Bone

The cuboid bone is part of the lateral column of the foot, articulating with the calcaneus proximally, the navicular and lateral cuneiform medially, and the fourth and fifth metatarsals distally. The peroneus longus travels through a groove on the plantar surface of the cuboid on its way to its insertion at the base of the first metatarsal. Injury to the cuboid bone is usually seen in conjunction with injury to the talonavicular or Lisfranc joints. Patients typically present with dorsolateral foot pain and swelling. In addition to foot series, stress radiographs and CT scan should be considered. MRI can be used to evaluate for stress fractures that are otherwise not seen on radiograph. Cuboid fractures without articular disruption or any loss of length can be treated closed and nonweightbearing in a boot for 6–8 weeks. If more than 2 mm of disruption of the articular surface is appreciated or the cuboid is compressed, than ORIF should be pursued. Calcaneocuboid fusion should be considered for fractures with residual articular displacement.

Tarsometatarsal (Lisfranc) Joint

Injury to the Lisfranc joint is relatively rare. However, given that up to 20% of the time this injury goes undiagnosed initially, suspicion should remain high, especially in the polytrauma patients with foot swelling or pain.

In the anteroposterior plane, the base of the second metatarsal is recessed between the medial and lateral cuneiforms, limiting translation. In the coronal plane, the middle three metatarsal bones have trapezoid-shaped bases that form a transverse arch, preventing displacement in the plantar direction. The second metatarsal base is a keystone, responsible for the inherent stability of the transmetatarsal joint. The Lisfranc ligament travels from the medial cuneiform to the base of the second metatarsal bone, providing additional stability. Of note, the dorsalis pedis artery travels between the first and second metatarsal bones at the Lisfranc joint; as a result, it is vulnerable to injury with disruption or manipulation of this joint.

There are three common mechanisms of injury: (1) twisting (forced abduction of the forefoot) such as is seen in equestrians who fall from a horse with their foot caught in the stirrup, (2) axial load, and (3) crush.

Clinical evaluation includes careful neurovascular documentation given the proximity of the dorsalis pedis artery to this joint. Additionally, compartment syndrome of the foot should be ruled out. Stress testing applying gentle forefoot abduction or pronation with the hindfoot stabilized may be performed.

Radiographic evaluation includes anteroposterior, lateral, and oblique views of the foot. Normally, the medial border of the second metatarsal should be collinear with the medial border of the middle cuneiform on the anteroposterior view; additionally, the medial border of the fourth metatarsal should line up with the medial border of the cuboid bone. Dorsal displacement of the metatarsals on the lateral view is also indicative of ligamentous injury. Weightbearing views should be performed to detect any displacement. CT scan can provide greater detail. Associated injuries to the cuneiforms, cuboid, and/or metatarsals are common and should be ruled out.

If no instability (displacement) is appreciated on standard and stress radiographs, a diagnosis of midfoot sprain may be considered with initial nonweightbearing treatment and progressive weightbearing as comfort allows. Repeat x-rays should be obtained once swelling has subsided. For any displacement of the tarsometatarsal joint greater than 2 mm, surgery should be pursued with screws and Kirschner wires.

▶ Fractures of the Forefoot

Fractures of the first metatarsal are rare because of its larger size and increased strength compared to the other metatarsals. Isolated fractures of the first metatarsal without instability may be treated with weightbearing as tolerated in a short-leg cast or removable boot for 4–6 weeks. If displacement is detected of the first metatarsal through the joint or fracture site, operative intervention is required.

Fractures of the second, third, or fourth metatarsals are much more common. Most isolated fractures can be treated closed with hard-soled shoes and progressive weightbearing. Operative indications include fractures with more than 10 degrees of deviation in a dorsal or plantar direction or 3–4 mm of translation in any plane.

Fifth metatarsal fractures usually result from direct trauma and are divided into two groups: proximal base fractures and distal spiral fractures. The proximal fifth metatarsal fractures are further subdivided: zone I (cancellous tuberosity, which is the insertion of the peroneal brevis), zone II (distal to the tuberosity), and zone III (distal to the proximal ligaments, without extension past the proximal 1.5 cm of the diaphyseal shaft). Zone I injuries are treated symptomatically with hard-soled shoe. The treatment of zone II injuries, or Jones fractures, is controversial because of healing difficulty. Some authors advocate weightbearing as tolerated; others recommend nonweightbearing in a short-leg cast or surgical intervention. Zone III injuries may be treated with nonweightbearing in a cast or with surgery. Fractures distal to the proximal 1.5 cm of the diaphyseal shaft are called dancer's fractures and are treated symptomatically with a hard-soled shoe.

4. Metatarsophalangeal Joint

Injuries to the first metatarsophalangeal joint are relatively common, especially in persons who participate in athletic activities such as ballet, football, or soccer. The metatarsophalangeal joint is composed of a cam-shaped metatarsal head articulating with the concave proximally articular surface of the proximal phalanx. The stability of the joint is provided by ligamentous constraints, which include the medial and lateral collateral ligaments as well as the dorsal capsule and plantar plate, which are reinforced by the extensor hallucis longus and flexor hallucis longus tendons, respectively. "Turf toe," which is a hyperextension injury of the first metatarsophalangeal joint, resulting in stretching of the plantar capsule and plate, may be treated with RICE, NSAIDs, and protective taping with gradual return to activity. Metatarsophalangeal dislocations are treated with closed reduction and a short-leg cast with toe extension for 3–4 weeks. Dislocations with displaced avulsion fractures require surgical intervention with lag screws or tension-band technique.

Injuries to the lesser metatarsophalangeal joints are common as well. Simple dislocations or nondisplaced fractures are managed with gentle reduction and buddy taping. Intra-articular fractures may be treated with excision for small fragments or ORIF with Kirschner wires or screws.

5. Fractures & Dislocations of the Phalanges of the Toes

Phalangeal fractures are the most common injury to the forefoot. The proximal phalanx of the fifth toe is the most common phalanx injured. Like the fifth digit, the first digit is also particularly vulnerable to injury because of its border position in the foot. Mechanisms of injury usually entails direct blow such as from a dropped heavy object or axial load resulting from a stubbing injury. Fractures and/or dislocations are diagnosed with foot series radiographs (anteroposterior, lateral, oblique). MRI or bone scan may aid in the diagnosis of stress fractures that are not visible on x-ray. Nondisplaced fractures are treated with stiff-soled shoe and protected weightbearing with advancement as tolerated. Buddy taping may be used as well. Fractures with clinical deformity require reduction. Operative intervention is performed only for those rare fractures with gross instability or persistent intra-articular deformity. Dislocated interphalangeal joints without fracture are usually amenable to closed reduction and buddy taping with progressive advancement of activity.

6. Fracture of the Sesamoids of the Great Toe

Fracture of the sesamoid bones is rare, occurring with hyperextension injuries in ballet dancers and runners. The medial sesamoid is more frequently fractured than the lateral sesamoid due to increased weightbearing on the medial side of the foot. Fractures of the sesamoids must be distinguished from bipartite sesamoids, which are relatively common, occurring in up to 30% of the general population (bilateral in 85% of cases). These fractures are initially treated closed with soft padding and a short-leg walking cast for 4 weeks followed by shoe with metatarsal pad for an additional 4–8 weeks. Sesamoidectomy is reserved for cases of failed conservative treatment.

Bucholz et al: *Rockwood and Green's Fractures in Adults,* 6th ed. Lippincott Williams & Wilkins, 2006.

Fischgrund JS: *OKU 9: Orthopedic Knowledge Update.* American Academy of Orthopaedic Surgeons, 2008.

Koval KJ, Zuckerman JD: *Handbook of Fractures,* 3rd ed. Lippincott Williams & Wilkins, 2002.

PEDIATRIC ORTHOPEDICS

CHILDREN'S FRACTURES & DISLOCATIONS

Children's skeletal injuries differ from those of adults in several significant ways. An important difference is the presence of the growth plate or physis, giving immature bone its potential for longitudinal growth. Bones increase in diameter by appositional growth from the periosteum. Injuries to the physis may disrupt skeletal growth. Children's bones heal rapidly, and nonunion is exceedingly rare. The periosteum is thick and strong, surrounding the long bone like a sleeve, and helps to minimize fracture displacement and promote healing.

When injury occurs in a young child, especially one under 3 years of age, a careful social history should be taken (see Chapter 43). State law in all jurisdictions requires that suspected cases of abuse be reported to local authorities.

Closed treatment is usually sufficient for children's fractures. Manipulation, also known as closed reduction under sedation, may be required for significant displaced fractures. Open fractures, fractures with articular surface displacement, and, less commonly, fractures that cannot be reduced by closed means require operative treatment.

Children's fractures heal rapidly, and immobilization rarely causes joint stiffness in children, so casts can be left on until union is achieved.

The bone in growing children is mechanically different from that in adults; immature bone is more porous and fails in compression as well as in tension. An example is the so-called buckle or torus fracture that occurs at the metaphysis of the distal radius. This stable injury should be protected in plaster for 3 weeks to control symptoms and prevent further trauma to the weakened bone.

Immature bone is less brittle than that of adults, and children's bones may therefore bend but not fracture. This plastic deformation may produce significant deformity that requires manipulation to restore alignment

Greenstick fractures are also a result of the plasticity of children's bones. Incomplete disruption of a long bone occurs such that the bone fractures on the tension side but the opposite cortex remains in continuity. The periosteum remains intact on the concave side, and typically, the intact cortex resists any significant angulation at the fracture site.

1. Growth Plate Fractures

About 15% of children's fractures involve a growth plate—most commonly the distal radius, distal tibia or fibula (or both), and distal humerus.

▶ Classification

Classification of physeal injuries helps to distinguish patterns that may disturb growth and also provides some guidance for treatment. It should be recognized that even "benign" injuries to the growth plate of the distal femoral and tibia can have clinically significant consequences.

Physeal injuries are classified according to the Salter-Harris system (Figure 40–22).

A. Type I

Type I injuries have fracture lines that follow the growth plate, separating the epiphysis from metaphysis. Without displacement, radiographs may appear normal. This is often a clinical diagnosis with tenderness localized over the physis confirming that a growth plate injury has occurred. Healing occurs rapidly, usually within 2–3 weeks.

B. Type II

In type II injuries, the fracture line traverses the epiphysis and exits in the metaphysic. The metaphyseal fragment is often referred to as the Thurston-Holland sign and is diagnostic of a growth plate injury. Type II injuries are the most common physeal fractures. Satisfactory alignment can often be achieved with gentle closed reduction and casting. If pin fixation is required, smooth pins can be safely used across the physis. The risk of growth disturbance is highest for distal femoral and distal tibial fractures.

C. Type III

Type III physeal injuries are those in which the fracture line exits through the epiphysis at the articular surface. Any displacement at the articular surface requires operative intervention.

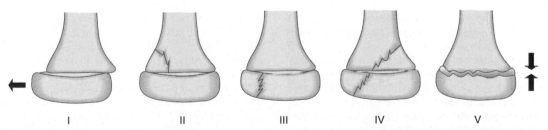

▲ **Figure 40–22.** Salter-Harris classification of physeal injuries occurring at the zone of provisional calcification of the growth plate.

D. Type IV

Salter-Harris type IV fractures cross both the metaphysic and the epiphysis. Because it involves the articular surface, anatomic reduction is essential to minimize the complications of type IV growth plate fractures, including growth disturbance, malunion, and articular incongruity. Even with perfect reduction, growth may be affected, and the prognosis is guarded.

E. Type V

Type V growth plate injuries are due to severe axial loading. Some or all of the physis is so severely compressed that growth potential is destroyed. Initial radiographs may appear normal, as in Salter-Harris type I injuries. A history of a significant mechanism with swelling and tenderness over the physis should suggest the possibility of such an injury. Subsequent follow-up radiographs are critical to watch for premature closure of the physis and/or progressive angular deformity due to asymmetric injury to the growth plate.

▶ Treatment

A. Conservative Treatment

Most fractures involving the physis may be managed nonoperatively. Nondisplaced fractures are protected in a cast until healed. Typically, 3–6 weeks is sufficient depending on the child's age and the site of injury. Displaced type I and type II injuries should be treated with a single attempt at closed reduction followed by immobilization as described previously. Because of the significant remodeling potential, acceptance of some deformity is better than repeated vigorous attempts at reduction, which causes additional damage to the physis. Attempts at reduction should be avoided if more than 7 days have passed since the injury.

B. Operative Treatment

Displaced type III and type IV injuries usually require ORIF. Fixation is ideally placed within the metaphysic or epiphysis. If it is necessary to cross the physis, only smooth pin fixation is recommended. Cast immobilization may be required to supplement fixation.

▶ Prognosis

All injuries that involve physes should be followed at least 12–18 months to confirm that growth has not been disrupted. The parents should be warned at the time of the injury of the possibility of altered growth. Physeal arrest may result in angular deformity and/or limb-length inequality. When a physeal bar is suspected, CT scan or MRI can be used to localize the area and estimate its size. If the bony bar is less than 50% of the physis and the child has at least 2 years of growth remaining, resection of the bar can be considered. Alternatively, the portion of the physis that remains open can be intentionally closed down to limit angular deformity.

Limb-length inequalities will occur if there is a complete physeal arrest. If the difference is less than 2 cm, no treatment is typically required. Differences of 2–5 cm are most frequently managed with an epiphysiodesis on the contralateral limb. Limb lengthening techniques can be considered with limb-length inequalities exceeding 5 cm.

2. Upper Extremity Fractures & Dislocations
▶ Proximal Humeral Fractures

Separation of the unossified proximal humeral epiphysis has been described following difficult delivery of an infant. The child is unable to use the arm, raising the concern for brachial plexus palsy. This "pseudoparalysis" resolves in 7–10 days, and radiographs demonstrate abundant callus, confirming the fracture. Older children most commonly sustain Salter-Harris II fractures. Significant displacement and angulation is well tolerated, and the child can be treated in a sling for 3 weeks. In the adolescent approaching maturity, displaced fractures are treated with closed reduction and pin fixation. There is so much potential for remodeling in the proximal humerus that the best obtainable closed reduction is preferable to open surgery. Residual deformity, loss of motion, and functional problems are exceedingly rare following sustain proximal humerus fractures.

▶ Supracondylar Fractures of the Humerus

Supracondylar fractures are among the most common injury in children ages 4–8 years. The typical mechanism is a hyperextension injury to the elbow. Type 1 undisplaced supracondylar fractures present with elbow pain, swelling, and tenderness at the site. Radiographs usually show a positive fat pad sign, indicating elbow hemarthrosis and a nondisplaced fracture of the distal humerus anteriorly. The fracture line may be subtle, so comparison radiographs of the uninjured elbow may be helpful. Cast immobilization for 3–4 weeks is recommended. Type II fractures are those in which there is posterior angulation of the distal fragment, with an intact periosteal hinge. The anterior humeral line no longer bisects the capitellum on the lateral radiograph. Closed reduction and pinning is advised to restore this relationship. Type III fractures are completely displaced. These are serious injuries that threaten the neurovascular structures. The radial pulse and the function of the radial, ulnar, and median (including anterior interosseous) nerves should be checked immediately. If ischemia is present initially, prompt reduction of deformity is the next step toward restoration of normal perfusion. If pulses cannot be restored with reduction, then an angiogram and vascular consultation is urgent. When the loss of pulses occurs following attempts at reduction, vascular entrapment should be suspected, and prompt surgical exploration of the brachial artery may be required.

Fracture reduction is secured with percutaneous pin fixation and splint immobilization for 4–6 weeks. Long-term problems include elbow stiffness, malunion, and growth arrest. Nerve injuries typically represent neuropraxias that resolve with observation over the subsequent 3–6 months.

Flexion-type supracondylar fractures are rare, but when they do occur, they are typically managed with open reduction and pin fixation. The ulnar nerve is most at risk with these injuries.

Subluxation of the Radial Head (Nursemaid's Elbow)

This common minor injury occurs in children under 4 years old. It is caused by a sudden pull on the extended pronated arm, usually by an adult tugging on a reluctant toddler. The pronated radial head slips partially under the annular ligament and displaces into the radiocapitellar joint. The child suddenly stops using the arm, holding it in a flexed and pronated position. Radiographs show no abnormalities, since positioning for elbow films will often reduce the subluxation. Reduction is achieved by firmly supinating the forearm and flexing the elbow while pressing down on the radial head. Often, a "click" is felt when reduction is achieved. Soon after reduction the child becomes less apprehensive and gradually resumes use of the arm.

Other Fractures & Dislocations of the Elbow

There are a few injuries unique to the pediatric elbow that warrant mention. Fractures of the distal humerus, including displaced lateral condyle fractures and displaced medial epicondyle fractures, require surgery to restore articular congruity. Radial neck fractures with angulation that inhibits forearm rotation require reduction and fixation. Displaced olecranon fractures, if not reduced by elbow extension, will also require internal fixation. Monteggia and Monteggia variant fractures represent a spectrum of injuries that include forearm fracture with radial head dislocation. Radiographs of the elbow are essential following any ulnar or radial shaft fractures to look for this injury.

Forearm Fractures

Fractures of the shafts of both the radius and the ulna occur frequently in children. The most common problem is malunion with angular or rotational deformity, which limits supination-pronation. Initial treatment is closed reduction. Because of the remodeling potential in the growing child, anatomic reduction is not essential. Side-by-side or "bayonet" apposition is acceptable, but angulation should be minimized. Radiographs are repeated weekly for 3 weeks to permit early remanipulation should the fracture displace. If displacement occurs, repeat reduction and possibly internal fixation with intramedullary nails or plates maybe required.

Galeazzi fracture combines dislocation of the DRUJ with fracture of the radial shaft. To avoid missing this injury, radiographs of the wrist and the elbow are obtained to confirm that normal bony relationships are present.

3. Lower Extremity Fractures & Dislocations
Traumatic Hip Dislocation

In children, traumatic dislocation is more common than fracture of the hip and has fewer complications. Prompt closed reduction under general anesthesia with good muscle relaxation is usually successful. Interposed soft tissue or bone fragments may necessitate open reduction. Following reduction, the hip should be protected for 4–6 weeks until soft tissue healing has occurred. With prompt reduction, avascular necrosis is rare, but radiographs should be followed for 18 months.

Fractures of the Proximal Femur

Proximal femur fractures are rare in children. This is fortunate, as displacement and injury to the growth plate and blood supply predispose to complications, including avascular necrosis, physeal arrest, and nonunion. Fractures involving the proximal femur are typically the result of high-energy trauma.

In children, most hip fractures involve the femoral neck. If there is no displacement, spica cast immobilization maintains alignment during healing, but close radiographic monitoring is required for prompt identification of any displacement. Displaced fractures of the femoral neck should be treated with anatomic reduction and screw fixation, preferably placed short of the physis. Satisfactory results are achieved in half or fewer cases, with avascular necrosis, varus malunion, and physeal arrest among the most common complications. Intertrochanteric and subtrochanteric fractures can generally be managed with ORIF. Late problems (eg, angular deformity, unequal limb lengths) are rare but do occur.

Femoral Shaft Fractures

Femoral shaft fractures are fairly common childhood injuries. They often result from significant trauma, so other injuries may also be present. Radiographs of the hip are required to ensure that fracture or dislocation is not present. The knee should also be x-rayed. Infants are treated with Pavlik harness. Children ages 1–6 are most commonly treated with closed reduction and spica casting for 4–6 weeks. Titanium elastic nails have become the mainstay of treatment for the older child. Standard antegrade femoral nails are reserved only for skeletally mature adolescents because of the risk of avascular necrosis when the physes remain open.

Fractures of the Tibia & Fibula

Fractures of the tibia and fibula are not unusual in childhood. An occult undisplaced spiral fracture may cause the toddler to refuse to bear weight ("toddler's fracture"). These fractures heal rapidly in a long-leg cast. Nerve and vessel damage may be present, especially with displaced fractures of the proximal metaphysis. Fractures of the tibial spine and tibial tubercle are unique to children. If displaced, these fractures require open reduction and fixation. Stiffness about the knee is common, and fracture healing must be balanced with restoration of joint motion to avoid long-term problems.

► Fractures of the Distal Fibula Physis & Transitional Fractures

Fractures of the distal fibular occur frequently in children. This injury is the equivalent of an ankle sprain in the skeletally mature individual. Physical examination localizes tenderness to the distal fibular growth plate, and radiographs will typically be interpreted as normal. Treatment is symptomatic, with resolution of symptoms expected in 3–4 weeks.

Children are at risk for transitional fractures of the distal tibia. These occur most commonly in kids ages 10–14 when a portion of the growth plate is closed but some portion still remains open. A Tillaux fracture is a fracture involving the anterolateral distal tibial epiphysis. Any displacement warrants open reduction and screw fixation. Triplane fractures of the distal tibia are identified as Salter-Harris III injuries on the anteroposterior radiograph and Salter-Harris II injuries on the lateral radiograph. Again, anatomic reduction and fixation is critical.

GAIT DISORDERS & LIMB DEFORMITY

Abnormalities of the lower extremities in children may be noticed by parents as the child learns to walk. The two most common areas of concern include rotational malalignment and angular deformity at the knees.

1. Intoeing

A normal foot progression angle with walking is 10 degrees external rotation. There are three common causes of the "foot turning in" in children. Metatarsus adductus represents adduction of the forefoot. This deformity is typically present at birth and passively correctable. Mild cases will resolve with stretching. If it persists beyond early childhood, surgical correction is an option.

Tibial torsion is an internal rotation deformity of the tibia. On physical examination, the ankle axis (a line connecting the tips of the medial and lateral malleoli) is internally rotated relative to the tibial tubercle. This developmental variant is common in children 1–3 years old and almost always corrects spontaneously with growth. Special shoes and orthotic devices have not been shown to change the natural history and are no longer recommended. Rarely, spontaneous correction does not occur (by age 6) and tibial derotational osteotomy can be considered.

Femoral anteversion is another common finding in children who walk with their feet turned in. Parents will report that the child is a "W" sitter. Observation reveals that the whole limb is internally rotated, so that the patella as well as the foot points medially. On clinical determination, internal rotation at the hip approaches 90 degrees. Femoral antever-

sion can correct spontaneously up until the age of 12. If functional limitations are noted, a femoral derotational osteotomy can be considered.

2. Angular Deformity of the Lower Extremities (Knock-Knees & Bowlegs)

Genu varum, or "bowlegs," is deviation of the knees away from midline. Genu valgum, or "knock-knees," is deviation of the knees toward midline. Children may develop bowlegs from about 12–18 months to 3 years. The majority of children will show spontaneous resolution and occasionally progression to slight valgus between ages 3 and 4 years. In young children, angular deformity of the knees requires radiograph evaluation after age 2 if it is asymmetric, associated with abnormally short stature, or progressing. The differential diagnosis includes infantile Blount disease and rickets. If metabolic bone disease is suspected, serum calcium, phosphate, and alkaline phosphatase should be measured. Operative treatment may be considered if deformity persists after the age of 3.

► Pathologic Genu Varum

It is important to distinguish physiologic tibia vara from pathologic conditions associated with varus, including rickets, Blount disease, and skeletal dysplasias. Blount disease (tibia vara) has both infantile and adolescent forms. Radiographs in infantile Blount disease typically show metaphyseal beaking and changes in the medial proximal tibial physis. The metaphysial-diaphysial angle (> 11 degrees) of the tibia helps to differentiate between physiologic bowing and infantile tibia vara. Progressive tibia vara should be treated with corrective osteotomy of the proximal tibia and fibula. Overcorrection into valgus alignment is recommended because recurrence is common. Adolescent Blount disease is most common in obese patients. Excessive stress on the medial tibial physis is thought to inhibit normal growth, leading to bowing. When the growth plates remain open, growth can be modulated using staples or plates to temporarily tether the lateral growth plate and allow for gradual correction. After skeletal maturity, proximal tibial osteotomy is recommended to restore normal mechanical alignment.

SYSTEMIC DISORDERS AFFECTING BONES & JOINTS IN CHILDREN

1. Juvenile Rheumatoid Arthritis

Rheumatoid arthritis is an autoimmune disorder whose exact cause remains elusive. There are three basic clinical forms of juvenile rheumatoid arthritis (JRA). Pauciarticular arthritis generally involves a single joint, most commonly the knee or the ankle but occasionally the hip or an upper extremity (mainly the elbow or the wrist). Clinical symptoms include the insidious onset of swelling and loss of motion at the affected joint. Systemic manifestations are absent. Iridocyclitis, or inflammation of the iris and ciliary body, is most common in this form of JRA, and an ophthalmology evaluation is necessary.

Polyarthritis is characterized by multiple joint involvement and minimal evidence of systemic disease. Fingers and toes, the neck, and the temporomandibular joints are more likely to be involved. The course is persistent, with periods of exacerbation.

Systemic rheumatoid disease (Still disease) usually presents with multiple (more than five) involved joints, fever, lymphadenopathy, hepatosplenomegaly, rash, subcutaneous nodules, and pericarditis. The course may be remitting or relentless, causing severe permanent disability. Inflamed joints develop synovial hypertrophy and pannus, which destroy articular cartilage. The associated hyperemia can stimulate the adjacent physes, with resulting overgrowth or with physeal arrest. Damage to underlying bone and ligament can produce severe deformity and joint subluxation. Musculoskeletal involvement may include the cervical spine, with spontaneous fusion of the apophysial joints, and result in C1–2 instability.

When a single joint is inflamed, it is necessary to exclude Lyme disease in endemic areas as well as septic arthritis and reactive synovitis. Polyarticular juvenile rheumatoid arthritis must be differentiated from rheumatic fever and leukemia.

Medical management is the first line of treatment: antiinflammatory agents and range-of-motion exercises as synovitis resolves and appropriate bracing to minimize stiffness and allow function. Synovial biopsy can be done percutaneously with arthroscopy to help confirm the diagnosis. Synovectomy is controversial, but some believe that it may slow the progression of arthritis.

2. Brachial Plexus Palsy

Brachial plexus palsy has three general patterns of involvement: (1) Erb palsy, involving C5 and C6 (upper trunk); (2) Klumpke paralysis, involving C8 and T1 (lower trunk); and (3) whole plexus. The first step in treatment is recognition. Physical therapy to maintain range of motion is started immediately and continued as the child is followed for recovery of function. Recovery of the biceps (elbow flexion and forearm supination) by 3–6 months is generally a good prognostic sign. If no spontaneous improvement is seen, neurosurgical evaluation/intervention is recommended. If muscle imbalance persists at the shoulder, transfer of the latissimus dorsi and teres major muscles, so that they become external rotators, is an option. Humeral osteotomy is typically reserved for the older child with residual internal rotation contracture.

SCOLIOSIS & SPINAL DEFORMITY

The spine is in balance when the head is aligned with the pelvis in the coronal and sagittal planes. Scoliosis is spinal curvature of more than 10 degrees in the coronal or frontal plane.

Scoliosis is a three-dimensional deformity with a concurrent rotational component that creates a rib and/or lumbar prominence. Deformity may also exist in the sagittal plane. Normal kyphosis is 20–40 degrees. Scheuermann kyphosis is defined as vertebral body wedging at 3 consecutive levels and greater than 40 degrees of kyphosis in the sagittal plane.

The etiology of spinal deformity in children may be congenital, neuromuscular, traumatic, or idiopathic (of unknown cause). The cause of deformity is an important determinant of the natural history, treatment options, and goals of management. Any family history of scoliosis should be elicited.

▶ Clinical Findings

A. Symptoms and Signs

Spinal deformity may be recognized in the perinatal period or during infancy in children with congenital anomalies of the spine. Most commonly, deformity of the spine is detected during the preadolescent growth spurt, when the spine is growing most rapidly. Spinal deformity is most commonly detected by family members, sports physicals, and primary care physicians. Routine school screening using the Adams forward-bending test has improved recognition. Scoliometer measurements of greater than 7 degrees are an indication for orthopedic evaluation.

Physical examination of the patient with spinal deformity includes both examination of the spine and a comprehensive examination. The location of the curve, deviation of the trunk from the midline (trunk shift), shoulder asymmetry, pelvic obliquity, and flexibility of the spine should be recorded. Clinical findings suggestive of intraspinal pathology, such as tethered cord or a syrinx, include asymmetric abdominal reflexes, clonus, muscle weakness or contractures, and foot deformities. Patients with congenital scoliosis may have associated chest wall deformity and sacral dimples. Scoliosis due to connective tissue pathology may present with joint hypermobility.

B. Imaging Studies

Spinal deformity occurs in three dimensions, and most imaging studies are limited by providing only a two-dimensional representation. Plain radiographs are useful for the detection of deformity and monitoring progression of deformity. The Cobb angle is used to measure deformity in the coronal and sagittal planes. An angular measurement is made between the end vertebrae that are most tilted from the horizontal at either end of the curve (Figure 40–23). Other radiographic measures may include trunk shift relative to the pelvis and overall sagittal and coronal balance of the spine measuring a plumb line between C7 and the sacrum.

MRI examination of the entire spine is an important imaging tool because of the association between intraspinal anomalies with certain types of spinal deformity. Congenital scoliosis may be associated with intraspinal abnormalities, including tethering of the cord, syringomyelia, diastematomyelia,

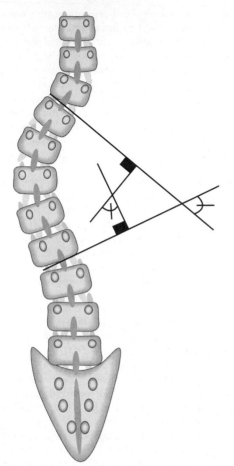

▲ **Figure 40–23.** Measurement of spinal deformity using the Cobb method.

diplomyelia, lipoma, teratoma, and neuroenteric cysts. MRI of the entire spine is indicated for patients with congenital scoliosis, patients with abnormal neurologic findings on physical examination, atypical curve patterns including left thoracic curves, as well as infantile and juvenile idiopathic scoliosis.

1. Idiopathic Scoliosis

Idiopathic scoliosis is the most common cause of spinal deformity in children and adolescents. The prevalence of adolescent idiopathic scoliosis is estimated at 2–3% by age 16. Curves larger than 20 degrees are present in 0.3–0.5% of adolescents. The ratio of affected males to females is equal in curves less than 15 degrees. However, for curves larger than 20 degrees, females are seven times more likely than males to be affected.

Nonoperative management of adolescent idiopathic scoliosis is intended to prevent progression of deformity during the growing years. Bracing is the only nonoperative treatment that has demonstrated efficacy in the management of progressive idiopathic scoliosis. Bracing is recommended for curves over 25–30 degrees in a child who remains skeletally immature. The efficacy of bracing is less predictable in larger curves.

▶ Treatment Options

Surgical management of adolescent idiopathic scoliosis is intended to prevent additional progression of deformity. Spinal fusion may be considered for curves greater than 45–50 degrees in patients when significant growth remains. The natural history studies of untreated idiopathic scoliosis suggest that curve size is a risk factor for curve progression once skeletally mature. Curves under 30 degrees at maturity are not thought to progress, curves 30–40 degrees progress 0.5 degrees per year, and curves over 40 degrees progress 1 degree per year on average.

2. Neuromuscular Scoliosis

Neuromuscular scoliosis presumably develops from a lack of trunk control. The term encompasses a spectrum of disorders, all of which result in some compromise of the patient's ability to control posture and trunk position. The severity of deformity is related to the severity of weakness or spasticity, the patient's age at presentation of neuromuscular pathology, and the rostral or caudal level of involvement within the spinal cord. A child with known neuromuscular disorder is monitored for progression of spinal deformity in concert with management of associated deformities involving the hips, feet, and upper extremities.

Neuromuscular scoliosis may present in patients with disorders involving upper motor neurons, lower motor neurons, or primary myopathies. Upper motor neuron disorders may include cerebral palsy, spinocerebellar degeneration (Friedreich ataxia, Charcot-Marie-Tooth disease, Roussy-Levy disease), syringomyelia, spinal cord tumor, and spinal cord trauma. Lower motor neuron disorders include poliomyelitis, spinomuscular atrophy, myelodysplasia, dysautonomia, and trauma. Primary myopathies that may lead to neuromuscular deformity of the spine include muscular dystrophy, arthrogryposis, and congenital hypotonia.

Neuromuscular scoliosis characteristically presents with long, sweeping curves involving the thoracolumbar spine. This may result in imbalance of the trunk relative to the pelvis. Pelvic obliquity is common in neuromuscular scoliosis, resulting in poor sitting balance and skin breakdown. Pulmonary compromise may be an important feature of neuromuscular curves due to the combination of thoracic deformity with intercostal and accessory muscle weakness. The child with neuromuscular scoliosis often has comorbidities and functional considerations that are distinct from the patient with idiopathic or congenital scoliosis.

▶ Treatment Options

In the neuromuscular patient, goals of treatment include sitting balance, prevention of sacral and ischial skin breakdown, and facilitating caregivers' ability to assist with patient transfers and mobility.

Orthotics—including molded body jackets and thoracolumbar orthoses—may be useful in preserving sitting balance and preventing or delaying surgical stabilization. Indications for surgery include curve progression, poor sitting balance, and respiratory compromise. In the patient who is nonambulatory, fusion of the spinal column to the pelvis can be performed to correct pelvic obliquity.

3. Congenital Scoliosis

Congenital anomalies of the spine are caused by defects in the embryologic formation and segmentation of spinal elements. The formation of the spine begins during the third week of embryonic development. Abnormalities of either the notochord or the neural arch may lead to congenital anomalies of the spine. Congenital anomalies may include unilateral failure of formation (hemivertebrae and wedge vertebrae), failure of segmentation, rib fusions, and mixed or complex anomalies. These anomalies of the spine appear to be sporadic events and not hereditary. Because the cardiac and renal systems are developing simultaneously, these organ systems may also be affected. Routine cardiac evaluation and ultrasound of the renal system is recommended in patients with congenital scoliosis.

Progression of deformity in congenital scoliosis is dependent upon the type of vertebral anomaly, the position of the vertebral anomaly within the spine, and the growth potential for that segment of the spine.

▶ Treatment Options

Bracing has not been effective for congenital scoliosis and is not recommended. If progression of deformity is noted, surgical intervention is recommended. The goal of surgery in young patients is to prevent the development of a severe, rigid deformity.

SEPTIC ARTHRITIS

▶ General Considerations

Infection is usually hematogenous and more frequent in infants exposed to invasive measures likely to cause bacteremia. The joint can be primarily involved, or secondary involvement may occur by spread of osteomyelitis from the proximal femur. Hip sepsis has also followed penetration of the joint during attempted blood aspiration from the femoral vein.

Staphylococcus aureus and *Streptococcus pyogenes* are the most common causative organisms.

▶ Clinical Findings

A. Symptoms and Signs

Refusal to bear weight and pain with hip motion are early signs. Fever is unlikely in very young children, but sepsis may be suggested by generalized irritability and failure to thrive. Another focus of infection should increase suspicion. The hip is typically held flexed in slight abduction and external rotation. Attempts to move the hip are resisted and especially painful.

B. Laboratory Findings

The sedimentation rate and C-reactive protein (CRP) are commonly elevated, but the white blood count may be normal. Leukocytes are abundant in the joint fluid, and Gram-stained smears of fluid show microorganisms as well.

C. Imaging Studies

The early radiographic signs are subtle, with obliteration of soft tissue planes and a suggestion of capsular distention (Figure 40–24). Ultrasound imaging provides an early indication of a joint effusion, and aspiration can be done under ultrasound guidance. Bone scan may initially be negative, especially in children under 6 months of age, but usually shows increased uptake around the involved joint before radiographic changes become evident. MRI may help identify associated osteomyelitis.

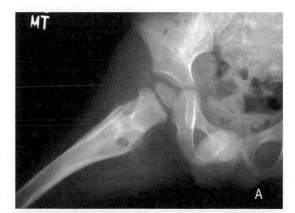
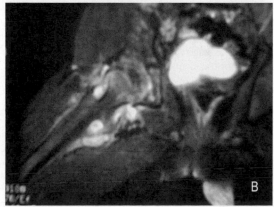

▲ **Figure 40–24.** Septic arthritis of the hip in a 2-year-old boy. **A:** Lateral radiograph shows signs of proximal femoral osteomyelitis. **B:** T2-weighted MRI showing large effusion in the hip joint and edema of the proximal femur.

Differential Diagnosis

Alternative diagnoses include fractures of the femur, acute osteomyelitis of the proximal femur, and iliopsoas abscess. Congenital hip dislocation is not painful, and limited abduction with limb-length inequality is noted. Transient synovitis typically presents with less severe symptoms and low-grade fevers, and it responds to anti-inflammatory agents.

Complications

Structural sequelae include pathologic dislocation and irreversible destruction of the femoral head and neck. Chronic persisting infection may also result.

Treatment

Emergent surgical drainage is required. Side effects from a negative arthrotomy are so few that an aspiration is warranted if the diagnosis is uncertain. Gram-stained smears of intra-articular fluid guide the initial choice of parenteral antibiotic, which is modified if necessary, according to the results of culture and sensitivity tests. Intravenous antibiotics are given until clinical improvement occurs, followed by oral antibiotics for 4 weeks.

Course & Prognosis

If the diagnosis is made and surgical drainage performed in a timely fashion, the long-term results are good. Delay and nonoperative treatment are predictably followed by the complications mentioned previously.

TRANSIENT SYNOVITIS OF THE HIP (TOXIC SYNOVITIS)

Transient synovitis is a common cause of a painful hip in young children. A respiratory illness often precedes the complaints of pain, which may be localized to the knee, thigh, or hip. The short duration of symptoms, absence of diagnostic radiographic signs, and nearly normal laboratory studies suggest a benign process. Children of any age may be affected; the average age is 6 years. Perhaps the most important aspect of transient synovitis is recognition.

Clinical Findings

A. Symptoms and Signs

When first evaluated, the child has rarely been symptomatic for more than a week. Pain in the lower extremity with activity (or even with rest) is the most common complaint. Limp and refusal to bear weight are also common. Passive range of motion of the hip must be checked and compared carefully with the opposite side. Normally, the child should be able to relax and motion should be free and easy without "guarding," which is especially noticeable with rotation or at extremes of flexion or extension. Low-grade fever may be present, but the child does not appear ill.

B. Laboratory Findings

Although the white blood cell count and erythrocyte sedimentation rate may be somewhat elevated, they are usually normal. Hip aspiration, if performed to help clarify a confusing case, reveals clear synovial fluid with a low white cell count, no organisms on Gram-stained smears, and negative cultures for all types of organisms.

C. Imaging Studies

Radiographs are essential to rule out other diagnoses. X-rays are usually normal with transient synovitis of the hip. Hip ultrasound will show little or no effusion.

Differential Diagnosis

Septic arthritis is the primary concern. Legg-Perthes disease (avascular necrosis), slipped capital femoral epiphysis, and, rarely, other forms of inflammatory joint disease such as rheumatoid arthritis or rheumatic fever must be considered.

Treatment

Hospitalization for observation and serial clinical examinations is often advised to ensure that an infection is not missed. The hip is placed at rest, and anti-inflammatory agents are initiated. This almost always relieves symptoms promptly and also helps confirm the diagnosis. The child should then be reexamined to make certain that normal hip motion and comfort have been achieved. Anteroposterior and lateral x-rays are repeated in 2–3 months to ensure that avascular necrosis has not developed. Occasionally, signs of systemic reaction are more pronounced or the child continues to guard the hip longer than usual. In such cases, needle aspiration confirmed by arthrogram should be performed to rule out infection.

Prognosis

Recurrent symptoms may develop after release from the hospital and resumption of activity but usually resolve with more rest.

DEVELOPMENTAL DYSPLASIA/ DISLOCATION OF THE HIP

ESSENTIALS OF DIAGNOSIS

▶ Mechanical instability of the hip.
▶ Limitation of abduction.
▶ Limb length inequality if unilateral.
▶ Abnormal gait once walking begins.

General Considerations

Developmental hip dysplasia may be detected at birth or develop early in life. The incidence of dislocation is 1 in 1000 infants. Both hips may be involved. Developmental hip dysplasia is more common in firstborn females and with breech positioning. It is rarely painful or disabling to the child but results in significant symptoms in adults if left untreated. The hip may be dislocated by reducible, reduced but dislocatable, or dislocated and not reducible.

Clinical Findings

A. Symptoms and Signs

The physical signs of developmental hip dysplasia are the key to diagnosis. They may be subtle, however, and can be missed by the most experienced examiner. This emphasizes the need for repeated evaluation of the hips during routine well-baby checks.

1. Dislocatable hip (Barlow positive)—The examiner attempts to displace the infant's femoral head posterolaterally from the acetabulum by means of a provocation test (Figure 40–25). In a positive test, the femoral head is felt to displace out of the acetabulum. Mechanical instability—not a "click"—is the essential finding.

2. Dislocated but reducible hip (Ortolani positive)—Ortolani described relocation of a dislocated femoral head when the examiner abducts the flexed hip and lifts the greater trochanter anteriorly.

The soft tissues surrounding the joint may not be lax enough to permit reduction. A fixed hip dislocation will result in limited abduction, apparent shortening of the affected side, and asymmetric thigh creases (if the dislocation is unilateral). As the child begins to walk, an abnormal gait becomes apparent. If dislocation is bilateral, the diagnosis is more challenging; the gait is "waddling," and lumbar lordosis is prominent.

B. Imaging Studies

Until the cartilaginous acetabulum and femoral head become substantially ossified, x-rays may fail to indicate the true condition of the hip joint. Obvious abnormalities must be considered significant, but apparently normal radiographs do not exclude hip dysplasia until a well-ossified femoral head is adequately contained by the acetabulum. Femoral head ossification is usually present by 6 months of age but may be delayed in developmental hip dysplasia. Figure 40–26 shows several of the many radiographic relationships that are important for evaluation of the hip joint in infants. In older children, the femoral head should be adjacent to the radiolucent triradiate cartilage that forms the medial wall of the acetabulum. Displacement of the femoral head confirms dislocation. A shallow acetabulum that poorly covers the femoral head is termed dysplastic. Ultrasonography is the best technique for assessing the infant's hip prior to ossification of the femoral head.

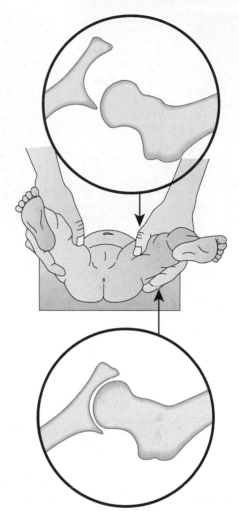

▲ **Figure 40–25. Upper window:** Subluxation provocation test. Holding the thighs of the relaxed infant as illustrated, the examiner stabilizes the pelvis with one hand while gently but firmly trying to displace the opposite femoral head posteriorly out of the acetabulum. Adduction of the thigh aids this maneuver. If mechanical instability of the femoral head is present, a "jerk" will be felt, indicating that the hip is subluxable. **Lower window:** In the Ortolani test, abduction and lifting with the fingers produces a corresponding jerk when the dislocated femoral head slides back into the acetabulum.

Differential Diagnosis

Proximal femoral focal deficiency and congenital coxa vara are rare conditions that produce shortening or instability in the hip region. Pathologic dislocation can occur rapidly in infected hips; the femoral head is displaced from a radiographically normal acetabulum. Hip dislocation may be

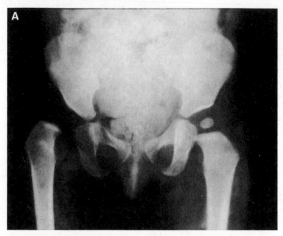

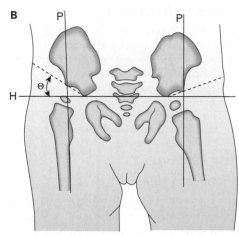

▲ **Figure 40–26. A:** X-ray of congenital dislocation of the right hip. **B:** Analysis of hip radiographs presupposes adequately exposed films of a properly positioned patient. Hilgenreiner horizontal line is drawn through both triradiate cartilages (H), and Perkins vertical line is drawn through the outer margin of each acetabulum (P). If the hip is located, the proximal femoral epiphysis will lie in the inferomedial quadrant formed by the two intersecting lines. Proximal or lateral displacement indicates dislocation. Abnormal acetabular development is suggested by lack of obvious concavity and by an acetabular index (Θ) greater than 30 degrees.

caused by muscle imbalance in children with cerebral palsy or myelomeningocele.

▶ Complications

Complications include inability to gain or maintain a stable reduction, avascular necrosis of the femoral head following operative or nonoperative treatment, and limitation of motion.

▶ Treatment

A. Dislocatable Hip

Neonates with confirmed dislocatable and reducible hips should be treated by means of abduction splinting (Pavlik harness) until stability is confirmed. It is important to flex the hips and abduct them no more than 60 degrees to avoid interfering with the blood supply and injury to the femoral nerve.

B. Dislocated Hip

1. Birth to 18 months—In this age group, closed reduction is usually possible. Reduction can be maintained with a spica cast. If closed reduction is not possible or cannot be maintained, open reduction is required. Arthrography and CT scan are used to confirm reduction.

2. Eighteen months to 4 years—Open reduction is more likely to be required in this group. If adequate reduction is obtained, satisfactory results are more likely. Acetabular remodeling is best until age 4.

3. Older children and adults—Treatment of newly diagnosed congenital hip dysplasia in this age group is difficult.

Acetabular remodeling through growth is minimal. Achievement of a concentric reduction does not ensure a stable, pain-free hip. Salvage osteotomies of the innominate bone have been described for improving acetabular coverage of the femoral head. Pain and limitation of motion will eventually necessitate total hip arthroplasty for many of these individuals.

SLIPPED CAPITAL FEMORAL EPIPHYSIS (SCFE)

During the period of rapid skeletal growth in early adolescence, the normal relationship of the femoral head with the femoral neck may become disturbed by a shearing displacement through the growth plate—known as slipped capital femoral epiphysis. The head remains within the acetabulum, while the femoral neck shifts anteriorly and laterally. This displacement may occur in response to minor trauma, or it can be gradual, as indicated by reactive bone formation and remodeling of the femoral neck adjacent to the growth plate. An acute SCFE may be superimposed upon a gradual "chronic" one. Involvement is bilateral in at least 25% of cases. SCFE are considered stable if the child can bear weight and unstable if weightbearing is not tolerated. The risk of avascular necrosis is reported to be near 50% for unstable SCFE. This condition can lead to severe deformity and may cause early degenerative joint disease.

▶ Clinical Findings

A. Symptoms and Signs

The patient typically reports pain in the knee or thigh and limps. Hip motion is limited, especially flexion and internal rotation, with obligatory external rotation found on examination.

B. Imaging Studies

Radiographs are diagnostic in all but the most minimal slips (Figure 40–27). The epiphysis is not centered on the neck but rather relatively displaced posterior and medial. Since posterior displacement is often more marked, the displacement is more evident on the lateral view. Bony callus, or widening of the metaphysis adjacent to the growth plate, indicates a chronic slip. A significant SCFE produces a bony prominence on the anterolateral femoral neck, restricting hip motion.

▶ Treatment

Surgical stabilization of the proximal femoral epiphysis is advised. In situ pinning of the epiphysis without reduction is then performed. The surgeon should make sure the screw does not enter the joint space. Gradual mobilization with protected weightbearing follows. The goal of in site pinning is to prevent further slip and gain closure of the physis. The opposite side must be watched until the physis closes as well. If severe deformity prevents hip motion, a subtrochanteric osteotomy or excision of the bony prominence on the femoral neck may be considered.

PERTHES (LEGG-CALVE-PERTHES) DISEASE

Legg-Calve-Perthes disease is an uncommon hip affliction that occurs in about 1 in 2000 children, generally between the ages of 4 and 10. Boys are affected five times as often as girls, but girls tend to have more severe involvement. About 10–15% of patients have bilateral disease. The etiology is unknown, but the hallmark is avascular necrosis of the proximal femoral epiphysis. Few patients achieve normal hip development. Others acquire permanent deformity of the femoral head, with limited motion and degenerative joint disease becoming symptomatic in middle age.

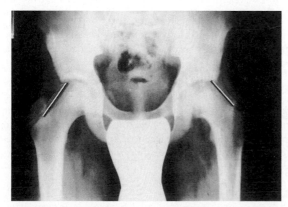

▲ **Figure 40–27.** Left slipped capital femoral epiphysis. Note that a line extended along the lateral side of the femoral neck misses the capital epiphysis. On the normal right side, this line enters the femoral head, which should overlap the neck on both anteroposterior and lateral views.

▶ Determinants of Final Outcome

A. Stages of Illness

The disease involves four stages: sclerosis, fragmentation, reossification and remodeling. The earliest clinical signs are pain in the thigh and limping. Radiographs show an apparent increase in density of the capital epiphysis. Later, a subchondral, crescent-shaped, radiolucent fracture may occur, and the metaphysis may widen. The epiphysis becomes irregular and flattened during fragmentation. Gradually, reossification occurs and symptoms subside. The ultimate shape will depend on the remolding of the proximal femur with growth. A spherical head correlates well with good long-term results.

B. Age of Patient

Younger patients have a better prognosis. Boys generally have less severe involvement than girls.

C. Severity of Involvement

The lateral pillar classification divides patients with Legg-Perthes disease into three groups according to the extent of involvement of the lateral pillar of the epiphysis relative to the central portion of the head: Group A has minimal involvement of the epiphysis, group B has a 50% decrease in height of the lateral pillar, and group C involves the entire head.

D. The "Head at Risk"

Catterall proposed certain clinical and radiographic criteria for determining whether the femoral head might deform in the course of the disease. The clinical criteria are (1) obesity, (2) decreasing range of motion of the involved hip, and (3) adduction contracture. The radiographic criteria are (1) lateral subluxation of the femoral head, (2) Gage sign (widening of the lateral part of the growth plate so that the superior portion of the femoral neck appears convex), (3) calcification lateral to the epiphysis in the cartilaginous femoral head, (4) diffuse metaphysial reaction, and (5) a horizontal growth plate.

▶ Clinical Findings

A. Symptoms and Signs

Insidious development of limp and sometimes pain in the groin, anterior thigh, or knee eventually bring the patient to a physician. An occasional case presents as acute synovitis. Examination shows antalgic gait, decreased hip motion (especially abduction and internal rotation), and sometimes flexion-adduction contracture. Passive motion is guarded rather than free.

B. Laboratory Findings

Bone scan may help with early diagnosis and assessment of the extent of head involvement.

C. Imaging Studies

Well-exposed radiographs in both anteroposterior and frog-leg lateral views are essential. Findings will depend on the stage and severity of disease, as discussed earlier, but initial films usually show increased density and deformity of the femoral head epiphysis, which may be flattened or fragmented (Figure 40–28).

▶ Differential Diagnosis

The early inflammatory stage of Legg-Perthes disease can be confused with toxic synovitis and septic arthritis. The epiphysial abnormalities are similar to those seen in epiphysial dysplasias, hypothyroidism, and avascular necrosis from other causes, notably sickle cell anemia, Gaucher disease, and chronic use of corticosteroid drugs.

▶ Treatment

Treatment requires categorization according to the stage of disease, the extent of head involvement, and the condition of the hip joint at the time of presentation. The mobility of the involved joint must be determined and then followed as an important indicator of need for intervention and prognosis.

A. Observation

Children under the age of 6 without at-risk signs typically do well with symptomatic treatment, including activity restriction, stretching, and anti-inflammatory agents. In older children, if the femoral head remains contained in the acetabulum and motion is maintained, observation is recommended.

B. Surgical Treatment

On occasion, surgery is necessary to reorient the acetabulum or the proximal femur to achieve containment. Both innominate osteotomy and varus proximal femoral osteotomy have been successful.

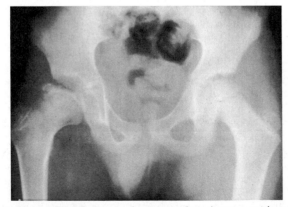

▲ **Figure 40–28.** X-ray of Legg-Perthes disease, with significant deformity of right femoral head.

▶ Prognosis

Prolonged follow-up is necessary to determine the outcome. Long-term results are best correlated with the shape of the femoral head at the completion of skeletal growth.

FOOT DEFORMITIES IN CHILDREN

Positional deformities of the foot are described with the following specific terms. Equinus refers to plantar flexion. Calcaneus is the opposite position, or dorsiflexion. The forefoot alone may be in adduction, known as metatarsus adductus. The hindfoot deformity may be varus or valgus.

The goal of treatment of any foot deformity is a pain-free, flexible, plantigrade foot during normal gait.

1. Clubfoot

Talipes equinovarus, or clubfoot, is the most common foot deformity, affecting approximately 1 in 1000 children. It occurs twice as often in boys and is bilateral half the time. There is a familial tendency, with a 5% chance that a sibling will also be affected. It can be idiopathic or associated with an underlying syndrome.

▶ Clinical Findings

In clubfoot, there is varus of the hindfoot, adduction of the forefoot, and equinovarus deformity. The exact etiology remains uncertain. The joints principally involved are both the subtalar and talonavicular joints. The adjacent ankle and midtarsal joints are affected to a lesser degree. The overlying soft tissues are contracted. Successful treatment requires serial casting with correction of the deformities, cavus-adduction-varus-equinus, in that order, as described by Ponseti. Surgical intervention is rarely required for clubfeet if treated early with casting.

▶ Treatment

Initial treatment is always nonoperative and should be started as soon as possible, preferably the day the infant is born.

A. Manipulation

Gentle manipulation into a corrected position should be done in order to stretch the contracted soft tissues—specifically, to align the calcaneus and navicular relative to the talus. Gentleness is required to avoid tissue trauma and to prevent overcorrection of the forefoot relative to persisting tarsal deformity.

B. Casting

After manipulation, a plaster cast is applied and molded to maintain the corrected position. Manipulation and cast application are repeated weekly, typically for 6 weeks. Often, a percutaneous tendoachilles lengthening is needed for residual equinus.

Casting is followed by application of a Denis-Browne bar with reverse last shoes worn at first full time and then at night and during nap times for 2 years. During this time, routine follow-up is required to monitor for recurrence.

C. Surgical Treatment

The traditional surgery involved a posteromedial release of the ankle and subtalar joints with realignment of the talonavicular and talocalcaneal joints. Surgery is rarely recommended for clubfoot.

2. Metatarsus Adductus

Metatarsus adductus is a common forefoot deformity that is often quite flexible. If passively correctable, there is an 85% chance of spontaneous correction by age 3 years. Easy passive correction also suggests that treatment is unnecessary. If the forefoot cannot readily be returned to a normal position, manipulation and casting can be recommended. Only a very rare, severe deformity will require surgical release or osteotomy and fusion of the tarsometatarsal joints.

Cook DA et al: Observer variability in the radiographic measurement and classification of metatarsus adductus. J Pediatr Orthop 1992;12:86.

3. Flatfoot

The normal newborn foot appears flat because subcutaneous fat fills the longitudinal arch. This fat deposit recedes over the first 4 years of life to reveal the typical adult appearance of a medial arch under the midfoot, which does not touch the floor with weightbearing. An inadequate bony arch, which permits the medial portion of the midfoot to bear weight, is the essential feature of true flatfoot. This deformity is further classified as rigid or flexible.

Rigid flatfoot is identified by the absence of normal mobility of the hindfoot. Rigid flatfoot presenting later in childhood is usually due to coalition of the tarsal bones. Associated episodic foot pain and spasm of the peroneal muscles are typical. Depending on the child's age and symptoms and the site of coalition, resection may be advisable or nonoperative treatment may suffice.

In flexible flatfoot, weightbearing obliterates the medial arch and also produces obvious valgus alignment of the calcaneus. Standing on tiptoes or sitting with the feet hanging free will restore the arch. Some patients with flexible flatfoot develop foot pain with weightbearing.

Treatment of asymptomatic flexible flatfoot in children is controversial. Parents distressed by the foot's appearance or by abnormal shoe wear often request treatment, but there is little evidence that treatment prevents future symptoms, and most children with flexible flatfoot have no symptoms in adulthood.

The child with painful flexible flatfoot deformity deserves treatment. Exercises to stretch tight gastrosoleus muscle groups or to strengthen intrinsic plantar muscles are usually

advised, and external support for the mediolongitudinal arch can be provided if necessary. If nonoperative treatment fails to control symptoms or if deformity precludes use of normal footwear, surgery may be considered.

Evidence-based care guideline for femoral shaft fractures. Cincinnati Children's Hospital Medical Center, 2006. Available at http://www.cincinnatichildrens.org/svc/alpha/h/health-policy/ev-based/femur.htm. Accessed February 14, 2009.

Evidence-based care guideline for loss of elbow motion following surgery or trauma in children aged 4 to 18. Cincinnati Children's Hospital Medical Center, 2007. Available at: http://www.cincinnatichildrens.org/svc/alpha/h/health-policy/ev-based/elbow.htm. Accessed February 14, 2009.

▼ SPORTS MEDICINE

PAIN SYNDROMES OF THE SHOULDER

1. Rotator Cuff Tendinitis & Subacromial Bursitis

▶ General Considerations

Inflammation within the glenohumeral joint is the most frequent cause of shoulder pain and limitation of motion. The patient is typically middle aged. Repetitive overhead activity from occupation or sports is a common cause. The most common site of inflammation at onset is the insertion of the rotator cuff tendons, particularly the supraspinatus tendon. The location of the supraspinatus tendon between the greater tuberosity of the humeral head and the overhanging acromion process renders it particularly vulnerable to mechanical compression. The subacromial space is another common site of inflammation with subdeltoid soreness frequently radiating along the lateral humerus to the deltoid insertion.

▶ Clinical Findings

Night pain is common. Active abduction becomes especially painful when the inflamed rotator cuff and overlying bursa are compressed beneath the acromion. The range of active abduction may be extended if the patient is instructed to rotate the arms so that the palms face upward. This rotates the greater tuberosity posteriorly, so that the attached rotator cuff tendons pass behind the acromion, resulting in diminished pain with continued abduction.

▶ Treatment

The initial treatment of rotator cuff tendinitis and subacromial bursitis is with anti-inflammatory agents (naproxen, ibuprofen) and physical therapy to preserve motion. Slings and shoulder immobilization should not be used for more than a few days, since capsular adhesions and prolonged stiffness may result. Gentle passive range-of-motion exercises should be started as soon as tolerated, followed by active pendulum exercises. Active exercise is gradually increased while passive range of motion is continued.

If pain does not respond to oral anti-inflammatory agents, relief may be obtained by injection into the subacromial bursa.

2. Biceps Tendinitis

ESSENTIALS OF DIAGNOSIS

▶ Localized tenderness over the bicipital groove.
▶ Pain during supination of the forearm against resistance.

▶ General Considerations

A common inflammatory process producing shoulder pain involves the biceps tendon in the bicipital groove. Biceps tendonitis usually affects individuals whose occupation involves repetitive biceps flexion against resistance or whose recreational activities include forceful throwing of a ball. Pain is prominent over the anterior aspect of the arm and is aggravated by shoulder motion. Symptoms are worse at night and improve with rest. Deltoid muscle spasm may be present and may limit both active and passive motion.

▶ Clinical Findings

Biceps tendinitis can be distinguished from rotator cuff tendinitis by localization of tenderness to the bicipital groove. Forearm supination against resistance with the elbow flexed at the patient's side elicits extreme tenderness in the region of the bicipital groove when the tendon is palpated near the shoulder. Instability of the tendon in the groove is occasionally manifested by a snapping sensation as the arm is abducted and externally rotated. Subluxation of the tendons can be provoked by the Yergason maneuver, in which the patient actively flexes the elbow against resistance while the physician rotates the humerus externally. An unstable tendon will "pop" out of the groove.

▶ Treatment

Treatment of bicipital tendinitis includes cessation of offending activities and short-term immobilization of the shoulder in a sling and a trial of NSAIDs. Surgery is occasionally required to stabilize a subluxating tendon. When discomfort has subsided, progressive mobilization is begun with exercises similar to those described for rotator cuff tendinitis.

3. Adhesive Capsulitis (Frozen Shoulder)

ESSENTIALS OF DIAGNOSIS

▶ Diffuse shoulder pain.
▶ Restricted shoulder joint motion.

▶ General Considerations

A common cause of shoulder pain in middle-aged and elderly patients is adhesive capsulitis, or frozen shoulder. This disorder may complicate other inflammatory shoulder ailments, particularly in individuals immobilized for prolonged periods. It may also occur without any identifiable inciting trauma and has been associated with cardiovascular disease, diabetes, rheumatoid arthritis, and degenerative cervical spine disease. Though the exact pathogenesis is unknown, the end result is a chronically inflamed, contracted capsule densely adherent to the humeral head, the acromion, and the underlying biceps and rotator cuff tendons. Normal bursae are obliterated by scarring.

▶ Clinical Findings
A. Symptoms and Signs

The onset of symptoms is usually gradual and heralded by complaints of diffuse tenderness with disproportionately severe restriction of active and passive motion. Motion is not improved by lidocaine or corticosteroid injection.

B. Imaging Studies

Arthrography reveals a contracted joint capsule and no bursal filling. X-rays may reveal osteopenia of the humeral head.

▶ Treatment

The natural history of adhesive capsulitis is occasionally spontaneous resolution. Subsidence of pain and return of nearly full motion can be obtained, though the process may persist for 6 months to several years. Efforts to speed return of function have included intensive physical therapy and anti-inflammatory agents. Rarely, surgical intervention is required to release the capsule, and this can be done arthroscopically. Clearly, the best treatment of this condition is prevention. Prolonged disuse or immobilization of a painful shoulder must be avoided. Early mobilization is stressed, with initiation of gentle range-of-motion exercises and guidance by the physician and the physical therapist.

4. Dislocation of the Shoulder Joint

The shoulder (glenohumeral) joint is the most commonly dislocated joint in the body because it is less constrained than other joints and motion is possible in multiple planes. The constraints that prevent instability include the labrum, negative pressure of the joint, and glenohumeral ligaments. The rotator cuff also provides dynamic stability by compressing the humeral head against the glenoid. These static and dynamic stabilizers create a delicate balance between motion and stability.

Dislocations are usually related to overhead trauma when the arm is in abduction, extension, and external rotation. Most traumatic dislocations are anterior, but posterior dislocations can occur. Shoulder instability is classified by several factors:

traumatic or atraumatic, initial or recurrent, acute or chronic, the direction of dislocation, and voluntary or involuntary.

Anterior Dislocations of the Shoulder Joint

Anterior dislocations can be diagnosed by history and physical examination. The arm is held in a position of slight abduction and external rotation. The anterior shoulder area appears full, and there is a vacant sulcus in the posterior shoulder area. Anteroposterior x-ray in the plane of the scapula and axillary x-ray are necessary to determine the direction of the dislocation and the presence of fracture. Humeral head impression fractures (Hill-Sachs lesion) and glenoid rim fractures are easily missed if the radiographs are inadequate. Dislocation may also be complicated by injury to the brachial plexus (most commonly the axillary nerve) and rotator cuff tear. The examiner should check for sensory changes over the deltoid to assess the axillary nerve.

Posterior Dislocation of the Shoulder Joint

Posterior dislocation is characterized by fullness beneath the spine of the scapula, flattening of the anterior shoulder, prominence of the coracoid, and restriction of motion in external rotation. The reported incidence of missed diagnosis is as high as 60%. The injury occurs either from direct or indirect force to the anterior shoulder, so that the humeral head is pushed out posteriorly. Common causes of posterior dislocation of the shoulder are seizures or electrical shock. Anteroposterior x-rays of the chest may look deceptively normal with posterior dislocation, but an axillary view and an anteroposterior x-ray in the scapular plane will show the true position of the head in relation to the glenoid. This dislocation may also be reduced by longitudinal and gentle transverse traction. The reduction may be held in a sling for 3–4 weeks with some external rotation if necessary.

Multidirectional Instability

Patients with congenital or acquired laxity may develop symptomatic shoulder instability in multiple directions. These patients should be initially treated with of rehabilitation and strengthening monitored by a physical therapist. Most of these patients recover stability with muscular strengthening of the rotator cuff and scapular stabilizing muscles.

Voluntary Dislocators

Patients who voluntarily dislocate their shoulders have a high recurrence rate after surgical procedures. Therefore, surgery is usually avoided in this population.

Treatment

The treatment of shoulder dislocations consists of closed reduction after careful examination and documentation of neurovascular status and good-quality x-rays. Many meth-

ods of closed reduction have been described, including gentle traction in the prone position and traction-countertraction with a sheet. All methods of reduction rely on adequate analgesia and relaxation. Forceful reductions should be avoided because they may cause brachial plexus injury, vascular injury, or fracture. Postreduction x-rays document a concentric reduction and rule out any associated fracture. Once reduced, the arm is placed in a sling for 3–4 weeks before protected motion exercises are initiated.

Surgical reconstruction is indicated for recurrent anterior traumatic instability. The incidence of recurrent instability approaches 80–90% for active young athletes. Therefore, the indication for surgery depends on age and activity level as well as the number of traumatic dislocations and associated fracture or soft tissue injury. After operative repair, the shoulder is usually immobilized in a shoulder immobilizer for 3–6 weeks before active motion is begun. Open and arthroscopic surgical repairs of the labrum for anterior dislocation are successful in preventing further episodes of dislocation in most patients.

Steinbach LS et al: Expert Panel on Musculoskeletal Imaging. Shoulder trauma. American College of Radiology, 2005. Available at http://www.acr.org/SecondaryMainMenuCategories/quality_safety/app_criteria/pdf/ExpertPanelonMusculoskeletalImaging/ShoulderTraumaDoc18.aspx. Accessed February 14, 2009.

5. Rotator Cuff Tears

Rotator cuff tears and rotator cuff impingement are common sources of shoulder pain. Four rotator cuff muscles (supraspinatus, infraspinatus, teres minor, and subscapularis) function to move the arm and stabilize the shoulder joint. There is a full spectrum of injury ranging from tendonitis to impingement and rotator cuff tears. The most severe condition is a massive, chronic rotator cuff tear that subsequently leads to proximal migration of the humeral head and arthritic changes of the humeral head known as rotator cuff arthropathy.

Patients with rotator cuff syndrome usually present with pain and weakness related to attempted overhead activities and active movements with the arm away from the body. Physical examination demonstrates impingement pain with certain overhead movements and rotator cuff weakness. Diagnosis is made by history and physical examination. Ultrasound and MRI are useful tests to evaluate rotator cuff tears and associated intra-articular pathology (Figure 40–29).

Treatment

The treatment of shoulder pain related to rotator cuff pathology (inflammation, degeneration, tear) depends on other patient variables such as age, activity level, hand dominance, and the chronicity and level of pain and dysfunction. Tears may result from single-event trauma (a fall on the outstretched hand), repetitive trauma (baseball pitchers), or degeneration of the rotator cuff in older patients.

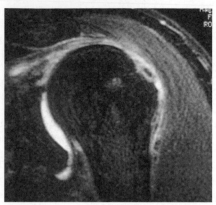

▲ **Figure 40–29.** T2-weighted MRI showing a massive rotator cuff tear.

Most cases of shoulder pain related to the rotator cuff tendonitis are initially treated nonoperatively. Activity modification, NSAIDs, and physical therapy can be beneficial. Some patients require a subacromial injection to control inflammation and pain. Rotator cuff tears can be treated with surgical repair. Acute traumatic rotator cuff tears should be repaired acutely in order to prevent rotator cuff atrophy and retraction. Acromioplasty and distal clavicle excision are performed at the same time if coracoacromial arch impingement contributes to the rotator cuff tear.

Ainsworth R, Lewis JS: Exercise therapy for the conservative management of full thickness tears of the rotator cuff: a systematic review. Br J Sports Med 2007;41:200.
Barfield LC, Kuhn JE: Arthroscopic versus open acromioplasty: a systematic review. Clin Orthop Relat Res 2007;455:64.
Grant HJ, Arthur A, Pichora DR: Evaluation of interventions for rotator cuff pathology: a systematic review. J Hand Ther 2004; 17:274.

6. Glenohumeral Arthritis

Arthritis of the glenohumeral joint may be caused by osteoarthritis, inflammatory disease, previous trauma, previous surgery, or arthritis of recurrent instability. Patients have pain with activities as in arthritis in other joints. They may also complain of stiffness, which is usually progressive over time. Physical examination discloses limited motion. Examination by proper shoulder x-rays shows the characteristic joint-space narrowing and humeral head osteophytes.

Before operative treatment is elected, a thorough course of conservative measures is indicated. Surgery becomes an option for patients with significant pain and limitation of activity because of their arthritis. Shoulder arthroplasty (hemiarthroplasty, total shoulder replacement) can provide pain relief; however, motion is rarely restored to normal. Contraindications to total arthroplasty are active or latent septic arthritis, paralysis of the shoulder musculature, and neuropathic joints.

PAIN SYNDROMES OF THE ELBOW

1. Tennis Elbow (Humeral Epicondylitis)

ESSENTIALS OF DIAGNOSIS

► Tenderness over the lateral humeral epicondyle.
► Pain at the elbow with resisted extension of the wrist.

► General Considerations

Though far more common in nonathletes, humeral epicondylitis is commonly termed tennis elbow. This overuse syndrome is uncommon before age 18 and most frequent in the fourth and fifth decades. Tennis elbow is commonly seen in nonathletes performing activities that require frequent rotary motion of the forearm, such as gardening, use of screwdrivers or wrenches, turning of doorknobs, and even operation of vehicles without power-assisted steering.

► Clinical Findings

Tennis elbow is characterized by tenderness and pain at the humeral epicondyle provoked by extension of the wrist. The origin of the inflamed common extensor muscle is the source of discomfort. The pain is readily reproduced with resisted extension of the wrist with the elbow extended.

Though the pathogenesis of tennis elbow is unknown, symptoms are usually attributed to inflammation of the origin of the common extensor muscle and, in some cases, to a tear in the origin of the extensor carpi radialis brevis. The tears are thought to be the result of repeated stress on degenerated tendon fibers. Elbow motion remains normal.

► Differential Diagnosis

Differential diagnosis includes radial nerve irritation at the elbow, which may often be delineated by electromyography.

► Treatment

A. Medical Treatment

Most patients with tennis elbow respond favorably to a brief period of rest and anti-inflammatory agents followed by a program of exercises to strengthen the forearm muscles. Subtendinous injection of soluble corticosteroids with lidocaine may be required in more severe cases. Repeated injections may further weaken tendons and should be avoided.

A nonelastic forearm band may be prescribed and worn near the elbow during occupational or recreational activities that aggravate the condition. The band is thought to be effective either because it limits full contraction of the tender muscles or because it slightly alters the position of the extensor tendons.

B. Surgical Treatment

Rarely, patients with severe or refractory symptoms may require operative treatment. Most surgeons repair the origin of the torn wrist extensor tendon after excision of granulation tissue and any rough subjacent bone. Lengthening of the short wrist extensor results in loss of strength.

2. Olecranon Bursitis

ESSENTIALS OF DIAGNOSIS

▶ Tenderness and swelling over the olecranon.
▶ Limited elbow flexion.

▶ General Considerations

Olecranon bursitis is a common cause of periarticular elbow pain. Like epicondylitis, this condition is often related to occupational activities, in this case prolonged periods of leaning on the elbow.

▶ Clinical Findings

The subcutaneous olecranon bursa becomes distended, sometimes to dramatic proportions. The skin of the extensor surface of the forearm may be edematous and pitted. Traumatic bursitis is often only mildly painful despite marked swelling.

▶ Treatment

Treatment of idiopathic or traumatic olecranon bursitis consists of protecting the bursa from further pressure or irritation. Compression dressings may be necessary if symptoms are prolonged. Recurrence is not uncommon. Excision of the bursa may be required for rare persistent cases. The bursa must be totally excised and the overlying skin sutured to the olecranon periosteum to ensure obliteration of the space.

INJURIES TO THE LIGAMENTS, MENISCI, & CARTILAGE OF THE KNEE JOINT

Internal derangement of the knee joint mechanism is usually caused by trauma but can also result from overuse. Injuries to the ligaments, cartilage, and meniscus commonly occur as combined lesions.

X-rays are often normal in suspected ligament or cartilage injury. MRI is a valuable imaging modality. MRI assists with preoperative confirmation of a clinical diagnosis.

Once a diagnosis is obtained, arthroscopy is a valuable diagnostic and therapeutic tool for the knee joint. The arthroscope is introduced into the knee joint through a small stab incision and allows examination of structures inside. Meniscus tears, ligament reconstruction, and chondral injury can all be addressed arthroscopically.

▶ Injury to the Menisci

Injury to the medial meniscus is the most frequent internal derangement of the knee joint. Clinical findings include swelling, pain, and varying degrees of restriction of flexion or extension. True locking (inability to fully extend the knee) is highly suggestive of meniscal tear. A marginal tear permits displacement of the medial fragment into the intercondylar region (bucket-handle tear) and prevents either complete extension or complete flexion. Motion may cause pain over the anteromedial or posteromedial joint line. Tenderness can often be elicited at the joint line. Weakness and atrophy of the quadriceps femoris may be present. Injury to the lateral meniscus is less common. Pain and tenderness may be present over the lateral joint line.

Initial treatment may be conservative. Swelling and pain can be relieved by aspiration. Isometric quadriceps exercises should be performed frequently throughout the day with the knee in maximum extension, and emphasis should be placed on restoring range of motion. Physical therapy and NSAIDs are helpful.

Arthroscopy with either meniscal debridement for central tears or meniscus repair for peripheral tears is recommended. Isometric quadriceps exercises and range-of-motion exercises are resumed and are gradually increased. As soon as the patient is able to perform these exercises comfortably, graded resistance maneuvers should be started. Exercises should be continued until motion and strength is equal to the healthy knee.

▶ Injury to the Ligaments

Ligaments in general prevent displacement or angulation beyond its normal arc of motion.

A. Medial Collateral Ligament

The medial collateral ligament is the primary restraint to valgus. Forced abduction of the leg at the knee causes injury varying from strain to complete rupture. The medial collateral ligament is attached to the medial meniscus at the joint line.

A history of a twisting injury or direct blow at the knee with valgus strain can usually be obtained. Pain is present over the medial aspect of the knee joint. In severe injury, joint effusion may be present. Tenderness can be elicited at the site of the lesion. When only an isolated ligamentous tear is present, x-ray examination may not be helpful unless it is made while valgus stress is applied.

Treatment of an incomplete tear consists of protection from further injury while healing progresses in a brace that allows motion but protects the knee from valgus injury. It may be helpful to bend the brace into varus to take load off of the ligament.

Tear of the medial collateral ligament is frequently associated with other lesions, such as tear of the medial meniscus and rupture of the anterior cruciate ligament.

B. Lateral Collateral Ligament

Tear of the lateral collateral ligament is often associated with injury to surrounding structures, including the popliteus muscle tendon and the iliotibial band. Avulsion of the apex of the fibular head may occur, and the peroneal nerve may be injured.

Pain and tenderness are present over the lateral aspect of the knee joint, and hemarthrosis may be present. X-rays may show bone avulsion from the fibular head.

The treatment of partial tear is similar to that described for partial tear of the medial collateral ligament. If complete tear is detected, healing is rare without surgical intervention, and exploration and reconstruction is required.

C. Anterior Cruciate Ligament

The function of the anterior cruciate ligament is prevention of anterior displacement of the tibia relative to the femur. Injury to the anterior cruciate ligament is often associated with injury to the menisci or the medial collateral ligament. The cruciate ligament may be avulsed with part of the tibial tubercle in children (Figure 40–30), but it usually ruptures within the substance of its fibers in adults.

The characteristic clinical sign of tear of the anterior cruciate ligament is a positive Lachman: the knee is flexed to 30 degrees and pulled forward, and excessive anterior excursion of the proximal tibia (in comparison with the opposite normal knee) is noted. MRI is helpful for identifying associated meniscal or chondral injury. Reconstruction is usually required for young, active patients who wish to participate in sports that call for sudden cutting or twisting movements. Reconstruction is delayed until full range of motion is obtained. With avulsion, displaced tibial bone is present, and attachment of the fragment in anatomic position by arthroscopy is necessary.

D. Posterior Cruciate Ligament

Tear of the posterior ligament may occur within its substance or by avulsion of a fragment of bone at its tibial attachment. Tear of the posterior cruciate ligament can be diagnosed by the posterior "drawer" sign: The knee is flexed at a right angle, and the upper tibia is pushed backward; if excessive posterior excursion of the proximal tibia can be noted, tear of the posterior ligament is likely. MRI is very accurate for diagnosis of these injuries.

Bony avulsion of the posterior cruciate ligament should be addressed surgically with reattachment. Isolated tears can be treated nonoperatively. Treatment is directed primarily at the associated injuries and maintenance of competency of the quadriceps strength.

▶ Cartilage Injury

Damage to the cartilage is common with trauma to the knee and should be differentiated from osteoarthritis. Developments in cartilage transplantation, including autograft and allograft reconstruction, have improved the prognosis for these injuries. Arthroscopy and MRI are required for accurate diagnosis (Figure 40–31). Cartilage can also be biopsied from the knee, cultured, and then implanted at a later date.

▶ Ligamentous Reconstruction of the Knee

Knee joint instability may be (1) single plane (medial, lateral, posterior, or anterior), (2) rotatory, or (3) a combination of the two.

Reconstructive procedures to replace the function of the anterior and posterior cruciate ligament include use of a portion of autograft or allograft tendon to recreate the native ligament. Indications for major reconstruction of knee ligaments depend on the patient's age and activity level and the status of the articular cartilage within the knee.

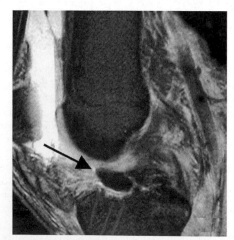

▲ **Figure 40–30.** Lateral T1-weighted MRI image showing an acute rupture of the anterior cruciate ligament (arrow).

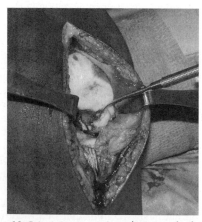

▲ **Figure 40–31.** Intraoperative photograph showing a full-thickness cartilage injury.

Bachmann LM et al: The accuracy of the Ottawa knee rule to rule out knee fractures: a systematic review. Ann Intern Med 2004; 140:121.

Cooper RL, Taylor NF, Feller JA: A randomised controlled trial of proprioceptive and balance training after surgical reconstruction of the anterior cruciate ligament. Res Sports Med 2005; 13:217.

The Diagnosis and Management of Soft Tissue Knee Injuries: Internal Derangements. New Zealand Guidelines Group, 2003.

Ryzewicz M et al: The diagnosis of meniscus tears: the role of MRI and clinical examination. Clin Orthop Relat Res 2007;455:123.

PAIN SYNDROMES OF THE HIP

1. Bursitis & Tendonitis of the Hip

Bursitis and tendonitis are frequent causes of pain around the hip area. These conditions most commonly affect middle-aged and elderly patients. Patients with a history of prior hip surgery, such as hip replacement or fixation of a hip fracture, may be especially prone to these conditions.

▶ Clinical Findings

A. Symptoms and Signs

A common complaint is the inability to sleep or rest on the affected side. The painful area is localized over the prominence of the greater trochanter, and the pain is reproduced by firm palpation. Hip bursitis may be associated with tendonitis of the hip abductors that insert onto the greater trochanter. Pain due to tendonitis may be reproduced with active hip abduction against resistance.

It is important to differentiate extra-articular sources of hip pain such as bursitis and tendonitis from intra-articular sources such as osteoarthritis. Intra-articular pathology is suggested by pain localized to the groin, limited internal rotation, and reproduction of the patient's pain at the extremes of rotation.

B. Imaging Studies

Plain radiographs are extremely useful in the evaluation of hip joint disorders.

▶ Treatment

Trochanteric bursitis often responds to rest, oral anti-inflammatory medications, and stretching. Corticosteroid injection is highly effective in refractory cases. Rapid relief of symptoms confirms injection of the proper area.

2. The Snapping Hip

The painful snapping hip is most commonly caused by the iliotibial band snapping over the prominence of the greater trochanter. Less commonly, the iliopsoas tendon may be the cause of pain as it snaps over the hip joint capsule.

Snapping due to the iliotibial band can be reproduced with passive flexion of the hip starting from an adducted position. Snapping of the iliopsoas tendon may be reproduced with passive extension and internal rotation of the hip starting from a flexed and externally rotated position. Fluoroscopy after injection of the iliopsoas bursa with contrast can help to confirm this diagnosis.

Treatment usually consists of stretching and strengthening exercises. In rare circumstances, surgical release may be indicated for refractory cases.

▼ JOINTS

ARTHRITIS

▶ General Considerations

Arthritis is an umbrella term for different inflammatory and noninflammatory disorders affecting synovial joints. Patients with advanced arthritis will experience pain, loss of motion, and joint deformity resulting in significant disability. Three major types of arthritis are discussed here: rheumatoid arthritis (RA), spondylarthritis, and osteoarthritis (OA).

1. Rheumatoid Arthritis

▶ General Considerations

RA is a chronic inflammatory autoimmune disease that attacks the synovial joints, causing a symmetric, erosive, deforming polyarthritis. RA is more common in women than in men, affecting approximately 75 of every 100,000 people. RA in many cases results in partial or total disability and is associated with a shortened life expectancy.

▶ Clinical Evaluation

Patients typically complain of joint pain, swelling, tenderness, and early morning stiffness that lasts more than 1 hour and improves with activity. The joints most commonly involved include the metacarpophalangeal, proximal interphalangeal, and metatarsophalangeal. The cervical spine is often involved as well. In later stages of RA, tendon subluxation, tendon rupture, and joint destruction occurs.

Currently, the most specific laboratory finding for RA is the presence of anticyclic citrullinated peptide antibodies. Approximately two thirds of RA patients will display these antibodies. Rheumatoid factor is a more sensitive but less specific laboratory finding, present in approximately 90% of patients with RA. Other common laboratory findings include antinuclear antibody (ANA) with homogenous pattern, elevated erythrocyte sedimentation rate (ESR), elevated cross-reacting protein (CRP), decreased hematocrit, and increased platelet count.

Radiographs typically show bony erosions and osteopenia. Joint-space narrowing, bone resorption, deformity, dislocation, and fragmentation occur as the disease process progresses. Protrusio acetabuli (medial migration of the femoral head through the acetabulum into the pelvis) is sometimes seen on x-ray.

Etiology

Currently, tumor necrosis factor alpha (TNF-α) and interleukin-1b (IL-1b) are considered to be the major proinflammatory cytokines responsible for the pathogenesis of RA. When these two cytokines are secreted, they stimulate synovial cells to proliferate and produce collagenase, which leads to cartilage degradation, bone resorption, and inhibition of proteoglycan synthesis. Additionally, these two cytokines induce other inflammatory cytokines and matrix metalloproteinases, which further contribute to and sustain the inflammatory cascade.

Treatment

In the past, treatment of RA was purely for symptom relief, consisting of splinting and rest of inflamed joints with oral NSAIDs. However, with the advent of disease-modifying antirheumatic drugs (DMARDs) and anticytokine medications, the actual progression of the disease has been curtailed in patients.

Currently, three TNF-α antagonists are approved for the treatment of RA in the United States: infliximab, etanercept, and adalimumab. When one of these three drugs is used in combination with methotrexate, patients experience better functional outcomes and less joint structural damage over the course of time when compared to patients who are treated with only one medication. Due to the increased risk of serious infection, especially tuberculosis reactivation, patients should be screened for TB prior to starting one of the TNF-α antagonists. Additionally, patients with demyelinating disease should not take one of these agents.

Glucocorticoids have also been used to treat active RA for several years. The immediate anti-inflammatory affects of glucocorticoids are well known. However, glucocorticoids have severe long-term side affects that make their continued use undesirable. At this time, treatment with low-dose prednisolone for the first 6 months of treatment in combination with a DMARD (eg, methotrexate) is an acceptable management plan. However, after 6 months, the prednisolone should be discontinued in favor of other therapy.

Other treatment medications for RA include anakinra (IL-1 receptor antagonist), abatacept (T-cell modulator), rituximab (B-cell modulator), doxycycline (matrix metalloproteinase modulator), and statins (anti-inflammatory). These medications may be considered when therapy with TNF-α antagonists is contraindicated.

For patients with severe arthritic change, joint replacement surgery can provide excellent pain relief and improved function. Joints that can be replaced include the hip, knee, shoulder, elbow, and metacarpophalangeal joints. Additionally, fusion may be considered for diseased joints of the hand and wrist that are not amenable to replacement.

2. Seronegative Spondylarthritis

General Considerations

Spondyloarthritis encompasses a group of inflammatory arthritides characterized by spinal and peripheral joint oligoarthritis and enthesitis (fibrosis and calcification at the point of attachment between muscle and bone). This family of diseases includes ankylosing spondylitis (AS), psoriatic arthritis, enteropathic arthritis (associated with inflammatory bowel disease), reactive arthritis, and undifferentiated spondyloarthropathy.

3. Ankylosing Spondylitis (AS)

AS is a chronic inflammatory disease of the axial skeleton characterized by back pain, prolonged morning stiffness, and progressive loss of motion of the axial spine. There can also be sacroiliac involvement, arthritis of the hips, and peripheral arthritis. This disease typically affects young adults, with peak onset usually between 20 and 30 years of age. Males are more commonly affected than females. Over time, there is increased flexion of the neck, increased thoracic kyphosis, and loss of lumbar lordosis leading to a stooped posture. Radiographs will show squaring of the vertebral bodies early on. With disease progression, bridging syndesmophytes, ankylosis of the facet joints, calcification of the anterior longitudinal ligament, and atlantoaxial (C1–C2) subluxation may be noted.

Laboratory values have little role in the diagnosis of AS. ESR and CRP are often elevated. HLA-B27 is the only genetic locus definitively linked to AS, but it is not specific.

Treatment with NSAIDs is very effective with significant improvement in back pain. Recently, TNF-α antagonists (infliximab, etanercept, and adalimumab) have been effective in the treatment of AS in clinical trials. As in patients with RA, tuberculosis screening should take place prior to the initiation of TNF-α treatment.

4. Psoriatic Arthritis

Psoriatic arthritis is chronic inflammatory disease characterized by skin lesions and arthritis of the peripheral joints. One third of patients have arthritis of the spine as well. Patients may experience nail pitting and onycholysis (painless separation of the nail from the nail bed).

Psoriatic arthritis is commonly treated with NSAIDs. DMARDs such as methotrexate are also used with success. Like RA and AS, recent success has been demonstrated with the use of anti-TNF-α agents.

5. Enteropathic Arthritis, Reactive Arthritis, & Undifferentiated Spondylarthropathy

Enteropathic arthritis is the spondyloarthropathy associated with ulcerative colitis and/or Crohn disease. Typically, the spondyloarthropathy in these patients progresses independently of the bowel pathology. Patients with reactive arthritis develop axial disease after exposure to an infectious agent such as *Salmonella, Shigella,* or *Chlamydia.* Undifferentiated spondyloarthropathy characterizes spinal disease without an adequate number of symptoms or signs to designate a specific type of arthritis. Treatment for these types of arthritides includes TNF-α inhibitors and NSAIDs.

6. Osteoarthritis (OA)

OA is a common age-related pathology characterized by damage to hyaline articular cartilage, synovitis, thickening of the joint capsule, and bony remodeling. In contrast to RA, patients with OA will complain of joint pain that worsens with activity and short-acting stiffness after inactivity. Female sex, prior joint injuries, family history, and obesity are additional risk factors for the development of OA. Radiographs will often show joint-space narrowing, sclerosis, and osteophytes.

Initial treatment includes NSAIDs or acetaminophen for pain relief and physical therapy to strengthen and improve the flexibility of muscles around the pathologic joint. A significant drawback to chronic NSAID treatment is the development of gastrointestinal toxicity, including ulceration. Cox-2 inhibitors, such as Celebrex, were introduced as anti-inflammatory alternatives without the same gastrointestinal side effects. However, because of concerns over possible increase in serious cardiovascular events, some Cox-2 inhibitors (rofecoxib and valdecoxib) were withdrawn from the market. At this time, there are Cox-2 inhibitors (celecoxib, etoricoxib, and lumiracoxib), that have been shown to have similar efficacy for treatment of OA compared to nonspecific NSAIDs with fewer gastrointestinal side effects and without significant increase in the rate of serious cardiac events.

Exercise and weight loss are two additional interventions that are critical for the management of osteoarthritis. Obesity is strongly associated with the development of OA. The average person's knee feels 3–6 times their body weight during activities such as walking and running. Moderate weight loss will reduce the pain and inflammation associated with OA as well as slow the progression of this disease. Also, improving the strength and flexibility of muscles around joints through exercise will lead to better functional outcome and pain ratings.

Other treatment options include intra-articular injection of glucocorticoids and hyaluronans. These injections appear to improve pain in the short term, without many significant side effects. However, these treatments do not provide significant long-term relief for most patients, nor do they alter disease progression.

Glucosamine and chondroitin sulfate result in improved pain and function for some patients and no effect for other patients. Given that side effects are minimal, treatment with these two products is reasonable for those who have an improvement in their symptoms.

For severe cases of OA, surgery including total joint replacement may be considered depending on the state of the disease and patient characteristics.

7. Hip Disorders and Reconstruction

▶ General Considerations

In the United States, 200,000 total hip replacements (THRs) are performed annually for hip arthritis. The incidence of THR will continue to increase as the population ages. The causes of hip arthritis include childhood disorders such as developmental dysplasia, Legg-Calve-Perthes disease, slipped capital femoral epiphysis, as well as inflammatory arthritis, osteonecrosis, trauma, and infection. Although arthritis is the most common cause of hip dysfunction, there are other causes as well, such as femoroacetabular impingement and "snapping" hip syndrome. Also, patients will often complain of "hip pain" when their pain is actually lower back pain or pain over the greater trochanter or lateral thigh. As a result, thorough history, physical examination, and radiographic studies are crucial for differentiating among these different entities and making the correct diagnosis.

▶ Clinical Evaluation

True intra-articular hip pathology typically presents as pain localized to the groin, exacerbated by internal rotation. Patients will often complain of difficulty with ambulation, climbing stairs, putting on shoes, and sexual intercourse.

Physical examination should include neurovascular documentation, hip range of motion, evaluation of the spine, and palpation for points of tenderness. Tenderness at the greater trochanter may be indicative of bursitis, which is often successfully treated with corticosteroid and lidocaine injection. True hip joint pathology should not result in pain that is reproducible with palpation.

Flexion contractures, asymmetric hip abductor weakness (Trendelenburg sign), and labral impingement signs (pain with flexion, adduction, and internal rotation, or FAI) should also be tested for. Leg-length discrepancy should be noted as well.

It is important to recognize that although groin pain and exacerbation of pain with internal rotation or the FAI maneuver is indicative of pathology specific for the hip joint, the exact cause of the patient's symptoms (arthritis, avascular necrosis, impingement) still requires further delineation with additional physical examination maneuvers and radiographic testing.

Younger patients with hip pain may specifically complain of a "snapping" or "catching" sensation. Also known as the "snapping hip," this may be caused by the iliotibial band (IT band) snapping across the greater trochanter or the iliopsoas tendon snapping across the iliopectineal prominence. The IT band is likely the source if pain or snapping is reproduced with adduction and rotation of the hip while the patient is standing. The iliopsoas tendon is tested with the patient supine, moving the hip from a flexed and internally rotated position to an extended and externally rotated position.

Standard radiographs of the hip include anteroposterior view of the pelvis, and anteroposterior and frog-lateral views of the pathologic hip. It is important to note any deformity of the femoral head, acetabulum, and joint space, as well as any signs that may be specific to a particular disease process. For example, patients with developmental hip dysplasia often display a shallow socket with decreased anterior and lateral acetabular coverage on radiographs. A false-profile view (true lateral view of the acetabulum) may be performed to evaluate the degree of acetabular dysplasia present.

When plain radiographs fail to reveal a diagnosis, additional diagnostic imaging, including MRI, CT, or bone scan, may detect osteonecrosis, stress fractures, neoplasms, or labral or hyaline cartilage pathology.

If the clinical picture remains unclear or is complicated by concomitant spine pathology, intra-articular diagnostic injection of the hip joint with anesthetic may be performed.

▶ Femoroacetabular Impingement

Femoroacetabular impingement describes abnormal tracking between the femoral head and neck and the acetabulum through a normal range of hip motion resulting in pain and/or bony deformity. There are two types of femoroacetabular impingement: cam-type and pincer-type. Cam-type impingement describes a femoral neck with prominent anterior bone that impinges on a normal acetabulum and labrum, resulting in damage to one or both. Pincer-type impingement results from an anterior acetabular osteophyte that abuts the anterior femoral neck during hip flexion.

Femoroacetabular impingement can be treated with resection of the offending osteophytes or prominent bone and debridement or repair of damaged labrum. These procedures can be performed through hip arthroscopy or an open approach.

▶ Avascular Necrosis of the Hip

Osteonecrosis of the femoral head can occur in young patients. Risk factors include steroid use, alcoholism, trauma, marrow-replacing diseases (such as Gaucher disease), high-dose radiation treatment, and hypercoagulable states (sickle cell disease, hypofibrinolysis, thrombophilia, protein S and C deficiencies). The disease course consists of decreased blood flow to the femoral head, resulting in osteonecrosis, subchondral fracture, and eventually collapse.

Standard anteroposterior and lateral radiographs of the hip often reveal the diagnosis. Of note, subchondral fracture of the hip is most clearly seen on the lateral radiograph. If radiographs are nondiagnostic for a patient for whom osteonecrosis is suspected, MRI is the next step. The lateral and anterior aspects of the femoral head are most commonly affected.

Avascular necrosis of the hip may be classified according the Ficat grading system: type I (no radiographic signs of avascular necrosis), type II (changes of the femoral head subchondral bone without collapse), type III (subchondral fracture with collapse), and type IV (collapse of the femoral head with changes on the acetabular side).

Unfortunately, without intervention, progression of osteonecrosis to collapse will occur in most patients. Patients with preclinical or asymptomatic osteonecrosis can be observed without surgical intervention. Symptomatic precollapse osteonecrosis may be treated with core decompression with or without bone graft, vascularized fibula grafting, or oral bisphosphonates. At this time, there is a paucity of data to definitively support one treatment over another.

Although some studies have demonstrated success with treating postcollapse osteonecrosis with vascularized fibula grafts or rotational osteotomies, arthroplasty is the more reliable method of treatment. Treatment with unipolar and bipolar arthroplasty is initially successful but often results in conversion to total hip arthroplasty due to eventual loss of acetabular cartilage and recurrent pain. Young patients who receive total hip arthroplasty with conventional polyethylene components experience a high rate of osteolysis and subsequent need for revision surgery. Currently, clinical trials are being performed to evaluate the use of alternative bearing surfaces and hip resurfacing surgery in this challenging patient population.

DeSmet AA et al: Expert Panel on Musculoskeletal Imaging. Avascular necrosis of the hip. American College of Radiology, 2005. Available at http://www.acr.org/SecondaryMainMenu Categories/quality_safety/app_criteria/pdf/ExpertPanelon MusculoskeletalImaging/AvascularNecrosisoftheHipDoc3.aspx. Accessed February 14, 2009.

Expert Panel on Musculoskeletal Imaging. Chronic hip pain. American College of Radiology, 2003. Available at http://www.acr.org/SecondaryMainMenuCategories/quality_safety/app_criteria/pdf/ExpertPanelonMusculoskeletalImaging/ChronicHipPainDoc8.aspx. Accessed February 14, 2009.

▶ Surgical Treatment Options for Hip Pathology

Surgical options for the hip include hip arthroscopy, osteotomies, resection, arthrodesis, and arthroplasty. Choice of treatment depends on the type of hip pathology being treated, patient characteristics, and the experience level of the surgeon.

A. Hip Arthroscopy

Hip arthroscopy typically involves the placement of two portals with the help of fluoroscopy. The arthroscope is inserted through one portal to visualize the hip joint and any pathology. The second portal serves as a "working portal" through which instruments such as debriders, shavers, or pincers are inserted to treat the pathology in question. This technique can be used to treat intra-articular and extra-articular hip pathology. Treatment of intra-articular pathology usually requires the aid of limb traction. Intra-articular indications include debridement of labral tears, loose body removal, chondral lesion debridement, osteophyte resection, biopsy, and synovectomy. Extra-articular pathology such as the snapping hip may be treated with lengthening or releasing the iliopsoas and/or IT band. Complications of hip arthroscopy, such as pudendal and sciatic nerve palsies, are becoming less frequent with improved patient positioning and surgical technique. More long-term studies are needed to assess the efficacy of this technique.

B. Osteotomy

Osteotomy of the adult hip involves the use of saws or osteotomes to make bone cuts on the femur or pelvis. The resulting pieces of bone are realigned and fixed with plates and/or screws to correct deformity. Osteotomy is used to treat dysplasia, residual deformity from slipped capital femoral epiphyses, cerebral palsy with hip instability, and avascular necrosis. Choice of femoral or acetabular osteotomy is dependent on the pathology present and patient characteristics.

C. Resection Arthroplasty

Resection arthroplasty, or the Girdlestone procedure, involves complete resection of the femoral head without replacement. This procedure is a salvage surgery reserved for severe hip infection resistant to antibiotic treatment, failed total hip arthroplasty with unreconstructible bone defects, previous high-dose pelvic radiation exposure that would limit healing of a complex reconstructive procedure, or patients with severe medical comorbidities and limited functional needs who may not tolerate a longer procedure. Patients treated with resection arthroplasty will have a significant limb-length discrepancy that will likely require the use of a shoe lift and/or other walking aides.

D. Arthrodesis

Arthrodesis of the hip may be indicated for patients with acquired (eg, trauma or infection) or developmental (eg, dysplasia) hip abnormalities. The optimal position for arthrodesis is 5–10 degrees of external rotation, 20–30 degrees of flexion, and neutral adduction. Although pain relief and function can be excellent, this procedure results in increased energy expenditure and late onset osteoarthritis of the lumbar spine and knee due to increased joint stresses resulting from changes in the patient's gait.

E. Hip Arthroplasty

Hip arthroplasty involves the replacement of the femoral head and/or the acetabulum with manufactured components. Hemiarthroplasty may be performed replacing the femoral head without treatment of the acetabulum. Total hip arthroplasty entails replacement of the femoral head and placement of an acetabular component.

Hemiarthroplasty typically entails replacement of native the femoral head with a metal femoral head and neck. Indications include hip fracture in the elderly patient, avascular necrosis of the femoral head, and arthritis of the femoral head without acetabular disease. Hemiarthroplasty

may be unipolar (one point of articulation between the metal femoral head and native acetabulum) or bipolar (two points of articulation: one between the femoral head and acetabulum and another between the femoral neck and femoral head). Due to development of acetabular disease, many hemiarthroplasties are often converted to total hip arthroplasties with placement of an acetabular component. Although bipolar hemiarthroplasties offers the theoretical advantage of improved range of motion and decreased acetabular wear compared to unipolar arthroplasty due to the second point of articulation, these effects have not been demonstrated in clinical studies. Due to the significantly higher cost, most authors do not advocate the use of bipolar hemiarthroplasty over unipolar hemiarthroplasty.

Total hip arthroplasty involves replacement of the femoral head and placement of an acetabular component (Figure 40–32). Conventional polyethylene acetabular components with metal femoral heads have performed well at 15–20 year follow-up in older patient populations (older than 60). However, in younger and or more active patients, polyethylene wear and associated osteolysis (bone breakdown) represent the most common cause of long-term failure. Alternative

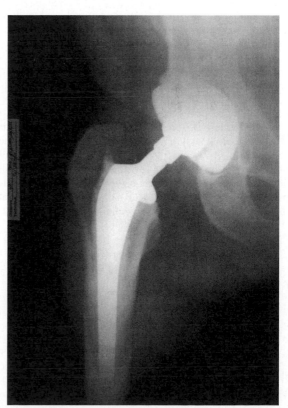

▲ **Figure 40–32.** Hybrid total hip replacement with porous coated acetabular shell and cemented femoral stem performed for osteoarthritis.

bearing options, such as ceramic-on-ceramic, metal-on–highly cross-linked polyethylene, and metal-on-metal designs, have been introduced to address these concerns.

Each of these bearing options has advantages and disadvantages. Ceramic-on-ceramic offers low wear rate without the production of metal ions; however, there is a reported 1–3% "squeaking" rate, and they can fracture, resulting in catastrophic failure. Metal-on-metal produces metal ions that can significantly increase their concentration in the blood. To date, no increase in cancer rates or other side effects have been noted due to the metal ions. Metal-on-metal prostheses do not cause the squeaking side effects and are unlikely to fracture. High cross-linked polyethylene is more forgiving with regard to the placement of the acetabular component. However, concerns regarding wear debris and subsequent osteolysis remain, although preliminary data suggests that the wear debris produced is significantly less than the regular cross-linked polyethylene.

F. Resurfacing Arthroplasty

Resurfacing arthroplasty is a type of total hip replacement that was first introduced in the 1970s. Resurfacing involves placement of an acetabular component in addition to replacing the surface ("resurfacing") of the femoral head without resecting the entire femoral head or femoral neck. The resurfacing is typically done with a metal femoral component. This prosthesis interface initially did quite poorly, with high early failure rates related to wear debris, osteolysis, and subsequent prosthetic failure. Due to advances in metallurgy and other aspects of total joint technology, the resurfacing arthroplasty has produced short-term successful results and gained popularity in recent years. Resurfacing is ideal for younger patients without any cyst or other pathology of the femoral neck. By preserving most of the femoral head and all of the neck, future total hip revision surgery, if needed, will be less difficult and demanding. Contraindications to this procedure include cyst or other pathology of the femoral neck, which can predispose to femoral neck fracture.

American Academy of Orthopaedic Surgeons clinical guideline on prevention of symptomatic pulmonary embolism in patients undergoing total hip or knee arthroplasty. American Academy of Orthopedic Surgeons, 2007.

Weissman BN et al: Expert Panel on Musculoskeletal Imaging. Imaging after total hip arthroplasty (THA). American College of Radiology, 2005. Available at http://www.acr.org/Secondary MainMenuCategories/quality_safety/app_criteria/pdf/ ExpertPanelonMusculoskeletalImaging/ImagingafterTotalHip ArthroplastyDoc12.aspx. Accessed February 14, 2009.

INFECTIONS ASSOCIATED WITH JOINT REPLACEMENTS

Infections that occur after total joint replacement may be caused by organisms introduced at the time of surgery or late hematogenous contamination. Medical providers should always maintain a high index of suspicion for infection in the patients with previous arthroplasty surgery. New onset pain or loosening of the prosthesis noted on x-ray is infection related until proven otherwise. ESR, CRP, and joint aspiration are part of the standard workup. Choice of treatment depends on when the infection occurs, the virulence of organism involved, and the stability of the prosthetic components. If the infection occurs within 3 weeks of the initial surgery, some authors advocate performing a wash-out with liner exchange. If infection occurs at a later time and/or loosening is noted radiographically, resection of the prosthesis is typically recommended with interval placement of an antibiotic cement spacer (methylmethacrylate with impregnated antibiotic) and intravenous antibiotic treatment for at least 6 weeks. Once the infection has cleared, reimplantation of a new prosthesis may be considered. For chronically infected prostheses, fusion or resection arthroplasty may be considered.

TOTAL KNEE REPLACEMENT

Reconstructive surgical options for the arthritic knee (Figure 40–33) include high tibial osteotomy, unicompartmental knee arthroplasty, and total knee arthroplasty. Indications for reconstructive surgery of the knee includes severe pain with or without deformity and radiographic evidence of arthritis for which conservative treatment (physical therapy, NSAIDs, corticosteroid joint injections) has failed. Choice of surgical treatment depends on patient characteristics in addition to the condition of the knee.

► Total Knee Arthroplasty

Total knee arthroplasty involves replacement of bone from the distal femur and proximal tibia with a metal component on the femoral side and polyethylene (or a metal tray with a polyethylene insert) on the tibial side. There are several types of total knee arthroplasty designs that vary in the degree to which they constrain knee motion. Choice of implant depends on the ligamentous stability of the knee and surgeon preference. A fully constrained prosthesis, which only allows flexion and extension, is typically used in knees with severe deformity and/or significant ligamentous instability. The literature reflects a significant success rate for total knee arthroplasty, with patients reporting good to excellent outcomes 85–90% of the time. Factors associated with poor outcome as perceived by the patients include obesity, female gender, age younger than 60, and previous history of depression.

► Unicompartmental Knee Arthroplasty

Unicompartmental knee arthroplasty may be considered in the elderly individual (> 60 years old), with isolated medial or lateral compartment arthritis. The advantages of unicompartmental over total knee arthroplasty include preservation of knee kinematics, decreased operative morbidity, and quicker rehabilitation time. However, unicompartmental

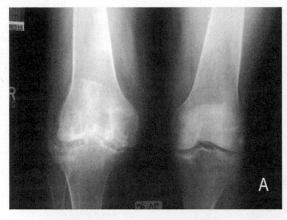
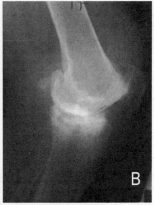
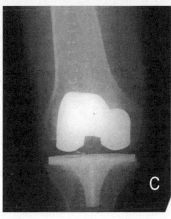
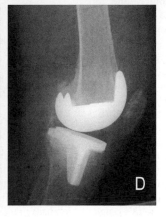

▲ **Figure 40–33. A–B:** Patient with rheumatoid arthritis and severe joint destruction of the right knee. **C–D:** Patient was treated with a cemented right total knee replacement.

knee arthroplasty is contraindicated in patients with an anterior cruciate ligament–deficient knee, range of motion less than 90 degrees or flexion contracture greater than 15 degrees, and patients with arthritic disease in more than one knee compartment.

▶ High Tibial Osteotomy

The high tibial osteotomy may be considered in the young, active patient with isolated medial compartment arthritis for whom total knee arthroplasty is an imperfect long-term solution. Patients with isolated medial compartment arthritis typically have varus deformity of the knee. The high tibial osteotomy will produce a valgus correction of this deformity and unload the diseased articular surface on the medial side. The short-term results of this procedure include reduction of pain levels and deformity correction; however, they typically deteriorate over time, resulting in the need for additional surgery.

AAOS Clinical Practice Guideline on Osteoarthritis of the Knee. American Academy of Orthopaedic Surgeons, 2003.
AAOS Clinical Guideline on Osteoarthritis of the Knee (Phase II). American Academy of Orthopaedic Surgeons, 2003.

GLENOHUMERAL ARTHRITIS & SHOULDER RECONSTRUCTION

Successfully treating the arthritic shoulder requires an understanding of the patient's functional demands as well as the severity and quality of the patient's symptoms. A careful history and physical examination, along with the appropriate diagnostic studies, will allow the treating physician to formulate an appropriate treatment plan.

History taking starts with determining the patient's primary complaint: Is it pain, weakness, or loss of motion? Patients with significant glenohumeral arthritis typically complain of anterior or superolateral shoulder pain that is worse with activity. Weakness with loss of motion due to inactivity may be noted as well. Posterior pain or radicular type symptoms (pain that radiates from the spine down the back of the shoulder) is concerning for disorder of the spinal cord and should initiate the appropriate workup. Prior treatment including physical therapy, injections, and any surgical procedures should be asked about as well.

Physical examination should note neurovascular status and the presence of any muscle atrophy. Particular attention should be paid to the integrity of the rotator cuff muscles (supraspinatus, infraspinatus, teres minor, and subscapularis) and deltoid muscles. The shoulder physical examination is described in greater detail in the Sports Medicine section of this chapter. Cervical range of motion is assessed as well, along with the Spurling maneuver (test for cervical radiculopathy).

Radiographic studies include anteroposterior and axillary views of the shoulder. Glenoid erosion resulting in decreased humeral head offset from the lateral border of the acromion may be noted. Patients with associated rotator cuff disease may have superior subluxation of the humeral head with associated decrease in the acromiohumeral distance.

Early stages of shoulder arthritis can be treated nonsurgically with NSAIDs, intra-articular steroid or hyaluronic acid injections, and a physical therapy program that focuses on maintaining range-of-motion and strengthening exercises.

Patients with mild arthritis that does not respond to conservative treatment measures may pursue arthroscopic surgery. Debridement of any chondral lesions and loose body removal may alleviate mechanical symptoms, while arthroscopic lavage removing inflammatory enzymes and proteins from the joint fluid often provides pain relief.

For patients with significant arthritis, shoulder arthroscopy may or may not provide relief. If successful, this surgery represents a temporary solution that may relieve symptoms for a short period of time. Shoulder reconstructive surgery, including humeral hemiarthroplasty, glenoid resurfacing, total shoulder arthroplasty, reverse total shoulder arthroplasty, and glenohumeral fusion, are the treatment options to consider. It is important to note that the primary indication for shoulder replacement surgery is debilitating pain. These surgeries may or may not improve the patient's range of motion and/or strength.

Patients with shoulder arthritis and an intact rotator cuff may be treated with total shoulder arthroplasty (replacement of the glenoid and humerus with prosthetic components) or hemiarthroplasty (resurfacing of the humerus) alone. Two recent prospective studies comparing the two procedures suggest that pain relief may be better and rate of revision surgery (conversion to total shoulder arthroplasty due to glenoid arthritis) may be lower for total shoulder arthroplasty than for hemiarthroplasty.

For patients with a deficient rotator cuff tear and arthritis, hemiarthroplasty is the preferred option, as superior humeral migration due to a deficient cuff leads to loosening of the glenoid component. Biologic resurfacing of the glenoid with interposition graft (anterior capsule, fascia lata autograft, allografts) may be performed as well to address any arthritic change of the glenoid.

Reverse total shoulder arthroplasty that involves a convex glenoid and concave humerus may be used in elderly (> 70 years), low-demand patients with a deficient rotator cuff and intact deltoid. This prosthesis places the center of rotation in the scapular neck, thereby increasing the lever arm.

Historically, shoulder fusion could be considered for the young laborer with severe arthritis due to long-term failure of

shoulder arthroplasty. With the advent of glenoid biologic resurfacing, shoulder fusion has become a less common surgical option reserved for deltoid deficient arthritic shoulders.

Ecklund KJ et al: Rotator cuff tear arthropathy. JAAOS 2007; 15:340.

Fischgrund JS: OKU 9: *Orthopedic Knowledge Update*. American Academy of Orthopaedic Surgeons, 2008.

Zeman CA et al: The rotator cuff-deficient arthritic shoulder: diagnosis and management. JAAOS 1998;6:337.

▼ ORTHOPEDIC SPINE

SPINE

Neck and back pain are two of the most common chief complaints in any outpatient clinic. Although most instances of these types of pain are related to muscular strain, neck and back pain may also be related to pathology of the spine. It is important for all health care providers to be able to distinguish between these two entities. True pathology of the spine requires timely referral to a spine surgeon for evaluation and treatment.

▶ History & Physical Examination

A chief complaint of neck or back pain should prompt a thorough history and musculoskeletal examination, including both the upper and lower extremities. Specific questions to ask regarding the pain include onset, characterization, intensity, radiation, and timing. Pain that radiates down a patient's arm or legs may qualify as a radicular symptom and is indicative of spine root pathology. Additionally, the patient should be asked about night sweats, fevers, nighttime pain, and weight loss, which are red flags for infection or cancer. The presence of numbness, tingling, motor weakness, or loss of bowel or bladder control is indicative of spine root pathology. Arm or leg pain that occurs during walking or activity and is relieved immediately with rest may be due to neurogenic claudication indicative of spinal stenosis. Patients with lumbar stenosis and resulting leg pain often state that their leg pain improves going upstairs or leaning over the grocery cart at the grocery stair (flexion of the lumbar spine opens up the canal, relieving the stenosis).

Physical examination includes strength, sensation, and reflex testing; gait observation; and documentation of vascular status. Strength of muscles is graded according to the 5-point scale described in the section on Fractures & Dislocations of the Spine. Neurosensory examination should also be carried out to evaluate the C5–T1 dermatomes for neck pain and the L2–S1 dermatomes for back pain. Reflex examination includes the documentation of the biceps, triceps, brachioradialis, patella, Achilles, and the presence or absence of a Babinski sign. Wide-based gait may be indicative of cervical spine pathology.

When neurologic testing is abnormal, distinction should be made between radicular (root pathology) and myelopathic (spinal cord pathology) symptoms/signs. Radicular symptoms include complaints of radiating pain from the spine down the arms or legs. Loss of bowel and/or bladder control and groin/perianal numbness is indicative of sacral rootlet pathology. Radicular signs on physical examination include a positive straight leg raise (pain shooting down the back of the leg extending below the knee with straight leg raise), positive Spurling test (radiating arm pain with neck extension and rotation toward the pathologic side), specific muscle weakness (eg, biceps weakness on the right side only), specific dermatome numbness, and specific decreased reflexes. Myelopathic signs include diffuse muscle weakness below a certain level, hyperreflexia, clonus, positive Babinski sign, positive Lhermitte sign (sensation of shooting pain down arms or legs with neck motion), and positive Hoffman sign (the patient's middle finger is flicked into extension by the examiner, resulting in unintended thumb and finger flexion).

1. Cervical Strain

▶ Clinical Findings

A. Symptoms and Signs

Cervical strain is characterized by paraspinous (next to the midline) neck pain with or without radiation to the shoulder. Patients often display limitation of neck motion as well. These symptoms typically appear after an episode of overexertion or prolonged tension or poor posture. Specific points of deep tenderness with reproducible pain with palpation, known as "trigger points," may be present. Pain is often characterized as deep aching or boring in sensation. Muscular spasm within the trapezius, levator scapulae, and paraspinous muscles may be palpable as a firm "knot." The patient may also complain of headache or dizziness. An important differentiating point from true spine pathology is that physical examination should not reveal any neurologic deficit.

B. Imaging Studies

Radiographic evaluation starts with anteroposterior and lateral x-rays of the cervical spine. Flexion-extension views should be considered in patients with precedent neck trauma, signs of rheumatoid arthritis, or Downs syndrome to examine for instability. X-rays may reveal degenerative change such as osteophytes, ankylosis of joints, or signs of instability. However, radiographs are often normal.

▶ Differential Diagnosis

One should consider cervical spondylosis and herniated cervical disk as part of the differential diagnosis. A patient with herniated cervical disk may complain of radicular symptoms in a specific dermatomal distribution, muscle weakness, and diminished sensation or paresthesias corre-

sponding to the pathologic disk level. Diminished reflexes may be noted as well. Pain arising from cervical spondylosis (degenerative change) is often indistinguishable from that due to cervical strain.

▶ Treatment

Acute cervical spine pain is initially treated with rest and immobilization. Bracing with a soft collar, analgesics, and muscle relaxants are used as needed. However, the collar should not be used for more than 1–2 weeks to avoid cervical muscle atrophy. Ice, heat, and other modalities such as ultrasound and massage may be helpful as well.

Neck pain related to cervical strain usually subsides within 1 week from onset. Once the pain has diminished, the patient should begin physical therapy exercises to strengthen cervical muscles, improve posture, and increase range of motion.

2. Whiplash Injury

▶ General Considerations

Whiplash is an acceleration-deceleration injury that occurs most commonly when the patient is rear-ended in a motor vehicle accident. Acute hyperextension occurs, causing injury to anterior soft tissue structures of the neck, including the anterior longitudinal ligament, the intervertebral disk, the strap muscles, and the longus colli and sternocleidomastoid muscles. When the vehicle decelerates, the head recoils into flexion, causing injury to the facet capsules, posterior ligaments, and paraspinal musculature.

▶ Clinical Findings

The symptoms after whiplash injury are often variable. Neck pain and stiffness are common. Occipital headaches and retroocular pain are also frequently noted. Spasm may manifest as decreased neck motion. Neurologic examination is normal. Radiographs are usually normal.

▶ Treatment

Management of whiplash injuries is similar for cervical strain: analgesics, rest, and immobilization in a soft cervical collar until the pain is controlled, followed by gradual mobilization. Physical therapy exercises are initiated when range of motion normalizes.

3. Degenerative Cervical Disk Disease (Cervical Spondylosis)

▶ General Considerations

The degenerative changes of the spine that typically occur with aging are collectively termed spondylosis. Most degeneration visualized on radiographs is asymptomatic. As a result, disk degeneration is considered a part of the natural aging process.

Cervical spondylosis is characterized initially by tears in the posterior annulus followed by fragmentation of the disk. The weakest area of the annulus is the posterolateral region, which is the most common site of bulging of the disk. With time, uncovertebral joints and ligamentum flavum can hypertrophy, which, along with prominent spurs and degenerative disk, may encroach onto the neural foramen and spinal canal, impinging on nerve roots and/or the spinal cord. Additionally, ossification of the posterior longitudinal ligament, which is particularly predominant in the Japanese population, can cause multisegmental cervical compression and myelopathy.

▶ Clinical Findings

A. Symptoms and Signs

Clinical symptoms may or may not accompany the degenerative changes of cervical spondylosis. Neurologic compromise may result from nerve root compression (cervical spondylotic radiculopathy) or compression of the cord itself (cervical spondylotic myelopathy) (Figure 40–34). Patients with cervical radicular symptoms typically complain of pain that radiates from the neck down into the shoulders and/or arms. A Spurling test may be positive. Patients with myelopathic symptoms may complain of Lhermitte sign (lightning pain down the spine with neck flexion) and/or difficulty with fine motor movements (buttoning a shirt) and balance.

Physical examination of patients with cervical radiculopathy may show muscle weakness and diminished reflexes. Physical examination of patients with spondylotic myelopathy may be characterized by spasticity and clonus. An inverted radial reflex and a scapulohumeral reflex may also be seen. Positive Babinski and Hoffman signs may be present. Fine motion of the fingers may not be present, and intrinsic muscle wasting may be noted. The patient may have an abnormal gait characterized by wide-based, shuffling movements.

B. Imaging Studies

Radiographic findings of cervical spondylosis include narrowing of the disk space (Figure 40–35), osteophyte formation at the vertebral body margins, and arthritic degeneration of the facet joints. MRI is used to evaluate for nerve root or spinal cord impingement. Electromyography may be used as an adjunct study to confirm diagnosis by demonstrating generalized motor impairment resulting from motor neuron involvement.

▶ Differential Diagnosis

In addition to arthritis, radiculopathy or myelopathy may also be caused by tumors and vascular malformations of the spinal cord, syringomyelia, amyotrophic lateral sclerosis, subacute combined degeneration, and multiple sclerosis. MRI is the most useful study, in addition to thorough history

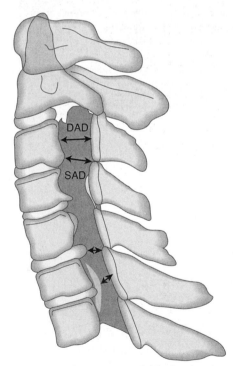

▲ **Figure 40–34.** The space available for the spinal cord in the subaxial cervical spine can be measured as the developmental anterior-posterior diameter (DAPD) in patients with developmental spinal stenosis and as the spondylolytic anterior-posterior diameter (SAPD) in patients with cervical spondylosis.

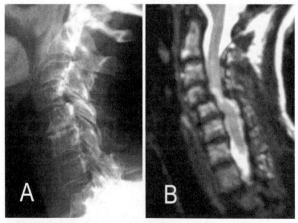

▲ **Figure 40–35. A:** Lateral radiograph of a 50-year-old man with neck pain and myelopathy. **B:** Sagittal T2-weighted MRI showing spinal cord compression at C4–5 at the level of the spondylolisthesis.

and physical examination, to distinguish between these different diagnoses.

▶ Treatment

A. Cervical Spondylotic Radiculopathy

Most patients with acute onset of cervical spondylotic radiculopathy have regression of symptoms over the course of 4–6 weeks. Progression to myelopathy is rare. Most patients achieve pain relief with rest, analgesics, and immobilization to relieve pain. Paresthesias and slight sensory changes may persist after neck and arm pain have subsided.

If pain continues, MRI of the cervical spine should be performed to investigate any areas of compression. If discrete herniation is present, surgical decompression with foraminotomy or diskectomy with or without interbody fusion may be considered.

B. Cervical Spondylotic Myelopathy

Initial management of cervical spondylotic myelopathy involves the use of NSAIDs and cervical collar to minimize symptoms.

When symptoms are progressive, are not relieved by the use of a collar, or occur in younger patients, operative treatment may be necessary. Treatment depends on the nature of the compression (disk, vertebral body, posterior osteophytes, hypertrophied ligamentum flavum, ossified posterior longitudinal ligament), the sagittal alignment of the cervical spine (kyphotic, neutral, or lordotic), and the number of levels involved. Compression confined to the intervertebral disks can be relieved by means of single-level or multiple-level anterior diskectomies and fusion. When the disease is limited to two vertebral body levels, or if there is a preexisting kyphosis greater than 15 degrees, anterior vertebrectomy, foraminotomy, and fusion with a strut graft achieves decompression and stabilization of the degenerative segments. When the compression involves more than two vertebral body levels, the morbidity associated with the anterior approach increases significantly. As a result, a posterior decompression via multilevel laminectomy with or without fusion is recommended (Figure 40–36).

▶ Course & Prognosis

Most cases of cervical spondylotic radiculopathy resolve in 4–6 weeks with conservative management. With regards to cervical spondylitic myelopathy, the results of surgical management are better when symptoms are mild and of shorter duration. However, complete postoperative resolution of symptoms is rare even in these cases. Of note, the natural evolution of spondylotic myelopathy will often result in at least partial spontaneous remission. Chronic myelopathy and multiple-level involvement are associated with poorer surgical results.

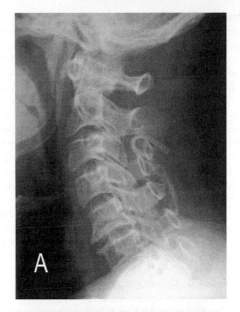

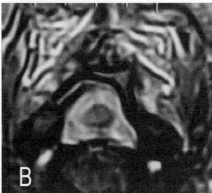

▲ **Figure 40–36.** **A:** Lateral postoperative radiograph of a patient who had multisegmental cervical stenosis and myelopathy treated with canal expansive cervical laminoplasty from C3 to C7. **B:** Postoperative axial MRI image showing significant canal expansion after the procedure.

Fischgrund JS. *OKU 9: Orthopedic Knowledge Update*. American Academy of Orthopaedic Surgeons, 2008.

PAIN SYNDROMES OF THE BACK

1. Low Back Pain

▶ General Considerations

In the United States, 400,000 workers are disabled by back pain each year. It has been estimated that 80% of the population suffers low back pain at some point during their lifetime. Due to its high prevalence, all physicians should be able to differentiate between the multiple different etiologies of back pain.

► Clinical Findings

A. Symptoms and Signs

The most common cause of low back pain is mechanical strain. Patients complain of pain related to overexertion. Often, patients in this group demonstrate poor conditioning, abdominal muscle tone, and posture.

Pain is often described as a deep-seated ache in the lumbosacral region. The pain is dull and somewhat diffuse, with or without radiation to the buttocks and hips. The pain is worsened by bending and relieved by inactivity. Palpation may reveal tenderness in the paraspinous area, with trigger points or knots. Spasm of the paraspinous muscles is a common finding.

Neurovascular examination, including strength, sensation, and reflexes, are usually within normal limits, and the straight leg raise test is normal. The straight leg raise test is performed with the patient supine on examining table; the examiner lifts the patient's leg, which is extended at the hip and knee, passively stretching the sciatic nerve with transmission of tension to the lumbosacral roots. Reproduction of pain down the legs is a positive test, indicating nerve root irritation.

B. Imaging Studies

Radiographic examination may reveal degenerative changes such as lumbar disk–space narrowing, and osteophytes or may be normal. X-rays should routinely be obtained. In persons over age 50, the presence of metastases should be evaluated. In patients under age 20, symptomatic congenital or developmental anomalies should be ruled out.

► Treatment

Management of lumbar strain includes anti-inflammatory medication and rest during the acute phase. Lumbosacral corsets may be considered for mechanical support. Abdominal conditioning and spinal muscle strengthening exercises are prescribed after the pain subsides. Typical exercises include bent-knee sit-ups and hamstring and spinal muscle stretching. Preventative measures should be presented to the patient, especially the correct manner of lifting objects while bending at the legs rather than at the spine.

► Course & Prognosis

The usual course of lumbar strain is spontaneous remission with time. Relapses of pain are common, often precipitated by heavy-duty activity. Patients with constant pain should be investigated for depression and or worker's compensation–related issues, which may be contributing factors. Patients who fail to respond to conservative treatment should be investigated for neurologic compression via MRI. If no pathology is found, patients should be encouraged to return to normal activity as soon as possible. Prolonged reliance on analgesics (especially opioids) should be discouraged.

2. Lumbar Disk Syndrome

► General Considerations

Patients may present with back pain and unilateral or bilateral leg symptoms. The back pain may be due to degeneration of the annulus fibrosis (outer layer of the disk), which contains many pain fibers. Degeneration of the annulus fibrosis may lead to herniation of the nucleus pulposus (central portion of disk) into the spinal canal impinging on neural elements, leading to leg symptoms. The posterolateral portion of the lumbar disk is the weakest and, as a result, the most common location for herniation These types of disk herniations are termed "paracentral" because they occur just lateral to the midline. Central disk herniations, which occur at the midline, occur less commonly.

The dural sac below L1 (conus medullaris) contains only nerve rootlets (cauda equina). In the lumbar spine, each nerve root emerges below its respective vertebra, just under the inferomedial border of its respective pedicle, and enters the neural foramen just above the intervertebral disk of that level. As a result, a paracentral disk herniation may compress the traversing root to the lower adjacent level. For example, an L4–5 paracentral disk herniation will compress the traversing L5 nerve root. In contrast, a far lateral disk herniation occurs near the exit zone of its respective neural foramen and therefore is most likely to compress the exiting root at that level (eg, a far-lateral disk herniation at L4–5 will impinge upon the L4 nerve root). Due to their transition point status between the lumbar and sacral spine, the L4–5 and L5–S1 disk levels correspond to the region of maximal mechanical stress in the lumbar spine. As a result, disk herniations are most likely at these two levels, and L5 and S1 nerve root pathology is most common.

► Clinical Findings

Back pain with sciatica (pain radiating down the posterior leg) is the most common presentation. The pain may be dermatome specific. The onset of leg pain is usually insidious, but pain may begin acutely when sudden disk herniation follows injury. Pain may be piercing, burning, or electrical in nature, accentuated by prolonged sitting or standing and relieved at least partially by rest.

Compression of nerve roots may produce objective sensory changes, with paresthesias and loss of sensation in the affected dermatome. With continued root compression, motor weakness may develop. Motor weakness corresponds to the specific myotomes innervated by the compressed nerve root. Muscle atrophy may accompany sensory and motor changes. The straight leg test may be positive.

► Radiographic Evaluation

Radiographs may show degenerative change, including osteophytes and loss of disk height. MRI or myelogram are very sensitive and should reveal disk herniation if present.

Care should be taken to specifically evaluate the location of the disk herniation, including the disk level and the relationship of the herniation to the midline (central, paracentral, or far-lateral).

▶ Treatment

Treatment of acute lumbar disk disease is controversial. If symptoms are produced by bulging rather than by extrusion of the herniated disk, conservative measures such as bed rest, analgesics, and anti-inflammatory medications often result in complete resolution of symptoms.

If symptoms continue or if neurologic symptoms progress or fail to respond to conservative measures, laminotomy and removal of the herniated disk may be required. Surgery is most successful in patients whose symptoms correlate with objective diagnostic study findings; that is, the patient who has L4–5 paracentral disk herniation and experiences L5 nerve root symptoms (extensor hallucis longus weakness, pain/paresthesias in the L5 dermatomal distribution) will most likely be helped by operation. Diskectomy can be performed via standard microdiskectomy techniques or though a "minimally invasive" endoscopic approach.

3. Lumbar Stenosis

In the presence of severe disk space degeneration and spondylosis, a generalized narrowing of the lumbar spinal canal (spinal stenosis) without specific disk herniation can also occur. The etiology of lumbar spinal stenosis is multifactorial, including facet joint hypertrophy, disk degeneration and loss of disk height, and hypertrophy and buckling of the ligamentum flavum.

Spinal stenosis usually affects people in their 50s and 60s. Symptoms include generalized backache and stiffness. Narrowing of the lateral recess can occur, causing unilateral nerve root symptoms and resulting in leg symptoms such as sciatica as well. Neurogenic claudication (back pain with radiating leg pain that is worse with activity and immediately relieved by rest) is a common complaint. This can be differentiated from vascular claudication by the immediacy of relief with rest (for vascular claudication, pain relief occurs only after minutes of rest).

For patients with spinal stenosis, extension leads to further narrowing of the canal exacerbating symptoms, while flexion of the spine provides symptom relief. Patients will often relate that it is easier to walk up stairs than down stairs (people have a tendency to lean forward or flex their spine when walking up stairs and lean backward or extend their spine when walking down stairs) and that walking hunched over a grocery cart helps their symptoms. On physical examination, diminished or asymmetric reflexes, specific motor weakness (extensor hallucis longus is most common), and decreased sensation in a specific dermatome may be noted.

X-ray examination may reveal degenerative changes, such as disk space narrowing and osteophytosis, or the results may

be entirely normal. A myelogram or MRI will confirm the diagnosis.

▶ Treatment

In the patient with persistent neurogenic claudication that fails to respond to conservative measures, foraminotomy or decompressive laminectomy is very effective in relieving symptoms and improving function. If spinal instability (degenerative spondylolisthesis) is also present, the spine should also be stabilized and fused over the affected levels.

4. Other Lower Back Conditions

In addition to the etiologies of back pain, one must also consider infection or tumor as possibilities. Additionally, conditions unrelated to the spine, such as abdominal aortic aneurysm, pancreatitis, and pyelonephritis, may also cause back pain and should be ruled out when suspicion is present.

The most common extradural tumors in the adult spine are metastatic, most often from breast carcinoma in women and prostate cancer in men. Multiple myeloma also frequently involves the spine and often causes pain via lytic lesions that weaken bone and lead to pathologic fractures. Intradural spinal tumors (neurofibromas, meningiomas, and ependymomas) are much less common than metastases in adults. A history of primary tumors elsewhere, back pain worse at night, night sweats, fevers, or persistent bilateral leg pain without back pain should arouse suspicion for cancer. Metastases of bone are often detected on routine x-ray studies. MRI should be ordered when radiographs are nondiagnostic.

Diskitis and vertebral osteomyelitis can cause back pain in the absence of significant neurologic symptoms. Vertebral osteomyelitis can arise from a number of sources, including direct inoculation from iatrogenic procedures (injections, diagnostic studies), contiguous spread from a local infection, and hematogenous seeding (from infected vascular sites or urinary tract infection).

Once the infection is established in the metaphysis, it can subsequently rupture through the endplate into the adjoining disk and infect the adjacent vertebral body. The disk material is relatively avascular and is rapidly destroyed by bacterial enzymes. Osteomyelitis of the spine can extend into the spinal canal, leading to epidural abscess or bacterial meningitis, or into the surrounding soft tissues, resulting in local abscess. Destruction of the vertebral body and intervertebral disk can lead to instability and collapse. In addition, retropulsion of infected bone and granulation tissue into the spinal canal can cause neural compression or vascular occlusion. If a spinal infection is suspected, the pathogenic organism must be identified with biopsy or aspiration before appropriate treatment with antibiotics (with or without surgical debridement) can be instituted. An MRI with gadolinium is the best test for delineating the location of the infection as well as investigating for the presence of an epidural abscess (Figure 40–37).

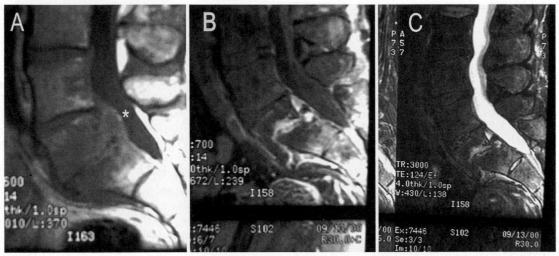

▲ **Figure 40–37.** Sagittal MRI images of a patient with low back pain due to L5–S1 diskitis, vertebral osteomyelitis, and a small anterior epidural abscess. **A:** T1-weighted image. **B:** T1-weighted image with gadolinium vascular contrast. **C:** T2-weighted image.

5. Acute Cauda Equina Syndrome

Rarely, acute posterior midline disk prolapse at the L2–3 level may cause compression of many nerve roots in the cauda equina. This is known as acute cauda equina syndrome. Symptoms include intense leg pain in one or both extremities, muscle weakness, urinary retention, and decreased rectal tone with subsequent loss of bowel/bladder control. An MRI of the lumbar spine will reveal the site of compression, which must be treated by emergent decompression.

6. Mechanical Back Pain

▶ General Considerations

People with longstanding lumbar disk disease may develop numerous degenerative changes in the involved segments. Collapse of the disk results in abnormal motion anteriorly between the vertebral bodies and posteriorly between the intervertebral facets, leading to osteophytosis.

▶ Clinical Findings

Symptoms arise from inflammation surrounding the abnormal facets and generally include diffuse aching that may or may not radiate into the buttock or posterior thigh. Patients may also complain of postural discomfort and "locking" of the lower back during stooping or attempts to straighten the back after forward bending.

▶ Diagnosis & Treatment

Radiographs may show osteophytes and narrowing of the disk spaces suggestive of degenerative change. Patients dem-

onstrating symptoms suggestive of facet syndrome should be initially treated conservatively with rest and anti-inflammatory agents. Fluoroscopically guided injection of the lumbar facets with corticosteroids and lidocaine may be diagnostic and therapeutic. For patients who fail conservative therapy, lumbar fusion by anterior or posterior techniques may be considered to eliminate abnormal motion. However, the results of these surgeries have been inconsistent.

Daffner RH et al: Expert Panel on Musculoskeletal Imaging. Chronic neck pain. American College of Radiology, 2005. Available at http://www.acr.org/SecondaryMainMenuCategories/ quality_safety/app_criteria/pdf/ExpertPanelonMusculoskeletal Imaging/ChronicNeckPainDoc9.aspx. Accessed February 14, 2009.

Fischgrund JS: *OKU 9: Orthopedic Knowledge Update.* American Academy of Orthopaedic Surgeons, 2008.

Neck and Upper Back Complaints. American College of Occupational and Environmental Medicine, 2004.

▼ ORTHOPEDIC ONCOLOGY

Bony lesions may be primary (of mesenchymal origin) or secondary (metastases, myeloma, lymphoma). Bony metastases and myeloma are significantly more common than primary bone tumors, particularly in older patients. Primary bony lesions can be grouped into three types: malignant tumors (sarcomas), benign tumors, and reactive or miscellaneous lesions. Sarcomas tend to spread hematogenously, most commonly to the lungs. Benign bone tumors vary widely and may be small and inconsequential or large and destructive.

PRESENTATION

Regardless of the type of lesion, most patients present with musculoskeletal pain, typically deep and dull in character. This may initially be intermittent and activity related but over time often becomes constant. Patients with a suspected bony lesion require careful physical examination. In the elderly, bony metastasis should be a significant concern and should prompt evaluation for a distant primary tumor. Standard anteroposterior and lateral views of the area of concern should be obtained. If concerned for malignancy, a chest x-ray should be obtained. CT scan and MRI are useful adjuncts for characterizing bony lesions.

RADIOGRAPHIC FEATURES OF BONY LESIONS

Plain radiographs can significantly narrow the differential diagnosis for bony lesions. Specific attention must be paid to the anatomical site of the lesion, the zone of transition between lesion and normal bone, and internal characteristics of the lesion. Benign lesions tend to be slow growing. While benign lesions can destroy cortical bone, a transitional rim of reactive periosteal bone is typically formed around the neoplasm. High-grade malignant lesions tend to grow rapidly, and host bone has little ability to wall off the lesion with a rim of periosteal bone. Correspondingly, aggressive lesions often have a poorly demarcated transitional zone. High-grade lesions frequently destroy cortical bone and can spread to adjacent soft tissue. Note should also be made of calcification or ossification within the lesion. Calcification appears more haphazard and frequently more dense than ossification and often denotes a cartilaginous tumor. Ossification indicates production of mineralized matrix, giving the appearance of organization or structure, and is more common in tumors of bony origin.

BIOPSY & SURGICAL TREATMENT

Biopsy is generally performed only after the lesion has been well characterized by physical and radiographic examination. If a lesion is found to be malignant, the entire biopsy tract must be removed at the time of tumor resection. As such, the biopsy site and tract should violate as few intrafascial compartments as possibly to prevent seeding adjacent compartments with tumor and limit the extent of necessary resection. Transverse incisions should be avoided. Frozen sections should be sent to confirm an adequate sample of the lesion has been obtained; samples should also be sent for culture as infection can masquerade as an aggressive-appearing lesion.

Surgical treatment is directed toward removing the entire lesion and preventing local recurrence. In general, more extensive resection confers a lower risk of local recurrence. Four types of tumor resection have been described:

Intralesional: dissection proceeds through the tumor itself (eg, curettage).

Marginal: resection through the reactive zone of the tumor, which contains inflammatory cells, fibrous tissue, and possible satellite metastases.

Wide: entire tumor is removed with a surrounding cuff of normal tissue.

Radical: removal of tumor and its entire surrounding fascial compartment.

STAGING

Staging for malignant musculoskeletal lesions is based on the histologic grade of the lesion, its location (intra versus extra-compartmental), and the presence of distant metastases. Grade (G) assesses the histologic characteristics of the tumor. G_1 lesions appear less aggressive and have a lower risk of distant metastasis. Increasing grade in G_2 and G_3 lesions denotes more aggressive cytologic features and increases the risk of distant metastasis. Tumor size (T) includes lesions within their capsule (T_0), extending through the capsule but within the compartment of origin (T_1) and beyond the compartment of origin (T_2). Metastasis (M) includes no metastases (M_0) and the presence of metastases (M_1).

CHEMOTHERAPY & RADIATION

A detailed discussion of chemotherapeutic and radiation regimens for various musculoskeletal neoplasms is beyond the limits of this text. Modern chemotherapeutic regimens offer significant benefits in disease-free survival for osteogenic sarcoma and Ewing sarcoma. Neoadjuvant (preoperative) chemotherapy is becoming more popular in treating these cancers. Radiation is effective in local treatment of Ewing sarcoma, osteosarcoma, lymphoma, myeloma, and metastatic bone disease.

METASTATIC BONE LESIONS

Metastases from remote primary tumors represent the majority of bone tumors seen in adults. Of these, most are derived from carcinomas from the breast, prostate, lung, kidney, thyroid, pancreas, and stomach. While breast and prostate cancer metastases commonly result from a known primary cancer, bony metastasis of unknown origin frequently stems from lung or renal cancer. The presence of a lytic bone lesion in an adult older than 40 without a diagnosis of a primary cancer should prompt the following investigation, which successfully identifies the primary tumor in 85% of cases:

- Plain radiographs of the affected limb, chest x-ray, CT scan of the chest, abdomen, and pelvis
- Technetium bone scan to detect multiple lesions
- Skeletal survey (if myeloma is suspected)
- Complete blood count, serum chemistry, liver function tests, erythrocyte sedimentation rate, and serum or urine immunoelectrophoresis.

Metastases are most commonly observed in the pelvis, ribs, vertebral bodies, and proximal limbs. These lesions typically have a lytic appearance on plain radiographs, although breast and prostate metastases can be sclerotic or mixed with lytic and sclerotic features. Metastases from renal cell carcinoma tend to be extremely vascular, and angioembolization is an important consideration prior to biopsy or definitive surgical treatment. Of note, bone destruction is not caused by the malignant cells but rather through induction of local osteoclasts by the metastasis. As a result, bisphosphonate therapy has come into common use in cancer patients.

Multiple myeloma is a common malignant tumors affecting bone. It is a plasma cell disorder most commonly affecting patients between 50 and 80. Patients most often present with bone pain or pathologic fracture. Vertebral and large bone involvement is most common. Radiographs commonly demonstrate multiple punched-out, lytic bone lesions. Patients with multiple myeloma should undergo a skeletal survey to evaluate for other lytic lesions as bone scan is frequently uninformative.

Surgical intervention for metastatic bone lesions is centered around reducing pain and maintaining functionality. Internal fixation is performed prophylactically if an impending fracture is observed. Risk factors for pathologic fracture include greater than 50% destruction of diaphyseal cortices, greater than 50–75% metaphyseal destruction, destruction of the subtrochanteric region of the femur, and persistent pain following radiation therapy.

COMMON PRIMARY MALIGNANT BONE TUMORS

Osteosarcoma

Osteogenic sarcoma is the most common primary malignant tumor of bone. It is more common in men and most commonly occurs in children and young adults about the knee (Figure 40–38). Other common locations include the proximal humerus and proximal femur. Histology demonstrates osteoid production with malignant stromal cells. Most lesions are high grade and penetrate the cortex, forming an extramedullary soft tissue mass. Plain films show a destructive lesion demonstrating some bone formation. Modern chemotherapy regimens have significantly increased survival and feasibility of limb-sparing approaches. Treatment consists of neoadjuvant chemotherapy followed by resection and maintenance chemotherapy. Less common subtypes of osteosarcoma include telangiectatic, parosteal, and periosteal.

Chondrosarcoma

Chondrosarcoma results from malignant cartilaginous cells with peak incidence in the fifth and sixth decades. It commonly occurs in the knee, shoulder, pelvis, and spine. Plain films demonstrate cortical thickening and stippling consistent with cartilage deposition. Determining malignancy in

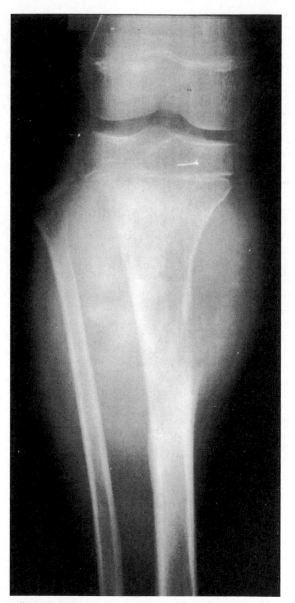

▲ **Figure 40–38.** Osteosarcoma with Codman triangle, a new area of subperiosteal bone formed when a tumor raises the periosteum away from the bone.

cartilaginous cells based solely on histologic examination is difficult; clinical history and imaging are essential for correct diagnosis. Chondrosarcomas tend to be grade 1 or 2 and less aggressive than osteosarcoma. Surgical resection with wide margins is the treatment of choice. Dedifferentiated chondrosarcoma is a subtype containing highly aggressive spindle-shaped cells. Prognosis is poor, and treatment consists of wide-margin resection and chemotherapy.

Ewing Sarcoma

Ewing sarcoma is a small blue cell tumor with a characteristic t(11:22) chromosomal translocation. It commonly occurs in children older than 5 years and in young adults. Children younger than 5 years with a small blue cell tumor should have leukemia and metastatic neuroblastoma excluded before the diagnosis of Ewing sarcoma is made. Likewise, metastatic carcinoma must be excluded in adults. Pain and fever are common presenting complaints, with many patients having elevated inflammatory markers and a leukocytosis (which can be confused with osteomyelitis). The pelvis, knee, proximal humerus, and femur diaphysis are the most common locations. Plain films demonstrate a destructive, frequently diametaphyseal lesion. The classic "onion-skin" appearance of multiple layers of reactive periosteum is uncommon; more commonly, the appearance is lytic with variable amounts of reactive bone. Treatment including chemotherapy, radiation, and surgical intervention can produce long-term survival approaching 70%.

Lymphoma of Bone

Lymphoma of bone can occur as a solitary focus, scattered through bone and soft tissue, or as a metastasis to bone. It can affect patients at nearly any point in life. Pain and a large soft tissue mass are common. The knee, pelvis, hip, shoulder, and vertebrae are commonly affected. Bony destruction with a variable degree of reactive bone is characteristic on plain film. Treatment centers around chemotherapy and radiotherapy. Surgical intervention is indicated for impending or pathologic fracture fixation.

COMMON BENIGN BONE LESIONS

Osteoid Osteoma

Osteoid osteoma is a benign bone lesion typically producing pain in patients from 5–30 years of age. Progressive pain, particularly at night, is characteristic. The lesion is commonly found in the proximal femur, spine, and tibial diaphysis. Plain films typically show a radiolucent nidus with a sclerotic, reactive rim. Bone scans are always positive. Often, pain is well relieved with NSAIDs, and 50% of lesions will "burn out" with conservative management. For persistent pain, percutaneous radiofrequency ablation of the nidus is highly effective.

Enchondroma

Enchondromas are benign cartilaginous tumors commonly found in the metaphyses of long bones and the hand, where pathologic fractures can be common. Plain films demonstrate a lytic lesion with a stippled appearance. Most enchondromas can be observed and followed with serial radiographs at 3 months and 1 year after presentation. Treatment, if necessary, consists of curettage and bone grafting. Malignant transformation to chondrosarcoma is exceedingly rare, except in two cases: Ollier disease is characterized by multiple enchondromas and confers a 30% risk of chondrosarcoma. Maffucci syndrome includes multiple enchondromas with associated soft tissue angiomas. Both diseases also confer increased risk of visceral malignancy.

Osteochondroma

Osteochondroma is a benign surface lesion of bone characterized by a cartilaginous cap connected to the medullary cavity of the underlying bone. It can be pedunculated or sessile. If asymptomatic, observation is sufficient. If painful, resection is appropriate. Multiple hereditary exostosis is an autosomal dominant condition in which patients have multiple osteochondromas. Although malignant transformation in isolated lesions is rare, multiple hereditary exostosis confers a higher risk (approximately 10%).

Giant Cell Tumor of Bone

Although benign, giant cell tumors can be locally aggressive. Giant cell tumor is more common in females and typically occurs in the epiphysis of long bones after the physis has closed. The knee, vertebra, distal radius, and sacrum are common sites. Plain films demonstrate a metaphyseal lytic lesion extending to the epiphysis (Figure 40–39). Treatment consists of cortical windowing, aggressive curettage, chemical cauterization with phenol, and bone grafting. If inoperable, radiation can be employed. Rarely, primary giant cell tumor can be malignant or can undergo secondary malignant degeneration (most often following radiation exposure).

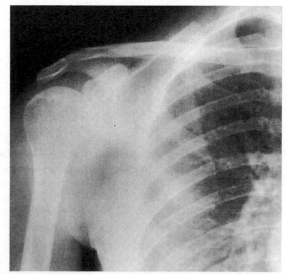

▲ **Figure 40–39.** Giant cell tumor of proximal humerus.

Aneurysmal Bone Cyst

Aneurysmal bone cysts are benign but can be associated with other tumors including giant cell tumor, chondroblastoma, and fibrous dysplasia. It can also be found within a malignant tumor. Seventy-five percent of patients are less than 20 years old. History consists of pain and swelling over months to years. Plain films demonstrate an expansile lesion with a thin rim of cortical bone. Aneurysmal bone cyst is characterized by a blood-filled interior without an endothelial lining. Occasional thin septae of bone may be present. Treatment is curettage with bone grafting, and recurrence commonly occurs if physes are open.

Unicameral Bone Cyst

Unicameral bone cysts are characterized by cystic expansion and cortical thinning. They are most commonly observed in the proximal humerus, proximal femur, and distal tibia. Patients commonly present with pain or pathologic fracture. Radiographs demonstrate a mildly expansile lytic-centered lesion with thin surrounding cortices and trabeculae (Figure 40–40). Active lesions border the physis, while latent lesions have interposed normal bone. First-line treatment consists of aspiration and cytologic examination of the fluid followed by methylprednisolone injection. Curettage and bone grafting are used if this proves ineffective.

Fibrous Dysplasia

Fibrous dysplasia is a developmental disorder of bone. It can be solitary (monostotic) or present in multiple locations (polyostotic). McCune-Albright syndrome is diagnosed when the polyostotic form is associated with café-au-lait spots and endocrine abnormalities. While nearly any bone can be involved, the proximal femur is the most common location. Plain films demonstrate a lucent lesion surrounded by a well-defined sclerotic rim; the lesions can range from purely lytic to having a ground-glass appearance. Most patients do not require surgical treatment; however, curettage, bone grafting, and internal fixation are appropriate in areas of high stress or pathologic fracture.

Osteomyelitis

Osteomyelitis can mimic bone tumors. Patients frequently present with bone pain, fevers, and chills. Constitutional symptoms, however, are not always present. Acute infections are typically lytic with periosteal elevation; chronic lesions can have a mixed lytic/sclerotic appearance. MRI can demonstrate changes in bone not easily seen on plain films early in the course of infection. In acute osteomyelitis, surgical treatment is initiated when an abscess is present, when patients have failed to respond to nonoperative management, and when soft tissues need debridement to prevent further destruction.

Chronic osteomyelitis can arise from incompletely treated acute osteomyelitis, in intravenous drug abusers, or in immu-

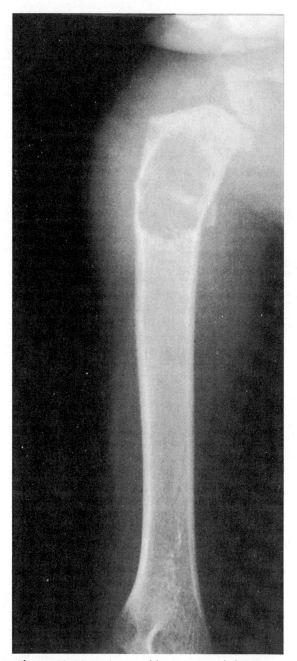

▲ **Figure 40–40.** Unicameral bone cyst with fracture.

nocompromised hosts. The disease course commonly follows a relapsing/remitting course with acute exacerbations in pain interspersed with periods of relative quiescence. Intravenous antibiotic therapy should be guided by deep cultures from the infected site. Surgical therapy consists of removal of all infected bone and soft tissue and removal of hardware (if present), followed by culture-directed intravenous antibiotic therapy.

Biermann JS et al: Bone cancer. J Natl Compr Canc Netw 2007; 5:420.

El-Khoury GY et al: Expert Panel on Musculoskeletal Imaging. Metastatic bone disease. American College of Radiology, 2005. Available at http://www.acr.org/SecondaryMainMenuCategories/quality_safety/app_criteria/pdf/ExpertPanelonMusculoskeletalImaging/MetastaticBoneDiseaseDoc14.aspx. Accessed on February 14, 2009.

Gibbs CP Jr, Weber K, Scarborough MT: Malignant bone tumors. Bone Joint Surg Am 2001;83:1728.

Manaster BJ et al: Expert Panel on Musculoskeletal Imaging. Follow-up of malignant or aggressive musculoskeletal tumors. American College of Radiology, 2006. Available at http://www.acr.org/SecondaryMainMenuCategories/quality_safety/app_criteria/pdf/ExpertPanelonMusculoskeletalImaging/FollowUpofMalignantorAggressiveMusculoskeletalTumorsDoc11.aspx. Accessed on February 14, 2009.

Miller MD: *Review of Orthopaedics*, vol. 4. Saunders, 2004.

Morrison WB et al: Expert Panel on Musculoskeletal Imaging. Bone tumors. American College of Radiology, 2005. Available at http://www.acr.org/SecondaryMainMenuCategories/quality_safety/app_criteria/pdf/ExpertPanelonMusculoskeletalImaging/BoneTumorsDoc4.aspx. Accessed on February 14, 2009.

▼ FOOT & ANKLE

PAIN SYNDROMES OF THE FOOT

1. Interdigital Neuritis

Interdigital neuritis is a common cause for pain in the foot. Originally described by Thomas Morton, the irritation of the interdigital nerve was believed to be due to compression between the metatarsal heads. However, it is now known that this is not the case given the location of the interdigital nerve lying plantar to the intermetatarsal ligament and metatarsal heads. Instead, it is now believed that interdigital neuritis is due to compression and tethering of a stretched nerve across the transverse metatarsal ligament.

▶ History & Physical Examination

Patients typically present with pain associated with burning or tingling on the plantar aspect of the foot near the web space of the affected nerve. This syndrome occurs most commonly in middle-aged women. Shoe wear, particularly wearing shoes with a tight toe box or high heels, appears to significantly exacerbate symptoms due to increased pressure on the plantar aspect of the foot and increased stretching of the nerve with dorsiflexion of the toes. Pain can be relieved with removal of the offending shoe and massage. Pain in the interdigital space may be reproduced on physical examination with pressure applied just proximal to the metatarsal heads by squeezing the forefoot between the examiner's thumb and index finger.

▶ Diagnosis

The differential diagnosis includes synovitis, bursitis, and metatarsalgia. In metatarsalgia, the pain is located directly under the involved metatarsal bone and often is accompanied with callous formation. The pain caused by synovitis is usually located immediately distal to the metatarsal head. Bursitis may present with swelling in the web space, which is not a typical finding associated with interdigital neuritis.

Interdigital neuritis is typically diagnosed with history and physical examination as described previously. Injection of the affected digital web space with 1 ml of lidocaine with successful relief of symptoms can provide diagnosis confirmation.

▶ Treatment

Treatment begins with nonsurgical management: avoidance of shoes with high heels or a tight toe box, use of a firm crepe sole to prevent hyperextension or dorsiflexion of the toes, and a metatarsal pad to relieve pressure on the plantar aspect of the foot. Steroid injection may improve symptoms, but the affect is usually short lived. If conservative measures fail, surgery with release of the transverse metatarsal ligament and/or neurectomy may be pursued.

2. Metatarsalgia

Metarsalgia is a disorder defined by pain located below the metatarsal heads that is worse with weightbearing. Mechanical factors such as laxity of the transverse intermetatarsal ligament appear to be the root cause. Plantar callosities, most commonly under the second metatarsal head, may also be present. Treatment starts with orthotics, such as felt or rubber pads below the metatarsal heads to relieve pressure. Surgery may be considered if conservative measures fail.

3. Hallux Valgus

▶ General Considerations

Hallux valgus is defined by subluxation of the first metatarsophalangeal joint, which results in first metatarsal head medial prominence and lateral deviation of the proximal phalanx on the first metatarsal.

▶ Etiology

Anatomic factors including varus alignment of the first metatarsocuneiform joint may predispose to hallux valgus. Women's shoes with a small toe box may also cause bunching of the toes, predisposing to the valgus deformity of the first metatarsophalangeal joint.

▶ Clinical Evaluation & Physical Examination

When evaluating hallux valgus, the patient's main complaint should be defined carefully because it may affect choice of treatment options. Chief complaints may be related to cosmesis, metatarsalgia, second-toe deformity, problems with shoe fit, or simply pain. The patient's occupational and recreational activities should be investigated as well. Professional dancers or high-performance athletes are not good candidates for certain surgeries.

Initially, the foot should be inspected for any deformity. Hallux valgus is present when there is medial prominence of the first metatarsal head, also known as a bunion. Limitation of dorsiflexion, pronation deformity of the big toe, synovial thickening, dorsal osteophytes, and medial deviation of the second metatarsophalangeal joint may be present as well. Neurovascular status of the foot should be documented.

► Radiographic Evaluation

Initially, weightbearing anteroposterior, lateral, and oblique radiographs of the foot should be obtained. The hallux valgus angle (the angle between the proximal phalanx and the first metatarsal; normal is < 15 degrees), the intermetatarsal angle (the angle between the first and second metatarsals; normal is < 9 degrees), and the distal metatarsal angle (angle between the distal metatarsal articular surface and the long axis of the first metatarsal; normal is < 10 degrees of lateral deviation) should be measured and recorded. Incongruence of the metatarsophalangeal joint (lateral deviation of the proximal phalanx from the metatarsal head) should be noted as well.

► Treatment

Initially, conservative treatment should be pursued with a wide, soft shoe with adequate toe box and insole padding. If conservative therapy fails, a number of surgical treatment options are available depending on the severity of the deformity, joint congruence, presence of arthritis, and other patient factors.

Coughlin MJ: Treatment of bunionette deformity with longitudinal diaphyseal osteotomy with distal soft tissue repair. Foot Ankle 1991;11:195.
Schoenhaus HD, Cohen RS: Etiology of the bunion. J Foot Surg 1992;31:25.

4. Hallux Varus

Hallux varus is subluxation of the medial proximal phalanx on the first metatarsal. Etiologies include trauma and iatrogenic (overcorrection via surgery for hallux valgus). Hallux varus may be defined as supple (correctable with physical manipulation) or rigid (fixed, not correctable via manipulation). If the deformity is supple, then tendon transfer with extensor hallucis longus or extensor hallucis brevis should be considered. If the deformity is rigid, then arthrodesis or fusion of the first metatarsophalangeal joint is the best surgical treatment.

5. Hallux Rigidus

Hallux rigidus entails significant arthrosis of the first metatarsophalangeal joint, resulting in significant pain and restriction of dorsiflexion. There may be increased bulk of the joint as well, resulting in difficulty wearing shoes. Marginal osteophytes may be present dorsally and laterally.

Forced dorsiflexion performed by the examiner often reproduces the patient's pain. Grind test should also be performed by holding the first metatarsal steady and applying an axial load with circumduction of the proximal phalanx. Significant pain with this maneuver indicates a positive grind test, which equates to significant loss of the plantar located cartilage. The dorsal medial cutaneous nerve may be sensitive as well.

Radiographic evaluation includes weightbearing anteroposterior, lateral, and oblique views of the foot. The extent of joint narrowing should be noted. Hallux rigidus may be classified as follows based on radiographs: grade I (preserved joint space), grade II (< 50% joint space–narrowing), and grade III (> 50% loss of joint space).

Initially, conservative management using a shoe with a large toe box to accommodate increased bulk of the first metatarsophalangeal joint and rigid rocker sole to minimize joint motion should be tried. If conservative measures fail, surgery may be considered.

Surgical treatment entails cheilectomy (removal of the osteophyte) or arthrodesis (fusion of the first metatarsophalangeal joint). Cheilectomy is indicated for grade I, grade II, and grade III pathology with a negative grind test. If cheilectomy fails to provide significant pain relief, arthrodesis may be performed. For grade III lesions on radiographs and a positive grind test (indicating lack of plantar cartilage), arthrodesis should be pursued. Although various arthroplasty (joint replacement procedures) are now available, the short-term to mid-term results of these procedures are not as successful as cheilectomy and/or arthrodesis.

6. Plantar Fasciitis

Plantar fasciitis is a degenerative process involving the plantar fascia origin. The typical patient with this disorder is the overweight 40–70 year old with significant plantar heel pain and localized tenderness at the plantar medial tuberosity of the calcaneus. An osteophyte (heel spur) may be visible on radiographs. Treatment entails stretching and massage of the plantar fascia and Achilles tendon, cushioned heel inserts, night splints, and/or a walking cast. If conservative measures fail, surgery with release of the medial third of the plantar fascia may be considered.

7. The Diabetic Foot

The pathology associated with the diabetic foot is complicated by neuropathy and angiopathy with varying degrees of severity. Diabetic ulceration and neuropathic arthropathy (Charcot foot) can result. Management of these two pathologic disorders depends on a number of factors.

► Diabetic Ulceration

Due to neuropathy, patients with diabetes have decreased sensation around their feet. As a result, injuries to the superficial layer of skin are not perceived, and progression to ulceration can occur. These patients should be initially evaluated with transcutaneous oxygen pressures and ABIs to determine healing potential. An ABI ratio higher than 0.6 and transcutaneous oxygen measurements greater than 40 mm Hg are usually indicative of adequate vascularity and necessary healing potential. Additionally, the character of the ulcer itself affects treatment choice. Localized, superficial ulcers that do not extend to tendon, bone, or ligament can be debrided at the bedside, followed by placement in an off-loading shoe or cast with serial physical examinations. Ulcers that extend to deeper tissues and/or bone may require debridement in the operating room and antibiotic therapy. Additionally, nutrition should be optimized to encourage healing. If appropriate blood flow is present, these ulcers will typically heal. If healing does not occur or gangrene is appreciated due to poor vascularity, amputation may be considered.

▶ Neuropathic Arthropathy (Charcot Foot)

Neuropathic arthropathy is characterized by osteopenia, joint subluxation or dislocation, and bony fragmentation that may progress to malunion at later stages. White blood cell–labeled scintigraphy with MRI can be used to differentiate this condition from osteomyelitis. Initial treatment includes nonweightbearing of the affected lower extremity with or without cast placement. Operative intervention is considered only in special cases.

Fischgrund JS. *OKU 9: Orthopedic Knowledge Update*. American Academy of Orthopaedic Surgeons, 2008.
Miller MD: *Review of Orthopaedics,* 4th ed. Saunders, 2004.

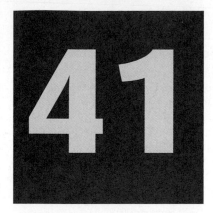

Plastic & Reconstructive Surgery

Henry C. Vasconez, MD

Ameen Habash, MD

Plastic surgery, although considered a technique-oriented and multiregional specialty, is in essence a problem-solving field. The training of a plastic surgeon allows him or her to see surgical problems in a different light and select from a variety of options to solve these surgical problems. Plastic surgeons have received broad training, and many have completed residencies in other fields such as general surgery, otolaryngology, orthopedics, urology, or neurosurgery. Other modalities of training have more recently integrated these and other surgical subspecialties into a more comprehensive training program.

The basic principles of plastic surgery are careful analysis of the surgical problem, careful planning of procedures, precise technique, and atraumatic handling of tissues. Alteration, coverage, and transfer of skin and associated tissues are the most common procedures performed. Plastic surgery may deal with the closure of surgical wounds—particularly recalcitrant wounds such as those occurring post radiation or poorly healing wounds in immunocompromised patients. Plastic surgery also deals with the removal of skin tumors, repair of soft tissue injuries including burns, correction of acquired or congenital deformities, or enhancement of undesirable cosmetic features. Craniofacial and hand surgery, also within the realm of plastic surgery, may require additional surgical training.

In the past quarter century, increased knowledge of anatomy and the development of many new techniques have brought about important changes in plastic surgery. It is now known that in many areas the blood supply of the skin is derived principally from vessels arising from underlying muscles and larger perforating blood vessels rather than solely from vessels of the subcutaneous tissue, as was formerly thought. One-stage transfer of large areas of skin, fascia, and muscle tissue can be accomplished if the axial pedicle of the underlying fascia or muscle is included in the transfer. With the use of microsurgical techniques, musculocutaneous units or combinations of bone, fascia, muscle, and skin can be successfully transferred and vessels and nerves

less than 1 mm in size can be repaired. These so-called free-flap transplantations are a major advance in the treatment of defects that were previously untreatable or required lengthy or multistaged procedures. More sophisticated knowledge of the blood supply to the skin has introduced the concept of perforator flaps whereby one perforating vessel is identified that may supply a large segment of overlying skin and subcutaneous tissue. Similarly, the concept of neurocutaneous flaps has given rise to the design of additional flap territories such as the sural flap in the lower leg and the sensate radial flap in the forearm.

The plastic surgeon, as a member of the craniofacial surgical team, is able to dramatically improve the appearance and function of children with severe congenital deformities. Children of normal intelligence who previously had been social outcasts are now able to lead relatively normal lives. Improved understanding of facial growth and abnormal development and diagnostic techniques such as the CT scan, MRI, and 3D computer-assisted imaging enable the reconstructive surgeon to develop a complex strategy for remodeling the deformed craniofacial skeleton. This may involve remodeling or repositioning of part or all of the cranial vault, the orbits, the mid face, and the mandible. These complex and at times formidable reconstructions are performed by moving specific skeletal units and adding autogenous bone grafts. These structures are kept in place using miniplate fixation; the miniplates are made of titanium or resorbable material.

A notable advance in craniofacial surgery was the introduction of distraction osteogenesis, which borrows from the Ilizarov principle of distraction. A cortical cut is made in the bone, and a distraction apparatus is applied so that in measured amounts (usually 1 mm per day) the bone is either stretched to offset a length discrepancy or transported to bridge a gap. In craniofacial surgery, it is more commonly brought to bear to enlarge or cause overgrowth of areas such as an underdeveloped mandible.

Additional areas of involvement for the plastic surgeon entail allotransplantation, particularly with the increasing number of clinical limb allotransplants, which unfortunately still require immunosuppression. It is hoped that immuno-tolerance will someday become a reality, allowing transplantation of nonessential organs with a minimum of dangerous immunosuppression. Transplantation of the hand with excellent functional recovery in some cases has been performed successfully but still requires a great deal of immunosuppression. Face transplants have been performed with some initial success. The first facial transplant was performed in France and consisted of a partial segment of the face. The functional recovery to date has been remarkable. The problems of facial animation still need to be refined. Additionally, a number of ethical issues with regard to facial identity and immunosuppression require further resolution.

Tissue engineering of bone, cartilage, and nerve is an area of ongoing research for plastic surgeons. Although encouraging experimental results have been reported in anatomic areas difficult to reconstruct, such as the external ear, the nose, or the larynx, there are as yet few clinical applications.

Fetal surgery for cleft disorders and scar considerations, an area pioneered by a number of plastic surgeons, appears to be in a quiescent stage, particularly because the persistent real and potential risks to the fetus and mother may not be warranted for disorders that are not life threatening. Significant technical advances in the postnatal treatment of cleft lip and cleft palate have also lessened the enthusiasm for fetal surgery for these disorders.

Devauchelle B et al: First human face allograft: early report. Lancet 2006;368:203.
Jones JW et al: Successful hand transplantation. One-year follow-up. Louisville Hand Transplant Team. N Engl J Med 2000; 343:468.
Rohrich RJ, Longaker MT, Cunningham B: On the ethics of composite tissue allotransplantation (facial transplantation). Plast Reconstr Surg 2006;117:2071.

▼ I. GRAFTS & FLAPS

SKIN GRAFTS

A graft of skin detaches epidermis and varying amounts of dermis from its blood supply in the **donor area** and is placed in a new bed of blood supply from the base of the wound, or

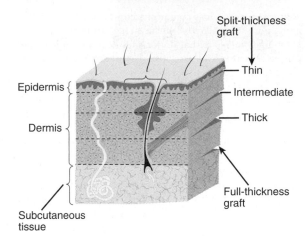

▲ **Figure 41–1.** Depths of full-thickness and split-thickness grafts.

recipient area. The way a skin graft survives or "takes" is first by diffusion of nutrient elements from the graft bed, known as imbibition; then after a period of 2–5 days, the graft actually revascularizes from the bed, a process known as inosculation. Although the technique is relatively simple to perform and generally reliable, definite considerations about the donor area and adequacy of the recipient area are important. Skin grafting is a quick, effective way to cover a wound if vascularity is adequate, infection is not present, and hemostasis is assured. Color match, contour, durability of the graft, and donor morbidity must be considered.

TYPES OF SKIN GRAFTS

Skin grafts can be either split-thickness or full-thickness grafts (Figure 41–1). Each type has advantages and disadvantages and is indicated or contraindicated for different kinds of wounds (Table 41–1).

A. Split-Thickness Grafts

Thinner split-thickness grafts (0.01–0.015 inch) become vascularized more rapidly and survive transplantation more reliably. This is important in grafting on less than ideal

Table 41–1. Advantages and Disadvantages of Various Types of Skin Grafts.

Type of Graft	Advantages	Disadvantages
Thin split-thickness	Survive transplantation most easily. Donor sites heal most rapidly.	Fewest qualities of normal skin. Maximum contraction. Least resistance to trauma. Sensation poor. Aesthetically poor.
Thick split-thickness	More qualities of normal skin. Less contraction. More resistant to trauma. Sensation fair. Aesthetically more acceptable.	Survive transplantation less well. Donor site heals slowly.
Full thickness	Nearly all qualities of normal skin. Minimal contraction. Very resistant to trauma. Sensation good. Aesthetically good.	Survive transplantation least well. Donor site must be closed surgically. Donor sites are limited.

recipient sites, such as contaminated wounds, burn surfaces, and poorly vascularized surfaces (eg, irradiated sites). A second advantage is that donor sites heal more rapidly and can be reused within a relatively short time (7–10 days) in critical cases such as major burns.

In general, however, the disadvantages of thin split-thickness grafts outweigh the advantages. Thin grafts exhibit the highest degree of postgraft contraction, offer the least amount of resistance to surface trauma, and are least like normal skin in texture, suppleness, pore pattern, hair growth, and other characteristics. Hence, they are usually aesthetically unacceptable.

Thicker split-thickness skin grafts (> 0.015 inch) contract less, are more resistant to surface trauma, and are more similar to normal skin than are thin split-thickness grafts. They are also aesthetically more acceptable but not as acceptable as full-thickness grafts.

The disadvantages of thick split-thickness grafts are relatively few but can be significant. They are less easily vascularized than thin grafts and thus result in fewer successful takes when used on less than ideal surfaces. Their donor sites are slower to heal (requiring 10–18 days) and heal with more scarring than donor sites for thin split-thickness grafts—a factor that may prevent reuse of the area.

Meshed grafts are usually thin or intermediate split-thickness grafts that have been rolled under a special cutting machine to create a mesh pattern. Although grafts with these perforations can be expanded from 1.5 to 9 times their original size, expansion to 1.5 times the unmeshed size is the most useful. Meshed grafts are advantageous because they can be placed on an irregular, possibly contaminated wound bed and will usually take. Also, complications of hemostasis are fewer because blood and serum exude through the mesh pattern. The disadvantage is poor appearance following healing (alligator hide look).

Donor sites for split-thickness grafts heal spontaneously by epithelialization. During this process, epithelial cells from the sweat glands, sebaceous glands, or hair follicles proliferate upward and spread across the wound surface. If these three structures are not present, epithelialization will not occur.

B. Full-Thickness Grafts

Full-thickness skin grafts include the epidermis and all the dermis. They are the most aesthetically desirable of the free grafts because they include the highest number of skin appendage elements, undergo the least amount of contracture, and have a greater ability to withstand trauma. There are several limiting factors in the use of full-thickness grafts. Since no epidermal elements remain to produce epithelialization in the donor site, it must be closed primarily, and a scar will result. The size and number of available donor sites is therefore limited. Furthermore, conditions at the recipient site must be optimal in order for transplantation to be successful.

Areas of thin skin are the best donor sites for full-thickness grafts (eg, the eyelids and the skin of the postauric-

ular, supraclavicular, antecubital, inguinal, and genital areas). Submammary and subgluteal skin is thicker but allows camouflage of donor area scars. In grafts thicker than approximately 0.015 inch, the results of transplantation are less reliable, except on the face, where vascularity is usually superior.

C. Composite Grafts

A composite graft is also a free graft that must reestablish its blood supply in the recipient area. It consists of a unit with several tissue planes that may include skin, subcutaneous tissue, cartilage, or other tissue. Dermal fat grafts, hair transplant grafts, and skin and cartilage grafts from the ear fall into this category. Obviously, composite grafts must be small or at least relatively thin and will require recipient sites with excellent vascularity. These grafts are generally used in the face.

D. Cultured Epithelial and Dermal Grafts

Epithelial cells, grown or cultured in a special medium in vitro, will coalesce into thin sheets that can be used to cover full-thickness wounds. Although these cultured epithelial sheets were first used in the treatment of burns, the result was somewhat unsatisfactory because the coverage was very fragile and disfiguring. More recently, success has been obtained with artificial dermis, which when placed in an appropriate bed will revascularize and can then be covered by a very thin (0.05 cm) split-thickness skin graft, cultured or otherwise. This artificial dermis is increasingly being used in the treatment of burns. Modifications of this concept have also been applied to the care of chronic ulcers, particularly in the leg. The artificial dermis is made out of a collagen matrix and has very low or no antigenicity.

▶ Obtaining Skin Grafts

Instruments used for obtaining skin grafts include razor blades, skin grafting knives (Blair, Ferris Smith, Humby, Goulian), manual drum dermatomes (Padgett, Reese), and electric or air-powered dermatomes (Brown, Padgett, Hall, Zimmer). The electric and air-powered dermatomes are the most widely used because of their reliability and ease of operation. A surgeon, even with only limited experience, can successfully obtain sheets of split-thickness skin grafts using the electric dermatomes.

▶ The Skin Graft Recipient Area

To ensure survival of the graft, there must be (1) adequate vascularity of the recipient bed, (2) complete contact between the graft and the bed, (3) adequate immobilization of the graft-bed unit, and (4) relatively few bacteria in the recipient area.

Because survival of the graft is dependent upon growth of capillary buds into the raw undersurface of the graft, vascularity of the recipient area is of prime importance. Avascular surfaces that will not generally accept free grafts are tissues with severe radiation damage, chronically scarred ulcer beds, bone or cartilage denuded of periosteum or perichondrium, and tendon or nerve without their paratenon or perineurium, respectively. For these surfaces, a bed capable of producing capillary buds must be provided; in some cases, excision of the deficient bed down to healthy tissue is possible. All unhealthy granulation tissue must be removed, because bacterial counts in granulation tissue are often very high. If bone is exposed, it can be decorticated down to healthy cancellous bone with the use of a chisel or power-driven burr, and a meshed split-thickness skin graft can be applied. If an adequate vascular bed cannot be provided or if the presence of essential structures such as tendons or nerves precludes further debridement, skin or muscle flaps are generally indicated for coverage.

Inadequate contact between the graft and the recipient bed can be caused by collection of blood, serum, or lymph fluid in the bed; formation of pus between the graft and the bed; or movement of the graft on the bed.

After the graft has been applied directly to the prepared recipient surface, it may or may not be sutured in place and may or may not be dressed. Whenever the maximum aesthetic result is desired, the graft should be cut exactly to fit the recipient area and precisely sutured into position without any overlapping of edges. Very large or thick split-thickness grafts and full-thickness grafts will usually not survive without a pressure dressing. In areas such as the forehead, scalp, and extremities, adequate immobilization and pressure can be provided by circular dressings. Tie-over pressure stent dressings are advisable for areas of the face, where constant pressure cannot be provided by simple wraparound dressings; areas where movement cannot be avoided, such as the anterior neck, where swallowing causes constant motion; and areas of irregular contour, such as the axilla. The ends of the fixation sutures are left long and tied over a bolus of gauze fluffs, cotton, a sponge, or other suitable material (Figure 41–2).

Grafts applied to freshly prepared or relatively clean surfaces are generally sutured or stapled into place and dressed with pressure. A single layer of damp or other nonadherent fine-mesh gauze is applied directly over the graft. Immediately over this are placed several thicknesses of flat gauze cut in the exact pattern of the graft. On top of these is placed a bulky dry dressing of gauze fluffs, cotton, a sponge, or other material. Pressure is then applied by wraparound dressings, adhesive tape, or a tie-over pressure stent dressing. An alternative dressing is to place a nonadherent fine-mesh gauze atop the graft followed by a negative-pressure dressing. The vacuum-assisted dressings may be useful for irregular contours, such as around digits and webspaces or joint surfaces, by maintaining wound-to-graft interface, immobilizing the grafted area, suctioning serosanguineous fluid, and possibly promoting neovascularization.

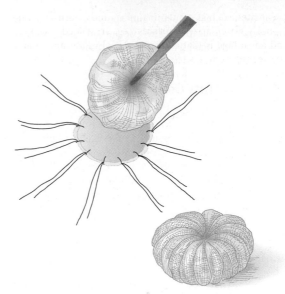

▲ **Figure 41–2.** Tie-over stent dressing.

In many cases, it is permissible—and sometimes even preferable—to leave a skin graft site open with no dressing. This is particularly true in slightly infected wounds, where the grafts tend to float off in the purulent discharge produced by the wound. These wounds are best treated with meshed grafts so that liquid forming between the graft and the wound bed can exude and be removed without disturbing the graft. This treatment can also be used for noninfected wounds that produce an unusual amount of serous or lymphatic drainage, as occurs following radical groin dissections.

In severely ill patients, such as those with major burns, where time under anesthesia must be kept to a minimum, large sheets of meshed split-thickness skin grafts are rapidly applied but not sutured. Skin staples may be used to fix the graft rapidly. Grafts need not be dressed if the area is small, but if the area is large or circumferential, a dressing should be applied. Meshed grafts should generally be covered for 24–48 hours to prevent dryness, because their dermal barrier has been partly disrupted.

Various biologic adhesives, in particular autologous fibrin glue, are being used to immobilize skin grafts. This is especially useful in the face or hands or in areas where bandaging is difficult or cumbersome.

Skin graft dressings may be left undisturbed for 5–7 days after grafting if the grafted wound was free of infection, if complete hemostasis was obtained, if fluid collection is not expected, and if immobilization is adequate. If any one of these conditions is not met, the dressing should be changed within 24–48 hours and the graft inspected. If blood, serum, or purulent fluid collection is present, the collection should be evacuated—usually by making a small incision through the graft with a scalpel blade and applying pressure with cotton-tipped applicators. The pressure dressing is then reapplied and changed daily so that the graft can be examined and fluid expressed as it collects.

► The Skin Graft Donor Area

The ideal donor site would provide a graft identical to the skin surrounding the area to be grafted. Because skin varies greatly from one area to another as far as color, thickness, hair-bearing qualities, and texture are concerned, the ideal donor site (such as upper eyelid skin to replace skin loss from the opposite upper eyelid) is usually not found. However, there are definite principles that should be followed in choosing the donor area.

A. Color Match

In general, the best possible color match is obtained when the donor area is located close to the recipient area. Color and texture match in facial grafts will be much better if the grafts are obtained from above the region of the clavicles. However, the amount of skin obtainable from the supraclavicular areas is limited. If larger grafts for the face are required, the immediate subclavicular regions of the thorax will provide a better color match than areas on the lower trunk or the buttocks and thighs. When these more distant regions are used, the grafts will usually be lighter in color than the facial skin in Caucasians. In people with dark skin, hyperpigmentation occurs, producing a graft that is much darker than the surrounding facial skin.

B. Thickness of the Graft and Donor Site Healing

Donor sites of split-thickness grafts heal by epithelialization from the epithelial elements remaining in the donor bed. The ability of the donor area to heal and the speed with which it does depends on the number of these elements present. Donor areas for very thin grafts will heal in 7–10 days, whereas donor areas for intermediate-thickness grafts may require 10–18 days and those for thick grafts 18–21 days or longer.

Because there is a normal anatomic variation in the thickness of skin, donor sites for thicker grafts must be chosen with the potential for healing in mind and should be limited to regions on the body where the skin is thick. Infants, debilitated adults, and elderly people have thinner skin than healthy younger adults. Grafts that would be split-thickness in the normal adult may be full-thickness in these patients, resulting in a donor site that has been deprived of the epithelial elements necessary for healing.

C. Management of the Donor Site

The donor site itself can be considered a clean open wound that will heal spontaneously. After initial hemostasis, the wound will continue to ooze serum for 1–4 days, depending on the thickness of the skin taken. The serum should be collected and the wound kept clean so that healing can proceed at a maximal rate. The wound should be cared for as described above for clean open wounds in either of two ways.

The more common method is the open (dry) technique. The donor site is dressed with porous, sterile fine-mesh or nonadherent gauze. After 24 hours, the dry gauze is changed but the nonadherent gauze is left on the wound and exposed to the air, a heat lamp, or a blow dryer. A scab will form on the gauze and will peel off from the edges as epithelialization is completed underneath. This method has the advantage of simple maintenance once the wound is dry.

The second method is the closed (moist) technique. Studies have demonstrated that the rate of epithelialization is enhanced in a moist environment. In contrast to the dry technique, pain can be reduced or virtually eliminated. Moist-to-moist gauze dressings that require frequent wetting have been replaced by newer synthetic materials. A gas-permeable membrane (OpSite, Tegaderm) that sticks to the surrounding skin provides an artificial blister over the wound. Occasionally, there is a break in the protective seal covering leakage of serum collected under the membrane. This increases the risk of infection, especially in a contaminated zone. Newer hygroscopic dressings actually absorb and retain many times their weight in water. They are permeable to oxygen yet impervious to bacteria. Infection is still a concern, however, because of occasional exposure of the wound during healing. Newer dressings with silver-impregnated ions are being used that control bacterial contamination and may hasten healing and reepithelialization. Silver ion is exquisitely antimicrobial and is used for burn dressing care as well as skin graft sites.

Demling RH, DeSanti L: The rate of re-epithelialization across meshed skin grafts is increased with exposure to silver. Burns 2002;28:264.
van Zuijlen PP et al: Graft survival and effectiveness of dermal substitution in burns and reconstructive surgery in a one-stage grafting model. Plast Reconstr Surg 2000;106:615.
Wang JC, To EW: Application of dermal substitute (Integra) to donor site defect of forehead flap. Br J Plastic Surg 2000;53:70.

FLAPS

The term "flap" refers to any tissue used for reconstruction or wound closure that retains part or all of its original blood supply after the tissue has been raised and moved to a new location. That part still connected through which the blood supply enters and exits is referred to as the flap base, or pedicle. With local skin flaps, a section of skin and subcutaneous tissue is raised from one site and moved to a nearby area, with the base remaining attached at its original location.

Flaps can be classified according to the pattern of blood supply to the skin into random or axial pattern. Flaps can further be classified according to their tissue content into muscle, musculocutaneous, fasciocutaneous, and others.

Random Pattern Flaps

Random pattern flaps consist of skin and subcutaneous tissue cut from any area of the body in any orientation, with no distinct pattern or particular relation to the blood supply of the skin of the flap. Such flaps receive their blood supply from vessels in the subdermal tissue. Although commonly used, this is the least reliable type of flap, and except when cut from facial and scalp skin, the ratio of length to width cannot safely exceed 1.5:1. Its use should be minimized. Presently, in any reconstructive effort, one should use a flap with known reliability and a predictable blood supply.

Axial Pattern Flaps

The axial pattern flap has a well-defined arteriovenous system running along its long axis. Because of good vascular supply, it can be made comparatively long in relation to width. Foremost among the axial flaps are the deltopectoral and the forehead flaps, which are based on perforating branches of the internal mammary artery and supraorbital and supratrochlear or superficial temporal vessels, respectively. Other axial flaps are the groin flap, based on the superficial circumflex iliac artery; the dorsalis pedis flap, based on the artery of the same name; the radial forearm flap; the scapular flap; the lateral upper arm flap; and various scalp and face flaps.

Muscle & Musculocutaneous Flaps

Musculocutaneous flaps consist of skin and underlying muscle, which provide reliable coverage with usually one operation. The use of musculocutaneous units has developed as surgeons have gained more knowledge of the way in which blood is supplied to the skin. The technique has revolutionized reconstructive surgery.

The subdermal plexus of vessels from which skin flaps derive their blood supply is augmented or directly supplied in many areas by sizable perforating vessels arising from underlying muscles. Many muscles receive their blood supply from a single axial vessel, with only minor contributions from other sources (Figure 41–3). The skin over these muscles can be completely circumscribed and elevated in continuity with the underlying muscle up to its major vascular pedicle. If the vessels in the pedicle are preserved, the unit can be moved in wide arcs to distant areas of the body while normal or near normal blood flow is continued to the skin island as well as to the muscle. The donor sites of such flaps can often be closed primarily.

Knowledge of the anatomy of muscles and their nerve and blood supply is necessary for the successful design of musculocutaneous flaps. Although almost any skeletal muscle can be used, muscles with a dominant arterial pedicle and reliable perforating vessels to the skin are most useful.

In addition to their reliability, musculocutaneous flaps clean up recipient sites that are heavily contaminated with bacteria better than skin flaps do. This is why muscle-containing flaps are the best choice for coverage of wounds caused by radiation or osteomyelitis or those that have a high probability of infection.

The most commonly used muscles and musculocutaneous flaps are the latissimus dorsi, pectoralis major, tensor fasciae latae, rectus femoris, rectus abdominis, trapezius, temporalis, serratus anterior, gluteus maximus, gracilis, and gastrocnemius muscles.

A. Latissimus Dorsi

The latissimus dorsi musculocutaneous unit is supplied by the thoracodorsal vessels. Use of this unit has been widely applied in the one-stage reconstruction of the breast following radical or modified radical mastectomy (see section on Rectus Abdominis). The entire latissimus dorsi muscle can be detached from its origin and transposed to the anterior chest. An island of skin can also be included in the center of the muscle to restore the skin lost on the anterior chest wall. Refinements in technique utilize only enough muscle to carry the skin island, thus leaving intact a good portion of

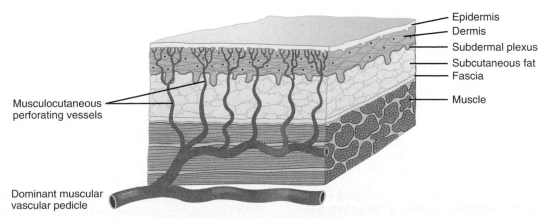

Epidermis
Dermis
Subdermal plexus
Subcutaneous fat
Fascia
Muscle

Musculocutaneous perforating vessels

Dominant muscular vascular pedicle

▲ **Figure 41–3.** Arterial supply to skin from main artery supplying muscles, as occurs in musculocutaneous flaps.

innervated, functional muscle. This unit is also useful for coverage of defects on the anterior chest, shoulder, head and neck, and axilla and even for restoration of flexion of the elbow. It is a popular muscle for free tissue transfer because of its long and relatively large and reliable vascular pedicle.

B. Pectoralis Major

The pectoralis major musculocutaneous unit obtains its vascular supply from the thoracoacromial axis of the subclavian artery just medial to the medial border of the pectoralis minor. It derives a dual blood supply from medial intercostal perforators branching from the internal mammary artery. The entire unit may be transposed medially, especially after disinsertion from the humerus, to cover defects of the sternum, neck, and lower face. Also, an island of skin can be outlined low on the chest and made to reach intraoral defects following cancer excision.

C. Trapezius

The trapezius musculocutaneous unit, based on the descending branch of the transverse cervical artery, is useful for covering defects in the neck, face, and scalp. When skeletonized as an island, the flap will reach the top of the head. When it is used in conjunction with a neck dissection, the transverse cervical artery must be preserved. Functional preservation of shoulder elevation may be accomplished by selectively sparing the transverse, superior fibers of the muscle.

D. Temporalis

The temporalis muscle extends from the temporal fossa to the coronoid process of the mandible. It is supplied by the deep and superficial temporal systems. It is commonly used to fill orbital defects. However, it can cover neighboring cranial, maxillary, palatal, and pharyngeal regions.

E. Tensor Fasciae Latae

The tensor fasciae latae musculofascial unit is supplied by the lateral femoral circumflex artery, a branch of the profunda femoris. It has a wide arc of rotation anteriorly and posteriorly. It is elevated with the fascia lata and thus can be used to reconstruct the lower abdominal wall. It has been used to cover defects following excision of osteoradionecrotic ulcers of the pubis or groin. It is also the method of choice for coverage of greater trochanteric pressure ulcers.

F. Rectus Femoris

The rectus femoris, a more robust flap than the tensor fasciae latae with a shorter arc of rotation, has supplanted the latter for reconstruction of the lower abdominal wall and for coverage to postradiation ulcers in the pubis and groin. It has a dual blood supply: a muscular branch from the profunda femoris and an axial branch from the superficial femoral artery to the overlying skin and fascia.

G. Rectus Abdominis

The rectus abdominis is supplied by the deep superior and inferior epigastric vessels that run in the undersurface of the muscle and anastomose with the segmentally arranged intercostal vessels to form the epigastric arcade. These vessels send perforating branches throughout the length of the muscle, perforating the anterior rectus sheath and supplying the overlying skin. The transverse rectus abdominis myocutaneous (TRAM) flap, when based on the superior epigastric vessel and including the infraumbilical skin, has become a workhorse for autologous tissue breast reconstruction. In situations of marked deformity, such as a radical mastectomy associated with radiation therapy or previous abdominal surgery, reconstruction of the breast can be accomplished reliably with infraumbilical skin and adipose tissue based on both rectus muscles. This superiorly based TRAM flap involves an abdominoplasty as well as reconstruction of the breast. It is a technically demanding operation but gives a very satisfying result. When based on the deep inferior epigastric vessel and using the supraumbilical skin (the "flag" flap), the flap can cover defects of the abdominal wall, flank, groin, and thigh. Using the inferior epigastric vessels to transport the skin and adipose tissue by means of microvascular surgery (see section on Free Flaps) has become a popular method of breast reconstruction. A small portion of the rectus muscle or just a main perforator vessel that supplies the overlying fat and skin is taken. This flap is known as the deep inferior epigastric perforator flap, or DIEP flap (see section on Perforator Flaps).

H. Gluteus Maximus

The gluteus maximus is useful as a muscle or musculocutaneous unit for covering pressure sores or traumatic defects over the sacrum and ischium. The muscle has a double blood supply from the superior and inferior gluteal arteries to the respective halves of the muscle. In ambulatory patients, it is advisable to perform a function-preserving operation by advancing the muscle medially and preserving its insertion laterally.

I. Gracilis

The gracilis muscle receives its dominant blood supply proximally from the medial femoral circumflex artery. Its arc of rotation makes it an excellent source of coverage for ischial pressure sores and vaginal reconstruction. Other recent uses have included transportation of the muscle alone for repair of a persistent perineal sinus following abdominal-perineal resection.

J. Gastrocnemius

The gastrocnemius musculocutaneous unit is based on either the medial or lateral head of the muscle. Each head is supplied by a sural artery, a branch of the popliteal artery that enters the muscle at its most proximal third near its origin. The flap is most useful to cover defects of the knee and proximal anterior tibia. Coverage of exposed bone in the middle and lower leg, where this unit cannot reach, can be accomplished by use of local muscle flaps such as the soleus. Complex bone and soft tissue injuries of the middle and lower leg may require reconstruction with free muscle flaps.

Fasciocutaneous Flaps

A plexus of vessels is located on top of the muscular fascia and is supplied from vessels that run within the intermuscular septa. These vessels tend to run axially along the fascia, sending perforators to the skin at intervals. Flaps can be designed that are safer than random flaps and that need not contain an entire muscle unit for their transfer. Furthermore, it is possible to make fasciocutaneous or septocutaneous flaps that safely exceed the traditional limits of a 1.5:1 ratio between length and width. Examples of fasciocutaneous flaps are those overlying the gastrocnemius, quadriceps, and rectus abdominis muscles. Other commonly used flaps are the radial forearm, lateral arm, scapular, and deltopectoral flaps.

Neurocutaneous Flaps

Anatomic studies have confirmed the presence of an arterial pedicle accompanying a sensory nerve such as the sural nerve. Consequently, one may be able to outline a skin territory over the trajectory of a sensory nerve with good viability of the overlying skin.

Free Flaps

Free flaps involve tissue transplantation using microvascular surgery. The term is actually incorrect, because the blood supply from the main axial pedicle of the flap is completely detached and then reattached at a distance to recipient vessels near the wound area.

An operating microscope with two viewing binocular lenses, specialized instruments, and swaged-on needles of 60–80 μm are required for microsurgery; 8-0, 9-0, and 10-0 suture is used to anastomose vessels as small as 0.5 mm in diameter.

Examples of free flaps in current use are axial pattern skin and fasciocutaneous flaps, such as scapular, groin, radial forearm, and anterolateral thigh, which are used when only skin and subcutaneous tissue are needed, and muscle and musculocutaneous flaps, such as latissimus dorsi, gracilis, and rectus abdominis flaps, which are used when the bulk and vascularity of muscle are needed. Composite free flaps such as the fibular flap with its overlying skin are most helpful free flaps for reconstruction of the mandible as well as the floor of the mouth following head and neck tumor extirpations.

The vascular pedicle areas of some flaps contain functional nerves, which can also be reattached with microscopic guidance. Examples are inferior gluteal, thigh, and tensor fasciae latae flaps, which contain sensory nerves. Attempts using sensory flaps to provide protective sensation in critical areas

such as the feet or the ischium in paraplegic patients have so far been clinically unsuccessful. More encouraging is the work being done to provide sensibility to the floor of the mouth with a sensory innervated radial forearm flap. Motor flaps can restore functions such as forearm flexion or facial expression.

Bone and functional joints can be transplanted as free flaps. Flaps from the ribs, fibula, and iliac crest have all been successfully transferred to areas such as the mandible and tibia. The toe-to-thumb transfer is an example of a complex transplantation, which includes bone with a functional joint, tendons, and nerves as well as skin.

Perforator Flaps

A sophisticated variation on the use of the musculocutaneous principle has been the development of perforator flaps. This usually entails taking a branch from the major vascular pedicle that may perforate the muscle to arborize and form a subcutaneous vascular plexus that will supply a considerable amount of overlying skin. Perhaps the greatest benefit from a perforator flap is decreased donor site morbidity. Structures such as the fascia, muscle, and associated nerves may be preserved while allowing the skin to be used for reconstruction.

The DIEP flap exemplifies this well for autologous tissue breast reconstruction. While maintaining the same skin territory as the TRAM flap, the perforating vessels are carefully dissected away from the rectus abdominis. By sparing the muscle, there is potentially a reduction in excessive abdominal wall weakness at the donor site.

The anterolateral thigh flap has become the mainstay for cutaneous flaps at some institutions. Based on musculocutaneous perforators from the vastus lateralis, it can be used when a relatively thin cutaneous flap is needed, such as in head and neck reconstruction. The donor site may be closed primarily depending on the flap width.

The perforator concept has been applied to further territories of skin over the perforator segments of the gluteal, thoracodorsal, and medial plantar arteries among others.

Blondeel N et al: The donor site morbidity of free DIEP flaps and free TRAM flaps for breast reconstruction. Br J Plast Surg 1997;50:322.

Coskunfirat OK et al: Reverse neurofasciocutaneous flaps for soft-tissue coverage of the lower leg. Ann Plast Surg 1999;43:14.

de Almeida OM et al: Distally based fasciocutaneous flap of the calf for cutaneous coverage of the lower leg and dorsum of the foot. Ann Plast Surg 2000;44:367.

Gill PS et al: A 10-year retrospective review of 758 DIEP flaps for breast reconstruction. Plast Reconstr Surg 2004;113:1153.

Imanishi N et al: Venous drainage of the distally based lesser saphenous-sural veno-neuroadipofascial pedicled fasciocutaneous flap: a radiographic perfusion study. Plast Reconstr Surg 1999;103:494.

Song YG et al: The free thigh flap: a new free flap concept based on the septocutaneous artery. Br J Plast Surg 1984;37:149.

Wei FC et al: Have we found an ideal soft-tissue flap? An experience with 672 anterolateral thigh flaps. Plast Reconstr Surg 2002;109:2219.

II. PRINCIPLES OF WOUND CARE

There are many types of wounds and many factors to consider when choice of coverage procedure is made. Skin type and color, glandular association, and hair-bearing characteristics must be considered. Avascular wound beds, such as exposed bone, cartilage, or tendon, will not accept skin grafts unless viable periosteum, perichondrium, or paratenon (respectively) is present. Other areas with poor vascularity are joint capsules, radiation-damaged tissue, and heavily scarred tissue. Exposed or implanted alloplastic material cannot be used as a graft bed. Such areas must be covered with tissue that is attached to its own blood supply. Skin flaps can be used but are sometimes inadequate because their blood supply is tenuous and the layer of subcutaneous fat is even less reliably vascular and may not attach to the underlying avascular surface. Muscle or musculocutaneous flaps are generally required for avascular areas.

The coverage tissue may need to have more bulk than the original tissue. Areas such as bony surfaces and prominences, weight-bearing surfaces, densely scarred areas, and areas of potential pressure breakdown may require thick, durable covering. Again, skin grafts or skin flaps may not be of adequate thickness even though they may survive and cover the wound. Musculocutaneous flaps are more successful. Bulkiness may be undesirable in areas such as the scalp, face, neck, or hand. Defects in these areas that for other reasons require a musculocutaneous flap for coverage may need to be debulked in a secondary procedure. Axial skin flaps or free axial pattern flaps may be a better choice than musculocutaneous flaps in some areas.

Contraction begins during the proliferative phase of healing and continues to a large degree in wounds covered only by split-thickness skin grafts. The grafted area may shrink to 50% of its original size, and both the graft and surrounding tissue may become distorted. Splinting of the area for 10 days or longer may favorably alter contraction. Full-thickness skin grafts rich in dermis, attached to a fresh wound bed, will considerably reduce contraction, and skin flaps will eliminate it altogether. In an orifice or tubular passageway, such as the nasal airway, pharynx, esophagus, or vagina, absence of contraction is critical.

The effects of atrophy and gravity should also be considered when technique of coverage is chosen. A denervated muscle will atrophy up to 60% of its regular size. The muscle tissue in a musculocutaneous flap will atrophy even when the nerve to the muscle is preserved in the pedicle, because the muscle's functional tension is generally not restored. Gravity will cause sagging of any tissue that does not have enough plasticity or muscle dynamics to counteract gravitational pull. Reconstructions in the face often tend to sag.

Wounds at risk for or known to have bacterial contamination also require certain types of coverage (eg, pressure sores, lower extremity defects, and wounds resulting from incision and drainage of abscesses). If the area can be skin grafted, meshed split-thickness grafts are most effective, because bacterial exudate will not collect under these grafts. Musculocutaneous flaps are associated with fewer residual bacteria over time than are random pattern skin flaps. This is probably due to the vastly superior vascularity of musculocutaneous flaps.

Contaminated wounds or wounds that are exuding a considerable amount of fluid can be treated by negative-pressure or vacuum wound dressings. This entails the application of a spongelike material connected to a suction device that keeps the wound dry as it suctions the excess exudates. The negative pressure on the wound also appears to have a positive effect on healing and increased revascularization. It has become a popular method of preparing a wound for definitive closure.

Wounds associated with nearby injuries that will probably require further surgery (eg, injuries to tendons or nerves) should be covered with flaps, because the flaps can be incised or undermined to allow for additional surgery. Skin grafts do not have sufficient vascularity to allow for these procedures.

► Excision & Primary Closure

The ideal type of wound closure is primary approximation of the skin and subcutaneous tissues immediately adjacent to the wound defect, producing a fine-line scar and the optimal aesthetic result in skin texture, thickness, and color match.

All excisions and wound closures should be planned with this ideal in mind. Obviously, large lesions cannot be excised and closed primarily. With invasive cancers, such as sarcomas, the primary goal is performance of adequate en bloc resection, with the type of wound closure being of secondary importance. Nevertheless, even larger excisions, such as mastectomies, can be planned with definite consideration for closure and subsequent reconstruction.

In most cases, minimal scars can be achieved only if the line or lines of incision are placed in, or parallel to, the skin lines of minimal tension. These lines lie perpendicular to the underlying muscles. On the face, they are obvious as wrinkles or lines of facial expression that become more pronounced with age, since they are secondary to repeated muscle contraction (Figure 41–4). On the neck, trunk, and extremities, the lines of minimal tension are most noticeable as horizontal lines of skin relaxation on the anterior and posterior aspects of areas of flexion and extension.

Langer lines, which were determined by cadaver study, probably show the direction of fibrous tissue bundles in the skin and are no longer considered accurate guides for placing skin incisions.

If the lines of expression cannot be followed, the line of incision should (if possible) be placed at the junction of unlike tissues such as the hairline of the scalp and the forehead, the eyebrow and the forehead, the mucosal and skin junction of the lips, or the areolar and skin margins of the breast. Scars will be partially hidden if incisions are placed in inconspicuous areas such as the crease of the nasal

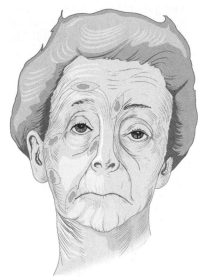

▲ **Figure 41–4.** Sites of elliptic incisions corresponding to wrinkle lines on the face.

ala and cheek, the auricular-mastoid sulcus, or the submandibular-neck junction. Lines of incision should never purposely cross flexor surfaces such as the neck, axilla, antecubital fossa, or popliteal space or the palmar skin creases of the fingers and hand, because of the risk of contracture formation. A transverse oblique or S incision should be incorporated when crossing these sites.

If a lesion is to be excised, an elliptic incision placed parallel to the skin lines of minimal tension will give the best result if the amount of tissue to be excised does not preclude primary closure.

If the ellipse is too broad or short, a protrusion of skin, commonly called a "dog-ear," will occur at each pole of the wound closure (Figure 41–5). This is most easily corrected by excising the dog-ear as a small ellipse.

A dog-ear may also be present if one side of the ellipse is longer than the other (Figure 41–6). In this case, it may be easier to excise a small triangle of skin and subcutaneous tissue from the longer side.

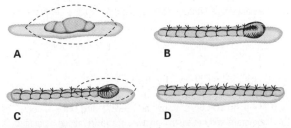

▲ **Figure 41–5.** Correction of dog-ear.

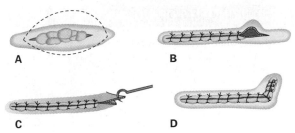

▲ **Figure 41–6.** Alternative method of correction of dog-ear.

A. Z-Plasty

One of the most useful and commonly used techniques in primary wound closure is the Z-plasty. The procedure is illustrated in Figure 41–7. The angles formed by the Z-shaped incision are transposed as shown in order (1) to gain length in the direction of the central limb of the Z or (2) to change the line of direction of the central limb of the Z. Ninety-degree angles would provide the greatest gain in length of the central limb, but smaller angles, such as 60-degree angles, are usually used, because the incision is easier to close and significant gain in length is still achieved. The Z-plasty is used for scar revision and reorientation of small wound incisions so that the main incision will be in a more ideal location. The lengthening function is used for the release or breakup of scar contractures across flexion creases. Frequently, many small Z-plasties in series rather than one large one are done. Occasionally, incisions will be placed under excessive vertical tension after the release of an underlying contracture, such as Dupuytren contracture in the hand.

B. Suture Technique

Suture technique in primary closure is important but will not compensate for poorly planned flaps, excessive tension across the incision, traumatized skin edges, bleeding, or other problems. Sometimes even a skillfully executed closure may result in an unsightly scar because of healing problems beyond the control of the surgeon.

The goal of closure is level apposition of dermal and epithelial edges with minimal or no tension across the incision and no strangulation of tissue between sutures. This is usually accomplished by placement of a layer of interrupted or running absorbable sutures in the superficial fascia and subdermal level at the base of the dermis. This suture prevents tension from forming in the upper dermis and epithelium and also causes the surface planes to be level. The epithelial edges can then be opposed with interrupted or running monofilament sutures of absorbable or permanent material. The absorbable suture is placed in the subcuticular or intradermal plane and is left in place. The permanent sutures are removed quickly according to the region of the body (within 3–4 days in the face), so the suture tracks can be avoided. Sterile

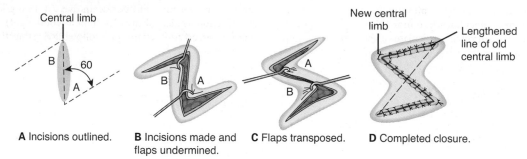

A Incisions outlined.　　B Incisions made and flaps undermined.　　C Flaps transposed.　　D Completed closure.

▲ **Figure 41–7.** Z-plasty.

adhesive tape (Steri-Strips) placed across the incision will also prevent surface marks and can be used either primarily or after surface sutures have been removed. Taping will not correct errors in suturing that have resulted in uneven edges or tension across the incision. Tape burns may occur if there is excessive tension or swelling around the incision.

The size and even the type of suture material are less important than careful suture placement and observance of previously mentioned factors. Almost any suture properly placed and removed early enough will provide closure without leaving suture marks. The use of monofilament nylon or polypropylene suture material is advised, however, because these types of sutures cause the fewest reactions of currently available suture materials, excluding stainless steel. Running subcuticular, pullout type monofilament sutures may be left in for up to 3 weeks without causing reactions. Even buried nylon sutures are well tolerated and generally cause fewer problems than braided or absorbable sutures.

An alternative to sutures is the use of skin adhesives such as 2-octylcyanoacrylate (Dermabond). It works well in small areas without much tension or shearing. It is also advisable in children. Further studies are needed to evaluate its wider applicability.

▶ **Choice of Coverage**

Table 41–2 shows some of the indications for choice of coverage in various types of wounds. Once a given type of flap is chosen, there are still at least two major considerations in the selection of the exact flap to be used. The most significant consideration is the degree of injury that will occur in the donor area. There is always a trade-off when tissue is taken from one area and used in another. This trade-off is minimal when a well-designed, well-placed skin flap leaves a donor defect that can be closed primarily, but the trade-off is great when the donor defect is as severe as the

Table 41–2. Indications for Various Types of Tissue Coverage.

Type of Wound	Type of Coverage	Reason for Choice
Mildly (< 10^5) infected wounds (including burns)	Thin split-thickness or meshed	Difficulty in obtaining successful take of thicker grafts. Donor sites may be reused sooner.
Significantly (> 10^5) infected wounds (osteomyelitis)	Thin split-thickness or meshed skin grafts or muscle or musculocutaneous flaps	Rich muscle vascular supply can sterilize an infected wound.
Wounds with poorly vascularized surfaces	Thin split-thickness skin grafts or flaps	Difficulty in obtaining successful take of thicker grafts. Flap with intrinsic blood supply may be required.
Small facial defects	Full-thickness skin graft or local flap	Produces best aesthetic result.
Large facial defects	Thick split-thickness skin grafts or flaps	Cannot use full-thickness graft, because of limited size of donor sites.
Full-thickness eyelid loss	Local flap or composite graft	Repair requires more than one tissue element.
Deep loss of nasal tip	Local flap or composite graft	Repair requires thicker tissue than present in split- or full-thickness grafts.
Avulsive wounds with exposed tendons and nerves	Flap	Requires thick protective coverage without graft adherence to tendons and nerves.
Exposed cortical bone or cartilage	Skin or muscle flap	Free grafts will not survive on avascular recipient site.
Wounds resulting from radiation burns	Muscle or musculocutaneous flap	Free grafts will not survive on avascular recipient site. Damaged tissue extends deeper than may be apparent.

original wound (eg, skin graft donor sites that become infected or musculocutaneous donor sites that fail to heal).

The patient can often participate in the choice of donor locations and should certainly be made aware of potential donor site scars and complications. The tendency has been to use muscle flaps instead of musculocutaneous flaps to permit easy primary closure of the donor site. The muscle can then be resurfaced with a split-thickness skin graft during the same procedure to give a satisfactory result. This provides for an acceptable donor site scar rather than risking disruption of a tight closure or an otherwise ugly donor site.

The second consideration in selection of a flap is that some or all of the graft or flap may be lost. In general, if the patient's overall condition is poor or the loss of a flap would result in a devastating defect, a very reliable type of flap should be chosen. For example, a microvascular anastomosis can be performed on a leg with one remaining arteriosclerotic vessel to the foot, but if the anastomosis fails, the vessel may thrombose and the leg may be lost. In this case, a flap that is safer, although more time-consuming to place, may be chosen, such as a cross-leg flap.

▶ Elevation & Transposition of Flaps

Additional considerations in reconstructive surgery involve the technique of elevating and transposing flaps. For random skin flaps, these considerations include proper length-to-width ratio, careful planning to allow for transposition with minimal tension and adjustments at the recipient site, accurate dissection in the subcutaneous plane to avoid injury to the subdermal plexus, and avoidance of folding or kinking of the flap. Surgical technique must be atraumatic, and hemostasis must be achieved. With axial pattern flaps, the surgeon must have knowledge of the important underlying blood vessels as well.

▶ Closure Technique

Closure technique is as important as elevation and transposition technique. Flaps should not be allowed to dry out. The wound bed should be irrigated. Closed-system, nonreactive suction drains are routinely used in both the wound bed and the donor defect for most flaps of any significant size. Suction evacuates blood or serum that may accumulate and keeps the flap firmly pressed against the wound bed. External pressure is both ineffective and detrimental for these purposes. Sutures should accurately and completely appose skin edges without strangulating the epithelium, particularly on the flap side. Buried half-mattress (flap) sutures are recommended (Figure 41–8). Dressings over flaps should be minimal and should not cause pressure or constriction. Emollient dressings, such as petrolatum gauze, antibiotic ointment, or silver sulfadiazine cream, have been shown to aid in preventing desiccation and subsequent necrosis of areas of marginal vascularity.

After a flap is at least temporarily tacked into its final position, adequacy of vascularity can be determined by intravenous injection of fluorescein dye, 10–15 mg/kg, and examination under ultraviolet light (Wood light). Areas that fluoresce within 10 minutes following dye injection can be expected to survive. Areas that do not fluoresce usually lack arterial inflow, which may be due to temporary arterial spasm but is often due to insufficient perfusion that will result in necrosis. A good clinical evaluation of the flap on the operating table is usually sufficient. Any sign of mottling or cyanosis or flap congestion that indicates a degree of venous obstruction warrants serious consideration of reexploration.

Avery C et al: Clinical experience with the negative pressure wound dressing. Br J Oral Maxillofac Surg 2000;38:343.
Switzer EF et al: Subcuticular closure versus Dermabond: a prospective randomized trial. Am Surg 2003;69:434.

▼ III. SPECIFIC DISORDERS TREATED BY PLASTIC SURGERY

DISORDERS OF SCARRING

HYPERTROPHIC SCARS & KELOIDS

In response to any injury severe enough to break the continuity of the skin or produce necrosis, the skin heals with scar formation. Under ideal circumstances, a fine, flat hairline scar will result. The details of wound healing are presented in Chapter 6.

However, hypertrophy may occur, causing the scar to become raised and thickened, or a keloid may form. A keloid is a true tumor arising from the connective tissue elements of the dermis. By definition, keloids grow beyond the margins of the original injury or scar; in some instances, they may grow to enormous size.

The tendency should be resisted to regard all thickened scars as keloids and to label as keloid formers all patients with unattractive scars. Hypertrophic scars and keloids are distinct entities, and the clinical course and prognosis are quite different in each case. The overreactive process that results in thickening of the hypertrophic scar ceases within a few weeks—before it extends beyond the limits of the original scar—and in most cases, some degree of maturation occurs and gradual improvement takes place. In the case of keloids, the overreactive proliferation of fibroblasts continues for weeks or months. By the time it ceases, an actual tumor is present that typically extends well beyond the limits of the original scar, involves the surrounding skin, and may become quite large. Maturation with spontaneous improvement does not usually occur.

Hypertrophic scars and keloids can be differentiated by histopathologic methods. Clinical observation of the course of the scar is also a practical means of differentiation.

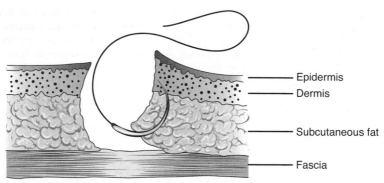

Epidermis
Dermis
Subcutaneous fat
Fascia

A. The strength of the closure lies in the dermis. Occasionally, the subcutaneous fat is incorporated to obliterate dead space.

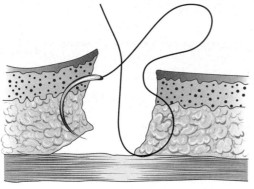

B. The suture is placed so that the knot will lie in the deepest part of the wound. Take care to avoid incorporating the epidermis with this suture, since epithelial cysts will form and result in suture extrusion.

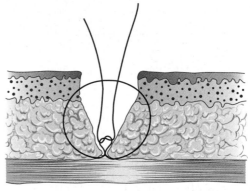

C. The dermal suture is tied just tightly enough to approximate the wound margins. Synthetic absorbable sutures are most commonly used for closure of the dermis.

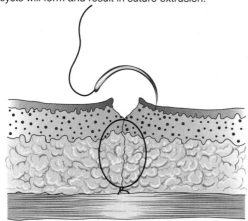

D. After the dermis is approximated, a fine "epidermal" suture is placed to align the wound edges. This suture adds little to the tensile strength of the wound closure.

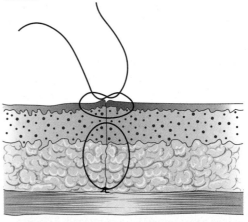

E. The epidermal suture is tied just tightly enough to approximate the epidermal edges of the wound. Since the strength of this closure lies in the dermis, the epidermal suture can be removed after 2–3 days. Skin tapes are often used to support the wound for an additional 7–10 days.

▲ **Figure 41–8.** Layered cutaneous closure (buried half-mattress [flap] sutures). (Reproduced, with permission, from Ho MT, Saunders CE [editors]: *Current Emergency Diagnosis & Treatment,* 4th ed. Originally published by Appleton & Lange. Copyright © 1992 by The McGraw-Hill Companies, Inc.)

▶ Treatment

Since nearly all hypertrophic scars undergo some degree of spontaneous improvement, they do not require treatment in the early phases. If the scar is still hypertrophic after 6 months, surgical excision and primary closure of the wound may be indicated. Improvement may be expected when the hypertrophic scar was originally produced by excessive endothelial and fibroblastic cell proliferation, as is present in open wounds, burns, and infected wounds. However, little or no improvement can be anticipated if the hypertrophic scar followed uncomplicated healing of a simple surgical incision. Improvement of hypertrophic scars across flexion surfaces such as the antecubital fossa or the fingers requires a procedure such as a Z-plasty to change the direction of the scar.

Pressure may help flatten a potentially hypertrophic scar. It is particularly useful for burn scars. A measured elastic garment or face mask (Jobst) is applied to the scarred area and provides continued pressure that causes realignment and remodeling of the collagen bundles. Pressure should be applied early, continuously, and for 6–12 months. Use of intermittent pressure (eg, only at night) or pressure applied after the hypertrophic scar is established (6–12 months) is of little value.

Additional methods of decreasing the thickness of hypertrophied scars include silicone sheeting applied early and continuously for weeks or months. More recently, early use of the potassium titanyl-phosphate (KTP) laser or the vascular pulsed-dye laser have been advocated to decrease scar redness as well as hypertrophy. These instruments appear to work by decreasing capillary supply to the scar. They appear to have a good effect on the pruritus of the scar, but more studies are needed to determine their effects on scar modification.

The treatment of choice for keloids and intractable hypertrophic scars is still injection of triamcinolone acetonide, 10 mg/mL (Kenalog-10 Injection), directly into the lesion. This will also help control itching associated with these lesions. In the case of larger lesions, injection is made into more than one site. There is evidence that keloids may respond better to early than to late treatment.

Lesions are injected every 3–4 weeks, and treatment should not be carried out longer than 6 months. The following dosage schedule is used:

Size of Lesion

1–2 cm²	20–40 mg
2–6 cm²	40–80 mg
6–10 cm²	80–110 mg

For larger lesions, the maximum dose should be 120 mg. The maximum doses for each treatment for children are as follows:

Age

1–2 years	20 mg
3–5 years	40 mg
6–10 years	80 mg

There is a tendency to inject the drug into the scar too often or in too high a dosage—or into the subjacent tissue, which may produce too vigorous a response, resulting in excessive atrophy of the skin and subcutaneous tissues surrounding the lesion and in depigmentation of darker skins. Both of these adverse responses may improve spontaneously in 6–12 months, but not necessarily completely. The response varies greatly; some lesions become flat after two or three injections, and some fail to respond at all. Topical corticosteroid therapy is of little or no value.

Before the advent of corticosteroid injection therapy, surgical excision and radiation therapy were the only methods of treatment of keloids. Both methods are disappointing; surgical resection usually leads to recurrence of a larger lesion; with very few exceptions, radiation therapy produces an unpredictable result and has obvious potential side effects, including neoplastic degeneration. At present, surgical excision is used only in conjunction with intralesional corticosteroid therapy. Excision is usually confined to the larger lesions in which steroid therapy would exceed safe dosages. (The wound is injected at the time of surgery and then postoperatively according to the schedule recommended above.) Care should be taken so that surgical incisions are not extended into the normal skin around the keloid, since the growth of a new keloid may occur in these scars. It has been reported that intramarginal excisions yield better results than extramarginal excisions.

Allison KP et al: Pulsed dye laser treatment of burn scars: alleviation or irritation? Burns 2003;29:207.

Mustoe TA: Evolution of silicone therapy and mechanism of action in scar management. Aesthetic Plast Surg 2008;32:82.

Niessen FB et al: On the nature of hypertrophic scars and keloids: a review. Plast Reconstr Surg 1999;104:1435.

Ziegler UE: International clinical recommendations on scar management. Zentralbl Chir 2004;129:296.

CONTRACTURES

Contraction is a normal process of wound healing. Contracture, on the other hand, is a pathologic end stage related to the process of contraction. Generally, contractures develop when wounds heal with too much scarring and contraction of the scar tissue results in distortion of surrounding tissues. Although scar contractures can occur in any flexible tissue, such as the eyelids or lips, contractures usually occur across areas of flexion, such as the neck, axilla, or antecubital fossa. The contracted scar brings together the structures on either side of the joint space and prevents active or even passive extension. Exceptions to this pattern of flexion contractures are extension contractures of the toes and MP (metacarpophalangeal) joints of the digits. Contraction is thought to occur via smooth muscle contractile elements in myofibroblasts, but the mechanism is not well understood. In one vertical abdominal scar there may be an area of normal scar formation and an area of hypertrophic scar formation with visible contracture. Contracture can occur in response to the presence of foreign material such as Silastic or saline breast implants. Overall, there is a 10% incidence of some form of breast capsular contracture. Myofibroblasts are thought to play an important role, but the actual cause is not known. Some patients have a soft, excellent result on one side but significant contracture on the other. Clinical practice with a newer type of implant by changing the surface from smooth to textured have yielded unclear results as to whether there is a decrease in capsular contracture with the textured surface. Polyurethane-coated silicone implants, which did show a decrease in the rate of capsular contracture, are no longer available for clinical use.

The best treatment of contractures is prevention. Incisions should not be made at right angles to flexion creases or should be reoriented by Z-plasties. Wounds in areas of flexion can be covered with flaps or grafted early with thick split-thickness or full-thickness grafts to stop the process of contraction. Such wounds should also be splinted in a position of extension during healing and for 2–3 weeks after healing is complete. Vigorous physical therapy may also be helpful.

Once a contracture is established, stretching and massage are rarely beneficial. Narrow bands of contracture may be excised and released with one or more Z-plasties. Larger areas must be incised from the medial to the lateral axis across the flexion surface and completely opened up to full extension. The resulting defect can be extensive and must be resurfaced with a skin flap or skin graft. In recurrent contractures a fasciocutaneous flap is the treatment of choice. If a skin graft is used, the area must be splinted in extension for approximately 2 weeks after the graft has healed. Less aggressive surgery is likely to result in recurrence.

Achauer GM, Spenler CW, Gold ME: Reconstruction of axillary burn contractures with the latissimus dorsi fasciocutaneous flap. J Trauma 1988;28:211.
Collis N et al: Ten-year review of a prospective randomized controlled trial of textured versus smooth subglandular silicone gel breast implants. Plast Reconstr Surg 2000;106:786.

SKIN TUMORS*

Tumors of the skin are by far the most common of all tumors in humans. They arise from each of the histologic structures that make up the skin—epidermis, connective tissue, gland, muscle, and nerve elements—and are correspondingly numerous in variety. Skin tumors are classified as benign, premalignant, and malignant.

BENIGN SKIN TUMORS

The many benign tumors that arise from the skin rarely interfere with function. Since most are removed for aesthetic reasons or to rule out malignancy, they are quite commonly

treated by the plastic surgeon. The majority are small and can be simply excised under local anesthesia following the principles of elliptical excision and wound closure discussed above. General anesthesia may be necessary for larger lesions requiring excision and repair by skin grafts or flaps or those occurring in young children.

When the diagnosis is not in doubt, most superficial lesions (seborrheic keratoses, verrucae, squamous cell papillomas) can be treated by simple techniques such as electrodesiccation, curettage and electrodesiccation, cryotherapy, and topical cytotoxic agents.

▶ Seborrheic Keratosis

Seborrheic keratoses are superficial noninvasive tumors that originate in the epidermis. They appear in older people as multiple slightly elevated yellowish, brown, or brownish-black irregularly rounded plaques with waxy or oily surfaces. They are most commonly found on the trunk and shoulders but are frequently seen on the scalp and face.

Because the lesion is raised above the epidermis, treatment usually consists of shave excision. Care should be exercised to avoid shaving a melanoma because if that is done it will interfere with the determination of the depth of invasion by the Breslow or Clark classifications. If there is any question about a pigmented lesion, it is preferable to do an excisional biopsy rather than to shave it.

▶ Verrucae

Verrucae (common warts) are usually seen in children and young adults, commonly on the fingers and hands. They appear as round or oval elevated lesions with rough surfaces composed of multiple rounded or filiform keratinized projections. They may be skin-colored or gray to brown.

Verrucae are caused by a virus and are autoinoculable, which can result in multiple lesions around the original growth or frequent recurrences following treatment if the virus is not completely eradicated. They may disappear spontaneously.

Treatment by electrodesiccation is effective but is frequently followed by slow healing. Repeated applications of bichloroacetic acid, liquid nitrogen, or liquid CO_2 are also effective. Surgical excision alone is not recommended, because the wound may become inoculated with the virus, leading to recurrences in and around the scar. However, surgical excision in conjunction with electrodesiccation, can be an effective form of treatment.

Recurrence remains a common problem; therefore, it is reasonable to delay treatment of asymptomatic lesions for several months to determine if they will disappear spontaneously.

Scheinfeld N, Lehman DS: An evidence-based review of medical and surgical treatments of genital warts. Dermatol Online J 2006;12:5.

---

*Melanoma is discussed in Chapter 44.

▶ Cysts

A. Epidermal Inclusion Cyst

Although sebaceous cyst is the commonly used term, these lesions more properly should be called epidermal inclusion cysts because they are composed of thin layers of epidermal cells filled with epithelial debris. True cysts arising from sebaceous epithelial cells are uncommon.

Epidermal inclusion cysts are soft to firm, usually elevated, and are filled with an odorous cheesy material. Their most common sites of occurrence are the scalp, face, ears, neck, and back. They are usually covered by normal skin, which may show dimpling at the site of skin attachment. They frequently present as infected cysts.

Treatment consists of surgical excision.

B. Dermoid Cyst

Dermoid cysts are deeper than epidermal cysts. They are not attached to the skin but frequently are attached to or extend through underlying bony structures. They may appear in many sites but are most common around the nose or the orbit, where they may extend to meningeal structures, necessitating CT scans to determine their extent.

Treatment is by surgical excision, which may necessitate sectioning of adjacent bony structures.

▶ Pigmented Nevi

Nevocellular nevi are groups of cells of probable neural crest origin that contain melanocytes that form melanin more rapidly upon stimulation than surrounding tissue. These cells migrate to different parts of the skin to give different types of nevi. They may also be distinguished by their clinical presentation.

A. Junctional Nevi

Junctional nevi are well-defined pigmented lesions appearing in infancy. They are usually flat or slightly elevated and light brown to dark brown. They may appear on any part of the body, but most nevi seen on the palms, soles, and genitalia are of the junctional type. Histologically, a proliferation of melanocytes is present in the epidermis at the epidermal-dermal junction. It was formerly thought that these nevi give rise to malignant melanoma and that all junctional nevi should be excised for prophylactic reasons. However, most investigators now feel that the risk is very slight. If there is no change in their appearance, treatment is unnecessary. Any change such as itching, inflammation, darkening in color, halo formation, increase in size, bleeding, or ulceration calls for immediate treatment.

Surgical excision is the only safe method of treatment.

B. Intradermal Nevi

Intradermal nevi are the typical dome-shaped, sometimes pedunculated, fleshy to brownish pigmented moles that are characteristically seen in adults. They frequently contain hairs and may occur anywhere on the body.

Microscopically, melanocytes are present entirely within the dermis and, in contrast to junctional nevi, show little activity. They are rarely malignant and require no treatment except for aesthetic reasons.

Surgical excision is nearly always the treatment of choice. Pigmented nevi should never be treated without obtaining tissue for histologic examination.

C. Compound Nevi

Compound nevi exhibit the histologic features of both junctional and intradermal nevi in that melanocytes lie both at the epidermal-dermal junction and within the dermis. They are usually elevated, dome-shaped, and light-brown to dark-brown in color.

Because of the presence of nevus cells at the epidermal-dermal junction, the indications for treatment are the same as for junctional nevi. If treatment is indicated, surgical excision is the method of choice.

D. Spindle Cell-Epithelioma Cell Nevi

These nevi, formerly called benign juvenile melanomas, appear in children or adults. They vary markedly in vascularity, degree of pigmentation, and accompanying hyperkeratosis. Clinically, they simulate warts or hemangiomas rather than moles. They may increase in size rapidly, but the average lesion reaches only 6–8 mm in diameter, remaining entirely benign without invasion or metastases. Microscopically, the lesion can be confused with malignant melanoma by the inexperienced pathologist. The usual treatment is excisional biopsy.

E. Blue Nevi

Blue nevi are small, sharply defined, round, dark blue or grayish-blue lesions that may occur anywhere on the body but are most commonly seen on the face, neck, hands, and arms. They usually appear in childhood as slowly growing, well-defined nodules covered by a smooth, intact epidermis. Microscopically, the melanocytes that make up this lesion are limited to (but may be found in all layers of) the dermis. An intimate association with the fibroblasts of the dermis is seen, giving the lesion a fibrotic appearance not seen in other nevi. This, together with extension of melanocytes deep into the dermis, may account for the blue rather than brown color.

Treatment is not mandatory unless the patient desires removal for aesthetic reasons or fear of cancer. Surgical excision is the treatment of choice.

F. Giant Hairy Nevi

Unlike most nevi arising from melanocytes, giant hairy nevi are congenital. They may occur anywhere on the body and may cover large areas. They may be large enough to cover the entire trunk (bathing trunk nevi). They are of special significance for several reasons: (1) Their large size is especially deforming from an aesthetic standpoint; (2) they show a predisposition for developing malignant melanoma; and (3) they may be associated with neurofibromas or melanocytic involvement of the leptomeninges and other neurologic abnormalities.

Microscopically, a varied picture is present. All of the characteristics of intradermal and compound nevi may be seen. Neurofibromas may also be present within the lesion. Malignant melanoma may arise anywhere within the large lesion; the reported rate of occurrence ranges from 1% to as high as 13.7% in one study. Malignant melanoma with metastases rarely arises in childhood or infancy.

The only full treatment is complete excision and skin grafting. Large lesions may require excision and grafting in stages. Some lesions are so large that excision is not possible and the most effective approach is using tissue expansion in combination with flaps. Split-thickness excision or dermabrasion has been successful when done in infancy.

The use of cultured epithelial autografts has been advocated for extensive lesions associated with multiple satellite nevi. Additionally, some have reported the use of laser photothermolysis of pigmented lesions that cannot be excised with favorable reconstructive outcomes. However, there is still concern over malignant transformation of remaining melanocytes, and close long-term follow-up is recommended when laser ablation is used.

Gur E, Zuker R: Complex facial nevi: a surgical algorithm. Plast Reconstr Surg 2000;106:25.

▶ Vascular Tumors & Vascular Malformations

Our understanding of vascular tumors and vascular malformations has evolved a great deal since the description by Mulliken and Glowacki in 1982 of the biologic classification of vascular anomalies based on their endothelial properties. In this way, infant hemangiomas appear within the first 3 weeks of life and have a proliferative endothelium that grows rapidly at first and commonly involutes usually in the first few years of life. Vascular malformations, on the other hand, have stable endothelium, grow proportionally with the child, and persist into adulthood. They can be associated with various complications, such as skeletal abnormalities, ischemia, coagulopathy, heart failure, and death.

The terminology of these vascular anomalies was previously based on anatomical, clinical, histologic, or descriptive features, contributing to much confusion in identifying the hemangioma. For example, the histologic term *capillary hemangioma* has been used for both the common involuting hemangioma of childhood that disappears by age 7 and the port wine stain that persists into adulthood. The term *cavernous* is used to designate several types of hemangiomas

that behave quite differently. Some hemangiomas are true neoplasms arising from endothelial cells and other vascular elements (such as involuting hemangiomas of childhood, endotheliomas, and pericytomas). Others are not true neoplasms but rather malformations of normal vascular structures (eg, port wine stains, cavernous hemangiomas, and arteriovenous fistulas).

Glucose transporter isoform 1 (GLUT1) has recently been discovered to be a distinguishing feature among various forms of vascular anomalies. It is an immunohistochemical marker that is normally restricted to endothelial cells with blood–tissue barrier function as in the brain and placenta. North and colleagues retrospectively studied specimens from vascular tumors for GLUT1. Specimens from infantile hemangiomas were universally positive. In contrast, biopsies of other vascular anomalies, including RICH, NICH, pyogenic granuloma, granulation tissue, vascular malformations, and tufted angioma and kaposiform hemangioendothelioma, were all negative. In addition to providing an early diagnostic assay for hemangiomas, GLUT1 can be useful in research and in trying to explain the pathophysiology.

The International Society for the Study of Vascular Anomalies proposed a classification in 1996 based on the pioneering work of Mulliken and Glowacki. It is now the most widely accepted among specialists and in the literature. Clear classification is vitally important so that proper communication regarding diagnosis and treatment can be established. Table 41–3 shows that classification.

A. Hemangiomas of Infancy (Involuting Hemangioma)

Involuting hemangiomas are the most common tumors that occur in childhood and constitute at least 95% of all the hemangiomas that are seen in infancy and childhood. They are true neoplasms of endothelial cells but are unique among neoplasms in that they undergo complete, spontaneous involution.

Table 41–3. International Society for the Study of Vascular Anomalies Classification.

Tumors
Juvenile hemangioma
Rapidly involuting congenital hemangioma (RICH)
Noninvoluting congenital hemangioma (NICH)
Kaposiform hemangioendothelioma
Tufted angioma
Vascular malformations
High-flow
Arteriovenous malformation
Low-flow
Venous malformation
Lymphatic malformation
Lymphatic-venous malformation
Capillary (or venular) malformation (port wine stain)

Typically, they are present shortly after birth or appear during the first 2–3 weeks of life. They grow at a rather rapid rate for 4–6 months; then growth ceases and spontaneous involution begins. Involution progresses slowly but in most cases is complete by 5–7 years of age.

Involuting hemangiomas appear on all body surfaces but are seen more often on the head and neck. They are seen twice as often in girls as in boys and show a predisposition for fair-skinned individuals.

Three forms of infantile hemangiomas are seen: (1) superficial, (2) combined superficial and deep (mixed), and (3) deep. Superficial involuting hemangiomas appear as sharply demarcated, bright-red, slightly raised lesions with an irregular surface that has been described as resembling a strawberry. Combined superficial and deep involuting hemangiomas have the same surface characteristics, but beneath the skin surface, a firm bluish tumor is present that may extend deeply into the subcutaneous tissues. Deep involuting hemangiomas present as deep blue tumors covered by normal-appearing skin.

The histologic findings in involuting hemangiomas are quite different from those seen in other types of hemangiomas. There is a constant correlation between the histologic picture and the clinical course. During the growth phase, the lesion is composed of solid fields of closely packed round or oval endothelial cells. As would be expected during the growth phase, cellular division with mitotic figures is seen, so that the lesion is sometimes called a hemangioendothelioma by the pathologist. This term should not be used, however, because it is commonly used to denote the highly malignant angiosarcoma that is seen in adults.

As the phase of involution progresses, the histologic picture changes, with the solid fields of endothelial cells breaking up into closely packed, capillary-sized, vessel-like structures composed of several layers of soft endothelial cells supported by a sparse fibrous stroma. These vascular structures gradually become fewer and spaced more widely apart in a loose, edematous fibrous stroma. The endothelial cells continue to disappear, so that by the time involution is complete the histologic picture is entirely normal, with no trace of endothelial cells.

Treatment is not usually indicated, since the appearance following spontaneous regression is nearly always superior to the scars that follow surgical excision. Surgical excision of lesions that involve important structures such as the eyelids, nose, or lips may sometimes be necessary in order to avoid serious functional disturbances of vision and airway. Complete excision is usually not necessary.

Partial resection of a portion of a hemangioma of the brow or eyelid is indicated when the lesion is large enough to prevent light from entering the eye—a condition that will lead to blindness or amblyopia. The same type of treatment may be necessary for lesions of the mucosal surfaces of the lips when they project into the mouth and are traumatized by the teeth. In these cases, surgery should be very conservative—only enough of the lesion should be resected to alleviate the problem, and the remaining portions should be allowed to involute spontaneously.

In approximately 8% of cases, ulceration will occur. This may be accompanied by infection, which is treated by the use of compresses of warm saline or potassium permanganate and by the application of antimicrobial powders and creams. Bleeding from the ulcer can occur if there is constant irritation and inflammation. When it occurs, gentle pressure should be applied. In some situations, such as the perianal region, specific measures may be needed to keep the area clean and dry including a diverting colostomy combined with judicious serial excision. In rare cases, the platelet trapping of these lesions leads to the clinical picture of disseminated intravascular coagulopathy called **Kasabach-Merritt syndrome.**

After involution of large lesions, superficial scarring may be present or the involved skin may be thin, wrinkled, or redundant. These conditions may require conservative plastic surgery procedures.

The application of local agents such as dry ice to the surface of these lesions has been popular. This type of treatment has no effect on the deep portions of the hemangioma. It will destroy superficial lesions but results in severe scarring. Injections of sclerosing agents have minimal effect. There is no place for radiation therapy in the treatment of these benign lesions. Corticosteroids given systemically or intralesionally have been used with varying success and should be considered if conservative measures are inadequate. Anecdotal evidence exists in favor of compression to speed up the involution process and give a better final result. Although surface laser therapy has little or no effect on these large hemangiomas, some have proposed the insertion of a laser probe deep into the lesion so that the heat generated by the laser produces contracture of the hemangioma. This may slow down the accelerated growth and trigger involution. In cases of life-threatening hemangiomas associated with Kasabach-Merritt syndrome or hemangiomas of the head and neck area that are obstructing the airway or vision, systemic interferon alfa has been shown to be extremely effective especially in those cases that are resistant to corticosteroids.

Ezekowitz RA et al: Interferon alfa-2a therapy for life-threatening hemangiomas of infancy. N Engl J Med 1992;326:1456.
Achauer BM et al: Intralesional photocoagulation of periorbital hemangiomas. Plast Reconstr Surg 1999;103:11.

B. Congenital Hemangiomas (RICH and NICH)

Congenital hemangiomas, as their name implies, are present at birth. They have undergone their rapid growth phase in utero, and in contrast to hemangiomas of infancy, they do not undergo rapid growth during the first 4–6 months of life Because of their natural history they are divided into two subtypes: rapidly involuting (RICH) and noninvoluting

(NICH) congenital hemangiomas. RICH are more common than NICH, although both are rare. The diagnosis of RICH is confirmed when they rapidly involute by 6–10 months of age. The NICH anomalies, on the other hand, persist into adulthood and may require surgical excision or other ablative measures. Imaging may be helpful (sonography or MRI) in order to evaluate location and extent of the tumor. Both RICH and NICH are GLUT1 negative in contrast to hemangiomas of infancy.

C. Capillary Malformations

Capillary malformations (ie, port wine stains) are by far the most common of the vascular malformations. They may involve any portion of the body but most commonly appear on the face as flat patchy lesions that are reddish to purple in color. When present on the face, they are located in areas supplied by the sensory branches of the fifth (trigeminal) cranial nerve. They usually start off light red in color yet have a propensity to deepen in color, as their name implies. Their growth is variable, but they persist into adulthood if not treated and become raised and thickened with nodules appearing on the surface (Figure 41–9).

Microscopically, port wine stains are made up of thin-walled capillaries that are arranged throughout the dermis. The capillaries are lined with mature, flat endothelial cells. In the lesions that produce surface growth, groups of round proliferating endothelial cells and large venous sinuses are seen.

Results following treatment of the port wine stain were uniformly disappointing. Because most lesions occur on the face or neck, patients seek treatment for aesthetic reasons, but as they progress in thickness and nodularity, they can become functionally disabling and can bleed spontaneously. The simplest method of treatment is camouflaging. Unfortunately, this is difficult because the port wine stain is darker than the surrounding lighter skin, and it does not affect the natural history of the lesion.

Superficial methods of treatment such as dry ice, liquid nitrogen, electrocoagulation, and dermabrasion have been tried but are ineffective unless they destroy the upper layers of the skin, which can produce severe scarring.

Radiation therapy, including the use of x-rays, radium, thorium X, and grenz x-rays, is to be condemned. If it is administered in doses high enough to destroy the vessels involved, it also destroys the surrounding tissues and the overlying skin, and the cancer incidence after radiotherapy for skin hemangioma increases.

The best treatment to date for early and intermediate port wine stains is with the pulsed dye laser. The pulsed dye laser produces a light with a specific wavelength of 585 or 595 nanometers. The method of treatment is termed selective photothermolysis. The beam is selectively absorbed by red-pigmented material such as hemoglobin in the blood vessels of the lesion. This produces selective heat destruction of these structures, and the treated area becomes whiter. When

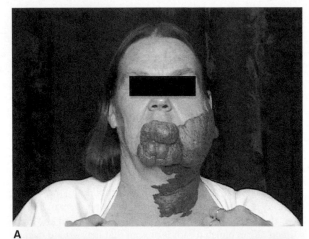

A

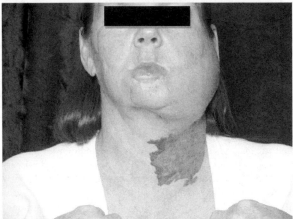

B

▲ **Figure 41–9.** 46-year-old white female with untreated port wine stain of left face. **(A)** Preoperative. **(B)** Status postexcision of facial portion and reconstruction with free tissue transfer.

started early, these treatments can be very effective. Multiple treatments are necessary to obtain a satisfactory result. In darker and more advanced nodular lesions, the laser is less effective because of the thickness of the lesion and the hyperpigmentation that may develop.

If the lesion is small, surgical excision with primary closure is possible. Unfortunately, most lesions are large. In the case of longstanding untreated lesions, surgical excision may be necessary, followed by skin grafting, locoregional flaps, or at times free tissue transfer. Certain fast-growing capillary or primarily arterialized hemangiomas have been managed successfully with superselective embolization, either alone or in conjunction with surgery. This is performed under fluoroscopic control and with an expert team. There have been reports of slough of large portions of the face as a result of misdirected embolizations.

D. Venous Malformations

Venous malformations (otherwise known as cavernous hemangiomas) are bluish or purplish lesions that are usually elevated. They may occur anywhere on the body but, like other vascular lesions, are more common on the head and neck. They are composed of mature, fully formed venous structures that are present in tortuous masses that have been described as feeling like a bag of worms.

Venous malformations are usually present at birth but do not usually grow except to keep pace with normal body growth. In many cases, growth occurs later in life and may interfere with normal function.

Microscopically, venous malformations are made up of large, dilated, closely packed vascular sinuses that are engorged with blood. They are lined by flat endothelial cells and may have muscular walls like normal veins.

Treatment is difficult. In only a few cases is the lesion small enough or superficial enough to permit complete surgical excision. Most lesions involve deeper structures—including muscle and bone—so that complete excision is impossible without radical surgery. Since most lesions are no more than aesthetic problems, radical surgery is rarely indicated. Occasionally, the injection of sclerosing agents directly into the venous channels may lead to some involution or may make surgical excision easier. Great care must be used so that areas of overlying skin do not slough.

E. Arteriovenous Malformations

Arteriovenous malformations are high-flow lesions having a direct connection between an artery and a vein, bypassing the capillary bed.

Arteriovenous malformations are typically recognized at birth but are misdiagnosed as capillary malformations or involuting hemangiomas. Periods of rapid growth are found after trauma and during periods when the body is under the influence of hormonal changes.

Clinical diagnosis can be confirmed with color Doppler examination, but this does not give information concerning extent of the lesion or relation to surrounding structures. This information can be obtained via MRI or angiography, which has the additional benefit of therapeutic embolization.

Treatment for arteriovenous malformations is based on clinical stage of the lesion. Smaller arteriovenous malformations can be primarily resected. Larger, more diffuse arteriovenous malformations are best managed with superselective arterial embolization followed by surgical resection 24–48 hours after embolization in order to minimize intraoperative blood loss.

Arneja JS, Gosain AK: Vascular malformations. Plast Recon Surgery 2008;121:195e.

Chang MW: Updated classification of hemangiomas and other vascular anomalies. Lymphat Res Biol 2003;1:259.

Enjolras O, Mulliken JB: Vascular tumors and vascular malformations (new issues). Adv Dermatol 1997;13:375.

Mulliken JB, Fishman SJ, Burrows PE: Vascular anomalies. Curr Probl Surg 2000;37:517.

Mulliken JB, Glowacki J: Hemangiomas and vascular malformations in infants and children: a classification based on endothelial characteristics. Plast Reconstr Surg 1982;69:412.

North PE et al: GLUT1: A newly discovered immunohistochemical marker for juvenile hemangiomas. Human Pathol 2000;31:11.

PREMALIGNANT SKIN LESIONS

▶ Actinic (Solar) Keratoses

Actinic keratoses are the most common of the precancerous skin lesions. They usually appear as small, single or multiple, slightly elevated, scaly or warty lesions ranging in color from red to yellow, brown, or black. Because they are related to sun exposure, they occur most frequently on the face and the backs of the hands in fair-skinned Caucasians whose skin shows evidence of actinic elastosis.

Microscopically, actinic keratoses consist of well-defined areas of abnormal epithelial cells limited to the epidermis. Approximately 15–20% of these lesions become malignant, in which case invasion of the dermis as squamous cell carcinoma occurs.

Since the lesions are limited to the epidermis, superficial treatment in the form of curette and electrodesiccation or the application of chemical agents such as liquid nitrogen, phenol, bi- or trichloroacetic acid, or fluorouracil is curative. The application of fluorouracil (5-FU) cream is of particular benefit in preventive treatment in that it destroys lesions of microscopic size—before they can be detected clinically—without causing damage to uninvolved skin.

▶ Chronic Radiation Dermatitis & Ulceration

There are two distinct types of radiation dermatitis. The first and most common follows the acute administration of relatively high dosages of ionizing orthovoltage radiation over relatively short periods—almost always for the treatment of cancer. Dermatitis is characterized by an acute reaction that begins near the third week of therapy, when erythema, blistering, and sloughing of the epidermis start to occur. Burning and hyperesthesia are commonly present. This initial reaction is followed by scarring characterized by atrophy of the epidermis and dermis along with loss of skin appendages (sweat glands, sebaceous glands, and hair follicles). Marked fibrosis of the dermis occurs, with gradual endarteritis and occlusion of the dermal and subdermal vessels. Telangiectasia of the surface vessels is seen, and areas of both hypopigmentation and hyperpigmentation occur.

The second type of radiation dermatitis follows chronic exposure to low doses of ionizing radiation over prolonged periods. It is usually seen in professional personnel who handle radioactive materials or administer x-rays or in patients who have been treated for dermatologic conditions such as acne or excessive facial hair. Therefore, the face and hands are most commonly involved. The acute reaction described above does not usually occur, but the same process of atrophy, scarring, and loss of dermal elements occurs. Drying of the skin becomes more pronounced, and deepening of the skin furrows is typically present. Fortunately, this second type of radiation dermatitis is rarely seen today.

In both types of radiation dermatitis, late changes such as the following may occur: (1) the appearance of hyperkeratotic growths on the skin surface, (2) chronic ulceration, and (3) the development of either basal cell or squamous cell carcinoma. Ulceration and cancer, however, are seen much less commonly in the first type of radiation dermatitis than in the second. When malignant growths appear, basal cell carcinomas are seen more frequently on the face and neck and squamous cell carcinomas more frequently on the hands and body.

Newer radiotherapeutic methods using megavoltage and electron beam techniques have a sparing effect on the skin. However, marked scarring and avascularity of deeper, more extensive areas may present more difficult problems.

Surgical excision is the treatment of choice. Excision should include all of the irradiated tissue including the area of telangiectasia, whenever possible, and the defect should be covered with an appropriate axial or musculocutaneous flap to provide a new blood supply.

Primary wound closure is feasible for only the smallest lesions, and even so, at some risk. Free-skin grafting is usually unsuccessful because of the damage to the vascular supply of the subcutaneous structures. Adjacent random flaps are unreliable because they depend on blood supply from the surrounding irradiated area.

MALIGNANT LESIONS

1. Intraepidermal Carcinoma

Intraepidermal carcinoma includes Bowen disease and erythroplasia of Queyrat.

▶ Bowen Disease

Bowen disease is characterized by single or multiple, brownish or reddish plaques that may appear anywhere on the skin surface but often on covered surfaces. The typical plaque is sharply defined, slightly raised, scaly, and slightly thickened. The surface is often keratotic, and crusting and fissuring may be present. Ulceration is not common but when present suggests malignant degeneration with dermal invasion.

Histologically, hyperplasia of the epidermis is seen, with pleomorphic malpighian cells, giant cells, and atypical epithelial cells that are limited to the epidermis.

Treatment of small or superficial lesions consists of total destruction by curette and electrodesiccation or by any of the other superficially destructive methods (cryotherapy, cytotoxic agents). Excision and skin grafting are preferred for larger lesions and for those that have undergone early malignant degeneration and invasion of the dermis.

▶ Erythroplasia of Queyrat

Erythroplasia of Queyrat is almost identical to Bowen disease both clinically and histologically but is confined to the glans penis and the vulva, where the lesions appear as red, velvety, irregular, slightly raised plaques. Treatment is as described for Bowen disease.

2. Basal Cell Carcinoma

Basal cell carcinoma is the most common skin cancer. The lesions usually appear on the face and are more common in men than in women. Since exposure to ultraviolet rays of the sun is a causative factor, basal cell carcinoma is most commonly seen in geographic areas where there is significant sun exposure and in people whose skin is most susceptible to actinic damage from exposure (ie, fair-skinned individuals with blue eyes and blond hair). It may occur at any age but is not common before age 40.

The growth rate of basal cell carcinoma is usually slow but nearly always steady and insidious. Several months or years may pass before the patient becomes concerned. Without treatment, widespread invasion and destruction of adjacent tissues may occur, producing massive ulceration. Penetration of the bones of the facial skeleton and the skull may occur late in the course. Basal cell carcinomas rarely metastasize, but death can occur because of direct intracranial extension or erosion of major blood vessels.

Typical individual lesions appear as small, translucent or shiny ("pearly") elevated nodules with central ulceration and rolled, pearly edges. Telangiectatic vessels are commonly present over the surface, and pigmentation is sometimes present. Superficial ulceration occurs early.

A less common type of basal cell carcinoma is the **sclerosing** or **morphea carcinoma,** consisting of elongated strands of basal cell cancer that infiltrate the dermis, with the intervening corium being unusually compact. These lesions are usually flat and whitish or waxy in appearance and firm to palpation—similar in appearance to localized scleroderma. They are particularly difficult to treat because it is difficult to clinically predict the extent of the margins of growth.

The superficial **erythematous basal cell cancer** ("body basal") occurs most frequently on the trunk. It appears as reddish plaques with atrophic centers and smooth, slightly raised borders. These lesions are capable of peripheral growth and wide extension but do not become invasive until late.

Pigmented basal cell carcinomas may be mistaken for melanomas because of the large number of melanocytes present within the tumor. They may also be confused with seborrheic keratoses.

▶ Treatment

There are several methods of treating basal cell carcinoma. All may be curative in some lesions, but no one method is applicable to all. The special features of each basal cell cancer must be considered individually before proper treatment can be selected.

Because most lesions occur on the face, aesthetic and functional results of treatment are important. However, the most important consideration is whether or not therapy is curative. If the basal cell carcinoma is not eradicated by the initial treatment, continued growth and invasion of adjacent tissues will occur, resulting not only in additional tissue destruction but also in invasion of the tumor into deeper structures, making cure more difficult. Adequate treatment of basal cell carcinoma by different modalities achieves a cure rate of approximately 95%.

The principal methods of treatment are curettage and electrodesiccation, surgical excision, and radiation therapy. Chemosurgery, topical chemotherapy, and cryosurgery are not often used but may have value in selected cases.

A. Curettage and Electrodesiccation

Curettage plus electrodesiccation is the usual method of treatment for small lesions. After infiltration with suitable local anesthetic, the lesion and a 2–3 mm margin of normal-appearing skin around it are thoroughly curetted with a small skin curette. The resultant wound is then completely desiccated with an electrosurgical unit to destroy any tumor cells that may not have been removed by the curette. The process is then repeated once or twice if necessary. The wound is left open and allowed to heal secondarily.

When used as treatment for superficial basal cell carcinoma, curettage and electrodesiccation is a simple, quick, and inexpensive procedure that will cure nearly all superficial lesions. However, this method of treatment should not be used in the deeper infiltrative and morphea type lesions. These lesions should be treated by surgical excision, x-ray therapy, or chemosurgery.

B. Surgical Excision

Surgical excision, following the principles outlined earlier in this chapter, offers many advantages in the treatment of basal cell carcinoma: (1) Most lesions can be quickly excised in one procedure. (2) Following excision, the entire lesion can be examined by the pathologist, who can determine if the tumor has been completely removed. (3) Deep infiltrative lesions can be completely excised, and cartilage and bone can be removed if they have been invaded. (4) Lesions that occur in dense scar tissue or in other poorly vascularized tissues cannot be treated by curettage and desiccation, radiation therapy, or chemosurgery, since healing is poor. Excision and flap coverage may be the only method for treatment in these conditions. (5) Recurrent lesions in tissues that have been exposed to maximum safe amounts of radiation can be excised and covered.

Small to moderate-sized lesions can be excised in one stage under local anesthesia. The visible and palpable margins of the tumor are marked on the skin with marking ink. The width of excision is then marked 3–5 mm beyond these margins. If the margins of the basal cell carcinoma are vague, the width of excision will have to be wider to ensure complete removal of the lesion. The lines of incision are drawn around the lesion as a circle. This tissue is excised, taking care to leave a margin of normal-appearing subcutaneous tissue around the deep margins of the tumor. Frozen sections may be obtained at the time of excision to aid in determining whether tumor-free margins have been obtained. This is minimized with experience. It is better to err on the side of removing more normal tissue than necessary rather than to risk including tumor at the margins. Closure of the wound is accomplished in the direction of minimal skin tension, usually along the skin lines. The dog-ears are removed appropriately.

Wounds resulting from the excision of some moderate-sized tumors and nearly all large tumors may require reconstruction of function and appearance with the use of local, regional, and free flaps. This can nearly always be performed in one stage with good frozen section control.

The disadvantages of surgical excision are as follows: (1) Certain large excisions and reconstruction require specialized training and experience to master the surgical techniques. (2) Whereas curettage and desiccation may be performed in the office, surgical excision often requires specialized facilities. (3) In lesions with vague clinical margins, an excessive amount of normal tissue may have to be excised to ensure complete removal even with the use of frozen section verification. (4) Reconstruction may need to wait until permanent pathologic diagnosis and margins are available in cases involving deep or specialized structures.

To overcome some of these objections, Mohs described in 1941 a new technique that allows for serial excisions and microscopic examination of chemically fixed tissue. Newer developments have obviated the cumbersome fixation techniques, but it may still take several hours to scan an area for suspected malignant cells. The procedure is nevertheless quite useful for recurrent lesions and in areas in which maximal preservation is desirable. Nonetheless, there are no prospective comparative studies to indicate that the microscopically controlled removal of tumor by the Mohs technique, which amounts to excision of the lesion with serial review by fresh frozen section, is superior to surgical excision. An additional problem is that there is no quality control because the excising physician is also the one who evaluates the pathology slides. Many of the more extensive lesions treated with the Mohs technique require complex reconstruction to rebuild noble structures that have needed resection.

Mohs FE: Mohs micrographic surgery. A historical perspective. Dermatol Clin 1989;7:609.

C. X-ray Therapy

X-ray therapy is as effective as any other in the treatment of basal cell carcinoma. Its advantages are as follows: (1) Structures that are difficult to reconstruct, such as the eyelids, tear ducts, and nasal tip, can be preserved when they are invaded by but not destroyed by tumor. (2) A wide margin of tissue can be treated around lesions with poorly defined margins to ensure destruction of nondiscernible extensions of tumor. (3) It may be less traumatic than surgical excision to elderly patients with advanced lesions. (4) Hospitalization is not necessary.

The disadvantages are as follows: (1) Only well-trained, experienced physicians can obtain good results. (2) Expensive facilities are necessary. (3) Improperly administered radiation therapy may produce severe sequelae, including scarring, radiation dermatitis, ulceration, and malignant degeneration. (4) In hair-bearing areas, epilation will result. (5) It may be difficult to treat areas of irregular contour (eg, the ear and the auditory canal). (6) Repeated treatments over a period of 4–6 weeks may be necessary.

X-ray therapy should not be used in patients under age 40 except in unusual circumstances, and it should not be repeated in patients who have failed to respond to radiation therapy in the past.

3. Squamous Cell Carcinoma

Squamous cell carcinoma is the second-most common cancer of the skin in light-skinned racial groups and the most common skin cancer in darkly pigmented racial groups. As with basal cell carcinoma, sunlight is the most common causative factor in whites. The most common sites of occurrence are the ears, cheeks, lower lip, and backs of the hands. Other causative factors are chemical and thermal burns, scars, chronic ulcers, chronic granulomas (tuberculosis of the skin, syphilis), draining sinuses, contact with tars and hydrocarbons, and exposure to ionizing radiation. When a squamous cell carcinoma occurs in a burn scar, it is called a **Marjolin ulcer.** This lesion may appear many years after the original burn. It tends to be aggressive, and the prognosis is poor.

Because exposure to the sun is the greatest stimulus for the production of squamous cell carcinoma, most of these lesions are preceded by actinic keratosis on areas of the skin showing chronic solar damage. They may also arise from other premalignant skin lesions and from normal-appearing skin.

The natural history of squamous cell carcinoma may be quite variable. It may present as a slowly growing, locally invasive lesion without metastases or as a rapidly growing, widely invasive tumor with early metastatic spread. In general, squamous cell carcinomas that develop from actinic keratoses are more common and are of the slowly growing type, whereas those that develop from Bowen disease, erythroplasia of Queyrat, chronic radiation dermatitis, scars, and chronic ulcers tend to be more aggressive. Lesions that arise from normal-appearing skin and from the lips, genitalia, and anal regions also tend to be aggressive.

Early squamous cell carcinoma usually appears as a small, firm erythematous plaque or nodule with indistinct margins. The surface may be flat and smooth or may be verrucous. As the tumor grows, it becomes raised and, because of progressive invasion, becomes fixed to surrounding tissues. Ulcer-

ation may occur early or late but tends to appear earlier in the more rapidly growing lesions.

Histologically, malignant epithelial cells are seen extending down into the dermis as broad, rounded masses or slender strands. In squamous cell carcinomas of low-grade malignancy, the individual cells may be quite well differentiated, resembling uniform mature squamous cells having intercellular bridges. Keratinization may be present, and layers of keratinizing squamous cells may produce typical round "horn pearls." In highly malignant lesions, the epithelial cells may be extremely atypical; abnormal mitotic figures are common; intercellular bridges are not present; and keratinization does not occur.

As with basal cell carcinomas, the method of treatment that will eradicate squamous cell carcinomas and produce the best aesthetic and functional results varies with the characteristics of the individual lesion. Factors that determine the optimal method of treatment include the size, shape, and location of the tumor as well as the histologic pattern that determines its aggressiveness.

The mainstay of treatment is surgery. Radiation has also been used in some circumstances. The advantages and disadvantages of each type of therapy are discussed earlier. Since basal cell carcinomas are relatively nonaggressive lesions that rarely metastasize, failure to eradicate the lesion may result only in local recurrence. Although this may result in extensive local tissue destruction, there is rarely a threat to life. Aggressive squamous cell carcinomas, on the other hand, may metastasize to any part of the body, and failure of treatment may have fatal consequences. For this reason, total eradication of each lesion is the imperative goal of treatment.

Because the overall incidence of lymph node metastasis is relatively low, most authorities agree that node resection is not indicated in the absence of palpable regional lymph nodes except in the case of very aggressive carcinomas of the genitalia and anal regions.

Alam M, Ratner D: Cutaneous squamous-cell carcinoma. N Engl J Med 2001;344:975.

Arbuckle HA, Morelli JG: Pigmentary disorders: update on neurofibromatosis-1 and tuberous sclerosis. Curr Opin Pediatr 2000;12:354.

Kanzler MH, Mraz-Gernhard S: Treatment of primary cutaneous melanoma. JAMA 2001;285:1819.

Lentsch EJ, Myers JN: Melanoma of the head and neck: current concepts in diagnosis and management. Laryngoscope 2001; 111:1209.

Stadelmann WK et al: Cutaneous melanoma of the head and neck: advances in evaluation and treatment. Plast Reconstr Surg 2000;105:2105.

SOFT TISSUE INJURY

The plastic surgeon is often involved in emergency room assessment and treatment of soft tissue injuries. Many aspects of wound management must be considered in even a relatively simple facial laceration.

Careful analysis of the soft tissue injury should include (1) the type of wound or wounds (abrasion, contusion, etc); (2) the cause of injury; (3) the age of the injury; (4) the location of injured tissues; (5) the degree of contamination of the injured area before, during, and after trauma; (6) the nature and extent of associated injuries; and (7) the general health of the patient (eg, any chronic or acute illnesses or any allergies; any medications being taken).

The location of the wound must be noted because different healing characteristics are present in various types of skin. The face and scalp are highly vascular and therefore resist infection and heal faster than other areas, but there are many important structures in and around the face, and scars and defects are noticeable. Skin of the trunk, upper arms, and thighs is fairly thick and heals more slowly than facial or scalp skin and is more susceptible to infection. Scarring is less noticeable. The hands are a critical area because there are important structures near the surface, and the destruction caused by infection can be devastating. The lower legs are a particular problem area because the relatively poor blood supply can cause skin loss, and infection is more likely to occur.

▶ Treatment

The type of wound must be determined so that proper treatment can be given. Contusions and swelling require ice packs for 24 hours, rest, and elevation. Abrasions should be cleaned and dressed in a sterile manner as for a skin graft donor site or must be washed daily until a dry scab forms or healing takes place. Ground-in dirt or gravel must be entirely scrubbed out or picked out with a small blade within 24 hours after injury, or foreign material will be sealed in and traumatic tattooing will result. Extensive local anesthesia may be required to accomplish this. Imbedded particulate matter from an explosion must be removed in a similar manner. Hematomas may be treated with ice bags and pressure until stable. Evacuation is then indicated if vital structures such as the ear or nasal septal cartilage are in danger of being injured or destroyed. Lacerations over bony prominences and various types of cuts require special care that will be detailed below. Treatment must be meticulous if optimal results are to be achieved. Puncture wounds and bites are notoriously innocuous in appearance but may result in severe destruction or tetanus or gas gangrene. Antibiotic coverage, irrigation, open treatment, and observation are indicated. Most bites on the face, however, can be cleaned and safely closed. Wounds that create flaps of skin or avulsions are difficult to manage. Careful debridement and judicious use of full-thickness or split-thickness grafts from the avulsed tissue are recommended. Timing is the first factor to consider.

Wound contamination can be caused by bacteria on the surface of the wounding agent, such as rust on a nail or saliva on a tooth, or bacteria that enter the wound when the skin is broken. Bacteria driven into tissue become more established

as time passes, and it is therefore important to know the age of the wound at the time of the presentation for treatment. Other injuries associated with cuts almost always take precedence in treatment. In general, wounds other than those on the face or scalp should not be closed primarily if they occurred 8–12 hours or longer before presentation unless they were caused by a very clean agent and have been covered by a sterile bandage in the interim. Delayed primary closure as described previously is an excellent and safe alternative. Nearly any facial wound up to 24 hours old can be safely closed with careful debridement, irrigation, and antibiotic coverage.

The surgeon must decide whether or not antibiotic treatment is indicated. In general, wounds treated appropriately and early do not call for antibiotic therapy. Antibiotics should be given for wounds with delayed presentation or those for which treatment is delayed by choice (eg, wounds with known contamination; wounds in compromised patients, such as very young or old persons, debilitated persons, or persons with general ill health; wounds in areas where infection may have serious consequences, such as the lower legs and the hands; and wounds in persons in whom bacteremia might have serious sequelae, such as those with prosthetic heart valves or orthopedic appliances). Antibiotics should be started before debridement and closure. Only a few days of coverage are necessary—usually until the wound is checked at 2–3 days and found to be free of infection. Penicillin or a substitute is appropriate for wounds involving the mouth, such as through-and-through lip lacerations and bites. Other wounds are usually contaminated by *Staphylococcus aureus*, and an antibiotic effective for penicillin-resistant *S aureus* is therefore appropriate. If gram-negative or anaerobic contamination is suspected, wound closure is risky, and hospitalization of the patient for treatment with parenteral antibiotics should be considered. Tetanus prophylaxis should be routinely given for patients who have not received current immunizations or who have wounds likely to lead to tetanus. Guidelines for this are detailed in Chapter 8.

Anesthesia is an important part of adequate soft tissue wound care and closure. Local anesthesia with either 0.5% or 1% lidocaine with epinephrine 1:200,000 or 1:100,000 is recommended for all wounds. Smaller amounts of lidocaine and epinephrine may be used in areas of appendages, such as earlobes, toes, and the penis. The injection may be given through the wound edge before debridement and irrigation for maximum patient comfort. Complete epinephrine vasoconstrictor effect occurs within 7 minutes. Overdose of epinephrine and lidocaine injection into vessels or use of the drugs in patients sensitive to these agents should be avoided.

The importance of irrigation cannot be overstated. Over 90% of bacteria in a recently sustained and superficially contaminated wound can be eliminated by adequate irrigation. Ideally, a physiologic solution such as lactated Ringer solution or normal saline should be forcefully ejected from a large syringe with a 19-gauge needle or from other equipment designed for this purpose such as a water-jet apparatus.

The wound is irrigated once to remove surface clots, foreign material, and bacteria and is then debrided and irrigated again. Detergents and antiseptic solutions are toxic to exposed tissue and should not be used.

Debridement must include removal of all obviously devitalized tissues. In special areas such as the eyelids, ears, nose, lips, and eyebrows, debridement must be done cautiously, since the tissue lost by debridement may be difficult to replace. Where tissues are more abundant, such as in the cheek, chin, and forehead areas, debridement may be more extensive. Small irregular or ragged wounds in these areas can be excised completely to produce clean, sharply cut wound edges which, when approximated, will produce the finest possible scar. Because the blood supply in the face is plentiful, damaged tissues of questionable viability should be retained rather than debrided away. The chances for survival are good.

Following adequate anesthesia, debridement, and irrigation, the wound is ready for final assessment and closure. Lighting must be adequate, and appropriate instruments should be available. The patient and the surgeon must be positioned comfortably. The skin surrounding the wound is prepared with an antiseptic solution, and the area is draped. A final check of the depth and extent of the wound is made, and vital structures are inspected for injury. Hemostasis must be achieved by use of epinephrine, pressure, cautery, or suture ligature. Important structures in facial wounds include the parotid duct, lacrimal duct, and branches of the facial nerve. These should be repaired in the operating room by microsurgical techniques.

Layers of tissue—usually muscle—in the depth of the wound should be closed first with as few absorbable sutures as possible, since sutures are foreign material within the wound. If possible, dead space should be closed with judicious use of fine absorbable sutures. If dead space cannot be closed, external pressure or small drains are sometimes effective. Skin closure should begin at the most important points of the laceration (eg, the borders of the ears and nose; the vermilion border or margins of the lip; the margins of the eyebrow [which should never be shaved]; and the scalp hairline). Subcuticular sutures are very helpful. Skin edges can be approximated without tension or strangulation with 5-0 or 6-0 monofilament suture material as outlined earlier under wound closure.

Complicated lacerations, such as complex stellate wounds or avulsion flaps, often heal with excessive scarring. Because of the associated subcutaneous tissue injury, U-shaped or trap-door avulsion lacerations almost always become unsightly as a result of wound contracture. Small lacerations of this type are best excised and closed in a straight line initially; larger flaps that must be replaced usually require secondary revision. Extensive loss of skin is generally best treated by initial split-thickness skin grafting followed later by secondary reconstruction. Primary attempts to reconstruct with local flaps may fail because of unsuspected injury to these adjacent tissues. The decision to convert avulsed tissues to free grafts that may not survive and thus delay healing requires sound surgical judgment.

Small or moderate-sized closures on the face may be dressed with antibiotic ointment alone. The patient may cleanse the suture lines with hydrogen peroxide to clear away crusts and dirt and then reapply the ointment. Elsewhere, closures benefit from the protection of a sterile bandage. Pressure dressings are useful in preventing hematoma formation and severe edema that may result in poor wound healing. Dressings should be changed early and the wound inspected for hematoma or signs of infection. Hematoma evacuation, appropriate drainage, and antibiotic therapy based on culture and sensitivity studies may be required. Removal of sutures in 3–5 days, followed by splinting of the incision with sterile tape, will minimize scarring from the sutures themselves.

The final result of facial wound repair depends on the nature and location of the wounds, individual propensity to scar formation, and the passage of time. A year or more must often pass before resolution of scar contracture and erythema results in maximum improvement. Only after this time can a decision be made regarding the desirability of secondary scar revision.

In wounds involving the major joints, the extracapsular soft tissue and the intracapsular structures should be considered individually to assess accurately the magnitude of the injury and to provide a prognosis. Open joint injuries that are single penetrating and without extensive soft tissue damage permit uncomplicated joint and wound closure. Injuries that are single or multiple penetrations with extensive soft tissue disruption (flaps, avulsions, degloving) often require secondary operations to attain closure. In injuries that show open periarticular fractures with extension through the adjacent intra-articular surface and with associated nerve or vascular injury requiring repair, the cornerstone for successful management is debridement, antibiotic therapy properly timed and performed, joint closure, and aggressive treatment of the bony injury. Newer techniques such as free-tissue transfer can expedite wound care, decrease morbidity, and spare some limbs from amputation.

FACIAL BONE FRACTURES

Because of the aesthetic and functional importance of the face, fractures of the facial bones—though rarely life threatening—are best treated by surgeons who have extensive experience with facial injuries and reconstruction. Operation is most successful when performed in the acute setting, usually within the first week, because reconstruction becomes much more difficult if surgery is delayed.

Facial bone fractures are usually caused by trauma from a blunt instrument, such as a fist or club, or by violent contact with the steering wheel, dashboard, or windshield during an automobile accident. Particularly in the latter case, the patient should be assessed for associated injuries. For example, cervical spine injuries are present in up to 12% of automobile accident patients and should be treated or stabilized before facial bone injuries are attended to. Injuries to the brain, eyes, chest, abdomen, and extremities must also be assessed and may require earlier treatment.

The diagnosis of facial fractures is made primarily on clinical examination. Ideally, the examination should be done immediately so that swelling will not obscure the findings. The mechanism and the line of direction of injury are important. If conscious, the patient should be asked about previous facial injuries, areas of pain and numbness, whether the jaw opens properly and the teeth come together normally, and whether vision in all quadrants is normal.

Most facial fractures can be palpated, or at least the abnormal position of bones can be noted. Beginning along the mandibular rims, one can feel for irregularities of the facial bones. The dental occlusion is noted. With bimanual palpation, placing the thumbs inside the mouth, one can elicit bony crepitus if there is an associated fracture. The maxilla and mid face can be rocked forward and backward between the thumb and the index finger in the presence of a midfacial fracture. Nasal fractures may be detected by palpation. Irregularities and step-offs along the infraorbital border, lateral orbital rim, or zygomatic arch regions indicate a depressed zygomatic fracture.

Radiologic studies are additional aids to the proper diagnosis of facial fractures. Rarely is a significant fracture seen on x-ray that is not also clinically evident. Helpful views include the Waters and submentovertex projections and oblique views of the mandible. The Panorex view of the mandible is very useful to look at the condyles. CT scans of facial bones, with appropriate biplanar and 3D reconstructions so that bones can be viewed through several planes, have essentially supplanted regular radiographs in the workup of the facially injured patient. They are helpful in assessing the extent of fractures, in particular in more posterior areas such as the ethmoid area, medial and inferior orbit, pterygoid plates, and base of the skull.

The bones of the nose are the most commonly fractured facial bones. Next in frequency are the mandible, the zygomatic-malar bones, and the maxilla.

NASAL FRACTURES

Fractures may affect the nasal bones, cartilage, and septum. Fractures occur in two patterns, caused by lateral or head-on trauma.

With lateral trauma, the nasal bone on the side of the injury is fractured and displaced toward the septum, the septum is deviated and fractured, and the nasal bone on the side away from the injury is fractured and displaced away from the septum, so that the upper part of the nose, as a whole, is deviated. Depending on the degree of violence, one or more of these displacements will be present, and the degree of comminution is variable.

Head-on trauma gives rise to telescoping and saddling of the nose and broadening of its upper half as a result of the depression and splaying of the fractured nasal bones. This of course produces severe damage to the septum, which usually buckles or actually suffers a fracture. The diagnosis of a fractured nose is made on clinical grounds alone, and x-rays are unnecessary except for medical-legal reasons.

Nasal fractures requiring reduction should be treated with a minimum of delay, for they tend to become fixed in the displaced position in a few days. The surgical approach depends on whether the fracture has resulted in deviation or collapse of the nasal bones. Local anesthesia is preferred; either topical tetracaine or cocaine intranasally or lidocaine for infiltration of the skin can be used. The nasal bones may be disimpacted with intranasal forceps or a periosteal elevator and aligned by external molding or pressure. Collapsed nasal fractures can be repositioned with Walsham nasal forceps, introduced into each nostril and placed on each side of the septum, which is then elevated to its proper position. A septal hematoma should be recognized and drained to prevent infection and subsequent necrosis of the cartilaginous septum with associated collapse of the entire nose. Compound fractures of the nose require prompt repair of the skin wound and, if possible, early reduction of the displaced nasal bones.

External splinting, which is essentially a protective dressing, and intranasal packing using nonadhering gauze are appropriate after reduction. The intranasal packing provides support for the septum in its reduced position and helps prevent development of a hematoma. It also provides counterpressure for the external splint immobilizing the nasal bones and prevents them from collapsing. The packing is usually removed within 48 hours.

In severe comminuted nasal fractures, the medial canthal ligaments, which are easily felt by applying lateral traction to the upper eyelid, may have dislodged. If they have been avulsed, they should be reattached in position to prevent late deformities. For these severe fractures involving the entire naso-orbital and ethmoid complex, the coronal approach, which offers wide exposure, allows for proper anatomic reduction of all small nasal fragments as well as repositioning of the canthal ligaments and correction and elevation of the telescoped bone fragments at the root of the nose and glabella.

The lacrimal apparatus is commonly disrupted in these injuries and should be repaired and stented appropriately.

MANDIBULAR FRACTURES

Mandibular fractures are most commonly bilateral, generally occurring in the region of the mid body at the mental foramen, the angle of the ramus, or at the neck of the condyle. A frequent combination is a fracture at the mental region of the body with a condylar fracture on the opposite side. Displacement of the fragments results from the force of the external blow as well as the pull of the muscles of the floor of the mouth and the muscles of mastication. The diagnosis is suggested by derangement of dental occlusion associated with local pain, swelling, and often crepitation upon palpation. Appropriate x-rays confirm the diagnosis. Special views of the condyle, including tomograms, may be required. Sublingual hematoma and acute malocclusion are usually diagnostic of a mandibular fracture.

Restoration of functional dental occlusion is the most important consideration in treating mandibular fractures. In patients with an adequate complement of teeth, arch bars or interdental wires can be placed. Local nerve block anesthesia is preferable for this procedure, though certain patients may require general anesthesia. Intermaxillary elastic traction will usually correct minor degrees of displacement and bring the teeth into normal occlusion by overcoming the muscle pull. When the fracture involves the base of a tooth socket with suspected devitalization of the tooth, extraction of the tooth should be considered. Particularly in the incisor region, such devitalized teeth may be a source of infection, leading to the development of osteomyelitis and nonunion of the fracture.

Patients with more severe mandibular injuries require anatomic reduction and fixation of the fracture by the open, direct technique. These include compound, comminuted, and unfavorable fractures. An unfavorable fracture is one that is inherently unstable because muscle pull distracts the fracture segments. In this situation, intermaxillary fixation alone is insufficient. Edentulous patients also benefit from the open technique, although proper dentures or dental splints are useful to maintain normal occlusion.

Metal wire fixation of fractured segments and intermaxillary fixation for 6 weeks was a proven and popular method of fracture treatment. The more recent resurgence in popularity of the screw-plate system is due to a number of advantages over wiring. The screw plate usually achieves rigid fixation in three dimensions, providing adequate stability; it eliminates the need for intermaxillary fixation in most cases; it is useful in complex, comminuted fractures; and it is quite easy to use after familiarity with the technique has been acquired.

With bilateral parasymphyseal fractures, anterior stabilization of the tongue may be lost, so that it may fall back and obstruct the airway. Anterior stabilization and splinting must be accomplished early in these cases.

Open reduction is rarely advised in condylar fractures; simple intermaxillary fixation for 4–6 weeks is sufficient. Indications for open reduction are severely displaced fractures, which may prevent motion of the mandible because of impingement of the coronoid process on the zygomatic arch. In children, the fracture may destroy the growth center of the condyle, resulting in maldevelopment of the mandible and gross distortion.

ZYGOMATIC & ORBITAL FRACTURE

Fractures of the zygomatic bones may involve just the arch of the zygomatic bone or the entire body of the zygoma (the malar eminence) and the lateral wall and floor of the orbit. The so-called tripod fracture characteristically occurs at the frontozygomatic and zygomaticomaxillary sutures as well as at the arch. It should be referred to as a tetrapod fracture because the anterior or posterior buttress of the maxilla is also involved in the fracture. Displacement of the body of the zygoma results in flattening of the cheek and depression of the orbital rim and floor.

Important diagnostic signs are subconjunctival hemorrhage, disturbances of extraocular muscle function (which may be accompanied by diplopia), and loss of sensation in the upper lip and alveoli on the involved side as a result of injury to the infraorbital nerve. Reduction of a displaced zygomatic fracture is seldom an emergency procedure and may be delayed until the patient's general condition is satisfactory for anesthesia. Local anesthesia will suffice only for reduction of fractures of the zygomatic arch. More extensively displaced fractures usually require general anesthesia. At least two-point fixation with direct interosseous wiring is necessary for these fractures. Here again, delicate miniplates have been used with success, providing anatomic reduction and rigid fixation.

Simple depressed fractures of the zygomatic arch can best be elevated using the Gillies technique. Through a temporal incision above the hairline, an instrument is passed beneath the superficial layer of the deep temporalis fascia and under the arch and the body of the zygoma. The fracture can also be elevated percutaneously with a hook or screw in conjunction with overlying palpation to achieve accurate reduction. If the fracture is complex or comminuted, as is often the case with high-velocity injuries, repair through a coronal scalp approach may be necessary to obtain an anatomic and stable result.

Extensive disruption should be suspected in conjunction with the zygomatic fracture when significant diplopia and enophthalmos and posterior displacement of the globe are present. Orbital fat and extraocular muscles may herniate through the defect and become entrapped, giving rise to the signs and symptoms. A "blowout" fracture is similar disruption of the orbital floor due to blunt trauma to the globe but not associated with a fracture of the zygoma or orbital rim. Treatment in both cases demands exploration, reduction of herniated contents, and repair of the floor. The most direct approach is through a lower lid subciliary incision, which provides excellent visualization. A buccal transantral (Caldwell-Luc) approach can be used, and blind antral packing for support has been described. This is quite hazardous, because bony spicules may be pushed into the ocular globe and perhaps cause injury or blindness. In cases of extensive communication or loss of bony fragments of the floor, use of local autogenous bone or cartilage as a scaffold may be performed. At times, in cases of extensive injuries to the floor, alloplastic material in the form of titanium mesh may be necessary.

Even with careful anatomic reduction and repair of the orbital floor, ocular problems—particularly enophthalmos—may persist, possibly due to an undiagnosed fracture, especially a medial ethmoidal blowout fracture. These can be properly evaluated with CT scanning. Treatment requires reduction and repair of the defect. The injury can at times cause ischemia of herniated soft tissue and subsequent atrophy and scarring. This may result in enophthalmos, which is almost impossible to resolve completely.

MAXILLARY FRACTURES

Maxillary fractures range in complexity from partial fractures through the alveolar process to extensive displacement of the midfacial structures in conjunction with fractures of the frontonasal bones and orbital maxillary region and total craniofacial separation. Hemorrhage and airway obstruction require emergency care, and in severe cases, tracheostomy is indicated. Mobility of the maxilla can be elicited by palpation in extensive fractures. "Dish-face" deformity of the retrodisplaced maxilla may be disguised by edema, and careful x-ray studies are necessary to determine the extent and complexity of the midfacial fracture. Treatment may have to be delayed because of other severe injuries. A delay of as long as 10–14 days may be safe before reduction and fixation, but the earliest possible restoration of maxillary position and dental occlusion is desirable to prevent late complications.

In the case of unilateral fractures or bilateral fractures with little or no displacement, splinting by intermaxillary fixation for 4 weeks may suffice. Fractures are usually displaced inferiorly or posteriorly and require direct surgical disimpaction and reduction and proper fixation with appropriate plates and screws. Early reduction may help control bleeding, as torn, stretched vessels are allowed to reestablish their normal tension. In certain severe cases, external traction may be necessary. Manipulation is directed toward restoring normal occlusion and maintaining the reduction with intermaxillary fixation to the mandible in association with direct plate fixation. Complicated fractures may require external fixation utilizing a head cap and intraoral splints in conjunction with multiple surgical incisions for direct plate fixation. Coexisting mandibular fractures usually necessitate open reduction and fixation at the same time.

Antonyshyn O, Gruss JS: Complex orbital trauma: the role of rigid fixation and primary bone grafting. Plast Reconstr Surg 1988; 7:61.

Krsarai L et al: A biomechanical analysis of the orbital zygomatic complex in human cadavers: examination of load sharing and failure patterns after fixation with titanium and bioresorbable systems. J Craniofac Surg 1999;10:400.

Thaller SR, Kawamoto HK: A histologic evaluation of fracture repair in the midface. Plast Reconstr Surg 1990;85:196.

Thaller SR, Mabourakh S: Pediatric mandibular fractures. Ann Plast Surg 1991;26:511.

Yaremchuk MJ: Vascularized bone grafts for maxillofacial reconstruction. Clin Plast Surg 1989;16:29.

CONGENITAL HEAD & NECK ANOMALIES

CLEFT LIP & CLEFT PALATE

Cleft lip, cleft palate, and combinations of the two are the most common congenital anomalies of the head and neck. The incidence of facial clefts has been reported to be 1 in every 650–750 live births, making this deformity second only to clubfoot in frequency as a reported birth defect.

The cleft may involve the floor of the nostril and lip on one or both sides and may extend through the alveolus, the hard palate, and the entire soft palate. A useful classification based on embryologic and anatomic aspects divides the structures into the primary and the secondary palate. The dividing point between the primary palate anteriorly and the secondary palate posteriorly is the incisive foramen. Clefts can thus be classified as partial or complete clefts of the primary or secondary palate (or both) in various combinations. The most common clefts are left unilateral complete clefts of the primary and secondary palate and partial midline clefts of the secondary palate, involving the soft palate and part of the hard palate.

Most infants with cleft palate present some feeding difficulties, and breast-feeding may be impossible. As a rule, enlarging the openings in an artificial nipple or using a syringe with a soft rubber feeding tube will solve difficulties in sucking. Feeding in the upright position helps prevent oronasal reflux or aspiration. Severe feeding and breathing problems and recurrent aspiration are seen in Pierre Robin sequence, in which the palatal cleft is associated with a receding lower jaw and posterior and cephalic displacement of the tongue, obstructing the naso-oropharyngeal airway. This is a medical emergency and is a cause of sudden infant death syndrome (SIDS). Nonsurgical treatment includes pulling the tongue forward with an instrument and laying the baby prone with a towel under the chest to let the mandible and tongue drop forward. Insertion of a small (No. 8) nasogastric tube into the pharynx may temporarily prevent respiratory distress and may be used to supplement the baby's feedings. Placement of an acrylic obturator or appliance has proved quite successful in alleviating the breathing difficulties by bringing the tongue down and permitting a better nasal airway. Several surgical procedures that bring the tongue and mandible forward have been described but should be employed only when conservative measures have been tried without success. Recently, the use of distraction of the mandible has shown some beneficial effects. However, it should be done with great caution in the neonate.

► Treatment

Surgical repair of cleft lip is not considered an emergency. The optimal time for operation can be described as the widely accepted "rule of 10." This includes body weight of 10 lb (4.5 kg) or more and a hemoglobin of 10 g/dL or more. This is usually at some time after the 10th week of life. In most cases, closure of the lip will mold distortions of the cleft alveolus into a satisfactory contour. In occasional cases in which there is marked distortion of the alveolus, such as in severe bilateral clefts with marked protrusion of the premaxilla, preliminary maxillary orthodontic treatment may be indicated. This may involve the use of carefully crafted appliances or simple constant pressure by use of an elastic band.

General endotracheal anesthesia via an orally placed endotracheal tube is the anesthetic technique of choice. A variety of techniques for repair of unilateral clefts have evolved over many years. Earlier procedures ignored anatomic landmarks and resulted in a characteristic "repaired harelip" look. The Millard rotation advancement operation that is now commonly used for repair employs an incision in the medial side of the cleft to allow the Cupid's bow of the lip to be rotated down to a normal position. The resulting gap in the medial side of the cleft is filled by advancing a flap from the lateral side. This principle can be varied in placement of the incisions and results in most cases in a symmetric lip with normally placed landmarks. Bilateral clefts, because of greater deficiency of tissue, present more challenging technical problems. Maximum preservation of available tissue is the underlying principle, and most surgeons prefer approximation of the central and lateral lip elements in a straight line closure, rolling up the vermilion border of the lip (Manchester repair).

Secondary revisions are frequently necessary in the older child with a repaired cleft lip. A constant associated deformity in patients with cleft lip is distortion of the soft tissue and cartilage structures of the ala and dome of the nose. These patients often present with deficiency of growth of the structures of the mid face. This has been attributed to intrinsic growth disturbances and to external pressures from the lip and palate repairs. Some correction of these deformities, especially of the nose, can be done at the initial lip operation. More definitive correction is done after the cartilage and bone growth is more complete. These may include scar revisions and rearrangement of the cartilage structure of the nose. Recent approaches involve degloving of the nasal skin envelope with complete exposure of the abnormal cartilage framework. These are then rearranged in proper position with or without additional grafts. Maxillary osteotomies (Le Fort I with advancement) will substantially correct the midfacial depression. A tight upper lip due to severe tissue deficiency can be corrected by a two-stage transfer of a lower lip flap known as an Abbe flap.

In utero repair of cleft lip deformities has recently become a topic of discussion. In utero repair affords the potential to provide a scarless repair and correct the primary deformity. Furthermore, scarless fetal lip and palate repairs may prevent the ripple effect of postnatal scarring with its resultant secondary dentoalveolar and midface growth deformities. While these suggestions make in utero repair attractive, the risk of fetal loss remains high. Preterm labor is a major complication and one that is directly related to the large hysterotomy required for fetal exposure. Due to the great risks associated with it, intrauterine fetal surgery is still largely reserved for severe malformations that cannot be helped significantly by postnatal intervention.

Palatal clefts may involve the alveolus, the bony hard palate, or the soft palate, singly or in any combination. Clefts of the hard palate and alveolus may be either unilateral or bilateral, whereas the soft palate cleft is always midline, extending back through the uvula. The width of the cleft varies greatly, making the amount of tissue available for repair also variable. The bony palate, with its mucoperiosteal lining, forms the roof of the anterior mouth and the floor of the nose. The posteriorly attached soft palate is composed of five paired muscles of speech and swallowing.

Surgical closure of the cleft to allow for normal speech is the treatment of choice. The timetable for closure depends on the size of the cleft and any other associated problems. However, the defect should be closed before the child undertakes serious speech, usually before age 2. Closure at 6 months usually is performed without difficulty and also aids in the child's feeding. If the soft palate seems to be long enough, simple approximation of the freshened edges of the cleft after freeing of the tissues through lateral relaxing incisions may suffice. If the soft palate is too short, a pushback type of operation is required. In this procedure, the short soft palate is retrodisplaced closer to the posterior pharyngeal wall utilizing the mucoperiosteal flaps based on the posterior palatine artery.

Satisfactory speech following surgical repair of cleft palate is achieved in 70–90% of cases. Significant speech defects usually require secondary operations when the child is older. The most widely used technique is the pharyngeal flap operation, in which the palatopharyngeal space is reduced by attaching a flap of posterior pharyngeal muscle and mucosa to the soft palate. This permits voluntary closure of the velopharyngeal complex and thus avoids hypernasal speech. Various other kinds of pharyngoplasties have been useful in selected cases.

Estes JM et al: Endoscopic creation and repair of fetal cleft lip. Plast Reconstr Surg 1992;90:743.
Lorenz HP, Longaker MT: In utero surgery for cleft lip/palate: minimizing the "ripple effect" of scarring. J Craniofac Surg 2003;14:504.

CRANIOFACIAL ANOMALIES

These are congenital deformities of the hard and soft tissues of the head. Particular problems of the brain, eye, and internal ear are treated by the appropriate specialist. The craniofacial surgeon often needs the collaboration of these specialists when operating on such patients.

Serious craniofacial anomalies are relatively rare, although mild forms often go undiagnosed or are accepted as normal variants. A classification is therefore difficult, although many have been proposed. Tessier has offered a numerical classification based on clinical presentation. He considers a cleft to be the basis of the malformation, which involves both hard and soft tissues (Figure 41–10).

Other classifications are based on embryologic and etiologic features. With greater understanding and continued investigation, classification efforts will no doubt be more satisfactory.

There are well-known chromosomal and genetic aberrations as well as environmental causes that can lead to craniofacial deformity. The cause in most cases, however, is unknown. Arrest in the migration and proliferation of neural crest cells and defects in differentiation characterize most of these deformities. We describe some of the more common ones in brief terms.

Crouzon syndrome (craniofacial dysostosis) and **Apert syndrome** (acrocephalosyndactyly) are closely related, differing in the extremity deformities present in the latter. Both are autosomal dominant traits with variable expression. Both present with skull deformities due to premature closure of the cranial sutures. The cranial sutures most affected will

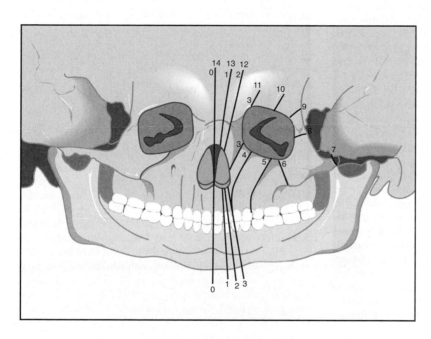

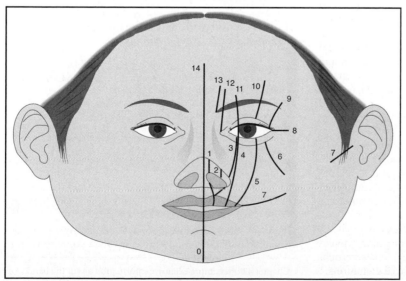

▲ **Figure 41–10.** Tessier classification of craniofacial clefts. The numbering system goes from 0 to 14, and the skeletal defects mimic the soft tissue presentation.

determine the type of skull deformity. Exophthalmos, midfacial hypoplasia, and hypertelorism are also features of these two syndromes.

The facial organs and tissues proceed in great measure from the first and second branchial arches and the first branchial cleft. Disorders in their development lead to a spectrum of anomalies of variable severity. **Treacher-Collins syndrome** (mandibulofacial dysostosis) is a severe disorder characterized by hypoplasia of the malar bones and lower eyelids, colobomas, and antimongoloid slant of the palpebrae. The mandible and ears are often quite underdeveloped. The presentation is bilateral and is an autosomal dominant trait. A unilateral deformity known as **hemifacial microsomia** presents with progressive skeletal and soft tissue underdevelopment. The Goldenhar variant of hemifacial microsomia is a severe form associated with upper bulbar dermoids, notching of the upper eyelids, and vertebral anomalies.

Some of these patients show mental retardation, but in most cases, intelligence is not affected. The psychosocial problems are serious and most often related to how the patients look. Within the past 2 decades, craniofacial surgery has progressed so that previously untreatable deformities can now be corrected. With the anatomic work of Le Fort as a basis—and guided by the incomplete attempts of Gillies and others—Paul Tessier, in the late 1960s, proposed a set of surgical techniques to correct major craniofacial deformities. Two basic concepts soon emerged from his work: (1) Large segments of the craniofacial skeleton can be completely denuded of their blood supply, repositioned, and yet survive and heal; and (2) the eyes can be translocated horizontally or vertically over a considerable distance with no adverse effect on vision. The tendency today is to operate at approximately 6–9 months of age (if possible not later than a year) for cranial vault remodeling and fronto-orbital advancement.

A bicoronal scalp incision is utilized to expose the skull and facial bones with an intracranial or extracranial approach. The cut bones are then reshaped, repositioned, and fixed with a combination of wires or miniplates and screws. The latter have the advantage of rigid fixation and less need to maintain large movements with bone grafts. Autogenous inlay and onlay bone grafts can be used to improve contour. The entire operation is usually completed in one stage, and complications are surprisingly few. Miniplates have been used extensively in the last few years. In infants, fixation with absorbable suture material or the newer absorbable plates and screws have provided effective and stable fixation. They commonly resorb at 6–9 months. They do not interfere with imaging techniques such as CT or MRI, and they seem to have less impairment of craniofacial growth and development.

Craniofacial surgery has improved the treatment not only of major congenital deformities but also of major complex facial fractures, chronic sequelae of trauma, isolated exophthalmos, fibrous dysplasia, and aesthetic facial sculpturing.

MICROTIA

Microtia is absence or hypoplasia of the pinna of the ear, with a blind or absent external auditory meatus. The incidence of significant auricular deformity is about one in 8000 births and is usually spontaneous. Ten percent of these defects are bilateral, and boys are afflicted twice or three times as commonly as girls. Because the ear arises from the first and second branchial arches, the middle ear is always involved, and many patients have other disorders of the first and second arches. The inner ear structures are usually spared.

Generally, correction of conductive hearing by an otologist has not been long lasting or helpful, and surgery for this problem is reserved for bilateral cases.

Reconstruction of the external ear usually involves a multistage procedure beginning at preschool age. Autogenous rib cartilage or cartilage from the opposite ear is used to construct a framework to replace the absent ear. The cartilage is imbedded under the skin in the appropriate area, and after adjustments are made in local tissue to reposition or recreate the earlobe and conchal cavity, the framework is elevated posteriorly and the resulting sulcus grafted to obtain projection. In cases in which local tissue is poor or unavailable, the neighboring superficial temporalis fascia is dissected and placed over the cartilage framework. This is then skin-grafted with adequate tissue. The opposite (normal) ear is occasionally altered to provide better symmetry. Excellent results have been achieved. Silastic frameworks for ear cartilage have also been used, and although their use eliminates donor site problems, rates of infection and extrusion have been unacceptable. More recently, a porous polyethylene construct has been used with better long-term results. A temporalis fascia flap is rotated to cover the allograft, and then a full-thickness skin graft is placed. They are quite useful in bilateral cases or when sufficient cartilage is not available.

Lesser deformities, such as overly large, prominent, or bent ears, are corrected by appropriate resection of skin and cartilage, "scoring" of the cartilage to alter its curve, and placement sutures to aid in contouring.

Cohen SR: Craniofacial distraction with a modular internal distraction system: evolution of design and surgical techniques. Plast Reconstr Surg 1999;103:1592.

McCarthy JG: The timing of surgical intervention in craniofacial anomalies. Clin Plast Surg 1990;17:161.

Nocini PF et al: Vertical distraction of a free vascularized fibula flap in a reconstructed hemimandible: case report. J Craniomaxillofac Surg 2000;28:20.

Romo T 3rd, Presti PM, Yalamanchili HR: Medpor alternative for microtia repair. Facial Plast Surg Clin North Am 2006;14:129.

ANOMALIES OF THE HANDS & EXTREMITIES*

The most common hand anomaly is syndactyly, or webbing of the digits. This may be simple, involving only soft tissue,

*Chapter 42 offers more extensive information about the hand.

or complex, involving fusion of bone and soft tissue. The fusion may be partial or complete. Surgical correction involves separation and repair with local flaps and skin grafts. Correction should be done before growth disturbance of the webbed digits takes place. Other anomalies, such as extra digits (polydactyly), absence of digits (adactyly), and cleft hand, also exist.

Flexion contractures of the hands or digits may require surgical release and appropriate skin grafting. Congenital ring constriction of the extremities may be associated also with congenital amputation. The ring constrictions are best treated by excision and Z-plasty.

Poland syndrome consists of a variable degree of unilateral chest deformity—usually absence of the pectoralis major muscle—associated with hand symbrachydactyly. The hand deformity is treated according to the severity. The latissimus dorsi muscles can be transposed to replace the absent pectoralis major, simulating the sites of origin and insertion. In more severe cases and in women requiring breast and chest reconstruction, the transverse rectus abdominis island flap can be used to replace the deficit.

POSTABLATIVE RECONSTRUCTION

HEAD & NECK RECONSTRUCTION

Many of the tumors discussed in Chapter 15 require surgical excision as a primary form of therapy. This often involves removal of large areas of composite tissue, such as the floor of the mouth, the maxilla, part of the mandible, or the lymph-bearing tissue of the neck. Reconstruction after such resections can be very challenging and may require special skill.

A salient advance in the complete treatment of the patient with a head or neck tumor is reconstruction, usually done in the same setting. Free flaps with microvascular techniques are the most appropriate methods even though they require a high level of skill and are time consuming. The free flaps most commonly used following ablative procedures in the head and neck include the anterolateral thigh flap or the radial forearm flap for resurfacing the floor of the mouth and the composite fibular flap, which includes fibula as well as skin, to reconstruct the mandible and the floor of the mouth. For larger defects, judicious use of the rectus abdominis muscle, latissimus dorsi, or other musculocutaneous flaps has also been helpful. For pharyngoesophageal reconstruction, either the tubed radial forearm flap or the free jejunum is most successful.

Since no two surgical resections for tumor in the head and neck are identical, the key to effective treatment is preoperative planning. Probable extent of resection, areas that will require preoperative or postoperative radiation therapy, incision and flaps created by neck dissections, and available donor areas must all be carefully assessed. Tissue attached to an adequate blood supply must be used to ensure early and watertight healing in the mouth and oropharynx, in areas of radiation injury, and over metal or other alloplastic implants.

Useful musculocutaneous flaps in the head and neck are the sternocleidomastoid, platysma, trapezius, pectoralis major, and latissimus dorsi muscles. Useful axial skin flaps can be obtained from the forehead, deltopectoral, and cervicohumeral areas. When these flaps are insufficient or unavailable for the reconstructive needs of the patient, free tissue transfer must be used. Although many flaps have been developed for bone and soft tissue reconstructions, the anterolateral thigh flap (cutaneous or myocutaneous), the radial forearm flap, and the osteoseptocutaneous fibula flap are the most useful free flaps for head and neck reconstruction. Healing is quick, so radiation, if necessary, may be started as early as 1 month after surgery.

Lutz BS, Wei FC: Microsurgical workhorse flaps in head and neck reconstruction. Clin Plast Surg 2005;32:421.

Pearl RM et al: An approach to mandibular reconstruction. Ann Plast Surg 1988;21:401.

Santamaria E et al: Sensation recovery on innervated radial forearm flap for hemiglossectomy reconstruction by using different recipient nerves. Plast Reconstr Surg 1999;103:450.

Yamamoto Y et al: Superiority of end-to-side anastomosis with the internal jugular vein: the experience of 80 cases in head and neck microsurgical reconstruction. Br J Plastic Surg 1999;52:88.

BREAST RECONSTRUCTION

Reconstruction of the female breast after mastectomy is available to all patients in the United States, and new techniques continue to be developed providing women with more options. The insurance carriers now pay for this procedure as part of the treatment for breast cancer, and this includes symmetry surgery of the contralateral breast. Even women with significant defects in the anterior chest wall as a result of radical mastectomy and radiation therapy can undergo reconstructive surgery if they are otherwise appropriate candidates.

Heightened awareness of breast cancer along with well-established screening guidelines has affected surgical treatment of the cancer and, subsequently, approaches to reconstruction of the breast. A skin-sparing, modified radical mastectomy, for example, may allow for an immediate reconstruction with autologous tissue that results in an aesthetically pleasing breast mound. Lumpectomy followed by irradiation, initially indicated for relatively small tumors, has now expanded to larger tumors and may thus result in considerable distortion and concavity in the treated breast. In the appropriate patient, concomitant bilateral reduction mammaplasty may allow for a large lumpectomy while maintaining symmetry.

The methods of reconstruction include the use of saline implants, tissue expanders, autologous tissue, or a combination of these methods. Following mastectomy, simple placement of an implant is usually unsatisfactory except in a few thin patients with relatively small contralateral breasts. The implant is usually placed in the submuscular position, utilizing the remaining pectoralis major muscle and occasionally the serratus anterior muscle for adequate muscle coverage. This results in a firm, rounded type of reconstruction and does not simulate the soft "teardrop" appearance of the normal breast. Even when adequate skin has been saved following a skin-sparing mastectomy, placement of an implant is unsatisfactory because of the high rate of complications due to skin necrosis of the saved overlying skin, which results in exposure of the implant. When doing an immediate reconstruction with implant following a skin-sparing mastectomy, it is preferable to transpose the latissimus dorsi muscle to provide another layer of cover for the implant so that if there is necrosis of the skin from the skin-sparing mastectomy, the implant will not be exposed.

The latissimus dorsi myocutaneous flap is used most often for reconstruction of the breast with an implant. The myocutaneous unit is outlined with a skin island transversely so that the scar will be transverse and covered by the brassiere. The unit is freed up completely except for its insertion at the humerus, thus preserving the neurovascular pedicle. It is transposed as a pendulum through the anterior chest wall. The superior portion of the latissimus dorsi is sutured to the pectoralis major muscle, and the lower edge is secured to the lower skin flap as far down as it will reach. The implant is then inserted, having been covered by the latissimus dorsi inferiorly and by two layers of muscle superiorly—the latissimus dorsi and the pectoralis major. The skin island is utilized in its entirety, if necessary, or is deepithelialized appropriately, maintaining only the skin portion that is needed. This method is most suitable for patients who do not have a large amount of abdominal skin, are relatively thin, and do not object to the use of implants, which sometimes may even be inserted in the opposite breast in an effort to achieve symmetry.

The use of tissue expanders is also a popular method of breast reconstruction. A partially filled silicone envelope with a separate valve is inserted under the chest skin and muscle, and at intervals over a period of 6 weeks to 3 months the bag is progressively inflated with saline percutaneously. The expander is inflated at least 25% more than the desired volume. A period of time—approximately 3 months—is advisable as a waiting period to prevent the "recall phenomenon," which is the shrinking that may occur following removal of the expander as it is replaced by a permanent implant. The disadvantages of this method include the rare occurrence of the hemispheric expansion of the skin, which may result in a hard, rounded breast mound; the necessity for a second operation; and problems with infection, deflation, exposure of the prosthesis, and occasional skin necrosis when expansion is too rapid.

The transverse rectus abdominis myocutaneous (TRAM) flap based on the superior epigastric vessel has been successfully used to provide adequate tissue so that an implant is not required in reconstructing the breast. This is the most versatile method of reconstruction in that one can usually obtain as much tissue as necessary to match the opposite breast and to contour it and position it to simulate the shape as well as the size of the opposite breast. The incision at the donor site is similar to that of an abdominoplasty operation along the lower abdomen. This method of reconstruction produces the most normal and natural breast in appearance and feel, but it requires a longer operating time as well as a longer period of hospitalization than reconstruction with tissue expanders and implants alone.

If the superior epigastric system has been violated (from surgery or trauma) or if there are other factors that would question the reliability of these vessels to adequately supply the volume and region of tissue required for the reconstruction, the surgeon may favor using the inferior epigastric system and transferring the TRAM as a free flap. Typical recipient vessels are the internal mammary or the thoracodorsal vessels. Again, past surgical history, previous (or planned) radiation, and anatomic variance may dictate reconstructive strategy regarding recipient vessels and whether to use the ipsilateral or contralateral inferior epigastric system.

Because successful breast reconstruction is common, many surgeons have sought to refine autologous reconstruction by decreasing donor site morbidity. Modifications of the free TRAM flap have been made so that the rectus abdominis muscle is mostly spared (muscle-sparing TRAM) or spared in its entirety. This latter technique is referred to as a deep inferior epigastric perforator (DIEP) flap. The same skin territory as the TRAM flap is used; however, the musculocutaneous branches that supply the skin are dissected away from the rectus abdominis muscle. In this manner the muscle itself is spared and left in situ in an effort to preserve muscular function and reduce abdominal wall weakness. The deep inferior epigastric vessels are then divided, the flap is inset into the thoracic defect, and the flap vessels are anastomosed to recipient vessels along the chest wall. Both techniques that spare the rectus abdominis and its innervation require more operative time and careful dissection. However, to some degree they seem to have a similar decrease in donor site morbidity with regard to avoiding an abdominal bulge and maintaining more muscle function.

In addition to reconstruction of the affected breast, many patients undergo procedures that alter the contralateral (noncancerous) breast so that volume and ptosis are comparable. Such symmetry procedures are considered stages in postoncologic breast reconstruction. The nipple-areola complex can also be reconstructed. Current techniques for nipple reconstruction utilize adjacent flaps from the area where the nipple is to be positioned, taking skin and variable amounts of underlying fat if a TRAM flap has been used or elevating skin and lesser amounts of subcutaneous tissue if an implant (with or without the latissimus dorsi flap) was used. The areola may be reconstructed with a full-thickness skin graft followed by tattooing at a later date for color match.

Bostwick J III: Breast reconstruction after mastectomy. Semin Surg Oncol 1988;4:274.

Hartrampf CR Jr: The transverse abdominal island flap for breast reconstruction: a 7-year experience. Clin Plast Surg 1988;15:703.

Lejour M, Jabri M, Deraemaecker R: Analysis of long-term results of 326 breast reconstructions. Clin Plast Surg 1988;15:689.

Nahabedian MY et al: Breast reconstruction with the DIEP flap or the muscle-sparing (MS-2) free TRAM flap: is there a difference? Plast Reconstr Surg 2005;115:436.

LOWER EXTREMITY RECONSTRUCTION

Probably one of the most difficult areas for which to provide wound coverage and closure is the lower extremity, particularly the distal leg and foot areas. Tenuous and unstable skin grafts or poorly vascularized local or cross-leg skin flaps were once the only tissues available for resurfacing of these parts of the body. When large segments of bone were exposed or missing or when infection had become established, these grafts or flaps often were inadequate and amputation was the only recourse. Use of musculocutaneous flaps, and particularly free flaps, has greatly improved coverage in the lower extremities.

Generally, wound problems in the lower leg, ankle, and foot involve orthopedic injuries, such as compound tibial or ankle fractures. Incisions and metal screws and plates associated with open reduction and fixation of fractures may lead to increased scarring and make coverage more difficult. Other injuries requiring reconstruction are avulsion loss of the skin of the leg, heel, or sole of the foot and ischemic or venous stasis skin loss.

Treatment depends on the extent of tissue loss and the depth of the wound. Fairly extensive wounds around the knee and upper third of the leg can be reconstructed with a gastrocnemius muscle flap (usually the medial head) and a split-thickness skin graft. Soft tissue defects of the middle third of the leg can be reconstructed in a similar manner by the soleus muscle in many cases. Large middle third and distal third soft tissue defects are more difficult to reconstruct. When they are complicated by extensive bone and soft tissue loss, free tissue transfer may be necessary. Although there are small muscles that end in tendons in the foot, such as the peroneus brevis, flexor hallucis longus, and extensor digitorum muscles, they can provide only limited coverage. If there is a suitable recipient artery remaining in the leg, better coverage is generally provided by a free muscle flap such as the gracilis muscle for small and medium-sized defects or the latissimus dorsi or rectus abdominis muscle for larger defects.

Large areas of the heel or the sole of the foot are difficult to replace because skin in these regions is specially adapted to bear the weight of the body without shearing or breaking down. Free muscle flaps surfaced with skin grafts have proven to be adequate, but protective sensation is missing. The use of free neurovascular axial skin flaps, such as the inferior gluteal thigh flap and the deltoid flap, may help provide coverage with some gross sensation. Neurosensory flaps—and specifically the sural flap, distally based on one of the lower septocutaneous perforators from the lateral aspect of the leg and supplied by the sural artery, which accompanies the sural nerve—have been used to resurface defects around the ankle and heel. The procedure provides good skin and fascia for a weight-bearing area such as the heel, but it usually does not provide protective sensibility.

Segmental defects of the tibia may be reconstructed with bone grafts or, if the gap is large, free bone flaps such as the contralateral fibula or iliac crest. It is also possible to reconstruct the soft tissue defect and then reconstruct the bony gap with a distraction osteogenesis technique (Ilizarov bone transport). This bone transport method consists of performing a cortical osteotomy proximal to the site of injury and then applying a distraction apparatus, which in effect lengthens the bone 1 mm per day by appropriate adjustment screws. Such lower extremity reconstruction requires a well-coordinated, cooperative effort between the plastic and orthopedic surgeons. While such limb salvage is possible, amputation may be recommended in cases where a constellation of complications are present, such as bony gaps greater than 8 cm, extensive vascular injury, greater than 6 hours of warm ischemia time, an insensate limb, loss of plantar flexion, or an overall medically unstable patient.

Osteomyelitis of the tibia or bones in the foot may be devastating and often uncontrollable. Probably because of poor vascularity in the area, even long-term antibiotic treatment has often failed to control bone infections in the leg. Recently, effective surgical treatment for bone infections has been developed. The bone is surgically debrided and covered with a microvascular free muscle flap such as the gracilis or rectus abdominis muscle. Apparently, the muscle tissue with its excellent blood supply not only covers the exposed bone but assists natural defenses in controlling infection. Antibiotics are also used, but the well-vascularized muscle flap appears to be the deciding factor in control of infection. Reconstruction of bony defects may be accomplished at a later date.

Erdmann MW, Court-Brown CM, Quaba AA: A five-year review of islanded distally based fasciocutaneous flaps on the lower limb. Br J Plastic Surg 1997;50:421.

Kuran I et al: Comparison between sensitive and nonsensitive free flaps in reconstruction of the heel and plantar area. Plast Reconstr Surg 2000;105:574.

May Jr JW et al: Foot reconstruction using fee microvascular muscle flaps with skin grafts. Clin Plast Surg 1986;13:681.

Vasconez HC et al: Management of extremity injuries with external fixator or Ilizarov devices: cooperative effort between orthopedic and plastic surgeons. Clin Plast Surg 1991;18:505.

PRESSURE SORES

Pressure sores—often less precisely called bedsores or decubitus ulcers—are another example of difficult wound problems that can be treated by plastic surgery. Pressure sores generally occur in patients who are bedridden and unable or unwilling to change position; patients who cannot change position because of a cast or appliance; and patients who have no sensation in an area that is not moved even though they may be ambulatory. The underlying cause of sores in these patients is ischemic necrosis resulting from prolonged pressure against the soft tissue overlying bone. There is also some evidence that local factors in denervated skin predispose to pressure breakdown because there is atrophy of the skin and subcutaneous tissue.

Absence of normal protective reflexes must be compensated for. Prevention is clearly the best treatment for pressure sores. Casts and appliances must be well padded, and points of pressure or pain should be relieved. Bedridden patients must be turned to a new position at least every 2 hours. Water and air mattresses, sheepskin pads, and foam cushions may help relieve pressure but are not substitutes for frequent turning. The introduction of the flotation bed system, which distributes pressure uniformly over a large surface area, has greatly aided in the management of these patients. The pressure on the skin at any time is less than the capillary filling pressure, avoiding many ischemic problems. Paraplegics should not sit in one position for more than 2 hours. Careful daily examination should be made for erythema, the earliest sign of ischemic injury. Erythematous areas should be freed from all pressure. Electrical stimulations, biomaterials, and growth factors are additional modalities to expedite wound repair, but the results are variable.

Once pressure necrosis is established, it is important to determine whether underlying tissues such as fat and muscle are affected, since they are much more likely than skin to become necrotic. A small skin ulcer may be the manifestation of a much larger area of destruction below. If the area is not too extensive and if infection and abscess due to external or hematogenous bacteria are not present, necrotic tissue may be replaced by scar tissue. Continued pressure will not only prevent scar tissue from forming but will also extend the injury. A surface eschar or skin may cover a significant abscess.

If the pressure sore is small and noninfected, application of drying agents to the wound and removal of all pressure to the area may permit slow healing. Wounds extending down to bone rarely heal without surgery. Infected wounds must be debrided down to clean tissue. The objectives at operation are to debride devitalized tissue, including bone, and to provide healthy, well-vascularized padded tissue as a covering. All of the original tissue that formed the bed of the ulcer must be excised.

When the patient's nutritional status and general condition of health are optimal, definitive coverage can be performed. Coverage is usually accomplished with a muscle, musculocutaneous, or, sometimes, an axial flap. Well-vascularized muscle appears to help control established low-grade bacterial contamination. The muscle flaps used for the more common bedsores are as follows: greater trochanter: tensor fasciae latae; ischium: gracilis, gluteus maximus, or hamstrings; sacrum: gluteus maximus. Occasionally, it is possible to provide sensibility to the area of a pressure sore with an innervated flap

from above the level of paraplegia. The most common example is the tensor fasciae latae flap with the contained lateral femoral cutaneous nerve from L4 and L5, which is used to cover an ischial sore. Rarely, an innervated intercostal flap from the abdominal wall may be used to cover an insensible sacrum. Unfortunately, attempts to provide protective sensibility with sensory flaps have not had good results. The tissue expansion techniques should not be the primary surgery treatment of decubitus ulcers but can be used in difficult cases where available tissue is insufficient to close the wound.

Postoperatively, the donor and recipient areas must be kept free of pressure for 2–3 weeks to allow for complete healing. This puts significant demands on other areas of the body that may be equally at risk or may already have areas of breakdown. The use of the air-fluidized bed has greatly aided such situations.

In spite of excellent padding provided by musculocutaneous flaps, recurrence of pressure sores is still a major problem, because the situation that caused the original breakdown usually still exists. Prevention of sores is even more important for these patients.

Bruck JC et al: More arguments in favor of myocutaneous flaps for the treatment of pelvic pressure sores. Ann Plast Surg 1991; 25:85.

Goodman CM et al: Evaluation of results and treatment variables for pressure ulcers in 48 veteran spinal cord-injured patients. Ann Plast Surg 1999;42:665.

AESTHETIC SURGERY

Aesthetic surgery is an integral part of plastic surgery. In fact, the two terms have become almost synonymous even though aesthetic surgery is only one band in a broad spectrum. Increased interest and curiosity about the specialty results in part from increased demands for its services by an aging population but also from the development of more predictable, lasting, and safer techniques. A number of specialists other than plastic surgeons have also performed and contributed to cosmetic surgery. A skilled surgeon can perform such cosmetic operations safely and with maximum benefit to the patient.

Patient selection is probably as important for success as any other factor. Not all patients are good candidates for aesthetic procedures, and such operations are contraindicated in others. Age or poor general health of the patient may be a reason for delay or avoidance of purely elective procedures. Two other major factors must be considered. The first factor is the anatomic feasibility of the procedure. Can the alterations be made successfully and safely? Which technique will best accomplish the goal? The second factor is the psychologic makeup of the patient. Does the patient fully understand the nature of the proposed procedure and its risks and consequences? Are the patient's expectations realistic? Cosmetic changes in appearance will generally not save a failing marriage, help to procure a new job, or substantially improve a person's station in life, and persons with such expectations should not undergo aesthetic surgery. Surgery should be postponed for persons experiencing severe stress, such as is associated with divorce, death of a loved one, or other periods of emotional instability.

The ideal candidate for cosmetic surgery is an adult or mature younger person who has a realistic idea of what is to be accomplished, is not under pressure from others to have the operation done, and does not expect major changes in interpersonal relations or career potential following surgery. Personal satisfaction is a valid reason for seeking aesthetic refinements.

The more common aesthetic procedures are discussed below. Some procedures involve correction of functional problems as well and are therefore not always considered purely cosmetic procedures.

RHINOPLASTY

Surgical alterations of nasal structures are done for relief of airway obstruction (usually secondary to trauma) and to reshape the nose because of undesirable characteristics, such as a prominent dorsal hump, bulbous or drooping tip, or overly large size. There is often a combination of problems.

Procedures are generally performed through intranasal incisions. The nasal skin is usually temporarily freed from its underlying bony and cartilaginous framework, so that the framework can be altered by removal, rearrangement, or augmentation of bone or cartilage. The skin is then redraped over the new foundation. The nasal septum and lower turbinate can also be altered to reestablish an open airway. A better understanding of nasal physiology has enabled surgeons to correct internal valve dysfunction by inserting spreader grafts—often following modification of the bony radix of the nose. Spreader grafts are small pieces of cartilage placed next to the septum and under the upper lateral cartilages. They serve to open up the internal valve in somewhat the same way as the external "breathe easy" appliances utilized by athletes.

Surgery can be done under local or general anesthesia; in either case, topical and injectable vasoconstrictors and anesthetic agents are commonly used. Hospitalization may or may not be indicated. Nasal packing is often used for hemostasis and support of the nasal mucosa during initial healing, as incisions are usually only minimally sutured with absorbable sutures. External nasal splints are placed to control swelling and provide some protection, particularly if osteotomy of the nasal bones is performed.

Convalescence requires 10–14 days before most swelling and periorbital ecchymosis subside; however, several months are often required before completely normal sensation returns, and all swelling resolves.

Nasal procedures are very commonly performed, generally quite safe, and usually effective. Complications include bleeding, internal scarring, recurrence of airways obstruction, and irregularities of contour. Infections are rare except with the use of alloplastic nasal implants.

RHYTIDECTOMY (FACELIFT)

The combined effects of gravity, sun exposure, and loss of elasticity due to aging result in varying degrees of wrinkles and sagging of skin along the cheeks, jawline, neck, and elsewhere in the facial area. These natural signs of aging can be removed to a great extent by a facelift procedure. Not all wrinkles can be removed, however; those in the forehead, around the eyes, in the nasolabial area, and around the lips are not significantly corrected without additional procedures.

Rhytidectomy is a major procedure requiring extensive incisions hidden in the scalp and in front of and behind the ears and occasionally in the submental region. The first such operations consisted of freeing up the skin and then stretching it and resuturing it as it was drawn cephalad and laterally. This gave a masklike and unnatural appearance. In the last few years, there has been a significant change in the concept of the facelift procedure, so that now it consists of elevation of the soft tissues—particularly the jowls and malar fat pads—to where they were at a younger age, giving more prominence to the cheek bones and better delineating the jawline. Undermining of the skin is done only to approach the soft tissues to be elevated, and the excess skin is now removed and reapproximated without tension. This approach to the mid face has given more natural and lasting results and provides also a 3D type of restoration of the soft tissues, giving a more youthful appearance.

For the double neck, extensive freeing up of the skin over the neck from the jawline down to the hyoid is performed, and the fat overlying the platysmal muscle is removed either by suctioning or directly with scissors. The platysma itself is tightened laterally as well as centrally to provide an effect similar to a hammock that will give a more defined neck and jaw angle.

Drains are used particularly in the neck, as well as a padded circumferential dressing to protect the face and provide light pressure during healing. The introduction of fat aspiration procedures (liposuction) has been adapted to the neck but is not recommended for the face since it may produce abnormal lines ("railroad tracks of demarcation"). In appropriate patients, liposuction in the neck does give fine definition to the chin and jawline and may substantially correct the double chin appearance.

Either local or general anesthesia may be used for this often lengthy (3–4 hours) procedure. Local vasoconstrictors are routinely used.

Complications include hematoma, skin slough, injuries to branches of the facial nerve or greater auricular nerve, scars, and asymmetry. Signs of aging often recur years later.

▶ Endoscopy

Endoscopy has become an integral part of plastic surgery, particularly for procedures involving the face or the breast. Smaller endoscopes are now utilized as well as different methods of achieving a desired optical field other than by distention of natural cavities with fluid or gases. In the face and in the breast, the optical cavity is usually obtained by tractioning the skin with appropriate elevators or sutures.

Endoscopy has been most effective for the forehead, where in appropriate circumstances it has replaced the coronal incision, which goes from ear to ear, peeling the scalp down to the supraorbital rims. By means of endoscopy, the forehead lift becomes a more physiologic operation in that one frees up the forehead skin at the subperiosteal level, dividing the periosteum at the supraorbital rim and then removing the depressors of the eyebrows (the procerus and corrugator muscles in the glabella region), thus allowing the frontalis muscle to act unopposed to elevate the eyebrows. The key to the procedure appears to be the division of the periosteum, which by itself frees up the eyebrows and elevates them for at least 5–10 mm. In addition, removal of the glabellar muscles seems to ameliorate in a lasting way the vertical wrinkles in the glabella region. For suspension of the elevated eyebrows, different methods have been advocated that include soft tissue to bony anchoring, the use of temporary screws in the skull as well as miniplates, or, most simply, by providing external traction tied in between staples with nylon sutures. It appears that it is only necessary to maintain that elevation for a short period of time (3–5 days) until the periosteum reattaches at the higher level.

Endoscopy has also been effectively utilized to do a midface lift, and this procedure is applicable to younger patients where there is no excess skin in the face or neck and where scars will be unattractive.

Endoscopy is also utilized for the breasts—particularly for insertion of breast implants in the submammary or subpectoral plane through an axillary incision. An endoscope attached to a right-angle retractor allows excellent visualization of the cavity where the implant is to be inserted, and it allows the development of a pocket inferiorly down to—and if necessary below—the submammary fold and also the division of the lower portion of the origin of the pectoralis major muscle from the sternum to permit insertion of a saline implant and to provide acceptable cleavage. Appropriate instruments for dissection as well as hemostasis have been developed for this procedure, which recently has gained in popularity.

BLEPHAROPLASTY

Blepharoplasty involves removal of redundant skin of the upper and lower eyelids and removal of periorbital fat protruding through sagging orbital septa. It is done alone or as part of a facelift procedure.

Incisions are made in the upper lids surrounding previously marked redundant skin, which is removed. A subciliary incision is generally used in the lower lids. The orbicularis oculi muscle may be altered if necessary. The periorbital fat compartments are opened, and protruding fat is removed.

The extent of redundant skin in the lower lid is gauged, and the skin is resected. External sutures are used. Minimal or no dressing is required.

Local anesthesia in the form of lidocaine with epinephrine is usually adequate. Swelling and ecchymosis subside in 7–10 days, and sutures are removed in 3–4 days.

Complications include bleeding, hematoma formation, epidermal inclusion cysts, ectropion, and asymmetry. Patients are usually satisfied with the results. Recurrence is much less of a problem than with facelift procedures.

In recent years there have been significant changes in the concept of the blepharoplasty procedure. For the upper lids, the change consists of the recognition of senile ptosis due to either disruption or stretching of the levator mechanism. This can be corrected by imbrication of the levator mechanism with sutures.

The lower eyelid operation has undergone even more changes. A general trend has been to do less surgery or dissection but still obtain the same satisfactory results. Less disruption of the orbicularis muscle and orbital septum with "no touch" techniques have become popular. Also, less removal of fat but rather redistribution has gained wider acceptance. The subconjunctival removal of fat has been advocated and is particularly applicable to young patients with congenital fat hernias. The subconjunctival approach is also utilized in conjunction with the laser, which has the effect of tightening the skin of the lower lid and ameliorating the periorbital wrinkles.

Another important concept is the recognition of the proper position of the lower lid, especially the lateral canthal area. A youthful appearance is restored by elevating this to a more normal level.

MAMMOPLASTY

Aside from procedures related to breast cancer, surgery of the female breast is generally done for one of the following reasons: to increase the size of the breasts (augmentation mammoplasty), to decrease the size of the breasts (reduction mammoplasty) or to lift the breasts (mastopexy). Augmentation, lifting of the breasts, and correction of asymmetry are nearly always done for cosmetic reasons. Reduction of hypertrophied breasts may, however, be done for functional reasons, since such breasts can cause poor posture, back and shoulder pain, and discomfort due to grooves from brassiere straps.

▶ Augmentation Mammoplasty

In procedures for augmentation of the breasts, a silicone bag filled with saline solution or silicone is placed beneath the breast tissue in the submammary or subpectoral plane. Incisions are concealed in the periareolar margin, inframammary fold area, or axilla. Dissection is then carried out above or below the pectoralis major muscle, and the implant is placed in the pocket created. Drains are not generally used, and a padded dressing providing light pressure is applied. The subpectoral plane is preferred by most surgeons for augmentation mammoplasty because it does not interfere with mammography, but it does necessitate division of the lower portion of the origin of the pectoralis major muscle up to approximately 3 o'clock in relation to the nipple to provide adequate cleavage.

After a prolonged investigation by the FDA, silicone gel–filled implants have recently become available again in the United States for cosmetic purposes. During the investigation, silicone gel–filled implants were found to be safe; however, long-term data concerning these implants (ie, capsular contracture, deflation and rupture rates) remains unknown. Nevertheless, patients and surgeons now have the opportunity to review the data and choose the type of implant used during breast augmentation.

The procedure can be done on an outpatient basis with local anesthesia, although this may not be satisfactory when subpectoral implants are used. General anesthesia is often used for augmentation procedures.

Although patient satisfaction is excellent in most cases, a significant rate of capsular contracture remains a problem in about 10%. Scar tissue around the implant may contract in variable degrees even in the same patient. Control of this process is difficult even though the best possible environment for healing is provided (ie, appropriate implants are used, infection is controlled, bleeding is not present, debris is removed, and movement is restricted). Implants placed in the subpectoral position appear to be associated with a lesser degree of capsular contracture and less severe deformity if contracture occurs. Deflation of saline implants occurs at a rate of 1% per year.

Other complications include hematoma, infection, exposure of the implant, deflation or rupture of the implant, asymmetry of the breasts, and external scars. Breast function and sensation are usually not altered in any way.

> Rohrich RJ, Reece EM: Breast augmentation today: saline versus silicone—what are the facts? Plast Recon Surg 2008;121:669.

Mastopexy

Mastopexy is another common procedure used for correction of sagging or ptotic breasts. Although some breasts develop in a ptotic manner, most cases are caused by normal relaxation of aging tissues, gravity, and atrophy after pregnancy and lactation. It is not clear whether use of a brassiere alters this process in any significant manner. The degree of deformity is defined by the relationship of the areola to the inframammary fold and the direction of the nipple. A ptotic breast will have a nipple that is below the inframammary line and pointing down towards the toes.

Correction may be done with simultaneous reduction or augmentation. An incision must be made around the areola, and the breast tissue itself is imbricated or, better still, an inferiorly based flap of breast tissue is designed and placed underneath the remnant superior part of the breast and over the pectoralis major muscle, serving as an autoaugmentation as one brings the lateral breast columns together. This procedure gives a more lasting effect than merely decreasing the skin envelope. Attempts at making more lasting corrections of ptosis of the breasts through the periareolar incision, which decreases the scarring, have included wrapping the breast with prosthetic material such as polyglycolic meshes or, more recently, by wrapping it around with segments of pectoralis major muscle.

Nonetheless, significant scarring may occur, particularly around the periareolar incision.

General anesthesia is usually necessary, and recovery from mastopexy may take 7–10 days. Complications include bleeding, infection, tissue loss, altered sensation or loss of function of the nipple and areolar areas, scars, and asymmetry of the breasts.

Patient satisfaction with the results is often not as great as with other procedures. Satisfaction often depends on how well the patient is prepared to accept the resulting scars.

Reduction Mammoplasty

Reduction mammoplasty is similar to mastopexy, since nearly all hypertrophic breasts are ptotic and must be lifted during correction. Enlargement can occur during puberty or later in life. Massive breasts can become a significant disability to the patient.

Although various techniques have been developed for breast reduction, nearly all require a pedicle to carry the nipple areola to its new position and a circumareolar incision as well as a vertical or inverted T incision beneath the areola. In gigantomastia, the nipple-areola is often removed as a free full-thickness graft and positioned appropriately. Most tissue is removed from the center and lower poles of the breast.

Vertical reduction mammoplasty has aroused considerable recent interest because of the decrease in amount of scarring. It can be accomplished through an incision made circumferentially around the areola and then a vertical incision that extends to and sometimes slightly below the inframammary fold. Resection of the breast tissue is done from below as well as from the lateral aspect of the breast. Considerable wrinkling of the skin occurs in an effort to avoid "T-ing off" the incision at the inframammary fold, but pleating of the skin usually resolves over a period of weeks. General anesthesia is nearly always required because dissection is considerable, but blood loss can be minimized by the use of epinephrine as a vasoconstriction agent. Transfusions are rarely indicated, and postoperative drains are often not used. The procedure can be done on an outpatient basis.

Although problems with nipple-areola loss, bleeding, infection, asymmetry of breasts, and scarring may occur; these women are generally among the most satisfied and appreciative of patients.

ABDOMINOPLASTY & BODY CONTOURING PROCEDURES

Other procedures usually classified as aesthetic are abdominoplasty and various body contouring procedures that serve to remove excess tissue from the lower trunk, thighs, and upper arms. Patients with sagging tissue due to aging, pregnancies, multiple abdominal operations, or significant or massive weight loss are usually good candidates for body contouring procedures. With the increased popularity of bariatric surgery, more people are seeking surgery to remove and correct large amounts of excess and redundant skin and soft tissue of the trunk and extremities. These types of procedures are not indicated as a treatment for obesity. This involves a complete regimen of diet, exercise, and lifestyle modifications.

Abdominoplasty usually involves removal of a large ellipse of skin and fat down to the wall of the lower abdomen. Dissection is carried out in the same plane up to the costal margin. The naval is circumscribed and left in place. After the upper abdominal flap is stretched to the suprapubic incision, excess skin and fat are excised. The fascia of the abdominal wall midline can be plicated and thus tightened. The umbilicus is exteriorized through an incision in the flap at the proper level, and the wound is closed over drains with a long incision generally in an oblique line or W shape just above the os pubis and out to the area below the anterior iliac crests (so-called bikini line). When the extent of excess abdominal tissue is severe, better results can be obtained with what is called a circumferential abdominoplasty. The incision is carried around the patient and this requires changing the position of the patient at least on one occasion. Proper markings preoperatively are essential in order to obtain a satisfactory and symmetrical result.

Spinal anesthesia may be used in some cases. Hospitalization is routinely required for up to a few days. Blood transfusions are rarely necessary. Proper deep vein thrombosis prophylaxis is important in these and other extensive procedures. Complications involve blood or serum collections beneath the flap, infection, tissue loss, and wide scars. Results are generally quite dramatic with excellent patient satisfaction in properly selected cases.

Various surgical procedures have been devised to remove excess skin and fat from the upper arms, buttocks, and thighs. These procedures commonly result in extensive incisions that can produce significant scarring, and there may be difficulty in achieving a smooth transition between the end point of the contour alteration and normal tissue. Careful planning and counseling of the patient is imperative in order to obtain a satisfactory result. The use of a suction-assisted lipectomy with appropriate cannulas to remove localized excess fat deposits has become widespread. It is clear, however, that patient selection and judicious use of liposuction are necessary to avoid complications, including hypovolemia due to blood loss, hematoma formation, skin sloughs, excess laxity of the skin and soft tissues and waviness and depressions in the operative site. Used with discretion, liposuction can offer definition to areas of the abdomen, flanks, thighs, and buttocks.

SUCTION-ASSISTED LIPECTOMY

Suction-assisted lipectomy, or liposuction, has now become the most common cosmetic surgical procedure performed in the United States. As presently practiced, it consists of infiltration of a "wetting" or "tumescent" solution to provide vasoconstriction and anesthesia to the operative sites. A common mixture consists in a solution of Ringer lactate with the addition of 1 mg of epinephrine per 1000 mL of Ringer and 250 mg of plain lidocaine—the former to provide vasoconstriction and the lidocaine to provide a certain amount of anesthesia and thus reduce the depth of general anesthesia. Some surgeons perform the entire operation under local anesthesia, necessitating the use of larger amounts of lidocaine.

Once the solution has been infiltrated sufficiently to produce the proposed effects, a small cannula is introduced through a small incision and suction is applied either with a syringe or with a suction machine. The fat layer that has been enlarged by the injection of tumescent solution dislodges easily and disrupts much faster than the blood vessels and the nerves.

Suction-assisted lipectomy is effective in removing abnormal bulges of localized fat throughout the body, particularly in the trochanters or the abdomen and flanks, but it is not considered a weight reduction technique.

The procedure is safe when done by well-trained surgeons respecting sterility and technique and in adequately equipped operating rooms. Safety in the use of up to 35 mg of lidocaine per kilogram has been established by clinical studies. Although fatalities have been reported with suction-assisted lipectomy—which is distressing in an entirely elective procedure—they are due to pulmonary embolization, perforation of the intestines, or severe infections of the abdominal wall. Fortunately, fatalities have markedly decreased since the American Society of Plastic and Reconstructive Surgeons established safety guidelines. High-volume liposuction (ie, over 5000 cc of aspirate) should be done in a hospital or accredited ambulatory facility and that combined procedures should be carefully monitored.

Complications of suction-assisted lipectomy include irregularities of contour, dimpling, and, rarely, local infection at the entrance points.

Ultrasonic liposuction, external and internal, has also been advocated. External ultrasonic liposuction has the effect of a massage to disperse the infiltrated tumescent solution. Internal ultrasonic liposuction, on the other hand, emulsifies the fat with ultrasonic energy, which produces heat, so that this emulsified fat needs to be suctioned with standard suctioning equipment. The problems with ultrasonic liposuction include seroma formation, the need for larger portals of entrance, the possibility of burns of the skin or perforations of the skin (end hits) if the cannula is misdirected.

Burk RW 3rd, Guzman-Stein G, Vasconez LO: Lidocaine and epinephrine levels in tumescent technique liposuction. Plast Reconstr Surg 1996;97:1379.

Cardoso de Castro C: The changing role of platysma in face lifting. Plast Reconstr Surg 2000;105:764.

Chajchir A: Fat injection: long-term follow-up. Aesthetic Plast Surg 1996;20:291.

Matarasso A, Hutchinson OH: Evaluating rejuvenation of the forehead and brow: an algorithm for selecting the appropriate technique. Plast Reconstr Surg 2000;106:687.

Pitanguy I: Facial cosmetic surgery: a 30-year perspective. Plast Reconstr Surg 2000;105:1517.

TELANGIECTASIAS (SPIDER VEINS)

When there is no trace of primary or secondary varicosities, most telangiectasias, or spider veins, are viewed as a cosmetic problem. However, one should be aware that in some cases spider veins may be an indication of deep venous valvular insufficiency. Factors that may play a role in the formation of spider veins include venostasis with decreased flow rate due to atony of the venous wall, chronic venous inflammation, trauma to the site, hormonal influences, or venous compression at the saphenofemoral valve.

Treatment of spider veins is with sclerosing agents, which may include hypertonic saline, sodium tetradecyl sulfate, and hydroxypolyethoxydodecan (Sclerovein). These agents are injected directly into the spider veins with the objective of creating intimal damage that will result in fibrosis and obliteration of the lumen. The technique is simple and effective, but when the sclerosing agent extravasates into the soft tissue, it might produce superficial skin necroses.

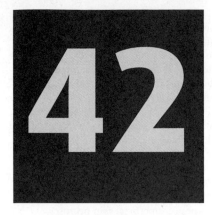

42

Hand Surgery

David M. Young, MD

Scott L. Hansen, MD

Both in industry and in the home, the hand is the most commonly injured part of the body. Disorders of the hand rarely jeopardize life but can significantly affect the ability to function.

▶ Introduction

The prime functions of the hand are feeling (sensibility) and grasping. Sensibility is most important on the radial sides of the index, middle, and ring fingers and on the opposing ulnar side of the thumb, where one must feel and be able to pinch, pick up, and hold objects. The skin on the ulnar side of the small finger and its metacarpal, upon which the hand usually rests, must register the sensations of contact and pain to avoid burns and other trauma.

Mobility is critical for grasping. The upper extremity is a cantilevered system extending from the shoulder to the fingertips. It must be adaptable to varying rates and kinds of movements. Stability of proximal joints is essential for good skeletal control distally.

The specialization of the thumb has allowed humans to have superior aptitudes for defense, work, and dexterity. The thumb has exquisite sensibility and is a highly mobile structure with well-developed adductor and thenar (pronating) musculature. It is the most important digit of the hand, and every effort must be made to preserve its function.

The **position of function** of the upper extremity favors reaching the mouth and perineum and achieves a comfortable, forceful, and unfatiguing grip and pinch. The elbow is held at or near a right angle, the forearm neutral between pronation and supination, and the wrist extended 30 degrees with the fingers flexed to almost meet the opposed (pronated) tip of the thumb (Figure 42–1A). This is the desired position of the extremity if stiffness is likely to occur, and it should be maintained when joints are immobilized by splinting, arthrodesis, or tenodesis.

Opposite to the position of function is the **position of rest,** in which the flexed wrist extends the digits, making grip and pinch awkward, uncomfortable, weak, and fatiguing (Figure 42–1B). The forearm is usually pronated, and the elbow may be extended. This habitus is assumed, without intention, after injury, paralysis, or the onset of a painful stimulus. For that reason, it is also called the **position of the injury.** Immobility in this position jeopardizes function.

ANATOMY

All references to the forearm and hand should be made to the radial and ulnar sides (not lateral and medial) and to the volar (or palmar) and dorsal surfaces. The digits are identified as the thumb, index finger, middle finger, ring finger, and small finger.

The skin is an elastic outer sleeve and glove of the arm and hand. Sacrifice of its surface area or elasticity by debridement and fibrosis can severely diminish the range of motion and constrict circulation. In the adult hand, the dorsal skin stretches about 4 cm in the longitudinal and in the transverse planes when the palm is flattened and spread. The long finger can have as much as 48 cm² of skin cover, and the whole hand (exclusive of digits) has 210 cm².

Fascia anchors the palmar skin to bone to make pinch and grip stable; the midlateral fibers of the Cleland and Grayson ligaments keep the skin sleeve from twisting around the digit (Figure 42–2). In the form of sheaths and pulleys, fascia holds tendons in the concavity of arched joints to convey mechanical efficiency and power. The fascial sleeve of the forearm, hand, and digits must sometimes be released along with skin to prevent or relieve congestion (eg, compartment syndrome). Any fascial compartment of the hand provides a space for infection or an avenue for its dissemination.

Each finger has three joints, the distal interphalangeal joint (DIP), the proximal interphalangeal joint (PIP), and the metacarpophalangeal joint (MCP). The thumb contains the interphalangeal joint (IP), the MCP, and the carpometacarpal joint (CMC). The wrist is the "key joint" of the hand, governing motion of the digits, and may need to be included

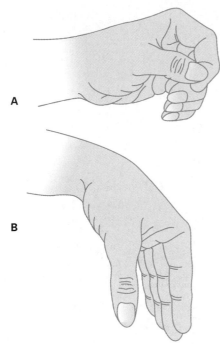

▲ **Figure 42–1.** Positions of function **(A)** and rest (injury) **(B).**

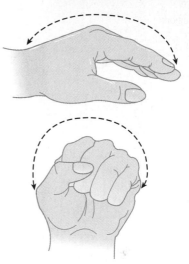

▲ **Figure 42–3.** Longitudinal *(top)* and transverse *(bottom)* arches.

in the immobilization required for a major finger or hand problem. The position of the wrist governs the efficiency of extrinsic muscle contraction. The wrist is composed of a proximal and distal row of carpal bones. The proximal row contains the scaphoid, lunate, triquetrum, and pisiform, while the distal row contains the trapezium, trapezoid, capitate, and hamate. The stability of the digital joints and their planes of motion are governed by the length of the ligaments and the anatomy of their articulating surfaces. The longitudi-

nal and transverse arches of the hand (Figure 42–3) are architectural prerequisites to gripping, pinching, and cupping and are maintained by the active contraction and passive tone of intact muscles. The arches create the position of function. When the arches are collapsed, the hand assumes the position of injury. Loss of these arches is most often initiated by edema. They may be preserved by splinting in the position of function, elevation without constriction, and early restoration of active joint motion.

Each MCP and PIP joint has a distally anchored volar plate (Figure 42–4) in addition to collateral ligaments stabilizing the joint on either side (Figure 42–5). The thickened lateral portions of the volar plate form the checkrein ligaments, which prevent IP hyperextension.

The extrinsic flexor tendons are contained in fibrous **sheaths** to prevent bowstringing and preserve mechanical efficiency as the digits flex into the palm. Pulleys (hypertrophied sections of the sheath) resist the points of greatest tendency to bowstring. The retinacular pulley system contains five annular bands and three cruciform bands. Sheaths are inelastic and relatively avascular. Therefore, they crowd and congest any swollen, inflamed, or injured tendons and curtail glide by friction, constriction, and the generation of inelastic adhesions. The A-2 and A-4 pulleys must be maintained to prevent tendon bowstringing. These are located over the proximal and middle phalanges, respectively. The A-1, A-3, and A-5 pulleys are located over the MCP, PIP, and DIP joints, respectively. Five flexor tendon zones have been described. Zone II, or **"no man's land,"** is the zone from the middle of the palm to just beyond the PIP joint, wherein the superficialis and profundus tendons lay ensheathed together and where recovery of glide is difficult after wounding (Figure 42–6).

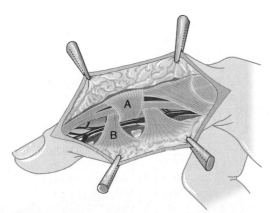

▲ **Figure 42–2. (A)** Cleland ligament. **(B)** Transverse retinacular ligament.

Extension

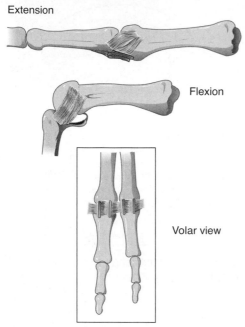

Flexion

Volar view

▲ **Figure 42–4.** Volar plate.

Across the wrist, the dense volar transverse carpal ligament closes the bony carpal canal (**carpal tunnel**) through which passes all eight finger flexors as well as the flexor pollicis longus and median nerve (Figure 42–6). The **ulnar**

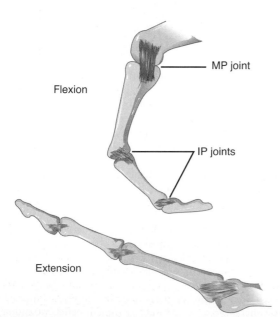

Flexion

MP joint

IP joints

Extension

▲ **Figure 42–5.** Collateral ligaments.

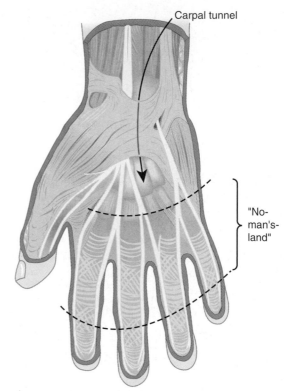

Carpal tunnel

"No-man's-land"

▲ **Figure 42–6.** Carpal tunnel and no man's land.

bursa is the continuation of the synovium around the long flexors of the small finger through the carpal tunnel, encompassing the other finger flexors which interrupted their separated bursa at the mid palm level. The **radial bursa** is the synovium around the flexor pollicis longus contained through the carpal tunnel. These two bursas may intercommunicate. **Parona space** is the tissue plane over the pronator quadratus in the distal forearm deep to the radial and ulnar bursas.

The extensor tendons are ensheathed in six individual compartments at the wrist beneath the extensor retinaculum (Figures 42–7 and 42–8), which predisposes to adhesions. Its role as a pulley is not as vital.

The nerves of greatest importance to hand function are the musculocutaneous, radial, ulnar, and median nerves. The importance of the musculocutaneous and radial nerves combined is forearm supination and of the radial nerve alone is innervation of the extensor muscles. The ulnar nerve innervates 15 of the 20 intrinsic muscles. The median nerve provides sensation to the thumb, index finger, middle finger, and the radial aspect of the ring finger; through its motor innervation, it maintains most of the long flexors, the pronators of the forearm, and the thenar muscles. Figure 42–9 shows the sensory distribution of the ulnar, radial, and median nerves.

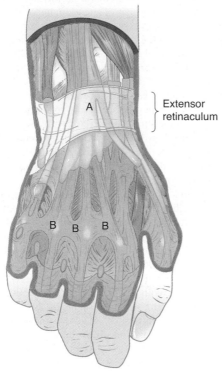

▲ **Figure 42–7. (A)** Extensor retinaculum over six tendon compartments. **(B)** Juncturae tendinum (conexus inter-tendineus).

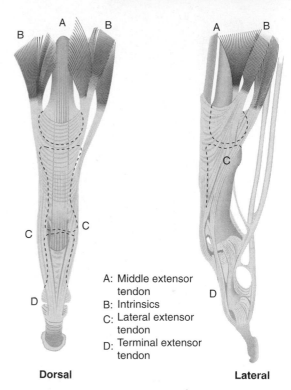

A: Middle extensor tendon
B: Intrinsics
C: Lateral extensor tendon
D: Terminal extensor tendon

Dorsal   **Lateral**

▲ **Figure 42-8.** Extensor hood mechanism.

CLINICAL EVALUATION OF HAND DISORDERS

The presenting complaint must be assessed in complete detail with regard to its mechanisms of onset, evolution, aggravating factors, and relieving factors. Age, sex, hand dominance, occupation, preexisting hand problems, and relevant matters pertaining to the patient's general health must also be noted.

The examination should follow an orderly routine. Observe the neck, shoulders, both upper extremities, and the action and strength of all muscle groups, and be certain that all parts can pass painlessly and coordinately through a normal range of motion, starting with the head and neck and working down to the fingertips. Compare both upper extremities and keep detailed notes, diagrams, and measurements. Having the patient reach for the ceiling and simultaneously open and close both fists and then spread and adduct the fingers and, finally, oppose the thumbs sequentially to each fingertip will immediately demonstrate any abnormalities.

Observe habitus, wasting, hypertrophy, deformities, skin changes, skin temperature, scars, and signs of pain (including when the patient attempts to bear weight on the palms). Feel the wrist pulses and the sweat of the finger pads, and test reflexes and the sensibility of the median, ulnar, and radial nerves.

Serial x-rays and laboratory studies may clarify a problem with an indolent evolution (eg, Kienböck avascular necrosis of the lunate, causing unexplained wrist pain). Contralateral and multiple-view x-rays in different planes are often helpful. In addition, CT scans, MRI, bone scans, or all of these may aid in diagnosis. This is especially true in patients who have persistent bone and joint pain or limited motion or in patients who have not attained adult growth. In the case of wrist problems, arthrograms and arthroscopy may be of diagnostic value. MRI can be quite helpful in the diagnosis of subtle carpal bone problems.

The diagnosis is often made by noting the response to therapy. This is particularly true in the case of local corticosteroids injected at the site of noninfectious inflammatory conditions (eg, carpal tunnel syndrome, trigger finger).

GENERAL OPERATIVE PRINCIPLES

A bloodless field (eg, by tourniquet ischemia) is essential for accurate evaluation, dissection, and management of tissues of the hand. This is achieved by elevating or exsanguinating the extremity and then inflating a padded blood pressure cuff around the arm to 100 mm Hg above systolic pressure. This is readily tolerated by the unanesthetized arm for 30 minutes and by the anesthetized arm for 2 hours.

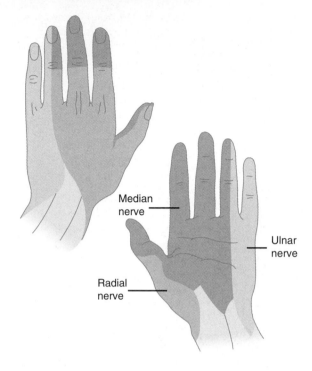

▲ **Figure 42–9.** Sensory distribution in the hand. Light shaded area, ulnar nerve; diagonal area, radial nerve; darker area, median nerve.

Incisions (Figure 42–10) must be either zigzagged across lines of tension (eg, must never cross perpendicularly to a flexion crease), termed Brunner incisions, or run longitudinally in "neutral" zones (eg, connecting the lateral limits of the flexion and extension creases of the digits), and whenever

possible, must be designed so that a healthy skin-fat flap is raised over the zone of repair of a tendon, nerve, or artery.

Proper evaluation and treatment of an acute injury often requires extension of the wound. Normal structures can then be identified and traced into the zone of injury, where blood and devitalized tissue can make their identification difficult or impossible.

Constriction and tension by dressings must be avoided. The dressing should be applied evenly to the skin without wrinkles. The wound should be covered with a single layer of fine-mesh gauze followed by a moist spongy medium (fluffs, Rest-On, Kling, or Kerlix). Moisture facilitates the drainage of blood into the dressing, which should be applied with gentle pressure to restrict dead space.

Splinting and immediate elevation are paramount in controlling swelling and pain postoperatively. In general, plaster (fast-setting) or fiberglass is preferred because of its adaptability to specific requirements. More often than not, the wrist requires immobilization along with any other part of the hand (Figures 42–11 and 42–12).

It must be appreciated that effective immobilization of a finger most often requires concomitant immobilization of one or more adjacent fingers, usually in the position of function. Straight splints such as tongue blades involve a hazard of digital stiffness and distortion and should not be used across the MCP joint.

Persistence of pain signifies inadequate immobilization and, if throbbing is present, congestion. Congestion must be promptly relieved by elevation and sectioning of the cast and dressing and, if necessary, the skin and fascia.

CONGENITAL ANOMALIES OF THE HAND

Major congenital hand anomalies are not rare, with approximately 1 in 700 live births affected. When minor deformities

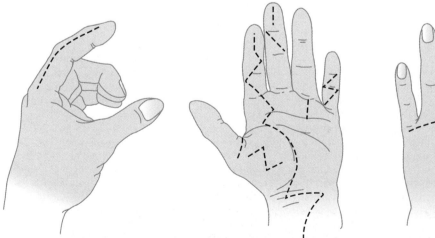
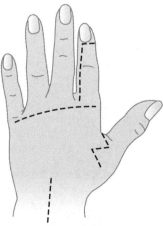

▲ **Figure 42–10.** Proper placement of skin incisions.

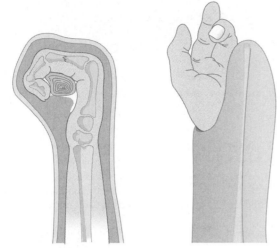

▲ **Figure 42–11.** Casting.

are included, approximately 3% of all births are affected. Camptodactyly (bent finger), polydactyly (more than five fingers), and syndactyly (two or more fingers are joined together) are the most common malformations. Newborns with hand anomalies should be carefully examined for other malformations because multisystem syndromes can be present in 5% of patients (eg, vertebral, anal atresia, cardiac, trachea, esophageal, renal, and limb [VACTERL] syndrome with radial head dysphasia).

Anomalies may be inherited, caused by environmental factors (drugs, viral infections, irradiation, alcohol), or idiopathic. Major genetic or major environmental causes are

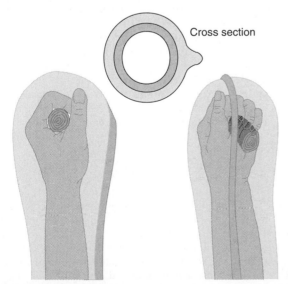

▲ **Figure 42–12.** Casting.

infrequently found, suggesting that the cause of most defects is multifactorial.

In order to simplify an extremely complex clinical problem, the American Society for Surgery of the Hand (ASSH) and all major international hand societies have adopted a single classification system that divides anomalies into six main categories: failures of formation (absent digits, phocomelia [seal limb]), failures of differentiation (syndactyly), duplication (polydactyly), undergrowth (brachydactyly), overgrowth (macrodactyly), and constriction ring syndrome (focal necrosis, intrauterine amputation). There is considerable overlap in the categories, as might be expected.

Ideally, surgery is performed early in the first 2 years of life, but timing is individually tailored to the problem.

McCarroll HR: Congenital anomalies: a 25-year overview. J Hand Surg [Am] 2000;25:1007.
Watson S: The principles of management of congenital anomalies of the upper limb. Arch Dis Child 2000;83:10.

▼ TENDON DISORDERS OF THE HAND

Movement of the muscles of the hand and arm are transmitted into finger and wrist motion by the tendons. The tendons are strong, compact units that glide within their individual compartments. Disruption of the tendon by trauma or loss of tendon gliding by inflammation hinders tendon excursion and therefore limits active motion of the joints. Passive motion of the joint is still possible with an isolated tendon problem and distinguishes tendon disorders from joint disorders when both active and passive motion are limited.

Tendon disruption can result from any penetrating injury and can be diagnosed by physical examination. A tendon injury should be suspected when the patient is unable to actively move a joint. Certain tendon lacerations, such as an isolated flexor digitorum superficialis disruption, may be masked because the profunda tendon can still move the entire finger. Blocking of profunda function by blocking flexion in the neighboring fingers (the profunda tendons are joined in the palm) reveals the injury to the superficialis when the injured PIP joint cannot be flexed.

The state of the wound and the complexity of the injury are the principal issues the hand surgeon must weigh in choosing between a primary or secondary tenorrhaphy. Clean wounds generally favor primary tenorrhaphy. Primary tenorrhaphy is defined as one that is done within 24–72 hours after injury. When wounds are unstable, contaminated, or complicated by fracture or ischemia, formal tenorrhaphy may have to be delayed for weeks or months until the tendon bed is more favorable to healing and glide. However, interim tacking of the tendons—together, to tendon sheaths, or to bone—to maintain the fiber length of a muscle may be done as a preliminary procedure.

Preoperative treatment of fresh lacerations consists of wound closure, immobilization, and prophylactic antibiotics.

Such cases can be deferred for definitive primary repair for 24 hours or more. The timing of delayed secondary procedures depends on the resolution of wound edema and fibrous callus (ie, how soft and pliable it is). After 6–8 weeks, tendons that retract over 2.5 cm may defy full excursion because muscle elasticity has been lost or because the tendon is recoiled and congealed in scar.

Tenorrhaphy must be done without surface trauma along the tendon or its bed. The repair is made end to end or by weaving one tendon with the other, using a 3-0 or 4-0 braided synthetic polyester material, Prolene or nylon sutures. A flexor tendon graft is anchored distally to bone (Figure 42–13). Tenodesis will occur if the surface of the tendon and the surface where adherence is desired are roughened. The position of immobilization should relieve tension on the tendon juncture. The duration of immobilization after tenorrhaphy is generally no more than 3–4 weeks. Controlled early, passive or active mobilization after tenorrhaphy may be initiated as early as 1 week to minimize excessive tendon scarring. This requires a very cooperative patient and close supervision by the hand therapist to avoid rupture of the repaired tendon.

Adhesions invariably form wherever tendons are even slightly inflamed or injured and can severely limit tendon function. Even so, adhesions are necessary for a tendon to reestablish continuity. With continuous active and passive movement over months, tendon glide can be increased with maturation and molding of the collagen in the adhesions. If the adhesions remain thick and tendon excursion is limited, surgical release of the tendon adhesions (tenolysis) needs to be performed. Successful surgery requires the release of all adhesions limiting tendon glide without rupturing the tendon repair. Movement of the tendon as soon as possible after surgery (within 24–48 hours) under the guidance of the hand therapist is critical to avoid recurrence of adhesions.

The access to tenolysis should be through an incision offering effective exposure and placed where the immediate active and passive joint motion that must follow will not jeopardize healing of the wound by undue stretching or direct pressure. Performing a concomitant procedure requiring immobilization such as a neurorrhaphy should be avoided. The patient must understand that joint mobilization after tendon surgery is a time-consuming process, often taking many weeks or months to achieve maximum recovery.

Mallet finger ("baseball" or "drop" finger) (Figure 42–14) is due to disruption of the extensor tendon to the distal phalanx. A distal joint that can be passively but not actively

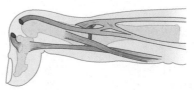

▲ **Figure 42–14.** Mallet finger with swan-neck deformity.

extended is diagnostic. The injury most commonly results from sudden forceful flexion of the digit when it is held in rigid extension. Either the extensor is partially or completely ruptured or the dorsal lip of the bone is avulsed. Less frequently, the injury is due to direct trauma such as a laceration. An x-ray should be taken to determine the presence and extent of any fracture.

Treatment requires 6–8 weeks of continuous splinting in full distal joint extension (not hyperextension) with or without 40 degrees of PIP joint flexion. Patient education and compliance are essential for good results. Joint fixation internally with a percutaneous Kirschner wire or externally with padded aluminum, plastic, or plaster splints are equally effective. A lacerated tendon should be repaired. When a significantly displaced fracture fragment represents one third or more of the surface of the joint, it should be reduced by wiring or pinning. If there is sufficient articular surface disruption, one may consider joint fusion.

Swan-neck deformity (Figure 42–14) is a frequent complication of mallet finger, but it may also be the result of disparity of pull between the extrinsic flexors and extensor hood with or without attenuation of the DIP joint extensor. It is seen in congenitally hypermobile joints, spastic and rheumatoid states, and following resection of the superficialis tendon. The dorsal hood acts to extend the distal joint but is held back by its insertion at the base of the middle phalanx, which it therefore hyperextends. This in turn increases the tension on the profundus, which hyperflexes the DIP joint. If the mallet deformity is 25 degrees or less and there is some active distal joint extension, it may be treated by undermining and elevating the extensor hood at the PIP joint and severing its insertion on the base of the middle phalanx. Otherwise, the deformity may be corrected by tethering PIP joint extension with one slip of the flexor digitorum superficialis threaded through the flexor pulley of the proximal phalanx with the PIP joint flexed 20 degrees.

The **boutonnière, or "buttonhole," deformity** (Figure 42–15) appears as the opposite of the swan-neck deformity: hyperextension of the DIP joint and flexion of the PIP joint. There is attenuation or separation of the dorsal hood, so that the middle extensor tendon becomes ineffective and the lateral extensor tendons shift volar to the PIP joint axis and the joint buckles dorsally. The entire extrinsic-intrinsic force on the hood passes onto the lateral extensor tendons, which flex the PIP joint and hyperextend the DIP joint. This deformity may develop suddenly or, more often, insidiously

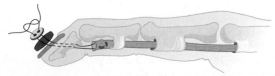

▲ **Figure 42–13.** Flexor tenorrhaphy by advancement or graft. Pulleys are saved.

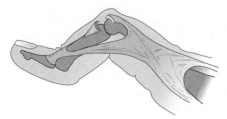

▲ **Figure 42–15.** Buttonhole deformity.

after closed blunt or open trauma over the dorsum of the PIP joint.

To avoid this complication, sutured extensor tendon lacerations and severe contusions over the PIP joint should always have the PIP joint alone splinted in extension for 3–4 weeks. Established deformities can be treated by such immobilization but more often require operative correction.

STENOSING TENOSYNOVITIS

In stenosing tenosynovitis, there is a disproportion between the clearance inside a tendon pulley or tunnel and the diameter of the tendon or tendons that must glide through it. Any pulley or tunnel may be implicated. The more common sites are as follows:

(1) The proximal digital (A1) pulleys in the distal palm, causing **trigger finger** or thumb. There is local tenderness of the pulley; pain, which may be referred to the PIP joint; and (usually but not always) locking of the digit in flexion with a painful "pop" as it goes into extension (ie, as the bulge in the tendon or tendons passes through the tight pulley).

(2) The pulley over the radial styloid housing the abductor pollicis longus and extensor pollicis brevis (first extensor compartment), causing **de Quervain tenosynovitis.** Local tenderness and pain occur if these tendons are actively stretched (eg, Finkelstein test). The Finkelstein test is performed by having the patient bend the thumb into the palm and grasp with the fingers. The wrist is then bent ulnarly, and the first extensor compartment palpated. Pain in this area suggests de Quervain tenosynovitis.

Relief of the symptoms can be achieved by local injections of triamcinolone mixed with lidocaine. Immediate surgery is justified if the constriction is so tight that the tendon is locked. Surgical section of the constricting tendon sheath is also indicated if symptoms persist or recur. When releasing the flexor tendon, care is taken not to resect more than the section of sheath restricting the tendon or else the tendon will pull away from the finger like a bowstring and weaken the grip.

Chan DY: Management of simple finger injuries: the splinting regime. Hand Surg 2002;7:223.

Finsen V, Hagen S: Surgery for trigger finger. Hand Surg 2003;8:201.

Hanz KR et al: Extensor tendon injuries: acute management and secondary reconstruction. Plast Reconstr Surg 2008;121:109e.

James R et al: Tendon: biology, biomechanics, repair, growth factors, and evolving treatment options. J Hand Surg [Am] 2008; 33:102.

Rozental TD, Zurakowski D, Blazar PE: Trigger finger: prognostic indicators of recurrence following corticosteroid injection. J Bone Joint Surg Am 2008;90:1665.

Thien T, Becker J, Theis JC: Rehabilitation after surgery for flexor tendon injuries in the hand. Cochrane Database Syst Rev 2004;CD003979.

▼ SKELETAL INJURIES OF THE HAND

Injuries to the bones and joints of the hand are the most common skeletal injuries treated by physicians. Recognition of the injury, appropriate diagnostic tests, and timely treatment are essential for minimizing the complications of these injuries. Some patients may neglect obvious fractures and dislocations in hope of spontaneous recovery. More subtle injuries to the wrist are more often neglected by the patient and sometimes even missed by physicians until further damage is done. The use of the fluoroscope, found in many offices, greatly enhances the surgeon's ability to diagnose fractures. The machine allows real-time assessment of the bones as part of the physical examination. A common late sequela of skeletal injury at the articular surfaces is osteoarthritis, which is difficult to treat. Patients with symptoms related to the hand or wrist but without a discernible cause should be referred early to a hand specialist.

METACARPALS & PHALANGES

▶ Fractures

Fractures of the metacarpal and phalangeal bones such as distal phalanx tuft of the fingers caught in closing doors and metacarpal shaft fractures of the ulnar side of the hand (boxer's fractures) create an obvious deformity and are easy to diagnose. Adequate x-rays of the specific site of the fracture with anteroposterior, lateral, and oblique views are essential for developing a treatment plan.

Fractures of the shaft can usually be treated with closed reduction and a cast or splint holding the hand in the position of function (Figure 42–1) for 3–4 weeks. Residual angulation of a metacarpal shaft fracture of up to 30 degrees in the fifth finger and 20 degrees in the fourth finger is functionally well tolerated, although a dorsal bump may be aesthetically unpleasant. However, even a small rotational misalignment of the fracture at the metacarpal bone results in scissoring of the fingers in flexion and causes severe dysfunction.

When fractures do not remain reduced, fixation with Kirschner pins placed through the skin is required. Placement of more than one pin is usually needed to keep the fracture reduced. The pins are removed after the fracture is healed. Displaced and comminuted fractures may require opening of the fracture site and reduction under direct visualization. Pins, lag screws, and small, low-profile metal plates and screws are used to maintain reduction. Metal plates provide strong support to the fracture site and allow earlier mobilization of the hand. However, plates are more invasive and occasionally interfere with tendon function due to excessive scar formation postoperatively.

Fractures through an articular surface need to be carefully evaluated. Nondisplaced fractures can be treated by casting. Displaced fractures require open reduction and accurate pin or lag screw fixation because discrepancies of the articular surface will eventually result in degenerative arthritis.

Fractures of the distal phalanx from crush injuries require attention to the disrupted nail bed. The nail is removed to decompress the painful subungual hematoma and provide irrigation of the open fracture and careful reapproximation of the nail matrix. Large disruptions in the nail matrix may result in deformity of the regenerating nail. The nail is replaced under the nail fold (eponychium) as a splint. A protective splint is placed over the finger to hold the distal fragment in extension.

An intra-articular fracture of the base of the thumb metacarpal bone with subluxation (displacement) of the metacarpal leaving a volar pyramidal shaped fragment attached to the trapezium is called a **Bennett fracture.** The anterior oblique ligament, responsible for stability of the thumb base, is left attached to the pyramidal fragment. The remainder of the thumb metacarpal is unstable and limits use of the thumb. The fracture must be reduced and stabilized with Kirschner pins, plate, or lag screws. Accurate reduction of the articular surface is crucial in reducing complications. Even despite adequate treatment, most patients eventually develop arthritis.

▶ Dislocations

Dislocations are most common in the PIP joint. Injuries are classified according to the position of the distal digit as hyperextension, dorsal displacement, or volar displacement. The type of dislocation determines which structures, such as the volar plate, collateral ligaments, and extensor tendon, are likely to be disrupted.

The MCP and CMC joints are better protected by surrounding soft tissue but can still be dislocated. The MCP joint of the thumb is most frequently injured by forced abduction. The ulnar collateral ligament is torn, as occurs with forced use of a ski pole or as historically described in gamekeepers when twisting the neck of birds ("gamekeeper's thumb"). Of the CMC joints, the fifth is most commonly injured. A fracture analogous to a Bennett fracture (reverse Bennett fracture) can occur. Examination to determine injury to the deep motor branch of the ulnar nerve in this area should be done.

Radiographs are occasionally useful for diagnosis, but the physical examination is most important. Since pain often limits the extent of the examination, regional anesthesia with a wrist or finger block allows a more detailed examination. Partial tears of ligaments without dislocation or instability

are treated by splints. Dislocations can usually be reduced, and the need for surgical therapy is determined by the stability of the joint after reduction. Stable reductions are treated with early mobilization to decrease stiffness.

Fracture dislocations usually require surgical repair. Instability after reduction can be treated by repair of the torn collateral ligament or volar plate. Severe dislocations of the PIP and MCP joints can result in interposition of disrupted soft tissue in the joint, making closed reduction impossible. The joint must be opened and the trapped soft tissue removed and repaired to correct the dislocation. A complete disruption of the ulnar collateral ligament in a gamekeeper's thumb injury can result in interposition of the adductor aponeurosis between the torn ends of the ulnar collateral ligament. The ends of the ligament must be reduced and repaired under direct vision.

WRIST & FOREARM INJURIES

▶ Fractures

Fractures in the wrist and forearm usually result from falls on the outstretched hand. The distal radius is most commonly fractured. Many classification systems and eponyms have been used based on the extent and displacement of the fracture and involvement of the articular surface. The hyperextended wrist also exposes the scaphoid bone to injury in a fall. Since the scaphoid is crucial to wrist motion, displacement of the fracture is poorly tolerated. In addition, the blood supply enters the distal part of the bone and makes ischemic necrosis of the proximal fragment a problem.

Diagnosis of distal radius fractures is not difficult, but scaphoid fractures can easily be missed. Special radiographic views of the wrist or CT or MRI scans may be needed in difficult cases. If the clinical picture is suspicious but the radiographs are inconclusive, the wrist should be immobilized. Repeat radiographs in 7–10 days may demonstrate the fracture. Untreated scaphoid fractures lead to debilitating arthritis and collapse of the wrist.

Distal radius fractures are treated by reduction and immobilization. As with other fractures, articular irregularities and unstable fractures need to be treated by open reduction and internal fixation. Use of bone grafting and external fixation devices to initially treat the fracture has been advocated. Scaphoid fractures require careful and prolonged immobilization. Displaced fractures or nonhealing fractures require operative treatment with screw compression, bone grafts, and/or scaphoid replacement.

▶ Dislocations & Sprains

Dislocations and ligamentous injuries of the wrist are the most difficult hand injuries to diagnose and treat. Wrist injuries often present as a painful wrist after minor trauma. Routine radiographs are often normal, and physical findings can be unimpressive. Still, these injuries can lead to chronic problems. Special stress radiographs, fluoroscopy, and physical maneuvers (scaphoid shift test) help delineate the injury.

The scaphoid lunate ligament is most often injured. Instability of the joint is best treated by repair or reconstruction of the ligament. Injury of the ligaments of the radiocarpal-radioulnar joint is likewise difficult to determine. Surgical treatment involves repair of the disrupted ligament.

Bhandari M, Hanson BP: Acute nondisplaced fractures of the scaphoid. J Orthop Trauma 2004;18:253.

Cohen MS: Fractures of the carpal bones. Hand Clin 1997;13:587.

Corley FG Jr, Schenck RC Jr: Fractures of the hand. Clin Plast Surg 1996;23:447.

Divelbiss BJ, Baratz ME: The role of arthroplasty and arthrodesis following trauma to the upper extremity. Hand Clin 1999; 15:335.

Kozin SH, Thoder JJ, Lieberman G: Operative treatment of metacarpal and phalangeal shaft fractures. J Am Acad Orthop Surg 2000;8:111.

Mack MG et al: Clinical impact of MRI in acute wrist fractures. Eur Radiol 2003;13:612.

Pao VS, Chang J: Scaphoid nonunion: diagnosis and treatment. Plast Reconstr Surg 2003;1666.

Wolf JM, Weiss AP: Portable mini-fluoroscopy improves operative efficiency in hand surgery. J Hand Surg [Am] 1999;24:182.

NERVE DISORDERS

Nerve disorders of the hands are conveniently organized into compression neuropathies, injuries of peripheral nerves, and various problems located more proximal to the upper extremities (spinal cord or central nervous system). For nerve dysfunction due to strokes, cerebral palsy, and spinal cord injury, readers are referred to more specific textbooks on hand surgery.

▶ Compression Neuropathies

Compression of the nerves of the upper extremities due to an increase in surrounding tissue pressure occurs in specific locations and causes predictable signs and symptoms. Tissue edema from a variety of causes such as crushing injuries, vascular disorders, and prolonged repetitive hand motions can compress nerves traveling within tight compartments of the arm and produce nerve ischemia. Prolonged ischemia results in axonal destruction and sensory and motor dysfunction.

The median nerve can be compressed by local structures at the elbow (pronator syndrome), the anterior interosseous branch, and the wrist (carpal tunnel syndrome). Compression of the median nerve at the elbow causes forearm pain and sensory changes in the radial four fingers. The anterior interosseous branch of the median nerve is purely a motor nerve, and lesions produce only weakness of thumb and index finger flexion and no pain. Carpal tunnel syndrome presents with weakness in the hand, sensory abnormalities of the fingers sparing the small finger and ulnar aspect of the ring finger, and exacerbation of symptoms on forced flexion of the wrist (Phalen sign) or tapping the nerve at the wrist (Tinel sign). Shoulder, elbow, and forearm pain is also common. Atrophy of thenar muscles occurs in longstanding cases.

The ulnar nerve can be compressed at the elbow (cubital tunnel syndrome) or the wrist (Guyon canal). Sensory abnormalities in the small finger and weakness of intrinsic hand muscles occur with compression in either area. Segmental nerve conduction velocity tests help to localize the abnormality to one site or the other. Compression of the radial nerve occurs most frequently from fractures of the humerus. Compression of the nerve along the proximal radius (radial tunnel syndrome) causes diffuse pain around the elbow but occurs rarely.

Abnormal findings on nerve conduction studies and clinical manifestations of nerve compression are adequate for diagnosis. Electromyography (EMG) demonstrating denervation patterns in the corresponding muscles or slowing of nerve conduction velocities indicates injury to the nerve. Although helpful, these tests only complement the physical examination, since electrodiagnostic tests can occasionally be inaccurate.

Early or mild cases of compression are treated by controlling tissue swelling. Resting the extremity with splints and using nonsteroidal anti-inflammatory medications as well as local injection of steroids often resolves the problem. If repetitive motions, such as typing, are thought to be the cause, changing the motion or hand position should help. If clinical manifestations are severe or if nonsurgical therapy fails, surgical decompression of the nerve is advocated.

Carpal tunnel syndrome is the most common type of compression neuropathy and one of the most common hand disorders. Surgical therapy of median nerve entrapment in the carpal tunnel or any of the compression neuropathies requires detailed knowledge of the anatomy. Division of the constricting structures results in partial or complete reversal of the symptoms. In the carpal tunnel, the median nerve is surrounded on three sides by carpal bones. Incision of the transverse carpal ligament, which forms the roof of the tunnel, decompresses the nerve. Occasionally, internal fibrosis of the nerve occurs and internal neurolysis with an operating microscope is required to allow the nerve to recover. Endoscopic release of the carpal tunnel through a smaller skin incision has been advocated.

▶ Nerve Injuries

Injury to individual peripheral nerves of the arm results in predictable and defined deficits. Proximal injuries involving the brachial plexus have more variable manifestations. Nerve conduction can be disrupted in the absence of structural changes due to compression, blunt injury, or ischemia (neuropraxia). More severe injury results in disruption of the axon with preservation of the epineurial covering of the nerve (axonotmesis). Both types of injury are followed by spontaneous recovery of function of good quality. Complete disruption of the nerve (neurotmesis), as with a laceration, requires surgical repair. Wallerian degeneration of the distal nerve occurs in both neurotmesis and axonotmesis, and recovery depends on the growth of the cut axon to the end organ. However, with neurotmesis, orientation of the proximal and distal axons are lost and recovery may be incomplete, especially in mixed motor and sensory nerves. Methods to differentiate sensory from motor fascicles have been used during repairs with some benefit.

A patient with loss of the radial nerve is unable to extend the fingers, wrist, and thumb. In addition, the patient will have sensory loss to the dorsum of the hand. Median nerve dysfunction causes problems with opposition of the thumb and grip of the fingers. Sensory loss is to the radial four digits and can significantly impair use of the hand. An ulnar neuropathy causes dysfunction of the intrinsic muscles of the hand, clawing of the ulnar two digits, and weakness in gripping smaller objects. Sensation is lost along the ulnar side of the hand.

Diagnosis of nerve injury is mainly by the physical examination. Understanding the functional anatomy of the peripheral nerves allows adequate evaluation of nerve loss. Electrodiagnostic studies are used to distinguish between partial and complete lesions and to follow functional recovery.

Obvious and complete disruption of the nerve is treated best by early surgical exploration and repair. An incomplete lesion or questionable disruption of nerve integrity is best treated with close observation, splinting to prevent contractures, and surgical exploration if no recovery occurs. Segmental loss of nerves requires nerve grafts, usually taken from a minor sensory nerve, such as the sural nerve, to bridge the gap. Results of primary repair are better than the results of grafts, and repairs done soon after injury are better than delayed repairs. Recovery of protective sensation of the hand is crucial for good functional recovery.

Motor dysfunction due to nerve damage can be treated by arthrodesis (stabilization of flail joints) and tendon transfers. Tendon transfers should utilize a muscle unit that is unaffected by the nerve injury, have direction of force and excursion similar to those of the damaged muscle, and produce no further deficits due to loss of the donor muscle. For radial nerve palsy, the pronator teres to extensor carpi radialis transfer provides wrist extension, the flexor carpi radialis to extensor digitorum communis transfer gives finger extension, and the palmaris longus or flexor digitorum superficialis of the fourth finger transfer to the extensor pollicis longus extends the thumb. Restoration of thumb opposition is most important with median nerve palsies, and the use of several donor muscles to achieve this result has been described including the extensor indices proprius and flexor digitorum superficialis from the middle or ring fingers. Tendon transfers to control claw deformity and strengthen key pinch are used for ulnar nerve palsies.

Brandsma JW, Ottenhoff-De Jonge MW: Flexor digitorum superficialis tendon transfer for intrinsic replacement. Long-term results and the effect on donor fingers. J Hand Surg [Br] 1992;17:625.

Dvali L, Mackinnon S: Nerve repair, grafting, and nerve transfers. Clin Plast Surg 2003;30:203.
Hentz VR: Surgical strategy: matching the patient with the procedure. Hand Clin 2002;18:503.
Ozkan T, Ozer K, Gulgonen A: Three tendon transfer methods in reconstruction of ulnar nerve palsy. J Hand Surg [Am] 2003;28:35.
Richards RR: Tendon transfers for failed nerve reconstruction. Clin Plast Surg 2003;30:223.
Tung TH, Mackinnon SE: Brachial plexus injuries. Clin Plast Surg 2003;30:269.
Verdugo RJ et al: Surgical versus non-surgical treatment for carpal tunnel syndrome. Cochrane Database Syst Rev 2002;2: CD001552.

▼ HAND INFECTIONS

Small breaks in the skin or nails of the hand can lead to widespread infection and abscess. The original injury often cannot be identified. Poor venous and lymphatic drainage of the upper extremity, especially when held in a dependent position, aggravate the situation. Immunocompromised patients (diabetics, HIV-positive patients) are prone to develop extensive infections very quickly and should be treated more carefully.

The hallmark of infection (pain, swelling, and erythema) may be widespread in the hand and make localizing the infection difficult. Swelling of the dorsum of the hand is common even with palmar infections, and knowledge of the tissue planes of the hand is crucial to understanding how infections spread. Lymphatic streaks (lymphangitis) extending up the arm indicate rapid extension of the infection and must be treated urgently.

Oral antibiotics effective against staphylococcus and common anaerobic organisms (ie, first-generation cephalosporins and penicillin) are adequate to treat most infections. Infections from animal bites (*Pasteurella multocida*) and human bites (oral flora) also respond to penicillin. The intravenous route is reserved for severe infections or for those not responsive to oral antibiotics. Once the situation improves, oral antibiotics are given for 7–10 days. Equally as important, the infected hand needs to be immobilized and elevated. Pillows and trapezes help to elevate the arm, but elbow slings aggravate the dependent position of the arm and should not be used. The best results are obtained when the patient is convinced that elevation of the extremity is beneficial.

Once treatment of a hand infection has begun, improvement within 24 hours is expected. If prompt improvement does not occur, an occult abscess may be present. Obvious abscesses should be drained at the point of maximum tenderness or the point of maximum fluctuance, where the overlying tissues are thinnest. The drainage wound should run parallel to and not across the paths of nerves, arteries, and veins. Wounds should be made long enough and should be zigzagged, when necessary, to avoid secondary contractures. Ultrasonography may be useful when a definite abscess cannot be located.

Pyogenic Granuloma

Pyogenic granuloma is a mound of granulation-like tissue 3–20 mm (or more) in diameter. It usually develops under a chronically moist dressing and may form around a suture. A small granuloma (6–7 mm in diameter) exposed to the air will soon dry up and epithelialize, whereas larger ones should be scraped flush with the skin under local anesthesia and covered with a thin split-thickness skin graft. If the granuloma is adjacent to the nail and the nail is acting as a foreign body aggravating the reaction, the nail must be removed.

Nail Infections

The nail fold is often traumatized and becomes secondarily inflamed, leading to a **paronychia** on the radial or ulnar side. The lesion is termed an **eponychia** if it involves the base of the nail, although the entire fold can be involved; and it is called a **subungual abscess** if pus develops and extends under the nail plate. Because of the early and unrelenting tissue tension that develops, these entities are quite painful. Early treatment before abscess formation consists of soaking, elevation, immobilization, and antibiotics. Most abscesses can be drained painlessly with a scalpel; the insensate necrotic skin cap should be cut through where it points (Figure 42–16). Sagittal incisions, which form a "trapdoor" of the eponychium, should be reserved for the longstanding case in which a dense fibrous callus of the nail fold must be excised. Occasionally, the nail must be basally excised or totally avulsed, after which the eponychial fold should be separated from the nail matrix by a thin, loose pack. Chronically wet nails of dishwashers may develop tissue changes and nail deformities, which are best treated by removing the nail plate. Fungal infections should be diagnosed and treated, and the fingers should be protected from water or excessive sweating.

Deep Space Abscess

A **felon** is an abscess in the pulp of the fingertip and is often deep and very painful. Untreated or inadequately drained abscesses may lead to osteomyelitis of the distal phalanx. Incision and drainage with disruption of the many vertical fibrous septa of the pulp space are required to adequately

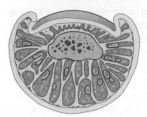

▲ **Figure 42–17.** Cross section of distal phalanx.

drain the abscess (Figure 42–17). The traditional fishmouth incision is no longer recommended for drainage since it may expose the underlying bone and because it often heals in a tender scar. Instead, lateral through-and-through incisions or direct incisions on the pulp, where the abscess points, have better results (Figure 42–18).

The **web spaces** are the path of least resistance for pus from infected distal palm calluses, puncture wounds, and infections of the lumbrical canals. Infection and abscess formation in the dorsum of the thumb web may be the result of extension from the volar thenar space (collar button). A dorsal incision is usually made between the fingers to drain both spaces. A dorsal incision in the web of the thumb may be zigzagged to prevent contracture (Figure 42–10).

The **midpalmar space** becomes infected by direct puncture or by extension of infections from the flexor sheaths of the index, middle, or ring fingers (Figure 42–6). Only the skin should be incised over the point of fluctuance. The rest of the dissection should be carried out by gentle spreading with a blunt clamp to avoid injury to arteries, nerves, and tendons. Infection spreads easily from this space along the lumbrical canals and to the thenar space.

A hypothenar space abscess is usually a product of a penetrating wound and should be drained at the point of greatest fluctuance. The same is true for a thenar space abscess, which may point in the palm rather than the thumb web.

Infection within the synovium of the flexor tendon is difficult to diagnose. **Pyogenic tenosynovitis** spreads easily down the tendon sheath to affect the other fingers. Untreated, the infection causes adhesions of the tendon to

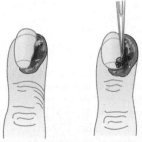

▲ **Figure 42–16.** Incision and drainage of paronychia.

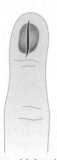

▲ **Figure 42–18.** Incision of felon (distal fat pad infection).

the surrounding soft tissues and permanently limits movement of the fingers.

The signs of flexor tendon infection described by Kanaval include fusiform swelling of the digit, severe pain on passive finger extension, a fixed flexed position of the finger, and most importantly, tenderness over the extent of the tendon sheath into the palm. Ultrasonography of the distal palm can also be helpful when the diagnosis is unclear. The probe is held across the palm and reveals swelling of the involved tendon and fluid around the tendon at the proximal flexor sheath.

Only unresponsive, tensely swollen, and toxic cases need immediate incision and drainage. With rest, elevation, and antibiotics, it is safe to observe most cases for several hours. The most common method of incision and drainage (Figure 42–19) is to make a short sagittal midline distal wound immediately over the tendon and introduce a small plastic catheter into the synovial bursa for irrigating with an antibiotic solution. The catheter should pass through the sheath and exit by a counterincision in the palm to allow for drainage of the fluid. Not all surgeons advocate placement of an irrigation catheter, however. When a catheter is placed, it should remain for only 24–48 hours. These incisions do not cross flexion creases. The hand should then be elevated and immobilized in the position of function and covered by a dressing. Phlegmonous tenosynovitis usually requires opening of the entire synovial sheath (often through a lateral midaxial digital incision or longitudinally across the wrist for extensor sheath infections) and, frequently, excision of necrotic tendon and sometimes amputation of a digit.

▶ Other Infections

Necrotizing soft tissue infections of the upper extremity are rare but devastating when they occur. The condition has been called many different names such as necrotizing fasciitis, Meleney ulcer, and streptococcal gangrene. The organisms responsible include clostridium species, *Streptococcus pyogenes,* and mixed infections. The hallmarks are the rapid spread of infection and the extensive necrosis of soft tissue. Treatment includes wide debridement of the necrotic tissue and intravenous antibiotics.

Human bite wounds of the hand occur most often during altercations when the fist strikes an opponent's tooth. The MCP joint can be entered. The injury is often ignored by the patient until infection of the joint has begun. The joint must be explored and cleaned and the patient treated with antibiotics to cover oral flora (penicillin). Once the infection reaches the joint, destruction of the cartilage often occurs despite all therapy.

An inordinate amount of pain, with little or no swelling or induration, predating and accompanying the appearance of multiple tiny vesicles, suggests **herpes simplex (herpetic whitlow).** The vesicles may appear cyclically. They contain clear fluid and not pus and should be distinguished from paronychias. Antibiotics are not indicated in this self-limited viral infection. Acyclovir 5% ointment applied topically for 7 days decreases the severity and duration of symptoms but is of no value in prophylaxis.

Tuberculous infection of the hand is usually chronic and may be relatively painless. Some cultures take months to become positive. Tuberculosis commonly involves only one hand, which may be the only focus of infection in the body. Bones and joints may be infected, but the process more commonly involves the tendon synovium, which becomes matted to the tendons. Treatment is by synovectomy and antituberculous drug therapy for 6–12 months.

Leprosy causes neuritis of the median and ulnar nerves, resulting in sensory and motor loss to the hand. Crippling claw deformities develop as a result of intrinsic muscle palsy. Open sores appear on the hands as a result of trauma to anesthetic digits. Reconstructive surgery and occupational training are required.

Fungal infections involve primarily the nails. Tinea unguium (onychomycosis) may be caused by many organisms, including *Epidermophyton floccosum,* trichophyton, and *Candida albicans.* Prolonged treatment with antifungal drugs—griseofulvin systemically or nystatin topically—may be necessary, along with daily applications of fungicidal agents such as tolnaftate. Removal of the nail is advocated for chronic intractable cases.

Jebson PJ: Infections of the fingertip. Paronychias and felons. Hand Clin 1998;14:547.

Lille S et al: Continuous postoperative catheter irrigation is not necessary for the treatment of suppurative flexor tenosynovitis. J Hand Surg [Br] 2000;25:304.

Perron AD, Miller MD, Brady WJ: Orthopedic pitfalls in the ED: fight bite. Am J Emerg Med 2002;20:114.

Spann M, Talmor M, Nolan WB: Hand infections: basic principles and management. Surg Infect (Larchmt) 2004;5:210.

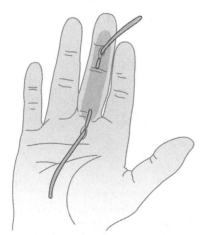

▲ **Figure 42–19.** Drainage and irrigation for septic tenosynovitis. The antibiotic solution drips in through the distal catheter and drains out through the proximal one.

INFLAMMATORY DISORDERS OF THE HAND

DUPUYTREN CONTRACTURE

▶ Palmar Fasciitis

The cause of Dupuytren contracture, which is common particularly among white populations of Celtic origin, is not known. It occurs in one of three types (acute, subacute, and chronic), predominately in males over 50 who have been in sedentary occupations, and is bilateral in about half of cases. There is a hereditary influence, and the incidence is higher among idiopathic epileptics, diabetics, alcoholics, and patients with chronic illnesses. The contracture may develop in people who do not work and (in laborers) in the hand that does the least work, so that it is not considered work related. It is frequently found in the plantar fascia of the instep and occasionally in the penis (Peyronie disease).

Dupuytren contracture manifests itself most commonly in the palm by thickening, which may be nodular, and therefore mistaken for a callosity, or may be cordlike, and therefore mistaken for a tendon abnormality because it passes into the digits and restricts their extension. This process typically involves the longitudinal and vertical components of the fascia but at times seems to exist apart from anatomically distinct fascia. The skin may fuse with the underlying fascia and become raised and hard, or it may be greatly shrunken and sometimes drawn into a deeply puckered crevasse. The disorder invades the palm at the expense of fat but is never adherent to vessels, nerves, or musculotendinous structures (though it may be adherent to flexor tendon sheaths). It has an unpredictable rate of progression, but the earlier it starts in life, the more destructive and recurrent it is apt to be.

Dupuytren fasciitis may involve any digit or web space, but it affects predominantly the ring and small fingers. In longstanding cases, the fingers may be drawn tightly into the palm, resulting in secondary contracture of joint capsule and ligaments, flexor sheaths, and atrophic muscles.

Surgery is indicated when the disorder has progressed sufficiently, especially when it causes more than 30 degrees of flexion at the MCP joint or any flexion contracture of the PIP joint. The patient must be warned about the increasing technical difficulty with progressive flexion and adduction contractures and the potential for recurrence after surgery. Fasciectomy is the surgical procedure that gives the best long-term results. In selected cases where only the longitudinal pretendinous fascial band is involved and the skin moves freely over it, subcutaneous fasciotomy done through a small longitudinal incision may release a contracture quite well with only a few days of postoperative disability. In the occasional case with acute and rapid onset of a tender nodule, local triamcinolone may be used for subjective and even objective relief.

Depending on the amount of cutaneous shrinkage, skin grafts may be required for wound closure after fasciectomy. The overlying dermis has been implicated as an inductive mechanism in this process. Thus, skin grafting may diminish the recurrence rate in severe cases. The hopelessly contracted little finger must sometimes be amputated.

Motion should be started within 3–5 days after surgery. Dynamic splints and postoperative injection of corticosteroids into joints and the zone of surgery may help the well-motivated patient.

The potential complications of surgery are wound breakdown (loss of skin flaps), hematoma, fibrosis and stiffness, digital nerve injury, recurrence of contractures and digital ischemia secondary to digital artery injury. Reflex sympathetic dystrophy, a painful, debilitating neurologic disorder of the hand, can occur after surgery and must be treated aggressively. In general, the functional reward for the patient is great at any age.

Draviaraj KP, Chakrabarti I: Functional outcome after surgery for Dupuytren's contracture: a prospective study. J Hand Surg [Am] 2004;29:804.
Shaw RB Jr et al: Dupuytren's disease: history, diagnosis, and treatment. Plast Reconstr Surg 2007;120:44e.
Skoff HD: The surgical treatment of Dupuytren's contracture: a synthesis of techniques. Plast Reconstr Surg 2004;113:540.

DEGENERATIVE & RHEUMATOID ARTHRITIS

Arthritis of the hand is divided into two categories. **Degenerative changes** are usually due to some trauma resulting in damage to the bone or cartilage or to the supporting ligamentous structures. The increased wear to the joint results in inflammation and damage to the cartilage or underlying bone followed by reactive new bone formation (spurs). The wrists, hips, and knees are most commonly affected. **Rheumatoid arthritis** is a systemic disease characterized by synovial inflammation. The diseased synovium destroys adjacent tendons and joints in a specific way, leading to characteristic deformities in the hand.

Patients with degenerative arthritis complain of pain, aching, and stiffness in the area of the affected joint. Progression of the problem leads to immobility of the joint that affects the entire hand. Radiographic studies demonstrate joint narrowing and periosteal thickening early in the problem, progressing to bone spurs, loss of the articular surface, and bone destruction later. Patients with rheumatoid arthritis often present with very severe deformities without pain. Nodules around the olecranon and dorsum of the hand are often found. Both flexor and extensor tendons at the wrist can be inflamed, limiting tendon movement and resulting in rupture of the tendon. Involvement of the tendons and ligaments at the digits and MCP joints results in ulnar deviation of the digits, MCP joint destruction and dislocation, and swan-neck and boutonnière deformities. Destruction of the wrist joint is also common.

Arthritis is common among older patients and usually treated by primary care physicians and rheumatologists with anti-inflammatory medications and modification of the patient's activities. In most cases, it is only when symptoms greatly hinder the patient's lifestyle that they are referred to a hand surgeon. Physical therapy, splints, and medications are often no longer effective for these patients.

Surgical treatment of painful joints includes replacement with a prosthetic joint and partial or full fusion. Prosthetic joints of metal or Silastic permit near-normal movement but can become unstable and dislocate or degenerate over time. For a durable solution to the problem, fusion of the joint is recommended. Motion is severely limited, but pain relief is complete. There are more therapeutic options for the wrist, such as replacement, local fusion of only the affected carpal bone, or complete excision of the proximal row of carpal bones, leaving motion and stability to the distal carpal bones and ligaments.

Therapy for synovial inflammation in rheumatoid disease includes excision of the synovium to increase tendon excursion and prevent rupture, repair of ruptured tendons, and excision of painful nodules. Tendon-balancing procedures can help ulnar deviation of the MCP joints and improve joint movement. The most important concept of treating patients with rheumatoid hand disease is that often the patients have adapted well to their functional deficits. Correcting a physical deformity in a well-compensated patient may actually result in more problems for that patient.

Adamson GJ et al: Flexible implant resection arthroplasty of the proximal interphalangeal joint in patients with systemic inflammatory arthritis. J Hand Surg [Am] 1994;19:378.

Alderman AK et al: Effectiveness of rheumatoid hand surgery: contrasting perceptions of hand surgeons and rheumatologists. J Hand Surg [Am] 2003;28:3.

Cavaliere CM, Chung KC: A systemic review of total wrist arthroplasty compared with total wrist arthrodesis for rheumatoid arthritis. Plast Reconstr Surg 2008;122:813.

Ferlic DC: Rheumatoid flexor tenosynovitis and rupture. Hand Clin 1996;12:561.

Wilson RL, DeVito MC: Extensor tendon problems in rheumatoid arthritis. Hand Clin 1996;12:551.

SCLERODERMA & LUPUS ERYTHEMATOSUS

These systemic diseases of unknown cause have distinctive—though not necessarily pathognomonic—manifestations in the hands.

Scleroderma initially produces joint stiffness, hyperhidrosis, and Raynaud phenomenon. Unchecked, it leads to marked tautness of skin and rigidity of joints with associated osteoporosis (even atrophy and ultimate resorption of the distal phalanges) and soft tissue calcifications.

Lupus erythematosus, which may be initiated or aggravated by certain drugs, foreign proteins, or psychic states, often causes polyarthritis indistinguishable from that of rheumatoid arthritis. It does not usually lead to similar joint destruction. Vasospasm in both lupus and scleroderma can cause severe ischemia of the hand and digits and may require therapy to prevent gangrene.

GOUT

Gout is a metabolic disorder of uric acid metabolism that affects about 1% of the population; approximately 50% of patients with gout have **cheiragra** (gouty hands).

The diagnosis is suggested by a rapid onset of severe pain and inflammatory signs about the joints and musculotendinous structure, simulating a phlegmonous infectious cellulitis with marked induration (most dramatically seen about the elbow). The usual duration of an attack is 5–10 days. The serum uric acid is elevated in 75% of cases. Gout may coexist with rheumatoid disease. The diagnosis is confirmed by identification of uric acid crystals in joint fluid or tissue biopsy.

In time, typical tophi form, consisting of toothpaste-like infiltrates of urate crystals, arising in multilobulated form about soft tissue structures that have been invaded. X-rays show characteristic punched-out lesions at the margins of articular cartilage.

Prophylactic treatment of gouty arthritis consists of diet, colchicine, allopurinol (a urate-blocking agent) or probenecid (a uricosuric agent), and avoidance of stress. Colchicine, 0.6 mg/h with a glass of water for 6–8 doses or to the point of gastrointestinal distress, is the time-honored means of interrupting an attack, but phenylbutazone, topical corticotropin gel, and systemic corticosteroids are also of value.

Surgical measures consist of drainage of abscessed tophi (seldom needed) and tophectomy. The latter procedure is more often of cosmetic rather than functional value. Tophectomy consists of removal of as much tophaceous material as can be fairly easily recovered. The surgeon should be careful not to destroy ligaments, tenoretinacular structures, nerves, and vessels in the process.

Gilbart MK et al: Surgery of the hand in severe systemic sclerosis. J Hand Surg [Br] 2004;29:599.

Nalebuff EA: Surgery of systemic lupus erythematosus arthritis of the hand. Hand Clin 1996;12:591.

Schuind FA et al: Gouty involvement of flexor tendons. Chir Main 2003;22:46.

BURNS & FROSTBITE OF THE HAND

▶ Thermal Burns

The hands are a common site of thermal (including frictional), electrical, chemical, and radiation burns. Function is imperiled in all instances by swelling and scar formation. Prompt measures to preserve existing function are often urgently required. Burns over other areas of the body may be more life threatening and require more urgent attention, but burns of the hand should never be neglected. Delay in therapy leads to irreversible impairment and deformity that are impossible to correct later.

As in other areas of the body, thermal burns are grouped into three degrees. Superficial (first-degree) burns are red and painful; partial-thickness (second-degree) burns develop blisters; and full-thickness (third-degree) burns are insensate and appear like leather or charred tissue. The prognosis and therapy depend on the location, depth, and extent of the burn.

All burns to the hand cause swelling of the tissues, and the need for elevation of the arm to relieve pain and prevent stiffness cannot be overemphasized. Tetanus immunization should be given. Cold compresses may help alleviate the pain in first-degree burns. Second-degree burns must be watched more carefully. Large blisters restricting motion are broken. Otherwise, since they are sterile, they should be left intact. Treatment with thrice-daily washing and silver sulfadiazine is usually adequate. Patients with third-degree burns or superficial burns that fail to heal and patients unable to care for their burns at home should be admitted to the hospital.

Deeper burns require close observation and more extensive treatment. In the first few hours after injury, circumferential or near-circumferential burns may cause ischemia in the extremity. Because evaluation of sensory function and capillary refill is nearly impossible in these limbs, escharotomies should be performed if compartment syndrome is suspected. If done correctly, escharotomies have few complications, since these burns usually require surgical debridement anyway. Incisions are placed to avoid exposure of neurovascular structures.

Partial-thickness burns heal spontaneously. Deeper burns on the dorsum of the hand are best treated with early excision of the eschar and placement of skin grafts to prevent contractures. Palmar burns are best left to heal spontaneously because skin grafts function very poorly in this area. Some hand surgeons believe that excision and grafting of superficial burns should be performed to prevent contractures. This is true if adequate therapy has not been available. In burn units with good rehabilitation services, surgeons are treating superficial second-degree burns without surgery and obtaining results as good as with skin grafting. Pigskin, cadaver homografts, or a number of commercially available biologic dressings can be used to cover the wounds temporarily, decreasing pain and keeping the wound moist until autologous skin grafts are placed.

Neglected burns of the hands result in contracture deformities that often require extensive surgery to restore function. Delayed healing and wound contractures often result in a claw hand with MCP hyperextension and fusion of the digits with loss of the web space (syndactyly). Burns on the volar surface leave flexion contractures. Some contractures can be treated with release and skin grafting of the tissue gap. Web space contractures and released contractures with exposed tendons or nerves must be covered with skin or muscle flaps. Web space release is done with skin flaps from the dorsum folded down to create the space. Large flaps can be obtained by attaching the hand to the groin, allowing the tissue to adhere and vascularize before cutting the flap away from the groin. Recently, free tissue transfer from other parts of the body using microsurgical techniques has allowed more extensive reconstruction of severely burned hands.

▶ Electrical Burns

Electrical burns of the upper extremity may not appear extensive on initial inspection. The skin may be burned only in a very small area of the entry point of the current or by ignited clothing. The current tends to spare the skin but damage underlying muscles, vessels, and nerves. Often, the extent of dead tissue is not evident for several days.

Initial treatment is the same as for thermal burns. Since muscle damage may be extensive, it is important to prevent renal failure from myoglobinuria by maintaining a high output of alkaline urine. Arteriography, fluorescein injections, and radionuclide studies may help delineate the extent of necrosis. Examination of the patient in the operating room is still the most accurate method of assessing the extent of tissue damage. All obviously dead tissue should be removed during the initial evaluation. Two or three days later, the patient is reexamined in the operating room and any additional debris is removed. The wounds are closed when only clearly viable tissue remains.

▶ Frostbite

Frostbite occurs most often in people under the influence of alcohol or with psychiatric illness. The lower extremity is affected more often than the upper. Freezing tissue causes cellular death and vascular thrombosis. Hypothermia of the entire body must first be treated. The frozen part should be quickly rewarmed by immersion in warm water (40 °C). Elevation of the extremity minimizes edema. Skin wounds are treated like burns with silver sulfadiazine cream. The extent of necrosis may not be obvious for several weeks, and debridement or amputation should be delayed until demarcation of the injury occurs. Sympathectomy may help ameliorate the sequelae of frostbite, such as cold sensitivity and pain. Children with frostbite may develop premature closure of phalangeal epiphyses, which creates growth disturbances of the bone.

Smith MA, Munster AM, Spence RJ: Burns of the hand and upper limb—a review. Burns 1998;24:493.

Su CW, Lohman R, Gottlieb LJ: Frostbite of the upper extremity. Hand Clin 2000;16:235.

Tredget EE, Shankowsky HA, Tilley WA: Electrical injuries in Canadian burn care. Identification of unsolved problems. Ann N Y Acad Sci 1999;888:75.

Umraw N et al: Effective hand function assessment after burn injuries. J Burn Care Rehabil 2004;25:134.

MASSES OF THE HAND

Only 2% of all masses in the hand are malignant lesions; the majority are benign neoplasms, cysts, or a myriad of other masses. Though the clinician must be ever vigilant to identify malignancy, a mass of the hand is highly likely to be benign—excisional biopsies are thus reserved for subcutaneous lesions that are rapidly growing or for skin lesions that may be carcinomas. Otherwise, masses can be observed over a period of time to determine that they are not growing. They may be removed for functional or cosmetic reasons.

Ganglions are formed by herniation of the synovial lining of joints or tendons into the surrounding soft tissue. These cysts are filled with a viscous fluid thought to be modified joint fluid. Trauma to the wrist or hand may cause extrusion of the synovium, but it is more likely that the ganglion was already present and that trauma to that area merely brought the lesion to the surgeon's attention.

Ganglions can arise from any joint of the hand but most commonly appear on the dorsal wrist over the scapholunate ligament and the volar wrist near the radial artery. Tendon ganglions are most common on the flexor sheath at the metacarpal head (A1 pulley). Pain and tenderness are due to compression of adjacent nerves by the mass.

Ganglions have a typical appearance, and diagnosis is simple. If any doubt exists, aspiration with a large-bore needle of the viscous fluid confirms the diagnosis and occasionally cures the lesions. Injection of the empty sac with steroids and lidocaine may help to keep the mass from reappearing, but the majority recur. Ganglions need not be treated unless they cause pain or interfere with hand function. Often, it is enough just to reassure the patient that the mass is benign.

Operative removal of ganglions should be done using loupe magnification and a tourniquet. The entire ganglion should be removed, including all attachments to the joint capsule and the underlying ligament, without injuring the surrounding structures. Prolonged splinting after removal of ganglions does not decrease recurrence rates but does cause hand stiffness. Unfortunately, despite careful surgical removal of the lesion, recurrence of ganglions is relatively common.

Epidermal cysts are rests of epidermis located in the subcutaneous tissue. Many are thought to be due to traumatic disruption of epidermal cells into the soft tissue (inclusion cyst). The cells proliferate just as skin does and form a cyst filled with creamy keratin, the remains of dead epidermal cells that usually desquamate from the skin. Infected cysts become inflamed and form abscesses. Removal of the entire cyst wall is required to prevent abscess formation.

Pyogenic granuloma may form in any chronic wound. Histologically, it consists of vascular tissue identical to granulation tissue. Just as for hypertrophic granulation tissue elsewhere on the body, excision or cautery of the material flush to skin level allows epidermis to migrate over the wound.

Giant cell tumors are benign, multilobulated, solid masses found on the lateral aspects of the finger. They are often attached to the tendon sheath. The mass may be quite complex and extend throughout the adjacent nerves, vessels, tendons, and ligaments. The entire lesion should be removed, but recurrence is relatively common.

The most common bone tumors are **enchondromas.** Multiple enchondromas (Ollier disease) are associated with other skeletal deformities. The lesion appears on x-ray as thinned cortical bone with speckled calcifications. Fractures through the tumors usually do not heal spontaneously. The tumor should be removed with a curette. Bone graft taken from the distal radius is used to fill the gap if needed.

A **carpal boss** is due to abnormal bone formation at the base of the second or third metacarpal bones and presents as a hard mass on the dorsum of the hand. The excess growth of bone can be removed if symptomatic.

Glomus tumors are composed of blood vessels and unmyelinated nerves of a heat-regulating arteriovenous malformation. They are usually found in the fingertip or under the fingernail and can be extremely painful. Local excision of the tumor is curative. Occasionally, when the tumor is large and disrupts the nail matrix, a split-thickness nail graft from another digit is needed to reconstruct the defect.

The most common malignant tumor of the hand is **squamous cell carcinoma,** though **basal cell carcinomas** and **melanomas** also occur. Subungual melanomas are often difficult to diagnose because they are difficult to examine. These tumors should be treated just the same as elsewhere on the body. Particular care should be taken to examine for spread of tumor in the lymphatic drainage at the supratrochlear and axillary nodes.

Other tumors include lipomas, fibromas, hemangiomas, arteriovenous malformations, neurofibromas, sarcomas, and various skin lesions. These tumors act no differently in the hand than elsewhere in the body. However, because of the close proximity of the nervous and vascular structures within the small spaces of the hand, these tumors cause compressive signs and symptoms sooner. CT scans or MRI help delineate the extent of soft tissue tumors and may help in preoperative planning.

Nahra ME, Bucchieri JS: Ganglion cysts and other tumor related conditions of the hand and wrist. Hand Clin 2004;20:249.
Peterson JJ, Bancroft LW, Kransdorf MJ: Principles of bone and soft tissue imaging. Hand Clin 2004;20:147.
Trigg SD: Biopsy of hand, wrist, and forearm tumors. Hand Clin 2004;20:131.

COMPLEX HAND INJURIES

▶ Crush Injuries & Amputations

Advances in microvascular surgery have greatly increased our ability to treat complex hand injuries. Mangled and amputated digits, hands, as well as entire upper extremities have been replanted or repaired. Complex nerve repairs, microvascular free tissue transfers of muscle flaps, and toe-to-hand reconstructions have made it possible to restore more function to severely injured hands. The end result must be a sensate, painless, and useful extremity. Patients who undergo multiple surgical procedures and prolonged rehabilitation with only marginal results would have benefited from early amputation. A surgeon with extensive experience can best assess the patient's injuries, occupational requirements, and psychosocial needs to determine if salvage is worthwhile.

Complex hand injuries often result from improper use or malfunction of machinery. Heavy machinery in the workplace or motorized cutting tools at home, such as rotary saws, are often cited as the mechanism of injury. Sharply amputated or partially devascularized parts are most likely to be saved. Severe crushing or avulsion of the part produces wider nerve and vessel injury. The extent of this type of damage is difficult to determine and often impossible to repair.

The decision to try to salvage a damaged part must be individualized to each situation, but some general principles apply. The thumb is crucial to hand function, and all efforts are made to save the entire digit or as much length as possible. When multiple digits or half of the hand is damaged or amputated, a greater effort is made to repair the part. Children can recover function in badly damaged extremities far better than adults can, and any amputated parts in children should be replanted. Replantation of the entire arm at the elbow and above is controversial. The usefulness of these replanted limbs is limited by the slow nerve regeneration, and some hand surgeons believe that amputations in these cases result in better function.

Patients with complex hand injuries should be immediately referred to a regional center with the staff and facilities to manage the problems. Occasionally, in the rush to transfer patients with these very obvious injuries, intra-abdominal, neurologic, and other less obvious injuries have been overlooked. The entire patient must be evaluated and stabilized prior to transfer. A clean, moist dressing should be placed on the wound and the extremity elevated. The amputated part is wrapped in a plastic bag and placed in ice water. The amputated part should never be frozen.

The accepting hand surgeon evaluates the patient's overall condition, potential for rehabilitation, and personal wishes before coming to a decision. To revascularize or replant a part, the patient must be taken urgently to the operating room. Ischemia over 6 hours is often associated with failure of revascularization, but—depending on the metabolic needs of the constituent tissues—extremities that have undergone periods of ischemia longer than this can be successfully replanted.

Bone must first be stabilized with Kirschner wires or metal plates before vascular repairs are performed. Arterial and venous repairs are done with microscopic magnification, and the ischemic tissue is reperfused. Failure of a replanted part is more often due to venous outflow problems than arterial inflow. Systemic and local anticoagulants help to maintain perfusion but are not always needed. Leeches placed on the part release a potent local anticoagulant and can decrease venous congestion. Nerve and tendon repairs must also be performed. When there is inadequate local soft tissue to cover the repaired structures, muscle or skin flaps from a distant site must be transferred using microsurgical methods to the area. Although these operations are not life threatening, blood loss can be extensive and transfusions are sometimes required.

Secondary procedures to free tendon adhesions, reduce bulky flaps, and transfer tendons in motor nerve injuries may need to be done. Reconstruction of unsuccessful replantations is being done more often. The original method using toes to reconstruct thumbs has also been used to make fingers. These reconstructions give patients the ability to grasp objects. Because these digits are sensate, they can even perform fine movement tasks not possible with prosthetic devices. Patients with loss only of the thumb are better treated with transfer of the index finger to the thumb position (pollicization).

Partial or total loss of a single digit is less critical. Hand function is better without a stiff or painful digit. When a decision is made to amputate a digit, care must be taken to leave a painless stump with good sensate soft tissue coverage. The flexor tendon must not be sutured to the extensor tendon for soft tissue coverage, since this will cause the tendons to pull each other rather than move the joint. Local flaps to cover the stump are preferred to skin grafts or cross-finger flaps, since they usually provide better sensation. A short amputation stump on the long or ring finger is often bothersome because small objects such as coins tend to fall out of the palm, and a ray amputation eliminates the problem. For cosmetic purposes, ray amputations are far less noticeable than partial amputations. The loss of hand breadth with a ray amputation can decrease grip strength, however.

The loss of part of all of the hand can be compensated both functionally and cosmetically by a variety of prostheses. Their use involves careful adaptation to the requirements of the patient, who must receive appropriate training to ensure success.

INJECTION INJURIES OF THE HAND

High-pressure devices used in industry to apply material such as air, grease, paint, and oil cause a unique hand injury. The typical case is injection of the material into the index finger of the nondominant hand of a factory worker. A pinpoint injection site may be the only external evidence of injury, and the hand appears discolored or pale, or swollen due to the injected material.

The examination should include a careful hand evaluation and an x-ray to demonstrate the distribution of material or gas in the hand. All such cases require continued, unrelenting scrutiny, even if the part seems completely normal. If there is any evidence of retained foreign material, swelling, or ischemia, early surgical exploration is advocated to release the tourniquet effect of the skin and fascia and to remove as much of the material as possible without injuring healthy tissue. Prophylactic antisludging agents (dextran 40), corticosteroids, and antibiotics may help.

Often, the pressure forces the material to spread along the tendon sheaths throughout the hand and even into the forearm. Expansion of the foreign material in a closed space and the chemical irritation cause congestion, inflammation, vascular thrombosis, and gangrene. The injected material is difficult to remove completely, and a foreign body response leads to fibrosis so extensive that it often destroys the function of the hand.

Buncke HJ Jr: Microvascular hand surgery—transplants and replants—over the past 25 years. J Hand Surg [Am] 2000; 25:415.

Chen HC, Tang YB: Replantation of the thumb, especially avulsion. Hand Clin 2001;17:433.

Christodoulou L et al: Functional outcome of high-pressure injection injuries of the hand. J Trauma 2001;50:717.

Del Pinal F et al: Acute hand compartment syndromes after closed crush: a reappraisal. Plast Reconstr Surg 2002;110:1232.

Freeland AE, Lineaweaver WC, Lindley SG: Fracture fixation in the mutilated hand. Hand Clin 2003;19:51.

Woo SH, Kim JS, Seul JH: Immediate toe-to-hand transfer in acute hand injuries: overall results, compared with results for elective cases. Plast Reconstr Surg 2004;113:882.

MINIMALLY INVASIVE HAND SURGERY

The goal of reconstructive hand surgery is return of normal function, including pain-free movement, normal active and passive range of motion, premorbid strength, and intact sensation. Yet the process of incising, dissecting, and sewing is associated with significant scarring and pain. Scarring is especially troublesome in the hand, since it leads to stiffness, ligamental tightening, and arthritis. As a result, any procedure in the hand that minimizes postoperative scarring or pain will contribute to an improved result.

Surgical care in the past decade has been revolutionized by the introduction and incorporation of minimally invasive surgical techniques. Laparoscopies and thoracoscopies have permitted the resection of hollow and solid organs through 1 cm incisions, reducing the need for laparotomies and thoracotomies. Likewise, urologists have employed cystoscopy for evaluation and treatment of bladder and kidney disorders, while orthopedic surgeons have used arthroscopy to similar effective ends in the knee, ankle, elbow, and shoulder.

Two areas of hand surgery incorporate minimally invasive techniques: Wrist arthroscopy has expanded the options for evaluating the chronically painful wrist, and endoscopic carpal tunnel release (ECTR) provides a less invasive method than open release for decompressing the median nerve. While ECTR theoretically allows for a faster recovery, it may in fact offer only limited advantages.

WRIST ARTHROSCOPY

Diagnostic wrist arthroscopy was first successfully used in 1970. Over the past 3 decades, it has taken its place among traditional imaging techniques as a low-morbidity method for evaluating chronic wrist pain. As the hardware for examining the wrist has become more sophisticated and as hand surgeons have become more familiar with the arthroscopic view of the wrist, increasingly aggressive attempts have been made to use the arthroscope to treat as well as to diagnose wrist problems.

▶ Indications & Contraindications

Diagnostic wrist arthroscopy is a useful technique to evaluate patients with wrist pain, whether chronic or acute. In patients with chronic pain, this technique can be used to augment information offered by plain radiographs, CT, MRI, or wrist arthrography. It can confirm an uncertain diagnosis or be used to reevaluate a patient who has failed other treatments. In contrast, patients with acute symptoms—such as those suffering from mechanical wrist pain—may complain of pain localized over the joint, catching and popping sensations, and relief with rest. Here, the wrist can be manipulated during arthroscopy to localize the source of the symptoms. In general, the technique is useful for evaluating articular cartilage, ligaments, the triangular fibrocartilage complex (TFCC), and the synovium. Interestingly, diagnostic wrist arthroscopy may provide too comprehensive an examination. Only some of the lesions that are visualized during an examination may be responsible for a patient's symptoms. The hand surgeon must critically correlate arthroscopic findings with the patient's examination to arrive at the appropriate diagnosis.

Therapeutic wrist arthroscopy is useful for the treatment of ligament tears, TFCC lesions, articular cartilage lesions, subtle distal radius and carpus fractures, dorsal wrist ganglions, removal of isolated carpal bones up to and including the proximal carpal row, and disorders of the distal radioulnar joint. It is useful also in the management of lesions arising from rheumatoid arthritis. It has been successfully used in completing synovectomies, proximal row carpectomies in the case of scaphoid nonunion or scapholunate collapse, radial styloidectomy, and isolated symptomatic chondral defects.

▶ Procedure

Equipment for diagnostic wrist arthroscopy includes an apparatus for elevating and distracting the wrist, an arthroscopic telescope, a video camera, a fluid infusion system, and both manual and powered instruments.

Either general or regional anesthesia may be used. A tourniquet is placed at the mid arm to provide a blood-free field during the operation. The distal forearm, wrist, and hand are prepared into the operative field. Traction is applied to the hand, usually via sterile finger traps, and a distraction force is applied across the wrist.

Individual skin incisions are then made at standard portal sites determined by the goal of the operation. Portal sites are described according to their relationship with the radius and ulna, the carpal bones, and the extensor tendons. The relationship to the extensor tendons is indicated by listing the extensor compartments on either side of the incision. Typical portals include the 3–4 radiocarpal, through which the scaphoid and lunate facets can be visualized; the 4–5 radiocarpal, through which the TFCC and the ulnocarpal ligaments can be seen; and the 6R radiocarpal, through which the extensor carpi ulnaris tendon and ulnar wrist are approached. The midcarpal joint is approached through any of three portals, including the midcarpal ulnar, the midcarpal radial, and the scaphotrapezial-trapezoid.

Once abnormalities are identified, therapeutic wrist arthroscopy can be used to effect repairs. Partial ligament tears and tears of the TFCC can be debrided arthroscopically using knife blades and motorized shavers. Carpal bone resections can be completed with miniature osteotomes and powered saw blades.

Outcomes

Operations employing diagnostic and therapeutic wrist arthroscopy typically result in less swelling, less postoperative pain, and less stiffness than comparable open wrist procedures. There is a concomitant earlier return to function and work. Therapeutic wrist arthroscopy even of dorsal wrist ganglia, the most superficial of wrist abnormalities, is followed by fewer—or no more—recurrences than the open technique.

Complications

The rate of complications associated with diagnostic and therapeutic wrist arthroscopy is estimated to be 2% and is due to a variety of causes. The continuous traction necessary to properly distract the wrist can cause problems, including ligamental strain at the MCP joints with concomitant joint edema and stiffness and stretching of peripheral nerves. Establishment of the operative portals can damage articular cartilage, ligaments, tendons, cutaneous nerves, the radial artery, and cutaneous and deep veins. Such injuries include abrasions, contusions, lacerations, and transections. A high proportion of complications of therapeutic wrist arthroscopy are associated with inadequate relief of symptoms or a diminished return of function. A now less common complication of therapeutic wrist arthroscopy results from the fluid infusion. Forearm compartment syndromes have resulted from extravasation of infusion fluid during endoscopic repair of distal radius fractures; this problem is now avoided by circumferential compression of the forearm during the procedure.

ENDOSCOPIC CARPAL TUNNEL RELEASE

Endoscopic release of the transverse carpal ligament is an increasingly popular method of treating carpal tunnel syndrome. Advocates of the procedure claim that it is associated with decreased postoperative morbidity and earlier return to work. Others caution that there is little if any short-term difference between endoscopic and open carpal tunnel release, no long-term difference, and that endoscopic carpal tunnel release is associated with an increased likelihood of significant nerve injury.

Indications & Contraindications

Endoscopic carpal tunnel release is easier to perform in patients with larger wrists. Ease of access to the carpal tunnel correlates with the wrist circumference and the height and age of patients. Surgeons should be aware that the procedure is likely to be more difficult in small patients with small wrists and are advised to maintain a lower threshold for conversion to the open technique to avoid neurologic complications.

Absolute contraindications to endoscopic carpal tunnel release include masses in the carpal canal and other space-occupying lesions, abnormalities in canal anatomy, and wrist stiffness that precludes proper positioning.

Procedure

In the United States, most surgeons use one of two techniques—either Chow or Agee. The two differ primarily in the number of incisions, or portals, needed to gain access. The Chow technique, first described in 1989, employs two portals, while the Agee technique requires only one.

Either operation can be performed under local anesthesia with a brachial tourniquet. An initial transverse incision is made proximal to the wrist flexion crease between the palmaris longus and flexor carpi ulnaris tendons. The space between the transverse carpal ligament and the flexor tendons is defined with a dissector. In the Agee procedure, the endoscope is advanced under the transverse carpal ligament, radial to the hook of the hamate along the axis of the ring finger. The ligament is incised along its entire length, with care taken to avoid the Guyon canal and the superficial palmar arch. In the Chow operation, a second transverse incision is made just distal to the transverse carpal ligament along the axis of the ring finger. The wrist is dorsiflexed, and a slotted cannula is advanced into the proximal incision, deep to the transverse carpal ligament, and out the distal incision. The endoscope is then used to visualize the ligament while the knife divides it. The wounds are closed, and the patient's wrist placed in dorsiflexion.

Outcomes

Several studies have compared open versus endoscopic carpal tunnel release, focusing on the incidence of recovery from symptoms, the time span until the patient returns to work, and the incidence of recurrence of symptoms. Overall, both techniques have equivalent outcomes.

Many of the most convincing studies are prospective randomized trials. One such study, comparing open and endoscopic carpal tunnel release among 32 hands in 29 patients, found no difference in postoperative recovery time or surgical result. The only significant difference noted by the authors was transient numbness on the radial side of the ring finger in three endoscopic carpal tunnel release patients.

In another study, the authors compared in a prospective randomized manner the early outcome of carpal tunnel release using either a conventional open carpal tunnel release procedure in 40 patients or a two-portal endoscopic release in 56 patients. They found no statistically significant difference between the groups in postoperative pain, recovery from paresthesias, or time taken to return to work. However, the endoscopic group demonstrated better grip strength recovery at 1 and 3 months. No surgical complications were observed in either group.

Nonrandomized studies have supported this trend. An analysis of 191 consecutive patients undergoing carpal tunnel release with an average 2-year follow-up showed that none of the patients undergoing open release had a recurrence, while 7% of patients undergoing endoscopic release had recurrences. Another study observed a higher incidence of incomplete release of the carpal tunnel with endoscopic techniques than with standard open releases.

The factors identified with poor outcomes in endoscopic carpal tunnel release are similar to those seen in open release. Less satisfactory results were present in workers' compensation cases; patients with normal motor latencies on nerve conduction studies; patients with preoperative hand weakness, widened two-point discrimination, myofascial pain syndrome, or fibromyalgia; and patients involved in litigation, those with multiple compressive neuropathies, and those with abnormal psychologic factors.

▶ Complications

Only a limited number of studies include a sufficient number of patients to compare complication rates and type between endoscopic and open carpal tunnel release. Overall, the types and rates of complications between the two forms of release are similar. Nonetheless, isolated but severe complications from endoscopic release over the past decade tend to dramatize its risk.

The study by Boeckstyns and Sorensen is perhaps the most comprehensive to date. These authors analyzed 54 published series of endoscopic and open releases comprising 9516 and 1203 patients, respectively. Irreversible nerve damage from the procedure occurred in 0.3% of endoscopic and 0.2% of open releases, including such injuries as transection of the median nerve. While reversible nerve injuries were more common with endoscopic release than with open release (4.4% versus 0.9%, respectively, among prospective controlled and randomized studies), tendon lesions, reflex sympathetic dystrophy, hematoma, and wound problems were equally common with either technique.

A less compelling analysis—a retrospective survey of hand surgeons who had performed either open or endoscopic carpal tunnel release over the preceding 5 years—found major complications with both approaches, including median nerve lacerations, ulnar nerve lacerations, digital nerve lacerations, vessel lacerations, and tendon lacerations. While the authors could not reach a conclusion about the rate of complications for one procedure versus the other, their results demonstrate the potentially devastating sequelae of carpal tunnel release even in experienced hands.

Carpal tunnel symptoms may persist or recur following either open or endoscopic release. In patients who have persistent symptoms following endoscopic release, many authors recommend open carpal tunnel release as definitive therapy.

Beredjiklian PK et al: Complications of wrist arthroscopy. J Hand Surg [Am] 2004;29:406.

Shih JT et al: Arthroscopically-assisted reduction of intra-articular fractures and soft tissue management of distal radius. Hand Surg 2001;6:127.

Slutsky DJ: Wrist arthroscopy through a volar radial portal. Arthroscopy 2002;18:624.

Thoma A et al: A systematic review of reviews comparing the effectiveness of endoscopic and open carpal tunnel decompression. Plast Reconstr Surg 2004;113:1184.

Pediatric Surgery

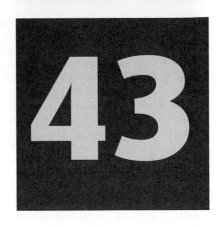

Craig T. Albanese, MD
Karl G. Sylvester, MD

Pediatric surgical patients are not merely small adults. The surgical care of children differs markedly from that of adults in many respects, including unique physiologic demands that vary according to age and development. The neonate's physiologic development is closer to that of a fetus, while adolescents' physiology is similar to that of adults, and infants and children have problems unique to their chronologic and developmental age. Infants and children also suffer from congenital abnormalities and diseases not seen in adults, and their management requires an intimate understanding of the relevant embryology and pathogenesis.

NEWBORN CARE

Neonatal Intensive Care

The newborn infant with a surgically correctable lesion often has other disorders that threaten survival. The care of these babies, particularly for premature and small-for-gestational-age (SGA) babies, has improved with the emergence of the intensive care nursery. Dramatic advances have been made in the technology of infant monitoring and respiratory support. Low-birth-weight infants can now receive ventilatory support from sophisticated infant respirators for prolonged periods in a precisely controlled microenvironment. Surfactant therapy and high-frequency ventilation has allowed a population of extremely premature infants to survive. Temperature is controlled by servoregulation, while pulse and blood pressure are continuously recorded. Ventilation is monitored by transcutaneous O_2 and CO_2 electrodes or by indwelling arterial catheters. The metabolic consequences of prematurity and intrauterine growth retardation are monitored by frequent measurement of glucose, calcium, electrolytes, and bilirubin in microliter quantities of blood. Nutritional requirements for growth and development can be provided by enteral or parenteral routes. This kind of specialized care of critically ill newborns requires trained personnel and specialized equipment. The care of such babies is best accomplished in designated regional centers capable of providing pediatric surgical and neonatal intensive care.

Phibbs CS et al: The effects of patient volume and level of care at the hospital of birth on neonatal mortality. JAMA 1996;276:1054.

Classification

Newborn infants can be classified according to their level of maturation (weight) and development (gestational age). A normal full-term infant has a gestational age of 37–42 weeks and a body weight greater than 2500 g. The gestational age of the infant is calculated from the date of the last normal menstrual period. However, clinical assessment of gestational age by morphologic and neurologic examination of the small infant can be more accurate than calculation from the menstrual history.

Four signs may be useful in assessing gestational age. Infants less than 37 weeks' gestational age have (1) fine fuzzy hair with thin, semitransparent skin, (2) ears that lack cartilaginous support, (3) a breast nodule less than 3 mm in diameter, and (4) few transverse creases on the balls of the feet anteriorly. In males, the testicles are incompletely descended and reside in the inguinal canal, and the scrotum is small with few rugae. In females, the labia minora are relatively enlarged and the labia majora are small.

Preterm infants are those born before 37 weeks' gestation. Several physiologic abnormalities may coexist in preterm infants. Apneic and bradycardic episodes are common and may represent an immature central nervous system or, conversely, may represent signs of physiologic instability, most notably with sepsis. The lungs and retinas of preterm infants are very susceptible to high oxygen levels. Retinopathy of prematurity from oxygen toxicity may lead to blindness. Relatively brief exposures to high oxygen concentrations, often coupled with barotrauma from the mechanical ventilator, may damage the lungs, resulting in hyaline membrane disease and respiratory distress syndrome. Shunting across a patent ductus arteriosus is not uncommon and may lead to pulmonary hemorrhage and congestive heart failure. The preterm infant has a friable choroids plexus and is thus susceptible to intraventricular hemorrhage when stressed in the first week of life. The premature infant may be unable to tolerate oral feeding because of a weak suck reflex. Tube feeds or total parenteral nutrition may be required. Preterm infants have increased requirements for glucose, calcium, and sodium as well as a propensity for hypothermia, impaired bilirubin metabolism, polycythemia, and metabolic acidosis. These problems are accentuated in very low-birth-weight infants or "micropremies" (birth weight less than 1000 g).

A SGA infant is one who is less than the 10th percentile in weight for their gestational age. An SGA infant is the product of a pregnancy complicated by any one of several placental, maternal, or fetal abnormalities. Although body weight is low, body length and head circumference are age-appropriate. Compared with the premature infant of equivalent weight, the SGA infant is developmentally more mature and faces different physiologic problems. Intrauterine malnutrition results in reduced body fat and decreased glycogen stores. Their relatively large surface area and high metabolic rate predisposes them to hypothermia and hypoglycemia. SGA infants also have an increased risk of meconium aspiration syndrome. Polycythemia (which may lead to complications of hyperviscosity syndrome) is common and necessitates close monitoring of their hematocrit. Because of their relatively mature organ development and function (compared to preterm infants), retinopathy of prematurity, intraventricular hemorrhage, and hyaline membrane disease are uncommon.

▶ Temperature Regulation

Infants and children are susceptible to heat loss because they have a relatively greater body surface area and a thinner subcutaneous fat layer compared with adults. Heat loss occurring by conduction, convection, evaporation, and radiation may be four times that of the adult and is further increased in the preterm infant. Infants are homeotherms and will expend metabolic energy to stay warm at the cost of other functions. Heat is generated not by shivering but by metabolizing brown fat reserves (nonshivering thermogenesis) in response to norepinephrine. This has practical consequences, since brown fat may be rendered inactive by some medications (pressors and anesthetic agents) and may be depleted by poor nutrition. Exposure to cold environments increases metabolic work and caloric consumption. Due to limited energy reserves and thin skin, prolonged exposure may rapidly cause hypothermia. Resultant catecholamine secretion increases the metabolic rate (particularly in the myocardium) and produces vasoconstriction with impaired tissue perfusion and increased lactic acid production.

Thus, it is important to maintain the sick newborn in an optimal thermal environment (thermoneutrality). This is the ambient temperature in which a baby, at a minimal metabolic cost, can maintain a constant and normal body temperature by vasomotor control. To attain such an environment, the gradient between the skin surface and the environmental temperature must be less than 1.5 °C. As the skin surface temperature averages 35.5 °C, the optimal environmental temperature is 34 °C (slightly higher for premature infants). The neonate's environmental temperature is best controlled by placing the infant in an enclosed incubator. An open radiant warmer is used when the infant is sick and frequent access is necessary. Either the ambient temperature of the incubator can be monitored and maintained at thermoneutrality or a servo system can be used. The latter regulates the incubator temperature according to the infant's skin temperature. Heat loss may be further reduced by wrapping the head, extremities, and as much of the trunk as possible in wadding, plastic wrap, plastic sheets, or aluminum foil.

In the operating room, the temperature of the infant must be continuously recorded by placing a thermistor in the rectum or esophagus. Body heat may be conserved by a heating pad, circulated warm air around the child (bear-hugger), infrared lamp, and warm irrigation fluids. The operating room should be prewarmed and the temperature kept at 20–27 °C. Wet sponges and drapes exaggerate evaporative heat losses. Plastic drapes contain body heat and keep the skin dry. One of the most effective means of regulating body temperature is to heat and humidify the inhalational anesthetic gases.

Albanese CT, Nour BM, Rowe MI: Anesthesia blocks nonshivering thermogenesis in the neonatal rabbit. J Pediatr Surg 1994; 29:983.

Nesher N et al: A novel thermoregulatory system maintains perioperative normothermia in children undergoing elective surgery. Paediatr Anaesth 2000;11:555.

Sauer PJ, Dane HJ, Visser HK: New standards for neutral thermal environment of healthy very low birth weight infants in week one of life. Arch Dis Child 1984;59:18.

▶ Ventilation

Assisted ventilation is often necessary because of underlying disease (eg, persistent fetal circulation and pulmonary hypertension), medications (eg, opioids, PGE_2), or physiologic changes imposed by a surgical procedure (eg, closure of an abdominal wall defect or diaphragmatic hernia). At birth, the pharynx should be aspirated of mucus, amniotic fluid, or meconium. Inadequate respiration should be assisted with a bag and mask or endotracheal tube. The diameter of an endotracheal tube (uncuffed) should approximate that of the fifth digit or the nares, usually between 2.5 and 4 mm. The full-term newborn usually requires a 3.0-mm tube. An orotracheal tube is preferred to a nasotracheal one to minimize trauma and subsequent infection in the nasal passages. The trachea from the glottis to the carina in the newborn is 7.5 cm long, and placement of the tube into the right or left bronchus must be avoided. For infants, optimal tube placement can be estimated as follows: 7 cm from the lips in a 1 kg infant; 8 cm in a 2 kg infant; and 9 cm in a 3 kg infant. Once placed, the endotracheal tube is firmly fixed in place and connected to an infant ventilator. A small air leak between the endotracheal tube and the airway is necessary to minimize laryngeal and tracheal trauma.

Most infant ventilators are time-cycled flow generators capable of delivering both continuous positive airway pressure (CPAP) and intermittent mandatory ventilation (IMV). IMV is a synthesis of simple mechanical ventilation and CPAP breathing that allows the baby to breathe independently between mandatory breaths provided by the ventilator while a continuous positive pressure is maintained on the airway. CPAP breathing helps keep the terminal airways open and is particularly useful when alveolar collapse develops, such as in hyaline membrane disease or with persistent atelectasis.

The gas mixture flowing into the system should be carefully controlled by an air-oxygen mixing device, and the inspired oxygen concentration should be regulated to maintain the arterial P_{O_2} at 60–80 torr. The gas should be humidified by using a heated nebulizer. Absorption of fluid in the lung may be considerable, and parenteral fluid may have to be restricted. When the arterial P_{O_2} exceeds 80 torr, the inspired oxygen concentration is gradually lowered toward room air; the end-expiratory pressure is incrementally lowered, as is the IMV rate. In this way, the baby is gradually weaned from oxygen and mechanical ventilation. Upon removal of the tube, the inspired oxygen concentration should be increased during the transition period.

In severe respiratory compromise (eg, congenital diaphragmatic hernia, meconium aspiration syndrome), more complex ventilatory strategies are needed. High-frequency ventilation (jet and oscillatory modes) utilizes low tidal volumes at high rates (up to 600 breaths/min) to minimize the deleterious effects of high airway pressure. Inhaled nitric oxide (iNO) can be administered via the ventilatory circuit and may help relax the small airways and pulmonary vasculature. There is a trend toward allowing higher P_{CO_2} levels (permissive hypercarbia) and lower P_{O_2} levels in order to lessen pulmonary trauma from pressure and oxygen. This has been termed "gentle ventilation." If gentle ventilation, permissive hypercapnia, and the high-frequency modes of ventilation are ineffective, oxygenation and gas exchange can be accomplished using extracorporeal membrane oxygenation (ECMO). This temporary bypass unit oxygenates the blood through an external circuit as the lungs are left to mature or recover from the underlying disease process. The clinical need for ECMO has diminished with the increased widespread use of iNO and adoption of permissive hypercapnia as a ventilatory strategy.

Boloker J et al: Congenital diaphragmatic hernia in 120 infants treated consecutively with permissive hypercapnia/spontaneous respiration/elective repair. J Pediatr Surg 2002;37:357.
Gerstmann DR, deLemos RA, Clark RH: High-frequency ventilation: issues of strategy. Clin Perinatol 1991;18:563.

Hemmila MR, Hirschl RB: Advances in ventilatory support of the pediatric surgical patient. Curr Opin Pediatr 1999;11:241.

▶ Fluids & Electrolytes

Effective fluid and electrolyte management involves (1) calculating the fluid and electrolyte requirements for maintaining metabolic functions, (2) replacing losses (evaporative, third space, external), and (3) considering preexisting fluid deficits or excesses. Taking these factors into consideration, a tentative program is devised for fluid and electrolyte administration. The patient's response is monitored, and the program is adjusted accordingly.

Monitoring fluid status and acid-base balance can be accomplished by both noninvasive and invasive means. Commonly used noninvasive devices include pulse oximetry, urine output, transcutaneous CO_2 monitoring, and sphygmomanometry. For critically ill infants, more invasive means are necessary to assess homeostasis. Blood gas analysis via heelstick (venous) or arterial catheter is frequently employed. Polyvinyl catheters may be placed via an umbilical artery into the distal aorta, with the tip positioned at the level of L4 (confirmed radiographically). Indwelling arterial catheters can also be placed in the radial, femoral, or temporal arteries, either percutaneously or by incision. Central venous access may assist in cases where prolonged venous access is needed or parenteral nutrition is necessary or when blood is frequently sampled. It may be obtained via the umbilical vein; a percutaneously inserted central catheter (PICC) via the saphenous, cephalic, median basilic, or temporal veins; or using a Broviac catheter via the femoral, internal jugular, facial, or subclavian veins.

A. Calculating Maintenance Needs

In the newborn infant, the basic maintenance requirement of water is the volume required for growth and replacement of losses from the skin, lungs, and stool. Requirements during the first day of life are unique because of the greatly expanded extracellular fluid volume in the newborn baby, which decreases after 24 hours. For example, infants born with intestinal obstruction (eg, intestinal atresia) are initially not hypovolemic as a result of fluid adjustments across the placenta. Up to 10% of a newborn infant's birth weight is lost in the first 3–7 days; the majority is water loss, with minor contributions from meconium and urine. During the first 24 hours of life, basic maintenance fluid should not exceed 90 mL/kg/d in preterm infants weighing less than 1000 g or of less than 32 weeks' gestation and should not exceed 65 mL/kg/d in larger infants. This requirement gradually increases to a minimum 80–100 mL/kg/d by 4 days of life in normal infants. For children and adolescents, the most commonly used method of calculating fluid requirements is based on body weight (Table 43–1). However, because of the many factors affecting maintenance requirements, there is no close or constant relationship between body weight and fluid and electrolyte needs.

Table 43–1. Calculation of Maintenance Fluid Requirements.

Body Weight	Fluid Volume per 24 h
1-10 kg	100 mL/kg
11-20 kg	1000 mL + 50 mL for each kg over 10 kg
> 20 kg	1500 mL + 20 mL for each kg over 20 kg

Reproduced with permission from Albanese CT: Pediatric surgery. in: *Surgery.* Norton JA (editor). Springer, 2000.

B. Perioperative Fluid Management

In the surgical patient, fluid, serum electrolyte, and acid-base abnormalities are corrected before operation, when feasible. Intraoperative fluid requirements consist of the estimated maintenance requirement plus replacement of preexisting deficits (if uncorrected) plus replacement of intraoperative losses, including blood.

Postoperatively, losses from intestinal drainage and fistulas are directly measured and replaced with an appropriate electrolyte solution (Table 43–2). In neonates, it is wise to measure the electrolytes in the fluid to more accurately guide replacement, especially for proximal intestinal stomas or fistulas. Protein-rich losses (eg, chest tube drainage of a chylothorax) can be replaced with colloid such as an albumin solution or fresh frozen plasma. Internal losses into body cavities or tissues (third space losses) cannot be measured; adequate replacement of these losses depends on careful monitoring of the patient's vital signs and urine output. Following an operation such as a laparotomy or thoracotomy, the fluid requirement may exceed 150 mL/kg/d for several days postoperatively.

C. Electrolyte Considerations

Basic electrolyte and energy requirements are provided by sodium, 3–4 meq/kg/d (up to 5 meq/kg/d for preterm infants)

in 5% or 10% dextrose, with the addition of potassium, 2–3 meq/kg/d, once urine production has been established. Calcium gluconate (200–400 mg/kg/d) may be added, especially in preterm infants. Additional electrolytes such as bicarbonate and magnesium are added, as needed.

Many stressed newborn infants develop low blood levels of potassium, calcium, magnesium, and glucose. A deficiency of any one of these will produce such signs as vomiting, abdominal distention, poor feeding, apneic spells, cyanosis, lethargy, eye rolling, high-pitched cry, tremors, or convulsions. Convulsions and tetany due to hypocalcemia should be treated with intravenous 10% calcium solution given at a rate of 1 mL/min while the electrocardiogram is carefully monitored. Although hypocalcemia can be largely eliminated by adding calcium salts to intravenous solutions, caution is required since subcutaneous infiltration may produce severe vasoconstriction and skin necrosis. If there is no response to correction of a documented calcium deficiency, hypomagnesemia should be suspected and a serum magnesium level obtained.

Rapid determination of the blood glucose level can be done in the neonatal unit with blood glucose reagent strips. This may be correlated at intervals with serum glucose determinations, the frequency depending on the stability of the infant. Intravenous fluids should contain a minimum of 10% dextrose, and if non-dextrose-containing solutions such as blood or plasma are being administered, close monitoring of the blood glucose level is essential. The treatment of hypoglycemia consists of giving 50% glucose, 1–2 mL/kg intravenously, followed by a continuous infusion of 10–15% glucose solutions at a rate equivalent to that needed for maintenance water requirements.

Coran A, Drongowski R: Body fluid compartment changes following neonatal surgery. J Pediatr Surg 1989;24:829.

Statter MB: Fluids and electrolytes in infants and children. Semin Pediatr Surg 1992;1:208.

Table 43–2. Replacement of Abnormal Losses of Fluids and Electrolytes.

Type of Fluid	Electrolyte Content				
	Na+ (meq/L)	K+ (meq/L)	Cl⁻ (meq/L)	HCO₃⁻ (meq/L)	Replacement
Gastric (vomiting)	50 (20–90)	10 (4–15)	90 (50–150)	...	5% Dextrose in half-normal (0.45%) saline plus KCl 20–40 meq/L
Small bowel (ileostomy)	110 (70–140)	5 (3–10)	100 (70–130)	20 (10–40)	Lactated Ringer
Diarrhea	80 (10–140)	25 (10–60)	90 (20–120)	40 (30–50)	Lactated Ringer with or without HCO₃⁻
Bile	145 (130–160)	5 (4–7)	100 (80–120)	40 (30–50)	Lactated Ringer with or without HCO₃⁻
Pancreatic	140 (130–150)	5 (4–7)	80 (60–100)	80 (60–110)	Lactated Ringer with or without HCO₃⁻
Sweat					
Normal	20 (10–30)	4 (3–10)	20 (10–40)	...	...
Cystic fibrosis	90 (50–130)	15 (5–25)	90 (60–120)	...	...

Nutrition

Newborns require a relatively large caloric intake because of their high basal metabolic rate, caloric requirements for growth and development, energy needs to maintain body heat, and limited energy reserve. An infant requires calories at a rate of 100–130 kcal/kg/d and protein at a rate of 2–4 g/kg/d to achieve a normal weight gain of 10–15 g/kg/d (Table 43–3). Thirty percent to 40% of the total nonprotein calories should be provided as fat. These requirements decline with age but increase with surgery, sepsis, and trauma or burns. Caloric requirements are increased 10–25% by surgery, more than 50% by infection, and 100% by burns.

A. Enteral Alimentation

The best means of providing calories and protein is through the gastrointestinal tract. If the gastrointestinal tract is functional, standard infant formulas, blenderized meals, or prepared elemental diets can be given by mouth, through nasogastric or nasojejunal feeding tubes, or through gastrostomy or jejunostomy tubes placed surgically. Gastric feeding is preferable because it allows for normal digestive processes and hormonal responses, a greater tolerance for larger osmotic loads, and a lower incidence of dumping. The use of nasoduodenal or nasojejunal tubes is reserved for infants who cannot tolerate intragastric feeding (eg, delayed gastric emptying, gastroesophageal reflux, depressed gag reflex).

The availability of nutritionally complete liquid diets of low viscosity allows continuous feeding through small-diameter catheters. Elemental diets made by mixing crystalline amino acids, oligosaccharides, and fats can be completely absorbed in the small intestine with little residue. Their use is limited because they cause diarrhea as a result of the high osmolality of full-strength formulas. This can be avoided by administering dilute solutions by continuous drip. Initially, the volume of dilute solution is gradually increased, and the concentration is then progressively increased in a stepwise

Table 43–3. Caloric Requirements of Various Age Groups per 24 Hours.

Age	kcal/kg per 24 h
Newborn term (0–4 days)	110–120
Low birth weight	120–130
3–4 months	100–106
5–12 months	100
1–7 years	75–90
7–12 years	60–75
12–18 years	30–60

Reproduced, with permission, from Albanese CT: Pediatric surgery. In: *Surgery.* Norton JA (editor). Springer, 2000.

fashion (ie, half strength, three-fourths strength, and full strength). Formulas that remain below 500 mOsm are best.

Small Silastic or polyethylene catheters such as those used for intravenous infusion can be passed through the nose or mouth into the stomach or jejunum. In more complex cases, a surgically placed gastrostomy or jejunostomy may be necessary for postoperative feeding. A variety of techniques and methods are employed in their construction. In the case of a gastrostomy, either a balloon catheter (ie, Foley) is used or a low-profile gastrostomy button is placed. Silastic is superior to other plastics because it does not become rigid when exposed to intestinal contents. Parenteral nutrition combined with enteral feeding is often necessary for infants with short bowel syndrome until intestinal adaptation occurs.

B. Parenteral Alimentation

The indications for parenteral alimentation include the following: (1) expected period of prolonged ileus (eg, following repair of gastroschisis or high jejunal atresia); (2) intestinal fistulas; (3) supplementation of oral feedings, as in intractable diarrhea, short bowel syndrome, or various malabsorption syndromes; (4) intrauterine growth retardation; (5) catabolic wasting states such as infections or tumors when gastric feedings are inadequate or not tolerated; (6) inflammatory bowel disease; (7) severe acute alimentary disorders (pancreatitis, necrotizing enterocolitis); and (8) chylothorax.

Concentrated solutions (12.5% glucose or more) thrombose peripheral vessels. Placement of a central venous catheter (PICC or Broviac) into the superior or inferior vena cavae allows the large blood flow to dilute the solution immediately, allowing more concentrated sugar solutions (15–30% glucose) to be administered. The catheter may be placed percutaneously through the subclavian or internal jugular vein or inserted by cutdown into the external jugular, anterior facial, internal jugular, cephalic, brachial, or saphenous veins. For long-term use, Broviac (single lumen) or Hickman (double lumen) catheters, with Dacron cuffs positioned near the exit site of the skin, are preferred to minimize infection and to prevent accidental dislodgement.

Intravenous alimentation solutions containing an amino acid source (2–5% crystalline amino acids or protein hydrolysate), glucose (10–40%), electrolytes, vitamins, and trace minerals are used. The electrolyte composition of the protein solution should be known so that the desired composition of the final solution can be adjusted by appropriate additives according to the individual patient's requirements. A standard solution suitable for infants and young children must contain calcium, magnesium, and phosphate to allow for growth. Trace minerals are also added to the basic solution (Table 43–4). These solutions should be infused at a constant rate with an infusion pump to avoid blood backing up the catheter and clotting and to prevent wide fluctuations of blood glucose and amino acid concentrations. If it is necessary to restrict the volume of infusion, more concentrated glucose solutions can be used to increase the caloric intake.

Table 43-4. Total Parenteral Nutrition Requirements.

Component	Neonate	6 mo to 10 yr	> 10 yr
Calories (kcal/kg/d)	90–120	60–105	40–75
Fluid (mL/kg/d)	120–180	120–150	50–75
Dextrose (mg/kg/min)	4–6	7–8	7–8
Protein (g/kg/d)	2–3	1.5–2.5	0.8–2.0
Fat (g/kg/d)	0.5–3.0	1.0–4.0	1.0–4.0
Sodium (meq/kg/d)	3–4	3–4	3–4
Potassium (meq/kg/d)	2–3	2–3	1–2
Calcium (mg/kg/d)	80–120	40–80	40–60
Phosphate (mg/kg/d)	25–40	25–40	25–40
Magnesium (meq/kg/d)	0.25–1.0	0.5	0.5
Zinc (μg/kg/d)	300	100	3 mg/d
Copper (μg/kg/d)	20	20	1.2 mg/d
Chromium (μg/kg/d)	0.2	0.2	12 mg/d
Manganese (μg/kg/d)	6	6	0.3 mg/d
Selenium (mg/kg/d)	2	2	10–20 mg/d

Reproduced, with permission, from Albanese CT: Pediatric surgery. In: *Surgery*. Norton JA (editor). Springer, 2000.

Complications of prolonged intravenous alimentation are numerous. The most frequent problem is catheter sepsis. Although catheter removal will quickly treat the problem, a trial of antibiotics effective against gram-positive and gram-negative pathogens is indicated. Catheter removal is indicated in the presence of worsening sepsis, three positive blood cultures, or documented yeast infection (with antifungal treatment after catheter removal). Clotting in the catheter may be controlled by adding 1 unit of heparin per milliliter of solution. Emphasis on a constant rate of infusion will minimize hyperglycemia or hypoglycemia. Analysis of serum electrolytes (including calcium and phosphate) may be necessary several times a week initially, but the interval is decreased to once a week when the patient is stable. Patients must be observed for hyperammonemia and for vitamin or trace mineral deficiency. Progressive hepatomegaly and jaundice of uncertain origin can occur after prolonged parenteral alimentation. This syndrome may subside when the parenteral solution is discontinued or when it is infused for a period of 12–16 hours and then the infusion is stopped for 8–12 hours (cycling) or when augmented with enteral feeding.

Amii LA, Moss RL: Nutritional support of the pediatric surgical patient. Curr Opin Pediatr 1999;11:237.

Holcomb GW 3d, Ziegler MM Jr: Nutrition and cancer in children. Surg Annu 1990;2:129.

Pereira GR: Nutritional care of the extremely premature infant. Clin Perinat 1994;22:61.

Reynolds RM, Bass KD, Thureen PJ: Achieving positive protein balance in the immediate postoperative period in neonates undergoing abdominal surgery. J Pediatr Surg 2008;152:63.

▶ Blood Loss

Total blood, plasma, and red blood cell volumes are higher during the first few postnatal hours than at any other time in an individual's life. Several hours after birth, plasma shifts out of the circulation, and total blood and plasma volume decrease. The high red blood cell volume persists, decreasing slowly to reach adult levels by the seventh postnatal week. Age-related estimations of blood volume are summarized in Table 43–5.

Although not clinically significant, both the prothrombin time (PT) and the partial thromboplastin time (PTT) may be slightly prolonged at birth because of relative deficiencies of clotting factors. Defects in the coagulating mechanism may occur in newborn infants as a result of vitamin K deficiency, thrombocytopenia, inherited disorders, and temporary hepatic insufficiency due to immaturity, asphyxia, or infection. It is standard to administer 1.0 mg of vitamin K intramuscularly to all newborns.

The blood lost during operation varies greatly according to the complexity of the operative procedure, the underlying disease, and the effectiveness of hemostasis. Mild blood loss, amounting to less than 10% of the blood volume, usually does not require transfusion. It is imperative to develop methods for closely monitoring the amount of blood lost during operations because significant blood loss is often underestimated in the newborn, especially the preterm infant. Dry sponges should be used and weighed shortly after use to minimize error from evaporation. The suction line, connected to a calibrated trap on the operating table, should be short to diminish the dead space of the tubing and to provide immediate data about accumulated blood loss. Visual observation may be used as a rough guide, but it tends to give a falsely low estimate of the loss.

Before operation, newborn infants should receive vitamin K, 1.0 mg intravenously or intramuscularly. If an extensive surgical procedure is anticipated, the patient's blood should be typed and crossmatched in case transfusion is required. In infants with hematocrits greater than 50%, blood loss may be replaced by infusing lactated Ringer solution or fresh frozen plasma to compensate for losses of up to 25% of total blood volume. Greater blood losses

Table 43-5. Blood Volume Based on Age.

Preterm infants	85–100 mL/kg
Term infants	85 mL/kg
Age > 1 month	75 mL/kg
Age 3 months to adult	70 mL/kg

should be replaced with fresh (< 3 days old) whole blood or packed red blood cells. A transfusion of packed red blood cells at a volume of 10 mL/kg usually raises the hematocrit 3–4%. The transfused blood should be prewarmed to body temperature by running it through coiled tubing immersed in water at 37 °C. With excessive blood loss, clotting factors and platelets can be depleted rapidly, and fresh frozen plasma and platelets of identical blood type should be available. A transfusion of 0.1 unit/kg of platelets raises the platelet count by approximately 25,000/μL.

▶ Perioperative Considerations

A. Gastrointestinal Decompression

The importance of gastric decompression in the surgical newborn cannot be overemphasized. The distended stomach carries the risk of aspiration and pneumonia and may also impair diaphragmatic excursion, resulting in respiratory distress. For example, oxygenation and ventilation in a neonate with congenital diaphragmatic hernia may become progressively impaired as the herniated intestine becomes distended with air and fluid. With gastroschisis, omphalocele, and diaphragmatic hernia, the ability to reduce the prolapsed intestine into the abdominal cavity is impaired by intestinal distention. It is critical to avoid bag-mask ventilation in these patients. A double-lumen (sump) tube, such as a 10F Replogle or Anderson tube, is preferred, utilizing low continuous suction. If a single-lumen tube is used, intermittent aspiration by syringe or machine is required. The correct position of the tube in the stomach is confirmed by carefully measuring the tube prior to insertion and by radiographs. Careful taping of the tube is essential to avoid displacement.

B. Preoperative Blood Sampling

Blood analyses should be restricted to those studies essential for diagnosis and management. The volume of blood drawn for laboratory tests should be documented because these small volumes cumulatively represent significant blood loss in a small infant. Generally, the only "routine" preoperative blood analyses for a neonate consist of a complete blood count and a blood specimen for type and crossmatch (in the case of major newborn surgery). Electrolytes in the first 12 hours of life simply reflect the mother's electrolytes. Coagulation studies (eg, PT, PTT, activated clotting time [ACT]) are rarely indicated.

C. Preoperative NPO Guidelines

The following are general guidelines, but institutional practices vary considerably. The guiding principles in setting a standard include risk of hypoglycemia associated with NPO status, tolerance or comfort level of the NPO child, and the desire to have an empty stomach upon induction of general anesthesia to mitigate aspiration risk.

1. Patients younger than 6 months—No solids, breast milk, or formula 4 hours prior to the procedure. Infants may have clear liquids (water, oral electrolyte mixtures, glucose water, or apple juice) until 2 hours prior to the procedure.

2. Patients from 6 months to 18 years—Nothing to eat or drink after midnight except clear liquids (water, apple juice, oral electrolyte mixtures, gelatin dessert, white grape juice), which can be continued until 2 hours prior to the procedure.

3. Patients older than 18 years—Nothing to eat or drink after midnight except clear liquids (water, apple juice, plain gelatin desserts) until 4–6 hours prior to the procedure.

D. Bowel Preparation Instructions

The bowel is mechanically cleansed for elective bowel resection. Opinion varies about whether a bowel preparation is needed for certain procedures as well as about what to use to accomplish it and whether to do it at home or in the hospital. An inpatient regimen begins the day before surgery and consists of polyethylene glycol-electrolyte solution (GoLYTELY), 25 mL/kg/h for 4 hours or until the effluent is clear. Metoclopramide (0.1 mg/dose intravenously) is given 1 hour before the GoLYTELY. Pedialyte can be given ad lib until the time to have nothing by mouth.

Outpatient preparations are reserved for patients over 1 year of age. Clear liquids are given the day before surgery. Bisacodyl (Dulcolax) suppositories and 8-oz lukewarm tap water enemas can be given in the morning and evening the day before surgery. For children over 5 years old, magnesium citrate is added (1 oz per year of age up to a maximum of 8 oz) and given orally in the morning and evening the day before surgery, along with 16-oz tap water enemas.

▼ LESIONS OF THE HEAD & NECK

DERMOID CYSTS

Dermoid cysts are congenital inclusions of skin and skin appendages commonly found on the scalp and eyebrows and in the midline of the nose, neck, and upper chest. They present as painless swellings that may be completely mobile or fixed to the skin and deeper structures. Dermoid cysts of the eyebrows and scalp may produce a depression in the underlying bone that appears as a smooth, punched-out defect on radiographs of the outer table of the skull. They do not extend intracranially. In contrast, cysts of the face and scalp that are located in the midline may represent an alternative diagnosis of encephalocele and would be handled much differently, so it is imperative to obtain an MRI or CT scan preoperatively. Dermoid cysts of the midline neck may be confused with thyroglossal duct cysts. However, dermoids do not move with swallowing or protrusion of the tongue, since they are not deep to the strap muscles, unlike thyroglossal cysts. All dermoids contain a cheesy material that is produced by desquamation of the cells of the epithelial lining. Care should be taken when planning the operative approach to facial dermoids to avoid both incomplete excision and unnecessary surgical scarring in cosmetically sensitive areas. Dermoids should be excised intact, since incomplete removal will result in recurrence. Those lesions arising near the eyebrows should be excised through an incision adjacent to the hairline. The eyebrows should not be shaved, nor should the incision go through any eyebrow follicles, since a permanent glabrous area will develop. Recently, tunneled endoscopic approaches originating from behind the hair line and performed through an operative endoscope have been described as an approach to avoid facial scarring.

Dutta S, Lorenz HP, Albanese CT: Endoscopic excision of benign forehead masses: a novel approach for pediatric general surgeons. J Pediatr Surg 2006;41:1874.

McAvoy JM, Zuckerbraun L: Dermoid cysts of the head and neck in children. Arch Otolaryngol 1976;102:529.

Steele MH et al: Orbitofacial masses in children: an endoscopic approach. Arch Otolaryngol Head Neck Surg 2001;128:409.

BRANCHIOGENIC ANOMALIES

During the first month of fetal life, the primitive neck develops four external clefts and four pharyngeal pouches that are separated by a membrane. Between the clefts and pouches are branchial arches. The dorsal portion of the first cleft becomes the external auditory canal; the other clefts are obliterated. The pharyngeal pouches persist as adult organs. The first pouch becomes the auditory tube, the middle ear cavity, and the mastoid air cells. The second pouch incompletely regresses and becomes the palatine tonsil and the supratonsillar fossa. The third pouch forms the inferior parathyroid glands and thymus; the fourth forms the superior parathyroid glands. Branchial anomalies are remnants of this fetal branchial apparatus.

A tract of branchial origin may form a complete fistula, or one end may be obliterated to form an external or internal sinus, or both ends may resorb, leaving an aggregate of cells forming a cyst (Figure 43–1). Fistulas that arise above the hyoid bone and communicate with the external auditory canal represent persistence of the first branchial cleft. These tracts are always lined by squamous epithelium. Cysts and sinuses of second or third branchial origin are lined by squamous, cuboidal, or ciliated columnar epithelium. Fistulas that communicate between the anterior border of the sternocleidomastoid muscle and the tonsillar fossa are of second branchial origin, and those that extend into the piriform sinus are derived from the third branchial pouch. Cysts developing from branchial structures usually appear later in childhood as opposed to sinuses and fistulas. Branchiogenic anomalies occur with equal frequency on each side of the neck, and 15% are bilateral. Second branchial cleft abnormalities are most common, occurring six times more frequently than first cleft anomalies.

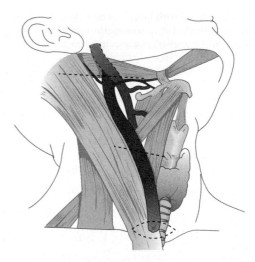

▲ **Figure 43–1.** Branchiogenic fistula from second branchial cleft origin. The fistula extends along the anterior border of the sternocleidomastoid muscle and courses between the internal and external carotid arteries and cephalad to the hypoglossal nerve to enter the tonsillar fossa.

▶ Clinical Findings

A sinus or fistulous opening along the anterior border of the sternocleidomastoid muscle may be noted at birth and usually discharges a mucoid or purulent material. The patient may complain of a foul-tasting discharge in the mouth upon massaging the tract, but the internal orifice is rarely recognized. Some may present with an acute infection. The cysts are characteristically found anterior and deep to the upper third of the sternocleidomastoid muscle, or they may be located within the parotid gland or pharyngeal wall, over the manubrium, or in the mediastinum. Sinuses and cysts are prone to become repeatedly infected, producing cellulitis and abscess formation. Incomplete branchial sinuses appear as a dimple that contain cartilage and do not drain or communicate with the deep structures of the neck.

▶ Differential Diagnosis

Granulomatous lymphadenitis due to mycobacterial infections may produce cystic lymph nodes and draining sinuses, but these are usually distinguishable by the chronic inflammatory reaction that precedes the purulent discharge. Suppurative lymphadenitis, most commonly due to *Staphylococcus aureus*, may resemble an infected branchial remnant. However, treatment and complete healing of the lymphadenitis is curative, whereas an identifiable branchial remnant will persist after the infection resolves. Hemangiomas and lymphatic malformations are soft, spongy tumor masses that might be confused with branchial cysts, but the latter have a firmer consistency. Lymphatic malformations may transilluminate, while branchial cysts do not. Carotid body tumors are quite firm, are located at the carotid bifurcation, and occur in older patients. Lymphomas produce firm masses in the area where branchial remnants occur, but multiple matted nodes rather than a solitary cystic tumor distinguish these lesions. Mucoid material may be expressed from the openings of branchial sinuses or fistulas, and a firm cordlike tract may be palpable along its course.

▶ Treatment

Nearly all branchial abnormalities should be excised early in life, since repeated infection is common, making resection more difficult. Asymptomatic, small cartilaginous remnants may be watched, but they are usually removed for cosmetic reasons as well as the smaller risk of infection, compared to the true cyst/fistula. Infected sinuses and cysts require initial incision and drainage. Excision of these tracts is staged and usually performed approximately 6 weeks later, when the acute inflammatory reaction has subsided. Every effort should be made to excise the entire cyst wall or fistula tract (including the skin punctum, if present), since recurrence and infection are common with incomplete removal. Excision should be undertaken cautiously because the tracts may lie adjacent to the facial, hypoglossal, and glossopharyngeal nerves as well as the carotid artery and internal jugular vein.

Al-Khateeb TH, Al Zoubi F: Congenital neck masses: a descriptive retrospective study of 252 cases. J Oral Maxillofac Surg 2007; 65:22242.

PREAURICULAR LESIONS

Preauricular sinuses, cysts, and cartilaginous rests arise from anomalous development of the auricle and are unrelated to branchial anomalies. The sinuses are often short and end blindly. They can be cosmetically unappealing and often become infected. Superficial skin tags and cartilaginous rests are easily excised without risk to other structures. Preauricular sinus tracts, however, may be very deceptive in their extent, and one should be prepared to proceed with extensive dissection that risks damage to branches of the facial nerve.

Tan T, Constantinides H, Mitchell TE: The preauricular sinus: a review of its etiology, clinical presentation and management. Int J Pediatr Otorhinolaryngology 2005;69:1469.

LYMPHATIC MALFORMATION (CYSTIC HYGROMA, LYMPHANGIOMA)

Lymphatic malformations (LM) are benign multilobular, multinodular cystic masses lined by lymph channel endothelial cells. They result from maldevelopment and obstruction of the lymphatic system. Since they are not proliferative lesions,

they should be distinguished from hemangiomas, hence the favored term *lymphatic malformation* is currently favored over the more frequently encountered misnomer lymphangioma. Cystic hygroma is another misnomer frequently encountered for cervical LM. Eventually, sequestrations of lymphatic tissue that do not communicate with the normal lymphatic system develop. LM appears at birth in 50–65% of cases and by the second year of life in 90%. They are located most commonly in the posterior triangle of the neck (75%) (Figure 43–2) and axilla (20%), with the remainder located in the mediastinum, retroperitoneum, pelvis, and groin.

▶ Clinical Findings

Cervical LMs may communicate beneath the clavicle with an axillary hygroma, mediastinal hygroma, or, rarely, both. The majority may be asymptomatic; however, the occult LM usually presents following an upper aerodigestive tract infection as a result of increased or infected lymph flow or following hemorrhage into the LM from a web of adherent

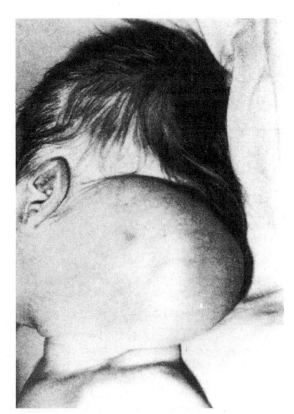

▲ **Figure 43–2.** Typical neonatal macrocystic lymphatic malformation arising from the posterior cervical triangle. (From Filston HC: Hemangiomas, cystic hygromas, and teratomas of the head and neck. Semin Pediatr Surg 1994; 3:147. Reprinted with permission from Elsevier.)

microvasculature. Occasionally, very large lesions occur with involvement of the floor of the mouth; these can cause in utero hydrops or asphyxiation at birth when associated with airway compromise. A recognized association between cervical LM and Turner syndrome exists. These lesions grow along fascial planes and around neurovascular structures; they are infiltrative but not invasive. Large lesions may be recognized prenatally using ultrasound or MRI examination.

▶ Treatment

The choice between two modes of treatment, sclerotherapy or excision, is based on imaging studies (CT, MRI). Intralesional injection of a sclerosing agent is most effective for unilocular or macrocystic lesions. Examples of agents that have been used are OK-432 (a lyophilized mixture of *Streptococcus pyogenes* and penicillin G potassium), bleomycin, and doxycycline. Excision is carried out with bipolar cautery to ensure a hemostatic dissection and decrease the incidence of lymph leak and nerve injury. Nevertheless, postoperative lymph leak is common and is treated by closed suction drainage for days to weeks. Intraoperative cyst rupture increases the difficulty of the dissection because the thin-walled cyst is difficult to identify and the margins are obscured. The persistence rate following surgery can be as high as 50%, since incomplete excision is the rule rather than the exception in order to avoid potential injury to adjacent neurovascular bundles. Given their infiltrative nature, persistence or symptomatic recurrence following surgical excision, and unavoidable surgical scarring, the trend has been increasingly toward sclerotherapy for cervical LMs.

Brown RL, Azizkhan RG: Pediatric head and neck lesions. Pediatr Clin North Am 1998;45:899.

Fonkalsrud EW: Congenital malformations of the lymphatic system. Semin Pediatr Surg 1994;3:62.

Nehra D et al: Doxycycline sclerotherapy as primary treatment of head and neck lymphatic malformations. J Pediatr Surg 2008;43:451.

Ogita S et al: OK-432 therapy in 64 patients with lymphangioma. J Pediatr Surg 1994;29:784.

THYROGLOSSAL DUCT REMNANT

During the fourth week of gestation, the thyroid gland develops from an evagination in the floor of the primitive pharynx located between the first pair of pharyngeal pouches. If the anlage of the thyroid does not descend normally, the gland may form at the base of the tongue or remain as a mass anywhere in the midline of the neck along its truncated path of descent. If the thyroglossal duct persists, the epithelial tract forms a cyst that usually communicates with the foramen cecum of the tongue. The thyroglossal duct descends through the second branchial arch anlage, which becomes the hyoid bone prior to its fusion in the midline. Because of this, the tract of a persistent thyroglossal duct often extends through the hyoid bone (Figure 43–3).

▶ Clinical Findings

The most common physical finding is a rounded cystic mass of varying size in the midline of the neck just below the hyoid bone. The acute inflammatory reaction of an infection may herald the presence of a cyst. The fluid in the cyst is usually under pressure and may give the impression of being a solid tumor. Cysts and aberrant midline thyroid glands move up and down with swallowing and with protrusion of the tongue, since they are deep to the cervical strap muscles. In contrast, lingual thyroid tissue is a rare clinical entity and may produce dysphagia, dysphonia, dyspnea, hemorrhage, or pain.

▶ Differential Diagnosis

Lymph nodes, dermoid cysts, and enlarged delphian nodes containing tumor metastases may be confused with thyroglossal remnants in the midline of the neck. Dermoid cysts do not move with swallowing. Lingual thyroids may be confused with a hypertrophied lingual tonsil or with a ranula, fibroma, angioma, sarcoma, or carcinoma of the tongue. These lesions and thyroglossal cysts may be distinguished from aberrantly located thyroid glands by needle aspiration or by radioiodine scintiscan.

▶ Complications

Thyroglossal cysts are prone to infection, and spontaneous drainage or incision and drainage of an abscess will often result in a chronically draining fistula. Excision of an ectopic thyroid may remove all thyroid tissue, producing hypothyroidism. There is a malignant potential of the dysgenetic thyroid tissue located in a thyroglossal duct cyst; carcinoma develops more frequently in ectopic thyroid tissue than in normal thyroid glands.

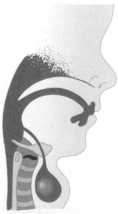

▲ **Figure 43–3.** Thyroglossal cyst and duct course through the hyoid bone to the foramen cecum of the tongue.

Treatment

Complete excision is indicated because of the risk of infection and the possibility of the development of papillary carcinoma later in life. Acute infection in thyroglossal tracts should be treated with antibiotics. Abscesses should be incised and drained. After complete subsidence of the inflammatory reaction (approximately 6 weeks), a thyroglossal cyst and its epithelial tract should be excised. The mid portion of the hyoid bone should be removed en bloc with the thyroglossal tract to the base of the tongue (Sistrunk procedure). Recurrences occur when the hyoid is not removed and when the cyst was previously infected or drained.

Housawa M et al: Anatomical reconstruction of the thyroglossal duct. J Pediatr Surg 1991;26:766.

Roback SA, Telander RL: Thyroglossal duct cysts and branchial cleft anomalies. Semin Pediatr Surg 1994;3:142.

TORTICOLLIS

Torticollis presents with a hard, nontender, fibrotic mass within the sternocleidomastoid muscle. It may be present at birth but is usually not noticed until the second to sixth weeks of life. The mass appears with equal frequency in both sexes and on each side of the neck. Rarely, there is more than one mass in the muscle or both sternocleidomastoid muscles are involved. A history of breech delivery is present in 20–30% of these children.

Clinical Findings

Torticollis is manifested when the sternocleidomastoid muscle is shortened and the mastoid process on the involved side is pulled down toward the clavicle and manubrium. As a result, the head is abducted to the ipsilateral side and rotated to the contralateral side (toward the opposite shoulder). The shoulder on the affected side is raised, and there may be cervical and thoracic scoliosis. Passive rotation of the head to the side of the involved muscle will be resisted and limited to varying degrees, and the muscle will appear as a protuberant band. Because of persistent pressure when the patient is recumbent, the ipsilateral face and contralateral occiput will be flattened. Facial hemihypoplasia and plagiocephaly (flattening of the ipsilateral posterior skull) occurs in untreated cases, usually within 6 months.

Treatment

Surgery is rarely necessary for this disorder. Torticollis is treated with active range-of-motion exercises. The child's shoulders are held flat to a table, and the head is tilted and rotated in a full range of motion. This procedure should be performed at least four times a day, usually for 2–3 months. The firm "tumor" often disappears well before the torticollis is cured. If the muscle continues to become progressively shortened, with facial and occipital skull deformity, both heads of the sternocleidomastoid muscle should be divided through a small transverse incision just above the clavicle. This procedure does not reverse the bony changes that have already developed but prevents progression of the process. Recently, endoscopic approaches have been described in order to avoid unsightly surgical scarring in the head and neck region.

Binder H et al: Congenital muscular torticollis: results of conservative management with long-term follow-up in 85 cases. Arch Phys Med Rehabil 1987;68:222.

Celayir AC: Congenital muscular torticollis: early and intensive treatment is critical. A prospective study. Pediatr Int 2000; 42:504.

Dutta S, Albanese CT: Transaxillary subcutaneous endoscopic release of the sternocleidomastoid muscle for treatment of persistent torticollis. J Pediatr Surg 2008;43:447.

CERVICAL LYMPHADENOPATHY

SUPPURATIVE LYMPHADENITIS

Infections in the upper respiratory passages, scalp, ear, or neck produce varying degrees of secondary lymphadenitis. Most of the causative organisms are streptococcal or staphylococcal species. In infants and young children, the clinical course of the suppurative lymphadenitis may greatly overshadow a seemingly insignificant or inapparent primary infection. Scalp or ear infections produce preauricular or postauricular and suboccipital lymph node involvement; submental, oral, tonsillar, and pharyngeal infections affect the submandibular and deep jugular nodes.

Clinical Findings

With significant lymphadenitis, the regional lymph nodes become greatly enlarged and produce local pain and tenderness. Enlargement of cervical nodes is most common, followed by occipital and submandibular nodes. Fever is high initially and then becomes intermittent and may persist for days or weeks. The regional nodes may remain enlarged and firm for prolonged periods, or they may suppurate and produce surrounding cellulitis and edema. Subsequently, the nodes may involute or a fluctuant abscess may form, resulting in redness and thinning of the overlying skin. Infected, matted nodes may become so hard as to be indistinguishable (on palpation) from a solid mass.

Differential Diagnosis

A smoldering lymphadenitis that neither resolves nor forms an abscess can be confused with granulomatous lymphadenitis, lymphoma, or metastatic tumor. Excisional biopsy is required to differentiate these lesions. After several weeks, there will usually be a reduction in the size and firmness of suppurative adenitis, especially after antibiotic treatment has been started. Recently, methicillin-resistant staph aureus

(MRSA) is being encountered at near epidemic levels as a causative agent of suppurative lymphadenitis in the ambulatory setting. A high suspicion of an MRSA infection should be entertained in all children presenting with either a first episode or, more certainly, with recalcitrant and recurrent cases.

▶ Treatment

In the acute phase, the patient should be treated with oral or intravenous antistaphylococcal antibiotics. In the subacute or chronic phase, the presence of pus in the node may be confirmed by needle aspiration of the mass. When an abscess is present, it should be incised and drained under general anesthesia. In those cases of MRSA infection, a prolonged course of either vancomycin or linezolid may be required for complete eradication even after drainage.

GRANULOMATOUS LYMPHADENITIS

Although typical tuberculous cervical adenitis is very rare in the United States, atypical mycobacteria (eg, *Mycobacterium avium-intracellulare*) is encountered and may present as a nonsuppurative area (usually cervical, axillary, or inguinal) of matted nodes with tenderness and a draining sinus. Granulomatous lymphadenitis and caseation may occur in the regional nodes draining the inoculation site of bacillus Calmette-Guérin (BCG). Cat-scratch disease causes a caseating lymphadenitis in regional lymph nodes (eg, epitrochlear and axillary nodes enlarge after an upper extremity cat scratch).

▶ Clinical Findings

Children under age 6 are most frequently affected. The initial manifestation is a painless, progressive enlargement of the lymph nodes in the deep cervical chain and the parotid, suboccipital, submandibular, and supraclavicular nodes. The duration of lymphadenopathy is usually 1–3 months or longer. The nodes may be large and mobile or, with progressive disease, may become matted, fixed, and finally caseate to form an abscess. Incision or spontaneous overlying skin breakdown will result in a chronically draining sinus. In tuberculosis, both sides of the neck or multiple groups of nodes are infected, and the chest radiograph indicates pulmonary involvement. In atypical mycobacterial lymphadenitis, pulmonary disease is rare and the cervical adenitis is unilateral. The tuberculin skin test is weakly positive in over 80% of patients with atypical mycobacterial infection. Skin test antigens from the various strains of atypical mycobacteria are available. A positive skin test helps differentiate granulomatous adenitis from malignant lymphadenopathy. A fluctuant node can be confused with a branchial cleft remnant or a thyroglossal duct cyst.

Cat-scratch disease is usually acquired by a bite or scratch from a kitten. It is caused by a pleomorphic gram-negative bacillus (*Bartonella henselae*) that is detected in tissues by a silver stain or via serologic testing. It is an acute illness characterized by fever, malaise, possible musculoskeletal manifestations, and occasionally a pustular lesion at the site of the scratch. Tender lymph node enlargement usually develops. Two to 4 weeks later, regional lymphadenitis persists, producing painful, fixed suppurative nodes that may develop into a chronically draining sinus.

▶ Treatment

Atypical tuberculous lymphadenitis may be treated with rifampin (10 mg/kg/d), though definitive treatment usually requires nodal excision. Trimethoprim-sulfamethoxazole may shorten the course of cat-scratch disease and prevent suppuration. When antibiotics are ineffective, the procedure of choice is excision of involved nodes before caseation occurs. Once the nodes become fluctuant or a draining sinus forms, a wedge of involved skin should be excised and the underlying necrotic nodes should be curetted out (rather than excised), taking care not to injure neighboring nerves. The wound edges and skin should be closed primarily. The value of continuing chemotherapy is influenced by sensitivity tests on the cultured material. Excision and primary closure usually result in excellent healing with good cosmetic results.

Beiler HA et al: Specific and nonspecific lymphadenitis in childhood: etiology, diagnosis, and therapy. Pediatr Surg Int 1997;12:108.

Bodenstein L, Altman RP: Cervical lymphadenitis in infants and children. Semin Pediatr Surg 1994;3:134.

Flint D et al: Cervical lymphadenitis due to non-tuberculous mycobacteria: surgical treatment and review. Int J Pediatr Otorhinolaryngol 2000;53:187.

Holley HP: Successful treatment of cat-scratch disease with ciprofloxacin. JAMA 1991;265:1563.

▼ CONGENITAL CHEST WALL DEFORMITIES

STERNAL CLEFT

Failure of fusion of the two sternal bars during embryonic development produces congenital sternal cleft, which may involve the upper, lower, or entire sternum. In its severe form, this defect is usually associated with protrusion of the pericardium and heart (ectopia cordis) and congenital heart lesions. Defects may be associated with extracardiac anomalies, including cleft lip, cleft palate, hydrocephalus, and other central nervous system disorders, or may be one component of the pentalogy of Cantrell. Operative correction is performed in the neonatal period when the chest wall is most pliable; it consists of simple suture approximation of the two sternal halves. More complex defects associated with ectopia cordis are often incompatible with life.

PECTUS EXCAVATUM

Pectus excavatum, a depression deformity, is the most common congenital chest wall abnormality, occurring in 1 in 300 live births, with a 3:1 male predominance. It is associated with other musculoskeletal disorders (Marfan syndrome, Poland syndrome, scoliosis, clubfoot, syndactyly), and 2% have congenital heart disease. There is a familial form. It results from the unbalanced posterior growth of costal cartilages that are often fused, bizarrely deformed, or rotated. The body of the sternum secondarily exhibits a prominent posterior curvature, usually involving its lower half (Figure 43–4). Commonly, the xiphoid is the deepest portion of the depression. The third, fourth, and fifth costal cartilages are usually affected, though the second to eighth costal cartilages may be involved. The severity of the defect varies greatly from a mild, insignificant depression to an extreme where the xiphoid bone is adjacent to the vertebrae. The depression may be symmetrical or asymmetrical with varying degrees of sternal rotation.

Clinical Findings

Patients with pectus excavatum are typically round-shouldered, with stooped posture, relative abdominal promi-

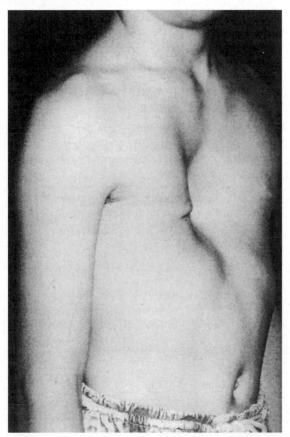

▲ **Figure 43–4.** Adolescent with a pectus excavatum deformity. Note that the most pronounced sternal curvature is in the lower half.

nence, flared costal margins, and an asthenic appearance. They may be withdrawn and refuse to participate in sports activities, particularly if their deformity might be exposed. Few patients complain of easy fatigability or inability to compete in exertional activities. Cardiopulmonary function studies rarely demonstrate impairments; this is predominantly a cosmetic deformity with potentially severe psychosocial sequelae.

Treatment & Prognosis

There is no standard age for repair. Undeniably, it is an easier operation in younger children than in adolescents. Drawbacks of an early operation include a higher risk of recurrence during the adolescent growth spurt and the inability of a young child to comprehend and assent to a predominantly cosmetic operation. Traditionally, an open repair (Ravitch technique) is performed in which the abnormal cartilages are resected; the sternum is often fractured and fixed in a corrected position (often with a Kirschner wire or steel strut). Recently, a minimally invasive technique (Nuss procedure) has been used in which a preformed sternal strut is passed, either blindly or with thoracoscopic assistance, under the chest wall muscles, into each hemithorax, and across the mediastinum under the sternum via two small incisions in the midaxillary line. The curved bar is passed upside down and "flipped" into position under the sternum, effectively lifting the sternum and chest wall into a corrected position. The bar is left in place for 2 years, and the patient can resume activity in 3 months. The recurrence rate for the open procedure is less than 3%; at present there is not enough long-term follow-up to assess the Nuss technique. The latest evolution in less invasive techniques involves placement of opposing magnetic field implants to draw the chest deformity forward and effect remodeling. In general, there is no cardiopulmonary benefit after chest wall repair except in rare instances when the deformity is excessive. Otherwise, the repair is performed solely to improve appearance. However, the psychosocial benefits of repair of this often embarrassing deformity cannot be minimized.

PECTUS CARINATUM

Pectus carinatum is a protrusion deformity, also called pigeon breast or chicken chest. It is approximately 10 times less frequent than pectus excavatum. It results from the overgrowth of costal cartilages, with forward buckling and secondary deformation of the sternum (Figure 43–5). Atypical and asymmetric forms with rotation are common. There is a familial form. It is associated with Marfan disease, neurofibromatosis, Poland syndrome, and Morquio disease. Unlike pectus excavatum, the deformity is typically mild or nearly imperceptible in early childhood and becomes increasingly prominent during the rapid growth in early puberty.

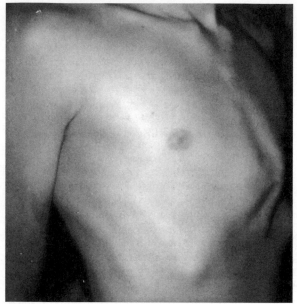

▲ **Figure 43–5.** Severe pectus carinatum deformity.
(Reproduced, with permission, from Albanese CT: Pediatric
surgery. In: *Surgery.* Norton JA [editor]. Springer, 2000.)
(Originally published in Shamberger R: Congenital chest wall
deformities. In: *Pediatric Surgery,* 5th ed. O'Neill JA, Rowe
MI, Grosted JL [editors]. © 1998 Mosby Co.)

▶ Treatment & Prognosis

As with pectus excavatum, there is no cardiorespiratory
compromise with this deformity, and repair is performed
solely to achieve an improved cosmetic appearance. Mild
deformities should be left alone and the patient followed to
observe for progression. Moderate to severe defects should
be repaired, particularly when the patient indicates a desire
for improvement. The deformed cartilages are resected,
leaving the costochondral membranes (perichondrium)
intact. Sternal fracture is usually not necessary. To ensure
that the costal cartilages grow back on a straighter line,
"reefing" sutures are placed in the perichondrium to shorten
them. The costal cartilages regenerate within 6 weeks. A
thorough procedure will provide an excellent cosmetic result
in nearly all cases. Recurrences are rare. An alternative
approach to operative repair is chest bracing via an orthotic
vest that needs to be fitted and worn by the affected child for
several hours daily over several years time.

Fonkalsrud EW, Beanes S: Surgical management of pectus carinatum: 30 years' experience. World J Surg 2001;25:898.
Harrison MR et al: Magnetic mini-mover procedure for pectus
excavatum I: development, design, and simulations for feasibility and safety. J Pediatr Surg 2007;42:81.
Kravarusic D et al: The Calgary protocol for bracing of pectus
carinatum: a preliminary report. J Pediatr Surg 2006;41:923.

Miller KA et al: Minimally invasive repair of pectus excavatum: a
single institution's experience. Surgery 2001;130:652.
Nuss D et al: A 10-year review of a minimally invasive technique
for the correction of pectus excavatum. J Pediatr Surg
1998;33:545.
Shamberger RC: Cardiopulmonary effects of anterior chest wall
deformities. Chest Surg Clin N Am 2000;10:245.

▼ SURGICAL RESPIRATORY EMERGENCIES IN THE NEWBORN

Certain aspects of respiration peculiar to the infant must be
appreciated. Except during periods of crying, the newborn
baby is an obligate nasal breather. The ability to breathe
through the mouth may take weeks or months to acquire.
Inspiration is accomplished chiefly by diaphragmatic excursion; the intercostal and accessory muscles contribute little
to ventilation. Impaired inspiration results in retraction of
the sternum, costal margin, and neck fossae; the resulting
paradoxical motion may contribute to respiratory insufficiency. The airway is small and flaccid, so that it is readily
occluded by mucus or edema, and it collapses readily under
slight pressure. Dyspneic infants swallow large volumes of
air, and the distended stomach and bowel may further
impair diaphragmatic excursion.

▶ Classification

A. Upper Airway Disorders

1. Micrognathia—Pierre Robin syndrome
2. Macroglossia—Muscular hypertrophy, hypothyroidism,
   lymphatic malformation, Beckwith-Wiedemann syndrome
3. Anomalous nasopharyngeal passage—Choanal atresia,
   Treacher-Collins syndrome, Apert syndrome, and Crouzon syndrome
4. Tumors, cysts, or enlarged thyroid remnants in the
   pharynx or neck
5. Laryngeal or tracheal stenosis, webs, cysts, tumors, or
   vocal cord paralysis
6. Epiglottitis
7. Tracheomalacia
8. Tracheal stenosis with or without complete tracheal rings

B. Intrathoracic Airway Disorders

1. Atelectasis
2. Pneumothorax and pneumomediastinum
3. Pleural effusion or chylothorax
4. Pulmonary cysts, sequestration, and tumors
5. Congenital lobar emphysema
6. Diaphragmatic hernia or eventration
7. Esophageal atresia with or without tracheoesophageal
   fistula

8. Anomalies of the great vessels (eg, double aortic arch, aberrant left subclavian artery, anomalous origin of left pulmonary artery)

9. Mediastinal tumors and cysts (foregut duplications, thymomas, substernal goiter, lymphoma)

PIERRE ROBIN SYNDROME

Pierre Robin syndrome is a congenital defect characterized by micrognathia and glossoptosis, often associated with cleft palate. The small lower jaw and strong sucking action of the infant allow the tongue to be sucked back and occlude the laryngeal airway and may be life threatening.

Infants with mild cases should be kept in the prone position during care and feeding. A nasogastric or gastrostomy tube may be necessary for feeding. Nasohypopharyngeal intubation is effective in preventing occlusion of the larynx. If conservative measures fail, prompt attention to maintaining an open airway by tracheostomy is indicated. Surgical treatment involves tongue placation in which the tongue is sutured forward to the lower jaw, but this frequently breaks down. In time, the lower jaw develops normally. These infants eventually learn how to keep the tongue from occluding the airway.

CHOANAL ATRESIA

Complete obstruction at the posterior nares from choanal atresia may be unilateral and relatively asymptomatic. It may be membranous (10%) or bony (90%). When it is bilateral, severe respiratory distress is manifested at birth by marked chest wall retraction on inspiration and a normal cry.

There is arching of the head and neck in an effort to breathe, and the baby is unable to eat. The diagnosis is confirmed by the inability to pass a tube through the nares to the pharynx. With the baby in a supine position, radiopaque material may be instilled into the nares and lateral x-rays of the head taken to outline the obstruction. A CT scan of the nasopharynx will define bony occlusion.

Emergency treatment consists of maintaining an oral airway by placing a nipple, with the tip cut off, in the mouth. The membranous or bony occlusion may then be perforated by direct transpalatal excision, or it may be punctured and enlarged with a Hegar dilator. The newly created opening must be stented with plastic tubing for 5 weeks to prevent stricture.

CONGENITAL TRACHEAL STENOSIS & MALACIA

There are three main types of congenital tracheal stenosis: generalized hypoplasia; funnellike narrowing, usually tapering to a tight stenosis just above the carina; and segmental stenosis of various lengths that can occur at any level. Tracheomalacia is a functional obstruction in a "soft" trachea that collapses with inspiration. It is often secondary to external compression by vascular anomalies or tumors or from a chronically dilated upper esophageal pouch in those with esophageal atresia.

▶ Diagnosis

The diagnostic approach to an infant with respiratory distress and possible distal tracheal obstruction must be carefully integrated with plans for management of the airway, since the compromised infant airway is easily occluded by edema or secretions. This is especially true in distal tracheal lesions, where an endotracheal or tracheostomy tube may not relieve the distal obstruction. The diagnostic value of every procedure must be weighed against the threat of precipitating airway obstruction. Tracheal lesions can be visualized using esophagography, angiography, or CT/MRI scans. Dynamic lesions such as tracheomalacia and vascular compression syndromes are best defined by videotape fluoroscopy or cineradiography with barium in the esophagus. Angiography may be necessary. Flow-volume curves can define the level of obstruction (intrathoracic versus extrathoracic) and the type of obstruction (stenosis versus malacia).

Although bronchoscopy often provides the best delineation of tracheobronchial lesions, it is an invasive procedure that can precipitate acute obstruction from edema or inflammation. A ventilating infant rigid bronchoscope with Hopkins optics should be kept above the critical area to avoid precipitating obstruction. Flexible transnasal awake bronchoscopy is most useful in demonstrating functional abnormalities (eg, malacia).

▶ Treatment

Noncritical stenotic and malacic lesions in infants and children should be managed as conservatively as possible, preferably without intubation. "Temporary" stenting of these lesions is seldom temporary, since the presence of the tube itself ensures continued trauma and irritation such that the tube cannot be removed without airway obstruction. If an infant or child cannot be managed without intubation, surgical correction must be considered. Tracheal reconstruction via resection or a variety of tracheoplasty techniques has proved to be the treatment of choice for tracheal lesions. Severe tracheomalacia is treated by addressing the underlying cause. Aortopexy or an endotracheal stent is often necessary. Tracheostomy is a last resort.

Acosta AC et al: Tracheal stenosis: the long and short of it. J Pediatr Surg 2000;35:1612.

Backer CL et al: Tracheal surgery in children: an 18-year review of four techniques. Eur J Cardiothorac Surg 2001;19:777.

deLorimier AA et al: Tracheobronchial obstructions in infants and children: experience with 45 cases. Ann Surg 1990;212:277.

Rutter MJ, Hartley BE, Cotton RT: Cricotracheal resection in children. Arch Otolaryngol Head Neck Surg 2001;127:289.

CONGENITAL DIAPHRAGMATIC HERNIA

Congenital diaphragmatic hernia is a highly lethal or morbid disease that affects 1 in 2000 live births (Figure 43–6). Anatomically, congenital diaphragmatic hernia results from an embryologic fusion defect, allowing herniation of intra-abdominal contents into the chest. Fusion of the transverse septum and pleuroperitoneal folds normally occurs during the eighth week of embryonic development. If diaphragmatic formation is incomplete, the pleuroperitoneal hiatus (foramen of Bochdalek) persists. Intestinal nonrotation is common because the bowel herniates into the thorax rather than undergoing its normal sequence of rotation and fixation. Severe defects cause pulmonary hypoplasia, pulmonary hypertension, and cardiac dysfunction. The larger the hernia and the earlier it occurs, the more severe the pulmonary hypoplasia.

► Clinical Findings

A. Symptoms and Signs

Infants with large diaphragmatic defects are usually symptomatic in the delivery room, with tachypnea, grunting respirations, retractions, and cyanosis, and may require urgent intubation. Smaller defects may not become symptomatic until the infant is several days or months old. Typically, the abdomen is scaphoid, since much of the abdominal viscera are in the hemithorax. The chest on the side of the hernia may be dull to percussion, but bowel sounds are not usually appreciated. The left side of the diaphragm is affected four or five times as frequently as the right, with a rate of associated anomalies of 20% (chromosomal abnormalities, neural tube defects, and congenital heart disease). When the hernia is on the left, the heart sounds may be heard best on the right side of the chest.

The development of symptoms with congenital diaphragmatic hernia correlates with the degree of pulmonary hypoplasia and pulmonary hypertension. Prenatal diagnosis is occurring more frequently and allows the mother and the fetus to be referred to an institution where sophisticated perinatal and pediatric surgical units are available.

B. Imaging Studies

A chest radiograph may demonstrate the following: a paucity of gas within the abdomen, radiopaque hemithorax if the bowel does not contain a significant amount of gas or if the left lobe of the liver occupies the majority of the hemithorax, loss of normal ipsilateral diaphragmatic contour, bowel in the thorax, contralateral mediastinal shift, and a coiled nasogastric tube in the hemithorax. Right-sided hernias can be difficult to distinguish from a diaphragmatic eventration. This can be differentiated by an MRI scan. MRI or CT scan can also distinguish between congenital diaphragmatic hernia and a cystic lung lesion (eg, congenital cystic adenomatoid malformation).

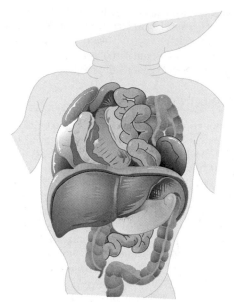

▲ **Figure 43–6.** Congenital posterolateral (Bochdalek) diaphragmatic hernia. Bowel, spleen, and liver sometimes herniate into the chest and severely compromise lung development in utero and ventilation after birth.

► Treatment

A nasogastric tube should be placed in the stomach to aspirate swallowed air and to prevent distention of the herniated bowel, which would further compress the lungs. Repair of the diaphragmatic defect is not a surgical emergency and should be performed once the infant has stabilized and has demonstrated minimal to no pulmonary hypertension. Early reduction (before 48 hours postnatally) and repair has been shown to transiently worsen pulmonary function by decreasing pulmonary compliance and increasing airway reactivity. A subcostal abdominal incision should be made and the herniated bowel reduced from the pleural space. Some surgeons prefer a thoracic approach, particularly for right-sided defects. The negative pressure between the bowel and the chest wall may make reduction difficult. Following reduction of the bowel, placement of a chest tube in the pleural space is optional; if used, it is connected to a water seal and not to vacuum. The diaphragmatic defect should be closed by nonabsorbable sutures. In many instances, a synthetic material is required to close large defects. The abdominal cavity may be too small and underdeveloped to accommodate the intestine and permit closure of the abdominal wall muscle and fascial layers. In such cases, abdominal wall skin flaps should be mobilized and closed over the protruding bowel or a silo created to allow for gradual visceral reduction with concomitant abdominal domain expansion and staged closure of the abdominal wall.

Respiratory support and treatment of hypoxemia, hypercapnia, and acidosis are required before and often after repair. Persistent pulmonary hypertension may result in right-to-left shunt and produce severe hypoxemia in the lower aorta. Nitric oxide added to the ventilation gases can induce pulmonary vasodilation, improve pulmonary perfusion, and reverse the right-to-left shunt. The persistent fetal circulation physiology may be treated successfully in many cases by extracorporeal membrane oxygenation and permissive ventilatory strategies (high-frequency ventilation). Hypoxemic myocardiopathy may require infusion of dopamine to enhance cardiac output. Prenatal treatment for severe congenital diaphragmatic hernia (temporary fetal tracheal occlusion to promote lung growth) has been extensively studied and presently offers no advantage over maximal postnatal care.

▶ Prognosis

The death rate for infants with congenital diaphragmatic hernia depends on the severity of pulmonary hypoplasia, the presence or absence of associated anomalies, and the quality of care provided for these critically ill infants. When diagnosed in utero, prognosis depends on the presence or absence of liver herniation into the left hemithorax, the gestational age at diagnosis, and an ultrasonographic estimation of lung size (the lung-to-head ratio). Long term, there are a number of likely clinically insignificant physiologic abnormalities such as a reduction in total lung volume, restrictive or obstructive lung disease, and abnormal lung compliance. However, a small subset of patients will survive as "pulmonary cripples" and remain oxygen-dependent or ventilator-dependent, often requiring tracheostomies. Since there may be deficient periesophageal muscular tissue or an abnormal orientation of the gastroesophageal junction, gastroesophageal reflux is common. It is most commonly treated nonoperatively, but refractory cases may require a surgical antireflux procedure. Recurrent diaphragmatic hernia occurs in 10–20% of infants and should be considered in any child with a history of congenital diaphragmatic hernia who presents with new gastrointestinal or pulmonary symptoms. Recurrence is most common when a prosthetic patch is used for the repair.

Surgical units that are immediately adjacent to obstetric services report death rates as high as 80%, because infants with severe pulmonary hypoplasia will be recognized and treated immediately. Infants who survive transfer to surgical centers remote from the delivery area usually have less severe disease, and the death rates reported from these facilities are usually under 40%.

With improvements in prenatal ultrasonographic imaging, many of these defects can be appreciated early enough so that planned delivery at a tertiary facility is possible. Excluding those infants with severe associated anomalies, the over-all survival rate using maximal medical therapy has been increasing over the past several years due to "gentle" ventilation strategies and is well over 70%.

FORAMEN OF MORGAGNI HERNIA

The foramen of Morgagni occurs at the junction of the septum transversum and the anterior thoracic wall. This anterior, central diaphragmatic defect accounts for only 2% of diaphragmatic hernias. It may be parasternal, retrosternal, or bilateral. Unlike Bochdalek hernias, children are typically asymptomatic and the defect is discovered later in life on a chest radiograph taken for reasons unrelated to the hernia. The lateral chest radiograph demonstrating an air-filled mass extending into the anterior mediastinum is pathognomonic. Repair is indicated in the asymptomatic patient due to the risk of bowel obstruction. The viscera are reduced and any associated hernia sac excised. The defect is closed by suturing the posterior rim of diaphragm to the posterior rectus sheath, since there is no anterior diaphragm. A prosthetic patch closure is frequently required given the tension that results with native tissue repairs because of the absence of anterior diaphragm. Laparoscopic approaches to this type of repair are increasingly being performed. There is no associated pulmonary hypoplasia or hypertension. This defect, when noted in newborns, can be associated with the pentalogy of Cantrell, a disorder with considerable morbidity and mortality that consists of the anterior diaphragmatic defect, distal sternal cleft, epigastric omphalocele, apical pericardial defect, and congenital heart disease (usually a septal defect). Excluding patients with the pentalogy of Cantrell, survival is nearly 100%.

EVENTRATION OF THE DIAPHRAGM

Diaphragmatic eventration is an abnormally elevated or attenuated portion of the diaphragm (or both). It may be congenital (usually idiopathic, but can be associated with congenital myopathies or intrauterine infections) or acquired (as a result of phrenic nerve injury during forceps delivery or surgery). In the congenital form, there is variable thinning or absence of diaphragmatic muscle, at which point its distinction from congenital diaphragmatic hernia with a persistent hernia sac is obscure. The elevated hemidiaphragm may produce abnormalities of chest wall mechanics with impaired pulmonary function. Respiratory distress and pneumonia are frequent presenting symptoms, although gastrointestinal symptoms such as vomiting or gastric volvulus have been reported.

The diagnosis is made by chest radiograph. It is confirmed by fluoroscopy or ultrasound, which demonstrates paradoxical movement of the diaphragm during spontaneous respiration. Incidentally discovered small, localized eventrations do not need repair. Eventrations that are associated with respiratory symptoms should be repaired by plicating the diaphragm using interrupted nonabsorbable sutures.

Congenital Diaphragmatic Hernia Study Group: Defect Size deter-mines survival in infants with congenital diaphragmatic hernia. Pediatrics 2007;120:3651.

Dutta S, Albanese CT: Use of a prosthetic patch for laparoscopic repair of Morgagni diaphragmatic hernia in children. J Lap-aroendosc Adv Surg Tech A 2007;17:391.

Harrison MR et al: A randomized trial of fetoscopic tracheal occlusion for severe fetal congenital diaphragmatic hernia. New Engl J Med 2003;349:1916.

Kizilcan F et al: The long-term results of diaphragmatic plication. J Pediatr Surg 1993;28:42.

Nobuhara K et al: Long-term outlook for survivors of congenital diaphragmatic hernia. Clin Perinatol 1996;23:873.

Pokorny W, McGill C, Halberg F: Morgagni hernia during infancy: presentation and associated anomalies. 1984;19:394.

Puri P: Congenital diaphragmatic hernia. Curr Probl Surg 1994; 31:785.

CONGENITAL LOBAR EMPHYSEMA

Congenital lobar emphysema results from hyperinflation of a single lobe; rarely, more than one lobe is affected. The upper and middle lobes are most frequently involved. Patho-logically, there are three forms: hypoplastic emphysema, polyalveolar lobe, and bronchial obstruction.

Hypoplastic emphysema is distinguished by a segment, lobe, or whole lung that has a reduced number of bronchial branches with a diminished number and smaller size of blood vessels. The number of alveoli is abnormally decreased, but the air spaces are too large. The hyperlucent region seen on chest radiograph is normal or small in volume, and since it does not affect the surrounding normal lung, surgical treatment is unnecessary.

Polyalveolar lobe is characterized by a normal size and number of bronchial branches, but there is an abnormal number of alveoli from each respiratory unit. These alveoli are prone to expand excessively, producing emphysema, which encroaches on the surrounding normal lung and therefore requires removal.

Bronchial obstruction may occur from deficient bron-chial cartilage support, redundant mucosa, bronchial steno-sis, mucous plug, or bronchial compression by anomalous vessels or other mediastinal lesions. With inspiration, the bronchus opens to allow air into the lung; but on expiration the bronchus collapses, trapping the air, and with each respiratory cycle there is progressive expansion of the lobe.

Clinical Findings

In one third of patients, respiratory distress is noted at birth; in only 5% of cases do symptoms develop after 6 months. Males are affected twice as frequently as females. The signs include progressive and severe dyspnea, wheezing, grunting, coughing, cyanosis, and difficulty feeding. An increased anteroposterior dimension of the chest and retractions may be seen. The chest is hyperresonant, and decreased breath sounds may be noted over the affected lobe. A chest radio-

graph may demonstrate radiolucency of the emphysematous lobe, with bronchovascular markings extending to the lung periphery. Compression atelectasis of the adjacent lung, shift of the mediastinum, depression of the diaphragm, and ante-rior bowing of the sternum can be seen. The emphysematous lobe may continue to expand, compressing adjacent lung and airways, producing progressively severe respiratory distress.

Treatment & Prognosis

Occasionally, the emphysema may be due to a mucous plug in the bronchus that may be aspirated by bronchoscopy. Compression of the bronchus by mediastinal masses may be relieved by removal of the tumor or repair of anomalous vessels. Treatment of mildly symptomatic cases may not be necessary.

Many patients with lobar emphysema are severely symp-tomatic, and pulmonary lobectomy is necessary. For those who are breathing spontaneously prior to operation, anes-thesia should not be started until all personnel are ready for a rapid thoracotomy, since positive-pressure ventilation may acutely enlarge the emphysematous lobe, thereby compress-ing the normal lung tissue and heart. The prognosis follow-ing surgical relief of the lobar emphysema is excellent. Rarely, patients may show residual disease in the remaining lung. At long-term follow-up, lung volumes are normal, but the airflow rates are diminished.

Martinez-Frontanilla LA et al: Surgery of acquired lobar emphy-sema in the neonate. J Pediatr Surg 1984;19:375.

Olutoye OO et al: Prenatal diagnosis and management of congen-ital lobar emphysema. J Pediatr Surg 2000;35:792.

GREAT VESSEL ANOMALIES

Tracheobronchial and esophageal compression by the great vessels may occur as a result of anomalies of the aortic arch or of abnormally located or enlarged pulmonary and subcla-vian arteries. While the most common abnormality is an aberrant right subclavian artery, the most important is the double aortic arch because it often causes serious respiratory distress in young infants (Figure 43–7). Affected infants have a characteristic inspiratory and expiratory wheeze, stridor, or crouplike cough. Echocardiography, CT, and MRI can dem-onstrate the anomalous anatomy. Esophagoscopy and bron-choscopy may be helpful in assessing the degree and level of compression. The surgical approach is through the left hemithorax. Following removal of the thymus, the aortic arch and its branches are skeletonized and the anatomy is identified. For the double aortic arch, the smallest arterial component is divided; an anomalous right subclavian artery is divided at its origin. The accompanying fibrous bands and sheaths constricting the trachea and esophagus must also be divided. The ductus arteriosus (or its fibrous remnant) is also divided.

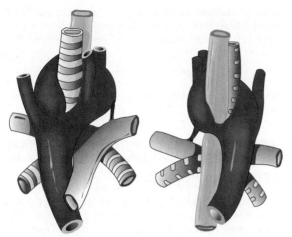

▲ **Figure 43–7.** Anterior (left) and posterior views of double aortic arch constricting the trachea and esophagus.

Sebening C et al: Vascular tracheobronchial compression syndromes—experience in surgical treatment and literature review. Thorac Cardiovasc Surg 2000;48:164.

Woods RK et al: Vascular anomalies and tracheoesophageal compression: a single institution's 25-year experience. Ann Thorac Surg 2001;72:434.

MEDIASTINAL MASSES

Mediastinal masses are relatively common in infants and children and can be classified according to the compartment of the mediastinum from which they arise. The mediastinum is classically divided into anterior, middle, and posterior compartments. Anatomically, the anterior mediastinum consists of the area between the sternum and the anterior aspect of the trachea and pericardium. The middle compartment contains the trachea, major bronchi, and paratracheal spaces. The posterior segment extends from the posterior aspect of the trachea to the spine.

Anterior masses make up one third and are most commonly teratomas and lymphomas. Teratomas may be cystic or solid and may also be found within the pericardium (middle compartment). Approximately 20% are malignant. Other masses include thymic cysts, thymomas, substernal goiters, and lymphangiomas. Middle mediastinal masses are rare but when present are most likely to be bronchogenic cysts. Sixty percent of mediastinal masses are located within the posterior compartment. Neurogenic tumors are most common and include neuroblastoma, ganglioneuroblastoma, ganglioneuroma, neurofibroma, and neurofibrosarcoma. Common symptoms include respiratory distress (via tracheal or lung compression), Horner syndrome, and pain. Enterogenous cysts or duplications are also commonly seen in the posterior compartment. They are termed neurenteric when there is an associated cervical or thoracic vertebral anomaly.

Grosfeld JL et al: Mediastinal tumors in children: experience with 196 cases. Ann Surg Oncol 1994;1:121.

CONGENITAL LUNG LESIONS

Congenital lung lesions, which arise from anomalous development of the foregut, are classified as follows: (1) bronchogenic cyst, (2) cystic adenomatoid malformation, (3) pulmonary sequestration, and (4) bronchopulmonary foregut malformation. Embryonic tissues that are destined to form bronchi and lung become anomalous isolated structures within or outside of the lung. These lesions produce symptoms from their size and position, resulting in compression of bronchi or lung parenchyma, or from infection and abscess formation within the cyst and surrounding normal lung.

BRONCHOGENIC CYST

Bronchogenic cysts are lined by cuboidal or ciliated columnar epithelium and are filled with mucoid material. Repeated infection in the cyst may produce squamous epithelial metaplasia. About half arise in the mediastinum and do not communicate with the bronchi. They appear as radiopaque masses on chest radiographs. When located within the lung parenchyma, the cysts usually communicate with the airways and consequently are prone to abscess formation. Bronchogenic cysts arise in the right lung three times more often than in the left. They are more common in the lower lobes but may be found in any lobe. Partial compression of bronchi produces hyperinflation of the involved lung, while complete obstruction produces atelectasis. Rupture of a cyst that communicates with bronchi may present as a tension pneumothorax. Treatment of a noninfected cyst is by excision. Infected cysts first require drainage (usually percutaneous) and intravenous antibiotic therapy followed by resection after the inflammation subsides (no sooner than 6 weeks after drainage).

CONGENITAL CYSTIC ADENOMATOID MALFORMATION

This lesion is considered a hamartoma in which multiple cysts are lined by a polypoid proliferation of bronchial epithelium surrounded by striated muscle and elastic tissue, but there is an absence of mucous glands and cartilage. They are most often lobar and are classified radiologically according to cyst size: type I are large (> 2 cm) cysts, type II are smaller cysts (< 2 cm), and type III have cysts that are so small as to import a solid appearance. These malformations occur with equal frequency in both lungs, with a slight predominance in the upper lobes. Associated renal and nervous system anomalies may be present.

▶ Clinical Findings

A large lesion can compress the fetal lung, resulting in pulmonary hypoplasia at birth, or may distort or obstruct the esophagus, producing polyhydramnios. In addition, compression of venous return to the heart with exudation of protein into the lung fluid may cause fetal congestive heart failure, hydrops fetalis, and death in utero. Large lesions that do not cause fetal hydrops can remain stable or involute during fetal life, producing little or no symptoms of respiratory distress at birth.

▶ Treatment

If prenatal ultrasound can recognize the presence of this disorder in association with hydrops, resection in utero is an option for select cases. Children in whom hydrops did not occur before birth may be born asymptomatic (small lesions) or may have variable degrees of respiratory distress due to compression of the ipsilateral normal lung. Asymptomatic children may be observed, but resection (pulmonary lobectomy) is recommended because these lesions often become infected, and there are case reports of malignant transformation occurring in untreated, longstanding cysts. Often, the plain chest radiograph does not demonstrate the small, asymptomatic lesion. A CT scan is indicated for those patients.

PULMONARY SEQUESTRATION & BRONCHOPULMONARY FOREGUT MALFORMATION

A sequestration consists of normally developed bronchioles and alveoli supplied by systemic rather than pulmonary arteries. Sequestrations occur in the lower chest, most commonly on the left, adjacent to the mediastinum. Rarely, sequestrations may occur in the upper or middle lobes or even below the diaphragm. They usually have a systemic arterial blood supply from the aorta, either above or below the diaphragm. On rare occasions, a sequestration will communicate with the esophagus or stomach, a condition termed bronchopulmonary foregut malformation. Sequestrations may be intralobar (typically in older children) or extralobar. Intralobar lesions drain through the pulmonary veins, are in communication with the tracheobronchial tree, and are prone to infection and lung abscess formation. Extralobar lesions drain into the azygous venous system, do not communicate with the lung, and are commonly asymptomatic. They are often found in association with congenital diaphragmatic hernia. Histologic evidence suggests that these lesions have embryologic origin similar to that of bronchogenic cysts and congenital cystic adenomatoid malformations. However, unlike the latter, sequestrations rarely grow large enough to produce hydrops and demise in utero. Treatment is by excision of the extralobar sequestration or lobectomy in cases of intralobar sequestration.

Adzick NS et al: Fetal lung lesions: management and outcome. Am J Obstet Gynecol 1998;179:884.
Albanese CT, Rothenberg SS: Experience With 144 Consecutive Pediatric Thoracoscopic Lobectomies. J Laparoendosc Adv Surg Tech A 2007;17:339.41

Cass DL et al: Cystic lung lesions with systemic arterial blood supply: a hybrid of congenital cystic adenomatoid malformation and bronchopulmonary sequestration. J Pediatr Surg 1997;32:986.
Neilson IR et al: Congenital adenomatoid malformation of the lung: current management and prognosis. J Pediatr Surg 1991; 26:975.
Nuchtern JG, Harberg FJ: Congenital lung cysts. Semin Pediatr Surg 1994;3:233.

▼ CONGENITAL GASTROINTESTINAL LESIONS

ESOPHAGEAL ANOMALIES

The trachea and esophagus are derived from the primitive foregut. Initially, they appear as a common ventral diverticulum at about the 19th day of gestation. Beginning several days later, elongation and separation of the diverticulum into the airway and esophagus occurs in a caudal to cephalad direction. Errors in this process result in esophageal atresia, tracheoesophageal fistula, and their variants (Figure 43–8).

▶ Classification

A. With Esophageal Atresia

1. There is a blind proximal pouch and a fistula between the distal end of the esophagus and the distal one third of the trachea (type C, 85% of cases).
2. There is a blind proximal esophageal pouch, no tracheoesophageal fistula, and a blind, short distal esophagus (type A, 10% of cases). This is referred to as "pure or long gap" atresia.
3. There are fistulas between both proximal and distal esophageal segments and the trachea (type D, 2% of cases).
4. There is a fistula between the proximal esophagus and the trachea and a blind distal esophagus without fistula (type B, 1% of cases).

B. Without Esophageal Atresia

1. There is an H-type tracheoesophageal fistula that is usually present in the low cervical region (type E, 4–5% of cases).
2. There is esophageal stenosis consisting of a membranous occlusion (often containing cartilage) between the mid and distal third of the esophagus (rare).
3. There is a laryngotracheoesophageal cleft of varying length, consisting of a linear communication between these structures (very rare).

▶ Clinical Findings

Shortly after birth, the infant with esophageal atresia is noted to have excessive salivation and repeated episodes of coughing, choking, and cyanosis. Attempts at feeding result in choking, gagging, and regurgitation. Infants with tracheoe-

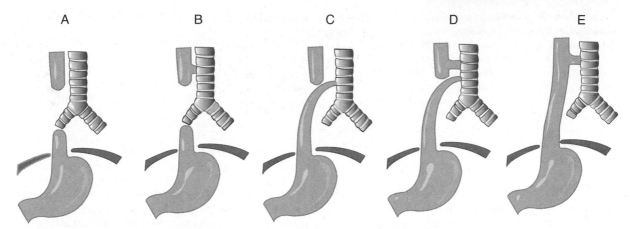

▲ **Figure 43–8. A:** Pure (long gap) esophageal atresia. **B:** Esophageal atresia with proximal tracheoesophageal fistula. **C:** Esophageal atresia with distal tracheoesophageal fistula. **D:** Esophageal atresia with proximal and distal fistulas. **E:** Tracheoesophageal fistula without esophageal atresia. (From Grosfeld JL: Pediatric surgery. In: *Textbook of Surgery.* Sabiston DC [editor]. Saunders, 1991. Reproduced with permission from Elsevier.)

sophageal fistula in addition to esophageal atresia will have reflux of gastric secretions into the tracheobronchial tree, with resulting pneumonia. Pulmonary infiltrates are usually noted first in the right upper lobe.

A size 10F catheter should be passed into the esophagus by way of the nose or mouth; if esophageal atresia is present, the tube will not go down the expected distance to the stomach and will coil in the upper esophageal pouch. If a tracheoesophageal fistula connects to the lower esophageal segment, air will be present in the stomach and bowel on plain radiographs. Absence of air below the diaphragm usually means that a distal tracheoesophageal fistula is not present.

Abdominal distention is a prominent finding because the Valsalva effect of coughing and crying forces air through a fistula into the stomach and bowel. The presence and position of the fistula can be determined by bronchoscopy.

Laryngotracheoesophageal cleft produces symptoms similar to those of tracheoesophageal fistula but of much greater severity. Laryngoscopy may show the cleft between the arytenoids extending down the larynx. Bronchoscopy is the best means of outlining the cleft.

There is a 50% incidence of associated anomalies: cardiac (patent ductus arteriosus, septal defects), gastrointestinal (imperforate anus, duodenal atresia), genitourinary, and skeletal. The VACTERL association (*v*ertebral, *a*norectal, *c*ardiac, *t*racheoesophageal, *r*enal, and *l*imb anomalies) is present in 25% of cases. Isolated esophageal atresia has been associated with various genetic abnormalities, including trisomy 18 and trisomy 21.

▶ **Treatment**

A sump-suction catheter should be placed in the upper esophageal pouch and the head of the bed elevated. An echocardiogram is required to determine the position of the aortic arch, since a right-sided arch makes the standard right thoracotomy (or thoracoscopic) repair difficult and is present in 5% of infants. If possible, aspiration pneumonia is treated before repair.

The goal of operative therapy is to divide and ligate the fistula and repair the atresia in one stage, if possible. This is usually performed using a right posterolateral thoracotomy with an extrapleural dissection, although a transpleural thoracoscopic approach is gaining popularity for stable, full-term infants. Also, thoracoscopic approaches are gaining acceptance as minimally invasive techniques continue to evolve. In those with an **H**-type tracheoesophageal fistula, the fistula is located above the thoracic inlet in two thirds of cases. These fistulas may be divided through a left transverse cervical incision. A feeding gastrostomy tube is no longer routinely inserted except when the esophageal repair is under extreme tension, when there is long-gap atresia not amenable to single-stage repair, and when there are severe associated anomalies (eg, congenital heart disease). A transanastomotic feeding tube is placed for postoperative feeding pending demonstration of a leak-free anastomosis by esophagogram obtained 7 days after surgery.

Staged operations are reserved for extremely premature babies, those who have severe aspiration pneumonitis, and those with severe anomalies or long gaps between the esophageal pouches. There are several strategies for repairing these defects. These include cervical esophagostomy, division of the fistula, and insertion of a gastrostomy tube. Several months later, a staged reconstruction by esophageal replacement with colon or stomach interposition can be undertaken. Another alternative is a gastrostomy tube alone with intermittent bougienage and stretching of the upper esophageal pouch, followed by primary esophageal anastomosis and immediate interposition grafting.

Esophageal narrowing or webs in the distal esophageal segment readily respond to esophageal dilation. This is usually accomplished with Hurst or Maloney mercury-weighted bougies. Dilations are repeated until healing occurs without recurrence of the web. Esophagoscopy and excision of portions of a tough or thick web, using biopsy forceps or the endoscopic laser, may be required in addition to dilation. A lower esophageal stricture containing cartilage will require excision and anastomosis.

▶ Prognosis

The survival rate for a full-term infant without associated anomalies is excellent. However, deaths occur as a result of pulmonary complications, severe associated anomalies, prematurity, and sepsis due to anastomotic disruption. Anastomotic leaks occur because of tension or poor blood supply. In performing the anastomosis, the extrapleural approach prevents the development of empyema and confines a leak and possible infection to a small localized area.

Swallowing is a reflex response that must be reinforced early in infancy. If establishment of esophageal continuity is delayed for more than 4–6 weeks, it may take many months to overcome oral aversion and learn to swallow. Babies with cervical esophagostomies should be encouraged to suck, eat, and swallow during gastrostomy feedings.

Dysphagia may occur for months or years following successful repair of esophageal atresia and is multifactorial. An anastomotic stricture is not uncommon and may require one or more dilations under anesthesia. Swallowed foreign bodies will lodge at the site of anastomosis and require removal with esophagoscopy. Another cause of dysphagia is poor peristalsis of the distal esophageal segment. This frequent problem improves with age.

Most of these infants have an alarming, barking cough and rattling sound on respiration from tracheomalacia. This results from in utero compression of the trachea by the dilated proximal esophageal pouch. This frequently improves with age and is rare after 5 years of age. Gastroesophageal reflux is common after successful repair and may result in recurrent aspiration pneumonia, dysphagia, failure to thrive, and recurrent anastomotic stricture. A surgical antireflux procedure may be necessary.

Choudhory SR et al: Survival of patients with esophageal atresia: influence of birth weight, cardiac anomaly, and late respiratory complications. J Pediatr Surg 1999;34:70.

Holcomb GW 3rd et al: Thoracoscopic repair of esophageal atresia and tracheoesophageal fistula: a multi-institutional analysis. Ann Surg 2005;242:422.

McKinnon LJ, Kosloske AM: Prediction and prevention of anastomotic complications of esophageal atresia and tracheoesophageal fistula. J Pediatr Surg 1990;25:778.

Rothenberg SS: Thoracoscopic repair of tracheoesophageal fistula in newborns. J Pediatr Surg 2002;37:869.

INTESTINAL OBSTRUCTION IN THE NEWBORN

Since fetuses continually swallow amniotic fluid into their gastrointestinal tracts and excrete it in their urine, intestinal obstruction may be noted on prenatal ultrasound by the presence of polyhydramnios (increased amniotic fluid level). The presence of polyhydramnios correlates with the level of the obstruction; it is most common with proximal gastrointestinal tract obstruction (eg, esophageal and duodenal atresia), is rarely noted with ileal atresia, and is never noted in association with anorectal obstruction.

After birth, vomiting is the principal symptom, and it is bile-stained if the obstruction is distal to the ampulla of Vater. It is important to note that bilious vomiting in the newborn is pathologic until proved otherwise. On physical examination, the presence and degree of abdominal distention depends on the level of the obstruction and should be noted. For example, there is no significant distention with duodenal obstruction versus massive distention with colonic obstruction (eg, Hirschsprung disease). A careful perineal examination should be performed to determine whether the anus is present, patent, and in the normal location. Meconium, the first newborn stool, passes in the first 24 hours of life in 94% of normal full-term infants and by 48 hours in 98%. Failure to pass meconium may be indicative of lower gastrointestinal tract obstruction. However, 30–50% of newborn infants with intestinal obstruction will pass meconium.

Depending on the pathology, the plain abdominal radiograph may demonstrate dilated bowel loops, air-fluid levels, calcifications (if in utero perforation occurred), or a gasless abdomen. Unlike in adult patients, one cannot differentiate small from large bowel by their usual markings on a plain radiograph of the newborn's abdomen. If a lower gastrointestinal tract obstruction is suspected, a contrast (usually water-soluble contrast) enema is the most useful study, since it can be both diagnostic and therapeutic in the majority of cases (see below). An upper gastrointestinal series is rarely indicated unless malrotation is to be ruled out. The CT, MRI, or ultrasound scans are virtually never indicated in the workup of newborn intestinal obstruction.

HYPERTROPHIC PYLORIC STENOSIS

Pyloric stenosis is the most common surgical disorder producing emesis in infancy. It results from hypertrophy of the circular and longitudinal muscularis of the pylorus and the distal antrum of the stomach with progressive narrowing of the pyloric canal (Figure 43–9). The cause is not known. The male-to-female incidence is 4:1. The disorder is more common in firstborn infants and occurs four times more often in the offspring of mothers who had the disease as infants than in those whose fathers had the disease. If one monozygotic twin is affected, the other will also have the disorder in two thirds of cases. A seasonal variation is noted in the occurrence of symptoms, with peaks in spring and fall.

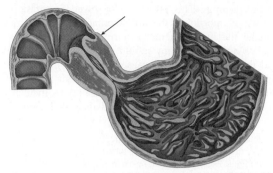

▲ **Figure 43–9.** Hypertrophic pyloric stenosis. Note that the distal end of the hypertrophic muscle protrudes into the duodenum (arrow), accounting for the ease of perforation into the duodenum during pyloromyotomy.

▶ Clinical Findings

A. Symptoms and Signs

Typically, the affected infant is full term when born and feeds and grows well until 2–4 weeks after birth, at which time occasional regurgitation of some of the feedings occurs. Several days later, however, the vomiting becomes more frequent and forceful. The vomitus contains the previous feeding and no bile. Blood may be seen in the vomitus in 5% of cases, and coffee grounds or occult blood is frequently present. Shortly after vomiting, the infant acts starved and will feed again. The stools become infrequent and firm in consistency as dehydration occurs. With dehydration, infants often have sunken fontanelles, dry mucous membranes, and poor skin turgor. Weight loss follows progressive feeding intolerance. Jaundice with indirect hyperbilirubinemia occurs in fewer than 10% of cases. Gastric peristaltic waves can usually be seen moving from the left costal margin to the area of the pylorus. In over 90% of cases, the pyloric "tumor," or "olive," can be palpated when the infant is relaxed. Abdominal relaxation may be accomplished by sedating the infant or by feeding clear fluids and simultaneously aspirating the stomach contents with a gastric tube.

B. Imaging Studies

An imaging study is indicated when the pyloric tumor cannot be palpated. Abdominal ultrasound, the most sensitive and specific test, will identify hypertrophic pyloric stenosis when the muscle thickness is greater than 4 mm and the length of the pylorus is greater than 16 mm. A contrast upper gastrointestinal series is indicated if an experienced ultrasonographer is unavailable or if there is a reasonable chance that the patient's symptoms are not due to pyloric stenosis (eg, a premature, 1-week-old baby), since this examination can demonstrate other entities in the differential, whereas the ultrasound can simply comment on the presence

or absence of a hypertrophied pyloris. A positive upper gastrointestinal series can include the following diagnostic signs: (1) outlining of the narrow pyloric channel by a single "string sign" or "double track" owing to folds of mucosa; (2) a pyloric "beak" where the pyloric entrance from the antrum occurs; (3) the "shoulder" sign, in which the pyloric mass bulges into the antrum; and (4) complete obstruction of the pylorus.

▶ Differential Diagnosis

Repeated nonbilious vomiting in early infancy may be due to overfeeding, intracranial lesions, pylorospasm, antral web, gastroesophageal reflux, pyloric duplication, duodenal stenosis, malrotation of the bowel, or adrenal insufficiency.

▶ Complications

Repeated vomiting with inadequate intake of formula results in hypokalemic hypochloremic alkalosis, dehydration, and starvation. Gastritis and reflux esophagitis occur frequently. Aspiration of vomitus may produce pneumonia.

▶ Treatment & Prognosis

The operative treatment is the Fredet-Ramstedt pyloromyotomy, in which the pylorus is incised along its entire length, spread widely exposing but not breaching the underlying mucosa. Surgery should be undertaken only after dehydration and the hypokalemic hypochloremic alkalosis have been corrected, heralded by a normal serum chloride and a urine output greater than 1 cc/kg/h. There are three approaches to the pyloromyotomy: a right upper quadrant transverse skin incision, a circumumbilical or intraumbilical skin incision, or a laparoscopic approach with the telescope in the umbilicus and the two working instruments placed directly through the abdominal wall. If, during the pyloromyotomy, the mucosa is inadvertently entered (usually on the duodenal side), it is closed with fine nonabsorbable sutures and an omental patch is placed. Large perforations are managed by closing the pyloromyotomy, rotating the pylorus 90 degrees, and repeating the myotomy. Successful repair is evident when the submucosa is seen to herniate out of the myotomy site.

Multiple postoperative feeding schedules have been described, ranging from immediate full feeds to delayed feeds with incremental advances in volume. This has stemmed from the observation that nearly all patients with pyloric stenosis vomit after surgery, presumably due to gastric ileus, gastritis, gastroesophageal reflux, or all of the above. An incomplete pyloromyotomy (usually on the antral side) is suspected when vomiting persists beyond 2 weeks postoperatively. This stems from a short myotomy or incomplete division of the muscle.

Pyloric stenosis never recurs, and there is a uniformly excellent outcome.

Forman HP et al: A rational approach to the diagnosis of hypertrophic pyloric stenosis. J Pediatr Surg 1990;25:262.

Leinwald MJ, Shaul DB, Anderson KD: The umbilical fold approach to pyloromyotomy: is it a safe alternative to the right upper-quadrant approach? JACS 1999;189:362.

Rothenberg SS: Laparoscopic pyloromyotomy: The slice and pull technique. Pediatr Endosurg Innov Tech 1997;1:39.

CONGENITAL DUODENAL OBSTRUCTION

The various causes of duodenal obstruction are atresia, stenosis, mucosal web (complete or variably perforate), annular pancreas, preduodenal portal vein, and peritoneal bands (Ladd bands) from malrotation. Duodenal atresia is distinguished from more distal gastrointestinal atresias because it is due to failure of recanalization of the duodenum early in gestation rather than due to mesenteric vascular abnormality late in gestation. Atresia of the duodenum is twice as common as in the jejunum or ileum. In about half of cases, multiple congenital anomalies are present, including Downs syndrome in 30% and congenital heart disease in 20%. Birth weight is less than 2500 g in half of these infants. Mucosal webs or stenoses occur as often as pure atresia. Annular pancreas is almost always associated with hypoplasia of the duodenum at the level of the ampulla. The cause is a developmental defect characterized by circumferential persistence of the gland around the duodenum at the site of the embryonic ventral anlage, leading to duodenal obstruction and an accessory pancreatic duct.

▶ Clinical Findings

In 75% of cases, duodenal obstruction occurs distal to the ampulla of Vater, causing bile to be diverted to the proximal duodenum and stomach. Bilious emesis occurs shortly after birth and during attempted feedings. The upper abdomen is rarely distended. Meconium is passed in over 50% of cases.

The plain abdominal radiograph demonstrates an air-distended stomach and duodenum (double-bubble sign). Gas in the small and large intestines indicates incomplete obstruction. Contrast upper gastrointestinal series is used to identify the presence or absence of malrotation in those cases with incomplete obstruction, since obstruction from intestinal malrotation is a surgical emergency.

▶ Treatment

Surgery is performed using a right upper transverse abdominal incision or via laparoscopy. A Kocher maneuver should be performed, with complete mobilization of the third and fourth portions of the duodenum. Obstruction from Ladd bands requires simple division of the bands and correction of the malrotation. Duodenoduodenostomy is performed for duodenal atresia and annular pancreas. A mucosal web is excised, taking care to avoid injury to the adjacent ampulla. Commonly, the duodenum is hugely dilated above the obstruction, which results in impaired aboral progression of ingested feedings. This problem is resolved by excision or plication of a portion of the antimesenteric wall of the bowel to make the lumen diameter normal (tapered duodenoplasty). Gastrojejunostomy should not be done because the blind duodenal pouch may cause repeated vomiting. In all cases, the distal bowel must be irrigated and assessed for associated intrinsic obstruction and atresia (1–3% incidence). Mortality is related to prematurity and associated anomalies.

Grosfeld JL, Rescorla FJ: Duodenal atresia and stenosis: reassessment of treatment and outcome based on antenatal diagnosis, pathologic variance, and long-term followup. World J Surg 1993;17:301.

Spigland N, Yazbeck S: Complications associated with surgical treatment of congenital intrinsic duodenal obstruction. J Pediatr Surg 1990;25:1127.

ATRESIA & STENOSIS OF THE JEJUNUM, ILEUM, & COLON

Atresia and stenosis of the jejunum, ileum, and colon are caused by a mesenteric vascular accident in utero, which may result from hernia, volvulus, or intussusception, producing aseptic necrosis and resorption of the necrotic bowel. Although atresia may occur in any portion of the intestine, most cases occur in the distal ileum or proximal jejunum. Colonic atresia is very rare, accounting for no more than 1% of all intestinal atresias. A short area of necrosis may produce only stenosis or a membranous web occluding the lumen (type I) (Figure 43–10). A more extensive infarct may leave a fibrous cord between the two bowel loops (type II), or the proximal and distal bowel may be completely separated with a V-shaped defect in the mesentery (type IIIa). Multiple atresias occur in 10% of cases (type IV). A type III variant (type IIIb) is commonly called apple-peel or Christmas tree atresia, in which there is a blind-ending proximal jejunum, absence of a long length of mid small bowel, and a terminal ileum coiled around its tenuous blood supply from an ileocolic vessel.

▶ Clinical Findings

Vomiting of bile, abdominal distention, and failure to pass meconium indicate intestinal obstruction. The plain abdominal radiograph will give an estimate of how far along the intestine the obstruction exists. A contrast enema may be indicated to detect the level of obstruction. In obstructions that occur in the distal bowel and appear relatively early in gestation, the colon is empty of meconium and appears abnormally narrow. When the obstruction is proximal or when it occurs late in pregnancy, meconium is passed into the colon. The contrast enema will then outline a more generous-sized colon with its contents (meconium). In older children with evidence of partial intestinal obstruction, a small bowel series may be indicated to identify intestinal stenosis.

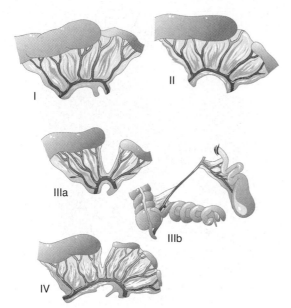

▲ **Figure 43–10.** The anatomic spectrum of intestinal atresia. Type I is a stenosis or mucosal web. Type II, a fibrous cord between two bowel ends. Type IIIa, blind-ending proximal and distal bowel loops with a V-shaped mesenteric defect. Type IIIb (apple-peel deformity, Christmas tree deformity) consists of a blind ending proximal jejunum, absence of a large portion of the midgut, and a terminal ileum that is coiled around its ileocolic blood supply. Type IV, multiple atresias of any kind. (From Grosfeld JL: Pediatric surgery. In: *Textbook of Surgery.* Sabiston DC [editor]. Saunders, 1991. Reproduced with permission from Elsevier.)

▶ Treatment

There are three main goals of operation: (1) to restore the continuity of the bowel, (2) to preserve as much intestinal length as possible, and (3) to retain the ileocecal valve if possible (the minimum length of bowel needed to sustain full enteral nutrition doubles in the absence of the ileocecal valve). A transverse upper abdominal incision is preferred. Infants with jejunal or ileal atresia usually have a segment of the proximal bowel adjacent to the atresia that is dilated out of proportion to the rest of the proximal bowel. This is referred to as the "club," and it lacks normal peristaltic activity. If left in or not tapered, it may become a source of persistent functional obstruction. It is tapered when it is a very proximal bowel segment, near the ligament of Treitz; otherwise it should be resected. A great discrepancy between the diameter of the segments of intestine proximal and distal to the atresia is the rule. Atresia of the proximal colon should be treated by resection of the dilated bowel and ileocolostomy. Atresia of the distal colon may be treated by proximal end colostomy or by a side-to-side colostomy. Later, the

continuity of the distal colon may be established by end-to-end anastomosis.

Infants born with extensive small bowel loss may benefit from a Bianchi procedure, whereby the entire greatly dilated bowel is divided longitudinally into two lengths of bowel. A recently described alternative bowel-lengthening procedure termed the STEP (serial transverse enteroplasty procedure) is quickly becoming the procedure of choice for gaining length from dilated and shortened intestine. The end of the jejunum in continuity with the duodenum is anastomosed to the proximal end of the divided bowel.

In contrast to duodenal atresia, associated anomalies are unusual in small bowel and colon atresia. Following repair, return of gastrointestinal function is prolonged (up to 10 days) with proximal atresia due to the overdistention of the duodenum.

Bianchi A: Autologous gastrointestinal reconstruction. Semin Pediatr Surg 1995;4:54.
Kim HB et al: Serial transverse enteroplasty (STEP): a novel bowel lengthening procedure. J Pediatr Surg 2003;38:425.
Modi et al: First report of the international serial transverse enteroplasty data registry: indications, efficacy, and complications. J Am Coll Surg 2007;204:365.
Puri P, Fujimoto T: New observations on the pathogenesis of multiple intestinal atresias. J Pediatr Surg 1988;23:221.
Sato S et al: Jejunoileal atresia: a 27 year experience. J Pediatr Surg 1998;33:1633.
Thompson JS et al: Experience with intestinal lengthening for the short-bowel syndrome. J Pediatr Surg 1991;26:721.

DISORDERS OF INTESTINAL ROTATION

The fetal intestine begins as a somewhat straight tube that grows faster than the abdominal cavity and thus herniates out into the body stalk (future umbilicus) at about 4–6 weeks' gestation. At 10–12 weeks, the bowel returns to the abdominal cavity, rotates, and becomes fixed to the retroperitoneum along a long diagonal axis extending from the level of the left of the T12 vertebra to the level of the right of the L5 vertebra. The duodenojejunal portion of gut rotates posterior (counterclockwise) to the superior mesenteric vessels for 270 degrees and becomes fixed at the ligament of Treitz and located to the left of and cephalad to the superior mesenteric artery. The cecocolic portion of the midgut also rotates 270 degrees, but clockwise (anterior) to the superior mesenteric artery. The cecum becomes fixed in the right lower abdomen (L5 level).

▶ Classification

Anomalies of rotation and fixation are twice as common in males as in females. They may be classified as (1) nonrotation, (2) incomplete rotation, (3) reversed rotation, and (4) anomalous fixation of the mesentery.

A. Nonrotation

With nonrotation, the midgut is suspended from the superior mesenteric vessels; the small bowel is located predominantly on the right side of the abdomen and the large bowel in the left abdomen. No fixation occurs, and adhesive bands are not present. This is the fetal anatomy prior to 10 weeks' gestation. Because its base is so short, the mesentery is narrow, which predisposes to volvulus, with clockwise twisting of the bowel about the superior mesenteric vessels. This anomaly is usually found in patients with omphalocele, gastroschisis, and congenital diaphragmatic hernia.

B. Incomplete Rotation

Incomplete rotation (commonly called malrotation) may affect the duodenojejunal segment, the cecocolic segment, or both. Adhesive bands (Ladd bands) are usually present. In the most common form, the cecum stopped rotating and fixed near the origin of the superior mesenteric vessels, and dense peritoneal bands extend from the right flank to the cecum and obstruct the second or third portion of the duodenum or other segments of the small bowel. The duodenojejunal segment also only partially rotates, usually stopping at or to the right of the vertebral bodies. The intestinal mesentery is fixed posteriorly but is very narrow, extending only the distance between the cecum and the duodenojejunal segment. This predisposes to volvulus (Figure 43–11).

C. Reversed Rotation

In reversed rotation, the bowel rotates varying degrees in a clockwise direction about the superior mesenteric axis. The duodenojejunal loop is anterior to the superior mesenteric artery. The cecocolic loop may be prearterial or may be rotated clockwise or counterclockwise in a retroarterial position. In either case, the cecum may be right-sided or left-sided. The most frequent anomaly is retroarterial clockwise rotation, which causes obstruction of the right colon.

D. Anomalous Fixation of Mesentery

Anomalies of mesenteric fixation account for internal mesenteric and paraduodenal hernias, a mobile cecum, or obstructing adhesive bands in the absence of anomalous bowel rotation. Excessive rotation of the duodenojejunal junction may result in superior mesenteric artery compression of the third portion of the duodenum.

► Clinical Findings

A. Symptoms and Signs

Anomalies of intestinal rotation may cause symptoms related to intestinal obstruction, peptic ulceration, or malabsorption. The majority of patients who develop intestinal obstruction are infants. Older patients may develop intermittent obstruction. The obstruction is in the duodenum or upper jejunum as a result of adhesive bands or midgut volvulus, respectively. Vomiting of bile occurs initially. Older patients may be thin and underweight because of chronic postprandial discomfort or malabsorption. Malab-

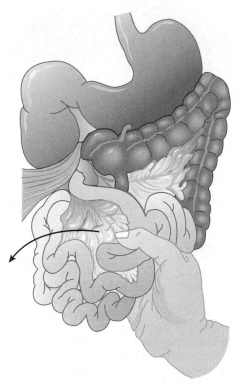

▲ **Figure 43–11.** Malrotation of the midgut with volvulus. Note cecum at the origin of the superior mesenteric vessels. Fibrous bands cross and obstruct the duodenum as they adhere to the cecum. Volvulus is untwisted in a counterclockwise direction.

sorption with steatorrhea may result from partial venous and lymphatic obstruction, which is associated with coarse rugal folds in the small bowel. With duodenal obstruction from bands, abdominal distention is not prominent. Midgut volvulus, however, produces marked abdominal distention. Bloody stools and signs of peritonitis are manifestations of intestinal infarction. Peptic ulcer occurs in 20% of patients, presumably as a result of antral and duodenal stasis.

B. Imaging Studies

With obstructing Ladd bands, plain abdominal radiographs may show a double-bubble sign that mimics duodenal stenosis. Distribution of gas throughout the intestines may be normal, although there may be a paucity of it. When volvulus occurs, the proximal bowel will be distended with gas early, but over time, a "gasless" abdomen may appear as the gas is resorbed in the ischemic bowel. The intestinal walls are thickened.

Upper gastrointestinal series demonstrates distention of the duodenum, abnormal positioning of the duodenojejunal segment (usually to the right of the midline), and narrowing at the point of obstruction. The small bowel is commonly visualized on the right side of the abdomen and the colon on the left. Contrast enema demonstrates abnormal position of the cecum, although the cecum can complete its rotation and fixation after birth, so the contrast enema is not a valuable diagnostic test for malrotation.

▶ Treatment & Prognosis

Through a transverse upper abdominal incision, the entire bowel should be delivered from the abdominal cavity to assess the anomalous arrangement of the intestinal loops. Volvulus should be untwisted in a counterclockwise direction. The Ladd procedure is used for incomplete rotation with obstruction of the duodenum by congenital bands. It consists of division of the bands between the proximal colon and the lateral abdominal wall that cover and compress (obstruct) the duodenum. The mesentery is often folded upon itself due to intermesenteric adhesions, and these are incised. The appendix is removed. The cecum is then placed in the left lower quadrant, and the duodenum dissected and straightened as much as possible with a final position to the right of the midline. In essence, one is creating nonrotated intestinal anatomy much like the anatomic situation in early fetal life (prior to 10 week' gestation). The Ladd procedure has increasingly been performed using laparoscopic techniques for those cases without suspected volvulus.

Approximately 30% of infants treated for volvulus die of complications of midgut ischemia and gangrene. If the anomaly is corrected before irreversible bowel damage occurs, the long-term results are good. Some patients tend to form adhesions that cause recurrent intestinal obstruction. Recurrent volvulus is rare after the Ladd procedure.

Bass KD, Rothenberg SS, Chang JH: Laparoscopic Ladd's procedure in infants with malrotation. J Pediatr Surg 1998;33:279.
Prasil P et al: Should malrotation in children be treated differently according to age? J Pediatr Surg 2000;35:756.
Rescorla F et al: Anomalies of intestinal rotation in childhood: analysis of 447 cases. Surgery 1990;108:710.
Torres AM, Ziegler MM: Malrotation of the intestine. World J Surg 1993;17:326.

MECONIUM ILEUS

In 10–20% of infants born with cystic fibrosis, the thick mucous secretions of the small bowel produce obstruction by inspissated meconium. This usually occurs in the terminal ileum. Although there is no clear correlation between pancreatic insufficiency and the development of inspissated meconium, meconium ileus also occurs in patients with pancreatic duct obstruction and pancreatic aplasia. Meconium obstruction with no apparent cause has also been described in newborn infants.

▶ Clinical Findings

A. Symptoms and Signs

The infant typically has a normal birth weight and very distended abdomen. No meconium is passed, and bilious emesis occurs early. Loops of thick, distended bowel may be seen and palpated.

B. Imaging Studies

Plain abdominal radiographs show loops of bowel that vary greatly in diameter; the thick meconium gives a ground-glass appearance. Air mixed with the meconium produces the "soap bubble" sign, which is usually located in the right lower quadrant. Radiographs taken shortly after the infant has been placed in an upright position may fail to show air-fluid levels because the thick, viscid meconium fails to layer out rapidly. Contrast enema will show microcolon with rare meconium flecks. Reflux of contrast medium through the ileocecal valve demonstrates a small terminal ileum containing "pellets" of inspissated mucus; more proximally, the bowel is progressively distended with packed meconium. Antenatal perforation may be detected by the presence of abdominal calcifications, since the meconium becomes saponified.

▶ Complications

Meconium ileus may be complicated by a segmental (not midgut) volvulus due to the heavy, distended loops of distal ileum. If this occurs early in fetal life, the volvulus may progress to gangrene of the affected bowel segment. This can heal completely, with abdominal calcifications as the only manifestation that it occurred. Conversely, it may heal in such a way that an intestinal atresia is formed. Perforation late in gestation may lead to meconium peritonitis or a large meconium pseudocyst at birth.

Other common complications of meconium ileus are related to the almost universal presence of cystic fibrosis. These infants are susceptible to repeated pulmonary infection with chronic bronchopneumonia, bronchiectasis, atelectasis, and lung abscess. Malabsorption due to pancreatic insufficiency requires pancreatic enzyme replacement. Rectal prolapse and intussusception may be produced by strained passage of inspissated stools. Nasal polyps and chronic sinusitis are frequent. Biliary cirrhosis and bleeding varices from portal hypertension are late manifestations of bile duct obstruction by mucus.

▶ Treatment & Prognosis

Nonoperative treatment is successful in 60–70% of cases. A nasogastric tube should be inserted and connected to suction. A contrast enema can be both diagnostic and therapeutic. It should be performed with a slightly hypertonic water-soluble contrast agent (never barium). The addition of N-acetylcysteine, which is mucolytic, may be necessary to disperse the meconium in uncomplicated cases. The infant must be well hydrated, and intravenous fluids must be continued during and after the procedure in order to prevent hypovolemia from the effects of the hypertonic contrast solution. If this treatment fails to relieve the obstruction, laparotomy is indicated. The ileum is opened and, if possible, flushed clear. The bowel can be reanastomosed or brought out as a double-barrel stoma. Alternatively, a T-tube may be placed in the bowel and brought out of the anterior abdominal wall for postoperative irrigations. Compromised intestine is resected, and appendectomy is performed because of the high rate of appendicitis in patients with cystic fibrosis.

All patients should be evaluated for cystic fibrosis. Pancreatic enzyme replacement may be required. A formula low in long-chain fatty acids and high in medium-chain triglycerides may give better absorption and growth than standard formulas. The patient must be placed in an environment with high humidity to keep tracheobronchial secretions fluid. Postural drainage with cupping of the chest should be taught to the parents so that they will continue to maintain tracheobronchial toilet indefinitely. Older children and adolescents may develop a meconium ileus–like syndrome termed distal ileal obstruction syndrome. This is ileal obstruction due to inspissated stool. It can occur when patients are not compliant with their medications or become dehydrated. Most often, it is successfully treated with hypertonic contrast enemas.

Mak GZ et al: T-tube ileostomy for meconium ileus: four decades of experience. J Pediatr Surg 2000;35:349.

Ziegler MM: Meconium ileus. Curr Probl Surg 1994;31:731.

HIRSCHSPRUNG DISEASE

Hirschsprung disease is due to failure in the cephalocaudal migration of the parasympathetic myenteric nerve cells into the distal bowel. Therefore, the absence of ganglion cells always begins at the anus and extends a varying distance proximally. The aganglionic bowel produces functional obstruction because the bowel fails to relax in response to distention. Short-segment aganglionosis involving only the terminal rectum occurs in about 10% of cases; the disease extends to the sigmoid colon in 75%, to more proximal colon in 10%, and to the entire colon with small bowel involvement in 5%. Extensive involvement of the small bowel is rare.

Males are affected four times more frequently than females when the disease is limited to the rectosigmoid. Females tend to have longer aganglionic segments. A familial association occurs in 5–10% of cases—more frequently when females are affected. The length of involvement tends to be consistent in familial cases. Downs syndrome occurs in 10–15% of patients.

▶ Clinical Findings

A. Symptoms and Signs

The absence of ganglion cells results in a functional obstruction because the affected area fails to relax due to unopposed sympathetic tone. The symptoms vary widely in severity but almost always occur shortly after birth. The infant passes little or no meconium within 24 hours. Thereafter, chronic or intermittent constipation usually occurs. Progressive abdominal distention, bilious emesis, reluctance to feed, diarrhea, listlessness, irritability, and poor growth and development follow. A rectal examination in the infant may be followed by expulsion of stool and flatus, with remarkable decompression of abdominal distention. In older children, chronic constipation and abdominal distention are characteristic. Passage of flatus and stool requires great effort, and the stools are small in caliber. Children with constipation from Hirschsprung disease do not exhibit soiling of their diapers or undergarments, distinguishing this form of constipation from idiopathic constipation (encopresis). These children are sluggish, with wasted extremities and flared costal margins. Rectal examination in older children usually reveals a normal or contracted anus and a rectum without feces. Impacted stools in the greatly dilated and distended sigmoid colon can be palpated across the lower abdomen.

B. Imaging Studies

Plain abdominal radiographs in infants show dilated loops of bowel, but it is difficult to distinguish small and large bowel in infancy. A contrast enema should be performed. There should be no attempt to clean out the stool before the fluoroscopic examination, for this will obscure the change in caliber between aganglionic and ganglionic bowel. The contrast enema often demonstrates a contracted (aganglionic) segment that appears relatively narrow compared with the dilated proximal bowel. The proximal aganglionic intestine can be dilated by impacted stool or enema, giving a false impression of the level of the normal colon. Irregular, bizarre contractions (sawtoothed pattern) that do not encircle the aganglionic portion of the bowel may also be recognized. The dilated proximal bowel may have circumferential, smooth, parallel contractions (similar in appearance to those of the jejunum) that are exaggerated contraction waves. The contrast enema may not show a transition zone in the first 6 weeks after birth, since the liquid stool can pass into the aganglionic bowel and the proximal intestine may not be dilated. Lateral projection radiographs should be taken to demonstrate the rectum, the transition zone, and the irregular contractions that may otherwise be obscured by a redundant sigmoid colon on anteroposterior views. Normally, the neonatal rectum is wider than the rest of the colon (including the cecum), and when the rectum is seen to be narrower than the proximal colon, then Hirschsprung disease is suspected. Radiographs of the abdomen and lateral pelvis should be repeated after 24–48 hours. The contrast agent will be retained for prolonged periods, and saline enemas may be required to evacuate it. The delayed film may show the transition zone and the bizarre irregular contractions more clearly than the initial study.

C. Laboratory Findings

Definitive diagnosis is made by rectal biopsy. Mucosal and submucosal biopsies may be taken from the posterior rectal wall with a suction biopsy capsule without anesthesia at the bedside. Serial sections may demonstrate the characteristic lack of ganglion cells and proliferation of nerve trunks in the Meissner plexus. If the findings are equivocal, it is necessary to remove a 1-cm or 2-cm full-thickness strip of mucosa and muscularis from the posterior rectum proximal to the dentate line under anesthesia. A sample of this size is sufficient for the pathologist to determine the presence or absence of ganglion cells in the Meissner plexus or in the Auerbach plexus. Manometric studies will show a failure of relaxation of the internal sphincter following rectal distention by a balloon, although this test is rarely performed except in older children.

Differential Diagnosis

Low intestinal obstruction in the newborn infant may be due to rectal or colonic atresia, meconium plug syndrome (see section on Neonatal Small Left Colon Syndrome), or meconium ileus as well as a variety of functional causes such as hypermagnesemia, hypocalcemia, hypokalemia, and hypothyroidism. Hirschsprung disease in patients who develop enterocolitis and diarrhea may mimic other causes of diarrhea. Chronic constipation due to functional causes may suggest Hirschsprung disease. Although functional constipation may occur early in infancy, the stools are normal in caliber, soiling is frequent, and enterocolitis is rare. In functional constipation, stool is palpable in the lower rectum, and a contrast enema shows uniformly dilated bowel to the level of the anus. However, short-segment Hirschsprung disease may be difficult to differentiate, and rectal biopsy may be necessary. Segmental dilation of the colon is a rare entity that causes constipation similar to that found in Hirschsprung disease.

Treatment

Traditionally, the surgical treatment was staged and consisted of a leveling colostomy followed several months later by resection of the aganglionic bowel and performance of a pull-through procedure. The trend recently has been toward performing a single-stage procedure (no colostomy) in the newborn period. This paradigm is as follows: bowel obstruction and enterocolitis (if present) may be relieved by placement of a large (30F) rectal tube and repeated warmed saline irrigations in 10 mL/kg aliquots preoperatively. Infants with moderate to severe enterocolitis should be treated with a diverting colostomy. At the time of surgery, frozen section analysis of the colonic muscle is required in order to establish the correct (ganglionic) level for the stoma. Infants who are not ill may undergo any one of three effective operative procedures: Swenson operation, Duhamel operation, or Soave operation. The main operative principles for these procedures are removal of most or all of the aganglionic bowel—while preserving the surrounding nerves to the pelvic organs—and anastomosing ganglionic bowel (confirmed by frozen section analysis) to the rectum 0.5 cm above the dentate line. In contrast to the Swenson and Soave procedures, the Duhamel operation leaves a cuff of aganglionic rectum along which the ganglionic bowel is stapled, creating a minireservoir. Historically, these operations have been performed via a low transverse abdominal incision. However, the laparoscopic approach has become the method of choice. A solely transanal mucosectomy has been used for those babies with short-segment disease. In total aganglionic colon, ileostomy is necessary. Nonoperative treatment with enemas is ineffective because it does not prevent further obstruction and enterocolitis.

Prognosis

The mortality for untreated aganglionic megacolon in infancy may be as high as 80%. Nonbacterial, nonviral enterocolitis is the principal cause of death. This tends to occur more frequently in infants but may appear at any age. The cause is not known but seems to be related to the high-grade partial obstruction, poor motility in the "normal" bowel, a frequently competent ileocecal valve, and hypertonic rectal sphincters. There is no correlation between the length of aganglionosis and the occurrence of enterocolitis. Perforation of the colon and appendix may result from distal bowel obstruction. Atresia of the distal small bowel or colon secondary to bowel obstruction due to Hirschsprung disease in utero has been reported.

Anastomotic leak with perirectal and pelvic abscess is the most serious complication following the pull-through procedure. This complication should be treated immediately by proximal colostomy until the anastomosis has healed. Necrosis of the pulled-through colon may occur if the bowel has not been mobilized sufficiently to prevent tension on the mesenteric blood supply.

Long-term patients who are properly treated for Hirschsprung disease do well. Incontinence and soiling may occur in a few cases despite a prompt diagnosis and a perfect operation. Episodic constipation and abdominal distention are more common, since the aganglionic internal anal sphincter is intact. Patients with these symptoms can respond to anal dilation. Occasionally, an internal sphincterotomy may be necessary. Smaller children may still develop enterocolitis after definitive treatment, and they should be treated with a large rectal tube and enemas. It is rare after age 5 years. Postoperative enterocolitis is more common in children with Downs syndrome.

Albanese CT et al: Perineal one-stage pull-through for Hirschsprung's disease. J Pediatr Surg 1999;34:377.

Coran AG, Teitelbaum DH: Recent advances in the management of Hirschsprung's disease. Am J Surg 2000;180:382.

Georgeson KE et al: Primary laparoscopic-assisted endorectal colon pull-through for Hirschsprung's disease: a new gold standard. Ann Surg 1999;229:678.

Langer JC et al: One-stage versus two-stage Soave pull-through for Hirschsprung's disease in the first year of life. J Pediatr Surg 1996;31:33.

NEONATAL SMALL LEFT COLON SYNDROME (MECONIUM PLUG SYNDROME)

This problem of newborn infants consists of low intestinal obstruction associated with a left colon of narrow caliber and a dilated transverse and right colon. The infants are in most cases otherwise normal, though approximately 30–50% are born to diabetic mothers and are large for gestational age. Most are over 36 weeks' gestational age and have normal birth weights. Two thirds are male. Hypermagnesemia has been occasionally associated when the mother has been treated for eclampsia by intravenous magnesium sulfate.

▶ Clinical Findings

Rectal examination may be normal or may reveal a tight anal canal. Little or no meconium is passed, and progressive abdominal distention is followed by vomiting. After thermometer or finger stimulation of the rectum, some meconium and gas may be evacuated. Contrast enema shows a very small left colon, usually to the level of the splenic flexure. Proximal to this point, the colon and commonly the small bowel are greatly distended. In about 30% of cases, a meconium plug is present at the junction of the narrow and dilated portion of the bowel, and the enema (using water-soluble contrast) will dislodge it.

▶ Differential Diagnosis

The small left colon syndrome may be confused with Hirschsprung disease or meconium ileus. These lesions rarely cause obstruction at the level of the splenic flexure, and when the colon readily decompresses without further obstruction, Hirschsprung disease is unlikely.

▶ Treatment

A nasogastric tube should be inserted and intravenous fluids started. A contrast enema is required to differentiate the various causes of low intestinal obstruction. When the left colon is narrow and contrast material refluxes into the dilated proximal colon, the diagnosis is most likely the small left colon syndrome. The contrast enema is usually followed by evacuation of copious meconium and decompression of the bowel. Incomplete evacuation of the meconium or persistent symptoms after the enema mandates a suction rectal biopsy to rule out Hirschsprung disease.

INTUSSUSCEPTION

Telescoping of a segment of bowel (intussusceptum) into the adjacent segment (intussuscipiens) is the most common cause of intestinal obstruction in children between 6 months and 2 years of age (Figure 43–12). The process of intussusception may result in gangrene of the intussusceptum. The most common form is intussusception of the terminal ileum into the right colon (ileocolic intussusception). In 95% of infants

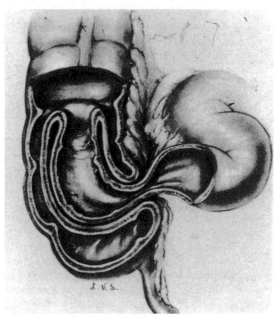

▲ **Figure 43–12.** Intussusception.

and children, it is idiopathic. The disease is most common in midsummer and midwinter, and there is a correlation with adenovirus infections. In most cases, hypertrophied Peyer patches are noted on the leading edge of bowel. Mechanical factors such as Meckel diverticulum, polyps, hemangioma, enteric duplication, intramural hematoma (Henoch-Schönlein purpura), and intestinal lymphoma are present with increasing frequency in patients over 2 years old. Postoperative intussusception can occur at any age, is usually ileoileal or jejunojejunal, and is due to differential return of bowel motility, often after retroperitoneal surgery. The ratio of males to females is 3:2. The peak age is in infants 5–9 months of age; 80% of patients are under the age of 2 years.

▶ Clinical Findings

The typical patient is a healthy child who suddenly begins crying and doubles up because of abdominal pain. The pain occurs in episodes that last for about 1 minute, alternating with intervals of apparent well-being. Reflex vomiting is an early sign, but vomiting due to bowel obstruction occurs late. Blood from venous infarction and mucus produce a "currant jelly" stool. In small infants and in postoperative patients, the colicky pain may not be apparent; these babies become withdrawn, and the most prominent symptom is vomiting. Pallor and sweating are common signs during colic. Repeated vomiting and bowel obstruction produce progressive dehydration. A mass is usually palpable along the distribution of the colon, most commonly in the right upper quadrant of the abdomen. Occasionally, intussusception is palpable on rectal examination. Prolonged intussusception produces edema and hemorrhagic or ischemic infarction of the intussusceptum.

Treatment & Prognosis

The contrast enema is diagnostic as well as therapeutic in 60–80% of cases (Figure 43–13). Contrast enema (using either barium or air) should not be attempted until the patient has been resuscitated enough to allow an operative procedure to be performed safely. It is contraindicated if peritonitis is present. If barium is used, the column of contrast should not stand more than 100 cm above the patient in order to minimize the risk of perforation. Air is pumped into the colon at a pressure of 60–80 mm Hg (never more than 120 mm Hg). A successful study reduces the intussusceptum and demonstrates reflux of barium or air into the terminal ileum. Several attempts should be made before taking the child to surgery. A contrast enema will not reduce gangrenous bowel.

Operation is required for unsuccessful enema reduction or signs of bowel perforation and peritonitis. The procedure may be performed either by laparotomy or laparoscopically. In the absence of gangrene, reduction is accomplished by gentle retrograde compression of the intussuscipiens, not by traction on the proximal bowel. Resection of the intussusception is indicated if the bowel cannot be reduced or if the intestine is gangrenous.

Intussusception recurs after 3% of barium enema reductions and 1% of operative reductions. Deaths are rare but occur if treatment of gangrenous bowel is delayed.

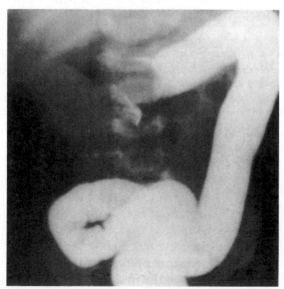

▲ **Figure 43–13.** Contrast enema demonstrating obstruction to retrograde flow of barium by a filling defect (intussusceptum) in the mid transverse colon. (Reproduced with permission from Albanese CT: Pediatric surgery. In: *Surgery,* Norton JA [editor]. Springer, 2000.)

DiFiore JW: Intussusception. Semin Pediatr Surg 1999;8:214.

Meyer JS et al: Air and liquid contrast agents in the management of intussusception: a controlled, randomized trial. Radiology 1993;188:507.

Ong NT, Beasley SW: The leadpoint in intussusception. J Pediatr Surg 1990;25:640.

ANORECTAL ANOMALIES (IMPERFORATE ANUS)

The normal continence mechanism for bowel control consists of an internal sphincter composed of smooth muscle and the striated muscle complex from the levator ani and external sphincter. The striated muscles assume a funnel shape, originating from the pubis, pelvic rim, and sacrum. These muscles converge at the perineum while interdigitating with the internal and external sphincters. Most of the striated muscle complex consists of horizontal muscles that contract against the wall of the rectum and anus while longitudinal muscle fibers run in a cephalocaudal direction and elevate the anus.

Anomalies of the anus result from abnormal growth and fusion of the embryonic anal hillocks. The rectum is normally developed, and the sphincter mechanism is usually intact. With proper surgical treatment, the sphincter will function normally. Anomalies of the rectum develop as a result of faulty division of the cloaca into the urogenital sinus and rectum by the urorectal septum. In these anomalies, the internal sphincter and striated muscle complex are hypoplastic. Therefore, surgical repair results in varying degrees of continence.

Classification

Physical examination of the perineum and imaging studies determine the extent of malformation of the anus or rectum. When an orifice is evident at the perineum or distal introitus, the anomaly is referred to as a low imperforate anus; the absence of an obvious orifice at the perineal level suggests a high imperforate anus (see Figures 43–14 to 43–17). In most instances, with high imperforate anus, there is a communication (fistula) of the rectum with the urethra or bladder in the male or with the upper vagina in the female. Distinguishing between a high and low anomaly may be possible radiologically by determining the position of the rectum in relation to the levator ani or pubococcygeal line.

A. Low Anomalies

In low anomalies, the anus may be ectopically placed anterior to its normal position or it may be in the normal position with a narrow outlet due to stenosis or an anal membrane. There may be no opening in the perineum, but the skin at the anal area is heaped up and may extend as a band in the perineal raphe completely covering the anal opening. A small fistula usually extends from the anus anteriorly to open in the raphe of the perineum, scrotum, or penis in the male or the vulva in the female. These babies often have well-developed perineal and gluteal musculature and rarely have sacral vertebral anomalies.

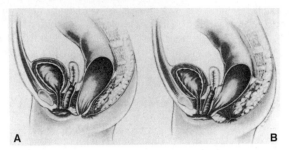

▲ **Figure 43–14. A:** Low female anomaly. Perineal fistula. **B:** Low female anomaly. Fourchette/vestibule fistula. (Reproduced, with permission, from Pena A: *Surgical Management of Anorectal Malformations.* Springer-Verlag, 1992.)

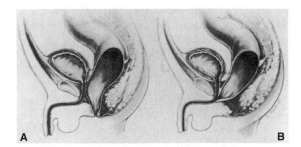

▲ **Figure 43–16. A:** Low male anomaly. Perineal fistula. **B:** Low male anomaly. Rectobulbar urethra fistula. (Reproduced with permission from Pena A: *Surgical Management of Anorectal Malformations.* Springer-Verlag, 1992.)

B. High Anomalies

In high anomalies, the rectum may end blindly (10%), but more commonly there is a fistula to the urethra or bladder in the male or the upper vagina in the female. In the female, a very high fistula may extend between the two halves of a bicornuate uterus directly to the bladder. Patients with high imperforate anus often have deficient pelvic and gluteal innervation and musculature, a high incidence of sacral anomalies (caudal regression), and a poor prognosis for continence after surgical repair. The most severe of the high deformities is a cloacal anomaly in which there is a common channel between the poorly developed pelvic structures (urogenital sinus and rectum) with a single perineal opening.

▶ Clinical Findings

A. Signs

The best means of establishing the type of anorectal anomaly is by physical examination. In low anomalies, an ectopic opening from the rectum can be detected in the perineal raphe in males or in the lower vagina, vestibule, or fourchette in females. A high anomaly exists when no orifice or fistula

can be seen upon examination of the perineum or when meconium is found at the urethral meatus, in the urine, or in the upper vagina. Absence of external sphincter contraction with cutaneous stimulation of the anus may also help differentiate between high and low lesions.

B. Imaging Studies

No single test is ideal in the evaluation of imperforate anus, so several studies are used to define the neonatal anatomy. Radiographs are sometimes useful when the clinical impression is unclear. A lateral film of the pelvis with the baby inverted (Wangensteen invertogram), once commonly used, is an inaccurate method of establishing the lower extent of the rectum because swallowed air may not have completely displaced the meconium from the rectum; or the striated muscle complex may be contracted, which obliterates the lumen and makes it look as if the gas in the rectum ends high in the pelvis. With crying or straining, the puborectalis muscle and rectum may actually descend below the ischium, giving a falsely low estimate of rectal height. Gas in the bladder clearly indicates a rectourinary fistula. Lower abdominal and perineal ultrasound, CT, and MRI have been

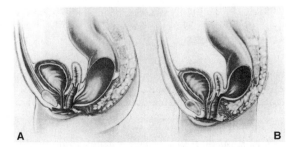

▲ **Figure 43–15. A:** High female anatomic anomaly. Low vaginal fistula. **B:** High female anomaly. High vaginal fistula. (Reproduced, with permission, from Pena A: *Surgical Management of Anorectal Malformations.* Springer-Verlag, 1992.)

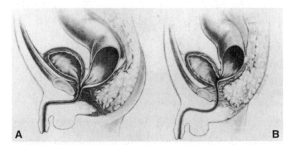

▲ **Figure 43–17. A:** High male anomaly. Rectoprostatic urethra fistula. **B:** High male anomaly. Rectovesical neck fistula. (Reproduced, with permission, from Pena A: *Surgical Management of Anorectal Malformations.* Springer, 1992.)

used to define the pelvic anatomy and location in relation to the rectal musculature. Anomalies of the vertebrae and the urinary tract occur in two thirds of all patients with high anomalies and in one third of male patients with low anomalies. Vertebral abnormalities in females invariably indicate a high imperforate anus. Anomalies of the sacrum warrant MRI of the lumbosacral area to identify spinal cord anomalies such as a tethered filum terminale.

Complications

Associated anomalies occur in up to 70% in those with a high anomaly. Imperforate anus is associated with the VACTERL syndrome (see Esophageal Anomalies). The possible constellation of anomalies includes esophageal atresia, anomalies of the gastrointestinal tract, hemivertebrae or agenesis of one or more sacral vertebrae (agenesis of S1, S2, or S3 is associated with corresponding neurologic deficits, resulting in neuropathic bladder and greatly impaired continence), genitourinary anomalies (up to 50% incidence with high imperforate anus), and anomalies of the heart and upper limbs/digits.

Delay in diagnosis of imperforate anus may result in excessively large bowel distention and perforation. The presence of a rectourinary fistula allows reflux of urine into the rectum and colon, and absorption of ammonium chloride may cause acidosis. Colon contents will reflux into the urethra, bladder, and upper tracts, producing recurrent pyelonephritis.

Treatment

The three main goals of treatment are (1) to allow passage of stool (ie, relieve obstruction), (2) to place the rectal pouch on the perineum in good position, and (3) to close the fistula.

A. Low Anomalies

Low anomalies are usually repaired from the perineal approach in the newborn period using a muscle stimulator to precisely determine the location of the sphincter complex. The anteriorly placed anal opening is completely mobilized and transferred to the normal position. After healing, the anal opening must be dilated daily for 3–5 months to prevent stricture formation and to allow for growth.

B. High Anomalies

Traditionally, a high deformity was treated by a three-stage repair consisting of colostomy and mucous fistula formation, a posterior sagittal anorectoplasty 4–6 weeks later, and closure of the colostomy several months after that. Recently, the staged approach has been challenged and a one-stage repair has been performed by both posterior sagittal and laparoscopic approaches. Because the anal sphincters are poorly developed—especially the internal sphincter—continence is most dependent upon a functioning striated muscle complex, which requires conscious voluntary contraction. Care must be taken to preserve the afferent and efferent nerves of the defecation reflex arc as well as the existing sphincter muscles. In all cases, the surgically created anus must be dilated for several months to prevent circumferential cicatrix formation.

Prognosis

Surgical complications include damage to the nervi erigentes, resulting in poor bladder and bowel control and failure of erection. Division of a rectourethral fistula some distance from the urethra produces a blind pouch prone to recurrent infection and stone formation, while cutting the fistula too short may result in urethral stricture. Erroneously attempting to repair a high anomaly from the perineal approach may leave a persistent rectourinary fistula. An abdominoperineal pull-through procedure performed for a low anomaly invariably produces an incontinent patient who might otherwise have had an excellent prognosis. Injury to the vas deferens and ureter is possible during repair of high anomalies.

Patients with imperforate anus tend to have varying degrees of constipation as an inherent part of the defect, believed to be due to poor inherent motility of the rectosigmoid. Patients with low anomalies usually have good sphincter function. Children with high anomalies do not have an internal sphincter that provides continuous, unconscious, and unfatiguing control against soiling. However, in the absence of a lower spine anomaly, perception of rectal fullness, ability to distinguish between flatus and stool, and conscious voluntary control of rectal discharge by contraction of the striated muscle complex can be achieved. When the stools become liquid, sphincter control is usually impaired in patients with high anomalies.

Albanese CT et al: One-stage repair of high imperforate anus in the newborn male. J Pediatr Surg 1999;34:834.

Georgeson KE, Inge TH, Albanese CT: Laparoscopically assisted anorectal pull-through for high imperforate anus—a new technique. J Pediatr Surg 2000;35:927.

Hendren WH: Management of cloacal malformations. Semin Pediatr Surg 1997;6:217.

Pena A, Hong A: Advances in the management of anorectal malformations. Am J Surg 2000;180:370.

GASTROINTESTINAL TRACT ABNORMALITIES

GASTROESOPHAGEAL REFLUX

Studies of esophageal motility, including manometric measurements of the cardioesophageal junction, show absence of the high-pressure zone (lower esophageal sphincter) in the terminal esophagus in most normal newborns. Evolution to the normal adult pattern of peristalsis and cardioesophageal sphincter function occurs after several months. Until this happens, many infants experience varying degrees of regurgitation after feeding. Rarely, repeated gastric reflux may produce peptic esophagitis and interfere with the development of a competent sphincter. Unlike adults, children rarely have a hiatal hernia as a cause of gastroesophageal reflux.

Clinical Findings

A. Symptoms and Signs

Symptoms consist of repeated effortless regurgitation of feedings, particularly when the baby is placed in a recumbent position. The baby will be hungry and will readily feed after regurgitating. Persistent regurgitation may result in poor weight gain (failure to thrive), peptic esophagitis with appearance of blood in the vomitus, or occult bleeding, producing anemia. One cause for apnea and acute life-threatening events is gastroesophageal reflux and aspiration. Lesser degrees of aspiration, particularly during sleep, may produce recurrent pneumonia. Stricture formation of the lower esophagus and metaplasia of the esophageal mucosa, producing Barrett esophagus, are possible late effects. Almost half of infants and children with gastroesophageal reflux have neurologic disorders related to perinatal asphyxia or congenital nervous system anomalies; seizure disorders are very common in this population. Abnormal motility of the esophagus and gastric dysmotility and impaired gastric emptying are frequently present. Gastroesophageal reflux is associated with esophageal atresia, congenital diaphragmatic hernia, and abdominal wall defects.

B. Imaging Studies

The standard diagnostic test is lower esophageal 24-hour pH monitoring. An upper gastrointestinal series is less sensitive but is useful to rule out other disorders (eg, intestinal malrotation) and to assess for esophageal stricture. Gastric emptying may be assessed by technetium pertechnate scan. There is virtually no role for esophageal manometric studies in young children except for those in whom one suspects the relatively rare achalasia or diffuse esophageal spasm.

Treatment

Nonoperative treatment is successful in most cases. Feedings should be thickened with rice cereal, and gastroesophageal reflux is lessened if the baby is maintained upright in an infant seat or in a prone position after feeding. Persistent symptoms mandate drug therapy with an antacid (eg, H_2-blocker or proton pump inhibitor) with or without a prokinetic agent (eg, metoclopramide). If a prolonged trial of nonoperative therapy fails or if complications of reflux can be documented (ie, esophagitis, stricture, asthma, recurrent aspiration pneumonia, failure to thrive), an antireflux procedure such as the Nissen or Thal fundoplication procedure is indicated. The open operation has been virtually replaced by the more cosmetic laparoscopic procedure that also provides for better visualization. Pyloroplasty may be required when there is associated impaired gastric emptying, though there is accumulating evidence suggesting that the "funneling" effect of the fundoplication promotes gastric emptying even in the face of documented delayed emptying.

Capito C et al: Long-term outcome of laparoscopic Nissen-Rossetti fundoplication for neurologically impaired and normal children. Surg Endosc 2007;22:875.

Georgeson KE: Laparoscopic fundoplication and gastrostomy. Semin Laparosc Surg 1998;5:25.

Johnson DG: The past and present of antireflux surgery in children. Am J Surg 2000;180:377.

Kazerooni NL et al: Fundoplication in 160 children under 2 years of age. J Pediatr Surg 1994;29:677.

Valusek PA et al. The use of fundoplication for prevention of apparent life-threatening events. J Pediatr Surg 2007;42:1022.

ACUTE APPENDICITIS

Acute appendicitis is one of the most common causes of an acute abdomen in childhood. This diagnosis must be considered in all age groups, but it is most common between the ages of 4 and 15 years.

Clinical Findings

The diagnosis is most often made by obtaining a careful clinical history and performing a thorough physical examination. In some patients, observation and periodic reexamination by the same physician may be necessary to confirm or exclude the diagnosis. In young children, the diagnosis of appendicitis can be difficult to arrive at, as the clinical history may be difficult to elicit. The classic presentation includes the onset of epigastric or periumbilical pain followed by anorexia, nausea, and vomiting. Anorexia is a significant finding, as the child will often refuse favorite foods. A fever will usually develop, and the pain then localizes to the right lower quadrant. Rovsing sign (right lower quadrant pain during palpation of the left lower quadrant), localized right lower quadrant tenderness, and involuntary spasm of the right hemirectus muscle indicate the presence of peritonitis.

A white blood count with differential and urinalysis should be obtained. The white blood cell count is greater than 10,000/μL (often with a left shift) in more than 80% of patients with appendicitis. Radiologic evaluation should include a chest film to exclude right lower lobe pneumonia. Findings on flat and erect abdominal radiographs are often nonspecific, though they may infrequently demonstrate the presence of a fecalith. Ultrasound (particularly in females) and CT scans are being used with increasing frequency, especially for those without the classic history and physical examination results.

Differential Diagnosis

Gastroenteritis is often confused with appendicitis. Vomiting follows periumbilical pain in appendicitis but often precedes abdominal pain in gastroenteritis. In addition, the patient with gastroenteritis commonly has diffuse abdominal pain and frequent copious watery diarrhea. Intussusception, intestinal obstruction and volvulus, mesenteric adenitis, Meckel diverticulitis, Henoch-Schönlein purpura, ruptured ovarian cyst, and Crohn disease must also be considered in the differential diagnosis for children. In adolescent girls, information regarding the menstrual cycle, previous episodes of pelvic inflammatory disease, and an accurate sexual history is important to exclude gynecologic causes of an acute abdomen.

▶ Treatment

Once the diagnosis is made, fluid resuscitation is performed and antibiotics are administered. Appendectomy is accomplished through a right lower quadrant incision or using the laparoscope. In cases of perforation, the peritoneal cavity is irrigated and aspirated dry but drainage is not performed unless there is a mature abscess cavity. The wound is closed in all cases. Antibiotics are continued for 3–7 days or until the white blood cell count and fever normalize. Overall, the morbidity and mortality of appendicitis in children have gradually decreased with the increased use of powerful broad-spectrum antibiotics. However, perforated appendicitis with abscess formation remains the variant with increased morbidity when compared to nonperforated cases. Still, many of the classic dogmas regarding risk of perforation upon presentation, relative to duration of symptoms in days, and initial operative versus nonoperative treatment for perforated appendicitis are currently being reexamined.

Henry MC et al: Matched analysis of non-operative management vs immediate appendectomy for perforated appendicitis. J Pediatr Surg 2007;42:19.

Henry MC et al: Risk factors for the development of abdominal abscess following operation for perforated appendicitis in children. Arch Surg 2007;142:236.

Madonna MB, Boswell WC, Arensman RM: Acute abdomen. outcomes. Semin Pediatr Surg 1997;6:105.

Pearl RH et al: Pediatric appendectomy. J Pediatr Surg 1995;30:173.

DUPLICATIONS OF THE GASTROINTESTINAL TRACT

Duplications may occur at any point along the gastrointestinal tract from the mouth to the anus. Duplications occur (in order of decreasing frequency) in the ileum (50% of cases), mediastinum, colon, rectum, stomach, duodenum, and neck. Intrathoracic and small bowel duplications are usually spherical; colonic duplications are commonly long and tubular (Figure 43–18). Characteristically, the intra-abdominal spherical duplications are on the mesenteric side of the intestine and do not share a common wall with the intestine.

Based on embryology, duplications have been categorized as foregut, midgut, and hindgut. Foregut duplica-

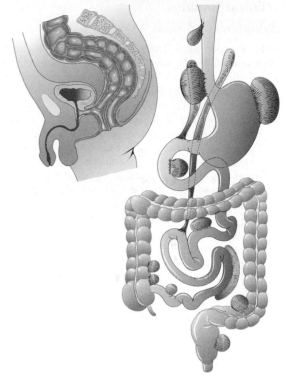

▲ **Figure 43–18.** Duplications of the gastrointestinal tract. Duplications may be saccular or tubular. They usually arise within the mesentery, having a common wall with the intestine. Thoracoabdominal duplications arise from the duodenum or jejunum and extend through the diaphragm into the mediastinum.

tions include the pharynx, respiratory tract, esophagus, stomach, and the first portion and proximal half of the second portion of the duodenum. Midgut duplications include the distal half of the second part of the duodenum, the jejunum, ileum, cecum, appendix, the ascending colon, and the proximal two thirds of the transverse colon. The hindgut is composed of duplications of the distal third of the transverse colon, the descending and sigmoid colon, the rectum, anus, and components of the urologic system. Combined thoracoabdominal duplications also occur in which the thoracic saccular component extends through the esophageal hiatus or a separate diaphragmatic opening to empty into the duodenum or jejunum. A thoracic duplication, associated with a cervical or thoracic vertebral anomaly, in which the duplication communicates with the subarachnoid space, is called a neurenteric cyst. Associated cardiovascular, neurologic, skeletal, urologic, and gastrointestinal anomalies occur in more than a third of cases. Carcinoma may arise within duplications of the colon.

▶ Clinical Findings

A. Symptoms and Signs

Two thirds of patients with duplications are symptomatic in the first year of life. Duplications of the neck and mediastinum produce respiratory distress by compression of the airway. Thoracic duplications may ulcerate into the lung and lead to pneumonia or hemoptysis. Intestinal duplications usually produce abdominal pain owing to spastic contraction of the bowel, excessive distention of the duplication, or peptic ulceration and bleeding resulting from ectopic gastric mucosa in the duplication. Intestinal obstruction due to intussusception, volvulus, or encroachment on the lumen by an intramural cyst also occurs. An isolated asymptomatic mass may be the only finding. Sixty percent of duplications are diagnosed by 6 months of life and 85% by 2 years.

B. Imaging Studies

Studies include radiographs of the chest and thoracolumbar spine, CT scan of the chest and abdomen, contrast enema, esophagography, and upper gastrointestinal series. If an intraspinal extension of a duplication is suspected, MRI is indicated. Ultrasonography may show a cystic or tubular mass within the mediastinum or abdomen. A Meckel scan (technetium pertechnetate) can also be used to visualize those duplications with ectopic gastric mucosa.

▶ Treatment

Duplications not intimately adherent to adjacent organs should be excised. Isolated spherical duplications can be excised with the adjacent segment of bowel and an end-to-end anastomosis of the bowel performed. Long, tubular duplications can be decompressed by establishing an anastomosis between the proximal and distal ends of adjacent bowel. Noncommunicating duplications, which would require radical resection of surrounding structures, should be drained by a Roux-en-Y technique. Duplications that cannot be removed completely and that contain gastric mucosa should be opened (without jeopardizing the blood supply of the normal bowel) and the mucosal lining excised. Extension of a mediastinal duplication into the spine or abdomen should be resected. An intra-abdominal extension is closed at the level of the diaphragm, and complete excision by laparotomy is accomplished.

Iyer CP, Mahour GH: Duplications of the alimentary tract in infants and children. J Pediatr Surg 1995;30:1267.

Merry C, Spurbeck W, Lobe TE: Resection of foregut-derived duplications by minimal access surgery. Pediatr Surg Int 1999;15:224.

Stern LE, Warner BW: Gastrointestinal duplications. Semin Pediatr Surg 2000;9:135.

Wilkinson CC et al: Fetal neurenteric cyst causing hydrops: case report and review of the literature. Prenat Diagn 1999;19:118.

OMPHALOMESENTERIC DUCT ANOMALIES

The omphalomesenteric (vitelline) duct is a remnant of the embryonic yolk sac. When the entire duct remains intact postnatally, it is recognized as an omphalomesenteric fistula. When the duct is obliterated at the intestinal end but communicates with the umbilicus at the distal end, it is called an umbilical sinus. When the epithelial tract persists but both ends are occluded, an umbilical cyst or intra-abdominal enterocystoma may develop. The entire tract may be obliterated, but a fibrous band may persist between the ileum and the umbilicus (Figure 43–19).

The most common remnant of the omphalomesenteric duct is Meckel diverticulum, which is present in 1–3% of the population. Meckel diverticulum may be lined wholly or in part by small intestinal, colonic, or gastric mucosa, and it may contain aberrant pancreatic tissue. Heterotopic tissue is

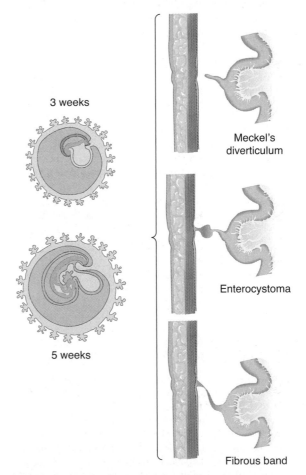

3 weeks

5 weeks

Meckel's diverticulum

Enterocystoma

Fibrous band

▲ **Figure 43–19.** Omphalomesenteric duct anomalies arise from the primitive yolk sac. Remnants include Meckel diverticulum, enterocystoma, and a fibrous band or fistulous tract between the ileum and the umbilicus.

found in 5% of asymptomatic and 60% of symptomatic cases. In contrast to duplications and pseudodiverticula, Meckel diverticulum is located on the antimesenteric border of the ileum, 10–90 cm from the ileocecal valve. Meckel diverticulum occurs with equal frequency in both sexes. It is usually asymptomatic and is seen as an incidental finding during operation for other disease. Of those with Meckel diverticulum, the lifelong risk of complications is 4%, and 40% of these cases occur in children under 10 years of age.

▶ Clinical Findings

Symptomatic omphalomesenteric remnants (male-to-female incidence 3:1) produce painless rectal bleeding in 40%, intussusception in 20%, diverticulitis or peptic perforation in 15%, umbilical fistula in 15%, intestinal obstruction in 7%, and abscess in 3% of cases. Rectal bleeding associated with Meckel diverticulum is due to peptic ulceration of the adjacent ileum caused by ectopic gastric mucosa. Over 50% of these patients are under 2 years of age. The blood is mixed with stool and is most often dark red or bright red; tarry stools are unusual. A history of a previous episode of bleeding may be elicited in 40% of cases. Occult bleeding from Meckel diverticulum is very rare. Younger patients tend to bleed quite briskly and may exsanguinate rapidly. Diverticulitis or free perforation will present with abdominal pain and peritonitis similar to acute appendicitis. The pain and tenderness occur in the lower abdomen, most commonly near the umbilicus. Periumbilical cellulitis may be present.

Intestinal obstruction may develop as a result of volvulus of the bowel about a persistent band between the umbilicus and the ileum or as a result of herniation of bowel between the mesentery and a persistent vitelline or mesodiverticular vessel. Obstruction is the most common presentation in adults. An infected umbilical sinus or omphalomesenteric fistula may present with mucoid, purulent, or enteric discharge; recurrent cellulitis; or a deep abdominal wall abscess about the umbilicus. This can be diagnosed by cannulation and contrast injection via the umbilical tract.

Upper and lower contrast studies rarely outline the primary defect. Technetium-99m (^{99m}Tc) pertechnetate may localize in gastric mucosa lining Meckel diverticulum and may identify the source of hematochezia or melena. Retention of dye in the mucous and parietal cells is enhanced by giving cimetidine, 30 mg/kg intravenously, 30 minutes before administration of the radiotracer nuclide.

▶ Treatment

Resection is accomplished by laparotomy or laparoscopy. An omphalomesenteric remnant with a narrow base may be treated by amputation and closure of the bowel defect (usually with a surgical stapler). In cases where the anomaly has a wide mouth with ectopic tissue or where an inflammatory or ischemic process involves the adjacent ileum, intestinal resection with the diverticulum and anastomosis may be necessary.

Fa-Si-Oen PR, Roumen RM, Croiset van Uchelen FA: Complications and management of Meckel's diverticulum and intestinal duplication—a review. Eur J Surg 1999;165:674.

Moore TC: Omphalomesenteric duct malformations. Semin Pediatr Surg 1996;5:116.

NECROTIZING ENTEROCOLITIS

Necrotizing enterocolitis is the most serious and frequent gastrointestinal disorder of predominantly premature infants, with a median onset of 10 days after birth. The incidence is increasing given the therapeutic advances in neonatal intensive care that have allowed ever more premature infants to survive. It is characterized by necrosis, ulceration, and sloughing of intestinal mucosa, which frequently progresses to full-thickness necrosis and perforation. This process progresses from the submucosa through the muscular layer to the subserosa. Gas-producing bacteria in the intestinal wall may lead to pneumatosis, a finding that may be noted on gross examination as well as on plain abdominal radiographs. The terminal ileum and right colon are usually affected first, followed in descending order of frequency by the transverse and descending colon, appendix, jejunum, stomach, duodenum, and esophagus. The most extreme case, pannecrosis, is defined as necrosis of 75% or more of the bowel. Eighty percent of cases occur in premature infants weighing less than 2500 g at birth, and 50% are under 1500 g. However, the disorder may also occur in full-term infants. Contrary to earlier impressions, there is no established relationship between necrotizing enterocolitis and stressful perinatal events such as premature rupture of membranes with amnionitis, breech delivery, intrauterine bradycardia, umbilical vessel catheterization with or without exchange transfusion, respiratory distress syndrome, sepsis, omphalitis, and congenital heart disease. An associated patent ductus arteriosus is common. In older infants and children, necrotizing enterocolitis is usually preceded by malnutrition and gastroenteritis. The clustering of cases in nurseries suggests that an infectious agent may be responsible.

▶ Clinical Findings

Clinical findings include increased gastric residual, bilious vomiting, abdominal distention, bloody stools, lethargy, and poor skin perfusion. When intestinal perforation occurs, guarding is evident on abdominal examination, but in weak premature infants, guarding may not be obvious. A variety of nonspecific clinical findings suggest physiologic instability such as apnea, bradycardia, hypoglycemia, and temperature instability. On examination, abdominal distention and fixed loops of intestine may be appreciated. The presence of abdominal wall erythema, edema, and crepitus may be a sign of bowel necrosis. Laboratory evaluation is nonspecific since the white blood cell count may be low or high, but thrombocytopenia and acidosis develop with perforation and sepsis.

Supine and cross-table lateral abdominal radiographs show small bowel distention early, followed by pneumatosis intestinalis. Gas within the portal venous system can be seen but it is fleeting. Serial examinations may show a loop or loops of bowel that are fixed in position and dilated. Perforation with peritoneal air develops in 20% of cases. Infants who develop ascites without pneumoperitoneum should have paracentesis and examination of the fluid for bacteria, which would signify perforation. Contrast studies are hazardous and contraindicated, as they may easily lead to perforation.

► Treatment

Treatment includes cessation of feedings, orogastric suction, systemic antibiotics, and correction of hypoxemia, hypovolemia, acidosis, and electrolyte abnormalities. The only absolute indication for intervention is pneumoperitoneum. Relative indications are portal vein air, clinical deterioration, a fixed intestinal loop on serial radiographs, erythema of the abdominal wall, an abdominal mass, and a paracentesis demonstrating bacteria. At laparotomy, necrotic bowel is resected and the proximal bowel is made into a stoma. Rarely is primary anastomosis safe. Severe disease may not be amenable to operation or require extensive bowel resection, resulting in short bowel syndrome. An alternative treatment option in very low-birth-weight infants (< 1500 g) that is gaining acceptance for documented perforation is bedside drainage of the peritoneal cavity in the right lower quadrant using local anesthesia. A recent prospective randomized trial comparing laparotomy to drain placement for very low-birth-weight infants demonstrated equivalent outcomes in mortality and short-term morbidity for these two modalities.

In one third of cases, the disorder resolves without further treatment, and the overall survival rate is more than 50%. Intestinal stricture may occur as a late complication following healing. For this reason, a contrast enema is used to evaluate the defunctionalized distal bowel before closing the stoma.

Andorsky DJ et al: Nutritional and other postoperative management of neonates with short bowel syndrome correlates with clinical outcomes. J Pediatr 2001;139:27.

Ladd AP et al: Long-term follow-up after bowel resection for necrotizing enterocolitis: factors affecting outcome. J Pediatr Surg 1998;33:967.

Noble HG, Driessnack M: Bedside peritoneal drainage in very low birth weight infants. Am J Surg 2001;181:416.

Moss RL et al: Laparotomy compared with peritoneal drainage in infants with necrotizing enterocolitis and intestinal perforation. New Engl J Med 2006;354:2225.

GASTROINTESTINAL BLEEDING

Significant gastrointestinal bleeding in children is rare. When it occurs, it can be alarming and anxiety provoking for caregivers and parents. The diagnostic approach used in the evaluation of these children is similar to that used in adults, but the causes vary depending on the age of the child. Rarely is the gastrointestinal bleeding massive, and the majority of causes are benign. A diagnosis can be established in over 85% of cases. Usual presenting symptoms include hematemesis, hematochezia, and melena. Depending on the amount of bleeding, the child may have sunken fontanelles, dry mucous membranes, and cool skin. Tachycardia, oliguria, and hypotension may be present. Intravenous access should be obtained, fluid and blood administered as needed, and an evaluation begun. Laboratory tests include serial hematocrit measurements and coagulation studies. Following stabilization and physical examination, evaluation should then proceed to the appropriate diagnostic tests.

► Upper Gastrointestinal Bleeding

Upper gastrointestinal bleeding originates above the ligament of Treitz. The presence of melena and the presence of blood on passage of an orogastric tube can help differentiate between upper and lower gastrointestinal bleeding. Upper gastrointestinal bleeding in infants and young children is most often associated with stress ulcers or erosions, but in older children it may also be caused by duodenal ulcer, esophagitis, and esophageal varices, particularly in children with underlying liver disease. Most of these diseases are benign. Evaluation following stabilization of the child begins with flexible esophagoduodenoscopy. Once the diagnosis is made, treatment is usually amenable to antacids (H_2-blockers, proton pump inhibitors). Variceal hemorrhage may require more aggressive intervention, including the use of octreotide, endoscopic varix sclerosis or band ligation, and, in extreme cases, transjugular intrahepatic portocaval shunt (TIPS), mesocaval shunt, or liver transplantation.

► Lower Gastrointestinal Bleeding

Although diverticulitis, cancer, and angiodysplasia are the most common causes of lower gastrointestinal bleeding in adults, those diseases are not present in children. The causes of lower gastrointestinal bleeding in infants and children can be categorized in diagnostic age groups whereby the age of the patient, the amount of bleeding, and the color of the blood passed provide some guidance to the probable source of bleeding.

Bleeding in the neonate may be caused by swallowing maternal blood at delivery, an anorectal fissure, upper gastrointestinal bleeding secondary to gastritis or ulceration, necrotizing enterocolitis, volvulus, and an incarcerated hernia. The Apt test for maternal blood, physical examination of the rectum and inguinal canal, and evaluation of the upper gastrointestinal tract can quickly rule out most of these causes. Bleeding from necrotizing enterocolitis is rarely life threatening, and the diagnosis is commonly made on the basis of the premature delivery of the infant and radiologic evaluation. If bleeding from malrotation with midgut volvulus is suspected, prompt laparotomy is indicated.

In infants, anal fissures continue to be the most common cause of rectal bleeding. Other causes include intestinal volvulus, intussusception, intestinal duplication, Meckel diverticulum, milk or formula protein allergy, and infectious diarrhea. Contrast studies and appropriate stool cultures guide treatment. Children have a differential diagnosis similar to that of infants with the addition of rectal prolapse and a variety of polyps of the colon (juvenile, Peutz-Jeghers, polypoid lymphoid hyperplasia, and, rarely, adenomatosis). These entities are diagnosed by physical examination and proctosigmoidoscopy. If no source of bleeding is identified, colonoscopy is indicated, while capsule endoscopy is gaining acceptance as a diagnostic modality for occult causes of gastrointestinal bleeding. Juvenile polyps are the single-most common cause of lower gastrointestinal bleeding in children (20–30%). Most juvenile polyps are single (80%) and often pass spontaneously without treatment. However, when bleeding continues to occur, the polyp can be snared and excised endoscopically. Adolescents may manifest signs and symptoms of inflammatory bowel disease (ulcerative colitis, Crohn disease), familial adenomatous polyposis, and small vascular lesions such as telangiectasias. Diagnosis is made by colonoscopy, and treatment is disease specific.

Arain Z, Rossi TM: Gastrointestinal bleeding in children: an overview of conditions requiring nonoperative management. Semin Pediatr Surg 1999;8:172.

Boyle JT: Gastrointestinal bleeding in infants and children. Pediatr Rev 2008;2:39.

El-Matary W: Wireless capsule endoscopy: indications, limitations, and future challenges. J Pediatr Gastroenterol Nutr 2008; 46:4.

GASTROINTESTINAL FOREIGN BODIES

Children aged 9 months to 2 years are at particular risk for the ingestion or aspiration of foreign bodies given their newly acquired mobility, curiosity, and the tendency to place objects in their mouths. The type of foreign body and the location in the airway or gastrointestinal tract dictate management.

▶ Esophagal Foreign Bodies

Typical foreign bodies found in the esophagus include coins, food, and small toys. The three most common sites of obstruction are at the level of the cricopharyngeus muscle, at the level of the aortic arch, and at the gastroesophageal junction. Previous areas of repair/anastomosis as in esophageal atresia or injury predispose to obstruction due to scar and narrowing. Common symptoms include drooling, feeding intolerance, dysphagia, and pain. Perforation is rare but is dictated by the ingested object's shape, composition, and time in the esophagus. The diagnosis is easily obtained by anteroposterior chest or lateral neck radiography if the ingested object is radiopaque. Otherwise, esophagoscopy or an upper gastrointestinal series is needed.

Because of the risk of erosion, aspiration, perforation, and late stricture, impacted objects should be removed. Extraction can be performed using balloon catheter retrieval under fluoroscopic control or under direct visualization using esophagoscopy with general anesthesia. The latter technique is generally preferred if the nature of the object is unknown, or is sharp, or the ingestion was 24–48 hours previously. A Hopkins rod lens endoscopy system allows visualization of the object and retrieval with specially designed forceps for grasping small objects.

Ninety-five percent of foreign bodies that pass beyond the gastroesophageal junction proceed uneventfully through the gastrointestinal tract. Operative retrieval is reserved for batteries, which must be removed, and for cases where ingested objects cause obstruction (bezoars) or intestinal injury or have been in place for more than 1 week.

▶ Tracheal Foreign Bodies

Children, particularly those 1–2 years of age, can occlude the airway by aspiration of a foreign body. The most common objects are peanuts and pieces of popcorn. Obstruction tends to occur at the level of the laryngeal inlet, the subglottis, or the right main stem bronchus. Because this can be a life-threatening problem, witnessed events should be treated with back blows, abdominal thrusts, or the Heimlich maneuver, which may dislodge the object.

Symptoms include coughing, choking, wheezing, dyspnea, and fever. Unilateral wheezing and rhonchi may be present. Air trapping may result when the foreign body forms a ball-valve obstruction leading to hyperinflation of the affected lung and mediastinal shift away from the affected side. On the other hand, complete obstruction may lead to loss of air volume with atelectasis and mediastinal shift to the ipsilateral side. Inspiratory and expiratory radiographs or bilateral decubitus films in infants may demonstrate air trapping; the foreign body is rarely noted on radiographs.

With a worrisome history, a foreign body suggested on a radiograph, or any symptoms, the child should undergo bronchoscopic evaluation under general anesthesia. Working in tandem with the anesthesiologist to allow ventilation during rigid endoscopy, the foreign body can be readily identified. Lighted grasping forceps made specifically for foreign body extraction are placed through the sheath of the bronchoscope; the foreign body is grasped; and the forceps, foreign body, and sheath are removed as one unit. Rarely, an unrecognized aspirated foreign body presents as chronic lung infection and can require removal of the affected lung.

Baharloo F et al: Tracheobronchial foreign bodies: presentation and management in children and adults. Chest 1999;115:1357.

Kaiser CW et al: Retained foreign bodies. J Trauma 1997;43:107.

LIVER & BILIARY TRACT DISORDERS

Jaundice in the first 2 weeks of infancy is usually due to indirect (unconjugated) hyperbilirubinemia. The causes include (1) "physiologic jaundice" due to immaturity of hepatic function (eg, that associated with breast-feeding); (2) Rh, ABO, and rare blood group incompatibilities, which produce hemolysis; and (3) infections. Jaundice that persists beyond the first 2 weeks in which the indirect and conjugated bilirubin levels are elevated should prompt a more thorough workup aimed at diagnosing potential surgical disorders. The most frequent cause (60%) of prolonged jaundice in infancy is biliary atresia; various forms of hepatitis occur in 35%; and choledochal cyst is found in 5% of cases of obstructive jaundice. Mild indirect hyperbilirubinemia occurs with pyloric stenosis and quickly disappears after pyloromyotomy. Intestinal obstruction can intensify jaundice by increasing the enterohepatic circulation of bilirubin. Finally, jaundice is an early and important sign of septicemia in the newborn.

BILIARY ATRESIA

Biliary atresia is the absence of patent bile ducts draining the liver. Familial cases and frequent association with the polysplenia syndrome indicate a congenital onset. However, biliary atresia probably develops after birth because jaundice is not usually remarkable in the newborn period but becomes evident more than 2 weeks later. Furthermore, conjugated bilirubin is not cleared by the placenta as unconjugated bilirubin is, and jaundice due to conjugated hyperbilirubinemia with biliary obstruction has not been recognized in newborn infants. The atretic ducts consist of solid fibrous cords that may contain occasional islands of biliary epithelium.

The extent of duct involvement varies greatly. There are three anatomic patterns of obstruction: (1) the proximal extrahepatic bile ducts are patent and the ducts distal to the cystic duct are obliterated; (2) the gallbladder, cystic duct, and common bile duct are patent and the proximal hepatic ducts are occluded; and (3) the entire extrahepatic ductal system is obstructed. Liver biopsy demonstrates proliferation of the bile canaliculi containing inspissated bile. Over time, the failure to excrete bile out of the liver results in progressive periportal fibrosis and obstruction of the intrahepatic portal veins, resulting in biliary cirrhosis.

▶ Clinical Findings

A. Symptoms and Signs

The infant with biliary atresia often has an uneventful neonatal course until jaundice is noted at 2–3 weeks of age. Stools may be normal or clay-colored, and the urine may be dark. The stools contain an increased quantity of fat but are of normal consistency and not frothy. The liver may be of normal size early, but it becomes enlarged with time. A hard liver may develop as a consequence of progressive cirrhosis.

Splenomegaly usually develops. Ascites and portal hypertension do not become manifest for several months.

B. Laboratory Findings

The workup of biliary atresia consists of analysis of liver function tests, complete blood count, and metabolic and serologic screening. The bilirubin levels may vary considerably from day to day, but direct bilirubin levels over 3 mg/dL are common. Alkaline phosphatase levels are often elevated to 500–1000 units/L, and γ-glutamyltranspeptidase levels are greater than 300 units/L.

C. Imaging Studies

Ultrasonography may demonstrate absence or inability to visualize a contracted gallbladder. Radionuclide scanning using technetium ^{99m}Tc-labeled iminodiacetate compounds (IDA, HIDA, PIPIDA, DISIDA) to observe the intensity of uptake within the liver and evidence of secretion into the bowel is valuable, usually preceded by a 2- to 3-day course of phenobarbital to promote tracer uptake. Core needle biopsy of the liver may be safely performed at any age if the clotting tests are normal. A diagnosis based on needle biopsy is accurate in 60%, equivocal in 16%, and erroneous in 24% of cases. Unless the workup has conclusively diagnosed another entity, all children suspected of having biliary atresia should undergo operative cholangiography with the intention of proceeding to exploration of the porta hepatis.

▶ Other Causes

Other causes of obstructive jaundice are choledochal cyst, inspissated bile syndrome, and any one of several neonatal hepatitides. A choledochal cyst is identified by the presence of a palpable mass in the right upper quadrant and ultrasonographic confirmation. Inspissated bile syndrome follows a hemolytic process in which a large bilirubin load is excreted into the bile ducts, where it becomes coalesced and impacted, or may occur after a prolonged period of bowel rest with total parenteral nutrition. The syndrome is recognized by abdominal ultrasound. Hepatitis is most commonly of unknown cause. It may be due to a variety of infections, often of maternal origin, such as toxoplasmosis, cytomegalovirus, rubella syndrome, herpes simplex, coxsackievirus, and varicella. Serum should be tested for elevated antibody titers to these agents. Neonatal physiologic jaundice is self-limited and also responds to phototherapy.

Genetic metabolic diseases producing jaundice include α_1-antitrypsin deficiency, galactosemia, and cystic fibrosis. Other rare causes include sepsis, parenteral alimentation cholestasis, Gilbert disease, and Alagille syndrome.

▶ Treatment

Surgical exploration for neonatal jaundice is indicated as early in infancy as possible, when biliary atresia is the likely cause. Delayed treatment will result in progressive cirrhosis. Fluoroscopy should be available in the operating room. The gallbladder is cannulated through a transverse abdominal incision or via laparoscopy. Water-soluble contrast should be gently instilled into the biliary tree. If the image shows a patent common bile duct but no reflux into the liver, a rubber-shod bulldog clamp may be placed on the distal common duct and the cholangiogram repeated. During development of the radiograph films, a core needle biopsy of each lobe is obtained.

Confirmed biliary atresia requires hepatic portoenterostomy (Kasai procedure). The scarred bile ducts and gallbladder are removed, and a Roux-en-Y limb of jejunum is sutured to an area of the hilum bounded laterally by the hepatic artery branches. Some surgeons utilize empiric postoperative antibiotic coverage to prevent cholangitis that can lead to scarring and ongoing occlusion of the bile canaliculi that may remain patent. Steroids have also been used both preoperatively and postoperatively in an effort to prevent ongoing biliary and hepatic fibrosis.

▶ Prognosis

A good long-term outcome is related to a meticulously performed procedure, age at operation less than 2 months, absence of cirrhosis at the time of operation, and establishment of adequate bile flow. In general, one third of the infants will have excellent bile flow and do not develop liver failure, one third never have bile flow and require early liver transplantation, and one third have initially good bile flow but months to years later develop progressive biliary cirrhosis requiring liver transplantation. The average life span for infants with uncorrectable biliary atresia without transplantation is 19 months. Death is due to progressive liver failure, bleeding from esophageal varices, or sepsis. For those with established bile flow postoperatively, the most common complication is cholangitis, which may recur. Most often, the cause is unknown and not readily correctable by surgical means.

Davenport M et al: Randomized, double-blind, placebo-controlled trial of corticosteroids after Kasai portoenterostomy for biliary atresia. Hepatology 2007;46:1821.

Narkewicz MR: Biliary atresia: an update on our understanding of this disorder. Curr Opin Pediatr 2001;13:435.

Nio M, Ohi R: Biliary atresia. Semin Pediatr Surg 2000;9:177.

Schreiber RA et al: Biliary atresia: the Canadian experience. J Pediatr 2007;151:659.

Tagge DU et al: A long-term experience with biliary atresia: reassessment of prognostic factors. Ann Surg 1991;214:590.

CHOLEDOCHAL CYST

A choledochal cyst is a dilation or diverticulum of all or a portion of the common bile duct. Estimates of incidence range from 1:2,000,000 to 1:13,000. There is a female predominance (3:1), and the lesions are more common in Asians, with a large majority of the reported cases from Japan. Numerous theories exist as to the cause of this abnormality, including infectious agents, reflux of pancreatic enzymes into the bile duct via a long common channel, genetic factors, and biliary autonomic dysfunction.

Choledochal cysts are classified into one of five subtypes. Type I is a fusiform dilation of the extrahepatic bile duct. Type II is a saccular outpouching of the common bile duct. Type III is referred to as a choledochocele and is a widemouth dilation of the common bile duct at its confluence with the duodenum. Type IV is cystic dilation of both the intrahepatic and extrahepatic bile ducts. Type V consists of lakes of multiple intrahepatic cysts with no extrahepatic component and, when associated with hepatic fibrosis, is termed Caroli disease. Type I and type IV are the most common lesions, with type I cysts accounting for 85% of these abnormalities. Caroli disease appears to be a congenital syndrome and often follows an autosomal recessive pattern of inheritance in association with various other anomalies such as polycystic kidney disease and renal tubular ectasia.

If left untreated, a choledochal cyst may cause cholangitis and cholangiocarcinoma. The risk of cholangiocarcinoma in the first decade of life is only 0.7%; however, this increases to 14% at 20 years and is postulated to increase even further throughout life.

▶ Clinical Findings

The clinical manifestations of a choledochal cyst are recurrent abdominal pain, episodic jaundice, and a right upper quadrant mass, though in most cases one of these features is missing. As children grow older, the cyst may become painful or infected. On rare occasions, children have been described with bile peritonitis secondary to perforation of a cyst. In adults, an abdominal mass is rarely appreciated, and patients present more commonly with symptoms of cholangitis or pancreatitis. Gallstones and cholangitis may develop due to biliary stasis.

The diagnosis is most often established by the clinical presentation and abnormal ultrasonography. ^{99m}Tc-labeled IDA scan, CT and MRI scans, endoscopic retrograde cholangiopancreatography, and operative cholangiography may be necessary. Ultrasonography is increasingly responsible for detecting choledochal cysts in the fetus.

▶ Treatment

In the past, the cysts were not removed but drained into a limb of intestine. However, many of these patients developed carcinoma in the cyst years later. Presently, the treatment is complete excision with Roux-en-Y hepaticojejunostomy. The duodenal end of the bile duct should be oversewn without injury to the anomalous entry of the pancreatic duct, limiting the amount of residual biliary tissue at risk for malignancy. Side-to-side choledochoduodenostomy is not recommended because it is followed by a high incidence of stricture of the anastomosis and recurrent cholangitis. Cholecystectomy is always performed. Biliary cirrhosis and portal hypertension, occurring from prolonged ductal obstruction, may be assessed with liver biopsy. The results of choledochal cyst excision with hepaticojejunostomy reconstruction are consistently excellent, but these children do require lifelong follow-up because of the risk of anastomotic stricture and intrahepatic stone formation. There is currently a trend toward laparoscopic approaches to the treatment of choledochal cyst disease.

Han S et al: Acquired choledochal cyst from anomalous pancreaticobiliary duct union. J Pediatr Surg 1997;32:1735.

Herman TE, Siegel MJ: Neonatal type I choledochal cyst. J Perinatol 2007;27:453.

Le DM et al: Laparoscopic resection of type I choledochal cysts in pediatric patients. Surg Endosc 2006;20:249.

Lipsett PA et al: Choledochal cyst disease: a changing pattern of presentation. Ann Surg 1994;220:644.

Miyano T, Yamataka A: Choledochal cysts. Curr Opin Pediatr 1997;9:283.

O'Neill J: Choledochal cyst. Curr Probl Surg 1992;29:365.

▼ INGUINAL & SCROTAL DISORDERS

INGUINAL HERNIA & HYDROCELE

Inguinal hernia is a common condition in infancy and childhood, occurring in 1–3% of all children. Unlike hernias in adulthood, these nearly always result from a patent processus vaginalis (indirect hernia) and not from a weakness in the floor of the inguinal canal (direct hernia). The processus vaginalis follows the descent of the testis into the inguinal canal. Failure of obliteration of the processus may lead to a variety of anomalies, including hernia, communicating hydrocele, noncommunicating hydrocele, hydrocele of the spermatic cord, and hydrocele of the tunica vaginalis (Figure 43–20).

The processus vaginalis remains patent in over 80% of newborn infants. With increasing age, the incidence of patent processus vaginalis diminishes. At 2 years, 40–50% are open, and in adults, 25% are persistently patent. Actual herniation of bowel into a widely patent processus vaginalis develops in 1–4% of children; 25% occur within the first year of life. Indirect inguinal hernia occurs four to six times more frequently in males. Direct and femoral hernias occur in children but are very rare.

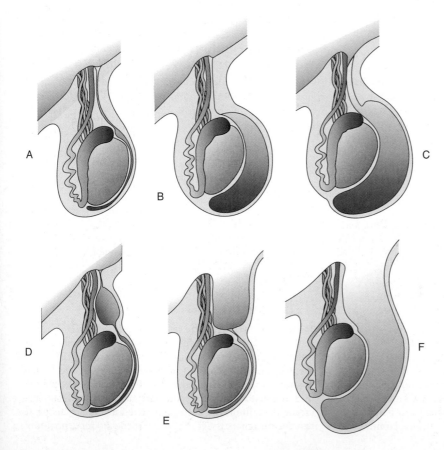

▲ **Figure 43–20.** Spectrum of inguinoscrotal disorders. **A:** Normal anatomy. The processus vaginalis is obliterated and there is a small remnant, the tunica vaginalis, adjacent to the posterior surface of the testis. **B:** Scrotal hydrocele. **C:** Communicating hydrocele. Note the proximal patency of the processus vaginalis. **D:** Hydrocele of the spermatic cord. **E:** Inguinal hernia. **F:** Inguinoscrotal hernia. (From Sheldon CA: Inguinal and scrotal disorders. In: *Essentials of Pediatric Surgery.* Rowe MI et al [editors]. Mosby, 1995. Reproduced with permission from Elsevier.)

Hernias are found on the right side in 60% of cases, on the left side in 30%, and bilaterally in 10%. Conditions associated with an increased risk of inguinal hernia include prematurity, family history, history of an abdominal wall defect (eg, gastroschisis), cryptorchidism, intersex anomalies, connective tissue disorders, and ascites. The processus vaginalis may be obliterated at any location proximal to the testis or labium.

Clinical Findings

The incidence of a clinically detectable inguinal hernia varies with gestational age: 9–11% in preterm infants and 3–5% for full-term infants. The diagnosis of hernia in infants and children can be made only by the demonstration of an inguinal bulge originating from the internal ring. The bulge can be elicited during times of Valsalva (crying, coughing, straining). Having an assistant hold the infant's arms over his or her head and legs straight will often elicit crying and straining that will aid in the physical examination. Indirect signs, such as a wide external ring and the "silk glove" sign (palpable thickening of the spermatic cord) are not dependable. One must always locate the position of the testis during examination for a hernia because an inguinal bulge due to an undescended or retractile testis may be mistaken for a hernia.

Incarcerated inguinal hernia accounts for approximately 10% of childhood hernias, and the incidence is highest in infants. In the majority of girls with incarcerated hernia, the sac contains the ovary and portion of the tube. These structures are usually a sliding component of the sac. In boys, small bowel, colon, or appendix can be within the sac.

A hydrocele is fluid within the remnant processus vaginalis. It is characteristically an oblong, nontender soft mass. It may be around the testicle only (testicular hydrocele), extend up from the testicle into the inguinal region (inguinoscrotal hydrocele), or be contained within a segment of the processus adjacent to the spermatic cord (hydrocele of the cord) or communicated with the peritoneal cavity (communicating hydrocele). With a noncommunicating hydrocele (the first three hydroceles described above), the processus vaginalis has closed proximally. The normal spermatic cord can usually be palpated above the level of the hydrocele. Transillumination is not reliable in the newborn because intestine and fluid transilluminate equally well. A communicating hydrocele is suspected by a history of size variation (smallest in the morning after sleep, largest during the day after the upright posture or repeated straining).

Differential Diagnosis

A hydrocele under tension may be confused with an incarcerated inguinal hernia. The sudden appearance of fluid confined to the testicular area may represent a noncommunicating hydrocele secondary to torsion of the testis or testicular appendage, epididymo-orchitis, panserositis from a recent viral syndrome, or idiopathic scrotal edema. Rectal examination and palpation of the peritoneal side of the inguinal ring may distinguish an incarcerated hernia from a hydrocele or other inguinoscrotal mass, but this is only reliable in the first 2–3 months of age because the internal ring is difficult to reach thereafter.

Complications

The principle risk of not treating an inguinal hernia is incarceration (viscus stuck in sac) and subsequent strangulation (ischemia of said viscus, usually the bowel, not the ovary). Compression of the spermatic vessels by an incarcerated hernia may produce hemorrhagic infarction of the ipsilateral testicle.

Treatment

In general, hydroceles that do not communicate with the peritoneal cavity are physiologic, and the vast majority resolve by 18 months of age. Those that persist after 1 year or those that demonstrate changes in size (communicating hydroceles) should be repaired.

Inguinal hernia in infancy and childhood should be repaired; they never resolve spontaneously. In premature infants under constant surveillance in the hospital, hernia repair may be deferred until the baby is ready to be discharged. High ligation of the hernia sac by obliteration of the internal ring (leaving enough space for the spermatic cord) is all that is required. Historically, it was recommended that all boys under 2 years of age and all girls under 5 years undergo operative exploration of the contralateral inguinal canal in search of a clinically silent patent processus vaginalis. This approach has been replaced, in large part, by laparoscopic exploration performed either through the ipsilateral hernia sac, through the umbilicus, or in-line with the internal ring (at the lateral border of the rectus muscle) using a needlescope. If a patent processus vaginalis is demonstrated, a second inguinal incision is made and the procedure is repeated as described previously. Recently, a completely laparoscopic repair has been advocated, which has the advantage of simultaneous exploration of the contralateral side and virtually no manipulation of the spermatic cord. The incidence of complications from uncomplicated inguinal hernia repair (recurrence, wound infection, and damage to the spermatic cord) should be 2% or less.

An incarcerated hernia in an infant can usually be reduced initially before operation. This is accomplished by sedation and by elevation of the foot of the bed to keep intra-abdominal pressure from being exerted against the inguinal area. When the infant is well-sedated, the hernia may be reduced by gentle constant pressure over the internal ring in a manner that milks the bowel into the abdominal cavity. This is a two-handed maneuver in which one hand "squeezes" the incarcerated mass while the other directs it posteriorly into the internal ring. If the bowel is not reduced within an hour, operation is required. If the hernia is reduced, operative repair should be delayed for 48 hours to allow edema in the tissues to subside. An incarcerated ovary may not be able to be reduced but is usually asymptomatic, and repair at the next available operating room time is sufficient, since torsion is rare and the blood supply, unlike that of the intestine, is not compromised by being trapped in the canal. Bloody stools and edema and red discoloration of the skin around the groin suggest a strangulated hernia, and reduction of the bowel should not be attempted. Emergency repair of incarcerated inguinal hernia is technically difficult because the edematous tissues are friable and tear readily. When gangrenous intestine is encountered, the bowel should be resected and an end-to-end intestinal anastomosis performed.

Dutta S, Albanese CT: Transcutaneous laparoscopic hernia repair in children: a prospective review of 275 hernia repairs with minimum 2-year follow-up. Surg Endosc 2009;23:103.

Fuenfer MM et al: Laparoscopic exploration of the contralateral groin in children: an improved technique. J Laparoendosc Surg 1996;1:S1.

Kapur P, Caty MG, Glick PL: Pediatric hernias and hydroceles. Pediatr Clin North Am 1998;45:773.

Yerkes EB et al: Laparoscopic evaluation for a contralateral patent processus vaginalis: part III. Urology 1998;51:480.

UNDESCENDED TESTIS (CRYPTORCHIDISM)

In the seventh month of gestation, the testicles normally descend into the scrotum. A fibromuscular band—the gubernaculum—extends from the lower pole of the testis to the scrotum, and this band probably acts by guiding the path for descent during differential growth of the fetus rather than by pulling the testes down. Undescended testis (cryptorchidism) is a form of dystopia of the testis that occurs when there is arrested descent and fixation of the position of the testis retroperitoneally, in the inguinal canal, or just beyond the external ring. Continued descent of the testes may progress after birth, but descent comes to a halt before 2 years of age.

Another form of dystopia is ectopic testis, in which the gubernaculum may have guided the testis near the pubis, penis, perineum, or medial thigh or to a subcutaneous position superficial to the inguinal canal. In these instances, the testis has descended beyond the external ring of the inguinal canal, and the vascular supply is sufficiently developed so as to pose little difficulty in operative repair.

Normal spermatogenesis requires the cooler temperature range provided in the scrotum. When the testis remains undescended and subjected to normal body temperature, degenerative changes in the seminiferous tubules occur in which the lining cells become progressively atrophic and hyalinized, with peritubular fibrosis. The degenerative changes begin to occur at 2 years of age. Unless the disorder is corrected, all bilaterally cryptorchid adult males become sterile.

The incidence of undescended or partially descended testis is 1–2% in full-term infants and up to 30% in premature babies. The right testis is affected in 45% of cases, the left

testis in 30%, and both testes in 25%. A patent processus vaginalis is present in 95% of patients with cryptorchidism, and approximately 25% develop a clinical hernia.

Anomalies associated with cryptorchidism occur in about 15% of cases and include a wide variety of syndromes such as Klinefelter syndrome, hypogonadotropic hypogonadism, the prune belly syndrome, horseshoe kidneys, renal agenesis or hypoplasia, exstrophy of the bladder, ureteral reflux, gastroschisis, and cloacal exstrophy.

▶ Clinical Findings

Physical examination demonstrates an "empty hemiscrotum" with absent rugae. Cryptorchidism must be differentiated from a retractile testis. Because of the very active cremaster of children under 3 years of age and the small size of the testis, the gonad can retract into the external inguinal ring or within the inguinal canal—this is called a retractile testis—and it is a variant of normal. The retractile testis can be manually manipulated into the mid to lower scrotum, and no therapy is required.

▶ Treatment

Operation is indicated after 12–18 months because degenerative changes begin to take place in these testes that may impair spermatogenesis and lead to malignant transformation. Additionally, cryptorchid testes are more susceptible to trauma and torsion, often have an associated inguinal hernia, and may cause adverse psychosocial effects. The incidence of testicular cancer in a cryptorchid testis is 30 times higher than in the normal population and is not lessened by repair. The role of repair is to allow reliable examination for a testicular mass later in life.

Orchidopexy is the surgical method for mobilizing the testis—based on the testicular vessels and the vas deferens—from its ectopic location into the scrotum. When the dystopic testis is not palpable preoperatively, 17% are absent, 33% are intra-abdominal, and 50% are in the inguinal canal or just beyond the inguinal ring. If the testis is not palpable when the child is anesthetized, laparoscopy should be performed before making an inguinal incision. Increasingly, the complete operation (diagnosis and intra-abdominal mobilization) is performed laparoscopically. This will allow for identification of an abdominal testis or the diagnosis of an absent testis (usually due to in utero torsion). Very high testes with a short blood supply can be brought into the scrotum by a two-stage repair (dividing the spermatic artery and vein with clips or laser followed by positioning in the scrotum 6–8 weeks later) based on collateral blood supply via the vas deferens and the gubernaculum. Testes confined in the inguinal canal (25% of cases) can usually be brought into the scrotum in one stage. Ectopic testicles located outside the inguinal canal, such as in the subcutaneous inguinal pouch, occur in over 50% of cases, and the testicular vessels are so well developed that scrotal placement is rarely a problem. The prognosis for fertility following orchidopexy in unilateral maldescent is 80%, whereas fertility after bilateral orchidopexy is about 50%. Due to variable degrees of tension and tenuous blood supply, the testis after an orchidopexy is often smaller than the contralateral one.

Docimo SG: The results of surgical therapy for cryptorchidism: a literature review and analysis. J Urol 1995;154:1148.

Gatti JM, Ostlie DJ: The use of laparoscopy in the management of nonpalpable undescended testes. Curr Opin Pediatr 2007; 19:349.

Humke U et al: Pediatric laparoscopy for nonpalpable testes with new miniaturized instruments. J Endourol 1998;12:445.

Mayr JM, Lawrenz K, Berghold A: Undescended testicles: an epidemiologic review. Acta Paediatr 1999;88:1089.

Pillai SB, Besner GE: Pediatric testicular problems. Pediatr Clin North Am 1998;45:813.

TESTICULAR TORSION

Testicular torsion is most frequent in late childhood and early adolescence, though the range can include the fetus and the adult. Anatomically, there are two forms of testicular torsion depending on where the spermatic cord is twisted with respect to the tunica vaginalis: intravaginal torsion (bell-clapper deformity), the most common form, and extravaginal torsion that occurs principally in neonates and in children with an undescended testis. Rarely, the testis may twist on a long epididymal mesentery. In children and adolescents, testicular torsion is either idiopathic or occurs after activity or trauma.

▶ Clinical Findings

Acute scrotal or testicular pain that may radiate to the lower abdomen is usually present. Progressive swelling, edema, and erythema of the hemiscrotum occur. The testis is exquisitely tender to palpation. The testicle may be foreshortened, the epididymis may lie anteriorly, and the cremasteric reflex may be absent—though these signs are difficult to elicit. Fetal or neonatal torsion is probably responsible for the "absent" testis noted during laparoscopy.

The diagnosis of testicular torsion is based mainly on clinical examination. Although one may utilize Doppler ultrasonography and radionuclide scanning to aid in the diagnosis, these tests are time consuming and, in the case of ultrasound, operator specific.

▶ Differential Diagnosis

Torsion of the testicular appendices (vestigial müllerian duct structures) and epididymitis may mimic testicular torsion. With epididymitis, there is often pyuria, voiding symptoms, and fever. Torsion of the testicular appendices often has a gradual onset, and careful palpation may reveal point tenderness rather than diffuse tenderness. There may be a visible necrotic lesion on scrotal transillumination (blue dot sign).

▶ Treatment

If the diagnosis is strongly suspected, the best "test" is operative scrotal exploration. The testicular salvage rate if detorsion is performed within 6 hours after onset of symptoms is up to 97%, versus less than 10% if delayed more than 24 hours. At operation, the torsion is corrected and the gonad, if viable, is fixed to the hemiscrotum in three places. Because the paired testicle is at risk for torsion, since the testicular anatomy tends to mirror itself, contralateral orchiopexy (suture fixation) should be performed in all cases. Torsion of the testicular appendices tends to be self-limiting, since necrosis and autoamputation usually occur. Treatment is with warm baths, limited activity, and an anti-inflammatory agent. If significant pain persists after 2–3 days and the appendix has not autoamputated, excision is indicated. Testicular salvage after neonatal testicular torsion is very rare.

Chiang MC et al: Clinical features of testicular torsion and epididymo-orchitis in infants younger than 3 months. J Pediatr Surg 2007;42:1574.

Kass EJ, Lundak BL: The acute scrotum. Pediatr Clin North Am 1997;44:1251.

▼ ABDOMINAL WALL DEFECTS

UMBILICAL HERNIA

A fascial defect at the umbilicus is frequently present in the newborn, particularly in premature infants. The incidence is highest in African American children. In most children, the umbilical ring progressively diminishes in size and eventually closes. Fascial defects less than 1 cm in diameter close spontaneously by 5 years of age in 95% of cases. When the fascial defect is greater than 1.5 cm in diameter, it seldom closes spontaneously. Unlike inguinal hernias, protrusion of bowel through the umbilical defect rarely results in incarceration in childhood. Surgical repair is indicated if the intestine becomes incarcerated, when the fascial defect is greater than 1.5 cm, and in all children over 4 years of age. Both open and laparoscopic approaches are associated with uniformly excellent results.

Albanese CA, Rengal S, Bermudez D: A novel laparoscopic technique for the repair of pediatric umbilical and epigastric hernias. J Pediatr Surg 2006;41:859.

OMPHALOCELE

This is a midline abdominal wall defect noted in 1:5000 live births. The abdominal viscera (commonly liver and bowel) are contained within a sac composed of peritoneum and amnion from which the umbilical cord arises at the apex and center (Figure 43–21). When the defect is less than 4 cm, it is termed a hernia of the umbilical cord; when greater than 10 cm, it is termed a giant omphalocele. Associated abnormali-

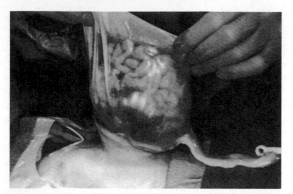

▲ **Figure 43–21.** Neonate with omphalocele. The liver and bowel herniated through a midline abdominal wall defect and are surrounded by a sac of amnion and chorion from which the umbilical cord emanates. (Reproduced, with permission, from Albanese CT: Pediatric surgery. In: *Surgery,* Norton JA [editor]. Springer, 2000.)

ties occur in 30–70% of infants and include, in descending order of frequency, chromosomal abnormalities (trisomy 13, 18, 21), congenital heart disease (tetralogy of Fallot, atrial septal defect), Beckwith-Wiedemann syndrome (large-for-gestational-age baby; hyperinsulinism; visceromegaly of kidneys, adrenal glands, and pancreas; macroglossia; hepatorenal tumors; cloacal extrophy), pentalogy of Cantrell, and prune belly syndrome (absent abdominal wall muscles, genitourinary abnormalities, cryptorchidism). Small omphaloceles are most often linked to chromosomal defects and Beckwith-Wiedemann syndrome, especially when the liver is not in the hernia sac.

▷ Treatment

The primary goal of surgery is to return the viscera to the abdominal cavity and close the defect. With an intact sac, emergency operation is not necessary, so a thorough physical examination and workup for associated anomalies is performed. An orogastric tube should be placed on suction to minimize intestinal distention.

The success of primary closure depends on the size of the defect and of the abdominal and thoracic cavities as well as the presence of associated problems (eg, lung disease). It is wise to leave the sac in situ, since primary closure may not be possible, and in this way, one has maintained the best biologic dressing for the viscera. Supplemental coverage with plastic wrap or a bowel bag can be used to prevent heat loss. If the viscera reduce but abdominal wall closure is not possible, there are three options: staged repair, prosthetic patch repair, or nonoperative compression dressing and orthotics for gradual return of domain. A staged repair aims to create a protective extra-abdominal extension of the peritoneal cavity (termed a silo), allowing gradual reduction of the viscera and gradual abdominal wall expansion using two

parallel sheets of reinforced Silastic sheeting sutured to the fascial edges or a preformed one-piece silo with a collapsible ring at its base for ease of insertion. A prosthetic patch repair bridges the fascial gap with a synthetic material (eg, polytetrafluoroethylene), and the skin is closed over the patch. The silo is progressively compressed to invert the amniotic sac and its contents into the abdomen and to bring the edges of the linea alba together by stretching the abdominal wall muscles. This usually requires 5–7 days, after which the defect is then primarily closed. The intra-abdominal pressure produced by the silo should not exceed 20 cm H_2O to avoid impairing venous return from the bowel and kidneys. When abdominal relaxation is sufficient to allow the rectus muscles to come together, the silo is removed, the amnion is left inverted into the abdominal cavity, and the defect is closed.

In rare cases, nonoperative management is advised for infants with severe associated anomalies or a giant omphalocele. The amnion is allowed to dry and form an eschar. The membrane becomes vascularized beneath the eschar, and contraction of the wound with skin growth covers the defect. This can be further facilitated by creation of a compression orthotic that allows for the gradual return of abdominal contents and recreation of abdominal domain. A ventral hernia results, which is repaired electively when the patient is stable. The survival rate for infants with small omphaloceles is excellent. Deaths associated with larger omphaloceles are principally from wound dehiscence with subsequent and ensuing infection or from associated anomalies.

GASTROSCHISIS

Gastroschisis is a defect in the abdominal wall that usually occurs to the right of a normal insertion of the umbilical cord (Figure 43–22). It is believed to arise at the site of involution of

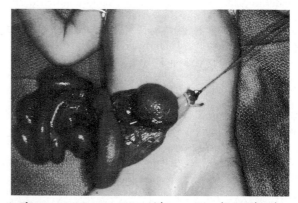

▲ **Figure 43–22.** Neonate with a gastroschisis. The defect is to the right of the umbilical cord, and the bowel has no investing sac. Note edema of the bowel wall and the dilated stomach adjacent to the umbilical cord. (Reproduced, with permission, from Albanese CT: Pediatric surgery. In: *Surgery.* Norton JA [editor]. Springer, 2000.)

the right umbilical vein, though a less popular theory holds there is some evidence that it results from rupture of an omphalocele sac in utero. It is twice as common as omphalocele and the defect is usually smaller. The remnants of the amnion are usually reabsorbed. The skin may continue to grow over the remnants of the amnion, and there may be a bridge of skin between the defect and the cord. The small and large bowel, stomach, and often the fallopian tube/ovary/testis herniate through the abdominal wall defect. Unlike an omphalocele, the liver is virtually never present in the defect. Having been bathed in the amniotic fluid and with compression of the mesenteric blood supply at the abdominal defect, the bowel wall is edematous and has a very thick, shaggy membrane ("peel") covering it. The loops of intestine are usually matted together, and the intestine appears to be abnormally short.

▶ Complications

Since the bowel has not been contained intra-abdominally, the abdominal cavity fails to enlarge, and it frequently cannot accommodate the protuberant bowel. Over 70% of infants with this disorder are premature, but associated anomalies occur in fewer than 10% of cases. Nonrotation of the midgut is present. Associated intestinal atresia occurs in approximately 7% because segments of intestine that have herniated through the defect become infarcted in utero.

▶ Treatment & Prognosis

Unlike omphalocele, urgent repair is necessary. Small defects may be closed primarily after manually stretching the abdominal cavity. A staged approach is frequently required using a silo, as described in the section Omphalocele. As bowel wall edema subsides, the bowel will readily reduce into the abdominal cavity. Reduction is aided by having the infant paralyzed and receiving endotracheal ventilation to relax the abdominal wall and allow it to stretch and accommodate the bowel. When the bowel has been completely reduced (usually 5–7 days), the silo is removed and the abdominal wall is closed. Most recently, the use of the umbilical remnant as a biological dressing has been described without primary fascial closure with good success.

The death rate for infants with gastroschisis is less than 5%. Poor gastrointestinal function and episodes of sepsis, presumably from compromised bowel, may occur. Prolonged postoperative ileus (more than 2 weeks) is the rule, and total parenteral nutrition is necessary. Primary repair of an associated intestinal atresia is rarely safe and possible. Either a proximal stoma is created or the atretic ends are reduced and repaired 6 weeks later when the intra-abdominal inflammation has subsided.

Langer JC: Gastroschisis and omphalocele. Semin Pediatr Surg 1996;5:124.

Lunzer H, Menardi G, Brezinka C: Long-term follow-up of children with prenatally diagnosed omphalocele and gastroschisis. J Matern Fetal Med 2001;10:385.

Molik KA et al: Gastroschisis: a plea for risk categorization. J Pediatr Surg 2001;36:51.

Sandler A et al: A Plastic sutureless abdominal wall closure in gastroschisis. J Pediatr Surg 2004;39:738.

▼ CUTANEOUS VASCULAR ANOMALIES

Cutaneous vascular anomalies comprise a group of congenital and acquired vascular malformations of the skin. They are present in 2.6% of all newborns. These anomalies are broadly divided into two categories: hemangiomas and vascular malformations. They are most precisely classified by the biologic activity of the endothelium.

HEMANGIOMAS

Hemangiomas demonstrate endothelial hyperplasia and are seen in children and adults but behave differently at different ages. Hemangiomas are much more common than vascular malformations. In the neonatal period, hemangiomas can be subclassified according to their growth phase. A rapid proliferating phase is usually seen during the first few years of life followed by an involuting phase that may last several years.

▶ Clinical Findings

The clinical appearance depends on the depth of the lesion. Superficial dermal lesions (capillary hemangiomas, strawberry hemangiomas) are raised and profoundly erythematous, with an irregular texture; deep lesions (cavernous hemangiomas) are smooth and slightly raised, with a bluish hue or a faint telangiectatic pattern on the overlying skin. Mixed lesions are often noted (capillary-cavernous hemangiomas). Twenty percent of patients have multiple lesions. Complications from hemangiomas consist of ulceration (during the proliferative phase), bleeding, thrombocytopenia (Kasabach-Merritt syndrome), consumptive coagulopathy, high-output heart failure, visual field encroachment, airway obstruction, and minor skeletal distortions.

▶ Treatment

Fifty percent of hemangiomas will involute without treatment by age 5 years and 70% by 7 years. The remainder will slowly resolve by age 10–12 years. Steroid therapy hastens the rate of proliferation of hemangiomas by 30–90% and is indicated for complicated lesions (ie, those causing severe physiologic or anatomic abnormalities).

CUTANEOUS VASCULAR MALFORMATIONS

Vascular malformations, in contrast to hemangiomas, have normal endothelial cell turnover and tend to grow proportionally with the child. These lesions are structural anomalies that are considered errors in vascular morphogenesis. They are usually visible at birth but may take years or even decades to become manifest. They are separated into low-flow and high-flow variants and further classified according to the type of vascular channel abnormality: capillary, venous, arterial, and mixed malformations. Capillary and venous malformations are low-flow variants; arterial and mixed arterial and venous ones are high-flow variants.

▶ Capillary Malformations

Capillary malformations are nevus flammeus (port wine stain), nevus flammeus neonatorum (angel's kiss), nevus flammeus nuchae (stork bite, salmon patch), angiokeratomas, and telangiectasias (spider, hereditary hemorrhagic telangiectasia [Rendu-Osler-Weber syndrome]). They are prone to infection and are treated aggressively with intravenous antibiotics. A compression garment should be used if anatomically feasible. Some lesions can be excised or injected with a sclerosing solution.

▶ Venous Malformations

Venous malformations have a wide spectrum of appearances ranging from simple varicosities to complex lesions that may be located in deeper tissues (eg, bone, muscle, salivary gland). Pain is often related to thrombosis within the lesion. Radiographic imaging delineates the nature and extent of the lesion (angiogram, CT, MRI). Photocoagulation or Nd:YAG laser may be effective for superficial lesions. Resection is the definitive treatment since it can reduce bulk, improve contour and function, and control pain. It is limited by anatomic boundaries, and multiple, staged procedures may be required.

▶ Arterial Malformations

Arterial and arteriovenous malformations are associated with multiple small fistulas surrounded by abnormal tissues and can cause high-output cardiac failure. They are most common in the head and neck region (especially intracerebral). There is pain and overlying cutaneous necrosis. Adjacent osseous structures are often destroyed. Selective embolization is used either as palliation or presurgically to limit hemorrhage. Excision, when possible, is the treatment of choice.

▶ Combined Malformations

Combined vascular malformations and hypertrophy syndromes consist of Klippel-Trenaunay-Weber syndrome (combined capillary-lymphatic venous malformation associated with lower limb hypertrophy), Parkes-Weber syndrome (upper limb arteriovenous shunting), Maffucci syndrome (low-flow vascular malformations and multiple extremity enchondromas with hypoplastic long bones), and Sturge-Weber syndrome (upper facial port wine stain and vascular anomalies of the choroid plexus and leptomeninges).

Low DW: Hemangiomas and vascular malformations. Semin Pediatr Surg 1994;3:40.

Mulliken JB, Fishman SJ, Burrows PE: Vascular anomalies. Curr Probl Surg 2000;37:517.

▼ TUMORS IN CHILDHOOD

NEUROBLASTOMA

Of all childhood neoplasms, neuroblastoma is exceeded in frequency only by leukemia and brain tumors. Approximately 60% of cases occur within the first 2 years of life and 97% within the first 20 years. This tumor is of neural crest origin and may originate anywhere along the distribution of the sympathetic chain. The most common site for primary disease is in the abdomen (adrenal), followed by the thorax, pelvis, and occasionally the head and neck. Neuroblastomas originate in the retroperitoneal area in 75% of cases; 55% arise from the adrenal gland. They may reach massive size and violate tissue planes such that they envelop major blood vessels, their branches, and other important structures (eg, ureters), making initial primary resection potentially hazardous. The biologic behavior varies with the age of the patient, the site of primary origin, and the extent of the disease.

▶ Clinical Findings

A. Symptoms and Signs

Symptoms are site specific. The most common symptom is pain (from primary or metastatic disease). Nonspecific symptoms include growth retardation, malaise, fever, weight loss, and anorexia. Children frequently appear ill at the time of diagnosis. Constipation and urinary retention are signs of pelvic disease. Orbital metastases commonly present with periorbital ecchymoses and proptosis ("raccoon eyes"). Spinal canal involvement may present with acute paralysis due to compression. Opsomyoclonus syndrome is an acute cerebellar encephalopathy characterized by ataxia, opsoclonus ("dancing eyes"), myoclonus, and dementia. It occurs in association with approximately 3% of all neuroblastomas and is usually associated with a good prognosis, though the neurologic abnormalities tend to persist after successful treatment of the primary tumor. Interestingly, it is not due to central nervous system metastases of neuroblastoma and is believed to be immune-mediated. Infants with stage IV-S disease may display cutaneous metastases ("blueberry muffin" lesions) or respiratory embarrassment secondary to massive hepatomegaly from tumor infiltration. Palpable lesions are often hard and fixed.

In infants, metastases confined to the liver or subcutaneous fat are frequent and cortical bone metastases unusual. In older children, metastases to lymph nodes and bone are found in over 70% of cases at diagnosis. Pain in areas of bony involvement and in joints with associated myalgia and fever mimics rheumatic fever. Eighty-five to 90 percent secrete high levels of the catecholamine metabolites vanillylmandelic acid and homovanillic acid. Hypertension and diarrhea may occur as a result of catecholamine and vasoactive intestinal peptide secretion.

B. Imaging Studies

Imaging is aimed at defining the extent of the tumor and determining the presence of metastases to distant sites (most commonly lymph nodes, bone, lung, and liver). Neuroblastoma is the most common abdominal tumor to demonstrate calcifications (50%) prior to chemotherapy. CT scan of the area of tumor involvement helps to identify the relationship to surrounding structures and determine resectability. MRI is useful in assessing tumor within the spinal canal and spinal cord compression. MRI is as sensitive as CT scanning in terms of assessing tumor size and resectability but has the added advantage of being superior to CT in assessing vessel encasement, vessel patency, and spinal cord compression. MRI can also demonstrate bone marrow involvement in selected cases. Metaiodobenzylguanidine (MIBG) scintigraphy is very sensitive in detecting tumors that concentrate catecholamines and has been useful in the diagnosis of primary, residual, and metastatic disease in patients with neuroblastoma. For retroperitoneal tumors, an intravenous urogram may show displacement or compression of the adjacent kidney without distortion of the renal calices. Bone scans may be useful in detecting osseous metastases.

▶ Prognostic Factors

Favorable prognostic factors include diagnosis before age 1, a thoracic primary lesion, and low stage. In addition, several molecular and cellular characteristics of neuroblastic tumors are prognostically important. The most important is the high incidence of amplification of the protooncogene N-*myc*, seen in approximately 30% of tumors. Amplification of N-*myc* (more than 10 copies) adversely correlates with prognosis independently of clinical stage. Using the histologic Shimada index, well-differentiated, stroma-rich tumors have a favorable prognosis. An elevated ratio of vanillylmandelic acid to homovanillic acid correlates with an improved outcome in patients with advanced disease. Other biochemical indicators of advanced disease include neuron-specific enolase, serum ferritin, and serum lactate dehydrogenase. Staging systems are surgically and anatomically based and have prognostic value. The most recent is the International Neuroblastoma Staging System (Table 43–6).

▶ Treatment

Diagnosis depends on demonstration of immature neuroblastic tissue obtained by tissue or bone marrow aspirate and biopsy. Tissue is obtained by biopsy (either by laparotomy or laparoscopically), which allows accurate determination of resectability and ensures that adequate tissue (1 g or 1 cm^3) is available for determination of tumor markers, cytologic

Table 43–6. Staging of Neuroblastoma.

	Survival
I. Tumor confined to site of origin.	100%
IIa. Unilateral tumor incompletely excised. Nodes negative.	80%
IIb. Unilateral tumor, complete or incomplete excision. Nodes positive.	70%
III. Tumor infiltrating across the midline, or a unilateral tumor with contralateral nodes positive.	40%
IV. Remote disease in bone, bone marrow, soft tissue, distant nodes.	15%
IVs. Infants with stage I or stage II primary and remote spread limited to liver, skin, or bone marrow.	85%

studies, and the special stains required for accurate diagnosis and staging.

A localized neuroblastoma should be excised, and the local area of the tumor should be irradiated only when gross tumor remains. Unresectable neuroblastomas should be biopsied and treated initially by chemotherapy and radiation therapy and then by surgical resection for residual tumor. Removal of all residual disease is the goal, and a more radical approach is warranted. Most neuroblastomas are radiosensitive and respond to 3000 cGy or less of radiation. Patients with disseminated disease should be treated with a combination of chemotherapeutic agents such as cyclophosphamide, vincristine, dacarbazine, doxorubicin, cisplatin, and teniposide. Patients with stage III or stage IV tumors who are at high risk by virtue of their age or of the stage and biologic characteristics of the tumor benefit from total body irradiation followed by either allogeneic or, more commonly, purged autologous bone marrow transplantation.

Chamberlain RS et al: Complete surgical resection combined with aggressive adjuvant chemotherapy and bone marrow transplantation prolongs survival in children with advanced neuroblastoma. Ann Surg Oncol 1995;2:93.

Grosfeld JL: Risk-based management: current concepts of treating malignant solid tumors of childhood. J Am Coll Surg 1999;189:407.

Maris JM et al: Neuroblastoma. Lancet 2007;369:2106.

Matthay KK: Neuroblastoma: a clinical challenge and biologic puzzle. CA Cancer J Clin 1995;45:179.

Shimada H et al: International neuroblastoma pathology classification for prognostic evaluation of patients with peripheral neuroblastic tumors: a report from the Children's Cancer Group. Cancer 2001;92:2451.

WILMS TUMOR (NEPHROBLASTOMA)

Renal neoplasms account for about 10% of malignant tumors in children. Nephroblastoma (Wilms tumor), which accounts for 80% of these, consists of a variety of embryonic tissues such as abortive tubules and glomeruli, smooth and skeletal muscle fibers, spindle cells, cartilage, and bone. Seventy-five percent of children with nephroblastoma are under 5 years of age; the peak incidence is at 2–3 years. With current multimodality treatment, the survival rate exceeds 85%.

The left kidney is affected in 50% of cases of Wilms tumor and the right kidney in 45%. In 5% of cases, the tumors are bilateral; 60% are synchronous and 40% are metachronous. Associated anomalies and their incidence per 1000 cases are aniridia, 8.5; hypospadias, 18; hemihypertrophy, 25; and cryptorchidism, 28. Beckwith-Wiedemann syndrome and neurofibromatosis occur together occasionally, and renal tumors may also occur in families. The constellation of Wilms tumor, aniridia, genitourinary anomalies, and mental retardation (WAGR syndrome) is associated with deletion of 11p13.

▶ Clinical Findings

A. Symptoms and Signs

In contrast to those with neuroblastoma, children usually appear healthy. Symptoms consist of abdominal enlargement in 60%; pain in 20%; hematuria in 15%; malaise, weakness, anorexia, and weight loss in 10%; and fever in 3%. Hypertension is noted in over half of patients. An abdominal mass, palpable in almost all cases, is usually very large, firm, and smooth, and it does not ordinarily extend across the midline.

B. Imaging Studies

Imaging is required to determine the extent of the mass; to assess for bilateral disease, venous invasion, and metastases; and to confirm contralateral renal function. This is accomplished with abdominal ultrasound (to assess venous invasion) and a CT scan of the chest and abdomen.

▶ Differential Diagnosis

Abdominal masses may also be caused by hydronephrotic, multicystic, or duplicated kidneys, and by neuroblastoma, teratoma, hepatoma, and rhabdomyosarcoma. Ultrasonography and CT scanning can usually distinguish nephroblastoma from these other tumors. Calcification occurs in 10% of cases of nephroblastoma and tends to be more crescent-shaped, discrete, and peripherally situated than the calcifications of neuroblastoma, which are finely stippled.

▶ Treatment & Prognosis

Surgical excision is often accomplished without any preoperative treatment unless significant inferior vena caval thrombus is present. The aim of surgery is to completely remove the tumor (nephrectomy) and ureter without spill and to determine the tumor stage by virtue of its extent and the presence of lymph node involvement (Table 43–7). Stage I is tumor confined to a kidney that has been completely excised; stage II is tumor extending beyond the kidney

Table 43–7. Wilms Tumor Staging System.

> **Stage I:** Tumor limited to kidney and completely excised. The surface of the renal capsule is intact, and the tumor was not ruptured prior to removal. There is no residual tumor.
> **Stage II:** Tumor extends through the perirenal capsule but is completely excised. There may be local spillage of tumor confined to the flank, or the tumor may have been biopsied. Extrarenal vessels may contain tumor thrombus or be infiltrated by tumor.
> **Stage III:** Residual nonhematogenous tumor confined to the abdomen: lymph node involvement, diffuse peritoneal spillage, peritoneal implants, tumor beyond surgical margin either grossly or microscopically, or tumor not completely removed.
> **Stage IV:** Hematogenous metastases to lung, liver, bone, brain, etc.
> **Stage V:** Bilateral renal involvement at diagnosis; each kidney should be staged separately.

(perirenal tissues, renal vein or vena cava, biopsy or local spill in the flank) and completely excised; stage III is residual, nonhematogenous tumor confined to the abdomen (lymph node metastases, preoperative or intraoperative diffuse peritoneal deposits, residual tumor at the surgical margins, or unresectable tumor); stage IV is hematogenous metastases (lung, liver, bone, and brain); and stage V is bilateral renal involvement.

Irradiation of the tumor bed is indicated if the tumor has extended beyond the capsule of the kidney to involve adjacent organs or lymph nodes or if intraoperative tumor spillage has occurred. Very large tumors may be treated with radiation therapy and chemotherapy preoperatively to reduce their size. A significant reduction in size usually occurs in 7–10 days, after which nephrectomy can be readily performed. Nephrectomy is accomplished through a long transverse or thoracoabdominal incision.

Palpation of the renal veins and inferior vena cava is performed to detect tumor thrombus. The contralateral kidney must be examined and palpated. Bilateral disease (6%) mandates nephron-sparing surgery. The treatment of bilateral disease is individualized with the goal of eradicating tumor while preserving the maximal amount of functional renal mass. It is a contraindication to primary nephrectomy. Suspicious lesions in the opposite kidney are biopsied. If the tumor is too large for safe resection, it is biopsied along with regional lymph nodes. Chemotherapy with or without radiation therapy will usually result in a significant reduction in tumor size and allow subsequent resection. Metastatic foci in the lung or liver may be resected or treated with radiation therapy. Any residual tumor following radiation therapy, including multiple lesions, should be resected.

Overall survival is 85%, and most patients are cured. Survival correlates with stage and histology. The 4-year survival with respect to stage and histology is shown in Table 43–8. Tumor rupture with gross spillage portends a sixfold increase in risk of local recurrence and requires the use of postoperative external beam radiation.

Table 43–8. Four-Year Survival for Wilms Tumor.

Stage I/FH: 98%
Stage I–III/UH: 68%
Stage II/FH: 90–95%
Stage III/FH: 85–90%
Stage IV/FH: 78–86%
Stage IV/UH: 52–58%

FH, favorable histology; UH, unfavorable histology.

Capra ML et al: Wilms' tumor: a 25-year review of the role of preoperative chemotherapy. J Pediatr Surg 1999;34:579.

Green DM et al: Wilms tumor. CA Cancer J Clin 1996;46:46.

Haase GM, Ritchey ML: Nephroblastoma. Semin Pediatr Surg 1997;6:11.

RHABDOMYOSARCOMA

Rhabdomyosarcoma is a childhood malignancy that arises from embryonic mesenchyme with the potential to differentiate into skeletal muscle. It is the most common pediatric soft tissue sarcoma and is the third-most common solid malignancy. It accounts for 4–8% of all malignancies and 5–15% of all solid malignancies of childhood.

The age distribution is bimodal, the first peak is between 2 and 5 years, and the second peak is between 15 and 19 years. Fifty percent present before 5 years, and 6% present in infancy. There is an increased incidence in patients with neurofibromatosis, Beckwith-Wiedemann syndrome, and Li-Fraumeni cancer-family syndrome.

Rhabdomyosarcoma is divided into distinct histologic groups: favorable, intermediate, and unfavorable. Favorable types (5%) include the sarcoma botryoides and spindle cell variants. Botryoid tumors typically present in young children from within visceral cavities (eg, vagina), while spindle cell types have a predilection for paratesticular sites. Intermediate-prognosis tumors (50%) are of the embryonal type. Unfavorable-prognosis tumors (20%) include alveolar and undifferentiated tumors. Alveolar tumors arise from the extremities, trunk, and perineum. Undifferentiated tumors arise from the extremity and head and neck sites. Thirteen percent cannot be adequately characterized and are labeled "small, round cell sarcoma, type indeterminate."

▶ Clinical Findings

The clinical presentation varies with the site of origin of the primary tumor, the patient's age, and the presence or absence of metastatic disease. The majority of symptoms are secondary to the effects of compression by the tumor or by the presence of a mass. The most common site is the head and neck region (35%). These are subdivided into orbital (10%), parameningeal (15%), and nonparameningeal (10%) sites. They are usually embryonal and present as asymptomatic masses or functional deficits. Genitourinary rhabdomyosarcoma (26%) are divided into two groups: bladder and pros-

tate (10%) and nonbladder and prostate, including paratesticular sites, perineum, vulva, vagina, and uterus (16%). The most common histologic type is embryonal, though botryoid tumors and spindle cell tumors are seen more frequently here than in any other site. These tumors may be so massive as to make determination of the primary tumor site impossible. There is a propensity for early lymphatic spread in genitourinary primary tumors. Bladder and prostate tumors frequently present with urinary retention or hematuria, while vaginal and uterine tumors present with vaginal bleeding or discharge or with a mass exiting the vagina. Extremity rhabdomyosarcoma (1%) are more common in the lower than in the upper extremity. These are usually alveolar varieties with a high incidence of regional nodal involvement and distal metastases. Other sites account for 20%. The most common are the thorax, diaphragm, abdominal and pelvic walls, and intra-abdominal or intrapelvic organs.

Staging is determined by the histologic variant, the primary site, and the extent of disease, since each has an important influence on the choice of treatment and on prognosis. CT scanning or MRI is essential to evaluate the primary tumor and its relationship to surrounding structures. A clinical grouping system was designed by the Intergroup Rhabdomyosarcoma Study Group to stratify different extents of disease in order to compare treatment and outcome results (Table 43–9). It is based on pretreatment and operative outcome and does not account for the biologic differences or the natural history of tumors arising from different primary sites.

▶ Treatment & Prognosis

The surgical management is site specific and includes complete wide excision of the primary tumor and surrounding

Table 43–9. Intergroup Rhabdomyosarcoma Study Clinical Group Staging System.

Group I: Localized disease, completely removed
   a. Confined to muscle or organ of origin
   b. Infiltration outside organ or muscle of origin; regional nodes not involved.

Group II: Total gross resection with evidence of regional spread
   a. Grossly resected tumor with microscopic residual
   b. Regional disease with involved nodes, completely resected with no microscopic residual
   c. Regional disease with involved nodes, grossly resected, but with evidence of microscopic residual and/or histologic involvement of the most distal regional node in the dissection

Group III: Incomplete resection, or biopsy with presence of gross disease

Group IV: Distant metastases

Reproduced, with permission, from Neville HL et al: Preoperative staging, prognostic factors, and outcome for extremity rhabdomyosarcoma: a preliminary report from the Intergroup Rhabdomyosarcoma Study IV (1991-1997). J Pediatr Surg 2000;35:317.

uninvolved tissue while preserving cosmetic appearance and function. Incomplete excision (beyond biopsy) or tumor debulking is not beneficial, and severely mutilating or debilitating procedures should not be performed. Tumors not amenable to primary excision should be amply biopsied and then treated with neoadjuvant agents; secondary excision is then performed and is associated with a better outcome than partial or incomplete excisions. Clinically suspicious lymph nodes should be excised or biopsied, while excision of clinically uninvolved nodes is site specific. Primary reexcision has been shown to improve outcome in patients when microscopic margins are positive, the initial procedure was not a formal "cancer" resection, or malignancy was not suspected preoperatively.

The 5-year survival for stage I tumors is 90%; for stage II, clinical group I or II, it is 77%; for stage II, clinical group III, it is 65%; and for stage III lesions (group I, II, or III), it is 55%. Stage IV tumors arising from favorable sites of origin are curable, while those from unfavorable sites have a very poor prognosis. The prognosis for recurrent disease is poor.

Andrassy RJ: Rhabdomyosarcoma. Semin Pediatr Surg 1997;6:17.
Neville HL et al: Preoperative staging, prognostic factors, and outcome for extremity rhabdomyosarcoma: a preliminary report from the Intergroup Rhabdomyosarcoma Study IV (1991–1997). J Pediatr Surg 2000;35:317.
Paulino AC, Okeru MF: Rhabdomyosarcoma. Curr Probl Cancer 2008;32:7.

TERATOMA

Teratomas are embryonal neoplasms derived from pluripotent cells containing tissue from at least two of three germ layers (ectoderm, endoderm, mesoderm). Approximately 80% are found in females. They are typically midline or paraaxial tumors and are distributed in the following regions: sacrococcygeal (57%), gonadal (29%), mediastinal (7%), retroperitoneal (4%), cervical (3%), and intracranial (3%). Other sites are rare. Nongonadal teratomas present in infancy; gonadal ones, in adolescence. Twenty-one percent are malignant.

The serum α-fetoprotein (AFP) level is elevated in tumors containing malignant endodermal sinus (yolk sac) elements. Serial AFP levels are markers for recurrence. β-Human chorionic gonadotropin (β-hCG) is produced from those containing malignant choriocarcinoma tissue. Rarely, enough β-hCG is produced to cause precocious puberty. Elevated AFP and β-hCG levels in histologically benign tumors indicate an increased risk of recurrence and malignant transformation, particularly with "immature" benign teratomas.

▶ Sacrococcygeal Teratoma

The majority of sacrococcygeal teratomas present in the newborn period and can be detected by prenatal ultrasound. Females predominate; a history of twins is common. Pregnancy may be complicated by fetal high-output cardiac failure via arteriovenous shunting within the tumor, maternal polyhydramnios, and hydrops fetalis leading to fetal demise. Fetal surgery has been utilized successfully in those with hydrops. The tumors are classified according to location: type I, predominantly external (46%); type II, external mass and presacral component (35%); type III, visible externally, but predominantly presacral (9%); and type IV, entirely presacral, not visible externally (10%).

Treatment is excision of the tumor and coccyx; type I and II lesions are resected from the perineal approach, and type III and IV lesions require a combined intra-abdominal and perineal resection. The majority (97%) of newborn sacrococcygeal teratomas are benign and do not require adjuvant therapy. Follow-up requires serial AFP levels and physical examinations, including digital rectal examination. Recurrent tumors are excised. The greatest risk factor for malignancy is age at diagnosis. The malignancy rate is approximately 50–60% after 2 months of age. Malignant tumors are often treated with surgery and chemotherapy. The 5-year survival for malignant germ cell tumors arising from a sacrococcygeal teratoma is approximately 50%.

▶ Mediastinal Teratoma

Mediastinal teratomas account for approximately 20% of all pediatric mediastinal tumors. They usually arise in the anterior mediastinum, though intrapericardial and cardiac lesions have been reported. Symptoms include respiratory distress, chronic cough, chest pain, and wheezing. Males with β-hCG-producing tumors may display precocious puberty. Cardiac failure may develop from compression or pericardial effusion. The chest radiograph demonstrates a calcified anterior mediastinal mass in over one third of cases. Ultrasonography delineates cystic and solid components. General anesthesia should not be induced until a CT scan evaluation of the airway has been obtained because the supine position coupled with a loss of airway tone from anesthetic agents may allow the anterior mass to obstruct the distal trachea, making rapid establishment of an airway all but impossible. If significant airway compression is present, an awake needle biopsy under local anesthesia followed by radiation therapy or chemotherapy is indicated. Complete resection is definitive treatment.

▶ Cervical Teratoma

Cervical teratomas are rare neonatal neck masses that by virtue of their large size frequently cause respiratory distress. Calcifications may be seen on a plain radiograph and a mixed cystic and solid appearance on ultrasound. These tumors are most commonly benign. The most common malignant type is the yolk sac tumor (endodermal sinus tumor). Serum AFP and β-hCG levels can be monitored to detect the presence of recurrent germ cell tumors. The rapid establishment of an endotracheal airway may be necessary. Tracheostomy is hazardous because of the distortion of landmarks by the large mass. Treatment is complete excision. Some malignant tumors respond to radiation therapy. Regardless of the stage of disease, these tumors behave aggressively and should be treated adjunctively with a combination of cisplatin, vinblastine, and bleomycin or with dactinomycin, cyclophosphamide, and vincristine.

Altman RP, Randolph JG, Lilly JR: Sacrococcygeal teratoma: American Academy of Pediatrics Surgical Section Survey-1973. J Pediatr Surg 1974;9:389.

Gabra HO et al: Sacrococcygeal teratoma—a 25 year experience in a UK regional center. J Pediatr Surg 2006;41:1513.

Kerner B et al: Cervical teratoma: prenatal diagnosis and long-term follow-up. Prenat Diagn 1998;18:51.

Rescorla FJ et al: Long-term outcome for infants and children with sacrococcygeal teratoma: a report from the Children's Cancer Group. J Pediatr Surg 1998;33:171.

LIVER NEOPLASMS

Tumors of the liver are uncommon in childhood (2% of all pediatric malignancies). More than 70% of pediatric liver masses are malignant. The majority of hepatic malignancies are of epithelial origin, while most benign lesions are vascular in nature.

1. Hepatoblastoma

Hepatoblastomas account for nearly 50% of all liver masses in children and approximately two thirds of malignant tumors. The majority are seen in children under 4 years of age, and two thirds are noted prior to 2 years of age. Beckwith-Wiedemann syndrome, hemihypertrophy, familial adenomatous polyposis syndrome, fetal alcohol syndrome, and parenteral nutrition administration in infancy all increase the risk of hepatoblastoma.

▶ Clinical Findings

A. Symptoms and Signs

The most common finding is an asymptomatic abdominal mass or diffuse abdominal swelling in a healthy-appearing child. There may be obstructive gastrointestinal symptoms secondary to compression of the stomach or duodenum or acute pain secondary to hemorrhage into the tumor. Physical examination reveals a nontender, firm mass in the right upper quadrant or midline that moves with respiration. Advanced tumors present with weight loss, ascites, and failure to thrive. Approximately 10% of males present with isosexual precocity secondary to tumor secretion of β-hCG.

B. Laboratory Findings

Laboratory studies reveal nonspecifically elevated liver function tests and a mild anemia. Thrombocytosis of unknown cause is occasionally seen. AFP is significantly elevated in 90–95%. This marker is also associated with other malignant lesions such as germ cell tumors, but levels are lower.

Serial serum AFP measurements are used to monitor patients for tumor recurrence. Levels fall to normal after curative resection.

C. Imaging Studies

Abdominal ultrasound demonstrates a solid, usually unilobar (right lobe most common) lesion of the liver but lacks sufficient detail to determine resectability. Abdominal CT scan using intravenous contrast is currently the imaging procedure of choice both for diagnosis and for planning therapy. The CT scan demonstrates the tumor's proximity to major vascular and hilar structures. The typical CT appearance is a solid solitary mass with lower attenuation levels than those of the surrounding liver. A novel technique, CT arterioportography, holds promise as a reliable means of assessing vascular invasion along with gross tumor distribution. MRI has proved to be very useful in defining the patency of vascular structures.

▶ Differential Diagnosis

One major management problem is the inability to differentiate adenomas from hepatocellular carcinoma. Because of this, hepatic adenoma, despite being a benign lesion, is often excised. Focal nodular hyperplasia is a well-circumscribed, nonencapsulated nodular liver mass. Ultrasonography and CT scan demonstrate a solid mass, but one cannot differentiate it from adenoma or malignancy without a biopsy. If the diagnosis can be made by biopsy (percutaneous or open), no further treatment is needed. Mesenchymal hamartoma is an uncommon benign lesion presenting in the first year of life as an asymptomatic large solitary mass usually confined to the right lobe of the liver. CT scan demonstrates a well-defined tumor margin and minimal to no contrast enhancement. The treatment is surgical wedge resection; lobectomy is rarely required.

▶ Treatment

The definitive diagnosis of hepatoblastoma requires tissue biopsy. Although this can be performed percutaneously, there are reports of seeding of the biopsy tract. It is preferable to perform open biopsy of the lesion with assessment of resectability. If the lesion is not primarily resectable, vascular access is obtained during the same anesthetic interval for subsequent chemotherapy. Table 43–10 outlines the surgical staging system for childhood hepatic malignancies.

Table 43–10. Hepatic Tumor Staging.

Stage I: Tumor localized and completely resected
Stage II: Tumor resected with microscopic residual disease
Stage III: Unresectable tumor or gross residual disease
Stage IV: Metastatic disease

Complete surgical resection is the major objective of therapy and represents the only chance for cure. Approximately 60% of patients will have primarily resectable lesions. Lobectomy or extended lobectomy (trisegmentectomy) is usual, but segmental (nonanatomic) resection of small isolated tumors may be possible. Careful preoperative evaluation and planning have made liver resection in children a safe procedure, with a mortality rate of less than 5%. Adequate exposure can be obtained via an extended subcostal or bilateral subcostal incision, although bulky lesions may require extension into the right hemithorax to gain adequate vascular control during dissection. Ascitic fluid is obtained for cytologic examination. If the lesion is deemed unresectable, the tumor is biopsied. If the lesion is made resectable following chemotherapy, lobectomy or trisegmentectomy is performed. Intraoperative cholangiography is helpful to verify the integrity of the remaining biliary tree.

Postoperative complications include bleeding, biliary fistula, subphrenic fluid collections or abscess, and inadvertent injury to the biliary tree. Hepatic regeneration occurs quickly, and hepatic insufficiency is rare if 25% or more of the liver parenchyma remains. Hepatic transplantation is used for unresectable disease when chemotherapy has failed to allow complete resection but no demonstrable metastases exist.

The overall survival for all children with hepatoblastoma is approximately 50%. The best survival (90%) is seen in patients with stage I tumors who receive adjunctive chemotherapy after complete excision. Survival decreases as the surgical stage increases, though long-term survival approaches 60–70% in patients with unresectable disease who receive chemotherapy.

Meyers RL: Tumors of the liver in children. Surg Oncology 2007;16:195.

Tagge EP et al: Resection, including transplantation, for hepatoblastoma and hepatocellular carcinoma: impact on survival. J Pediatr Surg 1992;27:292.

Wheatley JM, LaQuaglia MP: Management of hepatic epithelial malignancy in childhood and adolescence. Semin Surg Oncol 1993;9:532.

2. Hepatocellular Carcinoma

Hepatocellular carcinoma is less common than hepatoblastoma and typically presents in older children and adolescents (median age, 10 years). It is associated with preexisting chronic hepatitis, cirrhosis due to hepatitis B virus, and other causes of childhood cirrhosis (tyrosinemia, biliary cirrhosis, α_1-antitrypsin deficiency, type 1 glycogen storage disease, and long-term parenteral nutrition). Signs and symptoms consist of an abdominal mass or diffuse swelling, abdominal pain, weight loss, anorexia, and jaundice. The serum AFP level is elevated in 50%, though the absolute levels are lower than in patients with hepatoblastoma. Diagnostic studies, staging, and treatment are somewhat the same as for hepato-blastoma. Because of multicentricity, bilobar involvement, portal vein invasion, and lymphatic metastases, only 15–20% of hepatocellular carcinomas are resectable. Fibrolamellar hepatocellular carcinoma in younger patients is associated with a high rate of resectability and a better prognosis. The overall long-term survival is poor (15%), even for resectable disease. The role of liver transplantation is unclear.

3. Liver Hemangioma

This is the most common benign pediatric hepatic lesion. These tumors are solitary (cavernous hemangioma) or multiple (infantile hemangioendothelioma), involving the bulk of the liver. Isolated cavernous hemangiomas are not often associated with cutaneous hemangiomas, whereas infantile hemangioendotheliomas are commonly associated with hemangiomas in other parts of the body or integument. Patients with a solitary hemangioma frequently have no symptoms or present with a mass. Infrequently there is intratumor hemorrhage or rupture resulting in abdominal pain. Infants with hemangioendothelioma commonly present with massive hepatomegaly and high-output cardiac failure from arteriovenous shunting. Approximately 40% develop Kasabach-Merritt syndrome (thrombocytopenic coagulopathy due to platelet sequestration within the tumor). The diagnosis is made by red blood cell–labeled radionuclide or dynamic abdominal CT scanning. CT scan demonstrates increased filling and a rapid venous phase from arteriovenous shunting. Angiography is unnecessary, and percutaneous biopsy is contraindicated.

Treatment is not necessary in an asymptomatic child. Patients with congestive heart failure or thrombocytopenia are treated with corticosteroids, digoxin, and diuretics. Refractory patients benefit from hepatic artery embolization. External beam radiation reduces hepatic size and controls symptoms. Their large size and diffuse involvement often preclude resection. Indications for surgery include ruptured lesions with hemorrhage, masses with uncertain diagnoses, symptomatic lesions, or disease limited to one lobe. Hemangioendotheliomas may undergo malignant degeneration into angiosarcoma.

Newman KD: Hepatic tumors in children. Semin Pediatr Surg 1997;6:38.

Reynolds M: Pediatric liver tumors. Semin Surg Oncol 1999;16:159.

Stringer MD: Liver tumors. Semin Pediatr Surg 2000;9:196.

▼ BATTERED CHILD SYNDROME

Child abuse is any nonaccidental injury inflicted by a parent, guardian, or other supervising adult. It may be passive, in the form of emotional or nutritional deprivation, but is most readily recognized in the active form, characterized as "battered, bruised, beaten, broken, and burned." It is estimated that 1 million children per year in the United States suffer injuries that qualify for reporting to the National Center on Child Abuse and Neglect. About 20–50% of children are rebattered after the first diagnosis, resulting in death in 5% and permanent physical damage in 35% when the syndrome is not recognized.

The child abuser is usually a young, insecure, unstable person who had an unhappy childhood and who has unrealistic expectations of the child. Most of these individuals are of low socioeconomic status. The abuser may be a parent, guardian, baby sitter, neighborhood child, or other close associate. Active traumatic abuse is usually perpetrated by the father, but passive neglect with failure to thrive from nutritional or emotional deprivation is usually attributable to the mother.

Clinical Findings

In most cases, the battered child is under 3 years of age and is the product of a difficult pregnancy or premature labor, usually unwanted or born outside of a stable parental relationship. Many battered children have congenital anomalies or are hyperkinetic and colicky. In most cases, there is a discrepancy between the history supplied and the magnitude of the injury—or else a reluctance to give a history. Contradictory histories or delay in bringing the child to medical attention—or taking the child to many different emergency department visits in different hospitals for unusual reasons—should be regarded with suspicion. A past injury in the child or sibling and almost any injury in an infant less than 1 year of age should trigger a consideration of child abuse. The parents may be evasive or hostile. They may have open guilt feelings or may be capable of complete concealment. The innocent spouse is usually more protective of the abuser than of the child.

The child is usually withdrawn, apathetic, whimpering, and fearful and shows signs of neglect or growth retardation. Multiple forms of injury may be noted at varying stages of healing. The child should be completely disrobed to enable the clinician to look for welts, bruises, lacerations, bite or belt wounds, stick or coat hanger marks on the head, trunk, buttocks, or extremities, and similar evidence of mistreatment. Cigarette, hot plate, match, or scalding burns may be evident. Subgaleal hematomas may be caused by pulled hair. Retinal hemorrhage or detachment may follow blows to the head. Abdominal injuries may produce laceration to the liver, spleen, or pancreas or bowel perforation. Sexual abuse should be identified by determining whether the vaginal introitus or anus is bruised, lacerated, or enlarged and whether aspirated fluid contains sperm or prostatic acid phosphatase.

Even though no obvious fracture may be present, a skeletal radiographic survey should be performed. The bone most commonly fractured is the femur, followed by the humerus in the region of the diaphysis. Rib fractures and periosteal reactions in various stages of healing will be seen.

Skull fractures are most commonly seen in infants less than 1 year old. Suture separation of the skull may indicate subdural hematoma. Neurologic injury may require a CT or MRI scan.

Treatment

The child should be admitted to hospital to be protected until the home environment can be evaluated. Injuries should be documented radiographically and with photographs. The presence of sperm in the vagina or anal canal should be confirmed. Bleeding disorders should be evaluated by a platelet count, bleeding time, prothrombin time, and plasma thromboplastin test to make certain that multiple bruises are not due to coagulopathy. A serologic test for syphilis may be indicated as well as cultures (including pharyngeal) for gonorrhea.

Injuries should be treated. Consultation with ophthalmologists, neurologists, neurosurgeons, orthopedic surgeons, and plastic surgeons may be required.

It is required by law in every state for both the hospital and the physician to report child abuse (suspected as well as documented) to local child protection services, usually via the hospital's social work department. The physician is the protector of the child and a consultant to the parents and must not assume the role of prosecutor or judge. The most difficult task is to notify the parents without confrontation, accusation, or anger that battering or neglect is suspected. The physician must tell the parents that the law requires reporting injuries that are unexplained or inadequately explained in view of the nature of the injury. A written referral should then be made to other professionals, such as child welfare personnel, hospital social workers, or psychiatrists. The referral should describe the history of past injuries and the nature of current injuries, results of physical examination and laboratory and x-ray studies, and a statement about why nonaccidental trauma is suspected.

Prognosis

The abuser may require careful evaluation for possible psychosis by a psychiatrist. Child welfare personnel and social workers will have to assess the home environment and work with the parents to prevent future abuse. It may be necessary to place the child in a foster home, but approximately 90% of families can be reunited.

Berkowitz CD: New patterns of injury. Emerg Med Clin North Am 1995;13:321.
Duhaime AC et al: Nonaccidental head injuries in infants—the "shaken-baby syndrome." N Engl J Med 1998;338:1822.

REFERENCES

Andrassy RJ (editor): *Pediatric Surgical Oncology.* Saunders, 1998.
Ashcraft KW et al (editors): *Pediatric Surgery,* 3rd ed. Saunders, 2000.

Burg FD et al (editors): *Gellis & Kagan's Current Pediatric Therapy.* Saunders, 1999.

Gray SW, Skandalakis JE: *Embryology for Surgeons: The Embryological Basis for Treatment of Congenital Defects,* 2nd ed. Williams & Wilkins, 1994.

Harrison MR et al: *The Unborn Patient: The Art and Science of Fetal Therapy,* 3rd ed. Saunders, 2001.

Oldham KT, Colombani PM, Foglia RP (editors): *Surgery of Infants and Children. Scientific Principles and Practice,* Lippincott-Raven, 1997.

O'Neill JA et al (editors): *Pediatric Surgery,* 5th ed. Mosby, 1998.

Rowe MI et al (editors): *Essentials of Pediatric Surgery,* Mosby, 1995.

Rudolph C, Rudolph AM, Hostetter MK (editors): *Rudolph's Pediatrics,* 21st ed. McGraw-Hill, 2002.

Oncology

Michael S. Sabel, MD

Over 1.4 million individuals in the United States are diagnosed with invasive cancer each year. Currently, 1 in 4 deaths in the United States is due to cancer, ranking second only to heart disease as the leading cause of mortality in this country. Before age 65, among men and women combined, cancer is the leading cause of death.

The surgeon is intimately involved in the care of cancer patients, since the majority will require surgical therapy at some time. Surgeons are often the first specialists to see newly diagnosed cancer patients or are often called upon to make the diagnosis in patients suspected to have cancer. As such, they will be responsible for orchestrating the patient's care, including coordination with medical oncologists and radiation oncologists. It is imperative that they have an in-depth knowledge of the different types of cancer and the different modalities available for treatment.

TUMOR NOMENCLATURE

Neoplasms are defined as benign or malignant according to the clinical behavior of the tumor. Benign tumors have lost normal growth regulation but tend to be surrounded by a capsule and do not invade surrounding tissues or metastasize.

Benign tumors are generally designated by adding the suffix -oma to the name of the cell of origin. Examples include lipoma and adenoma. The term *cancer* normally refers to malignant tumors, which can invade surrounding tissues or metastasize to distant sites in the host. The nomenclature of malignant tumors is typically based on the cell's embryonal tissue origins. Malignant tumors derived from cells of mesenchymal origin are called *sarcomas*. These include cancers that derive from muscle, bone, tendon, fat, cartilage, lymphoid tissues, vessels, and connective tissue. Neoplasms of epithelial origin are called *carcinomas*. These may be further categorized according to the histologic appearance of the cells. Tumor cells that have glandular growth patterns are called adenocarcinomas, and those that resemble squamous epithelial cells are called squamous cell

carcinomas. Cancers composed of undifferentiated cells that bear no resemblance to any tissues are designated as "poorly differentiated" or "undifferentiated" carcinomas.

▶ Tumor Grade

Beyond the type of cancer, it is important to classify tumors by their behavior and prognosis in order to determine appropriate therapy as well as evaluate different treatment modalities. Grading of a tumor is a histologic determination and refers to the degree of cellular differentiation. Separate pathologic grading systems exist for each histologic type of cancer. Depending on the type of tumor, these systems are based on nuclear pleomorphism, cellularity, necrosis, cellular invasion, and the number of mitoses. Increasing grades generally denote increasing degrees of dedifferentiation. While the grade of the tumor typically has less prognostic value than its stage, tumor grade has great clinical significance in soft tissue sarcoma, astrocytoma, transitional cell cancers of the genitourinary tract, and Hodgkin and non-Hodgkin lymphoma.

▶ Tumor Stage

Tumor staging establishes the extent of disease and has important prognostic and therapeutic implications in most types of cancer. Clinical staging is based on the results of a noninvasive evaluation, including physical examination and various imaging studies. Pathologic staging is based on findings in surgical tumor specimens and biopsies and allows for the evaluation of microscopic disease undetectable by imaging techniques. Pathologic staging may reveal more extensive tumor spread than the clinical evaluation and is the more reliable information. Clinicians must be careful when attempting to compare clinically and pathologically staged patients, as the two groups may have dramatically different outcomes.

As with grading, the staging systems vary with different tumor types. Two major staging systems are currently in use, one developed by the Union Internationale Contre le Cancer

(UICC) and the other by the American Joint Committee on Cancer (AJCC). The UICC system is based on the TNM classification. *T* refers to the primary tumor and is based on the size of the tumor and invasion of surrounding structures. Tumors are characterized as T1 to T4 cancers, with the higher T stages for larger and more invasive tumors. *N* refers to regional lymph nodes, and classifications of N0 to N3 denote increasing degrees of lymph node involvement. Finally, *M* refers to distant metastatic disease, with M0 signifying no distant metastases and M1 and M2 indicating the presence of blood-borne metastatic disease. The AJCC system divides cancers into stages 0 to IV, with higher stages representing more widespread disease and a poorer prognosis. Regardless of the staging system or the tumor type, higher stages correlate with decreased survival.

▶ Cancer Epidemiology

Cancer epidemiology is the study of the distribution of cancer and its determinants among defined populations and is used to examine cancer etiology as well as the efficacy of prevention, detection, and treatment strategies. The most basic types of epidemiologic terms describe cancer rates or cancer deaths for specific populations over a certain period of time.

While absolute numbers of cancer cases may be useful for health care planning, they do not take into account the size or nature of the underlying population at risk. For this reason, the most commonly used population-based measures of cancer are incidence and mortality. **Cancer incidence rates** are defined as the number of new cancer cases diagnosed during a fixed time period divided by the total population at risk. **Cancer mortality rates** are defined similarly, with cancer deaths replacing new cancer cases. These rates are typically expressed as the number of events per 100,000 individuals per year.

Incidence and mortality rates are compared across populations or over time to identify causes as well as the effect of screening or treatment. However, other factors among populations may contribute to observed differences, and these must be taken into account. For most cancers, age is the strongest risk factor, and so comparison of cancer incidence between two populations must consider the age distributions of the two groups. Adjustment (or standardization) is the most common method used to account for such differences. Comparing age-adjusted cancer incidence rates ensures that any observed differences are not the results of differences in age distributions between the two populations. Incidence and mortality rates are often also adjusted for gender, race, or socioeconomic status.

Cancer incidence examines only those diagnosed with the disease during that time period; it does not include patients diagnosed earlier who are living with cancer. **Cancer prevalence** describes the number of people with the disease either at a single point in time (**point prevalence**) or within a defined period of time (**period prevalence**). Prevalence is more relevant to the public health burden of cancer because all prevalent cases involve accessing health care. The relationship among incidence, prevalence, and mortality is influenced by the fatality of the disease. If the disease is highly fatal and the interval between presentation and death is short, mortality rates will be similar to incidence rates. The number of deaths from cancer divided by the total number people diagnosed with the cancer is known as the **cancer fatality rate,** although this is somewhat of a misnomer because they are not technically rates (they do not include time as a parameter).

Examining the fatality of cancer is obviously important when comparing treatments meant to improve outcome. **Overall survival (OS)** is the most global endpoint and is defined as the proportion of people alive at a specified period after being diagnosed with the disease. Five years is conventionally used as the time period (ie, 5-year survival). However, overall survival may not always reflect the success of treatment. Over that period of time, some patients may die of disease, but others may die of other causes. In addition, some patient may have a local or regional recurrence that is successfully treated, while some may recur with distant metastases but not succumb to them. For this reason, survival rates in cancer are often qualified by the patient's disease status.

Disease-free survival refers to the proportion of patients alive and without disease over a specific period of time. A patient who developed metastases but is still alive would be included in the overall survival rate but not the disease-free survival rate. Disease-free survival and overall survival may provide different pictures of the success of treatment. A therapy that improves disease-free survival but not overall survival may still be important if quality of life is improved. In some cancers, local or regional recurrences can be readily treated with minimal impact on overall survival. In these cases, disease-free survival may present an overly pessimistic picture of outcome. Therefore, it may be more relevant to compare **distant disease-free survival,** which refers to the proportion of people alive and without distant metastases, regardless of local recurrence. In some cases, it is difficult to assess the efficacy of a treatment by looking at overall survival or disease-free survival if there are deaths from competing causes. It may be more helpful to compare **disease-specific survival,** which is the percentage of people who have survived a disease since diagnosis or treatment and does not count patients who died from other causes.

It is important for the surgeon to understand the different methods for describing cancer survival as well as the differences between the definitions, because the appropriateness of the comparison will vary with the biology of the disease and the clinical question being asked.

Cotran CS, Kumar V, Robbins SL (editors): *Robbins Pathologic Basis of Disease,* 6th ed. Saunders, 1999.
Greene FL: *AJCC Cancer Staging Manual,* 6th ed. Springer Verlag, 2002.
Jemal A et al: Cancer statistics, 2008. CA Cancer J Clin 2008;58:71.

ROLE OF THE SURGICAL ONCOLOGIST

The surgeon is often the first specialist to see a patient with suspected or newly diagnosed cancer and in many cases assumes responsibility for orchestrating the overall management of the cancer patient's care. The role of the surgeon involves not only the curative resection of the tumor but also obtaining tissue for diagnosis and staging, providing palliation for incurable patients, and preventing cancer by the prophylactic removal of organs. With improving imaging technologies, expanded use of neoadjuvant therapies, molecular staging, and increasing knowledge of the genetic predisposition to cancer, the role of the surgical oncologist is continuously evolving. It is therefore imperative for surgical oncologists to remain current on the newest approaches to cancer therapy and be prepared to adapt to the changing role of surgery.

▶ Diagnosis & Staging

A tissue diagnosis is critical to the care of all cancer patients. Depending on the type of tumor and its location, the method of biopsy will vary. Common diagnostic techniques include needle aspiration biopsy, core needle biopsy, incisional biopsy, and excisional biopsy.

Fine-needle aspiration biopsy (FNAB) is a rapid and minimally invasive technique for the biopsy of palpable superficial tumors. Deeper, nonpalpable lesions may also be sampled by this technique when FNAB is combined with various imaging modalities, such as ultrasonography or CT. FNAB involves aspiration of cells from a suspicious mass, followed by cytologic examination of the stained smear. FNAB is particularly useful in the diagnosis of enlarged lymph nodes, breast lumps, thyroid masses, and lung nodules.

Advantages to FNAB include the simplicity of the procedure and the low rate of complications. However, there are limitations to FNAB. FNAB cytology requires an experienced cytopathologist for accurate interpretation. Because cytology does not demonstrate architecture, it does not allow the cytopathologist to accurately grade tumors or to differentiate between in situ and invasive disease. If this information is necessary, FNAB may be inadequate. Sampling errors can lead to false-negative results, so a negative FNAB should be interpreted cautiously. In addition, though rare, false-positive results can occur, so confirmation may be needed before definitive surgical intervention. For example, a mastectomy should never be performed on the basis of an FNAB of a breast lump without confirming the diagnosis by either preoperative core biopsy or frozen section analysis at the time of surgery.

Core needle biopsy utilizes a needle that cuts a sliver of tissue for analysis. This technique provides more histologic information than FNAB because it allows the pathologist to see the histologic architecture of the sample rather than just the cellular characteristics. False-positive results are extremely rare. Although less so than with FNAB, sampling errors may occur, and a negative result must be weighed against clinical judgment. Core biopsies are frequently used for prostate, breast, and liver masses. Again, ultrasound and radiographic imaging may enable the clinician to sample deep-seated or nonpalpable masses. The technique may also be used during surgery to biopsy suspicious masses encountered at operation.

When a larger tumor sample is necessary for accurate grading or staging, an incisional or excisional biopsy is required. **Excisional biopsy** is the surgical removal of an entire gross lesion, while **incisional biopsy** involves sampling a representative portion of a suspicious lesion. In general, excisional biopsy is recommended whenever it is possible to excise the entire lesion without damage to surrounding structures. Incisional biopsy should be considered whenever a core biopsy fails to make the diagnosis but removing the tumor might compromise the subsequent operation (eg, a large [> 5 cm], deep soft tissue mass for which sarcoma is a possibility) or preclude delivery of neoadjuvant therapy.

Although biopsy techniques are usually simple, the surgeon must adhere to some specific principles when performing a biopsy for a suspected malignancy. The positioning of the needle tract or scar should be such that if further surgery is required, the biopsy site will be easily included in the excised specimen. Excisional biopsies of the breast should consider the possibility of a subsequent mastectomy, and the excision of skin or subcutaneous lesions on the extremities should be oriented in a way that allows for the following wide excision and lymphatic mapping if malignancy is discovered. Meticulous hemostasis is imperative, as the formation of a wound hematoma may make subsequent operation more difficult. The surgeon should also pay careful attention to the orientation of the pathologic specimen, which may prove important in curative surgical procedures.

Once a diagnosis is made, the next step is typically to determine the extent of the cancer, or **staging.** This step begins with a complete history and physical examination, looking for signs or symptoms of advanced or metastatic disease. Laboratory or imaging studies may follow to determine not only the extent of the primary tumor but the presence of regional or distant metastases. Patients with signs or symptoms of metastatic disease should undergo appropriate workup of their symptoms. For some tumor types, routine staging examinations are indicated. However, for many asymptomatic patients newly diagnosed with cancer, a full battery of staging studies is not necessary and not only will increase the cost of treatment but may lead to false-positive findings, unnecessary biopsies, and inappropriate changes in therapy.

Surgeons are often called upon to perform operations that provide staging information for various types of cancer. Such procedures are necessary when the clinical extent of the disease has a direct bearing on the choice of treatment modalities. Examples include laparoscopy for gastric or pancreatic cancer, a staging laparotomy for ovarian cancer, or mediastinoscopy for lung and esophageal cancer. Staging procedures can often help to avert highly morbid procedures in cases where there is little chance for cure.

Curative Surgery

Surgical resections with curative intent can be divided into three categories: resection of a primary lesion, resection of isolated metastases, and resection of metastatic deposits. In each case, the clinician must strive to reach a balance between the chance for cure and the morbidity of the procedure. Each situation must be evaluated individually, and the patient's wishes must be paramount.

The guiding principle of cancer surgery is to remove the entire tumor with adequate margins so as to prevent local recurrence and potentially distant recurrence. What constitutes an adequate margin varies among tumor types. Various tumors require different disease-free margins in order to achieve optimal chances for a cure. For a tumor that appears adherent or fixed to adjacent structures, **en bloc resection** is mandatory, and any attachment should be considered malignant in nature. Appropriate preoperative imaging of the tumor is often necessary to be prepared in the operating room for the possible resection of small or large bowel, bladder, or other adjacent organs.

It is important that the surgeon have knowledge of other modalities that may be integrated into the management plan to allow for a less ablative surgical procedure. Radiation and chemotherapy are commonly used in combination with surgery and are referred to as adjuvant therapies if used after complete resection with no demonstrable local or systemic disease. While their use has in some cases diminished the extent of resection necessary for local control (breast, sarcoma, head and neck), it is important to note that these modalities do not compensate for inadequate margins in controlling local disease. Every attempt should be made to achieve widely negative margins surgically, even if it requires a second operation, rather than assuming radiation will "clean up" residual disease.

If these modalities are used in the preoperative setting, they are called neoadjuvant therapies. In many cases, neoadjuvant therapy has dramatically improved outcomes, as with pediatric rhabdomyosarcoma or locally advanced or inflammatory breast cancer. In some cases, neoadjuvant therapy can convert an unresectable tumor to resectable, while in other cases, it can decrease the extent of surgery necessary to obtain control or decrease the likelihood of positive margins. Neoadjuvant therapy is commonly used in the treatment of esophageal cancer, rectal cancer, pancreatic cancer, breast cancer, and sarcoma. It is important the surgeon consider the possibility of neoadjuvant therapy when performing a biopsy, staging the patient, or planning surgery.

The regional lymph nodes represent the most prevalent site of metastases for solid tumors. For most cancers, involvement of the regional lymph nodes represents the most important prognostic factor. For this reason, the removal of the regional lymph nodes is often performed at the time of resection of the primary cancer. Besides staging information, a regional lymphadenectomy provides "regional control" of the cancer. More controversial is whether the removal of regional lymph nodes can improve survival. These controversies concern both the extent and the timing of the procedure. For example, the extent of lymphadenectomy at the time of gastrectomy for stomach cancer has been hypothesized to have an impact on improving overall survival. This has not, however, been borne out in prospective randomized trials. It may be that extended lymphadenectomy results in more accurate staging of patients at a cost of increased morbidity and minimal effect, if any, on overall survival. How extensive a lymph node dissection to perform at the time of definitive resection varies with tumor type and in many cases remains controversial.

For many nonvisceral solid tumors such as melanoma, breast cancers, and head and neck squamous cancers, the "elective" removal of clinically negative lymph nodes at the time of primary tumor resection (elective lymph node dissection) has been postulated to result in better survival outcomes compared to performing a lymphadenectomy only when the patient relapses in a nodal basin (therapeutic lymph node dissection). Prospective randomized clinical studies have yet to demonstrate a clear survival advantage for performing elective lymph node dissections, and this approach exposes a large number of node-negative patients to the morbidity of a dissection. The adoption of selective lymph node dissection based on the concept of the sentinel lymph node has dramatically improved our ability to stage the regional lymph nodes of certain cancers (helping guide adjuvant therapy decisions) and select patients with nodal metastases who may benefit from a complete lymph node dissection.

The surgeon plays a much more limited role when the patient has metastatic disease; nonetheless, the resection of "isolated" metastases in patients with solid malignancies is sometimes a consideration when technically feasible. The selection of candidate patients for surgical resection requires a thorough evaluation of the extent of known disease, likelihood of additional metastatic disease, medical status of the patient, and feasibility of resecting the metastatic site with a negative margin. Ultimately, this process identifies a small subset of patients who would be surgical candidates. Although there are no prospective randomized trials documenting the survival benefit of surgical resection of metastatic disease, there is considerable retrospective evidence indicating that this approach can result in long-term benefit. The resection of lung metastases in patients with osteogenic or soft tissue sarcomas has been associated with an approximately 20–25% overall survival rate greater than 5 years. There is also a large body of retrospective evidence documenting the benefit of resecting colorectal metastases to the liver, resulting in a 25–40% overall 5-year survival rate, depending on the extent of liver involvement. Other examples include an aggressive surgical approach to metastatic melanoma and the resection of isolated breast cancer metastases. One of the roles of the surgical oncologist is to know when it is appropriate to offer this option.

▶ Palliation

Surgical intervention is sometimes required in the patient with unresectable advanced cancer for palliative indications such as pain, bleeding, obstruction, malnutrition, or infection. The decision to operate must balance several factors, including the likelihood of adding significantly to the quality of life of the patient, the expected survival of the individual, the potential morbidity of the procedure, and whether there are alternative methods of palliation.

Malnutrition is a common problem in the cancer patient, especially one with advanced, unresectable disease. Commonly, the surgeon is involved in placement of vascular access for hyperalimentation, or if the gastrointestinal tract is functional, the placement of gastrostomy or jejunostomy tubes for enteral nutrition. Occasionally, the surgeon is involved in palliating pain due to a metastatic lesion compressing upon an organ or adjacent nerves. Examples include cutaneous or subcutaneous melanoma metastases, a large ulcerating breast cancer, or a recurrent intra-abdominal sarcoma mass. The surgeon must assess the relative risk-to-benefit ratio in resecting a symptomatic mass knowing that it will not impact the overall survival of the patient. If the quality of life of the individual can be improved at an acceptable operative risk, then the surgical intervention is warranted.

Finally, the surgeon may be called upon to manage oncologic emergencies. Acute hemorrhage and obstruction of a hollow viscus represent the most common potential oncologic emergencies. In these cases, surgeons may have to emergently intervene in the care of a cancer patient, or in some instances, use nonsurgical approaches (such as stents or angiography).

▶ Prophylaxis

With our improved understanding of inherited genetic mutations and the identification of patients who are predisposed to cancer, surgical therapy has expanded beyond the therapy of established tumors and into the prevention of cancer. Prophylaxis is not a new concept in surgical oncology. Patients with chronic inflammatory diseases are known to be at high risk of subsequent malignant transformation. This typically prompts close surveillance and surgical resection at the first identification of premalignant changes. One of the earliest examples of this is the recommendation for total proctocolectomy for subsets of patients with chronic ulcerative colitis.

The ability to perform genetic screening for relevant mutations has allowed for prophylactic surgery to be implemented prior to the onset of symptoms or histologic changes. Familial adenomatous polyposis (FAP) syndrome, defined by the diffuse involvement of the colon and rectum with adenomatous polyps, almost always predisposes to colorectal cancer if the large intestine is left in place. With the identification of the gene responsible for FAP, the adenomatous polyposis coli (APC) gene, members of families in which an APC mutation has been identified can have genetic testing prior to polyps becoming evident and be considered for prophylactic proctocolectomy. Medullary thyroid cancer (MTC) is a well-established component of multiple endocrine neoplasia syndrome type 2a (MEN 2a) or type 2b (MEN 2b). Mutations in the *RET* protooncogene are present in almost all cases of MEN 2a and 2b. Family members of MEN patients can be screened for the presence of a RET mutation, and those with the mutation should undergo total thyroidectomy at a young age (6 years for MEN 2a, infancy for MEN 2b). The role of prophylactic mastectomies has been greatly expanded with the identification of *BRCA1* and *BRCA2*, which can be associated with a lifetime probability of breast cancer of between 40% and 85%. Other prophylactic surgeries are listed in Table 44–1. However, potential benefits of prophylactic surgeries must be weighed against quality-of-life issues and the morbidity of the surgery. A detailed discussion must be held with each patient considering prophylactic surgery regarding the risks and benefits, so today's surgical oncologist needs a clear understanding of genetics and inherited risk.

Sabel MS, Sondak VK, Sussman JJ (editors): *Essentials of Surgical Oncology.* Mosby, 2007.

Table 44–1. Prophylactic Surgeries in Surgical Oncology.

Prophylactic Surgery	Potential Indications
Bilateral mastectomy	*BRCA1* or *BRCA2* mutation
	Atypical hyperplasia or lobular carcinoma in situ
	Familial breast cancer
Bilateral oophorectomy	*BRCA1* mutation
	Familial ovarian cancer
	Hereditary nonpolyposis colorectal cancer
	Hysterectomy for endometrial cancer
	Colon resection for colon cancer
Thyroidectomy	*RET* protooncogene mutation
	Multiple endocrine neoplasia type 2A (MEN 2A)
	Multiple endocrine neoplasia type 2B (MEN 2B)
	Familial non-MEN medullary thyroid carcinoma (FMTC)
Total proctocolectomy	Familial adenomatous polyposis (FAP) or antigen-presenting cell (APC) mutation
	Ulcerative colitis
	Hereditary nonpolyposis colorectal cancer (HNPCC) germ-line mutation

CYTOTOXIC CHEMOTHERAPY

The goal of chemotherapeutic regimens is to deliver pharmacologic agents systemically to eradicate all tumor cells. The ideal tumor drug would kill cancer cells without harming normal tissues. No such agent exists, and most drugs affect normal cells to some extent. The success of chemotherapy relies on the normal cell's greater capacity for repair and survival relative to tumor cells.

Even a single cancer cell can potentially reproduce to form a lethal tumor. For this reason, the goal of curative chemotherapy must be the complete eradication of all tumor cells. Tumor burden is important in chemotherapy. A large cancer may harbor more than 10^9 tumor cells. If a tolerable dose of an effective drug killed 99.99% of these cells, the tumor burden would still be 10^5 cells. The remaining cells, while clinically undetectable, are likely to continue to grow and lead to a clinical recurrence of cancer. For this reason, most chemotherapy protocols rely on repeated administrations of drugs in order to achieve maximal cell killing. Tumor cells may avoid the cell-killing effects of a particular drug because of their stage in the cell cycle, residence in an area protected from the drug (central nervous system), or an inherent resistance to the drug.

Drug resistance plays a large role in chemotherapy failures. Several mechanisms of tumor resistance are known. The multidrug resistance *(MDR)* gene encodes a protein that actively pumps drugs out of tumor cells. This gene confers resistance on a variety of antitumor drugs, including the antibiotics and plant-derived compounds. Other tumor mechanisms of resistance include the alteration of target enzymes, increased production of a target enzyme to overwhelm the drug, and an increased capability for DNA repair.

Tumor resistance to a given chemotherapeutic agent can often be overcome by the administration of multiple drugs.

▶ Principles of Chemotherapy Use

A. Curative Chemotherapy

Hematologic malignancies are typically treated by chemotherapy, radiation, or both, with surgery used primarily for diagnosis and staging. On the other hand, surgery is the primary treatment for nonhematologic malignancies, although there are some exceptions. Anal cancer is cured in approximately 80% of patients with the Nigro protocol—5-FU/mitomycin-C and radiation therapy—as first-line treatment. Testicular cancer, even when metastatic, is curable with bleomycin/etoposide/cisplatin in approximately 85% of patients.

B. Adjuvant Treatment

Although all visible tumor may be removed at the time of surgery, microscopic tumor deposits may still be present locally or may have spread to distant locations. Chemotherapy is most effective against very small tumors and microscopic tumor deposits. Therefore, adjuvant chemotherapy is often given to improve the likelihood of cure after surgical resection.

The benefit gained from adjuvant chemotherapy can be thought of in terms of absolute benefit or relative benefit (Figure 44–1). For example, after colectomy for stage III colon cancer, the chance of cure is approximately 50%. This can be increased to approximately 70% by adjuvant 5-FU/leucovorin. This represents a 40% relative benefit (40% more patients are cured with chemotherapy than without chemotherapy) but a 20% absolute benefit (20% of the patients who take the chemotherapy will have altered their

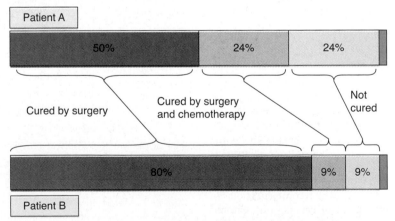

▲ **Figure 44–1.** Benefits of adjuvant chemotherapy. For 100 patients treated with adjuvant chemotherapy, some will be cured by surgery alone (dark red bar), some will die of other causes (gray bar), and some will die of their cancer (light red bar). Adjuvant therapy will prevent a cancer death in a portion of those patients (medium red bar). Adjuvant chemotherapy will result in a relative benefit of 50% for both patient A and patient B, meaning treatment will reduce the likelihood of dying of cancer by 50%. However, the absolute benefit is different for both patients. For patient A, who has a high likelihood of dying of disease, the absolute benefit is 24%. For patient B, who has a good prognosis, the absolute benefit is only 9%.

outcome). Another way to look at this is that with a 20% absolute benefit, 80% of patients experience the inconvenience and side effects of chemotherapy without gaining any improvement themselves. The decision to receive adjuvant chemotherapy is a balance between the expected benefit of treatment, the patient's comorbid conditions and general health, and the patient's wishes.

C. Neoadjuvant Treatment

Neoadjuvant chemotherapy is usually given to facilitate surgical resection by shrinking the primary tumor, or it may convert an unresectable tumor into a resectable tumor. In some cases, this treatment has been shown to prolong survival. Another advantage to neoadjuvant chemotherapy is that it allows the oncologist to observe the primary tumor to determine if it is sensitive to a particular chemotherapeutic regimen. During the course of cancer treatment, it is important to define the progress and outcomes resulting from therapy. The terms complete and partial response are often used as endpoints to evaluate the efficacy of a particular therapeutic regimen. A **complete response** is defined as the absence of demonstrable cancer. A **partial response** refers to a reduction of tumor mass by greater than 50%. The patient's response to neoadjuvant chemotherapy can be an important predictor of outcome.

D. Chemotherapy for Metastatic Disease

The majority of patients who are receiving chemotherapy have metastatic disease that is not curable. For these patients, treatment with chemotherapy is intended to prolong survival, improve quality of life, or both. Response rates range from 20% to 75% depending on the tumor type and chemotherapy regimen. However, even a complete remission is rarely durable. Most partial or complete remissions last only months.

As with all therapies, the decision to use chemotherapy must balance the potential benefits with the risks, toxicities, and the patient's general health and condition. There is little to be gained by treating an asymptomatic patient if no prolongation of survival is expected. A detailed discussion must be held with each individual patient; some patients are more willing than others to tolerate the side effects of chemotherapy. Since the disease is not curable, treatment with single agents, which are less toxic than combination chemotherapy, are often considered, with more willingness to reduce doses for toxicity.

▶ Classes of Chemotherapeutic Agents

With all forms of curative chemotherapy, the goal is elimination of all tumor stem cells. Cells that are incapable of further division cannot cause progression of a tumor, and the sterilization of a tumor cell is as good as a kill. Chemotherapeutic drugs are generally classified as cell cycle-specific (CCS) drugs, which are toxic to actively proliferating cells, or cell cycle-nonspecific (CCNS) drugs, which are capable of killing cells that are not dividing during drug exposure. These two classifications are not absolute, and many drugs may overlap between the two categories.

In order to achieve maximal cell killing, most therapeutic protocols use combination chemotherapy. Agents with differing mechanisms of action and different toxic side effects are used, allowing for relatively high doses of multiple agents. This method of combining agents helps to combat tumor cell resistance and increase the tumor cell killing while avoiding the compounding of toxic effects.

A. Alkylating Agents

These agents exert their effects by the transfer of alkyl groups to various cellular components, most importantly by the alkylation of DNA. Alkylators can cause DNA strand breaks, cross-linking of DNA strands, or miscoding of DNA during replication. The alkylating agents are considered cell cycle–nonspecific agents but tend to have their greatest effect on proliferating cells. Normal cells are able to avoid many of the lethal affects of alkylating agents because of their ability to repair DNA. The alkylating agents are effective in treatment of the hematologic malignancies and in a variety of solid tumors such as breast, melanoma, lung, and endometrial cancers. Included in this class are the nitrosoureas (eg, carmustine, semustine, lomustine), cyclophosphamide, chlorambucil, mechlorethamine, dacarbazine, and procarbazine.

B. Platinum Analogues

The platinum analogs are similar to the alkylating agents. They bind DNA to form interstrand and intrastrand cross-links, leading to inhibition of DNA synthesis and transcription. The mechanisms of cancer cell resistance are also similar to those of alkylating agents: decreased cellular uptake of the drugs, increased activity of DNA repair enzymes, and increased thiol-containing proteins. In addition, resistance to both cisplatin and carboplatin has been associated with a deficiency of mismatch repair (MMR) genes. It is not known why this mechanism of resistance appears to be specific to cisplatin and carboplatin, but the efficacy of the newest platinum analog, oxaliplatin, is not affected by MMR gene deficiency.

C. Antimetabolites

Rapidly dividing cells require increased synthesis of nucleic acid precursors. This increased synthesis can be exploited pharmacologically by the antimetabolites. These drugs are analogs of nucleic acids or nucleic acid precursors. The antimetabolites may be incorporated into the nucleic acids of a cell and serve as a false messenger. Antimetabolites can shut down the cellular synthetic machinery by binding to and inhibiting enzymes important in the production of nucleic acids. Since this class of drugs affects all rapidly proliferating cells, they are relatively toxic to normal tissues that have a high rate of cell turnover. Antimetabolites are most effective in the hematologic malignancies but are also used in the treatment of solid tumors such as breast and gastrointestinal cancers. They include methotrexate, mercaptopurine, thioguanine, fluorouracil, and cytarabine.

D. Antimicrotubule Agents

A variety of antitumor drugs are derived from natural plants (and are also known as plant alkaloids). Vincristine, vinblastine, docetaxel, and paclitaxel work by binding tubulin and poisoning the assembly of microtubules in the mitotic spindle. This leads to mitotic arrest in metaphase, and these compounds are effective only on rapidly dividing cell populations. The plant alkaloids are most useful for hematologic malignancies and breast, renal, testicular, and head and neck cancers.

E. Topoisomerase Inhibitors

These plant derivatives exert their antitumor effects by binding to and inhibiting various forms of the enzyme topoisomerase. Topoisomerases are responsible for the maintenance of DNA structure and are also important in the cleavage and religation of DNA strands. Inhibition of these enzymes leads to DNA strand breakage and structural damage. The topoisomerase inhibitors are also cell cycle–specific agents and have their greatest activity against rapidly proliferating cells. Examples include etoposide, teniposide, and topotecan. These drugs are used in the treatment of hematologic malignancies and lung, bladder, prostate, and testicular cancers.

F. Antibiotics

Most of the drugs in this class are derived from the soil fungus streptomyces. All the antibiotics exert their antitumor effects by interference with the synthesis of nucleic acids. Most of the drugs in this class intercalate in DNA, blocking DNA synthesis and inducing strand breakages. The antibiotics are considered cell cycle–nonspecific, and they have antitumor activity against a wide variety of solid tumors. Included in this class of drugs are doxorubicin, dactinomycin, plicamycin, mitomycin, and bleomycin.

▶ Side Effects of Chemotherapy

Most side effects from chemotherapeutic regimens are the result of toxicities to rapidly dividing normal cell populations—particularly bone marrow and epithelial cells. Bone marrow suppression is an adverse effect of many of these drugs, resulting in neutropenia, thrombocytopenia, and even anemia. Mucosal ulcerations and alopecia also occur in patients treated with cell cycle–specific agents. Intractable nausea and vomiting is another common side effect that can severely affect quality of life. Testicular or ovarian failure can result from chemotherapy, leading to sterility. Many of these drugs also are powerful teratogens and should be avoided in pregnant patients. Finally, many of the alkylating agents have been implicated in the development of secondary cancers, especially hematologic malignancies.

REGIONAL THERAPY

Systemic chemotherapy is limited by toxicity to the host. Regional delivery of chemotherapeutic agents via arterial cannulation allows for high levels of drugs in the region of the primary tumor while decreasing systemic toxicity.

Isolated limb perfusion is a technique for the delivery of chemotherapeutic agents to an extremity with locally advanced cancer and is of benefit primarily in the treatment of extremity melanoma and sarcoma. In this approach, a tourniquet is applied to the extremity to occlude venous outflow. The major artery perfusing the limb is then isolated, cannulated, and perfused with hyperthermic chemotherapeutic agents using a pump oxygenator as for cardiopulmonary bypass. The perfusion is done in the operating room and lasts for approximately 1 hour. The cannula is then removed. Most protocols involve only a single treatment. Melphalan, an alkylating agent, is the most common agent used today in the treatment of both sarcomas and melanomas. In patients with extensive in-transit melanoma confined to an extremity, isolated limb perfusion can provide regional control and palliation. In patients with unresectable extremity sarcomas, preoperative limb perfusion can often shrink the tumor and allow for a limb-sparing resection. While improving regional control, this therapy has yet to show a definitive survival benefit.

Another approach is isolated hepatic artery infusion for the treatment of colorectal cancer metastatic to the liver. Metastatic tumors derive nearly all of their blood supply from the hepatic artery, while the normal liver parenchyma derives more than two thirds of its blood supply from the portal system. This permits the delivery of higher doses of chemotherapeutic agents to the tumor relative to the normal hepatocytes. The drug most commonly used in this protocol is floxuridine, which is almost completely extracted on its first pass through the liver, resulting in relatively low systemic toxicity. Hepatic artery infusion requires the surgical placement of a catheter into the hepatic artery, which is connected to an implanted or external infusion pump for continuous treatment. Hepatic artery infusion has been used for unresectable colorectal metastases as well as an adjuvant to hepatic resection. While there are clearly improved tumor responses in comparison to systemic therapy, the data is less clear on overall survival benefits. Some studies, however, have suggested an improved survival and have stimulated further investigation.

TARGETED THERAPIES

An expanding knowledge of molecular biology is revolutionizing the field of oncology, truly personalizing care for each individual patient with cancer. Molecular diagnostics is increasingly allowing us to customize the selection and dosing of traditional agents to maximize benefit and minimize toxicity. Molecular oncology is changing the way we approach drug discovery and development, leading to the development of targeted therapies. One definition of targeted therapy is any drug in which there is a specific diagnostic test that must be performed before the patient can be considered eligible to receive the drug. An example is measuring Her-2/neu overexpression on breast cancer to determine if a patient is eligible for trastuzumab (Herceptin). A more oncologic definition is any drug with a focused mechanism that specifically acts on a well-defined target or biologic pathway. Inactivation of this target/pathway results in regression or destruction of the malignant cell. Targeted therapies are often considered "magic bullets."

Several targeted therapies have been FDA approved and are in clinical use; many others are being developed. The ideal target is one that is expressed (and can be measured) on cancer cells but not significantly expressed in vital organs and tissues. It is preferably crucial to the malignant phenotype, and its inhibition results in a clinical response in patients whose tumor expresses the target. Several methods for very specific targeting are being examined. The ability of therapeutic antibodies to bind with high affinity makes them excellent candidates for targeted therapy. While antibodies may induce an immune-mediated destruction of cancer cells (and be considered immunotherapy [see section on Immunotherapy]), they can also be used to target specific cell surface receptors to interrupt that pathway. For this latter function, it is important that the target, when bound by the antibody, is internalized by endocytosis to facilitate the intracellular mechanism of pathway inhibition and cell death.

Trastuzumab is an IgG antibody that binds to the juxtamembrane portion of the extracellular domain of the Her-2/neu receptor and has become an important option for patients with Her-2/neu–positive breast cancer. Her-2/neu is an epidermal growth factor receptor (EGFR) that has a functional intracellular tyrosine kinase and when overexpressed can lead to increased proliferation, increased metastatic potential, and resistance to therapeutic agents. While the binding of trastuzumab to the Her-2/neu protein may lead to antibody-dependent cell-mediated cytotoxicity, the more important function appears to be the disruption of the downstream signaling through the intracellular tyrosine kinase.

Cetuximab (Erbitux) binds to the EGFR with high affinity, blocking the subsequent signal transduction events leading to cell proliferation. It enhances the antitumor effects of chemotherapy by inhibiting cell proliferation and angiogenesis and promoting apoptosis. Cetuximab has been approved for use in combination with CPT-11 for the treatment of advanced colorectal cancer. **Bevacizumab** (Avastin) targets the vascular endothelial growth factor (VEGF), which regulates vascular proliferation and permeability and promotes angiogenesis. In contrast to trastuzumab and cetuximab, the use of bevacizumab does not include a diagnostic eligibility test, as the measurement of VEGF does not appear to correlate with the rates of response.

Another way to target cancer cells is through the use of small molecules. The development of **imatinib mesylate** (Gleevec) is the classic example of a small-molecule targeted therapy. Imatinib is an adenosine triphosphate-binding selective inhibitor of *bcr-abl*, and its use has been associated with durable, complete responses in the treatment of Philadelphia chromosome-positive chronic myelogenous leukemia as well as the treatment of gastrointestinal stromal tumors. The latter characteristically express an activating mutation in the c-kit receptor tyrosine kinase (RTK) gene. **Gefitinib** (Iressa) and **erlotinib** (Tarceva) are small-molecule drugs that target EGFR and have activity against lung, head and neck, breast, and pancreatic cancer. While these agents have been disappointing as single agents, they may have a role when combined with cytotoxic chemotherapy. **Sorafenib** (Nexxar) shows more broad-spectrum antitumor activity by inhibiting not only different isoforms of Raf serine kinase but also various RTKs such as VEGFR, EGFR, and platelet-derived growth factor receptor (PDGFR). **Sunitinib malate** (Sutent) is another multitargeted tyrosine kinase inhibitor of VEGFR, PDGFR, KIT, and FLT3.

Apoptosis-inducing drugs are also being studied. **Bortezomib** (Velcade) blocks proteasomes, which are important in regulating cell function and growth. It is presently approved in the treatment of multiple myeloma and is being investigated for non-Hodgkin lymphoma and a variety of solid tumors. **Oblimersen** (Genasense) targets the antiapoptotic gene *bcl-2* and is presently in clinical trial.

HORMONAL THERAPY

Hormones are normally involved in the differentiation, stimulation, and control of certain tissues, including but not limited to lymphoid tissue, the uterus, the prostate, and the mammary glands. Tumors arising from these tissues may also be stimulated or inhibited by hormones, and so manipulation of the hormonal balance can be beneficial in the systemic therapy of these cancers. In some cases, hormones themselves are used as cancer therapies. For example, the administration of estrogen to a man ultimately suppresses the production of testosterone, which is a useful effect in the treatment of prostate cancer. Corticosteroids, particularly the glucocorticoids, have a powerful suppressive effect on lymphoid cells, making them useful in the treatment of acute leukemias, lymphomas, myeloma, and other myeloproliferative disorders. In most cases, however, hormonal therapy involves blocking the effects of hormones that stimulate proliferation.

▶ Estrogen & Androgen Inhibitors

One approach to hormonal therapy is to block the hormone receptor on the cell. Selective estrogen receptor modulators (SERMs) are medications that mimic the structure of estrogen. Because the estrogen-receptor complex varies among tissue types, SERMs can have different effects on different tissues, sometimes inhibiting the actions of estrogen and sometimes behaving like estrogen. The most well-known

SERM is tamoxifen, which is used not only to treat estrogen-sensitive breast cancer but also to prevent breast cancer in high-risk individuals. Because it also has some proestrogen properties, side effects of tamoxifen can include an increased risk of uterine cancer and deep vein thrombosis. Raloxifene is a newer SERM that has been approved for prevention and treatment of postmenopausal osteoporosis and is presently being studied in the chemoprevention of breast cancer. Research is ongoing to identify related compounds that act like estrogen in desirable ways but do not act like estrogen in undesirable ways.

Flutamide is a testosterone antagonist used in the treatment of prostate cancer. It works by blocking translocation of the androgen receptor to the nucleus. Although hormonal therapy for prostate cancer is palliative, it can be quite effective in slowing the progression of disease. Hormonal therapy can add several years to the life expectancy of patients with unresectable or metastatic disease. Flutamide is most effective when used in combination with surgical or pharmacologic castration.

▶ Gonadotropin-Releasing Hormone Analogues

The most definitive way to block the production of testosterone and estrogen is by surgical castration. The pharmacologic equivalent of castration can be accomplished with leuprolide, an analog of gonadotropin-releasing hormone (GnRH). Normally, GnRH leads to the production of luteinizing hormone and follicle-stimulating hormone, the physiologic stimulators of sex hormone production. Constant stimulation with leuprolide actually inhibits luteinizing hormone and follicle-stimulating hormone release and leads to decreased synthesis of the sex steroids. Leuprolide is commonly used to decrease testosterone levels in the treatment of unresectable prostate cancer. In premenopausal women, estrogen levels fall to postmenopausal values with leuprolide administration. For this reason, the drug can be useful in the treatment of estrogen receptor-positive breast cancers in premenopausal women.

▶ Aromatase Inhibitors

Postmenopausal women have functionally inactive ovaries; however, estrogens are still produced to a lesser extent in extragonadal tissues, primarily the conversion of adrenal steroids in fat cells by the enzyme aromatase. Aromatase inhibitors can eliminate functional estrogen in this population of women and may be an effective hormonal treatment of breast cancer. The selective aromatase inhibitor, anastrozole, is approved for the treatment of metastatic breast cancer or as adjuvant therapy for postmenopausal women whose tumors possess estrogen or progesterone receptors. Another aromatase inhibitor, letrozole, has been shown to be beneficial as continued hormonal therapy in women who have completed 5 years of adjuvant therapy with tamoxifen.

Chang AE et al (editors): *Oncology: An Evidence-Based Approach.* Springer, 2006.

Chu E, DeVita VT: *Physicians' Cancer Chemotherapy Drug Manual.* Jones and Bartlett, 2003.

DeVita VT et al (editors): *Principles and Practice of Oncology,* 8th ed. Lippincott Williams & Wilkins, 2007.

Steeghs N, Nortier JW, Gelderblom H: Small molecule tyrosine kinase inhibitors in the treatment of solid tumors: an update of recent developments. Ann Surg Oncol 2007;14:942.

Zureikat AH, McKee MD: Targeted therapy for solid tumors: current status. Surg Oncol Clin N Am 2008;17:279.

RADIATION THERAPY

Radiation therapy may be used alone or in combination with surgery and chemotherapy and may be given with curative or palliative intent. Some tumors, such as head and neck cancers, prostate cancer, and Hodgkin disease, can often be cured by irradiation alone, eliminating the need for surgical resection or chemotherapy. More commonly, locoregional control of tumors involves surgical resection combined with localized radiation. The theoretical advantage of combining these two therapies is based on the mechanisms by which they fail to achieve their purpose. Surgical failures occur at the margins of tumors, while radiation therapy fails in the center of tumors, where the malignant cells are numerous and hypoxic conditions exist. Radiation failures are rare at the periphery of tumors, where cell numbers are low and oxygenation is high. Depending on tumor histology and location, radiation therapy can be used as a surgical adjunct either preoperatively or postoperatively. Preoperative radiation can shrink tumors and increase the chances for complete surgical resection in cancers such as sarcomas, rectal cancers, and superior sulcus lung cancers.

▶ Principles of Radiation Therapy

Ionizing radiation is defined as energy with sufficient strength to cause the ejection of an orbital electron from an atom when the radiation is absorbed. Ionizing radiation can take either an electromagnetic form, as high-energy photons, or particulate forms, such as electrons, protons, neutrons, alpha particles, or other particles. Most radiation therapies utilize either photons or electrons. Electrons interact directly with tissue, causing ionization, in contrast to photons, which affect tissues by the electrons that they eject. Electron beams deliver a high skin dose and exhibit a rapid fall-off after only a few centimeters and are therefore commonly used to treat superficial targets such as skin cancers or lymph nodes within a few centimeters of the surface of the body. More commonly, electromagnetic radiation (high-energy photons) is used to treat cancer. This consists of either gamma rays (photons created from the decay of radioactive nuclei) or x-rays (photons created by interaction of accelerated electrons with electrons and nuclei of atoms in an x-ray tube target).

To quantify the interaction of radiation on tissues, one must first measure the ionization produced in air by the beam of radiation. This quantity is known as **exposure** and is measured in Roentgens (R). One can then correct for the presence of soft tissue and calculate the **absorbed dose:** the amount of energy absorbed per unit mass. This quantity was previously measured in rads but today is typically measured as joules per kilogram, or gray (Gy) units: 100 rad = 100 cGy = 1 Gy. As photons enter tissue, the dose increases at first and then begins to fall off because radiation falls off with the square of the distance from the source (a law of physics known as the inverse-square law).

The effect on biological tissues when they encounter ionizing radiation comes from ejected electrons interacting either directly with target molecules within the cell or indirectly with water to produce free radicals (such as hydroxyl radicals) that subsequently interact with target molecules. During their brief life span, electrons and free radicals interact with molecules in a random fashion. If they interact with molecules that are not crucial to cell survival, the effect of the radiation will be harmless. If they react with biologically important molecules, the effect will be detrimental. Molecular oxygen prolongs the life of reactive radicals, increasing the likelihood that it will have a detrimental effect. This is why tumor hypoxia tends to increase resistance to radiation.

While ionizing radiation may damage many molecules with the cell, the most critical injury with respect to cell death appears to be DNA damage in the form of single-strand or double-strand breaks. Cells have relatively efficient repair mechanisms for single-strand breaks in DNA, but double-strand breaks in DNA are much more difficult for cells to repair, although not impossible. Therefore, the ability of ionizing radiation to kill cells is dependent not only on the generation of enough DNA double-strand breaks to overwhelm repair pathways but also on the time the cell has to repair those breaks prior to the next mitotic cell division.

This phenomenon is known as **sublethal damage repair** in which increased cell survival is observed if a dose of radiation is divided into two fractions separated by a time interval. As the time interval between the fractions increases, the surviving fraction of the cells also increases as the cells are able to repair double-strand DNA breaks. Of course, in clinical radiation therapy, the goal is to kill the cancer cells but spare the normal cells. Delivering a single large dose of radiation will have a high rate of tumor cell killing, but the concordant killing of the normal tissue cells may limit the clinical utility due to normal tissue toxicity. This has led to the development of multifraction regimens commonly used today, typically delivering daily fractions of 1.8–2.5 Gy. *Fractionation* of radiation dose spares normal tissues because of their greater ability to repair sublethal damage between dose fractions and repopulate with cells if the overall time is sufficiently long.

▶ Modes of Delivery

A. Teletherapy

Radiation is administered by two methods: an external machine (teletherapy) or the implantation of radioactive sources in or around the tumor (brachytherapy). In the past, teletherapy radiation was delivered using cobalt 60, a radioisotope produced in nuclear reactors. Although cobalt machines were very reliable, their usefulness is restricted by limited penetration to deep tumors without significant skin toxicity and difficulty in confining the dose to normal tissues. Today, external radiation is most often administered using a linear accelerator capable of producing higher energy photons without the geometric disadvantages associated with cobalt 60 units.

No matter the source, the beam of radiation needs to be modified to get optimal delivery of the desired dose to the tumor while minimizing dose to the normal tissues. Typically, the beam of radiation is rectangular. Collimators are thick shielding devices made from materials with a high atomic number. Primary collimators at the head of the machine create a rectangular beam, and additional devices such as wedges, compensators, blocks, or multileaf collimators are used to further modify the beam to desired specifications. Wedges or compensators can optimize the dose distribution if the treatment surface is curved or irregular in shape. The beam can also be shaped using individually fashioned blocks custom-made for each patient's anatomy and tumor size and shape. In modern linear accelerators, multileaf collimators have replaced handmade blocks and allow automated and precise field-shaping without the use of cumbersome handmade blocks.

B. Brachytherapy

Brachytherapy involves the placement of radioactive sources into or next to the target tissue. It takes advantage of the inverse-square law, which states that the intensity of electromagnetic radiation dissipates as the inverse square of the distance from the source. Thus, if radioactive sources can be placed so that the tumor is within a centimeter of the sources, the dose received by normal tissues just 2 cm distant from the source and 1 cm distant from the tumor would be one fourth of the dose received by the tumor. This can allow delivery of a high dose to the tumor with only a modest dose to normal tissue.

There are many implantation techniques for brachytherapy. The surgical approach to the target volume may be interstitial (such as prostate seed implantation), intracavitary (such as gynecologic applicators), transluminal (such as endoscopic applications), or surface mold techniques (such as eye plaques for ocular melanoma). The implants may be permanent or temporary, and the dose may be delivered using low, medium, or high dose rates. Many modern applications use afterloading techniques that place treatment applicators and load radioactive sources afterwards to reduce radiation exposure for therapy personnel.

▶ Complications of Radiation Therapy

A. Acute Radiation Effects

Acute radiation effects are those toxicities that occur within a few weeks to months of radiation therapy. They occur mainly in self-renewing tissues that are characterized by actively proliferating stem cells producing progeny that divide and differentiate into mature functioning cells. This includes bone marrow, skin and its appendages, and mucosal surfaces of the oropharynx, esophagus, stomach, intestines, rectum, bladder, and vagina. Once the normal life span of the mature cells expires, the normal turnover and replacement with new cells does not occur because of radiation killing of the dividing stem cells. Acute toxicity is influenced by both fraction size and the time interval between fractions. The more rapidly a given dose is delivered during the overall treatment period, the more severe the acute effects will be. A decrease in fraction size or prolongation of the interval between fractions allows the cell populations to repair and repopulate, decreasing the severity of acute toxicity.

Head and neck irradiation is among the most toxic in the acute period due to significant mucositis of the oral cavity, oropharynx, larynx, and cervical esophagus. Skin and the salivary glands are also affected. Mucositis, yeast superinfection, desquamation, pain, xerostomia, odynophagia, dysphagia, dehydration, and malnutrition are all common clinical scenarios that radiation oncologists manage when delivering head and neck radiotherapy. Other common acute effects observed during radiation therapy directed at other anatomic sites include dysphagia and cough from thoracic radiation, nausea, vomiting and diarrhea from abdominal radiation, and dysuria, proctitis, and perineal desquamation and pain from pelvic radiation.

B. Late Radiation Effects

Late effects are those toxicities that occur months to years after radiotherapy and are more commonly permanent. Mitotically inactive tissues without the capacity for self-renewal are commonly involved. The mechanism causing late effects may include direct damage to the parenchymal cells within an organ or indirect effects due to microvascular damage. Each organ is characterized by a **tolerance dose,** a radiation dose above which the risk of organ complications increases rapidly. These normal tissue tolerances are the true dose-limiting factors in clinical radiation therapy, because late complications can be permanent and in some cases life threatening.

The types of late complications induced by radiation can vary. For the brain, late toxicity may mean necrosis of the brain tissue, while in the kidney it may mean nephrotic syndrome and organ failure. The tolerance doses for different organs vary over a large range, from a few Gy for sterility from testicular irradiation to over 100 Gy for necrosis or perforation of the uterus. Late complications may include fibrosis, necrosis, ulceration and bleeding, chronic edema, telangiectasias and pigmentation changes, cataract formation, nerve damage, lung pneumonitis and fibrosis, pericarditis, myocardial damage, bone fracture, liver or kidney failure, sterility, intestinal obstruction, and fistula and stricture formation.

Perez CA, Brady LW (editors): *Principles and Practice of Radiation Oncology,* 5th ed. Lippincott Williams & Wilkins, 2007.

Tobias JS, Thomas PRM (editors): *Current Radiation Oncology,* vol 3. Oxford University Press, 1998.

IMMUNOTHERAPY

▶ Principles of Antitumor Immune Responses

Immunotherapy refers to treatments designed to kill tumor cells through immune mechanisms. There are two broad types of antitumor immune responses, one involving the humoral arm of the immune system and the other involving the cellular arm. Humoral immunity involves antibody production by mature B lymphocytes. Cell-mediated immunity involves stimulation of cytotoxic (CD8+) T cells through a major histocompatibility complex (MHC) class I-restricted process and stimulation of helper (CD4+) T cells through an MHC class II-restricted process. The humoral and cell-mediated immune responses overlap in that the activation of a B cell response usually requires the presence of helper T cells. Whether a humoral or a cell-mediated immune response is more important in generating antitumor immunity is still debated; however, patients who exhibit both responses appear to fare better than those who demonstrate only one type of response or no response.

Essential to the generation of an immune response through either arm of the immune system is the ability of antigen-presenting cells (APCs), such as monocytes, macrophages, B cells, and dendritic cells, to process and present tumor-related peptide antigens. Proteins are phagocytosed by APCs and partially digested into smaller polypeptides. These small peptide antigens are then bound to MHC molecules on the cell surface. These unique antigen:MHC complexes can then be recognized by naïve T lymphocytes through the T-cell receptor. When a naïve helper (CD4+) T cell recognizes the antigen being expressed on the MHC class II molecule and also recognizes costimulatory molecules present on the APC, it becomes activated, resulting in proliferation and differentiation. There are two types of helper T cells. The Th1 helper T cells produce cytokines to promote a cellular response (interleukin [IL]-2, interferon [IFN]-γ, tumor necrosis factor α, granulocyte-macrophage colony-stimulating factor). In the presence of these cytokines, naïve cytotoxic (CD8+) T cells that recognize antigen being presented on MHC class I molecules on the surface of an APC become activated. Once activated, cytolytic T cells destroy tumor cells via T-cell receptor recognition of tumor-specific antigen presented on MHC class I molecules at the tumor cell surface. Antigen-specific T cells bind to the MHC I receptor–tumor antigen complex and destroy the tumor cell via the release of granules containing granzyme B and perforin and via induction of the Fas/Fas ligand apoptosis. Cytotoxic T cells can only recognize antigen expressed on the tumor surface in the context of the MHC class I molecule.

The second type of helper T cell (Th2) secretes B-cell stimulatory cytokines (IL-4, IL-5, IL-10), which results in the proliferation and differentiation of plasma cells. As opposed to a cellular response, for an antibody response, the antigens do not have to be presented on class I MHC receptors. Tumor cells can then be killed by a variety of methods. Antibody-dependent cell mediated cytotoxicity involves the attachment of tumor-specific antibodies to tumor cells and the subsequent destruction of the tumor cell by the natural killer (NK) cell. Complement-dependent cell-mediated cytotoxicity involves the recognition and attachment of complement-fixing antibodies to tumor-specific surface antigens followed by complement activation. A third mechanism of tumor destruction, opsonization, results when tumor-specific antibodies attach to their target antigens on tumor cell surfaces, thus marking them for engulfment by macrophages.

There are several methods by which the immune system may be incorporated into cancer therapy. Immunotherapy can be categorized as either active or passive. With passive immunotherapy, the host need not mount an immune response; the therapeutic agent will directly or indirectly mediate tumor killing. Examples of passive immunotherapy include the use of monoclonal antibodies or adoptive (cellular) immunotherapy. Active immunotherapy, on the other hand, is the delivery of materials designed to elicit an immune response by the host. This can further be broken down to nonspecific and specific active immunotherapies. Nonspecific agents are those that stimulate the immune system globally but do not recruit tumor-specific effector cells. Active specific immunotherapy is designed to elicit an immune response to one or more tumor antigens, the prime example being the use of vaccines.

Passive Immunotherapy (Monoclonal Antibodies)

The development of monoclonal antibodies with unique specificity to tumor antigens has allowed for multiple attempts to utilize them as cancer therapy. In addition to their relative selectivity and minimal toxicity, they are easily mass produced for widespread application. In some cases, monoclonal antibodies work primarily through the immune system (antibody-dependent cell-mediated cytotoxicity), while in other cases, they behave more as targeted therapies (see earlier section on Targeted Therapies). Examples of monoclonal antibodies that are primarily immunotherapies include rituximab and alemtuzumab. Rituximab (Rituxan) is an anti-CD20 monoclonal antibody that is approved for the treatment of relapsed or refractory low-grade or follicular non-Hodgkin lymphoma (NHL). Alemtuzumab (Campath) targets CD52, which is present on both B and T cells, and is used in the treatment of B-cell chronic lymphocytic leukemia (B-CLL).

Adoptive Immunotherapy

Adoptive immunotherapy is the passive administration of cells with antitumor activity to the tumor-bearing host.

Tumor-infiltrating lymphocytes are lymphocytes that infiltrate growing tumors and can be isolated by growing single-cell suspensions from the tumor in the presence of IL-2. They have been isolated from virtually all types of tumors and can recognize tumor-associated antigens. These cells can also be manipulated ex vivo to increase their recognition of tumor antigen or cytolytic potential. Adoptive immunotherapy is presently under active investigation.

Nonspecific Active Immunotherapy

A. Immunostimulants

Before the mechanism by which the immune system can eradicate tumor cells was fully understood, early attempts at immunotherapy involved nonspecific stimulation of the immune system. The idea was that any increase in immune reactivity would be associated with a concomitant increase in the antitumor immune response. Probably the most widely embraced immunostimulant investigated has been the use of bacille Calmette-Guérin (BCG), a modified form of the tubercle bacillus. Initial trials suggested a possible benefit, but multiple prospective, randomized trials in various malignancies have failed to substantiate a survival benefit of BCG, either alone or in combination with other therapeutics. Local therapy with BCG in the bladder eliminates superficial bladder cancers and prevents tumor recurrences. It is one of several standard therapies for patients with bladder cancer. It is also being studied as an adjuvant to other immunotherapies, such as vaccines. Levamisole is an antihelminthic drug that was reported to have several immunomodulatory properties. Although the exact mechanism of action is unknown, it has been effective in the adjuvant therapy of colorectal cancer.

B. Cytokines

Cytokines are naturally occurring soluble proteins produced by mononuclear cells of the immune system that can affect the growth and function of cells through interaction with specific cell-surface receptors. There have been over 50 cytokines isolated to date, and several have subsequently been approved by the FDA for clinical use, including interferon-α and IL-2.

The interferons (IFN-α, IFN-β, IFN-γ) were originally described as proteins produced by virally infected cells that serve to protect against further viral infection through a variety of effects. These include the increased antigen presentation via increased expression of MHC and antigens, enhancement of NK cell function, and the enhancement of antibody-dependent cell-mediated cytotoxicity. In addition, the interferons exert direct antiangiogenic, cytotoxic, and cytostatic effects. While the anticancer effects of IFN-β and IFN-γ have been disappointing, several hematologic and solid tumors have proved responsive to IFN-α, including chronic myelogenous leukemia, cutaneous T-cell lymphoma, hairy cell leukemia, melanoma, and Kaposi sarcoma.

It is unclear whether the predominant effect of interferon is the direct antiproliferative activity or the immunologic actions.

IL-2 was originally described as the "T-cell growth factor" because it is required for the differentiation and proliferation of activated T cells. As such, it seems like an ideal choice for immunotherapy. The major drawback of IL-2 is the significant dose-related toxicity. IL-2 leads to significant interstitial edema and vascular depletion and lymphoid infiltration into vital organs, possibly resulting in severe hypotension and ischemic damage to the heart, liver, kidneys, and bowel, which limits the use of IL-2 to patients with excellent performance status, normal pulmonary and cardiac function, and no active infections. Despite these limitations, IL-2 has proved to be an effective therapy in patients with metastatic melanoma and metastatic renal cell carcinoma.

▶ Specific Active Immunotherapy (Vaccines)

The goal of cancer vaccines is to generate a host immune response to known or unknown tumor-associated antigens. Many different vaccine strategies are under investigation, each with advantages and disadvantages in regard to clinical feasibility, cost, the number of antigens available, and the mechanism of response (cellular, humoral, or both). Some vaccine strategies use specific peptide antigens. These are highly purified and therefore are easy to standardize, distribute, and administer. Unfortunately, immunizing a patient against a single antigen has several drawbacks that limit the potential clinical benefit. If a peptide vaccine does stimulate a response, it may not be the "right" peptide for many patients. Even commonly expressed tumor antigens are not present on all patients' tumors, or they may be present in varying degrees. In addition, the T cell's recognition of an antigen depends on the presentation of that antigen on a specific MHC molecule. Only certain human lymphocyte antigen (HLA) phenotypes can present any given peptide to induce an immune response, so they will function only on a limited subset of patients. A classic example is that of the MART-1/Melan-A antigen in melanoma. The antigen is expressed by 80% of melanomas, but the peptide only binds to HLA-A2. Because only about 45% of Caucasians have HLA-A2, only 36% (80% of 45%) of melanoma patients given a MART-1/Melen-A vaccine would see a benefit. Finally, a cancer can escape immune recognition rather simply if a population of cells stops expressing that antigen or the MHC molecule.

For many cancers, only a few tumor-associated antigens have been defined; these may not be present on a large percentage of patients. Using the patient's cancer as the vaccine precludes the need to identify specific antigens. Autologous tumor cell vaccines are created from cancer cells harvested from the patient, altered to be more immunogenic, and irradiated, before being returned to the patient to stimulate a tumor-specific immune response. This approach is limited to individuals with sufficient tumor to prepare a vaccine. Trials are restricted to patients with bulky nodal or accessible distant metastatic disease who have a poor overall prognosis to begin with. Furthermore, the technical complexities inherent in procuring tumor and preparing a vaccine have made it difficult to conduct multi-institutional trials to test the efficacy of these vaccines.

Since many tumor-associated antigens are shared among a large number of patients, it is possible that one could create a vaccine from cultured cell lines that would stimulate an antitumor immune response in any patient who shared some of those antigens. This is the principle behind allogeneic tumor cell vaccines. This approach offers several advantages over autologous vaccines: Allogeneic vaccines are readily available, even for patients who lack sufficient tumor to produce an autologous tumor cell vaccine, and can be standardized, preserved, and distributed in a manner akin to any other therapeutic agent.

▶ Tumor Induced Immunosuppression

It is becoming increasingly apparent that in addition to mechanisms to generate and propagate an immune response, the immune system has several mechanisms to limit an immune response. This immune regulatory function is necessary to prevent lymphoproliferative disorders and autoimmune diseases. Neoplasms, however, may take advantage of this, creating an immunosuppressive network within the tumor microenvironment that protects the tumor from immune attack and minimizes the efficacy of immunotherapy.

Several components of the immune system function to regulate or limit an immune response. While it was initially thought that dendritic cells were exclusively immunogenic, recent evidence suggests that they possess dual functions, and some subsets of dendritic cells possess a regulatory function. Myeloid-derived suppressor cells can also suppress the antitumor response to cancer by blocking the effects of cytotoxic T cells in the tumor microenvironment. In addition to cytotoxic and helper T cells, another T-cell population is the regulatory T cell, which also functionally suppresses immune responses. Immunosuppressive cytokines within the tumor microenvironment (IL-6, IL-10, TFG-β) may function to intensify these immunosuppressive components, augmenting tumor escape from immune recognition. It is also possible that many immunotherapies fail by augmenting not only immune stimulation but immune suppression, canceling out the effect. In some cases, these therapies may tilt the response toward immune suppression, for a detrimental effect. Newer immunotherapeutic strategies are focusing on not only increasing immune recognition of the tumor but blocking the suppressive mechanisms. These include pretreatment depletion of regulatory T cells, blocking suppressive pathways or neutralizing immunosuppressive cytokines.

Abbas AK, Lichtman AH, Pober JS (editors): *Cellular and Molecular Immunology,* 5th ed. Saunders, 2003.

Murphy KM et al (editors): *Janeway's Immunobiology,* 7th ed. Garland Science, 2007.

Pendergrast GC: *Cancer Immunotherapy: Immune Suppression and Tumor Growth.* Academic Press, 2007.

Zou W: Immunosuppressive networks in the tumor microenvironment and their therapeutic relevance. Nat Rev Cancer 2005;5:263.

SPECIFIC TYPES OF MALIGNANT NEOPLASMS

SOFT TISSUE SARCOMA

Soft tissue sarcomas account for approximately 1% of all new cancer diagnoses. Almost half of all patients diagnosed with the disease eventually die as a result of the cancer. Soft tissue sarcomas can occur anywhere in the body, but most originate in an extremity (59%), the trunk (19%), the retroperitoneum (15%), or the head and neck (9%). Soft tissue sarcomas originate from a wide variety of mesenchymal cell types and include malignant fibrous histiocytoma, liposarcoma, rhabdomyosarcoma, leiomyosarcoma, and desmoid tumors. While the histopathology of these tumors is highly variable, with some exceptions they tend to behave in a fashion dictated by tumor grade rather than the cell of origin.

Most soft tissue sarcomas arise de novo, and rarely do they result from malignant degeneration of a benign lesion. There are several familial syndromes in which patients are genetically predisposed to the formation of soft tissue sarcomas, including Li-Fraumeni syndrome, Recklinghausen disease, and Gardner syndrome. Other proven risk factors exist that may increase the chances of sarcoma formation. External radiation therapy can increase the incidence of sarcomas by 8-fold to 50-fold. Chronic extremity lymphedema also increases the risk for lymphangiosarcoma. A classic example is the development of upper extremity lymphangiosarcomas in the lymphedematous arm of women treated for breast cancer (Stewart-Treves syndrome). Other less clear associations link chronic tissue trauma and occupational chemical exposures with an increased risk for sarcoma formation.

The major features of the staging system for soft tissue sarcomas (Table 44–2) are the grade of the tumor, its size, and the presence of metastatic disease. Although the site of the tumor is not considered in staging, patients with retroperitoneal tumors tend to have a worse prognosis. Sarcomas generally metastasize by the hematogenous route, and the metastatic sites of sarcomas are related to the location of the primary tumor. The vast majority of metastases from extremity sarcomas are to the lung, while the majority of retroperitoneal tumors metastasize to the liver. Lymph node involvement is rare with most soft tissue sarcomas, although it may occur with epithelioid sarcoma, clear cell sarcoma, angiosarcoma, rhabdomyosarcoma, or synovial sarcoma.

Table 44–2. AJCC Staging System for Soft Tissue Sarcoma.

Primary tumor (T)	
T1	Tumor 5 cm or less
T1a	Superficial tumor
T1b	Deep tumor
T2	Tumor more than 5 cm
T2a	Superficial tumor
T2b	Deep tumor
Regional lymph nodes (N)	
N0	No regional lymph node metastasis
N1	Regional lymph node metastasis
Distant metastasis (M)	
M0	No distant metastasis
M1	Distant metastasis
Histopathologic grade (G)	
G1	Well differentiated
G2	Moderately differentiated
G3	Poorly differentiated
G4	Undifferentiated
Stage grouping	
Stage IA	G1-2, T1a-1b, N0, M0
Stage IB	G1-2, T2a, N0, M0
Stage IIA	G1-2, T2b, N0, M0
Stage IIB	G3-4, T1a-1b, N0, M0
Stage IIC	G3-4, T2a, N0, M0
Stage III	G3-4, T2b, N0, M0
Stage IV	Any G, any T, either N1 or M1

The most important prognostic variables for patients with soft tissue sarcoma are the size and grade of the primary tumor. Since grading is based on the cellular architecture and invasive nature of the tumor, FNAB is not a typically useful biopsy technique for the initial diagnosis of a sarcoma. If a tumor is small (< 3 cm) and superficial, excisional biopsy should be performed. All extremity biopsy incisions should be oriented longitudinally, as the biopsy incision scar should be excised in a subsequent definitive resection of the tumor. Core needle biopsies may be performed for large, palpable superficial tumors. For large, deep tumors or those adjacent to vital structures, incisional biopsy is usually the diagnostic method of choice. The incision should be centered over the mass, tissue flaps should not be raised, and meticulous hemostasis should be ensured, all to prevent the dissemination of tumor cells into adjacent tissue planes.

▶ Treatment of Extremity Sarcomas

MRI is the imaging modality of choice for any suspected extremity sarcoma because it is most accurate in defining the extent of the tumor and invasion of surrounding structures. MRI is also used for follow-up imaging to assess response in patients undergoing therapy, as well as for local and regional recurrence. A chest x-ray or chest CT should be obtained in order to evaluate for pulmonary metastases in patients with high-grade tumors.

Surgery remains the primary therapy for localized extremity sarcomas, but multimodality therapy is recommended to minimize the likelihood of recurrence or the need for amputation. Historically, amputation was the only form of curative surgical therapy for large extremity sarcomas, but multimodality therapy has allowed for a high rate of limb preservation. Today, fewer than 5% of patients with extremity soft tissue sarcoma require amputation, generally reserved for patients whose tumors do not respond to preoperative therapy and cannot be resected adequately, have no evidence of metastatic disease, and have a good prognosis for rehabilitation.

A pseudocapsule composed of tumor cells surrounds sarcomas, and local invasion along fascial planes and neurovascular structures is common. It is important not to dissect along the pseudocapsule, which is associated with high local recurrence rates, but rather obtain a wide (2-cm) margin of normal tissue. This may need to be compromised in the immediate vicinity of functionally important neurovascular structures. If the tumor involves these structures, nerve grafts and arterial reconstruction with autologous or prosthetic conduits may be required. Large soft tissue defects often require the construction of myocutaneous flaps to improve function and cosmesis. Soft tissue sarcomas rarely invade bone or skin, and wide resections of these structures are infrequently necessary.

Following wide local excision, metal clips should be placed at all margins of the resection in order to guide subsequent radiotherapy. For patients with T1 tumors located superficially in an area where it is not difficult to obtain widely negative margins, postoperative radiation therapy may not be necessary. For most other lesions, postoperative radiation is almost always recommended, with either external beam radiation or brachytherapy. Radiation should be started 4–8 weeks after surgery, as delay can result in a lower local control rate. Preoperative radiotherapy may have some advantages in patients with large tumors. Lower doses can be delivered to an undisturbed tumor bed, which may also have better oxygenation, and larger tumors may decrease in size, allowing for limb-sparing procedures. Preoperative radiation is associated with an increase in short-term wound complications but a decrease in long-term tissue fibrosis and edema. The optimal mode and sequence for treatment has yet to be defined and often requires a multidisciplinary approach.

Adjuvant chemotherapy remains controversial. Chemotherapy can be given either preoperatively or postoperatively.

The three drugs most effective in sarcoma are doxorubicin, dacarbazine, and ifosfamide. Preoperative chemotherapy is sometimes recommended because in addition to the early treatment of micrometastatic disease, it allows for assessment of tumor response, which helps avoid prolonged therapy in patients not responding. However, while disease-free survival may be improved, there are conflicting data on overall survival. A recent meta-analysis of randomized trials suggested there may be a small survival benefit for extremity sarcomas, and so its use has increased.

The vast majority of localized recurrences in soft tissue sarcomas occur in the first 2 years after resection, necessitating close follow-up during that period. A local recurrence is not indicative of systemic disease and, in the absence of evidence of metastases, should be treated aggressively in the same manner as a primary tumor. The resection of pulmonary metastases should be considered in patients who have fewer than four radiographically detectable lesions and who have achieved apparent local control following resection of the primary tumor. In such circumstances, disease-free survival can approach 25–35%.

▶ Treatment of Retroperitoneal Sarcomas

Retroperitoneal sarcomas comprise approximately 15% of all soft tissue sarcomas, with liposarcoma, malignant fibrous histiocytoma, and leiomyosarcoma the three most common types. They usually present as a large abdominal mass. Nearly half are over 20 cm in size at diagnosis. Once they compress or invade contiguous structures, they can cause symptoms such as abdominal pain or nausea and vomiting. Workup should include CT of the abdomen and pelvis to evaluate the mass as well as CT of the lung and liver to look for metastases. CT-guided core biopsy is the sampling technique of choice, with open or laparoscopic incisional biopsy reserved for inconclusive core biopsies.

As with extremity sarcomas, surgery represents the primary treatment, with the goal being en bloc resection with a rim of normal tissue. Although retroperitoneal tumors are generally large at presentation and often invade vital structures, the majority of these tumors are resectable. Retroperitoneal sarcomas rarely invade surrounding organs, but an intense desmoplastic reaction makes it difficult to assess the extent of tumor, so often these organs need to be resected rather than risk positive margins. The kidney, colon, pancreas, and spleen are the most commonly resected organs.

While adjuvant radiation therapy is standard in extremity sarcoma, evidence supporting its use in retroperitoneal sarcoma is less convincing. Because of the low tolerance to radiation of the abdominal and retroperitoneal organs, delivery of adequate radiotherapy is often difficult. There is encouraging evidence for intraoperative radiation therapy to the tumor bed, but this technique is still considered investigational and can be performed only in select centers. Although complex, preoperative radiation may be beneficial because it uses lower radiation doses, is less injurious to the small bowel, and can increase respectability by shrinking the tumor and creating a thickened capsular structure around the lesion.

Sabel MS: Sarcomas of bone and soft tissues. In: *Scientific Principles and Practice*, 4th ed. Mulholland MW et al (editors). Lippincott Williams & Wilkins, 2007.

Skubitz KM, D'Adamo DR: Sarcoma. Mayo Clin Proc 2007; 82:1409.

Weiss SW, Goldblum JR (editors): *Enzinger and Weiss's Soft Tissue Tumors*, 5th edition. Mosby, 2007.

MELANOMA

The incidence of melanoma is rising faster than any other cancer. The reasons for this rise are not clear but are most likely related to an increased exposure to ultraviolet radiation from sunlight. Individuals whose first sunburn occurred at an early age have an increased incidence of melanoma. Other risk factors include freckles, a fair complexion, reddish or blond hair, blue eyes, a first-degree relative with melanoma, and the presence of multiple or dysplastic nevi.

The best approach to melanoma is to prevent it from occurring, through sun avoidance and sun protection with sunscreens with a sun protection factor (SPF) of 30 or higher. Second to prevention, the most significant impact on melanoma comes from early recognition and diagnosis. The prognosis of melanoma is inversely and dramatically related to the depth of invasion at diagnosis (Breslow thickness), emphasizing the importance of early diagnosis of this disease. Lesions that are suspicious for melanoma can be identified by their clinical characteristics, often referred to as the ABCDs of melanoma (Table 44–3). Diagnosed early, well over 90% of primary melanomas can be cured with surgical excision alone. Patients presenting with thicker lesions or regional nodal metastases have a significantly poorer prognosis. The AJCC and UICC staging system is presented in Table 44–4.

There are several distinct categories of melanoma; the four most common are superficial spreading, nodular, lentigo maligna, and acral lentiginous melanoma.

Superficial spreading melanoma is the most common presentation, accounting for nearly 70% of all melanomas. These usually occur in sun-exposed areas of the body or in individuals with multiple dysplastic nevi. They generally arise in preexisting nevi and can occur at any age after puberty. The superficial spreading subtype tends to grow in a radial pattern

Table 44–3. Clinical Identification (ABCD) of Melanoma.

Asymmetry: Asymmetric shape, color, or contour
Borders: Irregular or ill-defined borders
Color: Black, brown, blue, red, gray, or white
Diameter: Larger than 5 mm *or*
Difference: Any lesion that has changed

Table 44–4. AJCC Staging System for Cutaneous Melanoma.

TNM classification		
T1	≤ 1.0 mm	a) Without ulceration and level II/III
		b) With ulceration or level IV/V
T2	1.01–2.0 mm	a) Without ulceration
		b) With ulceration
T3	2.01–4.0 mm	a) Without ulceration
		b) With ulceration
T4	> 4.0 mm	a) Without ulceration
		b) With ulceration
N0	No lymph node metastasis	
N1	Metastasis in 1 lymph node	a) Micrometastasis
		b) Macrometastasis
N2	Metastasis in 2–3 lymph nodes	a) Micrometastasis
		b) Macrometastasis
		c) In-transit metastasis with no nodal involvement
N3	Metastasis in ≥ 4 lymph nodes or matted lymph nodes or in-transit metastasis with nodal involvement	
M0	No distant metastasis	
M1	Distant metastasis	a) Skin, subcutaneous tissue, or lymph node metastasis, normal LDH
		b) Lung metastasis, normal LDH
		c) All other visceral or any distant metastasis with elevated LDH
Stage groupings		
IA	T1a, N0, M0	
IB	T1b, N0, M0	
	T2a, N0, M0	
IIA	T2b, N0, M0	
	T3a, N0, M0	
IIB	T3b, N0, M0	
	T4a, N0, M0	
IIC	T4b, N0, M0	
IIIA	T1–4a, N1a or N2a, M0	
IIIB	T4b, N1a or N2a, M0	
	T1–4a, N1b or N2b, M0	
	Any T, N2c, M0	
IIIC	T4b, N1b or N2b, M0	
	Any T, N3, M0	
IV	Any T, any N, M1	

during the earlier stages and converts to a vertical growth pattern during the later stages of development.

Nodular melanomas account for between 15% and 25% of all melanomas. These tend to occur in older individuals and are more common in men. Nodular melanomas generally develop de novo, not in a preexisting nevus. They usually are dome shaped with distinct borders and often resemble a blood blister. Nodular melanomas occur most commonly on the head, neck, and trunk. They lack a significant horizontal growth phase and tend to be deep at the time of diagnosis.

Lentigo maligna melanoma has less propensity to metastasize and thus has a more favorable prognosis relative to the other subtypes. However, it can be locally aggressive, with high recurrence rates after excision. These lesions account for 4–10% of melanomas and occur in an older population. Lentigo maligna lesions almost always develop in sun-exposed areas. They have a long horizontal growth phase and often have very convoluted borders.

Acral lentiginous melanomas account for between 2% and 8% of melanomas in Caucasians but for 30–60% of melanomas in blacks, Asians, and Hispanics. These lesions do not occur in sun-exposed areas; instead, they occur on the sole of the foot, the palm, beneath the nail beds, and in the perineal region. Acral lentiginous melanomas are often large, with an average diameter of 3 cm at the time of diagnosis. They develop relatively rapidly over the course of months to several years and tend to behave very aggressively. The clinical characteristics of these melanomas are often unmistakable, with variegations in color and convoluted borders. Ulceration of these lesions is common.

▶ Treatment of Primary Melanoma

Any suspected melanoma should be removed by punch or excisional biopsy. Given the importance of Breslow thickness, shave or curette biopsies are contraindicated. If the biopsy specimen reveals melanoma, a formal excision with adequate margins is required. Because microscopic tumor cells frequently surround primary melanomas, excision with narrow margins is associated with an unacceptably high rate of local recurrence. The current standard for lesions less than 1 mm in depth is excision with 1-cm margins. Melanomas between 1 mm and 2 mm in thickness should be excised with 2-cm margins, but a smaller margin (10–15 mm) may be acceptable in areas where it is difficult to get 2 cm without the need for a skin graft or exceptionally tight closure. Melanomas deeper than 2 mm should be excised with a 2-cm margin. The resection should be carried down to the underlying fascia, although the fascia need not be excised.

Melanomas generally metastasize by the lymphatic route in a predictable and orderly fashion. Any palpable nodes must be considered suspicious for metastatic involvement, easily verified with an FNAB. About 10% of patients have clinical evidence of nodal metastases upon initial presentation and should undergo a therapeutic lymph node dissection at the time of their wide excision. Many patients will have microscopic disease in the lymph nodes that will not be apparent on physical examination. In the past, substantial controversy surrounded elective lymph node dissection of the draining nodal basin for melanoma. The practice gained dramatic acceptance, however, with the advent of the sentinel lymph node biopsy, which is based on the anatomic concept that lymphatic fluid from defined regions of skin drains specifically to an initial node or nodes ("sentinel nodes") prior to disseminating to other nodes in the same or nearby basins. Sentinel node biopsy allows for a more detailed histologic examination of the sentinel lymph nodes and helps avoid the morbidity of lymph node dissection in patients who are pathologically node-negative. Patients with a negative sentinel node are over 6 times more likely to survive than those with a positive sentinel lymph node, making the predictive impact of sentinel node status much greater than any other prognostic factor. Evidence also suggests that early removal of micrometastatic disease from the lymph nodes, as compared with waiting for regional recurrence to perform a lymph node dissection, may improve survival.

The sentinel lymph node biopsy has become the standard of care in the staging and treatment of melanoma and should be performed at the time of the wide excision for primary melanomas thicker than 1.0 mm. It should be selectively applied for tumors between 0.75 mm and 1.0 mm when other worrisome features are present, such as ulceration, angiolymphatic invasion or a high mitotic rate. Melanomas less than 0.75 mm are very unlikely to have regional metastases and do not require sentinel lymph node biopsy. The dominant drainage basins can be identified by lymphoscintigraphy, which involves intradermal injection of technetium-99m (^{99m}Tc) sulfur colloid in the area around the tumor and a gamma camera to image the sites of lymph node drainage. In the operating room, blue dye (isosulfan or methylene) is injected in a similar fashion. Any lymph nodes that have evidence of ^{99m}Tc uptake on a handheld gamma probe, have evidence of blue dye, or are clinically suspicious should be excised. After removal of the nodes, they are analyzed by serial thin-sectioning, routine H&E staining, and immunohistochemical staining. Using these methods of analysis, the pathologist is able to detect even minute numbers of metastatic melanoma cells in the sentinel node. Patients with a positive sentinel lymph node biopsy should undergo formal lymph node dissection of the entire drainage basin.

Traditional chemotherapy regimens have proved largely ineffective in the treatment of melanoma; however, the cytokine IFN alfa-2b has been shown to improve disease-free and overall survival in high-risk patients with no evidence of systemic metastases. This treatment is not without controversy, however, as the duration of therapy is long (12 months), the toxicities are substantial, and some of the data regarding the overall survival benefit are conflicting. Even so, IFN alfa-2b remains the only approved adjuvant therapy of melanoma, and all patients with high-risk melanoma (node-positive melanoma or thick, node-negative melanoma) should have a balanced discussion of the potential risks and benefits. While melanoma is relatively radioresistant, there may be some benefit to regional control after node dissection with radiation in patients with gross extracapsular extension or multiple involved lymph nodes.

▶ Local Recurrence & In-Transit Metastasis

Although rare with appropriate surgery, an isolated local recurrence can be treated with a repeat wide excision with 2-cm margins. Approximately 2–3% of melanoma patients will develop in-transit metastasis, which is the appearance of metastasis along the path from the primary tumor to its regional nodal basin, and is lymphatic in nature. The management of in-transit metastasis is dictated by the number and the size of the lesions. If few in number, surgical excision with a margin of surrounding normal cutaneous and subcutaneous tissue is appropriate; however, this becomes unlikely with multiple lesions. Intralesional therapy with granulocyte-macrophage colony-stimulating factor can result in significant regression of melanoma deposits but requires multiple injections and is not always effective. Although melanoma is relatively radiation resistant, this therapy can provide palliation in unresectable lesions in many cases. Radiation therapy should be considered in those patients with a smaller volume of cutaneous or subcutaneous metastases.

Hyperthermic isolated limb perfusion is a way of isolating the blood circuit to the extremity and administering chemotherapeutic agents regionally at a concentration 15–25 times higher without resulting in systemic side effects. Melphalan has been used as a standard drug for hyperthermic isolated limb perfusion secondary to its efficacy and low regional toxicity. While this has not been shown to improve survival, the use of hyperthermic isolated limb perfusion provides a significant palliation of locoregional symptoms when other options are not available.

Regional and systemic recurrence of melanoma can be latent, and recurrence 10 years after the original diagnosis is not uncommon. This fact necessitates close lifelong follow-up of these patients. Patients with a past history of melanoma have a dramatically increased risk of developing a second primary lesion and require diligent screening for other lesions.

Balch CM et al: *Cutaneous Melanoma*, 4th ed. Quality Medical Publishing, 2003.

Blazer DG, Sondak VK, Sabel MS: Surgical therapy of cutaneous melanoma. Semin Oncol 2007;34:270.

Morton DL et al: Sentinel node biopsy or nodal observation in melanoma. N Engl J Med 2006;355:1307.

Sabel MS, Sondak VK: Pros and cons of adjuvant interferon in the treatment of melanoma. Oncologist 2003;8:451.

LYMPHOMA

Lymphomas are malignant neoplasms that originate from the lymphoid tissues. Two distinct categories of lymphoma

exist: Hodgkin and non-Hodgkin. The two types not only have different morphologic characteristics but differ also in their clinical behavior and their response to various therapeutic regimens. It is not possible to differentiate Hodgkin and non-Hodgkin lymphoma on clinical grounds; surgical biopsy is necessary. In the diagnosis of a suspected lymphoma, excisional biopsy of the entire lymph node or nodes is imperative, as the architecture has a bearing on the diagnosis and the subsequent treatment of the tumor.

1. Hodgkin Lymphoma

Hodgkin lymphoma may occur at any age but is generally a disease of young adults. Prevalence in women peaks in the third decade and then falls, while it remains fairly constant in men after this time. The diagnosis of Hodgkin lymphoma is based on the finding of Reed-Sternberg cells in an appropriate cellular background of reactive leukocytes and fibrosis. It is the pattern of the lymphocytic infiltrate that determines the classic subtypes of Hodgkin disease (see Table 44–5). All subtypes of classical Hodgkin lymphoma are presently treated in the same way, and modern therapy has allowed for cure of over 70% of patients with this malignancy.

The cause of Hodgkin disease is not well understood; however, epidemiologic studies have revealed certain patterns of disease clustering. The incidence appears to be higher with a lower number of siblings, early birth order, siblings with Hodgkin disease, a decreased number of playmates, certain HLAs, single-family dwellings, and patients who have undergone tonsillectomy. The incidence is increased also in persons with immunodeficiencies and autoimmune disorders. This pattern suggests that an oncogenic virus may cause Hodgkin disease. Nuclear proteins of the Epstein-Barr virus have been detected in about 40% of classical Hodgkin lymphoma, and alternative lymphotropic viruses may be involved in the pathogenesis of cases negative for Epstein-Barr virus.

Table 44–5. Classic Subtypes of Hodgkin Lymphoma.

Subtype	Characteristics
Lymphocyte-predominant	Uncommon (6% of Hodgkin lymphomas), diffuse lymphocytic infiltrate with few Reed-Sternberg cells, excellent prognosis
Lymphocyte-depleted	Rare (2% of Hodgkin lymphoma), abundant Reed-Sternberg cells, paucity of lymphocytes, occurs in older males, aggressive clinically
Mixed cellularity	Common (20–25% of Hodgkin lymphoma), histologically intermediate between above two forms, often presents with disseminated disease
Nodular sclerosis	Most common form (70% of Hodgkin lymphoma), fibrosis with Reed-Sternberg and lymphoid cells, more common in young women, presents with cervical or mediastinal disease

Most patients present with enlarged but painless lymph nodes, typically in the lower neck or supraclavicular region. On occasion, mediastinal masses are associated with cough or dyspnea or discovered on routine chest x-ray. About 25% of patients will have systemic symptoms, called B symptoms, including weight loss, pruritus, fever, and drenching night sweats.

Staging

With regard to therapy, the most important prognostic factor in Hodgkin lymphoma is the disease stage. The currently accepted classification for Hodgkin is the Ann Arbor staging system (Table 44–6).

As discussed earlier, excisional lymph node biopsy is essential to the diagnosis of Hodgkin lymphoma. Once the diagnosis is made, disease staging begins with a detailed history and physical examination, with attention to all lymph node beds, B symptoms, and symptoms related to extranodal involvement. CT of the chest, abdomen, and pelvis is the major means of staging intrathoracic and intra-abdominal disease. Bone marrow biopsy is also part of the staging evaluation of patients with bony symptoms or cytopenias. Fluorodeoxyglucose F 18 (FDG-PET) scan significantly adds to the staging of Hodgkin lymphoma and has become a standard staging tool both before treatment and at completion. In the past, a staging laparotomy (splenectomy, wedge liver biopsy, and dissection of the para-aortic, iliac, splenic hilar, and hepatic portal lymph nodes) was used to determine the extent of disease in the abdomen. Given the improved imaging studies and the inclusion of chemotherapy for patients even with favorable stage I disease, staging laparotomies are rarely, if ever, performed.

Treatment

The initial therapy for Hodgkin lymphoma is based on the stage of disease and the presence of constitutional symptoms. Patients with early-stage favorable disease (I-IIA) were previously treated by extended-field radiation therapy. However, high relapse rates and long-term complications have altered this approach. Today, short-term chemotherapy is often used to control occult lesions in combination with involved-field radiation therapy. Sometimes PET scanning is used to determine whether the radiation therapy is necessary, although this approach has not been tested in clinical trials. For patient with stage IA, nodular lymphocyte-predominant Hodgkin lymphoma may sometimes be observed or treated by involved-field radiation therapy only. On the other hand, patients with early-stage unfavorable disease are routinely treated by a combination of chemotherapy and radiation therapy, although the optimal agents, number of cycles, and field sizes of the radiation are controversial and vary among institutions. The typical treatment regimen involves 4 cycles of combination chemotherapy with involved-field radiation. For patients with advance disease, ABVD chemotherapy

Table 44–6. Modified Ann Arbor Staging System of Hodgkin Lymphoma.

Stage I	Involving one lymph node group or structure or extends locally to involve a single adjacent site (stage IE)
Stage II	Involving two or more lymph node groups on the same side of the diaphragm or involves one or more lymph node groups on the same side of the diaphragm, and there is localized involvement of the node(s) to one organ or site on the same side of the diaphragm (stage IIE)
Stage III	Involves lymph node groups on both sides of the diaphragm or has extended to an organ or site next to the lymph nodes and/or spleen (stage IIIE)
Stage III 1	With or without involved nodes of the spleen, hilum, abdomen, or liver
Stage III 2	With involved nodes of the aorta, iliac, or mesenteric arteries
Stage IV	Spread throughout the bloodstream to one or more organs or sites outside of the lymphatic system, with or without associated lymph node involvement

(doxorubicin, bleomycin, vinblastine, and dacarbazine) is the most widely used treatment, although other regimens are being studied, including high-dose chemotherapy with autologous stem cell transplantation.

Approximately 5–10% of patients are refractory to initial therapy, and 10–30% will relapse after complete remission. In this case, salvage therapy typically involves high-dose chemotherapy with bone marrow transplant. For patients who fail this approach or are not candidates for high-dose chemotherapy with autologous stem cell transplantation, there are unfortunately few good treatment options. Vinorelbine, gemcitabine, or rituximab (an anti-CD20 antibody) have shown high response rates but usually of short duration. New therapies are sorely needed.

2. Non-Hodgkin Lymphoma

Non-Hodgkin lymphoma encompasses a wide spectrum of lymphoid-derived tumors. This heterogeneous group of diseases includes more than 10 distinct tumor subtypes with variable biologic behavior and responses to treatment. As opposed to Hodgkin lymphoma, the prevalence of non-Hodgkin lymphoma rises with age. The incidence has been rising steadily over the past 20 years by about 3–5% per year, for unknown reasons. Several risk factors have been identified that predispose patients to the development of disease. Patients with congenital disorders such as ataxia-telangiectasia, Wiskott-Aldrich syndrome, and celiac disease have an increased incidence of lymphoma. Certain acquired conditions also predispose patients to lymphoma, including prior chemotherapy or radiotherapy, immunosuppressive therapy, Epstein-Barr infection, HIV infection, human T-cell lymphoma virus [HTLV]-1 infection, *Helicobacter pylori* gastritis, Hashimoto thyroiditis, and Sjögren syndrome.

Non-Hodgkin lymphoma may originate from B cells, T cells, or histiocytes. Morphologically, the tumors may appear as nodular clusters or diffuse sheets of lymphoid cells.

Classically, non-Hodgkin lymphoma presents as nontender enlargement of lymph nodes, but nearly one third of all cases originate outside the lymph nodes. These extranodal malignancies develop in organs that normally have nests of lymphoid tissue (mucosal surfaces, bone marrow, and skin).

▶ Staging & Classification

Although the Ann Arbor system was developed for Hodgkin disease, this staging system is also used in non-Hodgkin lymphoma. The goal of the staging evaluation is to distinguish patients who have localized disease from those with disseminated disease. After pathologic diagnosis, the staging evaluation for non-Hodgkin lymphoma consists of a detailed history and physical examination, routine laboratory tests, a bone marrow biopsy, and a CT scan of the neck, chest, abdomen, and pelvis. Evaluation of the cerebrospinal fluid should be considered in patients with diffuse large-cell non-Hodgkin lymphoma with bone marrow involvement, a high lactate dehydrogenase (LDH) level, or multiple extranodal sites of disease. It should also be considered in patients with high-grade lymphomas, HIV-related lymphomas, primary central nervous system lymphomas, and posttransplantation lymphoproliferative disorders. Finally, FDG-PET scans provide whole-body images that allow a comprehensive assessment of disease extent and, in conjunction with CT, provides complementary staging information. A pretreatment PET scan is often obtained so that PET can be used for monitoring of response to treatment. Normal PET at the end of therapy correlates with a highly favorable prognosis, while persistent abnormalities mandate close follow-up or biopsy to rule out residual disease.

Although helpful in assessing the anatomic extent of disease, the Ann Arbor system is of minimal clinical value in non-Hodgkin lymphoma. The International Prognostic Index (IPI) uses patient age, Ann Arbor stage, LDH level, number of extranodal sites, and ECOG performance status to categorize aggressive non-Hodgkin lymphoma. However, this system does not clearly stratify indolent lymphomas, so another prognostic factor model was devised for follicular lymphoma. The Follicular Lymphoma International Prognostic Index uses patient age, Ann Arbor stage, hemoglobin level, number of nodal areas, and serum LDH level to stage patients.

Scientists have made countless attempts to develop a universal, clinically relevant classification system for the subtypes of non-Hodgkin lymphoma, and the merits of the various classifications are an area of hot debate. The most widely accepted classification system is the Revised European-American Lymphoma/World Health Organization (REAL/WHO) classification (Table 44–7).

Table 44–7. REAL/WHO Classification of Non-Hodgkin Lymphoma.

B Cell
Precursor B-cell cancers (neoplasms)
Lymphoblastic lymphoma (LBL)
Peripheral B-cell neoplasms
B-cell chronic lymphocytic leukemia/small lymphocytic lymphoma
Lymphoplasmacytic lymphoma/immunocytoma
Mantle cell lymphoma
Follicular lymphoma
Extranodal marginal zone B-cell lymphoma of MALT type
Nodal marginal zone B-cell lymphoma
Splenic marginal zone lymphoma
Plasmacytoma/plasma cell myeloma
Diffuse large B-cell lymphoma
Burkitt lymphoma
T Cell and Natural Killer (NK) Cell
Precursor T-cell neoplasm
Lymphoblastic lymphoma (LBL)
Peripheral T-cell and NK-cell neoplasms
T cell granular lymphocytic leukemia
Mycosis fungoides/Sézary syndrome
Peripheral T-cell lymphoma, not otherwise characterized
Hepatosplenic gamma/delta T-cell lymphoma
Angioimmunoblastic T-cell lymphoma
Extranodal T-/NK-cell lymphoma, nasal type
Enteropathy-type intestinal T-cell lymphoma
Adult T-cell lymphoma/leukemia (HTLV1+)
Anaplastic large cell lymphoma, primary systemic type
Anaplastic large cell lymphoma, primary cutaneous type

In determining the therapeutic approach to patients with non-Hodgkin lymphoma, a simpler classification system can be utilized. For treatment purposes, these lymphomas can be functionally divided into two groups: indolent (low-grade) and aggressive (high-grade) lymphomas (Table 44–8).

Table 44–8. Indolent versus Aggressive Classification of Non-Hodgkin Lymphoma.

Indolent lymphomas
Follicular lymphoma
Small lymphocytic lymphoma
Lymphoplasmacytic lymphoma (Waldenström macroglobulinemia)
Extranodal marginal zone B-cell lymphoma (MALT lymphoma)
Nodal marginal zone B-cell lymphoma (monocytoid B-cell lymphoma)
Aggressive lymphomas
Diffuse large cell lymphoma
Burkitt lymphoma
Precursor B-cell or T-cell lymphoblastic lymphoma
Primary central nervous system lymphoma
Adult T-cell lymphoma
Mantle cell lymphoma
Polymorphic posttransplantation lymphoproliferative disorder
AIDS-related lymphoma
True histiocytic lymphoma
Blastic NK-cell lymphoma

Smaller, differentiated cells characterize the indolent lymphomas, and this class tends to have a follicular architecture. Although the course of these lymphomas is not very aggressive, they are very difficult to cure, and most patients eventually die of their disease. The natural history of indolent lymphomas often involves progression of the tumor cells to a more aggressive subtype. This progression is sometimes heralded by the onset of B symptoms and portends a dismal prognosis.

The aggressive lymphomas behave differently from the indolent ones and demand a different therapeutic approach. Histologically, the aggressive lymphomas spread more diffusely throughout the lymph nodes and consist of larger, less differentiated cell types. This class of lymphomas demonstrates a very rapid growth rate and an increased rate of early mortality. Despite this malignant behavior, this class of non-Hodgkin lymphoma is more often curable. The extranodal lymphomas develop outside of the lymph nodes and are not amenable to conventional classifications, so they are generally regarded as a separate entity. They can involve any organ but most commonly affect the oropharynx, paranasal sinuses, thyroid, gastrointestinal tract, liver, testicles, skin, and bone marrow.

▶ Treatment

A. Indolent Lymphoma

Patients with localized disease, although this is the minority, can be treated with radiation therapy only. Most patients have disseminated disease, which tends to be chronic relapsing and remitting. The current therapies for systemic indolent lymphomas are rarely curative, and the goal of treatment is generally directed at palliation of symptoms. At present, a "watch and wait" approach to treatment is recommended for asymptomatic patients. After diagnosis, asymptomatic patients are followed up clinically until they progress to more aggressive disease, major symptoms, or organ dysfunction. Withholding chemotherapy does not reduce survival in patients with non-Hodgkin lymphoma, and it probably improves quality of life.

For patients who have symptoms, a combination of rituximab and alkylator chemotherapy has high response rates and can alleviate symptoms. Rituximab is a monoclonal antibody that binds to the B-cell surface antigen CD20. CD20 is a cell-surface protein involved in the development and differentiation of normal B cells. It is found on the vast majority of B-cell lymphomas. Rituximab is well tolerated and has remission rates of 40–50% when used as single-agent therapy for relapsed indolent lymphoma. In younger patients with systemic indolent disease, or patients who had a short response to first-line treatment, high-dose chemotherapy with autologous bone marrow transplant may be considered, although the chance of cure should be balanced against the mortality of treatment, which can approach 10%.

B. Aggressive Lymphomas

Despite their aggressive nature, these lymphomas have a better chance for cure than their more indolent counterparts. The treatment is typically guided by the prognostic factors (IPI score). Patients with low-risk lymphoma respond well to CHOP (cyclophosphamide, doxorubicin, vincristine, and prednisone) chemotherapy plus rituximab. Radiotherapy may be used after chemotherapy for areas of bulky disease. Patients with high-risk lymphoma benefit from more intensive regimens of chemotherapy and rituximab and potentially high-dose therapy with autologous stem cell transplantation. This approach should also be considered for patients who relapse or fail to enter remission after induction chemotherapy. A promising immunotherapy is tositumomab, an anti-CD20 monoclonal antibody bound to ^{131}I (Bexxar). It can kill cells by antibody-mediated cellular cytotoxicity, activation of complement-mediated tumor cell lysis, and the tumor-specific delivery of radiation. Bexxar is currently indicated for the treatment of patients with CD20 antigen–expressing relapsed or refractory non-Hodgkin lymphoma.

C. Nonlymphoid Disease

There is no consensus about the proper management of localized nonlymphoid lymphomas because large-scale studies of therapy for this disease have not been conducted. With few exceptions, nonlymphoid disease is managed somewhat in the same way as systemic aggressive lymphomas, using combination CHOP therapy.

The CHOP regimen has the disadvantage of poor penetration of the blood-brain barrier and is thus ineffective in the treatment of primary central nervous system lymphomas. These lymphomas rarely metastasize, remaining localized to the central nervous system. Current regimens utilize steroids and whole-brain radiation with some form of adjuvant chemotherapy. Methotrexate is the most common adjuvant treatment in this patient population, and it can be effective when delivered either systemically or intrathecally. Central nervous system lymphomas have a poor prognosis, with approximately 20% 5-year survival rates in treated patients. The combined modalities, while providing modest survival benefits, have significant neurotoxicities, and as many as 50% of patients develop severe dementia. Given this morbidity, clinicians are currently attempting to improve the therapy for this disease, with most efforts directed toward using chemotherapy as the sole modality in the treatment of patients with primary central nervous system lymphomas. Extranodal lymphomas that have a predilection for metastases to the central nervous system, such as testicular, paranasal, and AIDS-related lymphomas, require systemic CHOP therapy combined with prophylactic intrathecal methotrexate treatments.

The treatment of gastric lymphomas has been controversial. Mucosa-associated lymphoid tissue–type gastric lymphomas (MALT-type gastric lymphomas) typically have an indolent behavior, and the most widely accepted initial therapy is the eradication of *H pylori* using regimens combining antibiotics and proton pump inhibitors. For patients with MALT-type gastric lymphoma who are *H pylori* negative or do not respond to antibiotic/proton pump inhibitor therapy, radiation therapy to the stomach and perigastric lymph nodes obtains high complete response rates and excellent long-term survival. While surgery had previously been used in the treatment of gastric lymphomas, there is now sufficient data to suggest nonoperative management permits a better quality of life with no impact on overall survival. When the disease has spread, the use of chemotherapy is similar to that used for other indolent, advanced lymphomas.

High-grade gastric lymphoma is treated with aggressive polychemotherapy, usually combined with rituximab. Again, surgery used to play a more prominent role but has greatly diminished. It was assumed that the increased risk of perforation and bleeding with chemotherapy could be prevented by pretreatment gastric resection, but modern series have failed to demonstrate that benefit and actually show a high degree of postsurgical complications that may delay the start of chemotherapy. Surgery is limited to patients who have complications or who cannot be managed by standard regimens.

Splenectomy in patients with lymphomatous splenic involvement has not demonstrated therapeutic benefit and should be reserved for patients with symptomatic splenomegaly, pain from recurrent splenic infarctions, and hematologic depression from hypersplenism.

Ansell SM, Armitage JO: Management of Hodgkin lymphoma. Mayo Clin Proc 2006;81:419.

Ansell SM, Armitage JO: Non-Hodgkin lymphoma: diagnosis and treatment. Mayo Clin Proc 2005;80:1087.

Marcus R, Sweetenham JW, Williams ME (editors): *Lymphoma: Pathology, Diagnosis and Treatment.* Cambridge University Press, 2007.

▼ PARANEOPLASTIC SYNDROMES

Many tumors develop the ability to elaborate hormones or cytokines that can have deleterious consequences for the host. Host antibodies to tumor antigens are also thought to play a role in the development of paraneoplastic syndromes. These immune effects probably result from cross-reaction with normal tissue antigens and immune complex deposition. Paraneoplastic syndromes can be systemic or can affect only a single organ system. Included in the paraneoplastic syndromes are the common cancer sequelae of hypercoagulopathy, cachexia, fevers, and anemia of chronic disease. More specific effects are summarized in Table 44–9.

Paraneoplastic syndromes occur in approximately 10% of all patients with advanced malignant disease. Rarely, these syndromes represent the earliest manifestations of an occult cancer. The presence of a paraneoplastic syndrome does not necessarily signify incurable disease, and treatment of the primary tumor can eliminate the related symptoms.

Endocrinopathies are familiar paraneoplastic syndromes, and they are readily understood because they result from the elaboration of true hormones or peptides that mimic naturally occurring hormones. The most common endocrinopathy is

Table 44–9. Paraneoplastic Syndromes.

Syndrome	Associated Cancers	Suspected Causal Mechanisms
Cushing syndrome	Lung, pancreatic, adrenal and neural tumors	ACTH or ACTH-like molecules
Syndrome of inappropriate ADH secretion	Lung and intracranial tumors	ADH secretion
Hypercalcemia	Lung, breast, parathyroid, renal, myeloma, prostate, and ovarian cancers	Osteolytic metastases or parathyroid hormone–related peptide
Hypoglycemia	Sarcomas, islet cell tumors, hepatocellular carcinoma	Insulin or insulinlike peptides
Myasthenia	Thymomas and lung cancer	Autoimmune
Encephalomyelitis	Lung, ovarian, and breast cancer	Autoimmune
Neuropathies	Myeloma, lung, breast, and ovarian cancer	Autoimmune
Cerebellar atrophy	Breast and ovarian cancer	Autoimmune
Acanthosis nigricans	Gastric, lung, and uterine cancer	Autoimmune
Dermatomyositis	Lung and breast cancer	Autoimmune
Venous thrombosis	Multiple cancers	Tumor products that activate clotting factors
DIC	Pancreas, lung, stomach, and prostate cancer	Tumor products that activate and consume clotting factors
Hypertrophic osteoarthropathy	Lung cancer	Unknown

Cushing syndrome, which results from tumor production of adrenocorticotropic hormone (ACTH) or an ACTH-like peptide. The production of these mediators leads to excessive cortisol production and its associated stigmas, including truncal obesity, moon facies, weakness, hypertension, and glucose intolerance. Bronchogenic carcinomas, thymomas, medullary thyroid cancers, and carcinoids are frequent causes of Cushing syndrome. Direct elaboration of cortisol from adrenal neoplasms may also lead to Cushing syndrome.

Hypercalcemia is another common paraneoplastic syndrome. Hypercalcemia of malignancy can generally be attributed to one of two causes. Multiple myeloma and cancers that metastasize to bone can raise serum calcium levels through lytic bone metastases. Solid tumors such as breast, lung, and renal cancers can secrete a molecule called parathyroid hormone–related peptide (PTHrP), which resembles parathyroid hormone. This molecule can bind parathyroid hormone receptors and mimic the action of parathyroid hormone. PTHrP is not subject to feedback inhibition like parathyroid hormone, and elaboration of large quantities of this molecule can cause severe hypercalcemia.

The neuromyopathic syndromes are presumed to result from cross-reaction of antitumor antibodies with neuronal cells. In some cases, neurologic deficits are the first manifestations of an occult cancer. The paraneoplastic syndromes can involve every level of the central and peripheral nervous system from the cerebral cortex to the neuromuscular junction. Individuals may present with symptoms predominantly affecting one particular element of the nervous system, or they may present with diffuse nervous system involvement. Common central nervous system syndromes include cerebellar degeneration, encephalitis, and myelopathies of the spinal cord. Peripheral involvement can manifest as polyneuropathy, myositis, or myasthenic syndromes similar to myasthenia gravis. The most common cancers causing neuromyopathic syndromes are small cell carcinoma of the lung, breast carcinoma, gynecologic cancers, and thymic tumors.

The etiology of the dermatologic syndromes is unclear, but they are theorized to result from either autoimmunity or tumor elaboration of growth factors. Acanthosis nigricans is characterized by the appearance of gray-black hyperkeratotic patches on the skin. Although these lesions may occur sporadically, they are often associated with neoplasms, including lung cancer, gastric carcinoma, uterine cancer, and melanomas.

Darnell RB, Posner JB: Paraneoplastic syndromes affecting the nervous system. Semin Oncol 2006;33:270.

Posner JB: Paraneoplastic syndromes: a brief review. Ann N Y Acad Sci 1997;835:83.

Thirkill CE: Immune-mediated paraneoplasia. Br J Biomed Sci 2006;63:185.

Organ Transplantation

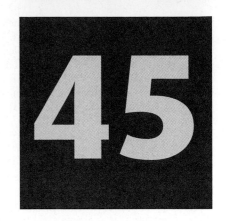

Jeffrey D. Punch, MD

The ability to transplant human organs successfully has developed in the span of a single generation of physicians and surgeons. This remarkable achievement is an excellent example of how animal models may be used to understand and develop treatments for human disease. Organ transplantation is now the preferred treatment modality for a variety of different types of organ failure. Transplantation offers not only improved long-term survival but also improved quality of life for many patients afflicted by renal, hepatic, cardiac, and pulmonary failure.

Enormous effort is currently being expended to develop methods of artificially replacing vital organ functions. Despite these efforts, the ability to replace organ function with mechanical or biomechanical devices remains elusive. While hemodialysis can replace renal function effectively, it offers neither a normal quality of life nor a normal life span. Despite major advances in artificial heart technology, current systems have not reached the point where they can be used routinely to restore normal cardiac function. To date, there are no effective replacements for hepatic or pulmonary function that are suitable for long-term use. Organ transplantation is frequently the only treatment modality that offers a normal lifestyle for patients with advanced organ failure. This chapter discusses the indications for organ transplantation as well as the limitations to the current state of the art.

KIDNEY TRANSPLANTATION

With the exception of organs from a genetically identical twin (**isografts**), all organs from genetically dissimilar individuals (**allografts**) will naturally be subjected to immunologic rejection. This fundamental biologic limitation has largely been overcome by the development of targeted immunosuppression therapies. These therapies are able to suppress the immunological reactivity that produces graft rejection while leaving intact sufficient immune competency to allow recovery from most infectious diseases. The same degree of success

has not been reached when transplanting organs between species (xenografts).

Once it was realized that allografts failed due to an active immunologic attack of the recipient's immune system on the donor organ, methods of suppressing the immune system were investigated. Early attempts at immunosuppression with substances such as nitrogen mustard and total lymphoid irradiation were unsuccessful because of the toxicity of the therapy. The first practical immunosuppressant was azathioprine, an antimetabolite inhibitor of DNA synthesis. When used in combination with corticosteroids, the first successful combination of immunosuppressants was born and the first boom in the number of transplants occurred. This combination remained the state of the art until it was realized that the cell type that exerts primary control over allograft rejection is the T lymphocyte. This led to the later development of agents able to specifically inhibit activation and proliferation of T cells. The result was immunosuppressants that were both more effective and much less toxic than the azathioprine/corticosteroids combination. These agents ushered in a further acceleration in the number of transplants occurring, because now it was possible to transplant organs between individuals who did not share human leukocyte antigens.

Almost all renal diseases responsible for renal failure can be treated by transplantation. Diabetes is the most common cause of chronic renal failure in adults and accounts for 45% of all renal failure in the United States. The second most common cause is hypertensive nephropathy (27%), followed by chronic glomerulonephritis (11%). The causes of renal failure in children are somewhat different, with congenital causes, including both nonobstructive and obstructive uropathies, predominating.

IMMUNOLOGIC RESPONSES

▶ HLA Histocompatibility Antigens

The **major histocompatibility (MHC)** antigens are the most antigenic proteins on donor organs, meaning that they cause the most intense immune responses when the donor and recipient do not share the same antigens. The MHC genes are coded by a single chromosomal complex of closely linked genes on the short arm of the sixth chromosome. This complex consists of at least seven loci that code for genes involved with histocompatibility: human lymphocyte antigen (HLA)-A, HLA-B, HLA-C, HLA-D, HLA-DR, HLA-DQ, and HLA-DP. Each HLA gene locus is highly polymorphic, so that as many as 50 or more discrete antigens are controlled by each locus. The collection of HLA genes in an MHC complex is termed a **haplotype.**

Histocompatibility antigens are grouped into class I (A, B, and C) and class II (DR, DQ, DP) antigens. Class I antigens are composed of a 45-kDa heavy chain with three globular extracellular domains ($\alpha1$, $\alpha2$, $\alpha3$) that confers HLA specificity, a transmembrane portion, and an intracellular domain. Class I antigens are stabilized by β_2-microglobulin, a 12-kDa protein that is not encoded in the MHC complex. Class I antigens are expressed on all nucleated cells and interact primarily with CD8+ T cells. Class II antigens are composed of two noncovalently linked chains: a 33-kDa α chain and a 28-kDa β chain. Each chain has two extracellular domains that confer HLA specificities. Class II antigens are only constitutively expressed on B cells and antigen-presenting cells (macrophages, monocytes, dendritic cells) but can be induced on activated T cells and endothelial cells. Class II antigens interact primarily with CD4+ T cells. The three most important antigens clinically in solid organ transplantation are A, B, and DR. Since each person has two MHC complexes, one on each copy of chromosome 6, everyone has a total of six HLA antigens that are relevant to organ transplantation.

The 3D structures of both class I and II molecules are similar. The extracellular domains form a β-pleated sheet with two looping α-helices that creates a groove facing away from the cell. Following ribosomal synthesis, during assembly of the HLA antigens, peptides are added to this groove. Intracellularly derived peptides are added to class I antigens in the endoplasmic reticulum, while extracellularly derived proteins are added to class II antigens. The end of the groove on class II antigens is open, allowing class II antigens to accommodate longer peptides. Antigenic determinants are found predominantly on the $\alpha1$ and $\alpha2$ chains of the class I molecule and on the β chain of the class II molecule. Some antigenic determinants are shared by many different HLA allotypes. These common determinants are called **public specificities.** Antigenic determinants that are only found on a unique HLA antigen are termed **private specificities.**

Lymphocytes are categorized as either B or T cells. B cells are responsible for antibody production. T cells are categorized into two functional subsets: helper cells that are CD4+ and cytotoxic T cells that are CD8+. Helper T cells preferentially recognize peptides displayed in the groove of class II antigens, while cytotoxic T cells preferentially recognize peptides displayed by class I antigens. A third type of T cell

called regulatory T cells has recently been identified and may be either CD4+ or CD8+. Helper T cells direct both the formation of cytotoxic T cells, which are able to cause graft destruction directly, and the maturation of B cells. Helper T cells can be further subdivided based on their cytokine secretion profile into type 1 and type 2 cells. Type 1 helper T cells secrete interleukin (IL)-2, interferon (IFN)-γ, IL-12, and TNF-α. These cytokines stimulate delayed-type hypersensitivity, cytolytic activity, and the development of complement-fixing IgG antibodies. Type 2 helper T cells secrete IL-4, IL-5, IL-10, and IL-13. These cytokines activate eosinophils and cause the production of IgE antibodies.

Allograft rejection begins when foreign antigen is taken up by an antigen-presenting cell, processed, and presented to helper T cells. The T cell is activated in response to properly presented antigen and secretes cytokines that in turn recruit and activate additional lymphocytes and cause them to begin to clonally proliferate. Cytokines released in the allograft milieu by other cells, including macrophages, contribute to the generation of the immune response as well. Helper T cells also stimulate the differentiation and proliferation of cytotoxic T cells and B cells.

B-cell activation induces the production of specific antibodies directed against donor antigens. This response is important, especially for class I antigens. Recipients who develop a primary immunological response to a particular antigen and produce cytotoxic antibodies directed against the donor HLA will often retain memory B cells and maintain the ability to produce antibodies that are directed against that particular HLA allotype. Upon reexposure to the same antigens, an immediate destructive reaction to the graft—called hyperacute rejection—occurs. Antibody directed against the donor vascular endothelium triggers fixation of complement, direct cellular damage, and the formation of platelet and fibrin plugs, leading to microvascular thrombosis and ischemic necrosis of the organ. Transplantation in the presence of cytotoxic anti-HLA antibody directed against a donor organ is prevented in practice by performing a complement-mediated cytotoxic crossmatch with pretransplant recipient sera against lymphocytes from the potential donor.

▶ Histocompatibility Testing, Crossmatching, & Blood Group Compatibility

Grafts between identical twins are rare but very successful because immunosuppressive therapy is not required when there is no antigenic difference between the donor and recipient. Grafts between HLA-identical siblings who share two HLA haplotypes give the next best results. One fourth of any given sibling pair will share both HLA haplotypes and thus share all of the same HLA antigens. Despite sharing HLA, immunosuppression is still required because of incompatibilities at minor histocompatibility loci. Parents, offspring, and half of siblings share one HLA haplotype. One fourth of siblings will not share an HLA haplotype and will therefore share antigens only by chance. The same is true for genetically unrelated donor/recipient pairs such as spouses and friends. At one time, HLA compatibility was considered to be crucial because there were large differences between graft survival depending on the degree of histocompatibility. Transplants between individuals who shared many HLA antigens were much more likely to avoid graft loss compared to donor/recipient pairs who did not share HLA antigens. This has changed due to the ability of modern immunosuppression to provide for excellent immunological outcome even in the setting of complete HLA mismatch. HLA testing is now of much lesser value than it once was. HLA histocompatibility testing is now primarily of value in determining which of several donors has the best histologic match to the intended recipient. Kidney allocation from deceased donors was once heavily influenced by HLA matching. This has now changed because of the realization that the degree of HLA match has a relatively unimportant effect on the odds of successful outcome. The newest allocation strategy relies more on waiting time and less on the degree of HLA match. Kidneys from donors who share all six HLA antigens with a recipient on the waiting list are still allocated first to any recipient who happens to be a "perfect match." This situation is uncommon, affecting fewer than 10% of the kidneys from deceased donors.

Regardless of the results of tissue typing and antigen matching, it is essential to determine whether a recipient has preformed antibodies against donor antigens, since their presence would result in a hyperacute rejection of the graft as described previously. Preexisting antibodies may develop because of prior exposure to foreign histocompatibility antigens in the form of blood transfusion, pregnancy, or previous organ transplants.

These antibodies are identified by performing a crossmatch between the patient's serum against the donor's lymphocytes. Multiple methods of performing the crossmatch are available with varying degrees of sensitivity and specificity. It is difficult to find an appropriate donor with a negative crossmatch for patients who have antibodies directed against multiple HLA specificities. Some of these patients can be treated with desensitization strategies to reduce their burden of circulating antibodies. Methods being currently investigated include plasmapheresis, infusion of random donor immune globulin, and anti–B cell monoclonal antibodies. Experience is accumulating with desensitization protocols suggesting that donor/recipient pairs with positive crossmatches can sometimes be successfully transplanted. The long-term outcome for these kidneys is unclear.

The ABO blood group antigens behave as strong histocompatibility antigens for kidney transplantation; therefore, ABO-incompatible kidney transplants have generally been considered an absolute impossibility. It is certainly true that ABO-incompatible kidneys will fail rapidly if nothing is done to reduce the amount of antibody directed against the incompatible antigen in the recipient's serum. Success is now being reported for AB-incompatible kidney transplants using combinations of anti–B cell therapy and plasmapheresis.

Klein J, Sato A: The HLA system. (Two parts.) N Engl J Med 2000; 343:702.

► Immunosuppressive Drug Therapy

Multiple immunosuppressive strategies are effective at preventing acute allograft rejection. Most strategies involve the use of more than one agent. Conceptually, using multiple immunosuppressive agents has the effect of blocking multiple targets in the immune response cascade, which allows relatively low doses of each drug to be used, thus avoiding toxicity associated with high doses of these powerful drugs. Thus, many patients are treated with "triple therapy" using corticosteroids, a calcineurin inhibitor, and either an antimetabolite or a TOR (target of rapamycin) inhibitor. A variant of this strategy, termed "quadruple therapy," involves the initial use of a very potent antilymphocyte agent and chronic administration of the same drugs used for triple therapy. The antibody treatment has two effects: It decreases the likelihood of rejection in the critical first few months after the transplant, and it allows there to be a delay before the introduction of the calcineurin inhibitor. This is advantageous because of the associated nephrotoxicity of calcineurin inhibitors. Since the risk of rejection is highest immediately after the transplant, it is typical to begin with relatively high doses of each agent and gradually taper down to a maintenance level over several weeks to months.

Rejection is diagnosed by biopsy. Patients are followed up with serial measurements of renal function in the form of serum creatinine. When a transplanted kidney begins to function, the serum creatinine will fall gradually over several days to reach a nadir level that becomes a new baseline for the patient. Any significant elevation above the baseline should prompt evaluation as to the cause, and once obstruction, dehydration, and infection have been ruled out, it is usually appropriate to biopsy the kidney graft. Rejection may be treated with high-dose "pulse" corticosteroid therapy over several days or with antilymphocyte antibodies. Rejection therapy is effective in more than 90% of cases.

Many drugs are available today for immunosuppression. All of these drugs share the common side effect of increasing susceptibility to infectious diseases. This is an intrinsic feature of currently available therapy, which aims to suppress natural immune responses against all foreign antigens. When the transplant recipient develops an infection, it is vital that a physician with experience prescribing immunosuppression is involved with the patient's care. In many cases, it is appropriate to temporarily reduce the degree of immunosuppression in order to allow recovery from the infection. Precisely how this is accomplished varies widely among practitioners, but it generally involves lowering the dosage or withholding one or more of the agents being used for maintenance immunosuppression. When the infection has resolved, immunosuppression is restored to an acceptable maintenance regimen. It is appropriate to individualize therapy because different individuals have different propensities to develop both rejection and infection.

Many long-term immunosuppressive therapies are associated with the development of malignancy, especially skin cancer and lymphomas. Patients receiving chronic immunosuppression should pay particular attention to minimizing direct exposure to ultraviolet radiation. Since many skin cancers are treatable with simple resection, it is also important that transplant physicians are careful to monitor for and treat skin lesions that develop in transplant recipients.

In the future, it may be possible either to modify the graft so that it is not viewed as foreign to the recipient's immune system or to modify the recipient's immune system so that it will not reject the graft without altering the immune response to other foreign antigens.

A. Antimetabolites

The antimetabolite drugs include azathioprine, cyclophosphamide, mycophenolate, and leflunomide. These drugs inhibit nucleic acid synthesis, which in turn limits the ability of activated lymphocytes to rapidly clonally expand. In general, these drugs are used to prevent rejection but are not effective at reversing active acute rejection.

Azathioprine, a purine analog, is the original member of this family. The effects of this drug are not specific to lymphocytes; therefore, the drug also frequently causes decreased levels of circulating neutrophils and platelets. This side effect is dose dependent.

Cyclophosphamide is an alkylating agent that is a common component of chemotherapy protocols. It is an effective immunosuppressant when given in high doses, but it has been used only very infrequently in clinical transplantation.

Mycophenolate is an inhibitor of inosine monophosphate dehydrogenase, a critical enzyme in the de novo synthesis pathway of purines. Lymphocytes uniquely depend on the de novo pathway to synthesize purines, while other cells are able to utilize a salvage pathway for synthesis. Mycophenolate is therefore more specific for lymphocytes than the other antimetabolites. It has largely replaced azathioprine for use in combination with a calcineurin inhibitor and corticosteroids since well-designed studies have shown it to have a superior ability to prevent rejection. Side effects are primarily gastrointestinal in nature.

Leflunomide is a selective inhibitor of de novo pyrimidine synthesis. It is thought to work by inhibiting the enzyme dihydroorotate dehydrogenase. It is used widely for treatment of rheumatoid arthritis. Clinical trials have demonstrated it to be efficacious in terms of preventing rejection, but it is difficult to use clinically because of its long half-life (15–18 days).

B. Corticosteroids

Corticosteroids used in combination with azathioprine was the first combination of immunosuppressants with the ability to prevent the development of allograft rejection, and high doses of corticosteroids was the first practical and effective means of reversing established rejection. Hence, over the past 40 years, corticosteroids have been a component of most successful immunosuppressive protocols. Typically, a high dose of intravenous corticosteroids is given at the time of engraftment, and the dose is tapered over weeks to months down to a maintenance dosage of 0.1–0.2 mg/kg of oral prednisone. In the recent past, there has been strong interest in discontinuation of corticosteroids—and even more recently, in developing protocols that do not require the administration of any corticosteroids. The evidence is accumulating that this treatment is appropriate and effective for some low-risk renal transplant recipients, but the use of corticosteroid-free protocols for higher-risk candidates—including those with known sensitization to HLA and patients undergoing second renal transplants—is more controversial.

Corticosteroid therapy is associated with many different side effects, including infection, weight gain, cushingoid features, hypertension, increased bruisability, hyperlipidemia, hyperglycemia, and acne. Daily corticosteroid therapy in children may inhibit somatic growth. This may be circumvented to some degree by alternate-day treatment, administering the drug once in the morning every other day.

Corticosteroids are standard therapy for a rejection episode, typically consisting of three or more daily doses of between 100 mg and 500 mg of intravenous methylprednisolone ("steroid pulses"). Depending on the severity of the rejection, steroid pulses will resolve 50–80% of allograft rejection episodes.

C. Calcineurin Inhibitors

Transplantation was revolutionized by the introduction of the first calcineurin inhibitor, cyclosporine, into clinical practice in the early 1980s. Cyclosporine is a cyclic undecapeptide isolated from a fungus. It is a potent immunosuppressant and the first compound identified that can inhibit immunocompetent lymphocytes specifically and reversibly. Cyclosporine was followed by the introduction of tacrolimus, another compound derived from a fungus that also inhibits calcineurin. The primary mechanism of these agents appears to be inhibition of the production and release of IL-2 by helper T cells. They also interfere with the release of IL-1 by macrophages as well as with proliferation of B lymphocytes. Blood levels must be carefully monitored because both drugs are nephrotoxic and neurotoxic at higher levels. They also both have chronic effects on renal function and lead to significant long-term renal dysfunction in many patients who take them chronically. Both cyclosporine and tacrolimus are also associated with an increased incidence of neoplasms, particularly lymphomas.

D. Inhibitors of Mammalian Target of Rapamycin

Sirolimus is a macrocyclic triene antibiotic produced by a species of *Streptomyces*. It was originally developed as an antifungal and antitumor agent but was found to have significant immunosuppressive properties. The effect of sirolimus is believed to relate to inhibition of lymphocyte transduction pathways through binding to the mammalian target of rapamycin. It functions as an antiproliferative and prevents not only expansion of lymphocyte clones but also smooth muscle proliferation. It is known to effectively prevent rejection in combination with a calcineurin inhibitor. The major advantages of this drug are that it does not cause renal dysfunction and its antiproliferative properties suggest that it will not be associated with the same risk of developing long-term malignancy. Side effects, in addition to the infections associated with immunosuppression, include oral ulcerations, wound healing problems associated with its ability to inhibit smooth muscle proliferation, and significant hyperlipidemias. An association with hepatic artery thrombosis has also been noted in patients receiving sirolimus therapy as part of their initial immunosuppression regimen following liver transplantation.

Everolimus is a derivative of sirolimus that also acts as a mammalian target of rapamycin inhibitor. It has a side effect profile similar to that of sirolimus but a shorter serum half-life.

E. Polyclonal Antithymoblast or Antilymphocyte Globulin and Antithymocyte Globulin

Antilymphoblast globulin and antithymocyte globulin are polyclonal antibody preparations derived by immunizing animals against some type of human lymphocytes and collecting and purifying the antibodies that animals develop in response to the foreign antigenic proteins. They are potent drugs that deplete circulating lymphocytes, an effect that can be measured and followed by flow cytometry or by simply following the complete blood count with differential. Because they are polyclonal, they not only are effective against T cells but also may have important effects against circulating B cells and natural killer cells.

These agents are particularly effective in induction of immunosuppressive therapy and in the treatment of established rejection that is either severe or resistant to pulse corticosteroid therapy. Therapy is typically given daily for 5–7 days. The effect of these agents is profound immunosuppression that lasts for weeks to months. They are associated with increased incidence of viral infections because of their effects on cellular immunity and also with a higher lifetime risk of developing malignancy, particularly B-cell lymphoma.

Side effects are many and include fevers and chills, neutropenia, and thrombocytopenia. Fever, chills, and malaise occur because of mediator release by T cells and circulating mononuclear cells, especially TNF-α, IL-1, and IL-6, that occurs when the antibody is bound to certain cell surface receptors. The symptoms are very similar to those associated with an acute viral infection. These effects are usually transient, often lasting less than 12 hours. They occur primarily following the first or second dose of the treatment and can be attenuated markedly by pretreatment with corticosteroids,

acetaminophen, and diphenhydramine. Neutropenia and thrombocytopenia occur because of direct antibody binding to these cell types, causing depletion. This effect is also transient and tends to resolve in 24–48 hours. It is necessary to monitor neutrophil and platelet counts during therapy and withhold doses of the treatment if the counts drop to dangerously low levels.

F. Monoclonal Antibody Therapy

The knowledge that the T cell is central to the development of allograft rejection led to the development of agents that selectively inhibit or deplete T cells, or both. The first example of such an agent is the monoclonal antibody OKT3 (muromonab-CD3), which is secreted by a hybridoma in culture. This agent may have some advantages over antilymphoblast globulin and antithymocyte globulin preparations in management of rejection because it specifically blocks T-cell generation and function. Because it is a monoclonal antibody and reacts with a defined antigen, it can be consistently produced with a defined activity and without unwanted reactivities against other cells like neutrophils and platelets. OKT3 is most effective in the treatment of steroid-resistant rejection, where more than 90% of rejection episodes are reversed, thus obviating further high-dose steroids. The downside of this antibody treatment is that since it is a murine monoclonal antibody, it may induce recipient antibody directed against the murine antibody molecule. This effect occurs in 5–10% of patients treated with OKT3 and may decrease the efficacy of the treatment if given a second or third time. Like the polyclonal antilymphocyte preparations, treatment is usually given daily for 5–7 days. Side effects due to cytokine release are typically more severe than those seen with polyclonal agents but may also be attenuated with appropriate pretreatment. Since the antibody does not bind to epitopes other than the CD3 molecule, which is found only on T cells, it does not cause cytopenias.

The success of OKT3 led to the development of a new generation of monoclonal antibodies that are "humanized." The monoclonal antibody molecule has been modified by genetic engineering to avoid the side effects seen with OKT3. The genetic code directing the production of the antibody molecule by the hybridoma has been altered by replacing most of the murine portion of the sequence with human antibody sequence. The antibody is thus chimeric, or "humanized" since only the highly variable portion of the antibody that binds to the antigenic epitope is foreign to the human recipient. Cytokine release therefore does not occur when the antibody is administered, nor is it likely that the recipient will develop neutralizing antibodies against the monoclonal preparation. Because the antibodies so closely resemble human immunoglobulin, they also have a long circulating half-life.

The first of these agents, daclizumab and basiliximab, bind to CD25, the high-affinity subunit of the T-cell receptor for IL-2. Since IL-2 is necessary for T-cell activation and proliferation, these agents have the ability to selectively inhibit the expansion of T-cell clones that are activated at the time of transplantation, without effecting existing T-cell immunity to other antigens. Existing cellular immunity to viruses, for example, is left intact. Induction treatment with anti-CD25 antibodies at the time of engraftment has been shown to reduce the incidence of future rejection episodes.

A more recent agent, alemtuzumab (Campath-1H), is a depleting humanized monoclonal antibody that binds to CD52, an antigen found on all peripheral blood mononuclear cells. Alemtuzumab administration causes a profound and sustained depletion of T cells from peripheral blood that lasts for many months. It similarly depletes B cells, natural killer cells, and monocyte, but to a lesser degree. Alemtuzumab is currently approved for treatment of patients with some forms of chronic lymphocytic leukemia. It is being used by some transplant centers for initial induction immunosuppression and for treatment of rejection.

Carpenter CB: Immunosuppression in organ transplantation. N Engl J Med 1990;322:1224.

Krieger NR, Emre S: Novel immunosuppressants. Pediatr Transpl 2004;8:596.

Levy G et al: Safety, tolerability, and efficacy of everolimus in de novo liver transplant recipients: 12- and 36-month results. [Erratum appears in Liver Transpl 2006;12:1726]. Liver Transpl 2006;12:1640.

Mourad G et al: Induction versus noninduction in renal transplant recipients with tacrolimus-based immunosuppression. Transplantation 2001;72:1050.

SOURCES OF DONOR KIDNEYS

The two sources of kidneys for renal transplantation are living donors and deceased donors. Approximately one third of patients who are acceptable candidates for transplantation will have a willing and medically suitable living donor. ABO-compatible donors are not absolutely required today because of the availability of treatments that can reduce the amount of antidonor antibody in the recipient. However, ABO-compatible donors are greatly preferred, because antibody reduction treatments are expensive and associated with infectious risk due to the depletion of protective antibodies.

At one time, only related living donors were acceptable because it was necessary to have closely matched HLA antigens between the donor and recipient in order to achieve acceptable graft survival rates. The graft survival rate for donor/recipient pairs who do not share any HLA antigens is now greater than 90%, leading transplant programs to accept increasing numbers of donors who are not genetically related to the recipients. It is now common practice to accept volunteer donors who are spouses, in-laws, friends, coworkers, and even members of the same community who may be only acquaintances. More controversial is a recent trend for patients and donors to meet through Internet web sites. Despite initial hesitancy to condone this method of finding a living donor, it has been difficult for the transplant commu-

nity to make value judgements about the relationship between living donors and recipients as long as both parties are fully informed and committed.

Recently, programs have begun arranging transplants between two or more pairs of living donors and recipients who participate in a paired exchange. Recipients with willing but incompatible donors are paired with another donor/recipient pair who have the same problem. The outcome from paired donation transplants has been similar to that seen with other living donor transplants.

Living donors should be in good health both physically and psychologically. Above all, the living donor should be a volunteer and must clearly understand the nature of the procedure so that informed consent to the operation can be given. Donors should generally be of legal age, but reasonable exceptions have been made in extenuating circumstances, particularly when an identical twin donor is available. In these circumstances, it is wise for the program to assign to the donor an outside advocate who has no relationship with either the recipient or the remainder of the family to ensure that the minor is not coerced into proceeding.

▶ Living Donors

Live kidney donors are now as common as deceased donors, although since each deceased donor can donate two kidneys, the total number of kidneys from deceased donors still far exceeds that obtained from living donors. Because of the biological ability of the body to compensate for the loss of one kidney, renal function tends to stabilize at approximately 75–80% of the original renal function a few months following donation. Follow-up studies on donors show that they have good renal function and do not appear to suffer ill effects from the procedure, either physically or psychologically. Women with one kidney do not have an increased incidence of urinary infections during pregnancy.

There are at least two methods of performing donor nephrectomy in common practice: open nephrectomy and laparoscopic nephrectomy. Open nephrectomy, long the standard method, involves a flank incision about 15 cm long below the 12th rib. The peritoneum is retracted medially, and the kidney is removed along with its vessels and ureter without disturbing the intra-abdominal contents. More recently, laparoscopic techniques have been developed to allow the removal of a kidney for transplantation. The donor is placed under general anesthesia, and the abdomen is insufflated with carbon dioxide to allow visualization of the abdominal structures. Some surgeons use a large port in the midline, just above the umbilicus, to insert their hand into the abdomen. The kidney is then withdrawn through the hand port once it has been dissected free from surrounding tissues and the vessels and ureter have been divided. It is also possible to remove the kidney using purely laparoscopic techniques without inserting a hand port. The kidney is removed by placing it in a bag inside the abdomen and withdrawing the bag through a low transverse incision. Laparoscopic nephrectomy tends to take longer than a nephrectomy through an open approach, but it is associated with somewhat less postoperative pain and a briefer period of convalescence. Prospective donors should be informed about the options for nephrectomy and the advantages and disadvantages of each technique as well as the associated risk and the known complications.

The main risk to a donor is the anesthesia and the operation itself. The mortality rate is estimated to be 0.03%, and most deaths are not judged to be preventable but appear to be intrinsic risks of having a major operation. The most common significant complications following nephrectomy are wound related, including infection and hernia formation. These complications occur in less than 1–3% of cases. Wound infections typically respond to dressing changes, and hernias require operative repair.

The evaluation of a living donor must be thorough and complete. It is first necessary to make sure that the donor is truly a volunteer and is not being coerced or unfairly influenced by the recipient or other family members. This often involves a careful evaluation by an individual with excellent understanding of the transplant process as well as excellent communication skills. It is advisable that this portion of the interview be conducted in private so that donors can be honest about their feelings. Transplant social workers, psychologists, and psychiatrists are typically involved with this aspect of donor selection. Once it is clear that the donor is genuinely seeking to donate of his or her own accord, a detailed history is taken, and a physical examination is performed. Factors that may affect operative risk as well as future risk of renal failure are carefully sought out. The routine workup includes chest x-ray, electrocardiography, urinalysis, complete blood count, fasting blood glucose, serum bilirubin, hepatic transaminases, serum creatinine, and blood urea nitrogen. If these are normal, the kidneys are imaged radiographically to make sure that two kidneys are present, to rule out intrinsic or structural renal disease, and to evaluate the vasculature of the kidneys. Angiography, CT, and MRI are all methods that can be used. Kidneys with multiple renal arteries may be transplanted, but care must be taken in the anastomosis of small accessory vessels, particularly when they come from the lower pole and may therefore provide the sole vascular supply to the ureter. When there are multiple renal veins, the smaller veins can often be ligated, since there is free communication of the veins within the kidney.

▶ Deceased Donors

Two thirds of eligible kidney recipients do not have a suitable living donor. These patients are placed on a waiting list for a kidney from a deceased donor. Since more patients are added to the list each year, the number of patients waiting for a kidney from a deceased donor grows longer each year and will exceed 100,000 in the United States by 2010.

Kidneys can be successfully transplanted from donors who are declared dead on the basis of brain death or from donors who die of cessation of spontaneous cardiovascular activity.

Brain death is now widely accepted in principle in the United States, and all hospitals have protocols to be followed to ensure that the diagnosis of brain death is confirmed without any doubt.

Consent for donation should always be obtained by individuals with training in how to approach the family of the donors. In this way, the family can be given time to grieve and express the inevitable sorrow and anger that accompanies the death of a loved one. Individuals who are not part of the team caring for the patient are best able to provide the emotional support that families need during this time. The discussion regarding donation can then occur separate from the discussion in which the family learns that their loved one has died.

Kidneys from brain-dead donors are removed operatively. The excision of the kidneys occurs operatively following in situ cold perfusion and exsanguination of the kidneys, often in concert with the removal of other transplantable abdominal and thoracic organs. The kidneys are perfused with specially designed preservative solutions and kept cold. Successful transplantation has been reported following cold storage of more than 72 hours, but optimal results are achieved if the kidney is transplanted as soon as possible following removal from the donor, preferable within 24 hours.

Kidneys may also be transplanted from deceased donors following cardiopulmonary death, a practice termed "donation following cardiac death." The most common circumstance under which this occurs in the United States is when medical therapy that is judged to be futile is withdrawn from an individual. Typically, patients have suffered profound, irreversible brain injury and have essentially no conscious awareness and no potential for meaningful recovery. Standard medical practice in this circumstance is to recommend withdrawal of life-sustaining support such as mechanical respiration and intravenous infusions, since the vast majority of people state that they would not want to be kept alive in such a hopeless state. Withdrawal of support always occurs with the consent and understanding of the family. The decision to donate organs should be made separate from the decision to withdraw medical therapy. Once consent is obtained and preparation for donation is completed, support is withdrawn by the primary care team. When cardiopulmonary activity ceases, the primary physician team declares death, and the organs are then excised as with brain-dead donors.

SELECTION OF RECIPIENTS

Patients with chronic renal failure should be considered for transplantation. Acute renal failure on the basis of acute tubular necrosis can usually be managed with temporary dialysis, and therefore kidney transplantation is not appropriate in this setting. It is not necessary for patients to be on dialysis at the time of transplantation. In fact, results for patients who receive kidney transplants prior to beginning dialysis have the best chance of graft survival, while patients who had long-term dialysis prior to transplantation have poorer success rates. It is therefore important to begin consideration for renal transplantation as soon as dialysis appears to be inevitable and imminent within the next year.

During the early years of renal transplantation, most of the patients accepted for transplantation were between 15 and 45 years old. In recent years, the age range has been extended in both directions—children younger than age 1 and adults who are over 70 years old have received transplants. For many years, the success rates for transplanting in young children was inferior to that achieved with adults, but this problem has now been corrected. Even children younger than 1 year of age at the time of transplantation can be expected to have an excellent chance of graft survival.

Historically, there has been reluctance to perform renal transplants in the elderly. However, as the practice of renal transplantation continues to improve, with less toxic and more effective immunosuppression and more effective methods of preventing posttransplant infections, this unwillingness appears less justified. Elderly individuals naturally have a shorter life span, but to date, patients over 60 years old who receive transplants appear to enjoy approximately the same degree of improvement in life expectancy as do younger patients.

This benefit has been quantified by comparing the mortality rate of suitable candidates awaiting kidney transplantation with the mortality rate following transplantation. Life expectancy appears to be approximately doubled by kidney transplantation in all age ranges that have been studied to date. The improved life expectancy following kidney transplantation is particularly dramatic for diabetic patients. Today, patients tend to be judged on the basis of their physiologic functional status rather than on their chronological age. It is nevertheless true that elderly patients are more commonly found to be poor candidates for transplantation because of either coexisting disease or poor functional status.

Candidates must be free of active infections at the time of transplantation. Chronically infected tissues such as chronic pyelonephritis or chronic osteomyelitis should be definitively treated prior to consideration for transplantation. Patients with active viral or bacterial infection at the time an organ is available for transplantation should usually be deferred until the infection has resolved. This is because it is unwise to initiate immunosuppression during an active infection, particularly given that the highest doses of immunosuppression are given around the time of the procedure.

Recipients with almost all types of primary renal disease have been successfully transplanted: glomerulonephritis, hypertensive nephropathy, chronic pyelonephritis, polycystic kidney disease, reflux pyelonephritis, Goodpasture syndrome, congenital renal hypoplasia, renal cortical necrosis, Fabry syndrome, and Alport syndrome. Successful transplants have been achieved in patients with certain systemic diseases in which the kidney is one of the end organs affected (cystinosis, systemic lupus erythematosus, and diabetic nephropathy). Renal transplantation is generally inadvisable in patients with oxalosis if high serum levels of oxalate are present because the disease recurs in the transplant quickly. However, liver transplantation corrects the enzymatic defect that leads to excessive oxalate accumulation. Therefore, combined liver-kidney transplantation may be an acceptable treatment option for these patients.

Patients who do not have normal bladder function may be acceptable kidney transplant candidates, but a plan for ureteral drainage should be made before transplantation occurs. Many patients with long-term defunctionalized bladders can still undergo ureteral reimplantation and then be treated with intermittent catheterization if necessary posttransplant. If the bladder is congenitally or surgically absent, a defunctionalized loop of small bowel can be created, brought out as a stoma, and used for a urinary conduit. Care must be taken in planning the positioning of the conduit so that the ureter from a transplanted kidney will reach it.

Transplant patients must be compliant with posttransplant care to achieve successful outcome. Patients with a history of poor compliance may be candidates for transplantation if they are regretful of past behavior and have established a compliant pattern. In some cases, especially in the adolescent age group, it is wise for the patient to experience dialysis prior to receiving a kidney transplant in order to foster a complete understanding of the differences in lifestyle that are afforded by a successful kidney transplant. It is also necessary that patients have a support network to help them manage following the transplant. They will need a way to reliably obtain immunosuppressive therapy as well as transportation to and from the transplant center that is continuously and reliably available. Fortunately, support services are often available to patients who lack social support, and it is rare to deny transplantation solely on the basis of inadequate social support.

In the early years of kidney transplantation, it was common to perform bilateral nephrectomy prior to transplantation, but this has recently become very uncommon. Most patients who have native nephrectomy have polycystic kidney disease with profound pain, recurrent infections, or recurrent hemorrhage. Other indications for native nephrectomy include recurrent infection, especially when associated with ureteral reflux, and occasionally profound hypertension attributable to an ischemic native kidney.

Wolfe RA et al: Comparison of mortality in all patients on dialysis, patients on dialysis awaiting transplantation, and recipients of a first cadaveric transplant. N Engl J Med 1999;341:1725.

OPERATIVE TECHNIQUES

The surgical technique of renal transplantation involves anastomoses of the renal artery and vein and ureter (Figure 45–1). The transplant kidney is placed in the iliac fossa through an oblique lower abdominal incision. The dissection is carried out by retracting the peritoneum medially so the kidney will lie in an extraperitoneal position. The iliac

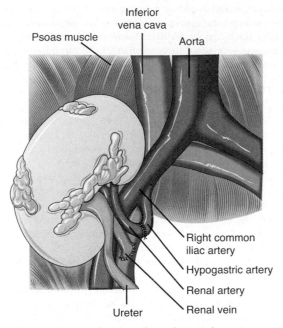

Psoas muscle — Inferior vena cava — Aorta

Right common iliac artery
Hypogastric artery
Renal artery
Renal vein
Ureter

▲ **Figure 45–1.** Technique of renal transplantation.

arteries and veins are mobilized as indicated for the proposed specific anastomoses. An end-to-side anastomosis is performed between renal vein and iliac vein; an end-to-side anastomosis is then performed between the renal artery and the iliac artery. An alternative technique is to connect the renal artery end-to-end to the internal iliac artery, but this technique is more difficult in most patients. When multiple arteries are present, there are several options. If the artery is very small (less than 2 mm), it can often be ligated, especially if it is an upper pole branch. If the kidney is from a deceased donor, it is often possible to use a large Carrell patch of donor aorta that encompasses all of the arteries. Other options include reimplanting multiple renal arteries into the iliac artery using multiple anastomoses; reimplanting a smaller artery into the side of the dominant renal artery and then using the larger artery for anastomoses to the iliac; and spatulating the ends of the two arteries together to form a single lumen for anastomosis.

In small children and infants, the kidney transplant can be performed either through a midline abdominal incision or by making a very large flank-type incision extending from the pubic symphysis to the costal margin and exposing the aorta and vena cava by reflecting the peritoneal contents medially and superiorly. End-to-side anastomoses of the renal vessels may be made to the iliac vessels if they are large enough, but often it is necessary to use the infrarenal vena cava and aorta for the anastomotic site.

Kidneys from small pediatric deceased kidneys function poorly when transplanted into small pediatric recipients.

However, many pediatric kidneys have often been transplanted en bloc with the donor aorta and vena cava anastomosed to the recipient's iliac vessels along with double ureteral anastomoses. The exact age at which it is best to transplant kidneys as a single unit is unclear, but certainly kidneys from children as young as 6 will function well and last a long time when transplanted into adults.

Urinary tract continuity can be established by pyeloureterostomy, ureteroureterostomy, or ureteroneocystostomy. The most common technique is ureteroneocystostomy. This technique can be performed by bringing the ureter into the bladder through a submucosal tunnel and suturing the mucosa of the ureter to the mucosa of the bladder from the inside of the bladder through a large cystotomy (Politano-Leadbetter method). Other techniques include an external neocystostomy, which avoids the need for a large cystotomy, and the "one stitch" technique, whereby the mucosa of the ureter is not directly sutured to the bladder mucosa, but rather the ureter is fixed into place in the interior of the bladder with a suture that traverses the full thickness of the bladder wall. A ureteral stent may be placed with any of the techniques discussed above. A 6Fr pediatric ureteral stent with a J shape at each end fits nicely across the anastomosis and goes from the interior of the renal pelvis into the bladder or other urinary conduit. The stent should be removed in the first month or two following the transplant to prevent stone formation and bladder infection.

POSTOPERATIVE MANAGEMENT & COMPLICATIONS

Recipients who have received a kidney transplant usually produce urine immediately, and the serum creatinine falls over the next 3–7 days. The magnitude of urine output is related to how hydrated the patient was before transplantation and to how much fluid is administered during the procedure. It is important that the patient is fully hydrated at the time the kidney is revascularized in order to achieve the best chance of immediate transplant kidney function. Transplanted kidneys frequently will have an obligate diuresis for a period of hours to days after they begin to function. During this phase, it may be necessary to replace urinary output in order to prevent the development of hypovolemia as a result of excess urinary output. Once this phase has passed, intravenous fluid can be discontinued. However, patients are encouraged to maintain generous fluid intake to prevent dehydration in the future, as transplanted kidneys appear to have a greater susceptibility to hypovolemia than native kidneys. Patients are usually able to eat the morning following the transplant procedure and should be encouraged to get out of bed with assistance. The urinary catheter can be removed as early as 2 days following the procedure, depending on the technique used for ureteral anastomosis. Some programs prefer to leave the urinary catheter in place for a longer period of time to allow sufficient healing of the anastomosis. Most recipients are able to be discharged from the hospital on the second or third postoperative day if there are no complications in their postoperative course once they are able to maintain oral hydration, have learned how to properly take their medications, and have received training about what to do, what not to do, and what to watch out for in the next few weeks.

Kidney transplantation can be followed by a variety of postoperative complications that must be recognized and treated early for optimal results. The most frequent complications are infection and rejection, reflecting the natural tension between too much and too little immunosuppression. Urinary infection is one of the most common complications and usually responds to antibiotic therapy. Bacterial pneumonia is the most common pulmonary complication and may be very serious if not promptly diagnosed and treated. Current immunosuppression protocols that focus on the T lymphocyte are associated with unusual, opportunistic types of infections including herpesviruses, the parasite *Pneumocystis carinii*, and fungal infections. These infections are seen much less often than previously because it is standard to prescribe prophylactic anti-infective therapy aimed at preventing the common types of infection. In particular, the availability of agents that are effective against cytomegalovirus (CMV) infection has almost eliminated clinical CMV infections. At one time, CMV infections were a frequent, expensive, and exceedingly unpleasant occurrence after many transplants.

In approximately 20% of kidney transplants from deceased donors, the kidney will fail to function immediately. This complication is termed delayed graft function and is due to acute tubular necrosis of the kidney. In some cases, there is a modest urinary output, but the serum creatinine does not fall. In other cases, there is profound oliguria. Delayed graft function can also occur following living donor transplantation, but it is much less common (less than 3%). Delayed graft function is associated with older donors and donors who had a rising creatinine at the time of donation. Long ischemic times are also known to increase the chance of delayed graft function. In most cases, the acute tubular necrosis will resolve and the renal function will recover. Most recovery happens within a week, but in some cases, the kidney will require several weeks before renal function is sufficient to support the patient without dialysis. Treatment is supportive with dialysis as necessary. If recovery takes more than a week, it may be wise to biopsy the kidney to rule out silent rejection.

Vascular complications of kidney transplants are uncommon, affecting 1–2% of renal transplants. Either renal artery or venous thrombosis of the kidney is devastating and almost uniformly results in graft loss. The incidence of acute graft thrombosis is higher in patients with high levels of circulating anti-HLA antibodies, suggesting that some of these cases are related to accelerated acute rejection. The incidence of graft thrombosis is also higher in patients with factor V Leiden and other physiologic derangements that cause a hypercoagulable state. Patients should be screened for factor V Leiden if they have a history of unusual thrombotic events

and receive anticoagulation perioperatively when it or other known hypercoagulable states are known. Renal artery stenosis, which may be associated with rejection involving the renal artery, is also a rare complication. It can present with severe hypertension. It may be treated surgically or in some cases by percutaneous transluminal balloon angioplasty.

Urologic complications occur in about 4% of patients, most often urinary extravasation from the cystotomy closure or ureteral obstruction. These complications can almost always be managed with percutaneous placement of a nephrostomy tube by an interventional radiologist and are not associated with a higher risk of graft loss.

A complication relatively unique to kidney transplantation is formation of a pelvic lymphocele in the transplant bed. Lymphatic fluid may come from either lymphatics in the hilum of the kidney or from lymphatics disrupted during exposure of the iliac vessels. Careful ligation of the adjacent lymphatics during preparation of the recipient blood vessels may decrease the incidence of this complication. Large lymphoceles may obstruct the ureter or the vasculature of the transplanted kidney, and they occasionally become infected. Sterile lymphoceles may be drained into the peritoneal cavity, while infected lymphoceles need to be drained externally.

Gastrointestinal complications may affect all levels of the intestine, but upper gastrointestinal symptoms, including nausea and abdominal pain, are most common. In many cases, the culprit is the large number of medications that the patient must take. Peptic ulceration was once a major problem for transplant recipients, but this complication has virtually disappeared because of routine use of medications like H_2-blockers and proton pump inhibitors to inhibit the production of gastric acid.

GRAFT REJECTION

Despite advances in immunosuppressive management, rejection is still a major hazard for the postoperative allograft recipient. Most episodes of rejection occur within the first 3 months. There are three basic kinds of rejection:

(1) **Hyperacute rejection** is due to preformed cytotoxic antibodies against donor antigens. Pretransplant crossmatch testing is designed to prevent this type of rejection. This reaction begins soon after completion of the anastomosis, and complete graft destruction occurs in 24–48 hours. Initially, the graft is pink and firm, but it then becomes blue and soft, with evidence of diminished blood flow. There is often no effective method of treating hyperacute rejection, but treatment with plasmapheresis and immunoglobulin infusion may be effective if the diagnosis is made immediately.

(2) **Acute rejection** is the most common type of rejection episode during the first 3 months after transplantation. It is primarily an immune cellular reaction against foreign antigens. The reaction may be predominantly cellular, or there may be a component of antibody-mediated inflammation. Typically, the patient is asymptomatic and the diagnosis of

rejection is suspected on the basis of serial measurement of serum creatinine levels. In severe cases, symptoms may include oliguria, weight gain, and worsened hypertension. Fever and tenderness and enlargement of the graft are uncommon with modern immunosuppressive protocols but used to be seen when only azathioprine and corticosteroids were available. This type of rejection process is usually treated with pulse steroid therapy. If this is unsuccessful, or in very severe cases of acute rejection, either a polyclonal or monoclonal depleting antilymphocyte preparation is used. The vast majority of acute rejection episodes are successfully reversed. Currently, grafts are only lost to rejection when patients are noncompliant or when rejection occurs together with a life-threatening infection, since it is unsafe to enhance the degree of immunosuppression in this setting.

(3) **Chronic rejection** is a late cause of renal deterioration. It is unclear precisely what causes chronic rejection, but the absence of cellular elements on biopsy and the association of antidonor antibodies with chronic graft loss have led to the assumption that it is mediated by humoral factors. It is most often diagnosed on the basis of slowly decreasing renal function in association with proteinuria and hypertension. Chronic rejection is resistant to all known methods of therapy and graft loss will eventually occur, though perhaps not for several years after renal function begins to deteriorate. It is unclear what the relationship is between this pathologic process and the damage produced by chronic calcineurin inhibitor use, which is seen in nonrenal transplant recipients as well. It has recently been uncovered that chronic graft loss is accelerated in patients who experienced rejection in the first year after a transplant, in patients who had delayed graft function, and in patients who received kidneys from marginal donors.

► Differential Diagnosis of Renal Allograft Dysfunction

An unexpected elevation in serum creatinine above baseline levels in a renal transplant recipient has a broad differential diagnosis list. Dehydration should be ruled out by history and physical examination. The medication the patient is taking should be reviewed, paying attention to over-the-counter medications, especially nonsteroidal anti-inflammatory drugs and herbal remedies. These drugs can cause renal dysfunction or can alter the metabolism of immunosuppressant medications and result in blood levels that are either too high or too low. Urinary infection should be ruled out with a urinalysis. If these simple evaluations do not disclose the cause of renal dysfunction, the next step is usually a renal ultrasound to rule out ureteral obstruction, followed by a renal allograft biopsy. This last step is crucial to arriving at the correct diagnosis. A biopsy may disclose acute rejection, or it may show calcineurin inhibitor toxicity. Since the treatment for these conditions is opposite, a biopsy is very important to guide appropriate therapy.

HEART TRANSPLANTATION

The first successful human heart allograft was performed in 1967 by Christiaan Barnard. At that time, however, the only available immunosuppressive therapy was azathioprine and steroids. This regimen was inadequate to safely prevent rejection in these patients. As a result, the procedure remained experimental and was limited to a small number of institutions worldwide. The introduction of cyclosporine in 1981 resulted in dramatically improved survival. As a result, heart transplantation was federally designated as no longer experimental in 1985. In 2003, there were about 2000 heart transplants performed in the United States at more than 100 centers. The 1-year survival rate is now over 85%, and the 3-year survival rate is over 75%.

SELECTION OF DONORS

At one time, deceased donors were considered suitable for cardiac donation only if they were men aged 40 years or younger or women 45 or younger. The large waiting list and the increasing number of patients who die on the waiting list has led surgeons to accept hearts from donors as old as 60, and more than one third of current donors are older than 40. Cardiac donors must be ABO-compatible with the recipient and should be within 20% of the recipient's ideal body weight. Ideally, there should be no history of preexistent or intercurrent cardiac disease. It is routine to obtain echocardiography to determine cardiac function, even in young donors. At many programs, it is routine to obtain cardiac catheterization in older donors to rule out silent coronary artery disease. Ideally, there should be no history of cardiac arrest, but if cardiac function is good, this factor alone does not usually rule out a cardiac donor. The donor should be receiving only moderate doses of pressor drugs.

At the donor operation, the chest is opened and the heart is inspected for evidence of contusion and observed to determine its overall function. If the heart is suitable, this information is relayed to the recipient operating team so that the timing of the recipient operation can be carefully coordinated. The heart is removed following cross-clamping of the aorta and infusion of cold cardioplegia, which results in cessation of electrical and mechanical cardiac activity. The heart is typically removed first, prior to the excision of kidney, liver, or pancreas. It is flushed with a preservative solution and stored aseptically at 4 °C. Optimal function is obtained when the heart is implanted within 4 hours of procurement. For recipients who have previously had cardiac procedures through a sternotomy, it is sometimes necessary to delay the procurement of the donor heart to make sure that the recipient will be ready to receive the heart when it arrives back at the transplant hospital. The same is true when recipients have left ventricular assist devices implanted and extra time is necessary to prepare the recipient to receive the donor heart.

SELECTION OF RECIPIENTS

Patients for cardiac transplantation should have end-stage cardiac disease for which there is no other surgical option and should have received maximal medical treatment. Most heart transplant candidates have idiopathic dilated cardiomyopathy or ischemic cardiomyopathy. Most patients are younger than 55 years of age, but successful transplantation has been reported on more elderly patients. Patients should not have systemic disease that will be worsened by the immunosuppressive regimen (infection, type 1 diabetes, severe peripheral vascular disease, poorly controlled hypertension), nor should they have underlying renal insufficiency that cannot be attributed to low cardiac output.

Patients should have pulmonary vascular resistance of less than 5 Wood units, since levels above this or a pulmonary artery systolic pressure of greater than 50 mm Hg or a transpulmonary gradient (mean pulmonary artery pressure–pulmonary capillary wedge pressure) of greater than 15 mm Hg are associated with inadequate donor heart function. As with other organs, a history of compliance with a complex medical regimen and a strong social support system are necessary for long-term success.

If the recipient has circulating antibodies directed against HLA antigens, it is necessary to perform a crossmatch between the recipient's serum and the donor lymphocytes to make sure that hyperacute rejection of the cardiac graft does not occur. Patients who have left ventricular assist devices in place may be particularly difficult to obtain hearts for because of the sensitizing effect that the device has on the immune system.

OPERATIVE TECHNIQUE

The operative technique originally developed by Lower and Shumway continues to be used and is shown in Figure 45–2. A median sternotomy is performed and the patient is placed on cardiopulmonary bypass. The recipient heart is removed, and the atrial cuffs trimmed. The left atrial anastomosis is performed first and then the right, each with one continuous suture. Before the left atrium is closed, it is filled with saline to avoid air embolism. The aortic and then pulmonary artery anastomoses are then performed. Topical cooling may be continued, and the addition of blood cardioplegia after the atrial anastomoses may be done in order to improve graft function. The implant time is generally 45–60 minutes. It is frequently necessary to provide chronotropic support for the denervated heart in the form of atrial pacing or isoproterenol.

IMMUNOSUPPRESSION

Triple immunosuppression with a calcineurin inhibitor, antimetabolite, and corticosteroids is typical of the standard immunosuppressive protocol at most heart transplant programs. Perioperative induction immunosuppressive therapy with either polyclonal or monoclonal antibody therapy directed at lymphocytes is sometimes used in order to avoid the renal toxicity associated with early high-dose calcineurin inhibition and to reduce the risk of later rejection. Rejection is diagnosed on endomyocardial biopsy, which is performed regularly, since rejection may occur in the absence of clinical symptoms. Rejection is treated with 3 days of pulse steroids and resistant rejection with antilymphocyte therapy.

FOLLOW-UP CARE

Transplant recipients must be carefully monitored for infection and rejection. Protocols for endomyocardial biopsies vary by center but are typically performed every other month for the first year, then every 3 months. The incidence of rejection episodes is 0.5–1.5 per patient for the first year. The major infection rate is 1.5 episodes per patient for the first year and then declines. Accelerated coronary atherosclerosis, believed to be a manifestation of chronic graft rejection, occurs in 30–40% of patients within 5 years after transplantation. There is no effective therapy for this condition except for retransplantation in highly selected, usually younger, patients. Progressive renal dysfunction may occur over time due to the cumulative effect of calcineurin inhibitor therapy.

Goldstein DJ, Oz MC, Rose EA: Implantable left ventricular assist devices. N Engl J Med 1998;339:1522.
Morrow WR: Cardiomyopathy and heart transplantation in children. Curr Opin Cardiol 2000;15:216.
Taylor DO: Immunosuppression therapies after heart transplantation: best, better and beyond. Curr Opin Cardiol 2000;15:108.

COMBINED HEART-LUNG TRANSPLANTATION

Combined heart-lung transplantation was first performed in 1981. Initially, it was felt that rejection of both organs would be evident in the myocardial biopsy. However, experience has shown that rejection is dissimilar in the two organs, with heart rejection occurring infrequently and lung rejection, evidenced by obliterative bronchiolitis and arteritis, being a more severe problem. Heart-lung transplantation is currently performed with gradually decreasing frequently. In 1994, there were 71 heart-lung transplants in the United States. This number had declined to 28 in 2003. The main indication for heart-lung transplantation is end-stage disease in both organs or end-stage disease in one with poor function in the other prohibiting single-organ transplantation. Examples are primary pulmonary hypertension, congenital heart disease with Eisenmenger physiology, fibrotic lung disease and cor pulmonale, and cystic fibrosis.

The operation consists of en bloc heart-lung transplantation with anastomosis of the trachea, right atrium, and aorta of the donor.

Immunosuppression parallels that of heart transplantation with the exception that steroids are avoided initially in

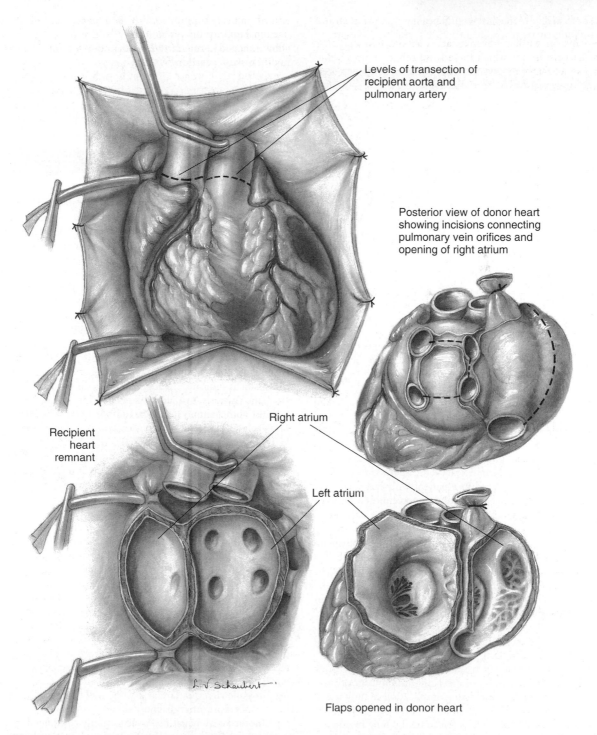

Levels of transection of recipient aorta and pulmonary artery

Posterior view of donor heart showing incisions connecting pulmonary vein orifices and opening of right atrium

Recipient heart remnant

Right atrium

Left atrium

Flaps opened in donor heart

▲ **Figure 45–2.** *Top left:* Recipient heart showing levels of transection across aorta and pulmonary artery. *Lower left:* Implantation site with recipient heart removed. *Top right:* Posterior view of donor heart showing lines of incision connecting pulmonary vein orifices and opening the right atrium in preparation for implantation. *Lower right:* Flaps opened in donor heart in preparation for implantation.

order to promote tracheal wound healing. Heart-lung transplantation currently results in a 70% 1-year survival rate.

LUNG TRANSPLANTATION

Single lung transplantation became clinically successful through a systematic approach by the Toronto Lung Transplant Group to the problem of bronchial disruption, which had made previous attempts unsuccessful. The addition of an omental wrap to the bronchial anastomosis and the avoidance of steroids during the first 3 weeks allowed bronchial healing and clinical success. Lung transplantation is currently performed for a myriad of indications, including emphysema, cystic fibrosis, idiopathic pulmonary fibrosis, α_1-antitrypsin deficiency, primary pulmonary hypertension, and congenital diseases. Candidates for lung transplantation have irreversible end-stage disease for which there is no other therapy, are oxygen dependent, and are likely to die of their disease within 12–18 months. Lung donors are scarce, but the use of one lung for transplantation does not preclude using the heart for another recipient. Long-distance procurement of lungs has been possible since institution of a regimen consisting of pulmonary artery flush with cold preservative solution following alprostadil (PGE_1) via the central venous line to promote pulmonary vasodilatation.

Patients with bilateral pulmonary sepsis, such as cystic fibrosis or bronchiectasis, or patients with emphysema and normal heart function may sometimes be eligible for double lung transplantation. The advantage is that the patient does not have the potential complications of heart transplant and rejection. Another innovative approach to the lung transplant patient with a normal heart is the operation whereby a heart-lung block is placed in a patient with end-stage lung disease and a normal heart, and the recipient's heart is extracted and donated to a patient in need of an isolated heart transplantation.

Immunosuppressive management of lung transplant recipients is very similar to that of heart recipients in that the cornerstone of therapy is a calcineurin inhibitor. The major difference is that steroids are omitted for several weeks in order to promote healing of the bronchial anastomosis. Postoperative management focuses on prevention of sepsis and detection and treatment of rejection. Bronchoscopy is performed liberally and transbronchial lung biopsy is used to diagnose lung transplant rejection. Acute rejection may be effectively treated with corticosteroid pulse therapy, or by enhancing the existing immunosuppressive regimen. The major long-term complication in lung transplant recipients is the development of bronchiolitis obliterans syndrome (BOS). BOS is felt to be the lung manifestation of chronic rejection. Episodes of acute rejection are risk factors for the development of BOS in the future. There is currently no effective therapy for BOS. A promising development that is currently experimental is aerosolized delivery of immunosuppression. It is hoped that directing immunosuppression preferentially to the lung itself may allow enhanced protection from rejection without increasing the risk of infection.

Tralock EP: Lung transplantation for COPD. Chest 1998;113:269S.
Yankaskas JR, Mallory GB: Lung transplantation and cystic fibrosis: consensus conference statement. Chest 1998;113:217.

LIVER TRANSPLANTATION

After many years of experimental effort, Dr Thomas Starzl performed the first successful human liver transplantation in 1967. Over the next decade and a half, the procedure was done only in low volumes, and outcomes were generally poor. As with other organs, the introduction of cyclosporine in the 1980s resulted in marked improvement in survival rates. Today, more than 5000 liver transplants are performed annually in the United States, and 1-year patient survival rates are more than 85%.

Since the introduction of clinical liver transplantation, the list of indications has rapidly expanded and the list of contraindications has diminished. The most common indication for liver transplantation is currently cirrhosis due to chronic hepatitis C infection. Other diseases for which liver transplant is indicated include cirrhosis due to hepatitis B, alcoholic cirrhosis, primary biliary cirrhosis, sclerosing cholangitis, autoimmune hepatitis, and cirrhosis secondary to nonalcoholic fatty liver disease. Less common indications are Wilson disease, α_1-antitrypsin deficiency, Budd-Chiari syndrome, and hemochromatosis. In children, the most common indication is biliary atresia. Other common diagnoses include α_1-antitrypsin deficiency, tyrosinemia, and other inborn errors of metabolism.

Alcoholic cirrhosis was once a subject of considerable controversy because of the self-induced nature of the disease. The world community rejected the notion that lifesaving therapy should be withheld from patients who could benefit from it merely because their disease is self-induced. It was pointed out that many, if not most, diseases are to some degree self-induced, whether it is diabetes and high blood pressure due to obesity or cancer and heart disease due to smoking. It is now recognized that alcoholic cirrhosis is an accepted indication for liver transplant if the patient has demonstrated the ability to abstain from alcohol and is clearly committed to continued abstinence. Overall results in alcoholic recipients have shown that patients transplanted for alcoholic cirrhosis fare at least as well as patients transplanted for most other diagnoses.

Chronic active hepatitis B was formerly considered to be a controversial indication for liver transplantation because recurrence was quite frequent and tended to result in rapid graft failure. This changed when effective strategies to prevent recurrence of hepatitis B using high-dose hepatitis B hyperimmune globulin infusions posttransplant were reported. Now hepatitis B is considered to be a standard indication, and results are equal to those obtained for other diagnoses. In contrast, the outcome for patients transplanted for hepatitis C was once considered to be equal to that of other diagnoses. Recent data, however, suggest that recurrence of hepatitis C in the new liver graft is virtually universal following transplantation, and 25% of patients will have developed cirrhosis in the graft within 5 years. It is not surprising that longer-term data are now appearing showing that the 10-year survival for patients transplanted for hepatitis C is significantly worse than for other diagnoses.

As with transplantation for hepatitis B and C, the consensus opinion has gone back and forth in recent years regarding whether liver transplantation should be used for the treatment of hepatocellular carcinoma in adults. Patients with cirrhosis are at risk for development of primary hepatocellular cancer. Since these patients usually die of liver failure, unlike patients with other forms of malignancy who usually succumb to widespread metastatic disease, it was reasoned that transplantation would be a curative therapy. Unfortunately, the initial results with transplantation for hepatoma were disappointing due to a high rate of tumor recurrence. These poor results prompted many programs to stop doing transplants for hepatoma. The group from Barcelona, Spain, then reported that survival rates are good if the tumor is small (less than 5 cm in diameter) but poor if the tumor is large or shows evidence of large vessel invasion. Numerous reports have confirmed this finding, and currently liver transplantation is considered to be a standard treatment for patients with small hepatomas. Results for liver transplantation for other malignancies remain poor, with the exception of several encouraging reports of reasonable survival rates for highly selected patients with cholangiocarcinoma who receive adjuvant radiation and chemotherapy.

Current contraindications are few and are primarily related to evidence of cardiopulmonary disease that prohibits safe liver transplantation. Examples are significant, uncorrected coronary artery disease; pulmonary hypertension with pulmonary artery systolic pressures greater than 70 mm Hg; and FEV_1 of less than 1 L on pulmonary function testing. Active substance abuse is also an absolute contraindication to transplantation. Diabetes increases the risks associated with transplantation and the incidence of posttransplant complications, but it is not an absolute contraindication to liver transplantation. Even infection with HIV, long considered a contraindication to transplantation, is no longer an absolute contraindications at some centers that are reporting good results in small numbers of carefully selected HIV-positive patients. Portal vein thrombosis, which at one time was a contraindication to transplant, is now managed by performing thrombectomy on the portal vein, by using vein grafts to bypass thrombosed vessels, or by using the infrahepatic cava for portal inflow.

Donor Selection

The number of patients listed for liver transplantation increases each year. This has led to a gradual increase in the number of patients who die while waiting and consequently to a relaxation of past standards for liver graft suitability. Livers are currently being transplanted from donors more than 80 years old with acceptable outcomes. It is important that the liver is a rough size match for the donor, but there is much leeway in this regard. Blood type compatibility is preferred but not an absolute requirement. Matching of tissue antigens does not appear to be relevant for liver transplantation, and a positive crossmatch is not a contraindication to proceeding with transplantation because it is not associated with a worse outcome posttransplant.

The technique of preserving the liver grafts after removal from the donor is based on decreasing metabolic requirements by keeping the graft cold. Blood is flushed from the organ to prevent vascular occlusion; preservation solution is infused; and the organ is kept on ice at 4 °C. Multiple preservative solutions are in common use worldwide. Most contain inert high-molecular-weight molecules that do not diffuse into the cell to prevent cellular swelling. Also, free oxygen radical scavengers, which are thought to prevent injury upon reperfusion of the graft, are frequently included. The introduction of Viaspan solution in the late 1980s revolutionized liver transplantation by extending the period of safe in vitro liver preservation from 10 hours to more than 24 hours. Despite this advance, it is clear that prolonged cold ischemia is bad for the liver graft, particularly if the graft contains a large amount of intracellular fat or is from an older donor. Transplant programs therefore continue to strive to minimize the cold ischemic time to whatever degree is feasible.

Operative Technique

In general, liver transplantation is an orthotopic procedure: The host liver is removed and the donor organ placed in an orthotopic position. The operation is performed in three phases: the dissection phase, during which the attachments of the diseased liver are dissected and the vascular structures are prepared for resection; the anhepatic phase, which extends from the time the host liver is removed until the time the donor liver is revascularized; and the reperfusion phase, during which blood is circulating through the new organ and the biliary tree is reconstructed.

Several techniques are available for handling the retrohepatic vena cava. Historically, the liver was removed en bloc with the vena cava and hemodynamic instability was avoided by using venovenous bypass to overcome decreased venous return when vena caval and portal vein flow was interrupted. The new liver was then sutured into place using a bicaval technique with end-to-end caval anastomoses being performed from donor to recipient both above and below the new liver. With careful anesthetic technique and preloading with fluid, venovenous bypass may be avoided in many cases. An alternative method of handling the retrohepatic cava is to dissect the liver off the cava and sequentially ligate the hepatic venous branches that enter the cava directly from the right and caudate lobes. This allows the liver to be removed by clamping the main hepatic veins without occluding the vena cava. The new liver is then sutured into place by connecting the suprahepatic cava of the donor to a common orifice created by connecting the right, middle, and left hepatic veins. This technique is called the piggyback technique because the donor cava sits directly on top of the recipient cava. The infrahepatic cava of the donor is occluded with either sutures or a vascular stapler. This method may preclude the need for venovenous bypass because caval flow is usually not completely interrupted. A third option for caval reconstruction is to connect the donor cava to the recipient cava using a side-to-side technique by making longitudinal incisions from the hepatic veins caudally, creating a very wide anastomosis. This technique is difficult when the donor liver is large relative to the size of the recipient's hepatic fossa.

The current methods of biliary reconstruction include primary choledochocholedochostomy (when the recipient duct is intact) or Roux-en-Y choledochojejunostomy if the recipient bile duct is not intact or if anatomically the donor and recipient duct cannot be approximated without creating tension on the anastomosis. It was once standard to place a T tube or another type of biliary stent across the biliary anastomosis, but many programs have now discontinued this practice because it is not clear that the presence of a stent influences the rate of biliary complications.

Although the liver can function normally with only portal venous flow, the bile duct is dependent on hepatic arterial flow. For this reason, the hepatic arterial anastomosis is crucial to postoperative graft survival. The arterial supply of the liver is quite variable, with nearly half of the patients having some form of aberrant circulation. The most common aberrancies are replacement of the right hepatic artery to the superior mesenteric artery and the presence of an accessory left hepatic artery that derives from the left gastric artery. When aberrant arterial vessels are identified on a deceased donor, it is important that they are carefully preserved so that reconstruction can occur when the liver has been perfused and cooled and is sitting in sterile ice slush. Multiple methods of reconstruction of aberrant vessels are available and, if necessary, a conduit of donor iliac artery may be used in the reconstruction.

► Living Donor Liver Transplantation & Split Liver Transplantation

The shortage of organs for small children in the late 1980s prompted the development of techniques to reduce the size of an adult liver graft by performing an anatomic resection of one or more lobes and transplanting the reduced graft. In this way, it was possible to transplant the left lobe or the left lateral segment from an adult liver into a child. This technique was successful and rapidly became a standard method of obtaining grafts for small children. The natural evolution of this technique was to apply the method used to reduce the size of a deceased donor liver graft to adult living donors. Broelsch at the University of Chicago popularized the transplantation of the left lateral segment from an adult into a child and showed that this technique could be at least as effective as using full-sized grafts from small children. It was hoped that living related liver transplantation would offer an immunologic advantage as it does with kidney transplantation, but this did not turn out to be the case. The major advantage of living donor liver transplantation appears to be the ability to allow transplant to occur prior to the deterioration of the recipient's condition into a poor state of health that is associated with a higher risk for transplantation.

The success of living donor liver transplantation from adult donors into children, together with the shortage of suitable adult donors, led to the development by Marcos and Tanaka of techniques to utilize the right lobe from a living donor to transplant into another adult. The donor operation is a major undertaking and is associated with appreciable morbidity as well as a mortality rate of approximately 0.5%. Nevertheless, living donor liver transplants have become a standard option when timely deceased donor liver transplantation is not possible.

By applying the living donor technique to deceased donors, two transplants can be obtained from a single adult liver from a deceased donor. This has been termed a split liver transplant. Typically, the lateral segment of the left lobe is used for a child or very small adult, while the remainder of the liver consisting of the right lobe plus the medial segment of the left lobe is used for an adult. Less commonly, the liver from an adult deceased donor can also be split into a right lobe graft and a left lobe graft and used for two adults.

► Immunosuppressive Therapy

The mainstay of immunosuppression for liver transplant recipients is a calcineurin inhibitor. An antimetabolite or corticosteroids, or both, may also be included but are not absolutely necessary. Induction therapy with antilymphocyte preparations was once considered standard but has now been abandoned by many liver transplant programs because it appears unnecessary.

Despite being one of the largest organs transplanted in terms of mass, the liver seems to require less immunosuppression for maintenance therapy compared to other organs. Corticosteroids can frequently be safely discontinued. Typically, monotherapy with a low dose of a calcineurin inhibitor is all that is required to suppress rejection long term. Spontaneous tolerance with normal graft function despite complete discontinuation of all immunosuppressants occurs in approximately 10–20% of liver transplant recipients. The liver is unique in this regard, since rejection is almost universal if immunosuppression is discontinued in recipients of renal, cardiac, pulmonary, and pancreatic grafts.

▶ Complications

Complications following liver transplantation are common, but most can be treated effectively. Coagulopathy is routinely present during liver transplant procedures, particularly during the anhepatic phase. For this reason, bleeding is common following the procedure, and 5–10% of liver transplant recipients will require reoperation because of continued bleeding following the procedure.

One of the most devastating complications is primary nonfunction of the liver. Primary nonfunction is a condition in which the new liver does not function and death results unless a second transplant is performed. Patients with primary nonfunction typically have profoundly elevated serum transaminases together with severe coagulopathy and acidosis. The incidence of this complication is between 5% and 10%. The cause of primary nonfunction is poorly understood, but multiple donor factors are known to be associated. Long cold ischemic times, poor perfusion of the graft with preservative solution, severe hepatic steatosis, and elevation of the donor serum sodium level above 165 meq/L are all known risk factors for primary nonfunction.

Vascular complications occur in 5–10% of transplant recipients. The hepatic artery is particularly prone to thrombosis, especially in children. If this is detected early, it is frequently possible to perform thrombectomy and restore hepatic arterial flow. If flow cannot be reestablished, necrosis of the intrahepatic and extrahepatic biliary tree usually occurs, resulting in death from sepsis if retransplantation is not performed.

The bile duct has been called the Achilles' heel of the liver transplant because it is so prone to anastomotic leakage or stricture. Fortunately, while as many as 20% of liver transplant recipients will experience a bile duct complication, it is uncommon for this complication to be lethal. Leaks tend to occur early and can often be managed by placing a biliary stent using endoscopic retrograde cholangiopancreatography (ERCP). If a large collection of bile develops because of a bile leak, it is usually necessary to drain the area either operatively or by placing a percutaneous suction drain. Biliary stenosis can occur early or late. Unlike the native liver, the transplanted liver will not always develop intrahepatic biliary dilatation when the bile duct is obstructed. It is therefore necessary to have a high index of suspicion. Patients with elevated bilirubin or elevated serum alkaline phosphatase levels (or both) should be evaluated with either ERCP or magnetic resonance cholangiography. Strictures can often be managed noninvasively with biliary stents and balloon cholangioplasty, but in some cases, operative correction is required. Patients who develop multiple intrahepatic strictures usually require retransplantation.

Rejection is a frequent complication of liver transplantation—it occurs in about 20–50% of patients. Rejection should be suspected whenever serum transaminases or bilirubin levels, or both, worsen or fail to gradually normalize following a liver transplant. The diagnosis of rejection is made histologically by the finding of a mixed portal cellular infiltrate together with injury to bile duct epithelium and inflammation of the central vein endothelium (endothelitis). When the condition is diagnosed early and treated aggressively, rejection rarely culminates in a need for retransplantation. Because the principal rejection target is the bile duct epithelium, severe, unrelenting rejection is often manifested by destruction and disappearance of bile ducts (vanishing bile duct syndrome). The treatment for rejection depends on its severity. Mild rejection is treated either with corticosteroid pulse therapy or by increasing the dosage of maintenance immunosuppressive therapy. Rejection that does not respond to these measures may require treatment with an antilymphocyte preparation.

Cytomegalovirus is a member of the herpes family of viruses. Prior to the availability of prophylaxis against this virus, as many as half of liver transplant recipients developed clinical CMV infection. Symptoms of this infection typically include fever, leukopenia, and malaise, but a more serious clinical syndrome with pneumonitis or hepatitis is possible. Patients at greatest risk for severe CMV disease are those without previous CMV exposure who receive a liver from a CMV-positive donor, but reactivation of CMV infection is possible in any patient with prior exposure to the virus. In order to prevent CMV infection, most liver transplant programs prescribe either ganciclovir or valganciclovir for a period of months following liver transplantation to all patients at risk for CMV infection.

Epstein-Barr virus is another common viral pathogen in these patients. Although the systemic illness with Epstein-Barr virus infection is usually mild, it may be associated with development of a lymphoproliferative disorder known as posttransplant lymphoma. This disorder can progress to frank malignancy, and the mortality rate is high. In many cases, the lymphoproliferation resolves merely be reducing immunosuppression. If the lymphoproliferative tissue expresses CD20, treatment with the monoclonal antibody rituximab may be helpful. Patients with lymphoproliferation that does not respond to these measures may require chemotherapy.

Immunosuppression predisposes to fungal infections, especially esophageal *Candida albicans* ("thrush"). The incidence of this infection is reduced by the use of prophylactic nystatin to decrease gastrointestinal fungal colonization.

Bussutil RW, Goss JA: Split liver transplantation. Ann Surg 1999;229:313.

Edwards EB et al: The effect of the volume of procedures at transplantation centers on mortality after liver transplantation. N Engl J Med 1999;341:2049.

Gridelli B, Remuzzl G: Strategy for making more organs available for transplantation. N Engl J Med 2000;343:404.

Neuberger J: Liver transplantation. Q J Med 1999;92:547.

▼ PANCREAS TRANSPLANTATION

Although pancreatic transplantation involves transplantation of a nonessential organ as compared with the liver, heart, or kidney, it has enormous potential in the management of patients with insulin-dependent diabetes. In many patients with type I diabetes—even though insulin and diet are carefully controlled—the complications of the disease progress relentlessly. Many patients develop severe retinopathy at an early age, leading to blindness and renal disease as well as severe neuropathy and peripheral vascular disease that ultimately results in limb loss. The goal of pancreas transplantation is primarily to prevent or delay end-organ damage by the complications of diabetes. Another important indication for pancreas transplantation is hypoglycemic unawareness. Diabetic nephropathy can cause loss of the autonomic nervous pathways that allow patients to sense hypoglycemia. These patients can lapse into a coma at any moment. For patients with severe hypoglycemic unawareness, pancreas transplantation can truly be a lifesaving procedure.

Currently, most pancreas transplants are whole-organ grafts from deceased donors. The pancreas is procured along with a cuff of the first, second, and third portion of the duodenum attached. The graft can be placed into the pelvis with the iliac artery supplying arterial supply to the pancreas and the iliac vein used for portal venous drainage of the graft. Alternatively, the graft can be placed in the mid abdomen and connected to the infrarenal aorta and the superior mesenteric vein. This allows insulin secreted by the pancreas to enter the portal circulation rather than the systemic circulation, which is more physiologic. The pancreatic exocrine secretions may be managed by anastomosing the duodenum to the bladder or to a loop of small bowel.

If the pancreas graft is successful, the patient will quickly become normoglycemic. As long as the graft functions normally, the patient will no longer require exogenous insulin because the pancreas graft responds normally by secreting insulin in response to rising blood glucose levels that occur following eating and ceasing insulin secretion when blood glucose levels fall to normal.

Much research has dealt with the transplantation of isolated pancreatic islet cells, which make up only about 2% of the pancreatic mass. This procedure is intuitively very attractive because it does not require an abdominal incision or general anesthesia. A team from Edmonton has reported successful transplantation of islets into the liver using a transhepatic injection into the portal vein. The patients in the original report all achieved insulin independence, although this often required more than one infusion of islets from more than one deceased donor pancreas. Immunosuppression consisted of rapamycin, tacrolimus, and induction treatment basiliximab, an inhibitor of IL-2R. The success at Edmonton has led to increased enthusiasm worldwide for islet transplantation, but to date, no other center has achieved the same degree of success. The critical factor appears to be the isolation procedure of the islets themselves. Nevertheless, it seems likely that in the long run, islet transplantation will eventually replace whole-organ pancreas transplantation.

Shapiro AM et al: Islet transplantation in seven patients with type 1 diabetes mellitus using a glucocorticoid-free immunosuppressive regimen. N Engl J Med 2000;343:230.

Sutherland DG et al: Lessons learned from more than 1000 pancreas transplants at a single institution. Ann Surg 2001;233:463.

Index

Page numbers followed by *t* and *i* indicate tables and illustrations, respectively. Drugs are listed under their generic names; when a trade name is listed, the entry is cross-referenced to the generic name.